YOUR GUIDE TO

Understanding Medical-Surgical Nursing

Everything you need to succeed...

in class, in clinical, on exams and on the NCLEX®

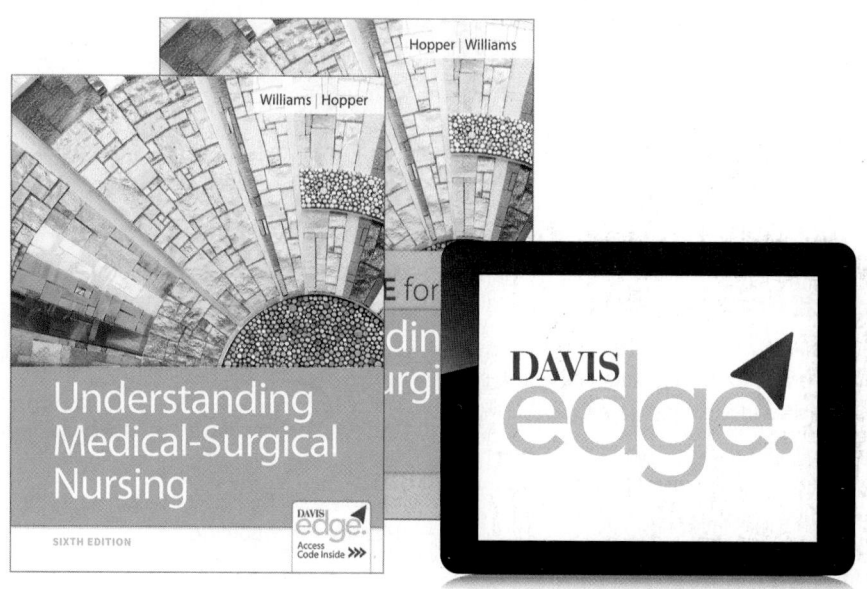

Your journey to success
BEGINS HERE!

Your text works together with Interactive Clinical Scenarios and Davis Edge to make the connections you need to master med-surg nursing.

Don't miss everything that's waiting online to make learning less stressful... and save you time. Follow the instructions on the inside front cover to use the access code to unlock your resources today.

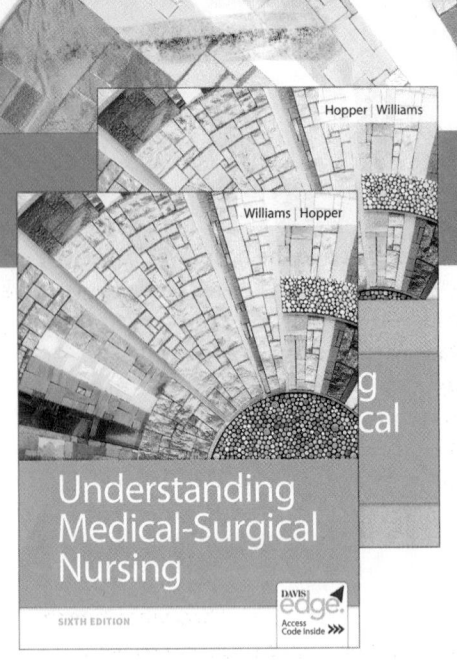

STEP #1
Build a solid foundation.

Gerontological Issues boxes prepare you to provide quality care to older adults.

Gerontological Issues

Arrhythmia Risk. The main factors that increase the risk of arrhythmias in older adults include the following:

- Digitalis toxicity (most common)
- Hypokalemia
- Angina
- Coronary insufficiency or cardiomyopathy (exercise, stress)
- Sleep apnea
- Hypothyroidism or hyperthyroidism

Arrhythmias that occur most often in older adults include the following:

- Atrial fibrillation (atria beating 400 to 700 times per minute)
- Sick sinus syndrome (alternating episodes of bradycardia, normal sinus rhythm, tachycardia, and periods of long sinus pause)
- Heart blocks (delayed or blocked impulses to the atria or ventricles)

Some of the common age-related effects of arrhythmias include the following:

- Bradycardia
- Confusion
- Dizziness
- Dyspnea or shortness of breath
- Fatigue
- Hypotension
- Palpitations
- Syncope
- Weakness

Older adults have less ability to adapt to sudden changes or stressors. They may not be able to tolerate tachycardia for very long. Any new-onset tachycardia in an older patient should be reported promptly.

Evidence-Based Practice

Clinical Question
Are probiotics effective in preventing *Clostridium difficile* (*C. difficile*)–associated diarrhea in the older adult?

Evidence
A systematic review and meta-analysis using five randomized control trials revealed that probiotics were not found to be more effective than a placebo in reducing the incidence of *C. difficile*–associated diarrhea in older patients hospitalized in the acute care setting (Vernaya, McAdam, & Hampton, 2017).

Implications for Nursing Practice
Probiotic administration is not effective for preventing *C. difficile*–associated diarrhea. Preventing *C. difficile* infection is important. Preventative measures include using standard precautions, hand hygiene, and disinfecting equipment and items in the patient's room.

Reference
Vernaya, M., McAdam, J., & Hampton, M. D. (2017). The effectiveness of probiotics in reducing the incidence of *Clostridium difficile* associated diarrhea in elderly patients: A systematic review protocol. *JBI Database of Systematic Reviews and Implementation Reports, 15*(1), 140–164.

Evidence-Based Practice boxes feature an in-depth look at research that supports the best care and how that knowledge applies in practice.

BE SAFE!

BE VIGILANT! Implement evidence-based practices to prevent central line–associated bloodstream infections. This requirement covers short- and long-term central venous catheters and peripherally inserted central catheters, per the 2018 National Patient Safety Goals (© The Joint Commission, 2017. Printed with permission.) Vascular catheter–related infections are considered "never events" because they can be prevented and should never occur. Hospitals will not be paid by Medicare for such infections acquired during hospitalization.

Be Safe! boxes emphasize and help students remember important aspects of safe care.

CRITICAL THINKING

Mr. Cheevers is admitted to the hospital for intravenous antibiotic therapy. He states that he has no allergies. One hour after the infusion begins, you happen to meet the nursing assistant coming down the hall with a blanket. He casually says, "Mr. Cheevers is very cold. I'm taking him a blanket. He is also restless and a bit short of breath." What is your responsibility in this situation?
Suggested answers are at the end of the chapter.

Critical-Thinking Exercises throughout each chapter help connect what you read to what you will see and do in the clinical setting, and include suggested answers at the end of the chapter to check comprehension.

STEP #2
Make studying easier.

Study Guide*

Corresponds to your text chapter by chapter to reinforce the "connections" each step of the way with exercises and activities that develop the critical-thinking and problem-solving skills essential to your success. Exercises for the Audio Case Studies are included.

eBook

Lets you access your text online anytime, anywhere for study, review, and reference. You can also add notes, highlights, and bookmarks.

Online Resources

Feature Audio Case Studies for each chapter and Interactive Clinical Scenarios to prepare you for real-world practice.

*Purchase separately.

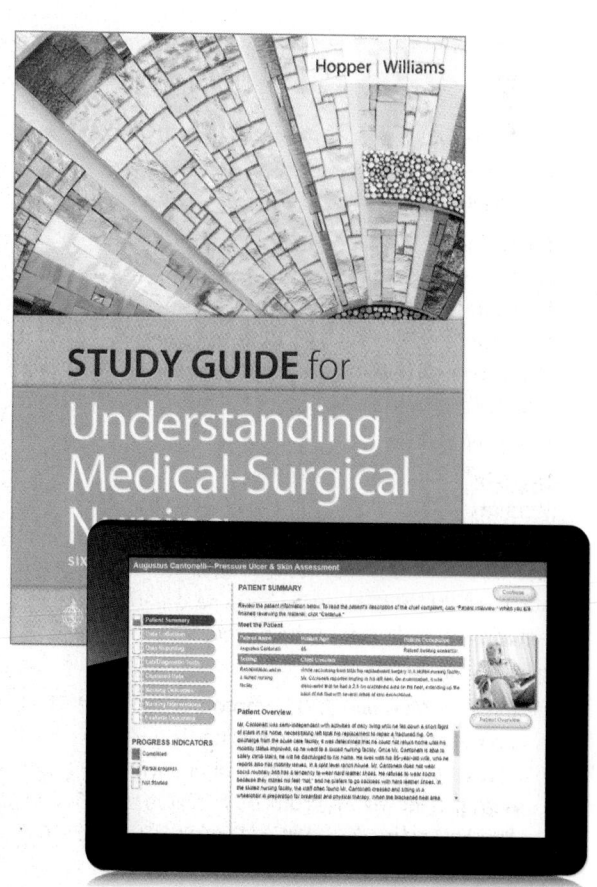

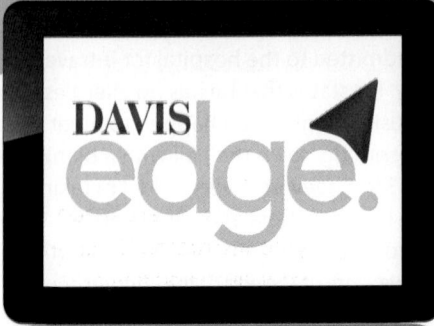

STEP #3
Study smarter, not harder.

Davis Edge is the interactive, online Q&A review platform that provides the practice you need to master course content and to improve your scores on classroom exams. Access it from a laptop, tablet, or mobile device for review and study on the go.

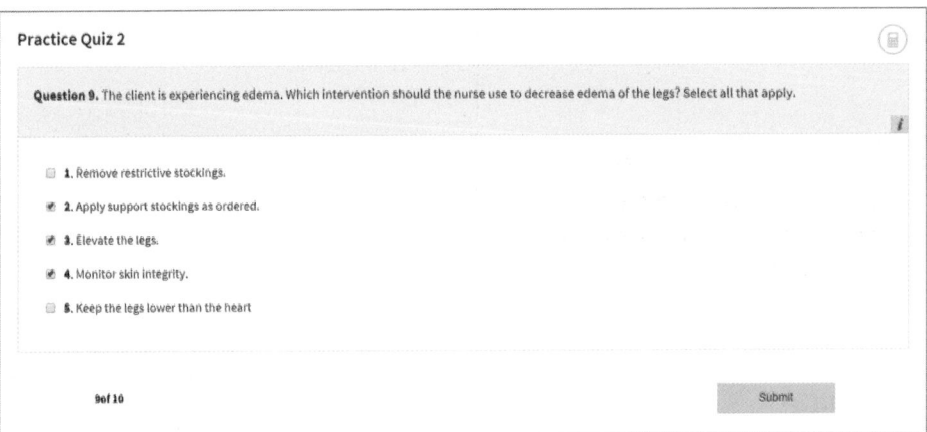

Practice Quiz 2

Question 9. The client is experiencing edema. Which intervention should the nurse use to decrease edema of the legs? Select all that apply.

☐ **1.** Remove restrictive stockings.

☑ **2.** Apply support stockings as ordered.

☑ **3.** Elevate the legs.

☑ **4.** Monitor skin integrity.

☐ **5.** Keep the legs lower than the heart

9 of 10

Submit

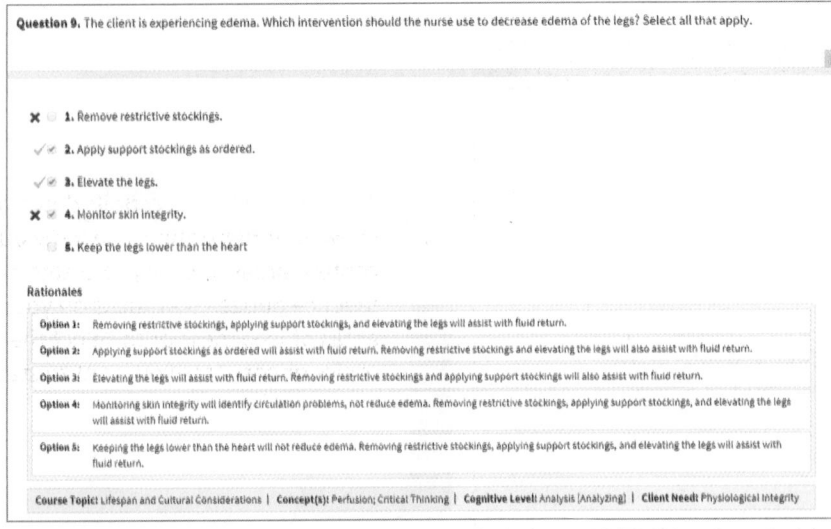

Question 9. The client is experiencing edema. Which intervention should the nurse use to decrease edema of the legs? Select all that apply.

✗ ☐ **1.** Remove restrictive stockings.

✓ ☑ **2.** Apply support stockings as ordered.

✓ ☑ **3.** Elevate the legs.

✗ ☑ **4.** Monitor skin integrity.

☐ **5.** Keep the legs lower than the heart

Rationales

Option 1:	Removing restrictive stockings, applying support stockings, and elevating the legs will assist with fluid return.
Option 2:	Applying support stockings as ordered will assist with fluid return. Removing restrictive stockings and elevating the legs will also assist with fluid return.
Option 3:	Elevating the legs will assist with fluid return. Removing restrictive stockings and applying support stockings will also assist with fluid return.
Option 4:	Monitoring skin integrity will identify circulation problems, not reduce edema. Removing restrictive stockings, applying support stockings, and elevating the legs will assist with fluid return.
Option 5:	Keeping the legs lower than the heart will not reduce edema. Removing restrictive stockings, applying support stockings, and elevating the legs will assist with fluid return.

Course Topic: Lifespan and Cultural Considerations | **Concept(s):** Perfusion; Critical Thinking | **Cognitive Level:** Analysis [Analyzing] | **Client Need:** Physiological Integrity

Comprehensive rationales explain why your responses are correct or incorrect. Page-specific references direct you to the relevant content in *Understanding Medical-Surgical Nursing*.

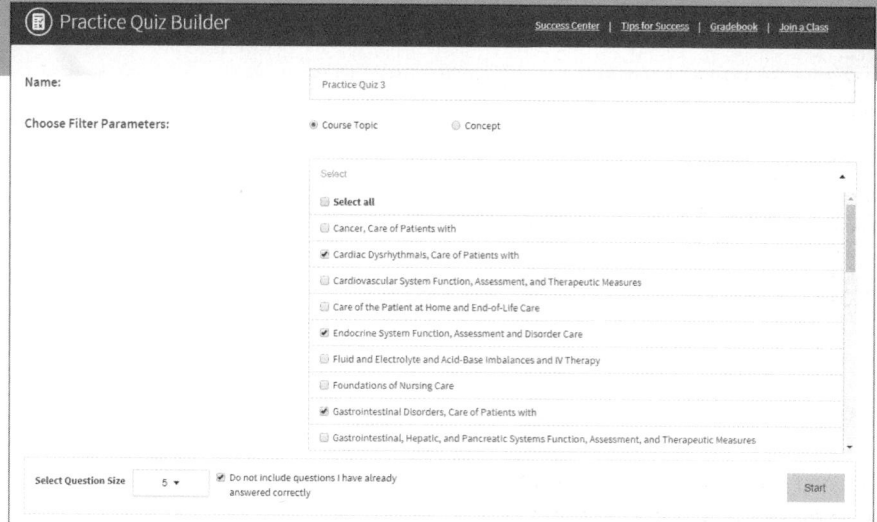

Assignments are made by your instructor. Or, create your own practice quizzes to review before an exam.

The Success Center offers a snapshot of your progress and identifies your strengths and weaknesses.

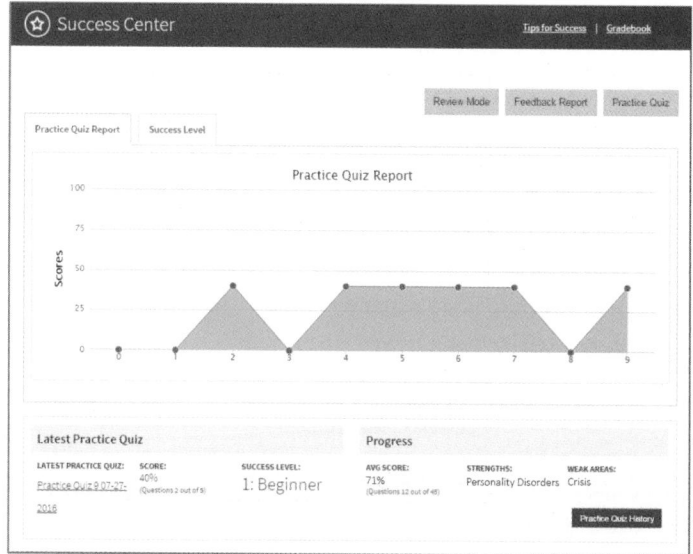

The Feedback Report drills down to show your performance in individual content areas. It's easy to create new practice quizzes that focus on your areas of weakness or to select the topics or concepts you want to study.

Feedback Report

Success Center | Tips for Success | Gradebook

Feedback Report

Create Practice Quiz On Weak Areas | Course Topic ▼

Strengths and Weaknesses will appear for a specific course topic or concept once you have answered a minimum of 10 questions in that area. Select to view by Course Topic or Concept from the drop down box above. Choose 'Create quiz on weak areas' above to begin creating a new quiz based on all weak areas.

Course Topic	Strength / Weakness	Number of Questions Answered	Success Level	Create Quiz
Anxiety, Obsessive-Compulsive and Related Disorders	● Needs More Practice	12	1: Beginner	Create Practice Quiz
Bereaved Individual, Mental Health Nursing of	● Needs More Practice	14	1: Beginner	Create Practice Quiz
Biological Implications	Strengths and Weaknesses will appear for a specific course topic or concept once you have answered a minimum of 10 questions in that area	22	1: Beginner	Create Practice Quiz

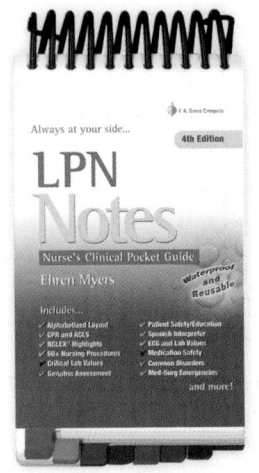
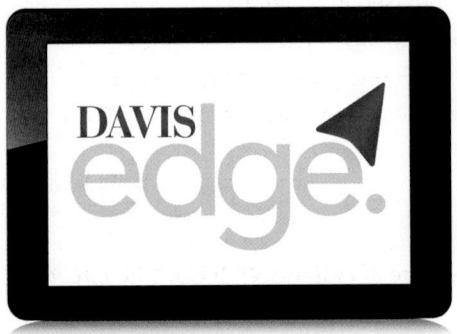

Brief Contents

Understanding Medical-Surgical Nursing

SIXTH EDITION

Linda S. Williams, MSN, RN
Master Adjunct Instructor & Professor Emeritus
  Jackson College
  Jackson, Michigan

Paula D. Hopper, MSN, RN, CNE
Adjunct Professor
  Spring Arbor University
  Spring Arbor, Michigan
Professor Emeritus
  Jackson College
  Jackson, Michigan

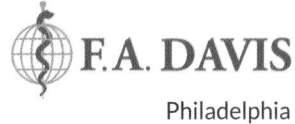

F.A. DAVIS

Philadelphia

F.A. Davis Company
1915 Arch Street
Philadelphia, PA 19103
www.fadavis.com

Printed in the United States of America

Last digit indicates print number: 10 9 8 7 6 5 4 3

Publisher, Nursing: Terri Wood Allen
Senior Content Project Manager: Elizabeth Hart
Art and Design Manager: Carolyn O'Brien
Digital Project Manager: Sandra Glennie

As new scientific information becomes available through basic and clinical research, recommended treatments and drug therapies undergo changes. The author(s) and publisher have done everything possible to make this book accurate, up to date, and in accord with accepted standards at the time of publication. The author(s), editors, and publisher are not responsible for errors or omissions or for consequences from application of the book, and make no warranty, expressed or implied, in regard to the contents of the book. Any practice described in this book should be applied by the reader in accordance with professional standards of care used in regard to the unique circumstances that may apply in each situation. The reader is advised always to check product information (package inserts) for changes and new information regarding dose and contraindications before administering any drug. Caution is especially urged when using new or infrequently ordered drugs.
ISBN: 978-0-8036-6898-0

Library of Congress Cataloging-in-Publication Data
Names: Williams, Linda S. (Linda Sue), 1954- editor. | Hopper, Paula D., editor.
Title: Understanding medical-surgical nursing / [edited by] Linda S. Williams, Paula D. Hopper.
Description: Sixth edition. | Philadelphia : F.A. Davis Company, [2019] | Includes bibliographical references and index.
Identifiers: LCCN 2018035783 (print) | LCCN 2018036302 (ebook) | ISBN 9780803694613 | ISBN 9780803668980 (pbk.)
Subjects: | MESH: Medical-Surgical Nursing | Nursing Process | Evidence-Based Nursing
Classification: LCC RT41 (ebook) | LCC RT41 (print) | NLM WY 150 | DDC 610.73—dc23
LC record available at https://lccn.loc.gov/2018035783

For practical and vocational nursing students: you are valuable members of the health care team. We trust this text will help you learn to think like nurses and become safe practitioners.

To my father, Richard, and sister, Lisa, for their ongoing encouragement and support.

—*Linda*

And for my first grandchild, Theo, who is the light of my life.

—*Paula*

Acknowledgments

Many people helped us make this book a reality. First and foremost are the students, who provide us with the inspiration to undertake this project. We hope that students everywhere continue to find this text worth reading.

The F.A. Davis Company is an exceptional publishing partner. We feel fortunate to have had their continued enthusiasm and confidence in our book. The staff at F.A. Davis has guided us through this project for six editions to help us create a student-friendly book that truly promotes understanding of medical-surgical nursing to provide safe, patient-centered care.

Terri Allen, Elizabeth Hart, Julia Curcio, Amy Reeve, and many others have been extremely patient and kind as we worked hard to provide a quality text.

Contributors from across the United States and Canada, including many well-known experts in their fields, brought expertise and diversity to the content. Their hard work is much appreciated. We are thankful to Gay Alcenius, PharmD, for her expertise in updating all of the medication information.

We wish to thank everyone who played a role, however large or small, in helping us to provide a tool to help students realize their dreams of becoming LPNs/LVNs. We hope this book will help educate nurses who can provide safe and expert care because we have helped them to learn to think critically and make sound clinical judgments.

Preface

Welcome to the Sixth Edition of *Understanding Medical-Surgical Nursing*! The material has been completely reviewed and updated. New evidence-based guidelines have been used wherever possible.

We continue to work hard to provide a text written at an understandable level, with features that help students understand, apply, and safely practice the challenging content required to succeed as practical/vocational nurses. We are thankful to the many faculty and students who tell us they find the book very readable and enjoyable. We have been overjoyed to hear from several nursing programs that their NCLEX® scores soared after adopting this textbook. We welcome and value your comments on this edition.

We continue to emphasize understanding, critical thinking, and the ability to make safe clinical judgments. We believe that a student who learns to think critically will be better able to apply information to new situations. We hope both students and instructors find this Sixth Edition a practical tool for learning and understanding the principles of medical-surgical nursing.

Content and Features

We have retained our most popular features from the first five editions and added new ones based on reader input and current practice.

New to the Sixth Edition:

• Concept list at beginning of each chapter
• Chapter 16 updated to "Patient Care Settings" with new content on Acute Care of Elders (ACE) hospital units, long-term care, and office nursing
• Health literacy information added to Chapter 2
• Human trafficking information added to Chapter 3
• Opioid crisis information added to Chapter 10
• Redesign of interior for easier readability

Based on feedback, we have retained, updated, and expanded the following:

• **Critical Thinking** case studies throughout each chapter. These exercises help students practice and think about what they are learning. **Suggested Answers to Critical Thinking** case studies are available at the end of the chapter. Research supports the importance of immediate feedback to reinforce learning, so we feel strongly that students should have access to correct answers while they are studying. Because there can be many answers to some of the critical thinking questions, we have provided sample answers to help stimulate students' thinking.
• **Review questions** at the end of each chapter. Questions have been updated and include application- and analysis-level questions, and more "select all that apply" alternate format items to reflect the NCLEX-PN®. Correct answers are provided with each chapter for quick reference. The

correct answers including rationales can be found online in the Davis Edge Student Resources.
• **Be Safe!, Nursing Care Tips,** and **Learning Tips** help make learning easy. The Joint Commission's National Patient Safety Goals are reflected in many of the safety tips.
• Boxed presentations of **Cultural Considerations, Evidence-Based Practice, Gerontological Issues, Home Health Hints,** and **Nutrition Notes.** Boxes have been updated where needed.
• **Nursing Care Plans** with gerontological considerations and a new, easier-to-read design.
• **Patient Perspectives** provide real patient experiences to bring life to theoretical material.
• **Pronunciation Guides** for new words at the beginning of each chapter.
• **Word Building** footnotes throughout the chapters.
• A comprehensive, updated **Glossary** is included in the back of the text.
• **Web links** in the text to help students do further research on topics of interest.

To Students: How to Use This Book

Learning Outcomes are provided for each chapter. Review them before reading and then go back and check to be sure you understand them.

You will find a list of key terms and their pronunciations at the beginning of each chapter. These words appear in bold at either their first use or most relevant use in a chapter, and they also appear in the glossary at the end of the book. By learning the meanings of these words as you encounter them, you will increase your understanding of the material. Many of these words are also broken down where they are used, so you can see how the parts of each word make up the whole.

Following the key terms, you will find a list of concepts covered in the chapter. At the end of each chapter, consider what you have learned about each concept and how it relates to what you already know about that concept.

You also will find learning tips to increase your understanding and retention of the material. You may want to develop your own memory techniques in addition to those provided. (If you think of a good one, send it to us at F.A. Davis and you may find it in the next edition!) Many of the learning tips have been developed and used in our own classrooms. We find them to be helpful in fostering understanding of complex concepts or as memory aids. However, we want to stress that memorization is not the primary focus of the text but rather a foundation for understanding and thinking about more complex information. Understanding an application will serve you far better than memorization when dealing with new situations.

Each chapter includes brief critical thinking case studies designed to help you apply material that has been presented.

A series of questions related to the case will help you integrate the material with what you already know. These questions emphasize critical thinking, which is based on a foundation of recall and understanding of material. Try to answer the questions before checking the answers.

Generic medication names are a must for you to know for the NCLEX-PN. We continue to provide both the generic and trade names for medications to help you prepare for both the NCLEX-PN and nursing practice.

Review questions and answers appear at the end of each chapter to help you prepare for chapter tests, and for the NCLEX-PN. To assess your learning, try to answer the questions before looking at the answers. Answers with rationales are provided in the Student Resources on Davis Edge.

The following are included in the back of the text for easy reference:

• Common Diagnostic Tests (Appendix A)
• Normal Adult Reference Laboratory Values (Appendix B)
• Glossary
• Common Medical Abbreviations
• Common Prefixes and Suffixes to help learn word-building techniques

Ancillaries

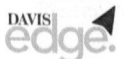

This online assessment platform integrates seamlessly with the textbook and course. Its interactive, question-based format provides the practice students need to build comprehension and improve scores on classroom exams and the NCLEX-PN through a series of quizzes that can be personalized to meet individual student needs.

The tool provides real-time analysis of:

• Comprehension. How well are students understanding and retaining the content?
• Participation. Are students engaging with their reading and keeping up with their assignments?
• Test-taking skills. Are students adapting to NCLEX-style questions and improving their skills?

Suggestions for implementing *Davis Edge* into the course are included in the Active Classroom Instructor's Guide. By incorporating assignments into a course, instructors are able to monitor engagement, participation, and areas of strength and weakness.

Study Guide

A Study Guide is available to provide additional practice with the material. Each chapter includes vocabulary practice, audio case study questions, objective exercises, a case study, and other critical thinking practice exercises. Review questions written in NCLEX-PN style include newly added hot spot questions. Study Guide answers are posted to the instructor's Davis Edge site.

Additional Online Resources for Students

There is an abundance of additional student resources for this edition of *Understanding Medical-Surgical Nursing* in the form of digital assets found on Davis Edge, including:

• **References.** Comprehensive list of chapter references, bibliographies, and web sites. Reference lists and bibliographies provide sources for content discussed in the chapter, as well as sources for additional reading material. Web sites have been included in the references for some chapters to aide in expanding information resources.
• **Audio Case Studies With Questions.** Students should listen to the chapter topic case scenarios on Davis Edge and follow-up with critical thinking questions for thought and discussion that are available in the Study Guide.
• **Animations.** Media enhancement of topics and concepts are included as relevant.
• **Procedures.** Selected LPN/LVN skills are provided for review.
• **Interactive Clinical Scenarios (ICS).** Hone critical thinking skills and make decisions for patient care based on the scenarios presented. Topics include dementia, chest pain, respiratory distress, and others.
• **Patient Teaching Guidelines.** Sample guidelines for disorders discussed throughout the text. These guidelines are printable for students to use in patient care settings while teaching patients.
• **NCLEX-PN prep guide.** A brief guide to help students understand the NCLEX-PN, including the types of questions to expect and tips on how to study.
• An **eBook** of the text

Instructor Resources on DavisPlus

Instructors have access to all student resources as well as materials specifically available to aid in the instruction of the content. Instructor Resources include the following:

• **NCLEX-Style Test Bank**
• **PowerPoint Slides**
• **Electronic Image Bank**
• *NEW* **Active Classroom Instructor's Guide** provides guidance on how to utilize and assign the text and ancillaries throughout the course. Abundant activities to promote an active classroom are included.
• A **PowerPoint Tutorial** and a **NCLEX-Style Item-Writing Tutorial** are provided to help you individualize our resources to your own needs.
• **Study Guide Answer Key** is posted on the instructor's Davis*Plus* site to allow instructors the option of providing answers to students for self-study or assigning the Study Guide exercises for grading.
• An **eBook** of the text

LPN/LVN Connections

F.A. Davis is pleased to introduce **LPN/LVN Connections,** a consistent and recognizable approach to design and content that will make it easier for students and instructors to use multiple F.A. Davis textbooks throughout the LPN/LVN curriculum. We have increased continuity whenever possible, without erasing the authors' autonomy or changing legacy content that has been popular in past editions. This makes it easier for instructors and students to move through the textbooks and ancillary products while recognizing shared themes and featured content.

Textbook Design, Style, and Pedagogy
- All textbook chapters include:
  - Numbered Learning Outcomes
  - Key Terms with phonetic pronunciations listed on the chapter opener and boldfaced where first defined in the chapter
  - Chapter Concepts
  - NCLEX-style Review Questions, with answers right on the page for student's ease of reference
  - Bulleted Key Points, available online
  - Chapter references, located online
- A Reading Level Evaluation is performed during the manuscript development, to ensure readability
- Word-Building Footnotes to help students build understanding of root terminology
- A uniform, space-saving internal design features special heads and colors that are shared across titles for features with similar content, to increase recognition

- Consistent and current terminology and laboratory values across titles; the authors followed *Davis's Comprehensive Handbook of Laboratory & Diagnostic Tests with Nursing Implications* by Van Leeuwen and Bladh for all values, and Taber's Cyclopedic Medical Dictionary for all pronunciations and terms

Standardized Student and Faculty Resources
For Students:

- *Davis Edge* personalized online quizzing to help master course content and prepare for the NCLEX-PN examination
- Gratis eBook with purchase of the print text, to allow flexibility in accessing course content
- Study Guide with perforated pages so that students can hand in assignments if requested; the Answer Key is provided to instructors online, to distribute if desired

For Instructors:

- *Davis Edge* pre-set quizzes and classroom management tools, with instructor reserve questions
- eBook
- Active Classroom Instructor Guide (ACIG) provides pre-, during-, and post-class suggestions for activities and assignments, focusing on the active classroom
- NCLEX-style test bank
- PowerPoint presentations
- Digital image collection

F.A. Davis LPN/LVN Advisory Board

Paula K. Mundell, MSN, RN
Coordinator, Nursing Program
Delaware Technical Community College
Dover, Delaware

Patricia Taylor, MSN-Ed, RN
Practical Nursing Coordinator
Kapi'olani Community College
University of Hawaii
Honolulu, Hawaii

Contributors

Gay Alcenius, PharmD
Pharmacist
Henry Ford Allegiance Health
Jackson, Michigan
Medication Tables

Kathy Berchem, DNP, RN, APRN
Associate Professor of Nursing
Lake Superior State University
Sault Ste. Marie, Michigan
Chapter 26: Nursing Care of Patients With Heart Failure

Terri Blevins, BSN, MSEd
Online Faculty
Tennessee Board of Regents
Elizabethton, Tennessee
Chapter 23: Nursing Care of Patients With Valvular, Inflammatory, and Infectious Cardiac or Venous Disorders

Michelle Block, MS, RN
Associate Professor of Nursing
Purdue University Northwest
Hammond, IN
Chapter 2: Evidence-Based Practice
Chapter 3: Issues in Nursing Practice
Evidence-Based Practice feature

Janice L. Bradford, MS
Associate Professor
Jackson College
Jackson, Michigan
Anatomy & Physiology

Linda K. Cook, PhD, RN, CNS, ACNP
Assistant Professor
University of Maryland School of Nursing
Baltimore, Maryland
Chapter 47: Neurologic System Function, Assessment, and Therapeutic Measures
Chapter 48: Nursing Care of Patients With Central Nervous System Disorders
Chapter 49: Nursing Care of Patients With Cerebrovascular Disorders
Chapter 50: Nursing Care of Patients With Peripheral Nervous System Disorders

Jaime Crabb, RN, MSN, BSN
PN Program Coordinator/Instructor
Northern Michigan University
Marquette, Michigan
Chapter 41: Genitourinary and Reproductive System Function and Assessment
Chapter 43: Nursing Care of Male Patients With Genitourinary Disorders

Michele Dickson, DNP, MS, RN, CNE
Professor of Nursing
Prince George's Community College
Largo, Maryland
Chapter 21: Cardiovascular System Function, Assessment, and Therapeutic Measures
Chapter 25: Nursing Care of Patients With Cardiac Arrhythmias

Kristy Gorman, MS, RN, OCN
Registered Nurse
University of Maryland Medical Center
Baltimore, Maryland
Chapter 16: Patient Care Settings
Chapter 18: Immune System Function, Assessment, and Therapeutic Measures
Chapter 19: Nursing Care of Patients With Immune Disorders

Marie Hedgpeth, MSN, MHA, RN
Nursing Faculty
Robeson Community College
Lumberton, North Carolina
Chapter 6: Nursing Care of Patients With Fluid, Electrolyte, and Acid–Base Imbalances

Alene Homan, MEd, RN, BSN, CSN, CPN
Practical Nursing Instructor
Clearfield County Career and Technology Center
Clearfield, Pennsylvania
Chapter 38: Endocrine System Function and Assessment
Chapter 39: Nursing Care of Patients With Endocrine Disorders

Dawn Johnson, DNP, RN, Ed
Director of Nursing
Great Lakes Institute of Technology
Erie, Pennsylvania
Gerontological Boxes

Cindy Leffel, PhD, MSN, RN-BC
Associate Professor
Trocaire College
Buffalo, New York
Chapter 12: Nursing Care of Patients Having Surgery
Chapter 45: Musculoskeletal Function and Assessment
Chapter 46: Nursing Care of Patients With
Musculoskeletal and Connective Tissue Disorders

Nancy Litch, MS, RD
Dietician, Retired
East Lansing, MI
Nutrition Notes

Bobbi M. Martin, MSN, RN
Executive Director
Galen Center for Professional Development
Louisville, Kentucky
Chapter 4: Cultural Influences on Nursing Care
Cultural Connections

Marina Martinez-Kratz, MS, RN, CNE
Professor of Nursing
Jackson College
Jackson, Michigan
Chapter 56: Mental Health Function, Assessment, and
Therapeutic Measures
Chapter 57: Nursing Care of Patients With Mental Health
Disorders

Laura L. McCully, MS, CNM
Certified Nurse Midwife
Women First Health Services
Clinical Adjunct, MSN FNP Program – OB/GYN
Michigan State University
Jackson, Michigan
Chapter 41: Genitourinary and Reproductive System
Function and Assessment
Chapter 42: Nursing Care of Women With Reproductive
System Disorders
Chapter 44: Nursing Care of Patients With Sexually
Transmitted Infections

Maureen McDonald, MS, RN
Professor, Department Chair – Nursing
Massasoit Community College
Brockton, Massachusetts
Chapter 24: Nursing Care of Patients With Occlusive
Cardiovascular Disorders
Chapter 36: Urinary System Function, Assessment, and
Therapeutic Measures
Chapter 37: Nursing Care of Patients With Disorders
of the Urinary System

Jennifer Mitchell, MSN, RN-BC
Assistant Professor
Tarrant County College District
Fort Worth, Texas
Chapter 9: Nursing Care of Patients in Shock
Chapter 27: Hematologic and Lymphatic System Function,
Assessment, and Therapeutic Measures
Chapter 28: Nursing Care of Patients With Hematologic
and Lymphatic Disorders

Betsy Murphy, RN, BSN, CHPN, FNP-Retired
Hospice Consultant
Round Hill, Virginia
Chapter 17: Nursing Care of Patients at the End of Life

Lazette V. Nowicki, RN, BS, MSN
Professor, Nursing
American River College
Sacramento, California
Chapter 33: Nursing Care of Patients With Upper
Gastrointestinal Disorders
Chapter 51: Sensory System Function, Assessment, and
Therapeutic Measures: Vision and Hearing
Chapter 52: Nursing Care of Patients With Sensory
Disorders: Vision and Hearing

Jennifer Otmanowski, RN, MSN
Clinical Coordinator/ Instructor
Baker College – Jackson
Jackson, Michigan
Chapter 16: Patient Care Settings
Home Health Hints

Sheria G. Robinson-Lane, PhD, RN
Assistant Professor
University of Michigan School of Nursing
Ann Arbor, Michigan
Chapter 10: Nursing Care of Patients in Pain

James Shannon, RN, JD, MHSA
Chief Nursing and Quality Officer
Mackinac Straits Health System
St. Ignace, Michigan
Chapter 3: Issues in Nursing Practice

MaryAnne Pietraniec Shannon, PhD, RN, GCNS-BC
Professor
Sault College
Sault Saint Marie, Ontario, Canada
Chapter 15: Nursing Care of Older Adult Patients

Gladdi Tomlinson, RN, MSN
Professor of Nursing
Harrisburg Area Community College
Harrisburg, Pennsylvania
Chapter 7: Nursing Care of Patients Receiving Intravenous Therapy

Rita Bolek Trofino, DNP, MNED, RN
Associate Dean, School of Health Sciences
Nursing Department Chair
Associate Professor
Saint Francis University
Loretto, Pennsylvania
Chapter 53: Integumentary System Function, Assessment, and Therapeutic Measures
Chapter 54: Nursing Care of Patients With Skin Disorders
Chapter 55: Nursing Care of Patients With Burns

April Hazard Vallerand, PhD, RN, FAAN
College of Nursing Alumni Endowed Professor of Nursing
Wayne State University
College of Nursing
Detroit, Michigan
Chapter 10: Pain

Kelli Verdecchia, MSN, RN
Assistant Professor
Lake Superior State University
Sault Sainte Marie, Michigan
Chapter 8: Nursing Care of Patients With Infections

Patrice Wade-Olsen, DNP, RN, AGPCNP-BC
Nurse Practitioner
Oakland Integrated Health Care Network
Waterford, Michigan
Chapter 20: Nursing Care of Patients With HIV Disease and AIDS

Patricia Williams, MSN, RN
Assistant Professor / PN Program Coordinator
Hagerstown Community College
Hagerstown, Maryland
Chapter 13: Nursing Care of Patients With Emergent Conditions and Disaster/Bioterrorism Response

Janet M. Yontas, MSNed, RN
Nurse Educator
Career Technology Center, Practical Nursing - Lackawanna County
Scranton, Pennsylvania
Chapter 11: Nursing Care of Patients With Cancer

Contributors to Previous Editions

We would like to acknowledge and thank the following individuals for their contributions to previous editions. All contributions have helped to make *Understanding Medical-Surgical Nursing* what it has evolved into today.

Betty Ackley, MSN, EdS, RN

Nancy Ahern, PhD, RN

Cynthia Barrere, PhD, RN

Lucy L. Colo, MSN, RN

Colleen Delaney, PhD, RN, AHN-BC

Sharon Gordon, MSN, RN, CNOR(E)

Karen P. Hall, RN-C, MSHSA, NE-BC

Wendy Hockley, BS, MA, LPN

Michelle Johnson, MSN, RN, CNE

Marty Kohn, BSN, MS, RN, FNP, CWOCN

Carroll A. Lutz, MA, RN

Diane Mayo, MSN, RN

Erin Mazur, MSN, RN, FNP-BC

Kelly McManigle, MSN, RN

Kelly Ann Morris, DNP, RN

Sharon M. Nowak, MSN, EdD (ABD), RN

Debra Perry-Philo, BSN, MSN, RN

Lynn D. Phillips, MSN, RN, CRNI

Deb Richardson, MS, RN, CNS

John Sturtevant, MSN, RN

Deborah L. Weaver, PhD, RN

Bruce K. Wilson, PhD, RN, CNS

Reviewers

Janice Ankenmann, RN, MSN, CCRN, FNP-C
Nursing Director
Napa Valley College
Napa, California

Linda Rogers Antuono, RN, MSN/Ed.
Nursing Program Manager
Charlotte Technical College
Port Charlotte, Florida

Kristen Bebeau, MA, RN
Nursing Faculty
Hennepin Technical College
Brooklyn Park, Minnesota

Ruth Fee Blackmore, MSN, RN, CNOR
Faculty of Nursing
Isabella Graham Hart School of Practical Nursing
Rochester, New York

Gretheline Bolandrina, MSN Ed, RN, CRRN
Program Director
Bay Path RVTHS Practical Nursing Program
Charlton, Massachusetts

Karla Cepeda, RN, BSN
Nursing Faculty
Kapi'olani Community College
Honolulu, Hawaii

Joan Eula Conde, MS, RN, AGCNS(c)
Nursing Faculty
Kapi'olani Community College
Honolulu, Hawaii

Denese Davis, RN, BSN, Med
Instructor
Wiregrass Georgia Technical College
Valdosta, Georgia

Christina Dent, PhD, RN
Assistant Professor
Abraham Baldwin Agricultural College
Tifton, Georgia

Deanna Dubay, MSN, RN
Nursing Instructor
Davenport University
Midland, Michigan

Penny Fauber, RN, BSN, MS, PhD
Director Practical Nursing Program
Dabney S. Lancaster Community College
Clifton Forge, Virginia

Gail Forrester, MSN, BSN, RN
Instructor, Practical Nursing
Lanier Technical College
Oakwood, Georgia

Louise S. Frantz, MHA, Ed, BSN, RN
Coordinator Practical Nursing
Penn State Berks
Reading, Pennsylvania

Jennifer Gazdick, RN, MSN
Nursing Instructor/Program Coordinator
Holy Name Medical Center School of Practical Nursing
Teaneck, New Jersey

Alice Gilbert, BSN, RN
Director/ Instructor
Ukiah Adult School Vocational Nursing Program
Ukiah, California

Janis Grimland, BSN, RN
Vocational Nursing Program Director
Hill College
Hillsboro, Texas

Theresa Hallowell, BSN, RN
Nursing Instructor
Lincoln Technical Institute
Allentown, Pennsylvania

Christy Henry, BSN, RN
Practical Nursing Coordinator
Texas County Technical College
Houston, Missouri

Susan Irvine, MS, RN
Faculty Program Director
Excelsior College
School of Nursing
AD Nursing
Albany, New York

Kathy A. Johnson, RN, BSN
Practical Nursing Instructor
Greater Lowell Technical School
Tyngsboro, Massachusetts

Cynthia L. Lapp, RN, BS
Nursing Instructor
Jefferson-Lewis BOCES
Watertown, New York

Kristin Madigan, MS, RN
Nursing Faculty
Pine Technical and Community College
Pine City, Minnesota

Nancy K. Maebius, PhD, RN
Education Consultant
Galen College of Nursing
San Antonio, Texas

Joann Maffeo, MSN, RN
Nursing Instructor
Lincoln Technical Institute
New Britain, Connecticut

Jennifer Mahnken, MS, RN, CNE
Adjunct Professor
Jefferson-Lewis BOCES
Watertown, New York

Ruth Martin, DNP, RN
Practical Nursing Coordinator
Somerset Community College
Somerset, Kentucky

Cinthia dos Santos Mesquita, BSN, RN
Faculty
Assabet Valley Practical Nurse Program
Marlborough, Massachusetts

Dianna Michael, MSN, RN
Assistant Director of Nursing
ECPI University
Greensboro, North Carolina

Paula K. Mundell, MSN, RN
Coordinator Nursing Department
Delaware Technical Community College
Terry Campus
Dover, Delaware

Karen O'Neil, MSN, RN
Practical Nurse Program Coordinator
Jefferson Community & Technical College
Louisville, Kentucky

Emilyn Ostrea, RN-BC, PHN, DSD, MBA
Nursing Faculty
City College of San Francisco
San Francisco, California

Judith Pahlck, MSN-Ed, RN
Dean of Nursing
Jersey College
Teterboro, New Jersey
The author also acknowledges her contribution to Chapter 45.

Amanda Perkins, RN, MSN
Assistant Professor of Nursing
Vermont Technical College
Randolph, Vermont

Thomas Petricini, MSN, RN
Nursing Instructor
Sharon Regional Health System
Sharon, Pennsylvania

Megan Pet, DNP, MSN, MBA, RN
Associate Professor, Program Coordinator
Moraine Valley Community College
Palos Hills, Illinois

Jennifer M. Rohr, RN, BSN, MS
Practical Nursing Faculty
Southeast Community College
Beatrice, Nebraska

Kristin Ruiz, MN, RN
Instructor Practical Nursing
Southeast Community College
Beatrice, Nebraska

Darla K. Shar, MSN, RN
Associate Director and Instructor
Hannah E. Mullins School of Practical Nursing
Salem, Ohio

Romona Smith, MSN-Ed, RN
Med/Surg Didactic and Clinical Instructor
Jersey College
Teterboro. New Jersey

Rhonda Stangl, DNP, RN
Nursing Instructor
Lake Area Technical Institute
Watertown, South Dakota

Elizabeth A. Summers, MSN, RN, CNE
Coordinator of PN Program
Cass Career Center
Harrisonville, Missouri

Sharon Weaver, EdS, MSN/Ed, BSN, RN
Practical Nursing Instructor
Lincoln Technical School
Allentown, Pennsylvania

Melanie Wynja, MSN, RN
Nursing Instructor/Simulation Coordinator
Northwest Iowa Community College
Sheldon, Iowa

Debbie Yarnell, BSN
Coordinator/Instructor
State Fair Community College
Eldon, Missouri

Contents

CHAPTER 1
Critical Thinking and the Nursing Process

Paula D. Hopper

KEY TERMS

assessment (ah-SESS-ment)
clinical judgment (KLIN-ih-kull JUDJ-ment)
collaborative (koh-LAB-rah-tiv)
critical thinking (KRIT-ih-kull THING-king)
data (DAY-tuh)
evaluation (e-VAL-yoo-AY-shun)
evidence-based practice (EV-ah-dens baste PRAK-tis)
intervention (in-ter-VEN-shun)
nursing diagnosis (NER-sing DY-ag-NOH-sis)
nursing process (NER-sing PRAH-sess)
objective data (ob-JEK-tiv DAY-tuh)
subjective data (sub-JEK-tiv DAY-tuh)
vigilance (VIJ-eh-lents)

CHAPTER CONCEPTS

Evidence-Based Practice
Patient-Centered Care
Safety

LEARNING OUTCOMES

1. Explain why good critical thinking is important in nursing.
2. Describe attitudes and skills that promote good critical thinking.
3. Describe the thinking that occurs in each step of the nursing process.
4. Identify the role of a licensed practical nurse/licensed vocational nurse in using the nursing process.
5. Differentiate between objective and subjective data.
6. Document objective and subjective data.
7. Prioritize patient care activities based on the Maslow hierarchy of human needs.

Excellence in the delivery of nursing care requires good thinking. Each day nurses make many decisions that affect the care of their patients. For those decisions to be effective, the thinking behind them must be sound.

 CRITICAL THINKING

Nursing students must learn to think critically—in other words, to think like a nurse. This means they must use their knowledge and skills to make the best decisions possible in patient care situations. Halpern (2013) says that "**critical thinking** is the use of those cognitive [knowledge] skills or strategies that increase the probability of a desirable outcome" (p. 4). Good thinking in nursing care has also been called *clinical reasoning* or *clinical judgment*. **Clinical judgment** can be defined as "the outcome of critical thinking and decision making" (Dickison

& Tillman, 2017). Good clinical judgment requires critical thinking attitudes and skills, which are described in this section. It also requires a good knowledge base, so that your thinking and decisions are based on correct, factual information. You will practice critical thinking skills and clinical judgment in clinical situations or simulations with your instructors. Our goal in this text is to provide you with evidence-based, solid medical-surgical knowledge on which to base good decisions.

Critical Thinking Traits
It is important for nurses to possess an attitude that promotes good thinking. The Foundation for Critical Thinking (2015) identifies eight traits associated with good critical thinking: (1) intellectual humility, (2) intellectual courage, (3) intellectual empathy, (4) intellectual autonomy, (5) intellectual

integrity, (6) intellectual perseverance, (7) faith in reason, and (8) fair-mindedness.

Intellectual Humility

Have you ever known people who think they know it all? They do not have intellectual humility. People with intellectual humility have the ability to say, "I'm not sure about that ... I need more information." Certainly, we want our patients to think we are smart and know what we are doing. However, patients also respect nurses who can say, "I don't know, but I'll find out." It is unsafe to care for patients when you are unsure of what you need to do.

Intellectual Courage

Intellectual courage allows you to look at other points of view even when you may not agree with them at first. Maybe you really believe that 8-hour shifts are best for nurses, and you have a lot of good reasons for your belief. But if you have intellectual courage, you will be willing to really listen to the arguments for 12-hour shifts. Maybe you will even become convinced. Sometimes you must have the courage to say, "Okay, I see you were right after all."

Intellectual Empathy

Consider the patient who snaps as you enter her room, "I've been waiting all morning for my bath. If you don't help me with it right now, I'm going to call your supervisor." The first response that comes into your head is, "I have five other patients. You're lucky I am here!" If you have intellectual empathy, however, you will be able to think, "If I were this patient, who is in chronic pain and is tired of being in the hospital, how would I feel?" Such thinking might change how you respond.

Intellectual Autonomy

Did your mom ever say, "Just because everyone is doing it doesn't make it okay!"? You may see some nurses cutting corners or doing things that you don't think are safe. If you have intellectual autonomy, you will think about what you observe and determine for yourself whether it is safe.

Intellectual Integrity

One of your patients asks a hundred questions when you bring her a medication that has been newly prescribed to lower her high blood pressure. Later, you notice she is taking an herbal remedy from her purse. It is good that she asks a lot of questions about her drug, which has been tested extensively by the Food and Drug Administration. In the United States, however, herbal remedies are not held to the same standards as are medications. Someone with intellectual integrity would want the same level of proof applied to both medications and herbal remedies to determine whether they are safe and effective before using them.

Intellectual Perseverance

Perseverance means you do not give up. Consider this scenario: You have concerns about some side effects that you noticed after giving a new drug to a patient. You mention it to the health care provider (HCP), who says not to worry about it. However, you are still concerned. If you have intellectual perseverance, you might do some research and then go to your supervisor or the pharmacist to further discuss your concerns.

Faith in Reason

If you have faith in reason, you believe in your heart that good clinical reasoning (i.e., critical thinking in clinical situations) will result in the best clinical judgments and, therefore, the best outcomes for your patients. And if you really believe, you will be more likely to attend a seminar or read an article on developing your clinical judgment skills.

Fair-Mindedness

A coworker wants to change the medication administration schedule on your unit. She says it will be better for the patients. However, you think it might be because it is a better fit for her coffee-break schedule. If you are fair-minded, you will be sure that your thinking is not biased by something that you just want for yourself, as seems to be happening with your coworker. You should examine your own motives as well as those of others when you are making decisions.

So, what does all this mean to you as a nursing student? The term *metacognition* means to "think about thinking." It is important for you to try to develop the attitudes of a critical thinker and learn to think clearly and critically about patient care. To do that, you need to constantly reflect on how you are thinking. Are you practicing intellectual humility? Are you trying to be courageous and empathetic? These attitudes create an excellent base on which to build nursing knowledge and develop further thinking skills.

> **LEARNING TIP**
> Each time you exit a patient's room, do a mini–critical thinking assessment. Ask yourself, "Did I ask the right questions? Was my thinking clear and logical? Is there anything I could have done better?" This 1-minute metacognition exercise will help you develop as a great thinker.

Nursing Knowledge Base

Nurses must have a solid knowledge base to safely care for patients. You would not drive a car without first learning the basics of how a car works and the rules of the road. In the same way, you must understand the human body in health and illness before you can understand how to take care of an ill patient. This is the reason you are going to school and studying this book.

Information is found in many places; some information is good, and some is not as good. For example, health information found on a web site may have been put there by a major university or other reputable source, or it may have been put there by a patient who has a particular disorder. While you may learn about a patient's experience by reading his or her web site, you certainly would not base your patient care on someone's personal story.

The best knowledge on which to base your practice comes from research. When nursing care is based on good, well-designed research studies, it is called **evidence-based practice.** You will read more about evidence-based practice in Chapter 2.

Critical Thinking Skills

Clinical Judgment

Clinical judgment involves solving problems effectively. Nurses solve problems every day. However, a problem can be handled in a way that may or may not help the patient. For instance, consider Mr. Frank, who is in pain and asks for pain medication. His analgesic is not due for another 40 minutes. You can choose to manage this problem in several ways. One approach is to tell Mr. Frank that it is not time for the pain medication and that he will have to wait. This may solve *your* problem (you can move on to the next patient), but it does not solve *Mr. Frank's* problem as he is still in pain. Another approach is to use a standard problem-solving method: (1) gather data, (2) identify the problem, (3) decide what outcome is desirable, (4) plan what to do, (5) implement the interventions in your plan, and (6) evaluate the plan of care.

1. Gather **data,** or factual information, to help you think critically about Mr. Frank's request for pain medication. As a good critical thinker, you can use intellectual empathy as well as your knowledge base about pain to decide what data you need. You decide to use a pain-rating scale on which the patient rates pain from 0 (no pain) to 10 (the greatest pain possible). Mr. Frank says that the pain is in his back and rates it at an 8 on the scale. He adds that his pain has gotten worse since he's been confined to the hospital bed. You check his history in the chart and find that he has spinal compression fractures. Your empathetic attitude tells you that waiting for 40 minutes to relieve his pain is not acceptable. You next go to the medication record and find that he has no alternative pain medications ordered.

2. Identify the problem. Here you use your knowledge base about compression fractures, pain, and medication administration to draw the conclusion that Mr. Frank is in acute pain and that the current medication orders are not sufficient to provide pain relief.

3. Decide what outcome (or goal) is desirable. Work together with the patient to determine the best outcome. The patient is intimately involved in this situation and deserves to be consulted. You may also collaborate with the registered nurse (RN) or HCP. You talk to Mr. Frank and determine that he needs pain relief now; he cannot wait until the next scheduled dose of medication. He states that he can tolerate a pain rating of 3 or less on the scale.

4. Plan what to do. Formulate and consider some alternate solutions. For example, you can tell Mr. Frank that he has to wait 40 minutes; however, this will not help him reach his desired outcome of pain control. You could give the medication early, but this would not be following the HCP's orders and may have harmful effects

for Mr. Frank. You could decide to try some nondrug pain-control methods, such as relaxation, distraction, or imagery. These might be helpful, but you recall from pharmacology class that complementary methods should be used in conjunction with, not in place of, medications. Another option is to report to the RN or HCP that Mr. Frank's pain is not controlled with the current pain-control regimen. Once you have several alternative courses of action, you can discuss options with the RN and together decide the best thing to do; in this case, you might decide to have the RN contact the HCP while you work with Mr. Frank on relaxation exercises. This would assure him that his pain is being taken seriously.

5. Implement the **interventions** in your plan. The RN enters the room and informs you and Mr. Frank that the HCP has changed the analgesic orders. You obtain and administer the first dose of the new analgesic, being sure to explain its effects and side effects to Mr. Frank. The RN also informs Mr. Frank that the HCP has ordered a consultation with the pain clinic.

6. Evaluate the plan of care. Did the plan work? As you recheck Mr. Frank 30 minutes later, he rates his pain level at 2 on the 10-point scale. He smiles and thanks you for your attentiveness to his needs. You think back to the desired outcome, compare it with the current data collected, and determine that your interventions were successful.

Can you see how using good thinking attitudes, a good knowledge base, and the problem-solving process led to a better outcome than simply choosing the first obvious option? You were able to achieve a desirable outcome: assisting Mr. Frank in relieving his pain. And you have earned Mr. Frank's trust in the process. Problem-solving is how nurses make decisions on a daily basis. In nursing, we call it the *nursing process.*

Other Critical Thinking Skills

Problem-solving is just one critical thinking skill. Another way you can use critical thinking in patient care is by anticipating what might go wrong, watching carefully for signs that a problem might be occurring, and then preventing it or notifying the RN or HCP in time to intervene. Nurses save many lives each year by anticipating and preventing problems. This is called **vigilance.** An example would be knowing the signs and symptoms of low blood glucose (because of your excellent knowledge base) and watching for them carefully (being vigilant) in a patient taking medication for diabetes. If early symptoms occur, you can intervene before the problem becomes severe. In addition, you could teach the patient and family about low blood glucose and how to prevent it, further reducing the risk to the patient.

There are many other thinking skills that are beyond the scope of this book. You can ask yourself the questions that follow as you continue to develop your thinking skills. These are not in any order nor would they all be asked for in a given situation. They are just some ideas to get you started.

• Have I thought this through?
• What information do I need?

- How do I know?
- Is someone influencing my thinking in ways I am not aware of?
- What conclusions can I draw from the information I have?
- Am I basing this decision on assumptions that may or may not be true?
- Am I thinking creatively about this, or am I in a rut?
- What do I need to watch for in order to prevent complications?
- Is there an expert I can consult who can help me think this through?
- Is there any supporting research or evidence that confirms this is true?
- Am I too stressed or tired to think carefully about this right now?

BE SAFE!

BE VIGILANT! Always ask yourself as you prepare for patient care each day, "What is the worst thing that could happen to this patient today? What are early signs I should recognize, based on the patient's diagnoses? What will I do if they occur?" Plan ahead to be vigilant and you can prevent many patient care disasters!

 ## NURSING PROCESS

You have just used the nursing process to solve Mr. Frank's problem. The **nursing process** is a clinical problem-solving process that links thinking with actions in nursing practice. The nursing process is used to determine patient needs by collecting data, formulating nursing diagnoses, and planning, implementing, and evaluating care. As a nursing student, you consciously apply the nursing process to each patient problem. With experience, you will internalize the nursing process and use it without as much conscious effort.

Role of the Licensed Practical Nurse/Licensed Vocational Nurse

The licensed practical nurse (LPN) or licensed vocational nurse (LVN) carries out a specific role in the nursing process, as described in Table 1.1. The role of the LPN/LVN is to provide direct patient care. The LPN/LVN often spends more time at the bedside than the RN, which allows the LPN/LVN to develop a therapeutic relationship and understand the patient's needs. The LPN/LVN and the RN collaborate to analyze data and develop, implement, and evaluate the plan of care (Fig. 1.1).

Data Collection

The first step in the nursing process is **assessment.** The LPN/LVN assists the RN in collecting data from a variety of sources to create a comprehensive assessment. Data are divided into two types: subjective data and objective data.

Table 1.1

Role of the Licensed Practical Nurse/Licensed Vocational Nurse in the Nursing Process

Steps of the Process	*Role of the Licensed Practical Nurse/Licensed Vocational Nurse*
Data Collection	Assists registered nurse (RN) in collecting data for assessment
Nursing Diagnosis	Assists RN in choosing appropriate nursing diagnoses
Planning Care	Assists RN in developing patient outcomes and planning care
Implementation	Carries out portions of the plan of care that are within the licensed practical nurse/licensed vocational nurse scope of practice
Evaluation	Assists RN in evaluation and revision of the plan of care

Note: There may be slight variations by state.

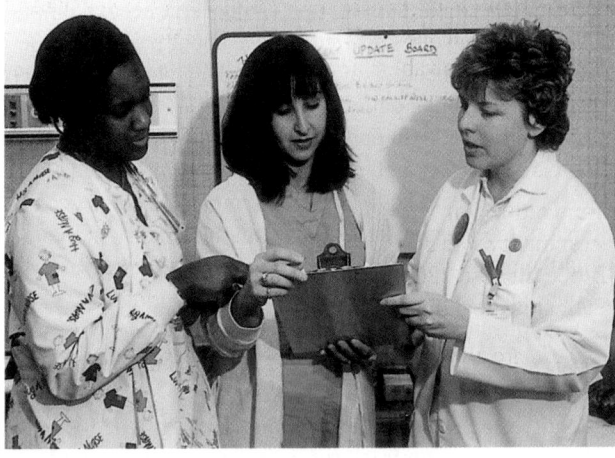

FIGURE 1.1 The nursing care team collaborating on a nursing care plan.

Subjective Data

Information provided verbally by the patient is called **subjective data.** Symptoms are subjective data. Anxiety or pain would be considered subjective data because only the patient can feel them. A nurse cannot objectively observe them. Often, subjective information is placed in quotes when documented, such as "I have a headache" or "I feel out of breath." You must listen carefully to the patient and understand that only the patient truly knows how he or she feels.

When collecting subjective data, start with the patient's main concern. Try asking, "What happened that brought you to the hospital [clinic, office]?" or "Do you have a specific concern today?"

Once the patient has identified the main concern, further questioning can reveal more pertinent information. Use the phrase **WHAT'S UP?** as a handy way to remember questions to ask the patient (Box 1.1). Asking the right questions can help you obtain better data with which to make the best decisions.

Next, obtain a patient history. Do this by asking the patient and family questions about the patient's past and present health problems, including specific questions about each body system, family health problems, and risk factors for health problems. The patient's medical record may also be consulted for background history information.

In addition to assessment of physiological function, ask the patient about personal habits that relate to health, such as exercise, diet, and the presence of stressors, according to institutional assessment guidelines. Finally, ask about the patient's family role, support systems, and cultural and spiritual beliefs.

> ### LEARNING TIP
> Practice assessing a symptom on a classmate. Ask the *WHAT'S UP?* questions.

Objective Data

Objective data are pieces of factual information obtained through physical assessment and diagnostic tests that are observable or knowable through the five senses. For example, a rash can be observed with the eyes and palpated with the fingers (with gloves on, of course). Objective data are sometimes called *signs*. Examples of objective data include the following:

- 3-cm red lesion
- Respiratory rate 36 per minute
- Blood glucose 326 mg/dL
- Patient is moaning

These are all observable or measurable by a nurse and do not need an explanation by the patient.

Box 1.1

WHAT'S UP? Guide to Symptom Assessment

W—Where is it?

H—How does it feel? Describe the quality (e.g., is it dull, sharp, stabbing?).

A—Aggravating and alleviating factors. What makes it worse? What makes it better?

T—Timing. When did it start? How long does it last?

S—Severity. How bad is it? This can often be rated on a scale of 0 to 10.

U—Useful other data. What other symptoms are present that might be related?

P—Patient's perception of the problem. The patient often has an idea about what the problem is or the cause but may not believe that his or her thoughts are important to share unless specifically asked.

Objective data are gathered through physical assessment. Inspection, palpation, percussion, and auscultation techniques are used to collect objective data (Fig. 1.2). You can find more on these techniques, as well as how to obtain a complete history, in a nursing assessment text. Pay special attention to problem areas identified by the patient.

Documentation of Data

Document all data in the patient's medical record. If you identify any significant problem, change in the patient's status, or variation from normal, first report it immediately to an RN or HCP and then document it. Recorded data should be accurate and concise.

When documenting subjective data, use what was stated by the patient or significant other. Use direct quotations whenever possible, such as, "I feel sad." Quotes accurately represent the patient's view and are least open to mistaken interpretation.

When documenting objective data, include exactly what you observed. Avoid interpreting the data and using words that have vague meanings. For example, "nailbed color is pink" gives clearer information than does "nailbed color is normal." "Normal" is an interpretation of data rather than true data. "Capillary refill is 2 seconds" is more precise than "capillary refill is good." The statement "the wound looks better" is not meaningful unless the reader has previously observed the wound. Stating that "the wound is 1 by 2 inches, red, with no drainage or odor" provides data with which to compare the future status of the wound and determine whether it is responding to treatment.

> ### LEARNING TIP
> Beginners may be tempted to use elaborate phrases or words to document, when simple, direct words are best. Simply state exactly what you saw or heard to provide the clearest and most accurate information.

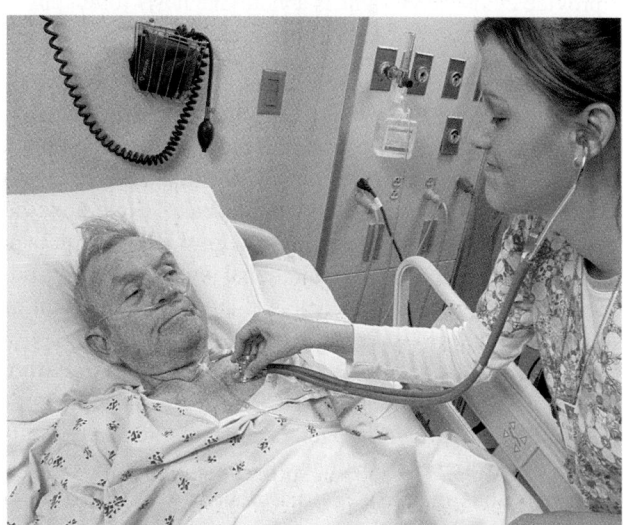

FIGURE 1.2 Nurse auscultating a patient's chest.

Nursing Diagnosis

Once data have been collected, the LPN/LVN assists the RN to compare the findings with what is considered normal. Data are then grouped, or clustered, into sets of related information that identify problems. Problems are then labeled as nursing diagnoses.

According to NANDA International (NANDA-I; formerly, the North American Nursing Diagnosis Association), a **nursing diagnosis** is a "clinical judgment concerning a human response to health conditions/life processes, or a vulnerability for that response, by an individual, family, group or community. A nursing diagnosis provides the basis for selection of nursing interventions to achieve outcomes for which the nurse has accountability" (NANDA International, 2017). Nursing diagnoses are standardized labels that make an identified problem understandable to all nurses.

A diagnosis is considered "medical" when the HCP directs most of the care. For example, pneumonia is a medical diagnosis and requires antibiotics, which are ordered by the HCP. A diagnosis is considered "nursing" if the interventions needed to treat the problem are mainly independent nursing functions.

One example of a NANDA-I nursing diagnosis is *Acute Pain.* In Mr. Frank's scenario, the nurse identified that pain was a problem, and a plan of care was developed to manage the pain. The HCP was contacted for analgesic orders, but independent nursing actions were also used, including relaxation and distraction. These independent nursing actions did not require an HCP's order.

A well-written nursing diagnosis helps guide development of a plan of care. The three parts of a diagnosis include the following:

- Problem: the nursing diagnosis label from the NANDA-I list
- Etiology: the cause or related factor (usually preceded by the words "related to")
- Signs and symptoms: the subjective or objective data that provide evidence that this is a valid diagnosis (often preceded by the words "as evidenced by")

The statement of **P**roblem, **E**tiology, and **S**igns and symptoms is called the *PES format.* Consider again Mr. Frank. A diagnosis using this format might read: "*Acute Pain* related to muscle spasms and nerve compression as evidenced by patient's pain rating of 8 on a 10-point scale." Note how the complete diagnosis gives you more helpful information than simply the label "pain." This additional information helps determine an appropriate outcome and guides the selection of interventions.

Many patient problems benefit from a **collaborative** approach—that is, the nurse, HCP, and other members of the health team all work together to reach the desired outcome. For example, a patient with pneumonia (a medical diagnosis) has many needs that depend on HCP orders, such as respiratory treatments and antibiotics. The role of the LPN/LVN is to collect important data on the patient's respiratory status and to provide nursing measures such as encouraging fluid intake, coughing, and deep breathing.

CRITICAL THINKING

Nursing Diagnoses: Which of the following are NANDA-I nursing diagnoses? Which are medical diagnoses?

1. *Impaired Physical Mobility*
2. *Ineffective Coping*
3. *Herniated Disk*
4. *Fractured Femur*
5. *Diabetes*
6. *Impaired Gas Exchange*
7. *Appendicitis*
8. *Activity Intolerance*

   Suggested answers are at the end of the chapter.

Planning of Care

Once nursing diagnoses have been identified, an individualized plan of care is designed to help meet the patient's needs. Planning involves setting priorities, establishing outcomes, and identifying interventions that will help the patient meet the identified outcomes. It is important to include the patient in the development of the plan of care. The plan will be most successful if the patient agrees with and understands the interventions.

Prioritize Care

Once you know what problems need to be addressed, you must decide which problem or intervention should be taken care of first. Because care should always be *patient-centered,* with the patient at the center of the health team, such decisions should involve the patient as well as the RN and LPN/LVN. The Maslow hierarchy of human needs can be used as a basis for determining priorities (Fig. 1.3). According to Maslow, humans must meet their most basic needs (those at the bottom of the triangle) first. They can then move up the hierarchy to meet higher-level needs.

Physiological needs are the most basic. For example, a person who is having difficulty breathing is not worried about love or self-esteem; he just wants to be able to breathe. Once physiological needs are met, the patient can concentrate on meeting safety and security needs. Love, belonging, and self-esteem needs are next; self-actualization needs are generally the last priority when planning care. Needs can occur simultaneously on different levels and must be addressed in a holistic manner, with prioritization guiding the care provided.

If several physiological needs are present, life-threatening needs are ranked first, health-threatening needs are second, and health-promoting needs, although important, are last.

LEARNING TIP

If you are stuck wondering which physiological need should take priority, ask yourself, "Which problem is most threatening to my patient's life?"

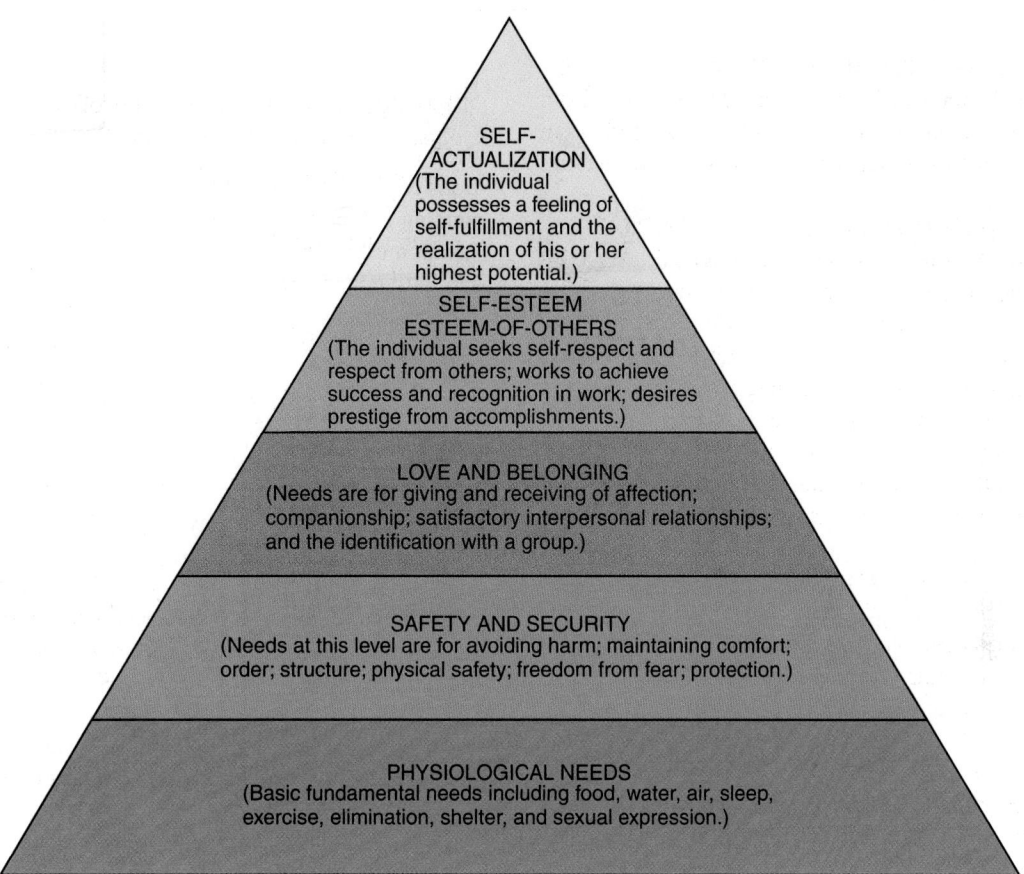

FIGURE 1.3 The Maslow hierarchy of human needs.

LEARNING TIP
If you are developing a plan of care for a patient with complex needs and are not sure where to start, go back to the assessment phase. Often, additional information can help you better understand the patient's needs and develop a plan of care individualized to the patient's specific problem areas.

CRITICAL THINKING

The Maslow Hierarchy of Human Needs: Based on the Maslow hierarchy of human needs, list the following nursing diagnoses in order from highest (1) to lowest (5) priority. Give rationales for your decisions.

____ *Deficient Knowledge*
____ *Constipation*
____ *Disabled Family Coping*
____ *Readiness for Enhanced Self-Concept*
____ *Ineffective Airway Clearance*

Suggested answers are at the end of the chapter.

Establish Outcomes
An outcome is a statement that describes the patient's desired goal for a problem area. It should be measurable, be realistic for the patient, and have an appropriate time frame for achievement. *Measurable* means that the outcome is objective or can be observed. It should not be vague or open to interpretation, with the use of subjective words such as "normal" or "large." Consider, for example, two outcomes:

1. The patient's shortness of breath will improve.
2. The patient will be less short of breath within 15 minutes as evidenced by the patient rating the shortness of breath at less than 3 on a scale of 0 to 10, having a respiratory rate between 16 and 20 per minute, and appearing relaxed.

Although the first outcome seems appropriate, in reality it is difficult to know when it has been met. There is nothing to objectively indicate when the problem has been resolved. The second outcome is objective. You can see that when the patient rates his or her shortness of breath at less than 3, is breathing at a rate of 16 to 20 per minute, and appears relaxed, the desired outcome will have been met. The outcome is realistic, and the 15-minute time frame ensures that the patient's distress is minimized. If the plan of care does not achieve the desired outcome in the given time frame, it should be evaluated and revised as needed.

When determining criteria for a measurable outcome, look at the signs-and-symptoms portion of the nursing diagnosis. The resolution of signs and symptoms identified in the nursing diagnoses is evidence that nursing interventions were effective. If the desired outcome is not achieved, the problem and interventions need reevaluation. Let's look again at Mr. Frank's nursing diagnosis:

- Nursing diagnosis: *Acute Pain* related to muscle spasms and nerve compression as evidenced by patient's pain rating of 8 on a 10-point scale
- Outcome: Patient will state his pain level is less than 3 on a 10-point scale within 30 minutes of intervention.

Identify Interventions

Interventions are the actions you take to help a patient meet a desired outcome. Therefore, interventions should be *goal directed.* Any intervention that does not contribute to meeting the outcome should not be part of the plan of care.

One way to create a care plan is to include interventions that can be categorized as "take, treat, and teach." In the first intervention category, "take," or identify, data related to the problem. Next, "treat" the problem by identifying deliberate actions to help reach the outcome. Last, identify what to "teach" the patient and family to promote self-care.

Look again at the nursing diagnosis of *Acute Pain.* A plan of care for this problem using the take, treat, and teach method might look like this:

Take: Assess pain level every 4 hours and as needed.
Treat: Provide pain medication as ordered.
Provide warm compresses as ordered.
Offer back rubs.
Teach: Teach the patient relaxation exercises.
Teach about the benefits of distraction such as music or television.

In addition to identifying interventions, it is important to understand how and why they will work. The "why" is called a *rationale.* For example, you should assess pain *because the patient is the only person who knows what his pain feels like.* You provide warm compresses *to bring blood to the tissues and promote muscle relaxation.* Sound rationales that are evidence based should guide the selection of each nursing intervention. You will find rationales with interventions throughout this book to help you understand why interventions will be effective.

Like nursing diagnoses, nursing interventions can be either independent or collaborative. Independent nursing actions can be initiated by the nurse. Examples of independent nursing actions include assessment, teaching the patient relaxation exercises, and giving a back rub for comfort. Collaborative actions require an HCP's order to perform. Examples of collaborative interventions include giving prescribed medications or applying a warm compress.

Implementation of Interventions

Once the plan of care has been identified, it must be communicated to the patient, family, and health team members and then implemented. One way a plan of care is communicated is by writing it as a nursing care plan. The nursing care plan is documented on the patient's medical record to communicate to all nurses the patient's priority problems, the desired outcomes, and the plan for meeting the outcomes. Many institutions have standardized care plans that are individualized for each patient by the nurse.

Implementation of the plan of care involves performing the interventions. The patient's response to each intervention is noted and documented. This documentation provides the basis for evaluation and revision of the plan of care.

Evaluation of Outcomes

The last step of the nursing process is **evaluation.** The nurse continuously evaluates the patient's progress toward the desired outcomes and the effectiveness of each intervention. So, if Mr. Frank's pain level is still at a level of 5 on the 10-point scale 30 minutes after intervention, the plan of care should be revised. Any part of the plan of care can be revised, from the diagnosis or desired outcome to the interventions. Acute care institutions require routine review and updating of the plan of care.

SUGGESTED ANSWERS TO CRITICAL THINKING

Nursing Diagnoses

1. *Impaired Physical Mobility* = nursing
2. *Ineffective Coping* = nursing
3. *Herniated Disk* = medical
4. *Fractured Femur* = medical
5. *Diabetes* = medical
6. *Impaired Gas Exchange* = nursing
7. *Appendicitis* = medical
8. *Activity Intolerance* = nursing

The Maslow Hierarchy of Human Needs

1. *Ineffective Airway Clearance:* physiological need that can be life-threatening
2. *Constipation:* physiological need that can be health-threatening
3. *Deficient Knowledge:* safety and security need
4. *Disabled Family Coping:* love and belonging need
5. *Readiness for Enhanced Self-Concept:* self-esteem need

Review Questions

1. In which of the following ways is critical thinking useful to the nursing process?
   1. It highlights the solution to a problem.
   2. It can lead to a better outcome for the patient.
   3. It simplifies the process.
   4. It helps the nurse arrive at a solution more quickly.

2. Which nurse is exhibiting intellectual humility?
   1. The nurse who is an expert at wound care
   2. The nurse who reports an error to the supervisor
   3. The nurse who tries to empathize with the patient
   4. The nurse who asks a coworker about a new procedure

3. Which of the following pieces of information is considered objective data?
   1. The patient's respiratory rate is 28.
   2. The patient states, "I feel short of breath."
   3. The patient is short of breath.
   4. The patient is feeling panicky.

4. The nurse is collecting data on a newly admitted patient who has an ulcerated area on his left hip. It is 2 inches in diameter and 1 inch deep, with yellow exudate. Which of the following statements best documents the findings in the patient's database?
   1. Wound on left hip, 2 inches diameter, 1 inch deep, infected
   2. Left hip wound, large, deep, with yellow drainage
   3. Pressure injury on left hip, yellow drainage
   4. Wound on left hip, 2 inches in diameter, 1 inch deep, yellow exudate

5. A 34-year-old mother of three is newly admitted to a respiratory unit because she has pneumonia. She has all the following problems. Based on the Maslow hierarchy of human needs, place the problems in order of priority.
   1. Frontal headache related to stress of hospital admission
   2. Anxiety related to concern about leaving children
   3. Shortness of breath related to newly diagnosed pneumonia
   4. Deficient knowledge related to discharge plan

6. Place the steps of the nursing process in correct chronological order of use. Use all options.
   1. Nursing diagnosis
   2. Evaluation
   3. Data collection
   4. Planning care
   5. Implementation

7. Which of the following parts of the nursing process can be carried out independently by a licensed practical nurse/licensed vocational nurse?
   1. Implementation of interventions
   2. Nursing diagnosis
   3. Analysis of data
   4. Evaluation of outcomes

8. The nurse teaches a patient the importance of stopping smoking. Which of the following patient responses provides the best evidence that the teaching was effective?
   1. "I have a brother who died of lung cancer. I know smoking is bad."
   2. "I tried to quit 5 years ago, and I really would like to, but it is very hard."
   3. "Thank you for the information. I will call the Smoke Stoppers organization today."
   4. "I know you are right. I should stop smoking."

Answer rationales available in your online resources.

ANSWERS 1. 2, 4; 2. 4; 3. 1; 4. 4; 5. 3, 1, 2, 4; 6. 3, 1, 4, 5, 2; 7. 1; 8. 3

Key Points

Find the chapter key points in your online resources available through Davis Edge.

Additional Resources

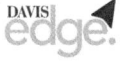 Use the scratch off code on the inside front cover of your book to access online quizzes that will help you to improve your scores on course exams and prepare for the NCLEX-PN®.

 Study Guide

CHAPTER 2
Evidence-Based Practice

Michelle Block, Betty Ackley

KEY TERMS

evidence-based practice (EH-va-dense based PRAK-tis)
evidence-informed practice (Eh-va-dense in-FORMD PRAK-tis)
health literacy (HELTH LIT-ur-AH-see)
numeracy (NEW-mer-ah-see)
randomized controlled trial (RAN-duh-mysd cun-TROLLD TRYUL)
research (re-SURCH)
systematic review (SIS-tem-AT-ik re-VIEW)

CHAPTER CONCEPTS

Evidence-Based Practice

LEARNING OUTCOMES

1. Define evidence-based practice (EBP) and evidence-informed practice.
2. Discuss benefits of using EBP.
3. Explain how to identify nursing evidence that should be put into practice.
4. Describe the EBP process.
5. List the six steps of EBP.
6. Identify who should give evidence-based nursing care, including when and where care should be given.
7. Explain health literacy.
8. Describe how the Quality and Safety Education for Nurses project can promote safe patient care.

Amanda, a licensed practical nurse (LPN), is caring for residents on Unit 4 in a long-term care facility. One of the residents, Mr. Samuel, suffers from dementia. He has difficulty carrying out activities of daily living. Upon inspection, his gums look red, and his tongue looks gray; he has halitosis. He currently receives oral care twice daily with oral foam swabs. Let's explore with Amanda what the evidence says should be done for oral care for Mr. Samuel. (See discussion and answers throughout the chapter.)

Evidence-based practice (EBP) is a systematic process that uses current evidence to make decisions about patient care. Sackett and colleagues (1996) define *evidence-based medicine* as the "conscientious, explicit and judicious use of current best evidence in making decisions about the care of individual patients" and "integrating individual clinical expertise with the best available external clinical evidence from systematic research" (p. 71). This EBP definition has been adapted to other disciplines, including nursing.

A newer term used to discuss the use of evidence in practice is **evidence-informed practice** (EIP). Peters, Hopkins, and Barnett (2016) adapted the work of Sackett and colleagues to define EIP as "conscientious, explicit and judicious use of best currently available evidence, integrated with

clients' values and professional expertise, in making decisions about the care of individuals" (p. 145). EIP stresses consideration of patient factors along with the use of evidence for shared decision making between the health care provider (HCP) and the patient.

EBP involves much more than simply evaluating **research** (scientific study, investigation, or experimentation) to determine which results apply to nursing care. Other factors include the context of care and the patient's preference for interventions and care. Because clinical reality can be very different from a research setting, it could be unrealistic or even unsafe to apply findings from a controlled laboratory research study to an actual clinical situation. Similarly, it could be unsafe to apply research results obtained on people of one age or medical diagnosis to those of another age or with multiple diagnoses. Using EBP is a complex process, but it is an important way to ensure quality care and optimal patient outcomes.

 REASONS FOR USING EBP

The use of EBP allows nurses to give patients the best care possible with improved patient outcomes, which is the goal of all caring nurses. The reasons given for nursing care used to be, "This is how it was taught in nursing school," "This is what they told us in orientation," or "That's the way it is done here." Now the rationale behind the best nursing care is, "Nursing care is based on evidence and how it applies to an individual patient in a specific setting." EBP is considered the gold standard of health care.

Evidence-based outcome measurement is built into the EBP process as a way to measure and confirm the value of a change in nursing practice. For example, nurses are measuring the number of new pressure injuries, new cases of pneumonia, and new urinary tract infections in health care settings. Measuring outcomes as a part of EBP reenergizes nursing by helping nurses see the results of their nursing care. Measured outcomes show nurses that they are giving the best care possible, based on the evidence available at the time.

Evidence comes from multiple sources. In addition to nursing research, medical research and research from many other professions, such as psychology, gerontology, and social work, are utilized to develop EBP nursing care guidelines.

 IDENTIFYING NURSING EVIDENCE

How do you identify nursing evidence that should be put into practice? It depends in part on the strength of the evidence. Evidence ranges from strong to weak, and levels can be assigned to rate its strength and quality. The rating scale used to label the quality of evidence ranges from Level I to Level IV (Table 2.1). Level I is the best evidence. It includes **systematic reviews** and analysis of many high-quality, **randomized controlled trials** (studies designed to assess the effects of a variable by randomly assigning subjects to experimental, placebo, or control groups). Level IV evidence is the weakest. It includes the nonresearch-based opinions of experts or published but nonresearch-based clinical articles. Two of the

best-known sources for Level I evidence are the Cochrane Database of Systematic Reviews (found at www.cochranelibrary.com) for medical evidence and the Joanna Briggs Institute's evidence-based resources (found at www.joannabriggs.org) for nursing practice.

 THE EBP PROCESS

Evidence that guides nursing care can be used in two ways, generally based on whether the evidence is a dependent or an independent nursing intervention. Dependent nursing interventions are those that are delegated by an HCP. Here, any change in practice must undergo committee review, such as the policy and procedure committee, to determine whether it is appropriate for adoption. If the intervention is independent, however, the nurse can implement an evidence-based change based on personal knowledge of the value of the intervention, as long as the change is safe and cannot harm the patient. An example of an independent intervention is reality orientation. Excellent research shows that the use of reality orientation can improve thinking ability in patients with dementia and delirium. The nurse can implement this intervention independently because it does not require an order. Other independent interventions include the use of hand massage, music therapy, and other anxiety-relieving interventions.

A simplified version of the EBP process is discussed next and shown in Figure 2.1. The acronym **ASKMME!** is designed to help you remember the six essential steps: **A**sk, **S**earch, thin**K**, **M**easure, **M**ake it happen, and **E**valuate (Ackley et al., 2008).

Step 1: Ask the Burning Question

EBP begins with questioning the status quo, trying to solve a problem, or learning about new evidence that should be used in nursing practice. The initial question nurses often ask is,

Table 2.1
Levels of Evidence

Level	Type of Evidence
Level I	*Systematic reviews, such as those through Cochrane Reviews and the Joanna Briggs Institute:* Evidence from a systematic review of all relevant randomized clinical trials or evidence-based clinical practice guidelines that are based on systematic reviews of randomized controlled trials. Three or more randomized controlled trials of good quality that have similar results also have been considered Level I evidence.
Level II	*Randomized controlled trials:* Evidence obtained from at least one well-designed randomized controlled trial. These are true experimental studies in which as many factors as possible that could falsely change the results are controlled.
Level III	*Quasi-experimental studies:* Evidence obtained from quasi-experimental research studies that do not control factors that could falsely change the results and, as a result, are less predictive of effectiveness of nursing care.
Level IV	*Expert opinion:* Evidence from the opinion of authorities and/or reports of expert committees or from nursing journal articles that are opinion based, not research based.

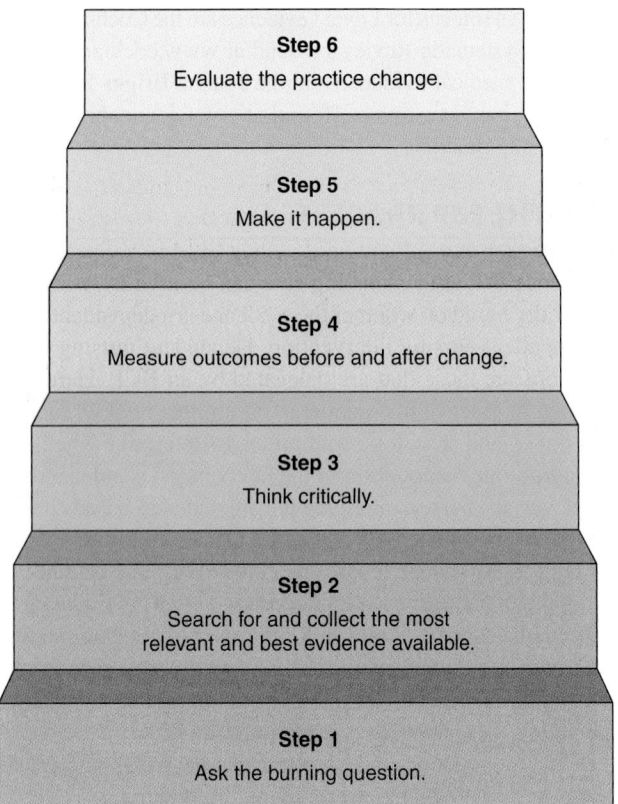

Step 6
Evaluate the practice change.

Step 5
Make it happen.

Step 4
Measure outcomes before and after change.

Step 3
Think critically.

Step 2
Search for and collect the most relevant and best evidence available.

Step 1
Ask the burning question.

FIGURE 2.1 The six steps of the evidence-based practice process.

"Why do we do it that way?" or "How could we do this better?" Questioning the existing way of doing things is part of critical thinking. It helps ensure that the patient receives the best care possible. As a student nurse, you can do this as well.

For Mr. Samuel, in the case study at the start of the chapter, Amanda was motivated to find the best way to give oral care, because her instincts told her the current care was not effective. Amanda took her clinical question to the policy and procedure committee. Together, they began the evidence-based process to find the best way to give oral care to patients at their agency.

Step 2: Search for and Collect the Most Relevant and Best Evidence Available

A thorough search of the literature in the subject area needs to be conducted. As a student nurse, you will find medical librarians most helpful. It is important that you learn basic computer skills so that you also have the ability to search the nursing and medical literature. To find the best available evidence, you must search multiple databases for systematic reviews, research studies, and journal articles.

One well-known database for nursing literature is CINAHL (Cumulative Index to Nursing and Allied Health Literature; https://health.ebsco.com/products/the-cinahl-database). CINAHL is available through college and hospital libraries. Evidence-based care sheets are available on CINAHL. These sheets summarize current best practice on a specific topic. For nursing evidence-based resources, visit the Joanna Briggs Institute web site (www.joannabriggs.org).

This may be available to access through your nursing library.

For biomedical literature, which includes nursing, the comprehensive PubMed/Medline database can be accessed at www.ncbi.nlm.nih.gov/pubmed. Cochrane Reviews are available at www.cochranelibrary.com.

Amanda worked with a medical librarian and other members of her agency's policy and procedure committee to conduct an EBP search on oral care. They then summarized the research articles they found in this area (Table 2.2).

Step 3: Think Critically

Always appraise the evidence you find for validity, relevance to the situation, and applicability. First, evaluate the quality of the evidence you find. It is helpful to determine the level of the evidence to make sure you have the best information available (see Table 2.1). For example, if you locate a systematic review, meta-analysis, or meta-aggregation, you have found a source of preappraised evidence using a prescribed step-by-step search of the best available evidence. Next, using critical thinking, evaluate the evidence as it applies to the individual patient or patient population, the clinical expertise of the nurse(s) involved, the values surrounding the situation, and agency policies that affect making a change in practice.

Amanda found many research articles on the value of oral care, and the results were exciting. When the research was analyzed, it became obvious that patients with dementia were at greater risk for periodontal disease and increased oral bacteria, leading to halitosis. Often, oral bacteria are noticeable as a coating on the tongue. In addition, Amanda discovered that increased severity of periodontal disease correlated with a decreased quality of life. Mr. Samuels had trouble swallowing, so it was important that suction be readily available when oral care was given. Amanda discovered that there are suction toothbrushes for patients such as Mr. Samuels (Fig. 2.2). Amanda felt a renewed sense of purpose when she realized that small changes to oral care could have a positive impact on the well-being of patients like Mr. Samuel.

Step 4: Measure Outcomes Before and After Change

Next, determine the patient outcomes that are likely to occur as a result of a change in nursing care. Usually, a small pilot study is done within the agency before any widespread change in practice is made. That way, it can be determined whether the change will be as effective as intended when the change is implemented across the agency.

The committee members decided to implement a halitosis scale and yearly evaluation for periodontal disease.

Step 5: Make It Happen

Institute the desired change in nursing practice based on evidence. This is done through education and by setting up quality systems to ensure that the desired change is happening.

The policy and procedure committee developed an evidence-based procedure guideline for oral care of all patients, with

Table 2.2
Summary of Research Findings for Patient Oral Care

Study	Key Findings
Ferreira, M. C., Dias-Pereira, A. C., Branco-de-Almeida, L. S., Martins, C. C., & Paiva, S. M. (2017). Impact of periodontal disease on quality of life: A systematic review. *Journal of Periodontal Research, 52*(4), 651–665.	Results showed periodontal disease can negatively impact quality of life. Moreover, more severe periodontitis was shown to have greater impact on quality of life than mild-to-moderate periodontitis.
Amou, T., Hinode, D., Yoshioka, M., & Grenier, D. (2014). Relationship between halitosis and periodontal disease-associated oral bacteria in tongue coatings. *International Journal of Dental Hygiene, 12*(2), 145–151.	Results suggest that periodontal disease-related oral bacteria are found in tongue coatings and are related to halitosis. In addition, cleaning the tongue during oral hygiene may be an effective method for improving halitosis and decreasing bacteria in the oral cavity. Recommendation was to brush the tongue once a day.
Gil-Montoya, J., Sanchez-Lara, I., Carnero-Pardo, C., Fornieles-Rubio, F., Montes, J., Barrios, R., ... & Bravo, M. (2017). Oral hygiene in the elderly with different degrees of cognitive impairment and dementia. *Journal of the American Geriatrics Society, 65*(3), 642–647.	Results showed that oral hygiene, bacterial plaque, and gingivitis were worse with increased cognitive impairment in this elderly population. It is recommended that those with cognitive impairment be given special preventive oral hygiene to help maintain oral health.
Schuch, H. S. (2016). Periodontal disease: Treatment [Monograph]. *Evidence Summaries*. Retrieved from Joanna Briggs Institute Library Database.	Recommendations from this evidence summary include the use of mouthwashes containing cetylpyridinium chloride; the use of chlorhexidine mouth rinses together with oral hygiene, which can have significant impact on oral plaque but can also cause enamel staining; Yag laser treatment, which significantly decreases halitosis; and flossing in addition to traditional tooth brushing to decrease gingivitis.

separate policies for those with dementia. The new policy and procedure were introduced and became a care requirement for patients at the agency. A quality audit was then done at intervals on selected patients to ensure the appropriate oral care was being given.

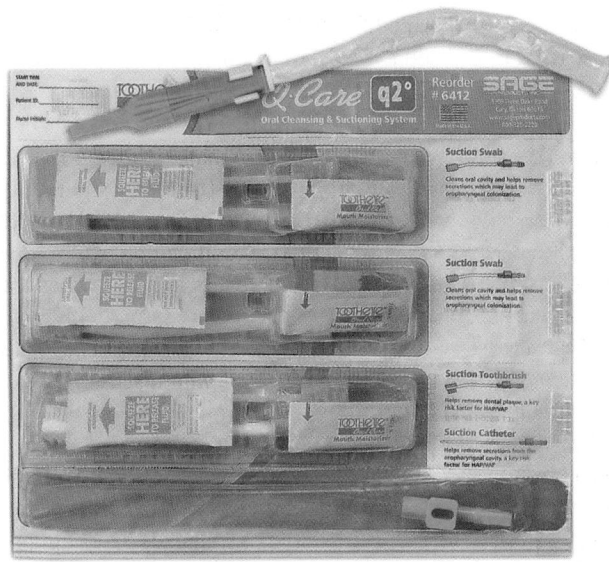

FIGURE 2.2 Oral suction toothbrush kit with thumb ports.

Step 6: Evaluate the Practice Change

Evaluation is the process used to determine whether the change made a significant difference. What were the results of the initial small study? Was the change in practice effective in improving patient outcomes? If it did make a difference, was the difference worth the extra cost or time it required?

Wow! Because of Amanda's concern about oral care, a policy change was made that upon evaluation showed a positive impact on the oral health for every patient. This was exciting and reinforcing to the committee, and especially to Amanda.

WHO SHOULD PROVIDE EVIDENCE-BASED NURSING CARE?

All nursing care should be based on use of appropriate evidence, including care provided by nursing assistive personnel such as competency evaluated nursing assistants (CENAs). Evidence-based care should be given at all times, if possible, and in all settings where nursing care is given. A good way to ensure that evidence-based care is provided by CENAs is to explain why the care should be given when the care is delegated.

Going back to the case study, Amanda asks a CENA to provide thorough oral care for each patient that includes brushing the teeth and tongue, flossing, and using mouth-wash. Along with the request, Amanda explains that research studies have shown that brushing both the teeth and the tongue decreases the bacteria that are responsible for halitosis and periodontal disease. She also explains that preventing periodontal disease increases a person's quality of life. With this knowledge, the CENA understands the importance of giving effective oral care.

HEALTH LITERACY

Health literacy is the degree to which a person has the capacity to obtain, process, and understand basic health information and services in order to make the best-informed health decisions (Institute of Medicine, 2004). Nine out of 10 people have difficulty understanding complex health information regardless of educational level (Centers for Disease Control and Prevention, 2016). Skills required for health literacy include basic literacy, knowledge of the body and health topics, and **numeracy** (ability to understand and use numbers in everyday life). These skills are needed to calculate health insurance costs, comprehend nutrition labels, prepare medications, and understand laboratory tests, including blood sugar levels.

Low health literacy leads to poorer health outcomes and higher health care costs. Increasing health literacy for everyone is a public health priority. The National Action Plan to Improve Health Literacy (U.S. Department of Health and Human Services, 2010) has two principles: first, that people have a right to health information for informed decision making and, second, that health services should be delivered so they are easy to understand and improve health, quality of life, and longevity. Excellent web sites for finding easy-to-understand health resources are www.healthfinder.gov and www.safecarecampaign.org/safe-care.html.

Healthy People 2020 objectives include improving health literacy. Objectives include increasing patients' reports of always receiving easy-to-understand instructions, being asked to explain how they will follow these instructions, and being offered help to fill out forms (Office of Disease Prevention and Health Promotion, 2017).

There are many things you can do to help patients understand health-related instructions. Use clear language and familiar words, concepts, and numbers understood by the patient. Provide easy-to-understand written materials, and use video or computerized learning and pictured medication instructions. Each health care professional must promote health literacy for their patients. This empowers patients to be partners in their care and make informed decisions. A new nursing diagnosis, *Readiness for Enhanced Health Literacy,* has been developed. Quality and safety increase when patients understand the care they are receiving.

EBP, QUALITY, AND SAFETY: THEY BELONG TOGETHER!

EBP is critical thinking at its finest, working to determine the best care for the patient based on the evidence. The evidence provides core information to direct safe, quality-driven, excellent patient care. Multiple quality initiatives are currently having a positive impact on health care. Insurance companies, businesses, patients, and the government are demanding quality care. All quality initiatives require collection of data. Data collection is greatly facilitated by the health care agency having an EBP framework. Some quality initiatives are required, such as those of The Joint Commission, to accredit health care agencies. Others are voluntary but desirable for the agency's well-being. All quality initiatives should begin with a literature search to determine the most effective interventions.

Quality and Safety Education for Nurses Project

The Quality and Safety Education for Nurses (QSEN) project focuses on nursing education that promotes the continual improvement of quality and safety in patient care. The goal is for students to develop understanding, attitudes, skills, and the desire to continually improve the quality and safety of patient care. Information on the QSEN project can be found at http://qsen.org/.

Teaching strategies for nursing students involve the following six areas of focus, which are supported throughout the book:

1. *Evidence-based practice:* Look for Evidence-Based Practice boxes throughout this book.
2. *Safety:* We all want our patients to be safe! Many interventions are available that can help us reach this goal. Look for Be Safe! boxes throughout the chapters and for a section on safety in Chapter 3.
3. *Teamwork and collaboration:* These are important aspects of providing safe, quality care. In Chapter 3, you are introduced to members of the health care team with whom you may work and collaborate. For example, you may talk with the pharmacist if you have a question about a patient's medication to ensure it is given safely, or you might alert the registered nurse to a change in a patient's vital signs so that the HCP can be informed for treatment orders.
4. *Patient-centered care:* When collaborating on the development of nursing care plans, it is important to individualize interventions to provide patient-centered care. As nursing interventions are performed, they should meet the patient's needs and preferred schedules rather than those of the institution or caregiver. You will find Nursing Care Plans throughout the chapters, but always remember that no plan fits all patients. Always evaluate each suggested intervention to see whether it fits with your patient's needs and then individualize it.

5. *Quality improvement:* Quality improvement (QI) is an ongoing process to improve patient care (see Fig. 3.3). You might participate in a QI project by collecting data, which is one aspect of a QI project.

6. *Informatics:* Informatics is a growing area in health care because of the increasing use of technology to provide safer care. Examples include electronic health records (EHRs), medication dispensing systems, medication barcoding systems, and computerized resources.

Concern for Patient Safety

Safety is being promoted for all patients in all care settings (visit www.safecarecampaign.org/safe-care.html). Guidelines to reduce errors in health care and to improve patient outcomes have been developed and based on evidence when available. The Joint Commission's 2018 National Patient Safety Goals can be found at www.jointcommission.org. As you will see at the web site, these goals address care in various types of health care settings.

You will find some 2018 National Patient Safety Goals featured in the Be Safe! boxes throughout this book. These goals are included to increase your awareness and understanding of patient safety. They address important areas of concern, such as administering medications safely, identifying patients correctly, identifying operative sites correctly, improving communication, reducing fall injuries, and reducing the risk of infection in institutionalized older persons, to name a few. Become familiar with them and look for updates at The Joint Commission web site. Of course, it takes critical thinking to use them at the right time and in the right circumstances. Using them appropriately helps you provide safer care with fewer errors.

BE SAFE!

Use at least two ways to identify patients or residents. For example, use the patient's or resident's name and date of birth. This is done to make sure that each patient or resident gets the correct medicine and treatment. (The Joint Commission's 2018 National Patient Safety Goals. © The Joint Commission, 2017. Reprinted with permission.)

Review Questions

1. The nurse requests the competency evaluated nursing assistant to help the patient with oral care. Which of the following methods requested by the nurse would be most appropriate to achieve evidence-based care?
   1. Instruct the competency evaluated nursing assistant to have the patient rinse the mouth with water after dinner.
   2. Instruct the competency evaluated nursing assistant to give oral care using oral swabs to clean the teeth and mouth.
   3. Ask the competency evaluated nursing assistant to instruct the patient to use a mouthwash rinse for the oral care.
   4. Explain that oral care is best done by brushing the teeth and tongue with a toothbrush and toothpaste.

2. The nurse is contributing to the plan of care for a patient. In considering appropriate care, the nurse bases the care on which of the following to provide excellent care?
   1. Content taught throughout a nursing educational program
   2. Orientation to the health care agency for new employees
   3. A nurse's personal judgment of what is best for each patient
   4. Evidence that is evaluated for the health care agency and each patient

3. A policy and procedure committee is reviewing evidence for a new policy. When considering the evidence, which of the following sources would generally be safest for a health care agency to implement?
   1. Joanna Briggs Institute evidence-based resource
   2. One randomized controlled trial
   3. Four quasi-experimental studies that show similar results
   4. The opinion of a national nursing expert on the subject

4. The nurse reads about a research study that affects nursing care and could lead to decreased wound infections. Which of the following actions should the nurse take regarding the information in the study?
   1. Put the information into practice while performing wound care.
   2. Discuss the research with a trusted coworker, and if the coworker agrees, put the information into practice at work.
   3. Present the proposed practice change to the policy and procedure committee for evaluation and possible adoption.
   4. Do a journal search to look for similar studies, and if three similar studies are found, incorporate the information into practice.

5. A policy and procedure committee is revising the nursing intervention of insertion of a urinary catheter. Where should the committee begin looking for evidence to write an effective policy and procedure on this intervention?
   1. In current nursing skills textbooks
   2. In nursing articles written by national nursing experts based on opinion
   3. In research articles, preferably systematic reviews of randomized controlled trials
   4. In the policies and procedures of other nursing facilities

Answer rationales available in your online resources.

ANSWERS 1. 4; 2. 4; 3. 1; 4. 3; 5. 3

Key Points

Find the chapter key points in your online resources available through Davis Edge.

Additional Resources

DAVIS edge.   Use the scratch off code on the inside front cover of your book to access online quizzes that will help you to improve your scores on course exams and prepare for the NCLEX-PN®.

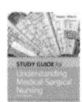   Study Guide

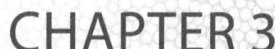

CHAPTER 3
Issues in Nursing Practice

Linda S. Williams, Michelle Block, James Shannon

KEY TERMS

administrative law (ad-MIN-i-STRAY-tive LAW)
autocratic leadership (AW-tuh-KRAT-ik
   LEE-der-ship)
autonomy (aw-TAWN-uh-MEE)
beneficence (buh-NEF-i-sens)
civil law (SIH-vil LAW)
confidentiality (KON-fi-den-she-AL-i-tee)
criminal law (KRIM-i-nuhl LAW)
delegation (DEL-a-GAY-shun)
democratic leadership (DEM-ah-KRAT-ik
   LEE-der-ship)
deontology (DEE-on-TOL-o-gee)
diagnosis-related group (DY-ag-NO-sis
   ree-LAY-ted GROOP)
ethics (ETH-iks)
fidelity (FAH-dell-eh-tee)
human trafficking (HEW-mun trah-FIK-ing)
informatics (IN-for-mat-iks)
justice (JUS-tis)
laissez-faire leadership (LAYS-ay-FAIR
   LEE-der-ship)
leadership (LEE-der-ship)
liability (LY-uh-BIL-i-tee)
limitation of liability (LIM-i-TAY-shun OF
   LY-uh-BIL-i-tee)
maleficence (ma-LEF-i-sens)
malpractice (mal-PRAK-tis)
moral distress (moh-Ral DIS-tres)
negligence (NEG-li-jens)
nonmaleficence (NON-ma-LEF-i-sens)
paternalism (puh-TER-nuhl-izm)
respondeat superior (res-POND-ee-et
   sue-PEER-ee-or)
summons (SUH-muns)
therapeutic privilege (ther-uh-PU-tik PRIV-uh-lej)
torts (TORTS)
utilitarian (yoo-TIL-ih-TAR-ee-en)
values (VAL-yooz)
veracity (VER-ah-sit-tee)

LEARNING OUTCOMES

1. Identify factors influencing changes in the health care delivery system.
2. Describe safe health care practices.
3. Explain the significance of hospital-acquired conditions.
4. Describe four leadership styles.
5. Discuss the licensed practical nurse/licensed vocational nurse's role in leadership and delegation.
6. Describe the importance of ethics in health care.
7. Discuss moral distress and its effect on nursing care.
8. List the steps of the ethical decision-making model.
9. Identify where the regulation of nursing practice is defined.
10. Explain mandatory reporting for health care professionals.
11. Describe human trafficking indicators to report.
12. Describe the Health Insurance Portability and Accountability Act of 1996.
13. Describe guidelines for professional use of social media.
14. Discuss how to provide quality care and limit liability.

CHAPTER CONCEPTS

Collaboration
Communication
Ethics
Health Care System
Leadership and Management
Legal
Professionalism
Quality Improvement
Safety

 ## HEALTH CARE DELIVERY

Health–Illness Continuum

The term *health–illness continuum* describes the continually shifting levels of health experienced by each person. One end of the continuum is high-level health. The other end is poor health and impending death. We all move back and forth on the continuum throughout our lives.

Health Care Delivery Systems

Health care systems provide health care services from birth to death, often over large geographic areas (Fig. 3.1).

Factors Influencing Health Care Change

Do you like change? Well, today's health care delivery is being influenced by many evolving changes. These changes will impact your career. The American population's increases in size, number of older adults, and cultural diversity are influencing health care delivery (U.S. Census Bureau, 2010). Additional changes include the use of evidence to guide practice (see Chapter 2); multidrug-resistant infectious organisms; newly emerging viruses; public awareness campaigns for human trafficking; electronic health records (EHRs); mobile health through the use of tablets, smartphones, and digital apps; telehealth through the use of telephones and online video; remote patient monitoring; and robotics. Nursing **informatics,** the study and use of information technology within nursing practice, is increasing as an area of expertise for nurses. You might consider educational programs in informatics as you continue your education. Change makes learning a continual need. We hope that you are flexible and embrace change throughout your career!

Safe Practice

Medication errors are of primary concern. The Institute for Safe Medication Practices has interventions to reduce medication errors. These include the lists containing Confused Drug Names, "Do Not Crush" Drugs, Drug Names Written With Tall Man Letters (distinguishes between similar looking drug names to prevent giving the wrong drug), Error-Prone Abbreviations, and High-Alert Medications (find these at www.ismp.org/tools). Successful ways to reduce medication errors include the use of tape in a bright color on the floor to outline an area that during medication preparation and administration is not to be entered, or wearing a bright-colored vest or sash that says, "Do Not Disturb Me While I Give Meds." Distractions during medication administration can increase errors, so you should always stay focused and avoid interruptions during this time. Promote a culture of safety. Ask your coworkers to avoid interrupting others during medication administration. Reducing errors requires everyone to be engaged and vigilant at all times during patient care.

There is also now a global initiative to prevent misconnections of medical tubing that have resulted in death. For example, a new type of enteral tubing connector, ENFit, has been designed that is *not* compatible with other types of tubing to provide safer care. Visit www.stayconnected.org for more information.

Preventing harmful, adverse events is of concern to organizations that promote safe health care practices. The Joint Commission's National Patient Safety Goals are updated annually (www.jointcommission.org). The Joint Commission's sentinel events are patient events that should never occur (www.jointcommission.org/sentinel_event.aspx). Specific interventions are suggested to prevent these events. Examples of sentinel events are surgery on the wrong body part or death/loss of function associated with a fall within a facility.

The National Quality Forum identifies 29 serious reportable events that should not occur in health care settings (www.qualityforum.org/Topics/SREs/List_of_SREs.aspx). As health information technology (HIT) use is expanding, the National Quality Forum (2018) has developed recommendations for HIT safety. Measuring performance in these areas is designed to improve HIT and patient safety (www.qualityforum.org/HIT_Safety.aspx).

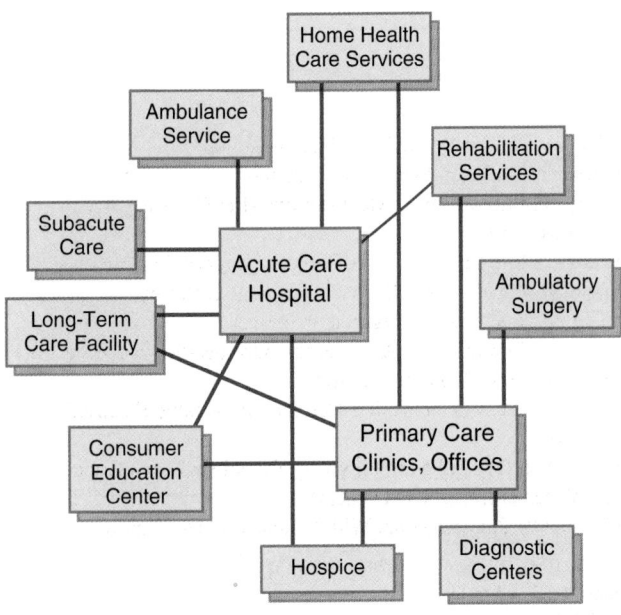

FIGURE 3.1 An integrated health care system.

> ### BE SAFE!
> Did you know that a medication is specifically made for only *one* type of administration route? It cannot be safely given by another route. For example, an intravenous medication cannot safely be given through a nasogastric (NG) or percutaneous endoscopy gastrostomy (PEG) tube. Serious effects, including death, can occur because the drug dosages or drug makeup is specific to its designated route. Request a medication order for an alternate route, if needed, to obtain the proper drug form for administration. Visit the Institute for Healthcare Improvement (www.ihi.org/IHI/Programs/IHIOpenSchool) to see examples of adverse effects when drugs were given incorrectly. Always keep your patients safe!

ECONOMIC ISSUES

Medicare and Diagnosis-Related Groups

Medicare was created in 1965 by the U.S. government to provide health insurance as part of the Social Security Act. It covers those aged 65 and older or those younger than age 65 who have disabilities. It is funded by a deduction from every paycheck that is matched by the government. Several Medicare plan options are offered, including original Medicare, prescription drug coverage for everyone with Medicare and supplemental Medicare health plans. There are two parts of coverage in the original Medicare plan. Part A covers inpatient hospital care, skilled nursing facilities, hospice services, and some home health care. There is no premium or deductible for Part A. Part B is medical insurance that covers physician costs, outpatient services, some home health care, supplies, and other areas not covered by Part A. Some preventive services may also be covered. A monthly premium and yearly deductible are paid for Part B coverage. For more information, visit www.medicare.gov.

Congress created the **diagnosis-related group** (DRG) payment system in 1983 for 470 diagnostic categories to help control costs in the Medicare program, which previously had no reimbursement limits. Today's DRG payment systems consider all populations, complications, and comorbidities to reflect medical severity. Hospitals lose money if the patient's costs exceed the DRG payment and make money if the costs are less than the payment.

Medicaid

The Medicaid payment system was also created in 1965 to provide health insurance as part of the Social Security Act for low-income or disabled persons younger than age 65 and their dependent children. Some low-income people older than age 65 also qualify. Benefits for Medicaid vary from state to state.

Hospital-Acquired Conditions and Present-on-Admission Reporting

In 2008, the Centers for Medicare & Medicaid Services implemented a change for Medicare Severity DRG payments to acute inpatient prospective payment system hospitals. This policy is called the Hospital-Acquired Conditions (HACs) and Present on Admission (POA) Indicator Reporting. Box 3.1 shows the 14 categories of HACs (for updates, see www.cms.gov/Medicare/Medicare-Fee-for-Service-Payment/HospitalAcqCond/icd10_hacs.html). At discharge, if certain conditions are not POA, hospitals do not receive additional payment for those conditions. For example, if a patient was admitted with a stroke (primary diagnosis) and then developed a pressure injury that was not POA (secondary diagnosis) and could have been prevented, the hospital would receive payment only for the primary diagnosis of stroke. The hospital would have to absorb the cost of care for the pressure injury.

With this requirement, nurses must carefully assess and document patient conditions that are POA to show that they did not occur during the hospitalization. Providing safe, quality care and educating patients to prevent complications, such as the need to do leg exercises, turn every 2 hours, or ambulate, are essential to prevent these conditions. Documenting interventions, education provided, and the patient's refusal to participate (if applicable) are essential to help ensure payment for secondary diagnoses.

Managed Health Care

Health maintenance organizations (HMOs) deliver health care services to individuals who enroll in this type of prepaid group practice health program. The purpose of an HMO is to reduce overlapping services and provide quality

---

Box 3.1

Categories of Hospital-Acquired Conditions

The Centers for Medicare & Medicaid Services identified the following 14 categories of hospital-acquired conditions as those that increase health care costs or that could have been prevented by using evidence-based guidelines:

• Foreign Object Retained After Surgery
• Air Embolism
• Blood Incompatibility
• Stage III and IV Pressure Ulcers
• Fall and Trauma Injuries (Burns, Crushing Injuries, Dislocations, Fractures, Intracranial Injuries, Other Injuries)
• Manifestations of Poor Glycemic Control (Diabetic Ketoacidosis, Nonketotic Hyperosmolar Coma, Hypoglycemic Coma, Secondary Diabetes With Ketoacidosis, Secondary Diabetes With Hyperosmolarity)

• Catheter-Associated Urinary Tract Infection
• Vascular Catheter-Associated Infection
• Surgical Site Infection, Mediastinitis After Coronary Artery Bypass Graft
• Surgical Site Infection After Bariatric Surgery for Obesity (Laparoscopic Gastric Bypass, Gastroenterostomy, Laparoscopic Gastric Restrictive Surgery)
• Surgical Site Infection After Certain Orthopedic Procedures (Spine, Neck, Shoulder, Elbow)
• Surgical Site Infection After Cardiac Implantable Electronic Device
• Deep Vein Thrombosis/Pulmonary Embolism (Total Knee Replacement, Hip Replacement)
• Iatrogenic Pneumothorax With Venous Catheterization

and cost-effective care. Healthy patients require fewer services, so preventive care is promoted. Preferred provider organizations (PPOs) are networks of providers who offer care to plan members at set discounted rates. PPOs are designed to reduce costs to businesses that insure employees. Hospitals and physicians develop a contract with employers to provide services at a negotiated fee.

Managed care has led to fewer hospitalizations and shorter lengths of stay. Patients are using home health care for more complex needs. Case management is helping to ensure that the best patient outcome is achieved while controlling costs.

> **LEARNING TIP**
> To understand what the term *managed care* means, reverse the words: care management.

NURSING AND THE HEALTH CARE TEAM

Nursing is an integral part of the health care network. Nurses work as *licensed practical nurses* (LPNs) or *licensed vocational nurses* (LVNs), *registered nurses* (RNs), or registered nurses with advanced education and practice skills, which includes *nurse practitioners* (NPs), *clinical nurse specialists* (CNSs), *certified nurse midwives* (CNMs), *certified registered nurse anesthetists* (CRNAs), and *doctors of nursing practice* (DNPs). *Certified nursing assistants* (CNAs) are trained to assist nurses in providing health care.

Collaborative Care
Nurses work in collaboration with other members of the health care team, which include the following:

- Licensed *physicians* provide medical care to patients after graduating from a college of medicine (MD) or osteopathic medicine (DO).
- *Physician assistants* (PA-C [certified]), after graduating from a physician's assistant program, work under the supervision of a physician and perform certain physician duties, such as history taking, physical examinations, and suturing of wounds.
- Licensed *pharmacists* complete 5 or 6 years of college and dispense medications from prescriptions, consult with physicians, and provide medication information to patients.
- *Social workers* usually have a master of social work (MSW) degree, can be *licensed clinical social workers* (LCSWs), and treat patients and their families with psychosocial issues.
- *Dietitians* provide nutrition information, analyze nutritional needs, and calculate special dietary needs.
- Licensed *physical therapists* complete a college physical therapy program and assist patients in reducing physical disability, bodily malfunction, movement

dysfunction, and pain through evaluation, education, and treatment.
- *Physical therapy assistants,* whose educational requirements vary, might complete 2 years of education and be licensed and then work under the supervision of a physical therapist.
- *Occupational therapists* (OTs) complete a bachelor's or master's program, can be registered (OTRs), and assist patients in restoring self-care, work, and leisure skills that have been diminished as a result of developmental deficits or injury.
- *Speech and language pathologists* typically complete a master's program and provide direct clinical services to those with communication or swallowing problems.
- *Respiratory therapists* (RTs) have a 2-year college degree, can be registered (RRTs), and work with patients who have respiratory problems.
- *Respiratory therapy technicians* (RTTs) have 1 year of education, can be certified (CRTT), and work under the supervision of a respiratory therapist to provide respiratory care.
- *Health unit coordinators* (*clerks, secretaries*) manage clerical work.
- *Student nurses* are enrolled in a nursing program and work under the supervision of nursing faculty in the clinical setting.

LEADERSHIP IN NURSING PRACTICE

A leader seeks to influence, motivate, and enable others to achieve goals. **Leadership** skills are necessary for the LPN/LVN to effectively guide patient care and achieve patient care goals.

Effective leaders in a health care setting must be knowledgeable about management and supervisory processes. They must use critical thinking and be able to make decisions. They should be role models and provide inspiration to others. A positive attitude and the use of humor are valuable assets of good leaders. Ultimately, leaders must earn the respect of their coworkers to be successful. To prepare for a leadership role, learning and applying the following principles of leadership, supervision, and management is helpful.

Leadership Styles
There are three traditional leadership styles: (1) autocratic, (2) democratic, and (3) laissez-faire. A fourth style, called *coaching,* is also used in health care settings.

Autocratic (Authoritarian) Leadership
An autocratic leader leads with a high degree of control. Almost no control is given to others. In **autocratic leadership,** the leader determines the goals and plans for achieving the goals. Others are told what to do and are not asked to provide input. The group usually achieves high-quality outcomes under this style of leadership. This is an efficient leadership style for emergency situations when decisions must be made

quickly, such as when evacuating a building or responding to a cardiac arrest.

Democratic (Participative) Leadership

A democratic leader has a moderate degree of control. Others are given some control and freedom. In **democratic leadership,** participation is encouraged in determining goals and plans for achieving the goals (Fig. 3.2). Decisions are made within the group. The leader assists the group by steering and teaching rather than dominating. The leader shares responsibility with the group. The group usually achieves high-quality outcomes and is more creative under this style of leadership. This is an efficient leadership style for most situations. With this type of leadership, group members have greater satisfaction and are motivated to achieve goals because they are active participants.

Laissez-Faire (Delegative) Leadership

A laissez-faire leader exerts no control over the group. The group, therefore, is given complete freedom for decision making. With **laissez-faire leadership,** no one is responsible for determining goals and plans for achieving the goals. This can produce a feeling of chaos. Often, little is accomplished under this leadership style. The quality of outcomes can be poor.

Coaching Leadership

By emphasizing active listening, clear communication, support, and accountability, coaching leaders work with others to develop problem-solving skills that facilitate critical thinking, prioritization, and effective communication. This leadership style helps direct-care employees feel more empowered, valued, and respected.

Management Functions

The five major components in the management process are (1) planning, (2) organizing, (3) directing, (4) coordinating, and (5) controlling.

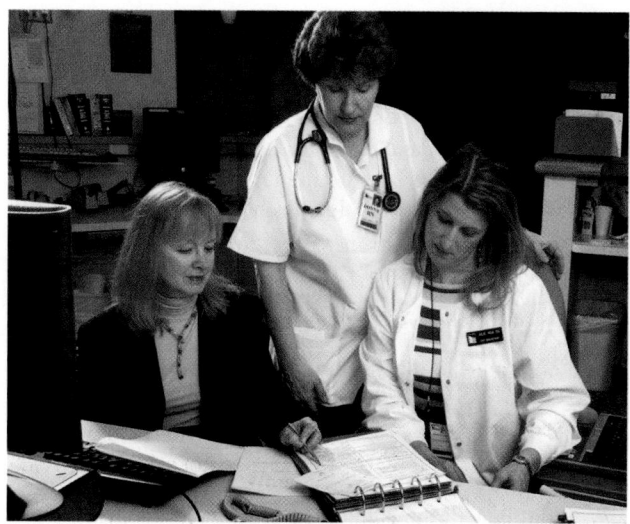

FIGURE 3.2 Group participation in decision making.

Planning

In the first step of the management process, a plan must be developed to ensure that desired patient care outcomes are achieved. To formulate the plan, desired outcomes or problems are identified and data about them are collected. Alternatives or solutions are considered using the collected data and input from others. A decision is then made about the best option or course of action. The leader should ensure that the choice is realistic and can be implemented. Involving others in the planning and decision-making process from beginning to end can increase acceptance at the time of implementation.

Organizing

The second step in the management process is organizing. The purpose of organizing is to provide an orderly environment that promotes cooperation and goal achievement. Providing a framework for goals and the activities that accomplish them is the initial step in organization. Policies and procedures provide this framework. They also provide guidance for those carrying out tasks designed to accomplish the organization's goals.

Directing

Making assignments is the primary function of directing. One person, usually the nurse in charge or the team leader, makes the assignments for patient care. The nurse practice act in each state defines who can make assignments and delegate care. Communication is important in directing. Assignments must be clearly and specifically stated. The person making assignments must be sure that each assignment is correctly understood and should seek out the receiving person for clarification. Effective directing can be accomplished by providing verbal and written assignment information, making requests rather than giving orders, and giving instructions as needed.

Coordinating

Coordination is the process of looking at a situation to ensure that it is being handled in the most effective way for the organization or coordinating services for a patient. The nurse might assess a particular activity or issues related to patient care assignments. In a long-term care facility, for example, the nurse might want to review skin assessment and care throughout the facility to see if it is being done consistently and uniformly. If a concern is found, problem-solving techniques are used.

Controlling

The final phase of the management process is controlling to evaluate the accomplishment of the organization's goals. Continuous quality improvement (CQI) is linked with controlling. If the organization's efficiency or ability to reach its goals is impaired, the use of the CQI model can facilitate correction of the concern (Fig. 3.3).

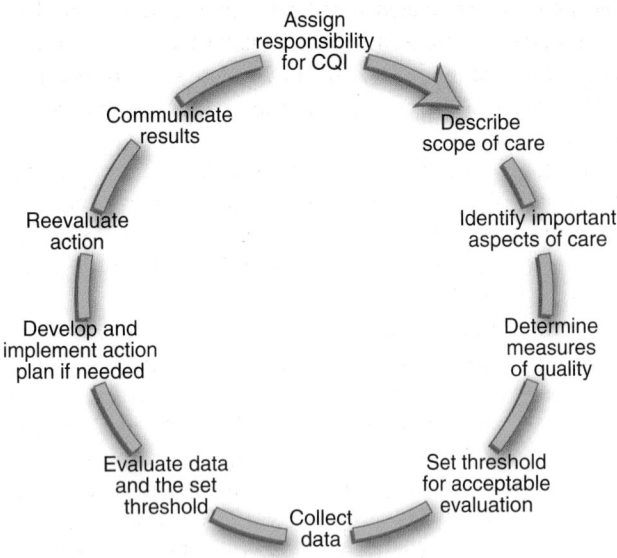

FIGURE 3.3 A continuous quality improvement (CQI) model.

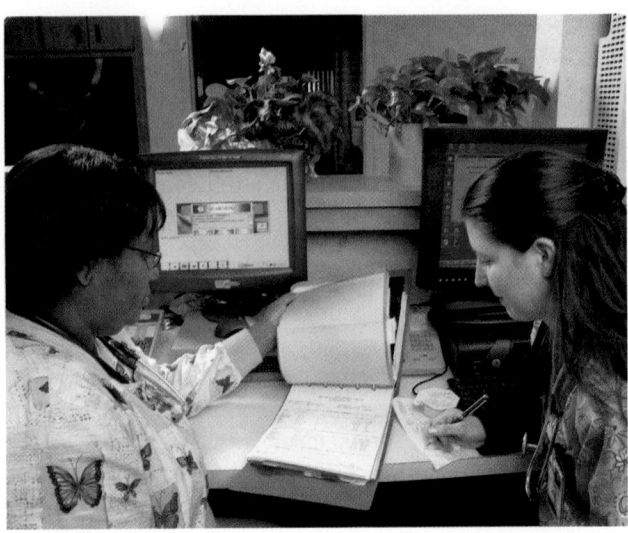

FIGURE 3.4 Communication of the patient's status by a team leader when transferring the patient's care to another team leader.

Leadership and Delegation for the LPN/LVN

LPNs/LVNs are leaders and managers of care for the patients to whom they are assigned, while under the supervision of an RN, health care provider (HCP), or a dentist as specified by each state nurse practice act. Beyond this application of a leader and manager role for the LPN/LVN, state nurse practice acts specify if the LPN/LVN can assume other leader or manager roles or delegate.

The LPN/LVN might function as a team leader or charge nurse, often in the long-term care setting, requiring some use of **delegation** to unlicensed assistive personnel (UAP). When the LPN/LVN acts as a team leader or charge nurse, an RN delegates the authority to provide supervision and delegation of tasks. Team leaders are responsible for the co-ordination and delivery of care to each of the patients assigned to the team. They assess the patients assigned to the team to plan appropriate care and contribute to the nursing care plan. Team leaders receive information from team members and communicate patients' needs to appropriate individuals. Because team leaders guide patient care provided by the team, they must be knowledgeable about safety policies, patients' rights, and the accountability of being a team leader.

All patients are entitled to quality care and treatment with dignity and respect. The team leader is accountable for all care provided by the team. Supervision involves initial direction for the task and then monitoring of the task and outcome at intervals. At the end of the team's work shift, team leaders are responsible for transferring patient care to the oncoming team in a way that prevents communication breakdowns that result in patient harm. This hand-off communication is accomplished by reporting the patient's condition, status, and needs to the oncoming team leader (Fig. 3.4). Institutional policy specifies whether the RN or LPN/LVN communicates the report.

Delegation is the act of empowering another person to act. RNs delegate to LPNs/LVNs and UAP. LPNs/LVNs, in certain circumstances, delegate to other LPNs/LVNs and UAP. When delegation occurs, responsibility for care is transferred to the delegatee, but accountability for the care remains with the delegator.

> **LEARNING TIP**
>
> Review your state nurse practice act. Does your state allow licensed practical nurses/licensed vocational nurses to delegate? If so, to whom and what can be delegated?

Within the leadership role, the LPN/LVN must decide when delegation would most benefit the situation and the patient. All nurses must follow their state nurse practice act and scope of practice when making any decisions regarding delegation. Consult the nurse practice act for your state, charge nurse, and team leader when deciding whether delegation is appropriate. Ultimately, you must ask several important questions to determine when delegation would best benefit the situation. These questions include the following:

• Does my state nurse practice act allow for delegation in this situation?
• Does the person to whom I am delegating have the knowledge and education to perform this skill, and is it documented for me to make the decisions regarding delegation?
• Would it benefit the patient if I delegated this skill to the support person?

Delegation Process

Delegation is a complex process encompassing the decision to delegate, what to delegate, and to whom:

1. Know your state nurse practice act rules for delegation. The LPN/LVN scope of practice usually does not provide legal authority for an LPN/LVN to delegate. However, some state board rules allow LPNs/LVNs to delegate tasks that are within the LPN/LVN's scope of practice as long as the RN has given the LPN/LVN authority to delegate the tasks.
2. Identify the skills of the person to whom you might delegate to determine whether he or she has the knowledge and ability to carry out the task. When selecting a team member to delegate tasks to, consider if there is potential for harm to the patient during the task, whether it is a complex task that will require problem-solving, how predictable the outcome is, and how much interaction with the patient is needed. Match the skills and talents of the team member to the task being delegated. Remember, nursing judgment can never be delegated.
3. Use the National Council of State Boards of Nursing's five rights of delegation (www.ncsbn.org/1625.htm). Following these rights provides a framework for your decision-making process and comfort in knowing you used them to make good choices.

Delegation requires trust. You should be comfortable with which tasks can be delegated and the team member to whom you are delegating the tasks. Also, it is important to know and understand each other's methods of communicating so that miscommunications do not occur. When you first begin your career, the process of delegating can seem difficult. As with any skill, it takes practice to feel confident in carrying out the process.

EDUCATIONAL OPPORTUNITIES FOR LPNS/LVNS

Many schools provide an accelerated educational tract for LPNs/LVNs seeking to become RNs. Advanced educational opportunities include a master's degree or a doctoral degree. Check with colleges/universities to see which program would best meet your needs to continue your education. Post-licensure certification for the LPN/LVN in intravenous therapy, long-term care, or pharmacology is offered by the National Association for Practical Nurse Education and Service (NAPNES).

ETHICS AND VALUES

The study and practice of ethics is grounded in philosophy and dates back to the time of Hippocrates. **Ethics** is a systematic approach not only to understanding an ethical dilemma but also to examining the best outcome for each situation (Butts & Rich, 2016). *Bioethics* is a branch of ethics that studies moral values in the biomedical sciences. It has come to be most closely associated with health care. Today more than ever, nurses are confronted with situations and variables that can contribute to clinical ethical dilemmas. Therefore, it is necessary to understand how to identify, process, and address ethical dilemmas.

Although the terms *ethics* and *morals* are often used interchangeably, morals refer more specifically to personally derived values, beliefs, and behaviors. We tend to think of these behaviors as "right and wrong" or "good and bad" (Butts & Rich, 2016).

Values are unwritten standards, ideals, or concepts that give meaning to a person's life. They often serve as a guide for making decisions and setting priorities in daily life. Values can change throughout a person's life based on individual experiences and life events. People make decisions based on their values; that is often how they solve conflicts that occur in everyday life. For example, a nurse who values both her career and her family might be forced to decide between going to work or staying home with a sick child. Similarly, a patient who values both his personal health and family may have to decide between filling a prescription or buying necessary items for his family.

There are many types of values, including personal, group, professional, and societal. Just as individuals have personal values that govern their lives and actions, so do groups. Group values represent the group as a whole but may or may not be identical to personal values. Examples of groups include professional groups, clubs, churches, and political parties. Society as a whole has values. As a member of a group, organization, or society/country, an individual accepts the values of that culture; however, he or she recognizes that those values may not be exactly the same as his or her personal values. The values of a profession are usually outlined in a code of ethics. This code is a comprehensive set of guidelines that outlines the behavioral expectations for the profession.

Ethical issues surround us constantly and may even change over time. Kangasniemi, Pakkanen, and Korhonen (2015) found that professional ethics are shaped by constantly changing influences within the profession. They are, therefore, not static. Bioethical issues are particularly prevalent in our professional lives for several reasons. To begin with, advances in technology and new treatment options both offer prolonging or saving life. However, in doing so, questions arise related to medical futility such as, Who should receive treatment? How long should treatment continue? Should a patient receive a treatment because it is available or because it will be effective? How many health care resources should be utilized for the treatment of terminal illnesses? Does quantity or length of life matter more than quality of life? Therefore, it becomes both difficult and important to decide how and when resources will be allocated.

Not all bioethical issues make headline news. In fact, many ethical dilemmas are regular occurrences in the clinical setting. Nurses are involved in decision making every day based on the traditional ethical principles of autonomy, beneficence, maleficence, and justice. Have you experienced any of the following examples? You are asked to consistently work on a unit that is understaffed. A patient asks you to keep his prognosis from his spouse. You overhear a coworker who is on break discussing a patient's status on the telephone, but you do not know who is on the line. Each of these examples prompts questions such as the following: What should be done? What ethical principles are involved? Whose wishes should be honored?

An ethical dilemma is a situation in which a person must choose between two options that will affect the outcome of the case. Although each option can be justified as "good," both have pros and cons. Therefore, when one option is selected or implemented, it creates uncertainty in the outcome of the case (Butts & Rich, 2016).

Decision making in the clinical setting is a complex process involving many members of the health care team. As a result of carrying out orders, nurses must handle consequences that arise from clinical problems. In addition, there is no one-size-fits-all solution for ethical problems. Even if dilemmas share a common thread, each has individual influences that make it unique.

When patients are conscious, their choices are usually respected, but on occasion, even that premise can be difficult to apply. Often, groups of individuals must work together to resolve a conflict if there is disagreement between an HCP and family, nurses and other HCPs, or family members. Nurses can experience moral distress as a result of being an integral part of this team. **Moral distress** can be defined as distress experienced when knowing the right thing to do but being unable to carry it out because of institutional constraints (Jameton, 1984). Moral distress can lead to job burnout. Therefore, finding ways to address moral distress is important. Lachman (2016) suggests that developing moral resilience can help nurses manage ethically difficult situations without the lasting effects of moral distress. Lachman defines *moral resiliency* as "the ability and willingness to speak and take right and good actions in the face of an adversity that is moral/ethical in nature" (p. 122). Using an ethical decision-making model can help a nurse build moral resiliency.

A basic mastery of several elements enhances your ability to perform competently when bioethical issues arise and decision making is the focus. Understanding the ethical component of your nursing role is the first step. Discovering how your personal value set influences your nursing practice is another. Acquiring knowledge about relevant ethical material is also essential. An ethical decision-making process is a useful tool for examining ethical dilemmas. Together, these elements provide a foundation from which you can begin to explore the meaning of bioethics in nursing practice today. For more information about bioethics, visit the Center for Bioethics & Human Dignity at www.cbhd.org.

Ethical Obligations and Nursing

As a nurse, you are an invaluable member of the health care team, contributing to patient care according to your educational preparation and assigned responsibilities. You are guided by the law and the standards of the profession as well as a professional code of ethics. In addition to practicing within the law, nurses have ethical obligations related to the law. First, if the law is considered unethical or has serious limitations, a basic moral obligation of the nurse is to make an effort to change that law. This might be done individually or through political activism guided by professional organizations.

Nursing Code of Ethics

Some of the major ethical obligations of nursing practice are addressed in a nursing code of ethics. A code of ethics has several purposes and serves to provide (1) guidance for appropriate decision making based on current laws and professional standards, (2) a method for professional self-evaluation and reflection, and (3) a way to hold the profession accountable. As a professional guide for ethical practice, the National Association of Licensed Practical Nurses has practice standards that include ethical practice and conduct (visit www.nalpn.org/wp-content/uploads/2016/02/NALPN-Practice-Standards.pdf). NAPNES also has standards of practice for LPNs/LVNs at www.napnes.org.

A code serves as a general guideline for professional practice and ethical issues. A code requires interpretation because the guidelines are generally broad. Although it is not a legal document, a code should not be in conflict with the law. The code is not enforced by any organization. Ethical codes are updated to reflect current practice, responsibilities, and obligations set forth by the profession.

Building Blocks of Ethics

An understanding of basic concepts, presented here in the form of ethical principles and ethical theories, helps specifically target the ethical components of the problem. Principles and theories offer frameworks for ethical problem-solving and ethical decision making. Knowledge about ethics can help us to systematically look at an issue and determine the best course of action.

Ethical Principles

Ethical *principles* act as guidelines or standards. They provide a framework for moral conduct as well as how to approach ethical dilemmas. Ethical principles can be found in many professional codes of conduct. They are key components of ethical decision making. The ethical principles widely used when examining bioethical and health care dilemmas include autonomy, beneficence, nonmaleficence, fidelity, veracity, and justice. Given the prominence of these ethical principles in the bioethical literature, a basic understanding of them is necessary.

AUTONOMY. According to ethicists (as well as behaviorists, social scientists, and psychologists), what makes human beings different from nonhumans is that people have dignity based on their ability to choose freely what they will do with their lives.

• WORD • BUILDING •

nonmaleficence: non—not + maleficentia—evil doing

Autonomy is the right of self-determination, independence, and freedom founded on the notion that humans have value, worth, and moral dignity. Autonomy in health care applies to all people capable of and competent in making health care decisions for themselves. HCPs do not need to agree with another person's decisions but must respect the autonomy of the person making the choice. **Paternalism** occurs when an HCP tries to prevent patients from making autonomous decisions or decides what is best for patients without regard for their preferences. Autonomy also encompasses the professional's self-determination and freedom. *Advocacy* occurs when patients are not capable of making their own decisions and, therefore, lack autonomy. In this case, the nurse may work to advocate for the patient's best interest ("Evidence-Based Practice").

Evidence-Based Practice

Clinical Question
What are nurses' experiences of advocating for patients?

Evidence
Nine qualitative studies were included in a systematic review that sought to identify the meaningfulness of perioperative nurses' experiences of advocacy. Thirty-one findings were aggregated into five categories and two synthesized findings, including safeguarding from harm through advocacy and that challenges of advocating can be alleviated by training and experience (Munday, Kynoch, & Hines, 2015).

Implications for Nursing Practice
Advocacy is at the core of ethics and nursing practice. It is important that it is outlined in various moral codes and codes of ethics. Advocating for patients can be complicated given the diversity of patient issues and complexity of the care environment. This review, although limited to perioperative nursing, showed that (1) nurses need to protect and safeguard vulnerable patients in their care, (2) advocacy preparation through education and role-modeling is required, and (3) models of nursing care promoting continuity of care enhance the nurse–patient relationship and support successful advocacy.

Reference
Munday, J., Kynoch, K., & Hines, S. (2015). Nurses' experiences of advocacy in the perioperative department: A systematic review. *JBI Database of Systematic Reviews and Implementation Reports, 13*(8), 146–189.

There are limitations to autonomy. Typically, these limitations arise when a person's autonomy interferes with the rights, health, or well-being of self or others. For example, patients generally have an autonomous right to make decisions regarding their care and level of independence. This autonomous right is guaranteed by federal legislation known as the Patient Self-Determination Act (visit www.nrc-pad.org/images/stories/PDFs/fedaddirectives2a.pdf). However, if a person is no longer capable of self-care upon discharge, a request to live independently will not be granted. When a person is unable to adequately care for him- or herself safely, the principle of autonomy cannot be upheld.

BENEFICENCE. The principle of **beneficence** proposes that actions taken and treatments provided will benefit a person and promote welfare (Butts & Rich, 2016). The provision of good care means the provision of not only technologically competent care but also care that respects the patient's beliefs, feelings, and wishes, as well as those of the patient's family and significant others. A common problem encountered when applying this principle is deciding what is good for someone else.

NONMALEFICENCE. Nonmaleficence is one of the oldest obligations in health care, dating back to the Hippocratic Oath (400 B.C.). Nonmaleficence is the obligation to "do no harm" (Butts & Rich, 2016). It is common to hear beneficence and **maleficence** talked about as being "two sides of the same coin."

HCPs are required to do no harm to their patients either *intentionally* or *unintentionally*. In current health care practice, the principle of nonmaleficence may be intentionally violated to produce a greater good in the patient's long-term treatment. For example, a patient might undergo a painful and debilitating or disfiguring surgery to remove a cancerous growth, thereby avoiding death and prolonging life.

By extension, the principle of nonmaleficence also requires a nurse to protect from harm those who are considered vulnerable. Vulnerable groups include children, older adults, and those who are mentally incompetent, unconscious, or too weak or debilitated to protect themselves.

FIDELITY. Fidelity is the obligation to be faithful to commitments made to self and others. In health care, fidelity includes faithfulness or loyalty to agreements and responsibilities accepted as part of the practice of nursing. It also means not promising a patient something that one cannot deliver or control. Fidelity is the main support for the concept of accountability, although conflicts in fidelity might arise because of obligations owed to different individuals or groups. For example, nurses have an obligation of fidelity to the patients they care for to provide the highest quality care possible as well as an obligation of fidelity to their employing institution to follow its rules and policies. Nurses can have an ethical dilemma when a hospital's policy on staffing creates a situation that does not allow nurses to provide the quality of care they believe is needed.

Maintaining a patient's privacy and **confidentiality** is related to fidelity (Fig. 3.5). Privacy and confidentiality may or may not be explicit promises. Nurses are obligated to discuss the patient only under circumstances in which it is necessary to deliver high-quality, holistic health care, such as

- When given specific instructions to do so by the patient.
- When there is the grave possibility of harm to either the patient or others.
- When legally mandated to do so.

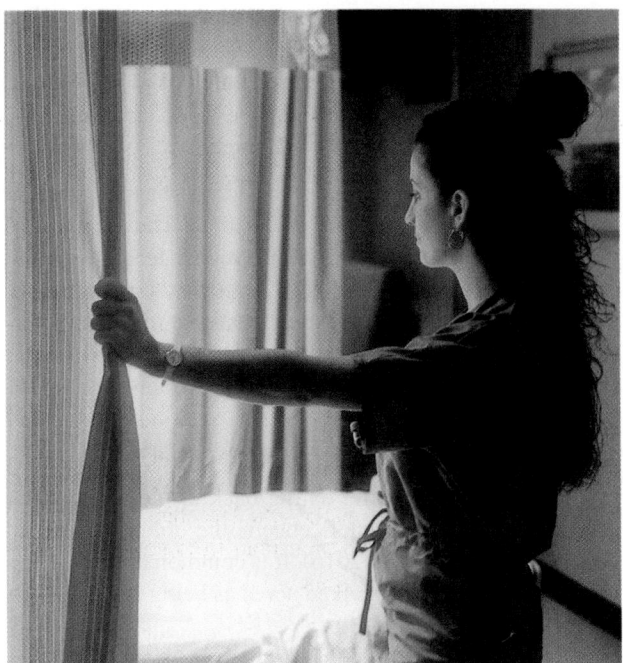

FIGURE 3.5 Maintaining privacy is a patient right and conveys caring to the patient.

Maintaining confidentiality also applies to the necessary communication of information through the posting of unit censuses and various schedules for tests, procedures, or special examinations (e.g., operating room, physical therapy, radiology); storage and access of patient information in computers; and the transmission of patient information via fax machines. Many people other than direct caregivers have legitimate access to a patient's chart: faculty members in the course of making student assignments, accrediting agencies, risk managers, quality assurance personnel, insurance companies, and researchers. Each is obligated to maintain patient confidentiality to the extent that concealing information

• Does not compromise mandated reports (communicable diseases or gunshot wounds).
• Considers various releases already granted by the patient (such as when insurance information was obtained).
• Ensures gathering data in the aggregate without identifying specific patients (research or institutional statistics).

Other forms of necessary communication include shift-change or transfer of care reporting and case conferences. Care must be taken to share this information in private.

VERACITY. Veracity is the virtue of truthfulness. Within health care, it requires HCPs, whenever possible, to tell the truth and not intentionally deceive or mislead patients. As with other rights and obligations, there are limitations to this virtue. The primary limitation occurs when telling patients the truth would seriously harm their ability to recover or when the truth can produce greater illness. This is known as

therapeutic privilege. It is exercised by HCPs in cases when (1) they are trying to protect patients from heartbreaking news, as in the initial stages of treatment; (2) they do not know the facts, making it better not to answer rather than instill false hope; and (3) they state what is true rather than state what is not true (Butts & Rich, 2016). As an example, consider a case of a new or experimental treatment. HCPs can say that, in certain clinical trials, patients benefited in specific ways. However, they might not be able to cite all of the possible side effects because the treatment has not yet been widely used.

Another difficult situation can be created in relation to diagnostic information. Although giving diagnostic information is the responsibility of the HCP or RN, LPNs/LVNs sometimes find themselves in situations in which they must deal with patients' questions. If LPNs/LVNs feel uncomfortable about reinforcing explanations given by the HCP or the RN, they might avoid answering patients' questions directly. However, patients do have a right to know this information. The LPN/LVN should inform the HCP or RN of the patient's request for information and follow the agency policy on patient information sharing.

JUSTICE. Justice is based on fairness and equality (Butts & Rich, 2016). Concerns for justice can focus on how we treat individuals and groups in society (psychologically, socially, legally, and politically). They can also focus on how we equitably distribute material resources, such as health care (distributive justice) and burdens (taxes), and the appropriate compensation to those who have been harmed. When a patient makes an appointment for 0900 at an outpatient clinic, the patient expects to be seen by the HCP at the designated time unless an emergency occurs. Unequal treatment would result if a walk-in patient who has no pressing problem is seen by the HCP in place of the patient with the 0900 appointment, forcing subsequent appointments to be delayed. Distribution of material resources can be complex because it involves not only benefits (what we receive) but also burdens (what we may be taxed for but then do not receive). Burdens are not just monetary but also include such factors as the unequal participation of individuals in medical research and the sacrifices family members make when caring for individuals with disabilities in the home.

USE OF PRINCIPLES. One of the most serious limitations of these principles is the lack of any built-in priority when applying them to an ethical dilemma. Autonomy is not automatically prioritized over justice, nor beneficence over nonmaleficence. However, these principles are helpful in categorizing various preferences and positions when examining a dilemma to clarify positions within it. Working with principles moves the discussion to a focus on ethics rather than on a particular personal viewpoint or feeling. Such a strategy can also avoid a power struggle between those who simply want to win the argument.

Ethical Theories

Ethical theories are concepts that are more complete than principles for analyzing ethical dilemmas. Theories are used to explain variables, guide inquiry, and provide a foundation with which to conduct decision making. A brief description of two of the major bioethics theories—utilitarianism and deontology—is provided here. Other theoretical approaches to ethical decision making exist. Theories are often combined to address ethical dilemmas. This section also explores the relationship of theology or religion to bioethics.

UTILITARIANISM. **Utilitarian** theory states that actions are judged "right" or "wrong" based purely on their consequences. Therefore, outcomes are the most important elements to consider when making decisions. The right actions are morally preferred if they produce more happiness or greater benefits than unhappiness or burdens. In utilitarianism, each person's happiness is equally important. This approach can be used by institutions and organizations under the guise of cost–benefit ratios. A hospital responsible for the care for hundreds of patients is not as concerned with the individual patient who unfortunately is caught in the bureaucracy of its functioning. This is not to say that all institutions operate on this theory at all times, but, in general, rules, policies, and procedures are developed with the majority in mind.

There are several major criticisms of the utilitarian theory. One is that an individual is often sacrificed for the good of the majority (often seen in wartime). The second is that it can be difficult to predict outcomes, especially when human nature is involved.

DEONTOLOGY. **Deontology** is based on duty, and the moral worth of an action (the result) should not be judged only in terms of its consequences. For example, HCPs might operate by a rule indicating that a moral person never lies. Therefore, we must tell the truth no matter how much the truth might hurt. Another rule might be never to use people as a means

to an end. In other words, we cannot "use" people to achieve an outcome. For example, it is an individual's right to voluntarily participate in research. Therefore, no matter how good our intentions are, we cannot "use" people or trick them into participating in research. A limitation of this theory is that it does not factor in consequences or take into account the role of the community.

THEOLOGICAL PERSPECTIVES. Theological perspectives include the many religious traditions represented in our culture. Religious teachings are key concepts for ethical decision making for some people. In fact, many consider these teachings a divine source of values and morals. Some examples include Jehovah's Witnesses' rejection of blood transfusions and religious-based opposition to abortion and euthanasia. One of the difficulties with religious traditions is that personal interpretation may vary from the actual teaching. Assessment of the importance of this dimension of the patient's life is important in an ethical analysis.

Ethical Decision Making

In its simplest form, ethical decision making is an informed, logical problem-solving process. Similar to the nursing process, as discussed in Chapter 1, the steps listed here assist in approaching a problem in an organized and systematic manner:

Step 1: Identify the ethical dilemma.
Step 2: Identify the stakeholders and their values.
Step 3: Gather and verify the information.
Step 4: Examine possible actions and the consequences of each action.
Step 5: Determine the ethical foundation for each action.
Step 6: Determine the best action with the strongest ethical support.
Step 7: Implement the action.
Step 8: Evaluate the outcome.

A sample case study using these steps is found in your online resources accessible through Davis Edge. Nurses applying the steps of the nursing process use critical thinking skills to be as logical and objective as possible. Ethical decision making is a similar process. The goal is to have a balanced perspective that does not let emotions overshadow the process or the outcome. The Nursing Ethics Network provides a host of links to information on ethical decision making for health care professionals (visit http://jmrileyrn.tripod.com/nen/nen.html).

CRITICAL THINKING

Ethical Decisions. Identify a health care–related ethical dilemma you have encountered as a student. How did you solve the dilemma? What expert resources did you use?

Apply the ethical decision-making steps to your ethical dilemma. How are your decision-making process and proposed actions different when using the steps?

LEGAL CONCEPTS

Regulation of Nursing Practice

Nursing is a licensed health care profession that is regulated by individual states. Nurses must be licensed by their state to practice nursing. The rationale for state licensure is to improve the quality of health care services and to protect the health, safety, and well-being of the residents of that state. Each state has a *board of nursing*. The board establishes requirements for nurses to be licensed and practice in that state.

Each state has laws that define the scope of a nurse's practice in that state. In most cases, these laws are contained in a *nurse practice act*. If a nurse violates the nurse practice act, his or her license can be sanctioned—that is, suspended or revoked. Unprofessional conduct, incompetence, conviction of a crime, or misuse of controlled substances are examples of circumstances that can result in sanctions against a nurse's license.

> ### BE SAFE!
> Do not go into work after drinking alcohol, even if it was the night before. It takes time to metabolize alcohol from your system. Most, if not all, organizations have a zero-tolerance policy for alcohol. Your employment could be terminated if random alcohol testing is done and your reading is not zero. Many factors affect alcohol metabolism rates. Men metabolize alcohol faster than do women, especially petite women. A woman's menses may increase the time required to metabolize alcohol. If you use a prescription medication, ensure you have a current prescription for a current condition. If you use controlled substances, even if legally prescribed, you cannot work when under their influence if the substance affects your ability to work safely.

Required Licensure Reporting

When you submit your application for state licensure, you must be honest and report any prior conviction for misdemeanors or felonies. Most states require a criminal background check for licensure, so they will find out! Briefly explain the conviction. Describe how you positively moved on in life (i.e., complied with the court's orders). Explain why criminal behavior will never happen again. Depending on the past criminal act and your explanation to the board, a past criminal conviction might not keep you from being licensed.

After you receive your license, address changes must be reported to the licensing board within 30 days. This ensures that you can always be contacted. Failure to do so is a violation of state law. It can also result in missing important communications, such as license renewal mailings. Any conviction (occurring anywhere, not just in your own state) must also be reported to your state board within 30 days. If in doubt, report! They *will* find out in time. If you haven't reported a conviction, you can be sanctioned not only for the conviction but also for not reporting.

Mandatory Reporting

A state's mandated reporting laws require licensed nurses to report known or suspected abuse of a person to state authorities. In their profession, nurses interact with vulnerable populations. These populations need additional eyes and ears looking out for their best interests. Whereas state laws protect all patient populations, older adults, children, and those with mental or developmental disabilities are the most vulnerable. Be sure to learn how your state's laws will affect your practice if you are obligated to report known or suspected abuse. Know how and when to notify the authorities.

Generally, *abuse* is defined as willful behavior that causes harm to an intended recipient. Abuse takes several forms: physical, sexual, verbal, emotional, financial/economic, or neglect. It can occur to anyone, of any age, and in any setting. Although neglect and abuse are related, the intent of neglect differs from the intent of abuse. Abuse occurs when the nurse acts with a desire to harm, whereas neglect occurs when a nurse's inaction produces harm regardless of the nurse's intent. For example, neglect potentially occurs when a nurse decides to place two adult briefs on a patient with heavy urination patterns to minimize the frequency of necessary changes. The nurse may try to rationalize the intervention as a benefit to the patient, but the neglectful behavior does not satisfy the needs of the patient and has the potential to cause harm, including skin breakdown, pain, and discomfort. Neglect produces harm unintentionally. Abuse is intentional. Abuse can be done in person and through use of technology. Older adults are especially vulnerable to financial abuse as well as physical abuse and neglect. In long-term care, the risk of abuse is higher for residents who have dementia and have directed unwelcome behaviors toward others. Other residents can willfully harm the dementia resident as payback for past behaviors. Licensed nurses must be aware of this potential for abuse to ensure safety of all residents.

Human Trafficking and the Nurse's Role

Human trafficking refers to the act of recruiting, harboring, transporting, providing, or obtaining a person for labor or as a sex worker though the use of force, fraud, or coercion (U.S. Department of State, 2015). Human trafficking is a worldwide problem. Some state boards of nursing are increasing awareness of the issue to help rescue victims. Nurses are being required when seeking licensure to obtain education on how to identify victims of human trafficking (Michigan Department of Licensing and Regulatory Affairs, 2017).

Human trafficking victims utilize the health care system to access emergency, inpatient hospital, or community-based services (Michigan Department of Licensing and Regulatory Affairs, 2017). The U.S. Department of Health and Human Services (n.d.) indicates that victims of human trafficking often lack access to quality health care for early treatment of health issues. Therefore, a victim may appear with late-stage issues that have gone untreated or have become chronic in nature. Victims seeking care often do not have identification or money. They are accompanied by someone in control. This person will not leave them alone and answers for them.

When providing care, licensed nurses have an opportunity to identify physical and psychological symptoms commonly seen in victims of human trafficking. Severe physical symptoms can develop over time. They can include headaches, fatigue, dizzy spells, back pain, and stomach or abdominal pain (Ottisova, Hemmings, Howard, Zimmerman, & Oram, 2016). Memory loss, depression, and anxiety are common psychological symptoms among human trafficking victims (Ottisova et al., 2016). Behaviors exhibited by human trafficking victims can resemble behaviors of sufferers of chronic abuse and neglect. Bruises, scars, and signs of physical abuse and torture, including malnutrition, should be noted. If you suspect a patient is a victim of human trafficking, discuss your suspicion with your clinical team (Box 3.2). After confirming the suspicion as a team, it must be reported to the appropriate authorities (Box 3.3).

Health Insurance Portability and Accountability Act (HIPAA)

The Health Insurance Portability and Accountability Act of 1996 (HIPAA) ensures privacy of a patient's protected health information (PHI) (visit www.hhs.gov/hipaa). All health care workers and students must follow HIPAA. This prevents illegal sharing of a patient's medical or billing information.

Nurses must be sensitive to all patient information that is learned during nursing care. HIPAA violations occur when PHI is shared without prior patient consent. An individual can be fined and/or sentenced up to 10 years in prison. They can also be sued individually and face possible employment termination. Some states, such as California, have enacted

---

Box 3.2

Indicators of Human Trafficking

Behaviors
Afraid, shy, or submissive
Coached dialogue
Sudden or dramatic change in behavior

Circumstances
Child involved with commercial sex acts
Controlled by someone who makes all decisions, will not leave the person alone, and speaks for the person
Evidence of poor housing conditions
Kept away from family, friends, school, public organizations, and church
Lack of personal possessions and adequate clothing
Movements restricted

Signs and Symptoms
Abuse signs: mental, physical, sexual, torture
Bruises (old and new)
Confusion or disorientation
Exhaustion
Malnourishment and/or dehydration
Minimal or no medical history
Poor hygiene

Box 3.3

Reporting Suspected Human Trafficking

U.S. Department of Homeland Security: Blue Campaign

The U.S. Department of Homeland Security is the voice of the federal government efforts to combat human trafficking. Blue is a color code used internationally for human trafficking awareness.

The Blue Campaign recommends safety first: Do not confront a suspected trafficker or alert a suspected trafficking victim. Report it!

To report suspected human trafficking, contact:
- Your local law enforcement
- The U.S. Department of Homeland Security Tip Line: 1-866-347-2423
- The National Human Trafficking Resource Center Hotline: 1-888-373-7888

   For additional information on human trafficking:
- Visit www.dhs.gov/blue-campaign or www.facebook.com/bluecampaign
- Follow on Twitter: #BlueCampaign
- Text HELP or INFO to BeFree (233733)

From U.S. Department of Homeland Security. (n.d.). Blue campaign: Indicators of human trafficking. Retrieved from www.dhs.gov/blue-campaign/indicators-human-trafficking.

---

laws ensuring the integrity of PHI. These state laws work in conjunction with HIPAA to deter unauthorized disclosure. If your agency reports an incident of unauthorized disclosure under federal or state law, a state agency may visit your organization to investigate. Review your employer's HIPAA compliance policies. Follow them.

Social Media and Protecting Privacy

With the pervasive nature of social media, health care agencies have increased their oversight of employees' social media activity. They are monitoring for unauthorized disclosures of PHI. HIPAA as well as state law can be violated by uploading photos to social media that were taken on a personal device in a patient care setting. Examples of social media include Facebook, Snapchat, and Reddit. Patient confidentiality and privacy must always be maintained. Only use PHI for intended purposes related to patient care. Nurses must afford dignity to patients and protect PHI in the virtual world. For more information and examples about using social media appropriately as a professional, see the National Council of State Boards of Nursing's guide at www.ncsbn.org/NCSBN_SocialMedia.pdf.

Nursing Liability and the Law

Nurses are expected to practice in accordance with the law. There are laws that establish **liability,** or responsibility for wrongful clinical decisions. For clinical nursing, there are three subcategories of the law: civil law, criminal law, and administrative law. **Criminal laws** regulate human behavior within society. **Civil laws** protect individual and personal property rights. **Administrative laws** license and regulate the practice of nursing.

Criminal and Civil Law

Criminal laws establish rules for social behavior and define the punishment for breaking those rules. Criminal laws relate to wrongs against society. Their violation can result in imprisonment and/or monetary fines. Violation of criminal laws can also produce civil liability. For example, a nurse acts maliciously in causing the injury or death of a patient. This nurse can be found criminally liable for the malicious act (being against societal norms) and civilly liable for the extent of injury and damages caused by the action. Examples of criminal actions include assault, battery, murder, and rape. Civil laws generally concern disputes among individuals. Actions that violate civil law do not commonly rise to violations of criminal law. Nevertheless, liability for violating a civil law may entail stiff penalties. This is done to deter similar behavior in the future.

A nurse's civil liability can arise from negligent patient care. Civil law provides a means for patients and families to recover from injuries that occur after receiving negligent care. Recovery in civil law requires the injured party to show causation between the licensed professional's action and the patient's injury. To show causation, the patient must demonstrate how the licensed professional's action or omission caused the injury. An injury can be physical, emotional, or financial in nature. Lawsuits involving personal injuries are called **torts.**

The process of a civil lawsuit begins with the filing of a complaint in a court by a *plaintiff.* Court systems have their own rules. They require the plaintiff to serve a copy of the complaint on the *defendant,* or the party defending the complaint. A **summons** acts as a notice of a lawsuit and should be attached to the complaint. Nurses served with a summons and/or complaint that arises from work-related duties should notify their employers immediately. An employer may choose to answer the summons. If the employer does not answer the summons, the nurse must seek legal counsel to answer it within the required time frame. Failure to answer the summons and complaint is harmful to a nurse's personal and professional life.

An employer may be liable for the acts or omissions of a nurse it employs. This theory of liability is called *respondeat superior.* Nurses must appreciate how their own behaviors can create civil liability for their employers. Always practice in accordance with your agency's policies and procedures.

Malpractice is a form of professional negligence. **Negligence** is a civil law claim that is presented when one's failure to exercise due care results in an injury to another. **Malpractice** arises when the resulting injury occurs as a result of the clinician–patient relationship. A nurse commits malpractice when the nurse fails to practice consistently within professional standards and the patient is injured as a result. For example, a nurse commits malpractice if the patient is injured because of a rough transfer performed inconsistently with organizational policy (e.g., to use lift sheets) and/or professional standards of practice. Professional standards of nursing practice are determined at the local and regional levels based on health care services and care and equipment offered there. Standards can vary by state. Licensed nurses are expected to use their knowledge learned through school and experience wisely when interacting with patients and families.

Limitation of Liability

Health care professionals should practice to limit liability. **Limitation of liability** reduces the actual and/or monetary responsibility for an undesired outcome. Prevention is the best way to limit liability. You can do this in the following ways: ensure patient rights, follow your employer's organizational policies, use current nursing practice standards, document accurately, and pursue continuing education.

Patient Rights

All patients are entitled to quality care that provides dignity, respect, and involvement in care planning. Ensure patient-centered outcomes. Question care directives that appear in conflict with patient rights. Rights are defined as something due an individual through legal guarantees or moral and ethical principles. Narrowly, the United States affords certain rights to patients who receive care at facilities reimbursed by the federal government through federal and state health insurance programs. Individual states may also enact laws that narrowly define rights for patients receiving care in that state. For example, Title 22 of the California Code of Regulations includes a bill of rights for patients at certain health care facilities operating under state licensure. Generally, patient rights promote a patient's individuality and decision-making capacity. Patient rights also prevent patients from experiencing abuse and unauthorized disclosure of PHI. Be aware of patient rights as you practice. Be courteous to your patient. Knock before entering a patient's room. Introduce yourself to promote a patient's right to privacy and limit liability in practice.

Appropriate Documentation

The medical record is a legal record in which nurses must document. Documentation must be clear, honest, and accurate. Always document according to agency policy. Failure to do so can create potential embarrassment and liability for you and your employer.

Malpractice Insurance

Individual malpractice insurance may not be essential. Often, an employer's corporate insurance covers the costs of civil liability arising from a nurse's care. If curious, ask your employer whether or how the employer's insurance provides coverage for malpractice complaints against persons with your position/title. Employer-provided liability insurance is not personal liability insurance. Its coverage may not cover the cost of defending actions brought by a state licensing agency against an individual nurse. LPNs/LVNs may opt to carry their own personal liability insurance. A cost–benefit analysis prior to purchase is recommended.

Quality of Care and the Survey Process

State agencies are charged by federal law with overseeing the quality of care and services provided in long-term care and skilled nursing facilities. On an annual basis, state agencies enter these facilities with a team of experienced evaluators. They assess the quality of care and review its environment and services. These surveys are stressful on the facilities and the surveyors. Teamwork is essential. Surveyors always appreciate honesty and candidness. The survey process is meant to ensure that quality is generated based on actual patient needs.

Acute care hospitals practice under a different method of quality oversight. Acute care organizations may seek quality accreditation from a private organization such as The Joint Commission. This type of accreditation requires a survey team to review care and services. It can shield an acute care organization from the more frequent quality assessments faced by long-term care and skilled nursing organizations.

State surveys and accreditation surveys are intended to review facility processes only. They are not intended to review an individual nurse's clinical practice methods.

Review Questions

1. The nurse is preparing a presentation on factors influencing health care changes. Which of the following would be a factor to include in the presentation? **Select all that apply.**
   1. Decreasing use of evidence
   2. Increasing older adult population
   3. Increasing cultural diversity
   4. Population size decline in the United States
   5. Campaign to stop human trafficking
   6. Technology advancements

2. Which of the following actions should the nurse take during admission and throughout a patient's hospitalization to help ensure payment to the agency for a secondary diagnosis occurrence? **Select all that apply.**
   1. Document patient education related to preventing complications.
   2. Document patient refusal of preventative interventions.
   3. Document interventions, such as turning and ambulating patients.
   4. Educate patients about methods used to prevent complications.
   5. Explain to the patient that participation in preventive interventions is optional.
   6. Photograph wounds that are present on admission.

3. Which of these actions would the nurse correctly interpret as falling within the scope of practice of the licensed practical nurse/licensed vocational nurse? **Select all that apply.**
   1. Performing a physical assessment on admission for a critical care patient
   2. Delegating to a registered nurse
   3. Ambulating a 1-day postoperative patient
   4. Developing the plan of care for a newly admitted surgical patient
   5. Administering medications to patients in a long-term care facility
   6. Obtaining vital signs of patients before medication administration

4. The nurse would like to suggest a new method for documenting intake and output to the nurse manager, who uses the autocratic leadership style. To approach the manager, the nurse would recognize that the autocratic leader makes decisions in which of these ways?
   1. Seeks information from all staff members
   2. Uses own knowledge
   3. Forms focus groups to gather information
   4. Forms a staff committee to provide input

5. During orientation, a newly hired licensed practical nurse/licensed vocational nurse reviews the agency job description for the position. Which of these situations would be an appropriate example of a leadership role for this position within the job description?
   1. Consulting with a registered nurse to modify care for an assigned patient
   2. Performing an annual employee evaluation for a nursing assistant
   3. Supervising the registered nurse and licensed practical nurse/licensed vocational nurse staff on a surgical unit
   4. Interviewing a new graduate registered nurse for a staff position

6. The nurse is caring for an adult patient admitted for an appendectomy who asks the nurse not to disclose any personal health information, including a positive human immunodeficiency virus status. The patient's mother arrives to visit and asks the nurse to explain why her child must take so many medications. Which of the following responses does the nurse use to apply the principle of veracity?
   1. "You will have to talk to the health care provider."
   2. "The medications are for recovery after a surgical procedure."
   3. "The medications are to treat an infection."
   4. "You will need to ask the patient directly about the medications."

7. A patient with cancer who is having chemotherapy has decided to stop receiving it because the patient has accepted mortality. What is the most ethical action by the nurse to address this situation?
   1. Explain to the patient that it would be silly to stop the last two treatments.
   2. Explain that this will be reported to a family member.
   3. Ensure that the patient understands the consequences of discontinuing treatment.
   4. Ensure that the patient knows that, without treatment, death will occur.

8. A patient with terminal cancer has an advance directive indicating that a feeding tube is not to be inserted. After the patient becomes unconscious, the patient's family requests that a feeding tube be inserted. Based on a deontological perspective and supporting the patient's autonomy, what action will the nurse anticipate the health care provider will take?
   1. Withhold the feeding tube.
   2. Insert the feeding tube.
   3. Order an electroencephalogram to determine if the patient will wake up.
   4. Place a "Do Not Resuscitate" bracelet on the patient's wrist.

9. The nurse is assisting in the health clinic in offering immunizations for school children. A mother asks the nurse why her children need to be immunized for communicable diseases. The nurse explains that when more children are immunized, more people are protected from the communicable diseases. Which ethical theory supports the nurse's reply?
   1. Deontological perspective
   2. Utilitarian perspective
   3. Theological perspective
   4. Autonomy perspective

10. A patient in a long-term care facility states that her family does not visit very often. She asks the nurse to give her extra medication so she can die. She says that she's old and no one will mind anyway. What is the nurse's best response?
    1. "Now that is just silly! Go to the activity room. They are playing bingo."
    2. "I'm sorry, but I cannot do that. Do you want to talk about how you are feeling?"
    3. "I can give you a sedative with lunch so that you can relax more."
    4. "My kids don't visit me often either. I understand how you feel."

11. The nurse is caring for a team of patients. Which of the following practice guidelines does the nurse follow to ensure appropriate patient care is provided? **Select all that apply.**
    1. An institution's policies
    2. A national organization's code of ethics
    3. State practice laws for nurses
    4. National association nursing standards
    5. Local nursing standards

12. The nurse provides nursing care to prevent liability. Which of these actions would the nurse take to prevent liability? **Select all that apply.**
    1. Breach the duty of care.
    2. Document accurately.
    3. Follow current nursing practice standards.
    4. Protect patient rights.
    5. Pursue continuing education.
    6. Utilize organizational policies.

13. Which action does the Health Insurance Portability and Accountability Act of 1996 require the nurse to take while caring for patients?
    1. Maintain continuing nursing education credit hours.
    2. Ensure the privacy of patients' protected health information.
    3. Limit nursing work hours to no more than 35 per week.
    4. Avoid membership in a union or collective bargaining agreement unit.

14. The nurse is collecting data on a patient in a health care clinic. Which of the following observed data contributes to the suspicion that the patient is a victim of human trafficking and not safe? **Select all that apply.**
    1. Physical bruising and marks
    2. Below normal weight range
    3. Emotionally depressed
    4. Unmanaged chronic health issues
    5. Personal identification available on request
    6. Excellent health history

Answer rationales available in your online resources.

ANSWERS 1. 2, 3, 5, 6; 2. 1, 2, 3, 4, 6; 3. 3, 5, 6; 4. 2; 5. 1; 6. 4; 7. 3, 8, 1; 9. 2; 10. 2; 11. 1, 3, 5; 12. 2, 3, 4, 5, 6; 13. 2; 14. 1, 2, 3, 4

Key Points

Find the chapter key points in your online resources available through Davis Edge.

Additional Resources

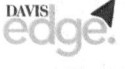 **Use the scratch off code on the inside front cover of your book to access online quizzes that will help you to improve your scores on course exams and prepare for the NCLEX-PN®.**

 Study Guide

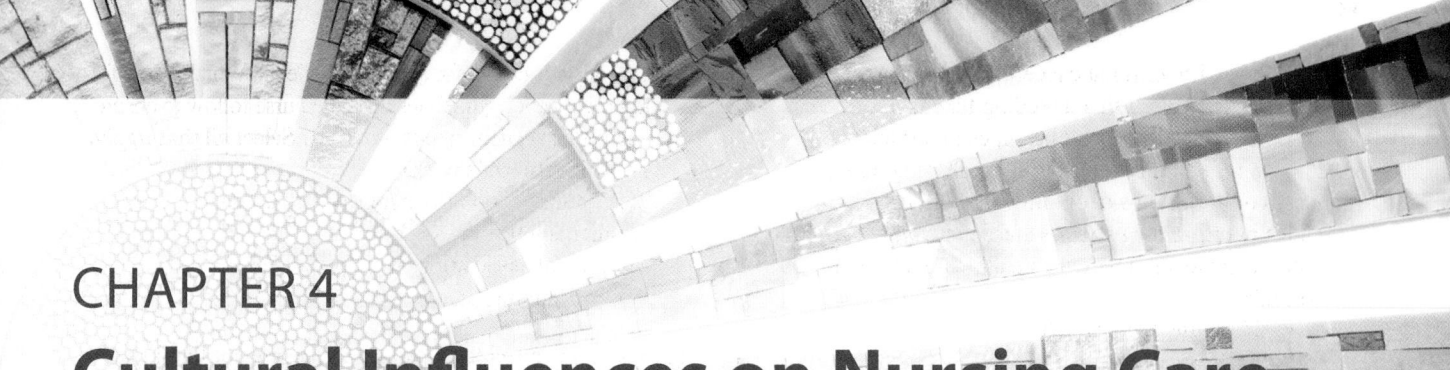

CHAPTER 4
Cultural Influences on Nursing Care

Bobbi M. Martin

KEY TERMS

acculturation (uh-KUL-chur-AY-shun)
belief (bee-LEEF)
cultural (KUL-chur-uhl)
cultural assimilation (KUL-chur-uhl uh-SIM-ih-LAY-shun)
cultural awareness (KUL-chur-uhl a-WEAR-ness)
cultural competence (KUL-chur-uhl KOM-pe-tents)
cultural conflict (KUL-chur-uhl KON-flikt)
cultural diversity (KUL-chur-uhl dih-VER-sih-tee)
cultural sensitivity (KUL-chur-uhl SEN-sih-TIV-ih-tee)
cultural shock (KUL-chur-uhl SHOK)
culture (KUL-chur)
customs (KUS-tums)
ethnic (ETH-nik)
ethnocentrism (ETH-noh-SEN-trizm)
practice (PRAK-tis)
spiritual (SPEER-ih-choo-AL)
spirituality (SPEER-ih-choo-AL-it-ee)
stereotype (STARE-ee-oh-TYPE)
traditions (tra-DISH-uns)
values (VAL-yooz)
worldview (WERLD-vyoo)

CHAPTER CONCEPTS

Communication
Culture
Family Dynamics
Grief and Loss
Patient-Centered Care
Spirituality

LEARNING OUTCOMES

1. Define common concepts related to culture and spirituality.
2. Describe attributes of culturally diverse patients and their families and how they affect nursing care.
3. Identify data you should collect from culturally diverse patients and their families.
4. Apply a holistic approach to patient care that respects cultural and spiritual characteristics and attributes.

Can you think of examples of cultural practices you have seen in your experience that were unique or different from your own? Cultural diversity in the United States is increasing. Figure 4.1 illustrates the racial and ethnic makeup in the United States as of 2017. According to the U.S. Census Bureau, by 2044 more than half of all Americans are projected to belong to a minority group (any group other than non-Hispanic white alone) (Colby & Ortman, 2015). Thus, **cultural, ethnic,** and **spiritual** differences between nurses and their patients are becoming more evident and must be recognized. More than ever, nurses must develop cultural awareness and recognize the patient as a full partner in providing compassionate care based on respect for the patient's preferences, values, and needs (Quality and Safety Education for Nurses, 2017). Healthy People 2020's goals include the need to "achieve health equity, eliminate disparities, and improve the health of all groups" (Office of Disease Prevention and Health Promotion, 2015). This chapter provides the basics of culture and spirituality as well as their impact on health promotion and wellness.

CONCEPTS RELATED TO CULTURE

Culture refers to the socially transmitted behavior patterns, beliefs, values, customs, arts, and all other characteristics of people that guide their view of the world (**worldview**). Cultural **beliefs, values, customs,** and **traditions** are primarily learned within the family on an unconscious level. They can also be learned from the communities in which we live.

As you try to understand more about culture, keep in mind that it contains a number of characteristics (Box 4.1). All individuals and groups have the right to maintain cultural **practices** that they feel are appropriate, as long as they do not infringe on the rights

Race and Hispanic Origin

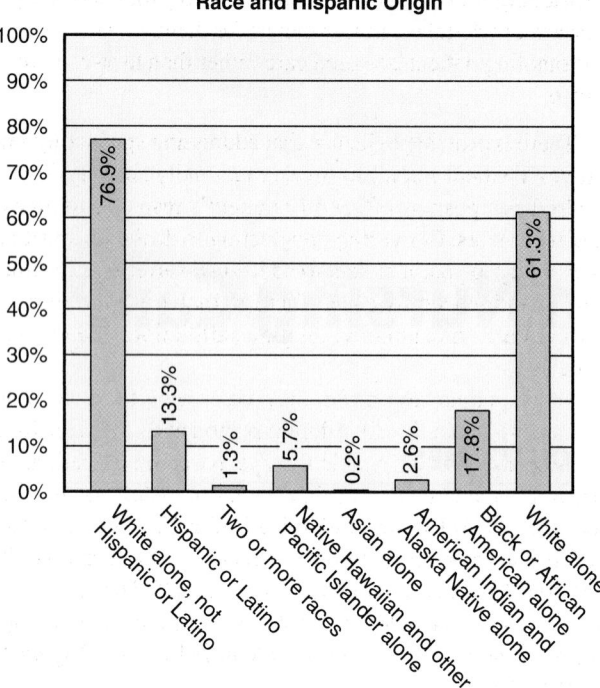

FIGURE 4.1 Percentage of the population of the United States, by race and Hispanic origin.

of others. However, as you will learn from this chapter, nurses must be aware of cultural health practices that can cause physical harm and require nursing intervention. To better meet the needs of your patients, you must understand how culture influences health behaviors (Fig. 4.2). As you learn more about cultural groups, you will be challenged to look at differences and similarities across cultures.

Although the terms *cultural sensitivity, cultural awareness,* and *cultural competence* are similar, they have different meanings. **Cultural sensitivity** is knowing culturally appropriate language and not making statements that may offend another person's cultural beliefs. **Cultural awareness** focuses on history and ancestry and emphasizes an appreciation for and attention to a culture's arts, music, crafts, celebrations, foods, and traditional clothing. **Cultural competence** refers to the skills and knowledge required to provide effective nursing care. To be culturally competent, you need to

- Have an awareness of your own culture and not let it have an undue influence on your patient care.
- Have specific knowledge about your patient's culture.
- Accept and respect cultural differences.
- Adapt your nursing care (when appropriate) to your patient's culture.

Although you may have knowledge about another culture, barriers such as ethnocentrism and stereotyping can keep you from appreciating cultural differences. **Ethnocentrism** is the tendency for us to think that our culture's ways of thinking, acting, and believing are the only right and natural ways, and

---

Box 4.1

Characteristics of Culture

- *Culture is learned.* Learning occurs through life experiences shared with other members of the culture.
- *Culture is taught.* Cultural values, beliefs, and traditions are passed down from generation to generation, either formally (e.g., in schools) or informally (e.g., in families).
- *Culture is shared by its members.* Cultural norms are shared through teachings and social interactions.
- *Culture is dynamic and adaptive.* Cultural customs, beliefs, and practices are not static but change over time and at different rates. Cultural change occurs with adaptation in response to the environment.
- *Culture is complex.* Cultural assumptions and habits are unconscious, which may make them difficult for members of the culture to explain to others.
- *Culture is diverse.* Culture demonstrates the variety that exists between groups and among members of a particular group.
- *Culture exists at many levels.* Culture exists at material (e.g., art, dress, and artifacts) and nonmaterial (e.g., language, traditions, customs, beliefs, and practices) levels.
- *Culture has common beliefs and practices.* Members of a culture share the same beliefs, traditions, customs, and practices as long as they continue to be adaptive and satisfy their needs. Some members do not always follow all of these, but many do.
- *Culture is all encompassing.* Culture can affect everything its members do and how they think.
- *Culture provides identity.* Cultural beliefs provide identity for members as long as there is no conflict with the dominant culture or lack of gratification by its members.
- *Culture shapes spirituality.* Spirituality gives meaning and purpose to our existence.

that beliefs that differ greatly from our own culture are strange or bizarre and, therefore, wrong. Additionally, you must be careful not to stereotype your patient. A **stereotype** is an opinion or belief about a group of people that is ascribed to an individual. For example, the statement "All Chinese people prefer traditional Chinese medicine" is a stereotype. This stereotype is not true. Although *some* Chinese people may prefer traditional Chinese medicine for some health conditions, *not all* Chinese people prefer traditional Chinese medicine.

The challenge is for you to understand the patient's cultural perspective. If you have specific cultural knowledge, you can improve therapeutic interventions by partnering with patients and their families. To do this, it is important to develop a personal, open style of communication and be receptive to learning from patients from cultures other than your own.

A few additional terms important for your understanding of culture relate to the socialization process of those who are learning to become a member of a society or group. When people immigrate to a new country, many gradually accept the new culture through a learning process. They learn to accept

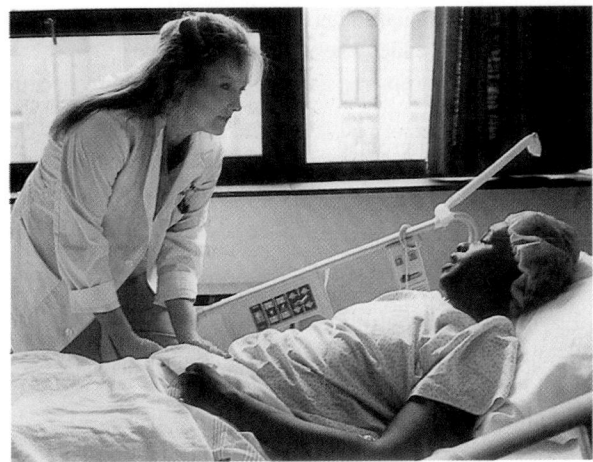

FIGURE 4.2 The nurse must assess patients' unique needs related to their cultural backgrounds.

their own beliefs as well as those of their new country. This is known as **acculturation.** Acculturation is commonly seen in second generation immigrants because they not only understand the necessity of learning their new culture but also see the value of it. Learning the new culture helps individuals survive and, more important, thrive in their new environment. **Cultural assimilation** occurs when a new member takes on the dominant culture's values, beliefs, and practices, sometimes at the cost of losing some of his or her cultural heritage. This process is often viewed as negative.

Imagine for a moment that you have moved to China. Initially, you try new foods and learn the language of your new country. Then, over time, you may learn to cook the food, speak the language, and perhaps blend some of the Chinese beliefs, traditions, and practices with your own. This is acculturation. However, this process is not always smooth. When one's own culture conflicts with a new culture, **cultural conflict** occurs. Worse than that, **cultural shock** can happen when values, beliefs, and practices sanctioned by the new culture are very different from the ones of the native culture.

 CONCEPTS RELATED TO SPIRITUALITY

Spirituality, simply defined, is the essence of being; it gives meaning and purpose to our existence (Rogers & Wattis, 2015). Although religion and spirituality are distinct, they may overlap. Some people view their faith in God or a higher being as the core of their spirituality. However, many would assert that one can be spiritual without being religious, and vice versa.

For many nurses, there is confusion between spirituality and religion. Knowing how to integrate spirituality into nursing care can be challenging. Exploring spirituality with patients may help them find hope and meaning during times of illness and crisis. A good starting point for being sensitive to the spiritual needs of patients is

• Being aware of your own spirituality and where your own sense of meaning, purpose, and values come from.

• Listening for cues and being attentive to patients raising issues of what their illness means for them.
• Promoting patient-centered care rather than task-centered care.

There is growing evidence that addressing spirituality improves a patient's comfort level emotionally and physically. It also has a positive effect on a patient's response to illness and treatments. Conversely, neglecting to deal with spiritual issues may expose a patient to additional suffering. Spiritual care is influenced by many factors, including the nurse's own culture and ethnicity, religious affiliation, and clinical experience.

When people are unwell, they may signal their desire to discuss spiritual issues. Being responsive and sensitive to these signals may enable therapeutic communications to occur. If a patient does not signal a desire to discuss spiritual matters, a sensitive and individualized approach is needed. Ask questions such as, "How has this illness affected you?" or "What has helped or might help you cope?" The discussion should result in a dialogue about how the patient can be supported in addressing his or her identified needs (Rogers & Wattis, 2015).

 HEALTH CARE VALUES, BELIEFS, AND PRACTICES

Cultural values, beliefs, and practices about the nature of disease and the human body are central in the delivery of health services, treatments, and preventive interventions (Agency for Healthcare Research and Quality, 2012). A *value* can be defined as a principle or standard that has meaning or worth to an individual (Purnell & Paulanka, 2008). Values help shape one's beliefs and practices. Do you know what your values are regarding health and illness? "Cleanliness" is an example of a value. A *belief* is something that a person accepts as true (e.g., "I believe that germs cause illness and disease"). A *practice* is a set of behaviors that one follows (e.g., washing your hands before eating). It is important for you to understand the differences between these concepts because we will be discussing them as they relate to cultural groups.

To provide culturally competent care, you need to know how the patients you encounter define health and illness. In general, people follow one of three major health belief systems: scientific (Western medicine or biomedical), spiritual, or holistic. You are already familiar with the scientific health system, which dominates health care in Western societies. Belief in supernatural forces dominates the spiritual system, which is considered by many to be an alternative health care system. The holistic belief system focuses on the need for balance and harmony of the body and spirit with nature.

Health care typically focuses on health promotion, illness prevention, and acute illness care while considering traditional, religious, and biomedical (scientific) beliefs. Additionally, individual responsibility for health, self-medicating practices, views toward mental illness, response to pain, and the sick role are shaped by one's culture. Most societies combine biomedical health care with traditional, folk, and religious practices. There are many examples of folk practices for curing or treating specific illnesses. Think for a minute about such practices that you may use. What do you do for a fever or a sore throat? Does chicken noodle soup come to mind? Many times, folk therapies are handed down from family members and may have their roots in religious beliefs. As you will see in Chapter 5, many people use complementary therapies such as acupressure or herbal remedies in addition to traditional Western therapies.

Often, folk practices are not harmful and can be added to the patient's plan of care. However, some therapies may conflict with prescription medications or cause a toxic effect. Other folk practices may actually cause physical harm to a patient. It is essential to inquire about the full range of therapies being used by your patients, such as foods, teas, herbal remedies, nonfood substances, over-the-counter medications, medications prescribed by others, and medications borrowed from others.

If patients sense that you do not accept their beliefs and practices, they may be less open to sharing information and less adherent to prescribed treatment. Your goal is to encourage your patients' practices that could be helpful and discourage those that may be harmful. Before encouraging or discouraging such practices, you will need to discuss them with the appropriate health care team member.

Before moving on, we need to discuss the topics of mental illness and cultural responses to pain and the sick role. Mental illness may be seen by some cultures as being unimportant compared with physical illness. Mental illness is many times culture bound. What may be perceived as a mental illness in one society may not be considered a mental illness in another society. Among some cultures, having a mental illness or an emotional difficulty is considered a disgrace and is taboo. As a result, a family may keep a person who is mentally ill at home as long as possible.

Responses to pain and the sick role can vary among cultures. For example, in some cultures, people are expected to openly express their pain. In others, people are expected to suffer their pain in silence. In some cultures, the sick role is readily accepted, and any excuse is sufficient for not fulfilling daily obligations. In other cultures, people minimize illness and make great efforts to meet obligations despite being ill.

 ## CHARACTERISTICS OF CULTURAL DIVERSITY

Primary and secondary characteristics of diversity affect how people view their culture. Primary characteristics of **cultural diversity** include nationality, race, skin color, gender, age, spirituality, and religious affiliation. Secondary characteristics include socioeconomic status, education, occupation, military experience, political beliefs, length of time away from one's country of origin, urban versus rural residence,

marital status, parental status, physical characteristics, sexual orientation, and gender roles.

Culturally appropriate care needs to take into account eight cultural phenomena that may vary with use but can be seen in all cultural groups:

1. Communication styles
2. Space
3. Time orientation
4. Social organization
5. Environmental control/health beliefs
6. Choice of health care providers (HCPs)
7. Biological variations
8. Death and dying issues

Communication Styles

Communication occurs both verbally and nonverbally. Verbal communication includes spoken language, dialects, and voice volume. Dialects include variations in grammar, word meanings, and pronunciation of spoken language. Nonverbal communication includes the use and degree of eye contact, the perception of time, and physical closeness when talking with peers and perceived superiors. In some cultures, people are expected to maintain eye contact without staring; this shows that they are listening and can be trusted. However, in other cultures, as a sign of respect, people should not maintain eye contact with superiors such as teachers and those in positions of higher status.

Nursing Assessment and Strategies

Ask the following questions of your patients:

- By what name do you prefer to be called?
- What language do you speak at home?
- Are you able to read and write in English? If not, what language is preferred?

  Be sure to do the following:

- Take cues from the patient regarding greetings and voice volume.
- Avoid appearing rushed.
- Speak slowly and clearly. Do not speak loudly or with exaggerated mouthing.
- Explain why you are asking specific questions.
- Provide written instructions in the patient's preferred language.
- Obtain an interpreter if needed.

Health care team members should refrain from relying on untrained individuals to interpret, especially family members. Although it may seem logical that a patient's best advocate is his or her family, it is risky to rely on family members to interpret medical or health information for the following reasons:

- Family members may not be proficient in medical terminology.
- They may unintentionally or intentionally omit or alter important information.

- Using family members to interpret may raise privacy issues protected by the Health Insurance Portability and Accountability Act of 1996 (HIPAA).
- If children are used, they may not be emotionally mature enough to handle the information being conveyed.

Space

Space refers to one's "personal space." Are you aware of your comfort zone? In other words, how close can someone get to you before you feel less safe and secure? Most people have such a comfort zone. Personal space tends to be different when speaking with close friends versus strangers. It also differs across cultures. For example, people from some cultures stand close together when talking. This might make those from cultures who prefer more personal space uncomfortable. The need for space is important for the patient's privacy, autonomy, security, and self-identity. Understanding what space means for your patients is important to patient-centered care.

Nursing Assessment and Strategies

Ask your patients whether they are comfortable. Be sure to do the following:

- Make sure your patients are comfortable before you interview them.
- Maintain appropriate physical distance (observe for cues).
- Make sure that the patient's physical environment is arranged to ensure safety, security, and familiarity.

Time Orientation

Time orientation can vary among people from different cultures. The perception of time has two dimensions. The first dimension is related to clock time versus social time. For example, some cultures have a flexible orientation to time and events; appointments take place when the person arrives. An event scheduled for 1400 may not begin until 1430 or when a majority of the participants arrive. In other cultures, time is less flexible; appointments and social events are expected to start at the agreed-on time. In some cultures, social events may be flexible, whereas medical appointments and business engagements start on time.

The second dimension of time relates to whether the culture is predominantly concerned with the past, present, or future. Past-oriented cultures maintain traditions that were meaningful in the past; this may include worshiping ancestors. Present-oriented cultures accept the day as it comes, with little regard for the past; the future is unpredictable. Future-oriented cultures anticipate a bigger and better future and place a high value on change. Some people balance all three views: They respect the past, enjoy living in the present, and plan for the future.

Hospitals, clinics, and HCP offices maintain a tight time schedule. It is, therefore, important that you understand patients' time orientation so you can prepare them for the timing of appointments, tests, and treatments. In addition, it is important that you assess their usual routines so that you can incorporate these as much as possible into their daily care.

Nursing Assessment and Strategies

Ask the following questions of your patients:

- Are you typically on time for appointments?
- Are there any routines that you prefer to follow?
- What time do you usually eat your meals? Take a shower or bath?

Be sure to do the following:

- Have a clock in the patient's room.
- Assess for orientation, and reorient to time as needed.
- Give time options when appropriate (e.g., "Would you like to take a walk now or in an hour?").

Social Organization

Family organization includes the perceived head of the household, gender roles, and roles of older and extended family members. The household may be patriarchal (male dominated), matriarchal (female dominated), or egalitarian (shared equally between men and women). An awareness of the family dominance pattern is important for determining which family members should be included when health care decisions must be made. Confidentiality issues can complicate this issue. Be sure to follow your institution's policies when communicating with family members. You may need to obtain the patient's permission before planning care with family members.

In some cultures, specific roles are outlined for men and women. Men may be expected to protect and provide for the family, manage finances, and deal with the outside world. Women may be expected to maintain the home environment and care for children. You must accept that not all societies have or even desire an egalitarian family structure.

Roles for older adults and extended family vary among cultures. In some cultures, older adults are seen as being wise, are deferred to for making decisions, and are held in high esteem. Their children are expected to provide for them when they are no longer able to care for themselves. In other cultures, although older people may be loved by family members, they may not be treated with the same regard. In many cases, they may be cared for outside the home when self-care becomes a concern.

The extended family is very important in some cultures. A single household may include several generations living together out of desire rather than out of necessity. The extended family may include both blood-related and non–blood-related persons who are given family status. In other cultures, each generation lives in a separate home or living space.

Nursing Assessment and Strategies

Ask the following questions of your patients:

- Who takes part in making decisions in your household?
- Who takes care of money matters, does the cooking, or is responsible for child care?
- Who decides when it is time to see an HCP?
- Who lives in your household? Are they all blood related?

Be sure to do the following:

- Observe the use of touch between family members.
- Let family members decide where they want to stand or sit for comfort.

Environmental Control

Environmental control consists of three major concepts: people's perception of their ability to control what happens to them and their health, people's beliefs about health and illness, and people's beliefs in alternative health care therapies such as folk medicine. For example, if a patient does not believe he or she has control of his or her health, the patient may not be receptive to nursing interventions that require self-confidence, such as self-administration of insulin. Also, if a patient believes that illness is due to a spiritual cause and not bacteria, he or she may not understand the need to take antibiotics. In addition, many people put great faith in folk medicine healing practices. Nurses need to consider the patient's cultural values and beliefs, especially if they are different from the dominant Western health care view.

Not all patients will turn to a Western health care system or provider. Many may try some form of alternative therapy before seeking treatment. Patients may also use alternative therapies and religious practices such as prayer in combination with the scientific medical system.

Nursing Assessment and Strategies

Ask the following questions of your patients:

- How do you define health? Illness?
- What do you do to keep well?
- When you feel ill, what is the first thing you do to get better?
- How do you deal with pain?
- How do you and your family express grief?
- Are there any cultural beliefs or practices that I need to know about to plan your care?

Be sure to do the following:

- Never stereotype based on what you know about different cultures; always ask for specific information.
- Perform a cultural assessment of all your patients.
- Ask whether patients have received treatment of any kind for their illness.
- Ask about religious beliefs and practices.
- Encourage helpful practices and discourage those that are harmful.

Choice of Health Care Providers

HCP choices are made based on the patient's perceived health status and previous use of traditional, religious, and biomedical HCPs. In some cultures, a highly educated HCP is the patient's first choice. However, patients in other cultures may prefer traditional healers because they are known to the patient, family, and community.

It is important to respect differences in gender relationships when providing care. Some people may be especially modest because of their culture or religion, seeking out same-gender nurses and HCPs for intimate care. Respect these patients' modesty by providing privacy and assigning a same-gender care provider when possible.

Nursing Assessment and Strategies

Ask the following questions of your patients:

- What HCPs besides physicians and nurses do you see when you are ill?
- Do you object to male or female HCPs providing physical care for you?

Be sure to observe for alternative care providers who may visit the patient in the health care facility.

Biological Variations

Biological variations refer to ways in which people are different from one another physiologically and genetically. These differences can make individuals more susceptible to certain illnesses and diseases. They may also influence the effectiveness of different medications. Biological variations can include differences in (1) body build and structure, (2) skin color, (3) vital signs, (4) laboratory values, (5) susceptibility to disease, and (6) nutrition. For example, darker skin color can challenge you to be more observant when you are assessing changes in the skin color of your patient. Laboratory test results can also be different in a number of cultures. For example, American Indians and Hispanic Americans tend to have higher blood glucose levels than do non-Hispanic whites.

Biological variations also include differences in nutritional practices, such as the personal meaning of food, food choices and rituals, food taboos, and how food and food substances are used for health promotion and wellness. Cultural beliefs may influence what people eat or avoid. In addition to being important for survival, food offers security and acceptance, plays a significant role in socialization, and can serve as an expression of love.

Culturally congruent dietary counseling, such as adapting preparation practices and including ethnic food choices, can reduce health risks. Whenever possible, determine a patient's current dietary practices. Counseling about food group requirements or dietary restrictions must respect an individual's cultural background. Most cultures have their own nutritional practices for health promotion and disease prevention. For many, a balance of different types of foods is important for maintaining health and preventing illness. A thorough history and assessment of dietary practices can be an important diagnostic tool to guide health promotion.

Nursing Assessment and Strategies

Ask the following questions of your patients:

- Are you at risk for any diseases or genetic disorders related to your culture or ethnicity?
- Are you satisfied with your weight?
- Are you active? What is your normal exercise pattern?

- Do you protect your eyes and skin from the sun? From possible injuries?
- Do you have any drug or food allergies?
- What do you eat to stay healthy?
- What do you eat when you are ill?
- Are there certain foods that you do not eat? Why?
- Do certain foods cause you to become ill? What are they?

Be sure to do the following:

- Teach about biological variations that may pertain to your patient.
- Determine and respect a patient's typical eating patterns whenever possible.
- Teach good nutrition habits, taking into account patient preferences. Refer to a dietitian if appropriate.

Death and Dying and End-of-Life Issues

Death rituals of cultural groups are the least likely to change over time. To avoid cultural taboos, become knowledgeable about rituals surrounding death and bereavement. In some cultures, the body should be buried whole. Therefore, an amputated limb may be buried in the amputee's future gravesite, and organ donation would probably not be acceptable. Cremation may be preferred in some culture; in others, it is taboo, and burial is the preferred practice. Views on autopsy vary. Some cultural groups have elaborate ceremonies that last for days in commemoration of the dead. In some cultures, these rituals appear celebratory, and, in a sense, they are a celebration of the person's life rather than a mourning of the person's death. If you are uncertain, find out from the family if there is anything that the health care team can do to facilitate cultural practices during the end-of-life phase.

The expression of grief in response to death varies among cultural and ethnic groups. For example, in some cultures, loved ones are expected to suffer the grief of death in silence, with little display of emotion. In other cultures, loved ones display elaborate emotions to show that they cared for the deceased. These variations in the grieving process may cause confusion, in that you may perceive some people as overreacting and others as not caring. You must accept that culturally diverse behaviors are associated with the grieving process. Bereavement support strategies include being physically present, encouraging reality orientation, openly acknowledging the family's right to grieve as they need to, helping the family express their feelings, and making referrals to other staff and spiritual leaders as appropriate.

At times, you may be involved with end-of-life decisions. Some of these may include advance directives, resuscitation status, and organ transplantation. Collaborate with the registered nurse or HCP to ensure cultural preferences are respected.

Nursing Assessment and Strategies

Ask the following questions of your patients:

- What are the usual burial practices in your family?
- What are your feelings about autopsy?

Be sure to do the following:

- Observe expressions of grief. Support the family in their expression of grief.
- Observe for differences in the expression of grief among family members.
- Offer to obtain a religious counselor/spiritual leader if the family wishes.

 ETHNIC AND CULTURAL GROUPS IN THE UNITED STATES

This section describes selected attributes of some cultural groups in the United States. These groups include European American (Census uses the term *white*), Spanish/Hispanic/Latino, African American (non-Hispanic black), American Indian/Alaskan Native, Arab American, Asian American, and Native Hawaiian or Other Pacific Islander. The groups described here by no means represent all the cultural groups in North America; they do, however, represent the largest population percentages in the United States. The terminology used in this section comes from the most recent U.S. Census in 2010.

Gerontological Issues

Aging and Cultural Diversity. By 2050, 39.1% of America's aging population will be a minority or ethnic group, up from 20.7% in 2012 (Ortman, Velkoff, & Hogan, 2014). To provide culturally competent care, remember that older adults need to be assessed within their personal cultural context. Always assess individual and family preferences.

European American

European American (or non-Hispanic white) describes people living in the United States whose heritage is from western, southern, and northern Europe. Many are descendants of European immigrants. Whereas *European American* comprises mostly white ethnic groups, there is much diversity in the primary and secondary characteristics within this cultural group. European Americans are more susceptible to heart disease, breast cancer, diabetes mellitus, thalassemia, and Tay-Sachs disease (Eastern European Jewish). Health screening and preventive health care strategies should be encouraged for European Americans as well as a low-fat, low-cholesterol, high-fiber diet.

Spanish/Hispanic/Latino

Spanish/Hispanic/Latino is used to describe people whose cultural heritage has a strong Spanish influence. People who identify as Spanish/Hispanic/Latino comprise approximately 17.6% of the U.S. population (U.S. Census Bureau, 2017). They recently became the majority–minority population. They live in all 50 states, with more than 90% living in and around cities.

Four of every five persons who are Spanish/Hispanic/Latino currently living in the United States were born and raised here. They are susceptible to lactose intolerance, diabetes mellitus, parasites, coccidioidomycosis, and gout.

African American (Non-Hispanic Black)

African Americans, or non-Hispanic blacks, are the third largest ethnic group in the United States and represent more than 100 racial strains. They make up 13.3% of the population (U.S. Census Bureau, 2017). Although African Americans live in all 50 states, more than half live in southern states. Common health problems for African Americans are high blood pressure, obesity, and diabetes, all of which can lead to heart disease and stroke.

American Indian/Alaskan Native

American Indians/Alaskan Natives are the original inhabitants of North America. There are more than 400 American Indian/Alaskan Native tribes in the United States, totaling 0.9% of the population (U.S. Census Bureau, 2017). Although there are similarities among American Indians, each tribe has its own unique perspective on health and illness.

Many American Indians/Alaskan Natives live on reservations while others live in urban areas. They are at greater risk for heart disease, liver disease, diabetes mellitus, tuberculosis, arthritis, and glaucoma.

Arab American

Arab Americans are a large and diverse population, with more than 3 million living in the United States. Arab Americans include people from Morocco, Algeria, Tunisia, Libya, Sudan, Egypt and the western Asian countries of Lebanon, occupied Palestine, Syria, Jordan, Iraq, Iran, Kuwait, Bahrain, Qatar, United Arab Emirates, Saudi Arabia, Oman, and Yemen. Many early Arab immigrants to the United States were Christians from Lebanon and Syria. Arab Americans are more prone to diabetes, hypertension, and hypercholesterolemia.

Asian American

The large Asian American group is far from homogeneous. The term *Asian,* as used in most references, includes 32 groups. It refers to a person having origins in the Far East, Southeast Asia, or the Indian subcontinent. Asian Americans as a group are composed of Asians, Indochinese, and other Asian groups. Asians include people from Korea, Japan, and 54 ethnic groups from China; Polynesians; Filipinos; Malaysians; and Guamanians. Indochinese populations include Cambodian, Vietnamese, Hmong, and Laotian. Other Asian groups include Asian Indian, Pakistani, and Thai. Although it is difficult to determine exact numbers of Asian Americans from specific countries because of the method of keeping population statistics, they are a significant and fast-growing population in the United States. Asian Americans are more likely to have lactose intolerance, thalassemia, liver and stomach cancers, hypertension, and coccidioidomycosis.

Native Hawaiian or Other Pacific Islander

Native Hawaiian or Other Pacific Islander refers to a person having origins in Hawaii, Guam, Samoa, or other Pacific Islands. The majority of the Native Hawaiian and the Pacific Islander population resides in Hawaii and California.

Native Hawaiian and Pacific Islanders have multiple health concerns. Native Hawaiians are more likely to have diabetes and have higher death rates due to cancer. Pacific Islander children have the highest rates of being overweight among all children. Together, both have the second highest rate of HIV infection and the second shortest AIDS survival rate of all Americans. Almost 20% live in poverty, and 18% live below the national poverty level (Wergowske & Blanchetter, 2010; White House Initiative on Asian Americans and Pacific Islanders, 2010).

CRITICAL THINKING

Ms. Waters is an older adult woman from a culture that is different from your own. She has had diabetes and hypertension (high blood pressure) for many years. She is admitted to the hospital for gangrene of her left foot. When you enter her room, you find Ms. Waters anxious and crying. As you approach her bed, she reaches out and takes your hand and holds it while you talk. When asked about her foot, she tells you that she has been applying a poultice to draw out the germs, but it has not worked yet. She adds that she has been praying for God to heal the infection. As you are collecting history information about her diabetes, Ms. Waters admits that her doctor advised her to follow a diabetic diet and to lose weight, but she doesn't like the foods on the diet. She quickly changes the subject, wanting to talk about her son and her grandchildren.

1. What does your interaction with Ms. Waters tell you about her time orientation?
2. What do you know about her spirituality and social organization?
3. Do you have any clues about Ms. Waters's personal space needs?
4. Whom might you involve in discussions with Ms. Waters about her health?
5. How might you learn more about the unique health practices Ms. Waters uses to address her health concerns?

   Suggested answers are at the end of the chapter.

CULTURALLY COMPETENT CARE

The American Nurses Association (2017) supports the need for nurses to understand cultural diversity and to become culturally competent. However, there is no real agreement as to how your knowledge, skills, and attitudes will best help these diverse populations. You certainly cannot achieve cultural competence overnight; it is a developmental process. Each time you care for a patient from a different culture, you learn more, become more aware and sensitive to individual needs, and move toward becoming culturally competent.

The following strategies for providing culturally competent care may be helpful:

- Consider each of your patients as unique, influenced but not defined by his or her culture.
- Know your own cultural values, beliefs, and practices and appreciate how they may be different from those of others.
- Never let your own biases about people and groups stand in the way of culturally competent care.
- Learn as much as you can about cultural groups in your community.
- Make an effort to include beliefs and practices from other cultures into your care when appropriate.
- Try to encourage helpful cultural practices and discourage harmful ones.
- Be aware of how you communicate with others; be aware of verbal and nonverbal patterns.
- Respect your patients regardless of their cultural backgrounds.
- Learn from your mistakes.

This list does not include everything you can do. Can you think of other strategies?

Rarely do practicing nurses have the luxury to assess each patient comprehensively on a first encounter. The essentials for culturally competent care are obtained as needed over time. As you meet patients from other cultures, continue to learn about these new cultures. Astute observations, openness to diversity, and willingness to learn from patients are essential for effective cross-cultural competence in clinical practice. Cultural competence is not a luxury; it is a necessity.

LEARNING TIP

Take a trip to BALI:

Be aware of your own cultural heritage.
Appreciate that your patient is unique and influenced but not defined by his or her culture.
Learn about your patients' cultural groups.
Incorporate your patients' cultural values, beliefs, and practices into their plan of care.

Home Health Hints

- The effects of a patient's cultural beliefs and practices related to health care are more evident when care is provided in the home. The nurse must adapt care to the patient's environment rather than the patient adapting to the nurse's hospital environment. The nurse is a guest in the patient's home.
- When scheduling a home visit, it is important to find out the primary language spoken in the home. The agency is required to inform the patient of his or her rights regarding language in a manner that the individual can understand. Check with your supervisor regarding the process for obtaining a translator. Avoid having children translate for parents.
- If you have a personal smartphone, you can download a language translator to assist with communication.

SUGGESTED ANSWERS TO CRITICAL THINKING

Ms. Waters

1. Ms. Waters may be present oriented. Her seeming lack of concern about her diabetes may reflect hesitance to worry about a future that is not yet here.
2. Family is important. She prays for healing.
3. Ms. Waters draws you close and holds your hand. This is a sign that she may not need a lot of personal space. Of course, you should ask her before you assume this.
4. Involving family members, both younger and older, might be helpful with Ms. Waters's permission. Because prayer is important to her, ask whether there is a minister or other religious person whom she might want to include in discussions and decision making. Contact the dietitian to suggest foods that fit Ms. Waters's preferences while she is in the hospital and to work with Ms. Waters to design a diabetes meal plan to be used at home that includes food she likes.
5. Ms. Waters is the expert on her own cultural practices. Do a thorough cultural assessment to learn whether any practices interfere with her health care. Work with the registered nurse to develop an appropriate teaching plan. Remember to include any cultural practices she already uses if they are safe and don't interfere with her care.

Review Questions

1. Which of the following characteristics is exhibited by a nurse who assumes that all patients have the same cultural beliefs as his or her own?
   1. Stereotyping
   2. Ethnocentrism
   3. Cultural sensitivity
   4. Cultural dominance

2. A 12-year-old patient is admitted for an appendectomy. The parents bring in a priest from their church to pray over the child. The prayers are continuing when it is time to take the child to surgery. How should the nurse respond?
   1. Gently tell the parents that they must stop praying so the child can be taken to surgery.
   2. Give the parents and priest as much time as they need for prayers before surgery.
   3. Tell the parents that the child could die of a ruptured appendix if surgery is delayed.
   4. Permit the parents and priest to stay and pray as the child goes into surgery.

3. A postsurgical patient is refusing a dinner tray, saying that it contains food not eaten in the patient's culture. Which response by the nurse is best?
   1. Take the tray away.
   2. Advise the patient that eating is essential to healing.
   3. Ask the patient whether there are other foods that would be acceptable.
   4. Leave the tray and hope that the patient gets hungry enough to eat the food.

4. A patient has been admitted for reconstructive orthopedic surgery of the knee. His wife brings jars of special blends of spices that the patient wants to use because the hospital food is too bland. The patient is on a general diet. What action should the nurse take?
   1. Check that the spices do not interact with the patient's medications and, if not, let the patient use them.
   2. Carefully explain that family cannot bring food items to the hospital.
   3. Have the dietitian provide spices from the hospital food services.
   4. Report the situation to the health care provider.

5. A nurse is collecting admission data from a hospitalized patient who does not speak English. The patient's 6-year-old daughter is in the room. How can the nurse obtain the needed information? **Select all that apply.**
   1. Have the daughter act as a translator.
   2. Ask the supervisor whether the hospital has a translation service.
   3. Provide an English translation dictionary to the patient.
   4. Use an electronic translation device.
   5. Wait for the patient's spouse to arrive.

Answer rationales available in your online resources.

ANSWERS 1. 2; 2. 4; 3. 3; 4. 1; 5. 2, 4

Key Points

Find the chapter key points in your online resources available through Davis Edge.

Additional Resources

DAVIS edge.   Use the scratch off code on the inside front cover of your book to access online quizzes that will help you to improve your scores on course exams and prepare for the NCLEX-PN®.

 Study Guide

CHAPTER 5

Complementary and Alternative Modalities

Paula D. Hopper, Cynthia Barrere, Colleen Delaney

KEY TERMS

acupuncture (ak-yoo-PUNGK-chur)
allopathic (AL-oh-PATH-ik)
alternative modality (all-TERN-ah-tiv
   moh-DAL-ih-tee)
Ayurvedic (AY-YUR-VAY-dik)
chiropractic (ky-roh-PRAK-tik)
complementary modality (comp-la-MEN-ta-ree
   moh-DAL-ih-tee)
homeopathy (HO-mee-AH-pa-thee)
naturopathy (NAY-chur-AH-pa-thee)
osteopathic (AHS-tee-ah-PATH-ik)

CHAPTER CONCEPTS

Evidence-Based Practice
Health Promotion
Collaboration

LEARNING OUTCOMES

1. Explain the difference between complementary and alternative modalities.
2. Describe systems of health care that have contributed to the development of new modalities.
3. Identify how selected modalities are classified.
4. Identify safety issues associated with complementary and alternative modalities.
5. Describe the role of the licensed practical nurse/licensed vocational nurse in assisting a patient with complementary and alternative modalities.

Health care in the 21st century requires that nurses recognize the shift toward the inclusion of complementary and alternative approaches in care. Nurses at all levels and in every area of practice are using new methods to care for those who are ill and enhance the health of those who are well.

Holistic nursing was a precursor to many of the now popular complementary and alternative modalities. It was introduced in the 1970s and has been growing ever since. *Holistic nursing* is simply defined as caring for the whole person—body, mind, and spirit—in a constantly changing environment.

COMPLEMENTARY OR ALTERNATIVE: WHAT'S THE DIFFERENCE?

The words *complementary* and *alternative* are sometimes used interchangeably, but they are not the same. A **complementary modality** refers to a therapy used *in addition* to a conventional modality. For example, a nurse might suggest guided imagery or relaxation techniques for pain control in addition to prescribed drug therapy. An **alternative modality** refers to a

therapy used *instead* of a conventional modality. An example is using acupuncture instead of analgesics for pain. The terms *therapy, modality,* and *medicine* can be used interchangeably. For consistency, this chapter uses the term *modality.*

A good resource for current information about complementary and alternative modalities is the National Center for Complementary and Integrative Health (NCCIH) at https://nccih.nih.gov. A good resource for nurses is the American Holistic Nurses Association at www.ahna.org.

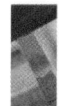

INTRODUCTION OF NEW SYSTEMS INTO TRADITIONAL WESTERN HEALTH CARE

In the United States, the primary system of medicine is just called *medicine,* although some people refer to it as **allopathic** medicine. Other schools of thought and philosophies are also

---

• WORD • BUILDING •
allopathic: allos—other + pathic—disease or suffering

being increasingly used. The most frequently seen new systems include Ayurvedic, traditional Chinese, chiropractic, homeopathic, naturopathic, American Indian, and osteopathic medicine. Each philosophical system can stand alone or, as in most instances in the United States, may be used in combination with other systems. Most of these recently introduced systems use complementary and alternative modalities, sometimes referred to as complementary and alternative medicine (CAM).

A survey conducted by the National Institutes of Health found that approximately 38% of adults in the United States and about 12% of children use some form of complementary and alternative modalities (Barnes, Bloom, & Nahin, 2008). It is, therefore, essential to ask your patients whether they use complementary and alternative modalities in their care, so you can incorporate these modalities when appropriate and safe to do so.

Gerontological Issues

Alternative Modalities. Many older adults use some form of an alternative modality but may not report the use of these therapies to their health care provider. Alternative modalities are commonly used to treat arthritis, back pain, heart disease, allergies, and diabetes. Be sure to ask specifically about complementary and alternative modalities at every visit. A good resource about alternative modalities and older adults is https://nccih.nih.gov/health/providers/digest/age-science.

Allopathic/Western Medicine

The most common name for allopathic medicine is *Western medicine.* Other commonly used terms are *conventional medicine* and *mainstream medicine.* Allopathy is a method of treating disease with remedies that produce effects different from those caused by the disease itself. For example, when a patient has a bacterial infection, a Western medical practitioner prescribes an antibiotic to eliminate the invading pathogen.

Practitioners of Western medicine are medical doctors, nurses, and allied health personnel. This system of medicine uses scientific data to determine the validity of a diagnosis and the effectiveness of treatment; this is called *evidence-based medicine* (see Chapter 2). Peer-reviewed medical literature is very important. In scientific investigations, results can be verified and reproduced through various types of studies and statistical analyses. Practitioners use a variety of therapies, including drugs, surgery, and radiation therapy. Western medicine practitioners have made most of the significant advances and developments in modern medicine.

Ayurvedic Medicine

Ayurveda is the ancient Hindu system of medicine that originated in India. **Ayurvedic** medicine's main goals are to maintain the health of well people and cure the illnesses of sick people. Ayurveda maintains that illness is the result of falling out of balance with nature. Diagnosis is based on three metabolic body types called *doshas.* An Ayurvedic doctor determines which *dosha* type is most appropriate for the patient: *vata, pitta,* or *kapha.* Treatment usually involves prescribing a diet, herbal remedies, breath work, physical exercise, yoga, meditation, massage, and a rejuvenation or detoxification program.

Ayurveda is rapidly becoming more popular in America. An introduction to Ayurveda can be found at https://nccih.nih.gov/health/ayurveda/introduction.htm.

Traditional Chinese Medicine

Traditional Chinese medicine is thousands of years old. It involves such practices as acupuncture, acupressure, herbs, massage, and qi gong. Chinese medicine involves diagnosis and treatment of disturbances of qi (pronounced "chee"), or vital energy.

Acupuncture is used commonly in the United States, most often for pain. To treat patients with acupuncture, practitioners insert one or more needles along the meridians (pathways) where qi flows (Fig. 5.1). Many acupuncturists prescribe herbal remedies as well. Find more information on how acupuncture is being integrated into Western medicine at https://nccih.nih.gov/health/acupuncture/introduction.

Chiropractic Medicine

Daniel David Palmer founded chiropractic therapy in 1895. **Chiropractic** medicine is based on the belief that illness is a result of neuromusculoskeletal dysfunction. The main treatment modality of chiropractors is manual adjustment and manipulation of the vertebral column and the limbs. The goal is to remove interference with nerve function so the body can heal itself. Chiropractors do not perform surgery or prescribe drugs. Learn more about chiropractic medicine at https://nccih.nih.gov/health/chiropractic/introduction.htm.

Homeopathic Medicine

Homeopathy was developed by Samuel Hahnemann in Germany in the early 19th century. Homeopathy is based on Hahnemann's principle that "like cures like," meaning that tiny doses of a substance that create the symptoms of disease in a healthy person will relieve those symptoms in a sick person.

Although schools and courses do exist for training homeopaths, no diploma or certificate from any school or

---

• WORD • BUILDING •
Ayurvedic: ayu—life + veda—knowledge or science
acupuncture: acus—needle + punctura—puncture
chiropractic: cheir—hand + pracktos—to do
homeopathy: homeo—like + pathos—disease

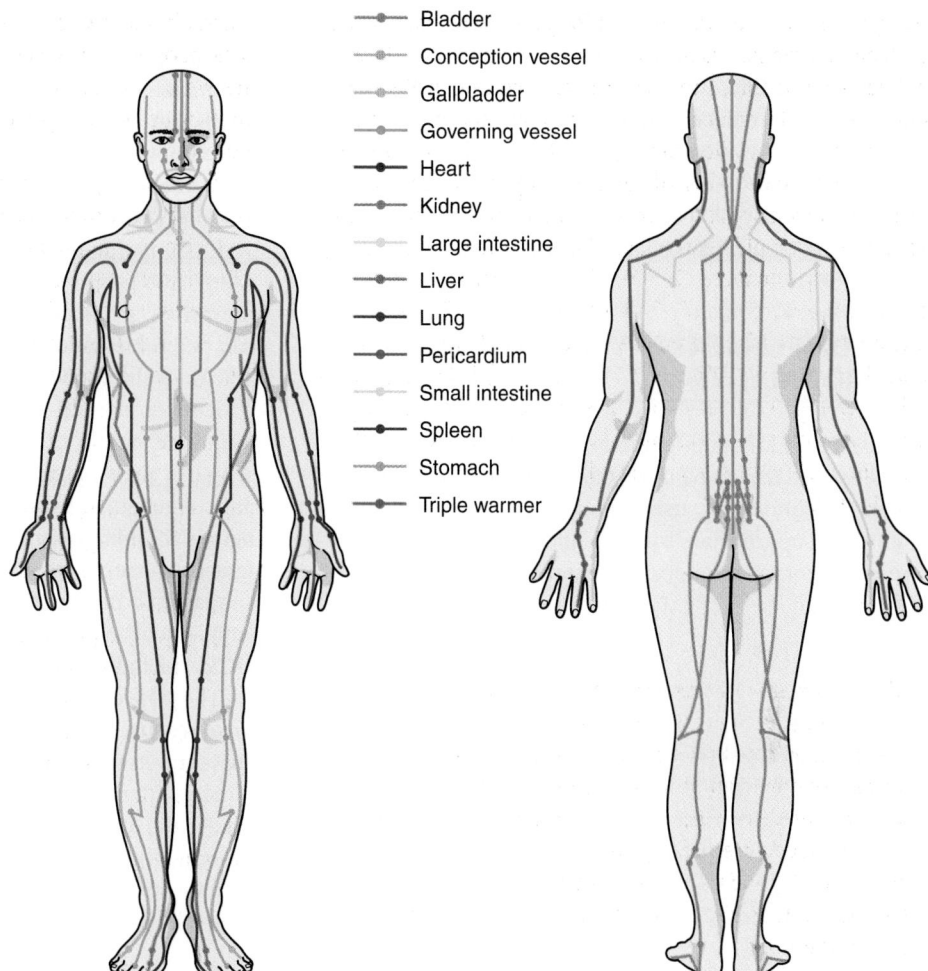

- Bladder
- Conception vessel
- Gallbladder
- Governing vessel
- Heart
- Kidney
- Large intestine
- Liver
- Lung
- Pericardium
- Small intestine
- Spleen
- Stomach
- Triple warmer

FIGURE 5.1 Qi meridians are used in the Chinese medicine techniques of acupressure and acupuncture.

program is a license to practice homeopathy in the United States. Medical doctors and doctors of osteopathy are granted national certificates of competency by the Council for Homeopathic Certification to practice homeopathy. There is very little evidence that homeopathy is safe or effective at this time. Learn more at https://nccih.nih.gov/health/homeopathy.

Naturopathic Medicine

Naturopathy primarily uses natural therapies such as nutrition, herbs, hydrotherapy (water-based therapy), counseling, physical medicine, and homeopathy to treat disease, promote healing, and prevent illness. Naturopathic physicians have a doctor of naturopathy (ND) degree and can be licensed in some but not all states. For more information about naturopathy, visit https://nccih.nih.gov/health/naturopathy and the American Association of Naturopathic Physicians web site at www.naturopathic.org.

American Indian Medicine

American Indian medical practices vary from tribe to tribe. In general, American Indian medicine is a community-based

system with rituals and practices such as the sweat lodge, herbal remedies, the medicine wheel, the sacred hoop, the "sing," and shamanistic healing. For example, an ill person may be placed in a small, enclosed sweat lodge while singing or chanting is done outside the lodge. It is believed that toxic substances are drawn out in the sweat of the person inside the lodge. After the ceremony, the ill person may be placed on a cot outside and be prayed over. Learn more at the Association of American Indian Physicians web site at www.aaip.org.

Osteopathic Medicine

Osteopathic medicine was founded in the United States in 1874 by Andrew Taylor Still, a frontier physician who was dissatisfied with the state of medicine at that time. This practice of medicine emphasizes the interrelationship of

• WORD • BUILDING •
naturopathy: naturo—nature + pathy—disease
osteopathic: osteo—bone + pathy—disease

the body's nerves, muscles, bones, and organs. The osteopathic philosophy involves treating the whole person, recognizes the body's ability to heal itself, and stresses the importance of diet, exercise, and fitness with a focus on prevention. Osteopathic physicians are fully licensed in all states and often work closely with traditional Western medicine providers. For more information about osteopathy, visit the American Osteopathic Association web site at www.osteopathic.org.

 ## COMPLEMENTARY AND ALTERNATIVE MODALITIES

Discussion of all complementary and alternative modalities is beyond the scope of this text. Table 5.1 summarizes the most commonly used modalities. It is important to note that appropriate training and skills are needed before using complementary and alternative modalities with patients.

Table 5.1
Categories and Types of Complementary and Alternative Modalities

Category of Therapy	Examples
Biologically based modalities	Herbal medicine Nutrition and special diet therapies Nutritional supplements
Mind–body modalities	Art therapy Guided imagery Hypnosis and hypnotherapy Meditation and relaxation Music/sound therapies Prayer Yoga
Manipulative and body-based modalities	Acupressure Chiropractic medicine Massage and related therapies Osteopathic manipulation
Energetic modalities	Biofeedback Magnet therapy Reiki Spiritual healing Therapeutic touch
Miscellaneous therapies	Aquatherapy/hydrotherapy Aromatherapy Chanting Kinesiology Light therapy Pet therapy

Herbal Therapy

Have you ever tried herbs for healing? Herbs should only be taken under the supervision of a health care provider (HCP). Herbs can aid in healing but can also do harm. Some of the more common herbs are described in Table 5.2. Figure 5.2 shows echinacea, an herb commonly prepared for use as an immune system booster.

It is important to note that herbal remedies are not foods. They have potent medicinal effects. They can interact with prescribed medications and even complicate surgery. This can be problematic. This is because herbs are readily available in health food stores and drugstores, and because many patients do not tell their doctors or nurses about their herb use. For example, the common herbs garlic, ginkgo, and ginseng can each increase the risk of bleeding when taken with anticoagulant or antiplatelet medications. Another popular herb is St. John's wort, widely used for depression. It can interact adversely with many drugs, including other antidepressant agents. Be sure to determine patients' use of herbs and supplements and to educate them about the need to inform HCPs, including their pharmacists, when using herbs.

The Mayo Clinic web site (www.mayoclinic.org) is a great resource for you and your patients to learn about herbs. Just type in the herb you want to know about in the search window for up-to-date information. It even has a section that grades the evidence of the herb's effectiveness for each disorder it is supposed to treat. Grades range from A, which indicates strong research evidence for the herb's use, to F, which indicates strong evidence against its use.

> **BE SAFE!**
> Teach your patients to do their research before trusting a specific brand of herbal supplement. The government does not regulate herbal supplements as it does drugs so they may not contain exactly what the manufacturer claims. Many emergency room visits each year are associated with indiscriminate use of herbal supplements!

Relaxation Therapies
Progressive Muscle Relaxation
Progressive muscle relaxation is a simple technique to learn. It involves the process of alternately tensing and relaxing muscle groups. Often this process is performed in a systematic manner, such as from the toes to the head. The purpose of the technique is to help the participant identify subtle levels of mental and physical tension that accompany mental and emotional stress. When our conscious awareness of the tensions increases, we can learn to relax and, thus, reduce the effects of stress and tension.

> **LEARNING TIP**
> Try using progressive muscle relaxation the next time you are anxious during a nursing examination.

Table 5.2

Common Herbs and Their Intended Uses

Herb	Purported Uses
Aloe vera	Soothing agent, used for skin lesions May absorb toxins
Bee pollen	May increase energy, stamina, and strength
Black cohosh	May ease menopausal symptoms
Capsaicin	May ease tenderness and pain of osteoarthritis, fibromyalgia, diabetic neuropathy, and shingles
Chamomile	May decrease anxiety, stomach distress, and infant colic
Echinacea	Has antiviral properties; may be effective for colds, flu, and other infections
Ephedra (ma huang)	A sympathomimetic agent used as a stimulant or weight loss supplement; banned by the Food and Drug Administration in 2004 because of deadly side effects, but patients may still obtain it outside the United States
Feverfew	Has anti-inflammatory properties; may help treat migraine headaches, stimulate appetite, promote menstruation, eliminate worms, and suppress fever
Garlic	Reduces low-density lipoprotein and raises high-density lipoprotein cholesterol May reduce blood pressure Suppresses platelet aggregation, increases arterial elasticity, and decreases atherosclerotic plaque formation
Ginger	May reduce nausea and vomiting, hypertension, and high cholesterol
Ginkgo biloba	May improve memory and help cognitive function in Alzheimer's disease
Ginseng	May reduce stress and increase alertness; also claims to lower cholesterol, balance blood glucose levels, slow the aging process, treat memory loss, and treat erectile dysfunction
Kava	May be effective for anxiety, insomnia, low energy, and muscle tension
Red yeast rice	May reduce cholesterol and triglycerides
St. John's wort	May help mild-to-moderate depression; may be effective against viral infections, including HIV and herpes

Warning: Herbs may have many side effects and may interact with many prescribed and over-the-counter medications. Urge patients to consult health care providers before self-prescribing.

Guided Imagery

Guided imagery involves using mental images to promote physical healing or changes in attitudes or behaviors. Practitioners may lead patients through visualization exercises or offer instruction in using imagery as a self-help tool. Guided imagery is often used to alleviate stress and to treat stress-related conditions such as insomnia and high blood pressure. People with cancer, AIDS, chronic fatigue syndrome, and other disorders can use specific images to boost the immune system.

A common guided imagery technique begins with progressive muscle relaxation. Guided imagery works best when all of the senses are used. The exercise in Box 5.1 is very basic but gives an idea of how the technique works. When used for healing, many more steps are involved. Find more on guided imagery at https://nccih.nih.gov; type "guided imagery" into the search window.

> **LEARNING TIP**
>
> When you are stumped on a test question, close your eyes and imagine yourself asking your favorite instructor the question. Imagine what his or her answer would be.

Biofeedback

Biofeedback could be considered the third tier of progressive relaxation. This technique is used especially for conditions that are aggravated by stress, such as asthma, migraines, insomnia, and high blood pressure. Biofeedback is a way of monitoring and controlling tiny metabolic changes in one's body with the aid of sensitive machines that provide feedback ("Patient Perspective").

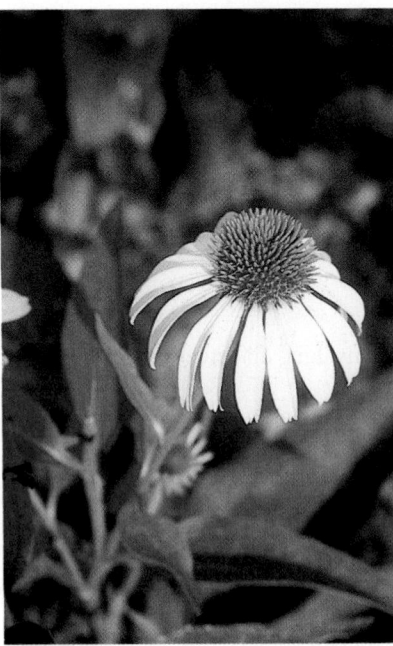

FIGURE 5.2 Echinacea is an herb commonly used to combat colds and flu.

Patient Perspective

Polly. I'm scared to death of flying. The minute I get on an airplane, I feel jittery, my heart races, and I can't calm down until we're safely back on the ground. Several years ago, I decided to try biofeedback therapy to overcome this fear.

My therapist immediately put me at ease and assured me I wasn't a crazy person to be afraid to fly. She listened to my fears and responses throughout all our sessions. At each practice session, she put a temperature sensor on my finger (my hands were usually pretty cold). In her calm, soft voice, she guided me through a relaxation exercise using imagery and progressive muscle relaxation. By the time we were finished, my hands would be several degrees warmer than when we started! This showed that my vessels were dilating, a sign that my sympathetic nervous system was slowing down its activity. So I felt calmer. The sensor gave me feedback that told me when my relaxation was working well. We did this every week for a couple of months, until I got really good at warming my hands and relaxing.

Now when I fly, I close my eyes, imagine a peaceful scene, and use my relaxation techniques. I still don't like flying much, but at least I feel a bit calmer!

Massage Therapy

Massage is the use of touch to achieve therapeutic results. It can include pressure, friction, and kneading of the body. Massage can be used to relax muscles, reduce anxiety, increase circulation, and reduce pain.

Massage also provides a caring form of touch. In the past, a back massage was a nightly routine for hospitalized patients,

Box 5.1

Guided Imagery

Assist your patient to progress through the following steps:
- Assume a comfortable position in a quiet environment.
- Close your eyes and keep them closed until the exercise is completed.
- Breathe in and out deeply to the count of four, repeating this step four times.
- When relaxed, think of a favorite peaceful place and prepare to take an imaginary journey there.
- Picture what this place looks like and how comfortable you feel being there.
- Listen to all the sounds; feel the gentle, clean air; and smell the pleasant aromas.
- Continue to breathe deeply and appreciate the feeling of being in this special place.
- Feel the sense of deep relaxation and peace of this place.
- As you continue to breathe deeply, slowly and gently bring your consciousness back to the setting in this room.
- Slowly and gently open your eyes, stretch, and think about how relaxed you feel.

helping them relax for sleep. Patients today are often not touched except during technical procedures.

You can learn basic massage techniques in nursing school. You may also choose to obtain formal massage therapy education to practice more advanced techniques. Try giving your patient an old-fashioned back massage, and see how delighted he or she is!

BE SAFE!
Do not use firm massage on a patient taking an anticoagulant or with a low platelet level. Tissue injury could cause bleeding. Check with the patient's health care provider before providing deep massage for any patient.

Aquatherapy

Sitting in a warm tub can feel good as aching, tired muscles relax and mental stress decreases. People who suffer from arthritis or other chronic pain understand how warm water can ease their discomfort. Relaxing in water feels good for three reasons: warmth, water movement causing massage, and buoyancy.

Long before analgesics were developed, the human body relied on its own naturally occurring, internally generated, pain-killing chemicals called endorphins. Endorphins are released in response to both acute and chronic pain. Through research, we now know that warm water also stimulates the release of endorphins.

Ultimately, blood flow is what brings nutrients to damaged cells and facilitates healing. When the body is immersed in warm water, the blood vessels nearest the skin relax, allowing more blood to flow. The results are faster tissue repair and relief of pain and fatigue. Be cautious with patients who have heart disease. Relaxing blood vessels can decrease blood pressure.

Heat and Cold Application

Local application of heat or cold provides additional skin stimulation. A warm compress can soothe sore muscles and dilate vessels in a localized area, bringing healing circulation as well as endorphin release. Ice or a cold gel pack can help numb an area. Cold can also cause overdilated vessels to constrict, yielding relief from pain and throbbing of overstimulated nerve endings. Ice can be helpful on an acute injury and for some types of headaches. Check institution policy before applying heat or cold; an HCP's order may be required.

Probiotics

Probiotics are considered beneficial bacteria. Their use is increasing in popularity. The Food and Drug Administration considers probiotics to be generally safe in healthy people. Common reasons for taking probiotics are to aid in healthy digestion or to treat constipation or infectious diarrhea. Nurses need to caution individuals to discuss plans to take probiotics with their HCPs. It is important to review the research available on a particular product because there are many strains available. It is essential to consider where the research was published (preferably in a peer-reviewed journal) and examine the findings on how safe the product is. Additional information on probiotics can be found at https://nccih.nih.gov; type "probiotics" into the search window.

SAFETY AND EFFECTIVENESS OF ALTERNATIVE MODALITIES

Safety generally means that the benefits outweigh the risks of a treatment or therapy. If a patient is interested in using complementary and alternative modalities, first counsel the patient to talk with the HCP. The patient also should ask the practitioner of the therapy about its safety and effectiveness. The patient should tell the HCP and alternative practitioners about all therapies they are using. This information may be important to consider in the safety of their overall treatment plan.

The patient should be as informed as possible and continue gathering information even after a practitioner or therapy has been selected (Box 5.2).

ROLE OF THE LICENSED PRACTICAL NURSE/LICENSED VOCATIONAL NURSE

Patients may ask you about the use of a complementary or alternative modality. Because the safety and effectiveness of many therapies are still unknown, advising patients presents a challenge. Collaborate with the HCP when discussing therapies with patients.

The following steps are suggestions for helping to advise patients regarding the use of these kinds of therapies. You should advise the patient to:

1. Discuss use of the modality with the HCP before trying it.
2. Take a close look at the background, qualifications, and competence of the proposed practitioner. Check

Box 5.2

Questions Patients Should Ask Before Starting a Complementary or Alternative Modality

1. What will this modality do for me?
2. What are its advantages and disadvantages?
3. What are its risks and side effects?
4. How much will it cost? Will my insurance cover the cost?
5. How long will it take? How many treatments will I need?
6. How will it interact with my other therapies and medications?
7. What research has been done on this modality?

credentials with a state or local regulatory agency with authority over the area of practice in which the patient is interested. Is the practitioner licensed or certified? By whom?
3. Visit the practitioner's office, clinic, or hospital, and evaluate the conditions of the setting.
4. Talk with others who have used this practitioner.
5. Consider the costs. Are the treatments covered by insurance, or will the patient have to pay?

NURSING APPLICATIONS

There are ways to gain confidence with complementary and alternative modalities:

- Begin by trying one or two of these modalities yourself. Start by choosing a basic therapy, such as massage, music, or guided imagery. Follow the guidelines listed in Box 5.2 to make sure it is a safe strategy. Not only will you encounter the possible benefits firsthand, you will also come away with a better understanding of what your patients might experience.
- Ask your patients if they use any complementary or alternative modalities and what their responses to them have been. Try to eliminate any preconceived ideas you might have. Your patients will feel more comfortable mentioning them to you if they feel you understand the treatment and why they decided to use it.
- If you decide to use these therapies, get instruction in the therapies before you administer them. Many universities and agencies offer continuing education courses on these therapies. Some nursing schools incorporate complementary and alternative modalities in their skills courses.

Before incorporating complementary and alternative modalities into practice, be sure to check your state's nurse practice act for any regulations. Discuss these therapies with the patient and the HCP before using them. If you work for a hospital or other health care institution, also check institutional policy. See "Evidence-Based Practice" for ways nurses are implementing various modalities in practice.

As the public learns more about complementary and alternative modalities, there is likely to be an even greater

Evidence-Based Practice

Clinical Question

How are complementary and alternative modalities used by nurses to improve health outcomes?

Evidence

The following are examples of how complementary and alternative modalities have been used by nurses to enhance health outcomes in various patient populations:

- In a meta-analysis by Kong and Park (2015), music therapy was found to reduce agitation in persons with dementia.
- In a meta-analysis by Huang and Liu (2015), the practice of Tai Chi Chuan was found to improve the balance control ability of older adults.
- In a meta-analysis by Youkhana, Dean, Wolff, Sherrington, and Tiedemann (2016), yoga-based exercise was found to improve balance and physical mobility in persons over 60 years of age.
- In a meta-analysis by Gong and colleagues (2016), mindfulness meditation was found to improve some sleep parameters in persons suffering from insomnia.

Implications for Nursing Practice

Complementary and alternative modalities such as music, aromatherapy, Tai Chi, and meditation can improve health outcomes in diverse patient populations. After learning these modalities, nurses can implement them in a variety of patient settings. Be sure to work within your institution's policies and procedures.

References

Gong, H., Ni, C. X., Liu, Y. Z., Zhang, Y., Su, W. J., Lian, Y. J., … Jiang, C. L. (2016). Mindfulness meditation for insomnia: A meta-analysis of randomized controlled trials. *Journal of Psychosomatic Research, 89,* 1–6.

Huang, Y., & Liu, X. (2015). Improvement of balance control ability and flexibility in the elderly Tai Chi Chuan (TCC) practitioners: A systematic review and meta-analysis. *Archives of Gerontology and Geriatrics, 60*(2), 233–238.

Kong, E. H., & Park, M. (2015). Effects of music therapy on agitation in dementia: Systematic review and meta-analysis. *Korean Journal of Adult Nursing, 27*(1), 106–116.

Youkhana, S., Dean, C. M., Wolff, M., Sherrington, C., & Tiedemann, A. (2015). Yoga-based exercise improves balance and mobility in people aged 60 and over: A systematic review and meta-analysis. *Age and Ageing, 45*(1), 21–29.

demand for them. Nurses have been in the forefront of developing the holistic philosophy that has now become an accepted standard of care.

CRITICAL THINKING

Mr. Jones asks whether he should stop his chemotherapy and try magnet therapy for his prostate cancer. How do you respond? What other health care team members might you collaborate with in helping Mr. Jones?

Suggested answers are at the end of the chapter.

Home Health Hints

- When taking a health history, ask the patient or caregiver about the use of complementary and alternative modalities because these may influence the effects or side effects of some prescription medications. Document and discuss concerns regarding potential interactions with the registered nurse or health care provider.
- Be mindful of the importance of complementary and alternative modalities to the patient's health care belief system.
- Consider the alternative practitioner as part of the patient's health care team.

SUGGESTED ANSWERS TO CRITICAL THINKING

Mr. Jones

As with all medical treatments, it is important to support the established therapy the health care provider has prescribed. Therefore, a good response might be the following: "Mr. Jones, chemotherapy is an established medical treatment for your condition. There is a lot of evidence for its effectiveness in the medical literature. If you want to supplement your therapy, there may be some other treatments you can add. I suggest that you discuss your feelings about seeking some additional treatments with your oncologist. If he agrees, then the registered nurse and I can share some information with you about how to stay safe while trying new things."

Review Questions

1. Which of the following statements best defines a complementary modality?
   1. An alternative treatment that is used in place of a conventional treatment
   2. A treatment that may be dangerous and should be avoided
   3. A treatment that can be used in addition to a conventional treatment
   4. A treatment that is used after conventional treatments have failed

2. Which of the following therapies is most likely to use research-based interventions?
   1. Naturopathy
   2. Osteopathy
   3. Allopathy
   4. Homeopathy

3. A patient who has high blood pressure tells the nurse he has been taking a ginger supplement in addition to his prescribed medications at home. What is the best response by the nurse?
   1. "Nonprescription supplements can interact with prescription medications. You should not take it any longer."
   2. "Ginger can be effective for hypertension. Be sure to monitor your blood pressure while you are taking it."
   3. "Ginger is a safe supplement because it is a food. It should not interact with your medications."
   4. "You should check with your health care provider to make sure the ginger doesn't interact with your other medications before you continue to take it."

4. Which of the following complementary modalities are considered relaxation therapies? **Select all that apply.**
   1. Progressive muscle relaxation
   2. Tai Chi
   3. Biofeedback
   4. Homeopathic therapies
   5. Guided imagery

5. Which of the following statements best describes the most important role of the nurse in complementary and alternative modalities?
   1. The nurse should become familiar enough to recommend at least one complementary or alternative modality.
   2. The nurse should become skilled at collecting and reporting data related to patients' use of complementary or alternative modalities.
   3. The nurse should discourage use of complementary or alternative modalities because they can interact negatively with conventional therapies.
   4. The nurse does not need to become involved in complementary and alternative modalities.

Answer rationales available in your online resources.

ANSWERS 1. 3; 2. 3; 3. 4; 4. 1, 3, 5; 5. 2

Key Points

Find the chapter key points in your online resources available through Davis Edge.

Additional Resources

DAVIS edge.   Use the scratch off code on the inside front cover of your book to access online quizzes that will help you to improve your scores on course exams and prepare for the NCLEX-PN®.

    Study Guide

CHAPTER 6

Nursing Care of Patients With Fluid, Electrolyte, and Acid–Base Imbalances

Bruce K. Wilson, Marie Hedgpeth

KEY TERMS

acidosis (as-ih-DOH-sis)
alkalosis (al-kah-LOH-sis)
anion (AN-eye-on)
antidiuretic (AN-ty-DY-yuh-RET-ik)
arrhythmia (uh-RITH-mee-ah)
cation (KAT-eye-on)
dehydration (DEE-hy-DRAY-shun)
diffusion (dih-FEW-shun)
edema (eh-DEE-mah)
electrolytes (ee-LEK-troh-lites)
extracellular (EX-trah-SELL-yoo-lar)
filtration (fill-TRAY-shun)
hydrostatic (HY-droh-STAT-ik)
hypercalcemia (HY-per-kal-SEE-mee-ah)
hyperkalemia (HY-per-kuh-LEE-mee-ah)
hypermagnesemia (HY-per-MAG-nuh-SEE-mee-ah)
hypernatremia (HY-per-nuh-TREE-mee-ah)
hypertonic (HY-per-TAWN-ik)
hypervolemia (HY-per-voh-LEE-mee-ah)
hypocalcemia (HY-poh-kal-SEE-mee-ah)
hypokalemia (HY-poh-kuh-LEE-mee-ah)
hypomagnesemia (HY-poh-MAG-nuh-SEE-mee-ah)
hyponatremia (HY-poh-nuh-TREE-mee-ah)
hypotonic (HY-poh-TAWN-ik)
hypovolemia (HY-poh-voh-LEE-mee-ah)
interstitial (IN-tur-STISH-uhl)
intracellular (IN-trah-SELL-yoo-ler)
intracranial (IN-trah-KRAY-nee-uhl)
intravascular (IN-trah-VAS-kyoo-ler)
isotonic (EYE-so-TAWN-ik)
osmolarity (OZ-moh-LAR-it-ee)
osmosis (ahs-MOH-sis)
osteoporosis (AHS-tee-oh-por-OH-sis)
semipermeable (SEM-ee-PER-mee-uh-bull)
transcellular (trans-SELL-yoo-lar)

CHAPTER CONCEPTS

Acid–Base Balance
Fluid and Electrolyte Balance

LEARNING OUTCOMES

1. Identify the purposes of fluids and electrolytes in the body.
2. List the signs and symptoms of common fluid imbalances.
3. Predict patients who are at the highest risk for dehydration and fluid excess.
4. Identify data to collect in patients with fluid and electrolyte imbalances.
5. Describe therapeutic measures for patients with fluid and electrolyte imbalances.
6. Identify the education needs of patients with fluid imbalances.
7. Categorize common causes, signs and symptoms, and treatments for sodium, potassium, calcium, and magnesium imbalances.
8. Identify foods that have high sodium, potassium, and calcium contents.
9. Give examples of common causes of acidosis and alkalosis.
10. Compare how arterial blood gases change for each type of acid–base imbalance.

Have you ever wondered why you get thirsty? The body is continually changing. Water supports these changes. Approximately 60% of a young adult's body weight is water. Older people are less than 50% water. Infants are between 70% and 80% water. Fat cells do not contain water. Therefore, people with a higher percentage of fat cells have a lower percentage of water.

In addition to water, body fluids also contain dissolved solid substances, called *solutes*. Some solutes are electrolytes; some are nonelectrolytes. **Electrolytes** are chemicals that can conduct electricity when dissolved in water. Examples of electrolytes are sodium, potassium, calcium, magnesium, acids, and bases; these are discussed in this chapter. Nonelectrolytes do not conduct electricity; examples include glucose and urea.

• WORD • BUILDING •
electrolyte: electro—electricity + lyte—dissolve

FLUID BALANCE

Fluids are located in various compartments within the body. Fluid inside the cells is referred to as **intracellular fluid (ICF)**. Fluid outside the cells is called **extracellular fluid (ECF)**. ECF can be further divided into three types: interstitial fluid, intravascular fluid, and transcellular fluid (Fig. 6.1).

Interstitial fluid is the water that surrounds the body's cells and includes lymph. **Intravascular** fluid, or blood plasma, is the fluid within arteries, veins, and capillaries. Fluids and electrolytes move between the interstitial fluid and the intravascular fluid. **Transcellular** fluids are those in specific compartments of the body, such as cerebrospinal fluid, digestive juices, and synovial fluid in joints.

Control of Fluid Balance

The primary control of water in the body is through pressure sensors in the vascular system that stimulate or inhibit the release of **antidiuretic** hormone (ADH) from the pituitary gland. A diuretic is a substance that causes the kidneys to excrete more fluid. ADH works in just the opposite way. ADH causes the kidneys to retain fluid. If fluid pressures within the vascular system decrease, more ADH is released, and water is retained. If fluid pressures increase, less ADH is released, and the kidneys eliminate more water.

Movement of Fluids and Electrolytes in the Body

Fluids and electrolytes move in the body by active and passive transport systems. Active transport depends on the presence of adequate cellular adenosine triphosphate

(ATP) for energy. The most common examples of active transport are sodium-potassium pumps. These pumps are located in the cell membranes. They cause sodium to move out of the cells and potassium to move into the cells when needed.

In passive transport, no energy is expended specifically to move the substances. General body movements aid passive transport. The three passive transport systems are diffusion, filtration, and osmosis.

Diffusion is the movement of a substance from an area of higher concentration to an area of lower concentration. If you pour cream into a cup of coffee, the movement of the molecules will eventually cause the cream to be dispersed throughout the beverage. If you stir the coffee, this process occurs at a faster rate. Body movement assists passive transport, like stirring the coffee. It causes diffusion to occur at a faster rate.

Filtration is the movement of both water and smaller molecules through a **semipermeable** membrane from an area of high pressure to an area of lower pressure. A semipermeable membrane works like a screen that keeps larger substances on one side and permits only smaller molecules to filter to the other side of the membrane. Filtration is promoted by hydrostatic pressure differences between areas. **Hydrostatic** pressure, sometimes called water-pushing pressure, is the force that water exerts. In the body, filtration is important for the movement of water, nutrients, and waste products in the capillaries. The capillaries serve as semipermeable membranes, allowing water and smaller substances to move from the vascular system to the interstitial fluid. Larger molecules and red blood cells remain inside the capillary walls.

Osmosis is the movement of water from an area of lower substance concentration across a semipermeable membrane to an area of higher concentration. The power to pull water toward an area of higher concentration is referred to as *osmotic pressure*. This process continues until the concentration is the same on both sides of the membrane. The term **osmolarity** refers to the concentration of the substances in body fluids. The normal osmolarity of blood is between 270 and 300 milliosmoles per liter (mOsm/L).

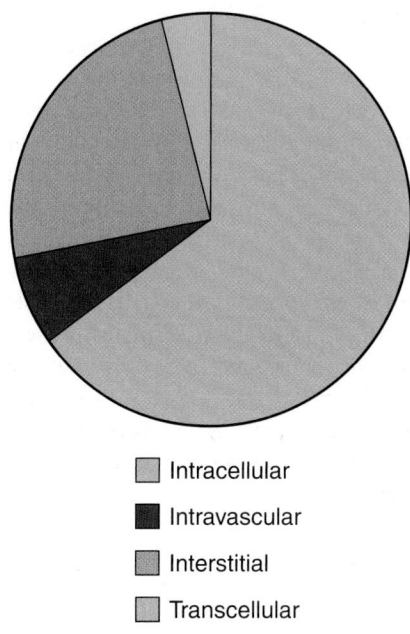

□ Intracellular

■ Intravascular

▨ Interstitial

▨ Transcellular

FIGURE 6.1 Normal distribution of total body water.

• WORD • BUILDING •

intracellular: intra—within + cellular—cell
extracellular: extra—outside of + cellular—cell
interstitial: inter—between + stitial—tissue
intravascular: intra—within + vascular—blood vessel
transcellular: trans—across + cellular—cell
antidiuretic: anti—against + diuretic—urination
diffusion: diffuse—spread, scattered
filtration: filter—strain through
semipermeable: semi—half or part of + permeable—passing through
hydrostatic: hydro—water + static—standing
osmosis: osmo—impulse + osis—condition

Another term for osmolarity is *tonicity*. Fluids or solutions can be classified as isotonic, hypotonic, or hypertonic. A fluid that has the same osmolarity as the blood is called **isotonic**. For example, a 0.9% (normal) saline solution is isotonic to the blood; it is often used as a solution for intravenous (IV) therapy. A solution that has a lower osmolarity than blood is called **hypotonic**. When a hypotonic solution is given to a patient, the water in the solution leaves the blood and other ECF areas and enters the cells. **Hypertonic** solutions exert greater osmotic pressure than blood. When a hypertonic solution is given to a patient, water leaves the cells and enters the bloodstream and other ECF spaces.

Fluid Gains and Fluid Losses

Water is very important to the body for cellular metabolism, blood volume, body temperature regulation, and solute transport. Although people can survive without food for several weeks, they can survive only a few days without water. Thirst is the major indicator that a healthy adult needs more water.

Water is gained and lost from the body every day. In addition to liquid intake, some fluid is obtained from solid foods. When too much fluid is lost, the brain's thirst mechanism tells the individual that more fluid intake is needed. Older adults are more prone to fluid deficits because they have a diminished thirst reflex and their kidneys do not function as effectively. An adult loses as much as 2,500 mL of sensible and insensible fluid each day. Sensible losses are those of which the person is aware, such as urination. Insensible losses may occur without the person recognizing the loss. Perspiration and water lost through respiration and elimination of feces are examples of insensible losses.

 FLUID IMBALANCES

Fluid imbalances are common in all clinical settings. Older people are at the highest risk for life-threatening complications that can result from either fluid deficit, more commonly called **dehydration,** or fluid excess. Infants are at risk for fluid deficit because they take in and excrete a large proportion of their total body water each day.

Dehydration

Although there are several types of dehydration, only the most common type is discussed in this chapter. Dehydration occurs when there is not enough fluid in the body, especially in the blood (intravascular area).

Pathophysiology and Etiology

The most common form of dehydration results from loss of fluid from the body, resulting in decreased blood volume. This decrease is referred to as **hypovolemia**. Hypovolemia occurs when the patient is hemorrhaging or when fluids from other parts of the body are lost. For example, severe vomiting and diarrhea, severely draining wounds, and profuse diaphoresis (sweating) can cause dehydration (Box 6.1).

Hypovolemia can also occur when fluid from the intravascular space moves into the interstitial fluid space. This

---

Box 6.1

Common Causes of Dehydration

Diarrhea
Diuretic therapy
Draining abscess or fistula
Fever
Gastrointestinal suction
Hemorrhage
Ileostomy
Long-term nothing-by-mouth (NPO) status
Profuse diaphoresis (sweating)
Systemic infection
Vomiting

---

process is called *third spacing*. Examples of conditions in which third spacing is common include burns, liver cirrhosis, and extensive trauma.

As described previously in this chapter, the body initially attempts to compensate for fluid loss by a number of mechanisms. If the cause of fluid loss is not resolved or the patient is not able to replace the fluid, dehydration occurs.

Prevention

You can help prevent dehydration by identifying patients who have the highest risk for developing this condition and intervening quickly to correct the cause. High-risk patients include older adults, infants, children, and any patient with one of the conditions listed in Box 6-1. Also see "Gerontological Issues: Dehydration."

Adequate hydration is another important intervention to help prevent dehydration. Encourage patients to drink adequate fluids. Adults need 30 mL/kg/day of fluids. If a patient is unable to take enough fluid by mouth, alternate routes may be necessary.

Gerontological Issues

Dehydration. As a person ages, total body water decreases from 60% to 50% of total body weight. This age-related decrease in total body water is secondary to an increase in body fat and a decrease in thirst sensation. These factors increase the risk of developing dehydration.

Manifestations of dehydration in an older adult are different from typical manifestations in a younger person. They may include altered mental status, light-headedness, and syncope (loss of consciousness). These occur because a patient with hypovolemia has an inadequate circulatory volume and, therefore, inadequate oxygen supply to the brain.

• WORD • BUILDING •

isotonic: iso—equal + tonic—strength
hypotonic: hypo—less than + tonic—strength
hypertonic: hyper—more than + tonic—strength
dehydration: de—down + hydration—water
hypovolemia: hypo—less than + vol—volume + emia—blood

Signs and Symptoms

Thirst is the initial symptom experienced by otherwise healthy adults in response to hypovolemia. As the percentage of water in the blood goes down, the percentage of other substances goes up, resulting in the thirst response. As the blood volume decreases, the heart pumps the remaining blood faster but not as powerfully. This results in a rapid, weak pulse; rapid, shallow respirations; and low blood pressure. The body pulls water into the vascular system from other areas. This results in decreased tear formation, dry skin, and dry mucous membranes.

A dehydrated person will have poor *skin turgor.* Turgor is considered to be poor if the skin is pinched and a small "tent" or wrinkle remains (called *tenting*). A dehydrated person's temperature increases because the body is less able to cool itself through perspiration. Temperature may not appear elevated in an older person because an older adult's normal body temperature is often lower than a younger person's. Urine output decreases. The urine becomes more concentrated as water is conserved. Dehydration should be considered in any adult with a urine output of less than 30 mL per hour. The urine may appear darker because it is less diluted. The patient becomes constipated as the intestines absorb more water from the feces. A major method of evaluating dehydration is weight loss. A pint of water (16 ounces or 473 mL) weighs approximately 1 pound. Symptoms of dehydration in older persons may be atypical (see "Gerontological Issues: Dehydration").

LEARNING TIP

Do you remember your grandmother saying, "A pint's a pound the world around"? It's a great way to remember how much fluid loss is represented by each lost pound.

Complications

If dehydration is not treated, lack of sufficient blood volume causes organ function to decrease and eventually fail. The brain, kidneys, and heart must be adequately perfused with blood to function properly. The body protects these organs by decreasing blood flow to other areas. When these organs no longer receive their minimum requirements, death results.

LEARNING TIP

The magic fluid number is 30: Healthy adults should drink approximately 30 mL of fluid per kilogram of body weight per day. They should urinate at least 30 mL per hour. This is just a basic rule of thumb and will vary based on individual circumstances.

Diagnostic Tests

A patient with dehydration usually has an elevated blood urea nitrogen (BUN) level and elevated hematocrit. Both values are increased because there is less water in proportion to the solid substances being measured. The specific gravity of the urine also increases as the kidneys attempt to conserve water, resulting in a more concentrated urine.

Therapeutic Measures

The goals of therapeutic measures are to replace fluids and resolve the cause of dehydration. In a patient with moderate or severe dehydration, IV therapy is used. Isotonic fluids that have the same osmolarity as blood, such as normal saline, are typically administered.

Nursing Process for the Patient Experiencing Dehydration

Nurses can play a major role in identifying and caring for patients who are dehydrated.

DATA COLLECTION. Assess the patient for signs and symptoms of dehydration. All the classic signs and symptoms may not be present.

When assessing an older patient for skin turgor (tenting), assess the skin over the forehead or sternum. The skin over these areas usually retains elasticity and is therefore a more reliable indicator of skin turgor. Also check mucous membranes, which should be moist.

Weight is the most reliable indicator of fluid loss or gain. A loss of 1 to 2 pounds or more per day suggests water loss rather than fat loss. The patient in the hospital setting should be weighed every day. The patient in the nursing home or home setting should be weighed at least three times a week if the patient is at risk for fluid imbalance. Weigh the patient before breakfast using the same scale each time. Intake and output (I&O) are also typically measured ("Cultural Considerations").

Cultural Considerations

Muslims who celebrate Ramadan traditionally fast for 1 month from sunup to sundown. Although the ill are not required to fast, adherents who are ill may still wish to do so. Fasting may include not taking fluids and medications during daylight hours. For a Muslim who is ill and is fasting, the nurse may need to alter times for medication administration, including intramuscular medication. Special precautions may need to be taken to prevent dehydration.

NURSING DIAGNOSES, PLANNING, AND IMPLEMENTATION.

Risk for Deficient Fluid Volume or Deficient Fluid Volume [Isotonic or Hypotonic/Hypertonic] related to fluid loss or inadequate fluid intake

EXPECTED OUTCOME: The patient will be adequately hydrated as evidenced by stable weight, moist mucous membranes, and elastic skin turgor.

• Monitor daily weights and I&O *so problems can be detected and corrected early.*

- Plan with the patient and other members of the health care team the type and timing of fluid intake. *Planning with the patient increases the likelihood that the plan will be followed.*
- Offer fluids often to the confused patient *because he or she may not drink independently.*
- Correct the underlying cause of the fluid deficit, *so it does not recur.*
- Be careful not to overhydrate the patient, *so fluid excess does not occur.*

See Box 6.2 for best practices for maintaining oral hydration in older people.

EVALUATION. The patient who is adequately hydrated will have elastic skin turgor, moist mucous membranes, and stable weight.

Patient Education

Teach the patient, family, and significant others the importance of reporting early signs and symptoms of dehydration to the health care provider (HCP). At home or in the nursing home, infections often cause fever and sepsis. Sepsis is a serious condition in which the infection invades the bloodstream. The body attempts to decrease the temperature through perspiration. The patient becomes dehydrated as a result and can become increasingly ill.

CRITICAL THINKING

Mrs. Levitt is a 92-year-old widow who has been living in the nursing home where you work for 4 years. Today, she mentions that her urine smells bad and that her heart feels like it is beating faster than usual. You suspect that she is becoming dehydrated. You check her urine and find that it is a dark amber color and has a strong odor. Her heart rate is 98 beats per minute, blood pressure 126/74 mm Hg, respiratory rate 20 per minute, and temperature 99.2°F (37.3°C).

1. What other data should you collect, and what results do you expect?
2. Which interventions should you provide at this time?
3. How should you document your subjective and objective findings?
4. What other team members should be informed of your plan for Mrs. Levitt?
5. How will you know if she is improving?

Suggested answers are at the end of the chapter.

Fluid Excess

Fluid excess, sometimes called *overhydration,* is a condition in which a patient has too much fluid in the body. Most problems related to fluid excess result from too much fluid in the bloodstream or from dilution of electrolytes and red blood cells.

Box 6.2

Maintaining Oral Hydration in Older People

Following are best practice recommendations for maintaining oral hydration in older people:

- A fluid intake sheet is the best method of monitoring daily fluid intake.
- Urine specific gravity may be the simplest, most accurate method to determine patient hydration status.
- Evidence of a dry furrowed tongue, mucous membranes, sunken eyes, confusion, and upper body muscle weakness may indicate dehydration.
- Regular presentation of fluids to bedridden older people can maintain adequate hydration status.
- Owing to the observation that medication time can be an important source of fluids, fluids should be encouraged at this time.

Source: From Oates, L. L., & Price, C. I. (2017). Clinical assessments and care interventions to promote oral hydration amongst older patients: A narrative systematic review. *BMC Nursing, 16,* 4. Retrieved from http://creativecommons.org/licenses/by/4.0/

Pathophysiology and Etiology

The most common result of fluid excess is **hypervolemia,** in which there is excess fluid in the intravascular space. Healthy adult kidneys can compensate for mild to moderate hypervolemia. The kidneys increase urinary output to rid the body of the extra fluid. Sometimes, however, the kidneys cannot keep up with the excess fluid.

Conditions that can cause excessive fluid intake are poorly controlled IV therapy or excessive ingestion of water. It can also occur secondary to excessive sodium intake, adrenal gland dysfunction, or use of corticosteroid drugs. Conditions that can result in inadequate excretion of fluid include kidney failure, heart failure, and the syndrome of inappropriate ADH. These conditions are discussed elsewhere in this book.

Prevention

One of the best ways to prevent fluid excess is to avoid excessive fluid intake. Monitor the patient receiving IV therapy for signs and symptoms of fluid excess. In at-risk patients, an electronic controller should be used to control the rate of infusion.

Also monitor the amount of fluid used for irrigations. For example, when a patient's stomach is being irrigated (gastric lavage), be sure an excessive amount of fluid is not absorbed.

Signs and Symptoms

Vital sign changes seen in the patient with fluid excess are the opposite of those found in patients with dehydration. Blood pressure is elevated, pulse is bounding, and respirations are increased and labored. Neck veins may become distended. Pitting

- WORD · BUILDING ·

hypervolemia: hyper—more than + vol—volume + emia—blood

dependent **edema** (excess water in tissues) in the feet and legs may be present. The skin is pale and cool. The kidneys increase urine output. Urine appears diluted, almost like water. The patient rapidly gains weight. In severe fluid excess, the patient develops moist crackles in the lungs, dyspnea, and ascites (excess peritoneal fluid).

Complications

Acute fluid excess typically results in congestive heart failure. As the fluid builds up in the heart, the heart is not able to properly function as a pump. The fluid then backs up into the lungs, causing a condition known as pulmonary edema. Other major organs of the body cannot receive adequate oxygen. Organ failure can lead to death.

Diagnostic Tests

In the patient experiencing fluid excess, BUN and hematocrit levels tend to decrease because the extra fluid dilutes the blood. The plasma content of the blood is proportionately increased compared with the solid substances. The specific gravity of the urine also diminishes as the urinary output increases.

Therapeutic Measures

Once the patient's breathing has been supported, the goal of treatment is to rid the body of excessive fluid and resolve the underlying cause of the excess.

POSITIONING. To facilitate ease in breathing, the head of the patient's bed should be in semi-Fowler or high Fowler position (Fig. 6.2). These positions allow greater lung expansion and thus aid respiratory effort. Once the patient has been properly positioned, oxygen therapy may be necessary.

OXYGEN THERAPY. Oxygen therapy is used to ensure adequate perfusion of major organs and to minimize dyspnea. Monitor pulse oximetry and respiratory rate carefully.

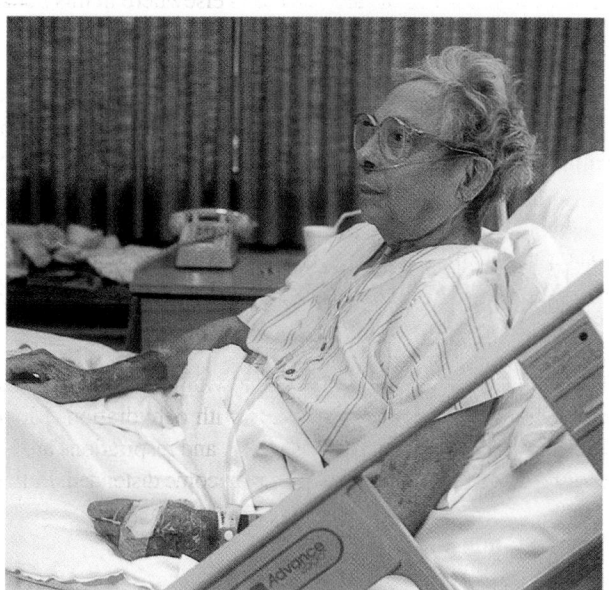

FIGURE 6.2 Patient in a high Fowler position with oxygen.

DRUG THERAPY. Diuretics are commonly administered to rapidly rid the body of excess water. A diuretic is a drug that increases elimination of fluid by the kidneys. The drug of choice for fluid excess when the patient has adequately functioning kidneys is usually a loop diuretic, such as furosemide (Lasix). Loop diuretics cause the kidneys to excrete sodium and water. Sodium (Na^+) and water tend to move together in the body. Potassium (K^+), another electrolyte, is also lost. This can lead to a potassium deficit, discussed later in this chapter.

Furosemide may be given by the oral, intramuscular, or IV route. The oral route is used most commonly for mild fluid excess. IV furosemide is administered for severe fluid excess. The patient should begin diuresis within 30 minutes after receiving IV furosemide. Strict I&O should be monitored, as well as daily weight, when a patient is receiving IV furosemide.

DIET THERAPY. Mild to moderate fluid restriction may be necessary as well as a sodium-restricted diet. In collaboration with the dietitian, an HCP prescribes the specific restriction necessary. This is usually a 1- to 2-g sodium restriction for severe excess. Different diuretics result in differing electrolyte elimination. Specific diet therapy depends on the medications the patient is receiving and the patient's underlying medical problems.

Nursing Process for the Patient Experiencing Fluid Excess

DATA COLLECTION. Observe a patient who is at high risk for fluid excess. Monitor fluid I&O carefully. If the patient is drinking adequate amounts of fluid (1,500 mL per day or more) but is voiding in small amounts, the fluid is being retained by the body.

Assess for edema; if it is pitting, a finger pressed against the skin over a bony area such as the tibia leaves a temporary indentation. For patients in bed, check the sacrum for edema. For patients in the sitting position, check the feet and legs. Also assess lung sounds. Excess fluid accumulation in the lungs can cause crackles (see Chapter 29).

As mentioned earlier, weight is the most reliable indicator of fluid gain. Weigh at-risk patients daily. A gain of 1 to 2 pounds or more per day indicates fluid retention, even though other signs and symptoms may not be present.

NURSING DIAGNOSES, PLANNING, AND IMPLEMENTATION.

Excess Fluid Volume related to excessive fluid intake or inadequate excretion of body fluid

EXPECTED OUTCOME: The patient will return to a normal hydration status as evidenced by return to weight that is normal for the patient, absence of edema, and clear lung sounds.

• Report increase in weight to the HCP. *Increased weight indicates fluid retention.*

• **WORD • BUILDING •**
edema: swelling

• Implement fluid restriction as ordered *to reduce excess intake.* Work with the patient and registered nurse (RN) to determine how it should be implemented. For example, if a patient is on a 1,000 mL per day fluid restriction, you might plan for 150 mL with each meal, 450 mL to be given to the patient to use as he or she likes during the day, and 100 mL to be used during the night. Be sure to include the patient in your planning. Remember to reserve enough fluid for swallowing medications. Post a sign in the patient's room so other caregivers know how much fluid the patient can have.

• Administer diuretics as ordered. Monitor patient response. Be sure to monitor potassium in patients receiving potassium-wasting loop or thiazide diuretics. *Diuretics promote diuresis.*

• Report urinary output below 30 mL per hour to the HCP or RN *because this may signify increasing renal complications.*

EVALUATION. If interventions have been effective, the patient will return to his or her normal weight with clear lung sounds and no edema. Many patients must remain on drug and diet therapy after hospital discharge to prevent the problem from recurring.

Patient Education

In collaboration with the dietitian, instruct the patient, family, or other caregiver about any fluid or sodium restrictions to prevent further problems ("Nutrition Notes"). Common foods that may have high sodium are listed in Table 6.1.

If a potassium-wasting diuretic is prescribed, teach the patient to eat foods that are high in potassium (Table 6.2). The patient's serum potassium level must be periodically monitored by an HCP or home health nurse. If it becomes too low, an oral potassium supplement is needed.

Teach the patient or caregiver common signs and symptoms of fluid excess that should be reported to the HCP. Of special importance is weight gain. A patient at high risk for fluid excess should be weighed at least three times a week in the home or nursing home at the same time each day and on the same scale. Weight gain should be reported.

 ## ELECTROLYTE BALANCE

Natural minerals in food become electrolytes or ions in the body through digestion and metabolism. Electrolytes are usually measured in milliequivalents per liter (mEq/L) or in milligrams per deciliter (mg/dL).

Electrolytes are one of two types: cations and anions. **Cations** carry a positive electrical charge. **Anions** carry a negative electrical charge. Although there are many electrolytes in the body, this chapter discusses the most important ones. These include sodium (Na^+), potassium (K^+), calcium (Ca^{2+}), and magnesium (Mg^{2+}). These electrolytes

---

Nutrition Notes

Reducing Sodium Intake. Whereas dairy products such as milk are naturally high in sodium, the major sources of dietary sodium are salt and processed foods, including baked goods, canned and packaged foods, and condiments. For example, American cheese has more sodium than does cheddar cheese, and cured ham has more than does fresh pork. Patients should be taught to read labels for sodium content on all packaged foods.

Drinking water may contain significant amounts of sodium, particularly if it is softened or mineral water. Because of the numerous hidden sources of sodium, patients on low-sodium diets benefit from education by a dietitian.

The adequate intake (AI) of sodium is:

• 1.5 g daily for adults through age 50
• 1.3 g daily for those aged 51 to 70
• 1.2 g daily for those aged 71 and older

The upper tolerable intake level (UL) for sodium is 2.3 g daily. This is contained in slightly more than a teaspoon of salt. None of these amounts applies to those losing large amounts of sweat daily or to unacclimatized persons exercising in a hot environment.

Specific definitions for reduced-sodium food products have been adopted. Note that serving size is an important variable:

• Salt or sodium free: Less than 5 mg sodium per serving
• Very low sodium: Less than 35 mg sodium per serving (per 100 g if main dish)
• Low sodium: Less than 140 mg sodium per serving (per 100 g if main dish)

CRITICAL THINKING

Mr. Peters is a 32-year-old man with a congenital heart problem. He has been recovering from acute congestive heart failure and fluid excess. Today, his blood pressure is higher than usual, and his pulse is bounding. He is having trouble breathing and presses the call light for your assistance.

1. What should you do first when you assess Mr. Peters's condition?
2. What questions should you ask him?
3. What objective data should you collect?
4. What should you do with your findings?

Suggested answers are at the end of the chapter.

• WORD • BUILDING •
cation: cat—descending + ion—carrying
anion: an—without + ion—carrying

Table 6.1
Common Food Sources of Sodium

Food	Sodium Range (in milligrams)
1 cheeseburger, fast food restaurant	710 to 1,690
5 oz pork with barbecue sauce (packaged)	600 to 1,120
3 oz turkey breast luncheon meat (deli or prepackaged)	450 to 1,050
1 cup canned pasta with meat sauce	530 to 980
1 cup chicken noodle soup, canned prepared	100 to 940
3 oz chicken strips, restaurant, breaded	430 to 900
4 oz slice restaurant pizza, plain cheese, regular crust	510 to 760
4 oz slice frozen pizza, plain cheese, regular crust	370 to 730
1 corn dog, regular	350 to 620
3 oz chicken nuggets, frozen, breaded	200 to 570
1 oz slice American cheese, processed (prepackaged or deli)	330 to 460
4 oz boneless chicken breast, fresh, skinless	40 to 330
1 slice of white bread	80 to 230
1 oz potato chips, plain	50 to 200

Source: Adapted from Centers for Disease Control and Prevention. (2017). Sodium and food sources. Retrieved from www.cdc.gov/salt/food.htm

are maintained in different concentrations inside the cell and outside the cell because of pumps in the cell wall (Fig. 6.3).

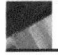 **ELECTROLYTE IMBALANCES**

At times, a patient may experience problems because of too much or too little of an electrolyte. In general, if a patient experiences a deficit of an electrolyte, the electrolyte is replaced either orally or intravenously. If the patient experiences an excess of an electrolyte, treatment focuses on getting rid of the excess, often via the kidneys. The underlying cause of the imbalance must also be treated.

The most important aspects of nursing care are preventing and assessing electrolyte imbalances. You must be vigilant in watching for signs of imbalance in high-risk patients. Serum electrolytes are measured on a regular basis. As a general rule, patients should be checked for electrolyte imbalance when

Table 6.2
Food Sources of Potassium

Food	Potassium (mg)
Potato, baked, flesh and skin, 1 medium	941
White beans, canned, ½ cup	595
Sweet potato, baked in skin, 1 medium	542
Salmon, Atlantic, wild, cooked, 3 oz	534
Plain yogurt, low-fat, 8 oz	531
Tomato juice, canned, 1 cup	527
Orange juice, fresh, 1 cup	496
Banana, 1 medium	422

Source: Adapted from Appendix 10. Food sources of potassium. In United States Department of Health and Human Services and U.S. Department of Agriculture. (2015). *2015–2020 Dietary Guidelines for Americans* (8th ed.). Washington, DC: Author. Retrieved from https://health.gov/dietaryguidelines/2015/guidelines/appendix-10/#table-a10-1

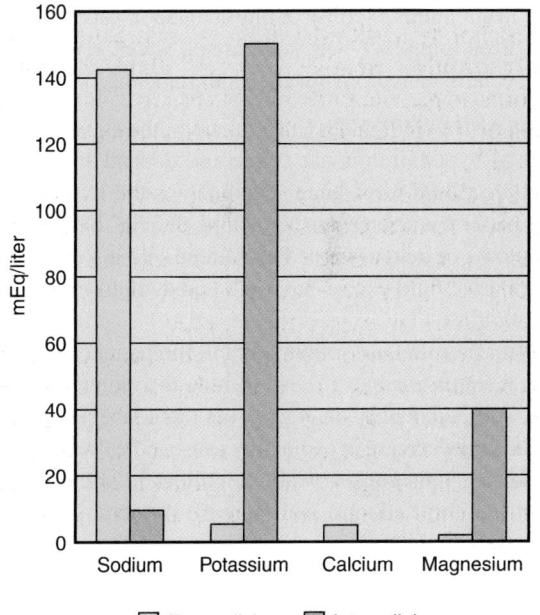

FIGURE 6.3 Extracellular and intracellular electrolytes.

there is a change in their mental status (either increased irritability or decreased responsiveness) or when muscle function changes. Patient education is another important nursing role.

Sodium Imbalances
The normal level of serum sodium is 135 to 145 mEq/L. Because sodium is the major cation in the blood, it helps maintain serum osmolarity. Therefore, sodium imbalances

are often associated with fluid imbalances, described earlier in this chapter. Sodium is also important for cell function, especially in the central nervous system. The two sodium imbalances are **hyponatremia** (sodium deficit) and **hypernatremia** (sodium excess).

Hyponatremia

Hyponatremia occurs when the serum sodium level is less than 135 mEq/L.

PATHOPHYSIOLOGY AND ETIOLOGY. Many conditions can lead to either an actual or a relative decrease in sodium. In an actual decrease, the patient has inadequate intake of sodium or excessive sodium loss from the body. As the percentage of sodium in the ECF decreases, water is pulled by osmotic pressure into the cells. In a relative decrease, the sodium is not lost from the body; instead, it may leave the intravascular space and move into the interstitial tissues (third spacing), where it becomes trapped and useless. Another cause of a relative decrease occurs when the plasma volume increases (fluid excess), causing a dilutional effect. The percentage of sodium compared with the fluid is diminished.

PREVENTION. Additional sodium is commonly administered to patients at high risk for hyponatremia (Box 6.3), usually by the IV route. Individuals who have high fevers or who engage in strenuous exercise or physical labor, especially in the heat, need to replace both sodium and water. Hyponatremia is especially dangerous for the older patient.

SIGNS AND SYMPTOMS. Unfortunately, the signs and symptoms of hyponatremia are vague and depend somewhat on whether a fluid imbalance accompanies the hyponatremia. The patient with sodium and fluid deficits has signs and symptoms of dehydration. The patient with a sodium deficit and relative fluid excess has signs and symptoms associated with fluid excess.

With more severe sodium deficit, the patient experiences mental status changes. These include disorientation, confusion, and personality changes. This occurs because the low sodium and decrease in osmolarity cause more "water-pushing pressure." This causes water to collect in and around the brain (cerebral edema) and increase intracranial pressure.

Box 6.3

High-Risk Conditions for Hyponatremia

The following conditions place patients at high risk for hyponatremia:
- Nothing by mouth (NPO)
- Excessive diaphoresis (sweating)
- Diuretics
- Gastrointestinal suction
- Syndrome of inappropriate antidiuretic hormone
- Excessive ingestion of hypotonic fluids
- Freshwater near-drowning
- Decreased aldosterone

Weakness, elevated body temperature, tachycardia, nausea, vomiting, and diarrhea may also occur ("Gerontological Issues: Confusion").

Gerontological Issues

Confusion. Often, older patients who experience a change in their electrolyte levels will present with sudden, unexplained confusion. Immediate identification and treatment may quickly relieve the confused state. The older patient's cardiovascular system is very sensitive to quick fluid shifts. It is important to remember intravenous infusions should only be provided at the rate prescribed by the health care provider.

COMPLICATIONS. In severe hyponatremia, respiratory arrest or coma can lead to death. The patient who also has fluid excess can develop pulmonary edema, another life-threatening complication ("Evidence-Based Practice").

Evidence-Based Practice

Clinical Question
How does hyponatremia affect hospital length of stay?

Evidence
A systematic review and meta-analysis using 46 randomized control trials revealed that hyponatremia occurred in approximately 20% of hospitalized patients in these studies. Patients with hyponatremia were hospitalized 3.3 days longer than those with normal sodium levels and were more likely to be readmitted (Corona et al., 2016). This may be an important factor in increased hospital-related costs as well.

Implications for Nursing Practice
Monitoring hydration status as well as fluid and electrolyte balance is an important part of caring for patients, no matter their age or health status. It is especially important to carefully monitor those at risk, such as older adults and those with comorbid conditions, since it can affect length of stay and readmission rates (see Box 6.3).

Reference
Corona, G., Giuliani, C., Parenti, G., Columbo, G. L., Sforza, A., Maggi, M., ... Peri, A. (2016). The economic burden of hyponatremia: Systematic review and meta-analysis. *American Journal of Medicine, 129*(8), 823–835.

· WORD · BUILDING ·

hyponatremia: hypo—less than + natr—sodium + emia—blood

hypernatremia: hyper—more than + natr—sodium + emia—blood

DIAGNOSTIC TESTS. The primary diagnostic test is a serum sodium level, which in hyponatremia registers below 135 mEq/L. The serum osmolarity also decreases in patients with hyponatremia. Other laboratory results may be affected if the patient experiences an accompanying fluid imbalance. Serum chloride (Cl^-), an anion, is often depleted when sodium decreases because these two electrolytes commonly combine as NaCl (salt in solution, or saline).

THERAPEUTIC MEASURES. Therapeutic measures focus on resolving the underlying cause of hyponatremia and replacing the lost sodium. The HCP may order IV saline for patients who have hyponatremia without fluid excess.

For patients who have a fluid excess, a fluid restriction is often ordered. Diuretics that rid the body of fluid but do not cause sodium loss may also be used. For patients with cerebral edema, steroids may be prescribed to reduce **intracranial** swelling. I&O are strictly monitored. The patient is weighed daily. Implement interventions to keep the patient safe if mental status is affected.

Hypernatremia

Hypernatremia occurs when the serum sodium level is above 145 mEq/L.

PATHOPHYSIOLOGY AND ETIOLOGY. A serum sodium increase may be an actual increase or a relative increase. In an actual increase, the patient receives too much sodium or is unable to excrete sodium, as in kidney failure. In a relative increase, the amount of sodium does not change, but the amount of fluid in the intravascular space decreases. Therefore, the percentage of sodium (solute) is increased in relationship to the amount of plasma.

In mild hypernatremia, most excitable tissues, such as muscle and neurons of the brain, become more stimulated. The patient becomes irritable and has tremors. In severe cases, these tissues fail to respond.

PREVENTION. Prevention of hypernatremia is not as simple as prevention of hyponatremia. Most patients have a sodium excess as a result of an acute or chronic illness. Patients with a potential for electrolyte imbalance must have their IV fluids carefully regulated.

SIGNS AND SYMPTOMS. Thirst is usually one of the first symptoms to appear. If you eat salty foods, such as potato chips, the amount of sodium in your body increases, and you become thirsty. Other signs and symptoms of hypernatremia are vague and nonspecific until severe excess is present. Like the patient with a sodium deficit, the patient experiencing sodium excess has mental status changes, such as agitation, confusion, and personality changes. However, this time the cause is too little fluid in the brain tissues. Seizures may also occur.

At first, muscle twitches and unusual contractions may be present. Later, skeletal muscle weakness occurs that can lead to respiratory failure if it affects the diaphragm. If fluid deficit or fluid excess accompanies the hypernatremic state,

the patient also has signs and symptoms associated with these imbalances.

COMPLICATIONS. A patient with severe hypernatremia may become comatose or have respiratory arrest as skeletal muscles weaken.

DIAGNOSTIC TESTS. The most reliable diagnostic test is the serum sodium level. This indicates an increase above the normal level. Serum osmolarity may also increase. If the patient has a fluid imbalance, other laboratory values, such as BUN, hematocrit, and urine specific gravity, are also affected (see earlier discussion).

THERAPEUTIC MEASURES. If a fluid imbalance accompanies hypernatremia, it is treated first. For example, fluid replacement without sodium in a patient with dehydration should correct a relative sodium excess. If the kidneys are not excreting adequate amounts of sodium, diuretics may help if the kidneys are functional. If the kidneys are not functioning properly, dialysis may be ordered (see Chapter 37). I&O and daily weights are strictly monitored.

The cause of hypernatremia is also treated in an attempt to prevent further episodes of this imbalance. For some patients, a sodium-restricted diet is prescribed.

Potassium Imbalances

Potassium is the most common electrolyte in the ICF compartment. Only a small amount, 3.5 to 5 mEq/L, is found in the bloodstream. Small changes in this laboratory value cause major changes in the body.

Potassium is especially important for cardiac muscle, skeletal muscle, and smooth muscle function. If the serum potassium level falls, the body attempts to compensate by moving potassium from the cells into the bloodstream.

The two potassium imbalances are **hypokalemia** (potassium deficit) and **hyperkalemia** (potassium excess). Hypokalemia is the most commonly occurring imbalance.

Hypokalemia

Hypokalemia occurs when the serum potassium level falls below 3.5 mEq/L.

PATHOPHYSIOLOGY AND ETIOLOGY. Most cases of hypokalemia result from inadequate intake of potassium or excessive loss of potassium through the kidneys. Hypokalemia most often occurs as a result of medications. Potassium-wasting diuretics (e.g., furosemide [Lasix] and hydrochlorothiazide), digitalis preparations (e.g., digoxin [Lanoxin]), and corticosteroids (e.g., prednisone) are examples of drugs that cause increased excretion of potassium

---

• **WORD** • **BUILDING** •

intracranial: intra—within + cranial—cranium (skull)
hypokalemia: hypo—less than + kal—potassium + emia—blood
hyperkalemia: hyper—more than + kal—potassium + emia—blood

from the body. Potassium may also be lost through the gastrointestinal (GI) tract, which is rich in potassium and other electrolytes. Severe vomiting, diarrhea, and prolonged GI suction cause hypokalemia ("Patient Perspective"). Major surgery and hemorrhage can also lead to potassium deficit.

Patient Perspective

Patricia. I take hydrochlorothiazide for my high blood pressure. Since it can make me lose potassium, I also take a potassium supplement. So, I thought I was all set. But recently I ate something that did not agree with me, and I had diarrhea for a couple of days. One morning as I was driving to work, I felt so weak it frightened me. I drove back home and asked my husband to drive me to work. I arrived safely, but as I walked down the hallway, I again felt so weak I had to sit down. I felt like I could not put one foot in front of the other. I kept thinking, "This is all in my head." I decided maybe I was dehydrated from the diarrhea, so I drank a bottle of Gatorade and a glass of orange juice. Slowly, I began to feel a bit better, and I made it through the day. After work, I had to take my daughter to the doctor, so I asked about my symptoms. I was sent to the lab where I had my potassium level checked, and it was 3.1! Normal is 3.5 to 5 mEq/L. Mine must have been even lower before I drank the juice and Gatorade. I learned that I probably lost a lot of potassium because of the diarrhea. I also learned that low potassium made my muscles weak and could have affected my heart function. Next time I have diarrhea, I plan to call my doctor.

PREVENTION. Most patients having major surgery receive potassium supplements in their IV fluids to prevent hypokalemia. For patients receiving drugs known to cause hypokalemia, potassium supplements or foods high in potassium may prevent a deficit (see Table 6.2).

SIGNS AND SYMPTOMS. Many body systems are affected by a potassium imbalance. Muscle cramping or muscle fatigue can occur with either a deficit or an excess of potassium. Vital signs change because the respiratory and cardiovascular systems need potassium to function properly. Diminished skeletal muscle activity results in shallow, ineffective respirations. The pulse is typically weak, irregular, and thready because the heart muscle is depleted of potassium. A major danger is an irregular heartbeat (**arrhythmia**), which can lead to cardiac arrest. Orthostatic (postural) hypotension may also be present.

The nervous system is usually affected as well. The patient experiences changes in mental status followed by lethargy. The motility of the GI system is slowed, causing nausea, vomiting, abdominal distention, and constipation. Vomiting may further increase potassium loss.

COMPLICATIONS. If not corrected, hypokalemia can result in death from arrhythmia, or respiratory failure and arrest. The patient must be treated promptly before these complications occur.

DIAGNOSTIC TESTS. The primary laboratory test is a serum potassium level. The patient's electrocardiogram (ECG) may show cardiac arrhythmias associated with potassium deficit. In addition to a decrease in the serum potassium level, the patient may have an acid–base imbalance known as metabolic **alkalosis.** This commonly accompanies hypokalemia. In metabolic alkalosis, the serum pH of the blood increases (more than 7.45) so that the blood is more alkaline than usual. Acid–base imbalances are discussed later in this chapter.

THERAPEUTIC MEASURES. The goal of treatment is to replace potassium in the body and resolve the underlying cause of the imbalance. For mild to moderate hypokalemia, oral potassium supplements are given. For severe hypokalemia, IV potassium supplements are given. Because the kidneys eliminate excess potassium, potassium should be administered only after the patient has voided, to be sure the kidneys are functioning. Potassium is a potentially dangerous drug, especially when administered intravenously. In too high a concentration, it causes cardiac arrest. Only IV solutions that are premixed and carefully labeled should be used. Potassium is *never* given by IV push. The patient's laboratory values must be monitored carefully to prevent giving too much potassium.

Teach the patient about the side effects of oral potassium and precautions associated with potassium administration. Box 6.4 summarizes the precautions the patient should be aware of when taking oral potassium supplements.

Hyperkalemia

Hyperkalemia is a condition in which the serum potassium level exceeds 5 mEq/L. It is rare in a person with healthy kidneys.

PATHOPHYSIOLOGY AND ETIOLOGY. Hyperkalemia may result from an actual increase in the amount of total body potassium or from the movement of intracellular potassium into the blood. Overuse of potassium-based salt substitutes or excessive intake of oral or IV potassium supplements can cause hyperkalemia. Use of potassium-sparing diuretics (e.g., spironolactone [Aldactone]) may also contribute to hyperkalemia. Patients with kidney failure are at risk for hyperkalemia because the kidneys cannot excrete potassium.

Movement of potassium from the cells into the blood and other ECF is common in massive tissue trauma and metabolic acidosis. Metabolic **acidosis** is an acid–base

• WORD • BUILDING •
arrhythmia: dys—bad or disordered + rhythmia—measured motion
alkalosis: alkal—alkaline + osis—condition
acidosis: acid—acidic + osis—condition

Box 6.4

Tips for Patients Taking Oral Potassium Supplements

- Do not substitute one potassium supplement for another.
- Take all forms of potassium with a full glass of water or juice.
- Dilute powders and liquids in water or juice exactly as directed.
- Do not crush extended-release potassium tablets, such as Slow-K or K-Dur tablets.
- Do not take potassium supplements if you take potassium-sparing diuretics such as spironolactone (Aldactone) or triamterene (Dyrenium).
- Tell your doctor if you use salt substitutes containing potassium.
- Take potassium supplements with meals.
- Report adverse effects, such as nausea, vomiting, diarrhea, and abdominal cramping, to the health care provider (HCP).
- Have frequent laboratory testing for potassium levels as recommended by the HCP.

imbalance commonly seen in patients with uncontrolled diabetes mellitus. Acid–base imbalances are discussed later in this chapter.

PREVENTION. For patients receiving potassium supplements, hyperkalemia can be prevented by monitoring serum electrolyte values and the patient's signs and symptoms and by adjusting the dose accordingly.

SIGNS AND SYMPTOMS. Most cases of hyperkalemia occur in patients who are hospitalized or undergoing therapeutic measures for a chronic condition. The classic manifestations are muscle twitches and cramps later followed by profound muscular weakness; increased GI motility (diarrhea); slow, irregular heart rate; weak pulse; and decreased blood pressure.

COMPLICATIONS. Cardiac arrhythmias and respiratory failure can occur in severe hyperkalemia, causing death.

DIAGNOSTIC TESTS. In addition to an elevated serum potassium level, ECG changes are also associated with hyperkalemia. If the patient has metabolic acidosis, the serum pH falls below 7.35.

THERAPEUTIC MEASURES. For mild, chronic hyperkalemia, dietary limitation of potassium-rich foods may be helpful. Potassium supplements are discontinued. Potassium-wasting diuretics are given to patients with healthy kidneys. For patients with kidney problems, a cation exchange resin, such as sodium polystyrene sulfonate, may be administered either orally or rectally. This drug releases sodium and absorbs potassium for excretion through the feces and out of the body.

In cases in which cellular potassium has moved into the bloodstream, administration of glucose and insulin can facilitate the movement of potassium back into the cells. During treatment of moderate to severe hyperkalemia, the patient should be in the hospital on a cardiac monitor.

Calcium Imbalances

Calcium is a mineral that is primarily stored in bones and teeth. A small amount is found in ECF. The normal value for serum calcium is 9 to 11 mg/dL, or 4.5 to 5.5 mEq/L. Minimal changes in serum calcium levels can have major negative effects in the body.

Calcium is needed for the proper function of excitable tissues, especially cardiac muscle. The two calcium imbalances are **hypocalcemia** and **hypercalcemia.**

Hypocalcemia

Hypocalcemia occurs when the serum calcium level falls below 9 mg/dL, or 4.5 mEq/L.

PATHOPHYSIOLOGY AND ETIOLOGY. Although calcium deficit can be acute or chronic, most patients develop hypocalcemia slowly as a result of chronic disease or poor intake. Postmenopausal women are most at risk for hypocalcemia. As a woman ages, calcium intake typically declines. The parathyroid glands recognize this decrease and stimulate bone to release some of its stored calcium into the blood for replacement. The result is a condition known as **osteoporosis,** in which bones become porous and brittle and fracture easily. The woman who is postmenopausal has a decreased level of estrogens, a hormone that helps prevent bone loss in the younger woman. Immobility or decreased mobility also contributes to bone loss in many patients. The patients at highest risk for osteoporosis are thin, petite, Caucasian women.

Hypocalcemia can also result from inadequate absorption of calcium from the intestines, as seen in patients with Crohn's disease, a chronic inflammatory bowel disease. Insufficient intake of vitamin D prevents calcium absorption as well. Conditions that interfere with the production of parathyroid hormone, such as partial or complete surgical removal of the thyroid or parathyroid glands, can also cause hypocalcemia.

Finally, patients with hyperphosphatemia (usually those with kidney failure) often experience hypocalcemia. Calcium and phosphate have an inverse relationship. When one of these electrolytes increases, the other tends to decrease.

PREVENTION. In the United States, the typical daily calcium intake is less than 550 mg. The Recommended Dietary Allowance (RDA) of calcium for adults aged 19 to 50 and

---

• **WORD • BUILDING •**

hypocalcemia: hypo—less than + calc—calcium + emia—blood

hypercalcemia: hyper—more than + calc—calcium + emia—blood

osteoporosis: osteo—bone + porosis—porous

men aged 51 and 70 is 1,000 mg; the RDA for women over age 50 and men over 70 is 1,200 mg.

Hypocalcemia can be prevented by consuming calcium-rich foods and by taking calcium supplements. These supplements can be purchased over the counter in any pharmacy or large food store. An inexpensive source of calcium for patients who do not require vitamin D supplementation is calcium carbonate (Tums), which provides 240 mg of elemental calcium in each tablet. Patients should be cautioned not to routinely take high doses of calcium without checking with their primary care provider.

Vitamin D supplementation may be required in addition to calcium for patients whose sun exposure is limited. The sun's ultraviolet light causes the skin to manufacture vitamin D.

SIGNS AND SYMPTOMS. Chronic hypocalcemia is usually not diagnosed until the patient breaks a bone, usually a hip. Acute hypocalcemia can occur after surgery or in patients with acute pancreatitis. Signs include changes in heart rate, decreased blood pressure, mental status changes, hyperactive deep tendon reflexes, and increased GI motility, including diarrhea and abdominal cramping. Two classic signs that can be used to assess for hypocalcemia are Trousseau sign and Chvostek sign.

To test for Trousseau sign, inflate a blood pressure cuff around the patient's upper arm for 1 to 4 minutes. In a patient with hypocalcemia, the hand and fingers become spastic and go into palmar flexion (Fig. 6.4). To test for Chvostek sign, tap the face just below and in front of the ear. Facial twitching on that side of the face indicates a positive test (Fig. 6.5). Trousseau sign is more specific for hypocalcemia than Chvostek sign.

LEARNING TIP

You can remember which sign is **CH**vostek sign because it causes spasm near the **CH**eek.

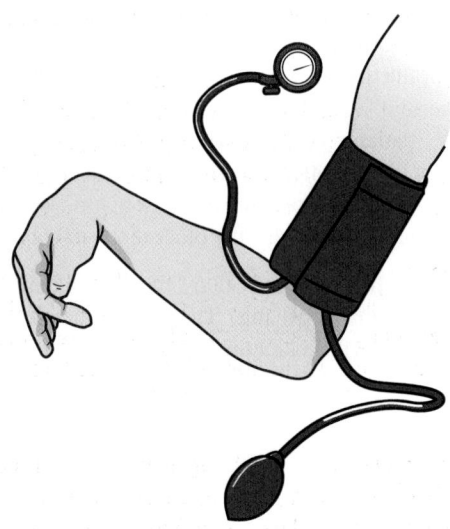

FIGURE 6.4 Trousseau sign.

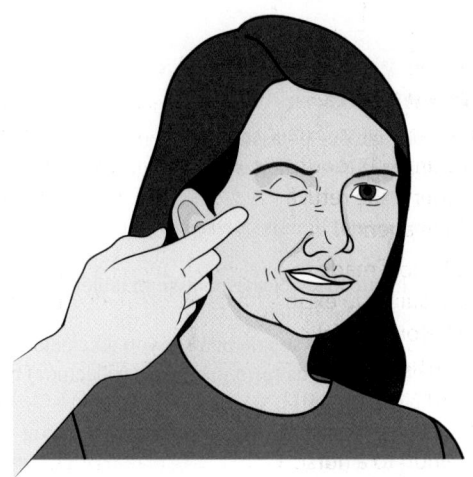

FIGURE 6.5 Chvostek sign.

COMPLICATIONS. In severe hypocalcemia, neuromuscular irritability can lead to *tetany,* or continuous muscle contraction. The patient may have a sudden laryngospasm that will stop air from entering the lungs. Seizures, respiratory failure, or cardiac failure can occur and lead to death if not aggressively treated.

DIAGNOSTIC TESTS. The patient with hypocalcemia has a low serum calcium level and an abnormal ECG. Parathyroid hormone level may be increased as it attempts to stimulate bone to release more calcium into the blood.

THERAPEUTIC MEASURES. In addition to treating the cause of hypocalcemia, calcium is replaced. For mild or chronic hypocalcemia, oral calcium supplements with or without vitamin D are given. Calcium supplements should be administered 1 to 2 hours after meals to increase intestinal absorption. Be sure to check compatibility when administering calcium with other medications.

For patients with acute or severe hypocalcemia, IV calcium gluconate or calcium chloride is given. When a patient has had thyroid or parathyroid surgery, there is a danger that parathyroid hormone will be decreased, causing serum calcium to drop. IV calcium must be readily available for emergency use if signs of hypocalcemia occur.

For patients with hyperphosphatemia, usually those with kidney failure, aluminum hydroxide is used to bind the excess phosphate for elimination via the GI tract. As the phosphate decreases, the serum calcium level begins to normalize.

Diet therapy is an important part of treatment. Teach the patient, family, or other caregiver which foods are high in calcium (Table 6.3). Many foods today are fortified with calcium. Vitamin D foods are also encouraged, especially milk and other dairy products. For patients experiencing difficulty digesting dairy products and those who choose not to use dairy products, special attention must be paid to including other dietary calcium sources in the diet.

CRITICAL THINKING

Mrs. Wright is a 77-year-old petite Caucasian woman who lives alone at home. She is on a fixed income and rarely eats calcium-rich foods. She recently fell and broke her hip. After surgery, she returned home under the care of a home health care agency.

1. What factors made the patient at high risk for a fracture?
2. What would you expect her serum calcium level to have been before the fall?
3. What patient teaching related to diet and calcium supplements should the home health nurse include during his or her home visits?
4. In addition to a nurse, what other home health care team members might be helpful for Mrs. Wright?

Suggested answers are at the end of the chapter.

Table 6.3
Food Sources of Calcium*

Food	Calcium (mg)
Fortified ready-to-eat cereals (various), ¾ to 1¼ cup	137 to 1,000
Parmesan cheese, hard, 1.5 oz	503
Plain yogurt, nonfat, 8 oz	452
Almond milk (all flavors), 1 cup	451
Tofu, raw, regular, prepared with calcium sulfate, ½ cup	438
Plain yogurt, low-fat, 8 oz	415
Soymilk (all flavors), 1 cup	340
Mustard spinach (tendergreen), raw, 1 cup	315
Low-fat milk (1%), 1 cup	305
Mozzarella cheese, part-skim. 1.5 oz	304
Skim milk (nonfat), 1 cup	299
Reduced fat milk (2%), 1 cup	293
Cheddar cheese, 1.5 oz	287
Whole milk, 1 cup	276

*Both calcium content and bioavailability should be considered when selecting dietary sources of calcium.
Source: Adapted from Appendix 11. Food sources of calcium. In United States Department of Health and Human Services and U.S. Department of Agriculture. (2015). *2015–2020 Dietary Guidelines for Americans* (8th ed.). Washington, DC: Author. Retrieved from https://health.gov/dietaryguidelines/2015/guidelines/appendix-11/

Hypercalcemia

Hypercalcemia occurs when the serum calcium is above 11 mg/dL, or 5.5 mEq/L.

PATHOPHYSIOLOGY AND ETIOLOGY. Chronic hypercalcemia can result from excessive intake of calcium or vitamin D, kidney failure, hyperparathyroidism, cancers, and overuse or prolonged use of thiazide diuretics, such as hydrochlorothiazide. Acute hypercalcemia can occur as an emergency in patients with invasive or metastatic cancers, especially cancers of the blood or bone.

PREVENTION. Although many causes of increased calcium cannot be prevented, a person receiving calcium supplements should be monitored carefully. Some patients believe that if two or three tablets a day are helpful, consuming twice as many will help even more. The result can be serum calcium excess. Educating the public about the proper amount of calcium needed each day and the danger of too much calcium is very important.

SIGNS AND SYMPTOMS. Patients who have mild hypercalcemia or a slowly progressing calcium increase may have no obvious signs and symptoms. However, acute hypercalcemia is associated with increased heart rate and blood pressure, skeletal muscle weakness, and decreased GI motility.

COMPLICATIONS. In some cases, the patient may experience kidney or urinary calculi (stones) resulting from excess calcium. In more severe cases of acute hypercalcemia, the patient may experience respiratory failure caused by profound muscle weakness or heart failure caused by arrhythmias.

THERAPEUTIC MEASURES. Patients with severe hypercalcemia should be hospitalized and placed on a cardiac monitor. Unless contraindicated by other conditions, the primary treatment is to give IV fluids and promote diuresis. Saline infusions are the most useful solutions to promote renal excretion of calcium.

The HCP also discontinues thiazide diuretics if the patient was receiving them and prescribes diuretics that promote calcium excretion, such as furosemide (Lasix). Drugs that slow calcium movement from bones to the blood may also be used, such as pamidronate disodium (Aredia), zoledronic acid (Zometa), or calcitonin.

If hypercalcemia is so severe that cardiac problems are present, hemodialysis, peritoneal dialysis, or ultrafiltration may be necessary to cleanse the blood of excess calcium. (See Chapter 37 for discussion of these procedures.)

Magnesium Imbalances

Magnesium and calcium work together for the proper functioning of excitable cells, such as cardiac muscle and nerve cells. Therefore, an imbalance of magnesium is usually accompanied by an imbalance of calcium.

The normal value for serum magnesium is 1.5 to 2.5 mEq/L. Magnesium imbalances are called **hypomagnesemia** and **hypermagnesemia.**

Hypomagnesemia

Hypomagnesemia occurs when the serum magnesium level falls below 1.5 mEq/L. It results from either decreased intake or excessive loss of magnesium. Causes of inadequate intake include malnutrition and starvation diets. Patients with severe diarrhea and Crohn's disease are unable to absorb magnesium in the intestines.

One of the major causes of hypomagnesemia is alcoholism. Alcohol causes both decreased intake and increased renal excretion of magnesium. Certain drugs, such as loop and osmotic diuretics, aminoglycosides (e.g., gentamicin [Garamycin]), and some anticancer agents (e.g., cisplatin [Platinol]), can increase renal excretion of magnesium.

The signs and symptoms of hypomagnesemia are similar to those for hypocalcemia, including positive Trousseau and Chvostek signs, described earlier in this chapter.

The goal of management is to treat the underlying cause and replace magnesium in the body. Magnesium sulfate is administered intravenously. If the serum calcium is also low, calcium replacement is prescribed. The patient is placed on a cardiac monitor because of magnesium's effect on the heart. Life-threatening arrhythmias can lead to cardiac failure and arrest.

Hypermagnesemia

Hypermagnesemia results when the serum magnesium level increases above 2.5 mEq/L. The most common cause of hypermagnesemia is increased intake coupled with decreased renal excretion caused by kidney failure.

Signs and symptoms are usually not apparent until the serum level is greater than 4 mEq/L. Then, the signs and symptoms include bradycardia and other arrhythmias, hypotension, lethargy or drowsiness, and skeletal muscle weakness. If not treated, the patient experiences coma, respiratory failure, or cardiac failure.

When kidneys are functioning properly, loop diuretics such as furosemide (Lasix) and IV fluids can help increase magnesium excretion. For patients with kidney failure, dialysis may be the only option.

ACID–BASE BALANCE

The cells of the body function best when the body fluids and electrolytes are within a narrow range. Hydrogen (H^+) is another ion that must stay within its normal limits. The amount of hydrogen determines whether a fluid is an acid or base.

An *acid* is a substance that releases a hydrogen ion. The stronger the acid, the more hydrogen ions that are released.

A common acid in the body is hydrochloric acid (HCl), which is found in the stomach. A *base* is a substance that binds hydrogen. A common base in the body is bicarbonate (HCO_3^-). *Alkali* is another word for "base."

Sources of Acids and Bases

Acids and bases are formed in the body as part of normal metabolic processes. Acids are formed as end products of glucose, fat, and protein metabolism. These are called fixed acids because they do not change once they are formed. Carbonic acid is a weak acid that can be formed when the carbon dioxide resulting from cellular metabolism combines with water. This acid can change to bicarbonate (a base) and hydrogen. It is, therefore, not a fixed acid.

The ECF maintains a delicate balance between acids and bases. The strength of the acids and bases can be measured by pH. The pH of a solution can vary from 0 to 14, with 7 being neutral, 0 to 6.99 being acid, and 7.01 to 14 being base, or alkaline. The normal serum pH level is 7.35 to 7.45, which is slightly alkaline. It must remain in this extremely narrow range to sustain life. An arterial pH lower than 6.9 or higher than 7.8 is usually fatal.

LEARNING TIP

The word *acid* has fewer letters and lower numbers (less than 7.35). *Alkaline* has more letters and higher numbers (greater than 7.45).

Control of Acid–Base Balance

The body has several ways in which it tries to compensate for changes in the serum pH. Three major mechanisms are used: cellular buffers, the lungs, and the kidneys.

Cellular buffers are the first to attempt a return of the pH to its normal range. Examples of cellular buffers are proteins, hemoglobin, bicarbonate, and phosphates. These buffers act as a type of sponge to "soak up" extra hydrogen ions if there are too many (too acidic) or release hydrogen ions if there are not enough (too alkaline).

The lungs are the second line of defense to restore normal pH. When the blood is too acidic (pH is decreased), the lungs "blow off" additional carbon dioxide through rapid, deep breathing. This reduces the amount of carbon dioxide

---

• WORD • BUILDING •

hypomagnesemia: hypo—less than + magnes—magnesium + emia—blood

hypermagnesemia: hyper—more than + magnes—magnesium + emia—blood

available to make carbonic acid in the body. If the blood is too alkaline (pH is increased), the lungs try to conserve carbon dioxide through shallow respirations.

The kidneys are the slowest to respond to changes in serum pH, taking as long as 24 to 48 hours to assist with compensation. The kidneys help in a number of ways, including regulating the amount of bicarbonate (base) that is kept in the body. If the serum pH lowers and becomes too acidic, the kidneys reabsorb additional bicarbonate rather than excreting it so that it can help neutralize the acid. If the serum pH increases and becomes too alkaline, the kidneys excrete additional bicarbonate to get rid of the extra base. The kidneys also buffer pH by forming acids and ammonium (a base).

Acidosis or alkalosis that is corrected for by the body is referred to as *compensated.* The pH is returned to normal or near normal, but the gases that monitor acid–base balance (Pco_2 and HCO_3^-) are abnormal.

ACID–BASE IMBALANCES

Acid–base imbalances are caused by a number of acute and chronic illnesses or conditions. The primary treatment for each of the imbalances is to manage the underlying cause, which corrects the imbalance. The role of the nurse is to identify patients at risk and monitor laboratory test values for significant changes.

The laboratory tests that are used to evaluate acid–base balance are called arterial blood gases (ABGs). As the name implies, the blood sample that is analyzed must be from an artery rather than a vein. The femoral, brachial, and radial arteries are most often used to obtain the sample. Table 6.4 lists ABG values and what they indicate.

The two broad types of acid–base imbalance are acidosis and alkalosis. Each of these imbalances can occur suddenly. This is called an *acute imbalance.* They can also develop over a long period, resulting in a *chronic imbalance.*

When the serum pH level falls below 7.35, the patient has acidosis because the blood becomes more acidic than normal. Too much acid or too little base in the body causes acidosis. Acidosis can be divided into two types: respiratory and metabolic. Respiratory acidosis is caused by problems occurring in the respiratory system. Metabolic acidosis is the result of problems in the rest of the body.

When the serum pH level increases above 7.45, the patient has alkalosis because the blood becomes more alkaline or basic. Alkalosis is caused by too little acid in the body or too much base. It can also be divided into two types: respiratory alkalosis and metabolic alkalosis.

See Figure 6.6 for details about respiratory and metabolic acid–base imbalances.

LEARNING TIP

Note the arrows in Table 6.4. In respiratory imbalances, the arrows are pointing in *opposite* directions. In metabolic imbalances, the arrows are pointing in the same or *equal* directions. So, simply remember "ROME": Respiratory Opposite, Metabolic Equal!

Table 6.4

Arterial Blood Gas Values and Changes in Acid–Base Imbalances

	pH	*Pco₂*	*HCO₃⁻*
Normal values	7.35–7.45	32–45 mm Hg	20–26 mEq/L
Respiratory acidosis	↓	↑	Normal
Respiratory acidosis with compensation	Nearly normal	↑	↑
Respiratory alkalosis	↑	↓	Normal
Respiratory alkalosis with compensation	Nearly normal	↓	↓
Metabolic acidosis	↓	Normal	↓
Metabolic acidosis with compensation	Nearly normal	↓	↓
Metabolic alkalosis	↑	Normal	↑
Metabolic alkalosis with compensation	Nearly normal	↑	↑

Acid-Base Imbalances

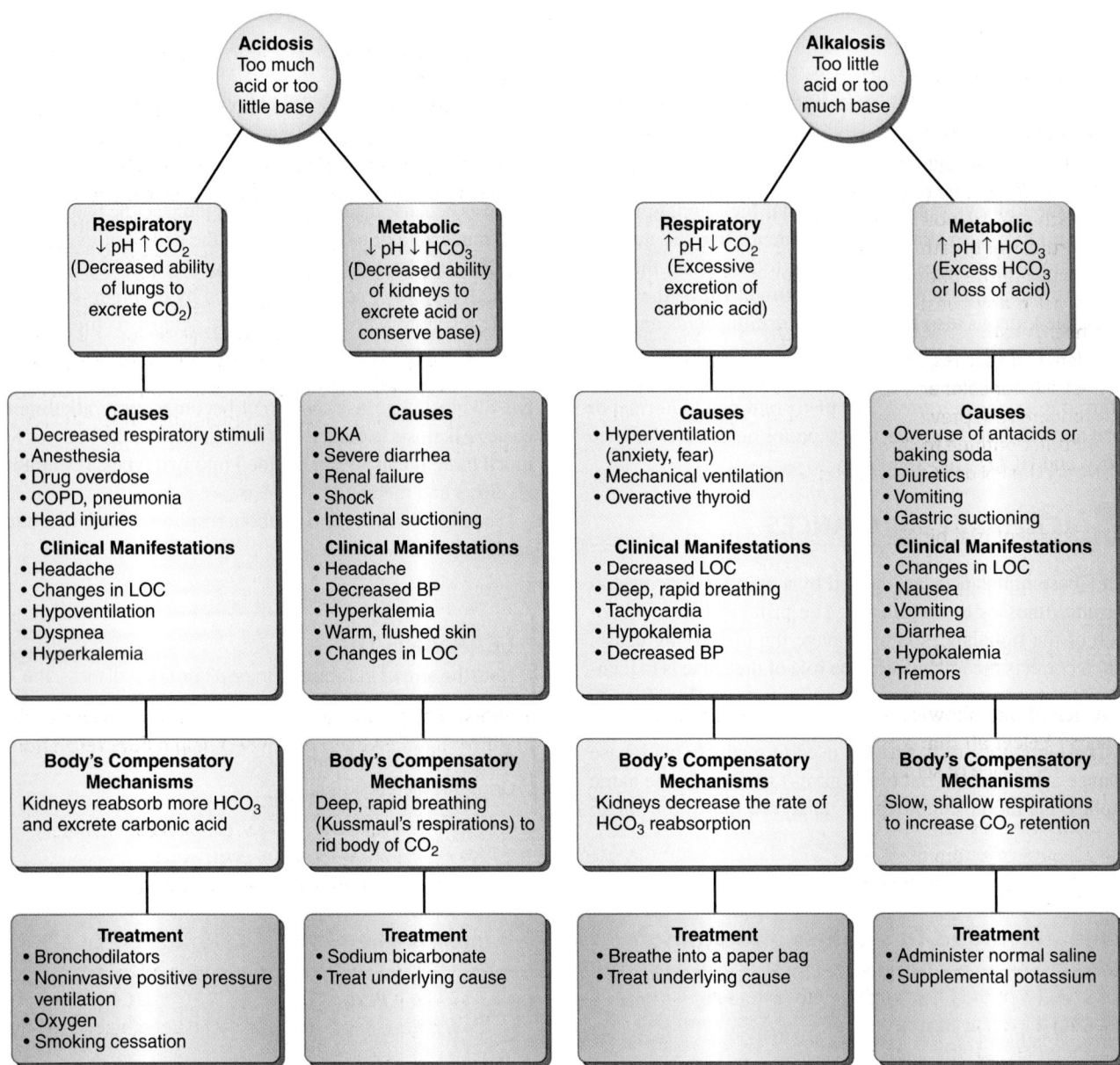

FIGURE 6.6 Mind map of acid–base imbalances.

SUGGESTED ANSWERS TO CRITICAL THINKING

Mrs. Levitt

1. Check her weight and compare it with her previous weights. Dehydration is associated with weight loss. Monitor mental status for disorientation. Check skin turgor for tenting. Compare vital signs to usual vitals. Continue to monitor vital signs.
2. Encourage increased fluid intake. Notify the registered nurse (RN) or health care provider (HCP) if Mrs. Levitt is unable to take in additional fluids or if the fluids do not normalize assessment findings.
3. Subjective: "My urine smells bad, and my heart is beating fast."; Objective: Pt's urine is dark amber

and strong smelling. Weight 112# (baseline 116#); skin tenting present. VS: P 98 beats per minute, BP 126/74 mm Hg, RR 20 per minute, T 99.2. Fluids encouraged. RN notified.

4. Notify the RN but also the nursing assistant, who can help with encouraging fluids during and between meals as well as monitoring skin condition. Contact the dietary department to obtain beverages Mrs. Levitt prefers that do not contain caffeine.
5. Watch for her weight to return to her normal, for her skin to feel more elastic, and for her urine to appear more dilute. Vital signs should also return to baseline.

SUGGESTED ANSWERS TO CRITICAL THINKING—cont'd

Mr. Peters

1. Raise the head of the bed to assist breathing.
2. Using the *WHAT'S UP?* format as a guide, ask the following questions: How are you feeling? Did anything aggravate your symptoms? When did your symptoms begin? On a scale of 0 to 10, how difficult is your breathing? Are you having any problems besides shortness of breath? What do you think might be happening? (If the patient is too dyspneic to answer, do not ask many questions.)
3. Check breath sounds for crackles, observe for dependent edema and ascites, observe for distended neck veins, assess skin for color and temperature, check weight and compare with previous weight, and monitor input and output. Continue to monitor vital signs.
4. Notify the RN or HCP of your findings.

Mrs. Wright

1. The patient is at high risk for osteoporosis and, thus, fracture because she is an older, petite, Caucasian woman. In addition, she does not get much calcium in her diet.
2. Her serum calcium levels would be low or low–normal because the body will mobilize calcium in the bones in an attempt to maintain serum calcium levels.
3. Teach her about consuming foods high in calcium, the need to be compliant with taking her calcium supplements, and to take the supplements 1 to 2 hours after meals for best absorption by the body.
4. She would benefit from physical therapy for ambulation and strengthening, occupational therapy for an evaluation of her home environment and possible assistive devices, and a dietitian for dietary counseling. Caution her to avoid taking more calcium than prescribed, because that can also be harmful.

Review Questions

1. Which of the following are functions of sodium in the body? **Select all that apply.**
   1. Maintenance of serum osmolarity
   2. Formation of bones and teeth
   3. Control of bronchodilation
   4. Control of serum glucose
   5. Maintenance of cellular function

2. A 93-year-old patient with diarrhea and dehydration is admitted to the hospital from a long-term care facility. For which of the following symptoms of dehydration should the nurse assess?
   1. Pale-colored urine, bradycardia
   2. Disorientation, poor skin turgor
   3. Decreased hematocrit, hypothermia
   4. Lung congestion, abdominal discomfort

3. Which patient is most at risk for fluid excess?
   1. An infant with pneumonia
   2. A teen with multiple injuries following an automobile accident
   3. A middle-aged man who has just had surgery
   4. An older adult patient receiving intravenous therapy

4. A patient gains 2 pounds in 24 hours, weighed on the same scale at 7 a.m. Approximately how much water weight is represented by the 2 pounds?
   1. 8 ounces
   2. 16 ounces
   3. 24 ounces
   4. 32 ounces

5. When caring for a patient with fluid excess, which of the following interventions will best help relieve respiratory distress?
   1. Elevate the head of the bed.
   2. Encourage the patient to cough and deep breathe.
   3. Increase fluids to promote urine output.
   4. Perform percussion and postural drainage.

6. A patient is being discharged following hospitalization for fluid imbalance. Which instruction by the nurse should take priority?
   1. "Weigh yourself at the same time three times a week and report changes."
   2. "Call your doctor immediately if you feel weak or fatigued."
   3. "Drink eight glasses of water a day."
   4. "Measure everything you drink, and measure how much you urinate each day."

7. A patient is being treated for hypokalemia. When evaluating response to potassium replacement therapy, which of the following assessment findings should the nurse observe for?
   1. Improving visual acuity
   2. Worsening constipation
   3. Decreasing serum glucose
   4. Increasing muscle strength

8. A patient is being placed on a potassium-losing diuretic. Which foods are high in potassium and should be recommended to the patient by the nurse? **Select all that apply.**
   1. Bread
   2. Potato
   3. Yogurt
   4. Banana
   5. Gelatin

9. Which patient is at risk for respiratory acidosis?
   1. The patient with uncontrolled diabetes mellitus
   2. The patient with chronic pulmonary disease
   3. The patient who is very anxious
   4. The patient who overuses antacids

10. Which pH value represents acidosis?
    1. 7.26
    2. 7.35
    3. 7.4
    4. 7.49

Answer rationales available in your online resources.

ANSWERS 1. 5; 2. 3, 4, 4, 5, 1; 6. 1; 7. 4; 8. 2, 3, 4; 9. 2; 10. 1

Key Points

Find the chapter key points in your online resources available through Davis Edge.

Additional Resources

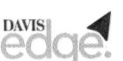 Use the scratch off code on the inside front cover of your book to access online quizzes that will help you to improve your scores on course exams and prepare for NCLEX-PN®.

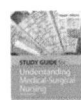 Study Guide

CHAPTER 7

Nursing Care of Patients Receiving Intravenous Therapy

Gladdi Tomlinson, Deb Richardson

KEY TERMS

cannula (KAN-yoo-lah)
extravasation (eks-TRAH-vah-ZAY-shun)
hematoma (HEE-muh-TOH-mah)
hypodermoclysis (HY-poh-DUR-moh-CLY-sis)
infiltration (in-fil-TRAY-shun)
intravenous (IN-trah-VEE-nuss)
macrodrop (MACK-roh-DROP)
microdrop (MIKE-roh-DROP)
parenteral (pah-REN-ter-ul)
phlebitis (fleh-BY-tis)

CHAPTER CONCEPTS

Fluid and Electrolyte Balance
Nutrition
Safety

LEARNING OUTCOMES

1. Discuss how the practice of intravenous (IV) therapy is regulated.
2. List indications for IV therapy.
3. Plan nursing interventions to prevent IV therapy complications.
4. Identify common complications associated with IV therapy.
5. Calculate flow and drip rates for IV solutions.
6. Differentiate characteristics of isotonic, hypertonic, and hypotonic solutions.
7. Explain the differences between peripheral and central venous access devices.
8. Describe types of central venous access devices.
9. List indications for subcutaneous infusions (hypodermoclysis).

Mrs. Brown, 85 years old, is admitted to the hospital with weight loss of 6% of her total body weight due to gastroenteritis and diarrhea. Her blood pressure is 102/80, pulse is 96 beats per minute, and respirations are 14 per minute. Her physical assessment shows decreased skin turgor over the sternum; dry, cracked lips; and a weak, thready pulse. The health care provider (HCP) has ordered an intravenous administration of 5% dextrose and 0.45% sodium chloride to be started at 100 mL per hour. As you read this chapter, reflect on the challenges of fluid volume deficit in older adults and initiation of infusion therapy.

Intravenous (IV) therapy is the administration of fluids or medication via a needle or catheter (also called a **cannula**) directly into the bloodstream. Each state's nurse practice act governs the practice of IV therapy in that state. Some states' nurse practice acts now include IV therapy within the licensed practical nurse/licensed vocational nurse (LPN/LVN) role.

The Infusion Nurses Society (INS; www.ins1.org) is recognized as a global authority in infusion nursing and publishes standards of practice for infusion therapy. The INS (2016) standards of practice address the infusion-related scope of practice for LPNs and LVNs. The Centers for Disease Control and Prevention (CDC, 2002; www.cdc.gov) provides guidelines for isolation precautions, hand hygiene, and prevention of intravascular catheter-related infections. The Institute for Healthcare Improvement (IHI, 2012; www.ihi.org) provides information related to central line care. The National Institute for Occupational Safety and Health (NIOSH; www.cdc.gov/NIOSH) oversees workplace safety, including safety issues related to IV therapy. The American Society for Parenteral and Enteral Nutrition (ASPEN; www.nutritioncare.org) provides resources related to IV nutrition.

LEARNING TIP

National organizations provide guidelines, but you must look at your state nurse practice act to decide which of those guidelines apply to you!

• WORD • BUILDING •

intravenous: intra—within + venous—vein

INDICATIONS FOR INTRAVENOUS THERAPY

A variety of substances can be administered via IV therapy, including fluids, electrolytes, nutrients, blood products, and medications. Why do patients receive IV therapy? Many medications are faster acting and more effective when given via the IV route. Fast action is especially important in an emergency. Medications can also be administered continuously via IV to maintain a therapeutic blood level. Patients with anemia or blood loss can receive lifesaving IV blood transfusions. Patients can receive life-sustaining fluids, electrolytes, and nutrition via IV when they are unable to eat or drink adequate amounts. Patients who are unable to eat for an extended period can have their nutritional needs met with parenteral nutrition. The term **parenteral** refers to any medication route other than the digestive tract.

TYPES OF INTRAVENOUS INFUSIONS

There are four primary administration modes for IV medications: (1) continuous, (2) intermittent, (3) direct injection/IV push, and (4) patient-controlled analgesia.

Continuous Infusion

A continuous infusion is a large-volume infusion of solution or medications (typically 250 to 1,000 mL) administered over 2 to 24 hours. For a continuous infusion, the HCP orders the infusion in millilitres (mL) to be delivered over a specific amount of time, such as 100 mL per hour or 1,000 mL over 8 hours. The infusion is kept running at the prescribed rate until ordered to be discontinued.

> ### BE SAFE!
> ***BE VIGILANT!*** Always verify that orders are complete and understandable. If you have any questions, contact the registered nurse, health care provider, or pharmacist.

Continuous infusions are used when a medication must be highly diluted, a constant plasma concentration of a drug must be maintained, or a large volume of fluids and electrolytes must be administered. Rate control is important in the delivery of continuous infusions. It can be achieved by using an electronic infusion device (EID), mechanical controller, or roller clamp.

Intermittent Infusion

Some IV medications, such as antibiotics, need to be infused over a short period of time. For example, an antibiotic may be mixed with 50 to 100 mL of 5% dextrose or 0.9% sodium chloride solution and infused over 30 to 60 minutes. This is often done as an intermittent infusion. As with any IV therapy,

the HCP orders must specify route, drug, dose, and amount to be infused over a specified time.

Primary Intermittent Infusion

Intermittent medications and solutions can be delivered using primary intermittent administration tubing that is connected and disconnected with each use. Access to the bloodstream can be provided by a short peripheral vascular access device, sometimes called a *saline lock,* in which an IV cannula is inserted and covered with a sterile needleless cap or valve that seals after each use.

> ### BE SAFE!
> ***BE VIGILANT!*** Each time a primary intermittent set is disconnected, the tip of the tubing must be kept sterile using a sterile end cap. The intermittent cannula is flushed with saline or heparin (10 u/mL or 100 u/mL) to keep it patent while it is not in use.

Piggyback (Secondary) Intermittent Infusion

If the patient already has a primary continuous IV infusing, the antibiotic (secondary) infusion can be "piggybacked" into the primary IV line. This piggyback set is left attached to the primary administration set. For the piggyback medication to infuse, it must hang higher than the primary infusion (Fig. 7.1). Piggyback medications can be infused using an EID, mechanical controller, or roller clamp.

> ### BE SAFE!
> ***BE VIGILANT!*** The medication in the piggyback tubing must be compatible with any other solution that is in the primary intravenous tubing. Check with your pharmacy for compatibilities.

NEEDLELESS CONNECTORS. Needleless connectors are devices that allow connection to IV catheters (such as piggybacking into a primary IV line), administration sets, and syringes without using a needle. They are important for avoiding needle stick injuries in nurses. Other terms used to describe such connectors are *injection cap, port,* or *injection valve.*

The hub or extension set of a peripheral cannula that is covered with a needleless connector is sometimes called a saline lock (Fig. 7.2). Intermittent IV lines can be "capped off" with a needleless connector. This makes them available for intermittent or emergency access. In addition, because the needleless connector does not have to be removed to allow access, a sterile closed infusion system is maintained.

• WORD • BUILDING •
parenteral: para—beside + enteral—intestines

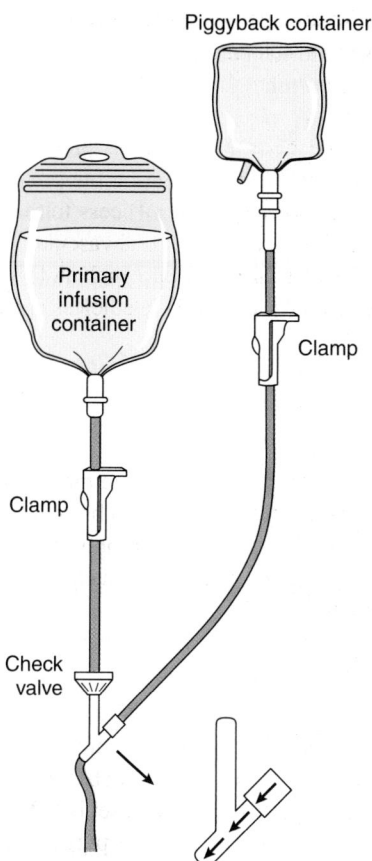

FIGURE 7.1 Gravity drip setup with piggyback infusion.

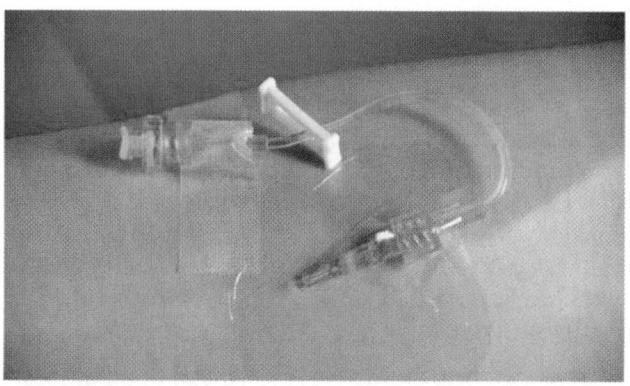

FIGURE 7.2 Peripheral IV with needleless connector attached to extension tubing.

The patency (unobstructed flow) of an intermittent cannula must be maintained by flushing at periodic intervals based on institution flushing policy and procedure. Always check for patency of an intermittent device before administering a medication. Do this by first scrubbing the hub. Attach the syringe and draw back to check for backflow of blood. If blood is seen in the syringe, the catheter is patent. Once patency is confirmed, flush with normal saline (0.9% sodium chloride). To maintain patency of a cannula, flush the cannula after each use or at least every 12 hours if not in use or

according to institution policy. In addition to ensuring patency, flushing with saline also prevents the mixing of incompatible medications and solutions. The INS recommends the use of sodium chloride for maintaining peripheral intermittent devices. Heparin, an anticoagulant, is recommended for flushing central venous access devices (CVADs). Remember that heparin is a medication and may be incompatible with other medications. Check your institution's policy for specific guidelines.

> **BE SAFE!**
> **BE VIGILANT! "SCRUB THE HUB"** for 10 to 15 seconds using friction before **each** access to prevent infection!

Positive pressure must be maintained in the lumen of the cannula during the administration of the flush solution. This prevents a backflow of blood or solution into the cannula lumen, which could lead to an occlusion. Positive pressure maintains a closed infusion system within the needleless connector.

If resistance is met while a cannula is being flushed, a clot may be occluding the cannula. Do not exert pressure on the syringe plunger in an attempt to restore patency. Doing so may dislodge the clot into the vascular system or rupture the cannula.

> **BE SAFE!**
> **BE VIGILANT!** Always check for cannula patency and follow manufacturer's guidelines for use before injecting any substance into the circulatory system. Forced flushing could cause a clot to dislodge from the cannula into the patient's circulatory system.

Direct Injection/Intravenous Push

An IV push, or direct injection medication, is injected slowly, between 1 and 10 minutes, via a syringe into an IV site or port. An IV push provides a rapid effect because it is delivered directly into the patient's bloodstream. IV push drugs can be dangerous if they are given incorrectly. A drug reference should always be checked to determine the safe amount of time over which the drug can be injected. IV push drugs are usually administered by registered nurses (RNs). They are not within the scope of practice of the LPN/LVN in some states. However, be aware of the drugs being given so you can assist in observing the patient for desired or adverse effects.

Patient-Controlled Analgesia

Patient-controlled analgesia (PCA) is used to deliver analgesic or pain medications. An EID or pump is used to deliver the analgesic drug. The EID is programmed to administer the prescribed amount to the patient when the patient presses a button. PCA administrations are usually done by RNs. They may not be within the scope of practice of the LPN/LVN. Verify with your state nurse practice act to determine whether PCA administration is within the LPN/LVN scope of practice. Again, be aware of the drugs being given so you can assist in observing the patient for desired or adverse effects.

METHODS OF INFUSION

Gravity Drip

Gravity can be used to administer a solution into a vein (see Fig. 7.1). The solution is positioned about 3 feet above the infusion site. If it is positioned too high above the patient, the infusion may run too fast. If positioned too low, it may run too slowly. Flow is controlled with a roller or screw clamp. A mechanical flow device can be added to achieve more accurate delivery of fluid.

Calculating Administration Rates

When using a gravity set, you must calculate the infusion rate and/or the drops (i.e., gtt, L. *guttae*) required per minute to deliver fluid at the ordered rate. Commercial parenteral administration sets vary in the number of drops delivering 1 mL of fluid. Sets typically deliver 10, 15, 20, or 60 drops per mL of fluid. Check the label on the administration set to determine how many drops per mL (known as the *drop factor*) are delivered by the set. Sets delivering 10, 15, or 20 drops per mL are called **macrodrop** sets. These are used for fluids that need to be infused more quickly. Sets delivering 60 drops per mL are called **microdrop** or minidrop sets. These are used for solutions that need to be infused more slowly.

To determine drops per minute for IV solution delivery, the nurse needs to know the amount of fluid to be given in a specified time interval and the drop factor of the administration set to be used. The formula for determining drops per minute is as follows:

$$\frac{mL}{hr \text{ or } hrs} \mid \frac{1 \text{ hr}}{60 \text{ min}} \mid \frac{gtt}{1 \text{ mL}} = gtt \text{ per minute}$$

LEARNING TIP
Always round to the nearest whole number when calculating drops per minute. You can't deliver a fraction of a drop!

The formula for determining milliliters per hour is as follows:

$$\frac{\text{Total \# of mL}}{\text{Total number of hrs}} = mL \text{ per hour}$$

SAMPLE PROBLEMS. Order: 125 mL of 5% dextrose and 0.45% sodium chloride per hour
Drop factor: 15 gtt/mL

$$\frac{125 \text{ mL}}{1 \text{ hr}} \mid \frac{1 \text{ hr}}{60 \text{ min}} \mid \frac{15 \text{ gtt}}{1 \text{ mL}} = 31 \text{ gtt per minute}$$

Order: Normal saline 1,000 mL over 8 hours

$$\frac{1000 \text{ mL}}{8 \text{ hours}} = 125 \text{ mL per hour}$$

Factors Affecting Flow Rates of Gravity Infusions

CHANGE IN CANNULA POSITION. A change in the position of the cannula's tip can affect the infusion flow rate. If the *bevel* (the slanted opening of the cannula) is against the wall of the vein, the flow rate will decrease; if it is away from the wall of the vein, the flow rate can increase. Placement of a peripheral IV (or PIV) in a joint area (wrist or elbow) can cause a kink in the cannula or change the tip position. This can cause a change in the flow rate. Securing the cannula carefully and avoiding areas of joint flexion will minimize this problem. Patients may need to be reminded to keep flexion to a minimum when an IV is placed near a joint.

BE SAFE!
BE VIGILANT! If the only useable vein is in an area of flexion, secure the peripheral IV (PIV) appropriately. Remind patients to keep flexion to a minimum. Closely monitor the PIV site and flow rate.

HEIGHT OF THE SOLUTION. Because infusions flow by gravity, a change in the height of the infusion bag or bottle or a change in the level of the bed can increase or decrease the flow rate. The flow rate increases as the distance between the solution and the patient increases. A patient may inadvertently alter the flow rate greatly simply by standing up. The ideal height for a solution is 3 feet above the level of the patient's heart.

PATENCY OF THE CANNULA. A small clot or fibrin sheath can occlude the cannula lumen and decrease the flow rate or stop the flow completely. A fibrin sheath begins developing within the first 24 hours of the cannula insertion. Clot formation can result from irritation, vein wall injury from the insertion or tip position, increased venous pressure, or backup of blood into the cannula. Avoid use of a blood pressure cuff on the affected limb because of the resulting transient increase in venous pressure. A regular flush schedule helps maintain patency.

• WORD • BUILDING •
macrodrop: macro—large + drop
microdrop: micro—small + drop

BE SAFE!

BE VIGILANT! **Never** exert pressure with a saline or heparin flush in an attempt to restore patency. Doing so could dislodge a clot into the vascular system or rupture the cannula.

Mechanical and Electronic Infusion Devices

Flow control devices, such as EIDs and mechanical controllers, regulate the rate of infusion and are used in all health care settings (Fig. 7.3). Mechanical controllers measure the amount of solution delivered and depend on gravity to deliver the infusion. EIDs, sometimes called pumps, use positive pressure to deliver the solution.

Pumps and controllers are used for infusing precise volumes and rates of solution. Institution policy often dictates use of controllers for infusion of potent medications, such as heparin, concentrated morphine, and chemotherapy solutions, and for very fast or slow rates. Some EIDs are portable and designed to be worn on the body. These are called ambulatory infusion devices. It is important to know the type of pump being used and to follow the manufacturer's guidelines.

Filters

Filters can either be add-on devices to administration sets or built into the set during manufacturing. Various types of filters are available. The INS (2016) standards address the use of inline filters to remove bacteria, fungi, particulate matter, air, and some endotoxins from IV fluids. Check institution policy and manufacturers' guidelines for use of filters.

TYPES OF FLUIDS

There are three basic types of IV solutions: isotonic, hypotonic, and hypertonic (see Chapter 6). Fluids and electrolytes administered via the IV route pass directly into the plasma space of the extracellular fluid compartment. They are then absorbed based on the characteristics of the fluid and the

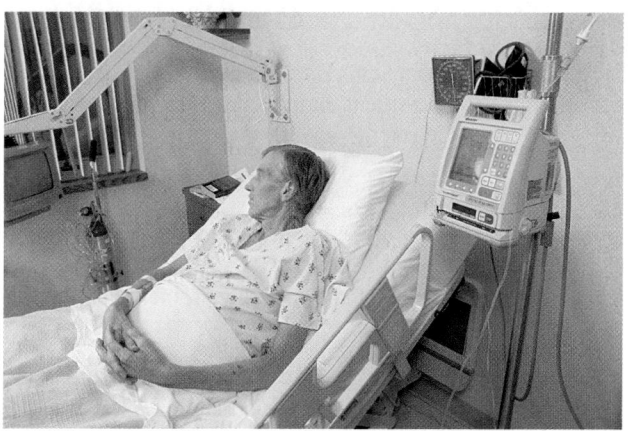

FIGURE 7.3 Infusion pump.

hydration status of the patient. The most commonly infused fluids are dextrose and sodium solutions. These are called crystalloid solutions.

Crystalloid Solutions

Dextrose Solutions

Dextrose in water is available in many concentrations (2.5%, 5%, and 10%). It is typically used for continuous peripheral infusions. Concentrations exceeding 10% and above must be infused via a central line into a large vein.

Advantages of dextrose solutions are as follows:

• They provide carbohydrates in a readily usable form for energy, reducing breakdown of glycogen and catabolism of protein to help prevent negative nitrogen balance.
• They act as a means for administration of medications.
• High concentrations can be used for treating hypoglycemia or in combination with parenteral nutrition because they supply a large number of calories.

Disadvantages of dextrose solutions are as follows:

• Vein irritation, damage, and thrombosis can result when hypertonic dextrose solutions are administered in a peripheral vein.

Sodium Chloride Solutions

Sodium chloride solutions are available in concentrations of 0.25%, 0.33%, 0.45%, 0.9% (normal saline), 3%, and 5%. Sodium chloride 0.45% and 0.9% solutions are used most commonly.

Advantages of sodium chloride solutions are as follows:

• They are useful for fluid replacement; treatment of shock, hyponatremia, and metabolic alkalosis; as a primer for blood transfusions; and during resuscitation after trauma. According to the American Association of Blood Banks, blood component administration sets can be primed only with 0.9% sodium chloride solution (Fung, Grossman, Hillyer, & Westhoff, 2014).
• Combination dextrose and sodium chloride solutions, such as 5% dextrose with 0.45% sodium chloride (often referred to as "D$_5$ and a half"), are commonly used for hydration and to check for kidney function before administration of potassium replacement therapy.

Disadvantages of sodium chloride solutions are as follows:

• They can cause circulatory overload if the prescribed rate is not monitored.
• If the patient is unable to excrete excess sodium (e.g., because of kidney disease or hormonal imbalance), hypernatremia can result.
• Acidosis can occur with continuous infusions.

Balanced Electrolyte Solutions

Electrolyte solutions are used to replace lost fluids and electrolytes. A variety of balanced electrolyte solutions are available commercially. Maintenance electrolyte solutions, such as lactated Ringer's solution, supply normal body electrolyte needs. Balanced solutions often contain lactate or acetate (yielding bicarbonate), which helps combat acidosis and provides a truly balanced solution. Potassium is an electrolyte that is commonly added to balanced solutions to replace potassium deficits. The patient must be monitored for signs and symptoms related to potassium imbalance (see Chapter 6).

BE SAFE!

BE VIGILANT! Be sure to review institution guidelines for potassium administration before administration of any potassium-containing solution. An inappropriate rate or amount can cause a life-threatening cardiac arrhythmia!

Osmolarity of Intravenous Solutions

The osmolarity of an IV solution refers to its osmotic activity. As noted previously, IV fluids may be classified as isotonic, hypotonic, or hypertonic. (See Chapter 6 to review these concepts.) Isotonic fluids have the same concentration of solutes to water as body fluids. Hypertonic solutions have more solutes (i.e., are more concentrated) than body fluids. Hypotonic solutions have fewer solutes (i.e., are less concentrated) than body fluids. Water moves from areas of lesser concentration to areas of greater concentration. Therefore, hypotonic solutions send water into areas of greater concentration (cells), and hypertonic solutions pull water from cells.

Isotonic Solutions

Normal saline (0.9% sodium chloride) solution is an isotonic solution that has the same tonicity as body fluid. When administered to patients requiring water, it neither enters cells nor pulls water from cells; it therefore expands the extracellular fluid volume. A solution of 5% dextrose in water (D_5W) is also isotonic when infused. However, the dextrose is quickly metabolized, making the solution hypotonic. Lactated Ringer's solution and 5% albumin are other examples of isotonic solutions. Isotonic solutions commonly treat dehydration, fluid loss, and hyponatremia.

BE SAFE!

BE VIGILANT! Since isotonic solutions expand the extracellular fluid volume, be vigilant for signs of fluid overload when infusing isotonic solutions.

Hypotonic Solutions

Hypotonic fluids are used when fluid is needed to enter the cells, as in the patient with cellular dehydration. They are also used as fluid maintenance therapy. Examples of hypotonic solutions are dextrose 2.5% water and 0.33% or 0.45% sodium chloride solution.

BE SAFE!

BE VIGILANT! Hypotonic solutions, because they enter cells, can worsen hypotension, cause cardiovascular collapse, and increase intracranial pressure.

Hypertonic Solutions

Examples of hypertonic solutions include 5% dextrose in 0.9% sodium chloride, 3% sodium chloride, calcium chloride 10%, 5% dextrose in lactated Ringer's solution, 10% dextrose in water, and albumin 25%. Hypertonic solutions are used to expand the plasma volume, for example, in a hypovolemic patient. They are also used to replace electrolytes.

BE SAFE!

BE VIGILANT! Monitor the patient receiving a hypertonic solution for circulatory overload.

INTRAVENOUS ACCESS

IV therapy can be administered into the systemic circulation via the peripheral or central veins. Peripheral veins lie beneath the epidermis, dermis, and subcutaneous tissue of the skin. They usually provide easy access to the venous system.

Central veins are deeper and located closer to the heart. A CVAD is a special catheter with a tip that ends in a large vessel (i.e., superior vena cava) near the heart. This chapter primarily focuses on short peripheral catheters. The definitions of the various types of CVADs are discussed briefly at the end of the chapter.

See "Initiating Peripheral Intravenous Therapy" under Procedures in your online resources for a detailed explanation of how to initiate a peripheral IV cannula.

NURSING PROCESS FOR THE PATIENT RECEIVING INTRAVENOUS THERAPY

IV therapy is a medical intervention. The nurse is responsible for appropriate assessment, monitoring, documentation, and reporting related to the therapeutic goals.

Data Collection

Some institutions require assessment as often as every hour. An INS position paper (Gorski et al., 2012) provides some guidance on frequency of site assessment, including the following recommendations:

- Assess at least every 4 hours for patients not getting an irritant or vesicant and who are alert and oriented.
- Assess every 2 hours for critically ill patients and adult patients who have cognitive sensory deficits, are receiving

sedative medications or unable to notify the nurse of any problems, or have an IV placed in a joint area or external jugular vein.
• Assess every hour for pediatric or neonatal patients.

Assessment should be systematic and thorough. It should include physiological and psychosocial data, critical laboratory values, allergies and environmental issues, and presence of adverse reactions or complications related to infusion therapy. Older adults are at increased risk for complications, making careful assessment essential ("Gerontological Issues").

Gerontological Issues

Care of the Older Adult Receiving Intravenous Therapy. When an older patient is receiving intravenous (IV) fluids, regularly assess the patient for potential fluid volume excess. Symptoms of fluid volume excess include the following:

• Elevated blood pressure
• Increasing weight (a weight gain of 2.2 lb is equal to the retention of 1 L of body water)
• Peripheral edema
• Full bounding pulse
• Shallow, rapid respirations
• Jugular venous distention
• Increased urine output
• Development of moist crackles in the lungs
• Cyanosis (a late symptom of pulmonary edema)

   If the above signs are present:

• Immediately notify the registered nurse (RN) or turn down the IV to a minimum drip rate (1 mL per minute); do not discontinue the IV because the health care provider (HCP) may want to order IV diuretics.
• Position the patient to maximize lung expansion.
• Check peripheral oxygen saturation with an oximeter.
• Apply oxygen by mask or nasal cannula if indicated and per institution guidelines.
• Closely monitor the patient's vital signs, level of consciousness, and oxygen saturation along with fluid output.
• Assist the HCP or RN with IV push administration of diuretic medication such as furosemide if ordered.

Physical assessments, such as daily weights and measurement of intake and output, help determine whether the patient is retaining too much fluid. Skin turgor, mucous membrane moisture, vital signs, and level of consciousness also indicate hydration status. New onset of fine crackles in the lungs can indicate fluid retention. Table 7.1 lists other symptoms of complications, along with prevention and treatment strategies.

Inspect the insertion site for redness or swelling, evaluate the integrity of the dressing, and document your findings.

Inspect the tubing to ensure tight connections and the absence of kinks or defects. Inspect the solution container and compare it with the HCP's order for type, amount, and rate. Report abnormal findings to the RN or HCP.

CRITICAL THINKING

Mr. Rick has blood backed up in his intravenous tubing. When you open the clamp to increase the flow, nothing happens. What should you do?
   Suggested answer is at the end of the chapter.

Nursing Diagnoses, Planning, and Implementation

Priority nursing diagnoses for IV-related issues may include the following:

Fluid Volume Excess related to IV fluid administration

EXPECTED OUTCOME: The patient will have stable fluid balance as evidenced by stable vital signs, stable weight, and clear lung sounds (see "Gerontological Issues").

Fear related to insertion of IV cannula

EXPECTED OUTCOME: The patient will have minimal fear as evidenced by cooperation with the procedure and verbalizing minimal fear.

• Explain the IV therapy (e.g., rationale for therapy, insertion procedure, care of the IV, and importance of reporting pain, swelling, or pump alarm) to the patient. *Lack of knowledge is associated with fear.*
• Use techniques to minimize discomfort. *Pain may increase fear.*

Impaired Physical Mobility related to placement and maintenance of IV cannula

EXPECTED OUTCOME: The patient will maintain mobility as evidenced by full range of motion and avoidance of complications related to immobility.

• Avoid insertion site close to joints if at all possible. *Joint areas are mobile, making it difficult to maintain an intact site.*
• If you must use a mobile site, such as the antecubital fossa or wrist area, immobilize the joint with arm board or other immobilizer *to reduce cannula movement. (Remember to get an order for this.)*
• If site must be wrapped to protect from movement, be sure to leave insertion site visible or remove wrapping to view site according to agency policy. *The site must still be visualized for complications even if it is covered.*
• Assist patient with activities of daily living (ADLs). *The patient may have difficulty with ADLs if movement is limited.*

Table 7.1

Complications of Peripheral Intravenous Therapy

Complication	Signs and Symptoms	Prevention	Treatment
Local Complications of Intravenous (IV) Therapy			
Hematoma	• Ecchymoses • Swelling • Inability to advance cannula • Resistance during flushing	• Use indirect method of venipuncture. • Choose smallest cannula appropriate. • Apply tourniquet just before venipuncture.	• Remove cannula. • Apply pressure with 2″ × 2″ gauze. • Elevate extremity. • Apply cold compress.
Thrombosis	• Slowed or stopped infusion • Fever/malaise • Inability to flush or aspirate cannula	• Use an electronic infusion device (EID). • Choose microdrop sets with gravity flow if rate is less than 50 mL/hr. • Avoid use of flexion areas for insertion site.	• Discontinue cannula. • Apply cold compress to site. • Assess for circulatory impairment. • Insert new cannula at another site.
Phlebitis	• Redness/warmth at site • Local swelling • Pain • Palpable cord along vein • Sluggish infusion rate	• Use larger veins for hypertonic solutions. • Choose smallest cannula appropriate. • Use good hand hygiene. • Add buffer to irritating solutions. • Change solutions and containers every 24 hours. • Assess peripheral IV (PIV) site per institution policy. • Remove cannula when clinically indicated.	• Discontinue cannula. • Apply cold compress initially; then warm. • Consult registered nurse (RN) or health care provider (HCP) if severe.
Infiltration or extravasation	• Coolness of skin at site • Taut skin • Edema above or below site • Absent backflow of blood • Sluggish infusion rate • Pain or burning • Blisters	• Place cannula in appropriate site. • Avoid antecubital fossa. • Stabilize cannula carefully. • Monitor PIV site per policy. • Instruct patient to notify RN immediately if any pain, burning, or swelling occurs.	• Discontinue cannula. • Apply cool/warm compress as indicated by solution type. • Elevate extremity. • Notify RN/HCP. • Follow agency infiltration/extravasation guidelines. • Have antidote available (if medication extravasates).
Local infection	• Redness and swelling at site • Possible exudate • Elevated white blood cell and T lymphocytes	• Inspect all solutions. • Use sterile technique during venipuncture and site maintenance.	• Discontinue cannula. • Culture site and cannula. • Apply sterile dressing over site. • Notify RN/HCP. • Administer antibiotics if ordered.
Venous spasm	• Sharp pain at site • Sluggish infusion	• Take thorough history. • Verify allergies. • Reduce infusion rate. • Dilute medications. • Keep IV solution at room temperature.	• Apply warm compress to site. • Restart infusion in new site if spasm continues. • Notify RN.

Table 7.1

Complications of Peripheral Intravenous Therapy—cont'd

Complication	Signs and Symptoms	Prevention	Treatment
Systemic Complications of Peripheral IV Therapy			
Septicemia	• Fever and chills • Profuse sweating • Nausea • Headache • Backache • Tachycardia/ tachypnea • Hypotension • Altered mental status • Decreased urine output	• Use good hand hygiene. • Use aseptic techniques for insertion/ maintenance of cannula, needleless connector, IV tubing, and solutions. • Carefully inspect fluids. • Cover infusion sites with appropriate dressings. • Follow standards of practice related to assessment and monitoring of PIV and hang time of infusions/IV tubing. • Use appropriate preparation solutions.	• Restart new IV system. • Obtain cultures. • Notify RN/HCP. • Initiate antimicrobial therapy as ordered. • Monitor patient closely.
Circulatory Overload	• Rapid weight gain • Puffy eyelids • Edema • Increased blood pressure and pulse • Changes in input and output (I&O) • Rise in central venous pressure • Shortness of breath • Crackles in lungs • Cough • Distended neck veins	• Monitor infusion. • Maintain flow at prescribed rate. • Monitor I&O. • Know patient's cardiovascular history. • Do not "catch up" infusion if behind schedule. • Be alert that older patients are more prone to this and monitor closely.	• **CALL FOR HELP!** • Decrease IV flow rate. • Place patient in high Fowler position. • Keep patient warm. • Monitor vital signs. • Administer oxygen. • Use an EID with dose-error reduction system and anti-free-flow administration set. • Notify RN/HCP.
Venous air embolism	• Light-headedness • Dyspnea, cyanosis, tachypnea, expiratory wheezes, cough • Chest pain, hypotension • Changes in mental status	• Remove all air from administration sets. • Use Luer Lock connections. • Follow protocol for catheter removal. • Check for cracks in tubing/catheter hub.	• **CALL FOR HELP!** • Place patient in Trendelenburg position on left side. • Administer oxygen. • Monitor vital signs. • Notify RN/HCP.
Speed shock	• Dizziness • Facial and neck flushing • Pounding headache • Tightness in chest • Hypotension • Irregular pulse • Progression of shock	• Use an EID. • Monitor infusion site and rate. • Give IV push medications over appropriate time.	• **CALL FOR HELP!** • Notify RN/HCP. • Stop infusion immediately. • Give antidote or resuscitation medications as ordered.

Source: Adapted from Phillips, L. D., & Gorski, L. A. (2014). *Manual of IV therapeutics: Evidence-based practice for infusion therapy* (6th ed.). Philadelphia, PA: F.A. Davis.

Risk for Infection related to broken skin or traumatized tissue

EXPECTED OUTCOME: The patient will be free from infection as evidenced by no redness, swelling, or purulence at IV insertion site; no fever; and normal white cell count.

- Watch for signs of infection *so the IV can be removed and/or site rotated and infection treated quickly if it occurs.*
- Use good hand hygiene and strict aseptic techniques during cannula insertion and maintenance care *to prevent introduction of pathogens.*
- Change tubing and solutions regularly according to agency policy *to prevent growth of microorganisms.*
- Change or remove cannula when clinically indicated *to reduce prolonged risk.*

Evaluation

The RN is responsible for evaluation of outcomes and thus monitors the patient for evidence that the goals of therapy are being met and that complications are avoided. The LPN/LVN collects data that contribute to the evaluation. For example, if antibiotic therapy is administered, monitor for signs that the infection is resolving. If IV therapy is ordered to correct dehydration, monitor for improved fluid balance. Document all findings and report them to the RN.

BE SAFE!

BE VIGILANT! To prevent infection, the Infusion Nurses Society (INS, 2016) standards of practice state, "In addition to routine changes, the administration set (tubing) is changed whenever the peripheral catheter site is changed or when a new central vascular access device (CVAD) is placed." The INS (2016) also instructs clinicians to replace or remove any peripheral intravenous cannula placed in an emergency situation within 48 hours of the insertion or as soon as possible.

 ## COMPLICATIONS OF IV THERAPY

Complications of infusion therapy fall into two categories: local and systemic. Any complication or unusual incident should be reported to the RN or HCP. A quality improvement report should be prepared according to institution policy.

The most common peripheral local complications are **hematoma, phlebitis,** or thrombophlebitis, **infiltration, extravasation,** and nerve injury (see Table 7.1). The INS (2016) lists the dorsal hand, radial wrist, and inner wrist as sites to avoid to prevent permanent nerve injury. Systemic complications can be serious. They include circulatory overload, septicemia, venous air embolism, and speed shock (a sudden reaction due to medication that is delivered too quickly). The nurse delivering infusion therapy must be knowledgeable in preventing, recognizing, and treating all complications of IV therapy (INS, 2016). See Table 7.1 for complications, prevention, and related care.

CRITICAL THINKING

Mrs. Gonzalez is receiving 5% dextrose in water at 83 mL per hour. One hour after the infusion starts, she reports pain at the site. The site is cool to the touch and swollen, and the infusion rate is sluggish.

1. What might be happening?
2. What additional data should you collect?
3. What action should you take?
4. How should you document your findings?
5. What other team members could be consulted to help in this situation?

Suggested answers are at the end of the chapter.

 ## CENTRAL VENOUS ACCESS DEVICES

The role of the LPN/LVN in CVA care in most states is limited to assisting the RN with assessments. Therefore, it is important for you to be familiar with the different CVADs so you can recognize and report problems.

Central venous catheter tips terminate in the superior vena cava near the heart (Fig. 7.4). They are used when peripheral sites are inadequate. CVADs can be used to deliver all types of solutions, medications, blood, or blood products when continuous infusion is required. They are also beneficial when irritant or vesicant medication must be given into a large vein. CVADs include tunneled and nontunneled catheters, peripherally inserted central catheters, and implanted ports. These devices can have one, two, or three lumens in the catheter or one or more port chambers. Each lumen of a multilumen device exits the site in a separate line, called a tail. Multilumen devices allow simultaneous administration of solutions while preventing mixing of incompatible solutions.

Be careful not to confuse a central catheter with a dialysis catheter. Dialysis catheters should be used only for dialysis and not for IV therapy. Also, they should be accessed only by HCPs or specially trained dialysis nurses. If you are not sure what type of catheter your patient has, be sure to ask the RN or HCP.

Nontunneled Central Catheter

A nontunneled CVAD is inserted by an HCP into the jugular, subclavian, or femoral vein. After insertion, correct placement

---

- **WORD · BUILDING ·**

hematoma: hemat—blood + oma—tumor
phlebitis: phleb—vein + itis—inflammation
infiltration: in—inside + filtrate—to strain through + tion—condition
extravasation: extra—outside + vas—vessel + tion—condition

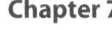

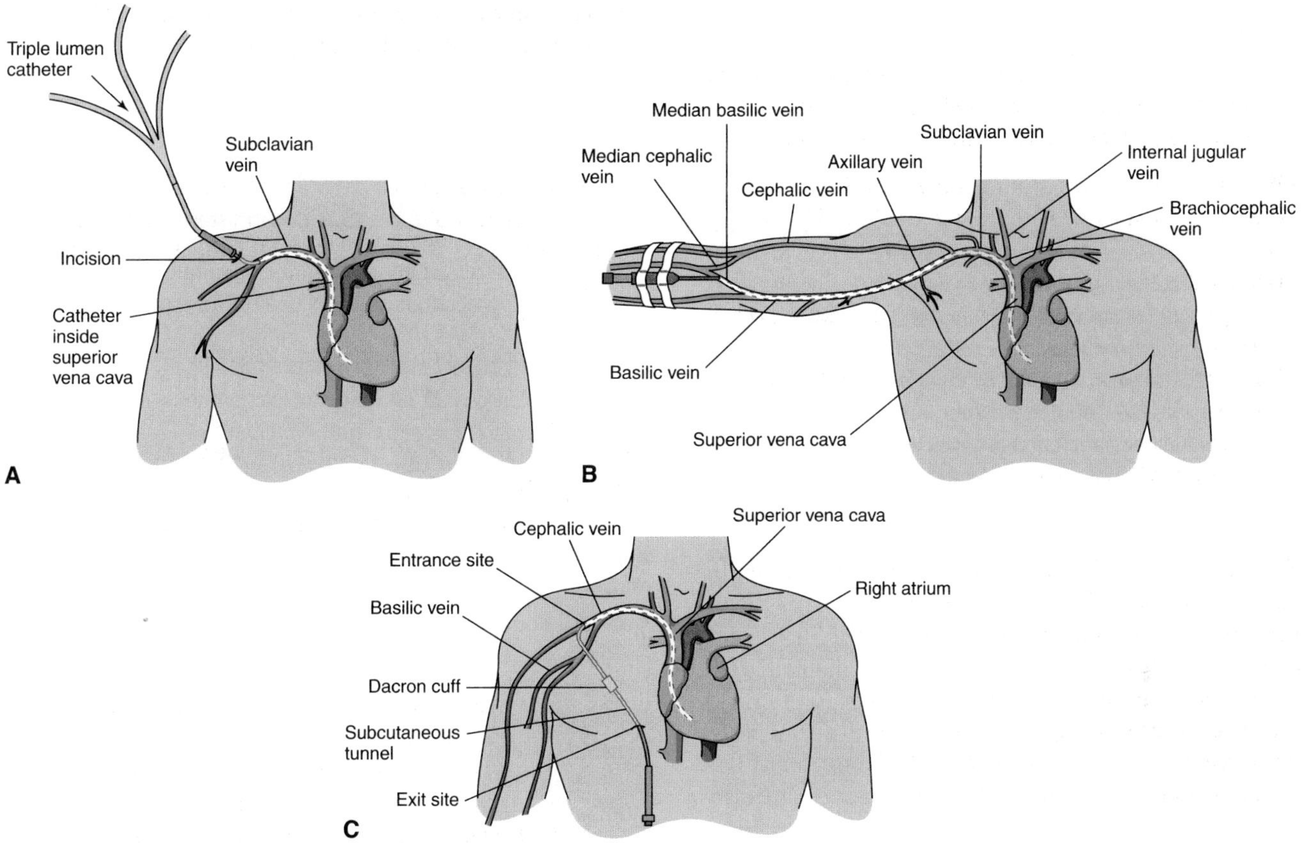

FIGURE 7.4 Central lines. (A) Triple-lumen subclavian catheter. (B) PICC line. (C) Tunneled catheter.

is determined by x-ray before the catheter is used. These short-term CVADs may remain in place up to several weeks, but placement time is typically about 7 days. Nontunneled CVADs can be inserted at the bedside or in an outpatient setting. They are cost effective for short-term CAV. Nontunneled CVADs can be used for many purposes and can be easily exchanged. However, there are disadvantages, such as ongoing maintenance care and body image issues.

Tunneled Catheters

Tunneled catheters are used when venous access is needed for months to years. These catheters are typically composed of polymeric silicone with a Dacron polyester cuff. The cuff not only anchors the catheter in place subcutaneously but also provides a barrier to prevent bacteria from migrating to the tip of the catheter. The catheter tip is commonly placed in the superior vena cava (see Fig. 7.4C).

Advantages of a tunneled catheter are that a break or tear in a catheter is easy to repair, and they can be used for many purposes. Disadvantages include such concerns as weekly site care, cost of maintenance supplies, and the effect on the patient's body image.

Peripherally Inserted Central Catheter

A peripherally inserted central catheter (PICC) is a long catheter that is inserted in the arm and terminates in the central vasculature (see Fig. 7.4B). A PICC can be tunneled or nontunneled. This device is used when therapy will last more than 2 weeks or the medication is too caustic for peripheral administration. Specially trained RNs can insert PICC lines. They can be left in place for long periods, minimizing the trauma of frequent IV insertions. Consult with the HCP for a PICC order if long-term therapy is anticipated.

It is important to follow the manufacturer's recommended guidelines for flushing the catheter and to be aware of your institution's PICC policy. A trained RN removes the PICC catheter when therapy is terminated. An LPN/LVN may assist the RN with this procedure if the state nurse practice act permits.

Ports

A port is a reservoir that is surgically implanted into a pocket created under the skin, usually in the upper chest. A catheter is attached to the reservoir and is tunneled under the skin into a central vein, such as the superior vena cava. An advantage of a port is that, when not in use, a dressing is not required. It can also be flushed and left unused for long periods. When the port is not in use, the patient can swim and shower without risk of contaminating the site.

Ports come in a variety of sizes and styles. They are now being placed in many areas of the body. Ports are suitable for long-term therapy. They can be used to administer all types of medications, including chemotherapeutic agents and antibiotics that are toxic to tissues. In addition, power injectable ports can be used for radiology imaging and procedures. Ports are usually accessed only by specially trained RNs. They require the use of noncoring needles that are specifically designed for port access and infusions.

BE SAFE!

BE VIGILANT! Implement evidence-based practices to prevent central line–associated bloodstream infections. This requirement covers short- and long-term central venous catheters and peripherally inserted central catheters, per the 2018 National Patient Safety Goals. (© The Joint Commission, 2017. Printed with permission.) Vascular catheter–related infections are considered "never events" because they can be prevented and should never occur. Hospitals will not be paid by Medicare for such infections acquired during hospitalization.

 OTHER THERAPIES

Parenteral Nutrition

Parenteral nutrition (PN) is complete IV nutrition that is administered to patients who cannot take adequate nutrients via the enteral route (by mouth or tube feeding). PN may be used to promote nutrition for wound healing, to help a patient achieve optimal weight before surgery, or to avoid malnutrition from chronic disease or after surgery. Patients with ulcerative colitis, trauma, or cancer cachexia (wasting syndrome) are candidates for PN. Every effort should be made to return a patient on PN to oral or tube feedings as soon as possible.

PN provides and maintains the essential nutrients required by the body. Solutions contain carbohydrates, amino acids, lipid emulsions, electrolytes, trace elements, and vitamins in varied amounts according to the patient's needs. Due to the components in PN, compatibility issues must be considered. Therefore, medications should not be piggybacked directly into PN solutions. PN requires filtration and an EID for administration. A 0.22 micron filter is required for lipid-free PN. PN solutions with lipids must have a 1.2 micron filter. Patients receiving PN in the home setting may use an ambulatory infusion device to allow for more mobility.

Initial assessment includes the patient's height, weight, nutritional status, and current laboratory values. Because of the high glucose concentration of PN, the patient is at risk for infection and blood glucose disturbances. Insulin therapy may be necessary during PN administration. Ongoing assessments include blood glucose levels according to institution policy and monitoring for signs and symptoms of infection, hyperglycemia, and hypoglycemia. When PN therapy is begun, the rate is increased gradually to the prescribed rate to help prevent hyperglycemia.

When nutritional solutions contain concentrations exceeding 10% dextrose or 5% protein, they must be administered via a CVAD. When concentrations are less than 10% dextrose or 5% protein, they may be administered through a peripheral vein. This is referred to as peripheral parenteral nutrition (PPN). PPN is a short-term intervention because it does not provide adequate nutrition over an extended period. Some states allow LVN/LPNs to initiate PPN.

The entire health care team must be involved in PN or PPN therapy. The pharmacist, dietitian, HCP, and nurse communicate in a team conference to discuss the assessment, plan, and outcome criteria. Many institutions have nutrition teams that assess the appropriateness of PN or PPN for individual patients.

Home Intravenous Therapy

As health care costs continue to rise, patients are using more alternatives to hospitalization. Subacute care, skilled nursing care in long-term care facilities, and home health care are growing. Home IV therapy allows many patients the benefit of early discharge and the ability to receive health care in the privacy and comfort of their own homes. Most patients requiring home infusion therapy will have a CVAD rather than a PIV. Some home health care agencies employ nurses to instruct patients and their families in the administration of home IV therapy (see "Home Health Hints"). Before discharge, the patient's benefits for reimbursement for home health care should be verified.

Home IV antibiotic therapy is becoming the method of choice for long-term treatment of certain infections, including bacterial endocarditis, osteomyelitis, and septic arthritis. Other patients with various diseases may choose to receive PN, chemotherapy, or IV pain medications at home. The health team can assess patients and their families for their ability to manage home IV therapy. Cleanliness of the home environment and the ability to safely store equipment in the home must be determined before discharge.

Home Health Hints

Before discharge:

- Obtain a referral for a home health nurse to coordinate intravenous (IV) therapy at home.
- Once the patient has selected a home health care agency, coordinate discharge from the hospital with the agency so that no IV doses will be missed.
- Provide home health care agency contact information to the patient.

At home:

- Instruct the patient to keep the IV site dry. If showering is permitted, instruct the patient to cover the IV with plastic (such as a grocery bag) and seal with tape on both ends to prevent water from entering the site.
- Assist the patient and caregiver to identify a safe place to store supplies. Note that some solutions or medications require refrigeration. Remind the patient to remove IV solution from the refrigerator 30 minutes prior to the arrival of the home health nurse.

Hypodermoclysis

An alternative option for administration of medications or fluids is subcutaneous infusion, or **hypodermoclysis.** This is becoming a more common route in pediatrics, palliative care, and hospice settings as well as for the elderly. Isotonic fluids and limited medications can be administered via this route (Arthur, 2015; Phillips & Gorski, 2014). Hypodermoclysis is recognized as a safe, low-risk, cost-effective route to treat dehydration and for use in patients with poor vein quality. Hypodermoclysis infusions were common in the 1950s, but complications and adverse reaction reports reduced the use of this infusion. Today, pharmacological companies are developing subcutaneous formulations of medications that will improve response, physiologic effect, and patient compliance. With new formulations, antiemetics, monoclonal antibodies, immunoglobulins, pain medications, and antibiotics are being studied as emerging therapies to be given via the subcutaneous route.

To access the subcutaneous route, a needle or catheter is placed below the dermis and epidermis in the fatty tissue. Fluid volume is limited at a site. To reduce the risk of edema, the administration rate is approximately 1 mL/minute. Fluids and medications administered via this route will pass through the extracellular matrix to be absorbed by the capillaries and the lymphatic system. Locations for subcutaneous access include the abdomen, thighs, upper arms, chest, and scapula area. Some advantages are slow absorption rate, decreased severity of infection, and minimal training. Site assessment and monitoring are crucial to limit complications. Patient education should include reporting pain, redness, swelling, or leaking at the site (Smith, 2014). Patients and caregivers can be taught how to obtain access and infuse the medications. Disadvantages include risk of edema, drug choice limitation, and less interaction with the home health nurse due to in-home self-administration (Arthur, 2015).

 REFLECTIONS ON MRS. BROWN

Think again about Mrs. Brown in the scenario at the beginning of the chapter. She will need monitoring of intake and output, daily weights, and close monitoring of her IV infusion. You should anticipate that serum electrolytes, blood urea nitrogen, and creatinine laboratory studies will be ordered. When initiating the infusion, use care in application of a tourniquet because older skin is thin and bruising can occur. Choose a number 20- or 22-gauge cannula to start the infusion. Once it is started, continue to monitor weights and lung sounds because older patients can quickly go from fluid depletion to fluid overload (see "Gerontological Issues").

• WORD • BUILDING •

hypodermoclysis: hypo – under + dermo—skin + clysis—infusion of fluid

SUGGESTED ANSWERS TO CRITICAL THINKING

Mr. Rick

Your patient's intravenous (IV) line is likely clotted. If it has been so for a long time, it will not be salvageable. Do not flush it because doing so can dislodge the clot into the circulation. Discontinue the IV line and insert a new cannula.

Mrs. Gonzalez

1. The IV fluid may be leaking at the insertion site and flowing into the subcutaneous tissue, a problem known as *infiltration* or *extravasation,* depending on the type of drug infusing.
2. Consider whether the pain could be caused by the buildup of fluid under the skin. Compare the insertion site with the opposite limb.

3. If the IV solution has infiltrated, stop the infusion, discontinue the cannula, and restart the cannula in a new site.
4. "Patient reports pain at IV site in right arm; area is cool to touch and edematous in 4.5-cm area around site. Flow rate sluggish. Infusion discontinued; IV restarted in left arm with 22-gauge cannula with good blood return. Infusing well with no signs of infiltration."
5. The registered nurse or IV therapy nurse would be good resources.

Review Questions

1. Which is the best resource for the nurse who has a question about the process and implementation of intravenous therapy for a specific patient?
   1. An experienced nurse
   2. Institution policy
   3. The physician
   4. Infusion Nurses Society standards of practice

2. Which patients have a need for intravenous therapy? **Select all that apply.**
   1. An 88-year-old man admitted to the hospital with dehydration
   2. A 21-year-old woman with an eating disorder and severe weight loss
   3. A 58-year-old woman with pneumonia who has been unresponsive to oral antibiotics
   4. A 37-year-old man recovering from a fall and broken arm
   5. A 4-year-old brought to the emergency room because of prolonged vomiting
   6. A patient with fluid overload who requires fast-acting diuretic therapy

3. A patient receiving intravenous therapy via a central line develops hypotension, cyanosis, and dyspnea. The nurse notes a crack in the intravenous tubing. After calling for help, what should the nurse do next?
   1. Raise the head of the bed.
   2. Clamp the tubing and administer oxygen.
   3. Monitor vital signs.
   4. Place tape over the tubing crack.

4. Which of the following solutions can be administered with a blood component?
   1. Lactated Ringer's solution
   2. 5% dextrose/0.2% sodium chloride (normal saline)
   3. 5% dextrose/0.45% sodium chloride (normal saline)
   4. 0.9% sodium chloride (normal saline)

5. A patient is receiving a subcutaneous infusion of 0.9% sodium chloride. While assessing the infusion, what infusion rate should the nurse expect to observe?
   1. 1 mL/minute
   2. 5 mL/minute
   3. 10 mL/minute
   4. 15 mL/minute

6. While assessing a patient, the nurse notes a silicone catheter taped to the patient's chest and can feel the catheter under the skin. Which type of catheter does the patient have?
   1. Peripherally inserted central catheter
   2. Implanted port
   3. Tunneled catheter
   4. Nontunneled catheter

7. The health care provider orders 5% dextrose in water at 100 mL per hour. What is the drip rate using tubing with a drop factor of 20? Round to the nearest whole number.
   Answer: _____ gtt per minute

8. A patient is to receive 1,000 mL normal saline over 12 hours. How many milliliters per hour should be set on the electronic infusion device?
   Answer: _____ mL per hour

Answer rationales available in your online resources.

ANSWERS 1. 2; 2. 1, 2, 3, 5, 6; 3. 2; 4. 4; 5. 1; 6. 3;
7. 33; 8. 83

Key Points

Find the chapter key points in your online resources available through Davis Edge.

Additional Resources

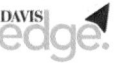 Use the scratch off code on the inside front cover of your book to access online quizzes that will help you to improve your scores on course exams and prepare for NCLEX-PN®.

 Study Guide

CHAPTER 8

Nursing Care of Patients With Infections

Kelli Verdecchia, Linda S. Williams

KEY TERMS

aerobic (air-OH-bik)
anaerobic (an-air-OH-bik)
antibodies (AN-ti-baw-dees)
antigens (AN-tih-jenz)
asepsis (ah-SEP-sis)
bacteria (bak-TEER-ee-ah)
Clostridium difficile (klo-STRIH-dee-um
   dih-fih-SEEL)
colonization (col-in-ih-ZAY-shun)
dormant (DOOR-mant)
fungi (FUNG-guy)
hand hygiene (HAND HY-jeen)
host (HOHST)
morbidity (more-BIH-dih-tee)
mortality (more-TAH-lih-tee)
pathogen (PATH-o-jen)
personal protective equipment (PUR-sun-al
   pro-TEK-tiv i-KWIP-ment)
phagocytosis (fay-go-sy-TOH-sis)
protozoa (pro-tow-ZOH-ah)
reservoir (REZ-er-vwar)
rickettsia (rah-KET-see-ah)
sepsis (SEP-sis)
standard precautions (STAN-derd
   pre-KAW-shuns)
Staphylococcus (staff-il-oh-KOCK-us)
trichinosis (TRIK-in-OH-sis)
vector (VEK-tur)
virulence (VEER-you-lence)
viruses (VY-rus-iz)

CHAPTER CONCEPTS

Infection

LEARNING OUTCOMES

1. List the links in the chain of infection.
2. Explain how to interrupt the routes of transmission for infections.
3. Describe the body's defense mechanisms to fight infection.
4. Describe the principles of anti-infective medication administration.
5. Describe nursing care for a patient with an infection.

THE INFECTION PROCESS

A **pathogen** is an organism that causes disease in a **host** (an infected person). **Colonization** occurs when pathogenic microbes are present in the body without causing symptoms or a detectable immune response. Infection occurs when a microbe multiplies in a host. Infection with only an immune response (increased antibody level for the microbe) and no symptoms is a *subclinical infection.* An infectious disease causes signs, symptoms, and injury to the host.

To prevent infection, the links in the chain of infection must be broken (Fig. 8.1). If an infection does occur, treatment focuses on breaking the chain of infection to prevent its spread to others.

Infectious Agents

Microorganisms that cause infection include bacteria, viruses, fungi, protozoa, helminths, and prions (Table 8.1). The organisms that occur naturally in or on a body part are known as normal flora. They are usually harmless (nonpathogenic). This is because they do not normally produce disease in a healthy person. Normal flora are helpful to the human host. For example, intestinal flora (i.e., bacteria) assist in vitamin K production. This is a nutrient needed for normal blood clotting. However, if these same bacteria get into another area of the body, such as the blood, they may produce disease. They are then referred to as pathogens.

• WORD • BUILDING •
pathogen: pathos—suffering + genes—producer of
protozoa: proto—first + zoon—animal

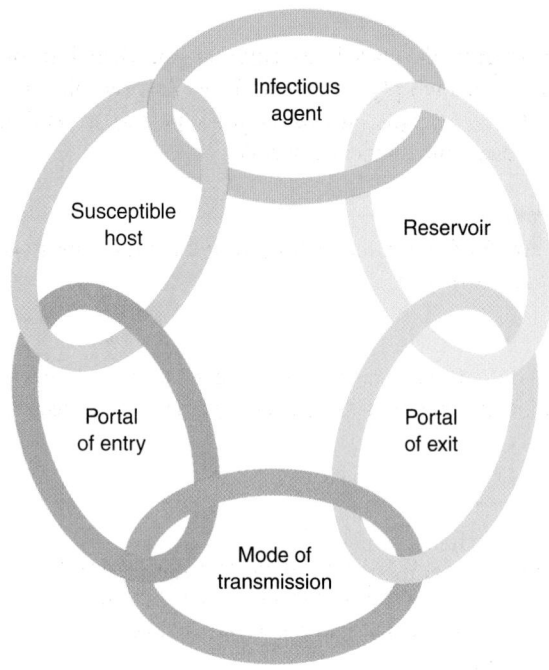

FIGURE 8.1 Chain of infection.

Bacteria

Bacteria are single-celled organisms. They may depend on a host. But they can also live and reproduce outside a host. Most bacteria produce cell walls that are susceptible to antibiotic effects. However, bacteria can mutate to survive.

Bacteria are named according to their shape: spherical (coccus), rod (bacillus), and spiral (spirillum). They are classified according to their staining properties (e.g., Gram method, acid-fast staining). Bacteria respond to stains in one of three ways. Gram-positive bacteria stain purple. Gram-negative bacteria lose purple stain when exposed to alcohol but stain pink with a second dye. Acid-fast bacteria keep purple stain when an acid is applied.

Bacterial growth depends on oxygen, nutrition, light, temperature, and humidity. **Aerobic** bacteria, such as those found on the skin, need oxygen to live. **Anaerobic** bacteria, such as bacteria in the gastrointestinal (GI) tract, live without oxygen. Most bacteria that inhabit humans grow best at a body temperature of 98.6°F (37°C).

Rod-shaped bacteria form spores that are thick walled. They are hard to kill. Spores remain in a resting state until favorable conditions exist to resume normal function. Prolonged exposure to high temperature destroys spores on surgical equipment. Bleach is used in patient rooms to kill spores from ***Clostridium difficile*** (*C. difficile*).

RICKETTSIA. **Rickettsiae** are tiny bacteria that must be inside living cells to reproduce. Rickettsia **vectors** (living organisms that transmit disease) are infected fleas, ticks, mites, and lice. They bite humans and cause disease. These diseases include typhus, scrub typhus, and Rocky Mountain spotted fever.

Table 8.1
Common Infections

Microorganism	Type or Site of Infection
Gram-Positive Bacteria	
Staphylococcus aureus	Pneumonia, cellulitis, peritonitis, toxic shock
Staphylococcus epidermidis	Postoperative bone/joints, intravenous (IV) line–related phlebitis
Staphylococcus pneumoniae	Pneumonia, meningitis, otitis media, sinusitis, bacteremia
Gram-Negative Bacteria	
Escherichia coli	Urinary tract, pyelonephritis, bacteremia, gastroenteritis
Klebsiella pneumoniae	Pneumonia, wounds
Legionella pneumophila	Pneumonia
Neisseria gonorrhoeae	Gonorrhea
Pseudomonas aeruginosa	Wounds, urinary tract, pneumonia, IV lines
Salmonella enteritidis	Gastroenteritis, food poisoning
Viruses	
Herpes virus group	Cold sores/fever blisters, genital herpes
Epstein-Barr	Infectious mononucleosis
Varicella-zoster	Skin (chickenpox and shingles)
Hepatitis (A, B, C, D, E)	Liver
Human immunodeficiency virus (HIV)	Acquired immune deficiency syndrome (AIDS)
Influenza (A, B, C)	Bronchiolitis, pneumonia
Rubella	German measles
Rubeola	Measles
Fungi	
Candida albicans	Nailbed, thrush, vaginitis
Histoplasma capsulatum	Pneumonia
Protozoa	
Giardia lamblia	Gastroenteritis
Trichomonas vaginalis	Trichomoniasis
Dientamoeba fragilis	Diarrhea, fever
Entamoeba histolytica	Amoebic dysentery
Toxoplasma gondii	Toxoplasmosis
Plasmodium falciparum	Malaria

Viruses

Viruses are organisms smaller than bacteria. They depend on host cells to live and reproduce (see Table 8.1). Invaded host cells make more of the virus material. The new viral particles are then released either by destroying the host cell or by forming small buds that break away to infect other cells.

When a virus enters a cell, it may immediately trigger disease or remain **dormant** (inactive) for years. An example of this is human herpesvirus 3 (varicella-zoster virus). It can cause disease quickly (e.g., chickenpox) or remain dormant for years. It can later erupt into the disease shingles. Antiviral drugs decrease viral symptoms and viral load (the number of viral cells in the patient's blood). Antibiotics are not effective against viruses.

Fungi

Fungi are organisms that include yeasts and molds. They can produce highly resistant spores (see Table 8.1). Fungi do not contain chlorophyll. They must obtain food from living organisms or dead organic matter. Normal flora of the mouth, skin, vagina, and intestinal tract include many fungi. Most fungi are not pathogenic. Serious fungal infections are rare. Antifungal medications treat fungal infections.

Protozoa

Protozoa are single-celled parasitic organisms. They have flexible membranes and live in the soil. Their nourishment comes from dead or decaying organic material (see Table 8.1). Protozoa infect humans through fecal–oral contamination, ingestion of food or water contaminated with cysts or spores, host-to-host contact, or the bite of a mosquito or other insect that has previously bitten an infected person.

Helminths

Helminths are wormlike parasitic animals. These include roundworms, flatworms, tapeworms, pinworms, hookworms, and flukes. Disease transmission occurs through skin penetration of larvae or ingestion of helminth eggs. **Trichinosis** (caused by the roundworm *Trichinella spiralis*) is a disease caused by eating raw or undercooked meat of pigs or wild animals that contain *Trichinella* larvae.

Prions

Prions are transmissible pathogenic agents. They cause abnormal folding of normal cellular proteins known as prion proteins. These prion proteins are found mainly in the brain. Brain damage results from the abnormal folding of prion proteins. Prion diseases have long incubation periods. They cause no inflammatory response. They progress rapidly and are fatal. In humans, they include classic and variant Creutzfeldt-Jakob disease. In animals, they include bovine spongiform encephalopathy (so-called mad cow disease) and chronic wasting disease.

Reservoir

A **reservoir** is the place in the environment where infectious agents live, multiply, and reproduce. A reservoir can be animate (e.g., people, insects, animals, plants) or inanimate (e.g., water, soil, medical devices).

Portal of Exit

The portal of exit is the path by which the infectious agent leaves its reservoir.

Mode of Transmission

Once the causative agent exits the reservoir, a direct or indirect means of transfer to a susceptible host is needed.

> **NURSING CARE TIP**
> Understanding the mode of transmission of a disease allows you to use the appropriate means of personal protection without using unnecessary supplies that increase costs.

Direct Transmission

Direct transmission occurs by direct contact or droplet spread. Direct contact occurs through touching, kissing, or sexual intercourse. Illnesses spread by this route include scabies, infectious mononucleosis, and sexually transmitted infections. Droplet spread occurs over short distances from spray during sneezing, coughing, or talking; pertussis and influenza spread this way. Protect yourself and your patients from direct transmission with **hand hygiene,** aseptic technique, and use of **personal protective equipment** (PPE). PPE includes gloves, goggles, gowns, masks, and foot covers (Fig. 8.2). For droplet precautions, wear a mask upon entry to the room if you will be within 6 to 10 feet of the infectious patient. PPE selection is based upon the task to be performed and the applicable isolation precautions (standard precautions and/or transmission-based precautions; see the Infection Prevention Guidelines discussion later).

Indirect Transmission

Indirect transmission is either vehicle-borne, vectorborne, or airborne. Vehicles indirectly spreading an infectious agent include biological products (e.g., blood, organs), soiled bedding, food, surgical instruments, toys, water, and wound dressings. Vehicle-borne illnesses include influenza, norovirus, and hepatitis. Methods to avoid vehicle transmission include hand hygiene, provisions for both clean water and food supplies, and cleaning of the patient environment and instruments per protocols.

Vectorborne transmission is the spread of infectious agents through a living source other than humans. This includes fleas, mice, mosquitos, rats, or ticks. Diseases spread through vectors include Lyme disease, malaria, plague, and Zika virus disease. Vector transmission can be reduced with avoidance of infested areas, use of insect repellents, and rodent control.

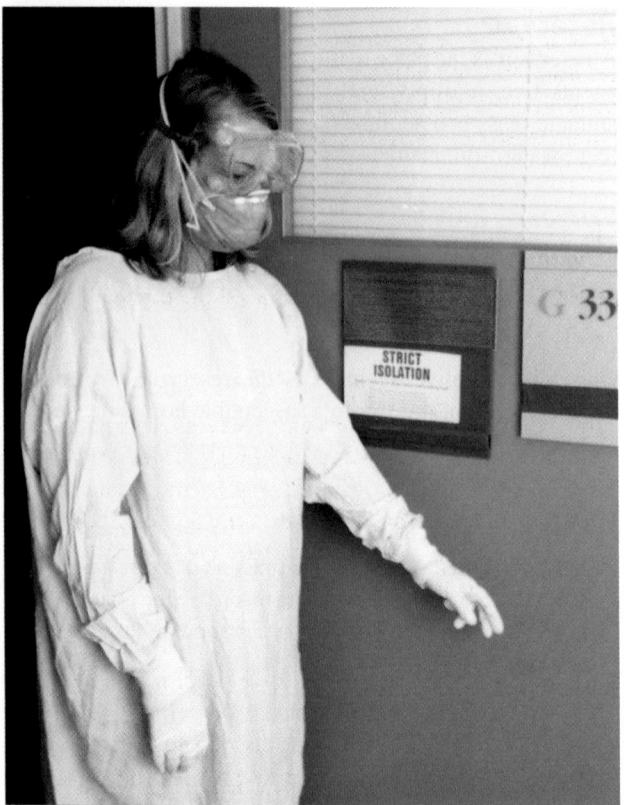

FIGURE 8.2 Personal protective equipment such as gloves, gown, mask, goggles, and face shield help prevent the spread of infection to health care workers and patients.

Airborne transmission occurs by dust or droplet nuclei carrying an infectious agent through the air. It is different from droplet transmission (see Direct Transmission, discussed earlier). The floating particles are much smaller, remain suspended in the air longer, and travel large distances. Airborne organisms can be inhaled or deposited on the mucous membrane of a susceptible host. *Mycobacterium tuberculosis* (TB), rubeola virus (measles), and varicella-zoster virus (chickenpox) are transmitted by airborne transmission. Airborne transmission is prevented with the use of a high-efficiency particulate air (HEPA) respirator. HEPA respirators filter the tiniest particles more effectively than simple isolation masks. This prevents particles from entering the respiratory system of a host.

BE SAFE!

• If you provide care for patients with suspected or confirmed diseases that are spread through airborne transmission, such as tuberculosis, you must have your own fit-tested National Institute for Occupational Safety and Health–approved N95 or higher-level respirator to wear. Institutions provide individual-fit testing and training for HEPA respirator use for each health care worker. Do not use other masks because they do not provide adequate protection. If you cannot obtain your own fit-tested mask, you should *never* enter the patient's room.

Multiple Modes of Transmission

Many diseases have multiple modes of transmission. This requires a variety of protective techniques. For example, chickenpox is transmitted by direct contact, indirect contact, and airborne transmission. So, it is no wonder that 80% to 90% of susceptible persons exposed to it develop the disease.

Portal of Entry

To produce disease, organisms enter a susceptible host through the blood, genitourinary tract, GI tract, mucous membranes, skin (usually nonintact), placenta, or respiratory tract. The condition of the host and other factors determine if the entry of the organism causes disease. This may include the **virulence** (ability to produce infection) of the organism.

Susceptible Host

The body has many defense mechanisms to prevent infection. A breakdown in these defenses increases the possibility of infection. Factors that increase susceptibility to infection are burns, chronic disease, being immunocompromised, invasive procedures, malnourishment, stress, and very young age or older age ("Gerontological Issues").

Gerontological Issues

Infection and Older Adults. Fever is not a common sign of an infection for an older adult. This difference among older adults may cause significant delay in providing appropriate treatment and care. Be alert for the following signs of infection in older patients:

• Behavioral change, such as pacing or irritability or new onset confusion
• Masking of the symptoms of infection by another condition such as the inflammation and pain of degenerative joint disease, making it difficult to recognize an infection in an affected joint

---

 ### THE HUMAN BODY'S DEFENSE MECHANISMS

Skin and Mucous Membranes

Intact skin and mucous membranes are the body's first line of defense against infection. Preventing skin dryness and cracking with lotion keeps the skin intact. This prevents an entry point for organisms. Oral mucous membranes have many layers. This makes it difficult for organisms to enter the body. The skin has acidic (pH less than 7) properties to make some organisms unable to produce disease. Many bacteria prefer an alkaline (pH more than 7) environment for reproduction. The body also has an abundance of normal flora impairing the growth of pathogens both on the skin and in the GI tract.

Cilia

Cilia are hairlike structures lining the mucous membranes of the upper respiratory tract that protect the lungs. Cilia trap mucus, pus, dust, and foreign particles to prevent them from entering the lungs. Cilia push the trapped particles up to the pharynx with wavelike movements to be expectorated.

Gastric Acid

Gastric acid (pH 1 to 5) destroys most organisms that enter the stomach.

Immunoglobulins

Immunoglobulins are proteins found in serum and body fluids. They act as antibodies to destroy invading organisms and prevent the development of infection. **Antibodies** are the proteins produced by B lymphocytes when foreign antigens of invading cells are detected. **Antigens** are markers on the surface of cells. They identify cells as being the body's own cells (autoantigens) or as being foreign cells (foreign antigens). Antibodies combine with specific foreign antigens on the surface of the invading organisms, such as bacteria or viruses, to control or destroy them. Antigens are neutralized or destroyed by antibodies in several ways. Antibodies can initiate destruction of the antigen, neutralize toxins released by bacteria, promote antigen clumping with the antibody, or prevent the antigen from adhering to host cells.

Leukocytes and Macrophages

Leukocytes, or white blood cells (WBCs), are the primary cells that protect against infection and tissue damage. There are five types of leukocytes in order of abundance:

- Neutrophils are phagocytic cells that focus on bacteria and fungi.
- Lymphocyte functions include antigen recognition and antibody production.
- Monocytes become macrophages and are mainly phagocytic on tissue debris and large particles.
- Eosinophils destroy parasites and respond in allergic reactions.
- Basophils are involved in inflammatory and allergic reactions.

After recognizing a foreign antigen, neutrophils and macrophages engulf and digest it. This is known as **phagocytosis.** The macrophages move the antigen fragments to their surface to be recognized by T lymphocytes to further stimulate action of the immune system. These phagocytes ingest and destroy bacteria, damaged or dead cells, cellular debris, and foreign substances.

Lysozymes

Lysozymes are bactericidal enzymes present in WBCs and most body fluids, such as tears, saliva, and sweat. These enzymes dissolve the walls of bacteria, destroying them.

Interferon

If an invading organism is a virus, WBCs and fibroblasts release interferon (a group of antiviral proteins). Interferon helps destroy infected cells, inhibits production of the virus within these cells, and may inhibit tumor cell growth.

Inflammatory Response

The inflammatory response occurs with any injury to the body. This response can be caused by pathogens, trauma, or other events causing injury to tissues. Infection may or may not be present.

Vascular Response

The first step of the inflammatory process is local vasodilation. This increases blood flow to the injured area. Pathogenic organisms can trigger the first step of the inflammatory process. Increased blood flow creates redness and heat at the injury. It also brings more plasma to the area to nourish tissue and carry waste and debris away.

Inflammatory Exudate

The second step of the inflammatory process is increased permeability of the blood vessels. This allows plasma to move out of the capillaries and into the tissues. Swelling occurs. This can result in pain from the pressure on nearby nerve endings.

Phagocytosis and Purulent Exudate

The final step of the inflammatory process is the destruction of pathogenic organisms and their toxins by leukocytes. During this process, a purulent exudate (pus) may form that contains protein, cellular debris, and dead leukocytes.

Immune System

The immune system is the body's final line of defense against infection (see Chapter 18). The immune system is a finely tuned network of specialized parts. When this network breaks down, infection can result.

Risk Factors for Infection

Risk factors for infection include:

- Aging (e.g., decreasing immune function, physical and functional aging-related changes)
- Being immunocompromised
- Chronic disease
- Dysphagia (e.g., risk of aspiration pneumonia, malnutrition)
- Environment (e.g., hospitals, long-term care facilities)
- Immobility
- Incontinence
- Instrumentation (e.g., central lines, endotracheal tubes, feeding tubes, intravenous lines, urinary catheters)

• WORD • BUILDING •

phagocytosis: phagein—to eat + cytos—cell + osis—condition

- Invasive procedures (e.g., cardiac catheterization, endoscopy, surgery)
- Malnutrition
- Medications (e.g., recent and/or multiple antibiotics, corticosteroids)

The older adult is most at risk for respiratory infections (e.g., influenza, pneumonia, TB), healthcare-associated infection, hepatitis, methicillin-resistant *Staphylococcus aureus* (MRSA), sepsis, and skin and urinary tract infections (UTIs).

 ## INFECTIOUS DISEASE

Localized Infection

Localized infection is caused by an increase of microbes in one area that triggers the inflammatory response. Manifestations of a local infection include pain, redness, swelling, and warmth at the site. Pain is most severe when the infection occurs in closed cavity areas. Redness and swelling are seen when surface structures are involved. Warmth may be felt at the site. Fever may occur to produce an antimicrobial effect.

Sepsis

Sepsis is defined as "life-threatening organ dysfunction caused by dysregulated host response to infection" (Singer et al., 2016). Septic shock can occur (see Chapter 9). Visit www.survivingsepsis.org.

Laboratory Assessment

A Gram stain, using gentian violet, allows bacteria to be better seen under a microscope for identification. Gram-positive bacteria turn purple. Gram-negative bacteria become pink. A culture and sensitivity (C&S) identifies an illness-causing organism. It also determines which antibiotic would be most effective for treatment. Organisms in the culture specimen are grown on a laboratory plate within 24 to 48 hours. The organism is then exposed to several antibiotics to determine to which antibiotics the organism is sensitive.

A serum antibody test measures the reaction to a certain antigen. A positive result for this test does not always mean that an active infection is present. It can simply mean there has been an exposure to the antigen. Therefore, it is not as accurate as a culture.

A complete blood cell count with differential (CBC with diff) is usually obtained when an infection is suspected. The levels of the five leukocytes are measured. Elevations in specific leukocytes occur based on the type and severity of the pathogen.

Erythrocyte sedimentation rate (ESR, sed rate) is an early screening test for inflammation. It is not a definitive test for infection. During the inflammatory process, red blood cells (RBCs) become heavier. The ESR measures in millimeters per hour the speed at which the RBCs settle in a tube: the faster the settling (due to heavier RBCs), the greater the inflammation.

Other tests such as x-rays, computed tomography (CT), and magnetic resonance imaging (MRI) are helpful in identifying abscesses (walled-off infections). Skin tests also diagnose infections. For example, the purified protein derivative (PPD) skin test screens for TB (see Chapter 31).

Immunity

Immunity is the ability of the body to protect itself from disease (see Chapter 18). There are several types of immunity:

- Natural immunity occurs in species and prevents one species from contracting illnesses found in another species.
- Innate immunity is genetic; hereditary immunity is that which a person is born with.
- Acquired immunity is obtained either actively or passively through exposure to an organism, from a vaccine, or from an injection of immunoglobulins (antibodies) or is passed from mother to baby. Visit www.cdc.gov/vaccines/schedules/easy-to-read.

Types of Infectious Diseases

Infectious disease examples are discussed next or in the chapters related to the body system they affect. For HIV, see Chapter 20; for respiratory diseases, see Chapter 31; for hepatitis, see Chapter 35.

Infectious Mononucleosis

Infectious mononucleosis (IM) is usually caused by the Epstein-Barr virus (EBV), a herpes virus. EBV is spread through contact with saliva or mucus of an infected person. IM is mainly symptomatic in teens or young adults. Most adults by age 40 have developed antibodies to it. EBV remains inactive in the body for life. The incubation period for IM is 4 to 6 weeks. Symptoms include fever, severe sore throat, and generalized lymphadenopathy (enlarged lymph nodes in two different sites other than inguinal nodes) that last 1 to 4 weeks. The spleen enlarges 50% of the time. Occasionally, a rash develops, similar to the rash seen with measles. Signs and symptoms as well as diagnostic tests confirm IM. A positive mononucleosis test and EBV antibody tests confirm IM. No specific treatment is needed. Antiviral drugs are not effective. Symptoms are treated with supportive care. Fatigue may last for months. Rest is important.

Ebola Virus Disease

In 1976, the Ebola virus was discovered near the Ebola River in the Democratic Republic of the Congo (Table 8.2). Beginning in 2014, the largest outbreak of Ebola virus disease in history occurred in West Africa. Survivors of the disease develop antibodies that last about 10 years.

Zika Virus Disease

The Zika virus is a single-stranded ribonucleic acid (RNA) virus. Its name is derived from the Zika Forest of Uganda where it was discovered in 1947 (see Table 8.2). It is transmitted to

Table 8.2

Ebola and Zika Infections

Infection	Ebola Virus Disease	Zika Virus Disease
Causative Organism	Ebola virus (*Zaire ebolavirus*) Sudan virus (*Sudan ebolavirus*) Taï Forest virus (*Taï Forest ebolavirus*) Bundibugyo virus (*Bundibugyo ebolavirus*)	Zika virus is a member of the *Flaviviridae* family.
Transmission	Direct contact via broken skin or mucous membranes with: • Infected blood, body fluids • Infected fruit bat or primate • Contaminated equipment (e.g., needles, syringes) • Semen from survivor	Via infected mosquito bite Sex with an infected partner Maternal-fetal
Prevention/ Isolation	Vaccine trial Meticulous hand hygiene Avoiding contact with infected blood, body fluids, objects, bats, primates, bodies of people who died of Ebola Isolation of patients Wearing specialized personal protective equipment Sterilizing equipment	Using Environmental Protection Agency–registered insect repellent, and emptying containers with stagnant water around the house Avoiding unprotected sex and not traveling to areas of risk with Zika virus if pregnant Meticulous hand hygiene Avoiding exposure to blood/bodily fluids, disinfecting household surfaces, washing contaminated clothing
Symptoms	Appear in 2 to 21 days (average 8 to 10 days) and include: • fever • headache • diarrhea • vomiting • abdominal pain • muscle pain • unexplained bruising/bleeding	Mild symptoms lasting several days to weeks include: • fever • headache • rash • muscle/joint pain • conjunctivitis
Diagnosis	After onset of fever: • Antigen-capture enzyme-linked immunosorbent assay (ELISA) testing • Immunoglobulin M (IgM) ELISA • Polymerase chain reaction • Virus isolation	Blood or urine test to detect neutralizing antibodies or virus-specific IgM
Complications	Long-term joint and vision problems	Guillain-Barré syndrome Microcephaly birth defect Severe fetal brain defects Miscarriage
Treatment	No antiviral drug exists Supportive care Maintain blood pressure/oxygen status Intravenous fluids/electrolytes	Supportive treatment including acetaminophen for fever Avoid aspirin/nonsteroidal anti-inflammatory drugs (NSAIDs) Fluids and rest

Sources: Centers for Disease Control and Prevention. (2016). Ebola (Ebola virus disease). Retrieved from www.cdc.gov/vhf/ebola/index.html; Centers for Disease Control and Prevention. (2017). Zika virus. Retrieved from www.cdc.gov/zika/index.html

humans by infected day and nighttime-active *Aedes* genus mosquitos. Once infected by the Zika virus, most people are protected from future infections of Zika.

INFECTION CONTROL IN THE COMMUNITY

Many levels of organizations work closely together to control communicable diseases. The World Health Organization (WHO) and the Centers for Disease Control and Prevention (CDC) teach standards to prevent, monitor, and control disease outbreaks. Local health departments teach prevention and control diseases. Immunization programs have helped reduce communicable diseases.

Although requirements vary from state to state, most elementary schools require some proof of childhood immunization. Many colleges require or recommend immunization to help control the outbreak of diseases such as measles and meningitis. Educating the public about the importance of hand hygiene, the CDC's respiratory hygiene/cough etiquette measures, immunization, clean water, safe food-handling techniques, and safer sex precautions in preventing the spread of disease is essential.

NURSING CARE TIP

For infection control, teach the Centers for Disease Control and Prevention *Cover Your Cough* campaign instructions to patients and family members who have a cough, congestion, rhinorrhea, or increased respiratory secretions:

- Cover your mouth and nose with a tissue when you cough or sneeze.
- Put your used tissue in the wastebasket.
- If you don't have a tissue, cough or sneeze into your upper sleeve or elbow, not your hands.
- Wash hands often with soap and water for 20 seconds; use an alcohol-based hand cleaner if soap and water are not available.
- Put on a facemask to protect others if asked.

Source: Centers for Disease Control and Prevention. (2016). Cover your cough. Retrieved from www.cdc.gov/flu/protect/covercough.htm

---

INFECTION CONTROL IN HEALTH CARE AGENCIES

If upon admission to a health care agency a patient already has an infection, it is referred to as a community-acquired infection. An infection that develops as a result of care provided in a health care agency is called a healthcare-associated infection (HAI). Living in a long-term care facility rather than at home can increase infection risk. The host's condition plays a major role in whether an infection is acquired. Patients in the hospital are often debilitated, malnourished, or immunocompromised.

Multiple antibiotic therapy also increases susceptibility to other types of infection. It also promotes the resistance of pathogens to antibiotics. Therefore, the risk of developing an HAI is high. Certain patient care areas tend to have an increased number of HAIs. These include burn, critical care, dialysis, neonatal, and oncology units. Patients in these units tend to undergo more invasive procedures and are more debilitated. An objective of Healthy People 2020 is to reduce invasive MRSA HAIs from 27.08 cases per 100,000 population to 6.56 (75% reduction). Data through 2014 reveal a reduction to 17.3 cases per 100,000 (Office of Disease Prevention and Health Promotion, 2017).

Several pathogens are commonly responsible for causing HAIs:

- *Escherichia coli* (*E. coli*) is the most common pathogen causing healthcare-associated UTIs. *E. coli* normally lives in the healthy intestinal tract of humans. *E. coli* can be spread by the patient, by the unwashed hands of a health care worker, or through contaminated food and water.
- *Staphylococcus aureus* (known as staph) is the most common pathogen causing healthcare-associated surgical wound infections. Staph usually lives in the nose and on the skin of healthy people.
- *Pseudomonas aeruginosa* is the most common pathogen in healthcare-associated pneumonia. It is found in soil, around water, and in the health care setting around sinks, water, irrigating solutions, and nebulizers on respiratory equipment.

Hand Hygiene

What is the single most effective way to prevent and control the spread of infection? Effective hand hygiene! Hand hygiene removes the transient organisms that cause most HAIs. Most of these organisms are transmitted via the hands of health care providers (HCPs). Hands must be cleansed before and after every patient contact to help prevent the direct transmission of organisms (Fig. 8.3). The use of gloves decreases the transmission of organisms. CDC guidelines require hand washing before and after glove use because hands may still become contaminated (view www.cdc.gov/handhygiene).

Hand hygiene can be performed with either hand washing or an alcohol-based hand rub. However, soap and water are needed to remove *C. difficile*. For visibly soiled hands, wash with soap and water rather than using a hand rub. An alcohol-based hand rub is preferred to kill bacteria in many cases. When using alcohol-based hand rubs, apply the specified amount of the hand rub to the palm of one hand. Rub both hands together, covering all surfaces until the hands are completely dry to ensure the alcohol has evaporated. Do not wash off hand rub.

Proper hand washing requires wetting the hands with warm—not hot—water, soaping, and lathering. Rub your hands together for at least 20 seconds (sing "Happy Birthday" twice), covering all surfaces. Interlace your fingers to cleanse between them. Rub your nails against your palms to clean under the nails. Then rinse your hands with fingertips pointed downward under running water. Dry your hands with clean disposable paper towels. Use the paper towel to turn off the

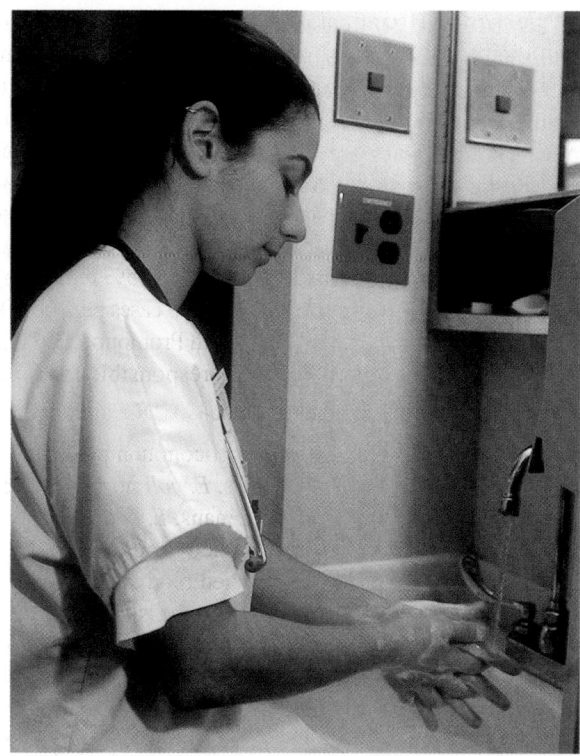

FIGURE 8.3 Frequent hand washing by health care workers helps reduce the spread of microorganisms.

CRITICAL THINKING

Mrs. Sampson has neutropenia from chemotherapy treatments.

1. Why is hand hygiene the most important intervention you can do to help prevent infection for Mrs. Sampson?
2. Who should perform frequent hand hygiene to reduce healthcare-associated infection?
3. What would be a priority nursing diagnosis for Mrs. Sampson?
4. What type of isolation could be beneficial to Mrs. Sampson?

Suggested answers are at the end of the chapter.

faucet. Use only facility-supplied lotions because others may reduce the effectiveness of soap or break down latex gloves (use water-based lotion only). Apply lotion to your hands to prevent drying and cracking in which infection could develop (CDC, 2017).

Patient Hand Hygiene

Did you know that patients may also transmit organisms with inadequate hand hygiene and that they are often never offered the opportunity to wash their hands? Research has shown that patient hand hygiene is a weak link in preventing HAIs. Offer and assist your patients with hand hygiene throughout the day! Teach them the importance of frequent hand hygiene before meals and after toileting, handling their own secretions, or leaving and returning to their room. If patients cannot get to a sink, make it easy for them to perform hand hygiene by placing hand sanitizer or disinfecting wipes at the bedside.

Asepsis

Asepsis is freedom from organisms. Be aware of patients at risk of developing infections. Protect them with aseptic techniques. For hospitalized patients, the most common sites for infection are the genitourinary tract, respiratory tract, bloodstream, and surgical wounds.

Medical Asepsis

Medical asepsis is referred to as clean technique. The goal is to reduce the number of pathogens or prevent the transmission of pathogens from one person to another. Frequent hand hygiene, use of PPE, patient rooms with special ventilation, disinfectants, and precautions as defined by the CDC help do this. As part of medical asepsis keep your own body, clothing, and shoes clean to prevent spread of infection to patients, yourself, and your family (Box 8.1).

Surgical Asepsis

Surgical asepsis (sterile technique) refers to an item or area that is free of all microorganisms and spores. Surgical asepsis is used in surgery and to sterilize equipment. Items can be subjected to intense heat or chemical disinfectants to destroy all organisms. The use of pressurized steam sterilizers, called autoclaves, kills even the most powerful organisms. Some equipment cannot be exposed to moist heat, so gas sterilizers are used instead. After these items are sterilized, they are dated, packaged, and sealed. Once a package is opened or outdated, it is no longer sterile.

Box 8.1

Guidelines to Prevent the Spread of Infection to Patients, Self, and Family

- Bathe daily and wear a clean uniform/clothing every day.
- Keep your natural fingernail tips less than ¼ inch long, and do not wear artificial nails. Studies have shown that long fingernails and artificial nails harbor harmful bacteria and have transmitted infections to patients that have sometimes resulted in death.
- Avoid wearing rings and bracelets at work because they harbor organisms.
- Cleanse your stethoscope at least daily and in between patient use with alcohol. Vancomycin-resistant enterococci have been cultured from stethoscopes in a hospital setting.
- Use hand hygiene between each patient contact. The use of an alcohol-based hand rub or hand washing is recognized as the single most important action to take to prevent spread of infection.
- Follow prescribed isolation precautions for your protection as well as that of the patient.
- Perform hand hygiene before going home to prevent transfer of bacteria to your home.
- Remove your uniform in a contained area of your home to launder it, and bathe/shower when you come home from work. This will decrease the spread of antibiotic-resistant bacteria to your home and your family. Keep your nursing shoes clean and stored away from the rest of the family.

Ultraviolet Environmental Disinfection

Health care agencies are using ultraviolet (UV) light to disinfect patient care areas and rooms after traditional cleaning. Portable robots that emit UV-C light are placed into empty rooms. The doorways are then blocked to prevent people from entering the room to protect them from the intense light. All surfaces are disinfected with bouncing and reflecting light waves in minutes. To see a robot, visit www.xenex.com.

Infection Prevention Guidelines

CDC guidelines for infection control and isolation precautions are used in policies at hospitals, long-term care facilities, and other health care agencies. CDC and agency guidelines are continuously updated. Follow them for your patients' and your own protection. Current CDC guidelines for isolation precautions in hospitals and long-term care facilities include two tiers of precautions: standard precautions and transmission-based precautions (Table 8.3).

Standard Precautions

Standard precautions are used in the care of all patients. These precautions require you to assume that all patients are infectious regardless of their diagnosis and to use PPE. Standard precautions apply to blood, secretions, excretions, open skin, mucous membranes, and all body fluids, excluding sweat. All patients with draining wounds or secretions of body fluids are considered infectious until an infection is confirmed or ruled out. Using PPE such as gloves, gowns, masks, goggles, and face

Table 8.3

Standard Precautions and Transmission-Based Precautions

Standard Precautions	
Use standard precautions for all patient care as appropriate. Use standard precautions along with *all* transmission-based precautions as needed based on the patient's illness and anticipated contact with the patient and environment.	
Hand hygiene	Use alcohol-based hand rub or wash hands with nonmicrobial soap, unless specifically contraindicated, before and after using gloves, between patients, and between procedures on the same patient.
Gloves	Wear gloves before contact with any body fluids or substances. Change gloves after each use.
Mask, eye protection, face shield	Use personal protective equipment for patient care if splashes or sprays of blood or body fluids are likely.
Gown	Wear gown to protect skin/prevent soiling of clothing for patient care if splashes or sprays of blood or body fluids are likely.
Occupational health and bloodborne pathogens	Dispose of sharps properly. Do not recap needles.
Patient care equipment	Clean reusable equipment before reuse. Dispose of single-use items properly.
Linen	Handle linen to avoid clothing contamination.
Patient placement	Use private room for infectious patients.

Table 8.3

Standard Precautions and Transmission-Based Precautions—cont'd

Transmission-Based Precautions	
Airborne Precautions	
Examples: *Mycobacterium tuberculosis* (TB), rubeola virus (measles), varicella-zoster virus (chickenpox)	
Patient placement	Provide private room with regulated airflow. Keep door closed.
Personal protective equipment (PPE)	
Respiratory protection	Do not enter room if susceptible to measles or chickenpox unless no caregivers who are immune are available. If susceptible, wear a fit-tested (N95) disposable respirator. Do not enter room of patient with TB unless wearing a N95 disposable respirator. Have patient with TB also wear surgical mask during times that care is performed. Offer visitors an N95 respirator per agency policy.
Standard precautions added as needed	Gloves, gown, goggles/face shield, foot covers.
Patient transport	Limit patient transport to essential purposes. Place surgical mask on patient (may not contain all TB organisms).
Droplet Precautions	
Examples: adenovirus, diphtheria (pharyngeal), *Haemophilus influenzae* (epiglottitis, meningitis, pneumonia), influenza, mumps, mycoplasma pneumonia, *Neisseria meningitidis* (meningitis, pneumonia, pertussis, pneumonic plague, rubella, group A streptococcus)	
Patient placement	Provide private room or separation greater than 3 feet between the infected patient and other patients and close privacy curtain.
PPE	
Respiratory protection	Wear mask upon entering patient area. Teach patient respiratory hygiene/cough etiquette.
Standard precautions added as needed.	Gloves, gown, goggles/face shield, foot covers
Patient transport	Limit patient transport to essential purposes. Place surgical mask on patient.
Contact Precautions	
Examples: cellulitis, *Clostridium difficile,* skin infections (cutaneous diphtheria, herpes simplex virus, impetigo, pediculosis, scabies), conjunctivitis, viral hemorrhagic infections (Ebola, Lassa, or Marburg), herpes zoster	
Patient placement	Provide private room or place with patient with same infection and no other infection.
PPE	Gloves, gown, and foot covers protect self and others from contaminated items.
Patient transport	Limit patient transport.
Patient care equipment	Dedicate the use of noncritical patient care equipment to a single patient.

Sources: Siegel, J. D., Rhinehart, E., Jackson, M., Chiarello, L., & the Healthcare Infection Control Practices Advisory Committee. (2017). *2007 guideline for isolation precautions: Preventing transmission of infectious agents in healthcare settings.* Washington, DC: Centers for Disease Control and Prevention. Retrieved from www.cdc.gov/infectioncontrol/pdf/guidelines/isolation-guidelines.pdf; Centers for Disease Control and Prevention. (2015). Infection prevention and control recommendations for hospitalized patients under investigation (PUIs) for Ebola virus disease (EVD) in U.S. hospitals. Retrieved from www.cdc.gov/vhf/ebola/healthcare-us/hospitals/infection-control.html

shields along with hand hygiene helps prevent the spread of infection to health care workers, other patients, and visitors.

Transmission-Based Precautions

Transmission-based precautions are used for patients with specific infectious diseases that can be transmitted to others. These precautions add an additional layer of protection to the standard precautions.

Prevention of Respiratory Tract Infections

Healthcare-associated pneumonia has been linked with the highest infection mortality rate. Patients who are at highest risk for pneumonia are those with endotracheal, nasotracheal, or tracheostomy tubes because these invasive tubes bypass the normal defenses of the upper respiratory tract. Strategies to prevent infections such as ventilator-associated pneumonia (VAP) are "bundled" together so nurses remember to use these strategies. For more information on VAP bundles, visit www.cdc.gov/hai/vap/vap.html.

Prevention of Genitourinary Tract Infections

The most common HAI is a UTI. Patients with urinary catheters are at greatest risk. The urinary tract is sterile. Insertion of a catheter into the bladder may allow organisms to enter it. Institutional policies on appropriate use of urinary catheters differ, so follow your agency's policy. Appropriate reasons for use of a urinary catheter may include urinary obstruction, a neurogenic bladder condition, shock, and palliative care.

Indwelling urinary catheters should be removed as soon as possible. For patients who need long-term catheterization, intermittent catheterization is preferred. This significantly reduces the risk of infection. Using strict aseptic technique while inserting and caring for the catheter in the health care agency is imperative. The catheter tubing must be securely anchored to the patient's leg, according to agency protocol, to prevent moving in and out of the urethra. This movement can encourage organisms to enter the sterile urinary tract.

The closed urinary drainage system seal should never be opened. (If intermittent irrigation is ordered, sterile technique must be used to protect both ends of the system from contamination.) The drainage bag should be positioned so it is never higher than the level of the bladder. This prevents backflow of urine into the bladder, which could contaminate the sterile urinary tract. If an indwelling urinary catheter and a drainage system are used long term, the catheter and the entire system should be changed regularly using sterile technique. All long-term indwelling urinary catheters are considered colonized. Standards in home health care can differ from institutional care. This is because patients are generally at lower risk of infection within their own environment.

The most crucial point at which bacteria may enter the patient is during insertion of the catheter. Excellent sterile technique is required. The urinary tract is highly vascular (many blood vessels close to the surface). Therefore, an infection can easily result in bacteremia (bacteria in the blood).

This can then progress to sepsis, a potentially life-threatening condition. For more information on prevention of UTIs in adults, visit www.kidney.niddk.nih.gov/kudiseases/pubs/utiadult/index.htm.

BE SAFE!

Catheters should be used only when necessary because of the **morbidity** (sickness) and **mortality** (death) associated with infections that can develop from them. The continued need for an indwelling catheter should be monitored daily. The catheter should be discontinued as quickly as it is no longer needed.

CRITICAL THINKING

Mr. Carson is being transported in a wheelchair by a nursing assistant to the activity room. He has a urinary catheter. The urine bag is hung on the arm of the wheelchair. What is your responsibility in this situation as a team member?
Suggested answers are at the end of the chapter.

Prevention of Surgical Wound Infections

The initial dressing for surgical wounds is applied in the operating room using sterile aseptic technique. Postoperative orders indicate when to change the dressing. Monitor the wound with each dressing change for signs of infection.

CRITICAL THINKING

Risk of Infection: Of the following patients, who is at greatest risk of infection and why?

1. Mr. Ashland, age 55, had an ambulatory hernia repair. He has adult-onset diabetes.
2. Mrs. Burrows, age 72, is hospitalized with a fractured hip. She is thin and frail, has dementia, and has undergone placement of a urinary catheter.
3. Jackson Dunn, age 22, underwent an appendectomy in the hospital. Jackson is underweight.

Suggested answer is at the end of the chapter.

 ANTIBIOTIC-RESISTANT INFECTIONS

Antibiotic-resistant infections, such as MRSA and vancomycin-resistant enterococci (VRE), are an urgent worldwide health concern. Currently, there are 12 organisms considered to be antibiotic-resistant by WHO. Resistant organisms are difficult to treat, can spread easily to others, and may result in death. It is up to each of us to understand how to prevent antibiotic resistance. The CDC's *Be Antibiotics Aware* campaign aims to educate health care providers and individuals on the appropriate use of antibiotics, including in long-term care (www.cdc.gov/antibiotic-use/index.html).

Methicillin-Resistant *Staphylococcus aureus* (MRSA)

MRSA is a serious, life-threatening antibiotic-resistant infection. It has resulted from long-term use of unnecessary antibiotics. People can be carriers of MRSA and spread it, even when they have no symptoms. MRSA occurs in health care settings and nursing homes. Symptoms include painful warm red bumps, fever, and drainage. MRSA can also be seen in the community among those who are healthy, starting as a skin boil. Treatment includes draining skin boils or antibiotics such as vancomycin hydrochloride. One study found that in long-term care targeted nasal and body decolonization, annual hand hygiene education, and bleach wiping of flat surfaces every 4 months significantly reduced MRSA (Peterson et al., 2016).

Vancomycin-Resistant *Enterococci* (VRE)

VRE infections are common. Although enterococci are normal flora in the GI and female genital tracts, VRE are a pathogenic strain. VRE are transmitted via direct or indirect contact. Patients at risk for VRE infections include those with indwelling urinary or central venous catheters, the immunocompromised or critically ill, those receiving multiple antibiotics or vancomycin therapy, surgical patients, and those with extended hospital stays. Preventive VRE measures focus on proper hand hygiene, education of HCPs, aggressive infection control methods, and restricting use of vancomycin. Patients with VRE should be isolated. Use PPE and follow CDC and agency infection control policies. Treatment involves combination antibiotic therapy.

THERAPEUTIC MEASURES FOR INFECTIOUS DISEASES

Once an infection-causing organism and the affected body system have been identified, the appropriate medication can be selected and treatment begun (Table 8.4). The drug of choice must be able to destroy (or control) the pathogen:

- Antibiotics treat bacterial infections, not viruses, fungi, helminths, or prions.
- Antiviral medications treat viral infections, but their use is aimed at symptom control rather than cure.
- Antifungal drugs are available for fungal infections, but cure may require extended use.

Antibiotics can be classified as either bactericidal or bacteriostatic. Bactericidal agents kill bacteria. Bacteriostatic agents inhibit or retard bacterial growth. The final destruction of the bacteria is done by the infected host's immune system. Bacteriostatic agents may be less helpful for the patient who is immunocompromised.

Many antibiotics are metabolized by the liver and excreted by the kidneys. Disorders of these organs may require lower doses. Antibiotic levels fluctuate greatly depending on organ function, age, sex, health, and other factors. Antibiotic serum peak level (highest level occurs right after drug administration) and trough level (lowest level occurs just before dose is due) are monitored per agency protocol to ensure therapeutic, nontoxic levels.

Antibiotic-Associated Diarrhea

Antibiotic therapy may cause antibiotic-associated diarrhea (AAD) because antibiotics upset the delicate balance of natural microbiota found in the intestine. Any antibiotic can cause AAD, but ampicillin, cephalosporins, and clindamycin are the most common. Antibiotics destroy helpful bacteria along with harmful bacteria. With fewer helpful bacteria, harmful bacteria increase. These bacteria produce toxins that harm the intestinal wall, cause inflammation, and result in watery bowel movements. When AAD occurs, the antibiotic therapy may be stopped. Then the diarrhea usually resolves. For severe diarrhea and colitis (colon inflammation), metronidazole (Flagyl) or vancomycin (Vancocin) is given.

Clostridium difficile

C. difficile is a gram-positive bacterium that can cause infection. It is sometimes found normally in the intestine. It can be one of the most serious causes of AAD. When normal gut microbiota has been destroyed, *C. difficile* can overgrow. This results in the release of toxins causing diarrhea of 20 or more stools daily, fever, bloating, and abdominal

(Text continued on page 102)

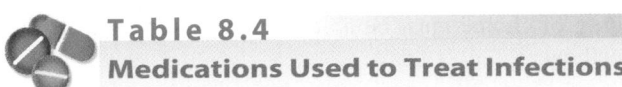

Table 8.4
Medications Used to Treat Infections

Medication Class/Action

Bactericidal Antibiotics

Penicillin
Antibacterial agent that inhibits cell wall synthesis most effectively for gram-positive organisms.

Examples	Nursing Implications
amoxicillin (Amoxil) ampicillin (Omnipen) penicillin G ticarcillin (Ticar)	Monitor for allergic reaction (rash, hives, itching) or anaphylactic shock (fever, chills, dyspnea, low blood pressure, tight throat, wheezing). Stop infusion for signs of allergic reaction. Notify health care provider (HCP) immediately. *Teaching:* Hold drug and call HCP for allergy signs, oral white patches, or vaginal irritation.

Carbapenems
Broad-spectrum antibacterial agent that inhibits cell wall synthesis for moderate-to-severe infection.

Examples	Nursing Implications
doripenem (Doribax) ertapenem (Invanz) imipenem/cilastatin (Primaxin) meropenem (Merrem)	Ertapenem: Check for lidocaine (intramuscular diluent) allergy. Monitor patient for seizures and, if applicable, serum valproic acid level.

Cephalosporins
Antibacterial agent inhibits cell wall synthesis.
First generation: more effective against gram-positive organisms.
Second and third generation: more effective against gram-negative organisms.
Fourth generation: more gram-negative coverage.
Fifth generation: methicillin-resistant Staphylococcus aureus *coverage.*

Examples	Nursing Implications
First generation: cefazolin (Ancef) Second and third generation: cefaclor (Ceclor); ceftriaxone (Rocephin) Fourth generation: cefepime (Maxipime) Fifth generation: ceftaroline (Teflaro)	Use caution with penicillin allergies or renal or hepatic dysfunction. *Teaching:* Take on empty stomach. Avoid excess sun exposure.

Aminoglycosides
Gram-negative antibacterial agent that inhibits protein synthesis.

Examples	Nursing Implications
amikacin (Amikin) gentamicin (Garamycin) tobramycin (Nebcin)	Check and report elevated creatinine levels before giving this nephrotoxic agent. Monitor peak/trough levels to keep drug in therapeutic range. *Teaching:* Report signs of allergy, tinnitus, vertigo, or hearing loss.

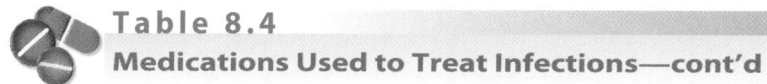

Table 8.4
Medications Used to Treat Infections—cont'd

Medication Class/Action

Fluoroquinolones
Broad spectrum antibacterial agent that inhibits bacterial deoxyribonucleic acid (DNA) replication for variety of infections.

Examples	**Nursing Implications**
ciprofloxacin (Cipro)	Boxed warning secondary to corrected QT interval (QTc) prolongation,
levofloxacin (Levaquin)	central nervous system (CNS) effects, peripheral neuropathy, tendon
moxifloxacin (Avelox)	rupture, tendonitis. Risk increased over age 60; in kidney, heart, and
norfloxacin (Noroxin)	lung transplant recipients; and concomitant steroid therapy.
ofloxacin (Floxin)	Contraindicated with history of myasthenia gravis.

Teaching:
Take on empty stomach with full glass of water.
Do not take with antacids.
Use sun protection.
Report joint or muscle pain, or tendon rupture immediately.

Nitroimidazoles
Inhibit nucleic acid synthesis in anaerobic bacteria and protozoa.

Example	**Nursing Implications**
metronidazole (Flagyl)	For sexually transmitted infection, treat partner as well as patient.

Teaching:
Take with or without food.
Avoid alcohol; abstain for a minimum of 48 hours following treatment
to prevent severe flu-like reaction.

Glycopeptides

Examples	**Nursing Implications**
Treat serious gram-positive infections.	Administer intravenous (IV) over 1 hour to prevent red man syndrome
Oral vancomycin given for *Clostridium*	(flushing, rash on upper body, neck, head).
difficile (C. difficile)-associated diarrhea:	Monitor drug levels.
vancomycin (Vancocin Hydrochloride,	Monitor IV site for thrombophlebitis.
Vancocin Hydrochloride Pulvules)	*Teaching*: Report sudden hearing or balance problems.
Treat gram-positive skin and skin structure	Not compatible with normal saline.
infections:	Infuse IV over 30 minutes to avoid reactions with rapid infusion.
dalbavancin (Dalvance)	
oritavancin (Orbactiv)	Dilute and flush IV line with D_5W only.
	Infuse IV over 3 hours.
telavancin (Vibativ)	Box warning for renal impairment.
	Infuse IV over 1 hour.

Bacteriostatic Antibiotics

Tetracyclines
Protein synthesis inhibitor for most gram-positive and gram-negative organisms.

Examples	**Nursing Implications**
tetracycline hydrochloride (Sumycin)	*Teaching:*
doxycycline (Vibramycin)	Do not take during pregnancy due to bone/teeth effects.
minocycline hydrochloride (Minocin)	Take on empty stomach.

Do not take with antacids or dairy products.
Avoid prolonged sun exposure, use at least sun protection factor (SPF)
30 sunscreen, and cover skin.

Continued

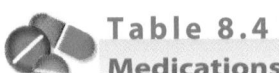

Table 8.4
Medications Used to Treat Infections—cont'd

Medication Class/Action

Macrolides
Protein synthesis inhibitor for many gram-negative and gram-positive organisms.

Example	Nursing Implications
azithromycin (Zithromax)	*Teaching:* Take on empty stomach with a full glass of water. Do not take with antacids. Avoid prolonged sun exposure, use at least SPF 30 sunscreen, and cover skin.
clarithromycin (Biaxin)	*Teaching:* Take with a full glass of water. Take time-release capsules with food.
erythromycin (E-Mycin, E.E.S.)	Administer IV slowly to decrease vein irritation. *Teaching:* Take orally on empty stomach with a full glass of water. Complete entire ordered treatment. If gastric distress occurs it is not a reason to stop the drug. Contact HCP if side effects are intolerable.
For *C. difficile* only: fidaxomicin (Dificid)	*Teaching:* Take tablets with or without food.

Lincomycins
Inhibit protein synthesis within bacterial cell for serious bacterial infection.

Example	Nursing Implication
clindamycin (Cleocin)	*Teaching*: Report foul-odor diarrhea, fever, and abdominal pain indicating possible *C. difficile* infection.

Streptogramins
Protein synthesis inhibitor for vancomycin-resistant Staphylococcus aureus and vancomycin-resistant Enterococci and severe skin infections.

Example	Nursing Implications
quinupristin/dalfopristin (Synercid)	After intravenous infusion, flush with D_5W solution (incompatible with saline or heparin).

Sulfonamides
Inhibit growth and multiplication for most gram-positive and many gram-negative organisms mainly in UTIs, Pneumocystis jiroveci *pneumonia, and otitis media.*

Example	Nursing Implications
trimethoprim sulfamethoxazole (Bactrim, Septra)	Administer IV drug over 1 hour. Monitor intake and output. Ensure fluid intake is 1,500 mL daily. *Teaching:* Take on empty stomach with a full glass of water. Avoid prolonged sun exposure, use at least SPF 30 sunscreen, and cover skin. Inform HCP for allergic reaction or bleeding.

Table 8.4
Medications Used to Treat Infections—cont'd

Medication Class/Action

Oxazolidinones
Synthetic protein synthesis inhibitor for complicated infections caused by gram-negative microorganisms.

Example	**Nursing Implications**
linezolid (Zyvox)	*Teaching:*
	Avoid tyramine (found in aged cheeses, smoked foods, draft beer, red wine, soy sauce, sauerkraut).

Antifungals

Amphotericin B
Interferes with the fungal cell wall structure for life-threatening fungal infections.

Examples	**Nursing Implications**
Amphocin	Monitor during first hour of infusion for febrile reaction.
Fungizone	Monitor injection site and for signs of kidney damage.
	Teaching:
	Drink 2,000 to 3,000 mL of fluid daily to flush drug.

Triazoles
Inhibit cell membrane ergosterol synthesis for yeast or fungus infections.

Examples	**Nursing Implications**
fluconazole (Diflucan)	Obtain cultures before giving drug.
itraconazole (Sporanox)	Monitor BUN and creatinine levels and liver function tests.
posaconazole (Noxafil)	*Teaching:*
voriconazole (Vfend)	Notify HCP at the first sign of yellow skin, dark urine, or pale stools.

Echinocandins
Disrupt fungal cell wall integrity for candidal infection.

Examples	**Nursing Implication**
anidulafungin (Eraxis)	Monitor liver function tests.
caspofungin (Cancidas)	
micafungin (Mycamine)	

Antivirals

Antiretrovirals
See Chapter 20

Anti-Influenza Virus
See Chapter 30

Anti-Hepatitis Virus
See Chapter 35

Anti-Herpes Virus and Cytomegalovirus
Inhibit viral DNA synthesis for viral infection.

Examples	**Nursing Implications**
acyclovir (Zovirax)	Use systemic preparations cautiously with CNS, hepatic, or renal disorders.
cidofovir (Vistide)	*Teaching:*
valacyclovir (Valcyte)	Maintain hydration with systemic preparations.
famciclovir (Famvir)	
foscarnet (Foscavir)	
valacyclovir (Valcyte)	

Continued

Table 8.4
Medications Used to Treat Infections—cont'd

Medication Class/Action

Other

Antimitotics and Acidic Agents
Antimitotics inhibit cell division; acidic agents slowly destroy virus-infected epidermis.

Examples	**Nursing Implications**
podophyllin/trichloroacetic acid (TCA)/ bichloracetic acid (BCA)	*Teaching:* Avoid medication contact with eyes or tissue surrounding lesion.

Antimitotic Agents
Inhibit cell division.

Examples	**Nursing Implications**
podofilox solution (Condylox)	*Teaching:* Apply to the genital wart only and allow to dry completely.

Antiviral/immune response modifier

Antivirals inhibit DNA synthesis; immune response modifiers stimulate the immune system.

Example	**Nursing Implications**
imiquimod (Aldara)	*Teaching:* Apply thin film to clean dry skin at bedtime, as ordered.

pain. *C. difficile* infection (CDI) often occurs after antibiotic therapy. It is seen in those who are hospitalized or in long-term care facilities as well as those in the community, which is a newer trend. Older adults are at greatest risk ("Evidence-Based Practice"). *C. difficile* overgrowth can lead to pseudomembranous colitis, a serious and sometimes life-threatening condition with fever, diarrhea, and abdominal pain. The bacteria are transmitted by the fecal–oral route from touching feces-contaminated surfaces. Lidless toilets increase the risk of *C. difficile* environmental contamination by spraying organisms during flushing, so their use is discouraged. Hand washing is essential to reduce its spread, as alcohol-based rubs are not effective. To treat diarrhea caused by CDI, the antibiotic treatment is stopped, and metronidazole (Flagyl) or vancomycin (Vancocin) given. Reoccurrence of the infection can occur. Vaccines are in trials to prevent CDI.

Fecal Microbiota Transplantation
Fecal microbiota transplantation can cure CDI, primarily when other treatments have failed. The purpose is to restore healthy bacteria in the intestine. Patients who have been gravely ill from recurrent CDI can be infection-free within days after the treatment. Donated feces from a screened healthy person is transplanted into a patient via oral capsules, colonoscopy, sigmoidoscopy, enema, nasogastric or

Evidence-Based Practice

Clinical Question
Are probiotics effective in preventing *Clostridium difficile* (*C. difficile*)–associated diarrhea in the older adult?

Evidence
A systematic review and meta-analysis using five randomized control trials revealed that probiotics were not found to be more effective than a placebo in reducing the incidence of *C. difficile*–associated diarrhea in older patients hospitalized in the acute care setting (Vernaya, McAdam, & Hampton, 2017).

Implications for Nursing Practice
Probiotic administration is not effective for preventing *C. difficile*–associated diarrhea. Preventing *C. difficile* infection is important. Preventative measures include using standard precautions, hand hygiene, and disinfecting equipment and items in the patient's room.

Reference
Vernaya, M., McAdam, J., & Hampton, M. D. (2017). The effectiveness of probiotics in reducing the incidence of *Clostridium difficile* associated diarrhea in elderly patients: A systematic review protocol. *JBI Database of Systematic Reviews and Implementation Reports, 15*(1), 140–164.

nasoenteric tube, or esophagogastroduodenoscopy (EGD). Understanding the role the gut microbiota play in our health is leading to the exploration of other uses for fecal transplant. Conditions such as Crohn's disease, ulcerative colitis, inflammatory bowel syndrome, and even rheumatoid arthritis are being explored for this treatment. Synthetic fecal substitutes are in clinical trials.

Nursing Care

Nurses are responsible for administering medications correctly and for teaching patients the importance of taking these medications properly (see "Patient Teaching Guide: Anti-infective Medications" in your online resources). Follow these general guidelines before giving anti-infectives:

- Note all patient allergies, and inform the HCP.
- Obtain ordered samples for culturing before starting ordered anti-infectives, so culture accuracy is not affected.
- Monitor and report to HCP any side effects or signs of allergic response, especially anaphylactic reactions, and peak and trough results.
- Observe and report to HCP any signs of superinfection (one that occurs as a result of antibiotic use). For example, oral thrush (white raised lesions on tongue) may develop because antibiotics disrupt the normal GI tract flora.

BE SAFE!

Always review medication doses. Compare them with the normal dose of the medications before giving them to keep your patient safe and protect your nursing license. You are responsible for any medication you give, even if the dose was ordered incorrectly and you followed the order. If the dose is outside the normal range, do not give the drug. Contact your supervisor or pharmacist for consultation with the ordering HCP for clarification.

NURSING PROCESS FOR THE PATIENT WITH AN INFECTION

General Infections
Data Collection

Early detection of signs and symptoms can help provide early treatment to prevent major complications and reduce costs. Providing emotional support to the patient is also important ("Patient Perspective"). Patients who are prone to infection because of immunosuppression should take special precautions to prevent infection (see "Patient Teaching Guidelines: Prevention of Infection in Older,

Frail, or Immunocompromised Patients" in your online resources).

Patient Perspective

Jeff. It was back! I wasn't sure I could deal with it one more time. I've been hospitalized four times with this same infection (cellulitis) in my leg. It feels like I've lost control of my life. I can't count on being able to do anything or go anywhere because the infection just keeps coming back.

My left leg is swollen, red, discolored, and very painful. I can tell when I'm infected. I feel weak and kind of spacey, and once I passed out. I'm tired of going to the emergency room—waiting forever to get admitted, having an IV [intravenous line] started and blood draws. With these infections, I've had a PICC [peripherally inserted central catheter] line twice. I've been sent home on IV antibiotics, sometimes for weeks at a time. I've learned how to hang my own IV antibiotics; in fact, I've learned much more than I ever wanted to know.

My cellulitis is associated with chronic lymphedema, causing swelling in my legs. I'm working hard to keep the swelling down so the infection doesn't recur. Wish me luck and keep giving me psychosocial support while you provide nursing care.

CRITICAL THINKING

Mr. Cheevers is admitted to the hospital for intravenous antibiotic therapy. He states that he has no allergies. One hour after the infusion begins, you happen to meet the nursing assistant coming down the hall with a blanket. He casually says, "Mr. Cheevers is very cold. I'm taking him a blanket. He is also restless and a bit short of breath." What is your responsibility in this situation?

Suggested answers are at the end of the chapter.

Nursing Diagnoses, Planning, and Implementation

Risk for Infection related to external factors

EXPECTED OUTCOME: The patient will remain free from symptoms of infection.

- Follow current hand hygiene guidelines *to reduce spread of infection.*
- Use standard precautions and transmission-based precautions *to prevent the transmission of organisms.*
- Observe and report signs of infection such as redness, warmth, and fever promptly, especially

for neutropenic patients *because they do not have normal inflammatory response and low-grade fever is often the only sign.*
• Monitor laboratory values of WBC counts and cultures *because they correlate to patient's immune function for planning care.*

Evaluation

If interventions have been successful, the patient remains free from symptoms of infection.

Deficient Knowledge related to disease process and treatment

EXPECTED OUTCOME: The patient will describe therapy and carry out treatment.

• Explain infection and how to prevent infection. *Patient understanding of how infections occur helps them in controlling their risk of infection.*
• Recommend responsible use of antibiotics *to prevent resistant organisms.*
• Explain medications, side effects, and symptoms to report *to promote adherence to treatment and safe medication use.*
• Teach patients how to participate in their own care and have them assist in the development of their plan of care *to promote adherence to treatment.*

Evaluation

If interventions have been effective, the patient will state understanding of therapy and plan and carry out treatment plan.

Respiratory Tract Infection
Data Collection

Patients with respiratory tract infections may have a cough, a congested or runny nose, a sore throat, chest congestion, or chest pain. The throat may be reddened or have white patches on the back. Lung sounds can include crackles, rhonchi, or wheezing. Ask patients whether they have a productive cough, and, if so, the amount, frequency, and color of the sputum. A sputum culture is obtained to identify pathogenic organisms for appropriate treatment.

Nursing Diagnoses, Planning, and Implementation

Risk for Infection related to external factors

EXPECTED OUTCOME: The patient will remain free from symptoms of infection.

• Encourage coughing and deep breathing *to keep airways clear and prevent atelectasis.*
• Provide oral care with toothbrush or suction-type toothbrush (see Chapter 2) and fluoride toothpaste regularly *to remove plaque, which has been found to contribute to pneumonia development.* (Toothettes do not remove plaque.)
• Encourage fluids if not contraindicated. *Dehydration is associated with dry, sticky secretions that are difficult to cough up.*
• Provide pain relief *so patient will take deep breaths.*
• Elevate head of bed 30 degrees or more when a tube feeding is infusing *to prevent aspiration pneumonia.*
• Use sterile water rather than tap water from faucet for oral care for immunocompromised patients *to prevent pneumonia.*

Evaluation

If interventions have been effective, oxygen saturation will be above 95%, with report of decreased dyspnea. Respirations will not be labored, and the patient will be free of signs and symptoms of infection.

Gastrointestinal Tract Infection
Data Collection

The symptoms of GI tract infections may include anorexia, cramping, diarrhea, nausea, and vomiting. Signs of dehydration from fluid loss are reported. Stool cultures may be ordered.

Nursing Diagnoses, Planning, and Implementation

Risk for Infection related to external factors

EXPECTED OUTCOME: The patient will remain free from symptoms of infection.

• Encourage fluid intake *to replace fluid lost during fever, vomiting, and diarrhea.*
• Follow standard and transmission-based precautions *to prevent the spread of* C. difficile.
• Teach hand hygiene with antimicrobial soap and water *because alcohols, chlorhexidine, iodophors, and other antiseptic agents are not effective in destroying* C. difficile *spores.*

Evaluation

Patient will be free of infection and nausea, vomiting, diarrhea, cramping, anorexia, and dehydration if interventions have been successful.

Genitourinary Tract Infection
Data Collection

Symptoms of a UTI include voiding urgency, frequency, burning, flank pain, change in urine color, foul urine odor, and confusion or change in mental status in older adults. Monitor frequency, amount, color, and odor of the urine. Urinalysis and urine cultures may be ordered.

Nursing Diagnoses, Planning, and Implementation

Risk for Infection related to external factors

EXPECTED OUTCOME: The patient will remain free from symptoms of infection.

- Do not request and avoid use of urinary catheters except for justifiable reasons *because patients are more likely to develop a UTI.*

- Use sterile technique for inserting urinary catheters *to prevent HAIs.*
- Avoid contamination when emptying urinary catheter bags *to prevent HAIs.*

Evaluation

If interventions have been effective, the patient will have normal urine output without symptoms of UTI.

SUGGESTED ANSWERS TO CRITICAL THINKING

Mrs. Sampson

1. Hand hygiene reduces the microorganisms on the nurse's hands to help reduce their transmission from patient to patient. This helps prevent exposure to pathogens and infection.
2. The nurse, the patient (whose hands often go unwashed even after toileting, as the patient may be unable to ambulate to the sink), and other health care workers.
3. *Risk for Infection.*
4. Reverse isolation, the goal of which is to protect the patient from exposure to organisms rather than to protect others from exposure to the patient.

Mr. Carson

Point out to the nursing assistant that the urinary bag is placed above the patient's bladder. Explain that the bag should always stay below the level of the bladder both for proper drainage and infection control. Assist the nursing assistant in repositioning the bag properly. Ensure that Mr. Carson is monitored for signs of a bladder infection due to the potential backflow of urine.

Risk of Infection

1. Mr. Ashland has two risk factors: chronic disease and invasive procedure. The procedure was done outside of hospital, which reduces healthcare-associated infection risk.
2. Mrs. Burrows has multiple risk factors: older age, dementia (unable to participate in preventive care such as coughing and deep breathing), frailty, hospitalization, immobility (risk of pneumonia increased), injury, malnourishment, and an invasive procedure. This patient is at greatest risk.
3. Jackson has three risk factors: hospitalization, invasive procedure, and malnourishment.

Mr. Cheevers

Mr. Cheevers may be experiencing signs of allergic reaction to the medication. If allergy is suspected, the intravenous line should be stopped. Notify your supervisor. After immediate evaluation, the health care provider must be notified. Epinephrine should be on hand in case of anaphylaxis. Later, the nursing assistant can be taught to report abnormal symptoms, as they may be a sign of an allergic response.

Review Questions

1. Place the links in the chain of infection in their order of occurrence to result in an infection.
   1. Portal of entry
   2. Infectious agent
   3. Mode of transmission
   4. Portal of exit
   5. Reservoir
   6. Susceptible host

2. Which of the following is the most important technique for the nurse to use during patient care to prevent infection transmission?
   1. Wear gloves.
   2. Wear a gown.
   3. Wash hands.
   4. Wear a mask.

3. The nurse is caring for a patient who is on bed rest. Which of the following nursing actions should the nurse include in the plan of care to help maintain the body's first line of defense against infection? **Select all that apply.**
   1. Help the patient cough and deep breathe.
   2. Apply lotion to clean skin.
   3. Give an antibiotic as ordered.
   4. Help the patient void.
   5. Turn patient every 2 hours.
   6. Keep skin clean and dry.

4. The nurse has taken patient temperatures. Which of the following patient temperature readings would be the priority for the nurse to report to the health care provider?
   1. Temperature 97°F (36.1°C) for an older patient with hypertension
   2. Temperature 98.9°F (37°C) for a first-day postoperative patient
   3. Temperature 99.6°F (37.5°C) for a patient with neutropenia
   4. Temperature 100°F (37.7°C) for a patient with appendicitis

5. The nurse is to give a newly ordered antibiotic to a patient with a wound infection. The nurse is to change the dressing and obtain a wound culture. Which of the following is essential to do before giving the medication? **Select all that apply.**
   1. Check all patient allergies.
   2. Check the patient's temperature.
   3. Change dressing.
   4. Give antibiotic with milk.
   5. Obtain ordered wound culture.
   6. Document wound appearance.

6. The nurse is caring for a patient with an indwelling urinary catheter. Which of the following is the most important action for the nurse to use to prevent a healthcare-associated urinary tract infection from developing in this patient?
   1. Ensure adequate hydration.
   2. Keep catheter tubing secured.
   3. Secure the drainage bag on the bedframe.
   4. Maintain a closed urinary drainage system.

7. The nurse is caring for a patient receiving an antibiotic. Which of the following statements indicates to the nurse that the patient understands the general principles of appropriate antibiotic use?
   1. "I'll take this until I start feeling better."
   2. "I have pills left over from the last time I had this infection to use."
   3. "I'll take all of this as directed on the medication label."
   4. "I can take only half of a pill to reduce the cost of the pills."

Answer rationales available in your online resources.

ANSWERS 1. 2, 5, 4, 3; 1, 6; 2. 3; 3. 2, 5, 6; 4. 3; 5. 1, 5; 6. 4; 7. 3.

Key Points

Find the chapter key points in your online resources available through Davis Edge.

Additional Resources

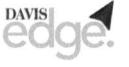 **Use the scratch off code on the inside front cover of your book to access online quizzes that will help you to improve your scores on course exams and prepare for NCLEX-PN°.**

 Study Guide

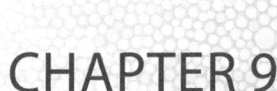

CHAPTER 9
Nursing Care of Patients in Shock

Jennifer Mitchell, Linda S. Williams

KEY TERMS

acidosis (AS-ih-DOH-sis)
acute pulmonary hypertension (ah-KEWT
   PULL-muh-NAIR-ee HY-per-TEN-shun)
anaerobic (AN-air-ROH-bik)
anaphylaxis (AN-uh-fih-LAK-sis)
arrhythmia (uh-RITH-mee-ah)
bronchospasm (BRONG-koh-spazm)
cardiac output (KAR-dee-ack OWT-put)
cardiogenic (KAR-dee-oh-JEN-ik)
cyanosis (SY-uh-NOH-sis)
distributive (dis-TRIB-yoo-tiv)
epinephrine (EP-ih-NEFF-rin)
hypoperfusion (HY-poh-per-FEW-shun)
hypotension (HY-poh-TEN-shun)
hypovolemic (HY-poh-voh-LEE-mik)
ischemia (is-KEY-mee-ah)
lactic acid (LAK-tik AS-id)
laryngeal edema (lah-RIN-jee-uhl eh-DEE-muh)
myocarditis (MY-oh-kar-DY-tis)
myocardium (MY-oh-KAR-dee-um)
neurogenic (NEW-roh-JEN-ik)
norepinephrine (NOR-ep-ih-NEFF-rin)
oliguria (ol-ih-GU-ree-ah)
perfusion (per-FEW-zhun)
pericardial tamponade (PER-ih-KAR-dee-uhl
   TAM-pon-AID)
sepsis (SEP-sis)
tachycardia (TAK-ih-KAR-dee-ah)
tachypnea (TAK-ip-NEE-ah)
tension pneumothorax (TEN-shun NEW-moh-
   THOR-raks)
toxemia (tock-SEE-mee-ah)
trauma (TRAW-mah)
urticaria (UR-tih-CARE-ee-ah)

LEARNING OUTCOMES

1. Explain the pathophysiology of shock and compensatory mechanisms.
2. Identify the etiology, signs, and symptoms for each of the four categories of shock.
3. Describe therapeutic measures for shock.
4. List data to collect when caring for patients in shock.
5. Plan nursing care for patients in shock.
6. Prioritize care for a patient in shock.
7. Identify findings that demonstrate a positive response to therapeutic measures for shock.

CHAPTER CONCEPTS

Acid/Base Balance
Fluid and Electrolyte Balance
Infection
Perfusion

Shock is defined as inadequate tissue **perfusion.** This means there is not enough oxygen being delivered to meet the metabolic needs of the tissues. An oxygen deficit leads to tissue hypoxia and **hypoperfusion** of vital organs and cell death. It is important to identify patients at risk for shock and to monitor them for early signs and symptoms of shock. Timely treatment of shock reduces injury to organs. Prolonged shock leads to cell death and potential organ failure.

PATHOPHYSIOLOGY OF SHOCK

Tissue perfusion and blood pressure are maintained by three mechanisms. The first is adequate blood volume. The second is an effective cardiac pump. Third is effective blood vessels. The body is able to compensate for a problem in one mechanism. It does so by making changes in one or both of the other mechanisms. Shock occurs when the compensatory mechanisms fail to maintain the blood pressure, leading to

• WORD • BUILDING •
hypoperfusion: hypo—low + perfuser—to pour over or through

poor tissue perfusion. Causes of shock include inadequate **cardiac output** caused by heart failure, hemorrhage, or a sudden decrease in peripheral vascular resistance due to **anaphylaxis** (a life-threatening allergic reaction), **sepsis** (a life-threatening condition caused by the body's response to an infection resulting in organ dysfunction), or neurologic alterations.

Metabolic and Hemodynamic Changes in Shock

When blood pressure falls, the sympathetic nervous system is activated. Compensatory mechanisms then begin. **Epinephrine** and **norepinephrine** are released from the adrenal medulla. This causes the heart to beat faster and stronger to increase cardiac output. Blood flow to the heart, brain, and liver is preserved by shunting blood from the intestines, kidneys, and skin. Epinephrine, cortisol, and glucagon raise blood glucose levels to increase cell fuel. The renin-angiotensin-aldosterone system is stimulated by decreased cardiac output. This results in vasoconstriction and retention of sodium and water to maintain fluid balance. Respiratory rate increases to deliver more oxygen to the tissues. Together, these compensatory responses produce the classic signs and symptoms of the first stage of shock: **tachycardia** (rapid heart rate), **tachypnea** (rapid breathing), **oliguria** (producing small amounts of urine), restlessness, anxiety, pallor, and cool, clammy skin. If blood pressure and oxygen delivery remain inadequate, signs and symptoms of progressive and then irreversible shock are seen (Table 9.1).

CRITICAL THINKING

Classic Signs of Shock: What is the cause and compensatory purpose of each of the classic signs of shock: tachycardia, tachypnea, oliguria, pallor, and cool, clammy skin?
   Suggested answers are at the end of the chapter.

LEARNING TIP

Tachycardia is a compensatory mechanism that is usually the first sign of shock. Sustained tachycardia is a signal that the patient's condition is changing. Older patients cannot tolerate tachycardia for very long. Report tachycardia to the registered nurse or health care provider. Consider the cause of the tachycardia. For example, a surgical patient who develops tachycardia may be hemorrhaging. Check for bleeding. Apply direct pressure to an area of hemorrhage. With internal hemorrhaging, there may not be visible bleeding. Vital sign changes may be the only sign. Take action!

When cells are deprived of oxygen, their energy production is affected. It moves from efficient aerobic metabolism to less efficient **anaerobic** metabolism. The energy needs of the cell can only be met by anaerobic metabolism for a brief time. If the oxygen deficiency is prolonged, the body's metabolic rate and temperature fall.

Anaerobic metabolism produces lactate. **Lactic acid,** a by-product of lactate buildup, accumulates. If the lactic acid is not cleared from the bloodstream, it causes acidosis (an acid-base imbalance). **Acidosis** (blood pH below 7.35) is one of the classic signs of shock.

CRITICAL THINKING

Anaerobic Metabolism: Why is anaerobic metabolism necessary and helpful if it produces the complication of metabolic acidosis?
   Suggested answers are at the end of the chapter.

Effect on Organs and Organ Systems

Why does prolonged shock cause extensive damage to organs (Table 9.2)? It does so because inadequate blood flow results in tissue **ischemia** and injury throughout the body. Early in shock, blood is shunted away from the kidneys to save fluid. This helps preserve blood pressure to provide oxygen to vital organs. The kidneys can tolerate reduced blood flow for about 1 hour. Then kidney cells begin to die from a lack of oxygen and nutrients. Acute kidney injury can result.

When the **myocardium** (the middle and muscle layer of the heart wall) receives inadequate oxygenation, pumping action and cardiac output decreases, and shock worsens. Acidosis, toxins released into the bloodstream from ischemic tissues, or ischemia-induced **arrhythmias** (abnormal heart rhythm) further reduce the pumping ability of the heart.

If the brain is deprived of blood flow for more than 4 minutes, brain cells die from a lack of oxygen and glucose. Brain death can result from prolonged shock.

Organs of the gastrointestinal system can be injured early in shock. Inadequate circulation to the intestines injures the mucosa. Paralytic ileus (intestine paralysis) can occur. If gastrointestinal bacteria or endotoxins move from the bowel into the circulation, **toxemia** can result.

The liver can be injured by ischemia. If liver function is affected by this injury, elevated serum levels of ammonia, bilirubin, and liver enzymes and decreased production of plasma proteins can occur. The immune system is weakened by shock, leaving the body vulnerable to infection. If the liver has been damaged, it cannot assist the immune system in providing defense.

• **WORD • BUILDING** •
anaphylaxis: an—without + phylaxis—protection
tachycardia: tachy—fast + cardia—heart
tachypnea: tachy—fast + pnea—breathing
oliguria: olig—few + uria—urine
anaerobic: an—without + aerobic—presence of oxygen
acidosis: acid—sour + osis—condition
arrhythmia: a—without + rhythmia—rhythm

Table 9.1

Characteristics of Shock Stages

Characteristics	Stages		
	• **Compensated** • Able to maintain blood pressure and tissue perfusion	• **Progressive** • Compensatory mechanisms start to fail	• **Irreversible** • No response to treatment • Death is imminent
Heart rate	Tachycardia	Tachycardia Greater than 150 beats/min	Slowing
Pulses	Bounding	Weak, thready	Absent
Systolic blood pressure	Normal	Below 90 mm Hg In hypertensive patient, 25% below baseline	Below 60 mm Hg
Diastolic blood pressure	Normal	Decreased	Decreasing to 0
Respirations	Increased rate, deep	Tachypnea, crackles, shallow	Slowing, irregular, shallow
Temperature	Varies	Decreased, can rise in septic shock	Decreasing
Level of consciousness	Anxious, restless, irritable, alert, oriented, sense of impending doom	Confused, lethargic	Unconscious, comatose
Skin and mucous membranes	Cool, clammy, pale	Moist, cold, clammy, pale	Cyanotic, mottled, cold, clammy
Urine output	Normal	Decreasing to less than 20 mL/hr	15 mL/hr, decreasing to anuria
Bowel sounds	Normal	Decreasing	Absent

COMPLICATIONS FROM SHOCK

Acute respiratory distress syndrome (ARDS), disseminated intravascular coagulation (DIC), and multiple organ dysfunction syndrome (MODS) are three critical conditions that can follow prolonged shock. MODS is a major cause of death following shock. When an organ has inadequate perfusion, it fails. This then contributes to the failure of other organs.

LEARNING TIP

To understand what disseminated intravascular coagulation (DIC) means, define each of the words:

• *Disseminated:* scattered or widespread
• *Intravascular:* intra = inside + vascular = vessel
• *Coagulation:* clotting

Put together, these definitions tell you that DIC is scattered, widespread clotting inside the vessel.

Hemorrhage does not seem likely when there is a clotting problem. But when many clots form throughout the body in response to stressors, few clotting factors remain available to form clots that are needed to prevent hemorrhage. As a result, hemorrhage is a risk in DIC.

CLASSIFICATION OF SHOCK

The four types of shock are classified by their cardiovascular characteristics (Table 9.3):

• Hypovolemic shock is caused by a decrease in the circulating blood volume.
• Cardiogenic shock is caused by cardiac pump failure.
• Obstructive shock is caused by a blockage of blood flow in the cardiovascular circuit outside the heart.
• Distributive shock is caused by excessive dilation of the venules and arterioles.

The classic sign in all forms of shock is a decrease in blood pressure below the level needed to provide sufficient blood flow to the tissues for adequate oxygenation.

Hypovolemic Shock

Hypovolemic shock can be caused by dehydration; internal or external hemorrhage; fluid loss from burns, vomiting, or diarrhea; or loss of intravascular fluid into the interstitial space from sepsis or **trauma** (physical injury caused by an external force). Heat exhaustion or heatstroke can also cause hypovolemic shock from excessive water loss through sweating. Signs and symptoms include restlessness; pale,

Table 9.2

Effect of Shock on Organs and Organ Systems

Organ or Organ System	Effect
Lungs	Acute respiratory failure Acute respiratory distress syndrome (ARDS)
Renal system	Renal insufficiency Acute kidney injury
Heart	Arrhythmias Myocardial ischemia Myocardial infarction
Liver	Decreased production of plasma proteins Impaired clotting Elevated serum levels of ammonia, bilirubin, and liver enzymes
Immune system	Depletion of defense components
Gastrointestinal system	Absorption of endotoxins and bacteria Mucosal injury Pancreatitis Paralytic ileus
Central nervous system	Ischemic damage, necrosis, and brain death

cool, clammy skin; tachycardia; tachypnea; flat, nondistended peripheral veins; decreased jugular vein circumference; decreased urine output; and altered mental status. The body is usually able to compensate for blood loss of less than 15%, or 750 mL. Tachycardia may be the only symptom. At 20% to 25% blood loss, tachycardia and mild-to-moderate **hypotension** are present. With a loss of 40% or greater (2,000 mL), all signs and symptoms of shock are present. Volume loss alone might not be the only contributing factor to hypovolemic shock. The patient's age, health status, and the time frame for fluid loss can also be factors.

NURSING CARE TIP

The Trendelenburg position, in which the body is supine with the feet raised higher than the head, was formerly used to try to increase cardiac output in hypovolemic shock. However, research has shown that it is not helpful in improving cardiac output for patients in shock and can have profound negative effects (Miller, Hayes, & Carey, 2015). Although you might still see this position being used, remember that evidence-based practice produces the best patient outcomes.

Cardiogenic Shock

Cardiogenic shock occurs when the heart fails as a pump and decreases cardiac output. It requires immediate treatment to prevent death. Signs and symptoms are like those of hypovolemic shock. Pulmonary edema may occur. This differentiates cardiogenic shock from other forms of shock. The main cause of cardiogenic shock is acute myocardial infarction. Other causes are traumatic injury to the heart, **myocarditis** (inflammation of the heart muscle), cardiomyopathy, heart valve defects, endocarditis, or arrhythmias.

Obstructive Shock

Obstructive shock occurs when there is a blockage of blood flow outside of the heart. **Pericardial tamponade** occurs when the pericardial sac fills with blood or fluid. This compresses the heart and limits its filling capacity. **Tension pneumothorax** compresses the heart because of an abnormal collection of air in the pleural space. **Acute pulmonary hypertension** is a sudden abnormally elevated pressure in the pulmonary artery. It increases resistance for the blood flowing out of the right side of the heart. All of these conditions decrease cardiac output. This can lead to shock. A pulmonary embolism or tumor blocking blood flow can also lead to shock. Signs and symptoms of obstructive shock are similar to those of hypovolemic shock, except that jugular veins are usually distended.

Distributive Shock

Distributive shock occurs when peripheral vascular resistance is lost because of massive vasodilation. In hypovolemic shock, there is an actual loss of blood volume. But in distributive shock, there is no loss of fluid volume; rather, the body's fluid distribution is altered within the body. There are three forms of distributive shock: anaphylactic, septic, and neurogenic.

Anaphylactic Shock

Anaphylactic shock is the most severe type of distributive shock. It occurs when the body has an extreme hypersensitivity reaction to an antigen. Death from anaphylactic shock can occur in minutes but is rare. Medical treatment must be sought immediately. Asthma or a delay in epinephrine injections can increase the risk of death. For safety, patients are taught allergen avoidance techniques (Box 9.1).

Anaphylaxis occurs most commonly from food allergies (e.g., shellfish or peanuts), insect stings, antibiotics (especially penicillin), anesthetics, contrast dye, and blood products. Symptoms specific to allergic reactions include **urticaria** (hives), pruritus, wheezing, **laryngeal edema** (swelling of the larynx), angioedema (edema of skin, mucous membranes, or internal organs), and severe **bronchospasm** (narrowing of bronchi in the lungs). Signs and symptoms similar to those of hypovolemic shock may also be seen. If conscious, patients can be extremely apprehensive and short of breath.

• WORD • BUILDING •
cardiogenic: kardia—heart + genesis—beginning

Table 9.3

Categories of Shock

Category	Causes	Signs and Symptoms
Hypovolemic Shock	Any severe loss of body fluid, including dehydration; internal or external hemorrhage; fluid loss from burns, vomiting, or diarrhea; or loss of intravascular fluid into the interstitium	Tachycardia, tachypnea, hypotension, cyanosis, oliguria, flat and nondistended peripheral veins, decreased jugular veins, altered mental status
Cardiogenic Shock	Myocardial infarction, traumatic cardiac injury, cardiomyopathy, endocarditis, myocarditis, arrhythmias, valvular disease	Arrhythmias, labored respirations, hypotension, cyanosis, oliguria, altered mental status, possibly distended jugular and peripheral veins, symptoms of heart failure
Obstructive Shock	Any block to the cardiovascular flow, such as pericardial tamponade, tension pneumothorax, intrathoracic tumor, massive pulmonary embolus, large systemic embolus	Tachycardia, tachypnea, hypotension, cyanosis, oliguria, altered mental status, possibly distended jugular veins
Distributive Shock	Any condition causing massive vasodilation of peripheral circulation, including the subcategories anaphylactic, septic, and neurogenic shock	*See below.*
• Anaphylactic shock	Reaction to an allergen, such as an insect sting, medication, peanuts, antibiotic, anesthetic, contrast dye, or blood product	• Tachycardia, tachypnea, wheezing, hypotension, cyanosis, oliguria, altered mental status • Can have urticaria, pruritus, angioedema, laryngeal edema, severe bronchospasm • If conscious, can be extremely apprehensive
• Septic shock	Loss of vascular autoregulatory control and loss of fluid into the interstitium caused by massive release of chemical mediators and endotoxins from pathogens	• *Early (warm) phase:* tachycardia; blood pressure, urine output, and capillary refill can be normal; skin warm and flushed; fever usually present; although temperature can be subnormal, fever may be absent in older or immunosuppressed people • *Late (cold) phase:* tachycardia; tachypnea; hypotension; oliguria; delayed capillary refill; cool, clammy skin; normal or subnormal temperature; altered mental status
• Neurogenic shock	Dysfunction or injury to the nervous system from spinal cord injury, general anesthesia, fever, metabolic disturbance, brain injury	• *Early phase:* hypotension; altered mental status; bradycardia; warm, dry skin • *Late phase:* tachycardia; tachypnea; cool, clammy skin

Box 9.1

Patient Education

Patients who have severe allergies and a risk for anaphylaxis should have a prescribed epinephrine autoinjector. It is important to have the epinephrine autoinjector available at all times for rapid onset, life-threatening reactions. Medical treatment must be sought immediately after using the epinephrine.

Septic Shock

Sepsis is defined as "life-threatening organ dysfunction caused by dysregulated host response to infection" (Singer et al., 2016). Septic shock is defined as "a subset of sepsis with circulatory and cellular/metabolic dysfunction associated with a higher risk of mortality" (Singer et al., 2016). Septic shock has a higher risk of death. With septic shock, there is extreme hypoperfusion. Early diagnosis and rapid treatment of sepsis are vital to increasing survival rates.

Sepsis cases have risen 5.7% per year from 2008 to 2012. However, mortality has decreased from 22.2% to 17.3% (Stoller et al., 2015). The goal of the Surviving Sepsis Campaign (www.survivingsepsis.org) is to reduce the sepsis mortality rate ("Evidence-Based Practice"). Factors that increase sepsis risk include being over age 65, having a chronic illness, having a weakened immune system, having severe burns, or being critically ill ("Gerontological Issues"). Infections of the gastrointestinal tract, lungs, skin, and urinary tract are more commonly associated with sepsis. Bacteria that commonly cause sepsis are *Escherichia coli, Staphylococcus aureus,* and *Streptococcus.*

Evidence-Based Practice

Clinical Question
What are the best ways to manage sepsis and septic shock?

Evidence
The International Guidelines for Management of Sepsis and Septic Shock: 2016 provide updated evidence-based interventions (Rhodes et al., 2017). Nursing care–related interventions include the following:

- Use screening protocol for sepsis on acutely ill and high-risk patients.
- Promptly obtain all ordered cultures (including two sets of blood cultures) prior to antimicrobial therapy so therapy is not delayed.
- Administer ordered broad-spectrum intravenous (IV) antimicrobials (often initially of two different classes) within 1 hour of sepsis or septic shock diagnosis.
- Administer and monitor ordered IV fluids (30 mL/kg of crystalloid fluid within first 3 hours for hypotension or lactate equal to or more than 4 mmol/L).
- Administer ordered vasopressors (norepinephrine first choice).
- Report ordered lab results (such as lactate level).
- Use ordered prone positioning for mechanically ventilated patients with sepsis-related acute respiratory distress syndrome (ARDS).
- Maintain ordered glycemic control (arterial blood may be more accurate for point of care testing).
- Provide ordered enteral nutrition (early initiation desirable).
- Assist with planning of care and the use of palliative care as appropriate.

Implications for Nursing Practice
Careful screening for sepsis and promptly carrying out ordered interventions included in the 2016 guidelines are vital to increasing patient survival rates from sepsis and septic shock.

Reference
Rhodes, A., Evans, L., Alhazzani, W., Levy, M. M., Antonelli, M., Ferrer, R., ... Dellinger, R. (2017). Surviving Sepsis campaign: International guidelines for management of sepsis and septic shock: 2016. *Critical Care Medicine, 45*(3), 486–552. doi:10.1097/CCM.0000000000002255

Gerontological Issues

Sepsis. The older adult population has less ability to fight infections, which places them at higher risk for sepsis. In a study of California hospitalizations from 2000 to 2010, the sepsis rate for those aged 85 and over was about 30 times the rate for those under age 65 (Gohil et al., 2016).

Neurogenic Shock
Neurogenic shock occurs due to nervous system injury or dysfunction that causes extensive dilation of peripheral blood vessels. Causes include spinal cord injury, general anesthesia, fever, metabolic disturbances, and brain contusions and concussions. Signs include hypotension and altered mental status and, during the early phases, bradycardia and warm, dry skin. As shock progresses, however, tachycardia and cool, clammy skin develops.

 ## THERAPEUTIC MEASURES FOR SHOCK

Because of the life-threatening nature of shock, immediate medical treatment is needed. The nature of the shock must be determined (Table 9.4) and interventions, including ventilatory and circulatory support, started. Life-threatening symptoms must be treated immediately (Table 9.5). If septic shock is identified, then current sepsis care guidelines are followed (visit www.survivingsepsis.org). Medications that are used in shock are listed in Table 9.6. The order of interventions and testing is guided by the stability of the patient. Interventions include the following:

1. Airway management
2. Breathing and respiratory support
3. Cardiovascular support
4. Maintenance of circulatory volume
5. Control of bleeding, if present
6. Assessment of neurologic status
7. Treatment of life-threatening injuries
8. Determination and treatment of the cause of shock

Table 9.4
Assessment of the Patient in Shock

Signs and Symptoms	Tachycardia, tachypnea, hypotension, oliguria, cyanosis, altered mental status
Laboratory Tests	Arterial blood gases, blood chemistries, blood typing and cross-match, cardiac isoenzymes, complete blood count, partial thromboplastin time, prothrombin time, serum lactate, serum osmolarity, urinalysis
Imaging	Chest x-ray, computed tomography, echocardiogram, spinal x-ray
Monitoring	Electrocardiogram, arterial pressure, hemodynamic monitoring

Table 9.5
Therapeutic Measures for Shock

Airway Management and Respiratory Support	Oxygen (nasal cannula, face mask, partial nonrebreather mask, assisted ventilations with bag-valve-mask, mechanical ventilator) SpO_2 over 95% Venous lactate less than 2.2 mmol/L
Cardiovascular Support	Vasopressor medication, if fluid resuscitation not effective Revascularization of heart in cardiogenic shock via angioplasty, with or without stent or fibrinolytic therapy Antiarrhythmics Positive inotropes
Adequate Circulatory Volume	Crystalloid fluids 30 mL/kg within first 3 hours for septic shock Blood or blood products Urine output greater than 30 mL/hr Hemoglobin greater than 10 g/dL
Control of Bleeding	Pressure dressings Surgical intervention
Treatment of Life-Threatening Injuries	Surgical intervention Medications
Medications for Types of Shock	Sepsis/septic shock: broad spectrum antimicrobials within 1 hour of diagnosis Cardiogenic shock: diuretics, nitrates, inotropics, vasopressors Anaphylactic shock: epinephrine, diphenhydramine (Benadryl), methylprednisolone (Solu-Medrol)

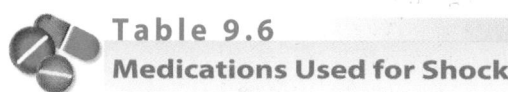

Table 9.6
Medications Used for Shock

Medication Class/Action

Autonomic Nervous System Agents and Alpha- and Beta-Adrenergic Agents

Examples	**Nursing Indicators**
To strengthen myocardial contraction, increase systolic blood pressure, and increase cardiac output: epinephrine (Adrenalin) dopamine (Intropin) norepinephrine (Levophed) phenylephrine hydrochloride (Neo-Synephrine)	Correct hypovolemia before giving medications Monitor vital signs often; vasopressor use should include arterial blood pressure monitoring; monitor intake and output
Examples	**Nursing Indicators**
To bronchodilate: epinephrine (Adrenalin)	First drug given in anaphylactic shock

Beta-Adrenergic Agent
Increases cardiac output in cardiogenic shock.

Examples	**Nursing Indicators**
dobutamine (Dobutrex)	Monitor vital signs often Monitor intake and output

Continued

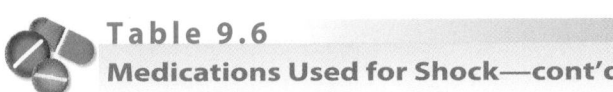

Table 9.6
Medications Used for Shock—cont'd

Medication Class/Action

Antihistamine
Inhibits histamine release.

Examples	**Nursing Indicators**
diphenhydramine (Benadryl)	Monitor vital signs
	May cause drowsiness

Anti-Inflammatory
Controls severe allergic reactions.

Examples	**Nursing Indicators**
methylprednisolone (Solu-Medrol)	Monitor patient for signs and symptoms of infection
hydrocortisone (Solu-Cortef)	
dexamethasone (Decadron)	

NURSING PROCESS FOR THE PATIENT IN SHOCK

Data Collection

Recognizing and reporting patients at risk for shock is vital for increased patient survival. Being vigilant and screening patients for sepsis is important. Early detection and prevention of shock in patients at risk for shock are the desired goals. Rapid response teams can be helpful in providing quick assessment and care of patients at risk of developing shock.

For the patient in shock, assessment must be carried out quickly and should always start with ABCD: airway, breathing, circulation, and disability.

*A*irway is checked for patency and opened as necessary. A compromised airway must be treated immediately with the head-tilt/chin-lift method, an oral or nasal airway, or endotracheal intubation.

*B*reathing is checked for rate, depth, and symmetry of chest movement. The patient is observed for use of accessory muscles. Lung sounds are auscultated. Wheezing can be present in the patient with anaphylactic shock. Crackles can be found in the patient with cardiogenic shock or in the patient who has received too much intravenous fluid.

*C*irculation is checked with blood pressure measurement. A narrowing pulse pressure can be present before a drop in systolic pressure. This indicates a decrease in cardiac stroke volume and peripheral vasoconstriction. Peripheral pulses are palpated. Tachycardia is the first sign of shock. However, patients on medications that block the sympathetic nervous system response will not exhibit tachycardia. The pulse is assessed for quality; commonly, it is weak and thready in a patient with shock. As shock progresses, the peripheral pulses become weaker or absent. A capillary refill greater than 3 seconds indicates inadequate circulation. However, it has been found to be an unreliable indicator of shock in adults, especially older adults. Other observations for circulation include distended neck veins; skin that is cool, pale, and diaphoretic; presence of **cyanosis** (bluish color of skin and mucous membranes from decreased oxygen in the blood); mucous membranes that are pale and dry; and thirst. Rapidly scan the entire body for evidence of bleeding or other injuries.

> **NURSING CARE TIP**
> There is usually a loss of peripheral pulses in the patient whose systolic blood pressure has dropped below 80. If you are able to palpate a radial pulse on your patient, the systolic blood pressure is usually at least 80.

*D*isability is determined by the patient's level of consciousness. A decrease in level of consciousness indicates disability. This disability can range from lethargy to coma.

All four limbs are checked for circulation, sensation, and mobility (remember as CSM). Bilateral responses are compared for equality. Circulation is assessed by palpating pulses for presence and quality. Sensation is determined by touching the patient's hands and feet and asking what the patient feels and if there is any numbness or tingling. Mobility (motor

• WORD • BUILDING •
cyanosis: cyan—blue coloring + osis—condition

ability) is assessed by having the patient move all four limbs and wiggle the fingers and toes. Have the patient push with his or her feet against your hands and squeeze two of your fingers to determine strength.

A head-to-toe approach can follow the primary ABCD assessment. The presence, severity, and location of pain or nausea and vomiting are noted. Body temperature is measured. Bowel sounds are auscultated to determine whether they are normal, absent, hyperactive, or hypoactive. With an indwelling urinary catheter, the color, rate, and amount of urine output are noted.

NURSING CARE TIP

To determine whether a patient is alert and oriented, ask his or her name, current place, and the date. If the patient correctly answers all three questions, he or she is "alert and oriented × 3 (person, place, time)."

CRITICAL THINKING

Mrs. Nabozny takes a beta blocker. What sign of shock do you understand will not be present?
Suggested answers are at the end of the chapter.

Nursing Diagnoses, Planning, Implementation, and Evaluation

See Table 9.7 for a summary of shock. Also see "Nursing Care Plan for the Patient Experiencing Shock."

Table 9.7
Shock Summary

Signs and Symptoms	Tachycardia Tachypnea Hypotension Oliguria Altered mental state Cyanosis
Diagnostic Tests	Increased lactate Decreased pH (metabolic acidosis) Decreased hemoglobin with hemorrhage Increased white blood cell count in sepsis
Therapeutic Measures	Oxygen Intravenous fluids Vasopressor medications Treatment of underlying cause
Complications	Acute respiratory distress syndrome (ARDS) Disseminated intravascular coagulation (DIC) Multiple organ dysfunction syndrome (MODS)
Priority Nursing Diagnoses	*Risk for Ineffective Tissue Perfusion (Cerebral, Peripheral)* *Decreased Cardiac Output*

Nursing Care Plan for the Patient Experiencing Shock

Nursing Diagnosis: *Risk for Ineffective Tissue Perfusion* (cerebral, peripheral) related to hypovolemia or inadequate cardiac output or changes in circulatory volume or inadequate vascular tone, possibly evidenced by altered level of consciousness, changes in skin color/temperature, tachycardia, reduced blood pressure, and decreased urine output
Expected Outcome: The patient will demonstrate adequate tissue perfusion as evidenced by warm and dry skin, strong peripheral pulses, vital signs within normal parameters of baseline, breath sounds without adventitious sounds, and balanced intake and output. The patient will be alert and oriented to person, place, and time within specified time frame.
Evaluation of Outcome: Is the patient's skin warm and dry? Are peripheral pulses present/strong? Are vital signs within the patient's normal range? Are lung sounds normal, intake/output balanced, edema absent, and pain/discomfort absent? Is the patient alert and oriented?

Intervention	Rationale	Evaluation
Maintain airway and provide oxygen as ordered.	*Ensures adequate oxygenation and tissue perfusion.*	Is Spo₂ over 95%? Are skin and mucous membranes pink? Are respirations between 12 and 20 per minute? Are lung sounds clear?
Monitor vital signs.	*Changes in vital signs, which indicate change in condition, can be detected early and treated promptly.*	Is heart rate between 60 and 100 beats per minute? Is heart rhythm regular? Are peripheral pulses strong? Is systolic blood pressure greater than 100 mm Hg? Is the patient alert and oriented × 3?

(nursing care plan continues on page 116)

Nursing Care Plan for the Patient Experiencing Shock—cont'd

Intervention	Rationale	Evaluation
Monitor intake and output.	*Adequate intake needed to maintain cardiac output. Urine output is an indicator of renal function.*	Is urinary output greater than 30 mL/hr?
Provide adequate fluid intake.	*Maintains volume.*	Are mucous membranes moist? Is skin turgor less than 3 seconds?
Maintain body temperature with warmed intravenous (IV) fluids, room temperature, and blankets.	*Recovery is aided by normal body temperature.*	Is body temperature within normal limits?
Provide a quiet, restful environment.	*Conserves energy and lowers tissue oxygen demands.*	Is patient resting comfortably without anxiety?
Monitor for pain, and provide pain relief measures.	*Pain increases tissue demands for blood and oxygen.*	Is patient pain free?

Geriatric

Intervention	Rationale	Evaluation
Change positions slowly.	*Age-related losses of cardiovascular reflexes can result in hypotension.*	Is systolic blood pressure greater than 100 mm Hg?

Nursing Diagnosis: *Decreased Cardiac Output* related to reduced circulating blood volume, structural damage, or decreased myocardial contractility as evidenced by abnormal vital signs and irregular cardiac rhythm
Expected Outcome: The patient will have adequate cardiac output as evidenced by vital signs and cardiac rhythm within normal limits within specified time frame.
Evaluation of Outcome: Are blood pressure, heart rate, and cardiac rhythm within normal limits? Are nailbeds and/or skin pink? Is skin warm, dry, and intact?

Intervention	Rationale	Evaluation
Monitor heart rate and cardiac rhythm with electrocardiogram, and report abnormalities.	*Changes in heart rate and cardiac rhythm can be detected immediately and treated appropriately.*	Are heart rate and rhythm normal?
Monitor skin/nailbed color, capillary refill, and peripheral pulses, and report abnormalities.	*Inadequate perfusion is first evident in skin/nailbeds and peripheral pulses.*	What color and temperature are the skin/nailbeds? Is capillary refill less than 3 seconds? Are peripheral pulses present?
Give cardiovascular medications and oxygen as ordered.	*Cardiac function can be supported with medications. Supplemental oxygen increases oxygenation of heart and tissues.*	Are heart rate and rhythm normal?
Monitor skin for pressure injuries and implement prevention interventions when vasopressors used.	*Vasopressors (e.g., norepinephrine and vasopressin) can cause unavoidable pressure injuries due to vasoconstriction.*	Is skin intact?
Provide comfort measures to alleviate pain and anxiety and maintain a normal body temperature.	*Pain, anxiety, and cold increase tissue demands for oxygen, which increases the heart's workload to supply it.*	Is patient free of pain and anxiety? Is body temperature within normal limits?

Nursing Care Plan for the Patient Experiencing Shock—cont'd

Geriatric

Monitor perfusion by methods other than capillary refill, such as skin temperature.	*Capillary refill is frequently delayed in the older adult population. Blood flow warms the body.*	Is body temperature within normal limits?

Nursing Diagnosis: *Deficient Knowledge* related to unfamiliar condition of shock as evidenced by verbalization of deficient knowledge (e.g., "I don't understand what's happening to me.")
Expected Outcome: The patient will explain shock and its treatment.
Evaluation of Outcome: Can the patient explain shock and how it is treated?

Intervention	Rationale	Evaluation
Identify patient's ability to learn and barriers to learning.	*For learning, patient must be stable and ready to learn.*	Is patient alert and stable? Does patient indicate willingness to learn?
Provide patient-centered information on shock and treatment.	*Giving individualized information on topics meets patient's need for understanding.*	Can patient explain shock and the purpose of treatment that the patient is receiving?
Allow time for questions and clarification.	*Clarification ensures accurate information is learned.*	Does patient state accurate information?

Geriatric

Involve family/caregivers in teaching.	*Family/caregivers can reinforce education provided.*	Do family/caregivers verbalize understanding of material presented?
Speak slowly and clearly in a low tone/pitch.	*Older adults have difficulty hearing high-pitched tones.*	Does patient acknowledge being spoken to?
Provide materials in large print.	*Visual changes that accompany aging can require a patient to need larger print materials.*	Can patient restate and/or read aloud information that has been given?

CRITICAL THINKING

Mr. Hall, who is 58 years old, had an acute myocardial infarction 2 days ago. He reports chest pain (rated 10 out of 10 on the pain rating scale) and difficulty breathing. His blood pressure is 96/40, pulse 110, respiration rate 22, and Spo_2 89%. Crackles are heard on auscultation of breath sounds. The electrocardiogram shows an irregular and rapid heartbeat. He is restless and apprehensive.

1. Name three priorities for Mr. Hall's nursing care.
2. With which members of the health care team does the nurse anticipate collaborating?
3. Are intravenous fluids appropriate for Mr. Hall now?
4. What signs and symptoms indicate Mr. Hall is in cardiogenic shock?

Suggested answers are at the end of the chapter.

CRITICAL THINKING

Mrs. Neal, aged 45, arrived at the emergency department in severe hypovolemic shock. She sustained several bleeding wounds in a motor vehicle accident. Her shock is resolving after receiving several transfusions and surgical repair of her injuries. She has just been admitted to your surgical unit for postoperative care.

1. What postoperative data collection should be done first?
2. How can patient-centered care be promoted during treatment?
3. What family-centered care can be provided to Mrs. Neal's family, who is alarmed by her condition?
4. What postoperative complications could develop in Mrs. Neal?
5. What nursing care documentation is appropriate for Mrs. Neal?

Suggested answers are at the end of the chapter.

SUGGESTED ANSWERS TO CRITICAL THINKING

Classic Signs of Shock

Tachycardia is caused by decreased cardiac output and reduced tissue oxygenation. Its purpose is to increase cardiac output and oxygen delivery with more heartbeats that pump blood out of the heart.

Tachypnea is caused by decreased tissue oxygenation. Its purpose is to increase respirations so that more oxygen is available for delivery to tissues.

Oliguria is caused by a reduced blood flow to the kidneys. Its purpose as a compensatory mechanism is to conserve as much fluid as possible to help maintain normal blood pressure.

Pallor is caused by reduced blood volume or flow. Peripheral vasoconstriction shunts blood from the skin to the vital organs.

Cool, clammy skin is the result of decreased blood flow to the skin and the release of moisture (sweat) from the skin. Sweating cools the body in anticipation of the fight-or-flight response, which generates body heat when it occurs.

Anaerobic Metabolism

Anaerobic metabolism is the source of nutrition and energy for the cell that prevents cellular death when oxygen is not available. It is a *short-term* compensatory mechanism to help save the cell until oxygen becomes available again.

Mrs. Nabozny

Tachycardia will not be present. Beta blockers block the cardiac response of the sympathetic nervous system activated in shock.

Mr. Hall

1. Nursing priorities for Mr. Hall include adequate tissue perfusion, relief of chest pain and anxiety, and stabilization of cardiac rhythm and vital signs.
2. The health care provider and case manager.
3. No. Because Mr. Hall's lung sounds reveal crackles, indicating fluid in the lungs, he should not be given intravenous (IV) fluids. He already has too much fluid within his body for his heart to handle and giving him more IV fluids could be life threatening. He should have an IV access for IV medications as needed.
4. Signs of cardiogenic shock include decreased blood pressure; increased heart and respiratory rates; cyanosis; decreased urine output; cool, pale nailbeds and/or skin; and decreased mental status.

Mrs. Neal

1. Data collection for respiratory and cardiovascular status, inspection of surgical wounds for bleeding, and noting mental status and the need for pain relief should be performed first.
2. Develop a pain management plan to meet Mrs. Neal's individualized needs. Identify her normal coping techniques to support their appropriate use. Provide explanations and teach as needed to keep the patient informed for decision making. Advocate for her individualized needs, such as nutritional needs.
3. Explain the cause of shock and all interventions, rationales, and desired outcomes. Keep the environment calm, provide for privacy, and answer all questions in a matter-of-fact and reassuring manner. Allow Mrs. Neal's family to visit.
4. Unrelieved pain, bleeding, infection, and respiratory complications are possible.
5. *Airway:* rate, depth, regularity of respirations, breath sounds, Spo_2. *Vital signs:* cardiac rhythm, quality of pulses, skin color, blood pressure, body temperature. *Urine output:* oral and IV intake, fluid balance. *Pain:* measures to relieve pain and evaluation of those measures. *Dressings:* drainage color and amount. *Bowel sounds:* presence.

Review Questions

1. The nurse is collecting data on a patient experiencing shock in the emergency department. The nurse would recognize signs of compensation for shock as resulting from which of these mechanisms?
   1. Peripheral nervous system depression
   2. Central nervous system depression
   3. Sympathetic nervous system stimulation
   4. Parasympathetic nervous system stimulation

2. Which of these findings during data collection would the nurse specifically anticipate in a patient experiencing anaphylactic shock? **Select all that apply.**
   1. Wheezing
   2. Hypertension
   3. Tachycardia
   4. Oliguria
   5. Urticaria
   6. Bronchospasm

3. The nurse would recognize which of these conditions as the cause for decreased level of consciousness, which is commonly found in patients experiencing shock?
   1. Severe pain
   2. Endotoxins
   3. Cerebral edema
   4. Cerebral hypoxia

4. The nurse is contributing to the plan of care for an older patient at risk for cardiogenic shock. Which of these interventions would the nurse include for the nursing diagnosis of *Deficient Knowledge* to aid the learning of this older patient about this condition? **Select all that apply.**
   1. Involve family/caregivers in teaching.
   2. Use a high-pitched tone when speaking.
   3. Provide materials in large print.
   4. Reinforce health promotion activities with the patient.
   5. Speak slowly and clearly.

5. The nurse is monitoring a patient experiencing shock who is being given crystalloid intravenous fluids. Which of these findings would indicate to the nurse that the treatment is effective?
   1. Decreased urine output
   2. Increased heart rate
   3. Clammy skin
   4. Increased blood pressure

6. The nurse is contributing to the plan of care for a patient experiencing shock. Which of the following nursing diagnoses is most appropriate to include in this plan of care?
   1. *Fatigue*
   2. Risk for *Ineffective Tissue Perfusion* (Cerebral, Peripheral)
   3. *Ineffective Health Maintenance*
   4. *Hopelessness*

7. A patient who is hemorrhaging from a leg incision is restless and confused. The nurse applies pressure to the incision and calls for help. Which of the following treatments for shock would the nurse anticipate being ordered first?
   1. Crystalloid intravenous fluids
   2. Oxygen
   3. Vasopressor medication
   4. One unit of packed red blood cells

8. The nurse is assigned to the nursing care team caring for the following patients. Which patient would be the priority for the nurse to see first?
   1. A patient who was in a motor vehicle accident with blood pressure 132/80 mm Hg, pulse 98 beats per minute, respirations 20 per minute
   2. A patient who has a migraine with blood pressure 108/68 mm Hg, pulse 84 beats per minute, respirations 16 per minute
   3. A patient who slipped and fell with blood pressure 112/74 mm Hg, pulse 68 beats per minute, respirations 14 per minute
   4. A patient who is 1 day post-op with blood pressure 88/58 mm Hg, pulse 152 beats per minute, respirations 24 per minute

9. Which of these objective data collection findings would indicate to the nurse that the therapeutic measures for a patient experiencing shock have been effective?
   1. Heart rate 110 beats per minute
   2. SpO_2 89%
   3. Systolic blood pressure 118 mm Hg
   4. Respiratory rate 22 per minute

10. The nurse is caring for a patient who is experiencing progressive shock. Place in correct order of occurrence the systolic blood pressure findings that the nurse obtained for this patient who progressed through the three stages of shock and is now in irreversible shock. Begin with compensated shock and use all options.
    1. 56 mm Hg
    2. 116 mm Hg
    3. 86 mm Hg

Answer rationales available in your online resources.

ANSWERS 1. 3; 2. 1; 5. 6; 3. 4; 4. 1, 3, 5. 4; 6. 2; 7. 2; 8. 4; 9. 3; 10. 2, 3, 1

Key Points

Find the chapter key points in your online resources available through Davis Edge.

Additional Resources

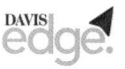 **Use the scratch off code on the inside front cover of your book to access online quizzes that will help you to improve your scores on course exams and prepare for NCLEX-PN®.**

 Study Guide

CHAPTER 10
Nursing Care of Patients in Pain

Sheria G. Robinson-Lane, April Hazard Vallerand

KEY TERMS

addiction (uh-DIK-shun)
adjuvant (ad-JOO-vant)
agonist (AG-un-ist)
analgesic (AN-uhl-JEE-zik)
antagonist (an-TAG-on-ist)
breakthrough (BRAYK-THROO)
ceiling effect (SEE-ling ee-FEKT)
endorphins (en-DOOR-fins)
enkephalins (en-KEFF-eh-lins)
equianalgesic (EH-kwee-AN-uhl-JEE-zik)
hyperalgesia (HYPER-al-JEE-zee-ah)
malingerer (muh-LING-gur-er)
neuropathic (NEW-roh-PATH-ik)
nociception (NOH-sih-SEP-shun)
opioid (OH-pee-OYD)
patient-controlled analgesia (PAY-shunt kon-TROHLD AN-uhl-JEE-zee-ah)
physical dependence (FIZZ-ik-uhl dee-PEN-dense)
prostaglandins (PRAHS-tah-GLAND-ins)
pseudoaddiction (soo-doh-uh-DIK-shun)
psychological dependence (SY-ko-LAW-jik-al dee-PEN-dense)
somatic (so-MAT-ik)
suffering (SUH-fur-ing)
tolerance (TAWL-ur-ens)
transdermal (trans-DER-mal)
visceral (VISS-er-uhl)

CHAPTER CONCEPTS

Addiction and Behaviors
Comfort
Patient-Centered Care
Safety

LEARNING OUTCOMES

1. Describe current definitions of pain.
2. Identify common myths and barriers to the effective management of pain.
3. Differentiate among addiction, physical dependence, and tolerance.
4. Explain current understanding about the basic physiology of the pain response.
5. Differentiate between nociceptive and neuropathic pain.
6. Perform a basic pain assessment.
7. Describe the three classes of analgesics and their uses.
8. Identify commonly used pain medication treatment modalities and their appropriate use.
9. Recognize appropriate use of nonpharmacological pain management techniques.

 ## THE PAIN PUZZLE

Pain hurts—and not just in a physical way. It can make us feel emotionally sad or angry, feel spiritually empty, and lead to social isolation. Having pain is an experience that can affect every aspect of a person's being and how he or she functions in the environment. Pain management is the most common reason patients seek medical advice. However, despite the widespread nature of the problem and the millions of dollars spent on care, pain often remains untreated or undertreated. Nurses can make a difference in pain management.

Nurses often worry about overmedicating patients and may think that they are "doing good" (beneficence) or "doing no harm" (nonmaleficence) by withholding medication from a patient whom they do not believe is in pain (see "Ethical Considerations: Controlling Pain" in your online resources). The questions then arise, how can we know what pain is, and how can we really tell when others are experiencing it?

 ## DEFINITIONS OF PAIN

According to McCaffery (1968), a well-known pain management expert, "Pain is whatever the experiencing person says it is, existing whenever the experiencing person says it does." This is a reminder to nurses to accept the patient's report of pain. The International Association for the Study of Pain (2017) describes pain in a bit more detail, as "an unpleasant sensory and emotional experience associated with actual or potential tissue damage or described in terms of such damage." This definition indicates that pain is a complex problem that is not just physical in nature or always a result of tissue injury.

Why does pain exist? It is a protective mechanism or a warning. In the presence of an injury, pain may help to prevent further injury. Consider the patient who has a fracture and holds it still to prevent further damage, or a child who touches a hot stove and pulls his or her hand away before a serious burn occurs. The immediate pain that often follows burns, surgery, or other trauma to the body is referred to as acute pain.

Acute pain prompts an inflammatory response in the body that subsides as healing takes place. This type of pain is often associated with short-term, objective, physical signs such as increased heart rate and blood pressure. As acute pain continues, the physiological responses that accompany acute pain cannot be sustained without harm to the body. As the body adapts, vital signs return to normal. When acute pain persists beyond the anticipated time of healing, it is referred to as chronic pain.

Chronic pain is typically diagnosed after a patient experiences 3 months or more of persistent pain. Examples include neck pain that continues years after an accident, pain that accompanies diseases such as arthritis, and phantom limb pain. Because of the body's ability to adapt, patients with chronic pain may not appear to be in pain. Guard against labeling such a patient a **malingerer** (someone who pretends to be in pain) or drug seeker. When pain is not treated effectively or lasts longer than expected, suffering can occur.

Suffering, or feelings of continuous distress, often accompanies pain. In a study of suffering, Ferrell and Coyle (2008) concluded, "Suffering is not synonymous with pain but is closely associated with it. Physical pain is closely related to psychological, social, and spiritual distress. Pain that persists without meaning becomes suffering" (p. 246). Persistent pain can diminish patients' quality of life. It can make them feel as though their health is getting worse and take away their motivation for self-care. Suffering can often be relieved if patients believe they can achieve comfort. A good assessment and individualized, culturally responsive approaches to care increase the likelihood of comfort.

 RISKS OF UNCONTROLLED PAIN

Why is untreated or undertreated pain a bad thing? Complications can occur when pain is experienced. The body produces a stress response to pain that causes harmful substances to be released from injured tissue. Reactions include breakdown of tissue, increased metabolic rate, impaired immune function, and negative emotions. In addition, pain prevents the patient from participating in self-care activities, such as

walking, deep breathing, and coughing. Consider the patient who has had chest surgery and then has to cough and deep breathe. It hurts! Pain may make the patient want to avoid coughing, turning, or even moving. Retained pulmonary secretions and pneumonia can develop. If the patient is less active, return of bowel function is delayed, and an ileus (disruption of normal propulsive gastrointestinal activity) can result. When pain is well controlled, complications can be avoided, and patients can participate fully in recovery activities. This will speed discharge as well as allow patients to do things that are meaningful and important to them when they get home.

 PAIN AND CULTURE

All individuals have learned patterns of behaviors, beliefs, and values that they share as members of particular social groups (Robinson, 2013). These cultural differences can affect responses to pain and expectations regarding treatment. For example, some patients may be dramatic and emotional when experiencing pain, while others may tend to be stoic and quiet. Be culturally responsive to the needs of patients by appropriately considering the unique attributes of the population you are working with. Also take time to understand the ways in which culture can affect a patient's health choices and care expectations (Robinson-Lane & Booker, 2017). Be mindful of your patients' language, family engagement, spirituality, and treatment preferences (see "Cultural Considerations"). It is important to evaluate a patient's pain care needs individually. In addition, pay careful attention to the ethical principles that influence patient care rather than making assumptions based on culture alone.

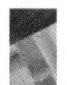 **WHO'S THE BOSS IN PAIN MANAGEMENT?**

The patient is at the center of the health care team. The patient also knows best how pain feels and affects him or her. Providing accurate information and offering relevant choices in pain management help patients to maintain autonomy. Just as risks, benefits, and alternatives to surgery and anesthesia are discussed with the patient, so too should pain management options be discussed in the process of obtaining informed consent. It is important to learn as much as you can about pain and pain management so you can effectively advocate for your patients and help with patient education.

The entire health care team is responsible for pain management. All members must provide care in the most cost-effective manner possible while continuing to provide the best quality. Effective pain management helps to improve patient function and reduces costs by minimizing the side effects of opioids, preventing complications related to inadequate pain control, and reducing the length of hospital/nursing home stay or period of recovery.

Various regulatory bodies recognize the importance of good pain management. Many have incorporated a review of

Cultural Considerations

Pain experiences may differ among cultures and individuals of various geographical regions; family structures; and ethnic, racial, or religious groups. Remember that people within groups vary (see Chapter 4).

Cultural Expression	Assessment	Intervention
Language	Listen for words or phrases the patient uses to describe discomfort, such as *achy, sore, fire, burning, shooting,* or *having a knot.* Observe use of nonverbal pain cues, such as moaning or crying, furrowed eyebrows, a clenched jaw, guarding or rubbing of body parts, and fetal positioning. Ask the patient about any nonverbal pain cues you see. Use standardized pain assessment scales.	Allow adequate time for the patient to respond to questions about pain. Use words the patient uses to discuss pain needs. Offer pain medications and interventions.
Family Engagement	Observe how involved the family is in the patient's care.	Teach the patient's family how to monitor the patient's discomfort. Engage the family to help with distraction and relaxation techniques.
Spirituality	Look for evidence of the patient's religious beliefs, such as clothing, jewelry, religious books or literature, clergy at the bedside, and patient engagement in prayer or meditation. Ask the patient whether he or she uses religion or faith as a part of healing.	Incorporate traditional healing methods as much as possible. Encourage the use of prayer, meditation, and relaxation as the patient desires. Offer and encourage pain medicines to promote healing. Support the patient's spiritual practices.
Treatment Preferences	Ask the patient how he or she usually treats pain at home. Ask the patient what he or she feels is needed to be comfortable.	Incorporate traditional home remedies, such as hot or cold packs and other practices, as permitted. Incorporate distraction and relaxation techniques. Administer medication promptly as requested.

organizational pain management practices into accreditation and review processes. These standards support the importance of appropriate and effective management of pain. They address assessment and the safe pharmacological management of pain as well as patient and family teaching, postoperative pain, management of opioid-induced side effects, discharge planning, and process improvement. Examples of these guidelines are available through The Joint Commission web site at www.jointcommission.org and the Centers for Medicare and Medicaid Services web site at www.cms.gov. For more information on pain management, visit the following web sites (for some sites, you may need to type "pain" in the search window):

- Agency for Healthcare Research and Quality, www.ahrq.gov
- American Cancer Society, www.cancer.org
- American Chronic Pain Association, theacpa.org
- American Pain Society, americanpainsociety.org
- American Society for Pain Management Nursing, www.aspmn.org
- Centers for Disease Control and Prevention, www.cdc.gov

- GeriatricPain.org, geriatricpain.org
- World Health Organization, www.who.int

The care of patients with pain is challenging. However, with a systematic and holistic approach to assessment and treatment, good pain management can be achieved. In this chapter, the difficulties of pain assessment and treatment are discussed. Some of the tools needed to effectively deal with these challenges are presented. Common myths and barriers that continue to affect nursing practice are clarified first.

 ## MYTHS AND BARRIERS TO EFFECTIVE PAIN MANAGEMENT

Many factors, including a nurse's personal experiences with pain, influence how patients with pain are treated. Why are some patients not believed when they report pain? Why do some nurses and other health care team members insist that patients behave a certain way before they are believed? Common myths about pain can impair a nurse's ability to be objective. This may create barriers to effective treatment. Because there are few objective measures for pain, many nurses rely on assumptions rather than facts. Note the following myths:

Myth: A person who is laughing and talking is not in pain.
Fact: A person in pain is likely to use laughing and talking as a form of distraction. This can be effective in managing pain, especially when used with appropriate drug therapies. Patients may be more easily distracted when they have visitors and may ask for pain medication as soon as their family or significant other goes home.
Myth: Respiratory depression is common in patients receiving opioid pain medications.
Fact: Respiratory depression is uncommon in patients receiving opioid pain medications when medications are taken as prescribed. If patients are monitored carefully when they are at risk, such as with the first dose of an opioid or when a dose is increased, respiratory depression is preventable. A patient's respiratory status and level of sedation should be routinely monitored and recorded using a level-of-sedation scale.
Myth: Pain medication is more effective when given by injection.
Fact: Oral administration is the first choice if possible or whenever the intravenous (IV) route is not an option. The IV route has the most rapid onset of action and is the preferred route for postoperative administration. Intramuscular injections are not recommended because they are painful, have unreliable absorption from the muscle, and have a lag time to peak effect and rapid falloff compared with oral administration.
Myth: Teenagers are more likely to become addicted to opioids than older patients.
Fact: Addiction to opioids is uncommon in all age-groups when taken for pain by patients without a prior drug abuse history. All patients using opioids should be monitored for medication effectiveness and taught how to appropriately discard unused medication.
Myth: Pain is a normal part of aging.
Fact: Although many older adults have medical conditions that cause pain, pain is not a normal or anticipated part of aging and should be treated proactively. Effective pain treatment for older people helps them to maintain their mobility longer and improve overall health.

CRITICAL THINKING

Mrs. Smithers had an abdominal hysterectomy and is sitting up in bed the morning after surgery, putting on her makeup. On morning rounds, she is smiling but reports that her pain is at 6 on a scale of 0 to 10. **Mr. Brown** has just been transferred from the surgical intensive care unit the day after surgery for multiple injuries. He is moaning and reports his pain at 6 on a scale of 0 to 10.

1. Which of these patients is really having as much pain as they say they are? How can you make this judgment?

Suggested answers are at the end of the chapter.

 OPIOID ADDICTION

In 2015 alone, more than 33,000 Americans died of opioid overdose (Kaiser Family Foundation, 2017). According to the Centers for Disease Control and Prevention (2017), a driving factor for the increasing numbers of opioid-related deaths is misuse of prescription medications such as oxycodone, hydrocodone, and methadone. Understandably, nurses often express concern about patients who need large amounts of opioid pain medication or know exactly when their next dose of pain medication is due. Nurses may worry that such patients are addicted or that they are "clock watchers." In truth, if a patient is watching the clock or asking for more medicine, the most likely reason is because he or she is in pain. Interestingly, patients are commonly taught to know the name, effects, and dosage of other medications, such as blood pressure medications and insulin; however, when they ask for a specific analgesic by name, concern that the patient is "drug seeking" is often raised.

Addiction is something that many patients fear—particularly today with increased media attention on opioid-related deaths. It is important to understand the differences between addiction, tolerance, and physical dependence. When talking with patients and their families about opioid medications, it is also important to verify that they understand these differences.

Tolerance is a normal biological adaptation to long-term use of a drug. The drug becomes less effective. Therefore, a larger dose is required to provide the same level of pain relief. **Physical dependence** is a normal physiological response that most people experience after a week or more of continuous opioid use. If an opioid is discontinued abruptly or if an opioid antagonist such as naloxone (Narcan) is administered, the patient experiences withdrawal syndrome. Withdrawal symptoms can include sweating, tearing, runny nose, restlessness, irritability, tremors, dilated pupils, sleeplessness, nausea, vomiting, and diarrhea. These symptoms can be prevented by decreasing the dose slowly over several days rather than stopping it suddenly.

According to the American Society of Addiction Medicine (2011), **addiction** (also known as **psychological dependence**) is a disease of the brain that causes the compulsive pursuit of a substance or behavior to obtain reward or relief from craving. Addiction is characterized by poor control over drug use, craving, reduced recognition of problem behaviors, and continued use despite harm. Patients with uncontrolled pain who desire treatment are not addicts. Sadly, patients with a history of addiction are more likely to have poor pain control due to medication tolerance and health care provider (HCP) bias. Careful assessment and monitoring of treatment are essential for *all* patients receiving treatment for pain—particularly patients who are prescribed opioid analgesics.

Pseudoaddiction has been described in patients who are receiving opioid doses that are too low or spaced too far apart

• WORD • BUILDING •

pseudoaddiction: pseudo—false + addiction—psychological dependence

to relieve their pain. Behavioral characteristics resembling psychological dependence, such as drug-seeking behaviors, develop in an attempt to get pain needs met. In contrast to the addicted patient, a patient with pseudoaddiction stops drug-seeking behaviors when the pain is reduced to a tolerable level.

CRITICAL THINKING

Janet is hospitalized with pancreatitis and has severe abdominal pain. She has a history of intravenous (IV) drug abuse. She is receiving IV morphine every 3 hours. Two hours after her last dose, she puts on her call light and says she is in severe pain, which she rates as 15 on a 0 to 10 scale. You feel that you have given her enough morphine to kill a horse, yet she keeps requesting more.

1. How is it possible for Janet to be in pain when she is receiving so much morphine?
2. It's not time for more medication. What should you do?
3. You speak to the health care provider, who prescribes acetaminophen (Tylenol) 1,000 mg for breakthrough pain (between morphine doses). When you take it to Janet, she rolls her eyes and says, "You must be kidding me." How do you respond?
4. What communication with Janet is important at this time?

Suggested answers are at the end of the chapter.

MECHANISMS OF PAIN TRANSMISSION

Pain is transmitted through four distinct processes:

1. *Transduction* represents the initiation of the stimulus and conversion of that stimulus into an electrical impulse at the time of the injury. Chemical neurotransmitters are released from damaged tissue. These substances include prostaglandins, bradykinin, serotonin, and substance P.
2. *Transmission* is the process of moving a painful message from the peripheral nerve endings through the dorsal root ganglion and the ascending tract of the spinal cord to the brain.
3. *Perception* is actually feeling pain. During perception, the hypothalamus activates, which controls emotional input and generates purposeful goal-directed behavior. Meanwhile, the cerebral cortex receives the pain message.
4. *Modulation* is the body's attempt to interrupt pain impulses by releasing endogenous (naturally occurring) opioids. **Endorphins** are endogenous chemicals that act like opioids, inhibiting pain impulses in the spinal cord and brain. Endorphins are the chemicals that stimulate the long-distance runner's "high." Unfortunately, they degrade too quickly to be considered effective analgesics. **Enkephalins** are one type of endorphin.

Pain Transmission: Nociceptive or Neuropathic?

Pain transmission can be nociceptive and neuropathic. **Nociception** refers to the body's normal reaction to noxious stimuli, such as tissue damage, with the release of pain-producing substances. Nociceptive pain may be somatic or visceral. **Somatic** pain is localized in the muscles or bones. Patients can often point to the exact location of pain and will describe it as throbbing or aching. Cancer patients may experience somatic pain when the cancer has spread to the bone or a tumor has invaded soft tissue. **Visceral** pain, or organ pain, is not well localized and is often described as cramping or pressure. Bowel obstructions and tumors in the lung can cause visceral pain symptoms. Pain may also be felt in parts of the body away from the pain source, such as low back/flank pain that often accompanies a bladder infection. This is called *referred pain* (Fig. 10.1).

Neuropathic pain is associated with injury to either the peripheral or central nervous system. Unlike nociceptive pain, neuropathic pain is poorly localized and may involve other areas along the nerve pathway. Neuropathic pain is common in cancer patients following chemotherapy or radiation therapy. It also occurs in patients who have fibromyalgia, diabetic neuropathy, and shingles. The pain is often described as numbing, tingling, sharp, shooting, or shocklike.

OPTIONS FOR TREATMENT OF PAIN

Medications that relieve pain are called **analgesics.** Analgesics make up the largest piece of the pain management puzzle. They encompass three main classes of medication: opioids, nonopioids, and adjuvants. **Opioids** bind to opioid receptors in the brain, spinal cord, and other areas of the body, inhibiting the perception of pain. *Nonopioids* include nonsteroidal anti-inflammatory drugs (NSAIDs) and acetaminophen (Tylenol). **Adjuvants** are different from opioid and nonopioids in that they include categories of medications that were originally approved by the Food and Drug Administration (FDA) for purposes other than pain relief (e.g., depression). Some patients may require a combination of opioids, adjuvants, and NSAIDs to effectively manage their pain. Nurses should have a good understanding of these pharmacological treatment options.

Nonopioid Analgesics

Nonopioids are typically the first class of drugs used to treat mild pain (Table 10.1). They can be useful for acute and chronic pain from a variety of causes, such as surgery, trauma, arthritis, and cancer. These drugs are limited in their use because they have a ceiling effect to analgesia. A **ceiling effect**

• WORD • BUILDING •

nociception: noci—pain + ception—reception
somatic: somato – body + ic – having to do with
neuropathic: neuro—nerves + pathy—disease, suffering
analgesic: an—not + gesia—pain

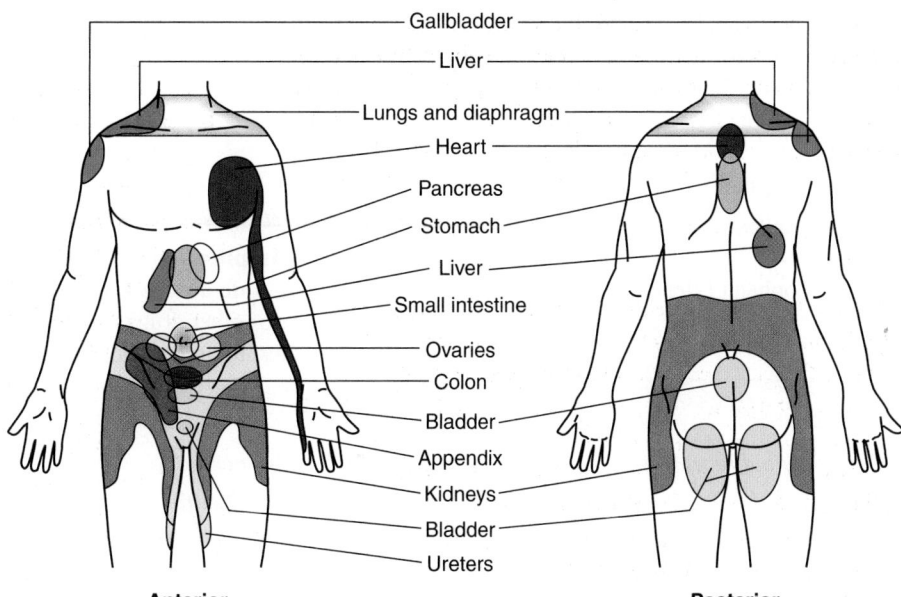

FIGURE 10.1 Sites of referred pain.   **Anterior**   **Posterior**

means that there is a dose beyond which there is no improvement in the analgesic effect, but there may be an increase in adverse effects. When used with opioids, the nonopioid dose must not exceed the maximum safe dose for a 24-hour period. For example, if a patient receiving two acetaminophen/hydrocodone (Norco) tablets every 4 hours continues to experience pain, the dose cannot be increased because of the potentially toxic effects of acetaminophen at that dosage. (See Table 10.1 for side effects and nursing implications.) Nonopioids do not produce tolerance or physical dependence.

Nonopioids work mainly peripherally, at the site of injury, rather than in the central nervous system, as opioids do. The exception in this class is acetaminophen, which is believed to act on the central nervous system. NSAIDs block the synthesis of **prostaglandins,** one of many chemicals needed for pain transmission. In general, it is helpful to include a nonopioid agent in any analgesic regimen, even if the pain is severe enough to require the addition of an opioid (see "Balanced Approach to Analgesia," later in this chapter).

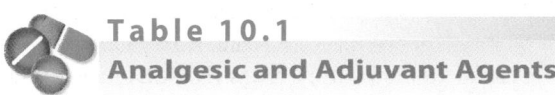

Table 10.1
Analgesic and Adjuvant Agents

Medication Class/Action

NONOPIOIDS

Salicylates
Peripherally acting analgesics; reduce pain, fever, inflammation.

Examples	Nursing Implications
aspirin	Give with food.
	Decrease platelet aggregation; watch for bruising or bleeding.

Nonsteroidal Anti-Inflammatory Drugs (NSAIDs)
Peripherally acting analgesics; reduce pain, fever, inflammation.

Examples	Nursing Implications
ibuprofen (Motrin)	Give with food.
ketorolac (Toradol)	Decrease platelet aggregation; watch for bleeding.
naproxen (Naprosyn, Aleve)	Do not give ketorolac for longer than 5 days.

COX-2 Inhibitors
Reduce pain and inflammation; no effect on platelet aggregation.

Examples	Nursing Implications
celecoxib (Celebrex)	Give with food.

Continued

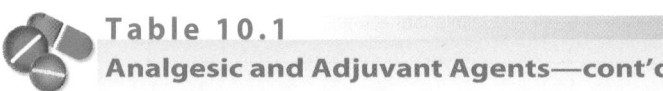

Table 10.1
Analgesic and Adjuvant Agents—cont'd

Medication Class/Action

Acetaminophen
Relieves pain and fever; no anti-inflammatory or antiplatelet effect.

Examples	Nursing Implications
acetaminophen (Tylenol, Ofirmev)	Maximum safe dose is 4 g per day; less for those who use alcohol. Be aware of other drugs that contain acetaminophen, such as cold remedies, to prevent accidental overdose.

Opioids and Opioid Combination Agents

Bind to opioid receptors in the central nervous system to alter perception of pain.

Examples	Nursing Implications
codeine (in Tylenol #2, #3, #4)*	May be combined with nonopioid (e.g., acetaminophen).
fentanyl (Sublimaze, Duragesic)	Monitor vital signs, level of sedation, and respiratory status.
hydromorphone (Dilaudid, Exalgo)	Avoid fentanyl patch in patient with fever; heat increases absorption.
methadone (Dolophine)	Encourage fluids and fiber to prevent constipation.
morphine (MS IR, MS Contin)	Codeine is contraindicated in pediatric patients.
oxycodone (Oxy IR, OxyContin)	Never crush extended-release tablets.
hydrocodone/acetaminophen (Norco, Lortab)	
tapentadol (Nucynta, Nucynta ER)	

Adjuvant Agents

Corticosteroids
Toxic to some cancer cells; reduce pain by decreasing inflammation.

Examples	Nursing Implications
prednisone	Administer with food.
prednisolone	
methylprednisolone	
dexamethasone	

Benzodiazepines
Treat anxiety or muscle spasms associated with pain.

Examples	Nursing Implications
midazolam (Versed)	Can cause sedation, which limits the amount of opioid that can be safely given at the same time.
diazepam (Valium)	

Tricyclic Antidepressants
Help relieve neuropathic pain.

Examples	Nursing Implications
amitriptyline	Often cause anticholinergic side effects (e.g., sedation, constipation, blurred vision, dry eyes, urinary retention).
imipramine	
desipramine	
doxepin	

Serotonin-Norepinephrine Reuptake Inhibitor
Effective for nerve pain and depression.

Examples	Nursing Implications
duloxetine (Cymbalta)	May take weeks before effect seen; teach patient to continue the medication even if it seems ineffective at first.

Table 10.1
Analgesic and Adjuvant Agents—cont'd

Medication Class/Action

Anticonvulsants
Treat neuropathic pain.

Examples	**Nursing Implications**
carbamazepine (Tegretol)	Must be taken regularly to get full benefit.
gabapentin (Neurontin)	

* Tylenol #2 = Tylenol 300 mg + codeine 15 mg; Tylenol #3 = Tylenol 300 mg + codeine 30 mg; Tylenol #4 = Tylenol 300 mg + codeine 60 mg

Opioid Analgesics

Opioids are drugs that have actions similar to those of morphine. Opioids are classified by how they affect receptors in the nervous system. They may be full **agonists** (stimulators), partial agonists, mixed agonists, or **antagonists** (blockers). Full agonists have a complete response at the opioid receptor site; a partial agonist has a lesser response. A mixed agonist or an antagonist activates one type of opioid receptor while blocking another.

Morphine, a full agonist, is often the drug of choice for treating severe pain. It is the standard against which all other analgesics are compared (see Table 10.2 for **equianalgesic** doses of medications). Morphine is long acting (4 to 5 hours) and available in many forms, making it convenient and affordable for patients. It also has a slower onset than many other opioids. Other examples of opioids include controlled-release drugs such as oxycodone (OxyContin), hydromorphone (Dilaudid, Exalgo), and tapentadol (Nucynta ER), which are effective for prolonged, continuous pain.

> **BE SAFE!**
> Never crush a controlled- or time-release tablet. Because the tablet is designed to deliver a dose of medication over time, crushing it could deliver the entire dose at once, resulting in overdose.

Opioids alone have no ceiling effect to analgesia. This means that doses can safely be increased to treat worsening pain if the patient's respiratory status and level of sedation are stable. However, inappropriate prescribing can lead to **hyperalgesia,** or increased sensitivity to pain. Patients with hyperalgesia have pain at the slightest touch, such as the moving of sheets, and require further medical intervention. Institutions must have policies and procedures in place related to opioids to prevent medication errors and reduce the risk of serious side effects. Other common side effects

include confusion and fatigue, which can increase a patient's risk for falls. See Table 10.1 for additional information and adverse effects of opioids.

Although opioids are important in pain management, they are also on a short list of "high-alert" drugs that can harm or even kill patients if they are not administered carefully (Institute for Safe Medication Practices, 2014). Institutions must have policies and procedures in place related to opioids to prevent medication errors and reduce the risk of serious side effects. It is especially important to be vigilant for side effects in patients unaccustomed to opioids. Such patients are sometimes called "opioid-naïve."

> **NURSING CARE TIP**
> Be vigilant for side effects in patients unaccustomed to opioids, particularly constipation. Patients taking opioids for three days or more should be on bowel management programs that include a stimulant laxative such as senna (ExLax, Senokot). In cases of severe constipation, the health care provider may prescribe a laxative specifically for opioid-induced constipation, such as naloxegol (Movantik) or methylnaltrexone (Relistor).

Opioids are added to nonopioids for pain that cannot be managed effectively by nonopioids alone. The use of a centrally acting opioid with a peripherally acting nonopioid can increase pain relief and reduce the amount of opioid needed.

Controlled-release opioids such as oxycodone (OxyContin) and morphine (MS Contin) are effective for prolonged, continuous pain. Whenever a controlled-release form of medication is used, it is important to have an immediate-release medication available for **breakthrough** pain (transient pain

· WORD · BUILDING ·
antagonist: ant—against + agonist—stimulates receptor site
equianalgesic: equi—equal + analgesic—relieving pain

Table 10.2
Equianalgesic Chart

Drug	Parenteral Dose*	Oral Dose
Morphine	5 mg	15 mg
Codeine	60 mg	100 mg
Hydromorphone	1.5 mg	4 mg
Methadone	5 mg	10 mg
Meperidine	50 mg	150 mg
Oxycodone	Not applicable	10 mg

*Intravenous, intramuscular, subcutaneous.

Note: Approximate doses of medications in milligrams to equal same amount of pain relief between drugs or same drug, different route. Consult pharmacist and health care provider before changing drugs or routes.

that arises during generally effective pain control), such as oral morphine solution, oxycodone immediate-release (Oxy IR), or hydromorphone immediate-release (Dilaudid).

CRITICAL THINKING

Mrs. Zales, a 32-year-old woman, is admitted for a hysterectomy after being treated for painful endometriosis for 12 months. After her surgery, she has a patient-controlled analgesia (PCA) pump with hydromorphone, which is effective in relieving her pain. Forty-eight hours after surgery, the surgeon discontinues the PCA pump and orders oral hydrocodone with acetaminophen. It is ineffective, so an order is added for hydromorphone 2 mg orally every 3 to 4 hours, as needed. The nurse gives only one dose of the hydromorphone and then, thinking that her pain should be lessening, switches Mrs. Zales back to the hydrocodone with acetaminophen. By the next morning, Mrs. Zales is in severe pain. The on-call health care provider orders intramuscular meperidine. Mrs. Zales's discharge is delayed until her pain can be controlled.

1. What do you think happened?
2. How could the delayed discharge have been avoided?
3. Who were the important team members in this scenario?

Suggested answers are at the end of the chapter.

Meperidine (Demerol) was at one time a commonly used synthetic opioid but is no longer recommended in most cases. Meperidine is an opioid agonist; when broken down in the body, it produces a toxic metabolite called normeperidine. Normeperidine is a cerebral irritant that can cause adverse effects, ranging from dysphoria and irritable mood to seizures. Normeperidine has a long half-life even in healthy patients, so those with impaired kidney function

are at increased risk. Meperidine use should be avoided in patients over age 65, patients with impaired kidney function, and patients taking a monoamine oxidase inhibitor (MAOI) antidepressant. In general, the use of meperidine should be limited to young, healthy patients who need an opioid for a short period and to those who have unusual reactions or allergic responses to other opioids. The effective dose of oral meperidine is three to four times the parenteral dose and is never recommended.

Fentanyl can be given parenterally or intraspinally (Sublimaze) or by **transdermal** patch (Duragesic). Fentanyl is commonly used via IV with anesthesia for surgery. It also is used to relieve postoperative pain via IV, patient-controlled analgesia pump, or epidural (discussed later in this chapter). IV fentanyl has a short duration of action and must be given more often than other opioids to maintain an effective level of analgesia. The transdermal fentanyl patch is useful for a patient with stable chronic pain. The patch lasts 48 to 72 hours after application.

CRITICAL THINKING

Mrs. Shepard is 92 years old and has undergone an open cholecystectomy. Her continuous epidural infusion of analgesic is discontinued at 1400 on her second postoperative day. The health care provider orders oral acetaminophen with hydrocodone every 3 to 4 hours as needed for pain. At 1700, Mrs. Shepard refuses to get out of bed because her pain is 7 on a scale of 0 to 10. The nurse checks the medication administration record and notes that she has not yet received a dose of acetaminophen and hydrocodone.

1. Why is Mrs. Shepard in so much pain?
2. What complications can occur as a result of her pain?
3. Each analgesic tablet contains 325 mg of acetaminophen and 5 mg of hydrocodone. The maximum daily dose of acetaminophen is 4 g. If she takes one tablet every 3 hours, is her dose safe?
4. What can be done to relieve her pain and better prevent it in the future?

Suggested answers are at the end of the chapter.

Opioid Antagonists

Naloxone (Narcan) is a pure opioid antagonist that reverses, or antagonizes, the effect of opioids. It is often used in emergency departments for treating the effects of opioid overdose, such as sedation and respiratory depression. Caution must be used when giving naloxone to a patient who is receiving opioids for pain control. If too much naloxone is given too fast, not only can it reverse the unwanted effects—such as respiratory depression and sedation—but the pain may return as well.

• WORD • BUILDING •
transdermal: trans—across + dermal—skin

Some antagonists are shorter acting than the opioid that is being used. If the antagonist is given because of respiratory depression, the dose may need to be repeated because its effect may wear off before the opioid wears off.

> **BE SAFE!**
> Although respiratory depression is not a common side effect, it is a life-threatening one, and respiratory rate should be monitored, especially when beginning opioid use or with dose increases. Always check the respiratory rate before administering an opioid and report any respiratory rate that is lower than 12 per minute or lower than normal for that patient. An additional sign of opioid overdose is pinpoint (very small) pupils.

Some analgesics are classified as combined agonists and antagonists or partial agonists. These drugs bind with some opioid receptors and block others. The most commonly used drugs in this class are butorphanol (Stadol), nalbuphine (Nubain), and buprenorphine (Buprenex).

How does this information translate into nursing practice? Consider, for example, a patient who receives sustained-release morphine every 12 hours to control metastatic bone pain, but the patient develops breakthrough pain between doses. You observe that butorphanol has been ordered for pain by another HCP and administer it. The butorphanol will antagonize, or counteract, some of the effects of the morphine, and the patient may experience acute pain. It is important to be informed about the actions of all drugs that are administered and to be aware of possible drug interactions that can interfere with patient care.

Analgesic Adjuvants

Adjuvants are classes of medications that are given in addition to other medications. Analgesic adjuvants can potentiate the effects of opioids or nonopioids, have analgesic activity themselves, or counteract the unwanted effects of other analgesics. Tramadol is an example of a commonly used adjuvant analgesic that acts very similar to an opioid. Some adjuvants are called *off-label* medications because they are being used in a way not specifically approved by the FDA; that is, they were not initially developed to treat pain. Adjuvants may have pain-relieving properties for certain conditions. Although the use of adjuvants is common, nurses must be mindful of the side effects of these medications, which often affect the central nervous system. Examples of adjuvants are corticosteroids, benzodiazepines, antidepressants, and anticonvulsants (see Table 10.1).

Balanced Approach to Analgesia

A balanced analgesia approach should be used, combining analgesics and adjuvants from different classes to minimize the adverse effects of opioids, such as nausea and vomiting or sedation, while maximizing pain relief. For example, an opioid and a nonopioid given together can provide pain relief with an overall lower dose of each medication than if each was given alone. Because these drugs have different mechanisms of action and different adverse effects, it is possible to safely use them together. If doses can be reduced in this manner, additional sedating medications such as antiemetics and antihistamines (to treat side effects) may not be needed.

Scheduling Options

Analgesics of any kind can be administered either as needed or on a scheduled basis. Intermittent, unpredictable pain may be best treated with as-needed doses. Pain that is predictable can be more effectively treated, or prevented, with scheduled doses of medication. Around-the-clock dosing is an effective way to schedule doses evenly over a 24-hour period to prevent pain from becoming unbearable. It is important to use around-the-clock dosing after surgery or trauma, with chronic pain, or in any other circumstance in which preventing pain will allow the patient to participate in daily or recovery activities.

Patient-Controlled Analgesia

Patient-controlled analgesia (PCA) involves an opioid on an IV controller. The patient has a button on a cord that can be pushed to receive a dose of IV medication. The registered nurse (RN) programs the pump to the dose and dosing interval ordered by the HCP. A "lockout" mechanism prevents the patient from receiving the medication more often than ordered. PCA is an excellent option after surgery because it gives the patient some control over pain management. Teach the patient and family that only the patient should push the button, never the nurse or a family member. If the patient is too sedated to push the button, a dose of opioid is not likely needed and could even be dangerous.

> **CRITICAL THINKING**
>
> **Ms. Jackson** had abdominal surgery 2 days ago. She has been receiving morphine via an intravenous patient-controlled analgesia pump at an average of 2.5 mg per hour for the past 6 hours. She rates her pain at 3 on a scale of 0 to 10. She is to be discharged today. Her health care provider has ordered codeine 30 mg with acetaminophen (Tylenol with codeine No. 3), one or two tablets every 4 hours as needed for pain at home.
>
> 1. Will Ms. Jackson be comfortable at home? Why or why not? (Check the equianalgesic chart).
>
>   *Suggested answers are at the end of the chapter.*

Other Interventions

Other pain treatments include topical local anesthetics, such as lidocaine/prilocaine cream (EMLA), which decrease the pain of procedures such as venipuncture and lumbar puncture. A lidocaine patch may be effective for patients with post-shingles or other nerve pain. In patients with osteoporosis, drugs that promote calcium uptake by the bones can aid in pain relief. These may include hormonal agents and medications that decrease calcium reabsorption from bone.

Placebos

Use of placebos involves the administration of an inactive substitute such as normal saline in place of an active medication. In the past, placebos were sometimes given in an attempt to determine whether a patient's pain was "real." This is unethical and inappropriate unless the patient has given written consent. The use of placebos is a denial of the patient's report of pain. If a placebo is ordered for a patient, discuss concerns with the HCP and nurse supervisor. Placebos are only to be used in drug studies (clinical trials) to compare a new drug with an inactive substance. In this situation, patients are informed that they may be receiving a placebo.

Routes for Medication Administration

Analgesics can be administered by almost any route. The oral route is desired in most instances because it is easy and painless for the patient and can be used at home. See Table 10.3 for a comparison of the various routes.

Nonpharmacological Therapies

Nonpharmacological treatments are usually classified as either cognitive-behavioral interventions or physical agents. The goals of these two groups of treatments differ. Cognitive-behavioral interventions can help patients understand and cope with pain and take an active part in its assessment and control. The goals of physical agents may include providing comfort, correcting physical dysfunction, or altering physiological responses. Nonpharmacological therapies should be used in conjunction with drug therapies. They are not expected to relieve pain on their own.

Table 10.3
Routes for Analgesic Administration

Uses	Advantages	Disadvantages	Nursing Considerations
Oral			
Preferred route in most cases.	Convenient. Less expensive than other forms. Immediate- and controlled-release forms available.	Slower onset than intravenous (IV) form.	Can provide consistent blood levels when given around the clock. Controlled-release form recommended for long-term use in chronic pain.
Rectal			
May be used to provide local or systemic pain relief.	Can be used when patient cannot take oral medication.	May be difficult for patient or family to self-administer.	Some oral preparations can be given rectally. (Place in empty gel cap for ease of use.) Check with health care provider or pharmacist.
Transdermal Patch			
Used for chronic pain.	Easy to apply. Delivers pain relief for several days without patch change.	May take up to 3 days before maximum effective drug level reached; delay in excreting once removed. Patient must be closely monitored; alternative routes may be needed when starting and stopping therapy.	May be less effective in smokers and very thin people. Absorption may be erratic. Absorption may be increased with fever. Avoid heat application over patch. Avoid touching medication when applying patch. Keep used patches away from pets and children.
Intramuscular Acute pain.	Rapid pain relief, although slower than IV.	Painful administration. Inconsistent absorption.	Use only if other routes cannot be used.

Table 10.3

Routes for Analgesic Administration—cont'd

Uses	Advantages	Disadvantages	Nursing Considerations
IV			
Preferred route for postoperative and chronic cancer pain in patients who cannot tolerate oral route.	Provides rapid relief. Continuous infusion to achieve steady drug level.	Difficult to use in home health care setting. Requires training and special equipment.	Follow drug manufacturer's instructions for administration.
Patient-Controlled IV			
Allows patient some control over administration schedule.	Patient pushes a button to administer a dose of opioid.	Requires special training. Pump must be pro-grammed correctly.	An hourly limit and lockout interval are programmed into the pump to keep the patient from receiving too much drug. Caution patient and family that only the patient should push the button.
Subcutaneous			
May be used if IV route is problematic.	Can deliver effective pain relief. Some opioids may be given as continuous infusion.	Injection may be painful.	May be effective for treatment of chronic cancer pain.
Intraspinal (Epidural or Subarachnoid)			
Catheter into epidural or subarachnoid space used for traumatic injuries or chronic pain unrelieved by other methods. May also be used for orthopedic, chest, and abdominal surgical procedures.	May be able to control pain with lower doses of opioid because relief is delivered closer to site of pain. Fewer systemic side effects.	Requires single or contin-uous injection in back. May be associated with intense itching. Motor function must be assessed especially when local anesthetic is used.	Steroids may be given with opioid to reduce pain by treating inflammation. Local anesthetic may be paired with opioid to enhance pain relief. Avoid use of anticoagulant and antiplatelet agents (including aspirin) because of risk of epidural hematoma.

Cognitive-Behavioral Interventions

Cognitive-behavioral interventions include educational in-formation, relaxation exercises, guided imagery, distraction (e.g., music, television), and biofeedback. These treatments require extra time for detailed instruction and demonstration. The use of these modalities must be acceptable to the patient to be useful. Educating patients about what to expect and how they can participate in their own care has been shown to decrease patients' reports of postoperative pain and anal-gesic use.

Relaxation can be accomplished through a variety of methods. The patient may prefer a scripted relaxation exer-cise that can be practiced and used the same way each time or simply the use of a favorite piece of music that allows a state of muscle relaxation and freedom from anxiety. Guided imagery uses the patient's imagination to take the patient away from the pain to a favorite place, such as a beach in Tahiti. The success of guided imagery does not mean that the pain is in any way imaginary. See Chapter 5 for more information on relaxation and imagery.

As noted earlier, distraction is commonly used by patients to focus their attention on something other than the pain. They may watch a favorite television program or laugh with visitors when they are in pain. When the program is over or the visitors leave, the patient may focus on the pain again and ask for a dose of pain medication.

Biofeedback is sometimes used in chronic-pain programs to teach patients how to train their bodies to respond to different signals. Biofeedback has been very useful in patients with migraine headaches. When an aura (a warning sign) occurs before a migraine headache, patients are prompted to begin the exercise that relaxes them, maybe allowing them to prevent the headache.

Physical Agents

Physical agents can contribute directly to the patient's comfort. Examples of physical agents include applications of heat or cold, massage, and exercise. Additional physical interventions, such as immobilization or transcutaneous electrical nerve stimulation (TENS), are also available.

APPLICATION OF HEAT. The application of heat to sore muscles and joints is effective for pain relief. Heat works to increase circulation, induce muscle relaxation, and decrease inflammation when applied to a painful area. Heat can be applied using dry or moist packs or wraps, or in a bath or whirlpool. Heat is contraindicated in conditions that would be worsened by its use, such as in an area of trauma, because of the possibility of increased swelling caused by vasodilation. To prevent burns, heat should not be applied directly to the skin or over areas of decreased sensation.

APPLICATION OF COLD. Cold can reduce swelling, bleeding, and pain when used to treat a new injury. It can also reduce the pain of an injection when applied prior to the injection, along with pressure, above the injection site. Cold can be applied by a variety of methods, such as cold wraps and cold packs as well as localized ice massage. Patients often choose heat over cold if they have the choice, because cold can be uncomfortable. Cold may be better tolerated over a small area. Alternating heat and cold therapies is most effective if not contraindicated.

MASSAGE AND EXERCISE. Massage and exercise are used to stretch and regain muscle and tendon length and to relax muscles. Massage pressure can be superficial or deep and may involve vibration. It is important that massage is acceptable and not offensive to the patient. Immobilization is used after a variety of orthopedic procedures as well as fractures and other injuries worsened by movement. Acupressure has also been shown to be beneficial for pain reduction (see "Evidence-Based Practice").

Physical agents are readily available and inexpensive and often require little preparation or instruction. But always remember, it is important to use nonpharmacological treatments as an enhancement of appropriate drug treatments, not as a substitute.

Evidence-Based Practice

Clinical Question
Can acupressure help relieve pain and reduce the need for pharmacological analgesics?

Evidence
Fifteen small studies were reviewed to determine the effectiveness of using finger and hand pressure to stimulate acupoints and relieve pain. The studies demonstrated a reduction in menstrual, labor, low back, headache, and other types of pain in diverse populations (Chen & Wang, 2014).

Implications for Nursing Practice
"Acupressure can be efficiently conducted by health care professionals as an adjuvant therapy in general practice for pain relief" (Chen & Wang, 2014). Nurses can be trained to perform acupressure.

Reference
Chen, Y., & Wang, H. (2014). The effectiveness of acupuncture on relieving pain: A systematic review. *Pain Management Nursing, 15*(2), 539–550.

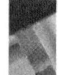

NURSING PROCESS FOR THE PATIENT EXPERIENCING PAIN

Data Collection

Accurate assessment of pain is essential to effective treatment. Without appropriate assessment, it is not possible to intervene in a way that meets the patient's needs. Because of regulatory requirements, most organizations require detailed pain assessments of patients at admission, with any change in condition, and at least every 3 months thereafter while in care. Nurses should verbally assess all patients under their care at least once per shift for pain and provide appropriate intervention as needed. The *WHAT'S UP?* format, introduced in Chapter 1, can help you perform a complete and effective assessment (Table 10.4). The following sections provide some additional key points for assessing pain and putting together more pieces of the pain puzzle.

Accept the Patient's Report of Pain

Pain is what the patient says it is, not what the HCP believes it is. When a member of the health care team distrusts the patient's report of pain, the patient can usually sense this. The patient may compensate by either underreporting pain or anxiously

Table 10.4

WHAT'S UP? Guide for Pain Assessment

Acronym	Key	Pain Assessment
W	Where is the pain?	Be specific. Use a drawing of the body if needed.
H	How does the pain feel?	Is the pain shooting, burning, dull, sharp, aching?
A	Aggravating and alleviating factors	What makes the pain better? What makes it worse?
T	Timing	When did the pain start? Is it intermittent? Continuous?
S	Severity	How bad is the pain on a scale of 0 to 10? Use a different tool, such as the FACES Pain Scale–Revised (see Fig. 10.2) or PAINAD Scale (see Fig. 10.3), if needed.
U	Useful other data	Are any other symptoms associated with the pain or pain treatment? Itching, nausea, sedation, constipation? How does the pain affect lifestyle (e.g., inability to eat, sleep, work, enjoy sex)?
P	Patient's perception	What is the patient's perception of what caused the pain? Is the patient experiencing suffering? Is the patient satisfied with pain control?

overreporting it. Patients may try to hide their pain for fear of being thought of as complainers or drug seekers.

Patient Perspective

Terry. I have had chronic back pain for 10 years. It is very real, related to multiple herniated discs in my thoracic and lumbar spine, arthritis, and degenerative disc disease. Because I've been dealing with it for 10 years, I have adapted. I never look like I am in pain. Sometimes I limp or move around a lot to find a comfortable position, but I don't have that pained look on my face, and my blood pressure doesn't go up like some people. I have tried many, many medications over the years and have become quite educated in pain treatments. I have tried antidepressants and anti-seizure medications (both are used for neuropathic pain), ice, heat, transcutaneous electrical nerve stimulation (TENS), relaxation, physical therapy, more physical therapy, exercises, more exercises, massage therapy, steroid injections, and nerve blocks. I had relief once for about a month following some injections, and I kept thinking something was wrong. "Wait, where's the pain? This doesn't feel right!" Sometimes I would like a big dose of morphine, but I know that opioids for chronic pain are a one-way street to dependence. I do have a prescription for hydrocodone/acetaminophen (Norco) that I take a couple of times a month when I feel desperate. I ration them because I am afraid of them.

My friend Joanne also has back pain, which started 20 years ago. When it started, she was writhing in pain. I am positive her blood pressure was sky high! She couldn't move because of muscle spasms. She was also diagnosed with a herniated disc, but she had surgery to fix it. She said the nerve pain relief was already evident in the recovery room. Of course, surgery causes pain, so opioids are needed for a short while. But once healing started for Joanne, no pain! She still has acute pain from time to time, when she experiences muscle spasms and can't move very easily for several days. She takes muscle relaxers and has to lay low until the spasms resolve.

Sometimes Joanne looks at me and says, "You don't look like you're in pain." At first this made me feel bad, like she is comparing her pain to mine. Then one day, I realized the difference—she experiences *acute* pain, and I have *chronic* pain. I've adapted. She is way more miserable than I am when she is in pain, but it is short-lived. My pain is not as severe, but after 10 years, it has worn me down.

When you are a nurse, please believe your patients when they say they are in pain, even if they don't look like they are. Maybe they've gotten used to it, but that doesn't mean they enjoy feeling pain. Do whatever you can to help them feel better.

Obtain a Pain History

Obtain information from the patient about the pain he or she is experiencing as well as the pain treatments used in the past. Letting the patient describe the pain in his or her own words helps establish a trust relationship between you and the patient. This is also the time to discover the effects the pain is having on the patient's quality of life. Does the pain prevent the patient from eating, sleeping, or participating in work or family activities? Are there adverse effects such as nausea and vomiting or constipation that need to be addressed? Also observe for emotional and/ or spiritual distress. Ask the patient about how he or she has coped with pain previously and what treatments have been effective and ineffective in the past. In nonverbal or cognitively impaired patients, information may be obtained from family members and the medical record. A painful diagnosis, such as arthritis, typically is a predictor of pain. A thorough history is essential so you can individualize pain interventions to fit the patient's needs.

PAIN ASSESSMENT TOOLS. Various tools are available to assist with accurate and complete pain assessment. You should become familiar with the tools used in your clinical practice setting and use them consistently. It is of utmost importance that all health care personnel caring for a particular patient use the same pain rating scale, whether it is a numerical scale (e.g., 0 to 10) such as a visual analog scale (Fig. 10.2) or the FACES Pain Scale–Revised (Fig. 10.3). There should also be consistent scales in place for nonverbal/cognitively impaired patients, such as the Pain Assessment in Advanced Dementia (PAINAD) Scale (Fig. 10.4; Warden, Hurley, & Volicer, 2003).

Whatever scale is used, it must be one that has been validated with research. The FACES Pain Scale–Revised was initially developed for use in children and has since been revised with faces that are more realistic for adults. The PAINAD Scale was developed for patients with advanced dementia but is an effective tool for patients with cognitive and communicative barriers. Longer questionnaires are useful in meeting regulatory requirements for the completion of comprehensive pain assessments (Fig. 10.5). These scales often contain examples of verbal pain descriptors—something many patients have difficulty verbalizing. A scale should also be used to monitor the patient's level of sedation after opioid administration (Fig. 10.6). Any unexpected increase in the patient's level of sedation should be reported promptly to the RN or HCP. Finally, keeping a pain diary helps patients to document pain ratings, interventions, and responses, which can help with the treatment plan.

Perform a Complete Physical Assessment
A thorough physical assessment is necessary to determine the effect of the pain and pain treatments on the body. It helps identify all of the pain sites and any medication side effects. It also helps prioritize the seemingly overwhelming

task of helping the patient achieve acceptable pain relief and quality of life. As discussed previously, the patient with acute pain may exhibit signs such as grimacing and moaning or elevated pulse and blood pressure. For patients with cognitive impairments, these indicators can be particularly important; however, these signs cannot be relied on to "prove" that a patient is in pain. The only reliable source of pain assessment is the patient's self-report. Even patients with cognitive deficits can provide important information about pain. They can often answer simple yes or no questions regarding comfort and may demonstrate favorable changes in behavior, such as diminished calling out, when pain is effectively controlled. Having accurate information regarding patient pain and activity levels before and after medications, particularly opioids, helps the HCP ensure that medications are prescribed as needed.

Gerontological Issues
Pain in Older Adults. Older adults frequently have unmet pain needs. Some believe that pain is an anticipated part of aging and may be hesitant to take strong medications such as opioids for pain. Nonsteroidal anti-inflammatory drugs (NSAIDs) are often contraindicated for older adults due to medication interactions and gastrointestinal side effects; however, patients should be evaluated for medications on an individual basis. Patients in long-term care facilities, particularly patients with cognitive deficits, should have medications for pain scheduled around the clock to ensure regular administration and effective pain control. Consider isolation, restlessness, confusion, aggression, and changes in appetite as possible signs of pain. Pulling at dressings, tugging at intravenous sites, and calling out can also be signs of discomfort. Any change in the patient's usual behavior should be considered a possible sign of discomfort. Remember to take more time when assessing pain in older patients because they may need more time to process what you are asking. Consider using the Pain Assessment in Advanced Dementia (PAINAD) Scale when assessing confused patients.

You can anticipate pain and provide relief measures to prevent severe pain. A trial dose of pain medication may help to determine if the patient's behavior is because of pain. Nagging achiness in hands and feet is often noted as a reason for decreased activity, inability to sleep, and altered functional ability. A hand or foot massage using lotion and gentle massage strokes is often a relaxing comfort measure.

Opioid analgesic doses may need to be decreased by 25% to 50% initially because they tend to work longer and stronger in the older patient.

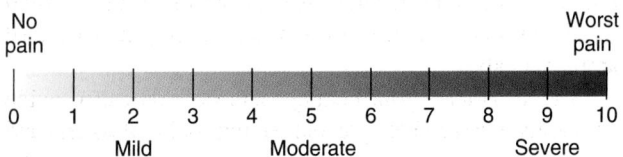

No pain   Worst pain

0   1   2   3   4   5   6   7   8   9   10
          Mild   Moderate   Severe

FIGURE 10.2 Analog pain scale.

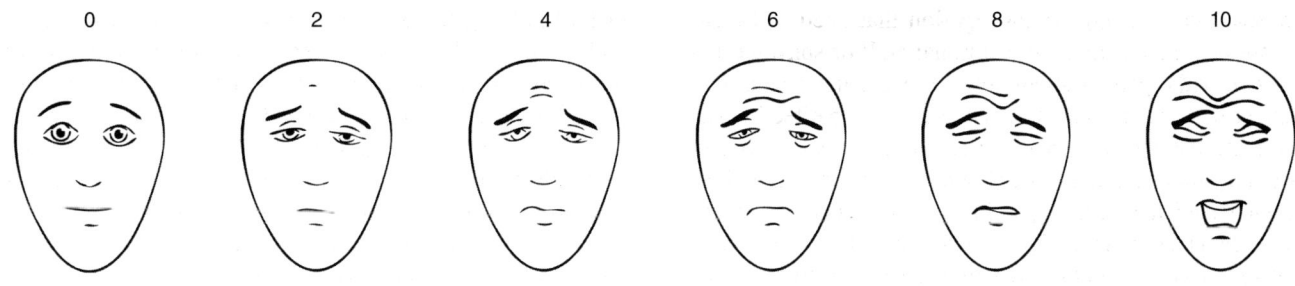

0   2   4   6   8   10

FIGURE 10.3 FACES Pain Scale–Revised.

Pain Assessment in Advanced Dementia Scale (PAINAD)

Behavior	0	1	2	Score
Breathing independent of vocalization	Normal	• Occasional labored breathing • Short period of hyperventilation	• Noisy labored breathing • Long period of hyperventilation • Cheyne-Stokes respirations	
Negative vocalization	None	• Occasional moan or groan • Low level speech with a negative or disapproving quality	• Repeated troubled calling out • Loud moaning or groaning • Crying	
Facial expression	Smiling or inexpressive	• Sad • Frightened • Frown	• Facial grimacing	
Body language	Relaxed	• Tense • Distressed pacing • Fidgeting	• Rigid • Fists clenched • Knees pulled up • Pulling or pushing away • Striking out	
Consolability	No need to console	• Distracted or reassured by voice or touch	• Unable to console, distract, or reassure	
			Total*	

* Total scores range from 0 to 10 (based on a scale of 0 to 2 for five items), with a higher score indicating more severe pain (0–"no pain" to 10–"severe pain")

FIGURE 10.4 The PAINAD Scale.

Nursing Diagnoses, Planning, and Implementation

See the "Nursing Care Plan for the Patient in Pain." Some additional principles to consider during planning and implementation follow.

Set Goals With Patients and Caregivers

Establish a pain control goal during the planning phase. Ask the patient to determine an acceptable level of pain if complete freedom from pain is not possible. Patients with cognitive deficits should also have pain goals established that include behavioral indicators. Education is important when helping patients and caregivers set realistic pain control goals. Although a pain goal of 0 is desirable, it may not be possible or safe. Conversely, a patient who chooses a pain goal of 6 may be unable to get out of bed and do daily or recovery activities.

Patients should also identify activity goals. After surgery, goals may include the ability to ambulate and achieve restful sleep. For patients with chronic pain, the goals may be different. For example, a patient with terminal cancer may want to be able to eat dinner with her family in the evening. You can assist the patient in reaching that goal by teaching her to conserve energy during the day for the activity that is most important to her. Instructing both types of patients in optimal timing of pain medications and appropriate use of nonpharmacological treatments will also assist them in reaching their desired activity goals.

Giving patients pain management options can provide autonomy and may help prevent feelings of helplessness and hopelessness. It is the nurse's responsibility to engage the patient and family in the pain management plan.

Pain Assessment Chart (For Admission and/or Follow-up)

1. Patient _____ 2. DX _____

Assessment on Admission

Date _____/_____/_____   Pain ☐   No Pain ☐   Date of Pain Onset _____/_____/_____

1. Location of Pain (indicate on drawing)

2. Description of Predominant Pain (in patient's words) _____

_____

_____

3. Intensity [Scale 0 (no pain) — 10 (most intense)] _____

_____

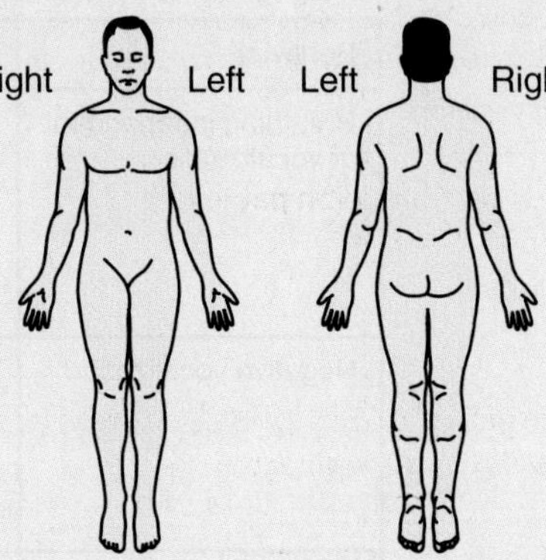

4. Duration and when occurs _____

_____

5. Precipitating Factors _____

_____

6. Alleviating Factors _____

_____

Right   [figure]   Left   Left   [figure]   Right

7. Accompanying Symptoms

   GI: Nausea ☐   Emesis ☐   Constipation ☐   Anorexia ☐

   CNS: Drowsiness ☐   Confusion ☐   Hallucinations ☐

   Psychosocial: Mood _____ Anger _____

   Anxiety _____ Depression _____

   Relationships _____

   _____

8. Other Symptoms

   Sleep _____ Fatigue _____

   Activity _____ Other _____

9. Present Medications _____

   _____

   _____

   Doses and times medicated last 48 hours _____

   _____

10. Breakthrough Pain _____

   _____

Signature: _____

FIGURE 10.5 Pain assessment chart (modified).

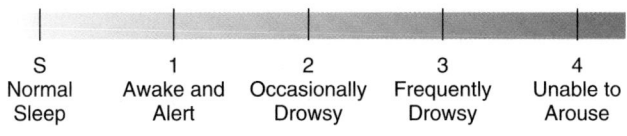

FIGURE 10.6 Level of sedation scale.

Understand That Pain Affects the Whole Family

It is important to include the whole family in the pain management plan. Understanding family dynamics helps in implementing an effective plan. Cultural influences are also important to consider (see Chapter 4 and "Cultural

Nursing Care Plan for the Patient in Pain

Nursing Diagnosis: *Pain (acute or chronic)*
Expected Outcomes: Pain will be at a level that is acceptable to the patient. The patient will be able to participate in activities that are important to him or her.
Evaluation of Outcomes: Is pain at a level that is acceptable to the patient? Is the patient able to participate in activities that he or she has identified as important?

Intervention	Rationale	Evaluation
Assess pain based on patient report. Use the *WHAT'S UP?* format.	*The patient's pain is defined as what the patient says it is and when the patient says it is occurring.*	Does patient verbalize his or her pain? Does patient use verbal or nonverbal messages that imply trust in the nurse's belief of the pain report?
Teach patient to use a pain rating scale. Use the same scales consistently.	*A rating scale is the most reliable method for assessing pain severity.*	Does patient understand the use of the scale and use it to report pain?
Have patient or caregiver keep a pain diary, documenting time of pain, interventions, and pre- and post-pain ratings.	*A diary can show patterns of pain and pain relief, and help in planning care.*	Does diary reveal patterns that help with planning?
Determine what is an acceptable pain level for the patient. Consider activities the patient should be able to perform.	*Only the patient can decide what pain level is acceptable.*	Is patient's pain at an acceptable level? Can they perform necessary activities of daily living with minimal pain?
Assess whether pain is nociceptive, neuropathic, or both.	*Nociceptive and neuropathic pain may present differently and may require different interventions.*	Has nociceptive versus neuropathic pain been identified? Are treatments appropriate?
Assess need for and offer emotional, spiritual, and social support for the experience of pain and suffering.	*Pain, as well as disease processes, can be accompanied by feelings of powerlessness, distress, and isolation.*	Does patient appear emotional, angry, or withdrawn? Does patient have difficulty making decisions? Does patient have a support system? Is patient-nurse relationship therapeutic?
Give analgesics before pain becomes severe. For persistent pain, give analgesics around the clock.	*Pain can be more difficult to relieve when it becomes severe.*	Is the analgesic schedule effective?
Combine opioid and nonopioid analgesics as ordered.	*Balanced analgesia provides optimum pain relief with fewer side effects.*	Is the analgesic combination effective?
Assess for pain relief approximately 1 hour after administration of oral analgesics or 30 minutes after intravenous analgesics.	*If pain is not relieved, additional measures will be needed.*	Does patient report an acceptable level of relief?
Observe for adverse effects of pain medication.	*Many pain medications cause nausea and fatigue. Both tend to subside after a few days.*	Are adverse effects occurring? Can they be managed? Does medication regimen need to be adjusted?

(nursing care plan continues on page 138)

Nursing Care Plan for the Patient in Pain—cont'd

Intervention	Rationale	Evaluation
If opioids and/or muscle relaxants are being used, assess for respiratory depression and level of sedation at regular intervals.	*Sedation and respiratory depression are risks if the patient is opioid-naïve or dose is increased. Sedation always precedes respiratory depression.*	Is patient's respiratory rate greater than 8 per minute or above the parameter ordered by the health care provider? What is patient's level of consciousness?
Institute measures to prevent constipation: 8 to 10 glasses of noncaffeinated fluid daily (unless contraindicated), stimulant laxatives, and exercise as tolerated.	*Opioid-induced constipation is a problem of gastrointestinal motility; stimulant laxatives are most effective. Caffeine can exacerbate constipation.*	Is patient easily passing soft feces in the expected amount every 1 to 3 days?
Teach patient to incorporate nonpharmacological pain relief interventions, such as using hot or cold packs and initiating relaxation techniques when taking medication.	*Nonpharmacological interventions can help the patient feel in control and may help reduce the perception of pain.*	Does patient use nonpharmacological interventions effectively?
Determine whether patient is taking pain medications appropriately, and if not, determine the reasons. Discuss how interventions may be modified.	*Pain medications must be taken appropriately to be effective.*	Is patient able to manage the pain control regimen? Does patient have concerns about medications? Are adjustments necessary?

Considerations"). It is difficult for family members to see loved ones in pain or in heavily sedated states. Including them in planning helps them feel that they can help make the patient more comfortable and recognizes the important role they have in the patient's care.

Recognize That Pain Is Exhausting

Pain may keep the patient from sleeping well. This cycle of sleeplessness and pain must be interrupted to help the patient. Fatigue is a common problem for the patient with chronic pain and can complicate the treatment process. Although older adults do not require as much sleep as younger adults, all patients must get at least 6 to 7 hours of uninterrupted sleep to be relaxed enough to break the cycle. Controlled-release opioids may help maintain pain relief throughout the night. If controlled-release medications are not used, it may be necessary to wake a patient to administer pain medication so that the pain does not get out of control. The addition of a sedative or sleep aid may be needed to allow the patient to sleep. Aromatherapy such as lavender, ensuring patient is comfortable, and limiting caffeine intake after 1500 can increase productive sleep.

Use a Team Approach to Pain Management

The interdisciplinary pain management team includes the patient and family, the licensed practical nurse/licensed vocational nurse, the RN, the HCP, therapists, spiritual advisers, social workers, and pharmacists. Communication among team members is essential. It is the important link that allows the team to be effective in creating a plan that works for the patient. As the nurse, you play a vital role in ensuring effective communication among team members, always remembering that the patient is at the center of the team.

Patient Education

Patients, and in some instances their family members, must be informed about the medications they are taking for pain management. This allows them to take an active role in their care. Patients who are informed about the goals of pain management and who are confident that their providers believe them are more likely to report unrelieved pain so that they can receive prompt and effective treatment. Goals include a satisfactory comfort level with minimal side effects and complications of pain and its treatment as well as a reduced period of recovery.

The patient should be provided with information about a drug's effects, common adverse effects, frequency of the dose and duration of action, and potential drug–drug and drug–food interactions, if indicated. There are many special considerations for medications, such as controlled-release oral agents and transdermal patches; care must be taken to include these considerations in the education plan for the patient taking these drugs at home. Drug-specific instructions are found in drug handbooks or databases. Education must be presented at a level that the patient can understand. Written information should be included when appropriate. Informed patients use their medications more effectively and safely.

Evaluation

The final phase of the nursing process is evaluation. Once the plan of care has been implemented, evaluate whether the patient's goals have been met. What is the patient's pain rating? Has the patient's identified goal for an acceptable level of pain been met? How were the pain treatments tolerated? Was the patient able to participate in activities that he or she identified as important? The plan should be continuously updated based on the evaluation.

CRITICAL THINKING

Mr. Sebastian is a 75-year-old man who has been diagnosed with lung cancer and is anxious about leaving the hospital to return home following surgery. The nursing assessment reveals the need for home health care for dressing changes and teaching about the medications he will need at home. While in the hospital, Mr. Sebastian has required 5 mg of intravenous morphine every 4 hours around the clock.

1. The morphine is available in syringes prefilled with morphine grains 1/6 per mL. How many milliliters should the nurse administer while Mr. Sebastian is in the hospital?
2. What discharge instructions must be given to Mr. Sebastian and his wife before sending him home?
3. How might his pain be managed at home to prevent unnecessary readmissions to the hospital?

Suggested answers are at the end of the chapter.

Home Health Hints

- Emotional or spiritual distress and fear related to dependence on family caregivers may alter the patient's perception or report of pain. Some patients may feel pain more intensely because of the influence of fear, and others may underreport if they are trying to protect family members.
- Pill boxes are useful to ease in administration of medications and for nurses to track usage.
- Medications should be locked up if there is a child or a teen in the home. A referral for palliative care may be appropriate for patients experiencing chronic pain.

SUGGESTED ANSWERS TO CRITICAL THINKING

Mrs. Smithers and Mr. Brown

1. It is important to accept both patients' pain reports. Assessment should be based on what the patient says rather than what is observed. Each patient copes with his or her pain in a unique way, and the nurse cannot judge whether one is in more pain than the other.

Janet

1. Remember, pain is whatever the experiencing person says it is, existing whenever the experiencing person says it does. You must assume that Janet is in pain. She has pancreatitis, which is commonly very painful. She has a history of intravenous (IV) drug abuse and is likely tolerant to the effects of the morphine. She may be experiencing "end-of-dose failure," when pain medication does not last as long as expected. If her vital signs are within normal limits, it should be safe to treat her pain.
2. Contact the registered nurse (RN) or health care provider (HCP) to explain the problem. Making Janet wait another hour in pain is not appropriate.
3. Tylenol works differently from morphine and may offer minimal relief but is not an appropriate order for severe pain. Talk to the RN or supervisor and explain the situation.
4. Listen to Janet and let her know that you understand she is in pain. Keep her updated at all times, and assure her that you will continue to advocate for her until she achieves adequate pain relief.

Mrs. Zales

1. Mrs. Zales may have been tolerant to opioids because of her need for medication for chronic pain during the past year. For this reason, she needed more medication than a nontolerant patient who does not usually use opioids. Intramuscular injections are not recommended because they are painful, absorption is not predictable, and there is a delay between injection and relief. A more rational approach to Mrs. Zales's pain management would have been regular pain assessment with around-the-clock treatment until the pain began to subside and a recommendation to the HCP to switch the meperidine to IV hydromorphone.
2. If her pain level had been better controlled, she might have been discharged on oral analgesics without the delay.
3. The most important team member here was Mrs. Zales— the patient should be the *center* of the team! If she had been listened to more carefully and her history considered, she might have been kept more comfortable.

Mrs. Shepard

1. Pain medication is most effective when given on a routine schedule around the clock to avoid breakthrough pain. Mrs. Shepard's epidural infusion should continue to relieve her pain for a time, up to several hours after it is discontinued, depending on the medication used. The oral medication is most effective when given at the time

Continued

SUGGESTED ANSWERS TO CRITICAL THINKING—cont'd

the epidural is stopped so that it is taking effect as the epidural effects wear off. See "Gerontological Issues" for special considerations for the older patient.

2. Pain prevents patients from moving freely. Postoperative complications such as retained pulmonary secretions and ileus can occur when patients are immobile. Effective pain management can help prevent these complications.

3. If she takes a dose every 3 hours, then she will receive eight doses in 24 hours: 325 mg × 8 = 2,600 mg or 4 g, which is below the maximum safe dose of 4,000 mg. Recall that older adult patients metabolize and excrete medications more slowly than younger patients. Always be mindful of the total acetaminophen dosages consumed.

4. Mrs. Shepard should be instructed about what her role will be when her pain management regimen is altered. Does she have to ask for the pain medication, or will it just be brought to her? Patient and family education are vital to success in management of a patient's pain.

Ms. Jackson

1. Using an equianalgesic conversion, we can determine whether Ms. Jackson is likely to have good pain relief based on her requirement with the patient-controlled analgesia (PCA) pump. Her current pain level of 3 shows that the morphine has been effective. Remember that the PCA pump keeps a history of what the patient uses, which is the best indicator of what the patient needs. Ms. Jackson has used 15 mg of morphine during the past 6 hours. An equianalgesic dose of codeine 30 mg with acetaminophen (Tylenol with codeine No. 3) would be almost 200 mg of codeine, but only 30 to 60 mg has been ordered. In addition, if Ms. Jackson takes enough Tylenol with codeine No. 3 to get 200 mg of codeine, she will receive a dangerous dose of both the codeine and the acetaminophen. The HCP needs to be contacted for different analgesic orders.

Mr. Sebastian

1. $\dfrac{5 \text{ mg}}{} \;\Big|\; \dfrac{1 \text{ grain}}{60 \text{ mg}} \;\Big|\; \dfrac{1 \text{ mL}}{\text{grains } 1/6} = 0.5 \text{ mL}$

2. Home instruction regarding around-the-clock administration of pain medication is indicated as well as effects and side effects to report. He will also need to implement measures to prevent constipation.

3. MS Contin, a long-acting oral form of morphine, may be an option for Mr. Sebastian, along with an immediate-release preparation for breakthrough pain. Make sure to check an equianalgesic chart to be sure his oral dose is adequate. Also, information about what to do and whom to contact if pain becomes unmanageable is necessary to help prevent readmissions to the hospital.

Review Questions

1. A patient is walking up and down the hall and visiting and laughing with other patients. When the nurse approaches, the patient reports a pain level of 6 on a scale of 0 to 10. Based on McCaffery's definition of pain, which of the following assumptions by the nurse is most likely correct?
   1. The patient is not really in pain but just wants medication.
   2. The patient is having pain at a level of 6 on a scale of 0 to 10.
   3. The patient is in minimal pain and should receive an oral analgesic instead of an injection.
   4. The patient is in pain but does not need pain medication yet.

2. A patient with terminal cancer has been requiring 5 mg of intravenous morphine every 1 to 2 hours to control pain. Yet, the patient is engrossed in a movie on television and appears to be in no pain. Which of the following explanations of this behavior is most likely correct?
   1. Denial of pain is common in patients with cancer.
   2. The cancer treatment is working and the pain is improving.
   3. The patient is hiding the pain to finish watching the movie undisturbed.
   4. Distraction can be an effective treatment for pain when used with appropriate drug treatments.

3. What action should the nurse take when a patient with cancer pain develops tolerance to opioid analgesics?
   1. Slowly wean the patient from opioids.
   2. Request a referral to an addiction specialist for the patient.
   3. Talk to the registered nurse or health care provider about increasing the dose of analgesic.
   4. Offer the patient nonopioid alternatives for pain control.

4. A patient has surgical site pain 24 hours after a total hip replacement. All the following medications are ordered. Which would be the most appropriate choice for the patient at this time?
   1. Ibuprofen (Motrin)
   2. Hydromorphone (Dilaudid)
   3. Acetaminophen (Tylenol)
   4. Gabapentin (Neurontin)

5. A patient is receiving duloxetine (Cymbalta) for neuropathic pain related to diabetes. Which symptoms of neuropathic pain should the nurse assess?
   1. Tingling, shocklike pain
   2. Dull, aching pain
   3. Deep, cramping pain
   4. Throbbing, aching pain

6. Which of the following methods is the most reliable way to assess the severity of a patient's pain?
   1. Ask the patient to describe the pain.
   2. Observe the patient for physical signs of pain such as moaning or grimacing.
   3. Ask the patient to rate his or her pain using a valid assessment scale.
   4. Ask a family member to rate the patient's pain.

7. A patient is hospitalized following a motor vehicle accident with multiple orthopedic injuries. The patient reports acute pain at an 8 on a 0 to 10 scale. An order is written for morphine 6 mg intravenously every 4 hours as needed as well as a nonopioid oral analgesic every 4 hours as needed. To reduce the risk of adverse effects and maintain an acceptable level of sedation and pain control, which of the following analgesic schedules will be most effective?
   1. Offer the opioid every 4 hours.
   2. Tell the patient to call when pain becomes severe and then give the drugs immediately.
   3. Give both the intravenous opioid and the oral nonopioid every 4 hours around the clock.
   4. Alternate the intravenous analgesic with the nonopioid oral analgesic as needed.

8. An 88-year-old patient is admitted with a broken hip after a fall. An order is written for meperidine 50 to 75 mg intramuscularly every 4 hours as needed for pain. Which of the following actions should the nurse take first?
   1. Give the meperidine every 4 hours around the clock.
   2. Offer the meperidine every 4 to 6 hours as needed.
   3. Administer a nonsteroidal anti-inflammatory drug with the meperidine for added pain relief.
   4. Discuss the order with the registered nurse or health care provider.

9. A patient is started on gabapentin (Neurontin) 300 mg by mouth three times daily for chronic low back pain related to lumbar disc herniation. Which instruction should the nurse provide?
   1. "Take the medication at the first sign of any pain, up to three times daily."
   2. "Take one capsule every 8 hours continuously to keep the pain under control."
   3. "Take the medication only when you need it, to prevent becoming addicted."
   4. "Take one capsule three times a day, then stop it when the pain is under control."

10. A nurse receives an order to administer 1 mL of sterile normal saline solution intramuscularly to a patient suspected of opioid abuse. Which response by the nurse is appropriate?
    1. Administer the saline and document the patient's response in the medical record.
    2. Inform the patient that the saline was ordered instead of an opioid.
    3. Discuss concerns about the order with the supervisor and health care provider.
    4. Administer an appropriate dose of opioid instead of the saline.

11. A nurse needs to administer morphine 10 mg intramuscularly. It is supplied as grains 1/4 per mL. How many milliliters should the nurse prepare for injection?
    Answer: _____ mL

Answer rationales available in your online resources.

ANSWERS 1. 2; 4. 3; 4. 3; 5. 1; 6. 3; 7. 3; 8. 4; 9. 2; 10. 3; 11. 0.7 mL.

Key Points

Find the chapter key points in your online resources available through Davis Edge.

Additional Resources

DAVIS edge.   Use the scratch off code on the inside front cover of your book to access online quizzes that will help you to improve your scores on course exams and prepare for NCLEX-PN®.

   Study Guide

CHAPTER 11
Nursing Care of Patients With Cancer

Janet Yontas, Lucy L. Colo, Janice L. Bradford

KEY TERMS

alopecia (AL-oh-PEE-shah)
anemia (uh-NEE-mee-ah)
anorexia (AN-oh-REK-see-ah)
benign (bee-NINE)
biopsy (BY-op-see)
cancer (KAN-sir)
carcinogen (kar-SIN-oh-jen)
chemotherapy (KEE-moh-THAIR-uh-pee)
contact inhibition (kon-takt in-huh-BIH-shun)
cytotoxic (SY-toh-TOK-sik)
desquamation (dee-skwa-MAY-shun)
in situ (in SY-too)
leukopenia (LOO-koh-PEE-nee-ah)
malignant (muh-LIG-nunt)
metastasis (muh-TAS-tuh-sis)
mucositis (MYOO-koh-SY-tis)
nadir (NAY-dur)
neoplasm (NEE-oh-PLAZ-uhm)
neutropenia (noo-troh-PEE-nee-ah)
oncology (on-CAW-luh-gee)
oncovirus (ON-koh-VY-rus)
palliation (pal-ee-AY-shun)
radiation therapy (RAY-dee-AY-shun THAIR-uh-pee)
stomatitis (STOH-mah-TY-tis)
thrombocytopenia (THROM-boh-SY-toh-PEE-nee-ah)
tumor (TOO-mer)
vesicant (VES-ih-kent)
xerostomia (ZEE-roh-STOH-mee-ah)

CHAPTER CONCEPT

Comfort

LEARNING OUTCOMES

1. Explain the structures and functions of the normal cell.
2. Describe changes that occur in a cell when it becomes malignant.
3. Identify commonly used chemotherapeutic agents.
4. Discuss the plan of care for the patient receiving chemotherapy and/or radiation therapy.
5. Identify data to collect when caring for a patient with cancer.
6. Recognize common oncological emergencies and related nursing care.
7. Discuss how you will know if your nursing interventions have been effective.
8. Describe the role of hospice in providing care for patients with advanced cancer.

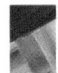

REVIEW OF ANATOMY AND PHYSIOLOGY OF NORMAL CELLS

Cells are the smallest living structural and functional subunits of the body. Although human cells vary in size, shape, and certain metabolic activities, they have many characteristics in common.

Cell Structure
Human cells have a plasma membrane, cytoplasm (cytosol, organelles), and a nucleus (Fig. 11.1). Organelles are specific in structure and function. Variations in the relative amounts of organelles and cell features allow great diversity in cells and, therefore, in tissues.

Nucleus
The nucleus of a cell is its control center, containing the individual's unique deoxyribonucleic acid (DNA) sequence (Fig. 11.2). Most cells have one central nucleus, although variations exist.

DNA coding regions are called *genes*; a gene is the code for one protein. Not all genes in a particular cell are active, rather only those needed for the proteins required to carry out their specific functions. These proteins may be structural, such as the collagen of connective tissue, or functional, such as the hemoglobin of red blood cells (RBCs). Important functional proteins are the enzymes that catalyze the specific reactions characteristic of each type of cell.

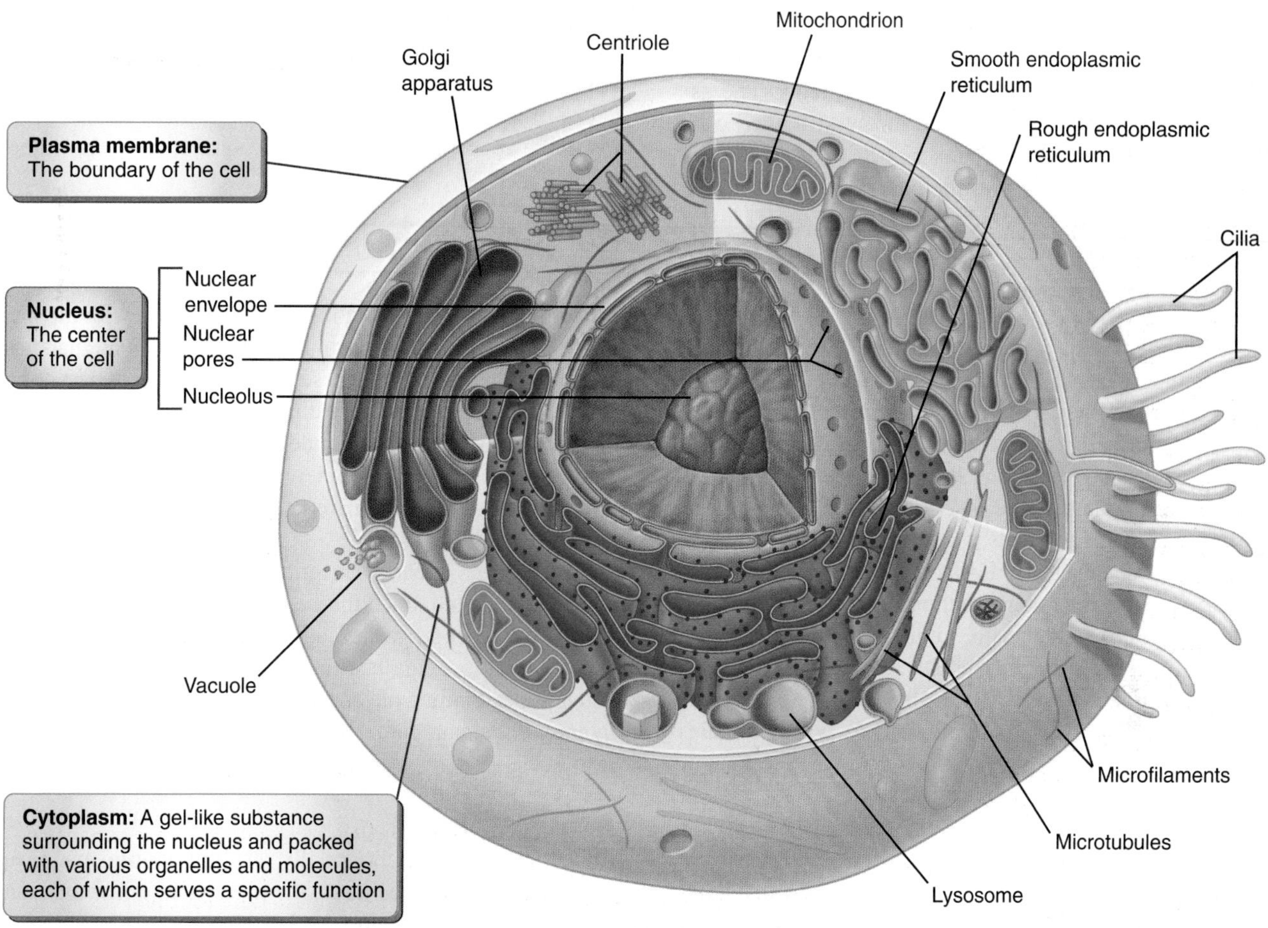

Golgi apparatus

Centriole

Mitochondrion

Smooth endoplasmic reticulum

Rough endoplasmic reticulum

Cilia

Plasma membrane: The boundary of the cell

Nuclear envelope

Nucleus: The center of the cell

Nuclear pores

Nucleolus

Vacuole

Microfilaments

Microtubules

Cytoplasm: A gel-like substance surrounding the nucleus and packed with various organelles and molecules, each of which serves a specific function

Lysosome

FIGURE 11.1 Schematic of a typical human cell.

A double-layered membrane called the **nuclear envelope** surrounds the nucleus.

Perforating the nuclear envelope are **nuclear pores.** These pores regulate the passage of molecules into the nucleus (such as those needed for construction of RNA and DNA), as well as out of the nucleus (such as RNA, which leaves the nucleus to perform its work in the cytoplasm).

Extending throughout the nucleoplasm (the substance filling the nucleus) are thread-like structures composed of DNA and protein called **chromatin.** When a cell begins to divide, the chromatin coils tightly into short, rod-like structures called **chromosomes**.

In the center of the nucleus is the **nucleolus.** The nucleolus manufactures components of **ribosomes**, the cell's protein-producing structures.

Ribosomes

Endoplasmic reticulum (attached to nucleus)

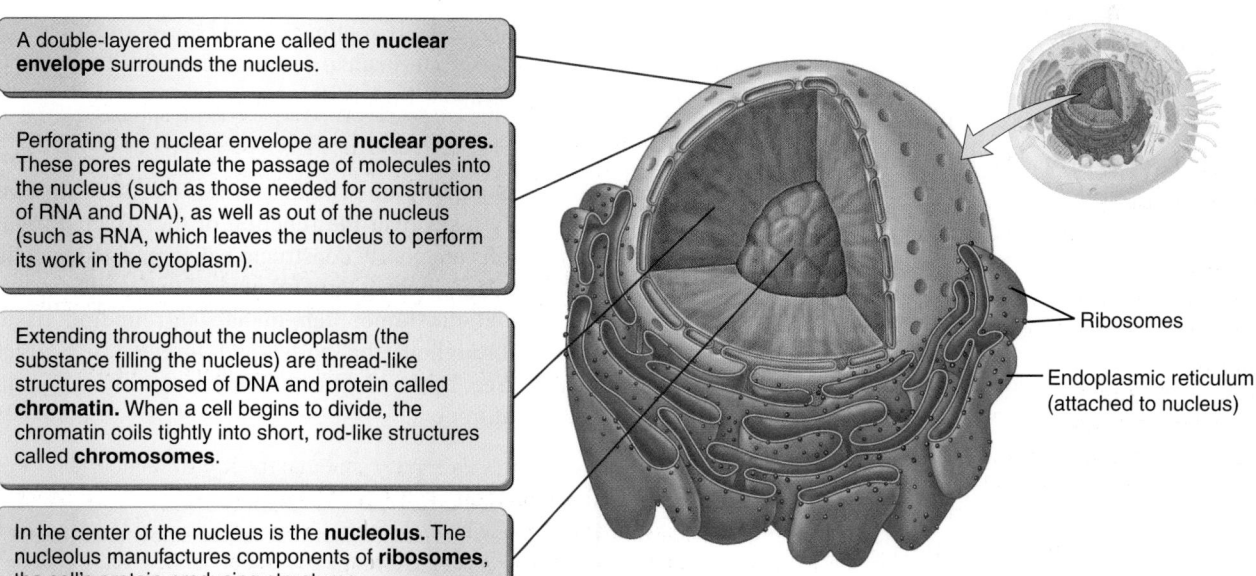

FIGURE 11.2 The nucleus.

Genetic Code and Protein Synthesis

The genetic code of DNA is the code for the amino acid sequences needed to synthesize a cell's proteins. The assembly of amino acids into the primary structure of a protein is a two-step process: transcription and translation. Transcription makes a copy of the code needed for a protein so DNA can remain guarded in the nucleus. Translation occurs at the ribosome where the nucleotide code of nucleic acids is translated into the amino acid code of protein (Fig. 11.3).

As with any complex process, mistakes are possible. If there is a mistake in the DNA code, the process of protein synthesis may continue. However, the resulting protein will not function normally; this is the basis for genetic diseases. DNA mistakes acquired during life are called *mutations.* A mutation is any change in the DNA code. Ultraviolet rays or exposure to certain chemicals may cause structural changes in the DNA code. These changes can kill the affected cells or may irreversibly alter their function. Such altered cells can become **malignant,** being unable to function normally. These cells actively replicate the mutated DNA during division, creating a mass of faulty cells. This is the basis of some forms of **cancer,** which is a general term for many types of malignant growths.

Mitosis

Mitosis is cell reproduction. After its 46 chromosomes have replicated, one cell divides into two cells, each with a complete set of chromosomes. Mitosis is necessary for the growth of the body and the replacement of dead or damaged cells. Not all cells are capable of mitosis; of those that are capable, the rate of division varies widely by tissue type. Some cells are capable of only a limited number of divisions; once that limit has been reached and the cells die, they are not replaced. Shortly after birth, almost all neurons lose their ability to divide, and muscle cells have limited mitotic capability. When such cells are lost through injury or disease, the loss of their functions in the individual is usually permanent.

Cell Cycle

The cell cycle involves a series of changes through which a cell progresses, starting from the time it develops until it reproduces itself. The duration of the cell's life, the time it takes for mitosis to occur, the growth ratio (percentage of cycling cells), the frequency of cell loss, and the doubling time (the time for a **tumor**—an abnormal mass—to double its size) are important concepts related to tumor growth and treatment strategies.

At any point in time, some cells are actively dividing, others leave the cycle after a certain point and die, and still others temporarily leave the cycle and remain inactive until reentry into the cycle. Inactive cells continue to synthesize (ribonucleic acid [RNA] and protein; Fig. 11.4).

Cells and Tissues

A tissue is a group of like cells of same structure and function, along with their intercellular substance. The four categories of human tissues are epithelial, connective, muscle, and nervous. Tissues organize into organs, organs construct systems, and systems form the individual. Because of this hierarchy, if a dividing mass of cells is mutated, the abnormality will produce symptoms at the higher levels.

 ## INTRODUCTION TO CANCER CONCEPTS

Oncology is the branch of medicine that deals with the prevention, diagnosis, and treatment of tumors or malignancies. Oncology nurses (cancer nurses) are an important part of the medical-surgical team, providing care for patients from prevention and detection to treatment, follow-up, and palliation. The American Cancer Society (ACS) reports more than 15.5 million Americans alive today have a history of cancer (ACS, 2017c).

The benefits of early cancer detection and treatment have been documented since the beginning of the 19th century. Today, microscopic technology, genetic testing, and continued research provide health care providers (HCPs) with a better understanding of cancer and means for early detection, interventions, and care. Box 11.1 lists some helpful cancer resources.

Benign Tumors

Cells that reproduce abnormally result in **neoplasms,** or tumors. The term *neoplasm* can be used to describe both cancerous and benign tumors. A **benign** tumor is a cluster of cells that is not normal to the body but is noncancerous. Benign tumors grow more slowly than cancer cells. They do not alter the cells of the original tissue. An organ containing a benign tumor usually continues to function normally. A neoplastic growth is difficult to detect until it contains about 500 cells and is about 1 cm in diameter.

Cancer

Cancer is a group of cells that grows out of control and eventually takes over the function of the affected organ. Cancer cells are poorly constructed, disorganized, and fast growing. *Malignant,* a term often used to describe cancer, means that the tumor can invade surrounding tissue, spread throughout the body, and threaten life unless treated. See Table 11.1 for a comparison of benign and malignant tumors.

> **NURSING CARE TIP**
> Teach patients and families that cancer is not contagious.

Pathophysiology

Cancer is not one disease but many diseases with different causes, manifestations, treatments, and prognoses. There

---

• WORD • BUILDING •

oncology: onco—mass + logy—word, reason
neoplasm: neo—new + plasm—form

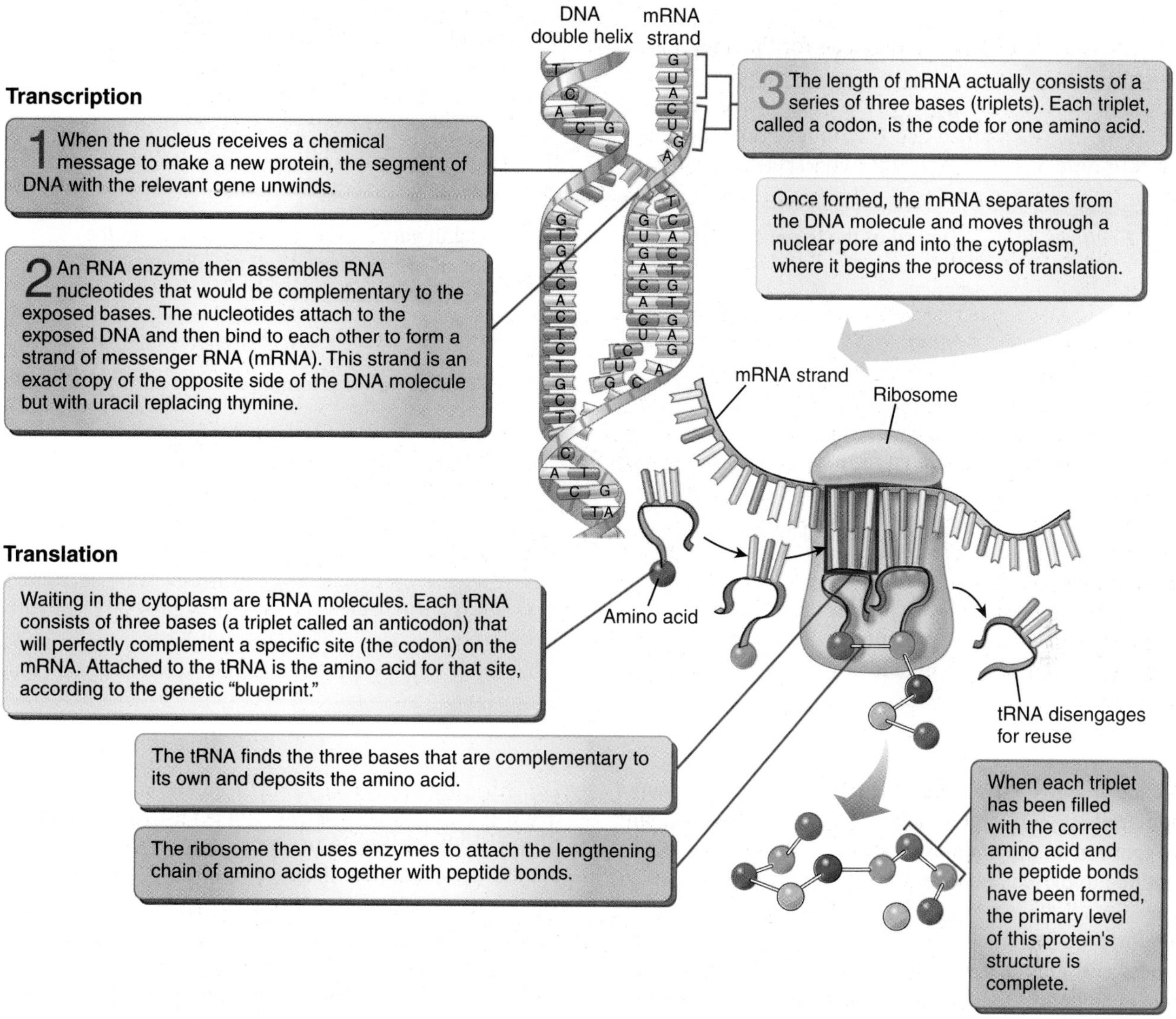

DNA double helix
mRNA strand
Transcription
1 When the nucleus receives a chemical message to make a new protein, the segment of DNA with the relevant gene unwinds.
2 An RNA enzyme then assembles RNA nucleotides that would be complementary to the exposed bases. The nucleotides attach to the exposed DNA and then bind to each other to form a strand of messenger RNA (mRNA). This strand is an exact copy of the opposite side of the DNA molecule but with uracil replacing thymine.
3 The length of mRNA actually consists of a series of three bases (triplets). Each triplet, called a codon, is the code for one amino acid.
Once formed, the mRNA separates from the DNA molecule and moves through a nuclear pore and into the cytoplasm, where it begins the process of translation.
mRNA strand
Ribosome
Translation
Waiting in the cytoplasm are tRNA molecules. Each tRNA consists of three bases (a triplet called an anticodon) that will perfectly complement a specific site (the codon) on the mRNA. Attached to the tRNA is the amino acid for that site, according to the genetic "blueprint."
Amino acid
tRNA disengages for reuse
The tRNA finds the three bases that are complementary to its own and deposits the amino acid.
The ribosome then uses enzymes to attach the lengthening chain of amino acids together with peptide bonds.
When each triplet has been filled with the correct amino acid and the peptide bonds have been formed, the primary level of this protein's structure is complete.

FIGURE 11.3 Protein synthesis.

Cell Division (Mitosis)
Organelle Duplication
Differentiation
Cell growth occurs
Resting phase
Cell Life Cycle
Point of Decision to Replicate or Differentiate
DNA Replication

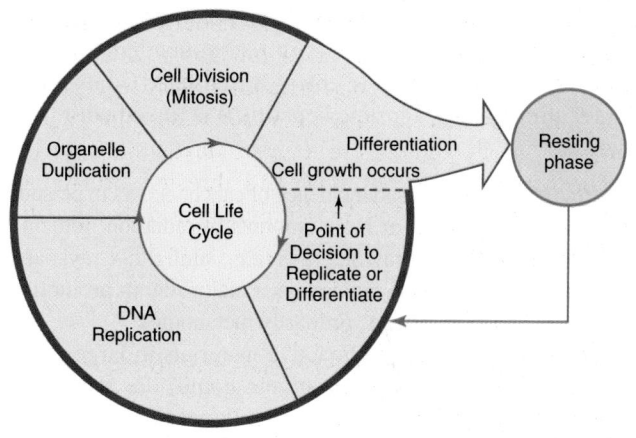

FIGURE 11.4 Cell cycle.

are more than 100 types of cancer. Normal cells are limited to about 50 to 60 divisions before they die. Cancer cells, however, do not have a division limit. They are considered to be immortal. They continue to grow out of control until they are destroyed.

Box 11.1

Cancer Resources

American Cancer Society: 800-227-2345; www.cancer.org
Cancer*Care*: 800-813-HOPE (4673); www.cancercare.org
National Cancer Institute: 800-4-Cancer (422-6237); www.cancer.gov
Oncology Nursing Society: 866-257-4ONS (4667); www.ons.org
Centers for Disease Control and Prevention: 1-800-CDC-INFO (800-232-4636); www.cdc.gov/cancer

The progression from a normal cell to a malignant cell follows a pattern of mutation, defective division, abnormal growth cycles, and defective cell communication. Cell mutation occurs when an alteration affects the chromosomes, causing the new cell to differ from its parent cell. The malignant cell's enzymes destroy the gluelike substance found between normal cells. This disrupts the transfer of information and communication used for normal cell structure and growth.

Table 11.1
Comparing Benign and Malignant Tumors

	Benign	Malignant
Growth Rate	Typically slow expansion	Often rapid growth; malignant cells infiltrate surrounding tissue
Cell Features	Typical of the tissue of origin	Atypical in varying degrees compared with the tissue of origin; altered cell membrane; contain tumor-specific antigens
Tissue Damage	Minor	Often causes necrosis and ulceration of tissue
Metastasis	Not seen; remains localized at site of origin	Often spreads to form tumors in other parts of the body
Recurrence After Treatment	Seldom recurs after surgical removal	Can be seen after surgical removal and following radiation and chemotherapy
Related Terminology	Hyperplasia, polyp, benign neoplasia	Cancer, malignancy, malignant neoplasia
Prognosis	Not injurious unless location causes pressure or obstruction to vital organs	Death if uncontrolled

Cancer cells also lack **contact inhibition.** Growth-regulating signals in the cells' surrounding environment are ignored as the abnormal cell growth increases. Cells continue to divide and invade surrounding tissues.

Etiology

Cancer cell growth and reproduction involve a three-step process: initiation, promotion, and progression. The first step, *initiation,* is the result of an alteration in the genetic structure of the cell (DNA). This occurs either spontaneously or following exposure to a **carcinogen** (a substance or agent that increases the risk of cancer). The cellular change primes the cell to become cancerous.

Promotion occurs after repeated exposure to carcinogens causes the initiated cells to mutate. During the promotion step, a tumor forms from mutated cell reproduction. During *progression,* further genetic mutations occur, leading to growth and metastasis. Scientists are now using their understanding of cancer cell growth to develop treatments aimed at harming the cancer cells at their various stages of formation.

A healthy immune system can often destroy cancer cells before they replicate and become a tumor. It is important to remember that any substance that weakens or alters the immune system puts the individual at risk for cell mutation with the potential to develop into cancer.

Risk Factors

VIRUSES. Certain viruses, such as **oncoviruses** (RNA-type viruses), are linked to cancer in humans. These viruses insert their own RNA into the host cell, causing a mutation with the ability to produce a cancer. Understanding oncoviruses has led to the development of vaccines to prevent these cancers.

The Epstein-Barr virus (EBV), which causes infectious mononucleosis, is associated with Burkitt lymphoma and nasopharyngeal cancer. Herpes simplex virus type 2 is associated with cervical and penile cancers. Human papillomavirus (HPV) is associated with cervical and vaginal cancer in women, penile cancer in men, cancer of the anus, and some head and neck cancers in both sexes. Vaccination against HPV (Gardasil) is recommended for girls and boys aged 11 to 12 (Centers for Disease Control and Prevention, 2017). Chronic hepatitis B is linked with liver cancer.

RADIATION. An increased incidence of cancer occurs in persons exposed to prolonged or large amounts of radiation. Ionizing radiation involving ultraviolet rays (e.g., sunlight; x-rays; and alpha, beta, and gamma rays) plays a major role in promoting leukemia and skin cancers, primarily melanomas.

Persons exposed to radioactive materials in large doses (e.g., a radiation leak or an atomic bomb) are at risk for leukemia and breast, bone, lung, and thyroid cancer. Controlled **radiation therapy** is used to treat cancer patients by destroying rapidly dividing cancer cells, but radiation can

• WORD • BUILDING •
carcinogen: karkinos—cancer, crab + genesis—birth
oncovirus: onco—mass + virus

Cultural Considerations

Many racial and ethnic groups in the United States have high rates of cancer. Although risk factors for the development of specific cancers are similar, barriers to prevention and nursing strategies to reduce risk factors vary among races and ethnicities because of differences in receiving or timeliness of recommended treatments.

Non-Hispanic White

Foreign-born and first-generation white men from Norway, Sweden, and Germany have an increased risk of stomach cancer. Be sure to assess for dietary risk factors.

Recent Eastern European immigrants may be at risk for thyroid cancer and leukemia because of industrial pollution and radiation exposure from the Chernobyl nuclear disaster in the former Soviet Union in 1986. Some contamination occurred in Estonia, Latvia, Lithuania, and Poland. It is essential for health care providers (HCPs) to carefully screen individuals for these cancers.

Non-Hispanic Black (African Americans)

The risk of death after a diagnosis of cancer is higher for non-Hispanic blacks for all cancers combined and for most cancer sites. In general, African Americans report later for treatment than non-Hispanic whites. Lower levels of thiamine, riboflavin, vitamins A and C, and iron may increase cancer risk.

Hispanic

Hispanic populations in the United States have an increased incidence for some types of cancer, most notably for leukemia. However, they have a lower risk of death after diagnosis for lung and cervical cancers.

Asian American/Pacific Islander

Although Asian Americans/Pacific Islanders have higher risk of death than non-Hispanic whites for all cancers, they have lower risk for some common cancers. Asian Americans/Pacific Islanders have higher risk of death for oral cavity cancer and for melanoma, non-Hodgkin lymphoma, and leukemia.

High rates of stomach, breast, colon, and rectal cancer common among the Japanese may be related to a genetic predisposition, hepatitis B, vitamin A deficiency, low vitamin C intake, and chronic esophagitis.

Arab American

Arab Americans are at risk for lung cancer and other cancers related to smoking. Rates of breast cancer screening and cervical Papanicolaou (Pap) smears are low among Arab American women.

American Indian

American Indian populations have an increased risk most notably for leukemia and thyroid cancer. Risk factors for the development of cancer include obesity, a diet high in fat, and high rates of alcohol consumption and smoking.

Reference

Jemal, A., Ward, E. M., Johnson, C. J., Cronin, K. A., Ma, J., Ryerson, A. B., ... Weir, H. K. (2017). Annual report to the nation on the status of cancer, 1975–2014, featuring survival. *Journal of the National Cancer Institute, 109*(1). doi:https//doi.org/10.1093.jnci/djx030

also damage normal cells. The decision to use radiation is made after careful evaluation of the tumor's location and vulnerability to other treatments.

CHEMICALS. Chemicals are present in air, water, soil, food, drugs, and tobacco smoke. Chemical carcinogens are implicated as triggering mechanisms in malignant tumor development. Length of time and degree of exposure intensity to chemical carcinogens are associated with risk for cancer development.

Smoking accounts for 30% of all cancer deaths in the United States and 80% of all lung cancer deaths (ACS, 2017a). Alcohol and tobacco together increase risk factors. They are the most frequent causes of cancers of the mouth and throat. Heavy use of alcohol has been associated with liver, breast, colon, and pancreatic cancers (ACS, 2017a).

Occupational exposures are associated with some cancers, such as bladder, liver, kidney, lung, and skin. The development of federal and state employee protection regulations has significantly reduced risk of occupational exposures.

IRRITANTS. Chronic irritation or inflammation caused by irritants such as snuff or pipe smoke often cause cancer in local areas. Nevi (moles) that are chronically irritated by clothing, especially clothing contaminated by chemical residue, can become malignant. Asbestos found in temperature and sound insulation has been proven to cause a particularly destructive type of lung cancer.

GENETICS. Genetics play a large part in cancer formation. Certain breast cancers are linked to a specific gene mutation. Skin, colon, ovarian, and prostate cancers have a genetic tendency. People with Down syndrome (a chromosomal abnormality) have a higher risk of developing acute leukemia.

DIET. Diet is a major factor in both cause and prevention of malignancies. People who eat high-fat, low-fiber diets are more prone to develop colon cancers. High-fat diets are linked to breast cancer in women and prostate cancer in men. Consumption of large amounts of pickled, smoked, and charbroiled foods has been linked with esophageal and stomach cancers. A diet low in vitamins A, C, and E is associated with cancers of the lungs, esophagus, mouth, larynx, cervix, and breast.

HORMONES. Hormonal agents that disturb the body's balance can also promote cancer. Long-term use of the female hormone estrogen is associated with cancer of the breast, uterus, ovaries, cervix, and vagina. It has been found that children born of mothers who took diethylstilbestrol (DES) during pregnancy have an increased incidence of reproductive cancers. DES is a synthetic hormone with estrogen-like properties that was used in the past to prevent miscarriage.

Tumors of the breast and uterus are tested for estrogen or progesterone influence. Treatment varies depending on test results.

IMMUNE FACTORS. A healthy immune system destroys mutant cells quickly on formation. An individual with impaired immunity is more susceptible to cancer formation when exposed to small amounts of carcinogens compared with someone with a healthy immune system. Immune system suppression allows malignant cells to develop in large numbers.

Altered immunity is noted in persons with chronic illness and stress. An increased risk of cancer follows a traumatic, stressful period in life, such as the loss of a mate or a job. Failure to decrease stress productively contributes to a higher incidence of chronic illnesses. Thus, a cycle of stress, illness, and increased cancer risk develops. People with AIDS have a compromised immune system and an increased risk for certain cancers. People on medication that reduces immune function are at risk. A decline in the immune system and increase in cancer risk are also noted as the body ages.

Cancer Classification

Cancers are identified by the tissue affected, speed of cell growth, cell appearance, and location. Neoplasms occurring in the epithelial cells are called *carcinomas*. Carcinoma is the most common type of cancer. It arises from cells of the skin, gastrointestinal (GI) system, and lungs (Figs. 11.5 and 11.6). *Sarcomas* are cancer cells affecting connective tissue, including fat, the sheath that contains nerves, cartilage, muscle, and bone. *Leukemia* is the term used to describe the abnormal growth of white blood cells (WBCs). Cancers involving cells of the lymphatic system, lymph nodes, and spleen are called *lymphomas*. See Table 11.2 for cancer types based on origin.

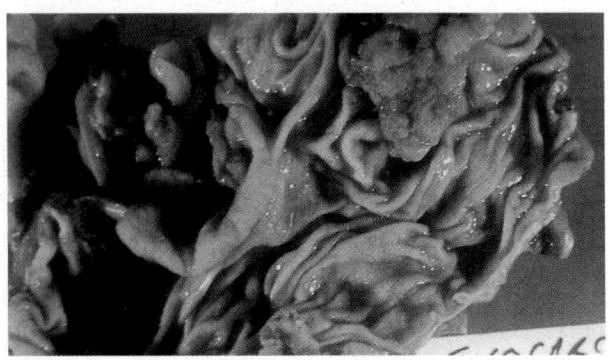

FIGURE 11.5 Adenocarcinoma of the cecum.

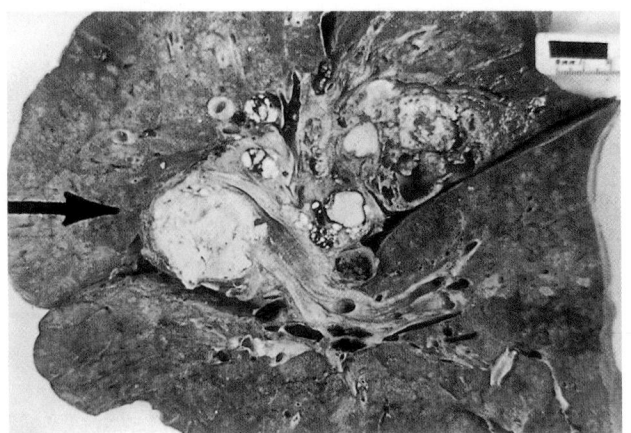

FIGURE 11.6 Lung cancer.

Table 11.2
Tumor Descriptions

Tumor Type	Character	Origin
Fibroma	Benign	Connective tissue
Lipoma	Benign	Fat tissue
Carcinoma	Cancerous	Tissue of the skin, glands, and digestive, urinary, and respiratory tract linings
Leukemia	Cancerous	Blood, plasma cells, and bone marrow
Lymphoma	Cancerous	Lymph tissue
Melanoma	Cancerous	Skin cells
Sarcoma	Cancerous	Connective tissue, including bone and muscle

Metastasis (Spread of Cancer)

Neoplastic cells that remain in one area are considered localized, or **in situ,** cancers. These tumors may be difficult to detect on clinical examination. They are identified through microscopic cell examination. In situ tumors are often removed surgically and may require no further treatment.

Metastasis is the term used to describe the spread of the tumor from the primary site into separate and distant areas (Fig. 11.7). Metastasis occurs mainly because cancer cells break away more easily than normal cells. Cancer cells can survive for a time independently from other cells. There are three steps in the formation of a metastasis: Cancer cells (1) invade blood or lymph vessels, (2) move by mechanical means, and (3) lodge and grow in a new location.

• WORD • BUILDING •
in situ: in—in + situ—position
metastasis: meta—beyond + stasis—stand

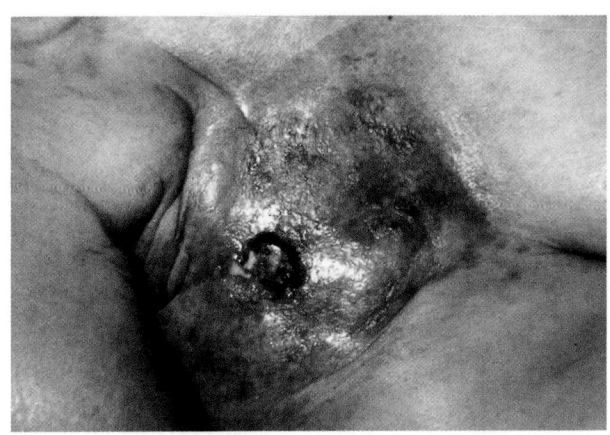

FIGURE 11.7 Invasive metastasis to skin area following mastectomy for breast cancer.

Metastatic tumors carry with them the cell characteristics of the original or primary tumor site. As a result, surgeons are able to determine the original tumor site based on metastatic cell characteristics. For example, lung tissue found in the brain suggests a primary lung tumor with metastasis to brain tissue. Common sites of metastasis are the lungs, liver, bones, and brain.

Incidence of Cancer

Cancer affects all age-groups but has the highest incidence in older people. In the United States, 87% of all cancers diagnosed are in people 50 years and older (ACS, 2017a). Men have a higher incidence of cancer than women. Cancer in people over age 50 is thought to occur from a combination of exposure to carcinogens and weakening of the body's immune system.

Acute lymphocytic leukemia and cancers of the central nervous system and brain are common cancers found in children aged 0 to 14 years. Causes of childhood cancer are not understood; therefore, prevention is difficult. Genetic predisposition is a factor.

The most common type of cancer in adults is skin cancer; it is also considered to be the most preventable. Exposure to ultraviolet radiation (sunlight) and indoor tanning increases the risk of skin cancer. Wearing protective clothing and sunscreen can greatly reduce the risk of skin cancer.

Lung cancer has the highest cancer mortality rate in both men and women. It also is commonly preventable. Cigarette smoking is the main cause, along with air pollution and exposure to radon and other chemicals.

Men have a high incidence of prostate cancer between ages 60 and 79. Cancer of the colon and rectum has been linked to consumption of high-fat, low-fiber diets. It ranks as the third highest cancer in men and women.

The highest incidence of cancer in women is in the breast. Women with a family history of breast cancer have a greater risk than those with no family history. Commercial testing for the oncogene linked with breast cancer is available and marketed for high-risk women, especially those in the Ashkenazi Jewish population. Genetic testing is done

through genetic counseling programs. Cost ranges from $400 to $4,000. It may be covered by some insurance plans if certain risk criteria are met. See Figure 11.8 for estimated new cancer cases and deaths for 2017.

Mortality Rates

Cancer survival rates have improved with the recognition of risk factors and improvements in early detection and treatment. A 5-year period is used to monitor cancer patients' progress following diagnosis and treatment. Survival statistics are based on those who live 5 years in remission. Remission is considered to have occurred when all signs and symptoms of cancer have disappeared, even though there may still be cancer in the body.

Early Detection and Prevention

Nurses play an important role in preventing and detecting cancer by educating patients about risk factors, self-examination, genetic testing, and cancer screening programs. Early diagnosis and treatment are important factors in fighting cancer.

EARLY DETECTION. Regular physical examinations help HCPs detect early warning signs of cancer. The ACS recommends mammography (a special x-ray of breast tissue used to detect a mass too small for palpation) every 1 to 2 years in women after age 45 (ACS, 2017b). Screening should continue as long as the woman is in good health and has a life expectancy of 10 years or more. Women should discuss individual risk factors and recommended screenings with their HCP.

Initial Papanicolaou (Pap) testing for cervical cancer is recommended to begin no later than age 21 and be performed every 3 years up to age 29. The preferred approach for women aged 30 to 65 is to have the Pap test with an HPV test every 5 years. However, it is acceptable to have just the Pap test every 3 years in this age-group (ACS, 2017b). After age 65, a woman who has had three normal Pap tests in a row within the past 10 years can choose to stop screening.

Some women choose not to be screened, even when they have access to health care. Barriers to screening include fear of health care personnel and testing procedures as well as lack of knowledge. Women who fear cancer but trust their HCPs and seek information are more likely to be screened. As a nurse, you can help by developing a trusting relationship and providing information to your female patients.

The ACS considers monthly breast self-examinations to be optional for women and testicular self-examinations to be optional for men. ACS guidelines encourage everyone to be familiar with their bodies and to report changes to their HCPs. Offer men and women instruction in breast and testicular self-examinations.

The ACS (2017b) recommends one of the following options to screen for colorectal cancer, beginning at age 50:

• Tests that find polyps and cancer
  • Flexible sigmoidoscopy every 5 years
  • Colonoscopy every 10 years

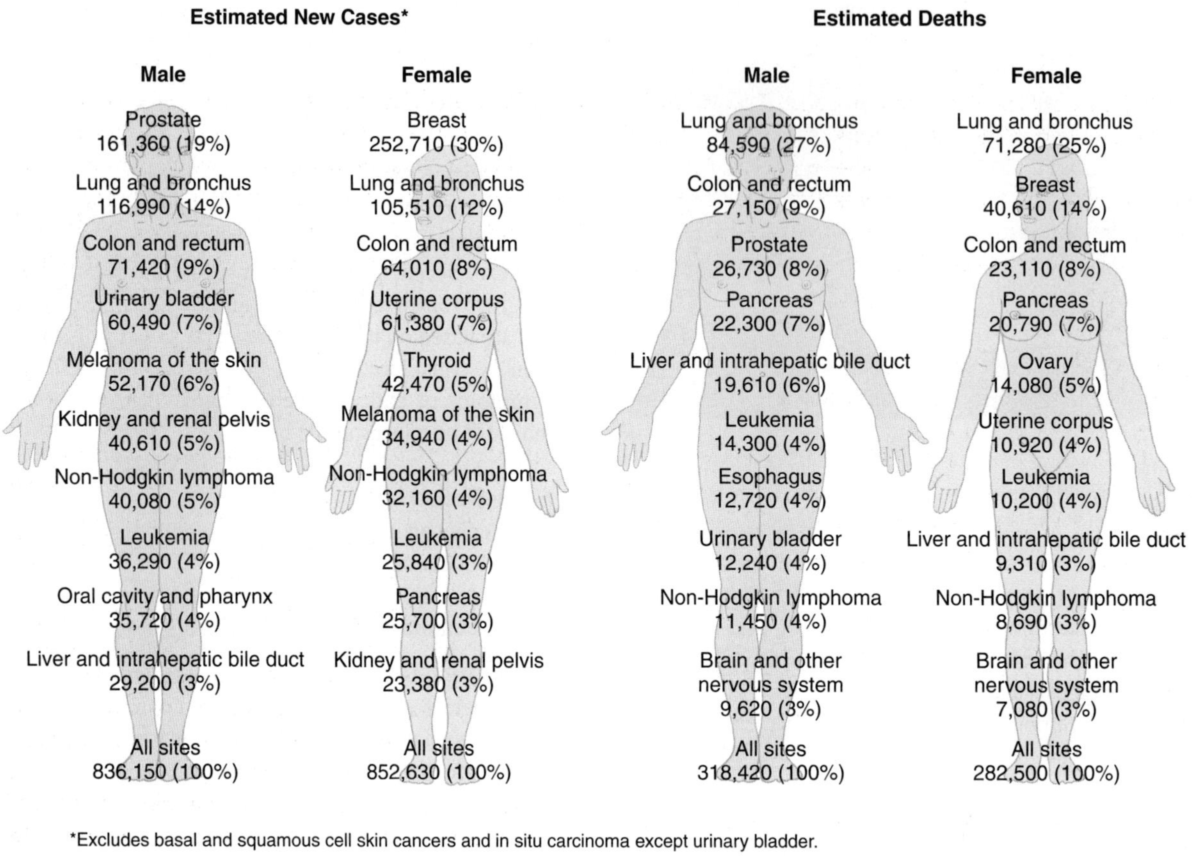

Estimated New Cases*

Male	Female
Prostate 161,360 (19%)	Breast 252,710 (30%)
Lung and bronchus 116,990 (14%)	Lung and bronchus 105,510 (12%)
Colon and rectum 71,420 (9%)	Colon and rectum 64,010 (8%)
Urinary bladder 60,490 (7%)	Uterine corpus 61,380 (7%)
Melanoma of the skin 52,170 (6%)	Thyroid 42,470 (5%)
Kidney and renal pelvis 40,610 (5%)	Melanoma of the skin 34,940 (4%)
Non-Hodgkin lymphoma 40,080 (5%)	Non-Hodgkin lymphoma 32,160 (4%)
Leukemia 36,290 (4%)	Leukemia 25,840 (3%)
Oral cavity and pharynx 35,720 (4%)	Pancreas 25,700 (3%)
Liver and intrahepatic bile duct 29,200 (3%)	Kidney and renal pelvis 23,380 (3%)
All sites 836,150 (100%)	All sites 852,630 (100%)

Estimated Deaths

Male	Female
Lung and bronchus 84,590 (27%)	Lung and bronchus 71,280 (25%)
Colon and rectum 27,150 (9%)	Breast 40,610 (14%)
Prostate 26,730 (8%)	Colon and rectum 23,110 (8%)
Pancreas 22,300 (7%)	Pancreas 20,790 (7%)
Liver and intrahepatic bile duct 19,610 (6%)	Ovary 14,080 (5%)
Leukemia 14,300 (4%)	Uterine corpus 10,920 (4%)
Esophagus 12,720 (4%)	Leukemia 10,200 (4%)
Urinary bladder 12,240 (4%)	Liver and intrahepatic bile duct 9,310 (3%)
Non-Hodgkin lymphoma 11,450 (4%)	Non-Hodgkin lymphoma 8,690 (3%)
Brain and other nervous system 9,620 (3%)	Brain and other nervous system 7,080 (3%)
All sites 318,420 (100%)	All sites 282,500 (100%)

*Excludes basal and squamous cell skin cancers and in situ carcinoma except urinary bladder.

FIGURE 11.8 Leading new cancer cases and deaths: 2017 estimates.

- Double-contrast barium enema every 5 years
- Colonography (virtual colonoscopy using computed tomography [CT]) every 5 years
- Tests that mainly find cancer
- Fecal occult blood test every year
- Fecal immunochemical test every year
- Stool DNA test every 3 years

If any tests are positive, a colonoscopy should be done.

Before 2009, the ACS recommended annual digital rectal examination and prostate-specific antigen (PSA) blood testing for men aged older than 50 years with a life expectancy of at least 10 years and for younger men at higher risk. The ACS currently recommends that men discuss the benefits of PSA testing with their HCP starting at age 50 (ACS, 2017b). It seems reasonable, however, to still offer these tests as options to men in these populations.

BLOOD TESTING. A new blood test called CancerSEEK was introduced in 2018 (Cohen et al., 2018). This test can help detect eight different cancers before any symptoms occur. It is unclear how this test will be used, but it is very promising because early detection can be critical for successful treatment.

GENETIC TESTING. Genetic testing is used to identify persons at risk for certain cancers. Genetic testing technology poses both legal and ethical questions concerning confidentiality and insurance cost issues. The cooperation of family members is important because genetic testing is done after a family member has been diagnosed with cancer. Family members may experience a variety of emotions surrounding the increased risk for themselves as well as guilt over the role they may have played in increasing risk for their children.

HEALTHY LIFESTYLE. Promotion of healthy lifestyles, including proper diet and exercise, helps strengthen the immune system and reduce cancer risk. Smoking is the most preventable cause of death from lung cancer. Smoking cessation is the subject of ongoing campaigns by the ACS. Secondhand smoke contributes to a significant increased risk of lung cancer in nonsmokers as well.

PROTECTANT FOODS. Much research related to diet and cancer risk is being conducted. Visit www.cancer.org and "Nutrition Notes: Reducing Cancer Risk" for additional dietary recommendations.

VACCINES. Preventive vaccines target viruses associated with certain cancers. Recombinant HPV vaccine (Gardasil), for example, prevents HPV, which is responsible for various cancers. Hepatitis B vaccine protects against the infection that increases susceptibility to liver cancer. Therapeutic vaccines are currently being researched and tested for various cancers. These vaccines stimulate the patient's immune system to destroy cancer cells. Currently, the only therapeutic cancer vaccines approved by the U.S. Food and Drug Administration

Nutrition Notes

Reducing Cancer Risk. The American Cancer Society (ACS) estimates that two-thirds of Americans are overweight or obese, increasing the risk of many types of cancer. The World Cancer Research Fund estimates that about 20% of all cancers diagnosed in the United States are related to body fatness, physical inactivity, excessive alcohol consumption, and poor nutrition. The ACS recommends that Americans:

- Achieve and maintain a healthy weight
- Eat a healthy diet, with an emphasis on plant foods:
  - Read food labels to be aware of portion sizes and calories
  - Choose whole, unprocessed fruits and vegetables
  - Limit intake of sugar-sweetened beverages
  - Limit processed and red meats; choose fish, poultry or beans
  - Eat a variety of at least 2½ cups of fruit and vegetables each day
  - Choose whole grains instead of refined grain products
- Limit alcohol intake to one drink for women and two for men per day (12 oz beer, 5 oz wine, or 1.5 oz distilled spirits)

Source: American Cancer Society. (2017). ACS guidelines for nutrition and physical activity. Retrieved from www.cancer.org/healthy/eat-healthy-get-active/acs-guidelines-nutrition-physical-activity-cancer-prevention/guidelines.html

are sipuleucel-T (Provenge) for the treatment of advanced prostate cancer and talimogene laherparepvec (T-VEC) for metastatic melanoma that cannot be surgically removed (National Cancer Institute, 2015).

Diagnosis of Cancer

A cancer diagnosis is a frightening experience ("Patient Perspective"). Often, people try to mask symptoms because they are so frightened of the disease. A physical examination along with careful and thorough assessment of the patient's current status, medical and surgical histories, and pertinent family history should be completed. The most conclusive information is obtained through tissue biopsy.

For explanations of the following tests, see Appendix A.

BIOPSY. Accurate identification of a cancer can be made only by **biopsy.** A biopsy can be done via an endoscopic procedure, surgical incision, or a small needle inserted into the site. Microscopic examination of a sample of suspected tissue or aspirated body fluid can confirm the presence of abnormal or cancerous cells. A biopsy is commonly done in an HCP's office or outpatient surgery department (Fig 11.9).

RADIOLOGICAL PROCEDURES. X-ray examination is a valuable diagnostic tool in detecting cancer of the bones and hollow organs. Chest x-ray examination is one diagnostic test used in detecting lung cancer. Mammography is a reliable

Patient Perspective

Nikki. When I was 27 years old, I went for a routine checkup. The doctor found a lump in my right breast. I had noticed it 6 months before, but I didn't think it was anything. When the doctor told me it was cancer, my reaction was, "Why me? I have such a healthy lifestyle!" I discussed treatments with my doctor, and he said I needed surgery, chemotherapy, and radiation. But because I was so young, I didn't want to lose my breast or my hair. The doctor said there was a new medicine that wouldn't make me lose my hair, but it is wasn't covered by insurance.

The doctor put a port in my chest for chemo. It was so painful, I cried. After two chemo treatments, I had surgery. They were able to remove all the cancer and still leave most of my breast. When I was in the hospital, all the young medical students had to look at my breasts. After a while, I stopped feeling embarrassed.

Fortunately, my father was able to help me pay for the medicine I needed. When I went for chemotherapy, everyone was together in a group. All the older people looked at me because I was always the youngest patient. They had all lost their hair and had hats on. I lost about 20% of my hair, but I was the only one who could tell. Also, my skin got very dark, and people would ask if I went to the beach. I am Taiwanese, and people in Taiwan value light skin. I didn't like being asked why I was so dark! I had four more chemo treatments and 30 radiation treatments. I started on tamoxifen to prevent the cancer from returning.

About 9 months later, when I was 28, I moved to Japan. I knew I wanted to have a baby someday, but I wasn't too worried at that time. Even the doctor wasn't sure whether I could have a baby. I met my husband, an American, when I was in Japan. I worried about telling him about the cancer, because I knew he wanted children someday. But he said it was okay and that we could adopt if I couldn't have a baby. After we married, I stopped taking tamoxifen and had to wait 6 months to try to get pregnant. Then, it only took 2 months to get pregnant! I now have a healthy baby, and I feel very lucky and happy.

I worried that I wouldn't be able to breastfeed my baby, and it turns out I can only feed him from my left breast. Now when my breast is full of milk, I am very lopsided! I have to put in a pad on the right side when I go out. My left breast makes more than enough milk for my baby. I am not sure how long I will breastfeed before I have to go back on the tamoxifen, but for now I am happy that everything is working just fine.

Nothing is more important to me than staying healthy and for my husband and baby to be healthy, too. Now I have a good life and healthy body, and I can take care of my family. To stay healthy, I am very careful to eat lots of fruits and vegetables, and not to eat unhealthy fats, and I try to exercise a lot.

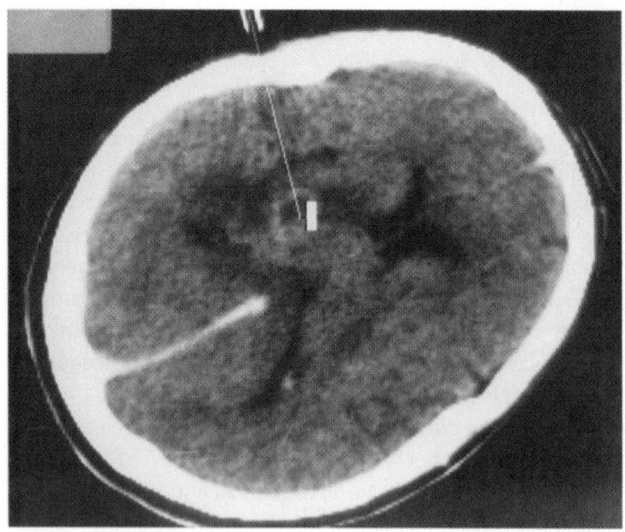

FIGURE 11.9 Stereotactic biopsy of a brain lesion.

and noninvasive low-radiation x-ray procedure for detecting breast masses (Fig. 11.10).

Contrast media x-ray studies are used to detect abnormalities that might not show up with regular x-rays. Barium is given orally for visualization of the esophagus and stomach. It can also be given rectally as a barium enema for visualization of the colon. Intravenous injection of contrast media is used for visualizing vessels, the urinary tract, or fallopian tubes.

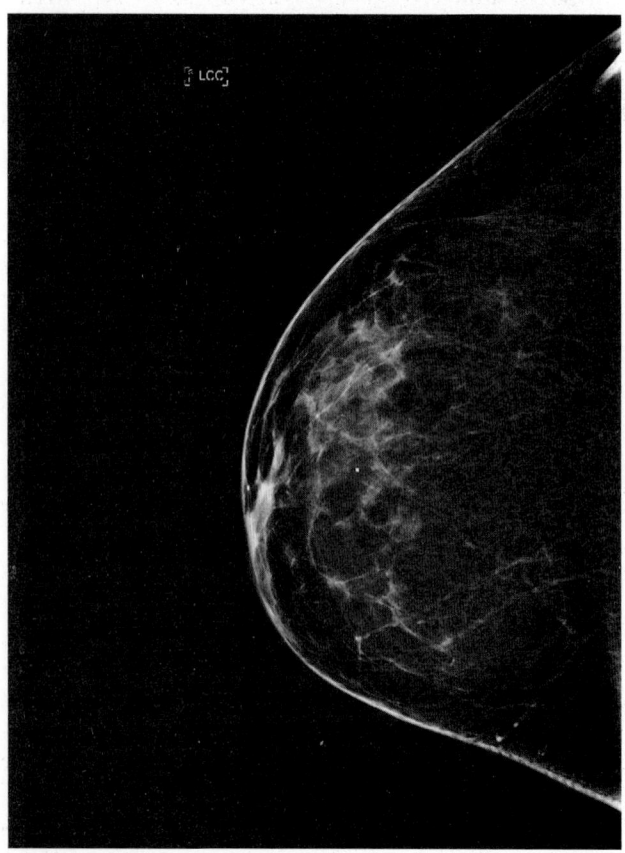

FIGURE 11.10 Mammogram.

CT scans are important in the diagnosis and staging of malignancies. They can detect minor variations in tissue thickness. The use of a contrast medium enhances the accuracy of an abdominal CT scan. CT scans are also used to improve the accuracy of inserting a fine needle for biopsy. Be sure to assess the patient for a history of allergic reaction to dyes and for kidney function. Dyes are excreted by the kidneys.

NUCLEAR IMAGING PROCEDURES. Nuclear medicine imaging involves camera imaging of organs or tissues containing radioactive media. Radioactive compounds are given intravenously or by mouth. These studies are highly sensitive. They can detect sites of abnormal cell growth months before changes are seen on an x-ray.

Positron emission tomography (PET) scanning provides information about cellular function. Patients are given biochemical compounds. Images are made of the tissue through gamma-camera tomography. PET scans have been useful in brain imaging as well as the detection of the spread of cancers of the lung, ovaries, colon, rectum, and breast.

ULTRASOUND PROCEDURES. Ultrasonography helps detect tumors of the pelvis and breast. Ultrasound also may be used to distinguish between benign and malignant breast tumors.

MAGNETIC RESONANCE IMAGING. Magnetic resonance imaging (MRI) is valuable in the detection, localization, and staging of malignant tumors in the central nervous system, spine, head, breast, and musculoskeletal system.

ENDOSCOPIC PROCEDURES. An endoscopic examination allows the direct visualization of a body cavity or opening. Endoscopy enables the surgeon to biopsy tissue. It is used to detect lesions of the throat, esophagus, stomach, colon, and lungs.

LABORATORY TESTS. For normal values for the following laboratory tests, see Appendix B. Blood, serum, and urine tests are important in establishing baseline values and general health status. An elevated WBC count is expected if the patient has evidence of infection; however, an increase in WBCs without infection raises suspicion of leukemia. Fifty percent of patients with liver cancer have increased levels of bilirubin, alkaline phosphatase, and glutamic-oxaloacetic transaminase.

Bone marrow aspiration is done to learn the number, size, and shape of RBCs, WBCs, and platelets. It is a major tool for diagnosis of leukemia. (See Chapter 27 for a description of this test and related nursing care.) Tumor markers, also called biochemical markers, are proteins, antigens, genes, hormones, and enzymes produced and secreted by tumor cells. Tumor markers help confirm a diagnosis of cancer, detect cancer origin, monitor the effect of cancer therapy, and determine cancer remission. Some examples of tumor markers are shown in Table 11.3.

CYTOLOGICAL STUDY. Cytology is the study of the formation, structure, and function of cells. Cytological diagnosis of cancer is obtained mainly through smears of cells shed from a mucous membrane (e.g., cervical, anal, oral). Test results

Table 11.3
Tumor Markers and Associated Cancers

Tumor Marker	Associated Cancer
Alpha-fetoprotein (AFP)	Hepatocellular cancer
Cancer antigen (CA) 15-3	Breast cancer (useful in monitoring patient response to therapy for metastatic breast cancer)
CA 125	Ovarian, cervical, liver, and pancreatic cancers
CA 19-9	Colorectal, pancreatic, and hepatobiliary cancers (used to aid diagnosis and evaluation)
Carcinoembryonic antigen (CEA)	Colon and rectal cancers
Prostatic acid phosphatase (PAP)	Prostate cancer
Prostate-specific antigen (PSA)	Prostate cancer

Table 11.4
Tumor-Node-Metastasis System for Cancer Staging

Primary Tumor (T)	
TX	Primary tumor cannot be evaluated
T0	No evidence of primary tumor
Tis	Carcinoma in situ (early cancer that has not spread to neighboring tissue)
T1, T2, T3, T4	Size and/or extent of the primary tumor

Regional Lymph Nodes (N)	
NX	Regional lymph nodes cannot be evaluated
N0	No regional lymph node involvement
N1, N2, N3	Involvement of regional lymph nodes (number and location of lymph nodes)

Distant Metastasis (M)	
M0	No distant metastasis
M1	Distant metastasis

Source: Data from American Joint Committee on Cancer. (2017.) Cancer staging system. Retrieved from https://cancerstaging.org/references-tools/Pages/What-is-Cancer-Staging.aspx

are based on the degree of cell abnormality. Slight cellular changes are considered normal, with a possible link to abnormal cells seen in infection. Significant cellular changes reflect a higher probability of precancerous or cancerous activity.

Staging and Grading

Tumor staging helps to describe the extent of cancer. This provides valuable information for the development of a treatment plan. The most common system used for staging is the tumor-node-metastasis (TNM) system, recommended by the American Joint Committee on Cancer (2017). This staging system classifies solid tumors by size and degree of spread (Table 11.4). For example, a breast cancer staged as T3 N2 M0 is a large breast cancer that has spread to regional lymph nodes, with no distant metastasis.

The TNM ratings correspond with one of five stages. However, ratings may differ based on the type of cancer. In this classification system, stages range from stage 0 (tumor in situ, no invasion of other tissues) to stage IV (distant metastasis to other sites). In general, a lower stage number means the cancer is less advanced and offers a better outcome. A higher number means a more serious situation exists, but treatment is possible. A rating system has also been established to define the cell types of tumors. Tumors are classified according to the percentage of cells that are differentiated (mature). If the tissue of a neoplastic tumor closely resembles normal tissue, it is called *well differentiated*. A *poorly differentiated* tumor is a malignant neoplasm that contains some normal cells, but most of the cells are abnormal. The better defined or differentiated the tumor, the

easier it is to treat. For more information on staging systems, visit www.cancerstaging.org.

Treatment for Cancer

There are three main types of treatment for cancer: surgery, radiation therapy, and chemotherapy. To find out more about cancer treatment options, visit the ACS web site at www.cancer.org.

SURGERY. Surgery can be curative when it is possible to remove the entire tumor. Skin cancers and well-defined tumors without metastasis can be removed without any additional intervention. For some tumors, as much of the tumor is removed as possible (debulking). Follow-up chemotherapy or radiation is used to treat the remaining tumor cells.

Prophylactic surgery is used to remove moles or lesions that have the potential to become malignant. Colon polyps are often removed to prevent malignancies from developing, especially if the polyps are considered premalignant. An extreme example of prophylactic surgery is a woman who elects to have a mastectomy (surgical removal of the breast) because of a high incidence of breast cancer in her family or positive genetic testing.

Surgery also may be done for **palliation** (symptom control). Surgical removal of tissue to reduce the size of the tumor mass is helpful, especially if the tumor is compressing nerves or blocking the passage of body fluids. The goals of palliative surgery are to increase comfort and quality of life.

Reconstructive surgery can be done for cosmetic enhancement or for return of function of a body part. Facial reconstruction is important for a patient's self-image after removal of head or neck tumors. Women can elect to have breast reconstruction after mastectomy.

Nurses should encourage patients to express their fears. Patients with a limited understanding of cancer may fear that tissues will not heal postoperatively. Provide information about wound care, including dressing changes and drainage tubes, to increase the patient's understanding and sense of control. Visual aids concerning tumor site and surgical procedures are valuable teaching tools. Include family members or caretakers in teaching when possible.

Patients who are undernourished are poor surgical candidates. They require intervention such as enteral or parenteral nutrition before and after surgery. Patients with cancer also are at increased risk for postoperative deep venous thrombosis (DVT). Preoperative teaching includes the importance of leg movement, early ambulation, wearing antiembolism stockings, and recognizing symptoms of DVT, such as calf redness, warmth, or pain.

RADIATION. Radiation may be used as a curative treatment if the cancer is localized. It can also be used in cancer control and palliation. Radiation destroys cancer cells by affecting cell structure and the cell environment. The decision to use radiation is commonly based on cancer site and size. Treatments use special equipment to send radiation to break up the cancer cells locally, causing little systemic effect; however, side effects can occur in the area being treated because of damage to normal cells. Radiation can be delivered in three ways: external radiation, internal radiation (brachytherapy), or systemic radiation (ACS, 2017a).

Radiation can be used before surgery to decrease the size of a large tumor. This makes surgical intervention more effective and less dangerous. It can also be used after surgery as adjuvant treatment. Palliative radiation is used to reduce the size of a large cancerous lesion and consequently reduce pressure and pain. Radioisotopes can be inserted into or near cancerous tissue (brachytherapy) during or after surgery to help destroy cancerous cells without removing the organ. Less skin damage occurs with brachytherapy.

Nursing Care of the Patient Receiving Radiation Treatment. Symptoms of tissue reaction to radiation can be expected about 10 to 14 days after treatment starts. Symptoms can continue for up to 2 to 4 weeks after treatment ends. Typical reactions and appropriate nursing interventions include the following:

• *Fatigue:* Encourage the patient to nap often and prioritize activities. Reassure the patient that the feeling will go away after the treatments are completed.

• *Nausea, vomiting, and anorexia:* Encourage the patient to take prescribed medication for nausea and vomiting. **Anorexia** can be eased by providing small amounts of high-carbohydrate, high-protein foods and avoiding foods high in fiber.

• *Mucositis* (inflammation of mucous membranes, especially of the mouth and throat): Urge the patient to avoid irritants such as smoking, alcohol, acidic food or drinks, extremely hot or cold foods and drinks, and commercial mouthwash. Advise the patient to perform mouth care before meals and every 3 to 4 hours. A neutral mouthwash can be made by using 1 ounce of diphenhydramine hydrochloride (Benadryl) elixir diluted in 1 quart of water or normal saline solution. Agents that coat the mouth, such as calcium carbonate (Maalox), are sometimes used. Lidocaine hydrochloride 2% viscous has an anesthetic effect on the mouth and throat.

• *Xerostomia* (dry mouth): Encourage frequent mouth care. Saliva substitute is available over the counter. It is helpful, especially at night when patients describe a choking sensation from extreme dryness.

• *Skin reactions:* These can vary from mild redness to moist **desquamation** (peeling skin) similar to a second-degree burn. Skin surfaces that are warm and moist, such as the groin, perineum, and axillae, are especially vulnerable. Prophylactic skin care includes keeping skin dry; keeping it free from irritants, such as powder, lotions, deodorants, and restrictive clothing; and protecting it from exposure to direct sunlight. Irradiated skin can be fragile during treatment. It is important to wash these areas gently with mild soap and water, rinse well, and pat dry. The skin may have markings or tattoos to delineate the treatment field. Take care not to wash off the markings.

• *Bone marrow depression:* Low blood cell counts occur with both radiation and chemotherapy. This is because they can attack all rapidly dividing cells, not just cancer cells. Weekly blood cell counts are done to detect low levels of WBCs, RBCs, and platelets. Transfusions of whole blood, platelets, or other blood components may be needed. See Table 11.5 for medications that can be used to stimulate production of blood cells.

Safety Considerations. Radiation may be administered externally or internally. External radiation is given by a trained medical specialist in a designated area of a hospital or clinic. Patients receiving external radiation therapy do not emit radioactive material. Therefore, they do not require any safety precautions before or after treatment.

• WORD • BUILDING •

anorexia: an—not + orexis—appetite
mucositis: muco—mucous (membrane) + itis—inflammation
xerostomia: xero—dry + stoma—mouth
desquamation: de—down, from + squamation—epidermis

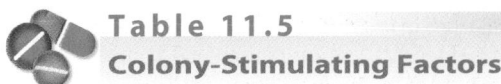

Table 11.5
Colony-Stimulating Factors

Medication Class/Action

Granulocyte–Colony-Stimulating Factor (G-CSF)
Stimulates proliferation of stem cells into granulocytes (neutrophils).

Examples	Nursing Implications
filgrastim (Neupogen) pegfilgrastim (Neulasta)	Monitor complete blood count (CBC). Teach subcutaneous administration if drug will be given at home.

Granulocyte Macrophage–Colony-Stimulating Factor (GM-CSF)
Stimulates proliferation of stem cells into neutrophils, monocytes, macrophages, and eosinophils.

Examples	Nursing Implications
sargramostim (Leukine)	Monitor vital signs and respiratory status during intravenous infusion. Monitor CBC. Teach subcutaneous administration if drug will be given at home.

Erythropoietin
Stimulates proliferation of stem cells into red blood cells.

Examples	Nursing Implications
epoetin alfa (Epogen, Procrit) darbepoetin alfa (Aranesp)	Black box warning for heart disease risk. Monitor blood pressure and hematocrit. Teach subcutaneous administration if drug will be given at home. Darbepoetin alfa (Aranesp) is long acting.

Interleukin-11
Stimulates production of platelets.

Examples	Nursing Implications
oprelvekin (Neumega)	Watch for fluid retention. Monitor CBC and platelet count. Teach subcutaneous administration if drug will be given at home.

Note: Because these drugs are proteins, they all require refrigeration, and you cannot shake them. Many thousands of dollars have been lost because a drug was not returned to the refrigerator when it was not used. Be sure to check package instructions.

Internal radiation is administered to patients admitted to a health care facility. Safety guidelines must be followed when caring for a patient with internal radioactive materials that have been implanted into tissue or body cavities or administered orally or intravenously, because the patient will be radioactive. Nursing responsibilities include knowledge about the following:

• Radiation source being used
• Method of administration
• Start of treatment
• Length of treatment
• Prescribed nursing precautions

Personnel involved with radiation therapy must follow three limitations to protect themselves: time, distance, and shielding. These three factors depend on the type of radiation used. *Time* involves the time spent administering care. *Distance* involves the amount of space between the radioisotope and the nurse. *Shielding* involves the use of a barrier such as a lead apron.

You must work efficiently when caring for patients who are receiving radioisotopes that are releasing gamma rays. Your exposure to radiation is proportionate to the time spent and the distance from the radiation source. For example, you will receive less exposure standing at the foot of the bed of a patient with radioisotopes inserted into the head than if you stand at the head of the bed (Fig. 11.11). Principles of time and distance are used to protect the nurse, visitors, and other personnel.

It is important to teach the patient and family members the reason nursing care focuses on providing only essential care. Speedy nursing encounters and visitor restrictions are better accepted and less likely to promote feelings of isolation when patients and family understand the reasons behind them.

Drainage from the site of a radioactive colloid injection is considered radioactive. The HCP must be informed

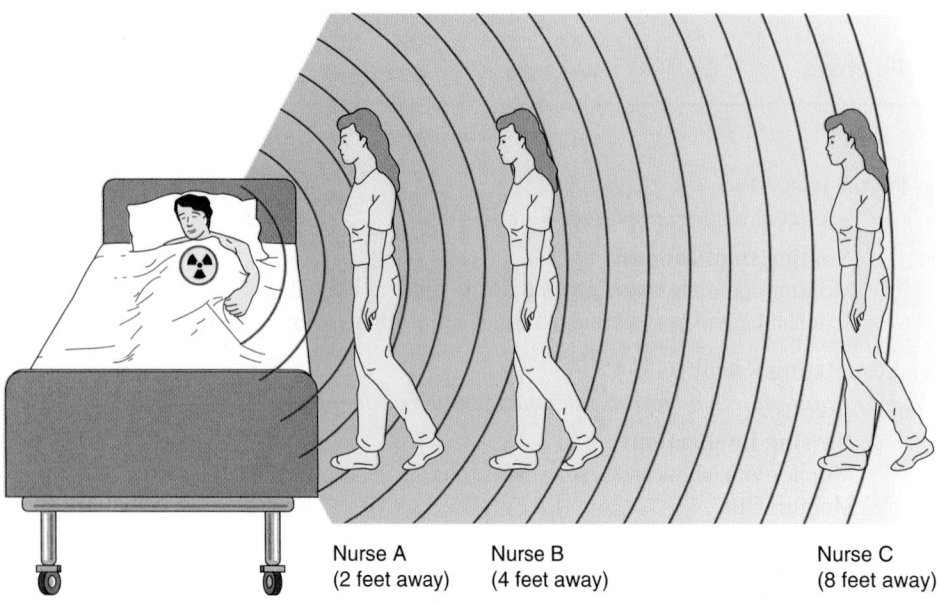

Nurse A
(2 feet away)

Nurse B
(4 feet away)

Nurse C
(8 feet away)

FIGURE 11.11 Radiation distancing. Nurse B receives less radiation than Nurse A, and Nurse C receives less radiation than Nurse B.

immediately if it occurs. Dressings contaminated with radioactive seepage must be removed with long-handled forceps. Radioactive materials must never be touched with unprotected hands; shielding is required to prevent exposure to radiation. Contamination from radioisotope applicators or interstitial implants cannot occur when the capsule it is contained in is intact; contamination occurs when the capsule is broken.

> **BE SAFE!**
> **BE VIGILANT!** Remember to use the principles of time, distance, and shielding to protect yourself from radiation exposure.

CHEMOTHERAPY. Chemotherapy is chemical therapy that uses **cytotoxic** drugs to treat cancer. Cytotoxic drugs can be used for cure, control, or palliation of cancerous tumors. They are classified according to how they affect cell activity. Examples of drugs are listed in Tables 11.6 and 11.7.

The effects of chemotherapy are systemic unless used topically for skin lesions. Chemotherapy is used preoperatively to shrink tumors and postoperatively to treat residual tumors. Tumor type and genetics influence the effectiveness of chemotherapy. Age is also a consideration; treatment should be based on physiological age rather than chronological age. That is, just because a patient might be 70 years old does not mean his body is the same as that of other 70-year-old patients.

Combination Chemotherapy. In this type of therapy, two or more antineoplastic agents are used together. This can expose a larger number of cells at different points in the cell cycle to chemotherapy. Combining drugs also allows for smaller doses of each drug. This decreases the side effects of individual drugs and decreases the possibility of the tumor becoming resistant to the therapy.

For drugs to be combined this way, several criteria must be met. Each drug must be effective when used alone to treat the cancer. Each must have a different toxicity that would limit its use. For example, if three drugs that are all toxic to the heart (cardiotoxic) are given, the patient is more likely to develop cardiotoxicity. Patients are still monitored for toxic effects from the treatment as well as improvement in their status.

Routes of Administration. Chemotherapy can be given by oral, intramuscular, intravenous (IV), or topical route. The dosage is determined by the size of the patient and the toxicities of the drug. IV administration requires specialized training and knowledge of antineoplastic drugs.

Vesicant drugs are given only by the IV route into a large vein. These drugs cause blistering of tissue that eventually leads to necrosis if they infiltrate (leak out of the blood vessel and into soft tissue; Fig. 11.12). Skin grafts may be needed if tissue damage is extensive.

Oral Chemotherapy Agents. The number of oral chemotherapy agents has increased in the past several years. Be aware that oral agents can be just as potent as chemotherapy administered via the IV route. Nursing considerations for oral chemotherapy include safe storage and handling as well as side effects to assess for. Some oral agents must be given

• WORD • BUILDING •
chemotherapy: chemo—chemistry + therapy—treatment
cytotoxic: cyto—cell + toxic—poison
vesicant: vesicate—to blister

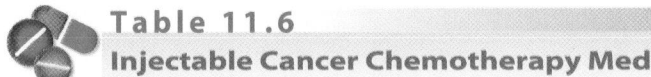

Table 11.6
Injectable Cancer Chemotherapy Medications

Medication Class/Action

Antitumor Antibiotics
Damage cells' deoxyribonucleic acid (DNA) and the ability to make DNA and ribonucleic acid (RNA).

Examples	Nursing Implications
doxorubicin (Adriamycin, Doxil)	Drug is a vesicant and should be given through a running intravenous (IV) or a central line if it is a continuous infusion. It turns urine red.
	Doxil is less irritating than Adriamycin.
	Monitor cardiac status.
	Lifetime dose is 550 mg/m².

Antimetabolites
Resemble normal metabolites needed for cell function. Once they gain entry into the cell, cell division becomes impaired.

Examples	Nursing Implications
cytarabine (Cytosar-U, Ara-C)	Check complete blood count (CBC) before each dose.
	Review the signs of infection or bleeding.
	Instruct patient to call primary health care provider (HCP) for any temperature increases greater than 100.0°F (37.8°C).
fluorouracil (5FU)	Check CBC before the dose. Nadir occurs in 10 to 14 days.
	Instruct about mouth care.
gemcitabine (Gemzar)	Check CBC before each dose.
	Premedicate with antiemetics.
	Instruct patient to report flu-like symptoms to primary HCP.

Alkylating Agents
Cause the DNA strands to bind together and prevent the cell from dividing.

Examples	Nursing Implications
cisplatin (Platinol)	Monitor neurologic status and kidney function studies.
	Premedicate with antiemetics.
	Monitor for signs of anaphylaxis.
	Nadir occurs in 2 to 3 weeks; check CBC before each dose.
	Ensure adequate hydration to prevent kidney failure.
cyclophosphamide (Cytoxan)	Check CBC before each dose.
	Monitor blood urea nitrogen and creatinine levels.
	Ensure adequate hydration to prevent kidney failure.
	Oral form should be taken early in the morning to keep drug from building up in the bladder at night.
ifosfamide (Ifex)	Monitor urine for blood.
	Given with Mesna (Mesnex) to prevent hemorrhagic cystitis.
	Ensure adequate hydration before and after each dose.
	Premedicate with antiemetics.
	Monitor CBC.

Antimitotic Agents
Come from plant sources. Prevent mitosis from occurring in the cell and then cells cannot divide.

Examples	Nursing Implications
docetaxel (Taxotere)	Patient must take dexamethasone starting 1 day before scheduled chemotherapy to prevent hypersensitivity.
	Monitor CBC; nadir occurs on day 7.
	Monitor weight.

Continued

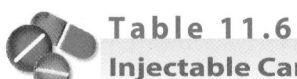

Table 11.6
Injectable Cancer Chemotherapy Medications—cont'd

Medication Class/Action

	Assess skin for changes.
	Watch for changes in neurologic status from baseline.
paclitaxel, nanoparticle albumin-bound (Abraxane)	Watch for signs of hypersensitivity.
	Monitor CBC and platelet counts.
	Watch for changes in neurologic status from baseline.
	Teach mouth care.
	Monitor vital signs for changes.
vincristine (Oncovin)	Drug is a vesicant and should be given through a running IV.
	Assess for neuropathies and changes in neurologic status from baseline.
	Monitor CBC and platelets.
vinorelbine (Navelbine)	Drug is a vesicant. When given through a running IV, use the port closest to the IV bag rather than the patient.
	Check CBC before each dose; nadir occurs in 7 to 10 days.
	Teach signs of infection and bleeding.
	Monitor neurologic status and changes from baseline.
	Teach mouth care.

Topoisomerase Inhibitors
Inhibit enzyme topoisomerase to interfere with DNA synthesis.

Examples	**Nursing Implications**
irinotecan (Camptosar)	Teach measures to control diarrhea and patient to contact primary HCP if it occurs.
	Dose of loperamide may be higher than normal; verify with HCP.
	Check CBC before each dose.
topotecan hydrochloride (Hycamtin)	Monitor CBC.
	Premedicate for nausea.

Hormones
Synthetic analog of luteinizing hormone-releasing hormone; causes decrease in testosterone levels.

Examples	**Nursing Implications**
leuprolide (Lupron)	Monitor prostate-specific antigen results.

Angiogenesis Inhibitors
Block formation of new blood vessels to slow growth and spread of cancer.

Examples	**Nursing Implications**
bevacizumab (Avastin)	Assess for pregnancy. Avoid administration after surgery.

Monoclonal Antibodies
Bind to receptor sites on cancer cells to inhibit proliferation.

Examples	**Nursing Implications**
alemtuzumab (Campath)	Watch for signs of allergic reaction.
trastuzumab (Herceptin)	
gemtuzumab (Mylotarg)	
cetuximab (Erbitux)	
ipilimumab (Yervoy)	

Table 11.7
Oral Cancer Chemotherapy Medications

Medication Class/Action

Tyrosine Kinase Inhibitor
Targets abnormal proteins on surfaces of some cancer cells to block the signals for cells to replicate.

Examples	Nursing Implications
imatinib mesylate (Gleevec) erlotinib (Tarceva)	Supportive care for nausea, diarrhea, and tumor lysis syndrome. Monitor lab studies for decrease in white blood cells and platelet counts. Tarceva: Should be taken on an empty stomach to prevent raising the level of the drug in the body.

Immunomodulating Agent
Affects immune system function; angiogenesis effect: prevents blood vessels from growing, which prevents tumor from growing.

Examples	Nursing Implications
lenalidomide (Revlimid)	Pregnancy must be avoided due to the risk for serious birth defects. Monitor labs and electrolytes.

Alkylating Agent
Interferes with the ability of the cells to replicate.

Examples	Nursing Implications
temozolomide (Temodar)	Monitor labs for white blood cell and platelet counts routinely. Supportive care for nausea and diarrhea.

Antimetabolite
Resembles normal metabolites needed for cell function. Once they gain entry into the cell, cell division becomes impaired. Used in metastatic breast, colon, or rectal cancer.

Examples	Nursing Implications
capecitabine (Xeloda)	Monitor labs for red blood cell, white blood cell, and platelet counts. Supportive care for diarrhea, nausea, and vomiting.

Hormones

Examples	Nursing Implications
Antagonizes effects of androgen: exemestane (Casodex)	Monitor prostate-specific antigen and liver function tests.
Synthetic analog of luteinizing hormone-releasing hormone, causes decrease in testosterone levels: leuprolide (Lupron)	Monitor prostate-specific antigen results.
Competes with estrogen for binding sites in breast and other tissues to reduce breast cancer recurrence: tamoxifen (Nolvadex)	Anticoagulants increase prothrombin time. Instruct patient not to take antacids within 2 hours of tamoxifen.
Reduces amount of estrogen produced to reduce breast cancer recurrence: anastrozole (Arimidex)	Should only be taken by postmenopausal women. Recommend regular bone density studies.

Miscellaneous Agent
Works by interfering with enzyme systems or metabolic pathways in the cells.

Example	Nursing Implications
hydroxyurea (Hydrea)	Monitor white blood cell count. Monitor metabolic panel for signs of tumor lysis syndrome. Monitor neurologic status and changes from baseline.

Note: Cyclophosphamide (Cytoxan) can also be administered by the oral route.

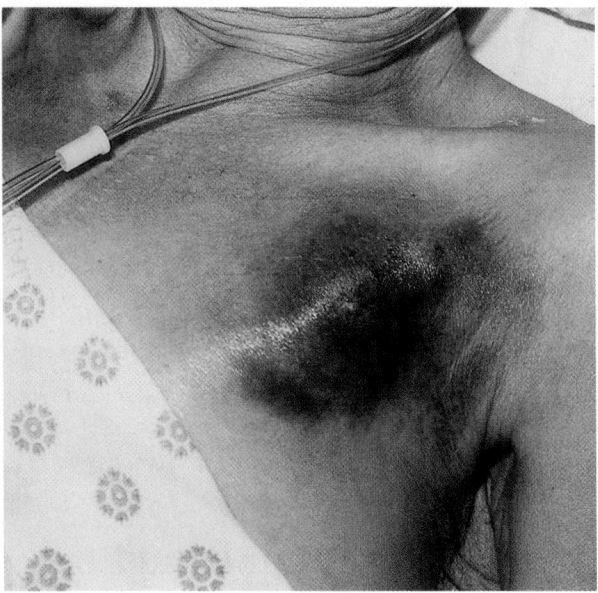

FIGURE 11.12 Necrosis of skin tissue resulting from administration of a vesicant chemotherapy drug.

concurrently with another treatment such as radiation, so timing is important. See Table 11.7 for sample oral chemotherapy agents.

> **BE SAFE!**
> **BE VIGILANT!** Oral chemotherapy pills should not be stored with other oral medications. They should never be crushed or broken. The nurse administering the pills should wear chemotherapy safety gloves.

Side Effects. Toxicities in patients receiving chemotherapy vary with the medications given; however, some general side effects are common to chemotherapeutic drugs because they affect all rapidly growing cells. Fast-growing epithelial cells, such as those of the hair, blood, skin, and GI tract, are usually the most affected by both chemotherapy and radiation.

Hematologic System. Chemotherapy is toxic to bone marrow, which is where blood cells are produced. The number of blood cells (especially WBCs) drops after approximately 7 to 14 days of chemotherapy, depending on the drug. This period when the cell counts are lowest is called the **nadir.** This is when patients are most at risk for complications. Patients may develop low WBC counts (**leukopenia**), increasing their susceptibility to infection and sepsis. Sometimes this is called **neutropenia** because neutrophils are the most plentiful white cells. A reduction in platelets (**thrombocytopenia**) increases the risk of bruising and bleeding. It can require platelet transfusions. Increased risk of **anemia** occurs with the reduction of RBCs and may require blood transfusions. See Table 11.5 for medications that can be used to stimulate production of these cells.

Gastrointestinal System. Because the lining of the GI tract is made up of rapidly dividing cells, it is susceptible to the toxicity of chemotherapy drugs. Patients often experience nausea, vomiting, and diarrhea. **Stomatitis** (inflammation of the mouth) is a common complaint and is discussed under side effects of radiation. These side effects can be controlled with medication.

Hair. Alopecia, or hair loss, is common with many, but not all, chemotherapeutic drugs. This is a temporary condition. Growth of new hair usually starts when the chemotherapeutic medication is stopped. Alopecia involves the entire body, including eyebrows, eyelashes, and axillary and pubic hair. Hair that regrows may be a different color or texture than the original hair. It is not uncommon for individuals who originally had straight hair to regrow curly hair.

Reproductive System. The effects of chemotherapy or radiation can cause temporary or permanent changes in the reproductive system. Chemotherapy can damage sperm and ova.

> **BE SAFE!**
> Some web sites promote icing the scalp to cause vasoconstriction and reduce the amount of chemotherapy agent affecting hair loss. Teach patients that this practice *may not be safe.* It may leave pockets of cancer cells in the brain and scalp that are not reached by the chemotherapy.

Issues concerning fertility should be discussed with the patient before treatment. Measures such as freezing ova and using a sperm bank can provide options for the patient and his or her partner. Patients should also talk to their HCPs before engaging in intercourse during chemotherapy and use protection against pregnancy.

Neurologic System. Drugs may affect the neurologic system. An adverse reaction to vincristine (Oncovin) is neurotoxicity. This can result in tingling or numbness in the extremities. In severe cases, it can cause foot drop from muscle weakness.

Other Systems. Less common complications include renal toxicities, such as pain and burning on urination, and hematuria. Doxorubicin (Adriamycin) has been associated with permanent heart damage. Bleomycin (Blenoxane) can cause pulmonary fibrosis.

Severe toxic side effects can be controlled by carefully limiting the amount of each medication given and constantly monitoring the patient for complications.

• WORD • BUILDING •
leukopenia: leuko—white cells + penia—lack
neutropenia: neutron—neutrophils + penia—lack
thrombocytopenia: thrombo—clot + cyte—cell + penia—lack
anemia: an—not + emia—blood
stomatitis: stoma—mouth + itis—inflammation

LEARNING TIP

When assessing patients with possible side effects of chemotherapy and radiation, use the mnemonic "BITES":

B—Bleeding suggests low platelet count.
I—Infection suggests low white blood cell count and a risk for infection.
T—Tiredness suggests anemia.
E—Emesis places the patient at risk for altered nutrition and fluid and electrolyte imbalance.
S—Skin changes may be evidence of radiation reaction or skin breakdown.

CYTOPROTECTIVE AGENTS. Cytoprotective agents protect healthy cells from some side effects of certain chemotherapeutic drugs. For example, dexrazoxane (Zinecard) helps prevent cardiac damage associated with doxorubicin. Amifostine (Ethyol) helps protect the kidneys from platinum-based chemotherapy. It also protects normal cells in parts of the body against damage from radiation treatments. Mesna (Mesnex) protects the bladder against chemotherapy drugs such as cyclophosphamide (Cytoxan).

New Treatments Being Researched

New therapies for cancer are constantly being researched. For example, hyperthermia has been used with radiation and chemotherapy. It has been beneficial in some types of cancer. However, it is typically used only in investigational studies.

Biological response modifiers (such as interferons) are drugs used to stimulate the immune system. These drugs are used commonly for specific types of cancer. They have produced some beneficial results. They are also being used in many investigational studies. Visit www.cancer.gov for information on current clinical trials.

NURSING PROCESS FOR THE PATIENT WITH CANCER

Data Collection

Thorough assessment of the patient with cancer will help the health care team build a plan of care relevant to the patient's needs.

The nurse should monitor laboratory studies. Potential for bleeding exists when the platelet count is $50,000/mm^3$ or less; risk for spontaneous bleeding occurs when the count is less than $20,000/mm^3$. Monitor the WBC count for risk of infection and the RBC count for anemia.

Monitor the patient's weight. Note reports of nausea, changes in taste, vomiting, and diarrhea related to either the disease or treatment. Monitor the oral mucosa for lesions or inflammation. Also watch for signs of dehydration. "Nutrition Notes: Assessing the Need for Nutritional Support" presents criteria for determining whether a patient needs nutritional support.

Psychosocial issues related to cancer are as varied as the persons afflicted with the disease. Help the patient explore perceptions about quality of life. Culture and age affect cancer perceptions. Assess the patient's ability to cope. Discuss coping strategies that have been effective in the past. Determine what information the patient has received and understands about his or her disease and prognosis.

Assess the roles of the patient and caregiver in the family. Be aware of whether the caregiver can be at home or whether he or she must work outside the home while also caring for the patient. Isolation can be either self-imposed or imposed by friends and family as issues surrounding terminal illness are confronted. It can be very distressing to see a loved one decline from cancer; often people say they are "afraid of saying or doing the wrong thing" so they "just stay away." Listen for cues from patients expressing self-blame, anger, or depression. It is important to recognize signs of depression and suicidal tendencies.

Nutrition Notes

Assessing the Need for Nutritional Support. The National Cancer Institute's Physician Data Query recommends that individuals who have any of the following findings may benefit from nutrition support. The dietitian or health care provider should be consulted about the need for nutritional support for:

• Weight less than 80% of ideal body weight or weight loss of more than 10% of usual body weight
• Intolerance of oral/enteral feedings for more than 5 days
• Malabsorption of nutrients due to disease, short bowel syndrome, or anticancer therapy
• Fistulas or draining abscesses
• Moderate or high nutritional risk status as determined by screening or an assessment tool

Source: National Cancer Institute. (2017). Nutrition in cancer care (PDQ)—Health professional version. Retrieved from www.cancer.gov/about-cancer/treatment/side-effects/appetite-loss/nutrition-hp-pdq

---

Assess for fatigue and anxiety in a patient being treated for cancer. A decline in sexual desire is not uncommon during cancer treatment. Assess for anxiety about sexual intercourse, including fears concerning contracting cancer from the patient and fears that sexual intercourse will make the cancer worse.

Assess the patient's feelings about any actual or perceived change in appearance due to surgery, radiation, or chemotherapy.

Nursing Diagnoses, Planning, and Implementation

See the "Nursing Care Plan for the Patient With Cancer" for top nursing care priorities. Additional nursing diagnoses are presented next. Remember to assess each patient before assuming a nursing diagnosis applies to that patient.

Nursing Care Plan for the Patient With Cancer

Nursing Diagnosis: *Ineffective Coping* related to the diagnosis and treatment of cancer as evidenced by behaviors such as denial, isolation, anxiety, and depression
Expected Outcomes: The patient will cope effectively as evidenced by identifying stressors related to illness and treatment; communicating needs, concerns, and fears; and use of appropriate resources to support coping.
Evaluation of Outcomes: Is the patient able to identify stressors and communicate concerns? Does the patient effectively draw on past coping mechanism? Does the patient have and appropriately use support systems?

Intervention	Rationale	Evaluation
Assess effective coping mechanisms used in the past and currently available to the patient.	*Coping mechanisms that worked in the past may be helpful again. The nurse can support appropriate choices.*	Is patient able to identify and draw on past coping mechanisms?
Use active listening skills to encourage patient to express feelings and fears.	*Patient must identify fears to be able to cope effectively with them.*	Does patient identify fears and concerns?
Assess the meaning of quality of life to patient.	*Once identified, the nurse can assist patient to achieve quality-of-life goals.*	Is patient able to identify the meaning of quality of life? Are there ways the nurse can assist the patient to reach quality-of-life goals?
Assess for suicide risks.	*A patient who feels hopeless may be at risk for suicide.*	Is patient at risk? Are suicide precautions necessary?
Explore outlets that promote feelings of personal achievement.	*Personal achievement promotes self-esteem.*	Does patient have creative outlets that promote feelings of achievement? Can the nurse assist in implementing these activities?
Consider the use of humor.	*Humor can be both distracting and therapeutic.*	Does patient use humor? Does it provide temporary distraction from concerns?

Nursing Diagnosis: *Acute Pain* or *Chronic Pain* related to tissue injury from disease process and treatment
Expected Outcomes: Pain will be prevented, and the patient will be comfortable at all times as evidenced by the patient stating pain is at an acceptable level on pain scale.
Evaluation of Outcomes: Does the patient state pain is controlled?

Intervention	Rationale	Evaluation
Assess the patient's pain based on *WHAT'S UP?* mnemonic.	*Assessment provides direction for the treatment plan.*	Is assessment complete and used to guide treatment?
Ask patient to rate pain on a scale from 0 to 10 (0 = absence of pain; 10 = worst pain).	*A pain rating should guide treatment and evaluate effectiveness of treatment.*	Does patient use pain assessment scale effectively? Is patient in pain?
Administer analgesics as ordered, around the clock.	*Using an around-the-clock schedule prevents pain from becoming severe.*	Is patient's pain kept under control at all times?
Check pain relief within 1 hour of administration of medication and then every 2 to 4 hours.	*Alternative short-acting medications may be necessary for breakthrough pain.*	Is breakthrough pain present? Does long-acting analgesic need to be increased to prevent pain?
Educate patient on use of patient-controlled analgesia (PCA).	*PCA allows patient to be in control of own pain relief.*	Does PCA keep patient pain-free and able to participate in desired activities?
Monitor level of sedation and respiratory status if opioid dose is increased.	*Patients who receive long-term opioid therapy develop a tolerance to the depressant effects of opioids.*	Is patient alert with respiratory rate between 12 and 20?

Nursing Care Plan for the Patient With Cancer—cont'd

Intervention	Rationale	Evaluation
Explain the use of nonpharmacological interventions, such as relaxation, once the pain is controlled with medications.	*Nonpharmacological interventions supplement but do not replace analgesics.*	Does patient use nonpharmacological interventions? Do they help?

Nursing Diagnosis: *Risk for Infection* related to diminished immunity and bone marrow suppression as a result of chemotherapy or radiation

Expected Outcomes: The patient will be free and safe from infection as evidenced by being afebrile and stating self-care measures to protect from infection. Signs and symptoms of infection are identified and treated early.

Evaluation of Outcomes: Are signs and symptoms of infection absent? If present, are they reported quickly? Can the patient identify self-care measures for preventing infection?

Intervention	Rationale	Evaluation
Promote good hand washing technique before interaction with patient.	*Appropriate hand hygiene can reduce the transmission of antimicrobial organisms.*	Are you careful with your hand washing? Have you also instructed the patient, family, and nursing assistants about careful hand washing?
Monitor body temperature every 4 hours.	*Elevated body temperature is an early sign of infection.*	Is body temperature within normal limits?
Monitor white blood cell (WBC) count daily.	*For the neutropenic patient, the WBC count will not be elevated. Neutropenia is a risk factor for infection.*	Is the WBC count 5,000 to 10,000/mm^3?
Assess for signs of inflammation or drainage at potential infection sites, such as old aspiration sites, venipuncture sites, oral and rectal mucosae, perineal area, axillae, incisions, pierced earlobes, under breasts, and between toes.	*Intact skin is the first line of defense against invading microorganisms.*	Are there any sites that need special care to maintain skin integrity?
Watch for signs of respiratory infection, such as sore throat, cough, shortness of breath, and sputum production.	*Hospital-acquired pneumonia has high morbidity and mortality rates.*	Are signs of respiratory infection present?
Assess for signs of urinary tract infection (UTI) including burning, pain, urgency, and blood in urine.	*Genitourinary tract is the most common site for hospital-acquired infection.*	Are signs of UTI present?
Teach administration of G-CSF (granulocyte–colony-stimulating factor) and GM-CSF (granulocyte macrophage–colony-stimulating factor) as ordered.	*These medications help the body produce more WBCs. Patient may need to administer it subcutaneously at home.*	Does patient or caregiver demonstrate correct administration? Is WBC count improving?
Limit visitors to only healthy adults.	*Viral infection in an immunosuppressed patient has a high mortality rate.*	Are patient and family aware of visiting restrictions and rationale? Is there a sign on the door reminding visitors?

(nursing care plan continues on page 164)

Nursing Care Plan for the Patient With Cancer—cont'd

Intervention	Rationale	Evaluation
Teach patient to ask health care provider about avoiding unwashed fruits and vegetables (see "Nutrition Notes: Treating Problems Related to Nutrition").	*Unwashed fruits and vegetables can carry pathogens.*	Are patient and family aware of the risks of eating unwashed fruits and vegetables?
Keep fresh flowers and potted plants out of the patient's room.	*Aspergillus is a fungus found in soil and water and can cause pneumonia.*	Is the room free from potential sources of infection?

Evidenced-Based Practice

Clinical Question
What educational measures are effective for cancer pain management?

Evidence
A review of 34 randomized controlled trials and eight systematic reviews revealed that educational interventions targeted at people with cancer can improve their knowledge about cancer pain as well as help them manage pain more effectively (Adam, Bond, & Murchie, 2015). When patients are knowledgeable about the origin of their pain, how to accurately report pain, how medications work, types of interventions, and how health care professionals evaluate the need for pharmacological interventions, patients can be more instrumental in managing effective pain relief.

Implications for Nursing Practice
It is important to focus on several areas when talking to patients about their pain, including how to report pain, pharmacological and nonpharmacological pain management strategies, and reassessment of pain after intervention.

Reference
Adam, R., Bond, C., & Murchie, P. (2015). Educational interventions for cancer pain: A systematic review of systematic reviews with a nested narrative review of randomized control trials. *Patient Education and Counseling, 98*(3), 269–282.

Ineffective Protection related to thrombocytopenia associated with chemotherapy and radiation

EXPECTED OUTCOME: The patient will be free of bleeding as evidenced by stable blood counts and the absence of bruising, petechiae, or frank bleeding.

- Monitor platelet counts. *A platelet count of less than 50,000 indicates potential for bleeding.*
- Teach self-administration of oprelvekin (Neumega) as ordered. *Oprelvekin stimulates production of platelets.*
- Test all urine and stool for occult blood *to detect the presence of blood.*

- Avoid giving intramuscular, subcutaneous, or rectal medications. *Medications given via invasive routes can cause bleeding.*
- Apply pressure for at least 5 minutes to venipuncture or injection sites. *Pressure for a longer time is needed at sites of invasive procedures to stop bleeding.*
- Teach the patient about gentle mouth care including no flossing, a soft toothbrush, and wearing properly fitting dentures *to help prevent trauma and bleeding.*
- Avoid trauma to rectal tissue by avoiding rectal temperatures and enemas. Teach importance of avoiding anal intercourse. *Trauma to rectal tissue can cause bleeding.*
- Instruct the patient not to take any salicylates or nonsteroidal anti-inflammatory drugs *because they can interfere with platelet function and cause bleeding in the GI tract.*
- Observe for bruising, petechiae, bleeding gums, tarry stools, and black or coffee-ground appearing emesis. *These are signs of bleeding.*
- Advise the patient to use an electric razor *to decrease risk for trauma and bleeding.*
- Teach the patient to avoid forcefully blowing his or her nose or inserting objects into the nose *to reduce trauma to nasal mucosa to prevent spontaneous bleeding.*
- Teach the patient to monitor for bleeding with intercourse *because of the risk of trauma to tissues.*

Imbalanced Nutrition: Less Than Body Requirements related to anorexia, nausea, or vomiting associated with disease, pain, and treatment

EXPECTED OUTCOME: The patient will have caloric intake that is adequate to meet body requirements and balanced intake and output, as evidenced by stable weight.

- Monitor food and fluid intake and output every 8 hours. *This will provide objective data for the amount of nutrients and fluids taken in.*
- Weigh the patient daily. *Weight is an objective measurement to determine if intake is adequate enough to maintain weight.*
- Consult a dietitian for dietary supplements. *Dietitians can calculate the calories needed for adequate nutrition and make recommendations for supplements.*

- Consult with the HCP for medications to control nausea, vomiting, and diarrhea. *If these symptoms are controlled, then the patient is better able to eat.*
- Keep the environment free of strong odors, such as disinfectants, perfumes, deodorizers, and body wastes. *Strong odors can induce nausea.*
- Provide room-temperature or cold foods and clear liquids. *These foods have fewer odors and may be more comfortable for the patient to eat.*
- Offer sour foods such as hard candy and lemon. *These can help control nausea.*
- Provide mouth care before meals. *Oral care allows for a better taste in the mouth, and saliva is needed for digestion of food.*
- Provide small, high-calorie meals. *Eating smaller, more frequent meals prevents the patient from feeling full and nauseated.*
- Administer pain medication before meals *to help reduce the impact of pain on appetite.*
- Instruct the patient to avoid fluids with meals *to prevent premature feelings of fullness.*
- Teach the patient to avoid exercise before meals. *If the patient is fatigued, he or she will not have the energy to eat and digest food.*

See "Nutrition Notes: Treating Problems Related to Nutrition" for additional nutrition interventions.

Nutrition Notes
Treating Problems Related to Nutrition
Early Satiety and Anorexia
- Present meals in a calm, comfortable environment, offering assistance as necessary.
- Provide small, frequent (every 2 hours) meals and snacks that are high in protein and calories.
- Arrange for assistance in preparing meals when at home.
- Dispense liquid supplements as recommended by a dietitian.
- Encourage regular exercise, which may promote appetite.

Changes in Taste and Smell
- Provide oral hygiene before meals.
- Cook in glass containers in a microwave oven.
- Use plastic utensils for eating (for metallic taste in mouth).
- Serve food cold or at room temperature.
- Offer lemon-flavored candy and beverages, or gum and mints.
- Provide eggs, fish, poultry, and dairy products instead of beef and pork.
- Promote foods with sauces and seasonings; sweet sauces and marinades may improve the palatability of meats. Offer high-protein vegetarian meals if meats are not tolerated.

Local Oral Effects
- *Ulcerations:* Offer soft, mild foods; cream sauces, gravies, and dressings for lubrication; cold foods (such as noncitrus popsicles) for numbing; and straws for liquids. Avoid hot items, salty or spicy foods, and acidic juices. If

an anesthetic mouthwash is prescribed, the mouth may be numb; caution the patient to chew carefully to avoid biting the lips, tongue, or cheeks.
- *Dry mouth:* Offer frequent sips of water or artificial saliva. Lubricate with gravies, butter, margarine, milk, cream, or bouillon. Sugarless hard candy, chewing gum, or popsicles may stimulate saliva production. Perform oral hygiene at least after each meal and before bedtime.
- *Dysphagia:* Have a speech pathologist evaluate the patient to determine the appropriate diet order, in consultation with the dietitian, and position for eating. Liquids may be modified in viscosity to enable the patient to safely swallow and reduce risk for aspiration.

Nausea and Vomiting
- Administer antiemetics on a regular prophylactic schedule.
- Rinse mouth before and after eating. Offer lemon or mint hard candies.
- Suggest dry crackers. Provide bland foods, avoiding spicy and greasy foods.
- Offer liquids between, instead of with, meals to reduce stomach volume. Offer low-fat meals to improve stomach emptying.
- Remove covers from food containers from the bedside if strong odors disturb the patient's appetite.
- Instruct the patient to chew thoroughly, eat slowly, and rest afterward, either sitting upright or reclining with the head raised for 1 hour after eating.
- Arrange meal schedule to take advantage of times when patient feels better.
- Avoid serving favorite foods when the patient is nauseous to avoid an association between these foods and vomiting.

Diarrhea
- Suggest a low-fiber diet; it should be individualized per patient's tolerance. Provide fluids, which may be tolerated better at room temperature. Limit the consumption of sugar substitutes (sugar alcohols) in beverages, candies, and gums; these may promote diarrhea.
- Limit milk to two cups per day or try a lactose-free diet for temporary lactose intolerance.
- Propose pectin-containing foods (apples, strawberries, citrus fruits) to absorb water in the bowel.
- Ask the health care provider or dietitian about probiotic therapy to repopulate the intestine.
- Consult with a dietitian about special feedings.

Altered Immune Response
- Observe strict procedures for food safety and sanitation to avoid bacterial exposure in foods. Keep foods within safe temperatures (cold: *under* 40°F, hot: *over* 140°F).
- Do not eat foods outside their expiration dates.
- Avoid undercooked and raw meats and eggs.
- Provide individually packaged foods, avoiding leftovers.
- Avoid salad bars and buffets when eating out.
- Wash fruits and vegetables before eating.

Source: National Cancer Institute. (2017). Nutrition in cancer care (PDQ)—Health professional version. Retrieved from www.cancer.gov/about-cancer/treatment/side-effects/appetite-loss/nutrition-hp-pdq

Social Isolation related to changing relationships

EXPECTED OUTCOME: The patient will manage social isolation as evidenced by (1) the ability to identify feelings of isolation and (2) the ability to participate in chosen activities.

- Observe the patient for signs of barriers to social interaction, such as incontinence, lack of transportation, or inadequate money or support system. *Why a patient feels isolated can vary from one person to another, but knowing the reason can help the nurse plan appropriate interventions.*
- Discuss causes of perceived or actual isolation. *How the patient is dealing with the illness will have an impact on how he or she manages the illness.*
- Promote opportunities for the patient to interact socially, such as at meal times or during therapy sessions. *The patient will feel less isolated if given an opportunity to participate in diversional activities.*
- Provide information about support groups, and encourage the patient to contact them. *Support groups can help the patient cope better with stressful events in life.*

Disturbed Body Image related to cancer and its treatment (e.g., surgical procedures such as mastectomy, ostomy, or loss of hair from chemotherapy)

EXPECTED OUTCOME: The patient will be able to accept the changes in body image as evidenced by willingness to participate in care and adjust to changes in lifestyle.

- Allow the patient to discuss feelings of anger or depression, and confirm that these feelings are normal when adjusting to body changes. *A patient may be better able to cope with body changes if he or she can talk about feelings and understand that they are normal.*
- Encourage the patient to select a wig before hair loss *so the patient can find one resembling his or her own hair color and style.*
- Provide education, and urge the patient to care for the ostomy site or surgical wound when ready *to promote independence.*
- Provide information about resources such as Reach to Recovery (http://www.cancer.org/treatment/support-programs-and-services/reach-to-recovery.html and Look Good Feel Better (www.lookgoodfeelbetter.org) support groups. *Support groups provide a forum for patients to share their experiences with others undergoing similar changes.*
- Provide information about community assistance and financial aid for programs or services. *Social workers can help with community resources that can provide equipment or supplies for the patient.*

Additional nursing diagnoses that might be appropriate include *Self-Care Deficit* related to weakness and fatigue, *Ineffective Sexuality Pattern* related to change in body functions, and *Grieving* related to diagnosis and potential disease outcome. Grieving and end-of-life care are covered in depth in Chapter 17.

Caregiver Role Strain related to needs of patient and anticipated outcome

EXPECTED OUTCOME: The caregiver will be prepared to provide care effectively as evidenced by (1) identification of resources available to assist in providing care for the patient and (2) maintenance of the caregiver's physical and emotional health.

- Observe the caregiver's ability to provide care for the patient. *The nurse needs to know if the caregiver will be able to handle the care needs.*
- Observe the quality of the relationship between the patient and caregiver. *The quality of the relationship impacts the care delivered.*
- Actively listen to the caregiver's concerns. *Doing so can assist the nurse in assessing the caregiver's ability to cope and can help in planning care.*
- Teach appropriate caregiving skills as needed. *The caregiver may not be aware of how to bathe a patient or how to provide basic or advanced care.*
- Assist the caregiver to identify available supports. *Assistance can provide a break and decrease the risk of exhaustion and depression in the caregiver.*
- Instruct the caregiver in the resources available in the community. *Support groups can help the caregiver by providing an outlet for sharing concerns and finding support.*
- Consult the multidisciplinary team to provide the services needed at time of discharge. *Preparing the caregiver for discharge needs/care with the proper resources will help the caregiver feel empowered to deliver the care.*
- Watch for signs of depression in the caregiver, and intervene to help coping. *The caregiver can develop a weakened immune system secondary to stress and depression.*
- Arrange for respite for the caregiver or encourage the caregiver to utilize this service. *Respite care can provide a break for the caregiver.*
- Assist the caregiver with ways to decrease stress. *Encouraging caregivers to take time to care for themselves will leave them with the energy they need to continue providing care.*

Evaluation

If the interventions have been effective, the patient will have no unusual bleeding or bruising. The patient and family will be knowledgeable about risk factors for bleeding and about signs of bleeding to report promptly. The patient will be nourished and maintain weight within normal limits. Caregivers will know how to provide care for the patient. They will make use of resources in the community to assist with patient care. The patient will be able to discuss feelings of isolation and seek out activities to participate in. Finally, the patient will adjust to changes in lifestyle and body image.

The patient will be able to openly discuss concerns regarding body changes and be able to maintain control of his or her body. The patient will know about community resources and support groups to assist with needs related to body image.

CRITICAL THINKING

Mrs. Jones is admitted to your unit after a simple mastectomy for breast cancer. The tumor was staged as a T2, N0, M0. A bone scan was negative for metastasis. She is scheduled for four chemotherapy treatments, 3 weeks apart. The medications prescribed are high doses of doxorubicin (Adriamycin) and cyclophosphamide (Cytoxan). A central line is inserted for chemotherapy.

1. What does the staging of Mrs. Jones's tumor mean?
2. What major side effects of her medications should you look for?
3. Why was a central line inserted?
4. What nursing diagnoses are appropriate for Mrs. Jones?

Suggested answers are at the end of the chapter.

SURVIVORSHIP

Millions of people around the world are no longer dying from cancer. Many are either disease-free or continuing treatments to reduce the risk of recurrence or to treat a chronic form of cancer. The need for medical and psychosocial interventions is ongoing as cancer survivors and their caregivers continue to deal with the emotional and physical effects of their disease and treatments. Continued reassessment of the patient's needs and creation of a survivorship plan are essential to maintaining a positive outcome. You can help your patients and families find local survivorship programs for needed assistance and counseling.

HOSPICE CARE OF THE PATIENT WITH CANCER

Hospice care is considered the model for quality compassionate care for patients and families facing a life-limiting illness. Hospice provides expert medical care, pain management, and emotional and spiritual support based on the patient and family's needs and wishes (National Hospice and Palliative Care Organization [NHPCO], 2017). Patients who have a life expectancy of 6 months or less are eligible for hospice care. The hospice approach includes an interdisciplinary team working together to develop a plan of care meeting the patient's individual needs for management of pain and symptoms. Hospice care is offered as an inpatient or outpatient

service. It may also be provided in nursing homes and assisted living facilities (see "Home Health Hints").

Home Health Hints

- The home health care or hospice nurse helps manage cancer pain in the home. Oral, transdermal, or intravenous analgesics are preferred. For moderate to severe pain, doses should be given around the clock with as-needed doses for breakthrough pain. The nurse is in contact with the interdisciplinary team to update plan of care as necessary.
- The nurse should anticipate constipation from opioid administration and treat prophylactically.
- Some patients are fearful of taking prescribed pain medications. Explain the importance of taking the medications as ordered. Explain that it is easier to maintain pain relief than to reverse severe pain.
- Home health care nurses are in key positions for making timely referrals for hospice care. Eligible patients are those who have a life expectancy of 6 months or less and who have a desire for supportive palliative care rather than continued treatments.

Inpatient services are used for symptom control and respite care for the family. Family and pets may be allowed to stay with the patient. Hospice care assists the family in crisis and continues for up to 1 year after the patient dies, with follow-up counseling, listening, nurturing, and referrals.

Outpatient care is given in the home with hospice staff educating family members in the care of the patient. Hospice staff also offers supportive care in pain management, psychosocial issues, bereavement, and symptom control as well as assistance during crisis (NHPCO, 2017). Hospice benefits are provided regardless of the ability to pay. They are covered by Medicare, Medicaid, and other insurances. In the home setting, a patient can maintain normal life patterns with familiar surroundings for as long as possible. See Chapter 17 for more information.

 ## ONCOLOGICAL EMERGENCIES

Superior Vena Cava Syndrome

Superior vena cava syndrome (SVCS) occurs in patients with lung cancer or cancers of the mediastinum when the tumor or enlarged lymph nodes block circulation in the superior vena cava. This results in edema of the head, neck, and arms. Symptoms include shortness of breath, cough, chest pain, facial redness, and swollen neck veins. Radiation therapy can be used to shrink the tumor and allow circulation to resume naturally. Nursing interventions for the patient with SVCS include removing rings and restrictive clothing, avoiding taking blood pressures and venipunctures in the arms, and elevating the head of the bed to decrease feelings of dyspnea.

Spinal Cord Compression

Spinal cord compression occurs when a malignant growth presses on the spinal cord. This is a painful problem and requires pain management while radiation is given to relieve the symptoms. Patients may develop some motor loss when this occurs. A myelogram or bone scan may be used for diagnosis. Nursing care includes providing a safe environment, assisting with activity, and watching for changes in neurologic status as well as changes in the location or intensity of pain. Patients at risk include those with cancers that spread to the bone and spinal cord, such as lung, breast, and prostate cancer.

Hypercalcemia

In hypercalcemia, the serum calcium level exceeds 11 mg/dL. Hypercalcemia can result from the release of calcium into the blood from bone deterioration or from ectopic secretion of parathyroid hormone by a tumor. It is common in patients with bone metastasis, especially metastasis from breast cancer. It can be treated with IV medication and hydration to lower the calcium level. Nursing care includes maintaining safety and monitoring intake and output, pain control, and changes in pulse rate and rhythm.

SUGGESTED ANSWERS TO CRITICAL THINKING

Mrs. Jones

1. Mrs. Jones's tumor is beginning to invade surrounding tissue. There is no lymph node involvement and no metastasis.
2. Doxorubicin (Adriamycin) is commonly associated with red urine. It also poses a risk for cardiac toxicity. Cyclophosphamide (Cytoxan) can cause blood in the urine and a risk for hemorrhagic cystitis. Therefore, the patient should take plenty of fluids and void often (every 2 hours). Both medications can cause nausea, vomiting, and alopecia. Both are vesicants.
3. Because the drugs are vesicants, it is important to inject them into a large vein.
4. Many diagnoses are appropriate, including *Acute Pain* related to surgical incision, *Disturbed Body Image* related to alopecia and loss of a breast, *Imbalanced Nutrition: Less Than Body Requirements* related to nausea and vomiting, *Risk for Injury* related to medication side effects, and *Deficient Knowledge* about cancer treatment and management of side effects. A thorough nursing assessment is needed to determine actual diagnoses.

Review Questions

1. A patient asks, "How do malignant tumors differ from benign tumors?" Which of the following statements by the nurse are correct? **Select all that apply.**
   1. "Malignant tumors invade surrounding cells and tissues."
   2. "Malignant tumors are generally encapsulated."
   3. "Malignant tumors remain localized."
   4. "Cells in malignant tumors stop dividing prematurely."
   5. "Cells in malignant tumors lack contact inhibition."
   6. "Malignant tumors have defective cell communication."

2. A patient has received vinorelbine (Navelbine) on day 1 of treatment. The nadir will occur in about 10 days. For which complication should the nurse be vigilant around day 10?
   1. Infection
   2. Hair loss
   3. Diarrhea
   4. Myalgia

3. A female patient is starting on doxorubicin (Adriamycin). Which of the following nursing interventions will be most helpful as she plans for hair loss?
   1. Obtain a prescription for a hair growth product.
   2. Massage her scalp to increase circulation and delay hair loss.
   3. Teach her to apply ice to her scalp to prevent hair loss.
   4. Help her choose a wig before her hair loss begins.

4. Which of the following nursing actions will best help the patient with cancer to control pain?
   1. Assess the patient's anxiety level.
   2. Assess the patient's understanding of the side effects of pain medication.
   3. Encourage the patient to use nonpharmacological methods for pain.
   4. Teach the use of a relaxation exercise to be used with prescribed analgesics.

5. The nurse notes that a patient undergoing treatment for bone cancer is having trouble walking. For which oncological emergency should the patient be assessed?
   1. Tumor lysis syndrome
   2. Hypercalcemia
   3. Spinal cord compression
   4. Thrombocytopenia

6. A nurse is intervening for a patient receiving radiation therapy with reddened skin over the treated area. How will the nurse know if nursing interventions have been effective?
   1. The patient will be able to describe a proper skin care regimen.
   2. The nurse will keep the skin clean and dry.
   3. The patient's skin will remain intact without breakdown or infection.
   4. The nurse will report the reddened area to the physician.

7. Which of the following patients will benefit from hospice care?
   1. A patient who has liver cancer and is expected to live 4 to 6 weeks
   2. A patient who is having multiple side effects from aggressive chemotherapy
   3. A patient who is trying to make a decision about cancer treatment
   4. A patient with uncontrolled pain related to cancer and radiation treatment

8. A patient is receiving internal radiation therapy for a gynecological malignancy. The patient expresses feelings of isolation in her private room. What intervention would be best on the part of the nurse?
   1. Encourage the patient's significant other to stay overnight.
   2. Move the patient into a semiprivate room so she can have a roommate.
   3. Teach the patient about the safety procedures for internal radiation therapy.
   4. Plan to spend more time with the patient.

Answer rationales available in your online resources.

ANSWERS 1. 1, 5; 6. 2, 1; 3, 4; 4, 5; 3; 6, 3; 7. 1; 8. 3

Key Points

Find the chapter key points in your online resources available through Davis Edge.

Additional Resources

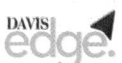 **Use the scratch off code on the inside front cover of your book to access online quizzes that will help you to improve your scores on course exams and prepare for NCLEX-PN®.**

 Study Guide

CHAPTER 12
Nursing Care of Patients Having Surgery

Cindy Leffel, Linda S. Williams

KEY TERMS

adjunct (AD-junkt)
anesthesia (AN-es-THEE-zee-uh)
anesthesiologist (an-es-THEE-zee-uhl-la-just)
aseptic (ah-SEP-tik)
atelectasis (AT-e-LEK-tah-sis)
débridement (da-breed-MAHNT)
dehiscence (dee-HIS-ents)
evisceration (EE-VIS-sir-ay-shun)
hematoma (HEE-muh-TOH-mah)
hypothermia (HY-poh-THUR-mee-ah)
induction (in-DUK-shun)
intraoperative (IN-trah-AW-pruh-tiv)
perioperative (PER-ee-AW-pruh-tiv)
postoperative (post-AW-pruh-tiv)
preoperative (pre-AW-pruh-tiv)
purulent (PURE-u-lent)
sanguineous (SANG-gwin-ee-us)
serosanguineous (SEER-oh-SANG-gwin-ee-us)
serous (SEER-us)
surgeon (SURGE-un)

CHAPTER CONCEPTS

Comfort
Patient-Centered Care
Safety
Tissue Integrity

LEARNING OUTCOMES

1. Describe factors that influence surgical outcomes.
2. Identify the role of the licensed practical nurse/licensed vocational nurse (LPN/LVN) in each perioperative phase.
3. Explain the role of the LPN/LVN in obtaining informed patient consent.
4. Develop a teaching plan to enhance learning for the older preoperative patient.
5. Identify nursing interventions used for common postoperative patient needs.
6. Describe how to evaluate effectiveness of nursing interventions.
7. List signs and symptoms of common postoperative complications.
8. List the criteria for ambulatory discharge.
9. Describe the role of the home health care nurse in caring for postoperative patients.

Surgery is the use of instruments during an operation. It treats injuries, diseases, and deformities. Surgical procedures are named according to (1) the involved body organ, part, or location and (2) the suffix that describes what is done during the procedure (Table 12.1). Surgery is performed by **surgeons** and other physicians trained to do certain surgical procedures. Advanced practice nurses with training may also perform minor surgical procedures. Surgery is scheduled based on the urgency required for a successful outcome for the patient (Table 12.2). Reasons for surgery to be performed are listed in Table 12.2.

 TYPES AND PHASES OF SURGERY

Laser, scope, and robotic technologies reduce the invasiveness of surgical procedures. Minimally invasive surgery is less damaging to tissues than traditional open incision surgery. This allows a faster and less painful recovery. Laser surgery uses a laser instead of a scalpel to cut tissue. It is often used for eye surgery. An endoscope is used for minimally invasive surgery. This is also called keyhole surgery. Minimally invasive surgery includes laparoscopic surgery (abdominal and pelvic cavity) and thoracoscopic surgery (chest and thoracic cavity). The endoscope is a flexible tube. A light, camera,

Table 12.1

Table 12.1
Surgical Procedure Suffixes

Suffix	Meaning	Word-Building Examples
-ectomy	Removal by cutting	crani (skull) + ectomy = craniectomy appen (appendix) + ectomy = appendectomy
-orrhaphy	Suture of or repair	colo (colon) + orrhaphy = colorrhaphy herni (hernia) + orrhaphy = herniorrhaphy
-oscopy	Looking into	colon (intestine) + oscopy = colonoscopy gastr (stomach) + oscopy = gastroscopy
-ostomy	Formation of a permanent artificial opening	ureter + ostomy = ureterostomy colo (colon) + ostomy = colostomy
-otomy	Incision or cutting into	oust (bone) + otomy = osteotomy thoro (thorax) + otomy = thoracotomy
-plasty	Formation or repair	oto (ear) + plasty = otoplasty mamm (breast) + plasty = mammoplasty

Table 12.2
Surgery Urgency Level and Purpose

Type	Definition	Examples
Urgency Level		
Emergency	Immediate surgery needed to save life or limb without delay	Ruptured aortic aneurysm or appendix, traumatic limb amputation, loss of extremity pulse from emboli
Urgent	Surgery needed within 24–30 hours	Fracture repair, infected gallbladder
Elective	Planned/scheduled, with no time requirements	Joint replacement, hernia repair, skin lesion removal
Optional	Surgery requested by the patient	Cosmetic surgery
Purposes of Surgery		
Aesthetic	Requested by patient for improvement	Blepharoplasty, breast augmentation
Diagnostic	To obtain tissue samples, make an incision, or use a scope to make a diagnosis	Biopsy
Exploratory	Confirmation or measurement of extent of condition	Exploratory laparotomy
Preventive	Removal of tissue before it causes a problem	Mole or polyp removal to prevent cancer
Curative	Removal of diseased or abnormal tissue	Inflamed appendix, tumor, benign cyst, hernia
Reconstructive	Correction of defects of body parts	Scar repair, total knee replacement, face lift, mammoplasty
Palliative	Alleviation of symptoms when disease cannot be cured	Debulking (removal of as much of tumor as possible) to relieve pain or pressure, colostomy for incurable bowel obstruction, insertion of gastrostomy tube to provide tube feedings for swallowing problem, rhizotomy (cuts nerve root to relieve pain)

and suction are attached to it. It is inserted through a small incision. An image is then projected on a screen for the surgeon to watch. Additional incisions are made for insertion of other instruments based on the type of surgery.

Robotic surgery, which uses robots, is growing in usage. The *da Vinci* Surgical System is one type of surgical robot. It has several moving arms. One arm is a camera. Two are robotic arms that act as the surgeon's hands. The fourth arm moves obstructions out of the way (Fig. 12.1). As the surgeon moves the controls, the robotic arms (inside the patient's body) translate the movements to cut, suction, or suture. Visit www.intuitivesurgical.com for more robotic information and videos.

There are three phases in the surgical process: **preoperative, intraoperative,** and **postoperative. Perioperative** refers to all three phases. It includes the time before, during, and after surgery. Each perioperative surgical phase has a defined time frame. Specific events related to surgery occur in each phase (Table 12.3).

PREOPERATIVE PHASE

Your primary role as a licensed practical nurse/licensed vocational nurse (LPN/LVN) in the *preoperative* phase is to:

- Assist in data collection and contribute to the patient's plan of care.
- Reinforce teaching and instructions given to the patient and family by the surgeon and registered nurse (RN).
- Provide emotional and psychological support for patients and families.

Other health care team members also assist in preparing the patient for surgery. The surgeon obtains a medical history,

Table 12.3
Perioperative Surgical Phases

Preoperative	Begins with decision for surgery and ends with transfer to the operating room
Intraoperative	Begins with transfer to operating room and ends with admission to perianesthesia care unit (PACU)
Postoperative	Begins with admission to PACU and continues until recovery is complete

performs a physical examination, and orders diagnostic testing. RNs perform a preoperative assessment, provide explanations and instructions, and offer patients and families emotional and psychological support to ease anxiety. They also develop a plan of care and verify the patient's name, surgical site (along with the patient), allergies, and related information when the patient arrives in the surgical area.

Factors Influencing Surgical Outcomes

When preparing a patient for surgery, the goal is to identify and implement actions that reduce surgical risk factors. The focus of preoperative care is to help the patient achieve the best possible surgical outcome. This is done by ensuring the patient is as healthy as possible for surgery.

Age

For older patients, surgery can promote quality of life. For healthy older patients, age alone does not mean that they are at greater surgical risk ("Gerontological Issues: Surgical

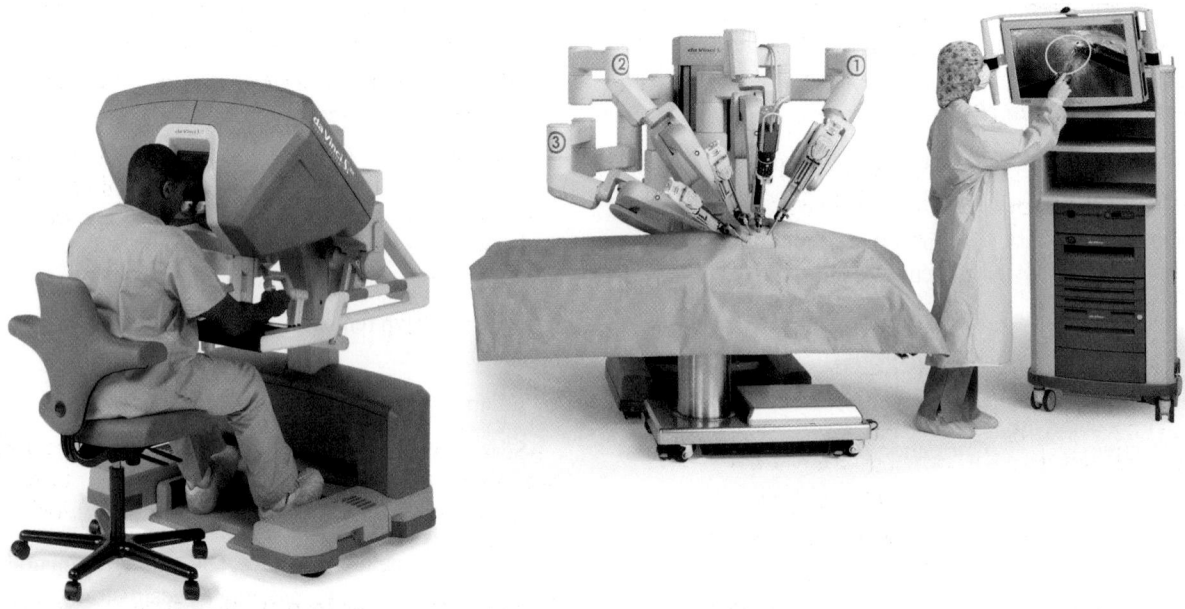

FIGURE 12.1 Operating room featuring the *da Vinci* Si Surgical System with a surgeon at the *da Vinci* robotic surgery console, the patient cart at the surgical table, and a nurse at the vision cart.

Gerontological Issues

Surgical Considerations for the Older Adult. Older adults have decreased ability to compensate for the stress of surgery due to declining physiological reserve (extra capacity of a body system or organ to carry out its function under stress). The risk for hemorrhage, anemia, fluid/electrolyte imbalance, infection, pressure injury, and acute kidney injury are increased in older adults. Nursing interventions before, during, and after the surgical procedure focus on reducing complications.

Preoperatively

• Pad bony prominences to protect against pressure injuries and muscle and bone discomfort.
• Reassure the patient and family by teaching what to expect before, during, and after surgery; diet changes; description and length of surgical procedure; activities in the recovery room; pain management; coughing and deep breathing exercises; procedures; and treatments (e.g., dressings, catheters).
• Ensure preoperative screening has been completed (e.g., blood work, radiographic studies, nutritional assessment, pulmonary function tests, electrocardiogram).

Intraoperatively

• Monitor patient for hypoxia (restlessness), hypothermia, hemorrhage, and balanced intake and output.

Postoperatively

Pain Control—Provide adequate pain relief so required postoperative activities, such as deep breathing, coughing, position changes, and exercise, can be performed more effectively.

Respiratory Function—Reduce respiratory complications by encouraging deep breathing and coughing:

• Perform after pain medication has begun to take effect to encourage deep breaths due to less pain. Assess the patient carefully when giving narcotics because they can cause respiratory depression.
• Use a pillow and instruct the patient to hold it firmly over abdominal or chest incisions to support the incision. Taking a deep breath increases chest expansion as well as abdominal pressure, which may pull or stretch an incision.
• Older adults perform deep breathing and coughing exercises better if you perform the exercises with them. For example, say the following: "Let's take a deep breath in through the nose. Hold it and count to three. Slowly blow it out completely through the mouth. When you blow the air out, shape your lips like they are going to whistle."

Mobility—Encourage mobility through the following nursing actions and observations:

• Use pillows to support the patient's body alignment. Assist the patient to ambulate as soon as possible after surgery. Regularly help the patient with passive or active range-of-motion exercises, along with flexion and extension exercises, for legs and feet.
• Monitor for unilateral swelling of the leg and calf or groin pain, which may indicate deep venous thrombosis (DVT). DVT is a risk related to venous pooling in the lower extremities. This risk is increased with postoperative inactivity.
• Assist the patient to change position at least every 2 hours. If patients lay in one position too long, pressure injuries can develop. When tissues are compressed between bones and the bed surface, blood supply is reduced to the tissue and cells begin to die. This can result in painful open wounds.

Bowel Function—It is common for patients to feel bloated after surgery. Increasing activity such as walking stimulates peristaltic action of the bowel. This helps expel flatus and reduce discomfort.

Urinary Function—Be aware of the following aspects of urinary function:

• Individuals often have difficulty emptying their bladder after surgery. Patients who are sleeping but restless should be evaluated for bladder distention. It is often difficult to void on a bedpan or in a urinal in a supine position.
• Older men with an enlarged prostate may have even greater difficulty voiding if they have received medications that have urinary retention side effects.
• Assisting patients to sit or stand to use urinals, use a bedside commode, or ambulate to the bathroom promotes bladder emptying and helps avoid the use of urinary catheters.
• Monitor urine amount, color, and odor. Older adults are prone to dehydration. Urine output provides an indication of their hydration status for intervention.

Delirium—Perform the following nursing actions to minimize delirium:

• Monitor level of consciousness routinely. Provide a calm environment and orient patients to their environment. Restraints should not be used because they can worsen delirium.
• Recognize that the presence of a urinary catheter can contribute to delirium. Avoid catheters if possible.

Considerations for the Older Adult"). Older adults may take longer to recover from anesthetic agents. This is due to aging changes related to drug metabolism and elimination.

Chronic Disease

Chronic diseases may increase the patient's surgical risk. A medical clearance for surgery may be needed from the patient's health care provider (HCP).

Emotional Responses

The word *surgery* causes a common anxious emotional reaction in patients and their families. *Anxiety* is a feeling of apprehension or uneasiness resulting from the uncertainties and risks associated with surgery. *Fear* is a feeling of dread from a source known to the patient. Assist patients in coping with these feelings. If patient fears are extreme, inform the surgeon. This includes a fear of dying. When fear is excessive, the surgeon may reschedule the surgery until the patient is better able to cope.

Surgical patients may experience various fears related to **anesthesia** (reversible loss of sensation). These fears include anesthesia awareness with general anesthesia (aware or conscious but not feeling pain during surgery), feeling loss of control, or not waking up. The patient should discuss these concerns with the anesthesia provider.

A growing trend is for surgery to be performed while the patient is awake. A form of anesthesia is used other than general anesthesia. Patients report feeling more comfortable when they are alert and aware of the surgical experience.

It is normal for patients to be concerned about pain. The anesthesia provider gives medications for pain during surgery. Nurses give prescribed analgesics after surgery. Complementary techniques are also used to help reduce pain. These include guided imagery or focused breathing.

Body image changes may be a fear for some patients. The thought of disfigurement, mutilation, bleeding, or having a scar may cause great anxiety for some patients. Allow the patient to discuss these fears.

Nutrition

Patients should be well nourished to adequately heal and recover from surgery ("Nutrition Notes: Screening and Nourishing the Preoperative Patient"). Higher levels of protein (for tissue repair and healing), vitamin C (for collagen formation), and zinc (for tissue growth, skin integrity, and cell-mediated immunity) are required. Obese patients may have more delayed healing and wound *dehiscence* (opening of the incision). Patients who are emaciated may have more infections and delayed wound healing

Smoking and Alcohol and/or Drug Abuse

Tobacco use and alcohol and/or drug abuse increase the surgical patient's risks. Smoking thickens and increases the amount of lung secretions. It reduces the action of cilia that remove the secretions. Patients are encouraged to avoid smoking for at least 24 hours before surgery. If they have a chronic lung disorder, avoidance should be for 3 to 4 weeks before surgery. Not smoking increases the action of the lungs' defense mechanisms, makes more hemoglobin available to carry oxygen, and improves wound healing.

Nutrition Notes

Screening and Nourishing the Preoperative Patient. Identifying and treating malnutrition before surgery may improve the patient's outcome. Unintended weight loss or decreased oral intake should prompt further nutritional assessment by a dietitian. Before elective surgery, the patient may have time to correct some nutritional deficiencies. If patients are overweight, they are often instructed to lose weight to reduce surgical risks, prevent respiratory problems, and promote wound healing. For anemia, an iron preparation may be administered. At least 2 to 3 weeks are required for objective evidence of the effectiveness of nutritional therapy. Before surgery on the gastrointestinal tract, a low-residue diet may be eaten for 2 to 3 days to minimize bowel contents.

The American Society of Anesthesiologists (2017) practice guidelines recommend a minimum of the following fasting time frames before anesthesia:

- Clear liquids: 2 hours
- Light meal (toast/clear liquid): 6 hours
- A meal containing meat or fat: 8 hours

Clinical judgment is required regardless of the guidelines, which do not apply to:

- Patients with gastromotility or metabolic disorders
- Those with potential airway problems

Long-term alcohol and/or drug abuse may cause nutritional deficiencies and liver damage. The damage can create bleeding problems, fluid volume imbalances, and medication metabolism alterations. In addition, alcohol and drugs that are abused can interact with administered medications and should be avoided before surgery for safety.

Preadmission Surgical Patient Assessment

Nonemergent surgical patients have a preoperative assessment. They have an interview with the **anesthesiologist,** or a preadmission telephone or face-to-face interview with RNs in the preadmission testing department under the direction of the anesthesia provider. The interview process includes a health history, identification of risk factors, patient and family teaching, discharge planning, and necessary referrals to social workers, support groups, and educational programs. Personal or family problems with anesthesia or malignant hyperthermia are identified (Box 12.1).

Preoperative diagnostic testing is based on the patient's age, medical history, assessment findings, and agency protocols (Table 12.4). A urine or serum pregnancy test as appropriate for female patients may be done. This is to prevent fetal exposure to anesthetics. Health information

Box 12.1

Malignant Hyperthermia

Malignant hyperthermia is a potentially fatal hereditary muscular disease. It can be triggered by some types of general anesthetic agents and/or succinylcholine. A history of anesthetic problems in the patient or family members indicates the potential for this condition. Precautions can then be taken. A muscle biopsy diagnoses this problem. Surgery can be safely done with planning. The anesthesia provider carefully chooses the anesthetic agents.

In malignant hyperthermia, metabolism in the muscles is increased. This produces a very high fever and muscle rigidity. In addition, tachycardia, tachypnea, hypertension, arrhythmias,

hyperkalemia, metabolic and respiratory acidosis, and cyanosis occur. Malignant hyperthermia is life-threatening. Immediate treatment is required to prevent death. Surgery is stopped. Anesthesia is discontinued immediately. Oxygen at 100% is given. The patient is cooled with ice and infusions of iced solutions. Dantrolene sodium (Dantrium) is a muscle relaxant that relieves the muscle spasms. It is the most effective medication for malignant hyperthermia. Dantrolene sodium is kept readily available in the operating room. It is given according to the treatment protocol of the Malignant Hyperthermia Association of the United States (www.mhaus.org).

Table 12.4

Preoperative Diagnostic Tests

Diagnostic Test	*Purpose*
Chest x-ray	Detect pulmonary and cardiac abnormalities
Oxygen saturation	Obtain baseline level and detect abnormality
Serum Tests	
Arterial blood gases	Obtain baseline levels and detect pH and oxygenation abnormalities
Bleeding time	Detect prolonged bleeding problem
Blood urea nitrogen	Detect kidney problem
Creatinine	Detect kidney problem
Complete blood cell count	Detect anemia, infection, clotting problem
Electrolytes	Detect potassium, sodium, chloride imbalances
Fasting blood glucose	Detect abnormalities, monitor diabetes control
Pregnancy	Detect early, unknown pregnancy
Partial thromboplastin time	Detect clotting problem
International normalized ratio	Detect clotting problem, monitor warfarin therapy
Type and cross-match	Identify blood type to match blood for possible transfusion
Urine Tests	
Pregnancy	Detect early, unknown pregnancy
Urinalysis	Detect infection, abnormalities

and diagnostic testing results are reviewed by anesthesia providers. Abnormal test results are reported to the surgeon for intervention.

Federal law requires patients to be asked before surgery if they have a signed advance directive (e.g., health care durable power of attorney or living will) for their medical record (see Chapter 17). Written information on an advance directive is offered if they do not have one.

Preoperative Teaching
Preoperative Routines

Preoperative teaching for common surgical routines includes:

• Date and time of admission and surgery
• Admission (e.g., arrive about 2 hours before surgery for preoperative preparation)
• Length of stay, and items to bring and wear

- Recovery after surgery
- Family information (e.g., waiting area and communication)
- Discharge criteria (e.g., responsible adult needed to take the patient home after outpatient surgery)

Preoperative Instructions and Preparation

Special preps are explained. Nasal cultures for *Staphylococcus aureus* screening and treatment may be done. Bathing or skin preps to reduce skin bacterial counts before surgery are explained. Their purpose is to reduce surgical site infections (World Health Organization, 2016). Enemas are ordered before abdominal or intestinal surgery to empty the bowel. This reduces fecal contamination intraoperatively. It also prevents distension or straining postoperatively.

Medications to take the morning of surgery are explained. They can be taken with an ounce of water. Food and fluids are restricted before surgery to reduce the risk of pulmonary aspiration during surgery. (The minimal fasting time guidelines of the American Society of Anesthesiologists are listed in "Nutrition Notes: Screening and Nourishing the Preoperative Patient.") Patients may brush their teeth or rinse their mouth without swallowing. Surgery may be canceled if the patient has not stopped eating or drinking as specified.

Instructions for postoperative care are given before surgery. This allows the patient to be alert for the teaching and have time for practice. Patients are informed that active participation in postoperative care helps their recovery. Patients are taught how to report their pain level using a pain rating scale (see Chapter 10). Pain relief methods are described. They can include parenteral or oral analgesics, an epidural catheter, or patient-controlled analgesia (PCA). Anticipated dressings, tubes, casts, or special equipment are also described. If needed, crutches are fitted to the patient. Their proper use is explained and demonstrated.

Postoperative exercises are taught to decrease complications. They include deep breathing and coughing, use of incentive spirometry, leg exercises, turning, and how to get out of bed. After an exercise is taught, the patient is asked to perform a return demonstration. This allows the nurse to evaluate if the exercise was done correctly.

Deep breathing expands and ventilates the lungs to prevent **atelectasis.** Atelectasis is the collapse of alveoli in one or more areas of the lung from hypoventilation or mucous obstruction. It reduces the lung's capacity to oxygenate the body. To deep breath, teach the patient to sit up, exhale fully, take in a deep breath through the nose, hold the breath and count to three, and then exhale completely through the mouth. This should be repeated hourly while awake, in sets of five, for 24 to 48 hours postoperatively.

Incentive spirometry can be ordered to prevent atelectasis. It increases lung volume, alveoli expansion, and venous return (Fig. 12.2). All patients can benefit from incentive spirometry. Keep the spirometer at the patient's bedside to use. (Do not store on the window sill or in a drawer where it cannot be reached by the patient.) Offer it to the patient

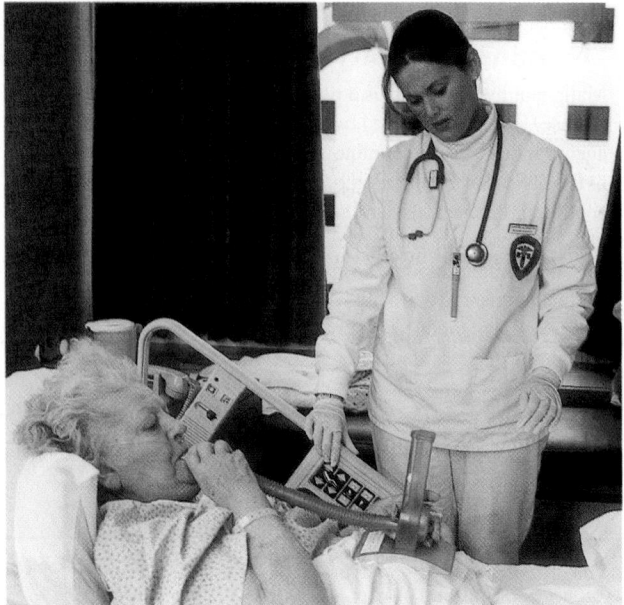

FIGURE 12.2 An incentive spirometer aids lung expansion.

as ordered to ensure that it is used. Teach patients to do the following:

- Sit upright, at 45 degrees minimum, if possible.
- Take two normal breaths. Place mouthpiece of spirometer in mouth.
- Inhale until target, designated by spirometer light or rising ball, is reached, and hold breath for 3 to 5 seconds.
- Exhale completely.
- Perform 10 sets of breaths as ordered.

Coughing moves secretions to prevent pneumonia. Reinforce teaching on how to cough effectively if not contraindicated by the patient's condition (such as hernia repair or head injury; Table 12.5). Give pain medication before asking the patient to cough. Reassure patient that coughing should not harm the incision. Splinting the incision with a pillow may be comforting. Several sets of coughing are performed every 1 to 2 hours while the patient is awake.

Leg exercises and foot circles should be done every hour while awake. Ensure they are not contraindicated. Leg exercises improve circulation. They help prevent emboli formation. Teach patients to do the following:

- For leg raises, lie down, raise leg, and bend leg at the knee.
- Flex foot, extend leg, and lower it to the bed.
- Do sets of five for each leg.
- For foot circles, raise a leg slightly off the bed with toes pointed.
- Draw a circle in the air with the great toe.
- Rotate to the right four times and then to the left four times.
- Repeat this five times and then repeat with the other foot.

· WORD · BUILDING ·

atelectasis: ateles—imperfect + ektasis—expansion

Table 12.5
Teaching Patients Coughing Techniques

Procedure	Rationale
Have the patient sit up and lean forward.	Promotes lung expansion and ability to generate forceful cough.
Show the patient how to splint incision with hands, pillow, or blanket.	Reduces incision pressure so it does not feel as if incision is opening.
Have the patient inhale and exhale deeply three times through mouth.	Helps expand lungs.
Have the patient take in a deep breath and cough out the breath forcefully with three short coughs using diaphragmatic muscles. Then have the patient take in a quick deep breath through the mouth, cough deeply, and deep breathe.	Generates forceful cough and expands lungs to help move secretions.

Reinforce teaching that turning from side to side in bed is easier if the leg that is to be on top is bent. Then, place a pillow between the legs to support the top leg. Unless contraindicated, have patients use the bed's side rail to pull themselves over to the side. To promote comfort, have patients deep breathe while turning instead of holding their breath.

To make it easier for patients to get out of bed and to reduce strain on the incision, instruct patients to:

• Turn on side without pillows between knees.
• Place hands flat against the bed.
• Push up while swinging legs out of bed into a sitting position.
• Sit for a few minutes after changing position to avoid dizziness and falling.
• Deep breathe while sitting to expand lungs.

Nursing Process for Preoperative Patients
Data Collection

HEALTH HISTORY. Patient data are collected on admission (Table 12.6). Have patients wear their contact lenses, glasses, or hearing aids to ensure accurate communication. Note the patient's emotional reaction to surgery (previously discussed).

Medications. All prescription and over-the-counter medications are reviewed. Herbal remedies or recreational drugs are reviewed. Anticoagulants such as warfarin (Coumadin) or nonsteroidal anti-inflammatory drugs (NSAIDS) including aspirin may need to be stopped several days before surgery. This is done to avoid bleeding problems during surgery. Herbal medicines can interfere with other medications. They can also increase bleeding times. Patients may be told to stop specific herbal medications 1 to 2 weeks before surgery.

Patients with diabetes who take insulin are given instructions. They are ordered to either hold their insulin or take half of their normal insulin dose on the day of surgery. After admission, blood glucose monitoring is done every 4 hours or as ordered. This ensures blood glucose levels are maintained within a desired range.

Patients on chronic oral steroid therapy cannot abruptly stop it. This is true even when they are taking nothing by mouth (nil per os; NPO). Circulatory collapse can develop if steroids are stopped abruptly. The surgeon should order a parenteral route for the steroids. Make sure parenteral steroid therapy is continued while the patient is NPO.

Patients should be asked about their use of alcohol or drugs. This includes cocaine, marijuana, or opioids. These drugs can interact with anesthesia and medications. To obtain honest, accurate information, tell patients of this potential interaction. Information and questions should be stated in a nonjudgmental manner. For example, ask, "How much alcohol do you drink daily or weekly?" instead of "Do you drink alcohol?" The first question assumes that people drink alcohol. This allows the patient who does not drink alcohol to indicate none. The patient who does drink alcohol can state an amount. They don't have to say yes and then give an amount upon further questioning. More accurate responses are given as this approach is viewed more positively by the patient who drinks alcohol. Another example would be to ask the patient, "What roles do drugs or alcohol play in your life?"

PHYSICAL ASSESSMENT. A physical assessment of body systems is performed. This information can identify risk factors for surgery and interventions to reduce them. Report a cough, cold, or fever to the surgeon. Surgery might be delayed until the acute infection is gone. Document dentures, bridges, capped teeth, and loose teeth. They can become dislodged during endotracheal (ET) intubation (insertion of breathing tube) for general anesthesia.

Nursing Diagnoses, Planning, and Implementation

Anxiety or Fear related to potential change in body image, hospitalization, pain, loss of control, and uncertainties surrounding surgery

EXPECTED OUTCOME: The patient will state reduced anxiety or fear before surgery.

• Inform patients about procedures and surgical routines, *which helps reduce anxiety.*
• Allow patients to express their concerns *to allow inaccurate information to be corrected.*

Table 12.6
Nursing Assessment of the Preoperative Patient

Subjective Data: Health History Questions	
Demographic information	Name, age, marital status, occupation, roles?
Condition for which surgery is scheduled	Why are you having surgery?
Medical history	Any allergies, acute or chronic conditions, current medications, pain, or prior hospitalizations?
Surgical history	Any reactions or problems with anesthesia? Previous surgeries?
Tobacco use	How much do you smoke? Pack-year history (number of packs per day × number of years)?
Alcohol use	How often do you drink alcohol? How much?
Drug use	Do you use recreational or street drugs?
Coping techniques	How do you usually cope with stressful situations? Support systems?
Family history	Hereditary conditions, diabetes, cardiovascular or anesthesia problems?
Female patients	Date of last menses and obstetrical information?

Objective Data: Physical Assessment	
Vital signs, oxygen saturation	
Height and weight	
Emotional status	Calm, anxious, tearful
Neurologic	Ability to follow instructions
Skin	Color, warmth, bruises, lesions, turgor, dryness, mucous membranes
Respiratory	Infection (cough, breath sounds); chronic obstructive pulmonary disease; respiratory rate, pattern, and effort; barrel chest
Cardiovascular	Angina, myocardial infarction, heart failure, hypertension, valvular heart disease, mitral valve prolapse, heart rate and rhythm, peripheral pulses, edema, jugular vein distention
Gastrointestinal	Bowel sounds, date of last bowel movement, abdominal distention, firmness, ostomy
Musculoskeletal	Deformities, weakness, decreased range of motion, crepitation, gait, artificial limbs, prostheses

- If patients express extreme anxiety or fear, inform the surgeon *because complications or even death could result.*
- Provide the opportunity to listen to music or use guided imagery, *which can help reduce patient's anxiety and fears.*

Deficient Knowledge related to lack of previous experience with surgical routines and procedures

EXPECTED OUTCOME: The patient will demonstrate understanding of surgical information and routines before surgery.

- Consider patient anxiety levels before providing explanations *because learning can be affected by high anxiety levels.*

- Identify knowledge deficiencies with patients *so they are motivated to learn.*
- Reinforce preoperative information and new information as *teaching is caring in action and empowers patients to be a participant in their care.*
- Include the patients' family or caregivers in teaching sessions *so they can assist patients through the surgical experience.*
- Use a variety of teaching methods (e.g., discussion, written materials and instructions, models, and videos) and individualize explanations *to allow for different learning styles and aging changes.* ("Gerontological

Issues: Considerations for Older Patient Teaching Sessions" describes methods to provide a positive learning experience for the older patient.)

• Document teaching and patient's understanding *as proof of teaching and the patient's level of understanding.*

Gerontological Issues

Considerations for Older Patient Teaching Sessions
Environmental Considerations
• Comfortable and safe: anxiety free, quiet, appropriate temperature
• Correctly lit: small, intense lighting with nonglare, soft white light (not fluorescent)
• Private: no distractions, no background noise

Presentation Considerations
• Identify readiness to learn.
• Plan learning based upon current knowledge.
• Use past experience and relate to new learning.
• Use simple, understandable words and avoid medical jargon.
• Use legible audiovisual materials (e.g., large print, black print on white nonglare paper).
• If using colors, remember that older adults see red, orange, and yellow best; blue, violet, and green are more difficult to see.
• Perform ongoing assessment of energy level of patient.
• Answer questions as they occur.

Presenter Considerations
• Have a positive attitude and belief in self-care promotion for older adults.
• Earn trust by being a credible, positive role model.
• Maintain a professional appearance.
• Use knowledge of aging changes in presentation.
• Sit in front of patients for best visibility.
• Speak slowly in a low tone.
• Ensure that prostheses are in place, such as glasses and hearing aids.
• Allow patients increased response time, and use memory aids such as pictures or diagrams.
• Use touch appropriately to convey caring.
• Teach most important information first.
• Present one idea at a time.
• Provide instruction using multiple senses (vision and hearing).
• Provide repetition and obtain feedback to ensure comprehension.
• Provide feedback and positive reinforcement.

Evaluation
The goal to decrease anxiety is achieved if the patient states and demonstrates that anxiety is relieved. The goal for increasing knowledge is met if the patient is able to correctly state or accurately demonstrate the information presented.

Preoperative Consent
Before performing surgery, the surgeon must obtain written informed consent. It gives legal permission for the surgery. Consent has two purposes: One is to protect the patient from unauthorized procedures; the other is to protect the surgeon, anesthesia provider, hospital, and hospital employees from claims of performing unauthorized procedures. Informed consent is needed for all invasive procedures. These include surgery, anesthesia, blood administration, and radiation or cobalt therapy. Consent is typically valid for 30 days after signing.

Informed consent involves three elements:

1. The surgeon must explain in terms the patient understands about the diagnosis, the proposed treatment and who will perform it, the likely outcome, possible risks and complications of treatment, alternative treatments, and the prognosis without treatment. If the patient has questions before signing the consent, the surgeon must be contacted to provide further explanation to the patient. It is not within the nurse's scope of practice to provide this information.
2. The consent must be signed before analgesics or sedatives are given. Patients must demonstrate to a witness that they are informed and understand the surgery.
3. Consent must be given voluntarily. No persuasion or threats can be used to influence the patient. The patient can withdraw consent at any time, even after the consent form has been signed.

It may be your role to obtain and witness the patient's or authorized person's signature on the consent form. As the patient's advocate, ensure that the person signing the consent form understands its meaning. Ensure that the patient has no further questions to be directed to the surgeon and that the consent is being signed voluntarily. If the patient is unable to read, read the entire consent to the patient before it is signed.

Patients can't give consent if they are unconscious, mentally incompetent, or minors. They also cannot give consent if they have received analgesics or drugs that alter central nervous system function within time frames specified by agency policy. Consent may be obtained in any of these cases in person or by phone from parents, next of kin, or legal guardians as specified by law. A court order can also be obtained in a medical emergency. If time does not permit this, the surgeon documents the need for treatment in the medical record as necessary to save the patient's life or avoid serious harm, according to state law and institutional policy.

NURSING CARE TIP
Your signature as a witness on a consent form indicates that you observed the informed patient or patient's authorized representative voluntarily sign the consent form. It does not mean that you informed the patient about the surgical procedure. That is the responsibility of the surgeon.

Preparation for Surgery
Preoperative Preparation Checklist

A preoperative checklist may be completed. The nurse signs it before the patient is transported to surgery (Fig. 12.3). The checklist provides the following guidelines for preoperative preparation of the patient:

• An identification band is placed on the patient. A hospital gown is given to the patient to wear. Underwear is removed, depending on the type of surgery.

• Vital signs are taken and recorded as baseline information of the patient's status.

• Makeup, nail polish, and artificial nails (if applicable) are removed to allow assessment of natural color and pulse oximetry for oxygenation status during and after surgery.

• Removal of hairpins, wigs, and jewelry prevents loss or injury. Rings, such as wedding rings, are taped in place if the patient does not want to take them off, except if the ring is on the operative side (arm or chest surgery), because edema may occur.

Pre-op Surgical Checklist   **Client Name**

_____ I.D. BAND ON   _____

_____ NPO AS ORDERED

_____ PRE-OP TEACHING COMPLETED

_____ INFORMED CONSENT SIGNED

_____ HISTORY AND PHYSICAL ON CHART

_____ ALLERGIES

_____ LAB RESULTS

_____   CBC: HGB _____ HCT _____ WBC _____ PLATELETS _____

_____   POTASSIUM _____

_____   URINALYSIS _____

_____   PREGNANCY TEST   SERUM _____ URINE _____

_____   PT _____ PTT _____ BLEEDING TIME _____

_____   TYPE AND SCREEN _____ CROSSMATCH _____-___ UNITS

_____ ECG ON CHART

_____ CHEST X-RAY REPORT ON CHART

_____ SHOWERED/BATHED

_____ HOSPITAL GOWN ON

_____ PREPS COMPLETED AS ORDERED

_____ ANTIEMBOLISM STOCKINGS

_____ JEWELRY TAPED/REMOVED: DISPOSITION _____

_____ VALUABLES: DISPOSITION _____

_____ DENTURES, PROSTHESIS REMOVED

_____ HAIR PINS, WIGS, MAKE UP, NAIL POLISH, ONE ACRYLIC NAIL REMOVED

_____ CONTACT LENSES REMOVED

_____ VOIDED

_____ VITAL SIGNS: T _____ P _____ R _____ BP _____

_____ PRE-OP MEDICATIONS GIVEN _____ SIDE RAILS UP _____

_____ IV STARTED _____

_____ EYE GLASSES AND HEARING AID(S) TO OR

_____ OLD CHART TO OR

_____ X-RAYS TO OR

_____ FAMILY LOCATION _____

_____ NEXT OF KIN _____

_____ CLIENT READY FOR SURGERY _____

        TIME _____   (NURSE SIGNATURE)

COMMENTS:

FIGURE 12.3 Sample preoperative checklist form.

- Dentures, contact lenses, and prostheses are removed to prevent injury. Some patients are concerned about body image and do not want family members to see them without dentures or makeup. Remove dentures after the family goes to the waiting room and insert them before the family sees the patient postoperatively.
- Glasses and hearing aids go with patients to surgery if they are unable to communicate without them. Label them with the patient's name and document where they go.
- All orders, diagnostic test results, consents, and history and physical (required in medical record) are reviewed for completion and documented on the checklist.

- Patient valuables are recorded and given to a family member or locked up per institutional policy by the nurse.
- Antiembolism devices are applied if ordered.
- Patients are asked to void before sedating preoperative medications are given, unless a urinary catheter is present, to prevent injury to the bladder during surgery.

Preoperative Medications

Preoperative medications are given at the time ordered or on call to surgery (i.e., surgery calls to instruct that it is time to give the drugs; Table 12.7). If sedatives or analgesics are

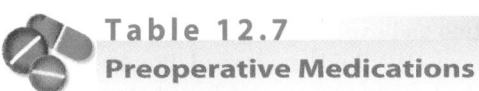

Table 12.7
Preoperative Medications

Medication Class/Action

Analgesic/Antipyretic
Relieves mild to moderate pain and reduces fever

Examples	**Nursing Implications**
acetaminophen (OFIRMEV)	Given intravenously as 15-minute infusion. Antipyretic effect may mask fever.

Antianxiety and Sedative Hypnotics
Sedation; anxiety reduction

Examples	**Nursing Implications**
diazepam (Valium) lorazepam (Ativan) midazolam (Versed)	Contraindicated for acute narrow-angle glaucoma. Monitor respirations.

Antiemetics
Control nausea and vomiting

Examples	**Nursing Implications**
metoclopramide (Reglan) ondansetron (Zofran) prochlorperazine (Compazine) promethazine hydrochloride (Phenergan)	Redness, pain, or burning at the site of injection. Increased drowsiness with opioids.

Antibiotics
Prevention of postoperative infection

Examples	**Nursing Implications**
Variety of antibiotics used	Give within 30–60 minutes of incision as prescribed for best effect.

Opioids
Bind to opioid receptors in the central nervous system to alter perception of pain and enhance postoperative pain relief

Examples	**Nursing Implications**
fentanyl (Sublimaze) hydromorphone hydrochloride (Dilaudid) meperidine (Demerol) morphine sulfate	Monitor vital signs, level of sedation, and respiratory status. Avoid meperidine use in older adult.

given, the bed rails are raised for safety per policy. Instruct the patient not to get up alone.

Transfer to Surgery Department

When the surgery department is ready, the patient is transported to the surgical holding area (Fig. 12.4). The patient's inhaler medications for those with asthma and glasses or hearing aids to aid communication are taken with the patient. Family members can go with the patient. During surgery, the family waits in the surgical waiting area, which is a communication center. The family can be called by cell phone or given a beeper. They are kept informed of the patient's status.

Post-Transfer to Surgery Department

After the patient goes to the surgery department, prepare the patient's room and necessary equipment to be ready when

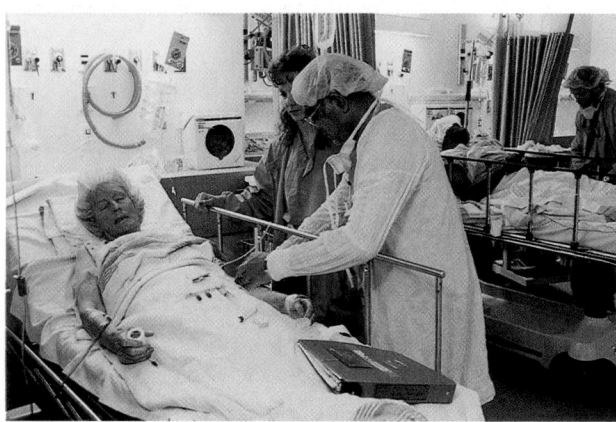

FIGURE 12.4 Surgical holding area.

the patient returns from the perianesthesia care unit (PACU; Table 12.8).

Patient Arrival in Surgery Department

The holding area nurse greets the patient. The nurse then verifies the patient's name, age, allergies, surgeon performing the surgery, informed consent, surgical procedure (correct site, especially right or left when applicable), and medical history. Next, the nurse answers questions and alleviates anxiety. The operative site is marked usually by the person most informed about the patient and procedure (surgeon), and confirmed by the patient. This helps ensure that the right surgery for the right patient on the correct section of the body is done.

The patient is introduced to the anesthesiologist and certified registered nurse anesthetist. They also verify patient information and explain the type of anesthesia to be used. Intravenous (IV) fluids are started. Prophylactic antibiotics may be timed to be given 1 hour before incision time. This timing has been shown to reduce surgical site infections.

Before entering the operating room (OR), the patient should be told what to expect:

- "If the room feels cool, you can request extra blankets."
- "There is a lot of equipment in the room, including a table and large, bright overhead lights."
- "Several health care team members will introduce themselves to you."
- "Your surgeon will greet you."
- "A safety checklist will be performed."

Table 12.8

Postoperative Patient Hospital Room Preparation

Preparation	Rationale
Bed With Wheels Locked	
Ensure bed linens are clean and changed if used by patient before surgery.	Reduces contamination of surgical wound.
Place disposable, absorbent, waterproof pads on bottom sheet if drainage is expected.	Protects linen from wetness and soiling so a patient in pain does not have to be disturbed for linen change.
Apply lift sheet on bed of patient needing assistance with repositioning.	Makes lifting and turning easier for patient and nurse.
Have warm blankets available.	Patient may be cold.
Fanfold top cover to end of bed or to side of bed away from patient transfer side.	Readies bed to receive patient on transfer and allows covers to be easily pulled up over patient.
Obtain extra pillows as needed for positioning, elevating extremities, and splinting during coughing.	Pillows help maintain position when patient is turned, splint an incision during coughing, or elevate operative extremities for comfort and swelling reduction.

Table 12.8
Postoperative Patient Hospital Room Preparation—cont'd

Preparation	*Rationale*
Equipment	
Have vital sign equipment available.	Promotes ability to promptly obtain vital signs.
Have intravenous (IV) pole/controller pump available.	Surgical patients have IV infusions postoperatively.
Have oxygen set up as needed.	After tracheostomy, patients wear humidified oxygen mask.
Prepare suction setup for tracheostomy, nasogastric tube, or drains as ordered.	Suction may be ordered related to surgical procedures: *Sterile suction:* tracheostomy *Nasogastric tube:* thoracic, abdominal, gastrointestinal surgery *T-tube:* cholecystectomy
Have emesis basin at bedside.	Nausea or vomiting may occur, especially after movement during transfer.
Have tissues and washcloths in room.	Promotes comfort (e.g., washing face or a cool cloth on forehead).
Have urinal or bedpan available in room.	Patients may be unable to get out of bed for first voiding.
Obtain special equipment as indicated by the surgical procedure.	Institutional policy and surgeon orders may require specialized equipment: *Jaw surgery:* suction, wire cutters, tracheostomy tray *Tracheostomy:* suction, extra tracheostomy set, tracheostomy care supplies

Preoperative Warming

Prewarming the patient's skin before anesthesia is helpful. This can help maintain normal body temperature (normothermia). It can also reduce intraoperative **hypothermia.** Associated complications can be prevented. A forced-air warming device used for 30 minutes may reduce hypothermia. Patients should be normothermic (body temperature within normal range) before transfer to surgery.

INTRAOPERATIVE PHASE

The next phase of the perioperative period is the *intraoperative* phase. It begins when the patient is transferred to the operating table (Figs. 12.5 and 12.6). Surgery can be done in a hospital or outpatient surgical center. Additionally, surgery is performed in HCP offices, cardiac catheterization laboratories, radiology centers, emergency rooms, and specialized units that perform endoscopy procedures.

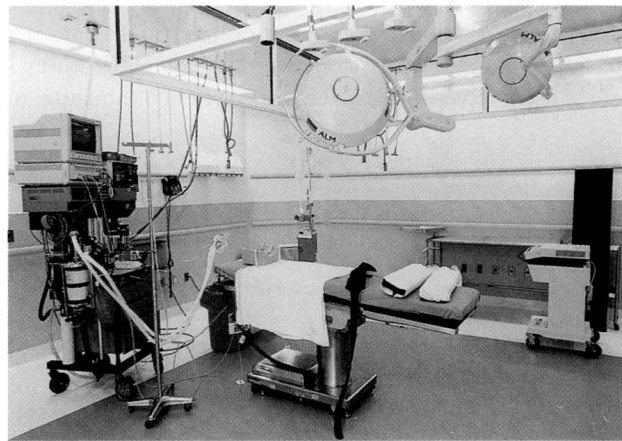

FIGURE 12.5 Operating room. Anesthesia equipment is on the left.

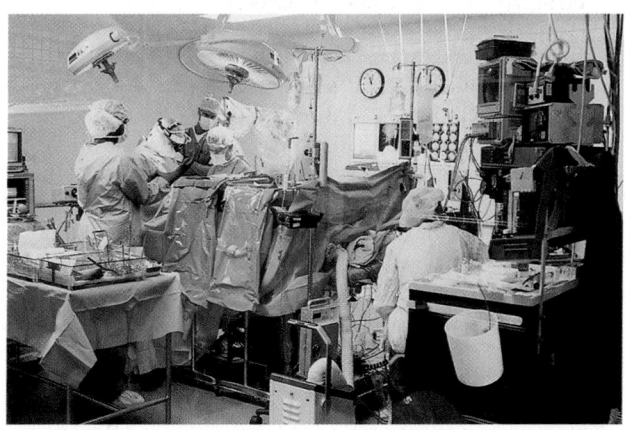

FIGURE 12.6 Operating room in use. Anesthesia equipment is on the right.

BE SAFE!

Prevent mistakes in surgery:

- Make sure that the correct surgery is done on the correct patient and at the correct place on the patient's body.
- Mark the correct place on the patient's body where the surgery is to be done.
- Pause before the surgery to make sure that a mistake is not being made.

(The Joint Commission's 2018 National Patient Safety Goals. © The Joint Commission, 2018. Reprinted with permission.)

The OR is designed to enhance **aseptic** (elimination of microorganisms) technique. Clean and contaminated areas are separated. Special ventilation systems control dust. They prevent air from flowing into the OR from hallways. The temperature and humidity in the OR is controlled to discourage bacterial growth. The OR temperature is recommended to be 68°F to 77°F (20°C to 25°C). This reduces patient hypothermia. Everyone entering the OR wears surgical scrubs, shoe covers, caps, masks, and goggles. This protects the patient from infection. It also protects the staff from bloodborne pathogens. Traffic in and out of the OR is limited. Strong disinfectants are used to clean the OR after each surgical case.

Prior to surgery, surgical team members (Box 12.2) must perform a sterile surgical hand scrub. This reduces the number of microorganisms on their hands and arms. Jewelry (e.g., watches, rings, bracelets) is removed. Fingernails are kept short and clean. Artificial nails and nail polish are not recommended. They may harbor microorganisms. If nail polish is worn, it should not be chipped. It should be removed and reapplied every 4 days. Sterile gloves are worn by the surgical team to keep the surgical field sterile.

A surgical case cart contains sterile instruments specifically for the patient's case. The LPN/LVN may assist with maintaining the sterile surgical field.

A nursing plan of care focusing on safety is prepared before the patient arrives in surgery (Box 12.3). It is developed with the patient's preadmission assessment data.

The LPN/LVN may help position the patient onto the operating table. A safety strap is carefully applied. A time-out is taken to verify all patient and surgical information to prevent mistakes. Then monitoring equipment is applied. Readings are recorded. The anesthesia provider begins anesthesia and says when to position the patient. Positioning is done carefully to prevent pressure points. These can cause tissue or nerve damage. Tubes that are needed, such as a nasogastric (NG) tube or urinary catheter, are inserted by the RN.

Patient allergies (e.g., to skin prep solutions) are rechecked. If the patient requires body hair removal, hair is removed with electric clippers. Shaving is avoided ("Evidence-Based Practice"). It can cause microabrasions that become colonized by microorganisms. Then the skin is cleaned with a skin prep solution such as povidone-iodine. A large area around the operative site is scrubbed. This allows the incision to be extended as needed. The scrub is completed in a circular motion from inner to outer edge. An allergic reaction to the solution can cause skin redness and blistering wherever the solution was used. After the skin is scrubbed, a sterile drape is applied. The incisional area is left exposed.

Box 12.3

Intraoperative Nursing Diagnoses and Expected Outcome

- *Risk for Injury* related to perioperative positioning, chemicals, electrical equipment, and effect of being anesthetized
  Is free from injury.
- *Risk for Impaired Skin Integrity* related to chemicals, positioning, and immobility
  Maintains skin integrity.

Box 12.2

Surgical Health Care Team Members and Roles

Members of the surgical health care team and their roles are as follows:

- *Surgeon:* medical doctor, doctor of osteopathy, oral surgeon, or podiatrist
- *Surgical (first) assistant:* another physician, a specially trained registered nurse (RN; such as a nurse practitioner or clinical nurse specialist), or a physician's assistant who assists the surgeon
- *Anesthesiologist:* physician who specializes in administering anesthesia and supervises certified registered nurse anesthetists (CRNAs) in the operating room
- *CRNA:* a certified RN with a master or doctorate degree in nurse anesthesia
- *RN:* circulates in the operating room; roles include being the patient's advocate, planning care, protecting patient safety, monitoring patient positioning, checking vital signs and patient assessment, reducing patient's anxiety, monitoring sterility during surgery, preparing skin before incision, managing equipment (e.g., making sponge counts), documenting the procedure, and aiding health team communications
- *Surgical (second assistant) technician:* assists surgeon (may be an RN, licensed practical nurse/licensed vocational nurse, or surgical technologist)

Evidence-Based Practice

Clinical Question

Does hair removal affect postoperative surgical site infection?

Evidence

A review of 14 studies (11 were randomized control trials) compared various hair removal methods including shaving, clipping, and depilatory creams amongst each other and with the option of not removing hair preoperatively. There were no significant differences between not removing hair and methods of hair removal (Shi, Yao, & Yu, 2017).

Implications for Nursing Practice

Unless it is necessary, it is recommended to avoid operative site hair removal from surgical sites. There is no advantage to shaving the operative site. In addition, patients expressed increased satisfaction when hair removal was avoided. When hair removal is necessary, it is recommended to clip hair rather than shave hair to avoid skin irritation and micro-irritation.

Reference

Shi, D., Yao, Y., & Yu, W. (2017). Comparison of preoperative hair removal methods for the reduction of surgical site infections: A meta-analysis. *Journal of Clinical Nursing,* *26*(19–20), 2907–2914.

BE SAFE!

Use medicines safely. Before a procedure, label medicines that are not labeled. For example, medications in syringes, cups, and basins. Do this in the area where medicines and supplies are set up.

(The Joint Commission's 2018 National Patient Safety Goals. © The Joint Commission, 2018. Reprinted with permission).

Anesthesia

Anesthesia is used during surgery mainly to prevent pain. The type of anesthesia and the anesthetic agents are ordered by the anesthesia provider with input from the patient and surgeon.

There are two types of anesthesia: general and local (regional). General anesthesia causes the patient to lose sensation, consciousness, and reflexes. It acts directly on the central nervous system. Local anesthesia blocks nerve impulses along the nerve where it is injected. This results in the loss of sensation to a region of the body. There is no loss of consciousness.

General Anesthesia

General anesthesia is given by IV or inhalation. It is used if the surgical procedure will take a long time and there is a need for muscle relaxation. It is also used when patients are anxious or do not want local anesthesia. In addition, it can be used for patients who are unable to cooperate, as with head injury, muscle disorders, or impaired cognitive function.

INTRAVENOUS AGENTS. To begin most general anesthesia, the patient is induced (meaning "to cause anesthesia"). A short-acting IV agent is used to provide rapid, smooth **induction** (the period from when the anesthetic is first given until full anesthesia is reached). These agents last only a few minutes and are used along with inhalation agents. After induction, the patient is intubated with an ET tube. This is used to provide anesthesia and mechanical ventilation (Fig. 12.7).

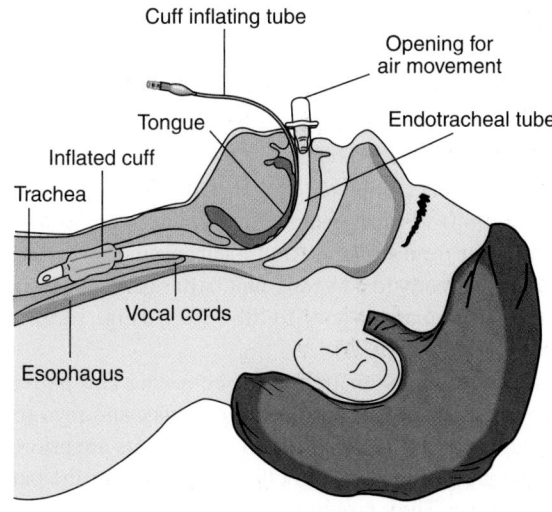

Cuff inflating tube

Opening for air movement

Tongue

Endotracheal tube

Inflated cuff

Trachea

Vocal cords

Esophagus

FIGURE 12.7 Endotracheal tube with cuff inflated.

INHALATION AGENTS. Inhalation agents maintain anesthesia during the surgery. These agents are delivered, controlled, and excreted via mechanical ventilation.

COMPLICATIONS. Side effects of general anesthesia are usually brief. They include nausea and vomiting, confusion (longer duration in older adult), sore throat, and shivering, likely from the body cooling. Serious complications occur rarely and include respiratory distress, malignant hyperthermia, and, more commonly in older adults, delirium (temporary) and cognitive dysfunction (e.g., long-term memory loss; difficulty learning, thinking, and concentrating). Inhalation agents and the ET tube can be irritating to the respiratory tract. Complications that can occur include laryngospasm (sudden violent contraction of the vocal cords), laryngeal edema, or injury to the vocal cords. When the tube is removed, closely monitor the patient. Be prepared to provide respiratory support. Assist with reintubation if needed.

ADJUNCT AGENTS. An **adjunct** agent is a medication used with the primary anesthetic agents. These medications include opioids to control pain, muscle relaxers to avoid movement of muscles during surgery, antiemetics to control nausea or vomiting, and sedatives to supplement anesthesia. Side effects related to a specific medication such as itching with narcotics can occur.

Local or Regional Anesthesia

Local or regional anesthesia is selected for the patient who wants to be awake, is not anxious, can tolerate the local agent, and is not required by the surgical procedure to be unconscious or have relaxed muscles.

A local agent can be placed directly on the surgical area or injected into the tissue where the incision is to be made to numb a small area. A regional block is done by injecting the local agent along a nerve that carries impulses in the region where anesthesia is desired. There are several types of regional blocks. A nerve block is the injection of a local agent into a nerve at a specific point. A Bier block is done by placing a tourniquet (cuff) on an extremity to remove the blood; the local agent is then injected into the extremity. A field block is a series of injections surrounding the surgical area.

SPINAL AND EPIDURAL BLOCKS. Injection of a local agent into the subarachnoid space produces spinal block (Fig. 12.8). Epidural block occurs when the local agent is injected into the epidural space. Spinal and epidural blocks are used mainly for lower extremity and lower abdominal surgery. Both motor and sensory function are blocked. The patient must be carefully monitored for complications. Hypotension results from sympathetic blockade. The blockage causes vasodilation and reduces venous return to the heart. Cardiac output is reduced. Respiratory depression results if the block travels too far upward. As the block wears off, patients feel

• WORD • BUILDING •
induction: inductio—to lead in

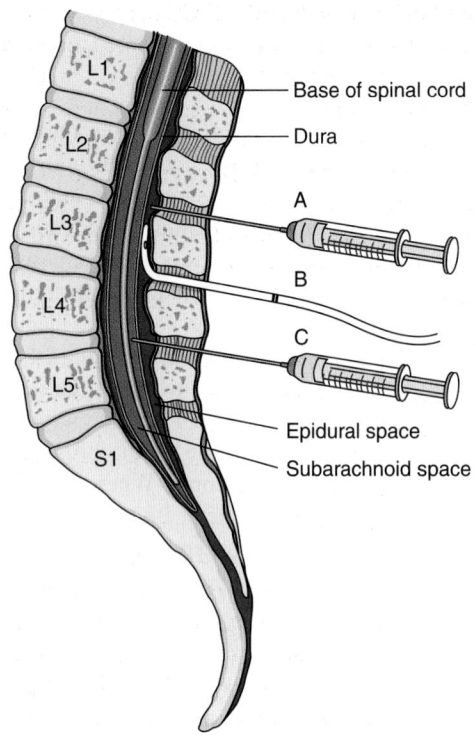

FIGURE 12.8 Injection of spinal anesthesia. (A) Epidural anesthesia. (B) Epidural catheter. (C) Spinal anesthesia.

as if their legs are heavy and numb. This is normal. Reassurance should be offered to the patient that this type of feeling does not last after the block wears off.

COMPLICATIONS. Back pain, urinary retention, hematoma, nerve damage, or postdural puncture headache can occur with regional anesthesia. Headache may occur from leakage of cerebrospinal fluid (CSF) out of the needle puncture hole in the dura. Pressure is then reduced on the spinal cord and brain. This causes a low-pressure headache, which can be severe. The headache can worsen with standing or sitting. The use of less than 25-gauge spinal needles helps prevent headache. Nausea, dizziness, tinnitus, and vision disturbances may be present.

The headache usually will resolve in 7 to 10 days. If symptomatic and conservative treatment is not effective, an autologous epidural blood patch can be used. This sterile procedure is done by the anesthesiologist. To create an epidural blood patch, approximately 15 mL to 20 mL of the patient's blood is injected into the epidural space one interspace below the previous puncture site.

Procedural Sedation and Analgesia

Procedural sedation and analgesia (formerly, conscious sedation) is purposeful, minimal sedation. It does not cause the complete loss of consciousness. The patient may fall asleep, but then arouse easily and respond. Patients remain in control of their own airway. They are comfortable and respond purposefully. Medications such as propofol (Diprivan), ketamine (Ketalar), midazolam (Versed), and opioids (fentanyl or morphine) are given to produce sedation. Selection of patients who

are eligible for this sedation is based on the procedure, the patient's general health, and patient or physician preference. Examples of short procedures for which this type of sedation is used are dental procedures, endoscopy, cardioversion, and closed fracture reduction. Procedural sedation can be administered by anesthesia providers or ordered by a physician and given by a specially trained RN.

The patient does not eat for 6 hours before the procedure. Clear liquids are allowed up to 2 hours before the procedure. A signed informed consent is obtained. Then an IV is started. Every 5 minutes, vital signs, electrocardiogram (ECG), and oxygen saturation are checked. Changes are reported to the HCP. Oxygen may be given by nasal cannula or mask. Emergency equipment (e.g., airway suction, defibrillator, drugs) is on standby.

After the procedure, the patient awakens quickly and remembers nothing or little about the procedure. The patient is monitored about every 15 minutes for response to the procedure and medications. Rare side effects include drowsiness, headache, and nausea. The patient is ready for discharge when vital signs return to baseline and are stable, oral fluids are retained, and voiding has occurred (if applicable). Written and oral discharge teaching must be given to both the patient and the responsible adult to whom the patient is being discharged. The responsible adult and the patient must sign the instructions. These state that an adult must drive the patient home and provide a safe environment. They also state that the patient must not and will not drive or operate heavy machinery or sign legal documents for 24 hours.

LEARNING TIP

In comparison with general anesthesia, procedural sedation and analgesia:

- Is less invasive.
- Requires less medication.
- Causes less depression of the cardiovascular and respiratory systems.
- Allows the patient to return more quickly to a wakeful state.

Transfer From Surgery

When surgery is completed and anesthesia stopped, the patient is stabilized for transfer. The patient is normothermic upon transfer from surgery. After local anesthesia, the patient may return directly to a nursing unit. After general and spinal anesthesia, the patient goes to the PACU (Fig. 12.9) or an intensive care unit (ICU).

Patient safety is an important concern. The patient is never left alone. Ensuring a patent airway and preventing falls and injury from uncontrolled movements are priorities. The anesthesia provider and OR nurses transfer the patient to the PACU. They monitor the patient until the perianesthesia nurse can receive the hand-off report and assumes

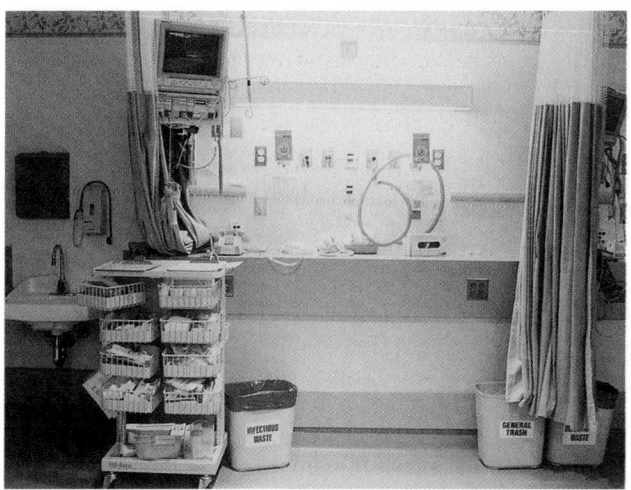

FIGURE 12.9 Perianesthesia care unit (PACU).

care of the patient. This promotes safe recovery from anesthesia. The family is updated on the patient's status by the surgeon.

POSTOPERATIVE PHASE

The *postoperative* phase is the final perioperative phase. It begins when the patient is admitted to the PACU or directly to a nursing unit. It ends with the patient's postoperative evaluation in the surgeon's office.

Admission to the Perianesthesia Care Unit

Responsibilities of perianesthesia nurses are listed in Box 12.4. It is essential for nurses to perform hand hygiene between patients in the PACU. When patients are admitted to the PACU, an admission assessment is done.

Oxygen by nasal cannula, mask, ET tube, or mechanical ventilation is given after general anesthesia. IV fluid infusion is maintained. Continuous monitoring is done at least every 5 to 15 minutes. This includes ECG, vital signs, ex-

Box 12.4

Perianesthesia Nursing Responsibilities

- Airway maintenance
- Vital signs including temperature, oxygen saturation (SaO_2), and exhaled end-tidal carbon dioxide ($EtCO_2$)
- Body systems assessment including surgical site
- Patient safety
- Monitoring anesthetic effects
- Pain management
- Accurate intake and output
- Identifying perianesthesia care unit discharge readiness
- Documentation
- Hand-off report to receiving nurse (includes name, allergies, procedure, type of anesthesia, status, complications, oxygen, dressing/drains/equipment, medications, postoperative orders, pertinent history, family, opportunity to ask questions)

haled end-tidal carbon dioxide ($EtCO_2$), and pulse oximetry. If the patient's temperature is normal, the temperature is monitored hourly and at discharge from PACU. Passive methods to maintain temperature are continued. Room temperature is kept at or above 75°F (24°C). A head covering and warm blankets are used. If shivering due to hypothermia occurs, the temperature is retaken. For hypothermia, active warming, usually with a forced-air warming system, is used. Body temperature is monitored every 15 minutes until normal. The patient must be normothermic before PACU discharge.

The surgical site incision or dressing is monitored. Drainage amount and color as well as **hematoma** formation are documented and reported to the HCP as needed. Tubes (e.g., chest, drains, NG, urinary catheter) and other equipment are checked for proper function.

IV analgesics or PCA are given for pain as needed. Antiemetics are administered for nausea or vomiting. Coughing and deep breathing are encouraged, unless they are contraindicated by the surgical procedure (e.g., hernia repair; eye, ear, intracranial, and jaw surgery; and plastic surgery). If the patient is no longer NPO, ice chips or sips of water are offered for a dry mouth when the patient is fully awake.

Nursing Process for Postoperative Patients in Perianesthesia Care Unit

Postoperative complications may occur due to the surgical procedure, anesthesia, blood and fluid loss, immobility, unrelieved pain, or other diseases the patient may have. Nursing care focuses on preventing, detecting, and caring for these complications.

Respiratory Function

DATA COLLECTION. Normal respiratory function can be altered in the immediate postoperative period by airway obstruction, hypoventilation, secretions, laryngospasm, or decreased swallowing and cough reflexes. Respiratory function assessment includes respiratory rate, depth, ease, and pattern. Breath sounds, chest symmetry, accessory muscle use, and sputum are also observed.

NURSING DIAGNOSES, PLANNING, AND IMPLEMENTATION

Ineffective Airway Clearance related to obstruction, anesthesia medications, and secretions

EXPECTED OUTCOME: The patient will have a patent airway at all times.

- Ensure that the patient maintains a patent airway *because airway obstruction may result when relaxed muscles allow the tongue to block the pharynx in patients with a decreased level of consciousness.*

• WORD • BUILDING •
hematoma: heimatos—blood + oma—tumor

• Use jaw-thrust method to manually open the patient's airway *if patient has snoring respirations and has not completely emerged from anesthesia.*

Ineffective Breathing Pattern related to anesthesia, pain, and analgesic/sedative medications

EXPECTED OUTCOME: The patient will maintain normal $EtCO_2$ and oxygen saturation (Sao_2) levels at all times.

• Maintain oxygen therapy as ordered *to prevent hypoventilation, which can be an effect of anesthesia medications, analgesics, or decreased level of consciousness.*
• Encourage deep breathing *to expand the lungs and expel anesthetic agents.*
• Maintain continuous positive airway pressure (CPAP)/bilevel positive airway pressure (BiPap) *to treat sleep apnea.* (Patients may bring their CPAP/BiPap machines with them.)
• Report respiratory depression or abnormal $EtCO_2$ to the anesthesiologist *to obtain prompt treatment.*

Risk for Aspiration related to depressed cough and gag reflexes and reduced level of consciousness

EXPECTED OUTCOME: The patient will have clear lung sounds with no signs of acute aspiration (coughing, wheezing, fever, respiratory distress, cyanosis, chest pain) at all times.

• Position the patient onto side, unless contraindicated, *to protect the airway until fully awake.*
• Use suction equipment as needed *to clear secretions or emesis.*

EVALUATION. The goal for ineffective airway clearance and aspiration is achieved if the patient's airway remains patent and lung sounds remain clear. The goal for ineffective breathing pattern is met if the patient's respiratory rate is within normal limits, no dyspnea is reported, and arterial blood gases are within normal limits.

Cardiovascular Function

DATA COLLECTION. Alterations in cardiovascular function can include hypotension, arrhythmias, and hypertension. Hypotension can be the result of blood and fluid volume loss, cardiac abnormalities, or a side effect of anesthesia or pain medication. Shock can result from the significant blood and fluid volume loss or from sepsis (see Chapter 9). Arrhythmias can occur from hypoxia, altered potassium or magnesium levels, hypothermia, pain, stress, or cardiac disease. New-onset hypertension can develop from pain, a full bladder, or respiratory distress.

Cardiovascular function assessment includes heart rate, blood pressure, ECG, and skin temperature, color, and moistness. Vital signs are compared with baseline readings to determine patient status. Tachycardia; hypotension; pale skin color; cool, clammy skin; and decreased urine output indicate hypovolemic shock. This requires reporting and prompt treatment.

Deficient Fluid Volume related to blood and fluid loss or NPO status

EXPECTED OUTCOME: The patient will maintain blood pressure, pulse, and urine output within normal limits at all times.

• Check dressings, incisions, and drains for color and amount of drainage *to detect fluid loss.*
• Maintain IV fluids at ordered rate *to replace lost fluids but avoid fluid overload.*
• Monitor intake and output *to detect imbalances.*

EVALUATION. The goal for deficient fluid volume is met if vital signs and urine output are within normal limits.

NURSING CARE TIP

Tachycardia is a compensatory mechanism designed to provide adequate delivery of oxygen in times of altered function. It is usually the earliest warning sign that an abnormality is occurring. It should be an indicator to assess the patient. Ask yourself what this particular patient is likely to be experiencing that is compromising oxygenation. This will allow you to begin prompt intervention.

Patient Condition	Possible Causes of Compromised Oxygenation
Postoperative	Hemorrhage, respiratory depression, pain
Myocardial infarction	Cardiogenic shock, pain, arrhythmia
Respiratory	Respiratory distress
Trauma	Hemorrhage, severe pain

Neurologic Function

Until its effects wear off, anesthesia can alter neurologic function. Patients may arrive in the PACU awake, arousable, or sleeping. Patients who are sleeping should become more alert during their stay in the PACU. As they emerge from anesthesia, they may become agitated or act wild for a short time; this is called *emergence delirium.* During this time, it is important to provide safety measures to prevent injury such as side rails and restraints—following restraint protocols—to protect IV lines and keep ET tubes in place. Once resolved, patients return to a calm state and have no recollection of the episode. Movement, sensations, and perceptions may also be altered by anesthesia. Movement is the first function to return after spinal anesthesia.

Confused patients may be agitated or frightened when they awaken. Review older adult patients' cognitive history. It is helpful to know how caregivers communicate with patients. If possible, have a familiar relative or caregiver with a patient in the PACU. They can calm the patient and help with communication. Watch for nonverbal pain cues (see the next section). Understand that postoperative patients will have pain and require pain relief interventions, even if they cannot report it.

DATA COLLECTION. A neurologic assessment includes level of consciousness; orientation to person, place, time, and event; pupil size and reaction to light; and motor and sensory function. Abnormalities are reported to the anesthesia provider.

Pain

DATA COLLECTION. If the patient is awake, ask the patient to rate the presence of pain using a pain scale. Document the location and character of the pain. If the patient is not fully awake, monitor vital signs and nonverbal indications of pain. Nonverbal indications of pain can include abnormal vital signs, restlessness, moaning, grimacing, rubbing, or pulling at specific areas or equipment.

NURSING DIAGNOSES, PLANNING, AND IMPLEMENTATION

Acute Pain related to tissue damage (mechanical [incision])

EXPECTED OUTCOME: The patient will report that pain is relieved at a satisfactory level within 15 to 30 minutes of the pain report.

- Monitor the patient for pain, *because pain may result from the surgical procedure, movement, deep breathing, anxiety, a full bladder, positioning during surgery, NG tubes, catheters, IVs, ET tubes, or prior medical conditions, such as arthritis, cancer, or back pain.*
- Give ordered IV opioid analgesics promptly *for their rapid onset.*
- Begin PCA as ordered, as *it is often initiated in PACU.*
- Reposition the patient, provide warmth, and assist to empty full bladder *to alleviate pain.*
- Play music (e.g., nature sounds or classical music) in the PACU, dim lights, and reduce room noise *to help alleviate pain.*

EVALUATION. The goal for pain is met if the patient reports a satisfactory decrease in level of pain. For example, the patient reports pain of 10 on a scale of 0 to 10. Thirty minutes after you medicate the patient, the patient rates pain as 2 on a scale of 0 to 10. The patient indicates that 2 is an acceptable pain level, so the goal is achieved.

Family Visitation

Family visitation in the PACU has been shown to be helpful to patients and their families. Allowing family visitation varies by hospital. Patients and families should be educated about the expectations for family visitation. During visitation, confidentiality of all patients in PACU must be ensured per the Health Insurance Portability and Accountability Act of 1996 (HIPAA). For example, some patients may not want

their surgical procedure revealed to their spouse or any family members.

Discharge From the Perianesthesia Care Unit

The length of stay in the PACU for a stable patient is about 1 hour. A postanesthesia recovery scale is used to score the patient's readiness to be discharged. The scale rates categories such as respiration, oxygen saturation, level of consciousness, activity, and circulation. The anesthesiologist discharges the patient for transfer to a nursing unit or home when discharge criteria are met (Box 12.5). The patient may be transferred to the ICU. This is done if the patient is unstable and/or frequent or invasive monitoring is needed.

Transfer to the Nursing Unit

The perianesthesia nurse provides a hand-off report to the unit nurse when the patient is transferred to the nursing unit. The patient is moved into a bed on the nursing unit unless the patient is being transferred in a bed, as may be done with major orthopedic procedures. Assistance is given to prevent dislodging of IVs, tubes, and drains. The following safety interventions are performed per agency policy to help prevent falls:

- The bed is placed in its lowest position with wheels locked, the side rails raised, and the call button within patient's reach.
- Instructions are given for the patient to call for assistance with ambulation.
- Assistance by one or two health care workers is given to help the patient get out of bed. The patient should be encouraged to sit on the side of bed prior to standing (Fig. 12.10). When the patient gets up postoperatively, especially for the first time, he or she may be weak or dizzy.

Box 12.5

Discharge Criteria for Perianesthesia Care Unit or Ambulatory Surgery

- Vital signs stable with temperature normal
- Patient awake or at baseline level of consciousness
- Drainage or bleeding not excessive
- Respiratory function not depressed
- Oxygen saturation above 90%

Additional Criteria for Ambulatory Surgery
- No nausea or vomiting
- No intravenous opioids within last 30 minutes
- Voided if required by surgical procedure or ordered
- Is ambulatory or has baseline mobility
- Understands discharge instructions
- Provides means of contact for follow-up telephone assessment
- Released to responsible adult

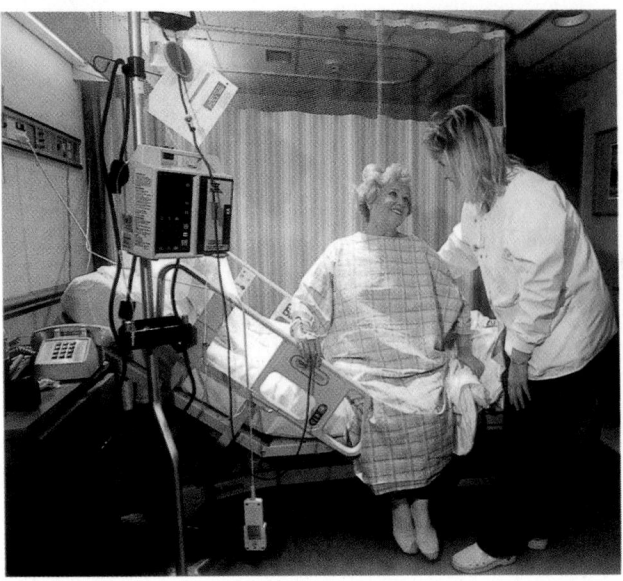

FIGURE 12.10 Postoperative patient sitting before standing.

Nursing Process for Postoperative Patients

A complete patient assessment is performed after transfer to the nursing unit. Respiratory status, vital signs (including temperature), level of consciousness, surgical site, dressings, and pain level are noted. IV site, patency, and IV solution and infusion rate are monitored. NG tubes are hooked to suction or clamped as ordered. Drains and catheters are positioned to promote proper functioning.

Interventions to promote recovery are implemented. They include monitoring for complications (e.g., respiratory depression, hemorrhage, and shock) and providing postoperative care. Additional interventions are reinforcing teaching to patients and their significant others and assisting with necessary referrals including providing home health care.

Respiratory Function

DATA COLLECTION. Regular monitoring of the patient's respiratory system is done. This includes rate, depth, and effort and breath sounds. Cough strength (if not contraindicated by the type of surgery, such as hernia repair or eye, ear, intracranial, jaw, or plastic surgery) is also noted. Postoperative patients are at risk for developing atelectasis. This can lead to pneumonia. They may have a weak cough from being drowsy from anesthesia or analgesics. Listen for fine crackles in the lung bases. If present, encourage the patient to deep breathe or cough. Listen again to see if the crackles have cleared. If the patient's airway is compromised, take immediate action to support the airway. Notify the surgeon.

NURSING DIAGNOSES, PLANNING, AND IMPLEMENTATION. See "Nursing Care Plan for the Postoperative Patient."

Nursing Care Plan for the Postoperative Patient

Nursing Diagnosis: *Ineffective Breathing Pattern* related to pain
Expected Outcomes: The patient will maintain normal arterial blood gases and oxygen saturation (Sao$_2$) levels at all times.
Evaluation of Outcome: Are arterial blood gases normal?

Intervention	Rationale	Evaluation
Give analgesics per pain scale rating as ordered.	*Promotes willingness to deep breathe as patient does not guard against deep respirations or coughing, especially if incision is near the diaphragm.*	Does patient perform deep breathing and coughing?

Nursing Diagnosis: *Ineffective Airway Clearance* related to ineffective cough and secretion retention
Expected Outcomes: The patient will maintain a patent airway at all times. Breath sounds remain clear at all times.
Evaluation of Outcome: Is the patient able to clear own secretions? Are breath sounds clear?

Intervention	Rationale	Evaluation
Monitor breath sounds.	*Abnormal breath sounds such as crackles or wheezes can indicate retained secretions.*	Are breath sounds clear?
Encourage deep breathing and coughing hourly and use of incentive spirometer as ordered while awake.	*Lung expansion and coughing helps prevent mucous plugs that block bronchioles, causing alveoli to collapse and atelectasis or infection to develop from stasis of mucus, resulting in pneumonia.*	Does patient perform deep breathing and coughing and use incentive spirometer?

Nursing Care Plan for the Postoperative Patient—cont'd

Intervention	Rationale	Evaluation
Ensure that patient's pain is relieved before activity.	*Movement can cause or increase pain.*	Does patient state pain is controlled before activity?
Encourage movement by turning every 2 hours and early ambulation as able.	*Movement promotes lung expansion and movement of secretions.*	Is patient moving?

Geriatric

Ensure adequate hydration.	*Older adults are prone to dehydration, making their secretions thicker and more difficult to clear.*	Does patient have balanced intake and output?

Nursing Diagnosis: *Acute Pain* related to tissue damage from surgery, muscle spasms, nausea, or vomiting
Expected Outcome: The patient will report that pain management relieves pain satisfactorily within 30 minutes of report of pain or when the patient awakens. The patient will describe pain management plan by first postoperative day.
Evaluation of Outcome: Does the patient report satisfactory pain relief? Is the patient able to describe pain management plan?

Intervention	Rationale	Evaluation
Explain pain relief interventions and set goals with the patient for pain management.	*Patients are partners in their pain management and need to understand the plan to collaborate on the goals.*	Does patient understand the plan and have a goal for acceptable pain level?
Monitor pain using a patient appropriate pain rating scale (self-report: 0 to 10; noncommunicative: pictogram, Pain Assessment in Advanced Dementia [PAINAD]; see Chapter 10).	*Self-report is the most reliable indicator of pain unless patient is unable to report pain.*	Is patient using the pain scale?
Provide ordered pain medication as needed.	*Analgesics along with other types of medications decrease pain along various pathways.*	Is patient's pain reduced after receiving medication?
Provide antiemetics as needed.	*Antiemetics relieve nausea and vomiting.*	Is patient's nausea and vomiting reduced after receiving medication?
Position patient comfortably.	*Incisions, drains, tubing, equipment, and bedrest can cause discomfort, which positioning can relieve.*	Does patient report positioning is comfortable?

Geriatric

Monitor patients who are cognitively impaired immediately at beginning of shift and then frequently.	*Cognitively impaired patients are vulnerable to undertreatment of pain and deserve excellence in pain relief management.*	Does patient exhibit signs of reduced or no pain per pain scale?
Use pain rating tools designed for cognitively impaired patients to assess pain regularly and observe nonverbal pain cues (e.g., restlessness, grimacing, moaning).	*The pain of older patients, especially if cognitively impaired, is often underreported and undertreated. Noting nonverbal cues can aid in pain treatment.*	Are nonverbal pain cues present in older patients, especially those who are cognitively impaired?

(nursing care plan continues on page 192)

Nursing Care Plan for the Postoperative Patient—cont'd

Intervention	Rationale	Evaluation
When monitoring pain, speak clearly and slowly so older patients can hear and understand.	*If older patients cannot hear or misunderstand, pain may not be reported accurately. Appropriate intervention would not be provided.*	Is patient able to report pain and relief accurately using pain scale?

Nursing Diagnosis: *Risk for Surgical Site Infection* related to inadequate primary defenses from surgical wound
Expected Outcome: The patient will remain free from infection at all times.
Evaluation of Outcome: Does the patient remain free from infection?

Intervention	Rationale	Evaluation
Observe incision for signs and symptoms of infection; report, if present.	*Redness, warmth, fever, and swelling indicate infection.*	Are signs and symptoms of infection present?
Maintain sterile technique for dressing changes.	*Sterile technique reduces infection development.*	Is incision free of signs and symptoms of infection?
Geriatric		
Monitor for and report low-grade temperature or new-onset confusion.	*Older adults may exhibit a low-grade temperature or new-onset confusion as indicators of infection requiring treatment.*	Does patient have low-grade temperature or new-onset confusion to report?

Circulatory Function

DATA COLLECTION. Monitor the patient's circulatory status to detect and prevent hemorrhage, shock, and venous thromboembolism. Vital signs, Sao₂, and skin temperature, color, and moistness are monitored (per institutional policy). Report abnormal findings. Check the incision or dressing for drainage or hematoma formation. Drainage may leak down the patient's side and pool underneath the patient. Turn the patient if able or, while wearing gloves, slide hands underneath the patient to check for bleeding. Report any signs of hemorrhage or shock promptly.

Observe the lower extremities of surgical patients. Check peripheral pulses and capillary refill. Tenderness or pain in the calf may be the first indication of a deep venous thrombosis (DVT). Leg swelling, warmth, and redness as well as fever may also be present. Bilateral calf and thigh measurements are taken daily if DVT is suspected or diagnosed.

NURSING DIAGNOSES, PLANNING, AND IMPLEMENTATION

Deficient Fluid Volume related to blood and fluid loss or NPO status

EXPECTED OUTCOME: The patient will maintain blood pressure, pulse, and urine output within normal limits at all times.

• Monitor dressings, incisions, drains, and tubes for color and amount of drainage, and report bright red drainage or excessive drainage amounts immediately *to detect hemorrhage.*
• Monitor intake and output *to detect imbalances.*
• Maintain IV fluids at the ordered rate *to maintain fluid volume.*

Ineffective Peripheral Tissue Perfusion related to interruption of blood flow during surgery, dehydration, and use of leg straps

EXPECTED OUTCOME: The patient will maintain normal tissue perfusion at all times.

• Encourage leg exercises hourly while the patient is awake *to prevent venous stasis and thrombosis.*
• Avoid pressure under the knee from pillows, rolled blankets, or prolonged bending of the knee and elevate legs *to help prevent venous stasis.*
• Use elastic stockings or an intermittent pneumatic compression device as ordered *to help prevent stasis of blood.* Thigh-length stockings are more effective than knee-length stockings in reducing the risk of thrombophlebitis.
• Assist with early postoperative ambulation as ordered *to prevent thrombosis.*
• Give anticoagulants as ordered *to reduce clot formation.*

EVALUATION. The goal for deficient fluid volume is met if vital signs and urine output are within normal limits. The goal for ineffective tissue perfusion is met if tissue blood flow remains normal.

Postoperative Pain

Pain is very common after surgery. Each patient's pain experience varies. Incisional pain and painful muscle spasms can occur. Nausea and vomiting, ambulation, coughing, deep breathing, and anxiety can increase postoperative pain. Unrelieved pain has negative physiological effects. It impairs deep breathing and coughing. Early ambulation is more difficult. Increased complications, length of hospital stay, and health care costs can occur. Pain should not be ignored or undertreated. Yet, it has been found that it often is.

Evidenced-based guidelines to manage postoperative pain have been developed (Chou et al., 2016). Increased use of multimodal therapies (e.g., different medications and routes, nonpharmacological therapies) is encouraged. This allows lower doses of opioids to be used and results in fewer side effects. Pain treated along various pathways provides better relief. Use of acetaminophen (Tylenol) and NSAIDS should be considered. Stay informed of advances in pain management. Make pain relief a priority in providing excellent patient care. It will reduce patient suffering and promote a quicker recovery (see Chapter 10).

DATA COLLECTION. Monitor nonverbal indications of pain for patients who are not fully awake ("Gerontological Issues: Postoperative Pain"). Nonverbal indicators of pain may include restlessness, moaning, grimacing, and rubbing or pulling at specific body areas or equipment. Ask patients who are awake about the location of the pain, to rate the presence of pain, and to describe the pain quality, such as sharp, aching, throbbing, or burning. Findings are documented.

Gerontological Issues

Postoperative Pain. Pain is not a normal part of aging. Careful identification of older patients' unique aging changes, chronic diseases, and pain relief needs is required to appropriately treat their postoperative pain.

Cognitively impaired adults are at risk for undertreatment of their postoperative pain. Make these patients a priority to observe, and provide pain relief at the start of your shift and then throughout it. Pain rating scales are available for use with those who are cognitively impaired to determine if they are experiencing pain. Refer to www.consultgeri.org for additional pain assessment tools.

NURSING DIAGNOSES, PLANNING, AND IMPLEMENTATION. See "Nursing Care Plan for the Postoperative Patient."

Urinary Function

DATA COLLECTION. Monitor the patient's urinary status. If the patient has a urinary catheter, note the amount, color, and consistency of the urine. Otherwise, monitor for the patient's first postoperative voiding within 8 hours of their last

CRITICAL THINKING

Mrs. Wood, age 42, returns to the surgical unit after a hysterectomy. Her postoperative vital signs and assessment findings are normal. Mrs. Wood rates her pain level at 9, and the nurse notes that she moans occasionally, repeatedly moves her legs, and pulls at her covers near her abdominal incision. She is drowsy but repeatedly says it hurts. In the perianesthesia care unit, a patient-controlled analgesia (PCA) pump was started. The last dose of medication was delivered 45 minutes ago.

1. What nonverbal pain cues does Mrs. Wood display?
2. How should the nurse document Mrs. Wood's pain?
3. What action should the nurse take to relieve Mrs. Wood's pain?
4. When should the nurse next monitor Mrs. Wood's pain level?
5. If Mrs. Wood indicates that her pain remains unrelieved with the PCA pump, what action should the nurse take? Which team members will the nurse collaborate with?

Suggested answers are at the end of the chapter.

NURSING CARE TIP

- Anticipate the postoperative patient's pain. Regularly assess pain level. Do not wait until the patient asks for the next dose of pain medication. This approach is essential to provide excellent pain relief.
- Monitor the patient using a patient-controlled analgesia (PCA) pump, including the patient's ability to use it, response to the medication, and relief obtained from the medication. Monitor for respiratory depression, hypotension, or other side effects. If PCA is not effective or if side effects occur, notify the surgeon.
- Promote comfort with positioning and warmth. Attention to environmental factors such as bright overhead lighting, excessive noise or visitors, and extreme room temperatures also helps promote comfort.
- Give antiemetics as ordered to relieve the discomfort of nausea and vomiting. If vomiting occurs, turn the patient onto one side to aid emesis removal and prevent aspiration.

voiding. This is to prevent urinary retention and bladder distention. Patients having urinary or gynecological procedures may need to void within 4 to 6 hours. This prevents increased pressure on the surgical site. Urinary catheterization may be needed if the patient is unable to void. Epidural anesthesia and narcotics may cause urinary retention. After outpatient surgery, patients may be required to void before being discharged.

If a patient reports the inability to void, palpate the bladder for distention. Perform a bladder volume measurement as ordered. This will determine the amount of urine in the bladder. Restlessness can be caused by discomfort from a full bladder. A distended bladder requires intervention to empty it. Efforts are made to promote voiding. Inserting a urinary catheter is the last option because of the risk of infection.

The sympathetic nervous system is stimulated by the surgical experience. Fluid is saved by reducing urine output. Initially, urine output may be reduced and concentrated. Then it should gradually increase. It will become less concentrated and lighter in color.

CRITICAL THINKING

Mrs. Owens returned from a bowel resection 2 days ago. She is receiving 1,000 mL of 0.9% normal saline solution over 10 hours on an intravenous (IV) controller pump.

1. At what rate will the IV controller pump be set?
2. How many milliliters should you record as intake for 12 hours?
   • Intake for 12 hours:
     • One 8-oz cup of coffee
     • 4 oz orange juice
     • 6 oz tomato soup
     • ¾ cup gelatin
     • Two cups of water
     • 1,200 mL of 0.9% normal saline solution IV
   • Output for 12 hours:
     • 1,700 mL of urine

Suggested answers are at the end of the chapter.

NURSING DIAGNOSES, PLANNING, AND IMPLEMENTATION

Acute Urinary Retention related to surgery, pain, anesthesia, and altered positioning

EXPECTED OUTCOME: The patient will completely and regularly empty bladder.

• Measure and record output on postoperative patients, especially those undergoing major procedures or urological surgery, older patients, and those with an IV or urinary catheter *to detect urinary elimination problems.*
• Report urinary output of less than 30 mL in 1 hour from the urinary catheter *because this is typically the minimum acceptable output.*
• Recognize that patients who are voiding small amounts frequently (30 to 50 mL every 20 to 30 minutes) or who dribble may have retention overflow and may not be emptying their bladder. This pattern may require catheterization *to empty the bladder and prevent complications.*
• Assist patients to the bathroom or bedside commode, and allow men to stand or sit to urinate if possible *to promote voiding.*

• Warm bedpans *to prevent reflexive sphincter tightening.*
• Use techniques to promote voiding before catheterization for patients who are unable to void (e.g., running water, pouring warm water over a female patient's perineum, or drinking a hot beverage to stimulate voiding) *because catheterization increases the risk of infection.*
• Provide privacy after safety is ensured *to promote voiding.*
• Have patients place their feet solidly on the floor to relax the pelvic muscles *to aid voiding.*
• Notify the surgeon if a patient is uncomfortable, has a distended bladder, or has not voided within the specified time frame *to obtain treatment orders.*

EVALUATION. The goal for urinary retention is met if the patient is able to void without pain or complications.

Surgical Wound Care

An incision is a wound made by a surgeon with a sharp instrument such as a scalpel. A puncture wound has a small opening and is made to insert a tube or drain. Incisions are closed with sutures, staples (Fig. 12.11), surgical adhesives, or adhesive strips. As the wound heals, sutures or staples are removed in 7 to 10 days.

Wounds can be clean or dirty. Clean wounds are surgical wounds that are not infected. Dirty (contaminated) wounds include accidental wounds or surgical incisions exposed to unsterile conditions. Infected wounds and dirty wounds contain microorganisms from trauma, ruptured organs, or infection. Necrotic and infected tissue is removed before infected wounds are closed. This is known as **débridement.**

WOUND HEALING. Wound healing occurs in phases (Table 12.9). Wounds can heal by first (primary) intention, second (secondary) intention, and third (tertiary) intention (Fig. 12.12). In first-intention healing, the edges of the wound are approximated with staples or sutures. This usually results in minimal scarring. For second-intention healing, the wound is usually left open. It heals by granulation. Scarring is usually extensive with prolonged healing. For

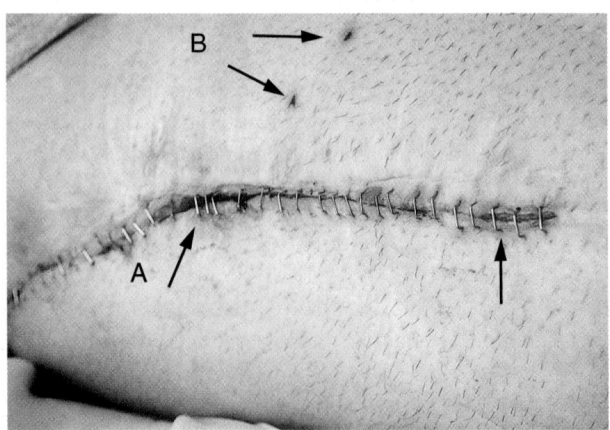

FIGURE 12.11 A stapled incision. (A) Note wound edges not approximated at arrows. (B) Arrows indicate puncture sites where drains were inserted.

Table 12.9

Wound Healing Phases

Phase	Time Frame	Wound Healing	Patient Effect
I	Incision to second postoperative day	Inflammatory response	Fever, malaise
II	Third to 14th postoperative day	Granulation tissue forms	Feeling better
III	Third to sixth postoperative week	Collagen deposited	Raised scar formed
IV	Months to 1 year	Wound contracts and heals	Flat, thin scar

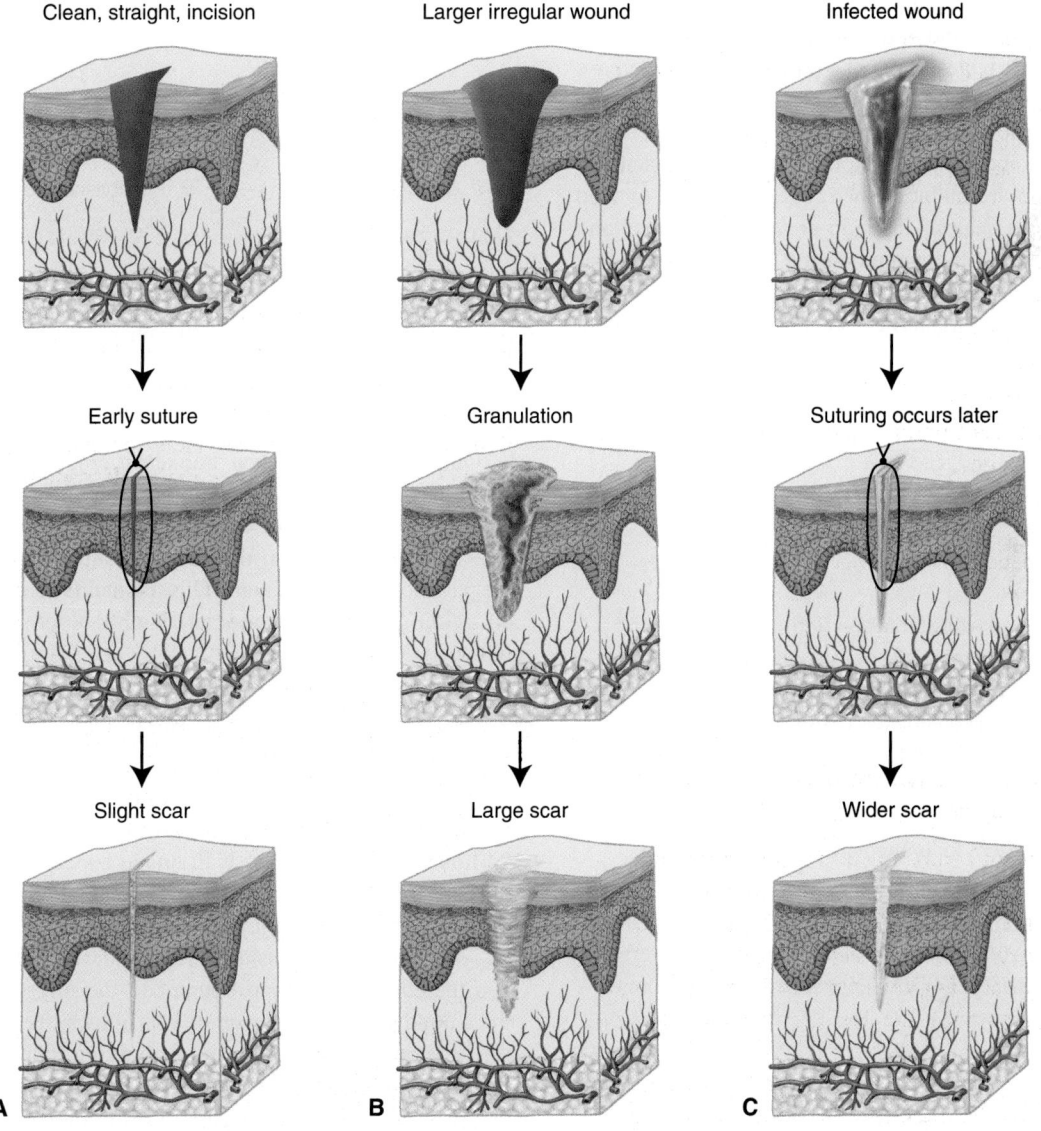

FIGURE 12.12 Wound healing. (A) Primary intention. Wound healing occurs in a clean wound, such as a surgical wound, for which edges are approximated, typically with staples or sutures. Healing occurs quickly with slight scarring. (B) Secondary intention. Large irregular or infected wounds are left open to allow healing to occur from the inside out. Pressure injuries or chronic wounds are often treated this way. Large scarring occurs with lengthy healing time. (C) Tertiary intention. Infected or contaminated wound is left open for a brief time period until wound is clean. Granulation tissue fills in for some wound healing, and then edges are approximated and closed surgically. Wider scarring occurs.

healing by third intention, an infected wound is left open until there is no evidence of infection. Then the wound is surgically closed.

WOUND COMPLICATIONS. Wound problems can include hematoma, infection, dehiscence, and evisceration. A hematoma occurs from bleeding in the wound and into the tissue around the wound. A clot forms from the bleeding. If the clot is large with swelling, the clot may need to be removed by the surgeon.

Infected wounds may be warm, reddened, or tender and have **purulent** drainage (pus). The drainage may have a foul odor. A fever and elevated white blood cell count may be present. Antibiotics are used to treat the infection.

Dehiscence and evisceration are serious wound complications (Fig. 12.13). Wound **dehiscence** is the sudden bursting open of a wound's edges. It may be preceded by an increase in serosanguineous drainage. **Evisceration** is the viscera spilling out of the abdomen. Dehiscence and evisceration often occur with abdominal incisions. Those at increased risk are patients who are malnourished, obese, or older or who have poor wound healing. To help prevent dehiscence and evisceration, support the wound during coughing and other activities that pull on the incision. Applying an abdominal binder can help reduce risk. If evisceration occurs, the patient may report that "something let loose" or "gave way." Pain and vomiting may occur.

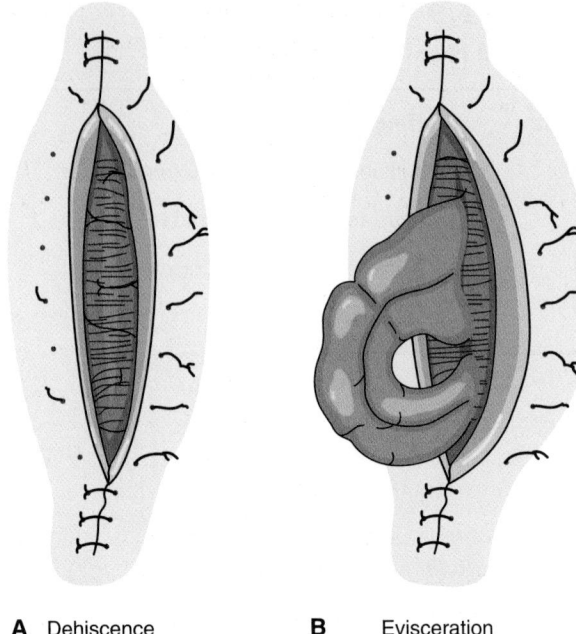

A Dehiscence   **B** Evisceration

FIGURE 12.13 (A) Wound dehiscence. (B) Wound evisceration.

> ### BE SAFE!
>
> If dehiscence or evisceration occurs:
>
> - Position the patient in low Fowler position with knees flexed.
> - Cover the wound with sterile dressings or clean towels moistened with warm sterile normal saline. Apply gentle pressure, and keep the patient still and calm.
> - Notify the surgeon immediately of this surgical emergency.
> - Monitor vital signs for evidence of shock (e.g., tachycardia, tachypnea, dyspnea, hypotension).
> - Infuse intravenous fluids as ordered.
> - Prepare the patient for immediate surgery to close the wound.
>
> For dehisced surgical incisions that resist healing, vacuum-assisted closure (VAC) aids in healing the incision and other wounds (see Chapter 54). VAC applies negative pressure to wound edges.

DATA COLLECTION.

Drains. Drains are inserted into wounds during surgery to prevent accumulation of blood, lymph, or necrotic tissue in wounds that can lead to infection or delayed healing. Drains may work by gravity or suction. Penrose drains are soft, flat, drains. Moderate, pink, **serosanguineous** (consisting of blood and serous fluid) drainage is expected from a Penrose drain. These drains may require frequent dressing changes.

Some drains use suction to gently enhance drainage. They include Jackson-Pratt and Hemovac drains (www.zimmerbiomet.com). These drains are closed systems. They may require periodic emptying.

Output is recorded when drainage is emptied. The amount of drainage expected varies with the type of surgery. Be alert for excessive amounts to report. Specialized drainage systems allow the transfusion of drainage containing blood back to the patient (autotransfusion). This maintains hemoglobin levels without the risks associated with blood transfusions (Chapter 27).

Dressings. Dressings protect the wound, absorb drainage, prevent contamination from body fluids, and provide comfort. They can also apply pressure to reduce swelling or bleeding as in a pressure dressing. The initial dressing is applied in surgery. It is then often removed by the surgeon about 24 hours postoperatively. If drainage appears on the initial dressing, reinforce it with another dressing. Follow surgeon's orders or institution policy.

After the initial dressing is removed, if the wound is dry and the edges intact (approximated), the surgeon can order the wound to be left uncovered. This allows easy observation of the wound and avoidance of applying tape to the skin. Draining wounds are dressed with several layers. They are changed as needed. When the old dressing is removed, it should be done carefully to prevent dislodging of tubes or drains. The condition of the wound is documented with each

---

• **WORD · BUILDING** •
evisceration: e—out + viscera—body organs
serosanguineous: sero—whey + sanguineous—bloody

dressing change. It is normal for the incision to be puffy and red from the inflammatory response. The surrounding skin should be the patient's normal color and temperature. Correct tape application over the dressing is done by gently laying the tape over the dressing and applying even pressure on each side of the wound. Pressure should not be applied on top of the wound by pulling on the tape from one side of the wound to the other side.

NURSING DIAGNOSES, PLANNING, AND IMPLEMENTATION

Risk for Infection related to inadequate primary defenses from surgical wound

See "Nursing Care Plan for the Postoperative Patient."

Impaired Skin Integrity related to surgical incision

EXPECTED OUTCOME: The patient will regain skin integrity within [specify individualized realistic time frame].

- Monitor skin color and temperature and report changes *to detect need for treatment.*
- Monitor dressings and note drainage color, amount, and consistency. *Surgical wound drainage initially is* **sanguineous** *(red). It changes to serosanguineous (pink) and then* **serous** *(pale yellow) after a few hours to days.*
- Promptly report drainage that is bright red, remains sanguineous after a few hours, or is profuse to the surgeon *because the patient may be hemorrhaging.*
- Use standard precautions when changing dressings *to protect yourself and others.*

EVALUATION. The goal for impaired skin integrity is met if the patient's wound heals and skin integrity is regained without delayed healing or complications.

Gastrointestinal Function

Nutritional intake and bowel function can be affected by surgery and anesthesia. Being NPO and having a bowel prep may occur preoperatively. After abdominal surgery, peristalsis, bowel sounds, and flatus usually stop (paralytic ileus). This may last for 24 to 72 hours. Flatus, bowel movements, and an appetite signal the return of gastrointestinal (GI) function. Interventions to shorten ileus time include the following:

- Minimally invasive surgery
- Alvimopan (Entereg) 12 mg given (in a hospitalized setting only) 30 to 90 minutes before surgery and twice daily for up to 15 doses only in 7 days (risk of myocardial infarction); this increases recovery of the functioning of the GI tract after partial small or large bowel resections
- Early ambulation as ordered
- Chewing gum
- Early feeding as ordered
- Avoidance of NG tubes, as complications and delayed feeding can occur

DATA COLLECTION. After abdominal surgery, monitor for the return of flatus and appetite, first bowel movement, nausea or vomiting, or signs of paralytic ileus. Paralytic ileus signs are distention, bloating, and cramps. Document the abdomen as being soft or firm, and flat or distended. The patient's abdominal girth is measured if distention occurs. Report abnormal findings to the surgeon.

Traditionally after GI surgery, bowel sounds were monitored by the nurse. The patient was kept NPO until flatus and bowel sounds returned. Studies show that bowel sounds are not correlated with bowel motility and the patient's ability to safely drink and eat postoperatively. In fact, patients can be hydrated and fed early. This promotes healing and faster recovery.

NURSING DIAGNOSES, PLANNING, AND IMPLEMENTATION

Imbalanced Nutrition: Less Than Body Requirements related to NPO, pain, and nausea

EXPECTED OUTCOME: The patient will resume normal dietary intake and maintain weight within normal limits.

- Maintain IV fluids, parenteral nutrition, or enteral feedings *until the patient resumes oral intake* ("Nutrition Notes: Nourishing the Postoperative Patient").
- Offer water and clear liquids first as ordered, then advance the diet *to promote tolerance.*
- Give antiemetics as ordered *to control nausea and vomiting.*

Constipation related to decreased peristalsis, immobility, altered diet, and opioid side effect

EXPECTED OUTCOME: The patient will return to normal bowel elimination patterns and report freedom from gas pains and constipation within 3 to 4 days postoperatively.

- Encourage early ambulation and exercise *to promote restoration of GI function.*
- Increase comfort by having patient lie prone and pull the knees up to the chest if gas pains occur *to relieve the pain.*
- Monitor elimination and document *to detect problems.*
- Provide stool softeners or laxatives as ordered *to prevent constipation.*

EVALUATION. The goal for imbalanced nutrition is met if patients are able to maintain their baseline weight and resume a normal dietary intake. The goal for constipation is met if patients are free from discomfort and establish a regular bowel elimination pattern.

Mobility

DATA COLLECTION. It is important for the patient to move as much as possible to prevent complications and promote healing. Pain, incisions, tubes, drains, dressings, and other equipment may make movement difficult. You should determine the patient's ability to move in bed, to get out of bed, and to walk. Pain levels that may interfere with movement are assessed. The

Nutrition Notes

Nourishing the Postoperative Patient. After surgery, 5% glucose in water given intravenously is commonly prescribed. Two liters of this solution contain 340 calories. This is insufficient to meet the patient's energy needs. However, it is enough to prevent ketosis from breakdown of adipose tissue. Previously well-nourished adults generally have nutrient reserves for 3 to 4 days of semistarvation. Prevent excessive muscle protein from being used for energy. Deliver adequate nourishment to the patient within 3 days. Boost Breeze and Ensure Clear are incomplete nutritional supplements. They have approximately 30 calories and 1 gram of protein per ounce. They can be used to supplement clear liquid diets as ordered.

To avoid abdominal distention, oral feedings traditionally have been delayed until peristalsis returns. Scientific evidence supporting this practice is lacking. Researchers are testing this practice.

Patients usually progress from clear liquids to a regular diet as soon as possible. If "diet as tolerated" is prescribed, the patient should be asked, "What sounds good?" Offering a full dinner when the patient doesn't feel well may "turn off" the appetite.

After gastrointestinal surgery, oral food and fluids are deferred longer than with other surgeries to allow healing. When specific amounts of intake are prescribed, those limits should be strictly implemented to preserve the suture lines. After oral and throat surgery, no red liquids are given. This is so bleeding can be seen and vomitus is not mistaken for blood.

Specific nutrients necessary for healing include the following:

- Vitamin C for collagen formation
- Vitamin K for blood clotting
- Zinc for tissue growth, skin integrity, and cell-mediated immunity
- Protein for controlling fluid balance and edema, for manufacturing antibodies and white blood cells, and for building scar tissue

patient's tolerance for activity is observed. Patient understanding of how to perform exercises is identified.

NURSING DIAGNOSES, PLANNING, AND IMPLEMENTATION

Impaired Physical Mobility related to surgery, decreased strength, and movement restriction

EXPECTED OUTCOME: The patient will resume normal physical activity.

- Position patients in bed with pillows *to support the body in good alignment.*

- Turn patients at least every 2 hours, alternating from supine to side to side if not contraindicated, *to prevent complications.*
- Encourage patients to move themselves *to increase circulation and promote lung expansion.*
- If ambulation is not possible, encourage hourly exercises (e.g., deep breathing, range of motion of all joints, and isometric exercises of the abdominal, gluteal, and leg muscles) while awake *to prevent complications.*
- If patients cannot perform active range-of-motion exercises, perform passive joint range of motion *to prevent complications.*
- Raise the head of the bed slowly *to let the circulatory system adjust to the position change.*
- If patients report dizziness or feeling faint, lower the head of the bed *to let the circulatory system adjust more slowly.*
- Ensure patients wear nonslip footwear *to ambulate safely.*
- Allow patients to sit on the side of bed prior to standing and pedal the feet to "wake up" the muscles controlling the arteries *to prepare for ambulation* (see Fig. 12.10).
- If a patient tolerates sitting, assist the patient to ambulate *to promote healing and reduce complications.* To rise, the patient should keep eyes forward and move slowly until feeling adjusted to being up. Usually the patient ambulates a short distance the first time and increases the distance as tolerated. One or two health care workers should assist the patient and use a gait (walking) belt for safety. Walkers with wheels and seats also may be used for support and for resting if the patient becomes dizzy or tired. If the patient feels faint or dizzy or if vital signs change, help the patient back to bed. A wheelchair may be needed for safe transport back to the room.

EVALUATION. The goal for impaired physical mobility is met if the patient can increase ambulation and resume normal activities.

Postoperative Patient Discharge

Discharge planning begins during preadmission testing. It is ongoing after admission. This ensures a timely discharge. When the patient meets discharge criteria, the surgeon discharges the patient.

Ambulatory Surgery

DISCHARGE CRITERIA. Usually, a patient is a candidate for discharge 1 hour after surgery if the PACU discharge scoring system or clinical discharge criteria are met (see Box 12.5). Clinical discharge criteria include stable vital signs, no bleeding, no nausea or vomiting, and controlled pain that is not severe. For certain surgical procedures (e.g., urological, gynecological, or hernia surgery), the patient may need to void before discharge. The patient should also be able to sit up without dizziness. Patients meeting discharge criteria are discharged by the surgeon. They are released to a responsible adult. Patients are not allowed to drive themselves home. This is because of the effects of anesthesia and medications.

DISCHARGE INSTRUCTIONS. Patients and their families are given written discharge instructions. The caregiver of an older patient should participate in the discharge instruction session. This promotes understanding for care and reporting of complications. The instruction form is signed by the patient or an authorized representative to indicate understanding. Send prescriptions and a copy of the instructions with the patient. Encourage the patient to rest for 24 to 48 hours. Instruct the patient to avoid operating machinery, driving, drinking alcoholic beverages, and making major decisions for 24 hours. The effects of surgery and anesthesia can alter energy levels and thinking ability. The surgeon will order fluid, dietary, activity, or work restrictions.

Patients are taught wound care, medication information (including side effects), and complications to report to the surgeon. Phone numbers for the surgeon, surgical facility, and emergency care are provided. Patients are told to call to make a follow-up appointment.

Inpatient Surgery

DISCHARGE CRITERIA. The surgeon determines the patient's readiness for discharge from the hospital. Before discharge, a complete assessment of the patient is performed and documented.

DISCHARGE INSTRUCTIONS. Patients and families are taught wound care, medication information, and signs and symptoms of complications to report to the surgeon. The surgeon orders fluid, dietary, activity, or work restrictions and the date for a follow-up visit to the surgeon. A copy of the signed written instructions and prescriptions are given to the patient. If further teaching or reinforcement is needed, a referral to a home health care nurse can be requested.

Home Health Hints

A referral for home health care is made when the patient who had surgery needs skilled nursing care at home after discharge. (See Chapter 16 for examples of skilled care.)

It is helpful for caregivers to keep a notebook in the hospital and continue it at home. Treatments, medicines, observations, procedures, health care provider and nurse visits, instructions, and therapies with dates and times can be recorded.

When the patient returns home, the home health care nurse can provide the following guidance to caregivers for setting up the living area, bathroom, and equipment the patient will use:

- It is helpful if the bedroom can be on the same floor as the bathroom and kitchen. This may require temporary use of a den or living room for sleeping.
- For the patient on bedrest, a hospital bed with full side rails helps with a variety of position changes and provides a better working height for the caregiver.
- Lift sheets made of folded twin sheets are needed as well as extra pillows for positioning and splinting.
- A bedside stand is needed for personal care items.
- A bedside commode can be placed near the bed if the patient cannot walk to the bathroom. A bedpan or urinal may be needed. A functional female urinal is easier to use than a bedpan.
- A handheld shower is convenient and allows the patient more independence in bathing.
- Installation of grab bars and tub stools as well as skid-proofing of a shower or tub are important safety measures to help prevent falls. Physical or occupational therapy can make specific recommendations.
- For the patient prescribed anticoagulants and/or elastic stockings, the importance of and instructions for using them to prevent deep venous thrombosis should be reinforced.
- Nutritional status should be monitored and reported to the registered nurse to aid wound healing.
- The patient and caregivers should be instructed on hand hygiene before and after wound care to prevent infection.
- For prescribed pain medication, pain management and potential side effects to report should be discussed.

SUGGESTED ANSWERS TO CRITICAL THINKING

Mrs. Wood

1. Moaning occasionally, moving legs restlessly, and pulling covers near abdominal incision are nonverbal pain cues.
2. Document pain levels by actual observations: occasional moaning, restless leg movements, and pulling of covers near abdominal incision. Also use the patient's statement: "It hurts." Because Mrs. Wood is too drowsy to use the pain scale, other data are used.

When Mrs. Wood is more awake, explanation of the pain scale should be reinforced and used.

3. Encourage patient to use patient-controlled analgesia (PCA) button if there is pain. Reinforce teaching on the PCA pump as able. Administer additional multimodality medications as ordered. Also, consider other pain relief measures such as patient warmth and positioning as well as environmental issues such as bright lighting, room temperature, and noise.

Continued

SUGGESTED ANSWERS TO CRITICAL THINKING—cont'd

4. After the PCA pump is pushed by the patient, monitor pain level in at least 30 minutes to determine pain relief. If Mrs. Wood is asleep, she should not be awakened unless it is necessary. Nonverbal cues should be observed. Count respirations and document. After Mrs. Wood is more alert, PCA monitoring is done hourly or per agency policy.

5. Document pain level such as on a scale of 0 to 10. Collaborate with the surgeon for report of inadequate pain relief.

Mrs. Owens

1. 100 mL per hour. Intravenous pumps are always set to deliver the amount of milliliters per hour. Divide the total volume of 1,000 mL by the total time of 10 hours = 100 mL per hour.

2. Intake = 2,400 mL
   To calculate this, remember these conversions:
   30 mL = 1 oz
   1 cup = 8 oz (don't supersize the cup!)
   Calculations:
   1 8-oz cup of coffee = $1 \times 8 \times 30$ = 240 mL
   4 oz orange juice = 4×30 = 120 mL
   6 oz tomato soup = 6×30 = 180 mL
   3/4 cup gelatin = $3/4 \times 8 \times 30$ = 180 mL
   2 cups of water = $2 \times 8 \times 30$ = 480 mL
   1,200 mL of 0.9 normal saline IV

   The patient's output does not affect the intake total, so it is not used for this calculation.

Review Questions

1. Which of the following should the nurse implement to reduce surgical risk factors for the preoperative patient? **Select all that apply.**
   1. Play music of patient's choice.
   2. Avoid discussion of fears.
   3. Reinforce pain control methods.
   4. Show use of incentive spirometer.
   5. Monitor blood glucose for a patient with diabetes.
   6. Teach to perform leg exercises hourly while awake.

2. Which of the following actions can the licensed vocational nurse take for a patient's care in the preoperative phase? **Select all that apply.**
   1. Assist in data collection.
   2. Explain the surgical procedure.
   3. Obtain preoperative orders.
   4. Conduct the preoperative anesthesia interview.
   5. Play requested music for patient.
   6. Reinforce teaching of leg exercises.

3. The licensed practical nurse is caring for a patient preoperatively who is to provide consent for surgery. Which of the following is within this nurse's scope of practice related to the patient giving consent for the surgery? **Select all that apply.**
   1. Answering surgical procedure questions
   2. Providing informed consent
   3. Witnessing minor patient's signature on the consent
   4. Requesting patient questions be referred to surgeon
   5. Reading the consent to a patient before it is signed
   6. Witnessing the patient's signature on the consent

4. The nurse is contributing to the teaching plan for an older adult. Which of the following should the nurse recommend using to improve the learning experience for the older adult? **Select all that apply.**
   1. Sit near a window with bright sunlight.
   2. Use large black-on-white printed materials.
   3. Sit in front of the patient for best visibility.
   4. Provide positive reinforcement.
   5. Provide background noise.
   6. Teach most important information first.

5. The nurse is contributing to the plan of care for a patient undergoing a cholecystectomy. Which of the following interventions should the nurse recommend including to help prevent atelectasis for this patient? **Select all that apply.**
   1. Ambulation
   2. Coughing and deep breathing
   3. Holding breath as turning
   4. Leg exercises
   5. Pain control
   6. Restricting fluids

6. The nurse is caring for a patient after thoracic surgery. Which of the following would the nurse evaluate as indicating that interventions to prevent respiratory complications have been effective? **Select all that apply.**
   1. Pain level "2"
   2. No abdominal distention
   3. Clear lung sounds
   4. Good appetite
   5. Arterial blood gases normal
   6. Airway patent

7. The nurse is caring for a patient who returned from surgery 3 hours ago. Which of these findings would the nurse recognize as being the most urgent to report to the surgeon?
   1. Fever
   2. Nausea
   3. Polyuria
   4. Tachycardia

8. The nurse is assisting with data collection on a patient following ambulatory surgery for a kidney biopsy. Which of the following criterion would the nurse evaluate as indicating patient readiness for discharge after ambulatory surgery? **Select all that apply.**
   1. Ability to drive an automobile
   2. Ability to ambulate 50 feet
   3. Absence of nausea or vomiting
   4. Being free of pain
   5. Presence of responsible adult
   6. Voided 350 mL of urine

Answer rationales available in your online resources.

ANSWERS 1. 1, 3, 4, 5, 6; 2. 1, 5, 6; 3. 4, 5, 6; 4. 2, 3, 4, 6; 5. 1, 2, 5; 6. 3, 5, 6; 7. 4; 8. 3, 5, 6

Key Points

Find the chapter key points in your online resources available through Davis Edge.

Additional Resources

DAVIS **edge.** Use the scratch off code on the inside front cover of your book to access online quizzes that will help you to improve your scores on course exams and prepare for NCLEX-PN®.

Study Guide

CHAPTER 13

Nursing Care of Patients With Emergent Conditions and Disaster/Bioterrorism Response

Patricia Williams

KEY TERMS

abrasion (ah-BRAY-zhun)
amputation (am-pew-TAY-shun)
anaphylactic shock (an-uh-fah-LAK-tik SHAWK)
anaphylaxis (an-uh-fah-LAK-sis)
anthrax (AN-thraks)
asphyxia (as-FIX-ee-ah)
bioterrorism (BY-oh-TARE-UR-is-um)
botulism (BOTCH-uh-liz-um)
capillary refill (KAP-ih-lar-ee REE-fil)
cardiac tamponade (KAR-dee-yak TAM-pon-AYD)
cardiogenic shock (KAR-dee-oh-JEN-ik SHAWK)
distributive shock (dis-TRIB-u-tiv SHAWK)
epinephrine (EP-ih-NEF-rin)
flail chest (FLAYL CHEST)
gastric lavage (GAS-trik la-VAHJ)
hypovolemic shock (HY-poh-voh-LEE-mik SHAWK)
laceration (las-ur-AY-shun)
obstructive shock (ub-STRUK-tiv SHAWK)
plague (PLAYG)
shock (SHAWK)
tachycardia (TAK-ih-KAR-dee-yah)
tachypnea (TAK-ip-NEE-ah)
tetanus (TET-nus)
triage (TREE-ahj)

CHAPTER CONCEPTS

Thermoregulation
Trauma

LEARNING OUTCOMES

1. Explain the components of the primary survey.
2. Plan nursing interventions for a trauma victim.
3. Identify the symptoms and care for an inhalation injury.
4. Describe the stages of hypothermia.
5. Describe the stages of hyperthermia.
6. Explain the priorities of care for poison overdose.
7. Describe the role of the licensed practical nurse/licensed vocational nurse in a disaster response.
8. Discuss bioterrorist agents and subsequent care if exposed or infected.

The ability to recognize an emergent condition is essential in nursing. This allows the nurse to prioritize and provide quick assessments and interventions. Upon arrival in the emergency department (ED), most patients are triaged by a registered nurse (RN). During this process, the RN evaluates the patient's condition. A rapid assessment of the patient is performed (Fig. 13.1). This allows the patient to be provided timely care. This chapter presents specific emergent conditions with application of the nursing process.

PRIMARY SURVEY

What do you think the nurse does first when a patient arrives in the ED? An initial assessment in order to recognize life-threatening conditions and determine priorities of care is done. The patient's airway, breathing, circulation status, and any disability are noted; the patient's area of distress is exposed (clothing removed) if necessary. This process is known as the primary survey:

• A=Airway
• B=Breathing
• C=Circulation
• D=Disability/central nervous system
• E=Exposure

A—Airway
The airway is the most important part of the primary survey. The neck should not be hyperextended, flexed, or rotated until a spinal injury is ruled out. Any movement can worsen a cervical spine injury.

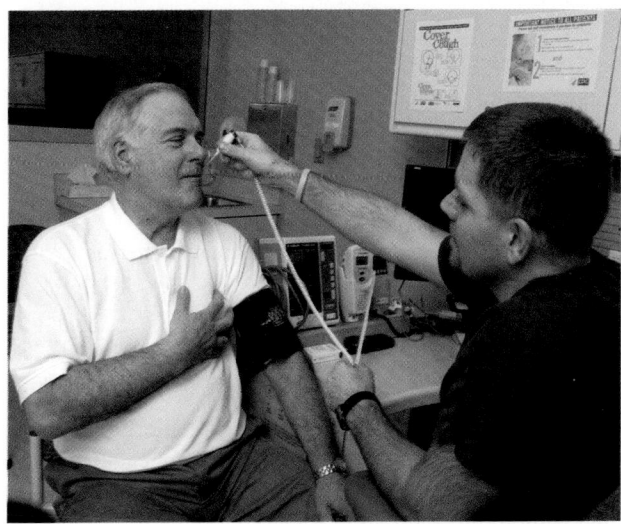

FIGURE 13.1 Triage nurse evaluating patient who has just arrived in the emergency department.

During cardiopulmonary resuscitation (CPR), if there is a possible or known spinal injury, the jaw-thrust maneuver rather than the chin-lift maneuver must be used (Fig. 13.2). This avoids movement of the head and neck. The airway is inspected for obstruction. This can be caused by loose teeth, foreign objects, bleeding, and vomitus. Any visible airway obstructions are removed using suction.

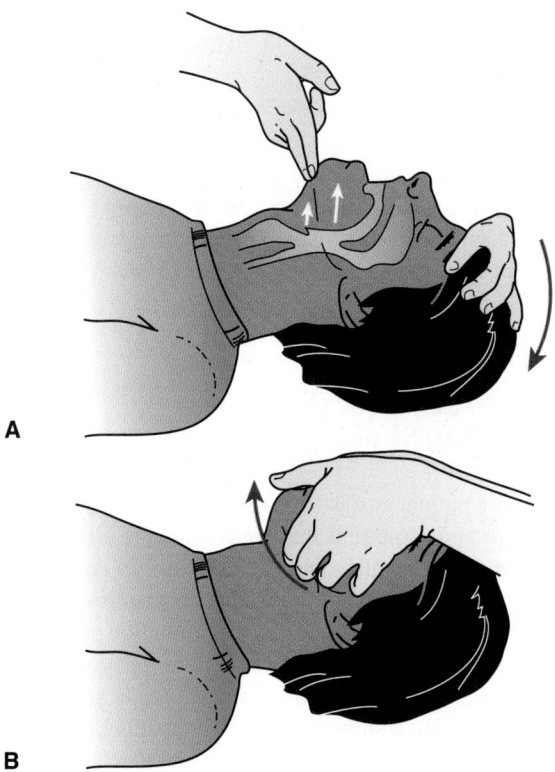

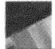

FIGURE 13.2 (A) Chin-lift maneuver is used to open the airway. (B) Jaw-thrust maneuver is used to open the airway if the patient might have a head or neck injury.

Airway adjuncts can be used to keep the airway open. These include nasopharyngeal or oropharyngeal airways. Additional airway support and mechanical ventilation may be required. Advanced airway adjuncts include endotracheal intubation or cricothyrotomy. These airway procedures are performed by specially trained emergency personnel or health care providers (HCPs).

B—Breathing

After the airway is opened, the patient is assessed for spontaneous breathing and respiratory rate and depth. The nurse observes whether the patient's chest rises and falls spontaneously. Breath sounds are auscultated bilaterally. If the patient is not breathing, interventions are performed. The patient can be ventilated with a mouth-to-face mask or a bag-valve face mask. For an unconscious patient, endotracheal intubation is the preferred method of establishing and maintaining an airway. It protects the lungs from aspiration (see Fig. 29.28).

C—Circulation

The carotid pulse is palpated for quality and rate. The skin is inspected for color and temperature. External bleeding is controlled by external pressure. Elevation is used as needed. Life-threatening conditions are noted that can compromise circulation. Interventions are provided. Conditions that can compromise circulation include internal bleeding, shock resulting from hemorrhage, or major burns. Large-gauge intravenous (IV) cannulas (16- or 18-gauge) are inserted for fluid resuscitation. If the patient does not have a pulse, CPR is started. If a pulse can be palpated, vital signs are taken and recorded.

D—Disability/Central Nervous System

To detect a serious central nervous system injury, a brief neurologic assessment is conducted. This determines level of consciousness. Levels of consciousness can include alert (A) and responds to verbal stimuli (V), responds to painful stimuli (P), or is unresponsive (U). To see response to painful stimuli, a painful stimulus is applied. This can include applying periorbital pressure or applying pressure with a pen to the lateral outer aspect of the second or third interphalangeal joint. The patient is observed for the type of response to the pain. The response is documented. Movement of each extremity is also noted.

E—Exposure

To allow for a complete visual assessment, clothing must be removed. Respect the patient's dignity as this is done. Keep the patient covered to reduce heat loss and prevent shivering. Look for injuries and medical alert jewelry.

SECONDARY SURVEY

For victims of severe trauma, a secondary survey is conducted. This identifies areas of injury or medical problems that are not life-threatening but do require treatment. Major body areas that can sustain serious injury are quickly examined to detect additional injuries (Table 13.1). These

Table 13.1
Components of the Secondary Survey

Head	Inspect for lacerations, bleeding from orifices. Check pupil size and response to light. Are pupils equal in size?
Chest	Auscultate for breath sounds in all lung fields. Inspect for lacerations, wounds, and foreign bodies.
Abdomen	Auscultate for bowel sounds in all four quadrants. Palpate for areas of tenderness and rigidity. Inspect for lacerations, wounds, and foreign bodies. Inspect for ecchymosis (bruising).
Extremities	Inspect for lacerations, wounds, and foreign bodies. Inspect for injuries and deformities. Note areas of tenderness. Palpate for pulses. Evaluate temperature and capillary refill, and compare the left to the right extremities.

include the head, spine, chest, abdomen, and musculoskeletal system. Each major body area is inspected and palpated. Deformity, bruising, open wounds, bleeding, and pain are noted.

SHOCK

Shock is a condition of progressively decreasing blood pressure. It results in inadequate tissue perfusion (see Chapter 9). There are three phases of shock: compensated, progressive, and irreversible. During the initial phase of shock (compensated), compensatory adjustments allow the body to adapt to the circulatory changes. In the second phase (progressive), compensatory mechanisms fail. This results in inadequate tissue and cellular perfusion. It causes cell death, if left untreated. In the third and last stage (irreversible), the patient no longer responds to treatment.

There are four types of shock. **Hypovolemic shock** signs and symptoms are caused by a decrease in the circulating blood volume. **Cardiogenic shock** signs and symptoms result from cardiac failure. **Obstructive shock** is caused by a blockage of blood flow in the cardiovascular circuit outside the heart. It results in signs and symptoms of reduced blood flow and oxygenation. **Distributive shock** is caused by excessive dilation of the venules and arterioles. It causes signs and symptoms of decreased blood pressure. Therapeutic interventions for shock are listed in Box 13.1.

Box 13.1
Guiding Principles for Treating Shock

- Maintain an open airway and give oxygen as ordered.
- Control external bleeding by direct pressure.
- Keep the patient supine if possible.
- Accurately record vital signs.
- Give intravenous fluids as ordered.
- Give the patient nothing to eat or drink until surgery is ruled out.

Anaphylaxis

Anaphylaxis is the response to a severe allergic reaction. The reaction can occur suddenly. It can happen after initial contact with an allergen or any subsequent exposure. Signs and symptoms result from a massive release of chemical mediators from mast cells and basophils (Box 13.2). Chemical mediators lead to vasodilation and capillary leakage. This results in hypotension. It eventually leads to vascular collapse.

Anaphylactic shock is a form of distributive shock. There is no loss of blood. Excessive vasodilation occurs. Bronchi constrict. This makes movement of air into the lungs increasingly difficult. Increased fluid and mucus enter the bronchial passages. The body becomes rapidly deprived of oxygen. The fluid and constricted bronchi cause wheezing. Signs of severe anaphylaxis include hypotension due to vasodilation, decreased level of consciousness due to decreased oxygenation, and respiratory distress with stridor and cyanosis due to airway constriction and fluid.

> ### NURSING CARE TIP
> One of the causes of anaphylactic shock is a latex allergy reaction. The use of latex-free products limits latex exposure. This reduces the risk of developing a latex allergy.

Nursing Process for the Patient Experiencing Shock
Data Collection

To monitor a patient at risk for shock, you will need to recognize signs and symptoms that are common to all types of shock (Box 13.3). Identify the patient's level of consciousness. A progressive decline in level of consciousness indicates an urgent need for intervention. Monitor the patient for any changes. Pulse indicates the strength of the heart's contractions. Because a pulse is an immediate indicator of the patient's condition, it should be taken frequently during any emergency condition. Blood pressure changes can occur

· WORD · BUILDING ·

anaphylaxis: an—without + phylaxis—protection

Box 13.2

Signs and Symptoms of an Allergic Reaction

- Generalized itching and flushing
- Urticaria (hives)
- Swelling of the lips, tongue, or uvula
- Dyspnea
- Bronchospasm, wheezing, and stridor
- Chest tightness and cough
- Crampy abdominal pain and vomiting
- Anxiety
- Hypotension

Box 13.3

Common Signs and Symptoms of Shock

- Restlessness and anxiety
- Thirst
- Pale skin color
- Cold and clammy skin
- Weak, rapid, thready pulse
- Shallow, rapid, labored breathing
- Gradually and steadily falling blood pressure
- Altered level of consciousness

rapidly. However, they do not usually change as swiftly as the pulse does.

Skin temperature and color changes can occur with shock. Severe blood loss activates the "fight-or-flight" response in the sympathetic nervous system. This causes the skin to become cool and clammy. This occurs when peripheral blood vessels constrict to shunt blood to vital organs. Skin color is influenced by the presence of circulating blood in the vessels of the skin. Insufficient circulation produces pale, white, or ashen skin. In patients with deeply pigmented skin, these color changes can be seen in the nailbeds, conjunctiva of the eye, or mucous membranes of the mouth.

Capillary refill is checked on the nailbeds to evaluate arterial circulation to an extremity. Compress the nailbed to produce blanching (lighter color change) and release. Count the seconds it takes for the color to return. Normally, nailbed color should return within 3 seconds after pressure is released. Older adults may typically have a longer refill time. Patients in shock can have a longer or absent capillary refill.

LEARNING TIP
Gently squeeze and release your own nailbed. Do you see the color change? Count the seconds until the color returns. That is your capillary refill time.

Nursing Diagnoses, Planning, and Implementation

Risk for Shock related to hypotension, hypovolemia, or hypoxia

EXPECTED OUTCOME: The patient will maintain vital signs within normal baseline range.

- Obtain frequent vital signs and oxygen saturation *to monitor patient status for intervention.*
- Monitor intake and output *to monitor fluid status.*
- Administer oxygen *to maintain Spo₂ (oxygen saturation) greater than 90%.*
- Maintain isotonic IV fluids as ordered *to maintain fluid volume and thus blood pressure.*

Risk for Ineffective Peripheral Tissue Perfusion related to decreased circulating blood volume secondary to internal and/or external bleeding

EXPECTED OUTCOME: The patient's bleeding will be controlled to maintain vital signs within limits normal for the individual.

- Apply direct pressure to external bleeding site *to stop the flow of blood and allow normal coagulation to occur.*
- Elevate a bleeding limb and combine with direct pressure *to help stop bleeding.*
- When direct pressure and elevation do not control hemorrhage, pressure-point control should be attempted *to stop the bleeding* (Fig. 13.3). The chosen artery for pressure-point control must be proximal to the injury site and must be over a bony structure.
- Monitor vital signs continually, record, and report to the HCP *to identify early changes in vital signs indicative of progressing shock.*

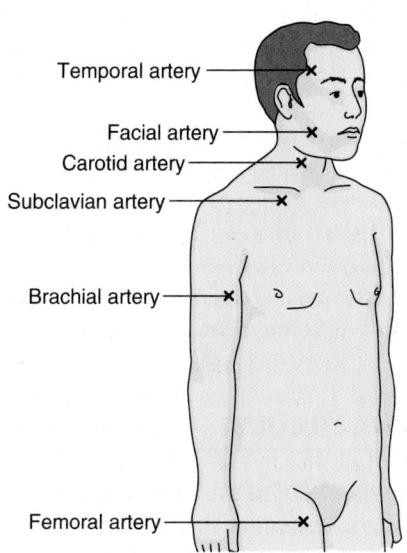

FIGURE 13.3 Arterial pressure points to control bleeding.

- Use blankets *to help keep the patient from getting cold;* however, the patient also should not be allowed to overheat *because this causes peripheral blood vessels to dilate, which draws blood away from vital organs.*
- Maintain IV fluids as ordered *to increase circulating volume* (IV fluid contraindicated in cardiogenic shock).

Risk for Allergic Reaction related to exaggerated immune response to substances

EXPECTED OUTCOME: The patient will implement the plan for treating an allergic reaction.

- Give **epinephrine** (Adrenalin; hormone secreted by adrenal medulla in response to stimulation of sympathetic nervous system) as ordered to *help reverse anaphylaxis and alleviate allergy symptoms.* The recommended route is intramuscular (Posner & Camargo, 2017).
- Seek immediate medical attention *because effects of epinephrine are temporary.*
- Give antihistamines and histamine-2 receptor antagonists (Zantac or Tagamet) as ordered for second-line therapy *to control rash, hives, and pruritus.*
- Give steroids as ordered, usually in gradually tapered doses, *to prevent return of symptoms.*

Ineffective Airway Clearance related to allergic airways

EXPECTED OUTCOME: The patient will maintain a patent airway and clear breath sounds at all times.

- Monitor breath sounds *to detect abnormal sounds such as wheezing.*
- Administer oxygen as ordered *to maintain the pulse oximetry at 95% or greater.*
- Position patient upright for optimal respiration *to allow maximal lung expansion.*
- Encourage patient to breathe deep and cough *to clear airways.*

Evaluation

If interventions have been effective, the blood pressure will improve to within normal limits for the patient. The patient will demonstrate a strong pulse and warm, dry skin. The patient will be less anxious. The patient should show an immediate reversal of shock symptoms. Breathing becomes easy. Blood pressure and pulse return to the normal range. Breath sounds become clear. Rash, hives, and pruritus subside.

MAJOR TRAUMA

Mechanism of Injury

It is important to determine the mechanism of injury for a victim of major trauma ("Gerontological Issues: Injuries Caused by Falls Versus Battery or Assault"). Injuries are classified as either penetrating or blunt. Penetrating (open) injuries can be caused by a sharp object (e.g., broken glass or a knife) or by projectiles traveling at high speed (e.g., bullets or fragments from an explosion). In blunt (closed) injuries, the skin surface is intact. An injury from blunt trauma may extend beyond the point of impact to surrounding and underlying structures. For example, a blow to the chest can cause rib fractures. These fractures could then cause a laceration or hematoma (collection of blood) of the spleen.

Damage caused by a gunshot wound and the trajectory of the bullet depends on the projectile mass, the type of tissue struck, the striking velocity, and the range. Entrance wounds are round or oval. They can be surrounded by a rim of abrasion. Powder burns are visible if the firearm was discharged at close range. Documentation of these wounds should include a clear description of their appearance. It should not include the words *entry* or *exit* as this is determined by trained experts. Patients with gunshot wounds near the level of the diaphragm are evaluated for both abdominal and thoracic injuries.

Surface Trauma

Surface trauma includes closed wounds (skin intact) and open wounds (skin open). Types of closed wounds include contusions (bruising) and hematomas. Types of open wounds include abrasions, punctures, lacerations, avulsions, and amputations.

Abrasions are a scraping away of the epidermal and dermal layers of the skin. They bleed very little. However, they can be extremely painful because of inflamed nerve endings. Dirt can become ground into abrasions. This increases the risk of infection, especially for large areas of skin.

Puncture wounds result from sharp, narrow objects such as knives, nails, or high-velocity bullets. They can often be deceptive. The entrance wound can be small with little or no bleeding. It is difficult to estimate the extent of damage to underlying organs as a result. Puncture wounds usually do not bleed profusely unless they are located in the chest or abdomen.

Lacerations are open wounds resulting from snagging or tearing of tissue. Skin can be partly or completely torn away. Lacerations vary in depth and can be irregular in shape. They can cause significant bleeding if blood vessels are involved.

Avulsions involve a full-thickness skin loss. The wound edges cannot be approximated. This type of injury is usually seen in machine, lawn-mower, or power-tool accidents.

An **amputation** is a partial or complete severing of a body part. In cases of complete amputation, the arteries usually spasm and retract into the tissue. This results in less bleeding than does a partial amputation, in which the lacerated arteries continue to bleed. If the patient has sustained an amputation, bleeding is controlled with direct pressure and elevation. A tourniquet is applied only as a last resort. If a tourniquet is needed, it should be made of wide material,

· WORD · BUILDING ·
epinephrine: epi—on + nephros—kidney

Gerontological Issues

Injuries Caused by Falls Versus Battery or Assault.
Older adults are at a high risk for falls. A fall can put them at risk for bruises, abrasions, cuts, and fractures. After a fall, patients must be evaluated for the reason for the fall. Arrhythmias, syncope, or neurologic issues can cause falls. Nurses can help the health care provider ask questions and perform assessments that identify an injury's cause in case the patient is a victim of abuse or neglect rather than a fall.

Injuries related to falls have a predictable injury pattern related to the history and report of the fall. When an older adult attempts to break a fall, there is bruising of the hands and knees. Additional bruising or injuries to the front of the body, arms, and head could be caused by hitting something during the fall. Skin tears on the arms are common with a fall. If someone sees the older adult starting to fall, they may try to steady the person by grabbing the arms that results in tearing the skin. Ask questions to be sure that the report of the fall incident is consistent with the presenting injuries.

Any unexplained bruises, burns, abrasions, cuts, fractures, evidence of old injuries or bruises, burns, and cuts that are in different stages of healing suggest abuse. The pattern of an injury can also suggest abuse: for example, cigarette burns in areas covered with clothing; bruises or friction burns in a ring around the neck, ankles, or wrists; welts, burns, or bruises in the outline of a hand or belt buckle; multiple similar injuries in an area, such as whip marks across the buttocks or back of the legs; defensive injury pattern of bruising; and trauma to the hands and forearms.

Abuse or the suspicion of abuse must be reported by health care professionals to a designated state agency. This agency will investigate the report of suspected abuse. It is not the nurse's responsibility to prove that there has been abuse or neglect. The nurse must only report the incident.

such as a blood pressure cuff. The wide material is less damaging to nerves and blood vessels. A dressing is applied to the amputated extremity, which is referred to as the stump. The stump is covered with sterile saline–moistened gauze followed by dry gauze. This is held in place with an elastic bandage for pressure. Amputated parts are sent with the patient for possible reattachment. At the ED, the amputated part is rinsed with saline solution. It is then wrapped in sterile gauze and placed in a sealed plastic bag. The bag is then placed on ice (not covered with ice or in ice water). The goal is to keep the body part cool without causing further damage from the cold ice.

When a patient is impaled by an object, it is vital that the object not be removed unless it is obstructing the airway. Removing an impaled object can cause additional trauma. It can also cause uncontrollable internal bleeding. Impaled objects should never be cut off, broken off, or shortened unless transportation to the ED is otherwise impossible. A bulky dressing is applied around the object to stabilize it and reduce motion.

Tetanus

Tetanus is a disease caused by the bacillus *Clostridium tetani*. Its spores enter the body through an opening in the skin or a wound. The spores produce toxins. The toxins affect the central nervous system by blocking inhibitor impulses. This causes muscle contraction and spasm. The first sign of tetanus may be jaw muscle spasms (lockjaw). Other signs include abdominal rigidity, difficulty swallowing and breathing, painful muscle stiffness, and seizures. Tetanus can cause death in 10% to 20% of generalized tetanus cases (Centers for Disease Control and Prevention, 2017). Emergency treatment includes hospitalization, airway maintenance, human tetanus immune globulin (intramuscular), muscle spasm control, wound care, and tetanus toxoid booster. Prophylactic tetanus vaccinations should begin at 2 months of age and be followed by a series of pediatric immunizations until age 15. Thereafter, booster vaccinations are recommended every 10 years in the absence of an open wound.

Head Trauma

Sharp blows to the head can cause shifting of intracranial contents. This leads to brain tissue contusion. The pathophysiology of head trauma can be divided into two phases. The first phase is the initial injury that cannot be reversed. The second phase involves intracerebral bleeding and edema from the initial injury. This causes increased intracranial pressure (ICP). Management of head trauma is directed at the second phase. It involves decreasing ICP. Early and late signs and symptoms of ICP are listed in Box 13.4.

Spinal Trauma

Spinal cord injury most often results from motor vehicle crashes, sports injuries, falls, and assaults. The cervical spine is especially vulnerable to traumatic injury. All trauma patients should be treated as though they have a spinal cord injury until proven otherwise. Moving a patient with a vertebral injury can cause displacement of the injured bones. This can damage the spinal cord. Patients should be moved only by trained professionals. Stabilizing the neck and back with a cervical collar and backboard is essential until a spinal cord injury is ruled out (Fig. 13.4).

> **BE SAFE!**
> Do not move a patient with suspected vertebral or spinal cord injury. Paramedics, emergency medical technicians, or health care providers should guide movement of the patient to prevent further injury to the spinal cord.

Box 13.4

Signs and Symptoms of Increased Intracranial Pressure

Early Signs and Symptoms
• Headache
• Nausea and vomiting
• Amnesia
• Changes in speech
• Altered level of consciousness or drowsiness

Late Signs and Symptoms
• Dilated nonreactive pupils
• Unresponsiveness
• Abnormal posturing
• Widening pulse pressure
• Decreased pulse rate
• Changes in respiratory pattern

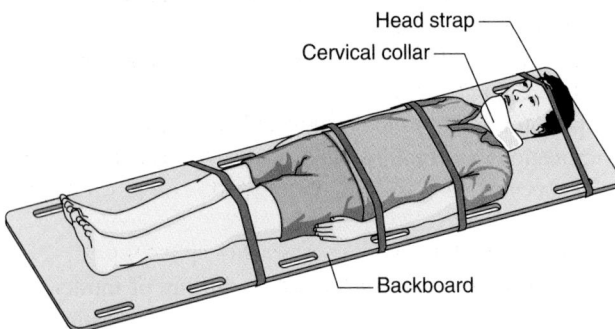

Head strap
Cervical collar
Backboard

FIGURE 13.4 Immobilization of a patient suspected of having a spinal cord injury using a backboard and cervical collar.

Chest Trauma

Chest trauma can damage the heart and lungs. It can cause life-threatening injuries. These can include pericardial tamponade, hemothorax, tension pneumothorax, and **flail chest** (condition of chest wall caused by two or more fractures on each affected rib, resulting in a segment of rib that is not attached on either end). Potentially life-threatening injuries can also occur. They include pulmonary and myocardial contusion, aortic and tracheobronchial disruption, and diaphragmatic rupture.

Chest trauma can lacerate lung tissue. Air or blood leaking into the intrapleural space collapses the lung. This results in a pneumothorax (air) or hemothorax (blood). Ineffective ventilation occurs. In a tension pneumothorax, air is trapped in the pleural space during exhalation. This puts pressure on the unaffected lung. The heart, great blood vessels, and trachea shift toward the unaffected side of the chest. Blood flow to and from the heart is greatly reduced. This decreases cardiac output. An uncorrected tension pneumothorax is fatal.

Chest trauma can also injure the heart and great blood vessels. It can reduce the amount of circulating blood volume. The heart can be bruised (myocardial contusion) or sustain direct trauma. **Cardiac tamponade** results when blood or fluid accumulates in the pericardial sac. This increases pressure around the heart. The increased pericardial pressure prevents the heart chambers from filling and contracting effectively. A patient with cardiac tamponade will have hypotension, **tachycardia** (rapid heart rate over 100 beats per minute), and jugular vein distention. It requires immediate intervention. Pressure must be reduced in the pericardial sac. This will restore normal filling and contraction of the heart chambers. Cardiac output will then increase.

Abdominal Trauma

The organs of the abdomen are vulnerable to injury. This is because of limited bony protection. Injury to organs such as the spleen and liver, which have a rich blood supply, can result in rapid loss of blood volume and hypovolemic shock. Abdominal organs can be injured from severe blunt or penetrating trauma. If hypotension is present, intra-abdominal hemorrhage may be the cause. If the urinary bladder ruptures, urine leaks into the abdomen. Blood can be seen at the urinary meatus or perineum. Penetrating trauma can cause lacerations to abdominal organs. This results in rapid blood loss and hypovolemic shock.

Orthopedic Trauma

Fractured bones can result in blood loss, compromised circulation, infection, and immobility. Unstable pelvic fractures can cause injury to the genitourinary system or disrupt pelvic veins. Fractures of large bones, such as the femur and tibia, can cause significant blood loss. Joint dislocations can cause neurovascular compromise. They do so by applying pressure on the nerves and blood vessels. Delayed fracture reduction (realignment or setting) can cause avascular necrosis. This leads to death of the affected tissue and bone.

LEARNING TIP
If a limb is fractured, splint it as it lies to prevent damage to blood vessels and nerves. If the distal circulation is severely compromised, the patient needs immediate medical intervention.

Nursing Process for the Patient Experiencing Trauma
Data Collection

The mechanism of injury is identified to determine the potential extent of the injury. Loss of consciousness immediately after an injury indicates that a concussion has occurred. The Glasgow Coma Scale (GCS) is used to rate a patient's level of consciousness (see Chapter 47). The highest score is 15. It indicates that the patient is alert and needs only observation. Scores lower than 13 can indicate the need for immediate treatment. Morbidity and mortality are highest for patients with GCS scores of 8 or lower. Pupil size and reaction are monitored and recorded. Dilated or nonreactive pupils indicate increased ICP. This

• **WORD** • **BUILDING** •
tachycardia: tachy—fast + cardia—heart condition

requires immediate intervention. Movement of extremities are also assessed and documented. Posturing and differences between limb movement on the right and left side can indicate increased ICP.

Spinal nerves in the spinal cord transmit sensory impulses to the brain. They also send motor impulses to the body. The higher a traumatic injury is on the spinal column, the more extensive the loss of muscle and sensory function (Table 13.2). A spinal cord injury at the C5 level or above interferes with diaphragm function and respiratory effort. Respirations must be carefully observed. Also, identify the patient's level of muscle control and ability to feel each limb.

Patients with major chest injuries can have dramatic symptoms. These include classic signs of shock with cyanosis, dyspnea, and restlessness. The patient's breathing pattern and effectiveness of respirations are assessed. The rise and fall of the chest is observed as well as symmetrical chest movement. Any bruising on the chest or upper abdomen is noted. Seat belts and restraint systems can cause significant bruising in high-impact crashes.

Vital signs are taken to detect shock. The shape of the abdomen is observed for distention from intra-abdominal hemorrhage. Skin color, bruising, open wounds, and penetrating trauma are noted. The abdomen is auscultated for bowel sounds. The perineum is inspected for blood from the urethra.

An injured extremity is inspected. Skin integrity, protruding bone, or deformity is noted. Skin color and capillary refill time are noted. Pulses distal to the injury are palpated. This identifies the quality of circulation distal to the injury. Motor function and sensation are checked to determine nerve injury. Respiratory function is monitored to detect a pulmonary embolism from a long bone fracture.

Nursing Diagnoses, Planning, and Implementation

Acute Pain related to tissue trauma

EXPECTED OUTCOME: The patient will experience relief within 30 minutes after measures are provided to relieve pain as evidenced by verbal and nonverbal expressions of pain relief.

- Apply ice and compression, elevate, and immobilize the affected area as ordered *to decrease swelling and relieve pain.*
- Provide analgesics as ordered *to relieve pain.*

Risk for Ineffective Cerebral Tissue Perfusion related to cerebral edema

EXPECTED OUTCOME: The patient will maintain adequate cerebral homeostasis without cerebral edema as evidenced by a GCS score of 14 or greater.

- Elevate the head of the patient's bed 30 to 45 degrees, as possible, *to reduce ICP.*
- Maintain the patient's head position at midline *to ensure unobstructed venous drainage to help reduce ICP.*

Table 13.2

Correlating Spinal Injury With Impairment of Motor Function

Injury Level	Impairment
S3 to S5 or above	Patient unable to tighten anus.
L4 to L5 or above	Patient unable to flex foot and extend toes.
L2 to L4 or above	Patient unable to extend and flex legs.
C5 to C7 or above	Patient unable to extend and flex arms.

- Give oxygen as ordered *to maintain adequate oxygenation of brain tissues and prevent cellular damage from hypoxia at the cerebral level.*
- Monitor neurologic checks and GCS score, and report changes *for intervention.*
- If the patient has an altered level of consciousness or deteriorating respiratory effort, anticipate and assist with endotracheal intubation as needed *to provide respiratory support to patient.*
- If the patient is agitated, provide calming measures *because agitation increases ICP.*

Ineffective Breathing Pattern related to spinal neck injury or unstable chest wall segment or lung collapse

EXPECTED OUTCOME: The patient will maintain effective respiratory rate and experience improved gas exchange in the lungs.

- If signs of respiratory distress are present, use the jaw-thrust or chin-lift maneuver, along with suction and airway adjuncts as needed, *to maintain patency of the airway.*
- Give oxygen as ordered *to improve tissue oxygenation.* Advanced adjunct airway equipment, including an endotracheal tube, must be readily available.
- Maintain cervical collar and backboard *to prevent further spinal injury.*
- Maintain chest tube drainage system if inserted *to help expand the lung.*

Ineffective Airway Clearance related to neck injury

EXPECTED OUTCOME: The patient will maintain clear lung sounds at all times.

- Suction the oropharynx and nasopharynx as needed *to clear secretions and prevent aspiration of secretions into the airway.*
- If the patient vomits, log roll the patient onto one side and use suction as needed *to prevent aspiration of emesis.*

Impaired Physical Mobility related to neck injury

EXPECTED OUTCOME: The patient will maintain movement of extremities normal for patient.

- Maintain neck immobility during initial treatment of a patient with head or neck trauma *to prevent serious spinal injury until trauma damage is identified.*

Decreased Cardiac Output related to compression of heart and great vessels

EXPECTED OUTCOME: The patient will maintain vital signs within baseline limits.

- Monitor the patient's vital signs and oxygen saturation continuously *to detect signs of shock.*
- Report unstable vital signs to HCP *because the patient may need immediate treatment or surgical intervention in the operating room.*
- Explain diagnostic testing for injury determination to patients who are alert with stable vital signs if radiographic studies are ordered *to reduce anxiety.*

Deficient Fluid Volume related to hemorrhage or abdominal organ injury

EXPECTED OUTCOME: The patient will maintain vital signs within baseline limits.

- Monitor for signs of shock *to detect hypovolemic shock.*
- Maintain IV fluids as ordered by 18- or 16-gauge IV cannulas *to restore circulating volume.*
- Assist with peritoneal lavage, if performed, *to detect intra-abdominal hemorrhage.*
- Assist with blood and blood product administration, as ordered and per agency policy, *to maintain circulating volume and improve tissue oxygenation.*

Risk for Infection related to tissue trauma

EXPECTED OUTCOME: The patient's wounds will remain free of infection.

- Cover abdominal wounds with a sterile dressing *to prevent infection.*
- If abdominal organs are exposed, cover with sterile saline–soaked dressings *to prevent tissue necrosis.*
- With open wounds, give tetanus immunization as ordered if it has been more than 5 years since the last one was given *to prevent tetanus infection.*
- Irrigate open wounds with sterile saline *to thoroughly remove dirt and debris and to clean exposed tissue to prevent infection.*
- Give antibiotics as ordered *to prevent infection.*

Impaired Physical Mobility related to bone injury

EXPECTED OUTCOME: The patient will maintain movement of extremities normal for patient.

- Remove all jewelry before applying a splint *to prevent constriction from swelling.*
- Immobilize the joints above and below the affected area using a folded towel or a pillow *to provide comfort and protection until the patient is evaluated by an HCP.*
- Maintain extremity in a splint in the position found, unless distal circulation is severely compromised. Keep it immobilized if there is severe pain or deformity. *Splinting promotes comfort and prevents further damage to surrounding tissue by preventing movement of broken bone ends.*
- Monitor skin color, temperature, distal pulses, capillary refill, movement, and sensation of the extremity after splint application *to detect abnormalities.*
- Elevate and ice extremity *to reduce edema and relieve pain.*

Evaluation

If interventions have been effective, a patient with trauma reports an acceptable pain level. A patient with head or spinal injury maintains a regular heart rate and rhythm, and pattern of breathing; clear lung sounds; intactness of mobility; and GCS score of 14 to 15. A patient with chest trauma maintains an open airway and effective breathing pattern. A patient with abdominal trauma has effective circulating volume as evidenced by vital signs within normal limits. A patient with altered tissue integrity has wounds that heal without infection. A patient with orthopedic trauma has strong and palpable pulses, normal blood pressure, normal skin color, skin that is warm and dry, capillary refill time of less than 3 seconds, pain controlled to a satisfactory level, and normal motor function and sensation in the extremity.

 BURNS

Skin function is impaired with a burn injury (see Chapter 55). It can lead to fluid and electrolyte loss, infection, and ineffective temperature regulation. The more extensive the burn injury, the greater the potential for complications and mortality, especially for those over age 60.

Assessment of the patient with burns begins with the ABCDE of the primary survey as well as F for "fluid resuscitation." The mechanism and time of the injury are noted. The presence of noxious chemicals or inhalation of smoke in an enclosed space is reported. The greatest threat to life in a patient with a major burn injury is smoke or heat inhalation, because it causes edema in the respiratory passages. Lung injury from a burn is diagnosed with a bronchoscopy. Continuous monitoring of respiratory status is essential for burns or soot on the face, singed nasal hairs, a hoarse voice, coughing, or restlessness.

Burns of the face can swell rapidly and compromise the airway. The head of the bed is elevated to 30 degrees to reduce edema. Oxygen is administered. Equipment for endotracheal intubation should be readily available. Large fluid losses occur in burn injuries. An IV infusion with large-bore cannulas is started. The patient's weight and the percentage of the body burned guide fluid resuscitation needs. The patient is kept warm, as a burn victim cannot maintain body heat. IV opioids are administered for pain.

Burn depth is described as superficial, partial thickness, or full thickness. Small partial-thickness burns are cleaned with sterile saline solution. They are then covered with a 1/8-inch layer of an anti-infective cream such as silver sulfadiazine (Silvadene, Flamazine) and dry, bulky, fluffed dressings. Major full-thickness burns are covered with dry, sterile dressings or linen. Patients with major burns are transferred to a specialized burn unit.

BE SAFE!

Be Vigilant! Is there anything you would want to check before applying silver sulfadiazine? Yes! Check allergies to sulfa medications. Look at the name of the medication to see that it contains "sulfa." A patient allergic to sulfa drugs should not be given this medication!

Gerontological Issues

Preventing Burns. Teach older adults to avoid wearing loose clothing that can catch on fire when cooking over open flames or with heating equipment, such as wood stoves or electric heaters. Teaching should also include not to use a heating pad with ointments on the skin, such as Bengay (methylsalicylate/menthol), as it can cause severe burns.

LEARNING TIP

Over-the-counter ointments, lotions, butter, and antiseptics are never used on a major burn. They can retain heat (causing further tissue injury), promote infection, and increase pain.

CRITICAL THINKING

Mr. Smith is a 28-year-old man who was welding close to a natural gas line. The flame of the welder caused the gas line to explode, throwing Mr. Smith 50 feet. He landed on his back. He is brought to the emergency department by paramedics. Mr. Smith is awake, alert, and oriented. He has soot around his mouth and nose. He sustained full-thickness burns to his neck, upper chest, and both forearms. He reports pain from his burns as well as thoracic back and hip pain. His pulse rate is 100 beats per minute, blood pressure is 160/90 mm Hg, and respiratory rate is 20 per minute.

1. What is the priority of care for Mr. Smith?
2. Is Mr. Smith at risk for respiratory burns? Why?
3. Are Mr. Smith's vital signs within normal limits?
4. Would wet or dry dressings be preferable for Mr. Smith's full-thickness burns? Why?
5. Mr. Smith is wearing a neck chain and a wedding ring. Should they be removed immediately, or should you wait until Mr. Smith's wife arrives to take them off? Why?
6. Mr. Smith continues to report hip and back pain. In reviewing his mechanism of injury, what other injuries could Mr. Smith have?
7. With what members of the health care team should you anticipate collaborating?

Suggested answers are at the end of the chapter.

 HYPOTHERMIA

Normally, the body maintains its temperature in a narrow range on either side of 98.6°F (37°C). This allows chemical reactions to work most efficiently. Heat loss is inversely proportional to body size and body fat. Fat insulates because it has fewer blood vessels that can vasodilate, resulting in heat loss. Hypothermia occurs when the core body temperature falls below 95°F (35°C). When this happens, the body is less able to regulate its temperature and generate body heat. This causes a progressive loss of body heat to occur.

Nursing Process for the Patient With Hypothermia
Data Collection

In cases of mild hypothermia (core temperature between 90°F and 95°F [32.2°C and 35°C]), the patient is usually alert and shivering. The patient may appear clumsy, apathetic, or irritable (Table 13.3). Hypoglycemia may occur. Glucose and glycogen stores are reduced by long-term shivering. Respiratory rate, heart rate, and cardiac output decrease.

More severe hypothermia occurs between 85°F and 90°F (29.4°C and 32.2°C). Shivering stops. Muscle activity decreases. Initially, fine muscle coordination ceases. Then, as core body temperature continues to drop, all muscle activity stops. Muscles become rigid. The patient becomes lethargic. There is less interest in fighting the cold environment. The patient's level of consciousness begins to markedly decrease at 89.6°F (32°C). The patient becomes lethargic and disoriented and begins to hallucinate. The pupils become dilated. As the core body temperature falls to 82°F (27.8°C), the patient becomes apneic, the pulse becomes slower and weaker, and cardiac arrhythmias occur. The profoundly hypothermic patient has a core temperature of less than 80°F (26.7°C) and usually appears dead, with no obtainable vital signs. Determination

Table 13.3

Defining Characteristics and Outcome Criteria for Hypothermia

Core Body Temperature	Defining Characteristics
Below 95°F (35°C)	• Skin cold to touch • Lack of coordination • Slurred speech • Vigorous shivering
Below 91.4°F (33°C)	• Cardiac arrhythmias • Cyanosis
Below 89.6°F (32°C)	• Shivering replaced by muscle rigidity • Hypotension • Dilated pupils
Below 82.4°F (28°C)	• Absent deep tendon reflexes • Hypoventilation (3 to 4 breaths per minute) • Ventricular fibrillation possible
Below 80.6°F (27°C)	• Coma • Flaccid muscles • Fixed, dilated pupils • Ventricular fibrillation to cardiac standstill • Apnea

Outcome Criteria
• Core body temperature is greater than 95°F (35°C).
• Patient is alert and oriented.
• Cardiac arrhythmias are absent.
• Acid–base balance is normal.
• Pupils react normally.

of death is made only after aggressive core rewarming to at least 90°F (32.2°C).

Nursing Diagnoses, Planning, and Implementation

Initial treatment of the hypothermic patient consists of rewarming the patient, stabilizing vital functions, and preventing further heat loss (see the "Nursing Care Plan for the Patient With Hypothermia"). The patient is removed from the cold environment. All wet clothing is removed to prevent further heat loss. The patient's core body temperature guides treatment. If body temperature is above 82.4°F (28°C), passive rewarming is preferred. The room temperature is set to 70°F to 75°F (21.1°C to 23.9°C). The patient is wrapped in warm, dry blankets. Heat loss from the head is reduced by covering the head with warm towels.

If core body temperature is below 82.4°F (28°C), active rewarming is needed. A heating blanket (carbon-fiber) and radiant heat lights are used. Warm, humidified oxygen is administered. Warm IV fluids are given. Body temperature is constantly monitored using a rectal probe. Heated **gastric lavage** (used to empty stomach when the contents are irritating), heated peritoneal lavage, or cardiopulmonary bypass can be used for profound hypothermia. Cardiac drugs are given sparingly. As the body warms, peripheral vasodilation occurs. Drugs that were trapped in the peripheral circulation are suddenly released during rewarming. This creates a bolus effect of the drug that can cause fatal arrhythmias.

Evaluation

Desired outcome criteria for the patient with hypothermia is a core body temperature higher than 95°F (35°C), no cardiac arrhythmias, pulse and blood pressure within normal limits, and being alert and oriented.

 FROSTBITE

The extremities are vulnerable to cold injury. *Frostnip* occurs when exposed parts of the body become very cold but not frozen. This condition usually is not painful. The skin becomes pale and blanched. Contact with a warm object such as someone's hand can be all that is needed to rewarm the part. During rewarming, the affected part might tingle and become red.

Frostbite occurs when body parts become frozen. The extremities are at increased risk because blood shunts away from them to maintain core body temperature. The affected tissue feels hard and frozen. Most frostbitten parts are white, yellow-white, or blue-white. When rewarmed, the skin appears deep red, hot, and dry to touch. The severity of a cold injury is determined by the duration of the exposure, the temperature to which the body part was exposed, and the wind velocity during exposure.

Interventions for frostbite protect the affected area from further damage. The frostbitten area is handled very gently and never rubbed. It is loosely covered with a dry, sterile dressing. The patient is not allowed to stand or walk on a frostbitten foot. The affected extremity is elevated to heart level. This minimizes edema and promotes blood flow.

 HYPERTHERMIA

The body's thermoregulation mechanisms usually work very well. This allows people to tolerate significant changes in temperature. To decrease body heat, sweating and dilation of blood vessels in the skin occur. When blood vessels dilate, blood comes to the skin surface. This increases radiation of heat from the body. If these mechanisms become overwhelmed, the consequences can be disastrous and irreversible. Those at greatest risk for heat illnesses include children, older people, and patients with cardiac disease.

Hyperthermia results when thermoregulation breaks down. This can be due to excess heat generation, an inability to dissipate heat, overwhelming environmental heat, or a

Nursing Care Plan for the Patient With Hypothermia

Nursing Diagnosis: *Hypothermia* related to exposure to cold environment
Expected Outcomes: The patient's body temperature and vital signs will be within normal limits.
Evaluation of Outcomes: Is the patient's body temperature greater than 95°F (35°C)? Is the patient alert and oriented? Is cardiac rhythm normal?

Intervention	Rationale	Evaluation
Monitor patient's core body temperature.	*Abnormal body temperature can be detected and treated.*	Is body temperature greater than 95°F (35°C)?
Monitor pulse and electrocardiogram (ECG) rhythm.	*Cardiac arrhythmias can occur at temperatures below 91.4°F (33°C).*	Is pulse rate and ECG rhythm normal?
Monitor patient's level of consciousness.	*Level of consciousness becomes markedly decreased at temperatures of 89.6°F (32°C).*	Is patient alert?
Institute rewarming passively or actively as ordered.	*Rewarming is necessary to return body temperature to desirable range.*	Is body core temperature rising to normal range?

combination of these factors. With a fever, the thermal set point is elevated; however, in a heat illness, the thermal set point remains normal. Hyperthermia occurs when heat builds up and cannot be lost. Antipyretics are of no use in hyperthermia. They can contribute to complications.

BE SAFE!

Be Vigilant! Recognize that older adults are vulnerable to hyperthermia. They do not readily perspire. In times of extreme summer temperatures, older people who live alone should be checked to make sure they are not experiencing hyperthermia. If they do not have fans or air-conditioning, they should be taken to a cooler environment.

Nursing Process for the Patient With Hyperthermia

Data Collection

Illness from heat exposure can take three forms: heat cramps, heat exhaustion, and heatstroke (Box 13.5). As heat illness progresses, circulating blood volume decreases, causing dehydration. Adequate fluid intake is crucial to prevent heat illness.

HEAT CRAMPS. Heat cramps are the mildest form of heat illness. They involve painful muscle spasms, usually in the legs or abdomen, that occur after strenuous exercise. Large amounts of salt and water can be lost as a result of excessive sweating. This causes stressed muscles to spasm. With adequate rest and fluid replacement, the body adjusts the distribution of electrolytes. Then the cramps disappear.

HEAT EXHAUSTION. Heat exhaustion occurs when so much water and electrolytes have been lost through heavy sweating

that hypovolemia occurs. Heat exhaustion is a manifestation of the strain placed on the cardiovascular system as it tries to maintain normothermia. Cerebral function is unimpaired. However, the patient can show minor irritability and poor judgment. The ability to sweat remains. The skin is usually cold and clammy, and the face is gray. Sodium and water loss cause dehydration. The body temperature is normal or slightly elevated, from 100.4°F to 102.2°F (38°C to 39°C). The patient may report feeling dizzy, weak, or

Box 13.5

Defining Characteristics and Outcome Criteria for Environmental Hyperthermia

Defining Characteristics

Early Signs
• Core body temperature 100.4°F to 102.2°F (38°C to 39°C)
• Diaphoresis
• Cool, clammy skin
• Dizziness
• Pulse rate greater than 100

Late Signs
• Increasing body core temperature of 106°F (41.1°C) or higher
• Hot, dry, flushed skin
• Altered mental status
• Coma or seizures possible
• Hypotension

Outcome Criteria
• Core body temperature less than 101°F (38.3°C)
• Patient alert and oriented
• Skin warm and dry to touch

faint, with nausea or a headache. Vomiting and diarrhea can be present.

HEATSTROKE. If symptoms of heat exhaustion are not treated, heatstroke can develop. Altered mental status and an inability to sweat are key symptoms in heatstroke. Some patients show confusion, irrational behavior, or psychosis. Others develop seizures or go into a coma. Because the sweating mechanism has been overwhelmed, many heatstroke victims have hot, dry, flushed skin. The body temperature rises rapidly to 106°F (41.1°C) or higher, and level of consciousness decreases. If heatstroke is not treated, death results.

Patients with heatstroke are treated in the intensive care unit. Late complications can appear suddenly. They require immediate management. Complications include seizures, cerebral ischemia, acute kidney injury, late cardiac decompensation, and GI bleeding. Prognosis varies with the length of time under heat stress and the patient's prior health status.

Nursing Diagnoses, Planning, and Implementation

Hyperthermia related to exposure to hot environment

EXPECTED OUTCOME: The patient will maintain body temperature within normal limits.

- For heat cramps, remove the patient from the hot environment *to allow cooling to begin and sweating to decrease.*
- Have the patient sit or lie down until muscle cramps subside *to prevent injury.*
- Remove the patient from the hot environment, and undress the patient *to allow the patient to cool more rapidly.*
- Mist-spray tepid water over the patient while maintaining a strong continual breeze from electric fans *because evaporative cooling is the most efficient method of cooling.*

Deficient Fluid Volume related to hypovolemia

EXPECTED OUTCOME: The patient will maintain blood pressure within normal limits.

- Give the patient oral fluids if the patient is fully alert as ordered *to replace lost fluids and electrolytes.*
- If the patient is hypotensive, maintain IV fluids as ordered *to restore fluid volume.*

Evaluation

Interventions have been successful if the hyperthermic patient has a core body temperature that is below 101°F (38.3°C); has warm and dry skin, a strong pulse, and blood pressure within normal limits; and is alert and oriented.

 ## POISONING AND DRUG OVERDOSE

Poisons enter the body by ingestion, inhalation, injection, absorption, or venomous bites. Poisons act by changing cellular metabolism, causing damage to structures, or disturbing body functions. Many toxins and poisons alter the patient's

mental status. This can make it difficult to obtain an accurate history.

Nursing Process for the Patient With Ingested Poisoning
Data Collection

After an ingested poisoning has occurred, the poison must be identified. The method of exposure is established. This allows the removal or interruption of the toxin. Most ingested poisons are drugs. About one-third of poisonings are caused by cleaners, soaps, insecticides, acids, or alkalis. Many household plants are poisonous if they are ingested. Some plants cause local irritation of the skin. Others can affect the circulatory system, GI tract, or central nervous system.

Empty medication bottles, scattered pills, or chemicals are examined by emergency medical personnel at the scene. This helps identify the poisonous substance. The patient's physical appearance also can give clues to the type of substance ingested. IV needle tracks, burns, erythema, and flushed skin may help identify the poison.

Nursing Diagnoses, Planning, and Implementation

Risk for Injury related to absorption of poisoning agent

EXPECTED OUTCOME: The patient will maintain normal vital signs and be free of injury.

- Administer naloxone (Narcan) as ordered *to treat an overdose. Narcan is available over-the-counter without a prescription in many states.*
- Contact the nationwide poison control center help line at 800-222-1222 or www.PoisonHelp.org *to access information concerning virtually all poisonous substances, available antidotes, and appropriate emergency treatment.*

NURSING CARE TIP

- The nationwide poison control center phone number (800-222-1222) should be kept near every home telephone and in cell phones. Text "POISON" TO 797979. This saves the poison control contact information in a smartphone.
- Syrup of ipecac is *not* recommended for at-home treatment of accidental overdose. Evidence shows that its use does not improve patient outcomes. For example, giving it to a person who has swallowed a caustic chemical results in greater tissue damage from the vomiting of the chemical. Also, after being given syrup of ipecac, a person who was poisoned may vomit the necessary antidote.
- Gastric decontamination, activated charcoal, and gastric lavage are no longer routinely recommended and should be reserved for the most severe cases.

Evaluation

Interventions have been successful if the patient has vital signs within normal limits and remains free from injury.

Inhaled Poisons

Inhaled poisons include carbon monoxide, chlorine, natural gas, pesticides, and other gases. Carbon monoxide is odorless. It can produce profound hypoxia by combining with hemoglobin molecules. This displaces oxygen in red blood cells. The patient's carboxyhemoglobin level is monitored to guide therapy. Inhalation of chlorine is irritating to the respiratory system. It can produce airway obstruction and pulmonary edema.

When an inhalation injury from a poison occurs, the patient must be moved into fresh air and away from the toxin. Supplemental oxygen is given as ordered. Prolonged inhalation of a poison can cause lung damage. Respiratory status must be closely monitored to detect complications.

Injected Poisons

Injected poisons pose problems because they are difficult to remove or dilute. Usually they result from drug overdose. However, they can also result from the bites and stings of insects or animals. Local swelling and tissue destruction can occur at the injection site. All jewelry is removed because swelling can occur. A cold pack is applied to decrease local pain and swelling around the injection site. The identity of the injected drug or toxin must be established so that adverse effects can be anticipated and managed.

Insect Stings or Bites

Insect stings or bites cause anaphylaxis in a small percentage of people (only 5% to 10% among adults). Symptoms in most people are limited to localized pain, swelling, heat, and redness. Potentially dangerous stings or bites can come from bees, wasps, yellow jackets, hornets, certain ants, or scorpions. Treatment involves applying ice to the site and elevating the affected part. Cellulitis can occur hours later and can require medical treatment.

When a patient has sustained a bee or wasp sting, examine the area for the stinger and remove it by gently scraping it off the skin. Tweezers or forceps are not used to remove the stinger. Squeezing the stinger can inject more venom into the patient. Placing ice over the injury site can help slow the rate of toxin absorption.

Snakebites

Only a small percentage of snakebites are caused by poisonous snakes. The most prevalent poisonous snakes are the coral snake and the pit vipers, which include rattlesnakes, copperheads, and cottonmouth moccasins. Envenomation occurs when the snake's hollow fangs puncture the skin and inject venom. Venom is stored in sacs located at the back of the snake's head. A poisonous snakebite leaves two small puncture wounds with surrounding discoloration, swelling, and pain. Envenomation by any pit viper snake produces burning pain at the site of the injury. Swelling and discoloration occur within 5 to 10 minutes after the bite.

Interventions are focused on decreasing the circulation of venom throughout the patient's system. This is done by keeping the patient calm and immobilizing the affected body part. An affected extremity should be positioned below the level of the heart. The site of the bite is cleaned with soap and water. It should not be irrigated or flushed. The wound should be covered with a loose, clean dressing. Ice should not be applied to the bite area. The patient is kept calm until antivenin can be given. Medical treatment of the patient with a poisonous snakebite should be directed by an experienced toxicologist.

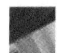 **NEAR-DROWNING**

Drowning is death from **asphyxia** (insufficient oxygen intake) after submersion in water. *Near-drowning* is submersion with at least temporary survival of the victim. When submersion occurs, conscious victims hold their breath until reflex inspiratory efforts override breath holding. As water is aspirated, laryngospasm occurs. In wet drowning, the laryngospasm is less prolonged. Fluid enters the lungs after the vocal cords relax. In dry drowning, cold water causes laryngospasm and vagal stimulation. This produces severe hypoxia. Most successfully resuscitated victims experience dry drowning. Risk factors for drowning include inability to swim, diving accidents, use of alcohol and drugs before swimming, exhaustion, and hypothermia. Factors that influence the outcome of near-drowning include the temperature of the water, length of time submerged, cleanliness of the water, and age of the victim. The younger the patient, the better the chance of survival.

After submersion, acute respiratory failure can occur. Symptoms of impaired gas exchange (known as secondary near-drowning) can be delayed as long as 72 hours after the incident. Contaminants in the water can irritate the pulmonary system and cause inflammatory reactions and impaired surfactant functioning. Metabolic acidosis is usually present. Hypoxemia and hypothermia predispose the patient to arrhythmias. Neurologic damage and cerebral edema can occur.

Aggressive resuscitative efforts are used for victims of cold-water drowning when submersion time is 1 hour or less. Hypothermia can decrease the metabolic needs of the brain. This can contribute to neurologic recovery even after prolonged submersion. Resuscitation should not be stopped until the body temperature is at least greater than 89.6°F (32°C). Supportive respiratory care is provided; this may include mechanical ventilation.

Nursing Process for the Near-Drowning Patient
Data Collection
Conduct ABCDE of the primary survey. Most near-drowning victims have mild dyspnea, a deathlike appearance with blue or gray skin color, apnea or **tachypnea** (breathing over 20 respirations per minute), hypotension, slow heart rate (possibly less than 10 beats per minute), cold skin temperature, dilated

• WORD • BUILDING •

tachypnea: tachy—fast + pnea—breathing

pupils, hypothermia, and vomiting. Vital signs are taken. Respiratory rate and pattern are observed. Dyspnea or signs of airway obstruction are reported. Skin color or cyanosis is noted. The patient's level of consciousness may be altered from anoxia.

Nursing Diagnoses, Planning, and Implementation

Risk for Ineffective Cerebral Tissue Perfusion related to severe anoxia

EXPECTED OUTCOME: The patient will maintain level of consciousness and vital signs within normal range, with clear breath sounds that are equal bilaterally.

• Give supplemental oxygen as ordered *to increase tissue oxygenation.*
• Ensure that adjunct airway equipment is available *because endotracheal intubation and insertion of a nasogastric tube to decompress the stomach may be needed.*

Evaluation

Interventions have been successful if the patient has normal respiratory rate and pattern, has normal vital signs, and is alert and oriented.

 ## PSYCHIATRIC EMERGENCIES

A psychiatric emergency occurs when a person no longer has the coping skills needed to maintain the usual level of functioning. The patient's moods, thoughts, or actions can be so disordered that the patient could harm self or others if the situation is not quickly controlled. If acute psychiatric episodes are not managed, they can result in life-threatening, suicidal, violent, or psychologically damaging behavior (see Chapter 57).

 ## DISASTER RESPONSE

A *disaster* is defined as any event that overwhelms existing personnel, facilities, equipment, and the capabilities of a responding agency, institution, or community. Potential sources of disaster include internal events such as fires and explosions; external events such as floods, storms, fires, earthquakes, and tornadoes; and created events such as motor vehicle accidents, plane crashes, and acts of terrorism.

External disasters involve a community-wide response of several agencies. These include first responders (i.e., emergency medical system [EMS] providers, fire departments, law enforcement) and hospitals. These agencies work together to coordinate communication, search, rescue, transportation, and treatment of multiple victims. Each agency and hospital involved in responding to a disaster follows a disaster plan. It outlines the role and responsibilities of the agency and its staff. It identifies procedures to follow when interacting with the casualties, families, media, or other agencies. Community-wide disaster drills are conducted on a regular basis to evaluate and rework plans.

Hospitals serve as the major treatment area for injured victims of a disaster (casualties). When a disaster occurs, the hospital activates its disaster plan. There are external and internal disaster plans. External plans respond to events occurring outside the hospital. Internal disaster plans are specific to an institution. They cover internal water, power, sewer, or computer issues that could cause harm. Specific duties for all staff and each department are outlined. You should be familiar with your agency's disaster plan. Know your role and responsibilities during a disaster.

Each nursing unit calls available off-duty staff to report to work. Units prepare for the influx of casualties by discharging noncritical patients. Each nursing unit is designated to receive specific types of casualties. These may include major trauma, burns, and medical, pediatric, or psychiatric issues. The ED serves as the **triage** (sorting for the purpose of assigning priorities) and stabilization area for casualties. A hospital disaster plan may assign one or more staff from other areas to work in the ED. These staff members assist in areas such as first aid, critical care, burn treatment, family room, or transportation. During a disaster, decision making and prioritization of patient care are guided by the personnel and resources available. Patients who are seriously injured but have the greatest chance of full recovery are treated first.

 ## BIOTERRORISM AGENTS

The Centers for Disease Control and Prevention (CDC) evaluates bacteria, viruses, and toxins on their risk for use in a **bioterrorism** attack (visit www.cdc.gov). Early recognition of a bioterrorism attack is vital. It allows for rapid implementation of preventive interventions, treatment, and public communication.

Anthrax

Anthrax is a disease caused by the spore-forming bacterium *Bacillus anthracis*. The organism is found worldwide in soil. Animals become infected by grazing in contaminated areas. Under natural conditions, humans can contract the disease. This occurs after close contact with infected animals or contaminated animal products (e.g., hides, meat, wool). The spores activate upon exposure to the tissues or blood of an animal or infected human. A vaccine is available.

Classification and Epidemiology

Anthrax occurs in three clinical forms in humans. These forms are inhalational, cutaneous, and GI. Aerosol exposure to anthrax spores is most likely in a biological attack. The 2001 U.S. mail anthrax attack showed that anthrax spores in envelopes or packages could cause illness. Inhalational anthrax and cutaneous disease occurred.

Cutaneous anthrax is the most likely way to develop anthrax. It results from injection of spores subcutaneously through a skin break. GI and oropharyngeal anthrax occur in rural parts of the world where anthrax is endemic. Those incidents result from eating meat contaminated with the spores.

Inhalational Anthrax

CLINICAL PRESENTATION AND DIAGNOSIS. Clinical symptoms develop rapidly after activation of anthrax spores. The incubation period is most commonly reported as 1 to 6 days.

Inhalational anthrax is a two-stage disease. The initial stage is a nonspecific, flu-like illness. It lasts from several hours to a few days. The early clinical presentation includes a combination of fever, myalgia, headache, cough, mild chest discomfort, weakness, abdominal pain, and chest pain. Profound malaise, fever, and drenching sweats are prominent symptoms. Nausea and vomiting are frequent. Classically, the initial stage is followed 1 to 3 days later, sometimes after brief improvement, by the rapidly progressive second stage. It is characterized by fever, dyspnea, diaphoresis, cyanosis, and shock.

There is no rapid screening test to diagnose inhalational anthrax in its early stages. The initial diagnostic tests for a suspected case are a chest x-ray, computed tomography scan, and culture of peripheral blood. Pleural fluid, cerebrospinal fluid, and biopsy of the pleura and lung are also useful for culture.

THERAPEUTIC INTERVENTION. Prognosis is poor. Early treatment is essential for survival of inhalational anthrax. Antibiotics (ciprofloxacin [Cipro] and doxycycline [Vibramycin, Oracea, Doryx]), antitoxins, and antibodies are used for treatment. Aggressive supportive care is important. This includes maintenance of fluid, electrolyte and acid–base balance, and drainage of pleural effusions.

Cutaneous Anthrax

There is an incubation period of approximately 7 days (the range is 1 to 12 days). The primary lesion of cutaneous anthrax then appears. It is a nondescript, painless, pruritic papule. It is usually on an exposed area such as the face, head, neck, or upper extremity (Fig. 13.5). The papule enlarges. It develops a central vesicle or bulla with surrounding brawny, nonpitting edema. The central vesicle enlarges and ulcerates over 1 to 2 days. It becomes hemorrhagic, depressed, and necrotic and leads to a central black eschar. Satellite vesicles can be present. Over the next 1 to 2 weeks, the eschar dries and falls off (Fig. 13.6). Tender regional lymphadenopathy, fever, chills, and fatigue can occur. Systemic disease has a mortality of 20% if untreated. Outpatient treatment with oral doxycycline or a quinolone antibiotic is used.

TRANSMISSIBILITY AND INFECTION CONTROL. Person-to-person transmission of anthrax is not known to occur. Therefore, patients can be hospitalized in a standard hospital room. Standard precautions can be used. No treatment is necessary for persons who come in contact with the patient.

Botulism

Botulism is caused by the most potent lethal toxin known, botulinum toxin. This neurotoxin is produced by *Clostridium botulinum,* an anaerobic, spore-forming bacterium. The toxin

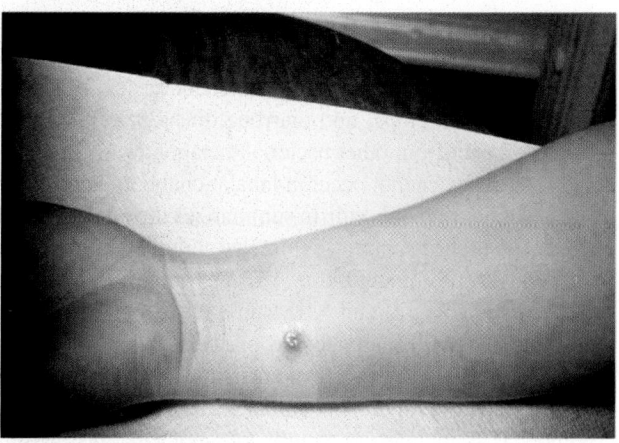

FIGURE 13.5 Cutaneous anthrax on right forearm in early stage of infection.

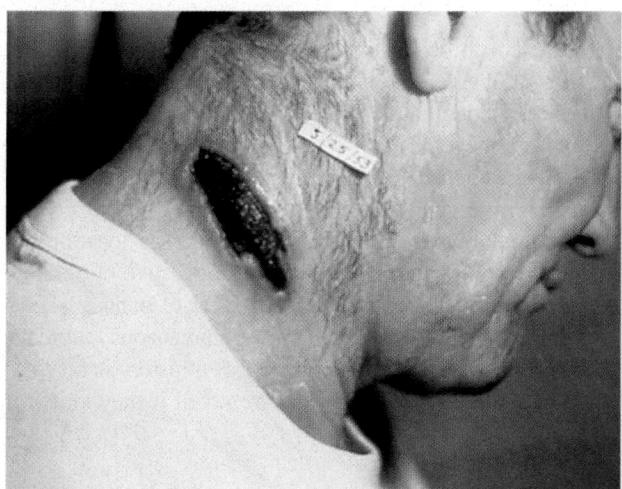

FIGURE 13.6 Cutaneous anthrax in later stage of infection.

is colorless, odorless, and likely tasteless. Botulinum toxin blocks neurotransmission. It binds to the presynaptic nerve terminal at the neuromuscular junction. This prevents the release of acetylcholine. Skeletal muscle weakness results.

Natural forms of the disease are foodborne botulism, wound botulism, and infant botulism. Foodborne botulism results from ingestion of improperly processed foodstuffs containing preformed toxin produced by *C. botulinum*. Botox is the trade name of a toxin made by *C. botulinum.* It reduces facial lines by blocking nerve impulses to the muscles whose action causes the lines. Wound botulism results from production of botulinum toxin by *C. botulinum* organisms in wounds. Infant botulism results from the colonization of the intestinal tract of infants after ingestion of spores. (Honey can contain the bacteria, so infants under 1 year of age should not eat honey.) Botulinum toxin has been developed as a biological weapon. An aerosol attack is considered the most likely use of botulinum toxin for bioterrorism.

Clinical Presentation

The typical incubation period for foodborne botulism is 12 to 72 hours (the range is 2 hours to 8 days). The incubation period for inhalational botulism has not been established. The neurologic features for types of botulism are similar. Although initial symptoms in foodborne botulism can include nausea, vomiting, abdominal cramps, and diarrhea, these symptoms are thought to result from other bacterial metabolites in contaminated food. They cannot occur in inhalational botulism.

The classic triad of botulism summarizes the clinical presentation: an afebrile patient, symmetrical descending flaccid paralysis with prominent bulbar palsies (impairment of cranial nerves IX, X, XI, and XII), and a clear mentation. Patients often have difficulty seeing, speaking, or swallowing. These symptoms can be mistaken for lethargy and central nervous system involvement. Anticholinergic symptoms are common. They include dry mouth, ileus, constipation, nausea and vomiting, urine retention, and mydriasis. Dizziness and sore throat may occur.

Diagnosis

Treatment with botulinum antitoxin should begin based on the clinical diagnosis without waiting for laboratory confirmation. For potential foodborne botulism, samples of stool, gastric aspirate, emesis, and suspect foods are submitted.

A bioterrorism attack is considered in any outbreak of botulism. It is especially considered when a cluster of cases occurs, when an outbreak has a common geographical location but there is no common dietary exposure (suggestive of possible aerosol exposure), when there is an outbreak of an unusual botulinum toxin type, or when multiple simultaneous outbreaks occur. A careful patient dietary and travel history is taken to help identify the source. Patients are asked if they know of others with similar symptoms.

Therapeutic Intervention

The mainstay of treatment for botulism is supportive care. This includes intensive care, mechanical ventilation, and parenteral nutrition. Frequent monitoring of the gag and cough reflexes, swallowing, oxygen saturation, vital capacity, and inspiratory force are critical. Airway intubation is needed for secretion control or impending respiratory failure. Morbidity and mortality are usually from:

- Pulmonary aspiration secondary to loss of the gag reflex and dysphagia, leading to inability to control secretions
- Respiratory failure secondary to inadequate tidal volume from diaphragmatic and accessory respiratory muscle paralysis
- Airway obstruction from pharyngeal and upper airway muscle paralysis

Trivalent (ABE) equine antitoxin is available from the CDC through state and local health departments. It should be administered as soon as possible. Antitoxin can prevent the progression of the disease. It does not reverse the effects of the already bound toxin. Therefore, antitoxin is not useful if the patient is no longer showing progression of disease or is already improving from maximum paralysis.

Transmissibility and Infection Control

Botulism is not spread from person to person. Standard precautions are used. Clothes of persons exposed to an aerosol release of botulinum toxin should be removed and washed. Exposed persons should then shower using soap and hot water. Exposed environmental surfaces can be decontaminated with 0.1% hypochlorite bleach solution.

Plague

Plague is caused by the gram-negative coccobacillus *Yersinia pestis.* Under natural conditions, plague is transmitted to humans by the bite of an infectious flea. It can also be transmitted by direct contact with infectious body fluids or tissues of an infected animal or by inhaling infectious droplets. Plague has a long history of use and development as a biological weapon. After a biological attack, primary pneumonic plague would most likely occur.

Clinical Presentation

Plague is a severe febrile illness. Pneumonic plague is the most fatal form of the infection. It can develop from inhalation of plague bacilli (primary pneumonic plague). The incubation period for pneumonic plague is typically 2 to 4 days (the range is 1 to 6 days). Signs and symptoms typically include the acute onset of malaise, high fever, chills, headache, chest discomfort, dyspnea, and cough with sepsis within 2 to 4 days. Hemoptysis is a classic sign that should suggest plague in the appropriate clinical context. Sputum can be watery or purulent. GI symptoms occur with pneumonic plague. They include nausea, vomiting, diarrhea, and abdominal pain. A cervical bubo (swelling of the lymph nodes) is infrequently present. The disease is rapidly progressive, with increasing dyspnea, stridor, and cyanosis. Rapidly progressive respiratory failure is typical of pneumonic plague.

Diagnosis

During a confirmed outbreak of pneumonic plague after a biological attack, a diagnosis can be made based on symptoms. The leukocyte count will be elevated with increased neutrophils. Platelets are normal or low. The international normalized ratio (INR), prothrombin time (PT), and partial thromboplastin time (PTT) are increased. Elevated liver function tests and abnormal renal function tests occur with systemic disease.

Therapeutic Intervention

When plague is suspected, antibiotic treatment should begin before laboratory confirmation. Levofloxacin (Levaquin) treats plague and reduces the risk of plague after exposure.

Smallpox/Variola Major

Smallpox is caused by the variola virus. It is an orthopoxvirus unique to humans. This virus is not known to be transmitted by animals or insects. Smallpox was declared eradicated in 1980. This was 3 years after the last naturally occurring case was reported. Smallpox is stable and highly infectious in the aerosol form. The risk for a smallpox attack currently is considered low but not zero.

SUGGESTED ANSWERS TO CRITICAL THINKING

Mr. Smith

1. The airway is the priority because edema from inhalation burns can occlude the airway.
2. Mr. Smith is at risk for respiratory burns because of the soot near his mouth and nose. He should be closely monitored. Assessment should include respiratory rate and pattern and the patient's ability to speak without a hoarse voice. Abnormal breathing sounds such as wheezing indicate partial upper airway occlusion.
3. The vital signs are within normal limits.
4. Full-thickness burns are covered with dry dressings. Because the skin can no longer protect the patient, wet dressings would provide a medium for bacterial invasion and could decrease body temperature because the skin can no longer maintain thermoregulation.
5. Jewelry, including wedding rings, should always be removed immediately before edema formation begins to save the digit (finger).
6. Mr. Smith was involved in an explosive incident and thrown 50 feet. He could have sustained fractures of the pelvis or back. He may also have internal organ injuries from blunt trauma.
7. The emergency department health care provider, registered nurse, and respiratory therapist.

Review Questions

1. Which of these assessments would the nurse include in a primary survey of a multisystem trauma victim? **Select all that apply.**
   1. Airway
   2. Breathing
   3. Chronic illness
   4. Circulation
   5. Deformity
   6. Vital signs

2. The nurse is caring for a trauma patient who is hemorrhaging from a puncture wound. Which of the following actions should the nurse use to control the bleeding?
   1. Application of a tourniquet
   2. Pressure dressing
   3. Pressure-point massage
   4. Pressure at the puncture site

3. A patient who was in a house fire is brought to the emergency department. Which of these findings would indicate to the nurse the potential for an inhalation injury? **Select all that apply.**
   1. Hoarse voice
   2. Jugular vein distention
   3. Increased capillary refill time
   4. Peripheral edema
   5. Singed nasal hairs
   6. Soot on lower face

4. The home health care nurse finds a patient experiencing potential hyperthermia. Which of the following actions should the nurse take first for this patient?
   1. Undress the patient.
   2. Use tepid water as a mist spray.
   3. Remove the patient from the hot environment.
   4. Place the patient in continual breeze from electric fans.

5. A patient is brought into the emergency department who has inhaled chlorine. The nurse should monitor the patient for the development of which of these? **Select all that apply.**
   1. Airway obstruction
   2. Dyspnea
   3. Increased capillary refill time
   4. Pulmonary edema
   5. Sacral edema
   6. Unequal pupils

6. A resident has fallen in the shower of an assisted living apartment and is found by the nurse. The resident is on the floor moaning with pain in the pelvic and right hip region. Place the following data to be collected in the correct order of priority:
   1. Pupil checks
   2. Breathing
   3. Distal pulses in both lower extremities
   4. Bleeding
   5. Exposure

7. Which one of the following patients should be treated first in a disaster situation?
   1. A 10-year-old with a closed leg fracture that is painful
   2. A 32-year-old with slight bleeding from a hand laceration
   3. A 45-year-old with an open head injury and no pulse or respirations
   4. A 62-year-old reporting chest pain and shortness of breath

8. The nurse is caring for a patient with an acute episode of anaphylaxis. Which one of the following conditions would the nurse recognize as the immediate threat to life?
   1. Hypotension
   2. Generalized itching
   3. Airway obstruction
   4. Tachycardia

9. The nurse is collecting data on a patient who is hypovolemic due to hyperthermia. Which of these signs and symptoms indicate that the patient is experiencing progressive shock? **Select all that apply.**
   1. Decreasing blood pressure
   2. Jugular vein distention
   3. Palpable, bounding pulse
   4. Sacral edema
   5. Thready, weak pulse

10. The nurse is to give penicillin G 500,000 units intramuscularly. The nurse has a 10-mL vial labeled "penicillin 400,000 units/mL." How many milliliters should the nurse give?
    Answer: _____ mL

Answer rationales available in your online resources.

ANSWERS 1. 1, 2, 4, 6; 2, 4; 3. 1, 5, 6; 4. 3; 5. 1, 2, 4; 6. 2, 4, 3, 5, 1; 7. 4; 8. 3; 9. 1, 5; 10. 1.25

Key Points

Find the chapter key points in your online resources available through Davis Edge.

Additional Resources

DAVIS edge. Use the scratch off code on the inside front cover of your book to access online quizzes that will help you to improve your scores on course exams and prepare for NCLEX-PN®.

 Study Guide

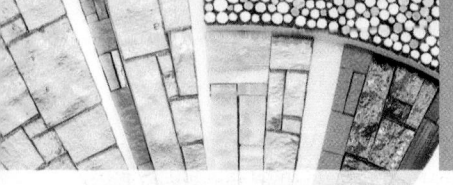

CHAPTER 14

Developmental Considerations and Chronic Illness in the Nursing Care of Adults

Linda S. Williams

KEY TERMS

chronic illness (KRAW-nick ILL-ness)
developmental stage (deh-vell-up-MEN-tal STAYJ)
health (HELLTH)
hopelessness (HOHP-less-ness)
illness (ILL-ness)
powerlessness (POW-er-less-ness)
reminiscence therapy (reh-meh-NISS-enss THAIR-a-pee)
respite care (RESS-pit CARE)
spirituality (SPEER-ih-chu-AL-ih-tee)

CHAPTER CONCEPTS

Family Dynamics
Growth and Development
Health Promotion
Patient-Centered Care
Safety
Sexuality
Spirituality

LEARNING OUTCOMES

1. List Erikson's eight stages of psychosocial development.
2. Identify the effects of chronic illness.
3. Describe special needs that caregivers have.
4. Explain health promotion methods.
5. Plan nursing interventions for a patient who is chronically ill.

 HEALTH, WELLNESS, AND ILLNESS

Have you ever known someone with what appears to be a small health problem who considers himself unwell or disabled? Or perhaps a person with major health problems who views himself as being well? Many factors play a role in a person's perception of **health.** These include the ability to perform activities of daily living (ADLs) and desired tasks, fulfilment of life roles (i.e., student, parent, or employee), and quality of life. *Wellness* is a term describing movement toward a higher level of functioning. Even though a person has a disabling illness, he or she may still achieve a higher level of wellness.

The concept of **illness** is one of imbalance or disharmony with the environment. Physical causes of illness are most easily recognized, such as a fall that breaks a bone. But illness can also result from a psychological, sociological, cultural, or spiritual imbalance. After the loss of a spouse, for example, one may experience loneliness, depression, and a loss of balance in the social and psychological aspects of life.

A hospitalization or long-term care stay may increase disharmony if cultural beliefs and practices are not understood or upheld by health care providers (HCPs). A person faced with a terminal diagnosis may lose hope and direction in life, causing anxiety and despair. So rather than being exclusive concepts, health and illness are dynamic and ever-changing states of being. A health crisis such as a myocardial infarction overwhelms a patient's ability to maintain a normal level of wellness. Two months after, however, the patient could be enjoying a higher level of wellness than before the myocardial infarction if he or she is following a healthy lifestyle.

THE NURSE'S ROLE IN SUPPORTING AND PROMOTING WELLNESS

The goal of nursing care is to help patients achieve their highest possible level of wellness. To do this, the patient's strengths and resources as well as weaknesses and disabilities must be considered. Working together, the patient, family, and members of the health care team develop a plan of care. The plan includes wellness goals and interventions to accomplish those goals. The plan of care focuses on six main areas:

- Mobilizing resources
- Providing a safe and adaptable environment
- Helping the patient learn about his or her health problem and treatment
- Performing and teaching the patient to perform health care procedures
- Anticipating problems and recognizing potential crises
- Evaluating the plan and progress toward the goals with the patient and family

Nurses assume a variety of roles in promoting the health of their patients, such as educator, advocate, caregiver, and consultant.

NURSING CARE TIP

Displaying photos, provided by family, in a patient's room of the patient at various ages when healthy and active allows caregivers to appreciate the patient in wellness roles.

DEVELOPMENTAL STAGES

There are many theories of developmental stages. The theory of Erik Erikson (1980, 1993), who described eight stages of psychosocial development, is discussed in this chapter (Table 14.1).

The **developmental stages** of life focus on the balance a person must achieve for high-level wellness within that stage. Each stage must be completed before accomplishing the next. The first five stages relate to the child and adolescent. The last three stages, discussed here, are young adulthood, middle adulthood, and late adulthood.

The Young Adult

Erikson's sixth psychosocial developmental stage, from ages 18 to 40, addresses intimacy versus isolation. The young adult's task is to develop relationships with a spouse, family, or friends that are warm, affectionate, and developed through fondness, understanding, caring, or love. The inability to do so results in isolation from others. Physically, growth is usually completed by age 20. Socially, young adults begin to move away from their parents to start their own families. The young adult begins to develop a place in society through school, work, and social activities. In this stage, intimacy or closeness develops with partners and friends. Having a pet, marrying, and having children shows the desire for intimacy. Challenges to intimacy are tasks that must be overcome in this stage. Blending one's traditions and customs with the traditions and customs of others is a major responsibility.

Common Health Concerns

The lifestyle choices of young adults may place their health at risk. Establishing lifelong positive health practices help prevent long-term health complications. Health promotion for this age group focuses on risk prevention through teaching. The importance of diet and exercise, sunscreen use to avoid increased risk of skin cancer, and avoiding tobacco use to prevent lung disease and cancer in later life should be explained.

In the early part of young adulthood, the individual is in the workforce or is preparing for a career with a college or vocational education. Being a novice in the work world and accepting new independence, freedom, and responsibilities

Table 14.1
Erikson's Stages of Psychosocial Development

Stage	Age Range	Developmental Task
Infancy	Birth to 18 months	Trust versus Mistrust
Toddler	18 months to 3 years	Autonomy versus Shame and doubt
Preschool	3 to 5 years	Initiative versus Guilt
School age	5 to 12 years	Industry versus Inferiority
Adolescence	12 to 18 years	Identity versus Role confusion
Young adulthood	18 to 40 years	Intimacy versus Isolation
Middle adulthood	40 to 65 years	Generativity versus Stagnation
Late adulthood	65 years to death	Integrity versus Despair

can introduce stressors into the young adult's life. Overeating, engaging in violence, and alcohol, drug, or tobacco use are risky lifestyle choices and poor coping mechanisms for stress. Young adults should be aware of their individual stressors and develop positive coping mechanisms such as exercise, music, and meditation.

Although marriage commonly occurs during this phase, this age group also has the highest rate of divorce. The blending of two people into a couple requires creative communication and loving care. When stressors overwhelm the couple's coping mechanisms or strategies, the relationship may be at risk.

Young adults may be sexually active with multiple partners. This puts them at risk for sexually transmitted infections. Safer sex guidelines and information on birth control should be available for the young adult.

Pregnancy commonly occurs for women in this age group. A woman's health practices affect the health of the fetus. Nutrition, drug and alcohol use, physical health, and stress coping mechanisms are lifestyle issues to discuss with every pregnant woman. Prenatal care should be encouraged for pregnant women.

The Middle-Aged Adult

In the middle adult years, ages 40 to 65, the psychological developmental stage is developing generativity versus self-absorption. Generativity includes a sense of productivity and creativity and is demonstrated by concern and support for others, along with a vision for future generations. The inability to develop generativity may be displayed as preoccupation with personal needs or self-absorption.

Physically, middle-aged adults may notice signs of intolerance for physical exercise if they have not maintained a healthy lifestyle. Traditionally, their children are adolescents or young adults who need assistance with entering adulthood and launching their own careers and families; however, people are having children later in life so this is not always the case. The term *empty nest* is used to describe the middle-aged couple's home after their children have left.

Today's middle-aged adult generation has been labeled the *sandwich generation*. This is due to caring for their children and their aging parents at the same time. Middle-aged adults look back over their lives and compare accomplishments versus unrealized goals. Midlife crisis may occur when a desire to change work, social, or family situations results. Planning for retirement occurs by developing interests outside of work. In addition, preparing for financial security is another important task during this stage.

Common Health Concerns

The need for immunizations continues into adulthood (visit www.cdc.gov). Unhealthy lifestyle choices often lead to serious health consequences during middle adulthood. These choices include smoking, use of alcohol or drugs, a sedentary lifestyle, a diet high in saturated fat, or overeating. Hypertension, heart disease, chronic bronchitis, emphysema, and lung cancer are major health concerns. Cardiovascular disease and cancer cause most deaths in this age group. However, middle adulthood is not too late for lifestyle changes to positively affect health. Helping adults in this age group recognize the benefits of positive lifestyle choices and empowering them to change is the major goal for HCPs.

CRITICAL THINKING

Mr. Paul, age 54, calls his health care provider's office for the fourth time this month to request medication for severe indigestion. He has refused to have diagnostic tests because he "can't fit them" into his schedule. Mr. Paul travels for work and eats fast food daily. His wife quit her job to supervise their 15-year-old son, who was not going to school every day. Their twin daughters are both in college.

1. What might be causing Mr. Paul to experience health problems?
2. What is affecting the developmental tasks Mr. Paul needs to perform?

Suggested answers are at the end of the chapter.

The Older Adult

The final psychological developmental stage affects adults from age 65 until death. Advances in living conditions and health care have allowed more people to live productive, fulfilling lives into their 80s, 90s, and 100s. Older adults are likely to be found gardening, hiking, exercising, or socializing (Fig. 14.1). Some may continue to work beyond retirement age or begin a second career after retiring.

Developmental work for older adults focuses on integrity versus despair. In this stage, older adults look back to see what they have done with their lives. Integrity refers to accepting responsibility for one's life thus far and reflecting on it in a positive way. Reaching this stage is a sign of maturity. Failing to reach this stage is an indication of unsuccessful completion of previous stages, causing feelings of despair that life has been lived in vain and also a fear of death. **Reminiscence therapy** may be one way to assist the older adult through this stage.

Aging is associated with role changes and transitions. Some roles, such as employee or child, are lost because of retirement or illness or death of a parent, causing sadness or depression. New roles may arise, such as grandparent, volunteer, or widow/widower. With retirement, household roles may need to change. If an older adult becomes ill and dependent and needs to be cared for by an adult child, the parent–child role may be reversed.

Life events such as decreased physical ability, retirement, illness, or death of a spouse are challenges that older adults face. The older adult's ability to cope with these stressors is

• WORD • BUILDING •

reminiscence: re—backward + minisc—mind + ens—action

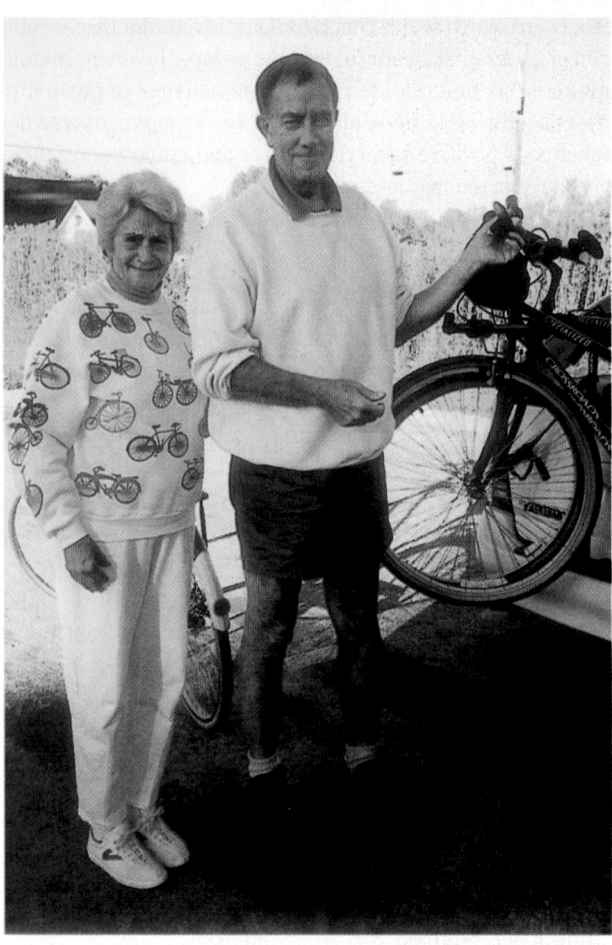

FIGURE 14.1 Socialization helps older adults maintain integrity.

essential for healthy aging and maintaining a sense of control. Coping with aging is influenced by the individual's cultural beliefs and the community's value of older adults. Sometimes the greatest loss for older adults is their lack of connection with the world and a lack of being part of a greater purpose. However, being alone is not the same as being lonely. For some older adults, being by oneself allows for reflection to better understand one's situation. Older adults who feel unwanted or unloved are more likely to develop anxiety and depression and fail to thrive.

Common Health Concerns

The focus of care for the older adult is assistance in meeting physical, psychological, cultural, sociological, and spiritual needs. Promoting self-care and encouraging the use of community services for seniors is important. Most older adults continue to live in their own residences. Impairment in mobility and the ability to carry out instrumental activities of daily living (IADLs) threaten their independence. IADLs include shopping for groceries, preparing meals, and cleaning and maintaining a home. Asking or paying others to perform tasks that they formerly could do themselves is a significant loss for many older adults. The loss of a spouse, death of friends, or lack of social contacts can further isolate an older

adult. This can lead to depression and a feeling of **hopelessness.** The accumulation of losses can overwhelm an older adult's resources and coping mechanisms. Hopelessness is related to a high rate of suicide, especially for older men. Suicide is the ultimate expression of hopelessness.

Older adults may need to be encouraged to remain active. Many cities have transportation services for older adults. Senior centers offer programs such as trips, dances, bowling leagues, and tax assistance. Older adults can also continue to work as volunteers for schools, nursing facilities, parks, museums, zoos, and youth groups. Colleges and universities may offer discounts for older adults. Elderhostel programs offer educational travel programs across the country. Topics include photography, Civil War history, nature survival, and bird watching.

Chronic diseases can limit an older person's ability to be independent in performing ADLs and IADLs. Hypertension, heart disease, and strokes are common in this age group. Managing these conditions helps keep the older adult active.

One of the most difficult tasks for the nurse who is interacting with an older adult is distinguishing normal age-related changes from pathological changes. Changes in mobility and chronic pain may limit an older person's activity and active lifestyle. Pain is not a normal part of aging and should always be investigated. It should not be attributed to aging and ignored.

CRITICAL THINKING

Mr. Klein, age 82, visits his health care provider. He reports left hip pain. The health care provider replies, "It can be common to experience pain as you get older." Mr. Klein thinks a minute and says, "But my right hip doesn't hurt, and it's as old as my left hip!"

1. What is occurring in this situation?
2. What actions could be taken to provide patient-centered care and improve the quality of life for Mr. Klein?

   Suggested answers are at the end of the chapter.

Falls are a serious concern for older adults. Data from Healthy People 2020, a national health promotion and disease prevention initiative, show that emergency department visits for falls for older adults are increasing (Office of Disease Prevention and Health Promotion, 2017). Falls result from multiple factors and can indicate the decline of the musculoskeletal system at the subcellular level that occurs with aging. Falls increase dependence and can be predictors of poor outcomes. Osteoporosis is a bone disease common among postmenopausal women and men over age 80, causing bone weakness and fracture risk. Fall prevention includes fall risk assessments and in-home safety assessments to alter the home environment for safety. Bathrooms should be equipped with grab bars, nonskid mats, and bath chairs or benches to make getting into a bath or shower safer. Removing clutter, throw rugs, and electrical cords near walkways decreases the risk of falls.

Hearing and vision loss can affect physical and psychological health in the older adult. Sensory input is needed to protect oneself from accidents, social isolation, and limitations in self-care. One of the most dramatic losses for many older adults is not being able to safely drive a car any longer. The loss of transportation can result in a loss of independence. Visual impairments (e.g., decreased peripheral vision, macular degeneration, cataracts, or glaucoma) can further isolate the patient. Many older adults continue to drive during the day but not at night because of night vision problems. Decreased hearing is also common in older adults. Loss of high-pitch discrimination and reduced ability to filter background noise causes older adults to hear the background noise more clearly than a one-to-one conversation when in a crowded room. Social stigmas related to memory changes such as forgetfulness and dementia are a serious worry for many older adults. They commonly confuse depression with memory changes and attempt to hide their symptoms rather than seek treatment.

 ## CHRONIC ILLNESS

A **chronic illness** is defined as an illness that is long lasting or that recurs and is never completely cured. It usually interferes with the person's ability to perform ADLs. The degree of disability a person has depends not only on the condition and its severity but also on the individual effects for that person. For example, both John F. Kennedy and Franklin D. Roosevelt would have been eligible for 100% disability benefits because of different chronic illnesses they suffered, but both were able to serve as presidents.

When caring for those with chronic illnesses, the goal of nursing care is to maintain and, when able, improve the patient's quality of life. A chronic illness also affects the family dynamics of the patient's family. Therefore, when planning patient care, also consider the family's needs.

Fostering hope is a primary foundation of care planning for people who are chronically ill. A chronic illness may appear to be a hopeless situation if no cure is possible. When recovery from an illness is not possible, it may be thought that nothing can be done for the patient. However, whenever there is life, there is potential for growth in areas such as developmental tasks, health promotion, knowledge, or spirit. Individuals have psychological developmental tasks to perform even as they cope with illness or prepare for a peaceful death.

Incidence of Chronic Illness

Incidences of chronic illness are rising for three reasons. First, people are living longer, and fewer people are dying from acute diseases. This is partly due to better hygiene, nutrition, exercise, vaccinations, antibiotic development, and new treatments. This has created a larger older population that is living longer and developing chronic illnesses. Second, medical advances have reduced mortality from some chronic illnesses. In turn, people are living longer with these illnesses. Third, today's technologically advanced and modern lifestyle contributes to the development of some chronic illnesses. Examples include a sedentary lifestyle; exposure to air and water pollution, chemicals, and carcinogens; substance abuse; and stress.

Types of Chronic Illnesses

Chronic illnesses have different causes (Box 14.1). One chronic illness can lead to development of other illnesses (e.g., hypertension can cause chronic kidney disease). Chronic illness can begin at any age. With age, there is an increasing likelihood of developing one or more chronic illnesses, such as arthritis, hypertension, and sensory losses.

CRITICAL THINKING

Mrs. Luce, age 87, lives alone and one day has a dizzy spell. Her daughter takes her to the emergency department, where her blood pressure reading is 170/88. She has blurred vision in the left eye that resolves after 1 hour. She is diagnosed with hypertension, which possibly contributed to a small stroke or transient ischemic attack. Mrs. Luce is started on metoprolol (Lopressor) 100 mg daily. She is discharged to her home with instructions on taking her medication, following a low-sodium diet, and home safety.

1. Why might Mrs. Luce have an increased risk of falling?
2. What patient-centered nursing interventions would help promote Mrs. Luce's independence and safety?
3. The nurse is to give metoprolol 100 mg, and 50-milligram tablets are available. How many tablets should the nurse give?

Suggested answers are at the end of the chapter.

Gerontological Influence

As people live longer, spouses or older relatives are increasingly being called on to care for chronically ill family members. Children of older adults who themselves are reaching their 60s and may have chronic illnesses of their own are

Box 14.1

Examples of Chronic Illnesses by Cause

Genetic
• Cystic fibrosis
• Huntington disease
• Sickle cell anemia

Congenital
• Heart defects
• Malabsorption syndromes
• Spina bifida

Acquired
• AIDS
• Arthritis
• Cancer
• Diabetes mellitus
• Emphysema
• Head/spinal cord injury
• Multiple sclerosis

being expected to care for their frail parents. A family in this situation is at great risk for ineffective coping or further development of health problems. Assessment of all older members of the family is essential to ensure that all their health and coping needs are being met.

Older adults are concerned about becoming dependent on others. They may become depressed and give up hope if they feel that they are a burden to others. Establishing short-term goals or self-care activities that allow them to participate or have small successes is an important nursing action that can increase their self-esteem. The nursing diagnosis *Frail Elderly Syndrome* may apply to older chronically ill patients.

When caring for a chronically ill older patient, barriers can exist for the patient. These include not understanding medications, being on special diets or treatments, and being unfamiliar with supportive services in the community. Share information with older patients and their families about meal programs or respite care. Also, provide a resource person for them to contact with questions.

Effects of Chronic Illness

Healthy People 2020's target goal for older adults with moderate-to-severe functional limitations is 26.4% (Office of Disease Prevention and Health Promotion, 2017). However, the data show that this percentage is instead rising. To cope with a chronic illness and resulting functional limitations, lifelong routines and habits may need to be changed. Treatment needs, such as going to therapy sessions, performing peritoneal dialysis exchanges, or monitoring blood glucose, can interrupt daily life and require adaptation into the daily routine.

Chronic Sorrow

Chronic sorrow is felt by those affected by a chronic illness. It is an intermittently occurring sadness in response to losses caused by a chronic illness. It can be felt by the patient or the patient's significant others. The nursing diagnosis *Chronic Sorrow* may apply to those with chronic illness. When chronic sadness occurs, nursing care should focus on active listening. Understanding the loss allows you to offer comfort, support, and information. Assistance with coping strategies includes fostering support systems.

Spiritual Distress

Patients with chronic illness can experience spiritual distress when faced with the limitations of their illness. Maintaining a patient's quality of life includes assisting with spiritual needs. Interventions that address **spirituality** might need to be performed first to promote later success with the patient's plan of care.

Several factors may make you uncomfortable in caring for a patient's spiritual needs. These include a lack of training, a lack of understanding of your own spiritual needs and beliefs, and not recognizing or believing that this is your role. Examine your own spiritual needs, and then

define a personal spiritual view. Doing this can help you develop insight into others' spiritual needs and resources. It will help you gain insight into issues surrounding your patients' spiritual needs. This can then make you more comfortable in addressing your patient's spiritual needs.

Many people use spirituality to cope with chronic illness. It gives them a sense of wholeness, hope, and peace during uncertain times. Spirituality empowers patients to handle their condition. It is a source of inner strength. A meditation room for quiet reflection or prayer, chaplain visits, or worship services can be used to support spirituality in the hospital.

Accreditation agencies require that the spiritual needs of patients are addressed and documented by nurses. Nursing diagnoses related to spiritual needs include *Spiritual Distress, Readiness for Enhanced Spiritual Well-Being,* and *Impaired Religiosity.*

NURSING CARE TIP

Spirituality is feeling connected to a higher power. It should not be thought of in only religious terms. Everyone has spiritual needs that involve hope, peace, and wholeness. Spiritual care goes beyond asking a patient's religion. It involves assessing the patient's perceptions of spirituality and then identifying ways to meet the person's spiritual needs.

Powerlessness

A chronic illness can be unpredictable. This leaves the patient vulnerable during the phases of a chronic illness: the diagnosis, the instability phase, an acute illness or crisis, remissions, and a terminal phase. Treatments that the patient undergoes may be painful, frightening, and invasive. A patient who does not understand what is happening can feel overwhelmed and alone. This contributes to a feeling of **powerlessness** because the patient cannot control the outcome (Fig. 14.2). This lack of control throughout an illness influences the patient's reactions to the illness. The nursing diagnosis *Powerlessness* may apply to chronically ill patients.

COPING. Patients can be helped to feel more in control of their illness if you remember to include them in their care. Listen to their feelings, values, and goals. Explain all procedures before they occur. Avoid using complex medical language when talking with patients to increase their understanding and feeling of being included in their care. Coping with a chronic illness can be aided if the patient develops a positive attitude toward dealing with the illness. This can be accomplished if the patient gains knowledge, uses a problem-solving approach, becomes motivated to continue adapting to the illness, and has resilience ("Evidence-Based Practice").

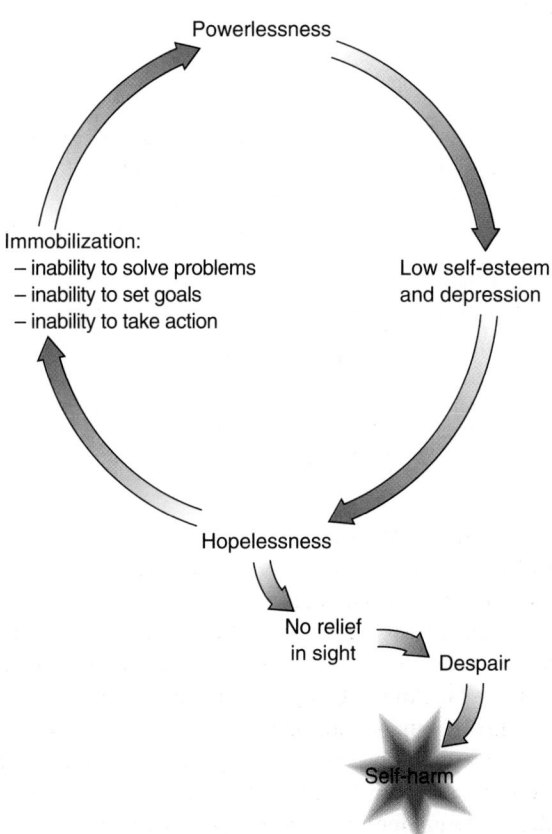

FIGURE 14.2 Powerlessness–hopelessness cycle.

Having a variety of coping techniques can be useful. Ask the patient about his or her perception of the illness and coping techniques that were previously used successfully. New coping resources may need to be added to help the patient effectively deal with the chronic illness. Offer community support service information to the patient and family. To cope effectively, help the patient learn to be comfortable with the newly defined person he or she is to become. The nursing diagnoses *Ineffective Coping, Compromised Family Coping, Disabled Family Coping,* and *Readiness for Enhanced Family Coping* may apply to those dealing with chronic illness.

HOPE. Before coping resources can be used, hope must be established in the patient. False hope is not beneficial and should be replaced with realistic hope. Providing patients with accurate knowledge regarding their fears helps do this. Hope should not be directed toward a cure that may not be possible but rather at living a quality life with the functional capacity that the patient has. Over the course of the illness, hope needs to be maintained for both the patient and family. Periodically assess if the patient is maintaining hope. Studies have shown that patients adapt better when hope is high. The nursing diagnoses *Readiness for Enhanced Hope* or *Hopelessness* may apply to chronically ill patients.

Encouraging patients to live each moment to the fullest helps them experience the joy of being alive. Using humor aids patients in being light-hearted and hopeful. Simple things, such as a cool breeze, the warm sun on the skin through a facility window, the clean scent of the air after it rains, or the scent of pine trees, allow one to appreciate the beauty of nature and inspire hope. Family members can be encouraged to foster hope in the patient. This can also make them feel hopeful as well. During times of acute illness, it is beneficial for the patient to maintain as much control as possible and be informed if any loss of control related to treatments is temporary. This prevents a continual feeling of loss of power. The use of music or inspirational reading material can reduce stress and help the patient find meaning in life. This in turn fosters hope. Hopeful patients are empowered and do not feel powerless.

Sexuality
Chronic illness can affect a patient's sexuality, which includes femininity and masculinity as well as sexual activity. Changes in the physical body affect the way patients view themselves and are viewed by others. Patients with a negative body image perception may withdraw and become depressed. When interacting with patients, be aware of your facial expressions, nonverbal cues such as appearing hurried or keeping a distance, use of or lack of touch, and amount of time spent with the patient. When patients believe they have lost their femininity or masculinity, their self-worth decreases. Interventions to enhance sexuality should be used. One example is obtaining a wig for patients undergoing chemotherapy.

CRITICAL THINKING

Mr. Webb, age 90, lives in his own home with his wife of 65 years. He is in good health except for limited vision and is very active physically and socially. Mr. Webb's wife is in the early stages of Alzheimer's disease. She cannot perform activities of daily living, so he has assumed the caregiver role. They complement each other's limitations because she has good vision and is helpful when she is not confused.

Over time, Mr. Webb's wife's health declines, and she enters a long-term care facility. Mr. Webb remains in his home alone, which concerns his family. They eventually convince him to move into senior housing. He is very reluctant to leave his home and does not actively participate in moving and selling his home. Mr. Webb rarely leaves his new apartment, sleeps 14 hours a day, and eats one daily meal. He tries to visit his wife by taking a bus but finds it difficult because of his limited vision, so he rarely sees her. Three months later, Mr. Webb develops pneumonia and dies.

1. Why do you think Mr. Webb behaved the way he did after he moved?
2. What patient-centered interventions could have been used to empower Mr. Webb?
3. Why might Mr. Webb have developed pneumonia and died?

Suggested answers at end of chapter.

Sexual intimacy can include touching, hugging, or sharing time together. Provide patients with the opportunity to discuss sexuality questions. Be professional and confidential. Sexuality counselors can help chronically ill patients cope with their sexuality needs.

Because sexuality is a part of a person's lifelong identity, ensure older patients' sexuality is addressed in their plans of care. Patients in long-term care facilities should be given private time with their significant other, as appropriate. Grooming methods can increase a patient's self-esteem and sexual identity. Women may want to get their hair and nails done; men can be shaved or get a haircut. Older patients' sexuality needs should be met just as younger patients' needs are. The nursing diagnoses of *Disturbed Body Image*, *Sexual Dysfunction*, or *Ineffective Sexuality Pattern* may apply.

Roles

Chronically ill patients usually are faced with altering their accustomed roles in life. These roles may include that of being a spouse, grandparent, parent, provider, homemaker, employee, or friend. Not only must the patient deal with these role alterations, but the family must adapt to them as well. Family members may have to take on new roles themselves to compensate for roles the patient can no longer perform. The nursing diagnosis of *Ineffective Role Performance* should be included in the plan of care for the patient and family.

The patient is faced with giving up aspects of old roles at the same time that new roles related to being chronically ill need to be assumed. Grieving accompanies the loss of old roles. If a patient is no longer able to participate in social activities, grief work needs to occur to help the patient accept the loss and maintain dignity. With other roles, only certain aspects of the role may change. For example, in the parenting role, patients may still function as a support system for a child, although they can no longer be the disciplinarian. Whatever the role loss, the patient needs to be allowed to grieve the loss. The nursing diagnosis of *Grieving* may help in planning care for the patient.

New roles for the patient who is chronically ill may include being a dependent, an ongoing health care consumer, and a chronically ill person. Patients need to be given understanding while they become familiar with these roles. For patients used to being independent before the illness, being dependent on others to meet ADLs can cause a loss in self-esteem. Navigating the complex health care and financial reimbursement systems can be overwhelming. Patient care navigators help patients in doing this. Transportation needs and waiting times for medical appointments can be difficult for patients who must deal with them on an ongoing basis. *Deficient Knowledge* and *Readiness for Enhanced Knowledge* are nursing diagnoses helpful for fostering learning for these new roles.

As patients live with chronic illness over time, they become experts on their own illness. Today, patients are being viewed as partners in their health care. Being sensitive to patients' knowledge and respecting it increases patients' self-esteem.

Family and Caregivers

Families are affected by the chronic illness of a family member in many ways. Most chronic illness care is provided in the home so that families can become involved in the management of the illness. Family members may have to take on new family roles or assume the role of caregiver. Decreased socialization, lost income, and increased medical expenses can increase family stress and tension.

Families must learn to cope with the stress of illness and its often-unpredictable course. Most families develop ways to cope with the patient's illness. They may become closer as a family unit. Families often deal with the illness on a day-by-day basis. They may take a passive approach to letting problems work themselves out. During times of exacerbation or crisis, however, the family may need coping assistance (Box 14.2).

Patients are often concerned about being a burden to their families. It is important to determine both the family's and the patient's feelings about the care required for the patient. The family's ability to provide this care adequately

Caregiver Resources

AARP: Family Caregiving, www.aarp.org/caregiving
Family Caregiver Alliance, www.caregiver.org
Eldercare Locator, www.eldercare.gov

must also be considered in care planning. If the family lacks the desire, skills, or resources to adequately care for the patient, alternative care options, such as home health care, adult foster care, or long-term care, must be explored.

Patients' caregivers often have certain ideas about the care that the patient should receive. Caregiver input into the patient's plan of care should be sought so that everyone has a clear understanding of the goals and expectations for the patient's care.

Caregivers can experience depression, role strain, guilt, powerlessness, and grieving related to caregiving. Awareness of this helps nurses detect indications that caregivers need help in dealing with these feelings. Chronic care coaches are available to provide caregivers with insight, encouragement, and support for caring for someone who is chronically ill. Nursing diagnoses for caregivers include *Risk for Caregiver Role Strain* and *Caregiver Role Strain.*

RESPITE CARE. When caregivers are required to provide 24-hour care for a patient, they can experience burnout, fatigue, and stress. If extreme, this may lead to patient abuse. Patients may not be able to be left alone, even briefly, because of wandering behaviors, confusion, or safety issues. Caregivers might find it impossible to get a normal night's sleep and suffer from sleep deprivation because of the patient's wandering or around-the-clock treatment needs. It is essential for caregivers to have periodic relief from caregiving to reduce the stress of always having to be responsible. Everyone requires private time for reflection or pursuing favorite hobbies or interests. Caregivers may need a night or weekend away simply to sleep soundly and be refreshed. **Respite care** is designed to provide caregivers with a much-needed break from caregiving by providing someone else to assume the caregiver role. Be familiar with your community's respite care services and share that information with caregivers.

CRITICAL THINKING

Mrs. Bow, age 64, is caring for her husband, who has Alzheimer's disease. He wanders at night and has been found outside in his pajamas in freezing winter weather. He tries to cook and burns the pans. He cannot express his needs. He disrobes frequently and is incontinent. Mrs. Bow quit her job to care for him. She no longer goes to lunch weekly with her friends. Her children live out of town. She places a chair and tin cans in front of the home's doors as

an alarm in case her husband opens the doors while she tries to sleep.

1. What indicates that Mrs. Bow is experiencing stress related to caregiving?
2. What nursing diagnoses should be included in a plan of care for Mrs. Bow?
3. What nursing interventions would be beneficial for Mrs. Bow?

Suggested answers are at the end of the chapter.

Finances

Managing a chronic illness can be expensive. Income can be lost if the patient is unable to work or caregivers are forced to stay home. Insurance may not cover all the patient's expenses. Family savings can quickly be used up and place a strain on families. This can lead to the nursing diagnoses *Compromised Family Coping, Disabled Family Coping,* or *Readiness for Enhanced Family Coping.* Social work referrals can be made to assist with financial aid.

Health Promotion

Health promotion is possible and necessary at all ages or levels of disability. Patients with chronic illness make daily lifestyle choices that affect their health. For example, the patient with chronic lung disease makes the choice to smoke or to quit smoking, and a patient with degenerative joint disease chooses whether to maintain an ideal weight to reduce wear and tear on the joints. Encourage health promotion efforts. Identify a patient's risk factors to plan methods of promoting health. Providing patients with the knowledge to make informed decisions empowers them to take control of their lives and reach their greatest potential.

Nursing Care

Because of the nature of chronic illness, nurses should understand the unique needs of patients and families experiencing chronic illness. These needs differ from those of patients experiencing acute care. In-depth knowledge is needed by the patient. Recognize that the wishes of the patient must be respected. This is true even if you do not agree with them. Patients have the right to establish their own goals along with the health care team. Patients are participating in their own daily bedside rounds with the health care team in institutions. This is true patient-centered care!

Most chronic illness care occurs in the home and community ("Home Health Hints"). Therefore, family members and caregivers, even more so than in acute care, must be included in the plan of care. As the numbers of those with chronic illness grow, increasing community support for chronically ill people and their caregivers is needed.

Home Health Hints

Patient-Centered Care

- Medicare requires that the home health care patient participates in the development of the plan of care. The patient has the right to be informed in advance about the care to be furnished and of any changes in care. Involve the patient in care planning by asking about care preferences and assisting the patient to set realistic and meaningful goals. Praise the effort the patient is making toward meeting his or her goals.
- Asking about displayed photos or mementos can increase a patient's self-concept.
- Reminiscing with the patient can show how the patient has coped with challenges in the past.
- Using appropriate humor can relieve stress and humanize care. Humor can also be irritating, however, if the patient is distraught, anxious, or angry.

Resources

- Encourage caregivers of bed-confined patients to use a portable nursery monitor to hear the patient.
- Occupational and physical therapists can recommend equipment, like a long-handled sponge or eating utensils, to increase patient independence.
- The home health care social worker should be informed of any patient concerns regarding cost of medicines or equipment.

A major focus of nursing care for the chronically ill is teaching. These patients and their families have tremendous educational needs if they are to learn to cope successfully with a long-term illness. The following are primary tasks that chronically ill patients need to perform:

- Be willing and able to carry out the medical regimen.
- Reorder time to meet demands caused by the illness, such as treatments, medication schedules, and pacing of activities.
- Understand and control symptoms.

- Prevent and manage crises.
- Adjust to changes in the disease over the course of time, whether positive or negative.
- Prevent social isolation as a result of physical limitations or altered body image.
- Compensate for symptoms and limitations in order to be treated as normally as possible by others.

Explain individualized interventions to deal with these tasks during teaching sessions. Provide dignity and show respect to all patients ("Patient Perspective"). Unique approaches are needed to positively assist chronically ill patients and their families on their long-term journey.

Patient Perspective

Mr. Lyman. A note to my nurse:

- Don't call me "sweetie" or "honey." My name is Mr. Lyman. If I want you to call me by my first name, I'll tell you.
- Be polite!
- Don't give me a huge glass of water; give me a small glass and don't fill it full. Otherwise, when I drink it, it spills all down the front of me.
- When you leave my meal tray, make sure I can reach it. Then when you take it away, don't leave a bunch of stuff on my table. There is not much room on those little tables.
- Ask how I like my blankets. Don't just fix them the way you do for anyone else.
- Make sure my call light is where I can reach it.
- Make sure my overhead light is working and that I can reach it.
- Keep a wastebasket where I can reach it.
- Ask whether I need anything before you leave the room.
- Try to talk quietly in the hallway, instead of being so loud.
- Thank you for preserving my dignity and showing me respect. I appreciate it!

SUGGESTED ANSWERS TO CRITICAL THINKING

Mr. Paul

1. Mr. Paul's physical health is being affected by poor diet choices and stress.
2. It is easy to recognize the psychological stress related to parenting skills when a child is in trouble. Decreased family income with increased family expenses (two children in college) can cause financial strains. With family problems and health problems, Mr. Paul may be questioning

why things are happening to him and his family, causing him spiritual distress.

Mr. Klein

1. Stereotypical misconceptions about older adults is occurring. This can lead to the belief that pain is part of the aging process. Therefore, Mr. Klein's issue may not be diagnosed and treated appropriately.

SUGGESTED ANSWERS TO CRITICAL THINKING—cont'd

2. Gathering data to assist with the diagnosis of the cause of the pain and possible treatment would improve Mr. Klein's quality of life. Taking him seriously would also convey that Mr. Klein is a valued member of society and increase his self-esteem.

Mrs. Luce

1. Falls could be caused by changes due to aging; things in the environment, such as throw rugs, clutter, or electrical cords in walking paths; lack of hand grips in the bathroom; or lack of nonskid mats in the shower or tub. Poor vision and altered depth perception can result in missing a stair step or obstacles. Weakness or orthostatic hypotension can cause an unsteady gait or fall.

2. Instruct the patient and family about home safety. Mrs. Luce may even benefit by using a cane or a walker if she is unsteady. Because Mrs. Luce lives alone, a portable emergency alert system would be beneficial. When activated, the transmitter alerts an answering service to contact designated individuals to check on the patient. Safety with medications is also an important consideration. Patients who take medications that lower blood pressure must be aware of the potential for orthostatic hypotension. Orthostatic hypotension is a drop in blood pressure that happens when a person moves from a lying to sitting or sitting to standing position. It is often accompanied by dizziness or light-headedness. Some people can even faint, causing a fall.

3. Give two tablets of 50 mg each.

Mr. Webb

1. Mr. Webb had lost control of his world and felt powerless. His environment, both home and outdoors, was shrinking. He had to give up his daily routines and interactions with others. His purpose in life was gone when he was no longer caring for his wife. He was separated from his loved one. His visual limitations made his new environment unfamiliar and frightening.

2. Options to keep him safely in his home could have been explored with his input. After the move, he should have been thoroughly oriented to his environment. He should have been asked to explain what he wanted his life to be like as he adapted to this new period. Hobbies and interests should have been continued. Visual support services should have been contacted for ideas. Transportation should have been arranged to allow him to visit his wife and continue golfing. It should have been determined whether phone calls to his wife were possible.

3. He was depressed and slept from a lack of interests. His lungs were at risk for pneumonia because of his long periods of immobility. He lost hope and gave up on living, which decreased his ability to fight the pneumonia.

Mrs. Bow

1. Mrs. Bow is at risk for sleep deprivation, fatigue, stress, and burnout.

2. Nursing diagnoses include *Disturbed Sleep Pattern, Fatigue, Social Isolation, Risk for Caregiver Role Strain,* and *Deficient Knowledge.*

3. Beneficial nursing interventions would include teaching her about Alzheimer's disease, recommending a chronic care coach, and providing a respite care referral, alarm devices for wandering, and stress management techniques.

Review Questions

1. The nurse is collecting data regarding a 68-year-old patient's developmental stage and finds that the patient is retired and that the patient's spouse died 4 months ago. The nurse identifies the patient as being in which of the following developmental stages?
   1. Generativity versus self-absorption
   2. Identity versus role confusion
   3. Integrity versus despair
   4. Intimacy versus isolation

2. The nurse is planning care for a patient with heart disease. Which of the following effects should the nurse consider is most likely to occur with a chronic illness when gathering further data collection?
   1. Hopefulness
   2. Increased socialization
   3. Powerfulness
   4. Spiritual distress

3. A 70-year-old man is the primary caregiver for his wife, who has moderately severe Alzheimer's disease. He becomes angry with her for spilling her dinner on the floor. He later feels guilty and begins to cry. The home health care nurse is developing a plan of care. Which of the following would be an appropriate nursing diagnosis for the nurse to include?
   1. *Caregiver Role Strain*
   2. *Hopelessness*
   3. *Powerlessness*
   4. *Risk for Caregiver Role Strain*

4. A 64-year-old patient goes to a clinic for a yearly physical. The patient has a history of hypertension and osteoarthritis. Which of the following would be a priority action for the nurse to take to promote wellness for this patient who has chronic illnesses?
   1. Demonstrate how to take a blood pressure.
   2. Explain hypertension and osteoarthritis.
   3. Encourage increased socialization.
   4. Evaluate goal progress with the patient and family.

5. The nurse is providing care for a patient who is chronically ill. Which of the following actions would the nurse take for the chronically ill patient? **Select all that apply.**
   1. Limit educational information.
   2. Encourage visits by family members.
   3. Include family members in teaching sessions.
   4. Set the goals for the patient.
   5. Limit visits from friends.
   6. Obtain patient input on plan of care.

6. Which of the following actions would be most appropriate for the nurse to take for a patient with a chronic illness who is experiencing chronic sorrow? **Select all that apply.**
   1. Provide quiet time.
   2. Make time to listen.
   3. Share information.
   4. Limit interactions.
   5. Use active listening.
   6. Encourage hope.

7. The nurse would evaluate the patient with a chronic illness as responding positively to interventions for chronic sorrow if the patient stated which of the following?
   1. "I have nothing left to accomplish."
   2. "Maybe tomorrow will be a better day."
   3. "I should not keep hoping for a cure."
   4. "There is nothing I can do."

Answer rationales available in your online resources.

ANSWERS 1. 3; 2. 4; 3. 1; 4. 2; 5. 2, 3, 6; 6. 2, 3, 5, 6; 7. 2

Key Points

Find the chapter key points in your online resources available through Davis Edge.

Additional Resources

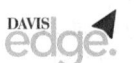 Use the scratch off code on the inside front cover of your book to access online quizzes that will help you to improve your scores on course exams and prepare for NCLEX-PN®.

 Study Guide

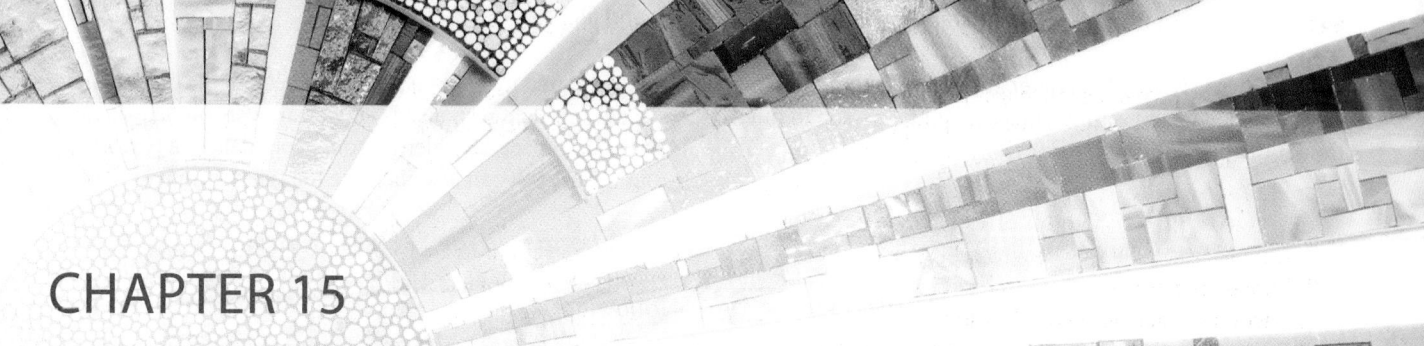

CHAPTER 15
Nursing Care of Older Adult Patients

MaryAnne Pietraniec-Shannon

KEY TERMS

activities of daily living (ack-TIH-vih-tees of DAY-lee LIH-ving)

aspiration (AS-pi-RAY-shun)

constipation (KON-sti-PAY-shun)

contractures (kon-TRAK-churs)

delirium (del-LEER-ee-um)

dementia (deh-MEN-cha)

depression (dih-PRESH-shun)

edema (eh-DEE-muh)

expectorate (ek-SPEK-tuh-RAYT)

extrinsic factors (eks-TRIN-sik FAK-ters)

holistic (hoh-LIS-tik)

homeostasis (HO-mee-oh-STAY-sis)

intrinsic factors (in-TRIN-sik FAK-ters)

nocturia (nok-TOO-ree-ah)

optimum level of functioning (OP-tih-mum LEV-uhl of FUNK-shun-ing)

osteoporosis (AWS-tee-oh-puh-ROH-sis)

perception (per-SEP-shun)

pressure injury (PRESH-ur IN-jer-ee)

range of motion (RAINJE of MOH-shun)

reality orientation (ree-AL-ih-tee OR-ee-en-TAY-shun)

sensory deprivation (SEN-suh-ree DEP-rih-VAY-shun)

sensory overload (SEN-suh-ree OH-ver-lohd)

urinary incontinence (YOOR-ih-NARE-ee in-KON-tih-nents)

CHAPTER CONCEPTS

Patient-Centered Care
Safety

LEARNING OUTCOMES

1. Define aging.
2. Describe basic physiological changes associated with advancing age.
3. Describe the psychological and cognitive changes associated with advancing age.
4. Plan nursing care for the physiological and psychological changes associated with advancing age.
5. Identify nursing practices that promote safety for the older patient.

 WHAT IS AGING?

Physical structures and body functions normally undergo changes and declines with advancing age. Although there is not one commonly accepted definition or theory to explain these declines, there is an understanding that aging is a universal and normal process that starts at conception and continues until death.

According to a 2016 report from the United States Department of Health and Human Services, the number of older people in the United States (65 years or older) increased from 36.6 million in 2005 to 47.8 million in 2015. The fastest growing group of older people continues to be adults 85 and older. Their numbers are projected to triple from 6.3 million in 2015 to 14.6 million in 2040 (U.S. Department of Health and Human Services, 2016).

In this chapter, *aging* is defined as a maturational process that creates the need for individual adaptation because of physical and psychological declines that occur throughout life. Even though aging truly begins at conception, the focus in this chapter is on the maturational process that is experienced after age 65 (older adult). People aged 85 and older are usually the frailest, although chronological age alone should never be the basis for determining health status. Functional age (health, independence, and functional abilities) should be used as the basis for determining individual care needs. In 2016, the federal government reported that about 9 million people in the United States received long-term care assistance through 4,800 adult day services centers, 12,400 home health care agencies, 4,000 hospices, 15,600 nursing homes, and 30,200 assisted living and similar residential care communities across the

United States (Harris-Kojetin et al., 2016). Quality nursing care provided in any setting allows the older person to function at the highest possible level.

NURSING CARE TIP

Aging is a unique experience. Placing older adults into one category titled "old" overlooks this. The concept of *functional age* recognizes that aging is individual. It promotes patient-centered care for the older adult.

Aging is a unique experience for everyone. Factors that contribute to aging fall within two categories. **Intrinsic factors** focus on genetic and physiological theories of aging. Genetic theories include the biological clock theory or programmed aging theory. Physiological theories include aspects of the wear-and-tear theory or stress adaptation theory. **Extrinsic factors** focus on environmental influences, such as pollutants, free-radical theory, and stress-adaptation theory.

Perception and attitude play key roles in how changes over time affect the individual. It is through the filter of perception and attitude that a person identifies, defines, and adapts to the changes that occur in body structure and function over time. Aging factors affect older patients and their families and the health care providers working with them.

PHYSIOLOGICAL CHANGES

Over time, cells change and do not function as efficiently as in earlier years. Compared with cellular changes, the physical changes seen when looking at an older person are slight. Cellular decline in structure and function increases in severity and extent over time. Although the body works hard to maintain **homeostasis,** it is often unable to fully adapt to many of the declines that result from aging. Some cells that die cannot regenerate themselves. As a result, structures are altered. The body then tries to make the revised structure meet functional demands.

Common Physiological Changes in Older Adults and Their Implications for Nursing Care

Key Changes in the Muscular System

Age-related changes in the muscular system include the following:

- Decreased elasticity of tendons and ligaments, resulting in restricted movements
- Decreased muscle mass, making muscles look smaller
- Slower muscle response, increasing response time
- Decreased muscle tone, making muscles flabbier

NURSING CARE. Changes in the muscular system impact movement, strength, and endurance. **Range of motion** (ROM)

can be limited in the arms, legs, and neck of the older patient. Because muscle response is slower, movement takes longer. This can impact the older person's confidence in performing routine tasks. It can also increase the risk for injury.

Key Changes in the Skeletal System

Age-related changes in the skeletal system include the following:

- Exaggerated bony prominences, increasing risk for skin breakdown
- Eroding cartilage, making joint movement painful
- Joint stiffening, decreasing flexibility
- **Osteoporosis,** thinning (decrease in density) and softening of the bone
- Water loss in the intervertebral disks of the spinal column and flexion of the spine associated with the influence of gravity over time, reducing height

NURSING CARE. Muscles and bones work together for movement. So, aging skeletal changes are most obvious when the older patient is moving. **Contractures** of the fingers and hands can limit the person's ability to perform self-care tasks. These tasks are referred to as **activities of daily living** (ADLs). Assist the patient with ROM exercises as needed. This can prevent long-term disabilities from contractures (Fig. 15.1). Performing ROM exercises in warm water can help prevent pain. If the person has arthritis, give prescribed anti-inflammatory medications so their action peaks when exercises are beginning. Older patients taking anti-inflammatory medicines should be monitored closely for gastrointestinal (GI) upset or bleeding. They should be taught the symptoms of bleeding to report to their health care provider (HCP).

Bone density is influenced by diet and weight-bearing exercise. Diets should be balanced and rich in calcium and vitamin D. Safe weight-bearing exercise programs should be encouraged. Tai-chi, an ancient Chinese gentle system of exercise and stretching, is very helpful in promoting balance and flexibility for the older adult to prevent falls. Patients should wear supportive shoes with nonskid soles. The environment needs to be safe for walking. Sturdy assistive devices such as handrails, canes, or walkers should be used as needed. Decreasing density of bones can cause fractures that result in falls or falls that cause fractures ("Evidence-Based Practice"). In both genders, severe pain and one or more chronic diseases are linked to falling. Gender differences exist for fall risk. Women are more likely to fall. Fall risk factors for women include frailty and incontinence. For men, risks include older age, symptoms of depression, and inability to perform a standing balance test (Gale, Cooper, & Sayer, 2016). Consider gender to plan fall risk interventions.

• WORD • BUILDING •

homeostasis: homios—similar + stasis—standing

osteoporosis: osteon—bone + poros—a passage + osis—condition

Evidence-Based Practice

Clinical Question
What are risk factors for falls in community-dwelling older adults?

Evidence
A systematic review of risk factors for adults living in the community included 62 studies. In all, 50 risk factors were identified in six categories for the adult: environment, medication, cognitive, physiological, psychological, and socioeconomic. Identified risk factors included the following:

- Adult: 65 or older, ambulatory assistive devices, fall history, female, living alone, wearing slippers
- Environmental: clutter, dim lighting, lack of nonslip bath material, no grab bars/handrails
- Medication: poly-medication, antihypertensives (diuretics, angiotensin-converting enzyme [ACE] inhibitors, calcium channel blockers, beta-adrenergic blockers), benzodiazepines
- Cognitive: change in function, diminished executive function
- Physiological: arthritis, gait difficulties, impaired balance, visual impairment, orthostatic hypotension, decreased leg strength, blood sugar changes, urinary urgency/incontinence, activities of daily living (ADLs)/instrumental ADLs decline, dizziness, chronic disease, insomnia, obesity
- Psychological: fear of falling, depression, anxiety
- Socioeconomic: low education/income

Implications for Nursing Practice
Fall prevention requires understanding of all fall risk factors to plan effective interventions to decrease falls.

Reference
Sousa, L. M., Marques-Vieira, C. M., Caldevilla, M. N., Henriques, C. M., Severino, S. S., & Caldeira, S. M. (2016). Risk for falls among community-dwelling older people: Systematic literature review. *Revista Gaúcha de Enfermagem, 37*(4), e55030. doi.org/10.1590/1983-1447.2016.04.55030

BE SAFE!
BE VIGILANT! Find out which patients and residents are most likely to fall. For example, is the patient or resident taking any medicines that might make them weak, dizzy, or sleepy? Take action to prevent falls for these patients and residents.

(The Joint Commission's 2018 National Patient Safety Goals. © The Joint Commission, 2018. Reprinted with permission.)

Key Changes in the Integumentary System
Age-related changes in the integumentary system include the following:

- Thin skin layers, making the skin more fragile
- Decreased subcutaneous fat layer, resulting in less insulation and less protective cushioning
- Water loss, causing increased dryness of the skin
- Decreased sebaceous and sweat glands, resulting in skin dryness and decreased temperature regulation.
- Increased pigmentation, causing aging spots
- Decreased melanin, resulting in gray hair
- Thinning scalp hair, resulting in baldness
- Harder and drier nails, making them more brittle

NURSING CARE. The skin is the first line of defense against infection and injury (Fig. 15.2). In the older adult, skin injuries take longer to heal. Healing times can be affected by the presence of multiple chronic diseases. These diseases include diabetes and circulatory disorders. The older person with limited mobility is at risk of developing **pressure injuries** (see Chapter 54). It is important to take time to check skin integrity daily, especially in high-risk areas of the body. To prevent accidental injury to the feet, instruct patients not to walk barefoot. Potential pressure points on the feet should be monitored. Referral to a podiatrist is made when there are concerns. People with neuropathy (decreased sensation) or diabetes should assess their feet daily to prevent injury.

BE SAFE!
BE VIGILANT! Find out which patients and residents are most likely to have bed sores. Take action to prevent bed sores in these patients and residents. From time to time, recheck patients and residents for bed sores.

(The Joint Commission's 2018 National Patient Safety Goals. © The Joint Commission, 2018. Reprinted with permission.)

BE SAFE!
BE VIGILANT! Shoes should be checked thoroughly before putting them on to ensure there is nothing in them that could cause injury. A person with severe foot neuropathy wore shoes for 8 hours without recognizing that a small toy was wedged in the toe of the shoe. Because he could not feel the irritation of the toy, he continued to walk. It was not until the end of the day when he removed that shoe that he saw a severe pressure injury on his toe that required hospitalization. Teach patients the importance of daily foot and shoe assessment for safety!

Skin care for the older adult should be gently performed. The New York State Department of Health details techniques for gentle bathing at www.health.ny.gov/diseases/conditions/dementia/edge/interventions/gentle/index.htm. These techniques include the towel bath, bag bath, and glove bath. These methods of bathing avoid the drying effects from using hot water and soap. Applying moisturizers regularly (except between toes); gently stimulating nonreddened, intact skin sites with massage; and avoiding use of heating pads that can burn all help to protect the skin. Nail care is also important for older people. Soaking

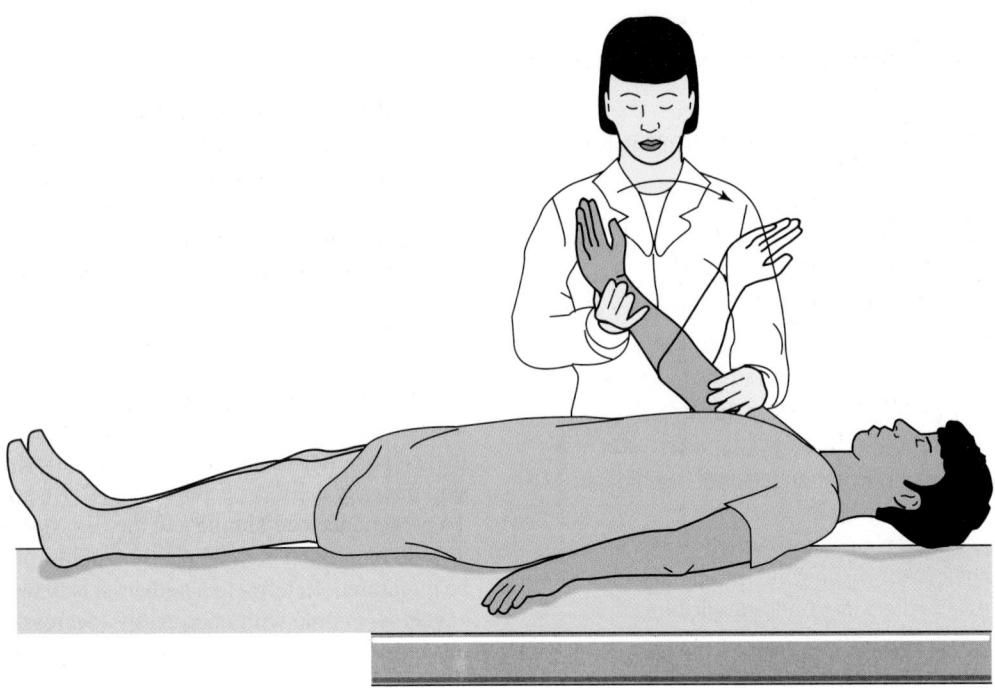

FIGURE 15.1 Nurse assists patient in range-of-motion exercises to prevent the development of contractures.

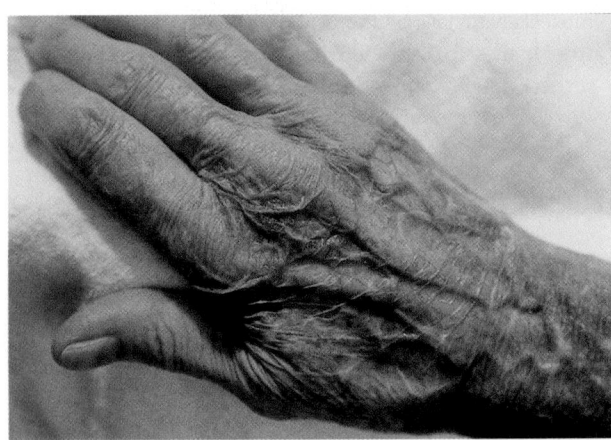

FIGURE 15.2 Thin, fragile skin of an older person.

nails in warm water helps soften nails. This makes it easier to trim them. It also promotes blood flow to these peripheral areas. Filing nails with an emery board is safer than cutting them.

Key Changes in the Cardiovascular System

Age-related changes in the cardiovascular system include the following:

- Decreased blood vessel elasticity, increasing blood pressure and cardiac workload
- Decreased cardiac output, causing less oxygen to body tissues
- Atypical classic symptoms of cardiac emergencies, delaying recognition and treatment
- Increased conduction time, possibly causing slower heart rate and making it unable to increase quickly

- Increased arrhythmias (irregular heartbeats), resulting in poor oxygenation of heart and heart failure
- Less efficient leg vein valves, creating fluid accumulation in tissues

NURSING CARE. Observe for early symptoms related to circulatory problems. They can be subtle. Cardiovascular disease causes half of all deaths in people over age 65. It is important to educate older patients on promoting healthy circulation and to take prescribed medications as ordered. Monitoring fluid balance is important. Thirst may be decreased. Oral fluids may need to be encouraged. Intravenous (IV) fluids must be carefully monitored to prevent fluid overload. If leg **edema** is present, the legs should be elevated higher than the heart. This promotes blood return to the heart for circulating. Compression stockings should be worn as ordered. Report circulation concerns for the older patient promptly to the HCP for treatment.

Changes in body position from lying to sitting to standing should occur gradually. Quickly changing body position can make the older patient feel weak and dizzy. Stand next to older patients as they dangle their legs over the side of the bed before rising to stand. For safety, use an ambulatory belt and provide a walker for unsteady older patients. Falls continue to be a leading cause of accidental death in older patients. A history of falls is a key predictor of future falls. Identify patients who are at risk of falling. Then implement interventions to prevent falls.

• **WORD** • **BUILDING** •
edema: oidema—swelling

Key Changes in the Respiratory System

Age-related changes in the respiratory system include the following:

- Reduced emptying of the lungs, causing carbon dioxide (CO_2) retention
- Decreased lung capacity, causing dyspnea with activity
- Decreased lung recoil strength or gag reflex, producing weaker cough and pulmonary **aspiration** risk
- Reduced tone of lung tissue, increasing shallow respirations to 16 to 25 per minute

NURSING CARE. The respiratory system is less efficient with advancing age. Older patients have a decreased tolerance for activity. It can take a longer amount of time for normal respiratory functioning to return when under stress. Help older patients pace their activities. Schedule rest periods to prevent overexertion. Rest periods should not outnumber activity sessions. This will help prevent the older adult from becoming immobile.

Cough, fatigue, and confusion can be early signs of inadequate oxygenation. Respiratory rates over 25 per minute can be an early indicator of a lower respiratory tract infection. Normally, the larger lower lobes of the lungs perform the oxygen (O_2) to CO_2 exchange. However, the older patient performs this exchange in the less efficient upper lobes of the lung. Because lung recoil strength is decreased, mucus is more difficult for the older patient to **expectorate** (cough up). With a weaker cough or gag reflex, there is a greater potential for lung problems.

Lifelong habits and exposures can contribute to respiratory sensitivity for the older patient. These include smoking, second- or thirdhand smoke exposure, work-related respiratory pollutant exposure, or paints and glues used in hobbies. It is important to include coughing, deep breathing, and position changes in the plan of care to stimulate all lobes of the older patient's lungs. Encourage the older adult to receive recommended pneumonia vaccinations and an annual flu shot. Influenza and pneumonia together are the fourth leading cause of death in people over age 65. Help prevent the spread of respiratory illnesses to older patients. Receive an annual flu shot, perform hand hygiene between patients, and do not work when ill. Your patients will appreciate it!

Key Changes in the Gastrointestinal System

Age-related changes in the GI system include the following:

- Delayed gastric emptying, reducing appetite
- Declining liver enzymes, reducing drug metabolism and detoxification
- Decreased peristalsis, causing constipation
- Decreased saliva production, causing dry mouth and altered taste
- Altered taste and smell, affecting eating enjoyment

NURSING CARE. Many factors can affect nutrition at any age. But age-related structural and functional changes put the older patient at greater nutritional risk ("Nutrition Notes"). This can result in illness.

Nutrition Notes

Older Adult Nutritional Needs. Changes in physiology and psychosocial conditions make older adults vulnerable to protein-calorie malnutrition. This negatively impacts their functional status. Decreased muscle mass, increase in fat stores, and nutrient deficiencies can cause anemia, cognitive function impairment, immune dysfunction, osteoporosis, impaired wound healing, and weakness. These conditions further impair the ability of individuals to shop, cook, and consume adequate calories and nutrients. Adequate nutritional intake can be further impaired by social isolation (Amarya, Singh, & Sabharwal, 2015).

Achlorhydria (low or absent gastric acid in the stomach) can occur as a result of aging or from chronic ingestion of stomach acid-reducing medications such as protein pump inhibitors (National Institutes of Health [NIH], 2016). In either case, protein digestion and absorption of iron and vitamin B_{12} can be impaired by the lack of gastric acid and intrinsic factor required for vitamin B_{12} absorption (see "Nutrition Notes" in Chapter 28). Malabsorption of iron and vitamin B_{12} can lead to anemia; however, sources of blood loss should also be considered. If test results demonstrate a vitamin B_{12} deficiency, fortified foods or supplements are recommended as the main sources of the vitamin (NIH, 2016).

Decreased visual acuity and impaired dexterity can make shopping for food and preparing it difficult or even hazardous. Arthritis can affect jaw movements so chewing can be problematic. Approximately 13% of U.S. residents aged 65 to 74 and 26% of adults over age 74 have lost all their teeth (edentulous) (Dye, Thornton-Evans, Li, & Iafolla, 2015; World Health Organization, 2017). They must then develop skill in the use and care of dentures. Proper fit and gum health should be monitored.

Older persons produce less saliva than younger people. The sense of taste and smell decline in most aging patients. As a result, they might increase their intake of salt and sugar to the detriment of a prescribed diet plan.

Many older patients are at increased risk for food, nutrient, and drug interactions. Situations associated with these interactions include polypharmacy, alcohol consumption, and chronic illness. Identification of any of these factors should prompt a thorough nutritional assessment by a registered dietitian.

Being knowledgeable and committed to helping meet the older patient's nutritional goals is important. Patients should be offered the opportunity for toileting before sitting down to eat. Providing enough time to eat is essential for the older patient to accomplish the task of eating. If the patient needs

• WORD • BUILDING •

expectorate: ex—out + pectus—breast

help with eating, be sensitive to the patient's pace. Give the patient as much control when eating as possible. Eating has a strong social component. Therefore, encourage the patient to be out of bed and to eat with others, as much as possible. However, it is also important to respect the patient's right of refusal to eat in a designated social setting. Some patients might not eat as well when seated next to agitated or confused residents in a common dining hall.

Offering a calm and comfortable environment helps food digestion. Seasonings can help stimulate a lagging appetite. Ask family members to bring in the older patient's favorite seasoning in shakers. Dietitians can provide other ideas to promote healthful eating.

Older people may wear dentures or partial plates. However, it is important not to assume that all older people wear dentures. Tooth loss is not a normal part of aging. With proper dental care, teeth should last a lifetime. For those with dentures, a significant change in body weight affects the fit and comfort of dentures. This can then affect nutritional intake. Ask the patient about denture fit and comfort regularly. Examine the mouth when assisting the older patient with oral care.

Medications can cause taste disturbances or problems with dry mouth. This can affect the older patient's ability to eat. Some medications reduce bowel motility. **Constipation** may occur. Stress, anxiety, or a change in routine can also cause constipation. Obtain baseline information about bowel routines unique for each older patient. Ask what the older person expects when it comes to "regular bowel movements." Identify what has worked for bowel elimination in the past. Over-the-counter and prescribed enemas, suppositories, and medications are often misused in this age-group. When overused, these products can create an unhealthy dependency. Teach the older patient realistic expectations for bowel elimination. Discuss the intake of fiber and water and exercise to promote safe elimination.

Key Changes in the Endocrine-Metabolic System

Age-related changes in the endocrine-metabolic system include the following:

- Altered adrenal hormone production, decreasing ability to respond to stress
- Slowing basal metabolic rate, requiring a 5% reduction in calorie consumption to maintain weight
- Decreased pancreatic insulin release and impaired glucose tolerance, increasing potential for hyperglycemia

NURSING CARE. Increased incidence of metabolic disease, such as diabetes, occurs with age. Encourage older adults to be screened for metabolic problems. With aging, there is also a notable decrease in the effectiveness and interaction of all hormones. It becomes more difficult for the older body to respond to stressful situations. Address the psychological needs of your older patients to reduce stressors affecting their care.

Typical symptoms of hyperthyroidism or hypothyroidism are not seen in older patients. It is important *not to assume* that cold sensitivity, constipation, fatigue, fluid retention, forgetfulness, and skin changes are only associated with "old age." These symptoms may be a result of an impaired thyroid gland. Blood tests can identify the thyroid problem.

Key Changes in the Genitourinary System

Age-related changes in the genitourinary system include the following:

- Benign prostate hypertrophy, causing difficult voiding
- Decreased bladder size and tone, increasing urinary frequency
- Decreased kidney filtration rate and tubular function, decreasing renal clearance of medications
- Weakened pelvic floor muscles, resulting in incontinence
- Increased incidents of urinary tract infections (UTIs), affecting mainly women
- Decreased urine concentrating ability, resulting in nocturia

NURSING CARE. Many older people have to urinate at night. This is referred to as **nocturia.** Changes within the kidneys, gravity, and medication effects contribute to nocturia. About 30 minutes after lying down, many older people need to urinate. This occurs because fluid held in the legs by gravity returns to the heart and is circulated through the kidneys. This produces urine and the urge to void after lying down. Review patient medications and personal medication practices. For example, the taking of diuretics late in the day can cause nocturia and sleep disruption. Adjusting the diuretic schedule can prevent this.

> ### NURSING CARE TIP
> With advancing age, older patients do not get the urge to void as early in the process as they did when younger. This aging change, accompanied with other normal aging changes in the urinary system (such as the pear-shaped bladder becoming funnel shaped), contributes to the older patient's voiding urgency. If the patient is not assisted to void promptly after making a request, incontinence can result. This can create a safety issue if the patient attempts to get up alone. A fall can occur, especially if the floor is slippery. Provide safe patient-centered care by planning for and meeting the patient's voiding needs *promptly.*

Urinary incontinence is *not* a normal condition of aging. It is usually a treatable condition that requires assessment. Urinary incontinence is socially embarrassing. It is one of the main reasons older people enter long-term care facilities. In older men, urinary incontinence results from benign prostate hypertrophy (enlargement). In older women, it is likely due to a short

• WORD • BUILDING •
nocturia: nocte—night + ouron—urine

urethra and weakened perineal muscles. Teaching pelvic floor muscle exercises is successful for some patients. All patients with urinary incontinence should be referred to a specialist.

Management of urinary incontinence is tailored to the need of the patient. Bladder training programs can be effective. They remind the older patient on a regular basis that it is time to urinate. Incontinence can result from problems that affect the toileting task itself. Ensure safe toileting for all older patients. Pathways to the toilet must be nearby and uncluttered. Toilets must be easy to access. Clothing must be easy to remove. Velcro fasteners can replace buttons or zippers. Urinary briefs can help instill confidence in older patients who fear urine leakage. Activities can be resumed. Ensure proper application of the correct type of brief. With use of an incontinence brief, assess for early signs of perineal skin breakdown.

Older patients might try to decrease urine leakage by severely limiting their fluid intake. This can result in dehydration. Acid–base and electrolyte imbalances can also occur. Over time, dehydrated patients can have problems with vomiting, diarrhea, weakness, and confusion. Fluid intake needs to be encouraged in older patients. Focus education on timing of liquid intake and beverage selection. Caffeine and alcoholic beverages should be avoided. They increase urinary output.

UTIs are more common in older people and often more serious. Monitoring the patient's intake and output to ensure hydration helps decrease UTIs.

Key Changes in the Immunological System

Age-related changes in the immune system include the following:

- Increased autoimmune response, increasing autoimmune diseases
- Declining immune response, increasing infection and cancer risk
- Decreased T cell number and function, leading to impaired ability to produce antibodies to fight disease

NURSING CARE. Older patients tend to have more chronic diseases. This can depress their immune responses over time. Older patients have few colds. However, they are at higher risk for influenza (flu) and other complications if they get a cold. It can take older adults longer to recover from infections. It is also important to screen visitors for illness before they visit a recuperating older patient.

Older patients are taught ways to prevent illness. The teaching plan includes obtaining age-appropriate immunizations. This includes a vaccine for shingles, or herpes zoster (Shingrix for age 50 and over, and Zostavax for age 60 and over). Shingles is a painful, contagious rash caused by the chickenpox virus (varicella-zoster virus). Additional teaching includes reducing stress, eating right, exercising, and maintaining a healthy lifestyle. Those who are immunocompromised (such as those who take steroids) need to take safety precautions around others who are ill. Teach older patients proper hand hygiene to help protect themselves.

CRITICAL THINKING

Mr. Jones, age 72, lives at home and is visited by a home health care nurse. His home has wood floors with throw rugs. The bathroom is located in the hall outside his bedroom. Mr. Jones has nocturia and is occasionally incontinent from urgency to void. He takes bumetanide (Bumex) 1 mg orally daily.

1. What additional data should be obtained about Mr. Jones regarding his urinary status and home environment?
2. Are safety concerns present in the home environment?
3. What nursing diagnoses should be included in Mr. Jones's nursing care plan?
4. What should be included in a teaching plan for Mr. Jones?
5. Mr. Jones is to take bumetanide 1 mg orally now. Bumetanide 0.5-mg tablets are available. How many tablets are required?

Suggested answers are at the end of the chapter.

Key Changes in the Neurologic System

Age-related changes in the neurologic system include the following:

- Decreased blood flow to the brain, causing short-term memory loss
- Decreased brain cells, although function occurs with remaining cells
- Decreased endorphins, increasing risk for depression
- Decreased equilibrium and motor coordination, resulting in fall risk
- Decreased hypothalamus function and regulation of body temperature, increasing risk of hyper/hypothermia
- Increased reaction times, increasing risk for injury
- Decreased sensitivity, increasing risk for injury

NURSING CARE. Changes in the nervous system of the older patient occur in both the peripheral and central systems. These changes have significant meaning for the older person. They impact safety. With normal aging, there is a slowed response to stimuli. There is a marked decrease in the speed of the psychomotor response to the stimuli. Stronger stimuli are needed to elicit a neurologic response. So, the older patient is unable to recognize early signs of danger. To protect from accidental skin burns, the thermostat on water heaters should be lowered, and electrical heating devices (heating pads, electric blankets, and mattress pads) should not be used.

Balance is a safety issue for the older adult. As one ages, it is more difficult to maintain balance. Musculoskeletal changes can also affect balance. Plan care to assist older patients to safely transfer and ambulate.

Fine tremors of the hand can be a normal finding with age. These movements tend to increase when the older patient is cold, excited, hungry, or active. Assistive devices can be provided by an occupational therapist. These devices help eliminate unsteadiness created by the fine tremors. This makes it easier to accomplish ADLs (Fig. 15.3).

Normal neurologic changes that arise with age usually occur on both sides of the body at the same time. One-sided weakness, sensory deficits, and performance problems should always be referred for further evaluation. Coarse tremors of the finger, forearm, head, eyelids, or tongue that occur when the body part is at rest can be a sign of a neurologic problem such as Parkinson's disease. These tremors typically occur on one side of the body first. Patients with these tremors should always be referred to an HCP for further evaluation.

Key Changes in the Sensory System

Age-related changes in the sensory system include the following:

- Decreased visual acuity
- Decreased elasticity of the eardrum
- Decreased sense of smell
- Decreased taste perception
- Decreased touch sensation

NURSING CARE. Sensory changes associated with age often occur gradually. Sensory losses can affect the older person's psychological health. Early diagnosis and treatment help to minimize the loss. Several eye disorders can affect the aging eye (see Chapter 52). Disorientation, withdrawal, or social isolation may occur from **sensory deprivation.**

Normal age-related changes within the eye affect the focus ability of the lens. This can affect near and far vision. It is especially difficult for older patients to read fine print. Reading glasses or bifocal lenses assist with this. When caring for a patient who wears glasses, remind the older patient to consistently wear the glasses as needed. Help the older patient keep them clean and in good repair. When glasses are not being worn, keep them accessible and in a protective, labeled case. The older patient has a more difficult time adjusting to changes between light and dark settings. Seeing in the dark is enhanced with the use of an amber or red nightlight. Red hued lighting is more easily detected by the cones and rods in the older patient's eye. Make every effort to reduce glare from bright sunlight. Sensitivity to glare occurs with normal changes in the aging eye. The glare from car headlights can impair night vision in older patients. This can create safety issues with night driving.

Hearing loss is common in older adults (see Chapter 52). Although the severity of age-related hearing loss is variable, the stigma it carries is the same. For older patients, the first difficult sounds to understand are the high-pitched tones. It is best to speak to a hearing-impaired patient in a moderate volume and a lower tone. It is also helpful to stand in front of hearing-impaired patients so they can see your face during communication. Using nonverbal gestures and cues can help as well (Box 15.1).

Patients should be referred to an audiologist for evaluation if hearing loss is suspected. Hearing aids are often not well accepted by older persons because they are visual signs of a loss. Because of this possible sensitivity, it is important to

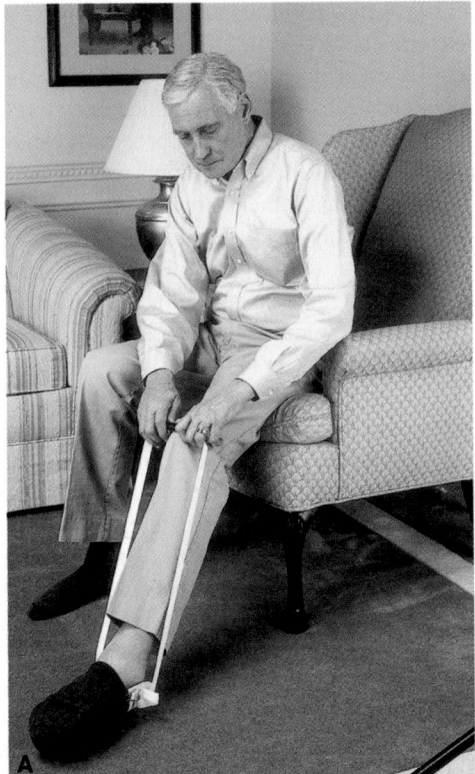

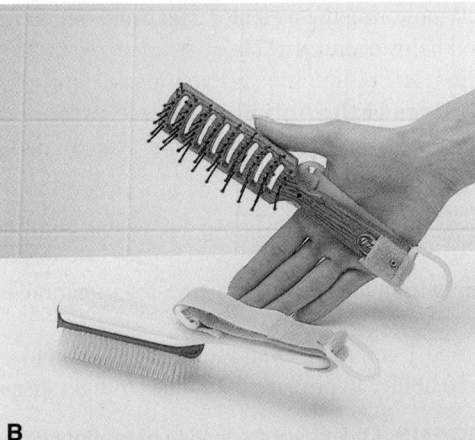

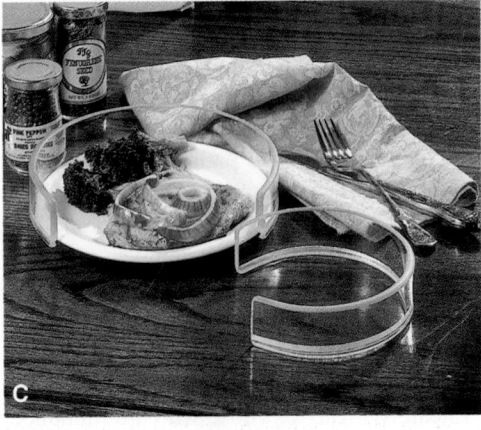

FIGURE 15.3 Assistive devices for activities of daily living. (A) Sock and stocking aid. (B) Easy-pull hairbrush. (C) Food guard.

Communicating With Patients Who Have Hearing Impairments

- Ensure that hearing aids are on with working batteries.
- Face the patient so your face (the speaker's) is visible.
- Speak toward the patient's best side of hearing.
- Speak in a clear, moderate-volume, low-pitched tone.
- Do not shout because doing this distorts sounds.
- Recognize that high-frequency tones and consonant sounds are lost first (e.g., *s, z, sh, ch, d, g*).
- Eliminate background noise because it can distort sounds.

maintain patient privacy if a referral for further evaluation is made. If the older patient has a hearing aid, keep it accessible at all times. The hearing aid should be kept clean and free of ear wax build-up. Store the hearing aid in a labeled protective container. Turn the battery turned off to conserve it. Have extra batteries available.

As discussed in the GI section of this chapter, the senses of taste and smell work closely together. Ill-fitting dentures and poor oral care can contribute to an alteration in the sense of taste. Some medications, tobacco products, and oral disease can also affect taste. A medication review and daily mouth inspections can help identify sources of the taste alteration. In some cases, the loss of smell can result from sinus problems, nasal obstruction, or allergies. If olfactory receptors are the primary cause for losing the sense of smell, little can be done. Teaching for safety related to the loss of smell is needed. Accidental ingestion of toxic substances, thought to be a food or beverage, that could not be smelled occurs. Teach patients to read all item labels, to ensure it is a food or beverage, before ingesting. Patients should use smoke alarms and natural gas alarms at home. Tell patients to report any sudden loss in taste or smell sensation to the HCP because it can signal other significant health care problems.

Decreased touch sensation can occur with age or disease. A reduction in the sensation of touch puts the older patient at risk of injury. Burns can occur when hot water is not felt. Electrical heating devices should not be used as the patient may not know if they become too hot on the skin. Teaching can help keep the patient free from injury.

Be aware of the environment you provide for the older patient. Overstimulation caused by **sensory overload** can create psychological and physical strain. This strain is difficult for an older patient to cope with. As a patient advocate, identify and minimize overload situations.

Key Changes in Sexuality
Age-related changes in sexuality include the following:

- Chronic illnesses, affecting sexual functioning
- Functional sexual changes in older men (e.g., altered ability to obtain or maintain an erection and to ejaculate), causing psychological concerns

- Functional sexual changes in older women (e.g., decreased vaginal lubrication causing painful intercourse and reduced vaginal acidity), resulting in risk for vaginal infection
- Increased nonintercourse intimacy behaviors, including various forms of touch
- Sexual problems caused by psychological factors, which are more common than physical ones in older adult patients
- Increased sexual arousal time, requiring more time for stimulation

NURSING CARE. The older patient's sexuality is an important aspect of **holistic** care. Sexuality is one of the basic physiological needs identified in the Maslow hierarchy of needs. This is true for everyone regardless of age. Become aware of your personal attitudes and values about sexuality, sex, and aging. Be careful that personal stereotypes and beliefs do not disrupt the older patient's sexual identity maintenance. Privacy remains a common problem for people in health care settings. This includes long-term care settings. Provide the patient with scheduled private time as desired. New sexual enhancement treatments are becoming more available to older people. This provides greater openness to discuss sexual expression with older patients. Many older patients have difficulty overcoming barriers to sexual expression. This can be due to cultural or religious beliefs, lack of a suitable partner, fear of failure, fear of consequences, illness, side effects of medications, or certain chronic diseases that can alter sexual function. It is important to address the older patient's sexual history sensitively, professionally, and completely (Box 15.2).

COGNITIVE AND PSYCHOLOGICAL CHANGES IN THE OLDER PATIENT

Cognition
Older patients can experience changes that influence cognition. Cognition involves abilities related to intelligence, judgment, learning, memory, orientation, and problem-solving. Cognition focuses on intake, storage, processing, and retrieval of information. Older patients store information without much conscious effort usually. When remembering becomes difficult, the older person can begin to worry. This worry needs to be addressed. If it is not, the patient's concern can result in psychological problems and fears.

Many factors can affect cognition. Sensory changes and diseases associated with age can cause misinterpretation of patient data. For example, pain from chronic diseases can limit cognition as pain takes over the body and mind. Sleep deprivation caused by worry or fear can make it more difficult to perform ADLs. Medications that cause drowsiness can also impair cognition.

Long-term memory retrieval is easier than short-term memory retrieval for the older adult. Plan methods to assist an older patient having short-term memory problems. Use written lists and visual cues to strengthen short-term memory skills.

Box 15.2

Sexuality Data Collection

As with any nursing skill, practice will increase your comfort in collecting sexuality data. This is important so that the older patient's concerns and needs are not ignored. It also can lead to the discovery of other health issues. Establish rapport with the patient by collecting other data first. Then, include sexuality data at the end. Older patients will often respond to sexuality questions but will not bring up the topic on their own. As you collect data, be aware of problems that were identified during data collection that could impact sexuality. They include angina, dexterity, elimination, medication side effects, mobility, pain, and surgeries.

Naturally, you should use a professional approach and manner. Tell the patient that you will be asking questions about sexuality. Start with questions that are likely to be more comfortable for the patient:

• Address roles first. For example: What concerns do you have or has your illness created in carrying out your roles with your spouse or sexual partner?
• Address relationship issues next. For example: What effect on your relationship with your spouse or sexual partner(s) has this illness, symptom, or chronic illness had?
• Address body image. For example: What effect has your (illness, surgery [mastectomy, prostate, ostomy], chronic illness, age-related changes) had on your self-concept of being a (man or woman)?
• Address safer sex practices. For example: How many sexual partners do you have? What type of protection do you use (condoms, female condoms or dental dams)?
• Address sexually transmitted infections. For example: Do you have any discharge or open sores (vaginal, penile)?

Intelligence does not decline as one ages. Cognitive abilities tend to slow down with advancing age, but they are not lost. Most of the subtle declines that occur with information processing and retrieval do not interfere with the older patient's abilities in performing ADLs.

It is common knowledge that health, good nutrition, and adequate sleep are important factors for brain function. The use of technology with guidance, such as an Internet-connected tablet, encourages curiosity and engagement. It can assist older adults to thrive. These factors should be included in planning care for the older patient.

Coping Abilities

People make choices in adapting to changes in functional ability over time. This impacts how a person will work through the entire maturational process called *aging*. In addition to normal aging changes, many older patients cope with chronic diseases. They are also dealing with societal and cultural losses associated with aging. Role changes in employment status, society, and family can create a shift from independence to dependence. This can have a strong psychological impact on them and their families. With all these losses, an older person's confidence level can be affected. Nurses may need to encourage self-care behaviors.

Personality, attitude, past life experiences, and the desire to adapt to change are all intrinsic influencing factors. They help the older patient cope with changes brought on by aging. Extrinsic factors include financial status and family and caregiver support. It is helpful for older people to have the energy, desire, determination, and support of their caregivers. This allows them to better utilize their cognitive function in maintaining health.

Depression

There are times when the psychological impact of change is too hard to cope with. Loneliness, grief, or sadness occur. This does not allow the older person to cognitively focus on health. **Depression** can result. This can disable the older person's mind and body. Depression is the most common psychiatric problem among older adults. It is a disturbance in mood. It increases the risk for suicide, physical health problems, and sleep disturbances.

The frequency and intensity of depression generally increase with aging. Depression can result from many factors. These include physical changes in the brain, a medication or a condition affecting neurotransmitters, or psychological changes on an emotional level. This could include ineffective coping to a perceived or actual loss. Depression may be reversed with prompt identification and treatment. It is important to be aware of what the older person is and is not saying during communications. If depression is suspected, a referral for treatment should be made. This can prevent maladaptive behaviors from occurring.

Dementia

Unlike depression, **dementia** involves a more permanent progressive deterioration of mental function (see Chapter 48). There are various types of dementia, with Alzheimer's disease being the main type. Dementia is often characterized by confusion, forgetfulness, impaired judgment, and personality changes. Refer any patient with confusion for a mental status examination to help determine whether the person has depression or dementia. It is essential that a sensory status examination be conducted before a mental status examination to help ensure the accuracy of the test results.

For patients with dementia, help them maintain an **optimum level of functioning**. Provide an environment with physical and emotional safety. To help the confused patient, if appropriate, use **reality orientation.** Orienting information (e.g., clocks, calendars) is presented to the older patient regarding time, place, and person. Sensory overload should be minimized. Speak calmly and slowly. Provide nonthreatening therapeutic touch, if accepted, by the patient. It is also important to address the education and support needs of the patient's family. They must learn to cope with changes in the older patient's behavior.

Delirium

Delirium reflects the patient's level of alertness and psychomotor activity. It is an acute, reversible state of disorientation and confusion with difficulty focusing attention, inability to sleep, and hyperactivity due to an underlying cause. It is commonly a complication of acute illness and treatments. It can occur in hospitalized patients at any age. However, it occurs most often in hospitalized older patients. It usually is documented as "confusion." The actual mechanism through which delirium occurs is not known. It is thought to occur from changes in brain neurotransmitters that control cognitive function, mood, and behavior. Unlike depression and dementia, delirium has a sudden onset. It tends to be worse at night. The patient appears to be disturbed or frightened. It can last for a few hours or a few weeks. Based on patient behaviors, delirium is classified as hypoactive, hyperactive, or mixed.

Delirium is different from depression and dementia. It is a cognitive state that can be easily reversed once the cause is identified and treated. The nurse must not always assume that the older patient's current mental status is his or her usual state. Know risk factors for this condition. They include acute illness, infection, alcohol or other drug abuse, surgery, hip fracture, and metabolic disturbance. Promptly report any patient abnormalities to help prevent delirium.

Sleep and Rest Patterns

The need for sleep does not decrease with age. However, the sleeping pattern of older adults usually changes from when they were younger. Lack of sleep leads to fatigue, irritability, increased sensitivity to pain, and increased likelihood of accidents. It is important to obtain a baseline sleep and rest history for the older patient. Ask about sleep patterns, bedtime rituals, rest and nap patterns, daily exercise patterns, stress level, dietary patterns, and lifestyle issues. Include caffeine, alcohol, and nicotine intake during data collection.

Circulatory problems can disrupt normal sleep patterns for the older adult. Disrupted sleep might be the only sign of an impending health problem. Use interventions to reduce stimulation and calm the anxious older patient who is unable to sleep. These can include back rubs, foot rubs, a warm towel bath, warm milk, or a glass of wine, if allowed. Sleep medications should generally be avoided. They can affect the quality and depth of sleep for the older adult. Side effects are also common.

Medication Management

Medication management is one of the most difficult tasks for older patients and their caregivers. Older patients are susceptible to drug-induced illness and adverse side effects. This happens for a variety of reasons previously addressed in this chapter. Always be aware of what medication the older patient is taking. Know how it is being taken and how it is affecting the older patient. The Beers Criteria (from the American Geriatrics Society Health in Aging Foundation) identifies potentially inappropriate medications for older adults (Table 15.1).

Older adults often have more than one chronic illness. As a result, they take multiple medications. Polypharmacy can cause side effects that can be dangerous. Duplication of medications with similar actions can occur. HCPs need to be aware of all prescribed medicines. They also need to review all over-the-counter medicines and self-prescribed extracts, elixirs, herbal remedies, herbal teas, cultural healing substances, and other home remedies being used by the older adult.

Older patients must understand how to take their medications correctly. An enteric-coated pill should not be crushed. This destroys the enteric protection. The stomach and intestines can then be damaged. Some older patients cut pills in half or skip medication doses to save money. When prescribed doses are not being taken as ordered, problems can result.

Be a patient advocate. Teach older patients and their families about their prescribed medications. Discuss the importance of adhering to the medication therapy. Explain the purpose of each drug, when a medication should be taken,

Table 15.1

Ten Medications Older Adults Should Avoid or Use With Caution

MEDICATION	REASON
USE WITH CAUTION **NonSteroidal Anti-Inflammatory Drugs (NSAIDs)** Used to reduce pain and inflammation. **AVOID regular, long-term use of NSAIDs** • When good alternatives are not available and NSAIDs are necessary, use a proton pump inhibitor such as omeprazole (Prilosec) or misoprostol (Cytotec) to reduce bleeding risk. • Use special caution if you are at higher risk of developing bleeding stomach ulcers. Those at higher risk include people more than 75 years old, people taking oral steroids, and people taking a blood-thinning medication such as apixaban (Eliquis), aspirin, clopidogrel (Plavix), dabigatran (Pradaxa), edoxaban (Savaysa), rivaroxaban (Xarelto), or warfarin (Coumadin). • Also use special caution if you have kidney problems or heart failure.	NSAIDs can increase the risk of bleeding stomach ulcers. They can also increase blood pressure, affect your kidneys, and make heart failure worse.

Continued

Table 15.1

Ten Medications Older Adults Should Avoid or Use With Caution—cont'd

MEDICATION	*REASON*
USE WITH CAUTION **Digoxin (Lanoxin)** Digoxin is used to treat heart failure and irregular heartbeats. • For most older adults, other medications are safer and more effective. • Avoid doses higher than 0.125 mg per day. Higher doses increase toxicity and provide little additional benefit. • Be particularly careful if you have moderate or severe kidney problems.	It can be toxic in older adults and people whose kidneys do not work well.
AVOID Certain Diabetes Drugs • Glyburide (Diabeta, Micronase) and chlorpropamide (Diabinese)	These can cause dangerously low blood sugar.
AVOID Muscle Relaxants • Such as cyclobenzaprine (Flexeril), methocarbamol (Robaxin), carisoprodol (Soma), and similar medications.	They can leave you feeling groggy and confused, increase your risk of falls, and cause constipation, dry mouth, and problems urinating. Plus, there is little evidence that they work well.
AVOID Certain Medications used for Anxiety and/or Insomnia • Benzodiazepines, such as diazepam (Valium), alprazolam (Xanax), or chlordiazepoxide (Librium) • Sleeping pills such as zaleplon (Sonata), zolpidem (Ambien), and eszopiclone (Lunesta)	They can increase your risk of falls, as well as cause confusion. Because it takes your body a long time to get rid of these drugs, these effects can carry into the day after you take the medication.
AVOID Certain Anticholinergic Drugs • Antidepressants amitriptyline (Elavil) and imipramine (Tofranil) • Anti-Parkinson drug trihexyphenidyl (Artane) • Irritable bowel syndrome drug dicyclomine (Bentyl)	They can cause confusion, constipation, dry mouth, blurry vision, and problems urinating (in men).
AVOID the Pain Reliever meperidine (Demerol)	It can increase the risk of seizures and can cause confusion.
AVOID Certain Over-the-Counter (OTC) Products • AVOID products that contain the antihistamines diphenhydramine (Benadryl) and chlorpheniramine (AllerChlor, Chlor-Trimeton). These medications are often included in OTC remedies for coughs, colds, and allergies. • AVOID OTC sleep products, like Tylenol PM, which contain antihistamines such as diphenhydramine.	Although these medications are sold without a prescription, they are not risk-free. They can cause confusion, blurred vision, constipation, problems urinating, and dry mouth.
If you are NOT being treated for psychosis, AVOID using Antipsychotics • Such as haloperidol (Haldol), risperidone (Risperdal), or quetiapine (Seroquel). These medications are commonly used to treat behavioral problems in older adults with dementia.	They can increase the risk of stroke or even death in older adults with dementia. They can also cause tremors and other side effects, as well as increase your risk of falls.
AVOID Estrogen pills and patches • Typically prescribed for hot flashes and other menopause-related symptoms	They can increase your risk of breast cancer, blood clots, and possibly dementia.

Used with permission from AGS Health in Aging Foundation. Ten Medications Older Adults Should Avoid or Use with Caution. (Sept. 2015).

how it should be taken, any food–beverage–medicine combinations that are not safe, and any early or late side effects of the drug to report to the HCP. Medication use, misuse, and abuse should be reviewed regularly with older adults. Older adults with a disability and with no or partial high school education tend to use inappropriate medication more than those who have a college education. Concerns need to be promptly addressed. Visual and verbal reminders that have meaning for the older patient are helpful. These factors along with promoting self-care and supportive independence help everyone involved in the older patient's medication management.

BE SAFE!

BE VIGILANT! For medication safety:

• Document a complete list of the patient's medications (prescribed, over-the-counter, herbal, and traditional) upon admission. Question the patient and family about anything the patient calls "my medicines."
• Ensure new medications are reviewed by a pharmacist.
• Use at least two patient identifiers unique to the patient (i.e., not the room number) when giving medications.
• Before the patient goes home, provide a complete written list of medicines and dosages to the patient and family/caregiver.

 HEALTH PROMOTION

To focus on health promotion and disease prevention, first determine the present health status of the older patient. When gathering holistic health data, focus on the older patient's mind, body, and spirit. Do this separately and in combination. Care must be taken to use valid and reliable data collection tools for the older adult. This allows a true picture of the older patient's condition, needs, and strengths. Listening and observing are two key nursing skills required to accurately obtain information from older patients. Know that symptoms often differ between younger and older patients with the same health conditions. For example, older patients can have confusion rather than chest pain during a heart attack.

Health education is the most important health promotion tool for older patients. Educational efforts must first focus on erasing stereotypes about aging. Erroneous associations between aging and illness must be corrected. As an example, research shows that urinary incontinence is not a normal sign of aging and is treatable. Yet, many still think it is inevitable with old age and do not seek treatment. Provide evidence-based health information. Do this at the right time, in the right amount, and in the right way to empower the older patient. This will help them value a proactive approach for wellness

in old age. Help the older patient with health screenings, immunization updates, safety program participation, and activity planning aimed at an optimal level of functioning and wellness (Table 15.2).

Gerontological Issues

Technology

• Video games: Playing Nintendo Wii games such as bowling can be an enjoyable activity for the older adult. It can provide socialization, exercise, and diversion to reduce boredom and loneliness. It is being used in settings such as long-term care.
• Robotic companion pets: Robotic pets (cat or dog) are being used as interactive companionship for older adults. Studies have shown they can reduce loneliness, bring joy, and promote health. They can also calm those with dementia. They have been found to be useful in long-term care settings.

Home Health Hints

Home Visits

• Schedule therapy visits and nurse visits on the same day, if possible, to decrease the risk of fatiguing the older patient.
• Because many older patients keep their homes warm, wear layers of clothing, removing a layer as needed, rather than adjusting the heat in the home.
• Place cell phones and pagers on a silent mode, if possible, to avoid startling or confusing the older patient.
• Do not assume that the older patient will remember the home health care nurses who come to the door. Each time, state your name and why you are there. Wear a large-letter, photo nametag that is in clear view.
• To enhance the effectiveness of a visit, in a quiet room, ask the older patient to talk with the main caregiver, invited in at the appropriate time. This can help the older patient stay more focused while ensuring privacy and fostering the person's ability to hear.
• Stressors in a patient's life, such as annoying visitors, chastisement by caregivers, and harassment by bill collectors, are often experienced firsthand by the home health care nurse. Document and share those with the home health care team, so a coordinated approach can be taken.

Home Environment

• Making a sign for the door of the home giving visitors instructions (e.g., ringing the doorbell several times, knocking loudly, or using another door) can be helpful to visitors of the older patient. Do not provide specific

information that would put the older person at risk for victimization.
- Assess the older patient's environment for safety hazards on each visit, and promote safety. Patients can easily trip on a scatter rug or fall trying to navigate around furniture. Urge the patient and caregiver to pack away scatter rugs and unneeded furniture.
- If the home is two stories, help the patient and caregiver consider how to relocate the bedroom to the first floor. Stairs are difficult to manage, especially if patients have visual disturbances or use an assistive device.
- Assist patients in obtaining a medical alert device that can be worn around the neck and activated in case of falls or other emergencies.

Medications
- Assist patients and/or caregivers with obtaining and setting up a weekly pill dispenser. These can be purchased at the local pharmacy. For patients who are forgetful, a pill dispenser with a timer can be purchased. An audible or visual alarm will go off when it is time for them to take medications.
- It is important for the home health care nurse to assess the patient's ability to follow instructions. During visits, check the medication dispenser to ensure that pills are being taken as prescribed. If there is a concern, inform the primary health care provider.

Nutrition/Fluids
- One of the first signs of dehydration is tachycardia. Instruct the patient regarding adequate hydration.
- If the older patient has dentures, assess if they are worn for eating. If not, assess why they are not worn (e.g., sores, improper fit from weight loss) and discuss solutions.
- Check the refrigerator for outdated food. Many older patients are on a limited budget and have been taught not to waste food. These factors, along with a decreased sense of smell and taste, can increase the risk of food poisoning.
- Encourage the uses of spices and herbs, such as parsley, oregano, lemon, garlic, and basil, instead of salt and sugar. Suggest keeping pared apples and segments of oranges in the refrigerator for snacks.
- If a Meals-on-Wheels program is available, ask whether the older patient would like to be placed on the service.
- Use a warming tray when feeding an older patient who takes a longer time to eat.
- When swallowing is difficult, freezing of liquids helps, so they can be eaten with a spoon or like a popsicle. Milkshakes, high-protein drinks, instant breakfast mix, or eggnog are thicker liquids that are easier to swallow.

Elimination
- If an older person wears perineal pads or adult briefs, ask how many are used in a 24-hour period to assess the degree of incontinency or amount of output. Have the patient keep a voiding diary to further assess the degree of incontinence.
- Suggest a bedside commode when a weakened older patient is on diuretics or has a history of falling or confusion. Placing it next to the bed at night helps reduce the risk of falls and eases caregiver burden.
- If the older patient reports constipation, review the diet and make suggestions regarding adequate fluid and fiber. A mixture of equal parts of applesauce, bran, and prune juice is often helpful to prevent or relieve constipation. Discourage the use of mineral oil because it will interfere with vitamin absorption.

Rest
- If the older patient seems fatigued early in the day, ask about sleeping patterns and things that disturb it, such as barking dogs, traffic noise, and visitors. Recommend earplugs or changing rooms to obtain a good night's rest. Check medications for insomnia listed as a side effect and suggest dosing of these medications early in the day if appropriate. A 15- to 30-minute nap in the early afternoon can be helpful.

Infection Symptom
- One of the first signs of infection in the older patient is confusion.

Education
- Suggesting that limiting visitors or not allowing persons with colds to visit can be helpful in preventing illness in the older patient.
- When auscultating lungs, ask the older patient to take deep breaths slowly in and out through the mouth. This can stimulate coughing, which is an opportune time to teach deep-breathing and coughing exercises.
- When teaching, it is important to acknowledge the patient's knowledge and life experiences. When given a chance, patients will tell you how they have maintained their health over the years. Use open-ended scenarios for teaching such as, "What would you do if you fell and you were alone?"
- Teaching should occur *with* patients, not *to* them. The nurse is in the patient's home, which is a personal place. Patient dignity should always remain intact during home health care visits and teaching sessions.

Lab Draws
- When drawing blood from the hand of an older patient, use the smallest needle possible and a butterfly device. Hold light pressure at the injection site for at least 2 minutes after the needle is removed.
- Do not use a bandage on the fragile skin of an older patient if the bleeding has stopped with pressure.

Table 15.2

Nursing Care Focus on Safety Alphabet for Older Patients

A is for ABILITIES	• Know your abilities. • Know your patient's abilities. • Base nursing actions on your abilities. • Seek out assistance when needed.
B is for BODY MECHANICS AND ALIGNMENT	• Use proper body mechanics. • Use appropriate assistive devices. • Ensure patient is in proper body alignment.
C is for COMFORT	• Ensure physical and emotional comfort during care. • Use pain scale during each assessment.
D is for DELIBERATE MOVEMENTS	• Plan ahead and communicate plans to patient. • Demonstrate confidence during care. • Alert patient to planned movements by saying, "Moving on three. One, two, three." • Ensure patient assists with moves as able.
E is for ENVIRONMENT	• Always place call light within reach. • Keep environment uncluttered and safe. • Ask patient's permission before moving items. • Put items back as patient prefers.
F is for FALLS	• Remember that falls are a primary concern for older patients. • Use interventions to prevent falls: assist patients with ambulation, use assistive devices, answer call lights promptly, provide accessible toileting facilities, use nightlights, avoid use of throw rugs.
G is for GIVING YOUR TIME	• Allow more time to perform actions. • Do not rush older patients. • Provide time for listening and observing, so concerns are addressed before becoming problems.
H is for HAND HYGIENE	• Use hand hygiene protocols and standard precautions to protect yourself and older patients. • Cleanse your stethoscope before and after each patient use.

SUGGESTED ANSWERS TO CRITICAL THINKING

Mr. Jones

1. Does he live alone? Does he have a history of falls? If so, does he wear a safety device to signal for help? What type of nightlight is used? How far is it to the bathroom? Does he take his bumetanide (Bumex) early in the day rather than at night? Does he void before going to bed? Does he anticipate needing to void 30 minutes after lying down?

2. Wood floors that are slippery when wet from incontinence are a safety hazard. Throw rugs can slide or cause tripping. An appropriate nightlight should be available.

3. Nursing diagnoses include *Functional Urinary Incontinence* related to distance to bathroom; *Deficient Knowledge* related to safety, medication administration, and nocturia; and *Risk for Injury* related to slippery floors from incontinence, use of throw rugs, and inadequate lighting.

4. A teaching plan should include the following:
   • *Safety:* Place urinal at bedside to prevent incontinence on the way to the bathroom. Consider a red nightlight to improve vision and prevent falls. Use an easily cleaned floor covering that is secure and absorbent to avoid falls. Consider the need for wearing a device that can send a signal for help.
   • *Medication administration:* Take diuretics early in the day to avoid having to get up frequently while sleeping at night.
   • *Nocturia:* Void before lying down. Anticipate the need to void after lying down by reclining in a chair for 30 minutes with legs elevated before going to bed and then void on way to bed.

5. Two 0.5-mg tablets.

Review Questions

1. When planning care for the older adult, the nurse understands the definition of aging as being which of the following?
    1. A disease state that results in the death of a person's body cells all at once
    2. A condition that starts for all people when they reach the age of 65
    3. A maturational process with individual adaptations for physical and psychological changes over time
    4. A state of accelerating decline in body functioning directly related to a disease process

2. The nurse is collecting data on a patient who is 77 years old and says, "I am shorter now." The patient asks the nurse why this is occurring. Which of the following would be a correct reply by the nurse?
    1. "Muscle contractions cause this."
    2. "Bone degeneration over time is occurring in your legs."
    3. "Hyperextension of your cervical spine has occurred."
    4. "Water is lost from the intervertebral disks of the spine with age."

3. Which of the following actions should the nurse take to protect skin integrity in the older adult? **Select all that apply.**
    1. Inspect skin daily.
    2. Apply moisturizer between toes.
    3. Use gentle bathing techniques.
    4. Massage nonreddened, intact skin sites gently.
    5. Use hot water for bathing.

4. Which of the following is the best approach for the nurse to make to encourage prescribed antihypertensive medication compliance?
    1. The nurse says, "It is important that you take your blood pressure pill every day. Do you understand this?"
    2. The nurse explains the medication and gives the patient a grid to record daily when the pill is taken. The nurse then asks, "How do you see this working for you?"
    3. The nurse asks the patient, "Do you have a relative or friend who can call you every day to remind you to take your blood pressure pill? It is really important that you take it, and as you get older it is harder to remember things."
    4. The nurse tells the patient, "If you don't take your blood pressure pill, you will probably have a heart attack or a stroke. You need to figure out a way that you don't forget to take it every day."

5. The nurse is caring for an older patient who has difficulty sleeping. Which of the following actions could the nurse take to promote rest for the patient? **Select all that apply.**
    1. Back rubs
    2. Encourage afternoon nap
    3. Foot rubs
    4. Set an alarm clock
    5. Warm towel bath
    6. Warm milk

6. The nurse is planning care for an older patient with a history of constipation. Which of the following actions should the nurse include in the patient's plan of care to help prevent constipation? **Select all that apply.**
    1. Increase dietary fiber intake.
    2. Decrease water intake.
    3. Encourage participation in activities of daily living.
    4. Review medication effects.
    5. Increase daily exercise.
    6. Decrease fresh fruit intake.

7. Which of the following topics should the nurse include in the teaching plan for safety for a patient who has a decreased sense of smell? **Select all that apply.**
    1. Carbon monoxide detector
    2. Flashing doorbell light
    3. Natural gas alarm
    4. Read labels before ingesting anything
    5. Security system
    6. Smoke alarm

Answer rationales available in your online resources.

ANSWERS 1. 3; 2. 4; 3. 1, 3, 4; 4. 2; 5. 1, 3, 5, 6; 6. 1, 3, 4, 5; 7. 3, 4, 6

Key Points

Find the chapter key points in your online resources
available through Davis Edge.

Additional Resources

 Use the scratch off code on the inside front
cover of your book to access online quizzes
that will help you to improve your scores
on course exams and prepare for NCLEX-PN®.

Study Guide

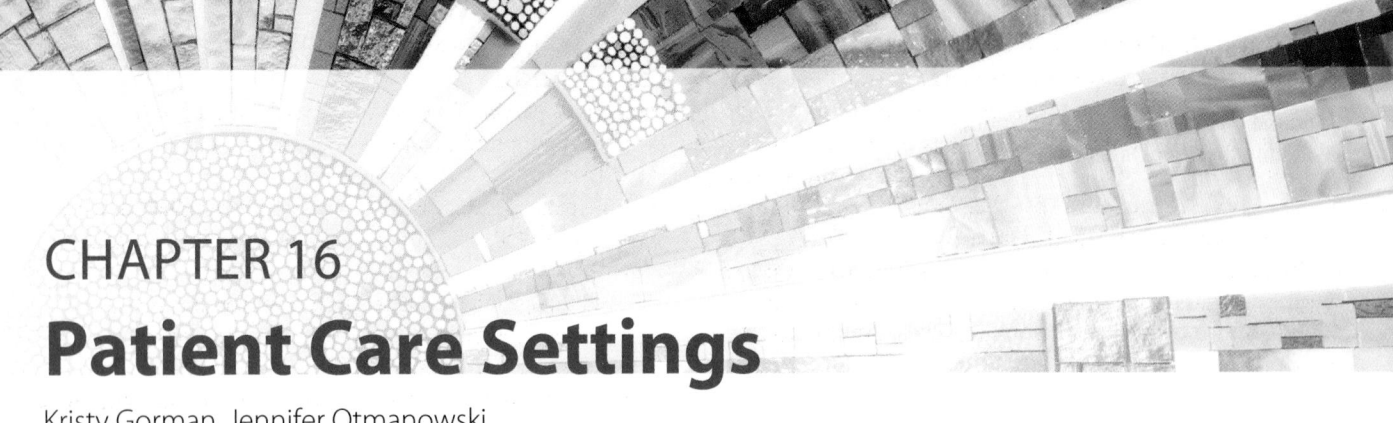

CHAPTER 16
Patient Care Settings

Kristy Gorman, Jennifer Otmanowski

KEY TERMS

autonomous (awe-TAH-nah-mus)
collaborative (kuh-LAB-er-uh-tiv)
elopement (ih-LOPE-munt)
respite (RES-pit)
telenursing (TEL-a-nurs-ing)
trauma-informed care (TRAW-muh in-FORMD care)

CHAPTER CONCEPTS

Health Care System
Patient-Centered Care

LEARNING OUTCOMES

1. Describe Acute Care for Elders units in hospitals.
2. Describe the role of the licensed practical nurse/licensed vocational nurse (LPN/LVN) in medical offices or clinics.
3. Describe the role of the LPN/LVN in correctional nursing.
4. Identify long-term care options.
5. Describe services offered in long-term care settings.
6. Describe the role of the LPN/LVN in long-term care settings.
7. Describe patient safety interventions in long-term care.
8. Describe home health care eligibility.
9. Explain differences in hospital versus home health nursing care.
10. Explain the steps involved in making a home health care visit.
11. Explain safety practices for the nurse while making home visits.
12. Identify home safety interventions for the patient.
13. Describe methods of infection control for the home health care nurse.
14. Identify documentation required for a home visit with a patient.
15. Plan nursing interventions for the home health care patient and caregiver.

The need for licensed practical nurses/licensed vocational nurses (LPNs/LVNs) is expected to grow 16% between 2014 to 2024. This growth is much faster than the average for all occupations (Bureau of Labor Statistics, 2017). Places LPNs/LVNs may work include child day-care centers, clinics (urgent care or addiction), correctional health care facilities, dentist offices, dialysis centers, home health care, hospices, hospitals, long-term care facilities, medical offices, occupational health departments such as in factories, rehabilitative facilities, or schools. The role of the LPN/LVN in acute care and Acute Care for Elders units, medical offices, correctional health care facilities, long-term care, and home health care are discussed in this chapter.

 ACUTE CARE

While hospital employment of LPNs/LVNs is declining, employment is growing in other settings. The employment of and types of roles for LPNs/LVNs vary by hospital. Some hospitals do not employ LPNs/LVNs. Others may, although the job title of LPN/LVN may not be used.

Acute Care for Elders Hospital Units

Acute Care for Elders (ACE) units began about 1993. They have slowly increased throughout the United States. These units are designed to meet the unique needs of hospitalized older adults. ACE units provide patient-centered care that meets the treatment goals and discharge needs of the older patient. Specifically, they utilize daily medical review, monitor polypharmacy to reduce unnecessary medications, and promote functional ability with early rehabilitation. These actions reduce adverse effects, decrease lengths of stay, and reduce costs and readmissions. In ACE units, health care team members are trained in geriatric care and work in an interdisciplinary team. The environment is designed to meet the special needs of the older adult to promote independence and ambulation and to prevent functional decline.

MEDICAL OFFICE NURSING

LPN/LVNs provide patient care in medical offices and work with patients of all ages. Following are the types of duties the LPN/LVN might perform:

- Greet, triage (assignment of degree of urgency to decide order of treatment of patients), and register patients.
- Escort patients to examination rooms.
- Follow the Health Insurance Portability and Accountability Act of 1996 (HIPAA) and advocate for patients.
- Obtain and document patients' vital signs, height, and weight.
- Obtain patients' medical and medication histories.
- Enter data into the electronic medical record.
- Contribute to the plan of care for patients.
- Provide patient care (e.g., wound care, dressings).
- Administer immunizations and other medication injections.
- Monitor patients after medications or treatments.
- Teach patients ways to promote health and use of new medications.
- Answer questions regarding patient care.
- Document understanding of teaching.
- Obtain prior authorization of medications.
- Assist with renewal of prescriptions.
- Communicate health information to patients.

CORRECTIONAL NURSING

Local, regional, and state correctional facilities hire LPN/LVNs to care for inmates and handle worksite wellness programs for correctional staff. In this practice setting, the LPN/LVN:

- Applies quality standards, procedures, and protocols as directed
- Demonstrates professionalism in providing health care delivery to inmates
- Demonstrates an interpersonal skill set, including high-quality oral and written communication skills

- Responds appropriately to situations and seeks supervision as needed
- Provides precertification and coordination for inmates admitted to and discharged from acute care facilities
- Implements the nursing process by following health care provider (HCP) orders regarding diet, medication, and treatments
- Is knowledgeable about and sensitive to cultural and socioeconomic differences among the populace related to health and behaviors
- Interviews, listens, and provides empathetic assistance to inmates during treatments
- Utilizes knowledge of nursing skills and therapeutic communication
- Utilizes knowledge of medications (e.g., actions, interactions, uses, and side effects)
- Responds to emergencies as part of the health care team
- Maintains institutional health records and provides required reports
- Works effectively and efficiently in conditions involving incarcerated patients

LONG-TERM CARE SERVICES

Over time, terminology to describe assistance with self-care for those who are disabled or frail has changed. Today, *long-term services and supports* or *long-term care services* are used. *Long-term care services* captures both health and nonhealth care services, and so this term will be used in this section.

In 2014, more than 9 million people were served by about 67,000 regulated long-term care services providers (Harris-Kojetin et al., 2016). Long-term care services can be provided in the home, via home health care (discussed later in this chapter), or hospice (see Chapter 17). Services can also be provided in community settings (e.g., adult day-care services), residential care settings (e.g., independent living, skilled nursing and memory care, adult foster care, assisted living facilities), and institutions (e.g., nursing homes) (Table 16.1). Some institutions specialize in care for people with chronic illnesses and physical impairments, such as those requiring mechanical ventilators. However, most long-term care is provided in the home setting.

Types of Long-Term Care Services

Long-term care services include daily personal care; dental care; physical, occupational, and speech therapies; pharmacist medication monitoring; podiatry; skilled nursing; intravenous therapy; intensive services such as dialysis; mechanical ventilator and tracheostomy care; and palliative or hospice care. Support services involve social workers, mental health professionals, and counselors.

Table 16.1

Long-Term Care Service Settings

Community	
Adult day-care service	Provide patient-centered assistance, supervision, socialization, and health care to older adults, adults with disabilities, and those with dementia during the day so that caregivers can work or receive respite. Services are provided by an interdisciplinary staff, including aides, nurses, social workers, and therapists (occupational, physical, and speech). Services may include assistance with activities of daily living (ADLs), meals, therapies, and transportation.
Residential	
Adult foster care	Private residences in which the owner lives with the residents to offer personal care, meals, supervision, and sometimes other supportive services. The number of residents allowed by each state varies from 1 to 20.
Continuing care retirement community	Residential care setting offering independent living, assisted living (assistance with ADLs, meals, medication assistance and supervision), skilled nursing, and memory care on site. Residents entering independent living pay an entrance fee and then a monthly fee for the various levels of care based on needs
Residential care community (semiassisted/ assisted living)	Residential care setting that combines housing, ADL assistance, supervision, support services, and limited health care for older adults. Residents are independent. Medication assistance and other treatments may be provided. Residents may have a kitchen to prepare meals and/or group meals may be provided.
Institution	
Nursing home	Provides the most comprehensive range of services, including housing, ADL assistance, nursing care, and 24-hour supervision. Short-term rehabilitation is also offered for physical, occupational, or speech therapy. *Skilled care:* Licensed nurses or therapists are required to perform medical care 24 hours a day, such as intravenous therapy, complex wound care, monitoring health status, tube feedings, or short-term rehabilitation services. A health care provider order is required. *Intermediate care:* ADL assistance and some (but not constant) nursing care is provided. *Custodial care:* Supervision and ADL assistance is provided. Nursing care is not required. This type of care is often provided for those with dementia. *Green House Project model:* This model for institutional long-term care represents a culture change toward long-term care in institutions that promotes natural living. Care is provided in a home environment in small houses on a campus with up to 12 residents per home. A great room, kitchen with dining, and outdoor access are open to everyone. Each resident has a bedroom and bathroom. A care team provides all patient-centered care and prepares meals. A nurse is available 24 hours a day. Up to an additional 30 minutes of direct care is given daily with this model. Residents are nurtured and may thrive as their individual needs are met.

Most long-term care that is provided is not medical or nursing care. It is primarily assistance with activities of daily living (ADLs) and instrumental activities of daily living (IADLs). ADL services include bathing, dressing, feeding, incontinence care, toileting, transferring (to or from bed or chair), and supervision for safety. IADL services include food prep, grocery shopping, money and bill management, housekeeping, laundry, pet care, and transportation.

Dementia Care

The physical environment is a key component in safe, patient-centered care for those with Alzheimer's disease or dementia. More than 60% of those with dementia will wander (Alzheimer's Association, 2017). There are positive benefits to wandering, in that movement by the resident results in exercise, more energy, improved appetite, pain control, and reduction of boredom and anxiety. However, there are negative effects, such as fatigue, risk of falls, and risk for **elopement** (leaving a facility unsupervised when unable to protect oneself). A long-term memory care unit must facilitate the positive benefits of wandering while protecting the resident (Galik et al., 2015).

Innovative thinking in the design of long-term memory care units stimulates the senses, reduces agitation, improves eating, and encourages safe wandering. Innovations include curvy or figure-8 hallways with seating areas and refreshment stations. Such elements encourage wandering, without agitating dead ends. Themed units provide sensory stimulation and use of color to help the resident recognize where he or she lives. Sensors also provide knowledge of the resident's location. The addition of fish tanks in dining areas can be calming and promote eating. Murals of peaceful rivers can discourage residents from going through a door. Memory stations can engage residents with activities during wandering. In addition, multisensory areas allow residents to use self-selected sensory stimulating items (e.g., aromas, sounds, textures) and interact with items used in the past by the resident for work or tasks. Encouraging residents' self-care ability (e.g., combing their own hair and brushing their teeth) reduces their anxiety and enhances their well-being.

Reducing noise levels in the long-term memory care environment increases quality of life for those with dementia. The Green House Project model of institutional long-term care (discussed in Table 16.1) has shown reduced verbal and overall aggression and agitation in residents with dementia (Chaudhury et al., 2017).

Role of the LPN/LVN in Long-Term Care Services

Licensed nursing hours per resident per day are higher in long-term care facilities than they are in residential care communities and adult day-care services centers (Harris-Kojetin et al., 2016). The LPN/LVN is responsible for patient safety and direct bedside care in nursing homes under the supervision of a registered nurse (RN). General LPN/LVN duties in long-term care facilities include administering medication, supervising, educating and mentoring nursing assistants, nursing care, contributing to the plan of care, communicating with the HCP, making rounds on residents, ensuring patient comfort, documentation, and reporting concerns to the supervising RN.

Common resident care tasks for the LPN/LVN include but are not limited to:

- Collecting the resident's history
- Monitoring vital signs and resident health status
- Monitoring fluid intake and output
- Monitoring nutritional intake
- Monitoring residents to prevent and detect pressure injury (see Chapter 54)
- Documenting resident information
- Giving medication (oral and injection) prescribed by the HCP
- Monitoring intravenous lines
- Monitoring for adverse effects of medications
- Assisting with ADLs
- Providing wound care, tube feedings, enemas, and insertion of urinary catheters
- Providing emotional support
- Teaching residents and families
- Assisting with end-of-life care

BE SAFE!

The Joint Commission has identified safety goals for residents in long-term care.

Identify residents correctly:

- Use at least two ways to identify patients or residents. For example, use the patient's or resident's name and date of birth. This is done to make sure that each patient or resident gets the correct medicine and treatment.

Use medicines safely:

- Take extra care with patients and residents who take medicines to thin their blood.
- Record and pass along correct information about a patient's medicines. Find out what medicines the patient is taking. Compare those medicines to new medicines given to the patient. Make sure the patient knows which medicines to take when they are at home. Tell the patient it is important to bring their up-to-date list of medicines every time they visit a doctor.

Prevent infection:

- Use the hand cleaning guidelines from the Centers for Disease Control and Prevention or the World Health Organization. Set goals for improving hand cleaning. Use the goals to improve hand cleaning.
- Use proven guidelines to prevent infections that are difficult to treat.
- Use proven guidelines to prevent infection of the blood from central lines.
- Use proven guidelines to prevent infections of the urinary tract that are caused by catheters.

Prevent residents from falling:

- Find out which patients and residents are most likely to fall. For example, is the patient or resident taking any medicines that might make them weak, dizzy, or sleepy? Take action to prevent falls for these patients and residents.

Prevent bed sores:

- Find out which patients and residents are most likely to have bed sores. Take action to prevent bed sores in these patients and residents. From time to time, recheck patients and residents for bed sores.

(2018 National Patient Safety Goals, © The Joint Commission, 2018. Reprinted with permission.)

Medicare and Medicaid Participation Requirements

Health and safety standards must be met for long-term care facilities to participate in Medicare or Medicaid programs. In 2016, revisions were made to the requirements for long-term care facilities in response to advances in knowledge and evidence-based practice to improve the quality of care and life of residents. Visit www.CMS.gov for current standards; see Table 16.2 for examples.

Table 16.2

Medicare and Medicaid Long-Term Care Facilities Reform Examples

Person-Centered Care	Develop and implement a baseline person-centered care plan for each resident, within 48 hours of the patient's admission. At discharge, planning must include resident's discharge goals to prepare residents to be active participants in their postdischarge care, transition, and prevention of readmission.
Quality of Care	Focus on care and services so residents achieve their highest possible physical, mental, and psychosocial well-being.
Quality of Life	Updated focus on special care issues that are based on an assessment of a resident and the person-centered plan of care and preferences. These include accidents, dialysis, incontinence, elimination ostomies, mobility, assisted nutrition and hydration, pain management, pharmacy (e.g., unnecessary medications, medication errors, antipsychotic medications, immunizations), restraints and bed rails, skin integrity, and **trauma-informed care** (e.g., special care to avoid traumatization triggers for trauma survivors, such as those of abuse, Holocaust survivors, veterans, or victims of large-scale disasters).
Alignment with U.S. Department of Health and Human Services Initiatives	Reduce avoidable hospitalizations and unnecessary hospital readmissions. Reduce incidences of healthcare–acquired infections. Improve behavioral health care. Safeguard nursing home residents from the use of unnecessary antipsychotic medications.

Source: Adapted from U.S. Department of Health and Human Services. (2016). Medicare and Medicaid programs; reform of requirements for long-term care facilities. *Federal Register, 81*(192). Retrieved from www.gpo.gov/fdsys/pkg/FR-2016-10-04/pdf/2016-23503.pdf

Patient Safety and Wellness in Long-Term Care Facilities

Activity and Exercise

For older adults to maintain health and independence in long-term facilities, activities and exercise should be promoted by the nursing staff. Strength, balance, and stretching exercises can assist residents in maintaining a normal weight, preventing falls, and improving freedom of movement. A recent study in nursing home residents with dementia demonstrated that exercise not only improves balance but also reduces apathy and symptoms of depression (Telenius, Engedal, & Bergland, 2015).

Fall Prevention

It is important to prevent residents from falling. In 2014, 74 older adults died from falls daily (U.S. Department of Health and Human Services, 2016). The U.S. Department of Health and Human Services (2016) recommends preventing falls through exercise to strengthen leg muscles and improve balance as well as keeping the environment clutter free and well lit. In addition, the National Institute on Aging (2017) recommends keeping bones strong with adequate vitamin D and calcium intake; annual vision checks and hearing tests; using properly fitting hearing aids, if needed; a medication review for side effects or interactions; adequate sleep; standing up slowly to prevent a drop in blood pressure; use of assistive walking devices; wearing nonskid, rubber-soled low-heeled shoes; and not walking in socks as they can be slippery.

As part of a fall prevention program, facilities may use a standardized fall risk assessment tool, such as the Morse Fall Scale (http://primaris.org/resource_library/morse-fall-scale/falls-morse-fall-scale-final-pdf), Hendrich II Fall Risk Model (http://uprightfallprevention.com/hendrich-ii-fall-risk-model), or St. Thomas's Risk Assessment Tool in Falling Elderly Inpatients (STRATIFY; www.ahrq.gov/professionals/systems/hospital/fallpxtoolkit/fallpxtk-tool3g.html). These scales can be used upon admission, after a fall, and when there is a change in the resident's status or medications to help quickly identify any risk of falling. To help prevent falls within the long-term care environment, monitor residents with cognitive impairment, balance problems, or incontinence closely. Ensure the environment is modified for safety by removing rugs or obstacles, installing grab bars and bath mats in the shower, checking on residents every 2 hours or more frequently for those at greater risk of falling, and encouraging residents to participate in activities outside of their rooms throughout the day.

Lighting

Older adults require more light for vision due to changes within the pupil and lens of the eye. They benefit from amber motion sensor nightlights and tunable lighting. Tunable lighting is adjustable lighting based on the desired intensity and color of light at various times of the day (e.g., brighter in morning and reduced over 24 hours) to promote normal circadian rhythms. This newly researched lighting has been shown to reduce falls, improve sleep with reduced need for psychotropic or sleep medication, and decrease agitation.

Restraints

The Centers for Medicare and Medicaid Services (CMS, 2016) defines *physical restraints* as "any manual method or physical or mechanical device, material, or equipment attached to or near your body so that you can't remove the restraint easily." *Chemical restraint* is the use of medication to restrict the freedom or movement of a resident in order to sedate the resident or control the resident's behavior. Federal law says restraints may not be used as discipline, as punishment, or for the convenience of staff. Restraints can only be used when the resident's behavior could cause harm to self or others. When used, the medical record must include an order for the restraint, a defined plan for the use, and the length of time it will be used. A new order for the restraint may be required every 24 hours. Restraint use is controversial and done as a last resort. The resident must be frequently monitored as restraint use can result in injury or death of the resident. A long-term care facility must have a plan in place to reduce restraint use (e.g., gradually increasing the time for ambulation and muscle strengthening activities). Restraint use regulations can vary by state.

HOME HEALTH CARE

Ask a patient in a hospital where he or she would choose to be, and chances are the answer will be "home." The number of home health care patients is growing as a result of the aging population in the United States as well as many older adults' desire to age in place. Home health care provides an affordable and convenient option for providing care in the community. Technological advances such as telehealth allow home health care agencies to provide high-quality complex care. The LPN/LVN is a valuable member of the home health care team. The LPN/LVN should understand the practice of delivering quality nursing care in the home. Much of the future job growth for LPNs/LVNs will be found in home health care.

Home Health Care Eligibility

The home health care patient must require skilled services that can only be provided by nurses, physical therapists, occupational therapists, and speech therapists (Box 16.1). Home health care aides are also available for patients that are receiving skilled care (care that cannot be provided by the patient alone and requires intervention of a qualified nurse). Depending on the patient's health insurance, a patient who is receiving home health care may be required to be homebound. For example, Medicare has very specific guidelines for determining homebound status. If the nurse suspects a patient is not homebound, the nurse needs to reinforce eligibility for home health care. The nurse should also suggest alternative options for health care to permit the patient to maintain independence. These options can include going to a clinic to have a blood pressure reading done, attending an outpatient physical therapy or occupational program, or having skilled needs (such as dressing changes) completed in an ambulatory surgery facility. Concerns about a patient should be discussed with the RN, who can work to assist the patient in receiving necessary health care.

Box 16.1

Skilled Activities for the Home Health Care Nurse

According to the Medicare Benefit Policy Manual (Centers for Medicare and Medicaid Services, 2015), to be considered as skilled nursing services, the services must require the skills of a registered nurse or a licensed practical nurse/licensed vocational nurse under the supervision of a registered nurse, and they must be reasonable and necessary to the treatment of the patient's illness or injury as discussed and must be intermittent. Examples of skilled nursing care include:

• Blood draws (only if the patient is receiving other home health care services)
• Dressing changes
• Intravenous medication administration
• Monitoring a patient's status following a change in medications or condition
• New feeding tube and tracheostomy management and monitoring
• New colostomy or urostomy management and monitoring
• Patient and family education
• Urinary catheter insertion and maintenance

If a family member is able to perform a skill part of the time, the nurse can teach that person how to perform the skill. The nurse can still complete skilled visits to monitor the patient's progress and provide care when family members are not available.

Home health care services usually are ordered after discharge from the hospital when there is a need for skilled care in the home. It is not uncommon, however, for an HCP's office to request home health care services after seeing a patient in the office. For example, a patient who is having difficulty controlling blood glucose levels could benefit from having a nurse visit to see how the patient uses a glucometer, observe what types of food are being purchased, monitor the glucose level, and teach the patient diabetic management. Another example would be a patient who cannot easily get to the HCP's office for weekly blood pressure checks after an antihypertensive medication adjustment. These types of home health care visits are usually short-term with the goal of facilitating independent care by the patient and/or family.

Home health care may be provided to residents in an assisted living facility. Because these facilities are not skilled nursing facilities, the facility staff is not trained to perform nursing skills. Home health care nurses need to understand the facility's policies when visiting a patient in assisted living. They must maintain communication with the facility staff regarding health care instructions for the patient.

Collaborative Home Health Care

Home health care is **collaborative**. Teamwork is facilitated through team meetings and communication promoted with communication notes to help ensure that patients and their families receive the care they need (Fig. 16.1).

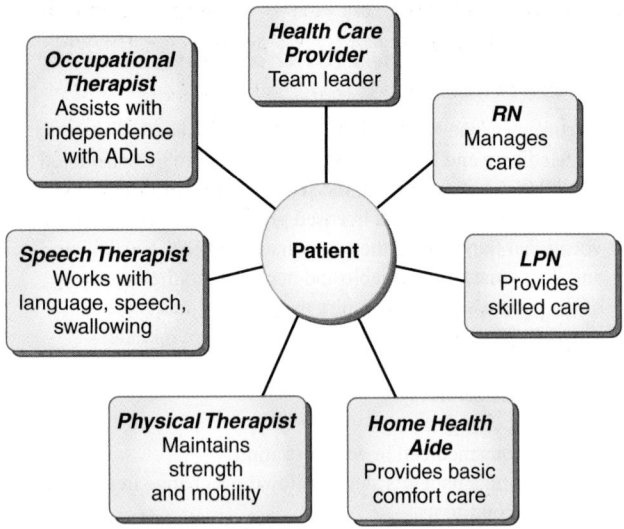

FIGURE 16.1 Home health care team members and their roles.

Based on recommendations from the RN or hospital case manager, the HCP may order a social worker to evaluate community resources to assist the patient. Social services can be helpful in creating a link between the patient and resources available within the community. These resources can include Meals on Wheels, safety resources, or outreach programs.

CRITICAL THINKING

Mr. Rosa, 75 years old, was discharged from the hospital following an acute exacerbation of heart failure with a referral for home health care. The home health care nurse notices that he has little food in his house. The house has not been cleaned recently and the clothes he is wearing are torn and soiled. Talking with him, the nurse learns that his wife died 6 months ago and that he has had a difficult time adjusting to this loss.

1. What are some community services that might be available to Mr. Rosa?
2. What information would be important to discuss with Mr. Rosa's health care provider?
3. Are there any other services that the home health care agency can offer Mr. Rosa for patient-centered care?

   Suggested answers are at the end of the chapter.

Transition From Hospital-Based Nursing to Home Health Care

Patients who enter the hospital are leaving behind the comfort of their own homes. They may be scared and isolated, trying to adjust not only to an illness but also to a new environment. The opposite is true in home health care nursing. In the patient's home, the nurse is the visitor and the surroundings are unfamiliar. This can be a difficult adjustment for a nurse. As confidence in being a home health care nurse grows, so does the comfort level with entering someone else's home. The nurse should recognize and consider cultural issues. Quick judgments about the home environment should not be made as patients may have values that do not match the nurse's values. If the home environment poses a health or safety risk, then it may be necessary to inform the RN.

When working in the hospital, the nurse has many staff and supply resources available. These resources are not always easily available when working in a patient's home. As such, the nurse must have a mastery of nursing skills. Home health care nursing requires an ability to adapt and remain flexible because, unlike the hospital environment, the home environment is unknown. Because of this, it is necessary to evaluate both the patient and the home setting.

For example, a patient has been referred for home health care after a fall at home that resulted in a fractured arm. During the initial evaluation at the patient's home, the nurse notes that the patient is lethargic and has very low blood pressure readings upon standing. Further data collection within the home environment leads the nurse to find that the patient was taking too much heart medication. The nurse then contacts the RN to obtain orders from the HCP to check the patient's blood for levels of the medication. Home health care nurses must evaluate the patient's case based not only on the referral diagnosis but also on what may be occurring within the home that is contributing to the diagnosis.

Families play an important role in the care of patients in the home. It is not surprising to walk into a home and find several anxious family members with a list of questions. Family members may be very involved in visits. Initially, this may be intimidating. When preparing for a visit, take the time to learn about an unfamiliar diagnosis or medication so you can answer their questions. In addition, be prepared for the unexpected. Carry extra common supplies, such as various sizes of urinary catheters, sterile dressing gauze, different types of tape, and alcohol wipes. Being prepared will help with developing a trusting relationship with patients and families.

Because of the **autonomous,** or independent, nature of home health care, most agencies require at least 1 year of medical-surgical nursing experience. This is to ensure that the nurse has the basic knowledge needed to work in home health care. Home health care agencies also hire nurses for specialty areas such as cardiac or wound care. See Box 16.2 for a review of liability issues.

The Role of the LPN/LVN in Home Health Care

The LPN/LVN's role in home health care is varied and complex. Skilled nursing care is similar to care performed in the hospital setting, only the setting is different (Fig. 16.2). The LPN/LVN works under the supervision of a home health care RN. The LPN/LVN role involves personal and patient safety, having necessary supplies, understanding and following infection control procedures, collecting patient data, providing

Liability Issues to Consider When Working in Home Health Care

When starting in home health care, review your state nurse practice act and scope of practice. The National Council of State Boards of Nursing (www.NCSBN.org) lists all the state boards of nursing web sites.

Understanding your scope of practice will ensure that you provide care that follows your state's guidelines. When in patients' homes, they might ask you to perform a skill or request something that is outside your scope of practice. It is important that you explain to them that it is outside your scope of practice but that you will notify your agency immediately about their request. For example, if a patient asks you whether it is okay to increase a medication, you should understand that, as a licensed practical nurse/licensed vocational nurse, you cannot prescribe medications. If you increased the medication, you would be altering the prescribed dose and, thus, practicing outside your scope of practice because only a health care provider can prescribe medications.

Always discuss your concerns with your supervisor and review your agency's guidelines, policies, and procedures. Know what you can and cannot do before you start, and never be afraid to question something that you feel or know violates your nurse practice act. Remember: It is your license, so follow your nurse practice act!

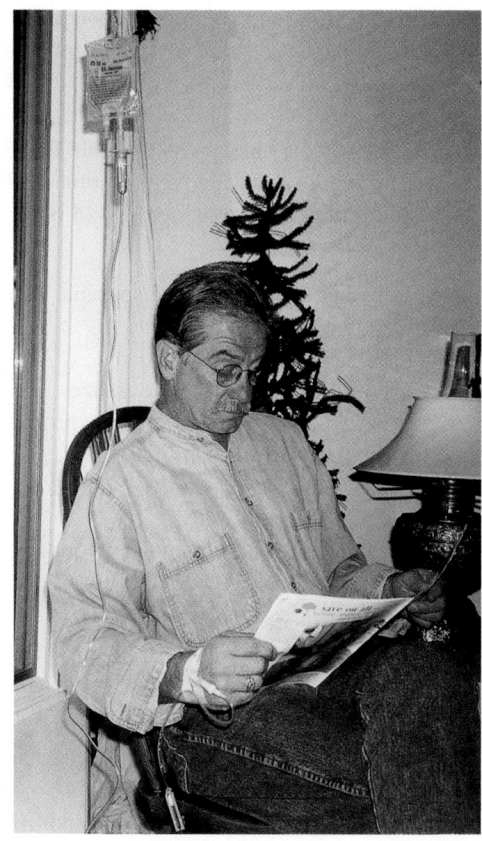

FIGURE 16.2 Patient receiving home intravenous therapy.

patient care, educating patients and caregivers, and documenting visits. Here is one LPN's personal testimonial:

Being a licensed practical nurse in a home health care setting requires many skills such as organization, excellent critical thinking skills, dedication, and the flexibility to adjust to patient and staffing needs. Being a home health care nurse allows you to focus on one patient at a time, to see patients in their homes, and to see the challenges they face day-to-day. It gives you the ability to change lives and possibly make a difference in someone's life.

Steps in the Home Health Care Visit
Preparing for the Visit

The typical day of a home health care nurse consists of six to seven home visits. These visits typically last 30 to 45 minutes. Most agencies try to arrange visits in the same geographical location for convenience. If visits are focused on a specialty, such as wound care, you may have to travel long distances between patients. In this case, you would be assigned less than seven visits. Agencies provide mileage reimbursement, so record mileage from house to house.

The day before your visit, develop a plan of action for how your visits will be structured. Sometimes, you will need to be at a certain place at a particular time, so factor this into your planning. Each patient must be contacted. Give the patient a 1- to 2-hour window for your arrival time. Remember, you cannot always anticipate what is going to happen during a visit. It is better to give your patients a time range as opposed to an exact time. If you are unsure how to locate your patient's home, ask for directions when you arrange the visit time. A global positioning system (GPS) or mapping application can help you arrive at your patient's home in a timely manner, thus improving patient satisfaction.

Many agencies utilize electronic documentation. You will likely be issued a laptop or tablet that allows you access to the patient's history and documentation from previous home health care visits. You can review the patient's diagnosis, pertinent medical information, and the reason for home health care prior to the visit.

Safety Considerations

A home health care nurses' travels can take them to areas that may be unsafe. It is important to be vigilant about personal safety. Box 16.3 lists tips on how to protect yourself before, during, and after a home health care visit.

Patient safety in the home is also of importance. Stay alert to things in the home that can pose a hazard to the patient. Teaching the patient how to prevent injuries in the home is an essential intervention. Physical or occupational therapy can help the patient build strength, learn how to use assistive devices, and maintain safety. (See "Gerontological Issues" for patient safety considerations in the home of older patients.)

Gerontological Issues

Safety. Older adults make up a significant proportion of home health care patients. Many items in older patients' homes can become potential safety hazards. The home health care nurse should always evaluate the patient's safety in the home. Things to consider are:

• Electrical cord safety
• Lighting
• Overcrowded spaces
• Pets
• Scatter/throw rugs
• Steps used to enter home
• Sturdy grab bars and a tub mat in the bathroom
• Supply access

Evidence-Based Practice

Clinical Question
What are the safety risks associated with providing in home health care to patients?

Evidence
A systemic review of 37 studies explored the safety risks associated with providing home health care to patients. Besides the more obvious safety risk findings, such as physical layout of the home, trip hazards, and inadequate or missing equipment or supplies necessary for care, other factors such as a lack of communication infrastructure or nonstandardized paperwork were also identified as possible sources of injury or resultant substandard care. In addition, lack of adequate time to provide care as well as lack of support for the caregiver were also identified (Hignett, Otter, & Keen, 2016).

Implications for Nursing Practice
It is important to use these findings that identify things that put either the patient and the caregiver (professional or family) at risk for injury to implement strategies that eliminate the risk for injury and promote safety.

Reference
Hignett, S., Otter, M. E., & Keen, C. (2016). Safety risks associated with physical interactions between patients and caregivers during treatment and care delivery in home care settings: A systematic review. *International Journal of Nursing Studies, 59*, 1–14.

Infection Control

Maintaining asepsis in the patient's home may be a challenge. The home health care agency will review infection control policies and procedures during agency orientation. In the hospital, everything is readily available for infection control.

Box 16.3
Safety Guidelines for Home Health Care Nurses

In general, providing home health care is a safe occupation. Most communities recognize the importance of the role of home health care nurses and are receptive to visits made to members of the community. However, it is still important to understand how you can protect yourself in case an unsafe situation arises.

Here are some tips for maintaining safety when completing a home health care visit:
• Always carry a map, whistle, and cell phone.
• Keep your gas tank filled.
• Complete recommended maintenance on your car and have the tires checked regularly.
• If possible, park on the street or road in front of the house. This prevents someone from blocking you in the driveway.
• When entering a home, be aware of where the exit doors are and any windows that will allow safe evacuation from the home.
• Be aware of your outside surroundings. When leaving the home, have your supplies packed up and keys out, ready to open the car door.
• If lost in an unknown area, leave and go to a familiar place and contact the patient for directions.
• If you need to complete a visit at night, request an escort. Many communities will have a police officer accompany you to and from the home. Discuss this option with your supervisor.
• Call your agency if you are concerned about your safety. Never complete a visit if you feel concerned for your safety.

However, in the home, the nurse is responsible for inventorying and bringing supplies provided by the home health care agency. It is always important to have extras of basic equipment, including the following:

• Personal protective equipment (e.g., disposable gowns, masks, goggles, shoe covers)
• Gloves, including latex-free gloves
• Biohazard bags and containers of various sizes
• Disposable underpads (which can be used to provide a clean field for supplies and for your bag)
• Antibacterial soap
• Hand sanitizer and sanitizing wipes
• Disinfecting spray to clean equipment and your bag after each visit
• Alcohol wipes for disinfecting thermometers and stethoscopes
• A small chemical spill kit

An important infection control measure is hand hygiene. It is important to wash your hands with soap and water before and after completing your patient care. If water is not available, use sanitizing liquid. Do not wash your hands in the patient's kitchen sink; always ask to use the bathroom for washing your hands.

CRITICAL THINKING

Mrs. Ambani was referred to your home health care agency after an appointment with her health care provider (HCP). During that visit, Mrs. Ambani was diagnosed as being anemic with dizziness, fatigue, and alterations in her blood pressure. The HCP requested home health care nurse visits for Mrs. Ambani to evaluate her safety and recommend appropriate safety devices.

1. What are hazards in the home you should look for?
2. What safety devices would assist Mrs. Ambani?

Suggested answers are at the end of the chapter.

Documentation

Because of reimbursement guidelines, the nurse must document specific things during the home visit. Home health care agencies receive their income based on a prospective pay system (predetermined rate), not per-visit payments. On admission, the RN fills out information that is entered into a computer system. This information is called the Outcome and Assessment Information Set, or OASIS (CMS, 2017). This tool is used to generate information about the home health care agency and patient outcomes. Home health care outcomes generated from OASIS are publicly reported via Home Health Compare (www.medicare.gov/homehealthcompare/search.html). OASIS allows the RN to implement a plan of care that is evidence-based, helping to eliminate potential complications, improve outcomes, and prevent unnecessary rehospitalizations. The LPN/LVN should be familiar with the general function of OASIS and its relevance to creating a plan of care.

For home health care agencies to be reimbursed, they need to demonstrate that a skill was completed. Documenting information is based on the patient's plan of care and the corresponding skill that was completed at the visit. For example, the HCP orders skilled nursing observation and medication management for a patient. In documenting the visit for this order, the nurse needs to state that this skill was completed. Documentation of the skill would include the following:

• The patient's response to medication (e.g., vital signs, level of consciousness, or other potential side effects)
• The patient's current understanding of medication regimen and the action the nurse took to improve that understanding
• The patient's response to that education and any areas in which the patient might continue to need assistance

Like hospitals, home health care agencies have different ways of documenting. The following items are typically included in all agencies' home health care documentation:

• Nurse's arrival and departure times
• Vital signs
• Data collection findings
• A narrative note, including patient education provided
• The patient's signature verifying that the nurse was present

Some agencies use the Clinical Care Classification System (www.sabacare.com) to facilitate documentation. This system was developed as a way to evaluate and classify home health care patients to determine what resources are required at the home. The system uses standardized codes similar to diagnosis codes to identify all of the elements of nursing practice that are utilized during the nursing process, including nursing interventions.

A folder with information is also kept at the patient's residence. It usually consists of relevant patient information and a communication form that all staff members complete at each visit. Similar to hospital charting, this documentation is important to ensure continuity of care.

Patient Education

A primary responsibility of nurses in home health care is educating patients about their illness and ways to effectively manage that illness at home. This is done with the intention of decreasing the need for hospitalization. Handouts are available from the home health care agency as well as other sources to help reinforce the verbal instructions the nurse provides. When teaching the patient or caregiver a procedure, always have the patient do a return demonstration before evaluating the patient as competent in performance of the procedure.

LEARNING TIP

An easy way to make sure you always have the handouts you need is to organize them into a three-ringed binder. You can organize the information in several ways (e.g., based on diagnoses or alphabetically). Have plenty of these handouts when making a visit. Many times, family members who do not live with the patient request copies so that they can have a copy at home.

Nursing Process for the Home Health Care Patient

Data Collection

Monitor and document patient and family adjustment to change and illness. Perform a complete patient evaluation during each visit. Monitor the home environment for potential safety hazards and the need for devices to assist with care.

Nursing Diagnoses, Planning, and Implementation

Ineffective Health Management related to deficient knowledge, complexity of medical needs, and limited access to social support

EXPECTED OUTCOME: The patient will demonstrate the changes in lifestyle needed to maintain health.

• Develop short- and long-term health goals with the patient *to ensure the patient's goals are being met.*

- Review the plan of care with the patient *to facilitate involvement and eventual independence.*
- Educate the patient on management of the health care regimen *to allow the patient to carry out the regimen.*
- Provide educational material in both written and verbal format *to promote understanding of complex issues.*
- Identify and work with social services *to meet the patient's needs.*
- Help the patient obtain needed supplies *to promote wellness.*
- Monitor the patient for changes in health status *to detect changes that can affect progress.*
- Praise small accomplishments *to motivate the patient's continued progress.*

Risk for Caregiver Role Strain related to management of a chronic illness and lack of understanding of resources available

EXPECTED OUTCOME: The caregiver will identify effective ways for dealing with the complexity of a chronic illness.

- Include the caregiver in the plan of care *to help develop an understanding of the management of the illness.*
- Request referral for a social worker *to facilitate contact with community resources such as respite care, Meals on Wheels, and support groups.*
- Discuss ways to help the caregiver deal effectively with feelings of anger and frustration *to allow resolution of the issues causing these feelings.*
- Discuss changes in family roles (e.g., a child taking care of a parent) and the challenges associated with this *to allow planning for the changes.*

Evaluation

Interventions have been effective if the patient and caregiver acknowledge acceptance and understanding of the change in health status, participate with goal setting, use community resources, maintain a safe home environment, and demonstrate ability to manage medical regimen.

Other Forms of Home Health Care Nursing
Telenursing

Technology makes it possible to provide care in the home to patients in remote or rural areas, or after office hours. **Telenursing,** a branch of telehealth, uses information technology and telecommunication (telephone, fax, e-mail, and video/audio conferencing) to provide nursing care. The nurse interacts with the patient via equipment set up in the patient's home. Because the nurse can see the patient, data collection can be obtained, including visualizing wounds. The nurse then plans care and educates the patient.

Private-Duty Nursing

This chapter has focused on home health care that is covered under the Medicare and Medicaid systems. The purpose of this type of home health care is to assist the patient with managing health needs on an intermittent basis. Additional types of home health care agency employment are available for nurses, including private-duty nursing and hospice nursing (see Chapter 17).

Private-duty nursing consists of scheduled care to assist patients with personal and homemaking needs as well as helping patients fill weekly medication dispensers. These services have been called home companion services, homemaker services, and private-duty care. They are generally not covered by insurance. They may focus mainly on companionship and **respite** care. Families who are taking care of a patient with complex needs, such as a patient with Alzheimer's disease, may need time away from the home to complete personal tasks or relax. Nurses may enjoy this type of work because of the long-term relationships that are formed with the patient and family.

SUGGESTED ANSWERS TO CRITICAL THINKING

Mr. Rosa

1. The loss of Mr. Rosa's wife and his subsequent health problems have affected his ability to properly care for himself. A nutritional diet is important for healing and maintenance of health. A referral to Meals on Wheels would be appropriate. This agency will deliver at least one healthy meal each weekday. The meal can be adapted to meet Mr. Rosa's dietary guidelines. Many communities offer older adult services to patients at a reduced cost to assist with housekeeping services. Helping the patient set up homemaker services will help him through this difficult time. Offering the patient information about grief counseling services in the community can be beneficial during this time. Once discharged from home health care, the patient can begin attending counseling services. Other community resources to consider

are neighborhood socials, church services if appropriate, and online communities that match the patient's values.

2. The health care provider needs to be contacted about the patient's withdrawn demeanor and lack of interest in self-care. Mr. Rosa may be experiencing situational depression because of the recent loss of his wife and his own health problems.

3. The nurse recognizes that Mr. Rosa needs extra help at this time. Consider a referral for a social worker to assist with community resources and grief counseling. Because heart failure is a chronic disease that can contribute to fatigue, an occupational therapist can work with the patient in developing energy-conserving techniques for completing activities of daily living. Also, the services of a home health care aide can help with personal care and provide additional emotional support.

SUGGESTED ANSWERS TO CRITICAL THINKING—cont'd

Mrs. Ambani

1. The home has many hazards. Important things to look for include scatter/throw rugs, overcrowded spaces, sharp edges along furniture, inadequate lighting, and stairs. Instruct the patient to keep frequently used kitchen appliances and foods on shelves that are easy to reach. The same is true for the bathroom and bedroom. Assist the patient with setting up a "command center" in the living room so that favorite items are kept in proximity and the patient does not have to get up too frequently.

2. Because anemia can cause extreme fatigue, it is important for Mrs. Ambani to have safety devices in the home to prevent falls. Equipment to consider includes a bath stool for the shower so she can sit while bathing, a detachable shower head, handrails in the shower and hallways, a bedside commode, an over-the-toilet seat, a reacher to assist with obtaining objects at a distance, a medical alert device that can be worn at all times, and, if fatigue is severe enough, a motorized wheelchair.

Review Questions

1. The nurse is caring for a patient who is a fall risk. Which of these interventions should the nurse implement to prevent a fall? **Select all that apply.**
   1. Ensure adequate vitamin D and calcium intake.
   2. Perform a medication review.
   3. Have resident stand quickly.
   4. Place socks on the patient for ambulation.
   5. Keep environment well lit and clutter free.
   6. Encourage exercise that strengthen leg muscles.

2. The nurse is caring for a resident who is confused, has become combative, and strikes out at the nurse. The nurse would demonstrate the appropriate legal use of restraints for the resident based on which of these? **Select all that apply.**
   1. The resident's plan of care identifies behaviors requiring restraints.
   2. The resident may harm others.
   3. The nurse cannot remain at the resident's bedside due to other tasks.
   4. The resident may cause self-harm.
   5. The resident's behavior requires discipline.

3. The home health care nurse is collecting data on a patient. Which of these is true about the nursing process step of data collection in home health care? **Select all that apply.**
   1. Data collection is done only while conducting the admission visit.
   2. Data collection is performed during every visit.
   3. Admission data collection may reveal problems unknown to the referrer.
   4. Data collection includes family roles.
   5. Environmental data is collected.
   6. Caregiver data is collected.

4. A patient is being seen by a home health care nurse for monitoring of weight and vital signs and education about medication changes following an acute exacerbation of heart failure. During this visit, which of these is a priority for the nurse to document?
   1. Food eaten by the patient for breakfast
   2. Education on keeping a daily weight log and when to inform the health care provider
   3. Explaining the role of the home health care aide in assisting the patient with personal care
   4. Distance the patient was able to ambulate while working with physical therapy

5. What steps does the home health care nurse take to ensure that a patient is not exposed to infectious materials in the home?
   1. Disinfect the home health care bag after each patient visit with a germicidal spray supplied by the home health care agency.
   2. Perform hand hygiene in the kitchen sink rather than the bathroom sink.
   3. Use the same red bag from patient to patient for disposing of soiled dressings.
   4. Place home health care bag on floor instead of furniture.

6. A licensed vocational nurse is preparing to interview for a position in a medical office and is reviewing the job description. Which of these tasks would be included in the job description? **Select all that apply.**
   1. Advocate for patients.
   2. Obtain and document patients' vital signs.
   3. Contribute to the plan of care for patients.
   4. Administer immunizations.
   5. Obtain informed consent.
   6. Assist with renewal of prescriptions.

7. A licensed practical nurse is offered a position in a correctional facility. The nurse is informed that the tasks will include which of these? **Select all that apply.**
   1. Demonstrates professionalism in providing inmate health care delivery
   2. Demonstrates sensitivity to cultural and socioeconomic differences related to health and behaviors
   3. Responds appropriately to situations and seeks supervision as needed
   4. Provides sympathy to inmates who are ill
   5. Responds to emergencies as part of the health care team

Answer rationales available in your online resources.

ANSWERS 1. 1, 2, 5, 6; 2. 1, 2, 4; 3. 2, 3, 4, 5, 6; 4. 2; 5. 1; 6. 1, 2, 3, 4, 6; 7. 1, 2, 3, 5

Key Points

Find the chapter key points in your online resources available through Davis Edge.

Additional Resources

 Use the scratch off code on the inside front cover of your book to access online quizzes that will help you to improve your scores on course exams and prepare for NCLEX-PN®.

Study Guide

The author acknowledges the contributions to this chapter by Anna Ricks, LPN, for the "Medical Office Nursing" section and Maryanne Pietraniec-Shannon, RN, PhD, for the "Correctional Nursing" section.

CHAPTER 17

Nursing Care of Patients at the End of Life

Betsy Murphy

KEY TERMS

advance medical directive (ad-VANSE MED-ih-kuhl dur-EK-tiv)
advocate (ADD-vuh-ket)
artificial feeding (ART-ih-FISH-uhl FEE-ding)
artificial hydration (ART-ih-FISH-uhl hy-DRAY-shun)
do not resuscitate (DNR) (DOO not re-SUSS-ih-TATE)
durable power of attorney (DUR-uh-buhl POW-ur OV uh-TUR-nee)
hospice (HOS-pis)
living will (LIH-ving WIL)
palliative (PAH-lee-uh-tiv)
postmortem care (pohst-MOR-tum CARE)

CHAPTER CONCEPTS

Collaboration
Comfort
Grief and Loss
Patient-Centered Care

LEARNING OUTCOMES

1. Identify characteristics of the patient who is approaching the end of life.
2. List necessary legal documents for patients with life-limiting illness.
3. Explain choices that are available to patients at the end of life.
4. Demonstrate appropriate communication with dying patients and their families.
5. Describe physical changes to expect during the dying process.
6. Plan nursing interventions for patients at the end of life.
7. Describe postmortem care.
8. Plan nursing interventions for the grieving patient and family.
9. Discuss the role of the licensed practical nurse/licensed vocational nurse in hospice care.

Mr. Moran, 89 years old, resides in a long-term care facility and has been losing weight and growing weaker for the past 6 months. Despite treatment for depression, he continues to grow weaker and more dependent on his caregivers. As you read this chapter, consider what decisions his family will face and what resources are available to them in their quest to provide appropriate care for him.

 A GOOD DEATH

Despite our best efforts, there will come a time when all our patients will die. Death is the expected end to a life well lived. In America, only 10% of us will die suddenly. The remaining 90% will experience a gradual decline over a period of months or years.

In the 21st century, most Americans die from chronic and acute illnesses such as cancer, heart disease, stroke, and dementia. We have the technology to prolong life, but sometimes this longer life can carry with it profound disability and reduced quality of life. Our patients sometimes tell us that this is not what they intended for the last phase of their life. So, what is the role of the nurse with patients nearing the end of life? Two priorities are to (1) help identify patients with life-limiting illnesses early so that they and their families have the opportunity to redefine their goals of care and (2) help our patients communicate their wishes to health care providers (HCPs), both orally and in writing, to ensure that their wishes are understood.

Perhaps the most important role for nurses is to give our patients support and validation as they move through the series of losses leading to a good death. Dying is, after all, the final phase of our growth and development. The developmental tasks associated with this phase involve reflecting on our lives, saying "goodbye;" saying, "I'm sorry;" and saying, "I love you." The goal of having a "good death" is a valid goal.

There have been multiple studies focused on identifying the needs of terminally ill patients and their families (Gardner & Kramer, 2010). The findings fit into five categories:

• Adequate pain and symptom management
• Ability to make their own decisions
• Avoidance of unnecessary life-sustaining treatment and prolongation of the dying process
• Reducing the emotional and financial burden on their families
• Ability to use remaining time to strengthen relationships with loved ones

This description of a good death helps nurses listen to what patients want and focus on how best to help them achieve their goals. Nurses who choose to provide care for the dying will experience personal growth in their own lives. Facing the inevitability of our own mortality can force us to look more deeply at our beliefs, values, and priorities in life. This can result in a richer, more focused life.

IDENTIFYING IMPENDING DEATH

Most Americans say that they want to die at home. Home for many patients will mean the place they are most comfortable, surrounded by caregivers who understand their needs and provide attentive care. Home can be where they live independently or with their families. It can also be in a continuing care retirement community, assisted living facility, or nursing home. In the United States, 30% to 40% of older adults die in long-term care facilities. A surprising 80% of older patients die within a year of admission to a nursing home (Kelly et al., 2010). Nurses who are working in long-term care and assisted living facilities will find themselves in a position both to identify patients who are likely to die soon and also to support these patients' families in planning for a good death. Because so many patients die within months of admission to long-term care facilities, their preferences should be identified soon after admission. Without proper documentation, should the patient become ill, he or she will be routinely transported to the hospital, possibly to receive unwanted treatments.

How can you identify patients who are nearing the end of their lives? Some patients die because of disease but others simply lose weight and grow weaker as they enter the final months of life. Research has shown that measuring both weight loss and increasing dependency in activities of daily living can help to identify patients who are dying. More than 5% loss of weight in 6 months is considered significant (Gaddey & Holder, 2014). Weight loss caused by depression

or acute illness may be reversed with aggressive treatment. But if neither depression nor acute illness is the cause of the patient's decline, he or she may be entering the final months of life.

Older patients who are having trouble swallowing and require treatment for aspiration pneumonia are likely to die within a year (Komiya et al., 2016). Aspiration risk is associated with recurrent pneumonia. Decreased respiratory muscle strength, lack of lung elasticity, and poor immune response make meaningful recovery unlikely. Older patients with poor renal and cardiac function are also at high risk for dying. The final truth is that, for some older patients with chronic illness, many aggressive treatments offer little benefit.

For most patients and their families, the transition from treating an illness to allowing the patient to die comfortably is a gradual process. Figure 17.1 shows the evolving relationship between treatments intended to cure and treatments intended to comfort as the patient approaches the end of life. As curative therapies are reduced, comfort care, also known as **palliative** measures, is increased. This chapter explores some of the choices people need to make at the end of life and the interventions you can use to help patients during this time.

ADVANCE DIRECTIVES, LIVING WILLS, AND DURABLE MEDICAL POWER OF ATTORNEY

The Patient Self-Determination Act, which took effect in 1991, ensures that every patient has the right to accept or refuse any medical treatment that is offered. The act also requires HCPs to ask patients entering a hospital if they have prepared **advance medical directives**. These directives include a living will and a durable power of attorney for health care. In preparing advance medical directives, patients are exercising their right to make their wishes known regarding

Simultaneous Care Model

Curative therapy

Presentation   Death

Palliative care   Hospice

FIGURE 17.1 The simultaneous care model.

specific medical treatments they would want—or not want—if they become unable to make decisions on their own. The directives require the signatures of two witnesses; neither can be a family member or HCP.

A **living will** is a document instructing HCPs about a patient's preferences (such as to withhold or withdraw life-sustaining procedures) if the patient is unable to communicate, found to be permanently unconscious, and/or has been declared "terminal." A **durable power of attorney** for health care specifies who will speak for a patient when he or she cannot speak. Many states provide standard forms to use and may require the patient to have both a durable power of attorney for health care and a living will to ensure the patient's wishes are followed. An attorney, although not required, may be helpful for some families.

Encourage patients not only to fill out the necessary forms but also to discuss their wishes with all family members. It is estimated that only about 30% of Americans have advance medical directives. Some patients are reluctant to complete them, concerned that they may change their minds about treatments in the future. It can be helpful to talk about advance care planning as a *process.* Patients can change their minds at any time about any treatment and write a new advance directive. If no advance directive is on record, the state law where the patient resides will dictate their proxy decision maker.

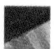 ## END-OF-LIFE CHOICES

Cardiopulmonary Resuscitation

During the 1960s, cardiopulmonary resuscitation (CPR) was developed as a method of rescuing healthy people who suffered a cardiac or respiratory arrest. Some of the early guidelines specified that CPR was not to be used in patients with terminal illnesses. Today, CPR has become standard in both hospitals and long-term care facilities. All patients receive CPR unless they have a do not resuscitate order.

Patients often have the misperception that CPR can save most lives. However, in reality, very few lives are saved by CPR: Patients of all ages who are not in a hospital have only a 7.6% chance of survival (Daya et al., 2015). One reason for the low survival rate is that CPR must begin within 3 to 5 minutes of collapse. The most successful cases are those in which CPR and an automatic external defibrillator are used within 3 to 5 minutes of collapse. In the hospital, the chance of CPR success declines with the patient's age. Patients who are 70 to 79 years old have an 18.7% chance of survival, while for patients over 90 years of age that rate drops to 11.6% (Van Gijn, Frijns, van de Glind, van Munster, & Hamaker, 2014).

A helpful way of presenting the DNR option to patients and families is to (1) provide them with the survival statistics; (2) help them to understand that, after receiving CPR, their medical condition will not improve and that it is likely that they will be more debilitated; and (3) reassure patients that

they will receive aggressive comfort care as they are dying a natural death.

Do Not Resuscitate Orders

A "No Code," or **do not resuscitate (DNR)** order, is written in a hospital or long-term care facility after collaboration with the patient, family, and the HCP, usually after it has been determined that the patient will not benefit from CPR. The patient will still have choices regarding all other treatments. A DNR order simply means that CPR will not be done. Some hospitals offer several options:

- DNR/Comfort Care Only
- DNR/Full Therapeutic Support
- Full Code

An advance directive or hospital DNR order does not cover patients' wishes in the home or nursing home. A durable DNR (also called an out-of-hospital or prehospital DNR) is a physician's order for emergency medical services workers to follow. The form varies by state and may be called Physician Orders for Life-Sustaining Treatment (POLST), Medical Orders for Life-Sustaining Treatment (MOLST), Medical Orders for Scope of Treatment (MOST), or Physician Orders for Scope of Treatment (POST). This document is signed by both the patient or the patient's decision maker and the patient's HCP. Emergency medical services workers are trained to look for such a document, often in a bright color and hanging on the patient's refrigerator.

Some patients fear that, in choosing DNR status, they will suffer and be alone at the time of their death. Patients and families may erroneously perceive DNR as withholding a treatment that could benefit the patient. It is important to tell patients that DNR does not mean *do not treat*. Patients who have a DNR/Comfort Care Only order will still receive oxygen, medications, and other comfort measures to aggressively manage their symptoms and ensure a comfortable death. A gentler way of discussing this choice may be to ask patients and families if they prefer to allow a natural death. All DNR orders and discussions with families should be documented on the patient's chart ("Patient Perspective").

LEARNING TIP

A Full Code order means that, if the patient's heart stops, everything possible will be done to save the patient, including cardiopulmonary resuscitation (CPR). Often, the patient will require artificial ventilation following CPR. A No Code/Full Therapeutic Support order means that everything possible will be done up to but not including CPR or ventilator. A No Code/Comfort Care Only order means that only medications and treatments that keep the patient comfortable will be done.

Patient Perspective

Anna. My mom, Anna, was diagnosed with cardiomyopathy and congestive heart failure when she was just 60 years old. At that time, she was still working and had recently remarried. She thought she had many years left in life. She did not have an advance directive—why would she?

Two years later, as her disease progressed, she decided she did not ever want to "live on machines." So, with the help of her doctor and our family, she wrote her living will and made her new husband her durable power of attorney for health care, with me as his backup person. Because she was still functioning well, with lots of medications and occasional hospitalizations, she chose a do not resuscitate (DNR) status, but with full therapeutic, aggressive interventions. She even took a tour of Europe during this time in her life, knowing she would not be able to do it later.

By age 67, she had a lot less energy to do things, and her heart failure really cramped her lifestyle. But she still enjoyed life, and her goal was to see my son, who was her oldest grandson, graduate from high school. She considered a heart transplant, but her doctor told her she was too old to qualify. She did have a new kind of valve surgery that was supposed to make her feel better, but it didn't help much.

Three months after my son's graduation, my mom was hospitalized several times with progressively worse outcomes. She weighed barely 100 pounds and could not eat much. She was only 70 years old and still looked and acted so young! Finally, she was in a semicoma in the hospital, and our family had to make the difficult decision to withdraw all therapeutic support. She was now a DNR, with comfort measures only. We were confident this would be what she wanted because we had talked about it with her. She was alert enough to let us know that she wanted to die at home.

She was discharged home with hospice care and died within a week. I moved in for her final days to help out. Between her husband, me, and her hospice nurse (who was a godsend), as well as frequent visits from family and her minister, she was well cared for. We kept her comfortable with lots of attention and morphine. She was alert and able to converse much of the time. She ate what and when she wanted, which amounted to one-quarter of a cheese and tomato sandwich one day, but she enjoyed it! She could finally enjoy a glass of grapefruit juice, which she had been unable to have for years because it interacted with one of her heart medications.

At the end, she died with me holding her left hand and her husband holding her right. We were telling her we loved her. It was a good death.

CRITICAL THINKING

Mrs. Hart has written a living will specifying her wishes should she become incapacitated. Because she has advanced disease, she tells you she would not want to be resuscitated if she has a cardiac arrest. She is currently hospitalized but will be discharged to her home in a few days.

1. What documents does Mrs. Hart need to have in place to ensure she will not receive resuscitation?
2. What health care team members should you collaborate with in helping Mrs. Hart through this process?

Suggested answers are at the end of the chapter.

Artificial Feeding and Hydration

Patients may be unable to eat or drink as a result of three conditions: an acute illness, a long illness with multiple medical problems, or simply the aging process. Otherwise healthy patients who are unable to eat while recovering from an acute illness will probably benefit from **artificial feeding,** for example, a cancer patient receiving parenteral nutrition (see Chapter 7) or tube feeding to prevent weight loss while receiving a treatment such as chemotherapy or radiation that is known to cause weight loss. In contrast, patients who are losing weight because of a life-limiting illness with multiple medical problems or the aging process itself will probably not benefit from artificial feeding. For terminally ill patients, research has shown that "no strong evidence exists supporting the use of parenteral hydration/nutrition" (Dev, Dalal, & Bruera, 2012). Terminally ill patients include cancer patients and those with life-limiting diseases such as Alzheimer's disease or other dementias, Parkinson's disease, and others.

It is now widely accepted that feeding advanced dementia patients via feeding tube does not prolong their life or enhance their quality of life. In fact, it increases rather than decreases their risk of aspiration. Despite this fact, many advanced dementia patients continue to receive feeding tubes because their families are not consistently provided with evidence-based information to make good decisions (Teno et al., 2011). Providing families with evidence-based information as part of advance care planning can help families make the best possible decisions for their loved ones. The Alzheimer's Association provides educational information for families of patients with end-stage dementia. It recommends that, instead of a feeding tube, these patients receive an effective program of hand feeding (visit www.alz.org for more information).

When a patient is recognized as having entered the dying phase, medical treatment should focus on comfort. Research suggests the benefits of artificial feeding and hydration may be limited and may not outweigh the burdens (Raijmakers et al., 2011). There are actually benefits to withholding artificial feeding and artificial hydration in the final weeks of life in actively dying patients. These benefits include the following:

- Fewer pharyngeal and lung secretions, which can reduce dyspnea
- Reduced swelling around tumors, which can reduce associated pain
- Less urination, resulting in dryer skin with less skin breakdown

It has been theorized that, as dehydration occurs, the body produces a form of endorphin that enhances comfort. As ketone levels rise from the breakdown of body fat, patients experience an anesthetic effect that creates a sense of well-being. Families often express concern that the patient will experience hunger or thirst. Thirst is prevalent in dying patients but unlikely to improve with **artificial hydration** (Zehm, Mullin, & Zhang, 2016). A recent study of dying cancer patients showed that patients who received 1 L of fluid daily did not live longer nor have fewer symptoms or experience improved quality of life (Bruera et al., 2013). See the nursing diagnosis *Impaired Oral Mucous Membrane Integrity* in the "Nursing Care Plan for the Patient at the End of Life" later in this chapter for suggestions about how to increase comfort in the patient unable to drink.

The issue of feeding is emotionally difficult for families. Often their loved one has been ill a long time. Bringing favorite foods may have been one of the ways family and friends showed love and communicated caring. The following are three ways you can support families in making decisions about feeding:

- Identifying goals of care and evaluating whether artificial feeding will help meet those goals
- Weighing the benefits and burdens of feeding
- Finding new ways (besides feeding) to communicate their love, such as skin care, mouth care, or reading to their loved one

For a different perspective on artificial feeding, see "Ethical Considerations" for Chapter 17 in your online resources found on Davis Edge.

Hospitalization

A hospital is where patients go to receive aggressive medical treatment. The goal of care in a hospital is to improve the patient medically and transfer him or her to an appropriate level of care that will better meet individualized needs. There are burdens associated with hospitalization for older adult patients approaching the end of life. They may actually decline more rapidly in a hospital setting. When removed from a setting with predictable routines and known caregivers, the older patient often loses weight. Research has shown that older adult patients suffer accelerated cognitive decline after hospitalization (Wilson et al., 2012). They enter a foreign environment and are cared for by health care workers who do not know them. Patients may be physically restrained as they become agitated and fearful while away from home. Frail patients with poor immunity risk developing infections. They

often enter the hospital with one infection and are discharged with other infections such as *Clostridium difficile* that may be resistant to antibiotics or caused by antibiotics.

Antibiotics are commonly prescribed in the final weeks of life. Their use is perceived by families as helpful, but the diagnostic process subjects the patient to testing and invasive treatments that can increase their distress while dying (Juthani-Mehta, Malani, & Mitchell, 2015). Helping families decide on goals for the patient's care will help with making decisions in the future. If the patient or family decides on comfort care only, then going to the hospital or receiving antibiotics may not meet their goal.

Patients living in nursing facilities with end-stage dementia who have severe cognitive impairment will benefit from having a "do not hospitalize" order. This will keep them in an environment that feels safe and preserves their chosen quality of life. Having hospice care in place (see next section) in nursing facilities reduces the chances of unwanted hospital and intensive care unit admissions (Obermeyer et al., 2014).

Hospice Care

Many people think of **hospice** as a place. It is actually a service. Hospice is provided in private homes ("Home Health Hints") or independent and assisted living facilities. It can also be provided in hospitals and nursing homes when there is a signed contract between the hospice organization and the facility. To qualify for hospice care, a patient must have an estimated prognosis of 6 months or less. Patients can receive hospice care longer than 6 months as long as their health continues to decline.

Home Health Hints

- Encourage discussion regarding advance directives with the patient and family/caregiver early in the care process. Decisions regarding resuscitation and the use of technology to prolong life are more difficult when the patient is in crisis.
- Allow time during your visit to sit quietly with the patient and caregiver. Sitting quietly lets the patient and caregiver know you are there to meet both physical and emotional needs.
- Encourage family involvement with care. Families need reassurance that they are not going to hurt the patient; take the time to teach them how to assist the patient with basic care.
- Prepare the family for what to expect as death approaches.
- When the patient is no longer conscious, encourage the family to continue to spend time at the bedside sharing personal thoughts and memories with the patient. For example, a spouse might talk about when they first met, or family members can play a favorite song.

Some indicators of a 6-month or less prognosis (regardless of diagnosis) are 10% unintentional loss of weight in 6 months, increased weakness, frequent hospital admissions, and recurrent infections. The goal of hospice care is holistic: to manage symptoms such as pain and nausea, to provide emotional and spiritual counseling for the patient and family, and to support the patient in achieving his or her goals of care. Each patient is assigned a multidisciplinary hospice team to assist with care (Table 17.1).

Most health insurance companies now provide a hospice benefit. Many are modeled after the Medicare hospice benefit. The Medicare benefit pays for both hospice care at home and inpatient hospice care provided in a contracted hospital, skilled nursing facility, or freestanding hospice unit. Medications, medical supplies, oxygen, and medical equipment are also covered if they are related to the terminal diagnosis.

Hospice care can help a family take care of a patient at home, but hospice nurses do not routinely provide 24-hour in-home health care. Rather, a nurse is on call for in-home visits 24 hours a day. Nurses and other team members make regular visits to support and teach the patient and family. In times of medical crisis, short-term inpatient hospice services or 24-hour in-home continuous nursing care may be provided under some hospice benefits.

COMMUNICATING WITH PATIENTS AND THEIR LOVED ONES

Terminal illness is a family experience. Family is defined by the patient and may include blood relatives, friends, significant others, or partners. The primary role of the nurse is to facilitate a comfortable death that honors the choices of the patient and family. The nurse, therefore, becomes the **advocate,** assuring that patient and family wishes are communicated to other members of the health care team. In addition, the nurse is often the professional caregiver and educator of the nonprofessional caregivers and family members.

To successfully work with dying patients and families, you must demonstrate empathy, unconditional positive regard, trustworthiness, and critical thinking. You are part of an interdisciplinary team (see Table 17.1). Each discipline has expertise and can lend support to the others in providing care. As illustrated in the earlier section on end-of-life choices, patients and their loved ones need support and evidence-based information to make good decisions. All members of the team can assist with this support.

Good communication requires that you take time to listen, answer questions honestly, help identify choices, and allow verbalization of fears. Eighty percent of communication is nonverbal, such as eye contact, body language, and tone of voice. Take time to identify your own communication barriers that will affect your ability to talk with families. Do you have fears about your own mortality or lack personal experience with death? Do you fear being blamed for decisions or disagree with decisions that were made? These barriers will affect your ability to sit with patients and families in crisis, sustain eye contact, and support them in their process. Practice attentive listening with patients and families. Allow them to talk. Be silent, don't change the subject, and know that you do not need to have all the answers. Your role can be to help them reflect on what they are trying to communicate and to clarify their goals of care so you can better advocate for them.

Set the stage for communication by sitting down to show you are not in a hurry (Fig. 17.2). Maintain eye

Table 17.1
The Hospice Team

Team Member	Role
Physician or other health care provider (HCP)	Works with the patient's primary HCP, offering suggestions to improve care. Directs team activities and often will make visits to the patient's home.
Nurse	Makes routine home visits, assessing patient needs and implementing plan of care. Nurses are available 24 hours per day to make visits as needed.
Social worker	Provides emotional counseling and long-term planning, assists patients with insurance issues, and helps identify community resources.
Chaplain or minister	Provides spiritual counseling or coordinates care of spiritual issues with the patient's chosen spiritual counsellor. May participate in funeral or memorial service.
Home health care aide	Provides personal care, linen changes, and light housekeeping.
Volunteers	Support caregivers by staying with the patient while they get out of the house. May also read to patient, run errands, etc.
Bereavement counselor	Provides counseling for family and significant others for 13 months after patient's death.

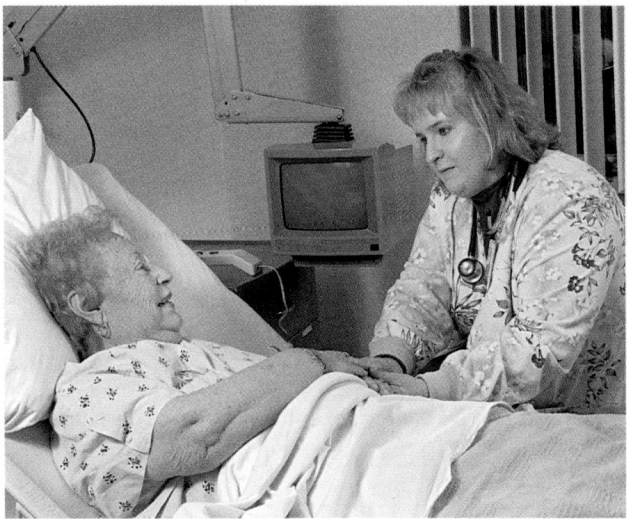

FIGURE 17.2 Nurses can be a comfort to patients and family members.

contact, encourage patients to speak, repeat what they say to gain clarification, and reflect on its meaning. Some things to say to facilitate good communication include the following:

- "Do you feel like talking?"
- "Tell me more about your fears of …"
- Repeat back what you hear: "You mentioned you were upset by …"
- Reflect: "So are you saying that …?"
- "How can I help you?"

From the patient's perspective, many factors influence the content and quality of communication with you. Some patients are so afraid that they cannot hear what they have been told about their illness. It can be helpful to ask what the HCP has told them to assess where they are in understanding their disease.

Patients may use denial as a mechanism to protect themselves from becoming overwhelmed by emotion. The denial is necessary to enable them to survive on a day-by-day basis. You do not need to correct their denial. Some patients remain in denial throughout the course of their illness. When patients in denial ask you a direct question about their condition, it can be an indicator that they are ready to hear the truth. It is essential that you always answer questions honestly and to the best of your knowledge. Dishonesty destroys trust and credibility.

Patients and their families may also feel angry. Allowing them to express their anger will validate it and enable them to progress emotionally. Comments such as "It is okay to be angry" will encourage them to continue to talk. Patients who fully understand their prognosis will express sadness and regret. Sitting with patients as they express sadness will allow them to share their feelings and give you an opportunity to offer emotional support. See "Evidence-Based Practice."

Evidence-Based Practice

Clinical Question

Do patients with a terminal diagnosis understand their prognosis? Do health care professionals benefit from end-of life communication training?

Evidence

A review of 34 studies including more than 11,000 patients with advanced cancer revealed that only approximately half of patients understood their disease status, prognosis, or treatment plan and, therefore, overestimated their expected survival (Chen, Keuo, & Tang, 2017).

In a separate systematic review of 20 studies, Chung and colleagues (2016) found that end-of-life communication training may increase health care professionals' knowledge, self-efficacy, and end-of-life communication scores.

Implications for Nursing Practice

It is important that all patients understand their disease status and prognosis. This may begin with health care professionals' ability to effectively communicate with those facing end-of-life issues. Successful communication between health care professionals and patients may help patients understand their conditions more clearly and increase their participation in end-of-life decision making.

References

Chen, C. H., Kuo, S. C., & Tang, S. T. (2017). Current status of accurate prognostic awareness in advanced/terminally ill cancer patients: Systematic review and meta-regression analysis. *Palliative Medicine, 31*(5), 406–418.

Chung, H. O., Oczkowski, S. J., Harvey, L., Mbuagbaw, L., & You, J. J. (2016). Educational interventions to train healthcare professionals in end-of-life communication: A systematic review and meta-analysis. *BMC Medical Education, 16,* 131.

 THE DYING PROCESS

This section discusses the expected changes in the days and hours before death. Assessing patients, planning and implementing treatments, and evaluating responses to interventions are all important. Nursing interventions are summarized in the "Nursing Care Plan for the Patient at the End of Life."

Educating family caregivers about what to expect is essential. Caregivers who anticipate the expected changes and understand the rationale behind the interventions are more successful in their caregiving and have fewer regrets or concerns after the death. The "Nursing Care Plan for the Patient at the End of Life" includes specific communications that may help caregivers understand what is happening and how they can help.

(Text continued on page 274)

Nursing Care Plan for the Patient at the End of Life

Nursing Diagnosis: *Impaired Gas Exchange* related to dying heart and lungs as evidenced by dyspnea, change in respiratory rate, and SpO_2 less than 90%
Expected Outcomes: The patient will state that breathing is comfortable. Respiratory rate is between 12 and 20 per minute, and SpO_2 will be 90% or greater.
Evaluation of Outcomes: Is the patient's breathing relaxed and rate between 12 and 20 per minute? Is SpO_2 90% or greater?

Intervention	Rationale	Evaluation
Monitor respiratory rate and effort.	*Increased rate and effort indicate distress.*	Is patient in distress? Are further interventions needed?
Intervention: Administer diuretics or antibiotics as ordered.	*Diuretics or antibiotics may be given to treat causes of dyspnea and promote comfort, not to prolong life.*	Do diuretics or antibiotics reduce dyspnea?
Explain to the family the rationale for medical interventions.	*Blood transfusions may be given to improve oxygenation and reduce dyspnea; a thoracentesis may promote lung expansion. These are not intended to prolong life but to promote comfort.*	Are additional interventions needed and effective? Does the family understand the rationale for their use?
Plan activities to conserve energy.	*Spacing rest with activity will help reduce oxygen consumption.*	Can patient tolerate spaced activities?
Place patient in a recliner with pillows to 45 degrees.	*An upright position allows lung expansion.*	Does positioning reduce dyspnea?
Offer alternative comfort measures, such as massage and muscle relaxation.	*Relaxation reduces anxiety and resulting dyspnea.*	Are alternative measures effective?
Administer oxygen as ordered.	*Oxygenation raises SpO_2 and reduces dyspnea.*	Does oxygen raise SpO_2 and relieve dyspnea?
Place a fan in room if patient desires.	*The feeling of a breeze may reduce subjective feelings of dyspnea.*	Does patient report increased comfort or appear more comfortable with a fan on?
Administer low-dose morphine as ordered.	*Morphine causes peripheral vasodilation, which can reduce pulmonary edema. It can also slow breathing and reduce anxiety.*	Are respirations less labored after morphine administration?

Nursing Diagnosis: *Ineffective Airway Clearance* related to excessive secretions and inability to swallow as evidenced by gurgling sound ("death rattle")
Expected Outcome: The patient's airway will be free of secretions.
Evaluation of Outcome: Is the patient's breathing quiet and unlabored?

Intervention	Rationale	Evaluation
Adjust patient's head to allow secretions to move down the throat.	*This will help patient swallow the secretions and decrease frightening noise.*	Is breathing quieter?
Place a humidifier in the room.	*Humidified air can liquefy secretions and help patient cough.*	Is patient able to cough up secretions?
If secretions are copious, administer hyoscyamine, glycopyrrolate, or scopolamine as ordered.	*These anticholinergic medications can dry secretions.*	Do medications help dry secretions?

Nursing Care Plan for the Patient at the End of Life—cont'd

Intervention	Rationale	Evaluation
Administer low-dose morphine as ordered.	*Morphine has an anticholinergic action that can help dry secretions.*	Does morphine help quiet breathing and help patient stay calm?
Suction patient as needed.	*If secretions are copious, suctioning may be needed.*	Is suctioning needed? Is it effective?
Explain to the family that, because the patient is unresponsive, a small amount of secretions is unlikely to be disturbing to the patient. The noisy breathing can often be reduced by repositioning patient's head.	*The informed family will be able to cooperate and assist with keeping the patient comfortable.*	Do patient and family understand reasons for care and feel secure that patient is receiving the best possible care?

Nursing Diagnosis: *Imbalanced Nutrition: Less Than Body Requirements* related to inability to swallow and lack of appetite as evidenced by refusing food and weight loss
Expected Outcomes: The patient will state satisfaction with amount and types of food offered. The patient will not aspirate food or fluid.
Evaluation of Outcomes: Does the patient appear content with foods and fluids offered? Does the patient swallow without aspirating?

Intervention	Rationale	Evaluation
Let patient choose when and what to eat. Do not force patient to eat if patient does not wish to.	*The goal is no longer providing adequate nutrition but keeping patient comfortable.*	Is patient receiving the foods and fluids the patient wants?
Sit patient upright to eat or drink.	*This can help patient swallow and prevent aspiration.*	Does patient swallow effectively?
Explain to family, as needed, that the patient is afraid to swallow now because swallowing is impaired and it causes the patient to choke. As the patient becomes dehydrated, the patient's comfort will increase as the body produces naturally occurring anesthesia.	*The informed patient and family will be able to cooperate and assist with keeping the patient comfortable.*	Do patient and family understand the reasons for care and feel secure that the patient is receiving the best possible care?

Nursing Diagnosis: *Impaired Oral Mucous Membrane Integrity* related to dehydration, not eating, and medication side effects
Expected Outcome: The patient's mucous membranes will be clean and moist.
Evaluation of Outcome: Are the patient's mucous membranes clean and moist? Does the patient indicate that the mouth is comfortable?

Intervention	Rationale	Evaluation
If patient is alert, offer ice chips or sips of water.	*These keep mucous membranes moist.*	Does patient indicate mouth feels comfortable?
Provide frequent mouth care with sponge-tipped Toothettes.	*This can keep mucous membranes moist when patient is not able to drink adequate fluids.*	Is the mouth clean and moist?
Apply lanolin to lips.	*Lanolin keeps mouth and lips from becoming dry and crusty.*	Are lips smooth and moist?

(nursing care plan continues on page 272)

Nursing Care Plan for the Patient at the End of Life—cont'd

Nursing Diagnosis: *Impaired Comfort* (pain, terminal restlessness) related to disease process, dying process, and medications
Expected Outcome: The patient will state that the patient feels comfortable or, if unable to speak, will appear calm and peaceful, not restless or agitated.
Evaluation of Outcome: Is the patient comfortable, calm, and peaceful?

Intervention	Rationale	Evaluation
Assess for reversible causes of agitation (e.g., pain or other discomfort, urine retention or fecal impaction, medications that are no longer beneficial, Spo_2 less than 90%).	*Often, agitation is a sign of discomfort. Identifying and removing the cause of the discomfort can help calm the patient.*	Can causes be identified? Are they removed?
Reposition patient in bed at least every 2 hours and as needed.	*Repositioning frequently can promote comfort and relieve pressure on bony prominences. When other medical interventions are discontinued, patient still needs to be repositioned regularly to prevent uncomfortable complications.*	Does repositioning promote comfort?
If Spo_2 is low, administer oxygen as ordered.	*Low Spo_2 causes dyspnea, which is not comfortable.*	Is Spo_2 raised to 90%? Is patient's breathing unlabored?
Discuss with the health care provider discontinuing all uncomfortable procedures, such as blood draws and finger sticks for blood glucose.	*Many procedures provide information to the staff but are not beneficial to the patient at the end of life. They should be discontinued.*	Are any uncomfortable procedures still being carried out that are not absolutely necessary?
If the cause of the agitation cannot be determined, try medication for pain, dyspnea, or anxiety as ordered.	*Medication may need to be administered based on objective observations if patient is unable to communicate.*	Does medication promote comfort?
Keep patient safe with one-on-one monitoring and side rails up.	*A fall would increase patient's discomfort.*	Is patient safety maintained?
Keep perineal area clean and dry, frequently checking adult briefs.	*A wet brief is not comfortable. Unchanged briefs can also lead to skin breakdown, another source of discomfort.*	Is patient clean and dry with intact skin?
Teach patient and family that restlessness can have many causes. It can be a sign of pain, bowel or bladder problems, or a medication issue. Tell them you will work with the health care provider to improve the situation.	*The informed patient and family will be able to cooperate and assist with keeping the patient comfortable.*	Do patient and family understand the reasons for care and feel secure that the patient is receiving the best possible care?

Nursing Care Plan for the Patient at the End of Life—cont'd

Nursing Diagnosis: *Hypothermia* or *Hyperthermia* related to dysregulation of central nervous system
Expected Outcomes: The patient's temperature will be maintained as close to normal as possible, and discomfort from temperature extremes will be managed.
Evaluation of Outcomes: Is temperature within normal limits? If unable to control temperature, does the patient appear comfortable?

Intervention	Rationale	Evaluation
Administer acetaminophen suppository as ordered.	*Acetaminophen is an antipyretic. It is given by suppository if patient cannot swallow.*	Does acetaminophen reduce fever?
Keep patient clean and dry. Change gown and bed linens as needed.	*A fever can cause diaphoresis (excessive sweating), and lying in damp sheets can be uncomfortable and cause skin breakdown.*	Is patient kept dry and comfortable?
If patient is cold, add blankets as needed. Do not use an electric blanket or heating pad.	*Blankets will warm patient without risking burns from electric heating devices.*	Are blankets helpful?

Nursing Diagnosis: *Acute Confusion* related to neurologic changes
Expected Outcomes: The family will voice understanding that confusion is not uncommon and will show appropriate responses if it occurs.
Evaluation of Outcomes: Does the family respond appropriately to the patient during times of confusion?

Intervention	Rationale	Evaluation
Assure families that some confusion is common.	*If family is prepared, confusion will be less disturbing.*	Is family informed? Do family members verbalize understanding of what to expect?
Do not correct patient but instead encourage patient to talk about what is happening.	*Sometimes patients talk about their fears in metaphor. Allowing them to express their fears will promote relaxation and decrease loneliness.*	Is patient less distressed after speaking?
Keep a dim light on in the room (but enough light to avoid shadows), and remind patient gently of who is present.	*Being able to see clearly helps keep the patient oriented if patient awakens during the night.*	Is the light on? Is patient able to orient on awakening?
Explain to the family that many patients don't make sense at times. It is as if "they are in two worlds at the same time." Patient will be less distressed if the family lets the patient talk about what the patient is experiencing.	*Family members will be less distressed if they understand what is happening.*	Does the family respond appropriately to patient's confused statements?

Nursing Diagnosis: *Fear* related to threat of death
Expected Outcome: The patient will be treated as still present and respected, and not as though the patient is already gone.
Evaluation of Outcome: Is communication respectful toward the patient?

Intervention	Rationale	Evaluation
When providing care, always speak as if the patient can hear you. When conversing with family members in the room, remember that the patient also can hear what you are saying.	*Patients may be able to hear even when they appear to be nonresponsive. Always assume the patient can hear you.*	Are caregivers and family members sensitive to patient's presence when communicating?

(nursing care plan continues on page 274)

Nursing Care Plan for the Patient at the End of Life—cont'd

Intervention	Rationale	Evaluation
When giving care, explain softly to patient what you are doing and why.	*Knowing what is happening can reduce anxiety and increase cooperation.*	Does patient appear calm? Does patient respond to your explanations?
Explain to the family that it is believed that hearing is the last sense to go in the dying patient. This can be a good time to say the things they have not been able to say.	*Continued communication can be comforting to both patient and family.*	Is communication appropriate?

Nursing Diagnosis: *Grieving* related to impending death
Expected Outcome: The patient and family will be able to openly communicate their feelings to each other and say goodbye.
Evaluation of Outcome: Are the patient and family able to communicate effectively and say goodbye to each other?

Intervention	Rationale	Evaluation
Be present with the patient. Just sit quietly and hold patient's hand for a period of time.	*This can help the patient feel less alone, especially if there are no family members present. Many patients fear dying alone.*	Is someone present with the patient as much as possible?
Show appropriate concern.	*This will promote trust and empower family members to ask for what they need.*	Is the family communicating openly with the health care providers?
Provide a quiet environment where loved ones can say goodbye in a way that will reflect their culture and values.	*These interactions will serve as valuable memories after the death and provide a feeling that all participants did what they needed to do for their loved one.*	Do family members appear satisfied with their participation in the process?
Consult a minister or religious counselor of family's choice.	*A minister often has special skills and training in communicating with people during difficult times. Talking about an afterlife may also be comforting to patient and family.*	Does the family appear to benefit from the presence of a minister or religious counselor?
Ask about the family's cultural and religious beliefs, and allow time for prayers and ceremonies.	*Providing a culturally familiar environment will reduce patient's and family's anxieties and give them more control over the process.*	Do family members feel free to carry out cultural and religious beliefs?

Eating and Drinking

As our bodies move toward death, there is less desire for food and fluids. Patients are conserving energy and often do not feel hunger. The swallowing reflex is impaired, so patients fear choking and may hold their mouth tightly closed when food or fluids are offered. This is normal, and the resulting dehydration will increase comfort due to endorphin production and rising ketone levels.

Changes in Breathing

About 50% to 70% of patients have dyspnea at the end of life. Patients who are not alert must rely on you to identify their distress. Signs of distress are tachypnea (respiratory rate greater than 24 per minute), facial grimacing, and use of accessory muscles to breathe. Untreated dyspnea can lead to fear and agitation, resulting in worsening shortness of breath. Dyspnea can be effectively managed without aggressive treatment (see "Nursing Care Plan for the Patient at the End of Life"). Some patients also will have episodes of apnea in the days or hours before they die.

Oral Secretions

Saliva that the patient is now unable to swallow may collect in the back of the throat, causing a sound sometimes called a *death rattle*. This can be disconcerting for the family.

Temperature Changes

As the body loses its ability to control temperature, the patient may become diaphoretic or feel cold all the time. Some patients have experienced fevers as high as 105°F (40.5°C). As death approaches, the feet and legs may become cool, cyanotic, and mottled. This is often an indicator that death will occur within hours.

Bowel and Bladder Changes

Most patients will become incontinent of bowel and bladder during the course of the dying process. Urine output will decrease as dehydration occurs. Urine often will darken in color and have a strong odor.

Sleeping

In the final weeks of life, patients may be sleeping for most of the day. They also begin to emotionally detach from families as part of their preparation to leave.

Mental Status Changes

As patients go through the process of dying, they often have episodes of confusion, possibly from electrolyte imbalance or medications. Some patients will say things like, "I have to catch a train" or "I need my passport." This metaphorical communication is well documented in the hospice literature (Kissane, Bultz, Butow, & Finaly, 2011).

Terminal Restlessness

Terminal restlessness is a syndrome observed in a significant number of patients with various diagnoses during the final days of life. The patient may be unable to concentrate or relax and may show nonpurposeful motor activities, such as picking at bed sheets. The patient may hallucinate or try to climb out of bed. Terminal restlessness can have many causes, including hypoxemia, metabolic abnormalities, and liver failure. Some physical causes may be reversible, so it is important to assess whether pain, urinary retention, or fecal impaction may be the cause.

Restlessness may also be caused by medications. As kidney and liver functions decline, medication levels rise in the body and cause toxicity. Consult with the HCP and pharmacist to determine if all the medications the patient is receiving are beneficial or necessary. Table 17.2 reviews medications that may be helpful at the end of life.

Unconsciousness

Most patients are unconscious for hours or days before they die. Before they lose consciousness, their ability to see may

be diminished. Hearing is the final sense to be lost. It is important for you to remember as you are caring for the patient and conversing with the family that your patient likely hears everything you are saying. Encourage the family to continue talking to the patient.

CRITICAL THINKING

Mr. Johnson is in the final hours of his life and has become increasingly short of breath throughout the day. With each inspiration, his respirations are moist and noisy. Currently, his respiratory rate is 30 per minute, and you notice he is using his accessory muscles to breathe.

1. What is the cause of his noisy breathing?
2. What can be done to lower his respiratory rate and decrease his dyspnea?

Suggested answers are at the end of the chapter.

 ## CARE AT THE TIME OF DEATH AND AFTERWARD

Death has occurred when you observe the absence of heartbeat and respirations. The skin becomes pale and waxen, the eyes may remain open, and pupils are fixed. Telling the family that the patient has died should be done with sensitivity, providing small amounts of information according to the family's level of understanding. Be sure to check and adhere to the policies in your health care setting and state regarding death pronouncement and organ donation. Document the general appearance of the body, including absent pulse and lung sounds. Your goal now is to provide a personal closure experience for the family.

After death has been pronounced, you will provide **postmortem care.** First, remove the tubes, medical supplies, and equipment. Bathing and dressing the patient and making him or her look presentable for the family shows respect. Some cultures dictate specific care of the body after death and who should provide that care (see Chapter 4 for more information). The nurse can assess and advocate for cultural practices requested by the family. Work toward providing a clean, peaceful impression of the deceased. Position the body in proper alignment, insert dentures, place dressings on leaking wounds, and use briefs as needed. Allow the family time with the body. Do not remove the body from the room until the family is ready. Covering or uncovering the face at removal should be done according to the family's preference. Additional activities, such as contacting the HCP or funeral home, should be carried out according to institution policy.

 ## GRIEF

Grief is the emotional response to a loss. Loss is a daily experience in everyone's life. Loss can occur due to divorce, children leaving home, loss of job, loss of possessions, or

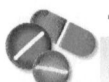

Table 17.2
Medications to Increase Comfort at the End of Life

Medication Class/Action

Opioids
Bind to opioid receptors to reduce pain and dyspnea.

Examples	**Nursing Implications**
morphine (MS, MS-IR, MS Contin, Roxanol) hydromorphone (Dilaudid) fentanyl (Duragesic, Sublimaze, Actiq, Fentora) buprenorphine patch (Transtec, BuTrans)	For pain and dyspnea. Longer acting agents must be given routinely to be effective. Give short-acting analgesia for 24 to 72 hours until longer acting agents take effect. Do not cut patches before application. Wear gloves when applying or removing patch because drug may be absorbed during handling. Do not apply heat over a patch. Heat increases drug absorption and may cause overdoses. Used patches may still contain drug. Dispose of used patches to prevent accidental exposure to others, especially children and pets.

Anxiolytics
Depress central nervous system to reduce anxiety.

Examples	**Nursing Implications**
lorazepam (Ativan) alprazolam (Xanax) diazepam (Valium)	Not first-line drugs for treating dyspnea. Effective for dyspnea caused by anxiety.

Neuroleptics
Reduce severe agitation and terminal restlessness.

Examples	**Nursing Implications**
haloperidol (Haldol)	Useful in treating anxiety or agitation when lorazepam ineffective.

Anticholinergics
Treat excessive pharyngeal secretions.

Examples	**Nursing Implications**
hyoscyamine (Levsin) atropine drops scopolamine (Transderm-Scop) glycopyrrolate (Robinul)	Place scopolamine patch behind the ear.

other losses, including death. People express grief in their own way according to their coping skills, life experiences, and cultural norms. In end-of-life care, grief is a process that begins before the patient's death and continues through a series of tasks that the survivors move through to resolve grief. Feelings associated with grief may include anger, frustration, regret, guilt, sadness, and many others. Although each person is different, the process commonly includes three general stages (Table 17.3).

Interventions for the grieving patient are addressed in the "Nursing Care Plan for the Patient at the End of Life."

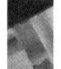

NURSING PROCESS FOR THE GRIEVING FAMILY

Data Collection
Some things to consider when assessing grief include the following:

- Where is the family in the grief process?
- Are family members experiencing physical problems, such as shortness of breath, sweating, or skin color changes?
- Is the stress of grieving worsening medical conditions?

Table 17.3
Stages of Grief

Stage	Tasks	Characteristics
Stage 1 Shock and disbelief	Acknowledge the reality of the loss. Recognize the loss.	Has difficulty with feelings of numbness, emotional outbursts, poor daily functioning, and avoidance.
Stage 2 Experiencing the loss	Work through the pain by expressing and experiencing the feelings.	Anger, bargaining, depression. May feel guilt over not preventing the death or not providing enough care. May feel angry at loved one who has "left them behind." May experience insomnia, loss of appetite, apathy, lack of interest in daily life.
Stage 3 Reintegration	Adjust to an environment without the deceased.	Finds hope in the future, participates in social events, and feels more energetic.

- What support systems are available to the family?
- What interventions might facilitate their grief process?

Nursing Diagnoses, Planning, and Implementation

Although many nursing diagnoses may be appropriate, the priority diagnosis is simply *Grieving*.

Grieving related to impending death or loss of loved one.

EXPECTED OUTCOME: Family members will be able to express feelings of anger, guilt, or sadness. They will be able to think about the future and perform activities of daily livings as needed.

- Simply be present. *Sitting with the bereaved, without having to have all the answers, is very powerful. If you don't know what to say, just be silent.*
- Actively listen and let the bereaved talk about the loved one and their feelings about the loss. Ask open-ended questions to encourage them to continue talking. *One of the greatest needs of the bereaved is to trust someone enough to share their pain.*
- Help family members identify their support systems (e.g., religious or spiritual affiliation, friends, family) and encourage them to use them. *Support systems can help in practical ways (e.g., meals, transportation) as well as lend emotional support.*
- Consider acknowledging the event by attending the memorial service or sending a card. *This simple act of caring is very important to families.*

Evaluation

Healing takes time. If interventions have been effective, however, family members will have the support to function effectively while they grieve.

 THE NURSE AND LOSS

Working with dying patients triggers awareness of your own losses and fears about death and mortality. Adapting to the care of the dying requires that you explore and experience your personal feelings toward death. Unresolved losses from your past can resurface and affect your ability to care for dying patients. You may find that you continue to think about patients who have died long after the event. Emotionally continuing to care about deceased patients takes energy away from the daily care you are providing to current patients and your own family. Unresolved grief can lead to symptoms that resemble burnout, such as insomnia, headaches, and fatigue.

If you find yourself distancing and withdrawing from your dying patients, it is an indicator that you need to attend to caring for yourself. Some nurses may find counseling helpful to effectively process losses from the past and learn healthy ways to process future losses.

Both formal and informal support systems should be in place to support staff through multiple losses. Informal support can be one-on-one sharing of experiences with coworkers, peers, pastoral counselors, and HCPs. Understanding and acknowledging your limitations, asking for help, and getting regular exercise and relaxation are important components. Some nurses find journal writing a helpful process; writing down feelings may allow you to release them. Formal support systems can be established in many ways:

- Preplanned gatherings where nurses can express feelings in a safe environment
- Postclinical debriefings after difficult deaths to alleviate anxiety and promote learning
- Ceremonies such as memorial services in facilities to allow both staff and residents to recognize and honor the loss of patients

In addition, many employers offer free employee assistance programs that provide counseling.

 REFLECTIONS ON MR. MORAN

Remember Mr. Moran from the beginning of the chapter? Clearly, he is approaching the end of life. Determine what he and his family want to happen in the final months of his life and where he wants to be. What are the goals of care? If comfort is the goal, how can this best be achieved? If keeping him in his familiar and safe environment is the goal, then help his family weigh the benefits and burdens of CPR, hospitalization, artificial feeding, and artificial hydration.

SUGGESTED ANSWERS TO CRITICAL THINKING

Mrs. Hart

1. Mrs. Hart will need a do not resuscitate (DNR) order in the hospital setting. When she goes home, she will need an out-of-hospital or prehospital, durable DNR (whatever the form is called, such as MOLST, MOST, POST, or POLST, in her state of residence). In addition, her family members should be aware of her wishes.
2. Her health care provider, hospital social worker, or case manager can be helpful. She may also wish to speak with the chaplain or her spiritual advisor.

Mr. Johnson

1. Mr. Johnson's noisy breathing may be caused by saliva collecting in the back of the throat or by pulmonary edema.
2. Mr. Johnson may benefit from oxygen, positioning, and suctioning oral secretions. Low-dose morphine will decrease his respiratory rate and improve his oxygenation. Morphine also has a drying effect on secretions. If morphine is unsuccessful, the addition of an anticholinergic medication may be helpful.

Review Questions

1. A 94-year-old patient is admitted from home to the hospital with pneumonia. What factors would lead the nurse to believe the patient is nearing the end of life?
   1. Distended abdomen and yellow skin tone
   2. Fever of 101.6°F (38.7°C) and a respiratory rate of 28 per minute
   3. Difficulty swallowing and weight loss
   4. Inability to cough and bring up secretions

2. What is a durable power of attorney for health care?
   1. A document that outlines a patient's wishes at the end of life
   2. A document that gives a patient a "do not resuscitate" status
   3. A document specifying the person who will make decisions for a patient once the document is signed
   4. A document specifying the person who will make decisions for a patient when the patient is no longer able to speak for himself

3. A patient's family member says, "I heard someone say my mother could have a 'good death.' What on earth is a good death?" Which response by the nurse is best?
   1. "We consider a good death to be one that follows the patient's wishes for care, is comfortable, and allows them to die where they choose."
   2. "In reality, no death is a good death, but we do our best to make sure patients are comfortable right up until they die."
   3. "A good death is when the patient is kept sedated so they don't really know what is happening during the last days until they die."
   4. "A good death occurs when the patient is kept alive as long as possible, so she can take care of all her unfinished business first."

4. A husband whose wife has just died cries, "What am I going to do? She is all I had." What is the best response the nurse can provide?
   1. "You are going to go on with your life. You still have your work and your children."
   2. "I am sorry you lost your wife, but I know she would not want you to be sad. You have to be strong for her."
   3. "I know how you feel. I lost my grandmother recently, and it was really hard."
   4. There is no need to say anything. Just be present and listen.

5. A dying patient has excessive secretions that are causing dyspnea. Which medications will best help dry the secretions and increase comfort? **Select all that apply.**
   1. Haloperidol
   2. Scopolamine
   3. Acetaminophen
   4. Morphine
   5. Guaifenesin

6. Which of the following nursing interventions should the nurse provide at the end of life? **Select all that apply.**
   1. Position the patient to increase comfort and prevent complications.
   2. Provide comfort measures such as massage.
   3. Research experimental treatments that may help the patient find a cure.
   4. Administer medications to control symptoms.
   5. Teach the family cardiopulmonary resuscitation for use if the patient dies when the nurse is not present.
   6. Sit quietly with the patient and family.

7. A patient has just died, and his family is waiting to see him. What postmortem care is essential first?
   1. Document the time and circumstances of the death.
   2. Place identification on the body according to hospital policy.
   3. Clean the patient up and make him look peaceful.
   4. Cover the patient's body and face with a sheet.

8. The wife of a hospitalized patient who died an hour ago is crying and unwilling to leave the hospital room. The rest of the family is in the waiting room. The admitting department just called and wants to have the room cleaned for a new patient. Which action should the nurse take?
   1. Allow the wife to stay in the room as long as she likes.
   2. Call a taxicab for the wife and gently guide her out of the room.
   3. Sit with the wife for a few minutes and then take her to the waiting room.
   4. Tell the wife that you are sorry for her loss but that another patient needs the room.

9. A patient who has been receiving hospice care for 3 months tells the nurse he has decided he wants to return to active treatment of his disease. What should the nurse do?
   1. Encourage the patient to discuss his desire with his health care provider.
   2. Tell the patient that he cannot change his goals once hospice care has been initiated.
   3. Check his medication supply for any leftover medications he was taking during treatment.
   4. Explain to the patient that, since he is terminal, treatment will not help the course of his disease.

Answer rationales available in your online resources.

ANSWERS 1. 3; 2. 4; 3. 1; 4. 5, 2, 4; 6. 1, 2, 4, 6; 7. 3; 8. 3; 9. 1

Key Points

Find the chapter key points in your online resources available through Davis Edge.

Additional Resources

CHAPTER 18

Immune System Function, Assessment, and Therapeutic Measures

Kristy Gorman, Janice L. Bradford, Sharon M. Nowak

KEY TERMS

active immunity (AK-tiv ih-MYOO-nih-tee)
anaphylactic (AN-uh-fih-LAK-tik)
antibody (AN-tih-bah-dee)
antigen (AN-tih-jen)
autoimmune (AW-toe-ih-mewn)
cell-mediated immunity (SELL mee-dee-ay-ted ih-MYOO-nih-tee)
humoral immunity (HYOO-mur-uhl ih-MYOO-nih-tee)
lymphocyte (LIM-fuh-site)
microbiota (MYK-row-by-ott-a)
neutrophil (NEW-troh-fil)
passive immunity (PASS-iv ih-MYOO-nih-tee)
white blood cells (WYTE BLUHD SELLS)

CHAPTER CONCEPTS

Immunity

LEARNING OUTCOMES

1. Identify the type of immunity that is obtained with a vaccine.
2. Describe the two mechanisms of immunity.
3. Discuss the function of each class of immunoglobulin and how each behaves in a particular immune response.
4. Describe how aging affects the immune system.
5. Explain subjective data that are collected when caring for a patient with a disorder of the immune system.
6. Explain objective data that are collected when caring for a patient with a disorder of the immune system.
7. Describe nursing care provided for patients undergoing diagnostic tests for the immune system.
8. Discuss common therapeutic measures used for disorders of the immune system.

NORMAL IMMUNE SYSTEM ANATOMY AND PHYSIOLOGY

Immunity is defined as the ability to destroy pathogens or other foreign material and to prevent further cases of infectious disease. Immunity is typically the body's response to foreign microorganisms such as bacteria, viruses, and fungi. However, immune responses can be directed toward other cells or substances that are identified by the body, correctly or incorrectly, as foreign. Malignant cells are considered foreign and are usually destroyed by the immune system after mutation but before they become malignant. Unfortunately, transplanted organs are usually perceived as foreign and, therefore, rejected. Occasionally, the immune system mistakenly reacts to self (**autoimmune** disease) or to a substance that should be tolerated (allergic reaction).

The immune system consists of lymphoid organs and tissues, **lymphocytes** and other **white blood cells** (WBCs),

and many chemicals that activate our own cells for the destruction of foreign antigens (Fig. 18.1). The lymphatic system includes lymphatic vessels that return lymph (tissue fluid) to the circulatory system; lymph nodes, nodules, and the spleen, where macrophages phagocytize (engulf and destroy) pathogens and where thymus-derived lymphocytes (T cells) and bone marrow–derived lymphocytes (B cells) carry out immune functions; and red bone marrow and the thymus (which functions primarily in childhood and atrophies with age). Lymph flows from vessels through lymph nodes, where pathogens are percolated out and destroyed. Lymph nodes are especially concentrated in the cervical, axillary, and inguinal areas. Lymph nodules, lacking encapsulation, are found under the surface of mucous membranes (e.g., tonsils).

- WORD · BUILDING ·
lymphocyte: lympho—lymph + kytos—cell

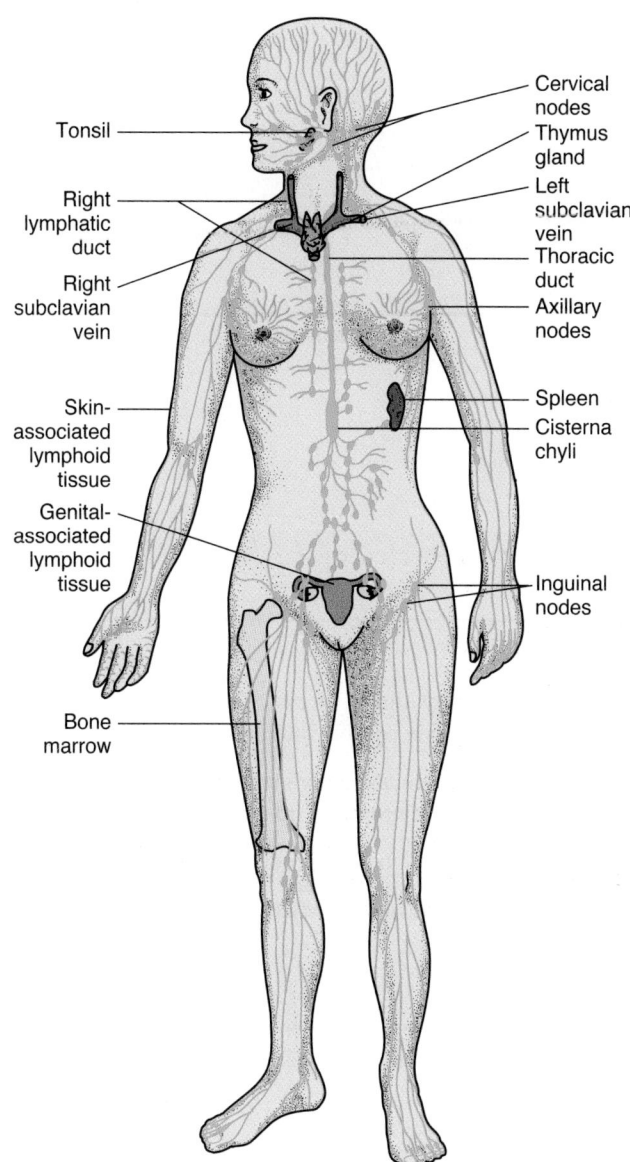

FIGURE 18.1 Immune system organs, lymph vessels, and major lymph nodes.

Antigens

Antigens are chemical markers that identify cells or molecules. Human cells have their own antigens—thousands of markers that identify the cell as "self." These are the major histocompatibility complex antigens, also called human leukocyte antigens, which are genetically determined. Major histocompatibility complex antigens are tolerated by the body's immune system, whereas foreign antigens will be destroyed in one of several ways.

Lymphocytes

There are three types of lymphocytes: natural killer (NK) cells, T cells, and B cells, each with different functions.

Natural Killer Cells

NK cells are found throughout the body and produce a quick immune response. They destroy a variety of foreign cells,

including altered self-cells (tumors) and infected cells. After binding with an abnormal cell, NK cells release perforins and granzymes, which cause cytolysis (destruction of cell). Cell fragments are then phagocytized by WBCs.

T Cells and B Cells

T cells and B cells are involved in specific immune responses; that is, each cell is programmed to respond to one kind of foreign antigen. Both T cells and B cells arise in the red bone marrow. T cells then migrate to the thymus, where the thymic hormones bring about their maturation. From the thymus, T cells migrate to the lymph nodes and nodules and to the spleen. B cells mature in the bone marrow and migrate directly to lymphatic tissue. When activated during an immune response, T cells perform a direct attack, whereas B cells differentiate into plasma cells that release antibodies for an indirect approach.

Antibodies

Antibodies are glycoproteins produced by plasma cells in response to foreign antigens. They are also called immunoglobulins (Ig). Antibodies do not themselves destroy foreign antigens but rather become attached to such antigens to label them for destruction. Each antibody is specific for only one antigen. B cells (which become plasma cells) are capable of producing millions of different antibodies. There are five classes of human antibodies, designated by letter names: IgG, IgA, IgM, IgD, and IgE (Fig. 18.2). Their functions are summarized in Table 18.1.

Mechanisms of Immunity

The two mechanisms of immunity are *cell-mediated immunity,* which involves T cells, and *humoral immunity,* which involves mainly B cells but is assisted by T cells. Although the mechanisms are different, invasion by a pathogen often triggers both.

Cell-Mediated Immunity

Cell-mediated immunity is effective against intracellular pathogens (such as viruses or fungi), malignant cells, and grafts of foreign tissue. A T-cell response results in cytotoxic T cells, which attack altered cells; helper T cells, which assist; and memory T cells, which retain knowledge of the pathogen in the event of future encounters with the same (Fig. 18.3).

Humoral Immunity

Humoral immunity involves antibody production. It is also called *antibody-mediated immunity.* It is effective against extracellular pathogens, which are usually bacteria but can also be viral or fungal infections (Fig. 18.4).

Although B cells are stationary, the antibodies produced by plasma cells circulate throughout the body and bond to the antigen, forming an antigen–antibody complex. This immobilizes

• **WORD • BUILDING •**

antigen: anti—against + gennan—to produce

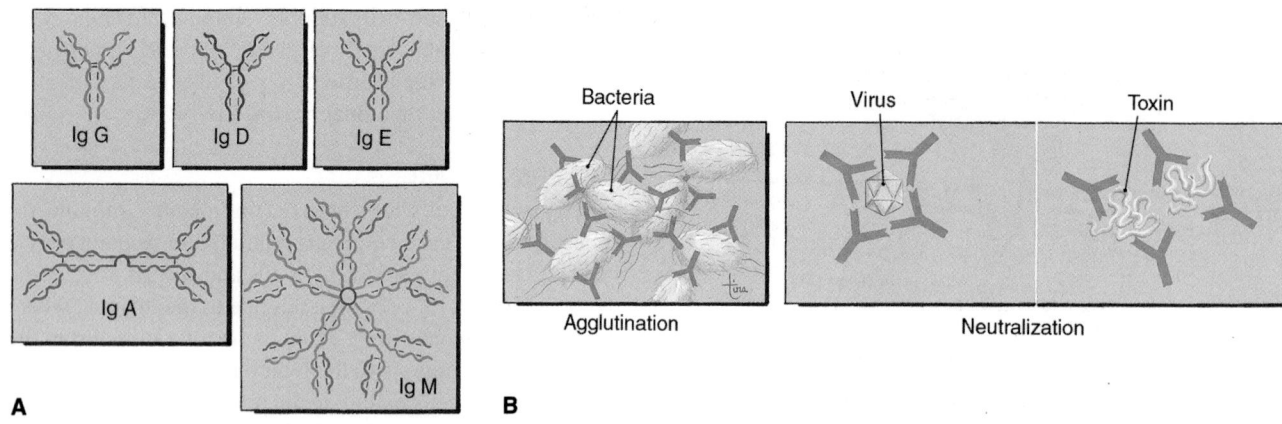

FIGURE 18.2 Antibodies. (A) Structure of the five classes of antibodies. (B) Antibody activity.

Table 18.1

Classes of Antibodies

Immunoglobulin (Ig)	Location	Function
IgG	Blood, extracellular fluid, lymph	Provides long-term immunity after a vaccination or illness recovery Crosses the placenta to provide passive immunity in newborns
IgA	External secretions (e.g., tears, saliva)	Found in secretions of all mucous membranes Provides passive immunity for breastfed infants
IgM	Blood, lymph	Produced first during an infection (IgG production follows)
IgD	B cells	Antigen-specific receptors on B lymphocytes
IgE	Mast cells or basophils	Important in allergic reactions Mast cells release histamine

Source: From Scanlon, V., & Sanders, T. (2018). *Understanding human structure and function* (8th ed.). Philadelphia, PA: F.A. Davis.

the bacteria; also, the antigen is now labeled for phagocytosis by macrophages or **neutrophils.** The antigen–antibody complex also activates the *complement cascade.*

Complement is a group of more than 30 plasma proteins that circulate in the blood until activated by either the presence of foreign bacteria or by an antigen–antibody complex. The activation of complement results in the formation of a protein cascade that lyses (causes disintegration of) the cell. Other complement proteins bind to foreign antigens and serve as further labels to attract macrophages.

ANTIBODY RESPONSES

The first exposure to a foreign antigen stimulates antibody production. However, the antibodies are produced too slowly to prevent the disease. With time, the person accumulates antibodies and memory cells specific for that pathogen. On second exposure to the antigen, the memory cells begin rapid production of large amounts of antibody, often enough to prevent a second occurrence of the illness (Fig. 18.5). This is the basis for the protection given by vaccines. A vaccine contains

an antigen that is not pathogenic. The vaccine stimulates the formation of antibodies and memory cells.

Antibodies may also neutralize viruses; that is, they attach to a virus and render it unable to enter a cell (see Fig. 18.2). Viruses cannot reproduce outside of living cells. Those coated with antibodies are phagocytized by macrophages. Interferon, another defense against viruses, is a chemical produced by cells infected with viruses. Although it does not help the infected cell, interferon protects surrounding cells by enabling them to resist viral replication.

Antibodies are also involved in allergic responses. During an allergic response, the immune system responds to foreign but harmless antigens (an allergen), such as plant pollen. IgE antibodies bond to mast cells, which break down and release histamine and other chemicals that contribute to inflammation. **Anaphylactic** shock is an allergic reaction, but massive

• WORD • BUILDING •

neutrophil: neutro—neuter + philein—to love
anaphylactic: ana—up + phylaxis—protection

1 The immune process begins when a phagocyte (such as a macrophage, reticular cell, or B cell) ingests an antigen.

2 The phagocyte, called an **antigen-presenting cell (APC)**, displays fragments of the antigen on its surface—a process called **antigen presentation**—which alerts the immune system to the presence of a foreign antigen. When a T cell spots the foreign antigen, it binds to it.

3 This activates (or sensitizes) the T cell, which begins dividing repeatedly to form clones: identical T cells already sensitized to the antigen. Some of these T cells become effector cells (such as cytotoxic T cells and helper T cells), which will carry out the attack, while others become memory T cells.

4 The cytotoxic T cell binds to the surface of the antigen and delivers a toxic dose of chemicals that will kill it.

5 Helper T cells support the attack by secreting the chemical **interleukin**, which attracts neutrophils, natural killer cells, and macrophages. It also stimulates the production of T and B cells.

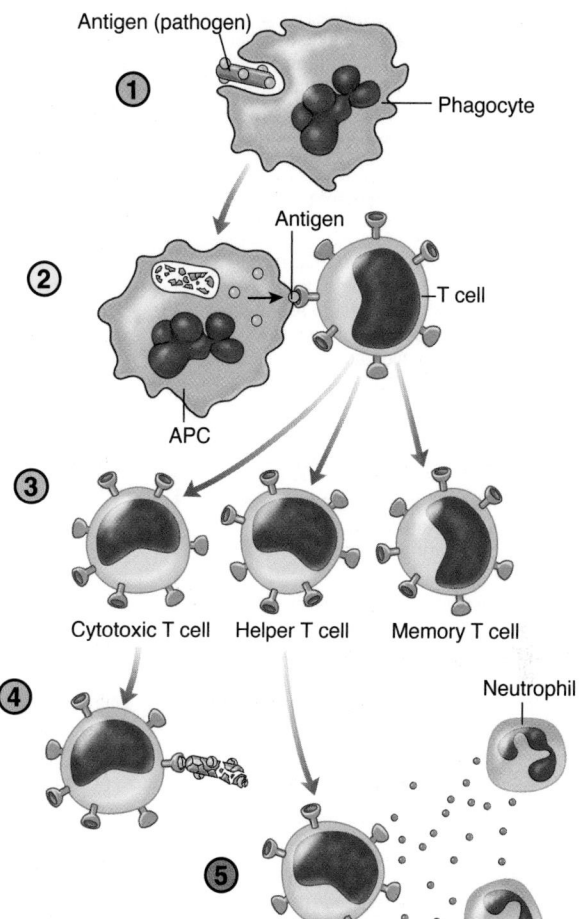

FIGURE 18.3 Cellular immunity.

in response. It is characterized by loss of plasma from capillaries (an effect of histamine) and a sudden drop in the intravascular blood volume and blood pressure.

TYPES OF IMMUNITY

Two categories of immunity are passive immunity and active immunity. In **passive immunity,** antibodies are not produced by the person but are obtained from another source. One form of *naturally* acquired passive immunity includes placental transmission of antibodies from mother to fetus and transmission of antibodies in breast milk. *Artificially* acquired passive immunity involves injection of preformed antibodies; this may help prevent disease after exposure to a pathogen such as the hepatitis B virus. Passive immunity is always temporary, in that antibodies from another source eventually break down.

   Active immunity means that the person produces his or her own antibodies. An example of *naturally* acquired active immunity occurs when a person recovers from an infection and then has antibodies and memory cells specific for that pathogen. *Artificially* acquired active immunity occurs as the result of a vaccine that stimulates production of antibodies and memory cells. The duration of active immunity depends on the particular disease or vaccine; some confer lifelong immunity, but others do not.

Aging and the Immune System

The efficiency of the immune system decreases with age (Fig. 18.6). As such, older adults are more susceptible to infections and autoimmune disorders ("Gerontological Issues"). The incidence of cancer is also higher; malignant cells that might once have been quickly destroyed by the immune system live and proliferate. The objective of Healthy People 2020 to reduce new invasive pneumococcal infections among adults over 64 has shown a decline from 40.7 cases per 100,000 people to 30.5 cases (Office of Disease Prevention and Health Promotion, 2017a). This is below the target of 31 cases. Another goal of Healthy People 2020 is to reduce invasive antibiotic-resistant pneumococcal infections among adults over 64 (Office of Disease Prevention and Health Promotion, 2017a). The target is 9.0. This has not been achieved yet, although there has been a decrease in cases from 12.2 to 10.2.

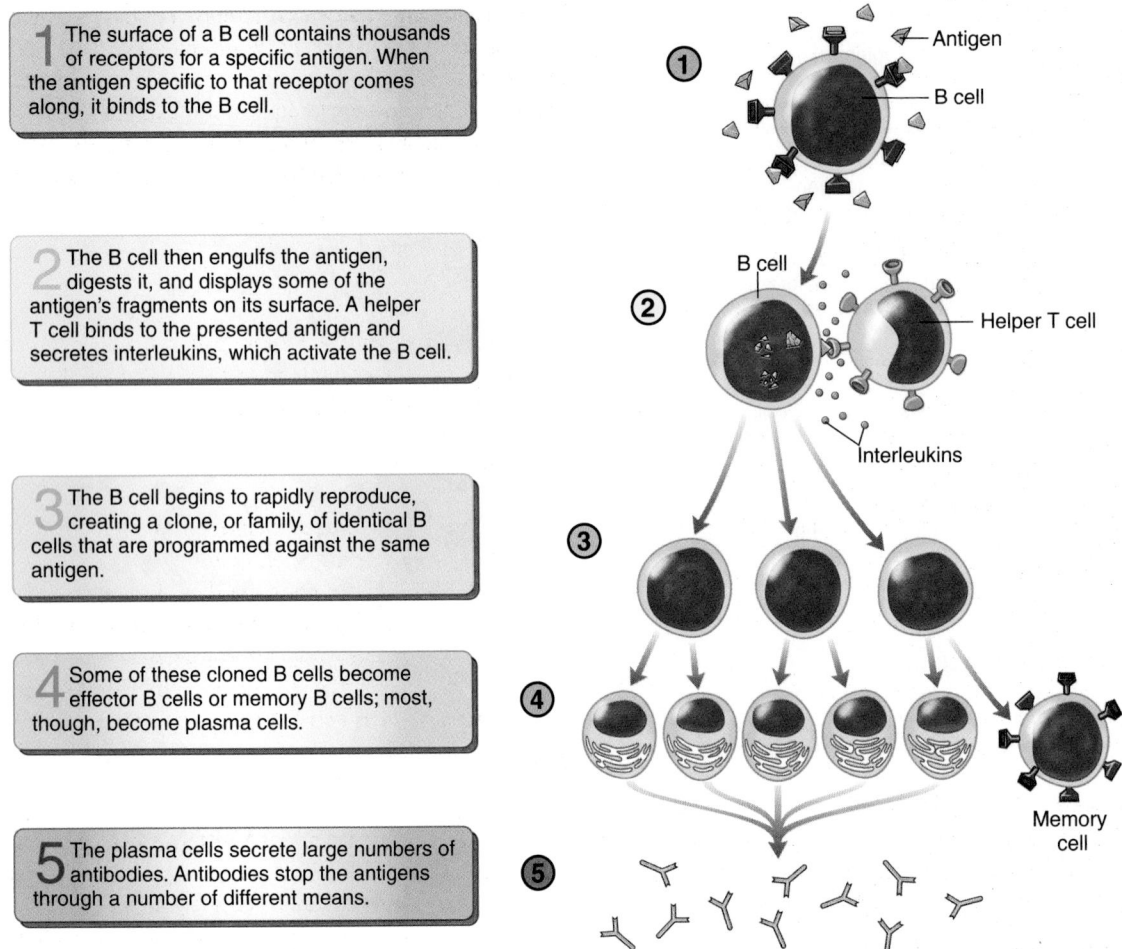

1 The surface of a B cell contains thousands of receptors for a specific antigen. When the antigen specific to that receptor comes along, it binds to the B cell.

2 The B cell then engulfs the antigen, digests it, and displays some of the antigen's fragments on its surface. A helper T cell binds to the presented antigen and secretes interleukins, which activate the B cell.

3 The B cell begins to rapidly reproduce, creating a clone, or family, of identical B cells that are programmed against the same antigen.

4 Some of these cloned B cells become effector B cells or memory B cells; most, though, become plasma cells.

5 The plasma cells secrete large numbers of antibodies. Antibodies stop the antigens through a number of different means.

FIGURE 18.4 Humoral immunity.

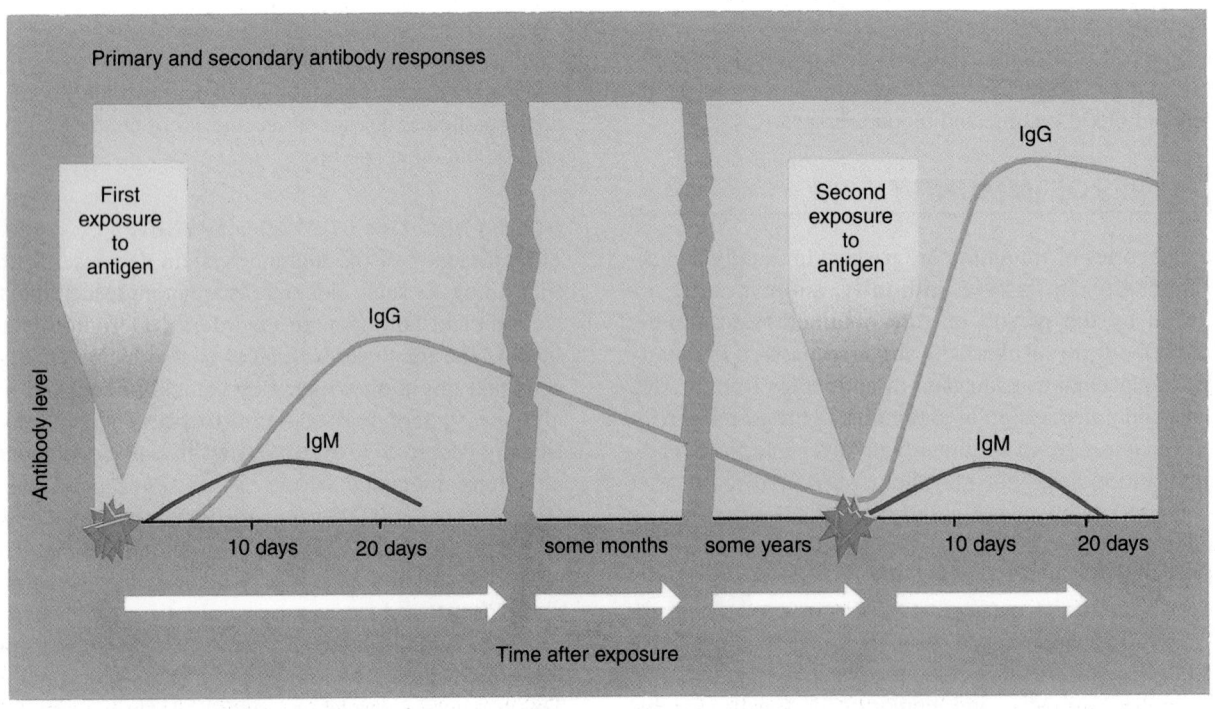

Primary and secondary antibody responses

First exposure to antigen

Second exposure to antigen

IgG

IgM

IgG

IgM

Antibody level

10 days   20 days   some months   some years   10 days   20 days

Time after exposure

FIGURE 18.5 Antibody responses to a first and then subsequent exposure to a pathogen.

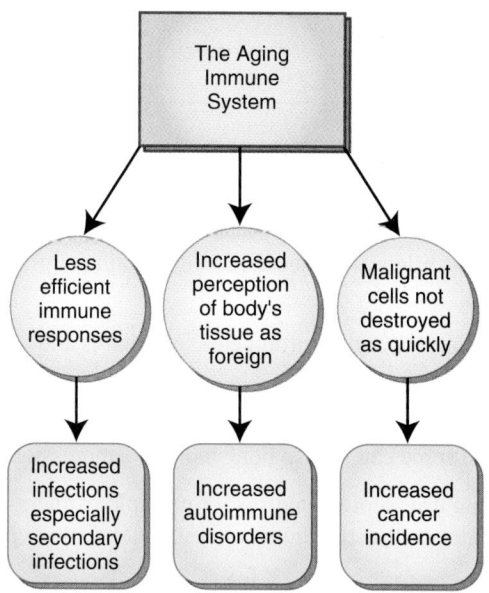

FIGURE 18.6 This concept map shows the effects the aging process has on the immune system.

Gerontological Issues

Immune System. Significant changes occur in the immune system of the older adult. These changes are known as *immune senescence,* which refers to a decline in immune system function. Some specific changes include the following:

- Thymus gland decreases in size, increases production of immature T cells, and has a subsequent decline in response to antigens.
- Age-appropriate immunizations for the older adult:
  - Herpes zoster (shingles) vaccine at age 50 or older (Shingrix, CDC recommended) or 60 or older (Zostavax)
  - Influenza vaccine (plus H1N1 flu vaccine if recommended) yearly, mid-October to mid-November, before influenza season
  - 13-valent pneumococcal conjugate vaccine (PCV13), then 23-valent pneumococcal polysaccharide vaccine (PPSV23) at least 1 year after PCV13
  - Tetanus and diphtheria booster every 10 years

  See Centers for Disease Control and Prevention immunization schedules at www.cdc.gov/vaccines/schedules/hcp/imz/adult.html.

Microbiota and the Immune System

Ongoing research suggests that microbes are essential for our immune system to work correctly. Microbiota is a collection or community of microbes that live in or on the body. The term *microbiome* refers to the genes within the microbes of the microbiota. Microbes affect metabolic pathways that provide the body nutrients. Some microbes can cause disease with their overgrowth, but most microbes are essential for

health. Lack of diversity and disruption of the microbiota are being studied as possible contributing factors in the development of some diseases (e.g., anorexia nervosa, cardiovascular disease, depression, irritable bowel syndrome, and immune disorders such as lupus and rheumatoid arthritis). Research findings may lead to new treatments for these diseases.

 ## NURSING DATA COLLECTION OF THE IMMUNE SYSTEM

Disorders of the immune system can affect every system in the body, so it is important to collect head-to-toe data as well as a patient history (Table 18.2).

Subjective Data
Demographic Data
Some diseases tend to be associated with a certain gender or ethnicity. For instance, systemic lupus erythematosus (SLE; see Chapter 19), an autoimmune disorder, occurs 10 times more often in women than in men and affects four times as many black women as white women (Paz, 2017). In addition, Hispanic, Native American, Asian, and African American women develop SLE two to three times more often than do Caucasian women.

Health History
Data are collected regarding the patient's health history and current health condition using the *WHAT'S UP?* format (see Chapter 1). A family history is also obtained. Many atopic (allergic) disorders, such as allergic rhinitis and asthma (see Chapter 31), and autoimmune disorders, such as ankylosing spondylitis (see Chapter 19), are thought either to be familial or to have a genetic predisposition in certain ethnic or cultural groups ("Cultural Considerations"). For example, four genes have been identified that are strongly associated with SLE and 10 others identified as risk factors. It is suggested that different genes may affect how the disease presents in individual patients. As an example, certain genetic mutations have been associated with lupus nephritis.

Cultural Considerations

The Navajo people have a high incidence of severe combined immune deficiency syndrome (SCIDS), an immunodeficiency syndrome unrelated to AIDS. SCIDS is a failure of the antibody response and cell-mediated immunity. Infants who survive are initially sent to tertiary care facilities. They must receive immunoglobulin on a regular basis until a bone marrow transplant can be performed. Thus far, studies indicate that SCIDS is unique to the Navajo population.

Ask about allergies. If the patient indicates a latex allergy, ask whether he or she has a latex service dog. Anaphylactic reactions can be caused by exposure to latex. Latex may be found in gloves and other medical products. Be aware of this

Table 18.2

Subjective Data Collection for the Immune System

Questions to Ask During the Health History	Rationale/Significance
Demographic Data	
Where were you born?	Determines ethnic and cultural background influences.
What is your ethnic or cultural background?	Some immune disorders are associated with certain cultural/ethnic groups.
Where have and do you currently live?	Shows ethnic, cultural, and environmental exposures and influences.
What is your occupation? Have you been exposed to hazardous chemicals, fumes, or radiation?	Chemicals can produce local reactions (skin) or systemic immune reactions, and some can lead to bone marrow suppression.
What risky behaviors do you engage in?	Intravenous drug use, unprotected sex, or multiple partners increase risk for contracting human immunodeficiency virus.
Allergies	
Do you have allergies to medications? Latex? Foods? Stinging insects? Environmental allergens? If yes, have you had a recent exposure to any of these? Describe the reaction.	Medication side effects are often inaccurately considered to be allergies by patients, which requires education. Recent exposure may provide cause for current symptoms.
What allergies do immediate relatives have?	If immediate family members have allergies, the patient may also be predisposed to the reaction.
Medications, Herbs	
What prescription or over-the-counter medications or herbal preparations do you take?	Corticosteroids and immunosuppressants suppress immune responses; anti-infectives and antineoplastics depress the bone marrow and white blood cells.
Medical Conditions	
What conditions have you been diagnosed with?	May provide insight into patient's current condition or symptoms.
Surgeries	
What surgeries have you had?	If any immune organs have been removed, this may reduce immune function.
Coping	
What do you do to cope with stress?	Identifying patient coping behaviors allows incorporation of them into the plan of care.
Who or what are your support systems?	Support systems can buffer stress that affects immune function.

potentially life-threatening allergy and know your agency's latex allergy protocol.

A surgical history can give clues to a patient's health status. For example, with thymus gland removal (thymectomy), T-cell production may be altered. This affects the cell-mediated immune response. If the spleen is removed (splenectomy), lymphocyte and plasma cell production may be altered. This affects the humoral immune response.

Objective Data

Physical data collection begins by observing the patient's general appearance, facial expression, hearing, vision, posture, gait, skin, and nailbeds. Rashes should be examined for size, shape, location, texture, drainage, and pruritus (itching). Additional objective data are collected (Table 18.3). Lymph nodes are not normally palpable by the health care provider (HCP; see Fig. 18.1). When they are enlarged, the following characteristics are noted: location, size, shape, tenderness, temperature, consistency, mobility, symmetry, pulsation, and whether red streaks, redness, or edema are present. The spleen if enlarged may be palpable by the HCP in the left upper quadrant of the abdomen. Enlargement occurs when there is an overproduction or excessive destruction of red blood cells.

Table 18.3

Objective Data Collection for the Immune System

Category	Normal Physical Examination Findings	Possible Abnormal Findings/Causes
Heart Sounds	Clear S_1 and S_2	Pericardial friction rub may be heard with rheumatoid arthritis or systemic lupus erythematosus (SLE) because of inflammation of the connective tissue surrounding the heart (pericardium).
Lung Sounds	Clear lung fields	Crackles with a dry cough may be indicative of *Pneumocystis jiroveci* pneumonia. Pleural effusion with tachypnea and diminished sounds in lungs can be seen in SLE or rheumatoid arthritis; pleural friction rub can occur. Wheezing may indicate an allergic response.
Lymph Nodes	Nonpalpable by health care provider and nontender	Painful, enlarged lymph nodes are associated with inflammation and infection. Enlarged lymph nodes that are painless, firm, and fixed are associated with cancerous lesions.
Gastrointestinal	Appropriate appetite No nausea or vomiting Regular pattern of brown, soft, formed stools	Anorexia, nausea, and vomiting may be associated with immune disorders. Diarrhea or diarrhea alternating with constipation is common with irritable bowel syndrome.
Musculoskeletal	Painless and nonswollen joints with full range of motion Overall strength, endurance, and coordination appropriate for age and physical fitness.	Swollen, painful joints and limited joint range of motion occur in rheumatoid arthritis. Decreased strength and coordination occur with multiple sclerosis. Strength and endurance lost during repetitive movements occur in myasthenia gravis.
Neurologic	Alert and oriented to person, place, time and environment. No muscle weakness or lack of coordination.	Confusion or lethargy are common in later stages of SLE and AIDS. Multiple sclerosis or myasthenia gravis can cause muscle weakness and coordination abnormalities.
Renal	An average of 30 mL per hour of clear, yellow/amber urine without presence of protein or pain.	Urine output of less than 30 mL/hour, the presence of protein in urine, and edema occur with SLE or serum sickness. Transfusion reactions can cause hematuria, flank pain, or oliguria. Glomerulonephritis may cause hematuria, flank pain, or oliguria.
Skin	Warm, dry, smooth, supple, even coloring, nonpruritic. Pink mucous membranes. Nail attached to nailbed.	Rash, erythema (redness), urticaria, pruritus, and pustules with many forms occur with allergic reactions. "Butterfly rash" (red rash over bridge of nose and cheek bones) occurs in less than 50% of patients with SLE. Onycholysis (nail detaches from nailbed) occurs with Hashimoto thyroiditis. Painless purple lesions occur with Kaposi sarcoma and are associated with HIV and AIDS. Pale edematous mucous membranes along with rhinorrhea and "allergic shiners" (dark circles under the eyes) occur with allergic rhinitis. Pale conjunctiva is associated with anemia. Periorbital edema can indicate hypothyroidism.

LEARNING TIP

A normally functioning immune system is required to trigger an inflammatory response and production of the signs of inflammation or infection (e.g., fever, redness, pain, swelling, and warmth). If the immune system is suppressed or functioning abnormally, this normal inflammatory response may not occur. Thus, the patient may have only a low-grade fever with none of the other signs of inflammation or infection.

Recognize patients who have suppressed immune systems so that low-grade fevers are reported to the health care provider for prompt treatment. This may be the only sign of a life-threatening infection that develops.

CRITICAL THINKING

Mrs. Sims is scheduled for a lymph node biopsy and is seen in preadmission testing before surgery. As the nurse prepares to draw blood specimens, he learns that Mrs. Sims is allergic to latex.

1. How can the nurse promote patient-centered care during this lab draw?
2. Why is this patient allergy information important?
3. What actions should the nurse take after learning of the allergy?
4. What precautions should the nurse use for drawing the blood specimen?

   Suggested answers are at the end of the chapter.

DIAGNOSTIC TESTS FOR THE IMMUNE SYSTEM

Table 18.4 describes the most common blood tests for patients with allergic, autoimmune, or immune disorders. Table 18.5 presents common noninvasive and invasive procedures for immune disorders. Chest x-ray, magnetic resonance imaging (MRI), and computed tomography (CT) scans might also be used.

Gene Testing

With human genome mapping data, scientists can test for numerous diseases, predisposition to diseases, and enzyme deficiencies that can alter immune response.

THERAPEUTIC MEASURES FOR THE IMMUNE SYSTEM

Allergies

For patients with allergies, medical identification jewelry or other readily available identification is essential. Allergies must always be verified before giving any medications or foods. All allergies must be taken very seriously.

Food allergies create serious management problems. A food allergen can be contained within other food such as baked goods. Food can be contaminated with an allergen from a previous batch of food made with the same equipment. Food allergies have become the most common cause

Table 18.4

Diagnostic Laboratory Tests for the Immune System

Test/Definition	Normal Value	Significance of Abnormal Findings
Red Blood Cell (RBC) Count—Number of RBCs per 1 mm of blood.	Adult male: $4.21–5.81 \times 10^6$ cells/microL Adult female: $3.61–5.11 \times 10^6$ cells/microL	Decreased in all forms of anemia, such as pernicious anemia that develops from the autoimmune form of gastritis or idiopathic autoimmune hemolytic anemia.
Differential—Each of these tests (MCV, MCH, MCHC, RDW) provides information about RBC size, shape, color, and intracellular structure.	See below.	Can help determine the cause of anemia. Pernicious anemia can develop because of the autoimmune form of gastritis.
• MCV	Adult male: 77–97 fL Adult female: 78–98 fL Older adult male: 79–103 fL Older adult female: 78–102 fL	

Table 18.4

Diagnostic Laboratory Tests for the Immune System—cont'd

Test/Definition	Normal Value	Significance of Abnormal Findings
• MCH	*Adult:* 26–34 pg/cell *Older Adult:* 27–35 pg/cell	
• MCHC	32–36 g/dL	
• RDWCV	11.6–14.8	
• RDWSD	38–48	
White Blood Cell (WBC) Count—Number of WBCs per 1 mm of blood.	*Adult:* 4.5–11.1 × 10^3/microL^3	Increased with immunosuppression and infection.
Differential—Percentage of each type of WBCs in 100 cell count. Absolute count is the actual number of specific types of WBCs present.	See below.	Eosinophils elevate with type I hypersensitivity reactions such as allergic rhinitis or anaphylaxis.

	%	**Absolute/microL^3**	
• Neutrophils	40–75	2.7–6.5	
• Lymphocytes	12–44	1.5–3.7	
• Monocytes	4–9	0.2–0.4	
• Eosinophils	0–5.5	0.05–0.5	
• Basophils	0–1	0–0.1	

Test/Definition	Normal Value	Significance of Abnormal Findings

Erythrocyte Sedimentation Rate (ESR)—A nonspecific test for generalized inflammation. Measures the RBC descent (in millimeters) in test tube after being in normal saline solution for 1 hour (Westergren method).	*Male under 50:*
	  0–15 mm/hr
	Female under 50:
	  0–25 mm/hr
	Male 50 and over:
	  0–20 mm/hr
	Female 50 and over:
	  0–30 mm/hr
		False negative may result if steroids or NSAIDs are taken when test is performed.

Rheumatoid Factor (RF)—An abnormal protein found in serum when IgM reacts with an abnormal IgG; ound in 80% of patients with rheumatoid arthritis and other autoimmune disorders.	Less than 14 IU/mL
	  (60 years and older
	  may be elevated)
		Increased in rheumatoid arthritis, SLE, leukemia, tuberculosis, older age, scleroderma, and infectious mononucleosis.

Antinuclear Antibody (ANA)/ Anti-ds DNA (ANA subset)—Measures autoantibodies that attack the cell's nucleus.	*Negative:* Less than 5 IU *Indeterminate:* 5–9 IU *Positive:* 9 IU	Presence strongly associated with SLE. Also indicates leukemia, scleroderma, rheumatoid arthritis, and myasthenia gravis; many medications influence levels.

Continued

Table 18.4

Diagnostic Laboratory Tests for the Immune System—cont'd

Test/Definition	Normal Value	Significance of Abnormal Findings
Complement—Specific serum proteins that help mediate inflammation. Measures the amount of each of the components in the complement system.	See below.	Deficiencies of specific complement proteins are seen in SLE.
• Total	25–110 CH_{50} units/mL	
• C3	83–177 mg/dL	
• C4	12–36 mg/dL	
C-Reactive Protein (CRP)—An abnormal protein found in plasma during acute inflammatory processes; more sensitive than sedimentation rate.	Less than 10 mg/L	Increased in rheumatoid arthritis, cancer, and SLE. Suppressed by aspirin and steroids.
Antigen/Antibody Combination Immunoassay—Detects both HIV-1 and HIV-2 antibodies and HIV-1 p24 antigen.	Negative	Shows established infection with HIV-1 or HIV-2 and acute infection for HIV-1. If positive, antibody immunoassay test is done to differentiate between HIV-1 and HIV-2 antibodies.
Antibody Differentiation Immunoassay—Differentiates between HIV-1 and HIV-2 antibodies.	Negative	Identifies infection with HIV-1 or HIV-2.
Nucleic Acid Test—Confirmation test for HIV-1 if antigen/antibody combination immunoassay is positive but antibody differentiation immunoassay is nonreactive or inconclusive.		Positive HIV-1 indicates acute HIV-1 infection.
Immunoglobulin Assay or Electrophoresis—Antibodies are made up of immunoglobulins, of which there are five different classes.	See below.	See below.
• IgG	650–1600 (mg/dL)	Increased in all types of infections, liver disease, rheumatoid arthritis, and dermatological disorders. Decreased in agammaglobulinemia, lymphoid aplasia, and Bence-Jones proteinuria.
• IgM	50–300 (mg/dL)	Increased in malaria, infectious mononucleosis, SLE, and rheumatoid arthritis. Decreased in lymphoid aplasia and chronic lymphoblastic leukemia.

Table 18.4

Diagnostic Laboratory Tests for the Immune System—cont'd

Test/Definition	Normal Value	Significance of Abnormal Findings
• IgA	40–350 (mg/dL)	Increased during exercise and obstructive jaundice. Decreased in familial inheritance, immunosuppressive therapy, and benzene exposure.
• IgE	Less than 100 units/L	Increased in allergic reactions and allergic infections.
• IgD	Less than 15 (mg/dL)	Decreased in agammaglobulinemia.
Radioallergosorbent Test (RAST)—Patient serum is mixed with a specific allergen, incubated with radiolabeled anti-IgE antibodies, and then the total amount of the specific IgE antibodies is measured.		A viable alternative to skin testing if the patient does not have multiple allergies.
CD4 Count—CD4 - Helper T lymphocytes are counted.	*Percentage:* 28%–51% *Count:* 332–1642 cells/ microL	Increased in allergy-proven patients. Decreased in patient with cancer, AIDS, and immunosuppression. Guides antiretroviral therapy.
CD8 Count—CD8-Suppressor T lymphocytes are counted.	*Percentage:* 12%–38% *Count:* 170–811 cells/ microL	Increased in viral infections. Decreased in SLE.

AIDS = acquired immune deficiency syndrome; HIV = human immunodeficiency virus; Ig = immunoglobulin; IU = international units; MCH = mean corpuscular hemoglobin; MCHC = mean corpuscular hemoglobin concentration; MCV = mean corpuscular volume; NSAIDs = nonsteroidal anti-inflammatory drugs; RDW = red blood cell distribution width; SLE = systemic lupus erythematosus.

Table 18.5

Diagnostic Procedures for the Immune System

Procedure	Definition/Normal Finding (if applicable)	Significance of Abnormal Findings	Nursing Management (if applicable)
Noninvasive *Gene Testing*	A sample of deoxyribonucleic acid (DNA), which can be taken as an oral or nasal swab, is examined and mapped for a variety of genetic disorders.	Abnormal findings may confirm a diagnosis or indicate patient may develop symptoms or pass on a disorder to children.	Identify patient support systems and need for counseling referral.
Invasive *Biopsy (of a Specific Organ)*	Biopsy tissue examined microscopically to confirm a diagnosis, determine a prognosis, or evaluate treatment. Specimen obtained through needle aspiration, incision, excision, or gavage, with or without endoscopy, fluoroscopy, stereotaxic, or needle localization.	Cancers, lymphomas, leukemias, and transplant rejections.	Ensure informed consent has been obtained. Monitor vital signs and site for bleeding as organs are very vascular with a higher risk for bleeding after the biopsy.

Continued

Table 18.5

Diagnostic Procedures for the Immune System—cont'd

Procedure	Definition/Normal Finding (if applicable)	Significance of Abnormal Findings	Nursing Management (if applicable)
Skin Testing	Done if immune system is intact. Testing is done for *Candida,* tetanus, tuberculosis (purified protein derivative [PPD] test), or specific allergens such as medications, food, or environmental factors.	If erythema (redness) or induration (firmness) occurs at the site within a prescribed time frame, test is positive. Indicates patient has been exposed to an organism, has an active infection, or has developed antibodies that stimulate an immune response.	Ask if patients have any allergies and the type of reaction or symptoms that occur.

of anaphylaxis in the community setting. Death from anaphylactic shock can result ("Nutrition Notes"). Occasionally, a food allergen may enter the body by inhalation or contact with skin or mucous membranes rather than eating.

Treatment for allergen exposure includes antihistamines, such as diphenhydramine (Benadryl), and an epinephrine auto-injector (Adrenaclick, AUVI-Q, EpiPen). An epinephrine auto-injector must always be carried when exposure to known allergens is possible. It must be checked routinely for discoloration or cloudiness and a past-due expiration date, all of which require replacement. The patient should also be instructed to obtain emergency medical care immediately after using the epinephrine auto-injector because the effect is brief (less than 15 minutes) and relapse can occur (Mustafa, 2017).

Nutrition Notes

Food Allergies. The Academy of Nutrition and Dietetics (2017) reports that more than 170 foods cause allergic reactions. The Food Allergen Labeling and Consumer Protection Act of 2004 requires food labeling for the eight foods that are responsible for 90% of all food allergies: eggs, milk, fish, peanuts, tree nuts, crustacean shellfish, wheat, and soybeans (U.S. Food and Drug Administration, 2017). If a food allergy is suspected, an in-depth medical history and physical examination should be conducted, along with other testing (e.g., skin testing).

Peanut allergies are estimated to affect 1% to 2% of children. To reduce allergies in adulthood, new guidelines for peanut consumption are based on studies in which infants either were exposed to or avoided peanut-containing food until age 5 (Togias et al., 2017). Infants who had a negative skin prick test at the start of the study had an 86% risk reduction for peanut allergy when peanut-containing food was introduced early. Those

with a positive skin prick test had a 70% risk reduction at age 5 for peanut allergy when peanut-containing food was introduced early.

Maternal diet should not be restricted during pregnancy or breastfeeding as an attempt at preventing the development of food allergies in infants. Infants should be fed peanut-containing foods after successful feeding of other foods at age 4 to 6 months per guidelines based on allergy risk to decrease peanut allergy development (Sicherer, 2017).

References

Academy of Nutrition and Dietetics. (2017). Food allergies and intolerances. Retrieved from www.eatright.org/resource/health/allergies-and-intolerances/food-allergies/food-allergies-and-intolerances

Sicherer, S. H. (2017, January 5). New guidelines detail use of "infant-safe" peanut to prevent allergy. *AAP News.* Retrieved from www.aappublications.org/news/2017/01/05/PeanutAllergy010517

Togias, A., Cooper, S. F., Acebal, M. L., Assa'ad, A., Baker, J. R., Jr., Beck, L. A., … Boyce, J. A. (2017.) Addendum guidelines for the prevention of peanut allergy in the United States: Report of the National Institute of Allergy and Infectious Diseases–sponsored expert panel. *Annals of Allergy, Asthma & Immunology, 118*(2), 166–173.

U.S. Food and Drug Administration. (2017). Food allergies: What you need to know. Retrieved www.fda.gov/Food/ResourcesForYou/Consumers/ucm079311.htm

Immunotherapy

Allergen immunotherapy, such as subcutaneous immunotherapy (SCIT) and sublingual immunotherapy (SLIT), aims to desensitize a patient with anaphylactic reactions or chronic allergic symptoms. SCIT involves preparing an extract of the allergen and injecting small amounts of it as a vaccine. The concentration of the allergen in the vaccine is increased over time until the desired hyposensitivity is reached. Anaphylactic reactions can occur during treatment. The HCP and emergency equipment should be readily available if a reaction occurs. The patient and family should be taught how to respond if a reaction occurs after discharge.

SLIT is the use of tablets or drops containing specific allergen extracts. These are placed under the tongue and swallowed. Studies have shown SLIT to be effective in dust mite allergy–related asthma as well as in demonstrating long-lasting symptom control for certain allergens. SLIT has significantly lower anaphylactic event occurrence when compared with SCIT.

Medications

Medications are one of the primary treatment options for immune disorders. General medication categories used include antibiotics, antihistamines, antivirals, corticosteroids, decongestants, epinephrine, histamine (H_2) blockers, hormone therapy, immunosuppressants, interferon, leukotriene antagonists, and mast cell stabilizers (see Chapter 19).

Surgical Management

In some cases, splenectomy is needed to control symptoms of an immune disorder. A significant side effect of this surgery is the reduced ability of the immune system to fight infections.

Monoclonal Antibodies

Monoclonal antibodies can be produced against a variety of antigens. A monoclonal antibody is made by cloning one specific antibody and then growing unlimited amounts of it in tissue cultures. Many uses are being found for these antibodies, such as in dealing with transplant rejections.

Recombinant DNA Technology

Recombinant deoxyribonucleic acid (DNA) technology combines genes from one organism with genes from another. This therapy is used to replace an abnormal or missing gene with the goal of producing a normal gene. The normal gene can then be injected into a patient to cure a disorder if the patient's body then reproduces the normal genes. T-lymphocyte-directed gene transfer and injection of stem cells into abnormal areas to produce normal cells have been performed successfully. For more information, visit www.nhgri.nih.gov or www.ncbi.nlm.nih.gov/guide.

SUGGESTED ANSWERS TO CRITICAL THINKING

Mrs. Sims

1. Review the patient's history and allergies to prevent complications. Explain the procedure, and allow the patient to ask questions or verbalize concerns.
2. The patient may have an anaphylactic reaction if exposed to latex, which can result in death for some patients.
3. The nurse should follow the agency's latex allergy protocol, enter this data into the patient's medical record,

notify surgery scheduling so latex precaution protocols can be planned for surgery, and ensure that the patient's health care provider is informed.
4. Following the agency's protocol, the nurse should wear nonlatex gloves and use nonlatex equipment to draw the specimens.

Review Questions

1. The nurse teaches a patient about vaccines. The nurse would evaluate the patient as understanding the presented information if the patient states that a vaccine provides which of these types of immunity?
   1. Naturally acquired passive immunity
   2. Artificially acquired passive immunity
   3. Naturally acquired active immunity
   4. Artificially acquired active immunity

2. Which of the following vaccines would the nurse correctly recommend be given annually during a teaching session on health maintenance with an older patient?
   1. Diphtheria tetanus
   2. Influenza
   3. Pneumococcal vaccine
   4. Polio

3. The nurse is assisting with data collection on a patient. Which of the following past surgeries found in the patient's history would alert the nurse to possible immune system dysfunction when planning care?
   Select all that apply.
   1. Appendectomy
   2. Parathyroidectomy
   3. Pneumonectomy
   4. Splenectomy
   5. Thyroidectomy
   6. Thymectomy

4. During data collection, the patient reports tenderness in the cervical lymph nodes. The nurse recognizes that enlarged and tender lymph nodes usually indicate which of the following problems?
   1. Arthritis
   2. Cancer
   3. Degeneration
   4. Infection

5. The nurse is caring for a patient who is suspected to be infected with HIV. The patient asks what type of test will be done first to diagnose it. Which response by the nurse would be appropriate?
   1. Antibody differentiation immunoassay
   2. Antigen/antibody combination immunoassay
   3. Lymphocyte count
   4. Nucleic acid test

6. Clarithromycin (Biaxin) 200-mg oral suspension is ordered for a patient. The nurse has 125 mg/5 mL available. How many milliliters should the nurse give? Fill in the blank.

   Answer: _____ mL

   Answer rationales available in your online resources.

ANSWERS 1. 4; 2. 3; 3. 4; 6; 4. 4; 5. 2; 6. 8

Key Points

Find the chapter key points in your online resources available through Davis Edge.

Additional Resources

DAVIS **edge.** ◀ Use the scratch off code on the inside front cover of your book to access online quizzes that will help you to improve your scores on course exams and prepare for NCLEX-PN®.

 Study Guide

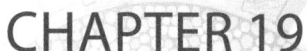

CHAPTER 19
Nursing Care of Patients With Immune Disorders

Kristy Gorman, Sharon M. Nowak

KEY TERMS

anaphylaxis (AN-uh-fih-LAK-sis)
angioedema (AN-gee-oh-eh-DEE-mah)
ankylosing spondylitis (ANG-kih-LOH-sing
   SPON-da-LY-tis)
histamine (HISS-tah-mean)
urticaria (UR-tih-CARE-ee-ah)

CHAPTER CONCEPTS

Immunity

LEARNING OUTCOMES

1. Explain the immunological mechanism for the four types of hypersensitivities.
2. Explain the pathophysiology of disorders of the immune system.
3. Identify the etiologies, signs, and symptoms of immune system disorders.
4. Plan nursing care for patients undergoing tests for immune system disorders.
5. Describe current medical treatment for immune system disorders.
6. List data collected when caring for patients with disorders of the immune system.
7. Explain factors that alter or influence the self-recognition portion of the immune system.
8. Plan nursing care for patients with disorders of the immune system.
9. Evaluate effectiveness of nursing interventions for disorders of the immune system.

Disorders of the immune system can be divided into three categories: hypersensitivity reactions (e.g., anaphylaxis), autoimmune disorders (e.g., systemic lupus erythematosus), and immune deficiencies (e.g., AIDS; see Chapter 20).

 HYPERSENSITIVITY REACTIONS

The immune system is an adaptive system that protects the body. However, sometimes this system can cause injury to the body because of its exaggerated response. One of these occasions is when a hypersensitivity reaction occurs. In 1963, Gell and Coombs developed a system of classifying hypersensitivity reactions as types I, II, III, and IV, according to the way the tissue is injured.

Type I Hypersensitivity Reactions
Type I hypersensitivity reactions involve the release of **histamine** and other mediators from mast cells and basophils. The reaction may lead to urticaria, eczema, angioedema,

conjunctivitis, allergic rhinitis, asthma, gastroenteritis, and anaphylaxis. Symptoms may range from mild to severe and life threatening. An anaphylactic reaction is an immediate reaction that occurs on exposure to a specific antigen (Fig. 19.1). The patient must have had previous exposure (sensitization) to the antigen. During this exposure, the immune system overreacts to the antigen and makes immunoglobulin E (IgE) antibodies that attach to mast cells throughout the body. When a subsequent exposure occurs, the antigen causes IgE to trigger mast cells to release their contents. When histamine is released, vasodilatation, bronchoconstriction, mucus secretion, and vascular permeability occur. If the exposure is localized, the reaction is mild and remains local. However, if the exposure is systemic, the reaction is massive and widespread.

Allergic Rhinitis
Allergic rhinitis is the most common form of allergy. When symptoms occur throughout the year, it is called perennial

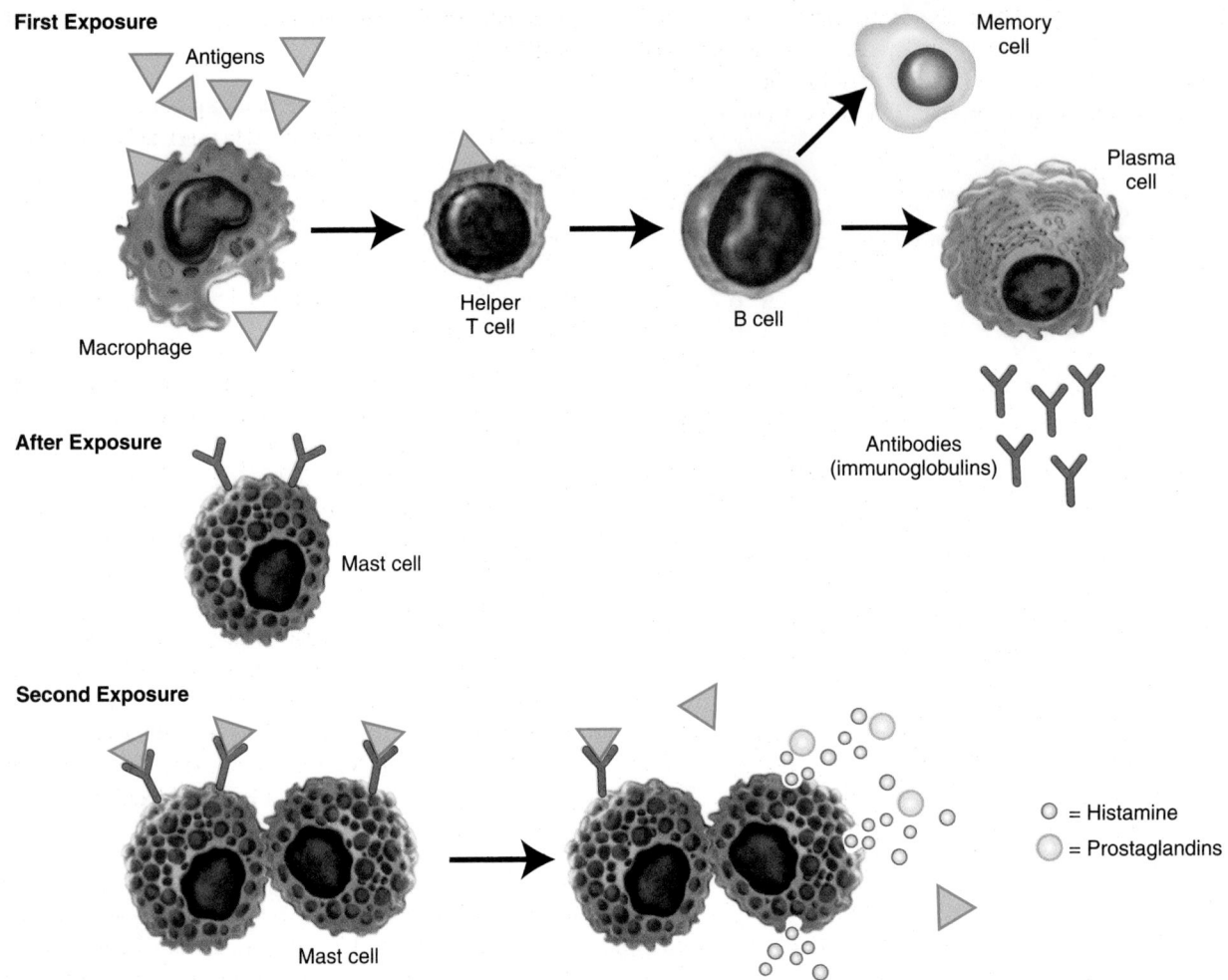

FIGURE 19.1 Type I hypersensitivity.

allergic rhinitis. If the symptoms occur seasonally, it is called hay fever. The causative antigens are environmental and airborne.

PATHOPHYSIOLOGY. Allergic rhinitis is the result of an antigen–antibody reaction. Ciliary action decreases and mucous secretions increase. Vasodilation and local tissue edema occur.

SIGNS AND SYMPTOMS. Signs and symptoms vary in intensity. They include sneezing, nasal itching, profuse watery rhinorrhea (runny nose), and itchy red eyes. The nasal mucosa is pale, cyanotic, and edematous. Frequently there are dark circles under the eyes, called allergic shiners, caused by venous congestion in the maxillary sinuses.

COMPLICATIONS. Sinusitis, nasal polyps, asthma, and chronic bronchitis can occur with repeated episodes of allergic rhinitis.

DIAGNOSTIC TESTS. Skin testing may be performed to identify the specific offending allergens to allow avoidance of the allergen. However, skin testing does not always identify the allergen. Testing also has limited usefulness for allergens that cannot be easily avoided once identified. The in-vitro allergy test, or radioallergosorbent test (RAST), can be a beneficial alternative to skin testing for some patients.

THERAPEUTIC MEASURES. Initial treatment involves eliminating the offending environmental stimuli. Antihistamines and nasal decongestants may be prescribed to relieve symptoms. If the symptoms are severe, corticosteroids may also be given via inhalation or nasal spray. Nasal corticosteroids should be used cautiously in the older adult because these medications can be drying to the nares. Intranasal saline irrigation can be an inexpensive and effective way to reduce nasal congestion.

Rhinophototherapy uses light waves to reduce the hyperimmune response seen in this disorder. The treatment is usually done three times a week for 3 weeks and relieves symptoms such as sneezing, itching, and runny nose.

Immunotherapy, known as allergy shots, is reserved for patients with severe or debilitating symptoms (see Chapter 18). This therapy continues until the patient no longer has symptoms when exposed to the environmental antigen.

Atopic Dermatitis (Eczema)

Atopic dermatitis, often called eczema, is a familial, chronic inflammatory skin response.

PATHOPHYSIOLOGY. Two theories exist regarding the pathophysiology of atopic dermatitis. One theory suggests the allergic response is mediated by IgE antibodies, because it is commonly found in patients with allergic rhinitis or allergic asthma. Another theory suggests atopic dermatitis is a defect in epithelial cells that damages the skin's protective barrier.

SIGNS AND SYMPTOMS. Initially, there is pruritus, edema, and extremely dry skin. This is followed by red, weeping lesions that break open, crust over, and scale off. The skin eventually thickens in the affected areas (lichenification).

DIAGNOSTIC TESTS. A diagnosis of atopic dermatitis is based on clinical examination and exclusion of other diseases with similar symptoms. Serum IgE levels will be elevated in patients with atopic dermatitis and tend to correlate with the severity of the disease. If an infection is present, culture and sensitivity tests may be ordered to determine the infecting organism and treatment.

THERAPEUTIC MEASURES. Treatment focuses on the symptoms of pruritus and dry and inflamed skin. Antipruritics are vital in reducing the itch–scratch cycle that predisposes the patient to lesion infections. Lukewarm soaks followed with application of emollients and oil-in-water lubricants tend to be the most effective for dryness (see "Home Health Hints" at the end of the chapter). Topical corticosteroids may be ordered for their anti-inflammatory properties. Topical calcineurin inhibitors such as tacrolimus and pimecrolimus also reduce the inflammatory response. They also relieve itching and rash when steroids are not effective. If skin lesions become infected, topical or systemic antibiotics are prescribed. Dilute bleach soaks may also be used twice a week to reduce severity of symptoms, especially those of infection. For long-term management of symptoms, it is important to identify and eliminate the triggers of the hypersensitivity, while controlling environmental temperature and humidity.

Anaphylaxis

Anaphylaxis is a severe systemic type I hypersensitivity reaction. Some causes of anaphylaxis are antibiotics such as cephalosporins, penicillin, and sulfonamides; anticonvulsants such as phenytoin (Dilantin); nonsteroidal anti-inflammatory drugs (NSAIDs) such as aspirin; foods such as eggs, nuts, shellfish, and wheat; latex; food additives such as monosodium glutamate (MSG) and bisulfites; and venom from insect bites or stings.

PATHOPHYSIOLOGY. IgE antibodies produced from previous antigen sensitization are attached to mast cells throughout the body. In this reaction, the antigen is introduced at a systemic level. This causes widespread release of histamine and other chemical mediators contained within the mast cells. The most profound complications of an anaphylactic reaction are respiratory and cardiac arrest. Immediate treatment is needed to prevent death.

SIGNS AND SYMPTOMS. Anaphylaxis produces sudden and life-threatening signs and symptoms (Table 19.1). Generalized smooth muscle spasms occur, causing bronchial narrowing and creating stridor, wheezing, dyspnea, and laryngeal edema, which can lead to respiratory arrest. Cramping, diarrhea, nausea, and vomiting also result from these spasms. Capillary permeability increases, allowing fluid to shift from the vessels to the interstitium. This causes hypotension, tachycardia, and an increase in respiratory symptoms. The blood volume in the vessels decreases while the blood vessels dilate, resulting in a further decrease in circulating blood volume. The dilation also causes diffuse erythema (redness) and warmth of the skin. Neurologic changes include apprehension, drowsiness, profound restlessness, headache, and possible seizures.

DIAGNOSTIC TESTS. The patient's history and signs and symptoms establish the diagnosis. Arterial blood gases may reveal hypoxemia, hypercarbia, and acidosis. Electrocardiogram (ECG) monitoring may show cardiac arrhythmias. After the patient's recovery, allergen testing may be considered for future prevention.

THERAPEUTIC MEASURES. Epinephrine is given IM. Intravenous (IV) access is a priority for administration of vasopressor drugs and fluids to increase blood pressure. Oxygen therapy is started. If respiratory symptoms are severe, a tracheostomy or endotracheal intubation may be needed, with mechanical ventilation. Antihistamines and corticosteroids may also be given.

Urticaria

PATHOPHYSIOLOGY AND ETIOLOGY. **Urticaria** (hives) is a type I hypersensitivity reaction. It is triggered by the antigen-stimulated reaction of IgE antibodies, which causes the release of mast cell contents, especially histamine. The causes of urticaria are numerous. In addition to various medicines and foods, chemicals, cold, local heat, pressure, and stress can also cause urticaria. Many patients with underlying chronic conditions, such as systemic lupus

• WORD • BUILDING •
anaphylaxis: ana—up + phylaxis—protection

Table 19.1

Anaphylaxis Summary

Signs and Symptoms	Generalized smooth-muscle spasms: • Bronchial narrowing, leading to stridor, wheezing, dyspnea, laryngeal edema • Abdominal cramping and diarrhea • Nausea and vomiting Increased capillary permeability (allowing fluid to shift from blood vessels to the interstitium): • Hypotension • Tachycardia • Increased respiratory symptoms Dilation of blood vessels: • Further decreasing circulating volume • Diffuse erythema (redness) • Increased skin temperature Apprehension Drowsiness Profound restlessness Headache Possible seizures
Diagnostic Tests	Testing to guide treatment: • Arterial blood gases • Electrocardiogram monitoring History and physical exam After recovery, allergen testing for prevention
Therapeutic Measures	Oxygen Intravenous (IV) access Epinephrine IM Vasopressor drugs IV (dopamine) Antihistamines (oral, IV, injection) Corticosteroids (oral, IV, injection) If severe respiratory compromise: • Tracheostomy or endotracheal intubation • Mechanical ventilation
Complications	Respiratory and cardiac arrest
Priority Nursing Diagnoses	*Impaired Gas Exchange* *Anxiety* *Ineffective Health Maintenance*

erythematosus, lymphoma, hyperthyroidism, or cancer, are susceptible to urticaria.

SIGNS AND SYMPTOMS. The lesions of urticaria are raised, pruritic, nontender, and erythematous wheals on the skin. They tend to be concentrated on the trunk and proximal extremities.

CRITICAL THINKING

Mrs. Barnes, a 32-year-old woman, was brought into the emergency department after having been stung multiple times by bees while gardening. She has numerous red welts over her body that she says are itchy. She is very anxious. Her temperature is 99.2°F (37.22°C), blood pressure is 102/58 mm Hg, pulse is 102 beats per minute, and respiratory rate is 26 breaths per minute.

1. What might be causing Mrs. Barnes's symptoms?
2. What additional information is needed?
3. What should the nurse do to help Mrs. Barnes?
4. With which members of the health team should the nurse anticipate collaborating?

Suggested answers are at the end of the chapter.

DIAGNOSTIC TESTS. Diagnosis is based on physical examination and history.

THERAPEUTIC MEASURES. Treatment depends on the degree of symptoms. In the most severe cases, epinephrine may be given to quickly resolve the urticaria. Corticosteroids may be given orally, topically, or via IV. Antihistamines and histamine (H_2) blockers may aid in resolution by blocking the release of histamine. Patients suffering with the chronic form of urticaria might require IgE monoclonal antibody therapy, such as with omalizumab (Xolair). Studies have found the use of acupuncture as an adjunctive measure may relieve symptoms (Yao, Li, Liu, Qin, & Liu, 2016).

Angioedema

PATHOPHYSIOLOGY AND ETIOLOGY. Angioedema is a result of vascular permeability that increases in the submucosal and subcutaneous layers. It may be acquired or hereditary. It may be caused by hypersensitivity (e.g., food, drugs, or insect stings), physical stimuli (e.g., cold), autoimmune disease or infection, angiotensin-converting enzyme (ACE) inhibitors, NSAIDs, or C1 esterase inhibitor (C1-INH) deficiency or dysfunction (hereditary and acquired). To learn more, visit the U.S. Hereditary Angioedema Association at www.haea.org.

SIGNS AND SYMPTOMS. Signs and symptoms include acute, localized swelling of the skin; mucosa; and submucosa due to vascular leakage. Depending on the location and extensiveness of the edema, angioedema eruptions are usually nonpruritic and painless. However, it can be life threatening if the upper airway is involved and obstruction of the airway develops. The eruptions usually last longer than with urticaria. They most commonly affect the face, eyes, and lips.

• WORD • BUILDING •

angioedema: angeion—vessel + oidema—swelling

DIAGNOSTIC TESTS. A comprehensive history and physical examination confirm the diagnosis. Skin testing may be performed to determine the specific antigen.

THERAPEUTIC MEASURES. The most basic treatment involves avoiding the antigen or allergen desensitization. Cinryze, a C1-INH, is for routine prophylaxis against angioedema attacks. Acute symptoms may be relieved with antihistamines, corticosteroids, or other medications. Berinert, also a C1-INH, treats angioedema of the abdomen, face, or throat. Haegarda is a human plasma-derived, concentrate prepared from donors. Ecallantide (Kalbitor), a plasma kallikrein inhibitor, and icatibant (Firazyr), a selective bradykinin B2 receptor antagonist, help control symptoms. Infusion of fresh frozen plasma reverses the angioedema symptoms associated with ACE inhibitor–induced angioedema, which tends to be resistant to standard treatments. Androgens, antifibrinolytics, and immunosuppressive therapy are useful in the long-term treatment of some acquired types of angioedema.

Nursing Process for the Patient With a Type I Hypersensitivity Disorder

DATA COLLECTION. Gather data about the patient's signs and symptoms. Immediately report any sudden dyspnea, shortness of breath, anxiety, restlessness, or chest or back pain. Identify any allergies the patient may have as well as signs and symptoms that occur with exposure to the allergen. Perform a thorough skin assessment, and carefully document any lesions or rashes. Note any changes in rashes or lesions or signs of infection, such as redness, warmth, and drainage. Identify the patient's knowledge of disease process, causes, treatment plan, and self-care.

NURSING DIAGNOSES, PLANNING, AND IMPLEMENTATION

Impaired Gas Exchange related to laryngeal edema

EXPECTED OUTCOME: The patient will maintain clear lung fields and remain free of signs of respiratory distress at all times.

- Monitor respiratory rate, depth, and effort, such as use of accessory muscles, nasal flaring, or abdominal breathing, *to identify problems early.*
- Monitor the patient for restlessness, changes in mentation, level of consciousness, changes in voice, or dysphagia *to identify problems and intervene early.*
- Position the patient in a high-Fowler or semi-Fowler position *to improve ventilation and decrease upper airway edema.*

Anxiety related to dyspnea or pruritus

EXPECTED OUTCOME: The patient will state that anxiety is controlled.

- Stay with the patient and speak calmly *to reduce fear or frustration.*

- Teach the patient to visualize the absence of anxiety, itching, or dyspnea *to decrease anxiety.*
- Teach the family to distinguish between anxiety or panic and a serious physiological problem *to make informed decisions regarding emergency medical care.*

Risk for Impaired Skin Integrity related to effects of allergic reaction

See "Nursing Care Plan for the Patient With Contact Dermatitis."

Ineffective Health Maintenance related to lack of knowledge to decrease inflammation and pruritus and reduce episodes of inflammation

EXPECTED OUTCOME: The patient or caregiver will state understanding and follow the mutually agreed-on plan of care.

- Identify the patient's knowledge of the disease and its causes *to provide a basis for teaching and evaluation.*
- Identify barriers to the patient's ability to carry out the plan of care, and plan interventions to decrease these barriers *to improve patient implementation of the plan of care.*
- Teach methods of avoiding the allergen, such as wearing a mask when mowing the lawn or working outdoors, having heating ducts cleaned, covering heat registers with filters, and frequent home vacuuming and dusting, *to promote an understanding of preventive methods and prevent allergen exposure and anaphylaxis.*
- Teach the patient to use medical identification for allergies *so prompt medical attention can be given if the patient is unable to give this information.*
- Teach the need to have a prescription for an epinephrine auto-injector, and teach the patient how to use it if the antigen is environmental (e.g., insect sting or foods; see Chapter 18).
- For atopic dermatitis, teach signs and symptoms of infection, use of humidification during the winter months *to prevent dryness,* wearing cotton clothing *to minimize irritation,* and cool soaks *to decrease pruritus.*
- For urticaria, teach stress management and relaxation techniques *to relieve urticaria* and to follow therapeutic regimen, including prescribed medications and their correct usage, *to reduce symptoms.*

EVALUATION. If interventions have been effective, there will be no signs of respiratory distress, and lung fields will be clear. The patient's posture, facial expressions, gestures, and concentration will reflect no anxiety. The skin will remain intact. If there are lesions, they will be reduced and healing. The patient will express knowledge of disorder and the treatment plan. The patient will verbalize no barriers to attaining treatment goals.

Type II Hypersensitivity Reactions

A type II hypersensitivity reaction involves the destruction of a cell or substance that has an antigen attached to its cell membrane, which is sensed by either immunoglobulin G (IgG) or immunoglobulin M (IgM) as being a foreign antigen (Fig. 19.2). When an antigen marker is sensed as foreign, an antibody attaches to the antigen on the cell membrane, causing lysis of the cell or accelerated phagocytosis (engulfing and ingestion). When a cell is foreign, such as a bacterium, this process is beneficial. However, sometimes antigens on the surface of a red blood cell (RBC) can be sensed as foreign for the different ABO blood types, which results in the RBC being destroyed.

Hemolytic Transfusion Reaction

PATHOPHYSIOLOGY. A hemolytic transfusion reaction is a type II hypersensitivity reaction in which incompatible surface antigens on RBCs are transfused. These antigens may be ABO or Rh [Rhesus] incompatible. (ABO and Rh are human blood group systems.) The recipient's antibodies attach to the foreign antigens on the transfused RBCs, causing rapid lysis (destruction) of the RBC. The rapid RBC lysis

results in a massive amount of cellular debris that blocks blood vessels throughout the body. This leads to ischemia and necrosis of tissue and organs. It can be life threatening.

ETIOLOGY. Occasionally, antibodies form after a bacterial or viral infection. However, prior sensitization is usually from a previous blood transfusion or pregnancy. ABO and Rh blood type must be matched for transfusions. The ABO blood types are A, B, AB, and O (Fig. 19.3). People with blood type O are universal donors because they do not have A or B antigens. However, those with type O blood can receive only type O blood. People with type AB blood are universal recipients, because they do not make A or B antibodies. Those with blood types other than AB cannot receive AB blood because they have A or B antibodies.

Rh antigens are present in people who are Rh⁺. A person who is Rh⁺ has the D antigen, which is the strongest antigen of the 50 possible antigens. Rh antibodies are present in those who are Rh⁻ after a sensitizing event. A person who is Rh⁻ does not have the D antigen. Those who are Rh⁺ can receive Rh⁻ blood, but those who are Rh⁻ cannot receive Rh⁺ blood because of the formation of antibodies to the Rh⁺ blood. If maternal and fetal blood Rh factors (RBC surface antigens) are different, the

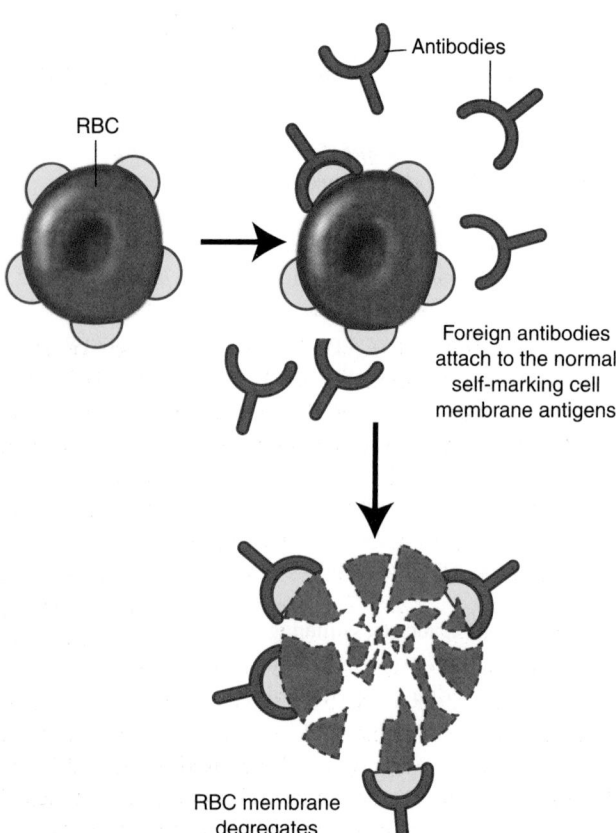

FIGURE 19.2 Type II hypersensitivity.

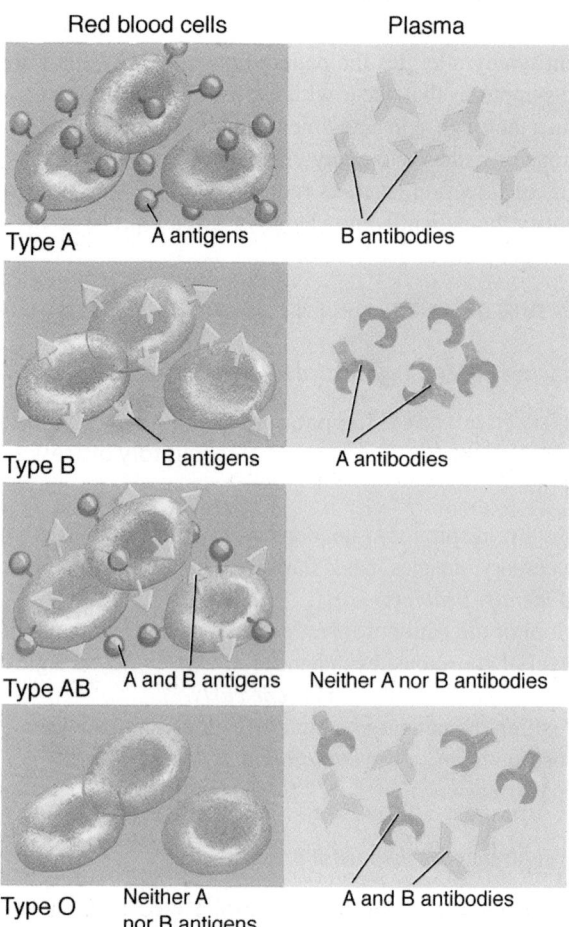

FIGURE 19.3 ABO blood types.

mother becomes sensitized by the fetal Rh type, which can affect future fetuses. For example, an $Rh_0(D)$-negative pregnant woman becomes sensitized by an $Rh_0(D)$-positive fetus. As a result, the blood cells of future $Rh_0(D)$-positive fetuses can be destroyed by maternal antibodies crossing the placenta.

CRITICAL THINKING

Blood Types: Consider the following scenarios:

1. A person with what blood type is the universal ABO Rh recipient?
2. A person with what blood type is the universal ABO Rh donor?
3. Can someone with an A Rh⁻ blood type safely receive O Rh⁺ blood?

Suggested answers are at the end of the chapter.

SIGNS AND SYMPTOMS. A hemolytic transfusion reaction is usually accompanied by a rather sudden onset of low back (flank) or chest pain, hypotension, fever rising more than 1.8°F (1°C), chills, tachycardia, tachypnea, wheezing, dyspnea, urticaria, and anxiety (Table 19.2). The patient also may report a headache and nausea.

DIAGNOSTIC TESTS. The direct Coombs test confirms this diagnosis. In the laboratory, a small amount of the patient's RBCs is washed to remove any unattached antibodies. Antihuman globulin is added to see if agglutination (clumping) of the RBCs results. If agglutination occurs, an immune reaction, such as a hemolytic transfusion reaction, is taking place.

THERAPEUTIC MEASURES. To prevent production of anti-$Rh_0(D)$ antibodies, an $Rh_0(D)$ immune globulin (RhoGAM) injection is given to $Rh_0(D)$-negative patients accidentally given $Rh_0(D)$-positive blood or exposed to $Rh_0(D)$-positive fetal blood by delivery, miscarriage, abortion, amniocentesis, or intra-abdominal trauma. When antibodies do not form, a hemolytic reaction can be prevented.

If a reaction occurs, medications are given to treat the reaction, including those listed in Table 19.3.

NURSING PROCESS FOR THE PATIENT EXPERIENCING A HEMOLYTIC TRANSFUSION REACTION.

Data Collection. Prevention of hemolytic reactions is crucial. Following strict institutional guidelines for blood transfusion administration helps ensure the patient's safety. After blood is released from the hospital blood bank, two nurses, designated per institutional policy, double-check specified data. At the bedside, transfusion guidelines include double-checking the patient's name and identification number in the medical record, unit of blood, and patient's identification bracelet as well as checking the patient's blood type in the medical record, on the unit of blood, and on the paperwork with the unit of blood.

Table 19.2

Hemolytic Transfusion Reaction Summary

Signs and Symptoms	Low back or chest pain
	Hypotension
	Fever rising more than 1.8°F (1°C)
	Chills
	Tachycardia
	Tachypnea, wheezing, dyspnea
	Urticaria
	Anxiety
	Headache
	Nausea
Diagnostic Tests	Direct Coombs test
	• Small amount of the patient's red blood cells are washed
	• Antihuman globulin is added
	• If agglutination (clumping) occurs, an immune reaction is occurring
Therapeutic Measures	Depends on severity of reaction and organs affected
	Antihistamines
	Corticosteroids
	Epinephrine
	Diuretics, to assist kidneys
Complications	If severe, shock, acute kidney injury
Priority Nursing Diagnoses	*Fear*
	Ineffective Peripheral Tissue Perfusion
	Risk for Injury

Agency policy is followed for taking vital signs during a blood transfusion. Minimally, vital signs are taken before the start of the blood transfusion, 15 minutes into the transfusion, and when the transfusion is completed. It takes only a small amount of blood to trigger a hemolytic transfusion reaction, so it is critical to stay with the patient at the bedside during the first 15 minutes of any blood transfusion.

If symptoms of a reaction are noted, the blood transfusion is immediately stopped. The agency policy for a suspected transfusion reaction is followed. A normal saline infusion with new tubing is started to keep the vein patent. The health care provider (HCP) and blood bank are immediately notified. Remain with the patient for reassurance and monitoring of symptoms and vital signs. The unused blood and blood tubing are returned to the blood bank for testing. A series of blood and urine specimens are collected and sent to the laboratory for analysis. The HCP's orders are followed to treat the patient's symptoms.

Table 19.3
Medications Used in Hemolytic Transfusion Reactions

Medication Class/Action

Antihistamines

Block histamine at histamine$_1$ receptors, thereby preventing or reversing the effects of histamine (capillary permeability, itching, and bronchospasms).

Examples	**Nursing Implications**
diphenhydramine (Benadryl)	*Teach:*
	• Take with or without food.
	• Avoid ethanol, central nervous system depressants, and over-the-counter antihistamines.
	• Avoid prolonged exposure to sunlight.
	• Use caution with activities requiring mental alertness.

Corticosteroids

Hormones with marked anti-inflammatory effects due to inhibition of prostaglandin synthesis and accumulation of macrophages and leukocytes at site.

Examples	**Nursing Implications**
dexamethasone (Decadron)	*Teach:*
hydrocortisone (Solu-Cortef)	• Take orally with food.
methylprednisolone (Solu-Medrol)	• ***Never*** stop taking suddenly.
prednisolone (Delta-Cortef)	*Monitor:*
prednisone (Deltasone)	• Weight
beclomethasone (Beconase)	• Edema, shortness of breath, jugular vein distention for heart failure development
	• Blood glucose level
	• Gastrointestinal bleeding

Sympathomimetics

Marked stimulation of alpha, beta$_1$, and beta$_2$ receptors, causing vasoconstriction, bronchodilation, and cardiac stimulation.

Examples	**Nursing Implications**
epinephrine (Adrenalin, EpiPen)	Teach patient to avoid exposing drug to heat or light.

BE SAFE!
Every unit of blood, even of the same blood type, is unique and can trigger a blood transfusion reaction. Careful monitoring with every transfusion is necessary.

Nursing Diagnoses, Planning, and Implementation

Fear related to serious threat to health status

EXPECTED OUTCOME: The patient will state reduced fear.

• Inform the patient about the procedures and treatments, and answer questions *to reduce fear.*

• Remain with the patient and allow significant others to visit *to offer emotional support.*

Ineffective Peripheral Tissue Perfusion related to arterial/venous blood flow exchange problems

EXPECTED OUTCOME: The patient will have adequate tissue perfusion as evidenced by palpable peripheral pulses, urinary output of 30 mL per hour, and no respiratory distress.

• Monitor and maintain airway, and provide oxygen *to promote oxygenation.*
• Monitor vital signs and intake and output *to detect changes for prompt treatment.*
• Have the patient rate pain using a pain scale, and provide pain relief measures *to reduce pain.*

Risk for Injury related to prolonged shock resulting in multiple organ failure or death

EXPECTED OUTCOME: The patient will remain free of injury at all times.

• Use two methods to identify the patient before giving blood products *to prevent incorrect administration of blood product.*
• Remain with the patient during the first 15 minutes of transfusion and then obtain vital signs *to detect signs of a reaction.*
• In case of a reaction, give medications such as epinephrine, steroids, or diuretics, as ordered, *to support affected tissues and organs.*

Deficient Knowledge related to lack of exposure to blood transfusions

EXPECTED OUTCOME: The patient will state understanding of blood transfusion options.

• Encourage the patient (in the case of elective surgery) to discuss the autologous (self-) blood donation option with the HCP *to avoid a transfusion reaction.*

• After a hemolytic transfusion reaction, explain to the patient the importance of informing future HCPs about the reaction *to ensure that specific blood tests are performed for less common antibodies if the patient is ever typed for a blood transfusion again.*

Evaluation. If interventions have been effective, the patient states reduced fear, has normal organ and tissue function, and reports understanding of how to help prevent transfusion reactions.

Type III Hypersensitivity Reactions

A type III hypersensitivity reaction involves immune complexes formed by antigens and antibodies, usually of the IgG type (Fig. 19.4). The patient is sensitized with an initial exposure to the antigen, and a reaction occurs with a later exposure. The reaction is localized and evolves over several hours. Symptoms range from a red, edematous skin lesion to hemorrhage and necrosis. The process involves formation of antigen–antibody complexes in the blood vessels as the antigen is absorbed through the vessel wall. Neutrophils are attracted to the area and release enzymes that ultimately lead to blood vessel damage.

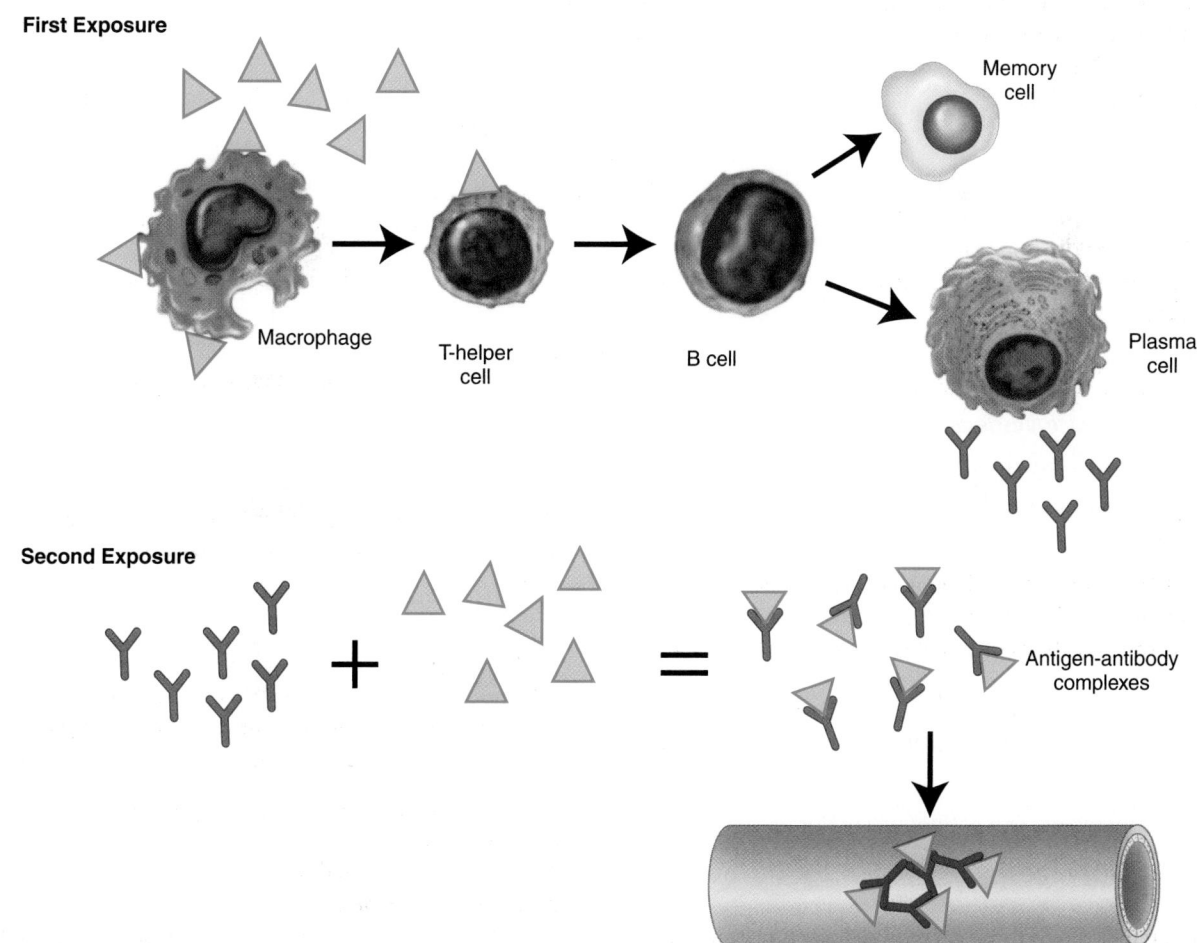

FIGURE 19.4 Type III hypersensitivity.

Serum Sickness

PATHOPHYSIOLOGY AND ETIOLOGY. Serum sickness is a type III hypersensitivity reaction in which antigen–antibody complexes form and lodge in small vessels. This leads to inflammation, tissue damage, and necrosis.

SIGNS AND SYMPTOMS. Signs and symptoms usually occur 7 days to 3 weeks after exposure. Most predominant is severe urticaria and angioedema. The patient may have a fever, malaise, muscle soreness, arthralgia, splenomegaly, and, occasionally, nausea, vomiting, and diarrhea. Lymphadenopathy may occur, especially in the lymph nodes closest to the antigen entry site.

DIAGNOSTIC TESTS. With serum sickness, there is often a slight elevation in the white blood cell (WBC) count, sedimentation rate, and C-reactive protein. IgG and IgM increase substantially, while the complement assay decreases. Plasma cells are seen on the peripheral blood smear.

THERAPEUTIC MEASURES. Because serum sickness tends to be self-limiting within about 10 days, treatment is focused on symptoms. Antipyretics may be given for fever, and analgesics and anti-inflammatories for arthralgia. Antihistamines and epinephrine may be given for urticaria and angioedema. If symptoms persist, corticosteroids may be ordered.

NURSING PROCESS FOR THE PATIENT WITH SERUM SICKNESS.
Data Collection. Symptoms and responses to prescribed medications are documented. The causative agent may be identified through the history-taking process. It is important for the patient to determine this to prevent a recurrence of the condition.

Nursing Diagnoses, Planning, and Implementation

Acute Pain related to muscle and joint soreness

EXPECTED OUTCOME: The patient will state pain is reduced to acceptable level within 30 minutes of report of pain.

- Monitor pain using a pain rating scale *to identify need for treatment.*
- Provide pain relief medications as ordered *to relieve symptoms.*

Risk for Deficient Fluid Volume related to fever and gastrointestinal fluid loss

EXPECTED OUTCOME: The patient will maintain blood pressure, pulse, and urine output within normal limits.

- Observe the patient for signs of hypovolemia, such as restlessness, weakness, muscle cramps, headaches, inability to concentrate, irritability, and postural hypotension, *to detect deficiencies to report to the HCP.*

- Monitor intake and output *to detect imbalances.*
- Provide antiemetics as ordered *to relieve nausea.*
- Encourage oral replacement therapy with glucose-electrolyte solutions, such as sports replacement drinks or ginger ale, *because they increase fluid absorption and correct deficient fluid volume.*
- Maintain IV fluids at ordered rate *to replace lost fluids but avoid fluid overload.*

Evaluation. Goals are met if the patient reports less pain and if vital signs and urine output are within normal limits.

Type IV Hypersensitivity Reactions

A type IV hypersensitivity reaction, also called a delayed reaction, occurs when a sensitized T lymphocyte comes in contact with the particular antigen to which it is sensitized (Fig. 19.5). The resulting necrosis is caused by the actions of macrophages and the various T lymphocytes involved in the cell-mediated immune response.

Contact Dermatitis
PATHOPHYSIOLOGY. When a substance or chemical comes in contact with the skin, it is absorbed and binds with special skin proteins called *haptens*. With the first contact, there is no reaction or symptoms, but within 7 to 10 days T memory cells are formed. Therefore, on subsequent exposures, the T memory

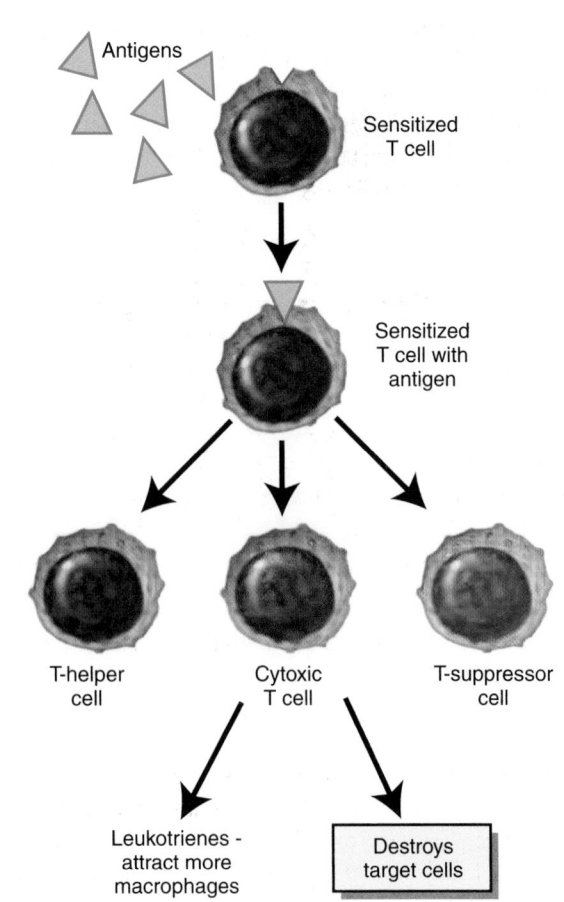

FIGURE 19.5 Type IV hypersensitivity.

cells quickly become activated T cells, which secrete the chemicals that may cause symptoms.

ETIOLOGY. Poison ivy and poison oak are the most common irritants that cause this reaction. Latex rubber also may cause contact dermatitis and can trigger type I anaphylactic reactions.

Latex Allergy. Latex allergy is a serious problem for those who work in health care. Anaphylactic reactions to latex can be fatal. Implementation of standard precautions and the use of latex gloves began in 1987 resulting in increased exposure to latex. Latex-free gloves are available. For patients who are allergic to latex, special protocols are followed using latex-free equipment. For information about latex allergy, visit the American Academy of Allergy, Asthma, and Immunology at www.aaaai.org. Also visit the U.S. Food and Drug Administration at www.fda.gov.

SIGNS AND SYMPTOMS. Within a number of hours of exposure, the area of contact becomes red and pruritic, with fragile vesicles. Secondary infections may develop. (See earlier discussion of atopic dermatitis.)

DIAGNOSTIC TESTS. Diagnosis is made by assessment of the skin and lesions through biopsy, culture or patch testing, and a detailed patient history.

THERAPEUTIC MEASURES. Treatment consists of controlling symptoms. Oral or topical antihistamines and topical drying agents may be used. Topical corticosteroids may be used and are most effective if sparingly applied after a bath or shower. If symptoms are severe, systemic corticosteroids or topical immunomodulators, such as tacrolimus (Protopic) and pimecrolimus (Elidel), may be prescribed.

NURSING PROCESS FOR THE PATIENT WITH CONTACT DERMATITIS.
Data Collection. Symptoms and the causative agent are noted. Patient recognition of the cause is important to prevent a recurrence of the condition. Special protocols are used for patients who are allergic to latex. Some agencies prepare special latex-free kits containing common supplies nurses use to care for patients. Ensure that latex allergy protocols are followed when a patient has a latex allergy to prevent development of life-threatening anaphylaxis (see "Home Health Hints" at the end of the chapter).

Nursing Diagnoses, Planning, and Implementation. See "Nursing Care Plan for the Patient With Contact Dermatitis."

Transplant Rejection

PATHOPHYSIOLOGY AND ETIOLOGY. Any form of transplanted living tissue is sensed as foreign material by the immune system. This is why lifelong immunosuppression is needed to help prevent transplant rejection, which can occur at any time. Lymphocytes become sensitized during an induction phase immediately after the tissue is transplanted. If immunosuppression is not effective, the sensitized lymphocytes invade the transplanted tissue and destroy it via the release of chemicals and macrophage activity. This results in varying degrees of transplant rejection.

SIGNS AND SYMPTOMS. Various signs and symptoms occur depending on the transplanted tissue or organ involved and the severity of the rejection (Table 19.4). Signs and symptoms reflect failure of the organ or tissue, such as renal failure for a rejected kidney.

COMPLICATIONS. The tissue or organ may be damaged from immunological reactions. It may not function at full capacity, or a total failure and loss of the transplanted tissue or organ can occur. The greatest cause of death following a transplant is infection. Immunosuppression therapy, which is needed to prevent tissue rejection after the transplant, is a major contributory factor for severe infection development. Because the immune system is suppressed, it may be unable to effectively fight infections.

DIAGNOSTIC TESTS. Biopsy, scans, blood tests, arteriography, and ultrasonography are tests that may be performed to aid in diagnosing a transplant rejection.

THERAPEUTIC MEASURES. Depending on the type of transplant, the body's immunological system is prepared before

Table 19.4
Transplant Rejection Summary

Signs and Symptoms	Dependent on: • Involved transplanted tissue or organ • Severity of reaction Reflect failure of the organ or tissue
Diagnostic Tests	Biopsy Scans Blood tests Arteriography Ultrasonography
Therapeutic Measures	Preventive preoperative preparation with medications, transfusions, or radiation to minimize the risk of rejection
Complications	Total failure and loss of transplanted organ or tissue Cause of death is most commonly due to infection, with immunosuppression therapy a contributory factor
Priority Nursing Diagnoses	*Grieving* *Fear* *Deficient Knowledge*

surgery with medications, transfusions, or radiation to minimize the risk of rejection. After the transplant, lifelong immunosuppression is needed. (However, studies are ongoing in which the same organ donor's bone marrow is transplanted to reduce or eliminate the need for antirejection drugs.) Improved specificity of immunosuppressants has reduced medication side effects while improving patient outcomes. If rejection occurs, medications may be used to attempt to reverse the rejection. Supportive care is provided based on the failing organ, such as hemodialysis if kidney rejection occurs.

NURSING CARE. Observing for signs of rejection is a priority after transplant. Teaching the patient signs and symptoms of transplant rejection to report is important before discharge. The patient will be afraid of transplant rejection and should be allowed to discuss these fears. If rejection occurs, nursing care depends on the type of transplant and signs and symptoms occurring.

Education. Rejection can take place weeks, months, or years after a transplant (with decreasing risk). The patient and family need to be educated about specific signs and symptoms of rejection and when to notify the HCP. Education regarding prescribed medications is a must because the long-term success of a transplant depends on compliance with immunosuppressant therapy (see "Home Health Hints" at the end of the chapter).

Nursing Care Plan for the Patient With Contact Dermatitis

Nursing Diagnosis: *Risk for Impaired Skin Integrity* related to effects of allergic reaction and pruritus
Expected Outcome: The patient's skin will remain intact.
Evaluation of Outcome: Is the patient's skin intact? If not intact, is the skin healing? Does the patient express a plan for preventing impaired skin integrity?

Intervention	Rationale	Evaluation
Identify and document skin and lesions.	*Provides a basis for intervention planning and evaluation of healing.*	Are lesions present? Are lesions healing?
Teach patient to keep fingernails short and clean.	*Short, clean nails cause less damage or infection if scratching occurs.*	Does the skin remain intact despite scratching?
Teach patient to apply clean, white cotton clothing (e.g., socks, gloves/mittens, undershirt) over affected area, especially at bedtime.	*Cotton allows air movement. White cloth is less irritating than those with dyes. Scratching is decreased during sleep with the use of gloves/mittens or by covering affected area.*	Are symptoms of skin irritation reduced?
Teach patient to use gentle rubbing or pressure instead of scratching.	*Use of gentle rubbing or pressure instead of scratching causes less skin trauma.*	Does skin remain intact despite itchy sensation?
Explain that tepid baking soda baths, colloidal oatmeal baths (e.g., Aveeno), and cool washcloths or cool baths reduce itching.	*These items help dry the vesicle and minimize the pruritus.*	Is itching reduced?

Nursing Diagnosis: *Ineffective Health Maintenance* related to lack of knowledge of methods to decrease inflammation and reduce episodes of inflammation
Expected Outcome: The patient or caregiver will follow the mutually agreed-on plan of care.
Evaluation of Outcome: Can the patient express knowledge of etiology, signs and symptoms, and treatment plan? Does the patient discuss any emotional, social, financial, or material blocks to attaining treatment goals?

Intervention	Rationale	Evaluation
Identify patient's knowledge of disease and causes.	*Provides a basis for the teaching plan.*	Does patient state baseline knowledge?
Identify barriers to patient's ability to carry out plan of care and plan interventions to decrease barriers.	*Barriers can prevent patient from carrying out plan of care.*	Are barriers identified? Are solutions to barriers planned?

Nursing Care Plan for the Patient With Contact Dermatitis—cont'd

Intervention	Rationale	Evaluation
Discuss methods of avoiding the allergen with patient.	*Understanding prevention methods can help prevent allergen exposure.*	Can patient state methods to help prevent allergen exposure?
Teach patient to wear medical alert identification for the allergen.	*With allergen identification, prompt medical care can be given in case the patient is unable to give this information.*	Does patient agree to use allergen identification?
Teach patient to wash with a brown soap (e.g., Fels-Naptha) or, if unavailable, any soap when contact with the offending agent is suspected.	*This removes offending agent.*	Does patient state understanding of the need to wash off the agent with exposure?
Teach patient not to scratch skin.	*Scratching can spread the dermatitis as well as cause infection.*	Does patient avoid scratching?

 ## AUTOIMMUNE DISORDERS

In autoimmune disorders, the immune system no longer recognizes the body's normal cells as self. Instead, antigens on these normal body cells are recognized as foreign material. The body then launches an immune response to destroy them.

Several factors either cause or influence this breakdown of self-recognition, including viral infections, drugs, and cross-reactive antibodies. Some microbes stimulate production of antibodies but are so closely related to normal cell antigens that the antibodies also attack some normal cells. Hormones also may influence this breakdown of self-recognition.

Some autoimmune disorders are discussed next, whereas others are discussed in chapters related to the body system most affected. Table 19.5 lists additional autoimmune disorders and the chapters in which they are discussed.

Table 19.5
Autoimmune Disorders

Disorder	*Refer to*
Idiopathic thrombocytopenic purpura	Chapter 28
Multiple sclerosis	Chapter 50
Myasthenia gravis	Chapter 50
Rheumatoid arthritis	Chapter 46
Ulcerative colitis	Chapter 34

Pernicious Anemia

PATHOPHYSIOLOGY. The body's immune system targets its own tissues. It then develops antibodies that destroy the parietal cells and disrupt intrinsic factor and hydrochloric acid production. These antibodies can alter the binding sites. This impairs the absorption of vitamin B_{12} in the ileum. A vitamin B_{12} deficiency may result. This leads to insufficient and deformed RBCs with poor oxygen-carrying capacity.

ETIOLOGY. There tends to be a familial tendency toward the autoimmune form of pernicious anemia. Causes of the acquired form of pernicious anemia (non–immune-related) include any type of gastric or small-bowel resections coupled with no or inadequate vitamin B_{12} or intrinsic factor replacement.

SIGNS AND SYMPTOMS. The patient experiences increasing weakness, loss of appetite, glossitis (inflammation or infection of the tongue), and pallor. Irritability, confusion, and numbness or tingling in the extremities (peripheral neuropathy) occur because the nervous system is affected.

DIAGNOSTIC TESTS. On microscopic examination of the patient's RBCs, macrocytic (enlarged cells) anemia is diagnosed. Macrocytic anemia and low vitamin B_{12} levels are indicators of pernicious anemia and folic acid deficiency. To determine if the diagnosis is pernicious anemia, intrinsic factor antibodies and parietal cell antibodies can be tested. Methylmalonic acid levels (when vitamin B_{12} is low) and homocysteine will be elevated. Serum cobalamin will be decreased.

Gastric secretion analysis is done to measure levels of hydrochloric acid. Low or absent hydrochloric acid may indicate pernicious anemia. A Schilling test (rarely performed today) is a 24-hour urine collection that may reveal decreased urinary excretion of vitamin B_{12}. Further studies such as radioimmunoassay or enzyme-linked immunosorbent assay may be performed to confirm an autoimmune etiology and specify which antibody is present, type I or type II.

THERAPEUTIC MEASURES. Corticosteroids may correct the problem if it is immunologically caused. Otherwise, vitamin B_{12} therapy is needed, usually for life.

NURSING CARE. Vitamin B_{12} is administered as ordered. Care related to fatigue and safety are important. Ambulation, frequent rest periods, and assistance with activities of daily living (ADLs) as indicated by the patient's activity tolerance are helpful for the patient with anemia.

Education. The patient and family need education regarding oral or parenteral medication therapy. If vitamin B_{12} injections are prescribed, the patient must understand that this is a lifelong need to prevent the return of symptoms. Patients should not miss injections, periodic vitamin B_{12} testing, or follow-up appointments.

Idiopathic Autoimmune Hemolytic Anemia

PATHOPHYSIOLOGY. In this disorder, autoantibodies, for no known reason, are produced that attach to RBCs and cause them to either lyse or agglutinate (clump). When lysis occurs, fragments of the destroyed RBCs circulate in the blood. If agglutination occurs, occlusions in the small blood vessels are followed by tissue ischemia.

SIGNS AND SYMPTOMS. Clinical manifestations vary from mild fatigue and pallor to severe hypotension, dyspnea, palpitations, headaches, and jaundice. Problems concentrating and thinking frequently occur.

DIAGNOSTIC TESTS. The RBC count, hemoglobin (Hgb) level, and hematocrit (Hct) level are low. Microscopic examination reveals fragmented RBCs. Lactate dehydrogenase and serum bilirubin levels are elevated because of RBC destruction and tissue ischemia. The direct antiglobulin test (also called the Coombs test) helps determine if the cause of hemolytic anemia is due to antibodies attached to RBCs.

THERAPEUTIC MEASURES. Supportive measures, such as supplemental oxygen, may be started. Folic acid may be prescribed to increase production of RBCs. IV immunoglobulin, immunosuppressant medications, and corticosteroids may be useful in obtaining remission. In more severe cases, blood transfusions and erythrocytapheresis (a process in which abnormal RBCs are removed and replaced with normal RBCs) may be instituted. For severe cases, a splenectomy may be performed to stop the destruction of RBCs.

NURSING CARE. The patient's signs and symptoms should be monitored and reported as needed. Frequent rest periods should be planned into the patient's daily routine to prevent fatigue. Blood products are administered as ordered to replace RBCs.

Education. The patient and family are instructed on the medical regimen, and their understanding is verified.

Hashimoto's Thyroiditis

PATHOPHYSIOLOGY. Autoantibodies for thyroid-stimulating hormone (TSH) form in Hashimoto's thyroiditis. However, instead of inactivating TSH, the autoantibodies bind with hormone receptors on the thyroid gland and stimulate the thyroid gland to secrete thyroid hormones. The thyroid gland enlarges as a result of this overstimulation (hyperthyroidism). It becomes infiltrated with lymphocytes and phagocytes, causing inflammation and further enlargement. Different autoantibodies then appear that destroy thyroid cells. This slows secretion activity, causing hypothyroidism.

ETIOLOGY. The exact cause is unknown, although it occurs in females eight times more often than in males. It is also more common in people aged 30 to 50 years and in patients with Down syndrome and Turner syndrome.

SIGNS AND SYMPTOMS. Initial signs and symptoms are those of hyperthyroidism, such as restlessness, tremors, chest pain, increased appetite, diarrhea, moist skin, heat intolerance, and weight loss.

These manifestations may go unrecognized and progress quickly into hypothyroidism. At this point, an enlarged thyroid gland (goiter) may be seen. Signs and symptoms may include fatigue, bradycardia, hypotension, dyspnea, anorexia, constipation, dry skin, weight gain, sensitivity to cold, facial puffiness, and a slowing of mental processes.

DIAGNOSTIC TESTS. Immunofluorescent assay, a test that detects antigens on cells using an antibody with a fluorescent tag, detects antithyroid antibodies. Serum TSH levels are elevated, whereas triiodothyronine (T_3) and thyroxine (T_4) levels are low. A thyroid scan is also done.

THERAPEUTIC MEASURES. Thyroid hormone replacement therapy of thyroxine is the primary means of treatment. Lifelong thyroid hormone therapy is needed.

NURSING CARE. If the patient has a goiter, a soft diet may be needed for comfort. Frequent rest periods may be needed as well as slowly increasing patient activity. Antiembolic stockings may help prevent venous stasis during the low-energy, decreased-activity phase. Daily weights and monitoring of intake and output when cardiac status is compromised are important to detect abnormalities such as fluid retention. Because weight gain and facial puffiness alter patients' self-image, patients need an opportunity to verbalize their feelings to help them adjust to this disease process.

Education. Patients taking thyroid hormone replacement therapy should avoid foods high in iodine. Their diet should also consist of large amounts of fiber to combat constipation. During the hyperthyroidism phase, a diet high in protein and carbohydrates encourages weight gain. Education regarding prescribed medications is also needed. Cholestyramine, ferrous sulfate, sucralfate, iron-containing multivitamins, calcium carbonate, and all other antacids interfere with the absorption of levothyroxine from the gastrointestinal tract. Therefore, levothyroxine should be taken a minimum of 4 hours after taking these medications.

Systemic Lupus Erythematosus

There are three types of lupus occurring in adults. (Another type is neonatal, a rare form that is passed on from a mother who has lupus to her fetus.) Drug-induced lupus erythematosus (DILE) affects approximately 10% of total lupus patients and rarely affects major organs. Research has identified about 80 prescription medications that have caused DILE (Box 19.1). A small percentage of lupus patients have the type that affects only the skin, a condition called discoid lupus erythematosus (DLE). This form is not life threatening and does not affect any internal organs. Most patients with lupus have systemic lupus erythematosus (SLE). SLE can be life threatening because it is a progressive, systemic inflammatory disease that can cause major body organ and system failure. Although this definition seems similar to the definition of rheumatoid arthritis, one distinct difference exists: Patients with SLE typically have more body organ involvement earlier in their disease than patients with rheumatoid arthritis.

PATHOPHYSIOLOGY. SLE is an autoimmune disease characterized by spontaneous remissions and exacerbations. In SLE, the body develops abnormal antibodies (antinuclear antibodies [ANAs]) against its own tissue, leading to the formation of immune complexes. These in turn activate the complement system, resulting in negative autoimmune effects on the patient's healthy connective tissue. Many of the manifestations result from recurring injuries to the patient's vascular system. The resulting immune complexes lodge in the blood and organs, leading to inflammation, damage, and possibly death.

ETIOLOGY. The cause of SLE is unknown, but the disorder tends to occur in families. Identified chromosomal markers indicate a genetic link. Environmental factors may also play a critical role in the development of SLE. Infections, high stress levels, various hormones and drugs (especially antibiotics such as sulfonamides and penicillin), and ultraviolet light have all been linked to triggering SLE. Exacerbation of symptoms, also called a *flare*, often occurs before the start of menstruation and during pregnancy, demonstrating the link hormones may have in triggering SLE. See Box 19.2 for a list of flare triggers.

African Americans, Hispanics, Native Americans, and Asians are two to three times more likely to develop SLE than others. Lupus most often affects women between the ages 15 and 40 and at a rate of 10 times more often than for men.

With improved therapy, the mortality rate for patients with SLE has improved greatly. The leading causes of death are kidney failure, heart failure, and central nervous system involvement.

SIGNS AND SYMPTOMS. Clinical manifestations vary from mild to severe (Table 19.6; "Evidence-Based Practice"); The classic feature of lupus is the characteristic reddened butterfly rash found over the bridge of the nose that extends to both cheeks, although less than half of patients develop the rash (Fig. 19.6). The rash is typically flat, is not painful or pruritic, and is photosensitive, worsening when exposed to ultraviolet light. Instead of the butterfly rash, some patients have discoid (coinlike) skin lesions on other parts of the body.

DIAGNOSTIC TESTS. Skin lesions can be biopsied and examined microscopically for signs of inflammation. Other tests include the erythrocyte sedimentation rate (ESR; to detect

---

Box 19.1

Medications Associated With Triggering Lupus Erythematosus*

- Adalimumab
- Chlorpromazine
- Diltiazem
- Etanercept
- Hydralazine
- Infliximab
- Isoniazid
- Methyldopa
- Minocycline
- Nitrofurantoin
- Phenytoin
- Procainamide
- Quinidine
- Rifampin

*Information is inconclusive and contradictory regarding some medications.

Box 19.2

Common Systemic Lupus Erythematosus Flare Triggers

- Sunlight (reflected off water and snow; window glass does not fully protect)
- Fluorescent and halogen lights
- Stress
- Emotional crisis
- Overwork
- Lack of rest
- Infection
- Surgery or injury
- Hormones
- Pregnancy and after delivery (postpartum)
- Stopping medications suddenly
- Environmental sensitivities or allergies
- Immunizations
- Certain prescription drugs
- Some over-the-counter drugs, such as cough syrups

Clinical Question

What effect does systemic lupus erythematosus (SLE) have on bone mineral density and risk for fracture?

Evidence

A meta-analysis was done by Wang and colleagues (2016) of 15 randomized studies on SLE patients' bone mineral density levels and six studies on SLE patients' fracture risk. Results showed that SLE patients had significantly lower bone mineral density levels than those in control groups within the entire body, including the femoral neck, lumbar spine, and total hip area. In addition, SLE was significantly associated with increased fracture risk for all these sites.

Implications for Nursing Practice

Because patients with SLE are at higher risk for fractures, teach them that bone mineral density testing is important. To reduce fracture risk, reinforce the need for adequate dietary calcium intake and adherence to prescribed calcium supplementations.

Reference

Wang, X., Yan, S., Xu, Y., Wan, L. Wang, Y., Gao, W., ... Xu, D. (2016). Fracture risk and bone mineral density levels in patients with systemic lupus erythematosus: A systematic review and meta-analysis. *Osteoporosis International, 27*(4), 1413–1423.

systemic inflammation) and ANA titers (to detect the presence of abnormal antibodies). There are also two subtypes of ANA: anti-double stranded DNA (anti-dsDNA) and anti-Smith (anti-Sm) antibodies. These are found only in patients with SLE and can be useful in confirming a diagnosis of SLE. A blood test involving serine/arginine-rich (SR) proteins also may aid in diagnosis of SLE. Although no laboratory test can confirm a diagnosis of SLE, the results of immunological tests may support the diagnosis.

THERAPEUTIC MEASURES. Treatment of SLE focuses on decreasing inflammation and preventing life-threatening organ damage (Table 19.7). The human monoclonal antibody belimumab (Benlysta) is the only medication directed at one of the underlying processes of SLE, overstimulated B lymphocytes (which produce an antibody-mediated response known as a humoral response). This medication decreases the activity of these cells. This in turn decreases the production of auto-antibodies. Many of the drugs used for SLE have serious side effects. Patients receiving them are carefully monitored.

Research is ongoing regarding the possible cause of SLE. Researchers have found about 50 genes that are associated with SLE or that, in combination, increase the risk for the development of lupus (Scofield, 2015). These genetic discoveries are enabling researchers to develop new methods of therapy, including gene therapy.

NURSING CARE. Prevention of exacerbations (flares) is important. Therefore, taking preventive measures is suggested.

Table 19.6

Systemic Lupus Erythematosus Summary

Signs and Symptoms	Discoid:
	• Patchy, crusty, sharply defined skin plaques
	• Tend to occur on face or sun-exposed areas
	Drug-induced:
	• Pleuropericardial inflammation
	• Fever
	• Rash
	• Arthritis
	Systemic:
	• Early symptoms are vague, then fatigue, fever
	• Dermatological: Butterfly rash (face), photosensitivity, mucosal ulcers, alopecia, pain, pruritus, bruising
	• Musculoskeletal: Arthralgia, arthritis
	• Hematologic: Anemia, leukocytopenia, elevated erythrocyte sedimentation rate (ESR), thrombocytopenia, false-positive venereal disease research laboratory test
	• Cardiopulmonary: Pericarditis, myocarditis, myocardial infarction, vasculitis, pleurisy, valvular heart disease
	• Renal: Renal failure, urinary tract infections, fluid and electrolyte imbalances
	• Central nervous system: Cranial neuropathies, cognitive impairment, mental changes, seizures
	• Gastrointestinal: Anorexia, ascites, pancreatitis, intestinal vasculitis
	• Ophthalmological: Conjunctivitis, dry eyes, glaucoma, cataracts, retinal pigmentation

Table 19.6
Systemic Lupus Erythematosus Summary—cont'd

Diagnostic Tests	Complete blood count Antinuclear antibody (ANA) Anti-Smith (a highly specific immunoglobulin for systemic lupus erythematosus [SLE]) Anti-nDNA positive in 60% to 80% of SLE patients Anti-Ro (SSA), an immunoglobulin, positive in 30% of SLE patients Anti-La (SSB), an immunoglobulin, positive in 15% of SLE patients Complement ESR and C-reactive protein (CRP) nonspecific 24-hour urine creatinine clearance If ruling out kidney involvement: • Urinalysis • Serum creatinine • Kidney biopsy
Therapeutic Measures	Symptom management Nonsteroidal anti-inflammatory drugs (NSAIDs) Immunosuppressants Corticosteroids Antimalarials Intravenous immunoglobulin
Complications	Emboli Mesenteric or intestinal vasculitis leading to obstruction, perforation, or infarction Myocarditis Osteonecrosis Renal failure Sepsis Thrombocytopenia Vasculitis
Priority Nursing Diagnoses	*Acute Pain* *Disturbed Body Image* *Fatigue* *Ineffective Health Maintenance*

Minimizing exposure to the sun and artificial ultraviolet light by wearing protective clothing and 70 sun protection factor (SPF) sunscreens will help those patients who are photosensitive. Fatigue during ADLs can be minimized using a daily personal schedule. The patient needs a minimum of 8 hours of sleep per night with naps as needed to combat fatigue. Because most patients with SLE develop transitory arthralgia (joint pain), maintaining fitness and joint range of motion through a regular fitness program while decreasing activity during flares is vital. Warm baths may help with morning stiffness, and application of heat and cold compresses, splints, assistive devices, and physical therapy may help soreness. Eating a well-balanced diet will also influence the level of fatigue and the corticosteroid-induced weight gain, which also can affect joint soreness. Additionally, it is recommended that patients keep immunizations up to date.

Finally, but most important, the patient's psychological state and support systems need to be addressed. The period from the onset of symptoms to the diagnosing of lupus is usually costly in terms of time, money, and emotions. Patients may face anger, frustration, and confusion before the diagnosis. For many, there is a sense of relief at diagnosis that may quickly be replaced with feelings of anger, fear, depression, or grief. This is when empathy, support, hope, and, most important, education for the patient, family, and significant others are vital for acquiring successful long-term coping skills. In addition, local support groups and educational and self-management programs available through the Lupus Foundation of America (www.lupus.org) can provide patients with avenues for attaining more specific knowledge and skills for coping and taking control of their lives.

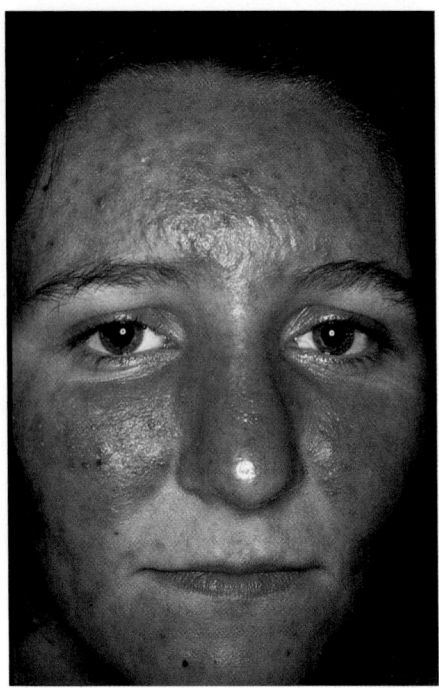

FIGURE 19.6 Lupus erythematosus: Red papules and plaques in butterfly pattern on face.

Education. Explain the signs of bleeding and of cardiac and vascular problems, such as myocardial infarction and thrombophlebitis. Encourage medical alert usage. Provide smoking cessation information to patients who smoke. Because kidney disease is a major complication of SLE, patients must learn the signs of impending problems that need to be relayed to the HCP immediately. These include facial puffiness and "foamy" or "cola-colored" urine, which are indicative of proteinuria and hematuria, respectively. Explain that regular ophthalmic examinations are needed for early detection and treatment of the complications that antimalarial drugs and corticosteroids can produce, such as retinal bleeding, glaucoma, and cataracts.

CRITICAL THINKING

Mr. Ellis is suffering from a flare of systemic lupus erythematosus. The health care provider has ordered intramuscular Solu-Cortef 80 mg to be given every 8 hours. Solu-Cortef 125 mg per 2 mL is available. How many milliliters will the nurse administer per dose?
Suggested answers are at the end of the chapter.

Table 19.7
Medications Used to Treat Systemic Lupus Erythematosus

Medication Class/Action

Nonsteroidal Anti-inflammatory Drugs (NSAIDs)

Reduce inflammation.

Examples	**Nursing Implications**
ibuprofen (Motrin)	*Teach:*
indomethacin (Indocin)	• Take with food and avoid alcohol.
naproxen (Naprosyn)	• Protect self from ultraviolet light.
	• Monitor for abnormal bleeding.

Antimalarials

Action is not clearly understood but can significantly help reduce inflammation and decrease platelet aggregation while lowering plasma lipid levels.

Examples	**Nursing Implications**
chloroquine (Aralen)	Obtain baseline physical assessment, including an ophthalmic
hydroxychloroquine sulfate (Plaquenil)	examination.
	Teach:
	• Administer either before or after meals at the same time of day.
	• That it may take weeks or months for effects to be noticed.

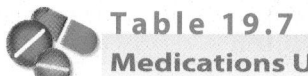

Table 19.7
Medications Used to Treat Systemic Lupus Erythematosus—cont'd

Medication Class/Action

Corticosteroids

Reduce inflammation and suppress immune response.

Examples
dexamethasone (Decadron)
methylprednisolone (Solu-Medrol)
hydrocortisone (Solu-Cortef)
prednisone (Deltasone)

Nursing Implications
Monitor for weight gain, elevated blood sugar, decreased urine output, pulse irregularities, increased blood pressure, edema, and temperature.
Teach:
• Take with food or milk.
• Do not miss doses.
• *Never* stop taking suddenly.
• Use methods to avoid infection.

Immunosuppressants

Target and damage auto-antibody-producing cells.

Examples
azathioprine (Imuran)
cyclosporine (Sandimmune)
methotrexate (Rheumatrex)

Nursing Implications
Monitor complete blood count, renal and liver function tests, abnormal bleeding, joint range of motion, edema, temperature, and erythema.
Teach:
• Take with food for gastrointestinal upset.
• Protect from infection.

Human Monoclonal Antibody

Only drug aimed at one of the underlying processes of systemic lupus erythematosus: overstimulated B-lymphocytes.

Examples
belimumab (Benlysta)

Nursing Implications
May have serious side effects; careful monitoring is needed.

Ankylosing Spondylitis

PATHOPHYSIOLOGY. Ankylosing spondylitis, also called rheumatoid spondylitis, is a chronic progressive inflammatory disease primarily of the spine and sacroiliac area. It can also affect the large limb joints. The inflammatory process begins in the lower region of the back and progresses upward. A specific histocompatibility antigen (antigen that identifies self), human leukocyte antigen (HLA) B27 is formed that stimulates an immune response. It can result in complete fusion of the spine. This causes complete rigidity in the spine, a condition known as "bamboo spine."

ETIOLOGY. There is strong evidence of a familial tendency, but no other specific causes are known. Ankylosing spondylitis tends to afflict men more than women. It is usually diagnosed between the later teens and age 40.

SIGNS AND SYMPTOMS. Ankylosing spondylitis causes an insidious onset of lower back stiffness and pain, which is worse in the morning. As the disease progresses, the pain worsens and there are spasms of the back muscles. The normal curvature of the lower back (lordosis) flattens, and the curvature of the upper back (kyphosis) increases. Patients may also experience fatigue, anorexia, and weight loss.

DIAGNOSTIC TESTS. Findings such as a positive family history, a positive HLA-B27 blood test, negative Rh, and radiographs of the joints showing spinal changes and fusion

• WORD • BUILDING •
ankylosing spondylitis: anayle—stiff joint + osing—condition + spondyl—vertebrae + itis—inflammation

(although these changes are a late finding) confirm a diagnosis of ankylosing spondylitis. There are no specific immunological tests to diagnose ankylosing spondylitis.

THERAPEUTIC MEASURES. Because there is no cure for ankylosing spondylitis, treatment consists of measures to minimize the symptoms. Analgesics and muscle relaxants for pain relief, anti-inflammatory agents to decrease joint inflammation, and physical therapy to maintain muscle strength and joint range of motion are used. Biological agents such as anti-tumor necrosis factor (TNF)-a, including etanercept (Enbrel), infliximab (Remicade), and adalimumab (Humira), have shown promising results in changing the disease progression. Surgery can be done to replace fused joints. For kyphosis, cervical or lumbar osteotomy can be performed. Physiotherapy and exercise can be beneficial in managing symptoms.

Klebsiella bacterium, found naturally in the gut, is found in high levels in the feces of patients with ankylosing spondylitis. It may be a trigger for the disease. This bacterium requires starch to grow, so it is thought that reducing starch in the diet might reduce symptoms. For more information, visit the Spondylitis Association of America at www.spondylitis.org.

NURSING CARE. Nursing care focuses on administration and evaluation of prescribed medications as well as patient education to help reduce pain and stiffness, including providing disease information. Teach proper posture, range-of-motion exercises, and changing positions frequently. Also teach patients to sleep on a mattress that is firm without a pillow or with a thin pillow. Pain management, rest periods, assistance with ADLs, and exercise promotion are provided.

CRITICAL THINKING

Mr. Beck, a truck driver who was recently diagnosed with ankylosing spondylitis, verbalizes concern about how this diagnosis will affect his ability to work.

1. How would the nurse answer his questions?
   a. "What is happening to me?"
   b. "Will I have to quit my job driving an interstate truck?"
   c. "Am I going to have really bad pain?"
   d. "Am I going to be dependent on someone?"
2. Mr. Beck plans to continue driving his truck and, therefore, has a need upon discharge for specific interventions that will help him maintain his independence. What will the nurse explain to Mr. Beck about the importance of each of the following interventions?
   a. Perform range-of-motion exercises daily.
   b. Do not stay in one position too long. Stop and walk around often.
   c. Sleep on a firm mattress without a pillow or with a thin pillow.
   d. Maintain good posture, even when driving the truck.

Suggested answers are at the end of the chapter.

IMMUNE DEFICIENCIES

Immune deficiencies occur when one or more components of the immune system are either completely absent or deficient in quantities sufficient to elicit or sustain an adequate immune response to combat an infectious agent.

Hypogammaglobulinemia

PATHOPHYSIOLOGY AND ETIOLOGY. Hypogammaglobulinemia is either a hereditary congenital disorder or acquired after childhood from unknown causes. It is characterized by the absence or deficiency of one or more of the five classes of immunoglobulins (IgG, IgM, IgA, IgD, and IgE) from defective B-cell function. The lack of normal function of these antibodies makes the patient prone to infections. The congenital form of this disorder affects males. Patients usually have a normal life span.

SIGNS AND SYMPTOMS. Recurrent infections occur, especially from *Staphylococcus* and *Streptococcus* organisms.

DIAGNOSIS. Immunoelectrophoresis, which measures the level of each immunoglobulin, can be performed.

THERAPEUTIC MEASURES. Treatment is aimed at minimizing infections while increasing immune system function through subcutaneous injections or IV infusions of immunoglobulin. Immunoglobulin mainly contains IgG, so fresh frozen plasma is given to replace IgM. IgA cannot be replaced, increasing the risk for frequent pulmonary infections. Gene therapy has been shown to be successful in stabilizing infant immune systems with severe combined immunodeficiency but has been less effective with older patients.

NURSING CARE AND EDUCATION. Monitor for infections. Any break in the skin must be cleansed immediately and monitored for infection development. Genetic counseling may be recommended. Education on signs and symptoms of various infections and seeking medical help promptly, avoiding crowds, the need for good nutrition, hydration, and hygiene is provided.

Home Health Hints

Atopic Dermatitis
- Encourage use of soaps for sensitive skin, oatmeal bath products, and a skin moisturizer without perfume to help prevent dryness.
- If a rash develops, encourage use of a mild laundry soap, such as Dreft.

Latex Allergy
- Always have latex-free gloves available.
- Use latex-free silicone urinary catheters.

Post-transplant
- Teach when taking immune-suppressing medications to avoid those who are ill with colds or flu.

SUGGESTED ANSWERS TO CRITICAL THINKING

Mrs. Barnes

1. Mrs. Barnes is most likely having an anaphylactic reaction to the bee stings with accompanying urticaria or possibly angioedema.
2. Further assessment might include identification of any previous allergies to food, medications, and environmental stimuli and what reactions occur with these allergies. Thorough respiratory assessment is needed, noting any adventitious sounds, particularly wheezing. Note any dysphagia, changes in her voice, or hoarseness.
3. Therapeutic measures to implement include monitoring vital signs, staying with the patient, using semi-Fowler to high-Fowler position, giving oxygen at 2 to 3 L per minute, and ensuring a patent intravenous access. Notify the registered nurse and/or health care provider right away. Anticipate administration of antihistamines, epinephrine, and fluids.
4. Health care provider, registered nurse, and respiratory therapist.

Blood Types

1. AB Rh+.
2. O Rh−.
3. No. Only type A Rh− or O Rh− blood is safe.

Mr. Ellis

1. 28 mL per dose.

Mr. Beck

1. a. "Human leukocyte antigen B27 is formed, stimulating a chronic immune (inflammatory) response specifically in the spine, sacroiliac area, and large limb joints. This leads to thickening of the joints, joint pain, and stiffness."
   b. "No, you shouldn't have to quit your job, but you may need to alter how you travel and drive."
   c. "No, you may not have severe pain with use of medication and exercise."
   d. "No, this disease may not affect your independence with proper treatment and rehabilitation."
2. a. "Range-of-motion exercises will help maintain joint mobility and a full range of motion and prevent contractures from forming."
   b. "Again, this frequent movement prevents stiffness and joint pain and contractures of joints."
   c. "Sleeping on a firm mattress without a pillow or with a thin pillow keeps the spine in correct alignment, which in turn helps prevent progressive changes in spine alignment (kyphosis, scoliosis) that affect various major body systems (respiratory, etc.)."
   d. "Again, good posture will aid in preventing bone deformities."

Review Questions

1. A patient asks the nurse how an allergy can develop to a medication that has been taken before without problems. Which of the following is the most appropriate response?
   1. "It probably is due to your age, because as we age, the body becomes more sensitive to environmental stimuli, which leads to hypersensitivities."
   2. "What have you eaten in the last 24 hours? Most medications are altered by food, thereby producing different effects in the body."
   3. "Viral illnesses and exposure to various chemicals and environmental substances can alter the immune system and its response to previously benign stimuli."
   4. "Patients who have autoimmune disorders such as lupus or arthritis tend to develop sensitivities to common medications."

2. The nurse is caring for a patient who asks what ankylosing spondylitis is. Which of the following responses from the nurse is appropriate?
   1. "It is a chronic progressive inflammatory disease of the spine and large limb joints."
   2. "Autoantibodies lyse red blood cells."
   3. "There is formation of antigen–antibody complexes leading to inflammation."
   4. "Production of immunoglobulin E antibodies occurs."

3. The nurse is collecting data on a patient with suspected pernicious anemia. Which of these signs or symptoms would the nurse expect to find for this patient? **Select all that apply.**
   1. Back spasms
   2. Glossitis
   3. Itching
   4. Kyphosis
   5. Pallor
   6. Weakness

4. A patient who has been diagnosed with systemic lupus erythematosus is being discharged. The patient reports she is leaving shortly for a 3-week tour of the Grand Canyon and whitewater rafting. Which of the following patient statements conveys the patient's understanding of the plan of care? **Select all that apply.**
   1. "As long as I wear sunscreen, I can be in the sun all day."
   2. "I will wear clothing on all exposed skin."
   3. "If I develop a rash, I should avoid the sun."
   4. "I will use sunscreen on exposed skin at all times."
   5. "The early morning sun presents the strongest danger."
   6. "I will wear a hat."

5. The nurse is caring for a patient with allergic rhinitis. Which of the following interventions should the nurse anticipate will be included in the treatment plan for this patient? **Select all that apply.**
   1. Antihistamines
   2. Anticholinergics
   3. Avoiding environmental stimuli
   4. Decongestants
   5. Immunotherapy
   6. Steroids

6. The nurse is collecting data from a patient with contact dermatitis. Which data is essential for the nurse to obtain?
   1. Date of gastric surgery
   2. Appearance of skin lesions
   3. Weight gain
   4. Appetite

7. A patient is admitted with an autoimmune disease and asks the nurse what autoimmune means. Which of the following responses by the nurse would be appropriate?
   1. "Immune cells produce too many antibodies."
   2. "Immune cells grow and multiply too rapidly."
   3. "Immune cells are not produced in sufficient amounts."
   4. "Immune cells are unable to distinguish between 'self' and 'not self.'"

8. A patient is receiving cefuroxime (Zinacef) intravenously. Fifteen minutes after the cefuroxime is started, the patient reports an uneasy feeling as well as feeling very warm. Which actions would the nurse take now? **Select all that apply.**
   1. Offer the patient ice water.
   2. Discontinue the angiocath.
   3. Stay with the patient.
   4. Turn off the intravenous infusion.
   5. Call for assistance.
   6. Monitor vital signs.

Answer rationales available in your online resources.

ANSWERS 1. 3; 2. 1; 3. 2, 5, 6; 4. 2, 4, 6; 5. 1, 3, 4, 5, 6; 6. 2; 7. 4; 8. 3, 4, 5, 6

Key Points

Find the chapter key points in your online resources available through Davis Edge.

Additional Resources

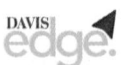 Use the scratch off code on the inside front cover of your book to access online quizzes that will help you to improve your scores on course exams and prepare for NCLEX-PN®.

  Study Guide

CHAPTER 20

Nursing Care of Patients With HIV Disease and AIDS

Patrice Wade-Olson

KEY TERMS

acquired immunodeficiency syndrome
  (uh-KWHY-erd im-yoo-noh-dee-FISH-en-see
  SIN-drohm)
cytomegalovirus (SY-tow-MEH-guh-low-vy-rus)
human immunodeficiency virus (HYOO-man
  im-yoo-noh-dee-FISH-en-see VY-rus)
personal protective equipment (PUR-sun-al
  pra-TEK-tiv ee-KWIP-ment)
pneumocystis pneumonia (new-moh-SIS-tis
  new-MOHN-yah)
undetectable viral load (un-dee-TECH-tah-bul
  VY-ruhl lohd)

CHAPTER CONCEPTS

Immunity

LEARNING OUTCOMES

1. Define human immunodeficiency virus (HIV) and acquired immunodeficiency syndrome (AIDS).
2. Explain how HIV is transmitted.
3. Explain tests for diagnosing HIV.
4. Describe the prognosis for HIV and AIDS.
5. Develop a teaching plan for prevention of an HIV infection.
6. Identify prevention measures used to decrease infection and opportunistic diseases for patients with HIV.
7. Develop a teaching plan for a patient with HIV receiving antiretroviral therapy.
8. Plan nursing care for patients with HIV and AIDS related to medications, coinfection prevention, and maintaining nutritional status.

Acquired immunodeficiency syndrome (AIDS) is the late phase of a chronic immune function disorder. This disorder is caused by infection with the **human immunodeficiency virus** (HIV). AIDS develops after a long period of untreated HIV infection and can be fatal. The Centers for Disease Control and Prevention (CDC) specifies the criteria for determining when HIV disease has developed into AIDS (Box 20.1).

In the United States, most people living with HIV who receive treatment do not develop AIDS. This is because antiretroviral medications suppress HIV replication. This improves immune function and reduces the risk of life-threatening opportunistic infections. The first antiretroviral (ARV) HIV drug was introduced in 1987. Highly active antiretroviral therapy (HAART) began in 1996. A newer term for HAART is antiretroviral therapy (ART). Both of the latter terms refer to the use of a combination of at least three ARV drugs that have different actions to suppress HIV replication.

> ### NURSING CARE TIP
>
> When caring for patients who are HIV positive or who have AIDS, it is important to be aware of and understand current information. Being informed helps you to provide competent, nonjudgmental care without fear (Table 20.1). Knowledge about HIV/AIDS and its treatment is continually evolving.

 ## HISTORY AND INCIDENCE

The HIV epidemic was first reported by the CDC in June 1981. Cases of HIV infection and AIDS increased rapidly through the 1980s. A decrease followed in the late 1990s and continues today. The CDC provides U.S. statistics on HIV cases (www.cdc.gov/hiv/statistics/overview/ataglance.html; Table 20.2). As of the end of 2015, it was estimated that

Box 20.1

CDC AIDS-Defining Opportunistic Conditions in HIV Infection

CD4 T-lymphocyte count below 200 cells/microL, or a CD4 T-lymphocyte percentage under 14% of total lymphocytes, or the presence of one of the following specified clinical conditions:
- Bacterial infections, multiple or recurrent
- Candidiasis of bronchi, trachea, or lung
- Candidiasis, esophageal
- Cervical cancer, invasive
- Coccidioidomycosis, disseminated or extrapulmonary
- Cryptococcosis, extrapulmonary
- Cryptosporidiosis, chronic intestinal (>1 month's duration)
- Cytomegalovirus disease (not including liver, spleen, or nodes; onset >1 month of age)
- Cytomegalovirus retinitis with loss of vision
- Encephalopathy attributed to HIV
- Herpes simplex, chronic ulcers (>1 month's duration) or bronchitis, pneumonitis, or esophagitis (onset >1 month of age)
- Histoplasmosis, disseminated or extrapulmonary
- Isosporiasis, chronic intestinal (>1 month's duration)
- Kaposi sarcoma
- Lymphoma, Burkitt
- Lymphoma, immunoblastic
- Lymphoma of the brain, primary
- *Mycobacterium avium* complex or *Mycobacterium kansasii,* disseminated or extrapulmonary
- *Mycobacterium* tuberculosis (any site), pulmonary, disseminated, or extrapulmonary
- *Mycobacterium,* other species or unidentified species, disseminated or extrapulmonary
- *Pneumocystis jiroveci* pneumonia
- Pneumonia, recurrent
- Progressive multifocal leukoencephalopathy
- Salmonella septicemia, recurrent
- Toxoplasmosis of brain (onset >1 month of age)
- Wasting syndrome attributed to HIV

Source: Selik, R. M., Mokotoff, E. D., Branson, B., Owen, S. M., Whitmore, S., & Hall, H. I. (2014). Revised surveillance case definition for HIV infection—United States, 2014. *Morbidity and Mortality Weekly Report, 63*(RR03), 1–10. Retrieved from www.cdc.gov/mmwr/preview/mmwrhtml/rr6303a1.htm

Table 20.1

Staying Current: HIV/AIDS Information Resources

AIDS InfoNet (drug fact sheets)	www.aidsinfonet.org
Association of Nurses in AIDS Care	www.nursesinaidscare.org (800) 260-6780
AVERT: AVERTing HIV and AIDS	www.avert.org
The Body: The Complete HIV/AIDS Resource	www.thebody.com
Centers for Disease Control and Prevention (CDC) National HIV, STD, and Hepatitis Testing	https://gettested.cdc.gov (800) CDC-INFO
CDC: HIV/AIDS	www.cdc.gov/hiv (800) CDC-INFO (888) 232-6348 (TTY)
CDC National Center for HIV/AIDS, Viral Hepatitis, STD, and TB Prevention	www.cdc.gov/nchhstp
CDC National Prevention Information Network	www.cdcnpin.org (800) CDC-INFO
HIV.gov (Gateway to federal domestic HIV/AIDS resources)	www.hiv.gov
HIV Prevention Trials Network	www.hptn.org
NAM AIDSMaps	www.aidsmap.com
Prevention Access Campaign	https://www.preventionaccess.org/
University of California, Los Angeles Clinician Consultation Center (Post-Exposure Prophylaxis hotline)	www.nccc.ucsf.edu (888) 448-4911
U.S. Department of Health and Human Services AIDSinfo (in English and Spanish)	www.aidsinfo.nih.gov (800) HIV-0440

Table 20.1
Staying Current: HIV/AIDS Information Resources—cont'd

U.S. National Library of Medicine	www.nlm.nih.gov (888) FIND-NLM
World Health Organization: HIV/AIDS info	www.who.int/hiv

Table 20.2
U.S. Adults With Stage 3 HIV (AIDS)

By Years of Age	*Cumulative Estimate 1981 to 2015*
20–29	195,725
30–39	471,722
40–49	348,340
50–59	133,845
60 and older	47,236
By Ethnicity/Race	
Asian/Pacific Islander	9,932
American Indian/Alaskan Native	3,543
Black/African American	506,163
Hispanic/Latino	222,227
Native Hawaiian/Other Pacific Islander	845
White	439,207
Multiple Races	35,000

Source: Centers for Disease Control and Prevention. (2016). *HIV Surveillance Report, 2015* (Vol. 27). Retrieved from www.cdc.gov/hiv/library/reports/hiv-surveillance.html

1.1 million people were infected with HIV. Of these, an estimated 15% were not aware of being infected. In 2016, an estimated 39,782 people were newly infected with HIV. Of those infected in 2016, 45% were African Americans and 19% were women (CDC, 2017b). Although HIV or AIDS can occur in a person of any age, this chapter focuses on adults with HIV or AIDS.

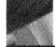

PATHOPHYSIOLOGY

Infection with HIV kills immune cells. A weakened immune system allows infections and cancers to take over. AIDS is the final phase of this immunodeficiency.

Two strains of HIV have been identified: HIV-1 and HIV-2. HIV-1 is found around the world; it is more pathogenic.

HIV-2 is found mainly in a small area in West Africa; it is less pathogenic. It is possible to become infected with both strains of HIV. Due to genetic differences, they require different types of diagnostic testing. They are transmitted in the same way, are incurable, and can progress to AIDS. Because HIV-1 is most common, reference to HIV in this chapter is to HIV-1, unless noted.

HIV is a retrovirus, which only has ribonucleic acid (RNA) for genetic material. HIV is attracted to immune cells with a surface-attaching site. This is the CD4 receptor. Cells with CD4 receptors include lymphocytes (called CD4 T lymphocytes, CD4+ T lymphocytes, T4 lymphocytes, or helper T lymphocytes) and macrophages (found in the brain). HIV hides in these latent reservoirs for infection flare-ups, which prevents a cure. The CD4 T lymphocytes are the main targets of HIV. CD4 T lymphocytes coordinate all immune functions. So, the destruction of these cells by HIV results in progressive impairment of the body's immune response. The study of macrophages and HIV has led to the discovery of how HIV enters these cells. This may help with a cure (Mlcochova et al., 2017).

There are seven steps in the HIV replication process: (1) The first is *binding* (attachment) to the CD4 receptor of the host cell (Fig. 20.1). Cellular chemokine receptor type 5 (CCR5) antagonist drugs act here to block HIV attachment. (2) Binding leads to fusion of the HIV envelope (membrane) and host cell membrane. Fusion inhibitor drugs act here. (3) After fusion, the HIV capsid (which encloses genetic material of the virus) is released into the host cell. HIV uses its enzyme *reverse transcriptase* to convert its RNA to HIV deoxyribonucleic acid (DNA). The new HIV DNA then enters the host cell's nucleus. Non-nucleoside reverse transcriptase inhibitors (NNRTIs) and nucleoside reverse transcriptase inhibitors (NRTIs) act here. Inhibitors of reverse transcriptase that act here were the first anti-HIV drugs developed. (4) HIV releases the enzyme *integrase*, which incorporates its HIV DNA into the host cell's DNA. Integrase inhibitors act here. (5) HIV then uses the machinery of the host cell to replicate long chains of HIV proteins for building more HIV. (6) Packaging of HIV RNA and HIV proteins within a viral envelope created from part of the cell membrane occurs next. (7) The immature, noninfectious HIV then buds from the host cell. It releases the enzyme *protease* to cut the HIV protein chains into their shorter functional forms. Mature, infectious HIV is then formed from these proteins. Protease inhibitors, which are potent antiviral medications, block this critical step.

HIV can persist in a latent (inactive) state for many years. There is no cure for HIV as the virus lies dormant in a small number of cells called viral reservoirs even when the virus is

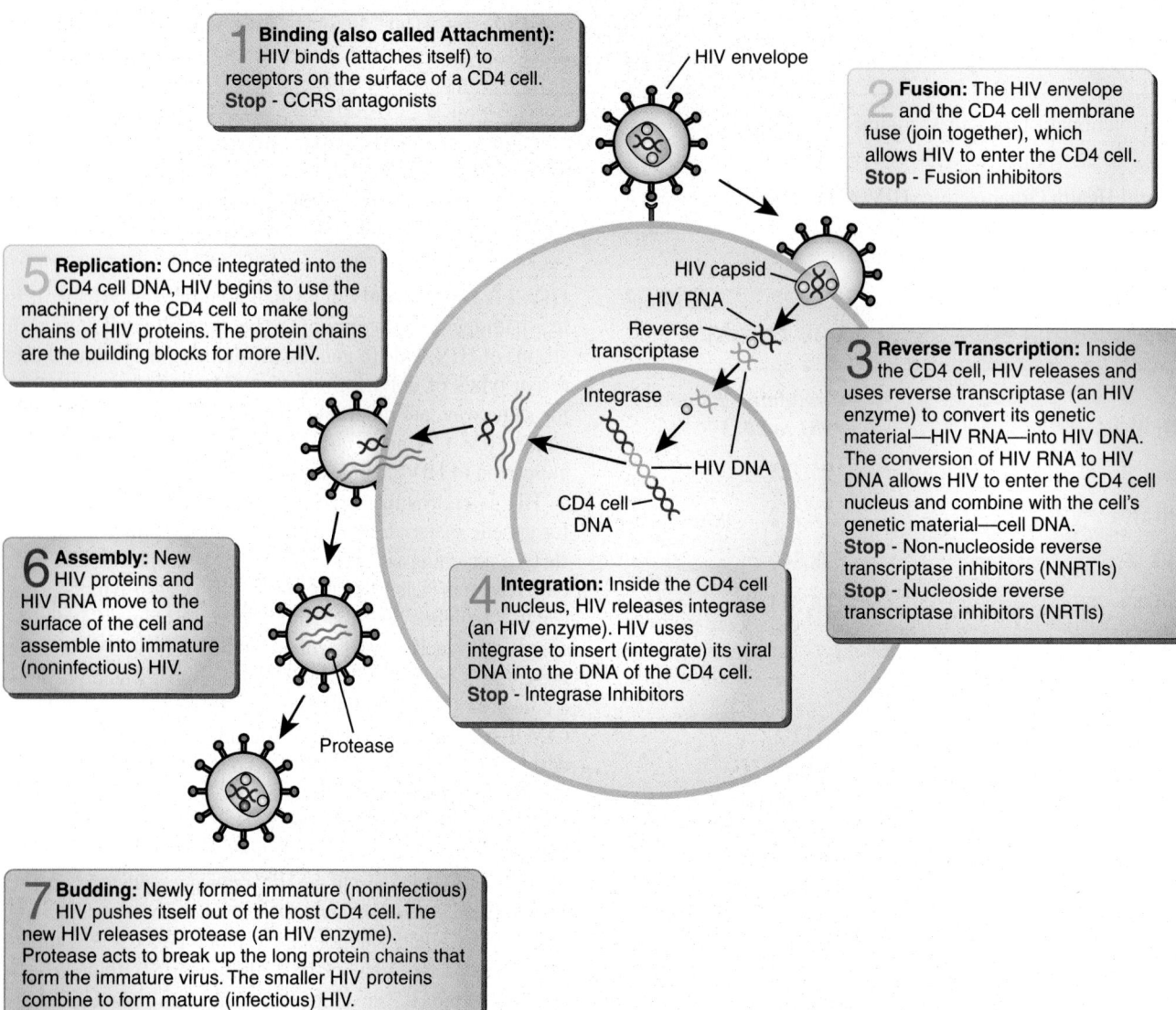

1 Binding (also called Attachment): HIV binds (attaches itself) to receptors on the surface of a CD4 cell. **Stop** - CCR5 antagonists

2 Fusion: The HIV envelope and the CD4 cell membrane fuse (join together), which allows HIV to enter the CD4 cell. **Stop** - Fusion inhibitors

5 Replication: Once integrated into the CD4 cell DNA, HIV begins to use the machinery of the CD4 cell to make long chains of HIV proteins. The protein chains are the building blocks for more HIV.

3 Reverse Transcription: Inside the CD4 cell, HIV releases and uses reverse transcriptase (an HIV enzyme) to convert its genetic material—HIV RNA—into HIV DNA. The conversion of HIV RNA to HIV DNA allows HIV to enter the CD4 cell nucleus and combine with the cell's genetic material—cell DNA. **Stop** - Non-nucleoside reverse transcriptase inhibitors (NNRTIs) **Stop** - Nucleoside reverse transcriptase inhibitors (NRTIs)

6 Assembly: New HIV proteins and HIV RNA move to the surface of the cell and assemble into immature (noninfectious) HIV.

4 Integration: Inside the CD4 cell nucleus, HIV releases integrase (an HIV enzyme). HIV uses integrase to insert (integrate) its viral DNA into the DNA of the CD4 cell. **Stop** - Integrase Inhibitors

7 Budding: Newly formed immature (noninfectious) HIV pushes itself out of the host CD4 cell. The new HIV releases protease (an HIV enzyme). Protease acts to break up the long protein chains that form the immature virus. The smaller HIV proteins combine to form mature (infectious) HIV. **Stop** - Protease inhibitors (PIs)

HIV envelope
HIV capsid
HIV RNA
Reverse transcriptase
Integrase
HIV DNA
CD4 cell DNA
Protease

FIGURE 20.1 The HIV life cycle and the medication classes that stop HIV in various life cycle stages.

at undetectable levels in the blood. However, it can be controlled with lifelong antiviral treatment. The goal of researchers is to use knowledge of the HIV life cycle to create a vaccine and develop a cure.

After a person has been infected with HIV, other immune system components form antibodies to fight HIV. These HIV antibodies typically become present within 3 months after infection. The time between infection and developing antibodies is called the window period. Testing for these antibodies can be done to diagnose HIV.

LEARNING TIP

Being HIV positive means that the person has been infected with the HIV virus. It does not mean that the person has AIDS.

Progression of HIV Infection

The initial infection is followed by a relatively symptom-free period. This is called the clinical latency stage. The virus remains in the lymph nodes, liver, and spleen and reproduces. If the infection is untreated, CD4 T lymphocytes gradually decrease. B lymphocytes also become dysfunctional and dysregulated by HIV progression. B and T lymphocytes normally work together in a healthy immune system. The period from infection to the beginning of the symptomatic stage varies for each person. It averages 8 to 12 years. During this stage, the person is considered to be HIV infected. In the early symptomatic stage of HIV disease, symptoms of the weakening immune system are seen. When the immune system is severely weakened, opportunistic infections and cancers can occur, resulting in a diagnosis of AIDS (see Box 20.1).

LEARNING TIP

Opportunistic diseases are referred to as such because they take advantage of the opportunity to attack a weakened immune system. A healthy immune system would be able fight off these infections and diseases.

PREVENTION

Education and prevention are the best ways to manage the HIV/AIDS epidemic. Education should begin with older school-age children and continue with adults of all ages ("Gerontological Issues").

Gerontological Issues

Older Adults and HIV. In 2014, the Centers for Disease Control and Prevention (2017a) reported that 17% of all persons living with HIV are aged 50 or over. Older adults are often diagnosed with an HIV infection when AIDS is already present. Ask older adults about their sexual and drug use history. Teach preventive measures. Share information on products to reduce transmission of HIV and sexually transmitted infections (STIs). At-risk adults over age 50 are less likely than younger at-risk adults to use condoms during sex. They tend to think of condoms only as a birth control measure. They are also less likely to be tested for HIV.

Erectile dysfunction treatments have contributed to more older adults being sexually active. They may have multiple partners. They are also contracting HIV through same-sex contact.

A decline in the older adult's immune system increases the risk for infection with HIV. Increased vaginal dryness and friability further increase an older woman's susceptibility to HIV infection. The rise in HIV infection among older adults is expected to continue due to a lack of preventative knowledge. With AIDS death rates dropping as a result of more effective treatments, the number of older adults living with HIV will increase.

Symptoms of HIV in older adults can be confused with commonly perceived problems of aging. These include fatigue, decreased endurance, and altered cognitive status. The brain effects of HIV can be mistaken for Alzheimer's disease. This can delay proper treatment.

Mode of Transmission

HIV is a fragile virus. It is only transmitted from person to person through certain body fluids from a person infected with HIV. These fluids include blood, semen, pre-seminal fluid, vaginal secretions, rectal fluids, and breast milk. HIV can be transmitted to others within 2 to 4 weeks of initial infection and then without treatment throughout all phases of HIV infection and AIDS (U.S. Department of Health and Human Services, 2017). HIV is not spread casually. It does not live long outside of the body. HIV needs a portal of entry into the body. Entry portals include a tear in a mucous membrane or nonintact skin, or direct injection into the bloodstream (via needle). Casual contact such as hugging, closed-mouth kissing, shaking hands, or sharing eating utensils, towels, or bathroom fixtures with an HIV-positive person does not transmit HIV. Transmission does not occur by air, water, food, or insects. Since 1985, donated blood has been tested for HIV antibodies. Donated organs are also tested. HIV infection is rare from blood transfusions or organ donation. Transmission within households from contact with HIV-infected blood or body secretions is also rare. Education for those living with someone infected with HIV is important (visit www.cdc.gov/hiv).

Pre-exposure Prophylaxis

Pre-exposure prophylaxis (PrEP), with an ARV, is an effective way to prevent HIV transmission for those who are at high risk of contracting the virus (Fonner et al., 2016). Emtricitabine/tenofovir disoproxil (Truvada) is approved for PrEP. It should be taken once daily consistently.

Counseling

Early knowledge of HIV status helps reduce the spread of HIV infection. The United States Preventive Services Task Force (USPSTF, 2016) recommends routine testing for those aged 15 to 65, pregnant females, or those who have been sexually assaulted. Testing is done either confidentially or anonymously. Permission is needed to release one's test results to others. Posttest counseling is available to help the patient understand the test results, assist with informing sexual partners and drug needle sharers, reduce risk factors, and provide care options, if needed.

Sexual Transmission

HIV can be transmitted through sexual contact with infected body fluids and mucous membranes. Some types of sexual contact carry a higher rate of transmission. Vaginal and anal sex have high rates of transmission for both males and females. Anal sex has the highest risk. It often results in tearing of the mucous membrane. This allows exposure to infected semen. Females have a greater risk for becoming infected. This is because the vagina has a greater area of mucous membranes than the penis. There is also a greater amount of HIV found in semen compared with vaginal secretions. Research has shown that starting early ART for HIV-1 infected individuals prevented HIV transmission to uninfected sexual partners when undetectable viral load was achieved and maintained (Cohen et al., 2016).

Safer Sex Practices

Abstaining from sexual intercourse is the only 100% way to prevent sexual exposure to HIV. A long-term, mutually monogamous sexual relationship is considered safest when both partners are known to be HIV negative. Limiting sexual partners, wearing latex gloves to protect hands during genital or anal contact, using latex condoms and dental dams (latex sheets) correctly and regularly as a barrier for the mouth and genitals or anus (Box 20.2), and understanding safer sex techniques reduce the risk of HIV transmission.

Parenteral Transmission

The best way to prevent parenteral transmission of HIV is to avoid or stop injecting drugs. If a person who injects drugs is unable or unwilling to stop, it is recommended that a new sterile syringe and needle, obtained from pharmacies, is used each time along with new sterile water and new or disinfected preparation equipment. Alcohol swabs should be used to clean the injection site. Afterward, the syringe should be disposed of safely. Drug injection equipment should never be shared or reused. Syringe exchange program availability varies by location, although these programs have been shown to decrease the risk of transmission of HIV and other blood-borne pathogens. If injection equipment is reused, it should be boiled or cleansed with bleach. Sexual activity should be discouraged when judgment is impaired by drug use because protective measures may not be used during this impairment. PrEP with an ARV for non-HIV-infected people who inject drugs can reduce HIV infection.

Autologous (one's own) blood transfusion, when possible, is the safest type of blood transfusion to prevent HIV infection. Donated blood is screened for HIV, but there is a very low chance of HIV transmission from donated blood that is infected but has not yet had time to develop antibodies.

Perinatal Transmission

Guidelines for HIV screening of pregnant women recommend that HIV counselling and testing be offered during routine prenatal care for all pregnant women and again in the third trimester for women at high risk (Panel on Treatment of HIV-Infected Pregnant Women and Prevention of Perinatal Transmission, 2017). All pregnant women who are HIV positive can reduce the risk of perinatal HIV transmission with ART during pregnancy, labor, and delivery. At the time of labor, pregnant women who have not been tested for HIV should be offered rapid HIV tests. Therapy should be started if HIV is confirmed.

Health Care Providers and HIV Prevention

Occupational HIV transmission is rare. Using standard precautions (see Chapter 8), appropriate hand hygiene, and safety devices to prevent needlesticks (e.g., needleless systems, protective covers, and *never* recapping used needles) reduce the risk of HIV exposure. It is essential to use these practices with all patients to protect yourself from exposure and transmission of HIV. If you are unsure of the appropriate **personal protective equipment** (e.g., gloves, gown, goggles, face shield) or isolation precautions to use for the situation, ask your instructor or the patient's nurse before providing care to a patient.

Know the occupational exposure protocol for the agency in which you are practicing. If exposure occurs, wash the exposure site with soap and water immediately. For mucous membrane exposure, flush with water. Then seek immediate medical care. The U.S. Public Health Service guidelines for occupational exposures can be viewed at www.jstor.org/stable/10.1086/672271. Visit www.cdc.gov/niosh/topics/bbp/guidelines.html for National Institute for Occupational Safety and Health guidelines.

HIV SIGNS AND SYMPTOMS

Each patient's HIV infection response is different. Initially, the patient may not have any symptoms but then may develop acute retroviral syndrome. Symptoms of this syndrome are extreme fatigue, headache, fever, lymphadenopathy (enlarged lymph nodes in two sites other than inguinal nodes), diarrhea, or a sore throat (Fig. 20.2 and Table 20.3). Symptoms typically develop 6 to 12 weeks after transmission of HIV. They can last a few days to weeks. The symptoms are usually mild. They are not usually associated with being infected with HIV.

An extended asymptomatic phase can occur. An untreated HIV infection then usually progresses to a symptomatic stage. This stage is seen when the virus has greatly impaired the immune system. The patient may have shortness of breath, fever, weight loss, fatigue, night sweats, persistent diarrhea, oral or vaginal candidiasis ulcers, dry skin, skin lesions, peripheral neuropathy, shingles (varicella zoster virus reactivation), seizures, or dementia. In the final stage of HIV infection, AIDS is diagnosed when the CD4 T-lymphocyte count is below 200 or opportunistic infections and diseases occur (see Box 20.1).

COMPLICATIONS

Complications from HIV and AIDS vary from patient to patient. With ART, fewer complications are seen than in the past. Some, such as Kaposi sarcoma (a connective tissue tumor), are rarely seen anymore.

Box 20.2

Patient Education

Condom Use to Prevent HIV Transmission

Condoms should be:
- New for each sex act.
- Made of latex (highly effective) because other materials have large pores that allow HIV to pass.
- Undamaged and used before expiration date.
- Applied before partner is touched. (Tip of condom is held while unrolling over erect penis, allowing room at tip for semen collection.)
- Used with adequate amounts of only water-soluble lubricant. (Petroleum or oil-based lubricants such as petroleum jelly, cooking oil, shortening, or lotions can damage latex condoms.)
- Replaced if broken. (If ejaculation occurs before replacement, immediate use of a spermicide can give some protection.)
- Withdrawn from partner by holding condom against base of erect penis to avoid semen leakage.

CD4+ T-lymphocyte Count During HIV Disease and AIDS

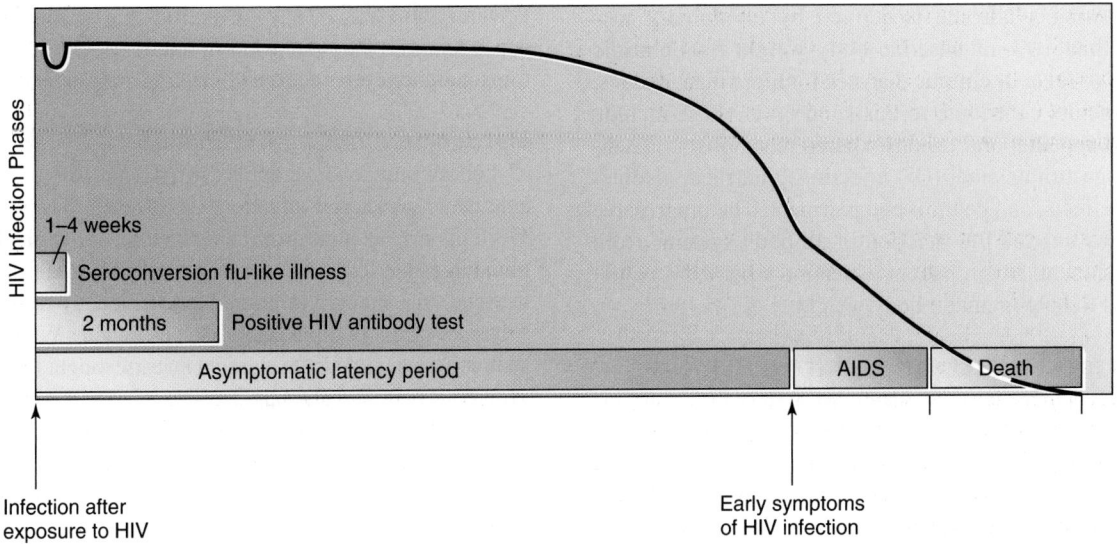

FIGURE 20.2 Typical phases of HIV infection, AIDS development, and CD4+ T-lymphocyte counts without treatment. Length of latency period varies but is usually many years. As CD4+ T-lymphocyte counts drop, symptoms, AIDS, opportunistic infections, and then death can result.

Table 20.3

HIV/AIDS Summary

Signs and Symptoms	Initially vary; none or acute retroviral syndrome
	Asymptomatic phase
	Immune system impairment (e.g., dyspnea, fever, weight loss, fatigue, night sweats, persistent diarrhea, oral or vaginal candidiasis ulcers, dry skin, skin lesions, peripheral neuropathy, shingles, or dementia)
	AIDS diagnosed when CD4 T-lymphocyte count is below 200 or opportunistic infections and diseases occur
Diagnostic Tests	HIV antibody/antigen combination immunoassay nucleic acid test
	Antibody differentiation immunoassay
	Complete blood cell count/lymphocyte count
	CD4 T-lymphocyte count
	Viral load testing
	Genotyping
Therapeutic Measures	Cellular chemokine receptor type 5 (CCR5) antagonists
	Fusion inhibitors
	Integrase inhibitors
	Non-nucleoside reverse transcriptase inhibitors (NNRTIs)
	Nucleoside reverse transcriptase inhibitors (NRTIs)
	Post attachment inhibitors
	Protease inhibitors
Complications	AIDS wasting syndrome
	Opportunistic infections and cancer
	AIDS dementia complex
Priority Nursing Diagnoses	*Ineffective Protection*
	Risk for Injury
	Ineffective Coping

AIDS Wasting Syndrome

AIDS wasting syndrome is defined by involuntary loss of more than 10% of baseline body weight plus chronic weakness or fever or chronic diarrhea for more than 30 days. Several factors contribute to this syndrome. These include decreased appetite, oral lesions, altered metabolism, malabsorption, gastrointestinal (GI) infections, diarrhea, medication side effects, and cognitive impairment. The progressive weight loss impairs the function of all body systems from malnourishment. Begin patient education when HIV is first diagnosed to help maintain body weight.

HIV-Associated Neurocognitive Disorder

HIV infection in the brain or other parts of the central nervous system (CNS) results in varying CNS conditions. Examples include asymptomatic neurocognitive impairment, minor neurocognitive disorder, and HIV-associated dementia (HIV encephalopathy or AIDS dementia complex). Symptoms range from mild to severe and can include memory impairment, personality changes, hallucinations, leg weakness, loss of balance, and slower responses. In advanced AIDS, with ART, minor cognitive motor disorder is most common. When CNS changes occur, patient safety is an important consideration.

NURSING CARE TIP

AIDS wasting syndrome is challenging. Do not give up! Develop interventions to help increase the patient's appetite and calorie intake. Small, frequent meals are usually helpful. A registered dietitian can be a helpful member of the care team for HIV patients.

Cancer and Opportunistic Infections

Why does a person with HIV or AIDS have increased risk for cancer and opportunistic infections? With an impaired immune system, cancer incidence rises because the abnormal cancer cells are not being destroyed. Opportunistic infections, which a healthy immune system should fight off, cannot be fought. Opportunistic infections can be viral, bacterial, mycobacterial, fungal, protozoal, or parasitic. Some opportunistic infections can now be prevented with prophylactic treatments.

Candida Albicans

Candida albicans is a fungus normally found in the GI tract. It does not cause infection in a person with a healthy immune system. In a person with AIDS, overgrowth of this fungus occurs. Candidiasis of the mouth or esophagus is common in AIDS. Signs and symptoms of candidiasis include oral or esophageal pain, dysphagia, and yellow-white plaques that look like cottage cheese in the mouth and throat. Nutrition can be affected by oral or esophageal candidiasis. Recurrent vaginal candidiasis, with severe itching and a white discharge, is common in women with AIDS.

Cytomegalovirus

Cytomegalovirus (CMV) infection can be serious. It can cause retinitis. This can result in blindness. Signs and symptoms include fever, fatigue, diarrhea, GI upset, and hepatitis.

Mycobacterium Avium Complex

Mycobacterium avium complex (MAC) is a serious nontuberculous mycobacterial infection. Occurrence rises when CD4 T-lymphocyte counts drop below 50 cells/microL. MAC is found in water, foods like raw or partially cooked fish or shellfish, and soil. A prophylactic antibiotic may be given when CD4 T-lymphocyte counts fall below 50 cells/microL. With infection, symptoms can include fever, night sweats, weight loss, fatigue, abdominal pain, and diarrhea. Treatment includes a combination of antibiotics for at least 12 months. These might include clarithromycin or azithromycin, with ethambutol and rifabutin.

Pneumocystis Pneumonia

Pneumocystis pneumonia (PCP) is caused by the fungus *Pneumocystis jiroveci* in immunocompromised persons. PCP develops slowly and produces shortness of breath, fever, and dry cough. When CD4 T-lymphocyte counts fall below 350 cells/microL, prophylactic oral trimethoprim-sulfamethoxazole (TMP-SMX [Bactrim, Septra, Cotrim]) is recommended. PCP is less likely to occur than in the past with TMP-SMX. However, it remains a concern for those with HIV or AIDS. The preferred treatment agent for PCP is TMP-SMX. If not tolerated, other possible agents are listed in Table 20.4. Oxygen can be used, and steroids help reduce lung inflammation.

Tuberculosis

Tuberculosis is a bacterial infection caused by the mycobacterium tuberculosis. Symptoms include dyspnea, cough, chest pain, fever, night sweats, and weight loss. A Mantoux tuberculin skin test with tuberculin-purified protein derivative should be performed at least yearly in people with HIV infection. Induration of 5 mm or more is defined as a positive result in patients with HIV infection (see Chapter 31). This defines the onset of AIDS.

 ## DIAGNOSIS

HIV screening is recommended for people from 15 to 65 years of age at least once (USPSTF, 2016). Those with increased risk outside of this age range should be screened. For those at high risk, screening should occur more frequently.

Finger stick blood, oral fluid (e.g., OraQuick Rapid HIV test, which tests a swab of complete upper and lower outer gums), and serum specimens can be used for HIV testing. Urine can also be tested but is slightly less accurate and rarely used. Results can be available in less than 20 minutes with the Multispot HIV-1/HIV-2 Rapid Test or in 1 hour for immunoassay testing. Consumer-controlled test kits (home sample collection devices) can be purchased at drug stores. The blood sample for this testing is mailed to a laboratory as directed. The person then anonymously calls for the results, counseling, and referral, if needed.

After infection with HIV, HIV antigen can be detected within 2 weeks of the exposure. Antibodies form usually within 3 weeks to 3 months. It can be longer in some cases (visit www.cdc.gov/hiv/basics/testing.html). Early-detection HIV tests are available that detect HIV infection as soon as 1 week after potential exposure.

HIV Antibody and Antigen Tests

In 2014, the CDC updated their algorithm recommendations for HIV testing and diagnosis (Branson et al., 2014). They recommend beginning with a U.S. Food and Drug Administration (FDA)-approved antigen/antibody combination (fourth generation) immunoassay that detects both HIV-1 and HIV-2 antibodies and HIV-1 p24 antigen. Established infection with HIV-1 or HIV-2 and acute infection for HIV-1 is determined. If the test is positive, an antibody immunoassay test to differentiate between HIV-1 and HIV-2 antibodies should be done. If the combination immunoassay is positive but the antibody differentiation immunoassay is nonreactive or inconclusive, an FDA-approved HIV-1 nucleic acid test should be done for confirmation. The updated algorithm has allowed earlier detection of HIV and fewer false positives for those within the "window period" (visit www.cdc.gov/hiv/testing/laboratorytests.html).

Complete Blood Cell Count/Lymphocyte Count

Patients with HIV are susceptible to leukopenia, lymphopenia, anemia, and thrombocytopenia. This is due to the HIV infection and as a complication of ART. A complete blood cell count (CBC) with a lymphocyte count should be obtained. The CBC is repeated as needed.

CD4 T-Lymphocyte Count

The CD4 T-lymphocyte count is essential for initial evaluation of the status of the immune system and the need for ART. In healthy adults, CD4 levels range from 332 to 1,642 cells/microL. In people with HIV disease, CD4 levels drop. After ART is begun, a rapid CD4 increase occurs during the first 3 months, with an increase of 50 to 150 cells/microL per year. This is followed by an annual increase of 50 to 100 cells/microL until stabilization occurs, which is considered a satisfactory response. CD4 T-lymphocyte counts should be performed before ART begins, 3 months after ART is begun, every 3 to 6 months for the first 2 years, and then annually for consistently suppressed viral load with a CD4 count at 300 to 500 cells/mm³ (Panel on Antiretroviral Guidelines for Adults and Adolescents, 2017).

Viral Load Testing

Viral load testing measures the amount of HIV RNA in the plasma. It shows the risk of the disease progressing without treatment, the risk of opportunistic infections, and, most importantly, response to ART. ART usually produces a 50% decrease in total-body HIV levels within just a few days. Viral load testing should be performed before starting ART and then within 1 month afterward, continuing every 1 to 2 months until viral load is suppressed to < 200 copies/mL, then every 3 to 4 months for the first 2 years. After 2 years, monitoring for consistently suppressed viral load is done every 6 months or for detectable viremia every 3 months (Panel on Antiretroviral Guidelines for Adults and Adolescents, 2017). The goal of ART is to obtain and maintain an ultrasensitive, **undetectable viral load**. With ART, an optimal viral load would be less than 20 to 75 copies/mL or below the level of detection, which is under 40 copies/mL. Failure to respond to ART is considered to be a viral load above 200 copies/mL. Drug resistance testing is recommended for a viral load greater than 1,000 copies/mL.

Genotyping

Genotyping measures resistance to currently available ARV treatments. This guides health care providers (HCPs) in choosing treatment that will be most effective against a person's virus.

General Tests

Standard serological testing for syphilis is recommended annually in patients who are sexually active. Hepatitis A, B, and C serologies and liver chemistry panels are done because of the high incidence of concurrent hepatitis coinfection in HIV-positive patients. Coinfections can influence the course of either the patient's HIV or the coinfection. Coinfections can also affect HIV treatment options.

THERAPEUTIC MEASURES

The goal of HIV therapy is to suppress the virus to protect health and prevent or delay development of opportunistic diseases and an AIDS diagnosis. In 2016, the federal Guidelines for the Use of Antiretroviral Agents in Adults and Adolescents Living With HIV was updated (Panel on Antiretroviral Guidelines for Adults and Adolescents, 2017). It is recommended that all patients with HIV be started on ART, regardless of their CD4 T-lymphocyte count. To increase life expectancy and treatment cost effectiveness, prophylactic treatment for certain opportunistic infections is recommended. These include hepatitis A and hepatitis B, herpes simplex virus, MAC, and PCP (Table 20.4). Other opportunistic infections are treated if they occur.

Antiretroviral Therapy

ARV medications inhibit reproduction of HIV but do not kill it. ARV medication classes have been developed to act on processes specific to HIV (see "Pathophysiology" section). Use of these medications in combination is referred to as antiretroviral therapy, or ART. Each ARV medication class affects HIV in a different stage of its life cycle. Usually, at least three medications in at least two classes of treatment categories are used in ART (Table 20.5). This makes medication therapy more effective and reduces drug resistance. Most people treated with ART achieve undetectable viral loads

Table 20.4

Treatment for AIDS-Related Conditions

Opportunistic Infection/ Complication	Treatment
Candidiasis	amphotericin B (Fungizone), fluconazole (Diflucan), isavuconazole (Cresemba), ketoconazole (Nizoral), nystatin (Nyamyc)
Cytomegalovirus retinitis	ganciclovir (Cytovene)
Hepatitis B virus	Hepatitis B virus vaccine when HIV infection diagnosed, unless already infected with hepatitis B
Hepatitis C virus	interferon, lamivudine, tenofovir for infection; pegylated interferon and ribavirin
Herpes simplex, herpes zoster, varicella zoster	acyclovir (Zovirax), valacyclovir, famciclovir, foscarnet
Influenza	annual influenza vaccine
Mycobacterium avium complex (MAC)	azithromycin, clarithromycin, ethambutol
Pneumococcal pneumonia	pneumococcal vaccine when HIV infection diagnosed
Pneumocystis pneumonia (PCP)	trimethoprim-sulfamethoxazole (Bactrim, Septra, Cotrim), dapsone, atovaquone, pentamidine isethionate
Tuberculosis	Tuberculosis skin test; drug therapy per Centers for Disease Control and Prevention guidelines: pyrazinamide, isoniazid (Laniazid, Isotamine), ethambutol (Myambutol)
AIDS wasting syndrome	*Patient education:* Eat frequent small high-calorie and high-protein meals with snacks daily. Eat low-residue diet for diarrhea control. Control odors if they cause nausea. Develop easy meal plan (e.g., favorite foods, meal programs, frozen dinners, cold food to control nausea). Use antiemetics, appetite stimulants, and/or testosterone. Rest or listen to music. Numb painful oral sores with ice, popsicles, or topical analgesic; avoid spicy foods. Use artificial saliva for dry mouth. Use nutritional supplements. Use Supplemental Nutrition Assistance Program, community food pantries, or free meal programs as needed. Exercise to increase muscle mass. Take medications prescribed to treat wasting.

within six months or less. Having a durably undetectable viral load (viral load is undetectable for at least 6 months after first undetectable test result) prevents transmission of HIV. It also allows CD4 T-lymphocyte counts to rise to protect health and promote quality of life.

The major cause of drug resistance is not taking medications as directed. *Adherence* is the term used to describe taking medications exactly as directed. Teaching adherence is important. Drug resistance can occur when a person with resistant HIV exposes someone else with HIV to the resistant HIV. This can happen with unprotected sex or shared injected drug use.

NURSING CARE TIP

Teach patients that it is essential to take every medication every day as ordered. Missing just 10% of medication doses (1 out of 10) decreases effectiveness to about 80%, depending on the drug. This means that, if a patient is taking three to seven pills each day, missing one to two pills a week will decrease the medication's effectiveness by 20%. When ART is interrupted, HIV can reemerge and multiply again to detectable levels in the blood.

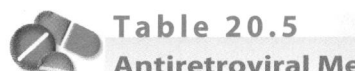

Table 20.5
Antiretroviral Medications for HIV Infection

Medication Class/Action

Non-Nucleoside Reverse Transcriptase Inhibitors (NNRTIs)

Block reverse transcriptase enzyme activity to prevent conversion of HIV RNA to HIV DNA.

Examples	Nursing Implications
delavirdine mesylate (Rescriptor) efavirenz (Sustiva) etravirine (Intelence) nevirapine (Viramune, Viramune XR) rilpivirine (Edurant)	Monitor for rash (especially first month); Stevens-Johnson syndrome can occur, requiring discontinuation of the drug. Can be life-threatening. *Teach:* Report rash immediately. Monitor white blood cell count, liver tests, especially with history of hepatitis B or C.

Nucleoside/Nucleotide Reverse Transcriptase Inhibitors (NRTIs/NtRTIs)

Block reverse transcriptase enzyme by binding to the enzyme to prevent conversion of HIV RNA to HIV DNA.

Examples	Nursing Implications
abacavir sulfate (Ziagen)* abacavir sulfate/lamivudine (Epzicom) didanosine (Videx, Videx EC) emtricitabine (Emtriva) lamivudine (Epivir) lamivudine/zidovudine (Combivir) stavudine (Zerit, Zerit XR) tenofovir disoproxil fumarate (Viread)** abacavir sulfate/lamivudine/zidovudine (Trizivir) emtricitabine/tenofovir disoproxil fumarate (Truvada) zidovudine (Retrovir)	Monitor for peripheral neuropathy, bone marrow suppression, lactic acidosis, and kidney and liver function. *Report flu-like symptoms immediately as a life-threatening condition can develop. **Monitor for hepatomegaly with steatosis and for lactic acidosis, which can be fatal, especially in women. ***Teach:* Take 2 hours before or 1 hour after didanosine.

Protease Inhibitors

Bind to active site of HIV protease enzyme (cuts reproduced HIV strands), interrupting formation of mature viral particles.

Examples	Nursing Implications
atazanavir sulfate (Reyataz) darunavir (Prezista) darunavir/cobicistat (Prezcobix) fosamprenavir calcium (Lexiva)* indinavir sulfate (Crixivan)** lopinavir/ritonavir (Kaletra) nelfinavir mesylate (Viracept) ritonavir (Norvir) saquinavir mesylate (Invirase) tipranavir (Aptivus)	Manage gastrointestinal symptoms. Monitor lab results. Watch for increased bleeding in patients with hemophilia. *Report rash. *Should not be given if patient is allergic to sulfa. ***Teach*: Importance of hydration (at least 48 oz of liquids in 24 hours).

Continued

Table 20.5

Antiretroviral Medications for HIV Infection—cont'd

Medication Class/Action

Fusion Inhibitors

Block HIV-1 fusion with the CD4 cell membrane to prevent cell entry.

Examples	Nursing Implications
enfuvirtide (Fuzeon)	*Teach*:
	Subcutaneous injection technique and injection site rotation.
	If dizzy, do not drive.

Cellular Chemokine Receptor Type 5 (CCR5) Antagonists

Block CCR5 receptor preventing HIV-1 entry into CD4 cells.

Examples	Nursing Implications
maraviroc (Celsentri, Selzentry)	Monitor for liver problems.

Post-Attachment Inhibitors

Blocks binding to CCR5 and CXCR4 coreceptors after HIV-1 binds to CD4 receptor. For adults with multidrug resistant HIV-1 infection failing current antiretroviral regimen.

Examples	Nursing Implications
ibalizumab (Trogarzo)	Monitor post intravenous infusion for side effects.

Integrase Inhibitors

Block HIV from combining with its genetic code so more copies of itself cannot be made.

Examples	Nursing Implications
dolutegravir (Tivicay)	*Teach*:
elvitegravir (Vitekta)	Side effects to report.
raltegravir (Isentress, Isentress HD)	

Combination Agents

Multiclass single tablet regimens; cobicistat: Inhibits metabolizing liver enzymes; combined with HIV agents, enhances their effect with fewer side effects.

Examples	Nursing Implications
dolutegravir/abacavir/lamivudine (Triumeq)	See individual agents above.
efavirenz/emtricitabine/tenofovir disoproxil fumarate (Atripla)	Patient compliance is key to efficacy. Combination medications increase patient compliance with fewer tablets to take.
efavirenz/lamivudine/tenofovir disoproxil fumarate (Symfi, Symfi Lo)	
elvitegravir/cobicistat/emtricitabine/tenofovir alafenamide (Genvoya)	
elvitegravir/cobicistat/emtricitabine/tenofovir disoproxil fumarate (Stribild)	
lamivudine/tenofovir disoproxil fumarate (Cimduo)	
rilpivirine/emtricitabine/tenofovir disoproxil fumarate (Eviplera)	
rilpivirine/tenofovir alafenamide/emtricitabine (Odefsey)	

Anti-HIV drugs can have side effects. If they occur, the drug regimen can be changed or interventions can be used to help control the side effects. Teach the patient about potential side effects. Instruct them to report them immediately. Rashes (e.g., from TMP-SMX [trimethoprim-sulfamethoxazole]) or abdominal pain (e.g., from AZT [Retrovir]) can be serious or life-threatening.

When someone with a suppressed immune system (very low CD4 T-lymphocyte count) is started on ART, the person can experience immune reconstitution syndrome. The patient's immune system can be greatly improving, but the patient feels worse. This is because, when the patient's immune system was severely damaged, immune responses were too weak or absent to produce the signs of an existing infection. When immune function improves, the immune system begins to fight off infections already present in the body. Symptoms then occur. This can be a serious, sometimes fatal condition that can occur a few weeks after ART starts. Educate the patient to report immediately any symptoms of opportunistic infections after starting therapy. This allows for prompt diagnosis and treatment of the infection. It can save the person's life.

Treatment as Prevention

Research has shown that antiretroviral therapy (ART) that results in undetectable blood levels prevents transmission of HIV sexually. So those infected with HIV that take ART as prescribed and achieve and maintain an undetectable viral load have effectively no risk of sexually transmitting the virus to an HIV-negative partner (Centers for Disease Control, 2017). It takes 1 to 6 months of ART to achieve undetectable viral loads plus 6 months of maintained undetectable viral levels after the first undetected test result (known as durably undetected) to effectively have no risk of transmitting HIV sexually (National Institutes of Health and Infectious Disease, 2017; see www.niaid.nih.gov/news-events/10-things-know-about-hiv-suppression).

The Undetectable=Untransmittable (U=U) Campaign (Prevention Access Campaign, 2016; see www.preventionaccess.org/undetectable) was developed to promote this important information that is giving hope to those with HIV that they can live healthy lives without fear of transmitting HIV. Many worldwide health organizations are publicly sharing this message to reduce the stigma associated with being HIV positive. This may encourage more people to be tested and treated to prevent the transmission of HIV.

Nursing Process for the Adult Patient With HIV/AIDS

Data Collection

Ongoing monitoring is important for the patient with HIV/AIDS to detect problems early. Health history information is obtained (Box 20.3). Determining the patient's understanding of HIV/AIDS information is necessary for planning and teaching. A physical examination provides data on the

Patient Perspective

Jennifer. As a productive, single mother of three, I never expected to hear the term HIV infected, but at 45 years old that diagnosis became my reality. In February 2016, I had viral symptoms that progressively manifested into AIDS and my world turned upside down in a split second. I was immediately consumed with shame and fear, but most importantly a small glimpse of hope. Within weeks of my diagnosis, my body responded as expected to treatment and my psychological state healed at literally the same pace.

What I eventually discovered is that an 8-month-long sexual relationship was with a high-risk individual. He was diagnosed with HIV shortly after we ended our relationship and left "the call" up to the clinic that helped him. They never called. Almost 3 years later, I was on my deathbed. My HIV doctor confirmed that I would have died had it been 10 to 15 years earlier, before effective therapies became available.

What I would like for people to learn from my story is that if they are at high risk, or if they have been exposed to someone who is at high risk, they should be tested for HIV every year. People with HIV, whose antiretroviral therapy is effective and who continue to take their medication as prescribed, can not only become undetectable (virus undetected in blood), but they are also no longer able to transmit the virus sexually. (U=U, Undetectable= Untransmittable). It's imperative that medical professionals treat people living with HIV as human beings. We are not contagious in every aspect of casual contact. We feel small nuanced stigma and it's a human rights failure on every level when our treatment is handled in any other manner. With today's medical advancements in HIV treatment, I take one pill a day, my virus is undetectable, and I'm back to doing things that I love like surfing and skateboarding. Life is good!

LEARNING TIP

Key points to remember:

- HIV and AIDS are disease labels, not people labels.
- Each person reacts to an HIV or AIDS diagnosis differently.
- It is not the HIV that ultimately causes death; it is an opportunistic infection or disease that the compromised immune system is unable to fight off, even with medical intervention.
- With today's antiretroviral therapy, HIV has changed from being a life-ending infection to a chronically managed disease.
- With ART, a person who achieves and then maintains an undetectable viral load for 6 months and continues to do so is effectively unable to transmit HIV sexually, thus reducing the fear and stigma of being HIV positive.

Box 20.3

Data Collection: Health History Information for HIV/AIDS

- Demographic data (e.g., gender, age, marital status, occupation, residence, pets)
- Date of diagnosis of HIV or AIDS
- Height/weight (also weight loss)
- Allergies
- Current health status and concerns
- Immunizations
- Past medical history and surgeries
- Infections/cancers (see Box 20.1)
- Family history
- Medication history of antivirals used with reason for discontinuing

- Current prescribed medications, over-the-counter medications, supplements
- For females, gynecological history, last Pap test
- Sexually transmitted infections and treatments
- Social and sexual history, risk behaviors, safe sex practices
- Needlestick/blood exposure, injection drug use, blood transfusions/treatment for hemophilia
- Lifestyle (e.g., nutrition, exercise, sleep)
- Tobacco use
- Drug and alcohol use
- Occupational history

effects of HIV/AIDS and ART. Monitoring the patient's level of pain is ongoing. Many patients with HIV do not have pain related to their HIV. Signs and symptoms of opportunistic infections are also noted.

Nursing Diagnoses

See "Nursing Care Plan for the Patient With HIV/AIDS." Additional nursing diagnoses are individualized to the patient's presenting symptoms.

Nursing Care Plan for the Patient With HIV/AIDS

Nursing Diagnosis: *Ineffective Protection* related to deficient immunity and inadequate nutrition
Expected Outcomes: The patient will remain free of infection. The patient and/or caregiver explains precautions to take to prevent infection.
Evaluation of Outcomes: Is the patient free of infection? Does the patient and/or caregiver explain precautions for preventing infection?

Intervention	Rationale	Evaluation
Identify patient's risk factors, such as CD4 T-lymphocyte counts, skin condition, portals of entry for infections, and presence of infections.	*Status of risk factors provides input for plan for care.*	Does patient have risk factors present?
Use hand hygiene, standard precautions, and strict aseptic technique as required for procedures.	*Protect patient from microorganisms. Transmission of microorganisms can occur in both directions between the patient and caregiver.*	Are correct hand hygiene, standard precautions, and strict aseptic technique utilized?
Inform patient and caregiver of techniques to avoid transmission of microorganisms, including excellent hand hygiene and avoiding those who are ill or keeping others away from the patient if ill.	*It is difficult for the weakened immune to fight infections.*	Does patient and caregiver demonstrate correct hand hygiene? Does patient and caregiver state understanding of remaining apart when ill?
Monitor and report signs of infection or sepsis, including elevation of temperature or change in mental status.	*Fever may be the only sign of infection in an immunosuppressed patient; mental status changes are also a sign of sepsis. These are signs of a medical emergency.*	Is patient's temperature normal?

Nursing Care Plan for the Patient With HIV/AIDS—cont'd

Intervention	Rationale	Evaluation
Avoid invasive procedures, if able.	*Invasive procedures can be an entry portal for pathogens.*	Are invasive procedures avoided?
Promote skin integrity with frequent turning, optimum mobilization, use of specialized mattress and chair pads, gentle washing/drying of skin, application of emollients as needed to keep skin dry, and prompt treatment of any skin injury.	*Skin is the body's first line of defense.*	Does patient's skin remain intact and infection free?

Nursing Diagnosis: *Ineffective Coping* related to potentially terminal disease and progressive debility
Expected Outcome: The patient will use effective coping skills.
Evaluation of Outcome: Does the patient report an increase in psychological comfort?

Intervention	Rationale	Evaluation
Establish and maintain an open and trusting therapeutic relationship.	*Effective communication is based on trust—assurance of confidentiality is essential.*	Does patient talk about concerns with the caregiver?
Ask patient to describe prior coping mechanisms used.	*Prior effective coping mechanisms can be encouraged and utilized during patient care.*	Does patient state coping mechanisms are effective?
Encourage patient to express feelings and concerns, and use active listening during interactions. Contact a counselor, chaplain, or AIDS support worker if patient wishes.	*Talking about feelings and concerns helps defuse anger, clarify needs, and relieve tension.*	Does patient verbalize concerns?
Offer patient information about support groups and then arrange it, if desired.	*Social support can help patient cope.*	Does patient utilize and state satisfaction with coping resources?

Nursing Diagnosis: *Risk for Injury* related to impaired mobility, weakness, fatigue, electrolyte imbalances, neurologic impairment, and sedative effects of pain medications
Expected Outcome: The patient will remain free from injury.
Evaluation of Outcome: Is the patient free from injury?

Intervention	Rationale	Evaluation
Evaluate patient for fall risk and take precautions to prevent falls, such as assisting an unsteady patient with ambulation.	*Falls from weaknesses can cause injury.*	Is patient free from fall injuries?
Identify potential hazards in patient's environment and eliminate or modify them.	*Elimination of hazards decreases accidents and injuries.*	Are hazards removed from the environment?

(nursing care plan continues on page 332)

Nursing Care Plan for the Patient With HIV/AIDS—cont'd

Intervention	Rationale	Evaluation
Institute safety measures as required, such as close observation, frequent reorientation, two staff members for ambulation, use of side rails, bed motion alarm, or a room near nurse's station.	*Protection of patient against inadvertent removal of tubes or equipment, falls, and other injuries can require extraordinary measures due to neurologic damage.*	Are safety measures effective for patient?
Instruct patient on avoiding hazards.	*Patients can help avoid injury if they understand hazards.*	Is patient effectively avoiding hazards, or is patient a danger to self?

Planning and Implementation

HIV/AIDS can affect every system of the body and every aspect of a person's life. Nurses can positively influence a patient with HIV/AIDS by providing a nonjudgmental approach, empathy, and psychological support. All patients will need protection from infection and teaching. Other types of care will depend on a patient's condition.

INEFFECTIVE PROTECTION. Caregivers should use excellent hand hygiene to protect the patient. Those with an infection, such as a cold, should not care for the patient with HIV/AIDS. To help reduce infection risk, extensive patient education is needed (Table 20.6). The patient is taught signs of infection to report to the HCP immediately (see Patient Teaching Guidelines, "Signs and Symptoms of Opportunistic Infections to Report," on Davis Edge). Treatment of opportunistic infections is most effective when begun early.

DEFICIT KNOWLEDGE. Extensive teaching is needed for patients to understand the chronic, potentially life-threatening nature of HIV (see previous "Prevention" section). Understanding medication regimens is vital to prevent drug resistance and reduce the risk of disease progression.

MEDICATIONS. Encourage the patient to take medications exactly as instructed. It is important to stress that medication doses must not be missed. Use memory aids such as alarm watches to assist the patient to remember to take medications on time. Teach that if a dose is missed it should be taken as soon as possible, unless it is close to the time of the next dose. Doses should not be doubled. Missing doses of medication could cause therapy failure because viral loads can rise and resistance to treatment can develop. HIV/AIDS medications can potentially cause severe reactions. Encourage the patient to contact the HCP promptly for side effects or questions.

IMPAIRED GAS EXCHANGE. PCP is a potential respiratory infection that occurs in AIDS (see Table 20.4). With a respiratory condition, the goal is to maintain oxygenation within normal limits and reduce dyspnea. Monitoring the patient's vital signs, including respiratory rate, depth, rhythm, and oxygen saturation, is important. Oxygen therapy may be ordered. Elevating the head of the bed may aid breathing. Assisting with activities will help reduce patient fatigue.

DIARRHEA. Diarrhea can be caused by HIV infection, opportunistic infections, or ART. An antimotility agent can be prescribed. Consulting a dietitian for dietary changes helps reduce diarrhea (e.g., low-residue diet, no dairy products, no spicy foods, no caffeine or alcohol). Thorough cleansing of the anal area after each stool is a must. Ointments can be applied to protect and soothe the anal area from excoriation. Sitz baths can also be soothing.

FATIGUE. Some patients with HIV experience fatigue. Other causes of fatigue include infections, medications, anemia, dehydration, depression, and poor nutrition. The patient can manage fatigue by alternating periods of activity and rest. Tasks that use more energy should be planned at times when the patient will be most energetic.

FOOD AND WATER SAFETY. Ensuring food and water safety are vital to an immunocompromised patient (see Table 20.6). For symptoms of foodborne or waterborne infection (e.g., diarrhea, nausea, vomiting, abdominal cramps, headache, fever), teach the patient to report them to the HCP immediately.

IMBALANCED NUTRITION: LESS THAN BODY REQUIREMENTS. Maintaining nutrition is vital but challenging ("Nutrition Notes"). Along with adequate nutrition, exercise helps maintain muscle mass ("Evidence-Based Practice"), promotes relaxation, aids sleep, and gives the person a sense of control and well-being.

IMPAIRED ORAL MUCOUS MEMBRANE. Oral or esophageal candidiasis is more common in the late stage of AIDS. The painful lesions interfere with swallowing and nutrition. In

Table 20.6

Patient Teaching: Preventing Opportunistic Infections

Environmental/Occupational

To protect from:	*Consider risk and prevent exposure to infectious agents from:*
Tuberculosis	Health care settings, correctional facilities, homeless shelters
Cytomegalovirus (CMV), cryptosporidiosis, hepatitis A, giardiasis	Child-care settings: wash hands after diaper changing/body fluid contact.
Cryptosporidiosis, toxoplasmosis, salmonellosis, campylobacteriosis	Animal contact: exposure possible from veterinary work, pet stores, farms.
Cryptosporidiosis, toxoplasmosis, histoplasmosis, coccidioidomycosis	Gardening/soil contact: avoid gardening/houseplant care or bird-roosting site or soil, cleaning chicken coops. Wear gloves and mask and wash hands after soil contact.

Food/Water Safety

To prevent or protect from:	*General measures for home or restaurants:*
Foodborne and waterborne infections caused by bacterial, viral, protozoal, or parasitic pathogens	Food handlers must practice excellent hand hygiene. Discard food past expiration date and dented or swollen cans. Control insects and rodents to prevent food contamination. Disinfect kitchen counters and food preparation appliances (e.g., cutting boards, can openers). Avoid cross-contamination of foods with uncooked meat on food preparation surfaces. Do not thaw foods at room temperature as freezing does not kill bacteria in foods. Maintain adequate refrigeration and cooking temperatures. *Foods to avoid:* Buffets and salad bars Cheese (e.g., soft cheeses, which can harbor bacteria, such as feta, brie, camembert, blue veined, queso fresco) Dairy (e.g., unpasteurized milk/dairy products and fruit juice, raw seed sprouts) Eggs (e.g., raw/undercooked eggs and foods with raw eggs, such as hollandaise sauce, Caesar dressing, mayonnaise, uncooked batters, ice cream, eggnog) Meat if not cooked until internal temperature is 180°F (82.2°C) for poultry or 165°F (73.8°C) for red meats with no trace of pink Seafood raw or undercooked
Cryptosporidiosis, giardiasis	Foods to avoid or cook until steaming hot: delicatessen foods, leftovers, meat spreads, ready-to-eat, and refrigerated pâtés.
Hepatitis A, campylobacteriosis, *Escherichia coli,* giardiasis, leptospirosis, norovirus, rotavirus, shigellosis	*Water safety:* Use safe water supply or, when unsure, boil water for 1 minute for drinking or making ice cubes. Drink bottled water purified from reverse osmosis, filtration through absolute 1-micrometer filter, or distillation (only safe methods) in areas where water sources are known not to be safe. (For information, visit www.bottledwater.org.) Bottled or canned carbonated soft drinks, commercially packaged unrefrigerated beverages, pasteurized beverages, and beers are safe. Avoid beverages made from tap water in public places in areas where water sources are known not to be safe. Avoid public drinking fountains and water directly from lakes or rivers.

Continued

Table 20.6

Patient Teaching: Preventing Opportunistic Infections—cont'd

Sexual Relations	
To protect from:	*General measures:*
Sexually transmitted infections, herpes simplex virus, CMV, human papillomavirus, resistant HIV strain	Always use latex (if no allergy) condom for every sex act.
Intestinal infections: amebiasis, hepatitis A, cryptosporidiosis, shigellosis, campylobacteriosis, giardiasis	Avoid oral-anal contact or use dental dams; use latex gloves for hand-anal contact; wash hands and genitals with warm soapy water after contact.
Hepatitis A	Get hepatitis A vaccine.
Hepatitis B	Get hepatitis B vaccine

Injection Drug Use	
To protect from:	*General measures:*
Hepatitis A, hepatitis B, hepatitis C, resistant HIV strain	Get hepatitis A and B vaccines. Stop using injection drugs and enter substance abuse treatment. If unable to stop, never reuse or share syringes, needles, water, or drug preparation equipment. If shared, use bleach and water to clean equipment. Use sterile syringes from pharmacies or community syringe exchange programs and dispose of safely. Use clean water and equipment and new alcohol swab.

Pet-Related Issues	
To protect from:	*General measures:*
Cryptosporidium, Salmonella, Campylobacter spp. infection	Avoid pet feces/diarrhea; seek veterinary treatment for pet's diarrheal illness. Counsel on pet contact risks but recognize emotional benefits of pets and do not suggest parting with pet. Immunize pets. For new pets, avoid those younger than 6 months old (and cats younger than 1 year old); obtain pets from known sanitary source; avoid strays; wash hands after handling pets.
Toxoplasmosis, *Bartonella* spp. infection, salmonellosis, campylobacteriosis	Cat ownership increases risk from litter box cleaning, scratches, bites, licking, and fleas. If patient must clean litter box daily, wear gloves and wash hands well afterward. Keep cats indoors to avoid hunting infected prey.
Cryptococcus neoformans, Mycobacterium avium, Histoplasma capsulatum infection	Unhealthy birds can transmit infectious organisms.
Salmonellosis	Avoid reptiles, turtles, chicks, and ducklings.
Mycobacterium marinum infection	Wear gloves for cleaning aquariums.

Table 20.6

Patient Teaching: Preventing Opportunistic Infections—cont'd

Travel	
To protect from:	*General measures:*
Opportunistic pathogens, foodborne and waterborne infections	Consult health care providers on travel to developing countries. Traveler's diarrhea prophylaxis is not recommended. Carry supply of antimicrobial agent to take for diarrhea. Consider prophylaxis for other types of exposures. Avoid raw fruits, vegetables, raw/undercooked seafood or meat, tap water, ice from tap water, unpasteurized milk/dairy products, and items from street vendors. Safe items include steaming-hot foods, self-peeled fruits, bottled (especially carbonated) beverages, hot coffee/tea, beer, wine, and water boiled 1 minute. Avoid soil/sand contact by wearing shoes, using beach towels.

Source: Panel on Opportunistic Infections in HIV-Infected Adults and Adolescents. (2018). Guidelines for the prevention and treatment of opportunistic infections in HIV-infected adults and adolescents: Recommendations from the Centers for Disease Control and Prevention, the National Institutes of Health, and the HIV Medicine Association of the Infectious Diseases Society of America. Retrieved www.aidsinfo.nih.gov/contentfiles/lvguidelines/adult_oi.pdf

Nutrition Notes

Nourishing the Patient With HIV or AIDS. Nutrition has preventive and therapeutic functions for patients with HIV or AIDS. Those who are well nourished stay healthier. They are better able to resist opportunistic infections and tolerate the side effects of treatment. Visit www.nal.usda.gov/fnic/aidshiv for nutrition information relating to HIV and AIDS.

Many factors can interfere with nutrition during an HIV infection or AIDS. Anorexia is common, perhaps due to an oral infection or lesions. Diarrhea from damage to intestinal cells affects absorption of nutrients. These factors, along with nausea and vomiting from medications, can lead to weight loss and a lean body mass.

A dietitian should be consulted for nutritional care of the patient with HIV or AIDS. Interventions to optimize nutrition include (U.S. Department of Agriculture, 2017; Wolfram, 2016):

- Assessing nutritional status (baseline and weight changes, bioelectrical impedance analysis, and serum nutrient deficiencies) and monitoring body composition changes for treatment
- Maintaining a nutritionally balanced diet (see 2015–2020 Dietary Guidelines for Americans at www.health.gov/dietaryguidelines/2015)
- Managing factors that affect nutrition such as anorexia, oral sores, or diarrhea, and maintaining food safety due to a weakened immune system (see Nutrition Notes "Treating Problems Related to Nutrition" in Chapter 11)

- Consulting a social worker for food access resources (e.g., food pantry, Meals on Wheels)

Every effort should be made to provide nourishment orally. Helpful strategies include the following:

- Offering small, frequent feedings
- Serving food cold or at room temperature
- Using a variety of seasonings
- Adding powdered milk to mashed potatoes or puddings to increase calories and protein
- Modifying texture to accommodate chewing difficulty or oral lesions
- Providing nutritional supplements (e.g., Boost or Ensure)

Studies have found that the use of a nutritional supplement delayed the onset of advanced disease in HIV positive patients (Friis, Olsen, & Filteau, 2015).

References

Friis, H., Olsen, M. F., & Filteau, S. (2015). Nutritional support to HIV patients starting ART. *Journal of Acquired Immune Deficiency Syndromes, 70*(2), 68–69.

U.S. Department of Agriculture. (2017). Food and nutrition information center: AIDS/HIV. Retrieved from www.nal.usda.gov/fnic/aidshiv

Wolfram, T. (2016). Nutrition tips to keep the immune system strong for people with HIV-AIDS. Academy of Nutrition and Dietetics. Retrieved from www.eatright.org/resource/health/diseases-and-conditions/hiv-aids/nutrition-and-hiv-aids

Evidence-Based Practice

Clinical Question

Is progressive resistance exercise (PRE) safe and beneficial for persons with HIV infection?

Evidence

A systematic review of 20 studies examined the effectiveness of PRE for persons with HIV (O'Brien, Tynan, Nixon, & Glazier, 2017). Results showed that it is not only safe for persons with stable HIV to perform PRE three times per week but also beneficial for overall cardiorespiratory fitness (maximum oxygen consumption, exercise time), maintenance of weight, body muscle composition, and strength. In addition, CD4 T-lymphocyte counts and viral load remained stable.

Implications for Nursing Practice

It is important for persons with HIV to maintain stable health. Medically stable patients with HIV should be encouraged to discuss an exercise program with their health care provider that includes PRE and aerobic exercise.

Reference

O'Brien, K. K., Tynan, A. M., Nixon, S. A., & Glazier, R. H. (2017). Effectiveness of progressive resistive exercise (PRE) in the context of HIV: Systematic review and meta-analysis using the Cochrane collaboration protocol. *BMC Infectious Diseases, 17*(1), 268. doi:10.1186/s12879-017-2342-8

---

patients with AIDS who smoke, there is an increased incidence of oral thrush (candidiasis). Therefore, patients should be encouraged to quit smoking. Antifungal medication is given. Mouth care with a soft toothbrush is important. A numbing agent, such as lidocaine viscous (Xylocaine Viscous), can be given to decrease pain during eating.

PAIN. Pain can occur from a variety of causes. Treatment is focused on the cause to achieve pain control and relief. Medications can be given as ordered. Timing medication administration before planned activities is helpful in increasing ability to function. Complementary therapy can be used by patients (see Chapter 5). Measures such as heat or cold, massage, and frequent position changes can be helpful.

IMPAIRED SKIN INTEGRITY. Varied skin conditions can occur with HIV infection. Some medications can cause skin infections that can be life-threatening. Report skin rashes immediately.

RISK FOR SITUATIONAL LOW SELF-ESTEEM. Changes in self-esteem and self-concept occur from several of the effects of HIV infection. Patients often experience changes in their relationships with others and in day-to-day activities

such as work. Major weight loss and changes in fat distribution from ARV medications, a condition called *lipodystrophy,* can cause dramatic changes in appearance that alter body image and reduce self-esteem. Tesamorelin (Egrifta), a synthetic growth hormone–releasing hormone, is used to treat lipodystrophy. Nurses can assist patients in maintaining self-esteem and self-concept by ensuring a climate of acceptance and promoting a trusting relationship. Patients should be encouraged to express feelings, if ready, and to identify positive aspects of self. Receiving emotional and spiritual support can help improve the patient's self-esteem.

SOCIAL ISOLATION. People with HIV/AIDS continue to face discrimination, rejection, and isolation, even from relatives and friends. The Americans with Disabilities Act makes discrimination toward patients with HIV/AIDS illegal. Being knowledgeable about the transmission of HIV allows appropriate interaction with the patient. This reduces feelings of isolation. Providing patient education to reduce fear of HIV transmission also decreases isolation. Taking care to maintain confidentiality is essential. It is important to be aware that many patients with HIV do not share their diagnosis with family or friends.

CRITICAL THINKING

Zoe Sampson, age 22, is diagnosed as HIV positive. She is tearful and asks many questions.

1. How would you answer the following questions?
   a. "Am I going to die?"
   b. "How is AIDS diagnosed?"
   c. "Can my boyfriend get it?"
2. What food and water safety methods would you teach her?
3. Years later, Zoe loses weight and becomes malnourished. What interventions can you use to promote adequate nutrition?

   Suggested answers are at the end of the chapter.

RESOURCES. Financial resources may need to be addressed so that food and medications can be obtained. Treatment can be expensive, and the patient may be unable to work. With ART, many people are able to continue working. The Ryan White Comprehensive AIDS Resources Emergency Act provides funding for some services and treatment-related needs. Knowledge of local resources and referrals to financial resources and support groups are very important.

COMMUNITY AND HOME HEALTH CARE. If an HIV infection progresses, the patient may need more care from caregivers and home health care nurses ("Home Health Hints"). Support services should be identified, such as community AIDS organizations, Meals on Wheels, respite care services, community mental health services, and Internet support groups. Respite care provides the caregiver time away from the caregiver role to reduce stress. When a patient is terminal, comfort care and emotional support for the family are essential. Hospice care can be helpful at this time.

Evaluation

Patient goals are met if the patient remains free from infection and maintains desired quality of life and activities as long as possible. If the disease should progress, goals are met if the patient's needs are being met and the patient's dignity is maintained.

Home Health Hints

- When providing patient care, perform hand hygiene and wash hands frequently; follow standard precautions.
- Observe caregivers for caregiver role strain.
- Teach the family of a patient with AIDS which signs and symptoms to report to the health care provider or nurse immediately. These include fever; increased dyspnea; pain; change in sputum production; upper respiratory tract infection; pneumonia; respiratory distress syndrome; diarrhea five times a day or more for 5 days; uncontrolled weight loss greater than 10 pounds in the past month; persistent headaches; falling; seizures; mental status changes, including memory loss and personality changes; rashes and skin changes; difficulty swallowing; and problems with urination.
- Teach patients with HIV/AIDS and their families how to properly clean and disinfect the home to prevent infection:
  - The least expensive recommended disinfectant is a diluted bleach mixture that contains 1 part household bleach to 10 parts water. However, this solution must be mixed daily to be effective. Many spray-type disinfectants are available and can be easier for patients/families to use.
- Flush body fluids, solid body waste, and contaminated solutions down toilet.
- Use disinfectant to (1) disinfect body fluid spill areas, (2) clean toilet seats and bathroom fixtures, and (3) clean inside the refrigerator to avoid mold growth.
- Rinse clothing and then wash separately from other clothes with 1 cup of bleach if soiled with blood, urine, feces, or semen.
- Wash dishes and silverware in hot, soapy water, and rinsed thoroughly or placed in dishwasher. Patients with HIV/AIDS do not require separate sets of dishes or silverware.
- To dispose of sharps (e.g., needles, lancets, razors), use a red biohazard container if provided. If not, use a rigid labeled container such as a tin can with a sealable lid. Add 1:10 bleach solution to disinfect the sharps. Tape the lid. Place in a bag and dispose of in the trash.
- Dispose of contaminated articles by sealing them in a plastic bag and placing in the trash.

SUGGESTED ANSWERS TO CRITICAL THINKING

Zoe Sampson

1. a. "There is no cure for HIV/AIDS; however, medications are available that make an HIV infection a manageable chronic illness. Research continues in the search for a cure."

   b. "AIDS is diagnosed when CD4 T-lymphocyte counts are below 200 cells/microL, or the CD4 T-lymphocyte percentage is under 14% of total lymphocytes, and/or an opportunistic clinical disease, as defined by the Centers for Disease Control and Prevention, is present in an HIV-infected person."

   c. "If you do not have durably undetectable viral loads, then your boyfriend could become infected through exposure to your blood and vaginal or rectal secretions. You can learn about preventive measures and discuss them with him. If you have had unprotected sex, he should be tested for HIV."

2. Food handlers must maintain good hand washing and hygiene practices. Discard food that is past the expiration date and dented or swollen cans. Ensure adequate refrigeration and cooking. Control insects and rodents to prevent food contamination. Drink purified bottled water if you live in areas with unsafe drinking water. Use a safe water supply or boil water for 1 minute when unsure. Avoid unpasteurized milk, other dairy products, fruit juice, and raw seed sprouts. Avoid raw and undercooked eggs, meats, and seafood.

3. Eat three to four high-calorie, high-lean protein meals and snacks daily. Eat a low-residue diet if diarrhea is present. Develop an easy meal plan. Use antiemetics, if needed. Numb painful oral sores. Refer for food stamps/free meal programs if necessary. Engage in regular exercise.

Review Questions

1. The nurse would evaluate the patient as understanding modes of HIV transmission if the patient stated that the modes of HIV transmission for a person who has a detectable viral load include which of the following? **Select all that apply.**
   1. Saliva and tears
   2. Fecal-oral contact
   3. Sharing towels and eating utensils
   4. Unprotected sex
   5. Mosquito bites
   6. Contact with infected blood products

2. The nurse is teaching a patient about HIV testing. Place HIV diagnostic tests in the sequential order in which they are performed.
   1. HIV-1 nucleic acid test
   2. HIV antibody immunoassay differentiation test for HIV-1 and HIV-2
   3. HIV antigen/antibody combination immunoassay

3. A patient who is newly diagnosed with HIV infection asks what to expect for future health status. The best response for the nurse to give is based on the understanding that HIV disease is characterized as which of the following?
   1. An acute disease
   2. A life-ending disease
   3. A chronically managed disease
   4. A disease with remissions and exacerbations

4. The nurse is planning to teach a patient about HIV prevention. What should the nurse include in a teaching plan to prevent HIV infection? **Select all that apply.**
   1. Caregiver should recap used needles.
   2. Abstain from sexual intercourse.
   3. Avoid injection drug use.
   4. Avoid use of female condoms.
   5. Plan for autologous blood transfusion.
   6. Test for HIV at time of labor.

5. The nurse is contributing to the teaching plan for a patient with HIV on reducing infection risks. Which of the following should the patient with HIV be taught to do to decrease risk of infections? **Select all that apply.**
   1. Wash hands before eating.
   2. Wash toothbrush.
   3. Reuse dishes.
   4. Buy prepared deli foods.
   5. Report signs of infection.
   6. Share razor if no visible blood.

6. The nurse would recognize that the patient needs further reinforcement of knowledge if the patient stated that the goals of antiretroviral therapy are which of these? **Select all that apply.**
   1. "To increase viral load."
   2. "To improve survival rates."
   3. "To decrease CD4 T lymphocytes."
   4. "To delay progression of HIV disease."
   5. "To reduce HIV load to undetectable levels."
   6. "To suppress the immune system."

7. The nurse would recognize that the patient is having a reaction to abacavir sulfate (Ziagen) if which of the following occurred?
   1. Edema
   2. Flu-like symptoms
   3. Abdominal pain
   4. Blurred vision

Answer rationales available in your online resources.

ANSWERS 1. 4, 6; 2. 3, 2, 1; 3. 3; 4. 2, 3, 5, 6; 5. 1, 2, 5; 6. 1, 3, 6; 7. 2

Key Points

Find the chapter key points in your online resources available through Davis Edge.

Additional Resources

 Use the scratch off code on the inside front cover of your book to access online quizzes that will help you to improve your scores on course exams and prepare for NCLEX-PN®.

 Study Guide

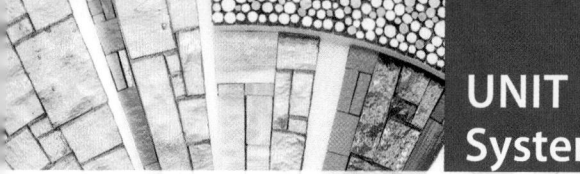

CHAPTER 21

Cardiovascular System Function, Assessment, and Therapeutic Measures

Michele Dickson, Janice L. Bradford

KEY TERMS

arrhythmia (uh-RITH-mee-ahs)
atherosclerosis (ATH-er-oh-skleh-ROH-sis)
bruit (brew-EE)
claudication (KLAW-dih-KAY-shun)
clubbing (KLUH-bing)
endothelium (EN-DOE-thee-lee-um)
hyperkalemia (HY-per-kuh-LEE-mee-ah)
hypokalemia (HY-poh-kuh-LEE-mee-ah)
hypomagnesemia (HY-poh-MAG-neh-SEE-mee-ah)
ischemic (is-KEY-mik)
murmur (MUR-mur)
pericardial friction rub (PEAR-ih-KAR-dee-uhl FRIK-shun RUB)
poikilothermy (POY-kih-loh-THER-mee)
point of maximum impulse (POYNT OF MAKS-ih-muhm IM-puls)
preload (PREE-lohd)
pulse deficit (PULS DEF-ih-sit)
Starling's law (STAR-ling's law)
sternotomy (stir-NAW-tuh-mee)
thrill (THRILL)

CHAPTER CONCEPT

Perfusion

LEARNING OUTCOMES

1. Identify the normal anatomy of the cardiovascular system.
2. Explain the normal function of the cardiovascular system.
3. List data to collect when caring for a patient with a disorder of the cardiovascular system.
4. Identify diagnostic tests commonly performed to diagnose disorders of the cardiovascular system.
5. Plan nursing care for patients undergoing diagnostic tests for cardiovascular disorders.
6. Describe current therapeutic measures for disorders of the cardiovascular system.
7. Describe preoperative and postoperative care for patients undergoing cardiac surgery.

NORMAL CARDIOVASCULAR SYSTEM ANATOMY AND PHYSIOLOGY

The cardiovascular system consists of the heart, blood, and vessels (including arteries, capillaries, and veins). Its function is to perfuse the organs and tissues with blood.

Heart

Cardiac Structure and Function

LOCATION OF THE HEART. The heart is located in the mediastinum within the thoracic cavity. It is enclosed by three membranes. The outermost is the fibrous pericardium, which forms a loose-fitting pericardial sac around the heart. The second, or middle, layer is the parietal pericardium, a serous membrane that lines the fibrous layer. The third and innermost layer, the visceral pericardium or epicardium, is a serous membrane on the surface of the heart muscle. Between the parietal and visceral layers is serous fluid, which prevents friction as the heart beats.

STRUCTURE OF THE HEART AND CORONARY BLOOD VESSELS. The walls of the four chambers of the heart are made of cardiac muscle (myocardium) and are lined with endocardium. Endocardium is smooth epithelial tissue that prevents abnormal clotting. The epithelium also covers the valves of the heart and continues into blood vessels, at which point it is called the **endothelium.** Coronary circulation provides oxygenated blood throughout the myocardium and returns deoxygenated blood to the right atrium via the coronary sinus. The two main coronary arteries are the first branches of the ascending aorta, just outside the left ventricle (Fig. 21.1).

The superior chambers of the heart are the thin-walled right and left atria, which are separated by the interatrial septum. The lower chambers are the thicker walled right and left ventricles, which are separated by the interventricular septum. Each septum is made of myocardium that forms a common wall between the two chambers.

CORONARY BLOOD FLOW. The right atrium receives deoxygenated blood from the coronary sinus, from the upper body by way of the superior vena cava, and from the lower body by way of the inferior vena cava (see Fig. 21.1). This blood flows from the right atrium through the tricuspid valve into the right ventricle. Backflow during ventricular systole (contraction and emptying) is prevented by the tricuspid, or right atrioventricular (AV) valve (Fig. 21.2). The right ventricle pumps blood through the pulmonary semilunar valve to the lungs by way of the pulmonary trunk and arteries. The pulmonary semilunar valve prevents backflow of blood into the right ventricle during ventricular diastole (relaxation and filling).

The left atrium receives oxygenated blood from the lungs by way of the four pulmonary veins. This blood flows through the mitral, or left AV valve (also called the bicuspid valve) into the left ventricle. The mitral valve prevents backflow of blood into the left atrium during ventricular systole. The left ventricle pumps blood through the aortic semilunar

valve to the body by way of the aorta. The aortic valve prevents backflow of blood into the left ventricle during ventricular diastole.

The tricuspid and mitral valves consist of three and two cusps, respectively. These cusps, or flaps, are connective tissue covered by endocardium. They are anchored to the floor of the ventricle by the chordae tendineae and papillary muscles. The papillary muscles are columns of myocardium that contract along with the rest of the ventricular myocardium. This contraction pulls on the chordae tendineae and prevents hyperextension of the AV valves during ventricular systole (see Fig. 21.2).

Although each ventricle pumps the same amount of blood, the much thicker walls of the left ventricle pump with approximately five times the force of the right ventricle to distribute the blood throughout the body. This difference in force is reflected in the large difference between systemic and pulmonary blood pressure.

Cardiac Conduction Pathway and Cardiac Cycle

The cardiac conduction pathway is the pathway of electrical impulses that generates a heartbeat. The sinoatrial (SA) node in the wall of the right atrium is autorhythmic and depolarizes about 100 times per minute, initiating each heartbeat. (While at rest, parasympathetic fibers dominate and slow the SA node to about 75 beats per minute.) For this reason, the SA node is called the pacemaker, and a normal heartbeat is called a normal sinus rhythm. From the SA node, impulses travel on a specific path (Fig. 21.3). If

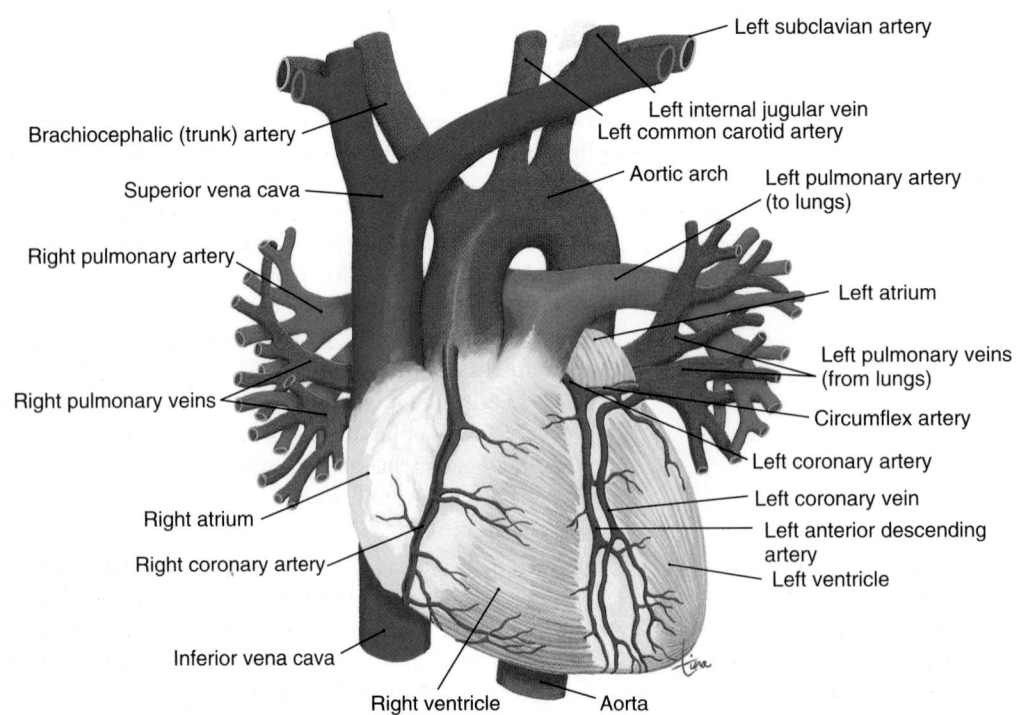

FIGURE 21.1 Anterior view of the heart and major blood vessels.

Left subclavian artery

Left internal jugular vein
Left common carotid artery

Brachiocephalic (trunk) artery

Aortic arch

Left pulmonary artery (to lungs)

Superior vena cava

Right pulmonary artery

Left atrium

Left pulmonary veins (from lungs)

Right pulmonary veins

Circumflex artery

Left coronary artery

Left coronary vein

Right atrium

Left anterior descending artery

Right coronary artery

Left ventricle

Inferior vena cava

Right ventricle   Aorta

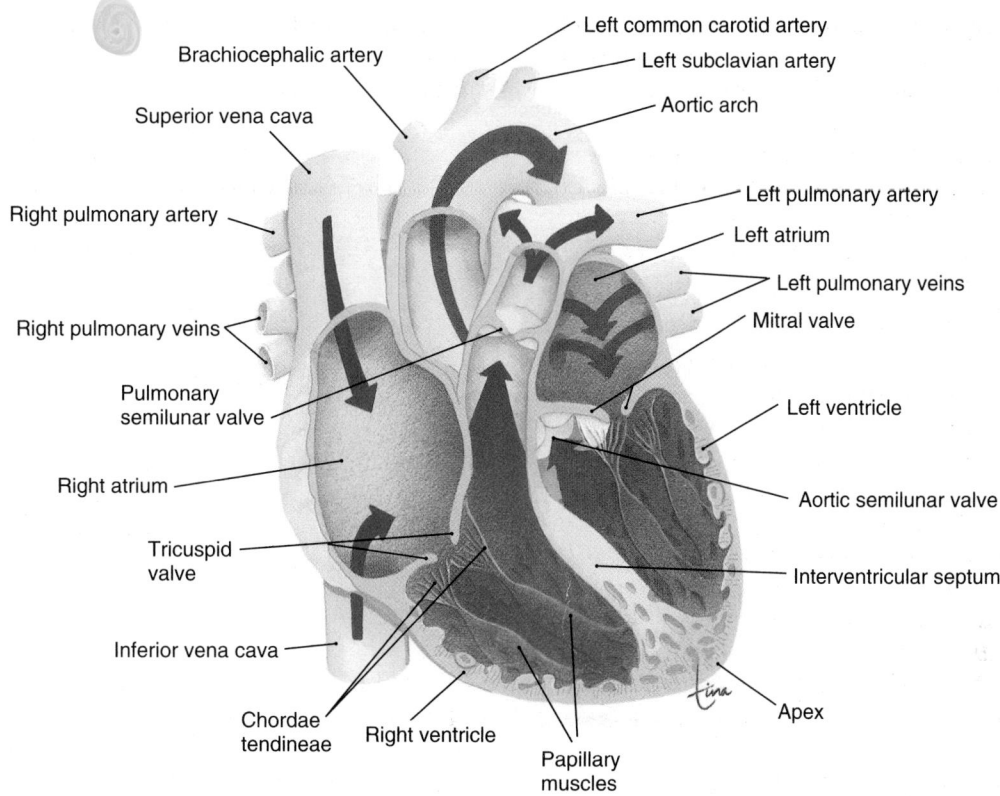

Brachiocephalic artery

Superior vena cava

Right pulmonary artery

Right pulmonary veins

Pulmonary
semilunar valve

Right atrium

Tricuspid
valve

Inferior vena cava

Chordae
tendineae

Right ventricle

Papillary
muscles

Left common carotid artery

Left subclavian artery

Aortic arch

Left pulmonary artery

Left atrium

Left pulmonary veins

Mitral valve

Left ventricle

Aortic semilunar valve

Interventricular septum

Apex

FIGURE 21.2 Frontal section of the heart showing internal structures and cardiac blood flow.

the SA node becomes nonfunctional, the AV node can initiate each heartbeat, but at a slower rate of 40 to 60 beats per minute. The *bundle of His* is capable of generating the beat of the ventricles, but at the much slower rate of about 20 to 35 beats per minute.

A cardiac cycle is the sequence of mechanical events that occurs during each heartbeat. Simply stated, the two atria contract simultaneously, followed by the simultaneous contraction of the two ventricles (a fraction of a second later). The contraction (emptying), or systole, of each set of chambers is followed by relaxation (filling), or diastole, of the same set of chambers.

The events of the cardiac cycle create the normal heart sounds. The first of the two major sounds (the "lub" of "lub-dub") is caused by the closure of the AV valves during ventricular systole. The second sound is created by the closure of the aortic and pulmonary semilunar valves.

Cardiac Output

Cardiac output is the amount of blood ejected from the left ventricle in 1 minute (the right ventricle pumps a similar amount). It is determined by multiplying stroke volume by heart rate. Stroke volume is the amount of blood ejected by a ventricle in one contraction. It averages 60 to 80 mL/beat. With an average resting heart rate of 75 beats per minute, average resting cardiac output is 5 to 6 L (approximately the total blood volume of an individual that is pumped within

1 minute). Ejection fraction is a measure of ventricular efficiency. It is normally 55% to 70% of the total amount of blood within the left ventricle that is ejected with every heartbeat.

During exercise, venous return increases and stretches the ventricular myocardium, which in response contracts more forcefully. This is known as **Starling's law** of the heart, and the result is an increase in stroke volume. More blood is pumped with each beat. At the same time, the heart rate increases, causing cardiac output to increase by as much as four times the resting level (or more for fit athletes).

Regulation of Heart Rate

The heart generates its own electrical impulse, which begins at the SA node. The nervous system, however, can change the heart rate in response to environmental circumstances. In the brain, the medulla oblongata receives sensory input and alters heart function (Fig. 21.4).

Hormones and the Heart

The hormone epinephrine is secreted by the adrenal medulla in stressful situations. It is sympathomimetic in that it increases the heart rate and force of contraction and dilates the coronary vessels. This in turn increases cardiac output and systolic blood pressure.

Aldosterone is a hormone produced by the adrenal cortex. It is important for cardiac function because it helps

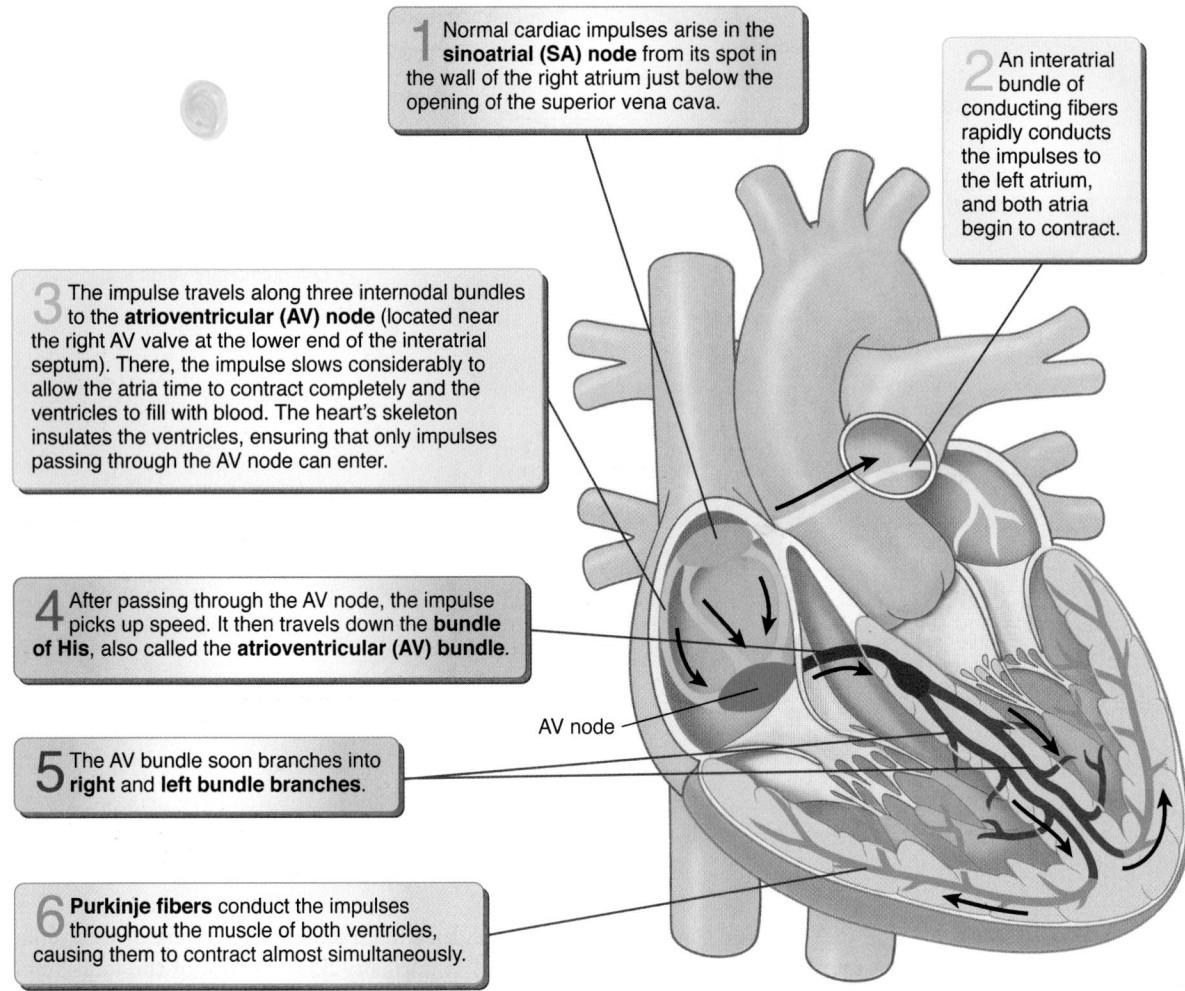

1 Normal cardiac impulses arise in the **sinoatrial (SA) node** from its spot in the wall of the right atrium just below the opening of the superior vena cava.

2 An interatrial bundle of conducting fibers rapidly conducts the impulses to the left atrium, and both atria begin to contract.

3 The impulse travels along three internodal bundles to the **atrioventricular (AV) node** (located near the right AV valve at the lower end of the interatrial septum). There, the impulse slows considerably to allow the atria time to contract completely and the ventricles to fill with blood. The heart's skeleton insulates the ventricles, ensuring that only impulses passing through the AV node can enter.

4 After passing through the AV node, the impulse picks up speed. It then travels down the **bundle of His**, also called the **atrioventricular (AV) bundle**.

AV node

5 The AV bundle soon branches into **right** and **left bundle branches**.

6 **Purkinje fibers** conduct the impulses throughout the muscle of both ventricles, causing them to contract almost simultaneously.

FIGURE 21.3 Conduction pathway.

regulate blood levels of sodium and potassium, both of which are needed for normal electrical activity of the myocardium.

The atria of the heart secrete a hormone of their own, called atrial natriuretic peptide or atrial natriuretic hormone. As its name suggests, atrial natriuretic peptide increases the excretion of sodium by the kidneys by inhibiting secretion of aldosterone by the adrenal cortex. Atrial natriuretic peptide is secreted when a higher blood pressure or greater blood volume stretches the walls of the atria. The loss of sodium is accompanied by the increased loss of water in urine. This decreases blood volume and, therefore, blood pressure as well.

Blood Vessels
Arteries and Veins

Arteries and arterioles carry blood from the heart to capillaries. Their walls are relatively thick and consist of three layers. Arteries carry blood under high pressure. The outer layer of fibrous connective tissue prevents rupture of the artery. The middle layer of smooth muscle and elastic connective tissue contributes to the maintenance of normal blood pressure, especially diastolic blood pressure, by changing the diameter

of the artery. The diameter of arteries is regulated primarily by the sympathetic division of the autonomic nervous system. By use of the smooth muscle, the arteries can also alter where the greatest volume of blood is directed. The inner layer, or lining, of the artery is simple squamous epithelium, called endothelium, which is very smooth to prevent abnormal clotting.

Veins and venules carry blood from capillaries to the heart. Their walls are relatively thin because they have less smooth muscle than arteries. However, sympathetic impulses can bring about extensive constriction of veins. This becomes important in situations such as severe hemorrhage. The lining of veins is, like arteries, endothelium that prevents abnormal clotting; at intervals, it is folded into valves to prevent backflow of blood. Valves are most numerous in the veins of the extremities, especially the legs, where blood must return to the heart against the force of gravity.

Capillaries

Capillaries carry blood from arterioles to venules and form extensive networks in most tissues. The exceptions are cartilage, covering/lining epithelia, and the lens and cornea of the

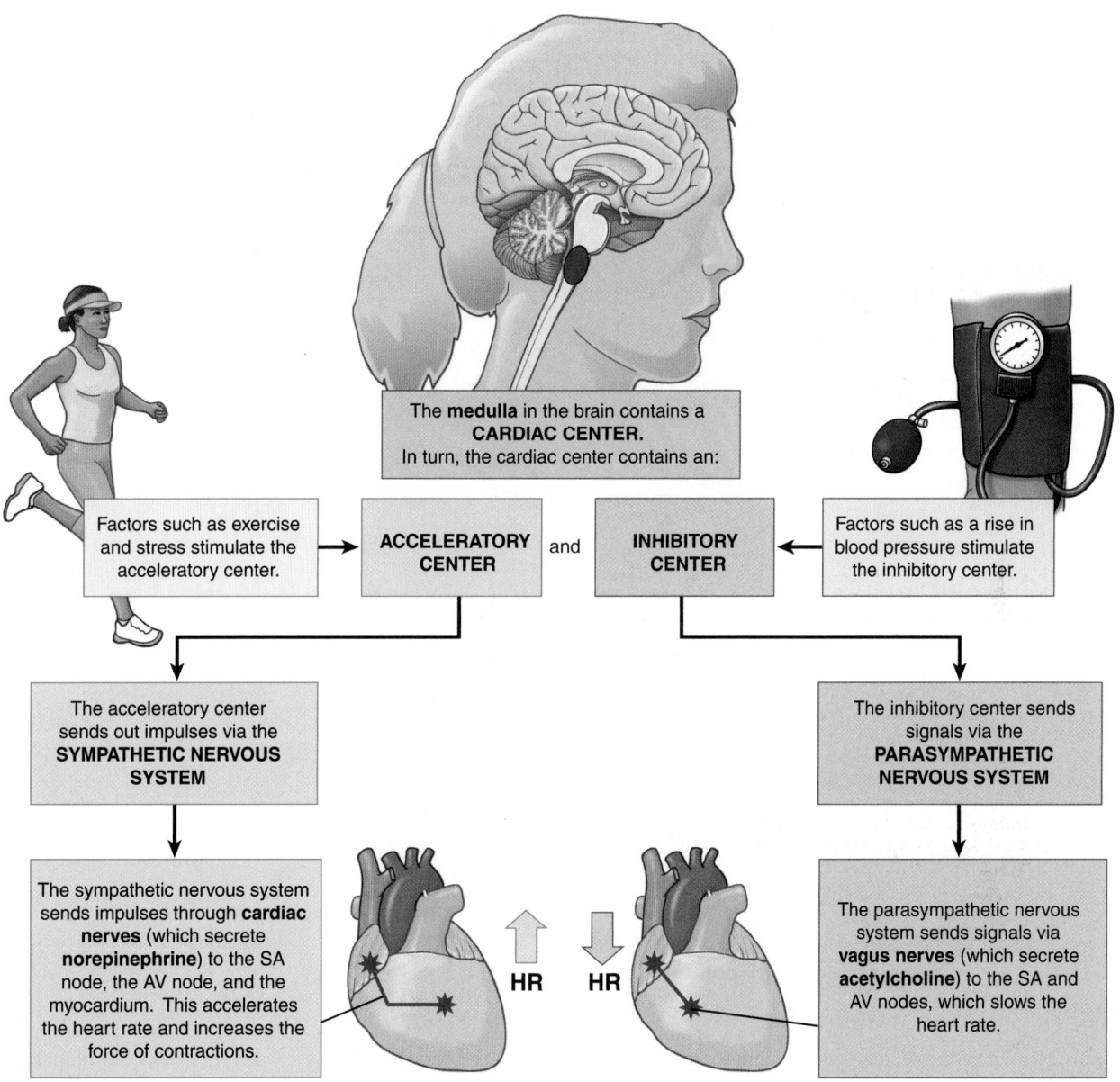

The **medulla** in the brain contains a **CARDIAC CENTER.** In turn, the cardiac center contains an:

Factors such as exercise and stress stimulate the acceleratory center.	**ACCELERATORY CENTER**

and

INHIBITORY CENTER	Factors such as a rise in blood pressure stimulate the inhibitory center.

The acceleratory center sends out impulses via the **SYMPATHETIC NERVOUS SYSTEM**

The inhibitory center sends signals via the **PARASYMPATHETIC NERVOUS SYSTEM**

The sympathetic nervous system sends impulses through **cardiac nerves** (which secrete **norepinephrine**) to the SA node, the AV node, and the myocardium. This accelerates the heart rate and increases the force of contractions.

HR   HR

The parasympathetic nervous system sends signals via **vagus nerves** (which secrete **acetylcholine**) to the SA and AV nodes, which slows the heart rate.

FIGURE 21.4 Factors affecting heart rate.

eye. Capillary walls are a continuation of the lining of arteries and veins. They are one-cell thick to permit the exchange of gases, nutrients, and waste products between the blood and tissues (Fig. 21.5). Blood flow through a capillary network is regulated by a precapillary sphincter, a smooth muscle fiber ring that contracts or relaxes in response to tissue needs. In an active tissue such as exercising skeletal muscle, for example, the rapid oxygen uptake and carbon dioxide production cause dilation of the precapillary sphincters to increase blood flow. At the same time, precapillary sphincters in less active tissues constrict to reduce blood flow. This is important because the body does not have enough blood to fill all of the capillaries at once; the fixed volume must constantly be shunted or redirected to where it is needed most.

Exchange between blood and tissue fluids occurs primarily due to diffusion and/or filtration at the capillaries.

Diffusion is important to gas exchange. Filtration is a vital mechanism for homeostasis of extracellular fluids. Some of this tissue fluid returns to the capillaries, and some is collected in lymph capillaries. Lymph is returned to the blood by lymph vessels. Should blood pressure within the capillaries increase, more tissue fluid than usual is formed, too much for the lymph vessels to collect. This may result in tissue swelling, called *edema*.

Blood Pressure

Blood pressure is the force of the blood against the walls of the blood vessels. It is measured in millimeters of mercury (mm Hg), systolic over diastolic. The normal average of systemic arterial pressure is 120/80 mm Hg. Blood pressure decreases in the arterioles and capillaries, and the systolic and diastolic pressures merge into one pressure. As blood enters

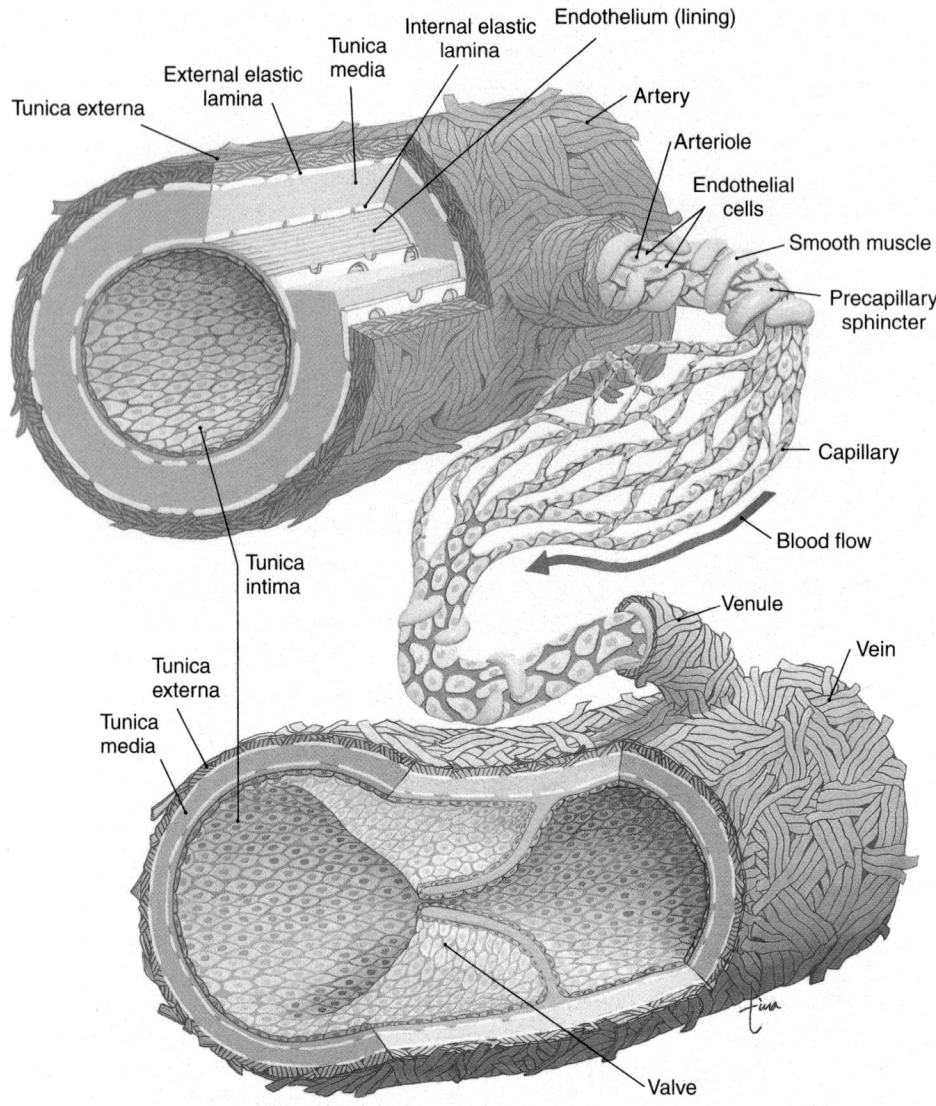

FIGURE 21.5 Structure of an artery, arteriole, capillary network, venule, and vein.

the veins, blood pressure decreases further and approaches zero as it flows into the right ventricle. As mentioned previously, the blood pressure in the capillaries is of great importance. Normal blood pressure is high enough to permit filtration for nourishment of tissues but low enough to prevent rupture.

The arterioles (and veins during increased sympathetic stimulation) are usually in a state of slight constriction that helps to maintain normal blood pressure, especially diastolic pressure. This contributes to peripheral resistance; it is regulated by the vasomotor center in the medulla, which receives input via the glossopharyngeal and vagus nerves.

Blood pressure is also affected by many other factors. If heart rate and force increase, blood pressure increases within limits. If the heart is beating very fast, the ventricles are not filled before they contract, cardiac output decreases, and blood pressure drops. The strength of the heart's contractions depends on adequate venous return, which is the amount of blood that flows into the atria. Decreased venous return results in weaker contractions.

Venous return depends on several factors: constriction of the veins to reduce pooling, the skeletal muscle pumping to squeeze the deep veins of the legs, and the diaphragm's downward pressure during inhalation to compress the abdominal veins as the thoracic veins are decompressed. The valves in the veins prevent backflow of blood and thus contribute to the return of blood to the heart.

The elasticity of the large arteries also contributes to normal blood pressure. When the left ventricle contracts, the blood stretches the elastic walls of the large arteries, which absorb some of the force. When the left ventricle relaxes, the arterial walls recoil, exerting pressure on the blood. Normal elasticity, therefore, lowers systolic pressure, raises diastolic pressure, and maintains normal pulse pressure. Pulse pressure is the difference between the systolic and diastolic pressures. The usual ratio of systolic to diastolic to pulse pressure is 3:2:1.

Renin-Angiotensin-Aldosterone Mechanism

The kidneys are of great importance in the regulation of blood pressure. If blood flow through the kidneys decreases, renal filtration decreases and urinary output decreases to preserve blood volume. Decreased blood pressure stimulates the kidneys to secrete renin, which initiates the renin-angiotensin-aldosterone mechanism, raising blood pressure (Fig. 21.6).

Other hormones that affect blood pressure include those of the adrenal medulla, norepinephrine and epinephrine, which increase cardiac output and cause vasoconstriction in skin and viscera. Antidiuretic hormone is released from the posterior pituitary. It directly increases water reabsorption by the kidneys, thus increasing blood volume and blood pressure. Atrial natriuretic peptide is secreted by the atria of the heart. It inhibits aldosterone secretion and thereby increases renal excretion of sodium ions and water, which decreases blood volume and subsequently blood pressure.

Circuits of Circulation

The two circuits of circulation are pulmonary and systemic (see Fig. 21.2). Pulmonary circulation begins at the right ventricle, which pumps deoxygenated blood toward the lungs for gas exchange at the alveoli. Oxygenated blood returns to the left atrium by way of the pulmonary veins. Low pressure in the pulmonary capillaries prevents filtration in pulmonary capillaries. This keeps tissue fluid from accumulating in the alveoli of the lungs, which can otherwise result in pulmonary edema.

Systemic circulation begins in the left ventricle, pumping oxygenated blood into the aorta, the many branches of which eventually give rise to capillaries within the tissues. Deoxygenated blood returns to the right atrium by way of the superior and inferior vena cava and the coronary sinus. The hepatic portal circulation is a special part of the systemic circulation in which blood from the capillaries of the digestive organs and spleen flows through the portal vein and into the sinusoids in the liver before returning to the heart. This pathway permits the liver to regulate the blood levels of nutrients such as glucose, amino acids, and iron and to remove potential toxins such as alcohol or medications from circulation.

Aging and the Cardiovascular System

The aging of blood vessels, especially arteries, is believed to begin in childhood, although the effects are not apparent until later in life (Fig. 21.7). **Atherosclerosis** is the deposition of lipids in the walls of arteries over a period of years. The deposited lipids can narrow the arteries' lumens and form rough surfaces that may stimulate intravascular clot formation. Atherosclerosis decreases blood flow to the affected organ. With age, the heart muscle becomes less efficient, and maximum cardiac output and heart rate both decrease, although resting levels may be more than sufficient ("Gerontological Issues: Orthostatic Hypotension"). Valves may become thickened by fibrosis, leading to heart murmur.

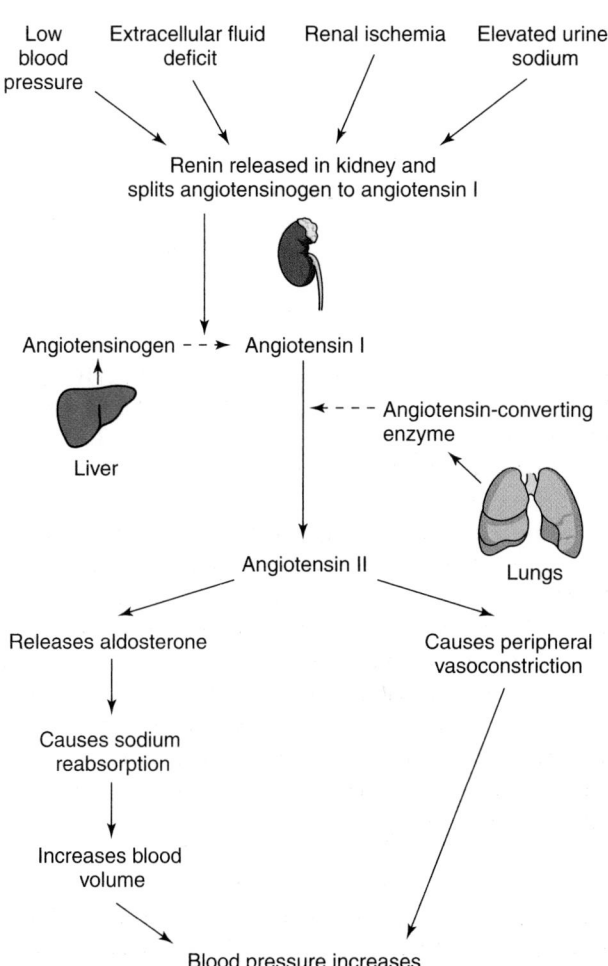

FIGURE 21.6 The renin-angiotensin-aldosterone mechanism.

Low blood pressure · Extracellular fluid deficit · Renal ischemia · Elevated urine sodium

Renin released in kidney and splits angiotensinogen to angiotensin I

Angiotensinogen - - ► Angiotensin I

Liver

◄ - - - Angiotensin-converting enzyme

Angiotensin II

Lungs

Releases aldosterone

Causes peripheral vasoconstriction

Causes sodium reabsorption

Increases blood volume

Blood pressure increases

Gerontological Issues

Orthostatic Hypotension. The older adult is at increased risk for developing orthostatic hypotension, which could precipitate a fall. This is often due to a combination of age-related changes, immobility, chronic illnesses, and medications. It is important to assess blood pressure and pulse while the patient is lying, sitting, and standing and to teach the patient to sit up and stand slowly before walking.

CARDIOVASCULAR DISEASE

An estimated 92.1 million American adults have one or more types of cardiovascular disease (Benjamin et al., 2017) ("Cultural Considerations"). Lifestyle plays a leading role in risk factors for cardiovascular disease. Americans continue to be sedentary and eat excess calories. Ways to improve cardiovascular health include not smoking, exercising, eating healthy, and maintaining normal blood pressure, blood glucose, total cholesterol levels, and weight. In women, the greatest cause of death is cardiovascular disease. The movement Go Red for Women (www.goredforwomen.org) gives women encouragement and tools to prevent cardiovascular disease and live healthy.

• WORD • BUILDING •

atherosclerosis: athere—porridge + sklerosis—hardness

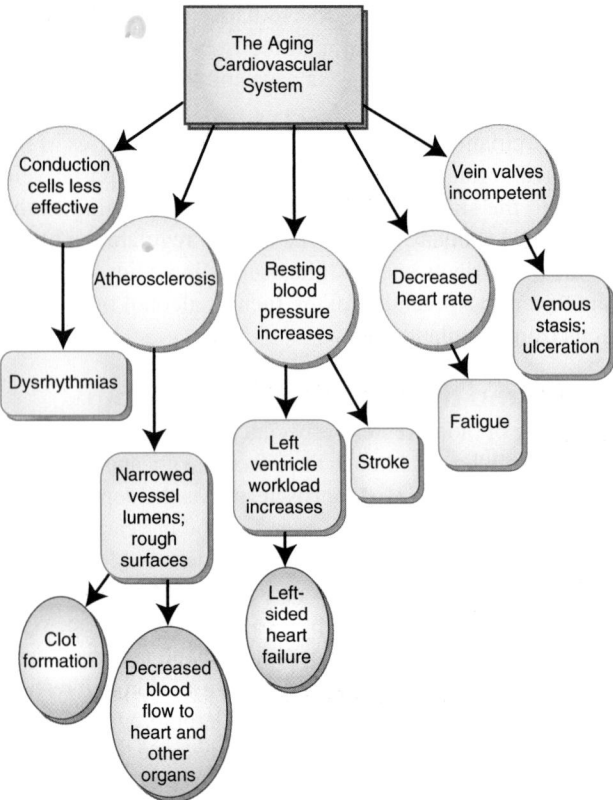

FIGURE 21.7 Aging and the cardiovascular system concept map.

Cultural Considerations

Adults in the United States are more likely to die of heart disease than any other cause, regardless of their racial or ethnic heritage. However, certain minority groups face a greater risk than others. Many intertwined factors likely contribute to these high heart disease rates, including lower average income, which affects where people live, and access to healthy food, safe places to exercise, and quality health care.

Certain racial and ethnic groups have higher rates of hypertension, tend to develop hypertension at an earlier age, and are less likely to undergo treatment to control their high blood pressure. Following are some examples:

• Mexican American men and women tend to have higher rates of elevated blood pressure.
• Obesity continues to be higher for African American and Mexican American women.
• Only 50% of Native Americans, 44% of Asian Americans, and 38% of Mexican Americans have had their cholesterol checked within the past 2 years.
• Coronary heart disease mortality is higher for African Americans.
• Stroke is the only leading cause of death for which mortality is higher for Asian American males.

Strategies to improve disparities should focus on culturally competent engagement in health promotion and disease prevention education.

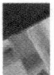

NURSING ASSESSMENT OF THE CARDIOVASCULAR SYSTEM

Nursing assessment of the cardiovascular system includes a patient health history and physical examination ("Gerontological Issues: Atypical Symptoms"). If the patient is experiencing an acute problem, focus on the most serious signs and symptoms and physical data until the patient is stabilized (Table 21.1).

Gerontological Issues

Atypical Symptoms. Older adults commonly have signs and symptoms that are not typical of a myocardial infarction. For example, the only symptom of myocardial infarction in an older patient may be dyspnea. Chest pain, a typical symptom, may not be present. It is important for the older adult to have a complete assessment for this reason.

Health History

For cardiovascular problems, data collection focuses on the areas listed in Table 21.2. Patient allergies, medications, medical disorders, and surgeries are documented. Functional limitations that are related to cardiovascular problems, such as difficulty performing activities of daily living, walking, climbing stairs, or completing household tasks, are noted.

Physical Examination

The patient's general appearance is observed. Height, weight, and vital signs are recorded.

Blood Pressure

Normal blood pressure is considered less than 120/80 mm Hg (see Chapter 22). Readings in both arms are done for comparison (Box 21.1). A difference in the readings is reported to the health care provider (HCP). The arm with the higher reading is used for ongoing measurements. If necessary, blood pressure may be measured in the leg with a larger blood pressure cuff. The reading in the leg is normally 10 mm Hg higher than in the arm.

ORTHOSTATIC BLOOD PRESSURE. Measurements are taken with the patient lying, sitting, and standing to detect abnormal variations with postural changes. When the patient sits or stands, a drop in the systolic pressure of up to 15 mm Hg and either a drop or slight increase in the diastolic pressure of 3 to 10 mm Hg is normal. In response to the drop in blood pressure, the pulse increases 15 to 20 beats per minute to maintain cardiac output. Orthostatic hypotension (postural hypotension) is a drop in systolic blood pressure greater than 15 mm Hg, a drop or slight increase in diastolic blood pressure greater than 10 mm Hg, and an increase in heart rate greater than 20 beats per minute in response to the drop in blood pressure. It indicates a problem that should be investigated by the HCP (Box 21.2). The patient often reports light-headedness or syncope because the drop in blood pressure decreases the

Table 21.1

Data Collection for Acute Cardiovascular Disorder

History	Significance
Allergies	For medication administration, diagnostic dyes
Smoking history	Risk factor for cardiovascular disorders
Medications	Toxic levels; influencing symptoms
Pain: location, radiation, description	Possible angina, myocardial infarction, thrombus, embolism
Dyspnea	Left-sided heart failure; pulmonary edema or embolism
Fatigue	Decreased cardiac output
Palpitations	Arrhythmias
Dizziness	Arrhythmias
Weight gain	Right-sided heart failure

Physical Examination	Possible Abnormal Findings
Vital signs	Bradycardia, tachycardia, hypotension, hypertension, tachypnea, apnea, shock
Heart rhythm	Arrhythmias
Edema	Right-sided heart failure
Jugular vein distention	Right-sided heart failure
Breath sounds	Crackles, wheezes with left-sided heart failure
Cough, sputum	Acute heart failure—dry cough, pink frothy sputum

Table 21.2

Subjective Data Collection for the Cardiovascular System

Questions to Ask During Health History	Rationale/Significance
Pain: WHAT'S UP? Format	
Where is your pain? Does it radiate?	Vascular disorders cause extremity pain. Cardiac pain may radiate to shoulders, neck, jaw, arms, or back.
How does it feel? Discomfort, burning, aching, indigestion, squeezing, pressure, tightness, heaviness, numbness in chest area? Fullness, heaviness, sharpness, throbbing in legs?	Pain can be associated with angina or myocardial infarction. The quality of pain varies. Arterial pain is sharp or throbbing. Venous pain is a fullness or heaviness.
Aggravating/alleviating factors that increase/relieve your pain?	Activity may cause or increase angina. Rest or medications may relieve angina. Leg activity pain, intermittent claudication, results from decreased perfusion that is aggravated by activity. Rest pain, from severe arterial occlusion, increases when lying. Dangling reduces the pain as blood flow is increased by gravity.

Continued

Table 21.2

Subjective Data Collection for the Cardiovascular System—cont'd

Questions to Ask During Health History	Rationale/Significance
Timing of your pain: onset, duration, frequency?	Pain may be continuous, intermittent, acute, or chronic. Arterial occlusion causes acute pain.
Severity of pain?	Pain is rated, such as on a scale of 0 to 10.
Useful data for associated symptoms?	Accompanying symptoms and their characteristics guide diagnosis and treatment.
Perception of your problem?	Patient's insight to problem is helpful in planning care.
Dyspnea Are you short of breath? What increases or relieves your shortness of breath?	Dyspnea can be present with heart failure that reduces cardiac output, on exertion in angina pectoris or from a pulmonary embolus resulting from thrombophlebitis, heart failure, or arrhythmias.
Palpitations Are you having palpitations or irregular heartbeats? Does your heart race, pound, or skip beats?	Palpitations can occur from arrhythmias resulting from ischemia, electrolyte imbalance, or stress. Dizziness can be associated with arrhythmias.
Fatigue Have you noticed a change in your energy level?	Fatigue occurs from reduced cardiac output resulting from heart failure.
Are you able to perform activities that you would like to?	Functional abilities can be limited from fatigue.
Edema Have you had swelling in your feet, legs, or hands? Are rings, shoes, or gloves tighter?	Right-sided heart failure can cause fluid accumulation in the tissues.
Have you gained weight?	Fluid retention causes weight gain.
Paresthesia Any numbness, tingling, or other abnormal sensations in your extremities?	Numbness and tingling, pins and needles, and crawling sensations are paresthesia.
Childhood Diseases Did you have rheumatic fever or scarlet fever?	These childhood illnesses can lead to heart disease.
Risk Factors What is your typical diet? Do you exercise, smoke? Any recent stressors?	Modifiable risk factors include diet, being sedentary, smoking, and stressors.
Family History Do your parents, siblings, or grandparents have cardiovascular disorders?	Many cardiac problems are hereditary.

amount of oxygen-rich blood traveling to the brain. Factors that may cause orthostatic hypotension include deficient fluid volume, diuretics, analgesics, or pain.

Pulses

The apical pulse is auscultated for 1 minute to assess rate and rhythm. Normal heart rate is 60 to 100 beats per minute. In athletic people, the heart rate is often slower, around 50 beats per minute, because the well-conditioned heart pumps more efficiently. Apical pulse rhythm is documented as regular or irregular. The apical rate can be compared with the radial rate to assess equality. If there are fewer radial beats than apical beats, a **pulse deficit** exists and should be reported to the HCP.

Box 21.1

Taking Accurate Blood Pressure Measurements

- Instruct the patient to avoid exercise, caffeine, and smoking for 30 minutes before the blood pressure measurement.
- Instruct the patient to void before the reading.
- Use the auscultatory method with a properly calibrated and validated blood pressure instrument.
- Seat the patient quietly for at least 5 minutes in a chair (not on an examination table) with feet on the floor and arm supported at heart level before the blood pressure measurement.
- Use the appropriate-sized cuff so that the cuff bladder encircles at least 80% of arm when placed 1 inch above the antecubital fossa.
- Ask the patient to remain still without talking during measurement, as motion alters reading.

- Determine the patient's baseline blood pressure by inflating the cuff and noting the reading when the radial pulse is no longer felt. When taking blood pressure, inflate the cuff to 20 numbers above the obtained baseline reading. (Overinflation may cause inaccurate reading.)
- During measurement, deflate the cuff slowly at rate of 2 mm Hg/second.
- Take at least two blood pressure measurements and average.
- Remember that systolic blood pressure is the first of two or more sounds heard and that diastolic blood pressure is the final sound before the disappearance of sounds.
- Provide patients, verbally and in writing, with their specific blood pressure reading.

Box 21.2

Orthostatic Hypotension Assessment

To assess orthostatic hypotension:
1. Explain the procedure to the patient; determine whether the patient can safely stand.
2. Tell the patient not to exercise, eat, or smoke 30 minutes before readings.
3. Have the patient lie flat in bed at least 5 minutes before readings.
4. Use the correct size blood pressure cuff.
5. Tell the patient not to talk during readings and to sit up with legs uncrossed while sitting.
6. Take the patient's lying blood pressure and heart rate.
7. Assist the patient to sitting position. Ask if dizzy or light-headed with each position change. If yes, ensure safety from fainting or falling. A gait or walking belt can be used. With any position change, if the patient experiences additional symptoms with the dizziness and decreased blood pressure and increased heart rate, assist the patient to lie down, take blood pressure, and notify the health care provider (HCP). Consider the possible cause of the orthostatic hypotension (e.g., hemorrhaging, dehydration, diuretics) to plan patient care.

8. Wait 3 minutes and then take the patient's sitting blood pressure and heart rate. If the patient is dizzy or light-headed, continue sitting position for 5 minutes if tolerated. Do not attempt to bring the patient to standing. Repeat sitting blood pressure. If blood pressure has increased and the patient is no longer dizzy, assist the patient to stand.
9. After the patient is standing, take blood pressure and pulse immediately. Repeat in 3 minutes. If blood pressure drops and the patient is dizzy or light-headed, do not attempt to ambulate the patient.
10. Document all heart rate and blood pressure measurements, including extremity used and patient position when reading was obtained (e.g., right arm: lying 132/78 mm Hg, sitting 118/68 mm Hg, standing 110/60 mm Hg). Also document patient tolerance, symptoms, and nursing interventions if symptomatic.
11. Report abnormal findings to HCP.

Arterial pulses are palpated for volume and pressure quality. They are palpated bilaterally and compared for equality. A normal vessel feels soft and springy. A sclerotic vessel feels stiff. The quality of the pulses is described on a four-point scale as follows: 0 absent; 1+ weak, thready; 2+ normal; and 3+ bounding. An absent pulse is not palpable. A thready pulse is one that disappears when slight pressure is applied and returns when the pressure is removed. The normal pulse is easily palpable. The bounding pulse is strong and present even when slight pressure is applied. When the normal vessel is palpated, a tapping is felt. In the abnormal vessel that has a bulging or narrowed wall, a vibration is felt, which is called a **thrill.** When auscultating an abnormal vessel, a humming is heard that is caused by the turbulent blood flow through the vessel. This is referred to as a **bruit.**

> **BE SAFE!**
> Anticipate potential drops in blood pressure with position changes. Orthostatic hypotension can be found in patients of any age but is most commonly found in the older patient. The blood pressure drop increases the risk of fainting and falling. Use fall precautions such as a walking belt or two-person assist for patients at risk of or with orthostatic hypotension.

Respirations

The rate and ease of respirations are observed. Breath sounds are auscultated. Sputum characteristics such as amount, color, and consistency are noted. Pink, frothy sputum is an indicator of acute heart failure. A dry cough can occur from the irritation caused by the lung congestion resulting from heart failure.

Inspection

During the health history, inspection begins by noting shortness of breath when the patient speaks or moves. The patient's oxygenation status is noted through skin, mucous membrane, lip, and nailbed color. For those with dark skin, oxygen deficiency appears as a whitish or gray color around the mouth and conjunctiva that are blue or gray. For those with yellowish skin, a grayish-greenish color is seen. For those with light-skin, it appears as dark blue skin and mucous membranes, also referred to as cyanosis. Pallor may indicate anemia or lack of arterial blood flow. A dependent rubor (red) found in the lower extremities occurs from decreased arterial blood flow. Brown discoloration and purple skin when the extremity is dependent may be seen in the presence of venous blood flow problems. Hair distribution on the extremities is observed. Decreased hair distribution; thick, brittle nails; and shiny, taut, dry skin occur from reduced arterial blood flow. Venous blood return is assessed by inspecting extremities for varicose veins, stasis ulcers, or scars around the ankles and signs of thrombophlebitis such as swelling, redness, or a hard, tender vein.

The patient's internal and external jugular neck veins are observed for distention in a 45- to 90-degree upright position. Normally, the veins are not visible in this position. Distention indicates an increase in the venous volume, often caused by right-sided heart failure.

Capillary refill time is normally 3 seconds or less and shows arterial blood flow to the extremities. The patient's nailbed is briefly squeezed, causing blanching, and then released. The time that it takes for the color to return to the nailbed after release of the squeezing pressure is the capillary refill time. Longer times indicate anemia or a decrease in blood flow to the extremity.

Clubbing of the nailbeds occurs from oxygen deficiency over time. It is often caused by congenital heart defects or long-term use of tobacco. The distal ends of the fingers and toes swell and appear clublike. With clubbing, the normal 160-degree angle formed between the base of the nail and the skin is lost, causing the nail to be flat (Fig. 21.8). Later, the nail base elevates, the angle exceeds 180 degrees, and the nail feels spongy when squeezed. This should be reported to the HCP. To check for this, touch your index fingers together at the nailbeds and first joint. Look through the space created at the nailbeds. Do you see a diamond? If so, that is normal. If there is not a diamond, this indicates the nailbeds are clubbed and therefore filling that space.

> ## LEARNING TIP
> Six Ps characterize peripheral vascular disease:
> - Pain
> - Paresthesia (decreased sensation)
> - Pallor
> - Pulselessness
> - Paralysis
> - Poikilothermia (assumes temperature of the environment)

Palpation

In addition to palpating the arteries, the thorax can be palpated at the **point of maximum impulse** (PMI). The PMI is palpated by placing the right hand over the apex of the heart. If palpable, a thrust is felt when the ventricle contracts. An enlarged heart may shift the PMI to the left of the midclavicular line.

The temperature of the extremities is palpated bilaterally for comparison. Palpation begins proximally and moves distally along the extremity. In areas of decreased arterial blood flow, the **ischemic** area feels cooler than the rest of the body because it is blood that warms the body. In the absence of sufficient arterial blood flow, the area becomes the temperature of the environment (**poikilothermy**). A warm or hot extremity indicates a venous blood flow problem.

Edema is palpated in the lower extremities or dependent areas such as the sacrum for the supine patient (Fig. 21.9). Edema can occur from right-sided heart failure, gravity, or altered venous blood return. Severity of the edema is identified by applying pressure for 5 seconds over the bone where the edema is. If the finger imprint or indentation remains, the edema is pitting. Measuring the leg circumference is an accurate method for monitoring the edema.

Auscultation

Normal heart sounds are produced by the closing of the heart valves. See the figure in the "Learning Tip" that follows for the areas to auscultate to best hear these sounds. Erb's point is where S_2 is best heard. In blood-flowing vessels, sound is transmitted in the direction of the blood flow. The first heart sound (S_1) is heard at the beginning of systole as "lub" when the tricuspid and mitral (AV) valves close (Fig. 21.10). The

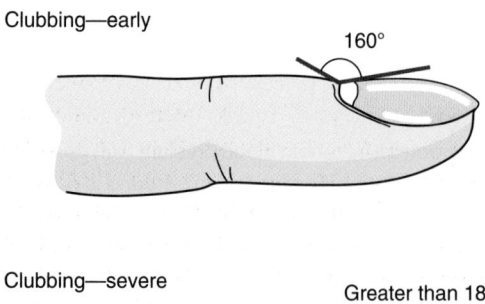

Clubbing—early

160°

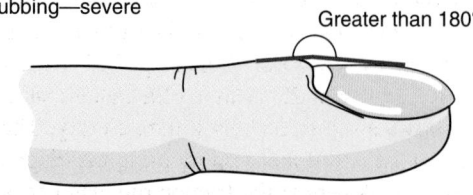

Clubbing—severe

Greater than 180°

FIGURE 21.8 Clubbing of the fingers.

• WORD • BUILDING •

ischemic: ischein—hold back + haima—blood
poikilothermy: poikilos—varied + therme—heat

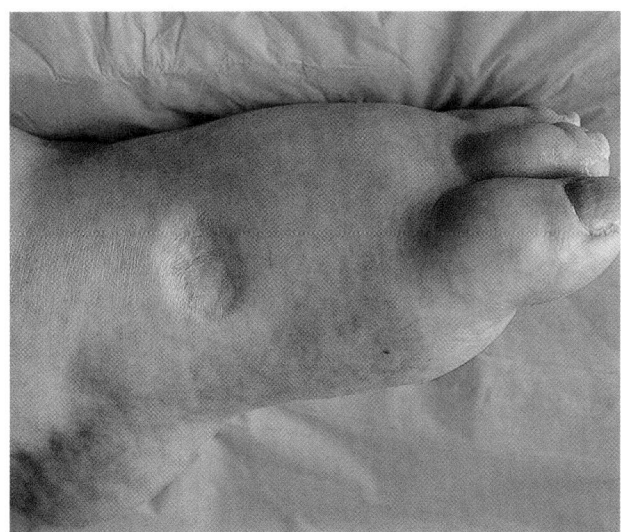

FIGURE 21.9 Pitting edema. Application of pressure over a bony area displaces the excess fluid, leaving an indentation or pit.

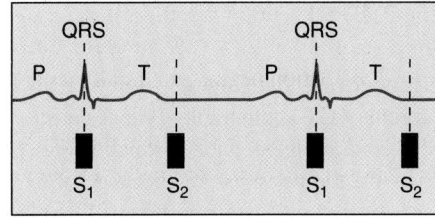

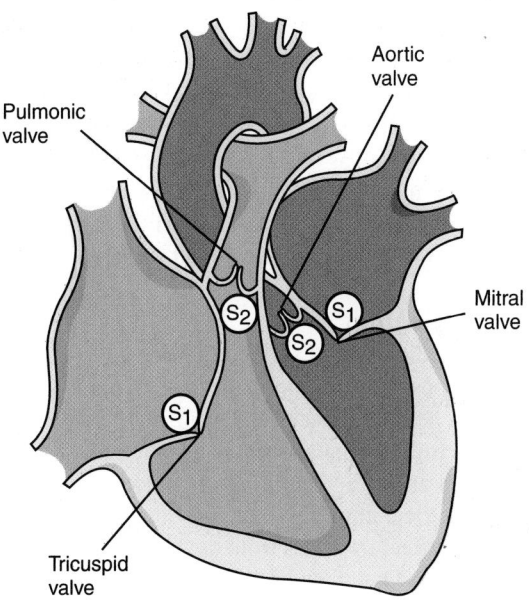

FIGURE 21.10 Heart sounds shown on electrocardiogram: S_1 is heard at the beginning of systole, and S_2 is heard at the beginning of diastole.

second heart sound (S_2) is heard at the start of diastole as "dub" when the aortic and pulmonic semilunar valves close. The diaphragm of the stethoscope is used to hear the high-pitched sounds of S_1 and S_2. Normally, no other sounds are heard between S_1 and S_2. With the bell of the stethoscope placed at the apex, a third heart sound (S_3) or a fourth heart sound (S_4) may be heard. Having patients lean forward or lie on their left side can make the heart sounds easier to hear by bringing the area of the heart where the sound may be heard closer to the chest wall. The S_3 heart sound is normal for children and younger adults. It sounds like a gallop and is a low-pitched sound heard early in diastole. In older adults, S_3 may be heard with left-sided heart failure, fluid volume overload, and mitral valve regurgitation. The S_4 heart sound is also a low-pitched sound, similar to a gallop but heard late in diastole. It occurs with hypertension, coronary artery disease, and pulmonary stenosis.

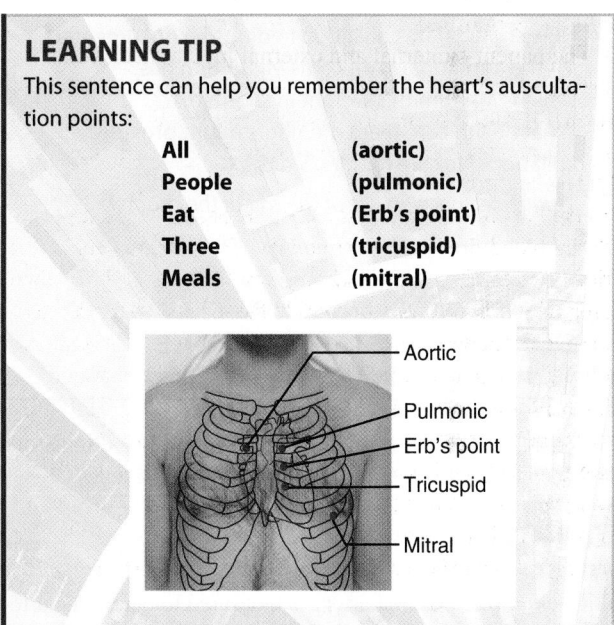

LEARNING TIP

This sentence can help you remember the heart's auscultation points:

All	**(aortic)**
People	**(pulmonic)**
Eat	**(Erb's point)**
Three	**(tricuspid)**
Meals	**(mitral)**

Murmurs are caused by a narrowed valve opening or a valve that does not close tightly. A **murmur** is a prolonged, swishing sound that ranges in intensity from faint to very loud.

A **pericardial friction rub** occurs from inflammation of the pericardium. The intensity of a rub can range from faint to loud enough to be audible without a stethoscope. A rub has a grating sound, like that of sandpaper being rubbed together, that occurs when the pericardial surfaces rub together during a heartbeat. (See the "Learning Tip" on pericardial friction rub in Chapter 23.) Having the patient sit and lean forward allows a rub to be heard more clearly. The rub is best heard to the left of the sternum using the diaphragm of the stethoscope. A pericardial friction rub may occur after a myocardial infarction (MI) or chest trauma.

CRITICAL THINKING

Mrs. Smith, age 78, baseline weight 162 pounds, is admitted to the hospital with shortness of breath. Initial data collection findings are blood pressure 152/88 mm Hg, pulse 104 beats per minute, respirations breaths 26 per minute, and temperature 99.4°F (37.2°C). She has shortness of breath at rest that increases with activity, ankle edema, distant heart tones, pale nailbeds, and no pain. She has not eaten well for 2 weeks but has had a 6-pound weight gain in 1 week. She sleeps on three pillows, and her jugular veins are visible bilaterally. A diagnosis of acute myocardial infarction (MI) with heart failure is made by her health care provider.

1. Why might Mrs. Smith not be having chest pain with a diagnosis of acute MI?
2. How should ankle edema data be collected to provide complete and measurable data?
3. What data should be documented for the ankle edema, and how should the findings be documented?
4. How should data collection findings be documented for the additional symptoms Mrs. Smith has?
5. What is Mrs. Smith's weight in kilograms?
6. What health care team members might provide collaborative care for Mrs. Smith?

Suggested answers are at the end of the chapter.

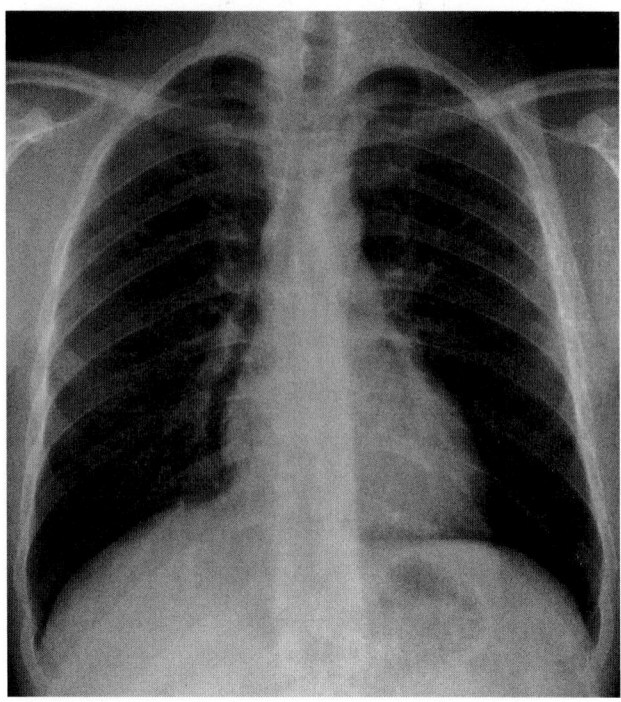

FIGURE 21.11 Normal chest x-ray film. Note white outline of heart borders in center.

DIAGNOSTIC TESTS FOR THE CARDIOVASCULAR SYSTEM

Diagnostic test results are combined with the health history and physical assessment to plan care for the patient.

Noninvasive Studies

Arterial Stiffness Index

Stiffness of the brachial artery is measured to determine arteriosclerosis and cardiovascular disease risk. The brachial artery correlates with the coronary arteries in regard to the extent of atherosclerosis. The arterial stiffness index test is done with a device that has a blood pressure cuff hooked to a computer that maps the waveforms during the blood pressure reading.

Chest Radiograph (X-Ray)

A chest x-ray can reveal heart enlargement, calcifications, fluid around the heart, heart failure, and placement of pacemaker leads and pulmonary artery catheters (Fig. 21.11). Fluoroscopy uses a luminescent x-ray screen to guide cardiac catheter or pacemaker lead placement. Visit www.radiologyinfo.org for more information.

Computed Tomography

Computed tomography (CT) is used for calcium scoring of calcified plaque in the coronary arteries. The body deposits calcium to harden plaques, which are not normally found in the coronary arteries. CT angiography (views body blood vessels) and coronary CT angiography (views coronary arteries) use an iodine contrast agent. Kidney function (i.e., glomerular filtration rate, creatinine) must be checked before the test to help prevent contrast-induced nephropathy (see Chapter 36).

Coronary Magnetic Resonance Imaging and Angiography

Two- or three-dimensional still or moving images of the beating heart are produced with magnetic resonance imaging (MRI). Cardiac MRI is useful for identifying ischemia and heart damage as well as other conditions affecting the heart. For coronary magnetic resonance angiography (MRA), a non–iodine-based contrast, gadolinium-DTPA, may or may not be used to view the coronary blood vessels.

Electrocardiogram

The electrocardiogram (ECG) records electrical activity of the heart in various views. Abnormalities related to conduction, rate, rhythm, heart chamber enlargement, myocardial ischemia, MI, and electrolyte imbalances may be reflected on an ECG.

To obtain an ECG, electrodes are placed on the skin to transmit electrical impulses to the ECG machine for recording. The electrical impulses from the heart appear as waves on graph paper. One view of the heart using a combination of the electrodes to obtain the view is called a lead. The standard 12-lead ECG provides 12 views of the heart. In addition, 15- and 18-lead ECGs can be done.

SIGNAL-AVERAGED ECG. The signal-averaged ECG uses a computer to record electrical heart signals for 20 minutes to capture undetected low-level signals that are averaged. This can identify if a patient is at risk for ventricular **arrhythmias** (abnormal heart rhythms; also known as *dysrhythmias*).

HOLTER MONITORING (AMBULATORY ECG). A Holter monitor is worn and continuously records an ECG in one lead for up to 48 hours as a patient goes about his or her daily activities. The patient records a diary of activities and symptoms and pushes the event button if symptoms occur. Symptoms are documented for later correlation with the ECG recordings. Recordings are scanned by a computer and interpreted by an HCP. Arrhythmias or myocardial ischemia that occur infrequently can be detected.

Echocardiogram

An echocardiogram is an ultrasound that records the motion of the heart structures, including the valves and chambers, as well as the heart size, shape, and position. Three-dimensional images of the heart and four-dimensional (real-time) heart imaging is possible. Color Doppler can record blood flow through the heart valves. This test transmits ultrasonic sound waves across the chest wall (transthoracic) and through lung and rib tissue into the heart so that the returned echoes can be recorded. An ECG is recorded at the same time. Examples of echocardiograms include the following:

• A strain echocardiogram shows changes in the shape of the heart (deformation). It is used for heart failure, in cardiomyopathy, to guide treatment, or to evaluate cardiac surgery or transplant.
• An exercise stress echocardiogram shows exercise-induced cardiac ischemia to diagnose coronary artery disease. If the patient is unable to exercise, dobutamine (a cardiac inotrope and chronotrope) is given as the heart responds to it as it does to exercise. A transesophageal echocardiogram (TEE) produces clear images using a transducer on a probe placed in the esophagus because lung and rib tissue does not have to be penetrated by the sound waves. Patients take nothing by mouth (NPO) for about 6 hours before the test and receive a sedative. The patient's throat is anesthetized with a local anesthetic.

BE SAFE!
Whenever a patient's throat is anesthetized for a procedure, the patient must not take anything by mouth (NPO) until the nurse has verified (by touching the back of the throat with a cotton tip swab) that the gag reflex has returned. The patient could aspirate or choke while drinking or eating if the gag reflex is not present.

Exercise Stress Test

The exercise stress test measures cardiac function or peripheral vascular disease during a defined exercise protocol (Fig. 21.12). If the patient is unable to exercise, a coronary vasodilator such as adenosine or dipyridamole

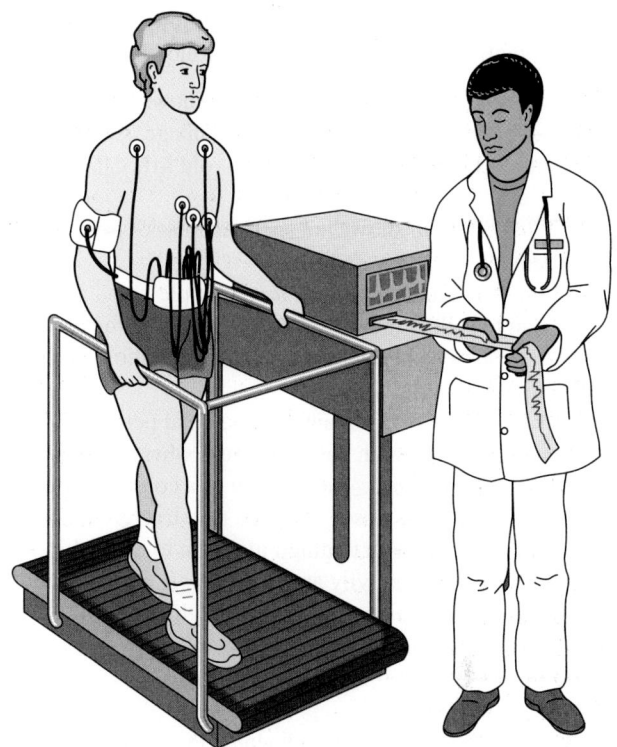

FIGURE 21.12 Performance of exercise stress test.

can be given to increase blood flow in healthy vessels and show unhealthy areas with reduced blood flow. Test instructions include an explanation of the test; not smoking, eating, or drinking for 2 to 4 hours before the test; and wearing comfortable walking shoes, a loose top, and, for women, a supportive bra.

Before the test, baseline vital signs are obtained. Then, while the patient exercises on a treadmill, on a stationary bicycle, or by climbing stairs, vital signs, oxygen saturation, skin temperature, physical appearance, chest pain, and ECG are monitored to help ensure patient safety. The test is completed when the patient reaches his or her peak heart rate (patient's age subtracted from 220), experiences chest pain or other symptoms, is unable to exercise further, or develops abnormal vital sign or ECG changes. Vital signs and ECG continue to be monitored after the test until they return to baseline.

For a peripheral vascular stress test, the patient walks for 5 minutes at 1.5 miles per hour on the treadmill. Pulse volume measurements are taken at baseline resting, during the test, and at final resting after the test. If intermittent **claudication** (pain in the legs with activity) occurs, the test is stopped.

Nuclear Radioisotope Imaging

For nuclear radioisotope imaging, small amounts of radioisotopes are given via intravenous (IV) route. The patient is then scanned with a gamma camera to produce a radionuclide image. Radiation exposure is similar to that of other x-ray examinations. These tests can provide information about myocardial ischemia, MI, cardiac blood flow, and ventricle size and motion. Examples include the following:

- Technetium (TC-99m) pyrophosphate shows hot spots in areas of ischemia or myocardial cell damage. Acute MI size and location can be detected, but old MIs cannot be detected.
- TC-99m sestamibi shows hot spots in areas of myocardial cell damage.
- TC-99m pertechnetate is used in a multiple-gated acquisition scan to follow the flow of radioactivity in the bloodstream to show ventricular function, wall motion, and the ejection fraction of the heart.
- Thallium-201 detects impaired myocardial perfusion and ischemia or MI through cold spot areas where the thallium was not absorbed. The patency of a coronary artery graft may also be assessed with this test. Exercise testing may be combined with thallium injection to detect blood flow changes with activity and after rest. If patients are unable to participate in exercise for the thallium stress test, coronary vasodilators can be given.

Tilt Table Test

The tilt table test is used to help diagnose the cause of syncope (fainting spells). Heart rate and blood pressure are monitored during a change in position from lying down to standing up.

Doppler Ultrasound

In a Doppler ultrasound test, sound waves bounce off moving blood cells in the peripheral blood vessels and return a sound frequency in relationship to the amount of blood flow. With decreased blood flow, the sounds are reduced. This test requires no patient preparation, takes about 20 minutes to complete, and is painless.

BE SAFE!

Identify patients correctly. Use at least two ways to identify patients. For example, use the patient's name and date of birth. This is done to make sure that each patient gets the correct medicine and treatment. (2018 National Patient Safety Goals, © The Joint Commission, 2018. Reprinted with permission.)

Blood Studies
Cardiac Biomarkers

Proteins and enzymes released into the blood by damaged cardiac cells are known as cardiac biomarkers. These biomarkers help identify whether a patient is having or has had a recent MI.

CARDIAC TROPONIN. Cardiac muscle contains proteins called troponin I and troponin T, which control the muscle fibers that contract or squeeze the heart muscle. They detect minor myocardial damage not detected by creatine kinase-MB, so it is the more commonly done test to diagnose MI. Levels elevate within 4 to 6 hours of damage. These levels peak in 10 to 24 hours and remain elevated for 10 to 14 days. Troponin T appears slightly earlier than troponin I and remains elevated longer after cardiac damage.

CREATINE KINASE. Creatine kinase (CK) is an enzyme found in the brain, skeletal muscle, and heart muscle. Isoenzymes of CK contained in these tissues are CK-BB (brain), CK-MM (skeletal muscle), and CK-MB (heart muscle). CK-MB helps diagnose an MI because its level rises within 4 to 6 hours after cardiac cells are damaged, peaks in 12 to 18 hours, and returns to normal in 24 to 36 hours. Invasive procedures such as IV and intramuscular (IM) injections are avoided before drawing the first CK to prevent elevation in the CK levels from cell trauma caused by the procedure.

MYOGLOBIN. Myoglobin is a protein found in skeletal and cardiac muscle. It is not site specific so it can only indicate that muscle damage has occurred. However, it rises before CK-MB or troponin so it can detect an MI earlier for prompt treatment. Myoglobin levels elevate within 1 hour of an acute MI. Peak levels are reached 4 to 12 hours after an MI, and levels return to normal within 18 hours after the onset of chest pain.

C-Reactive Protein

C-reactive protein is an acute-phase protein that increases during the inflammatory process. A highly sensitive C-reactive protein (hs-CRP) test can predict heart attack risk. With elevated hs-CRP levels, nurses have the opportunity to help patients understand and reduce cardiac risk factors.

Homocysteine

Homocysteine is an amino acid in the blood that may damage the lining of arteries and promote blood clots. Elevated levels are associated with increased cardiovascular disease risk. Folic acid, vitamin B_6, and vitamin B_{12} break down homocysteine. Green leafy vegetables and grains fortified with folic acid as well as vitamin B can help reduce homocysteine levels.

Lipids

Lipids include triglycerides, cholesterol, and phospholipids. Lipoproteins carry these lipids attached to proteins. Triglycerides are found in very low-density lipoproteins. Cholesterol is mainly found in low-density lipoproteins (LDLs). High-density lipoproteins (HDLs) are a mixture of one-half protein and one-half phospholipids and cholesterol.

A lipid profile can screen for increased risk of coronary artery disease. Patients fast for 12 hours and avoid alcohol for 24 hours before the test. Water is not withheld. High levels of LDLs are linked to an increase in coronary artery disease because they circulate cholesterol in the arteries. HDLs play a protective role against coronary artery disease because they carry cholesterol to the liver to be metabolized. Controlling lipids is important in reducing coronary artery disease.

Magnesium

Magnesium, an electrolyte, is important to many functions in the body. Among these is control of the heartbeat and regulation of blood pressure. A normal magnesium level is 1.6 to 2.6 mg/dL. **Hypomagnesemia,** a low level of magnesium in the blood, can cause cardiac arrhythmias, hypertension, and tachycardia. Many things can contribute to low magnesium levels, including diuretic therapy, digitalis, some antibiotics, diabetes mellitus, and MI.

> **BE SAFE!**
>
> *Improve staff communication.* Get important test results to the right staff person on time. (2018 National Patient Safety Goals, © The Joint Commission, 2018. Reprinted with permission.)

Potassium

A normal potassium level of 3.5 to 5.0 mEq/L is essential for normal cardiac function (see Chapter 6). **Hypokalemia** (low potassium level) can cause the pulse to become weak, irregular, and thready. **Hyperkalemia** (high potassium level) can result in muscle twitches and cramps followed by muscular weakness and a slow, irregular heart rate; weak pulse; and reduced blood pressure. Hypokalemia is more common. An abnormal potassium level can be dangerous. Arrhythmias can occur, which can lead to cardiac arrest. Report abnormal potassium levels to the HCP.

Invasive Studies

Angiography

Arteriography and venography are the two types of angiography (Fig. 21.13). Arteriography examines arteries. Venography studies veins. Angiography uses dye injected into the vascular system to visualize the vessels on radiographs. This test is used to assess blood clot formation, peripheral vascular disease, and test vessels for potential grafting use.

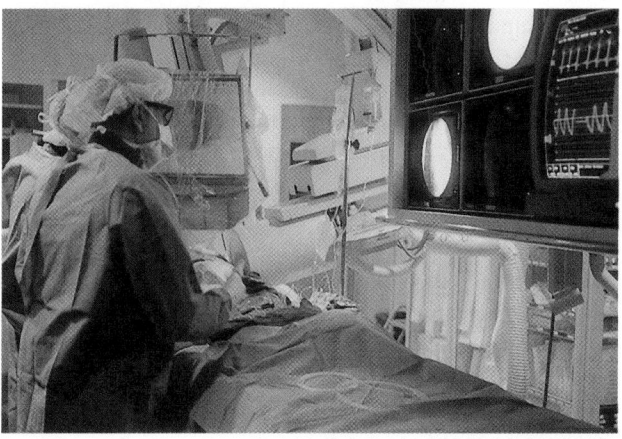

FIGURE 21.13 Coronary angiography and cardiac catheterization.

The patient must be assessed for allergies, give informed consent, be NPO for about 4 hours before the test, and be informed that the dye produces a hot, burning feeling when injected. After the procedure, vital signs, allergic reaction signs, hemorrhage at the injection site, and pulses are monitored for several hours.

Cardiac Catheterization

Cardiac catheterization allows the heart's anatomy and physiology to be studied or therapeutic procedures to be done. As an invasive diagnostic procedure, it measures pressures in the heart chambers, great blood vessels, and coronary arteries. It provides information on cardiac output and oxygen saturation. Fluoroscopy is an x-ray procedure that produces real-time images of internal organs in motion on a video monitor. It is used to guide the insertion of the catheter into the heart. Dye can be injected once the catheter is in place to visualize the heart chambers and vessels. This procedure is often done before heart surgery.

An informed consent must be obtained. Allergies to contrast agents are identified. The patient will be NPO for about 8 hours before the test. IV hydration may be given before the procedure while the patient is NPO. Patients should be told that during the test that they will be awake; a local anesthetic, which may sting, will numb the catheter insertion site; a warm, flushing sensation may be felt when the dye is injected; the room has a lot of equipment; a movable table is used; the patient's vital signs and ECG are monitored constantly; and the length of the procedure is 2 to 3 hours.

In right-sided catheterization, a catheter with or without a fiber optic tip may be inserted into the internal jugular vein (neck), the femoral vein (leg), or an arm vein and advanced into the vena cava. It is then moved through the right chambers of the heart and into the pulmonary artery. The catheter can be wedged momentarily in the artery by inflating the balloon at the tip of the catheter. This position provides the pulmonary artery wedge pressure, which reflects pressures in the left side of the heart. Other pressures obtained with right-sided cardiac catheterization are right atrial pressure, which reflects central venous pressure; pulmonary artery systolic and diastolic pressures; cardiac output; and mixed venous oxygen saturation (SvO_2) if a fiber optic catheter is used.

The left side of the heart can be directly assessed by inserting a catheter into the radial, brachial, or femoral artery. It is advanced against the flow of blood into the aorta, through the aortic valve, and into the left ventricle. Coronary angiography, which visualizes the coronary arteries with dye, can be done with this approach. The catheter is inserted into the opening of the coronary arteries, the dye is injected, and x-ray films are taken. Coronary artery disease can be assessed with coronary angiography.

• WORD • BUILDING •

hypomagnesemia: hypo—low + magnes—magnesium + emia—in blood

After the procedure, the catheter is removed. Firm pressure must be applied to the insertion site for 15 to 30 minutes to prevent hemorrhage, retroperitoneal bleeding or hematoma formation which are the most common complications. Manual pressure, a clamp or artery closure device is used. Vital signs, the puncture site, and peripheral pulses are monitored. The patient is on bedrest without moving or flexing the leg for a few hours to prevent bleeding if the groin was used. For comfort, modified positioning and use of a pillow may be used without complications as ordered. Patients can eat and are encouraged to drink fluids to help eliminate the dye from the body. If the patient is stable and no significant findings are found, the patient may be discharged.

Complications of cardiac catheterization can be allergic reaction, breaking of the catheter, hemorrhage, thrombus formation, emboli of air or blood, arrhythmias, MI, cerebrovascular accident (stroke), and puncture of the heart chambers or lungs.

Hemodynamic Monitoring

A catheter attached to a transducer and monitor, called an arterial line, can be inserted into the radial or femoral artery to measure continuous arterial blood pressure. Ongoing monitoring of central venous pressure, cardiac pressures, and cardiac output can be done with either a central catheter inserted into the vena cava or a pulmonary artery catheter. Central venous pressure reflects **preload** (pressure stretching the ventricle of the heart from fluid returned to the heart).

Electrophysiological Study

To study the heart's electrical system, one or more catheters with electrodes are inserted via the femoral vein into the right side of the heart. Two to three electrodes are usually inserted. The heart's electrical impulses are then recorded and pacing can also be done. Arrhythmias can be triggered to help the HCP diagnose why they are occurring. A consent is obtained, and the patient is NPO 6 to 8 hours before the test.

THERAPEUTIC MEASURES FOR THE CARDIOVASCULAR SYSTEM

Health Promotion and Lifestyle Changes

To reduce risk factors or promote recovery from cardiovascular disease, lifestyle changes are often needed. Long-standing habits are difficult to change. Support groups can offer encouragement that is helpful in promoting a healthy lifestyle. Patients should be referred to community support groups as needed.

Diet

A healthy, balanced diet is important to help reduce the risk for coronary artery disease. Weight reduction, if needed, is encouraged. Eating at least five servings of fruits and vegetables daily, increasing fish intake, eating poultry without skin, and limiting saturated fats and sodium are parts of a healthy diet.

Exercise

A prescribed walking program helps promote blood flow by contracting the skeletal muscles and may reduce symptoms of peripheral vascular disease. Exercise is very important for optimum cardiac functioning.

Smoking Cessation

Smoking causes vasoconstriction that can last up to 1 hour after smoking one cigarette. For patients with cardiac or vascular disease, blood flow is reduced, which can exacerbate symptoms. Patients should be encouraged to stop smoking and be provided with information on cessation programs and support groups (see www.americanheart.org).

Antiembolism Devices

Antiembolism devices improve arterial blood flow and venous return to prevent the formation of blood clots. They are used for patients with peripheral vascular disease, on bedrest, or after surgery or trauma.

Elastic Stockings

Antiembolism stockings apply compression to the leg to promote the movement of fluid and prevent stasis of fluid. These stockings may be knee or thigh length. They must be applied correctly so that a tourniquet effect is not produced by the stockings. For ease in application, the stocking is turned inside out to the heel, the foot portion is placed on the patient up to the heel, and then the remaining stocking is pulled up over the leg. Knee-length stockings should be 1 to 2 inches below the bottom of the kneecap. They should not roll down, or they will cause stasis rather than prevent it. Some patients may require assistance in applying the stockings if they have impaired manual dexterity. Devices are available that aid in applying the stockings, such as the Sigvaris Doff N' Donner.

Intermittent Pneumatic Compression Devices

An intermittent pneumatic compression device consists of plastic inflatable stockings that are filled intermittently with air by an attached motor. This device simulates the contraction of the leg muscles, promoting fluid movement, which helps to prevent thrombosis development. The compartments in the stockings inflate to 35 to 55 mm Hg of pressure, beginning in the ankle compartment and progressing next to the calf compartment and finally the thigh compartment. Monitor the device for proper pressure inflation.

Oxygen

Supplemental oxygen is administered to patients with chest pain to help ensure that the heart receives sufficient oxygen to function. Oxygen may be delivered via a nasal cannula or facemask. Teach the patient safety precautions necessary for home use of oxygen, such as avoiding open flames and not smoking when the oxygen is in use.

Medications

The primary cardiovascular drugs are antihypertensives, antiarrhythmics, antianginals, anticoagulants, cardiac glycosides, thrombolytics, and vasodilators. They are discussed in further detail where the disorders they are used to treat are discussed (see "Nutrition Notes").

Nutrition Notes

CYP Enzymes and Fruit. Cytochrome P450 (CYP450) is a superfamily of more than 50 enzymes found mainly in the liver but also in the gastrointestinal tract, lungs, placenta, and kidneys. The isoenzyme CYP3A4, found in the small intestine, plays a major role in regulating the oral bioavailability of many drugs, a function that may have evolved to protect the body from toxins. After uptake by the intestinal epithelial cells (enterocytes), many substances are metabolized by CYP3A4 or returned to the intestinal lumen by a transporter protein, P-glycoprotein (P-gp). This provides repeated opportunities for CYP3A4 enzymes to metabolize the drug. The amount of the drug available for absorption is, therefore, limited.

Grapefruit, Seville oranges (often used to make marmalade), and tangelos appear to inhibit intestinal CYP3A4, causing more drug to be absorbed into the bloodstream (Food and Drug Administration, 2017). Adverse effects can result. Consult a pharmacist for specific drug information. These fruits, whether in whole or juice form, should be avoided when taking the following medications: statins to lower cholesterol, including simvastatin (Zocor), atorvastatin (Lipitor), and pravastatin (Pravachol); antihypertensives, including nifedipine (Nifediac, Afeditab); and antiarrhythmics, including amiodarone (Cordarone, Nexterone).

Reference

U.S. Food and Drug Administration. (2017). Grapefruit juice and some drugs don't mix. Retrieved from www.fda.gov/ForConsumers/ConsumerUpdates/ucm292276.htm

---

Cardiac Surgery

As heart disease symptoms increase in severity and frequency or the disease process worsens, cardiac surgery may be used as treatment.

Preparation for Surgery

A nursing assessment is important to provide baseline data that can be used for postoperative comparison and early discharge planning. In addition to common admission testing, patients with chronic obstructive pulmonary disease may have baseline arterial blood gases and pulmonary function tests (Box 21.3). Patients with carotid bruits have carotid studies to determine the amount of occlusion in the carotid artery. If the occlusion is significant, a carotid endarterectomy, which removes the plaque on the lining of the blocked

---

Box 21.3

Cardiac Admission Testing

- Twelve-lead electrocardiogram
- Chest x-ray
- Complete blood cell count
- Coagulation studies
- Chemistry profile
- Blood crossmatch

---

or diseased carotid artery, is performed, usually several weeks before having cardiac surgery.

Medications that may increase bleeding or reduce fluid volume may be ordered to be held before surgery by the HCP. Drugs that increase bleeding include aspirin, often stopped 3 to 7 days preoperatively; warfarin (Coumadin), often stopped 4 to 5 days preoperatively; and heparin, usually stopped 4 hours preoperatively. During surgery, fluid volume and blood pressure may be decreased by blood loss or medications. Therefore, diuretics, which could further reduce fluid volume and blood pressure, are withheld up to 2 days before surgery. The patient is NPO as specified before surgery. For this reason, patients with diabetes have insulin and oral hypoglycemic agents reduced or withheld the morning of surgery. Blood glucose monitoring is done. The anesthesiologist assesses the patient before surgery and orders preoperative medications.

Patients recover more quickly and have less postoperative stress with thorough preoperative teaching on coughing and deep breathing exercises; incision care; pain management; equipment, including the endotracheal tube and ventilator, and methods of communicating while intubated; chest tubes; IV lines; the urinary catheter; and equipment alarms. It should be emphasized to the patient and family that the patient will not be able to talk while the endotracheal tube is in place. Additionally, a preoperative family tour of the patient's postoperative unit and the waiting area helps prepare them for the surgical experience. A referral to pastoral care, if desired, can be comforting to the patient and family.

Cardiopulmonary Bypass

Cardiac surgeries may use a cardiopulmonary bypass pump in which blood is temporarily diverted away from the heart and lungs to the special pump (Fig. 21.14). This diversion allows for a bloodless and motionless surgical field while the function of the heart and lungs is maintained by the pump (Fig. 21.15).

Before going on the pump, the patient is anticoagulated with heparin until the partial thromboplastin time is five to six times greater than normal. Immediately before the patient comes off the pump, the effects of the heparin are reversed with protamine sulfate (antidote for heparin). Heparin is absorbed and stored in organs and tissue and can be sporadically released hours after surgery. As a result, the patient may have

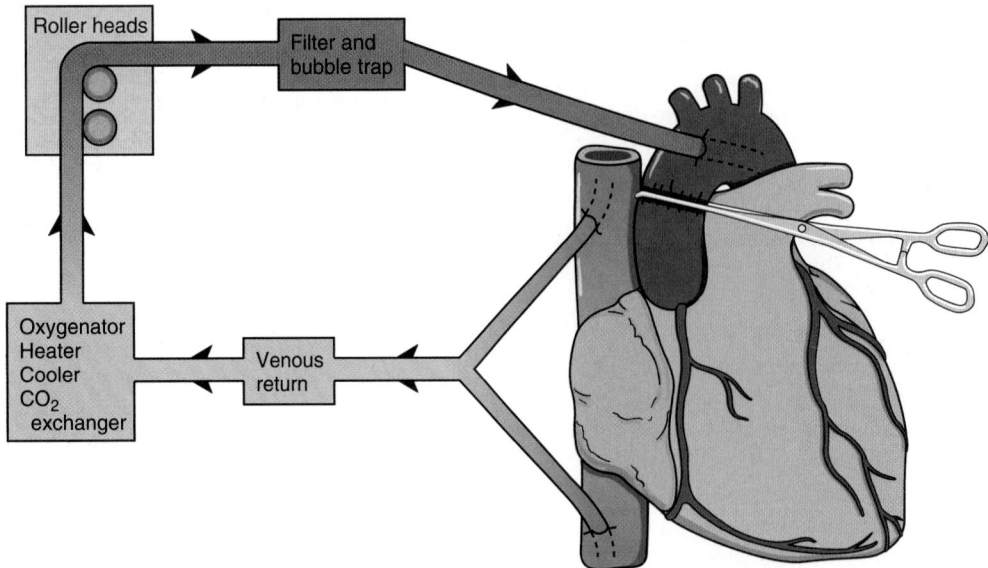

FIGURE 21.14 Cardiopulmonary bypass pump components.

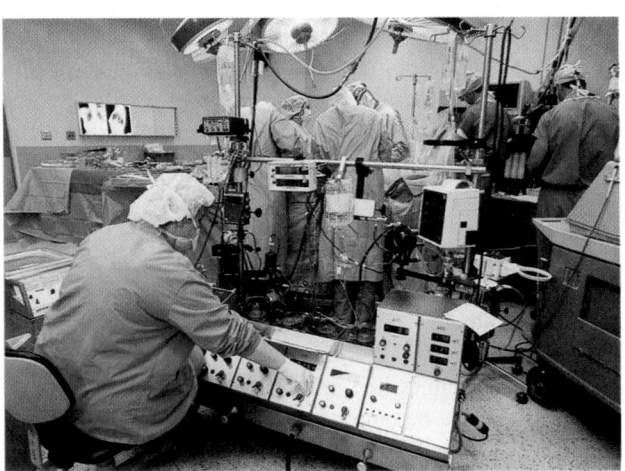

FIGURE 21.15 Cardiopulmonary bypass pump in use.

excessive bleeding. The risk of an air embolism is minimized by priming the pump with lactated Ringer's solution. The priming solution increases circulating volume, which then results in a shifting of fluid into the interstitial tissue and edema formation. These fluid shifts can continue up to 6 hours after surgery and can cause hypotension.

General Procedure for Cardiac Surgery

After the patient is placed on cardiopulmonary bypass, a cardioplegic solution is infused into the aortic root along with iced saline to cause cardiac standstill. When the surgery is completed, the patient's blood is warmed in the cardiopulmonary bypass circuit, and the patient is slowly weaned from bypass. The heart starts beating again after it is warmed and defibrillated. Temporary pacing wires are attached to the heart before the cardiopulmonary bypass pump is discontinued, so an external temporary pacemaker can be used if bradycardia develops. Once the heart is beating, bypass is stopped. Mediastinal chest tubes are placed to drain remaining blood and fluid from the chest. The **sternotomy** is closed with wires through the sternum and then sutures for the layers of tissue and skin. While still under anesthesia, the patient is transferred to a cardiac care unit. Cardiac universal beds may be used, in which patients stay in the same room during their entire hospitalization to receive care.

For patients recovering from cardiac surgery or an MI, activity is gradually increased. A cardiac rehabilitation program is usually prescribed, and individualized exercise goals are determined. After discharge from the hospital, exercise three times a week for 20 to 30 minutes is encouraged.

Minimally Invasive Cardiac Surgery

Minimally invasive direct visualization coronary artery bypass is a technique that is done without the use of cardiopulmonary bypass. Port-access coronary artery bypass combines peripheral cardiopulmonary bypass with minimally invasive heart access (see Chapter 24). Risk for complications associated with these surgeries is much lower than with the traditional procedure, and the recovery time is often weeks less.

• WORD • BUILDING •

sternotomy: stern—sternum + otomy—incision into

SUGGESTED ANSWERS TO CRITICAL THINKING

Mrs. Smith

1. An older person may not experience typical myocardial infarction (MI) symptoms. Chest pain is often not present in MI because of reduced nerve sensitivity with aging. Dyspnea is the classic symptom of MI in the older patient.

2. Inspect both legs to determine edematous areas. Determine location and severity of edema by pressing for 5 seconds over the medial malleolus and moving up the leg along the tibia until no edema is found. Palpate bilaterally. Measure leg circumference.

3. Document location of edema and whether edema is nonpitting or pitting for both legs. Documentation would state "Bilateral pitting ankle edema" with the leg circumference measurement number.

4. Additional symptoms should be documented as follows: dyspnea at rest that increases with exertion, heart tones clear and distant, nailbeds pale, pain free, poor appetite for 2 weeks, 6-pound weight gain in 1 week, three-pillow orthopnea, bilateral jugular venous distention.

5. Unit analysis method:

$$\frac{162 \text{ pounds}}{} \; \left| \; \frac{1 \text{ kilogram}}{2.2 \text{ pounds}} \; \right| = 73.6 \text{ kilograms}$$

6. Health care provider, nurses, pharmacist, respiratory therapist, dietitian, and social worker or case manager.

Review Questions

1. The nurse is contributing to the plan of care for a patient with heart disease. Which of the following is a modifiable cardiovascular risk factor identified during patient data collection that should be included in the teaching plan? **Select all that apply.**
   1. 56 years old
   2. Male
   3. Asian
   4. Tobacco use
   5. Obesity
   6. Sedentary lifestyle

2. The nurse checks capillary refill on a patient and finds it is 4 seconds. The nurse would inform the health care provider since which of the following could be indicated?
   1. Decreased arterial flow to the extremity
   2. Increased arterial flow to the extremity
   3. Decreased venous flow from the extremity
   4. Increased venous flow from the extremity

3. The nurse is to obtain orthostatic blood pressure measurements. Which of the following safety interventions should the nurse use during this procedure? **Select all that apply.**
   1. Reality orientation
   2. Gait or walking belt
   3. Liquids at bedside
   4. Standing patient quickly
   5. Asking whether dizzy before standing
   6. Standing near patient

4. The nurse is caring for a patient on bedrest who is on diuretic therapy. Which action should the nurse take to check for the presence of edema? **Select all that apply.**
   1. Press on sternal area.
   2. Ask patient to perform ankle pumps.
   3. Turn patient onto side.
   4. Inspect sacrum.
   5. Perform sternal rub.
   6. Press on sacrum.

5. The nurse is providing teaching for a patient undergoing a coronary angiography. Which of the following would the nurse include in the teaching plan for a coronary angiography with femoral catheter insertion site? **Select all that apply.**
   1. Dye injection causes a hot, flushing sensation.
   2. General anesthesia is administered.
   3. Claustrophobia may be experienced.
   4. Ambulation is not possible immediately after procedure.
   5. Allergies are assessed before testing.
   6. Firm pressure must be applied to the insertion site.

6. The nurse is reinforcing teaching about a high-fiber diet for a patient with angina. The patient asks what the purpose of the diet is. Which of the following replies by the nurse would be appropriate?
   1. "To increase absorption of the nutrients in your intestine."
   2. "To prevent straining to reduce your heart's workload."
   3. "To prevent ankle edema development."
   4. "To reduce your appetite."

7. A patient is scheduled for vascular surgery. The patient is taking digoxin (Lanoxin), furosemide (Lasix), warfarin (Coumadin), and famotidine (Pepcid). Which medication would the nurse question the possible need to stop several days before surgery?
   1. digoxin (Lanoxin)
   2. furosemide (Lasix)
   3. warfarin (Coumadin)
   4. famotidine (Pepcid)

Answer rationales available in your online resources.

ANSWERS 1. 4, 5, 6; 2. 1; 3. 2, 5, 6; 4. 3, 4, 6; 5. 1, 4, 5, 6; 6. 2; 7. 3

Key Points

Find the chapter key points in your online resources available through Davis Edge.

Additional Resources

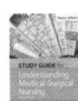 Use the scratch off code on the inside front cover of your book to access online quizzes that will help you to improve your scores on course exams and prepare for NCLEX-PN®.

Study Guide

CHAPTER 22

Nursing Care of Patients With Hypertension

Linda S. Williams

KEY TERMS

cardiac output (KAR-dee-yak OWT-put)
diastolic (dy-uh-STAH-lik)
essential hypertension (ee-SEN-shul HY-per-TEN-shun)
hypertension (HY-per-TEN-shun)
hypertensive emergency (HY-per-TEN-siv ee-MUR-gen-see)
hypertensive urgency (HY-per-TEN-siv UR-gen-see)
hypertrophy (hy-PER-truh-fee)
peripheral vascular resistance (puh-RIFF-uh-ruhl VAS-kyoo-lar ree-ZIS-tense)
plaque (PLAK)
primary hypertension (PRY-mare-ee HY-per-TEN-shun)
secondary hypertension (SEK-un-DAR-ee HY-per-TEN-shun)
systolic (sis-TALL-ik)
viscosity (vis-KAW-sih-tee)

CHAPTER CONCEPT

Perfusion

LEARNING OUTCOMES

1. Define classifications of hypertension in adults.
2. Explain the pathophysiology of hypertension.
3. Identify causes and risk factors for hypertension.
4. List signs and symptoms of hypertension.
5. Describe therapeutic measures for hypertension.
6. Define hypertensive emergency.
7. List common complications of hypertension.
8. Plan nursing care for patients with hypertension.
9. Evaluate effectiveness of nursing interventions.

Hypertension, or high blood pressure (BP), is a primary risk factor for cardiovascular disease (CVD) and stroke. Its prevalence remains high. Visit www.heart.org for hypertension statistics from the American Heart Association (AHA). The American College of Cardiology (ACC) and the AHA redefined normal and abnormal BP for adults aged 18 and older, which is provided in Table 22.1 (Whelton et al., 2017). The United States Preventive Services Task Force's (2017) recommendation for screening for those aged 18 to 39 with a normal BP is every 3 to 5 years. Annual screening is recommended for those who are over 39 or at increased risk. Those at increased risk include people who have an elevated BP (130 to 139 millimeters of mercury [mm Hg] **systolic** or 85 to 89 mm Hg **diastolic**), are overweight, or are African American.

Lifestyle interventions to reduce cardiovascular risk are identified in the 2013 AHA/ACC Guideline on Lifestyle Management to Reduce Cardiovascular Risk (Eckel et al., 2013). The 2014 Evidence-Based Guideline for the Management of High Blood Pressure in Adults by the Eighth Joint National Committee (JNC 8) defines pharmacologic treatment thresholds, recommends drug therapy, and supports the 2013 AHA/ACC lifestyle modifications guidelines (James et al., 2014). Counseling patients with brief messages about diet can be effective in changing diet behaviors (e.g., "Eat whole foods as they are found in nature" and "Avoid added sugars except for special occasions") (Fleming, Aspry, Resnicow, & Kris-Etherton, 2016).

• WORD • BUILDING •
hypertension: hyper—excessive + tensio—tension
systolic: systole—concentration
diastolic: diastole—expansion

Table 22.1
Blood Pressure (BP) Categories*

BP Category	Systolic BP		Diastolic BP
Normal	<120 mm Hg	and	<80 mm Hg
Elevated	120-129 mm Hg	and	<80 mm Hg
Hypertension			
Stage 1	130-139 mm Hg	or	80-89 mm Hg
Stage 2	≥140 mm Hg	or	≥90 mm Hg

*Individuals with SBP and DBP in 2 categories should be designated to the higher BP category. BP indicates blood pressure (based on an average of ≥2 careful readings obtained on ≥2 occasions.

Reprinted with permission
Hypertension.2017;HYP.0000000000000065
©2017 American Heart Association, Inc.

Evidence-Based Practice

Clinical Question
Does diet affect high blood pressure?

Evidence
A systematic review and meta-analysis using 24 randomized control trials revealed that adopting healthful dietary modifications, including low-sodium, low-calorie, the Dietary Approaches to Stop Hypertension (DASH), and Mediterranean diets, led to significant reductions in both systolic and diastolic blood pressure. The effects were similar across the types of diets examined and among the subgroups included in the studies (Gay, Rao, Vaccarino, & Ali, 2016).

Implications for Nursing Practice
Teach patients that diet is an important part of a healthy lifestyle to help control blood pressure. Even small decreases in blood pressure can reduce cardiovascular disease and mortality.

References
Gay, H. C., Rao, S. G., Vaccarino, V., & Ali, M. K. (2016). Effects of different dietary interventions on blood pressure: Systematic review and meta-analysis of randomized controlled trials. *Hypertension, 67*(4), 733–739.

PATHOPHYSIOLOGY OF HYPERTENSION

Normally, the heart pumps or perfuses blood through the body to meet the cells' needs for oxygen and nutrients. As it pumps, the heart forces blood through the blood vessels. The pressure exerted by blood on the walls of the blood vessels is measured as BP. BP is determined by **cardiac output** (CO), **peripheral vascular resistance** (PVR; the ability of the vessels to stretch), the **viscosity** (thickness) of the blood, and the amount of circulating blood volume. Decreased stretching ability of blood vessels, increased blood viscosity, and/or increased fluid volume may cause an increase in BP.

Several processes influence BP. These include nervous system regulation, arterial baroreceptors and chemoreceptors, the renin-angiotensin-aldosterone mechanism, and the balance of body fluids. One way BP is influenced is through adjustment of CO, which is the amount of blood that the heart pumps each minute. The heart rate rises to increase CO in response to physical or emotional activities that increase the need for oxygen in the organs and tissues. PVR also influences BP; it is the opposition that blood encounters as it flows through vessels. Anything causing blood vessels to become narrower increases PVR. Any time PVR is increased, more pressure is needed to push the blood through the vessels, so BP increases as a result. If PVR is decreased, less pressure is needed. Increased arteriolar PVR is the main mechanism that elevates BP in hypertension.

Factors that impair normal regulation of BP may lead to hypertension. Many of these factors are not well understood. Sympathetic nervous system overstimulation, which causes vasoconstriction, can contribute to hypertension. Alterations in baroreceptors and chemoreceptors may also influence the development of hypertension. For example, baroreceptors may become less sensitive from prolonged increases in vessel pressure. They may then subsequently fail to stimulate vasodilation through vessel stretching. Additionally, increases in hormones that cause sodium retention, such as aldosterone, lead to increased fluid retention. Changes in kidney function that alter the excretion of fluid also result in an increase in overall body fluid that may contribute to hypertension.

Types of Hypertension
Primary Hypertension
Primary hypertension (or **essential hypertension**) is chronic elevation of systolic and/or diastolic BP from an unknown cause.

Secondary Hypertension
Secondary hypertension has a known cause. It is a sign of another problem, such as a kidney abnormality or a tumor of the adrenal gland. When the cause of secondary hypertension is treated before permanent structural changes occur, BP usually returns to normal.

• **WORD • BUILDING •**
viscosity: viscous—sticky

SIGNS AND SYMPTOMS OF HYPERTENSION

Hypertension often causes no signs or symptoms other than elevated BP readings. As a result, hypertension is referred to as the "silent killer." Patients with hypertension are often first diagnosed when seeking health care for reasons unrelated to hypertension. In a small number of cases, a patient with hypertension may report a headache, bloody nose, severe anxiety, or shortness of breath (Table 22.2).

DIAGNOSIS OF HYPERTENSION

Diagnosis of hypertension considers a patient's risk factors for hypertension, presence of signs and symptoms, history of kidney or heart disease, and current use of medications. Confirmation of hypertension is recommended with an ambulatory BP monitoring device over 12 or 24 hours. Home BP monitoring may also be done.

RISK FACTORS FOR HYPERTENSION

A combination of genetic (nonmodifiable) and environmental (modifiable) risk factors is thought to be responsible for the development of hypertension, although the cause remains unknown. Nonmodifiable risk factors—those that *cannot* be changed—include a family history of hypertension, age, and ethnicity. Modifiable risk factors—those that *can* be changed—include blood glucose level, activity level, smoking, salt and alcohol intake, and insufficient sleep (less than 5 hours per night). Managing these risk factors can help to decrease BP.

Nonmodifiable Risk Factors
Family History of Hypertension
Hypertension is more common among people with a family history of hypertension. Indeed, people with a family history have almost twice the risk of developing hypertension as those with no family history and should have their BP checked regularly.

Age
People age differently because of their genetic and environmental risk factors and lifestyle habits. Thus, the results of the aging process may be reflected in wide variations of BP among older adults. With age, **plaque** builds up in the arteries. Blood vessels become stiffer and less elastic, causing the heart to work harder to force blood through the vessels. These vessel changes increase the amount of work required by the heart to maintain blood flow into the circulation. Consequently, BP increases.

Race and Ethnicity
African Americans have a higher risk of developing hypertension. Hypertension among African Americans is usually caused by increased renin activity, resulting in greater sodium and fluid retention. Thus, African Americans respond well to diuretics such as hydrochlorothiazide (HydroDIURIL) and furosemide (Lasix).

Modifiable Risk Factors
Lifestyle
Lifestyle modifications are used along with antihypertensive drugs to control hypertension. Modifications include adoption of the Dietary Approaches to Stop Hypertension (DASH) or Mediterranean diet, reduction of dietary sodium, and increased physical activity ("Nutrition Notes"). A dietitian can help the patient develop a healthy diet plan.

Table 22.2
Hypertension Summary

Signs and Symptoms	Often none Increased blood pressure Headache, bloody nose, severe anxiety, or shortness of breath
Diagnosis	See Table 22.1
Therapeutic Measures	Lifestyle modification Medication
Complications	Heart failure Kidney disease Myocardial infarction Stroke
Priority Nursing Diagnoses	*Readiness for Enhanced Health Literacy* *Ineffective Health Management* *Risk for Unstable Blood Pressure*

Nutrition Notes

Reducing Blood Pressure With Diet. The Dietary Guidelines for Americans 2015–2020 recommend a sodium intake of 2,300 mg for adults and children 14 or older. For adults with elevated blood pressure or hypertension, the recommendation is to limit sodium to 1,500 mg per day. The average sodium intake of Americans is more than 3,400 mg per day. Examples of low-sodium diet plans include the Dietary Approaches to Stop Hypertension (DASH) diet as well as the Healthy U.S., Mediterranean, and Vegetarian eating patterns described in the Dietary Guidelines (https://health.gov/dietaryguidelines/2015/guidelines). On a 2,000-calorie diet, a person following the DASH diet would consume the following:

Food Group	Number of Servings	Example of One Serving
Grains	7–8	• 1 slice of bread • ½ cup cooked cereal or pasta

Food Group	Number of Servings	Example of One Serving
Vegetables	4–5	• 1 cup raw leafy • ½ cup cooked, nonstarchy
Fruits	4–5	• 1 medium fresh • ½ cup canned or frozen • ¼ cup dried
Dairy, low-fat or nonfat	2–3	• 8 ounces of milk • 1½ ounces of cheese
Lean meat, poultry, or fish	2 or fewer	• 3 ounces cooked
Fats and oils, preferably monounsaturated (e.g., canola, olive, peanut)	2½	• 1 teaspoon
Nuts, seeds, legumes	4–5 weekly	• ⅓ cup of nuts • 2 tablespoons of seeds • ½ cup cooked beans

Diabetes Mellitus

Many adults who have diabetes mellitus also have hypertension. The risk of developing hypertension with a family history of diabetes and obesity is greater than when there is no family history. Lifestyle modifications and adherence to therapy are crucial to prevent heart attacks, strokes, blindness, and kidney disease associated with high blood glucose and BP levels.

CRITICAL THINKING

Ms. Miller, age 54, visits a health care clinic because she has a headache every morning. The nurse collects data on Ms. Miller and finds that she is an office manager, smokes a pack of cigarettes a day, and eats fast food for lunch at her desk. She has two adult children, is recently divorced, and has two to three alcoholic drinks every evening. Ms. Miller has been in good health and takes two aspirin tablets daily for her headaches.

1. What are Ms. Miller's risk factors for hypertension?
2. What is the most significant patient information identified? Why?
3. Why is hypertension referred to as the "silent killer"?
4. Why should Ms. Miller be told of the need for lifelong therapy if she is diagnosed with hypertension?

   Suggested answers are at the end of the chapter.

THERAPEUTIC MEASURES FOR HYPERTENSION

Treatment begins with lifestyle modifications and then individualized consideration of antihypertensive medication therapy. See Table 22.3 for examples of medications used to treat hypertension.

The treatment plan of lifestyle modifications and medications is effective only when patients are motivated to accept

Table 22.3
Medications Used to Treat Hypertension

Medication Class/Action

Diuretics

Increase urine output by inhibiting sodium and water reabsorption by the kidney.

Examples	**Nursing Implications**
thiazide and thiazide-like diuretics loop diuretics potassium-sparing diuretics	Give with food to prevent gastrointestinal upset. Monitor intake and output (I&O) and weight to determine fluid loss. Check for improvement of edema in patients with heart failure and reduced blood pressure (BP) in hypertension. Electrolyte imbalances may occur quickly. *Teach:* Take during waking hours to prevent excessive urination during sleeping hours.

Thiazide and Thiazide-Like Diuretics

Increase urine output by promoting sodium, chloride, and water excretion; cause loss of potassium, sodium, and magnesium; calcium saved; no immediate effect; most effective in normal kidney function.

Examples	**Nursing Implications**
Thiazide: hydrochlorothiazide (HydroDIURIL) chlorothiazide (Diuril)	Hypercalcemia could be hazardous to patient on digoxin. Monitor potassium level for hypokalemia. Blood glucose may increase in diabetics.

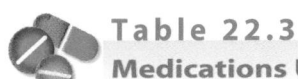

Table 22.3

Medications Used to Treat Hypertension—cont'd

Medication Class/Action

Thiazide-like:
chlorthalidone (Hygroton)
indapamide (Lozol)
metolazone (Zaroxolyn)

Teach:
Wear sunscreen and protective clothing to prevent photosensitivity.

Loop Diuretics

Act on ascending loop of Henle in kidney to cause sodium and water loss; also causes loss of potassium, magnesium, and calcium.

Examples	**Nursing Implications**
bumetanide (Bumex)	Contraindicated if allergic to sulfonamides.
furosemide (Lasix)	Monitor potassium level for hypokalemia.
torsemide (Demadex)	*Teach:*
	Take with food or milk to prevent gastrointestinal upset.
	Use sunscreen to prevent photosensitivity.

Potassium-Sparing Diuretics

Mild diuretic; can be used as combination therapy; promote sodium and water excretion and potassium retention by the kidney.

Examples	**Nursing Implications**
amiloride (Midamor)	Check potassium level for hyperkalemia before administration.
spironolactone (Aldactone)	Check BP before administration.

Sympatholytics (Beta Blockers)

Decrease sympathetic nervous system response, resulting in decreased BP, heart rate, contractility, cardiac output, and renin activity.

Examples	**Nursing Implications**
atenolol (Tenormin)	Check heart rate and BP before administration as causes bradycardia and orthostatic hypotension.
metoprolol (Lopressor)	
metoprolol extended release (Toprol XL)	Check daily I&O and weight.
nadolol (Corgard)	Monitor for bronchospasm.
propranolol (Inderal)	*Teach:*
propranolol long-acting (Inderal LA)	Rise slowly.
	Do not stop drug abruptly to avoid rebound hypertension, angina, or arrhythmias.

Alpha-1 Blockers

Block effects of sympathetic nervous system on smooth muscle of blood vessels, resulting in vasodilation and decreased BP.

Examples	**Nursing Implications**
prazosin (Minipress)	Check heart rate and BP before administration; causes hypotension and tachycardia.
terazosin (Hytrin)	*Teach:*
	Rise slowly.

Combined Alpha and Beta Blockers

Block alpha-adrenergic receptors, causing vasodilation and reduced BP; decrease sympathetic nervous system response, resulting in decreased heart rate and contractility.

Examples	**Nursing Implications**
carvedilol (Coreg)	Check heart rate and BP before administration as causes bradycardia and hypotension.
labetalol (Normodyne)	Check daily I&O and weight.

Continued

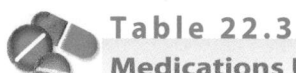

Table 22.3

Medications Used to Treat Hypertension—cont'd

Medication Class/Action	
	Monitor edema, neck vein distention, and lung sounds.
	Teach:
	Rise slowly.
	Do not stop drug abruptly to avoid rebound hypertension, angina, or arrhythmias.

Central-Acting Alpha₂ Agonists

Block effects of sympathetic nervous system centrally.

Examples	**Nursing Implications**
clonidine (Catapres)	Check for decreased BP and edema.
guanfacine hydrochloride (Tenex)	*Teach:*
	Rise slowly.
	Do not stop drug abruptly to avoid rebound hypertension, angina, or arrhythmias.
	Suggest gum or hard candy for dry mouth.

Angiotensin-Converting Enzyme (ACE) Inhibitors

Block production of angiotensin II, a potent vasoconstrictor; reduces peripheral arterial resistance and BP.

Examples	**Nursing Implications**
benazepril hydrochloride (Lotensin)	Monitor patient for edema with heart failure, decreased
captopril (Capoten)	BP with hypertension, and new-onset cough.
enalapril maleate (Vasotec)	*Teach:*
fosinopril (Monopril)	Rise slowly.
lisinopril (Prinivil, Zestril)	Report new-onset cough.
moexipril (Univasc)	Use sunscreen to prevent photosensitivity.
perindopril (Aceon)	Understand angioedema can occur anytime during therapy.
quinapril (Accupril)	Do not stop drug abruptly to avoid rebound hypertension,
ramipril (Altace)	angina, or arrhythmias.
trandolapril (Mavik)	

Angiotensin II Receptor Blocker (ARB)

Blocks angiotensin II receptors, causing vasodilation and reduction in BP.

Examples	**Nursing Implications**
candesartan (Atacand)	Monitor patient for edema with heart failure and
eprosartan (Teveten)	decreased BP with hypertension.
irbesartan (Avapro)	*Teach:*
losartan (Cozaar)	Report new-onset cough.
olmesartan (Benicar)	Use sunscreen to prevent photosensitivity.
telmisartan (Micardis)	
valsartan (Diovan)	

Aldosterone Receptor Antagonist

Blocks binding of aldosterone at receptor site to reduce sodium reabsorption and then BP.

Example	**Nursing Implication**
eplerenone (Inspra)	Monitor potassium for hyperkalemia before and during therapy.

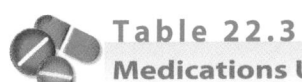

Table 22.3
Medications Used to Treat Hypertension—cont'd

Medication Class/Action

Calcium Channel Blocker (CCB)

Prevents movement of extracellular calcium into the cell causing vasodilation.

Examples
amlodipine (Norvasc)
diltiazem (Cardizem)
felodipine (Plendil)
isradipine (DynaCirc)
nicardipine hydrochloride (Cardene, Cardene SR)
nifedipine (Procardia)
nisoldipine (Sular)
verapamil (Calan SR, Isoptin SR)

Nursing Implications
Check BP (for hypotension), heart rate (for bradycardia), arrhythmias, and angina.
Might increase blood levels of digoxin.

Direct Vasodilators

Relax smooth muscles of blood vessels, causing vasodilation and decreased BP.

Examples
hydralazine (Apresoline)
minoxidil (Loniten)

Nursing Implications
Monitor BP for hypotension/hypertension and increasing heart rate.
Treat headache with acetaminophen.
Often given with diuretic to reduce edema resulting from water and sodium retention.

Combination Agents

See individual agent for action.

Examples
losartan (Cozaar)
 + hydrochlorothiazide (HydroDIURIL) = Hyzaar
telmisartan (Micardis) + hydrochlorothiazide
 (HydroDIURIL) = Micardis HCT

Nursing Implications
See individual agent.

the diagnosis of hypertension and include lifelong treatment in their daily routine. Empathy and trust can increase patient motivation. Patients should be instructed that antihypertensive therapy typically must be continued for the rest of their lives. Remind them that, although they may feel better with lifestyle modifications and medications, the hypertension condition is still present even if it is well controlled. Patients should be told not to stop taking their medications unless instructed to do so by their health care provider (HCP).

Antihypertensive medications can have unpleasant side effects. Patients should be told what these side effects are and to report them if they occur, so that medications can be altered if possible. Erectile dysfunction can be one of the side effects of these medications. Men may be reluctant to discuss this side effect and instead choose to stop the medication. The nurse should be proactive and inform male patients about this

side effect so they will understand that, if it occurs and is reported, the HCP can make medication changes.

Gerontological Issues

Managing Antihypertensive Therapy
• For safety, teach older adults who take antihypertensive drugs to rise slowly to prevent the effects of orthostatic hypotension. Dizziness may increase the risk of falling.
• Deficiencies in fluid volume can be a common problem for older adults as well. Diuretics can contribute to them. Careful monitoring of fluid balance is important to prevent dehydration.
• Older adults may be more sensitive to medications and need lower dosages. Monitor them carefully for adverse effects.

BE SAFE!

Clonidine, an alpha-adrenergic agonist, and clonazepam, a benzodiazepine, have look-alike and sound-alike drug names. Be aware of drug names that look alike and sound alike to prevent errors involving these drugs.

COMPLICATIONS OF HYPERTENSION

Common complications of hypertension include coronary artery disease, atherosclerosis, myocardial infarction (MI), heart failure (HF), stroke, and kidney or eye damage. High BP levels may also increase the size of the left ventricle, referred to as **hypertrophy.** The severity and duration of the increase in BP determine the extent of the vascular changes causing organ damage. Over time, elevated BP damages the small vessels of the heart, brain, kidneys, and retina. The results are a progressive functional impairment of these organs, known as target-organ disease.

LEARNING TIP

Walking for 30 minutes is an effective way to lower blood pressure (BP), as is listening daily to 30 minutes of classical, Celtic, or raga music while practicing slow abdominal breathing. Transcendental meditation also helps control high BP.

Here are additional, important lifestyle modifications arranged in an easy-to-remember mnemonic:

L—Limit salt, caffeine, and alcohol.
I—Include daily potassium and calcium.
F—Fight fat and cholesterol.
E—Exercise regularly (e.g., walking).
S—Stay on your BP regimen.
T—Try to quit smoking.
Y—Your medications are to be taken daily.
L—Lose weight.
E—End-stage complications will be avoided!

SPECIAL CONSIDERATIONS

BP should be well controlled before the patient has an invasive procedure. Hypertensive patients are at greater risk for strokes, MI, HF, kidney disease, and pulmonary edema. These patients should be instructed to continue to take their BP medications as directed by their HCP. Antihypertensive medications should be resumed as soon as possible after the procedure, as directed by the HCP.

CRITICAL THINKING

Mrs. Bell, 80 years old, is seen in her physician's office. She lives a sedentary lifestyle alone in her own home with a bathroom down the hall from the bedroom. Mrs. Bell's son lives in the same city and visits her often. She has wood floors with throw rugs in the hall and a tile floor in the bathroom. She wears glasses and has a cataract. She has an unsteady gait and nocturia. She is 40 pounds overweight and has a 10-year history of hypertension for which she is taking hydrochlorothiazide (HydroDIURIL) and lisinopril (Zestril), when she remembers to take them.

1. What are Mrs. Bell's modifiable and nonmodifiable risk factors for hypertension?
2. What are the actions of hydrochlorothiazide and lisinopril?
3. What teaching methods could be used to help ensure that Mrs. Bell will understand and follow her treatment plan?
4. Why should patient safety needs be addressed in the nursing care plan?
5. What patient-centered safety interventions should the patient and family be taught?
6. Lisinopril 20 mg by mouth is ordered now because Mrs. Bell forgot to take her medication. The nurse has on hand lisinopril 10-mg tablets. How many tablets should the nurse give?

Suggested answers are at the end of the chapter.

HYPERTENSIVE URGENCY

Hypertensive urgency occurs when the BP is as elevated as in a hypertensive emergency (described next) but without progression of target-organ dysfunction. A patient with hypertensive urgency may have severe headaches, nosebleeds, shortness of breath, and severe anxiety. Appropriate treatment is implemented with a follow-up visit within several days.

HYPERTENSIVE EMERGENCY

Hypertensive emergency is a severe type of hypertension. Systolic BP higher than 180 mm Hg or diastolic BP higher than 120 mm Hg occur (National Heart, Lung, and Blood Institute, 2004). There is a risk for or progression of target-organ dysfunction (such as MI, HF, and dissecting aortic aneurysm). These patients require immediate BP treatment in a critical care unit. Gradual reduction of BP is often desired to prevent decreased blood flow to the kidneys, heart, and/or brain. An intravenous (IV) medication such as nitroprusside (Nipride) may be given to reduce BP during the crisis. The nursing diagnosis *Risk for Unstable Blood*

Pressure is applicable to the patient with hypertensive emergency.

NURSING PROCESS FOR THE PATIENT WITH HYPERTENSION

Data Collection

Data collection for a patient with hypertension includes the patient's health history, BP measurements, medications, along with physical assessment (Fig. 22.1). Determining what hypertensive patients and their families know about hypertension and associated risk factors is essential for planning patient and family education and subsequent lifelong lifestyle modification needs.

Nursing Diagnoses, Planning, Implementation, and Evaluation

See "Nursing Care Plan for the Patient With Hypertension."

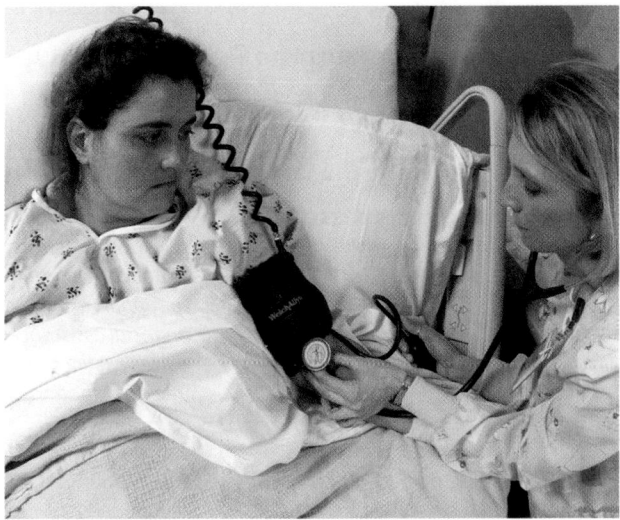

FIGURE 22.1 Nurse obtaining BP measurement. Correct size cuff use is essential for accurate reading.

Nursing Care Plan for the Patient With Hypertension

Nursing Diagnosis: *Readiness for Enhanced Health Literacy* related to desire to learn about hypertensive disease process and treatment regimen
Expected Outcome: The patient will verbalize understanding of disease process and treatment regimen.
Evaluation of Outcome: Is the patient able to discuss and explain hypertension disease process, including its risk factors, complications, and treatment regimen?

Intervention	Rationale	Evaluation
Verify patient's readiness and ability to learn and preferred method of learning.	*Patient must express the desire to enhance understanding of the hypertension diagnosis and be able to receive and understand information given.*	Does patient verbalize readiness to learn about hypertension? Does patient demonstrate ability to read, write, and retain information presented in the preferred learning method?
Provide patient with information concerning disease process, including risk factors, complications, and treatment regimen.	*Patient is better able to participate in treatment regimen when the patient understands need for changes in behavior.*	Is patient able to accurately state information explained about hypertension?
Explore patient's feelings about the hypertension diagnosis and answer patient's questions.	*Understanding of the patient's perception and knowledge allows the opportunity to provide accurate information and make helpful referrals as needed.*	Is patient able to participate in discussion concerning hypertension disease process including risk factors, complications, and treatment regimen?

Nursing Diagnosis: *Ineffective Health Management* related to complexity of therapy, cost of medications, lack of symptoms, side effects of medications, and need to alter long-term lifestyle habits
Expected Outcome: The patient will verbalize ability and willingness to adhere to treatment.
Evaluation of Outcome: Is the patient able to state how lifestyle will include therapy? Does the patient identify and problem-solve barriers for therapy?

Intervention	Rationale	Evaluation
Identify patient's modifiable risk factors and lifestyle modification needs.	*Identifying risk factors is the first step in planning therapy. Patient must understand the relationship of these risk factors with hypertension and complication development.*	Can patient state rationale for modifying risk factors to prevent development of complications?

(nursing care plan continues on page 370)

Nursing Care Plan for the Patient With Hypertension—cont'd

Intervention	Rationale	Evaluation
Develop plan to overcome identified barriers to patient adhering to therapy. Make referrals as needed.	*Identified barriers can be overcome with planning and intervention, such as instructions provided at level of patient's learning ability, referral to support groups, referral for financial assistance or prescription delivery service, or simplifying to one combination medication.*	Have barriers been eliminated? Can patient self-administer medications accurately on daily basis?
Teach patient to take medications as prescribed and not to skip dosages.	*Older patients may skip dosages to save money, reduce side effects, or reduce need to void from diuretics.*	Does patient take dosages as prescribed? Does patient express concern over cost, side effects, or frequent voiding?
Teach patient to change positions slowly to prevent falls.	*Antihypertensive medications can cause hypotension, resulting in dizziness and weakness, possibly leading to falls.*	Does patient understand how to change positions slowly? Does patient experience dizziness or weakness?

Home Health Hints

Medications

- Discuss medication usage with the patient and count the number of remaining pills in the patient's pill bottles, if needed, to determine compliance.
- Instruct patients to take medication as prescribed even if they feel fine and have no symptoms; instruct them to report side effects if they occur. Medication compliance may be a challenge for the older adult patient.
- Monitor carefully for symptoms of heart failure if the patient takes a beta blocker. This is a side effect that needs to be caught early and reported to the health care provider (HCP).
- Teach the patient or caregiver to take the patient's pulse and to call the nurse if it is below 60 beats per minute or the parameters defined by the HCP. Many antihypertensive medicines can cause bradycardia.
- Teach the patient or caregiver proper use of a home blood pressure monitoring device and recording of the date, time, and reading obtained. The home health care nurse should review the log on each visit.
- Teach patients to weigh themselves every morning after voiding, in the same amount of clothing, and to keep a log for the nurse to review.
- Note on a calendar medication refills and medical appointment dates to remind the patient.
- Check with the HCP and pharmacist for less expensive alternatives if medicines are found to be too expensive for the patient.
- Teach patients who are traveling to refill medicines ahead of time to make sure they do not run out. The HCP can write a prescription for the patient to have for emergency refills.

Nutrition

- Discuss with the dietitian if the Dietary Approaches to Stop Hypertension (DASH) eating plan would be appropriate for the patient (www.nhlbi.nih.gov/files/docs/public/heart/dash_brief.pdf).
- Request consultation with a dietitian to teach patients how to read food labels for fat and salt content; to avoid prepackaged convenience foods that tend to be high in sodium; to encourage the consumption of fresh, frozen (without sauces), and no-salt-added canned vegetables; and to provide recommendations of spice mixes that are low in sodium and potassium to enhance the flavors of foods.

Lifestyle

- Provide the following suggestions to help a patient decrease or stop smoking: use cinnamon mouthwash on waking; put away all ashtrays but one, and keep it in a place not normally used for smoking; and find ways to keep hands busy at times when usually holding a cigarette, such as when drinking coffee or alcohol.
- Encourage patients to put "No Smoking" signs on their entrance door to prevent second- and thirdhand smoke.
- Promote home exercise if cleared by HCP. Weights for exercising can be improvised using canned goods and bags of sugar. The amount of weight being used is easily identified for documentation by the food label.

SUGGESTED ANSWERS TO CRITICAL THINKING

Ms. Miller

1. Risk factors include gender; age; smoking; a diet high in fat, salt, and calories; consumption of two to three alcoholic drinks per evening; and possibly her morning headaches.
2. Morning headaches. Ms. Miller may be experiencing an episode of hypertensive urgency and should be evaluated immediately by a health care provider (HCP).
3. "Silent killer" refers to the fact that there are often no signs or symptoms associated with hypertension.
4. Lifelong therapy is required because there is no cure for hypertension, and complications need to be prevented.

Mrs. Bell

1. Nonmodifiable risk factors include age, gender, and history of hypertension. Modifiable risk factors include weight and adherence to antihypertensive therapy.
2. Diuretics remove excess salt and water to decrease blood volume and lower blood pressure. The angiotensin-converting enzyme (ACE) inhibitor lisinopril blocks production of angiotensin II, a potent vasoconstrictor, to reduce peripheral arterial resistance and blood pressure.
3. Identify patient's reading level and primary language. Provide patient with written instructions in large letters about medications. Include family members and enlist their support in reinforcing the importance of adhering to the treatment plan.
4. Patient is 80 years old, makes frequent trips to the bathroom related to diuretics, and has vision problems, and a side effect of lisinopril is fatigue.
5. Discuss with the HCP a combination medication to reduce the number of pills to be remembered. Make arrangements for a bedside commode to reduce the distance and urgency to get to the bathroom. Encourage the patient and family to place nightlights in the bedroom, hall, and bathroom. Explain that throw rugs increase the risk of falling and that wood or tile floors can be slippery when wet and hard if a fall occurs. Encourage removal of throw rugs, and suggest carpeting these areas if possible. Suggest the use of safety bars in the hall and bathroom for support or other walking aids as needed. If incontinence is a concern, suggest wearing an adult brief to prevent a wet, slippery floor. Suggest discussing with the HCP an exercise program to increase strength, such as lifting small, lightweight objects (e.g., soup cans); squeezing a rubber ball; or riding an exercise bike, if able. These exercises can be done while sitting so they are not fall-risk activities.
6. Unit analysis method:

$$\frac{20 \text{ mg}}{} \cdot \frac{1 \text{ tablet}}{10 \text{ mg}} = 2 \text{ tablets}$$

Review Questions

1. The nurse provides a teaching session for a newly diagnosed patient with primary hypertension. Which of the following statements about the cause of primary hypertension if stated by the patient would indicate the need for further teaching? **Select all that apply.**
   1. "It is caused by a tumor of the adrenal gland."
   2. "There are no tests to identify the cause."
   3. "An arteriogram will show why the hypertension is occurring."
   4. "The cause is unknown."
   5. "The cause can be identified with magnetic resonance imaging."

2. Which of the following would the nurse reinforce after a teaching session on hypertension control as the most important lifestyle modification for the patient with hypertension who is age 59, 71 inches tall, 127 kilograms, and eats a vegetarian diet?
   1. Reduce weight.
   2. Restrict salt intake.
   3. Increase potassium intake.
   4. Avoid use of alcohol.

3. The nurse is reinforcing teaching on hypertension for a patient. Which of the following statements if made by the patient after a teaching session would indicate understanding of what is often the only sign of hypertension?
   1. "Sacral edema."
   2. "Elevated blood pressure level."
   3. "Tachycardia."
   4. "Jugular venous distention."

4. The nurse is participating in a teaching session on diet for a patient with hypertension. Which of the following statements if made by the patient would indicate understanding of the teaching? **Select all that apply.**
   1. "Canned fruit and vegetables are best to eat."
   2. "Add salt to food during cooking."
   3. "Increase foods high in saturated fat."
   4. "Choose fresh or frozen fruits and vegetables."
   5. "Read food labels."
   6. "Be aware of potassium in salt substitutes."

5. The nurse is obtaining blood pressure readings for people aged 18 to 39 during a community health fair. For which of the following blood pressure readings would 3- to 5-year screenings be recommended? **Select all that apply.**
   1. 108/92 mm Hg
   2. 110/88 mm Hg
   3. 112/78 mm Hg
   4. 118/74 mm Hg
   5. 142/90 mm Hg
   6. 160/88 mm Hg

6. During a health screening, a patient's blood pressure is confirmed by two nurses to be 220/120 mm Hg. Which of the following actions should the nurse recommend to the patient?
   1. "Return to work and have your blood pressure rechecked in 2 days."
   2. "Take two doses of blood pressure medication right now."
   3. "Sit quietly while we call 911 to request an ambulance."
   4. "Take off work for the rest of the day and rest."

7. The nurse is reinforcing medication teaching for a patient. The nurse would include which of the following instructions to a patient taking a diuretic?
   1. Change position slowly.
   2. Eliminate salt in your diet.
   3. Take your medication before bed.
   4. Empty your bladder after taking the first dose.

8. At a follow-up visit, which of the following data would best indicate to the nurse that the patient's blood pressure therapy has been successful?
   1. Weight decreased by 3 pounds.
   2. Diary of dietary intake is within suggested diet.
   3. Blood pressure is 118/74 mm Hg.
   4. Patient reports walking 30 to 40 minutes daily.

Answer rationales available in your online resources

ANSWERS 1. 1, 3, 5; 2. 1; 3. 2; 4. 4, 5; 5. 3, 4; 6. 3; 7. 1; 8. 3

Key Points

Find the chapter key points in your online resources available through Davis Edge.

Additional Resources

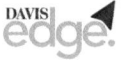 Use the scratch off code on the inside front cover of your book to access online quizzes that will help you to improve your scores on course exams and prepare for NCLEX-PN®

 Study Guide

CHAPTER 23

Nursing Care of Patients With Valvular, Inflammatory, and Infectious Cardiac or Venous Disorders

Terri Blevins

KEY TERMS

allograft (AL-oh-graft)
annuloplasty (AN-yoo-loh-PLAS-tee)
autograft (AW-toh -graft)
beta-hemolytic streptococci (BAY-tuh-HEE-moh-LIT-ik STREP-toh-KOK-eye)
bioprosthesis (by-oh-prahs-THEE-sis)
cardiac tamponade (KAR-dee-yak TAM-pon-AYD)
cardiomegaly (KAR-dee-oh-MEG-ah-lee)
cardiomyopathy (KAR-dee-oh-my-AH-pah-thee)
chorea (core-REE-ah)
commissurotomy (KOM-ih-shur-AHT-oh-mee)
Dressler syndrome (DRESS-ler SIN-drohm)
emboli (EM-boh-ly)
heterograft (HET-er-oh-graft)
homograft (HOH-moh-graft)
infective endocarditis (in-FEK-tive EN-doh-kar-DY-tis)
insufficiency (IN-suh-FISH-en-see)
international normalized ratio (IN-ter-NASH-uh-nul NOR-muh-lized RAY-she-oh)
murmur (MUR-mur)
myectomy (my-EK-tuh-mee)
myocarditis (MY-oh-kar-DY-tis)
pericardial effusion (PEAR-ih-KAR-dee-uhl ee-FYOO-zhun)
pericardial friction rub (PEAR-ih-KAR-dee-uhl FRIK-shun RUB)
pericardiectomy (PEAR-ih-kar-dee-EK-tuh-mee)
pericardiocentesis (PEAR-ih-KAR-dee-oh-sen-TEE-sis)
pericarditis (PEAR-ih-kar-DY-tis)
petechiae (peh-TEE-kee-eye)
regurgitation (ree-GUR-jih-TAY-shun)
rheumatic fever (roo-MAT-ik FEE-vur)
stenosis (steh-NOH-sis)
thrombophlebitis (THROM-boh-fleh-BY-tis)
valvotomy (val-VAW-tuh-mee)
valvuloplasty (VAL-vyoo-loh-PLAS-tee)
xenograft (ZEE-no-graft)

LEARNING OUTCOMES

1. Explain the pathophysiology, etiology, signs and symptoms, diagnostic tests, therapeutic measures, and nursing care for each of the valvular disorders.
2. Compare and contrast the differences between commissurotomy, annuloplasty, and valve replacement.
3. Identify postoperative complications that can occur following any type of cardiac valve replacement.
4. Explain the pathophysiology, etiology, signs and symptoms, diagnostic tests, therapeutic measures, and nursing care for infective endocarditis, pericarditis, and myocarditis.
5. Explain the pathophysiology, etiology, signs and symptoms, complications, diagnostic tests, therapeutic measures, and nursing care for dilated, hypertrophic, and restrictive cardiomyopathy.
6. Explain the pathophysiology, etiology, signs and symptoms, prevention, complications, diagnostic tests, therapeutic measures, and nursing care for thrombophlebitis.

CHAPTER CONCEPT

Perfusion

CARDIAC VALVULAR DISORDERS

Within the normal heart, blood flows in one direction because of the presence of heart valves. There are four valves in the heart: mitral, tricuspid, pulmonic, and aortic (see Fig. 21.2). The chordae tendineae and papillary muscles are attachment structures for both the mitral and tricuspid valves. They ensure that these valves close tightly.

Damage to the valves or their surrounding structures can result in abnormal valvular functioning (Fig. 23.1). The valves of the left side of the heart are more commonly affected. There are two major types of valvular dysfunction: **stenosis** and **insufficiency.** Forward blood

• WORD • BUILDING •
stenosis: stenos—narrow
insufficiency: in—not + sufficiens—sufficient

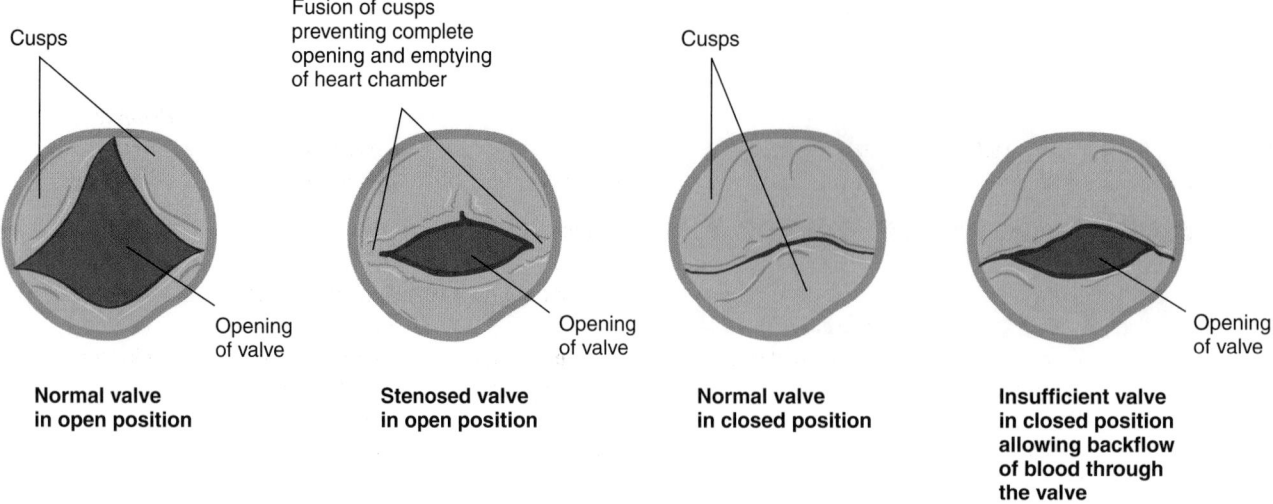

Cusps

Fusion of cusps preventing complete opening and emptying of heart chamber

Cusps

Opening of valve

Opening of valve

Opening of valve

Normal valve in open position

Stenosed valve in open position

Normal valve in closed position

Insufficient valve in closed position allowing backflow of blood through the valve

FIGURE 23.1 Openings of stenosed and insufficient valves compared with a normal valve.

flow is hindered if the valve is narrowed (*stenosed*) and does not open completely. If the valve does not close completely, blood backs up; this is referred to as **regurgitation** or *insufficiency*. Either type of valve damage increases the heart's workload and increases pressure in the affected heart chamber due to a backup of blood flow. These conditions may result from congenital defects, infections, or rheumatic fever. Valvular disorders are summarized in Table 23.1 and discussed in more detail in the following sections.

Rheumatic Fever

Rheumatic fever is an autoimmune reaction 2 to 3 weeks after an upper respiratory infection due to a group A **beta-hemolytic streptococci** infection. Although rheumatic fever can occur at any age, it typically occurs between ages 5 and 15. Rheumatic fever and subsequent rheumatic heart disease and valvular damage can be prevented by detecting and treating streptococcal infections promptly with penicillin. It is a rare complication of strep throat in the United States. A throat culture is used to diagnose a streptococcal infection. Signs and symptoms include polyarthritis, subcutaneous nodules, **chorea** (brief, rapid, uncontrolled movements), carditis, fever, arthralgia, and pneumonitis. Rheumatic heart disease may not be evident for years after rheumatic fever; however, when manifested, the valves are most commonly affected.

Mitral Valve Prolapse
Pathophysiology and Etiology
During ventricular systole, as pressure in the left ventricle rises, the flaps of the mitral valve normally remain closed and stay within the atrioventricular junction. In mitral valve prolapse (MVP), however, one or both flaps bulge backward into the left atrium (like a parachute) during systole. This can happen when one flap is too large or if a defect occurs in the chordae tendineae that secure the valve to the heart wall. If the bulging flaps do not fit together, blood can leak

backward into the left atrium (mitral regurgitation). Increased pressure on the papillary muscles results in ischemia within the muscle, causing further dysfunction of the mitral valve.

MVP can be due to a hereditary collagen tissue disorder, with unknown etiology; an infection damaging the mitral valve; ischemic heart disease; or cardiomyopathy. It is the most common form of valvular heart disease, typically occurring in women, aged 15 to 30, who are thin and have slight chest deformities.

Signs and Symptoms
Most patients with MVP are asymptomatic and have a good prognosis (see Table 23.1). MVP severity ranges from having a **murmur** (caused by blood leaking backward) to chordae tendineae rupture with mitral regurgitation. The murmur is best heard at the heart apex. It begins in the middle of systole (*midsystolic*) and becomes more intense until the end of systole. Symptoms may include anxiety, atypical chest pain not related to exertion, arrhythmias causing palpitations, dizziness or syncope (fainting), fatigue, and dyspnea (shortness of breath), especially when lying flat or during activity.

Complications
Rare complications include mitral regurgitation, arrhythmias, heart failure (HF), emboli, or infective endocarditis (IE).

Diagnostic Tests
Auscultation for a murmur or a click caused by the stress on the chordae tendineae or valve leaflets when they prolapse is the first diagnostic step for MVP. A normal electrocardiogram (ECG) is common, although inverted (downward) T waves (indicating ischemia) may be seen (see Fig. 25.6).

• WORD • BUILDING •
regurgitation: re—again + gurgitare—to flood

Table 23.1

Cardiac Valvular Disorders Summary

Valve Disorder	Signs and Symptoms	Diagnostic Tests	Complications	Therapeutic Measures	Priority Nursing Diagnoses
Mitral valve prolapse	None Murmur Atypical chest pain Palpitations Arrhythmias Dizziness Syncope Fatigue Dyspnea Anxiety	Echocardiogram Electrocardiogram (ECG) Cardiac catheterization	Emboli Infective endocarditis Mitral regurgitation Arrhythmias Heart failure (HF)	None Beta blockers Antiarrhythmics Aspirin or anticoagulants Valvuloplasty Valve replacement	*Activity Intolerance* *Decreased Cardiac Output*
Mitral stenosis	None Murmur Chest pain Palpitations Dizziness Syncope Fatigue Edema Exertional dyspnea Cough Hemoptysis Respiratory infections	ECG Chest x-ray Echocardiogram Doppler ultrasound Transesophageal endoscopy (TEE) Cardiac catheterization Magnetic resonance imaging (MRI)	Emboli HF	None Anticoagulants Antiarrhythmics Valvuloplasty Valve replacement	*Activity Intolerance* *Decreased Cardiac Output*
Mitral regurgitation	None Murmur Chest pain Palpitations Syncope Fatigue Exertional dyspnea Cough Hemoptysis Peripheral edema *Acute:* Pulmonary edema Shock	ECG Chest x-ray Echocardiogram Doppler ultrasound TEE Cardiac MRI Cardiac catheterization	Arrhythmias Emboli HF	None Angiotensin-converting enzyme (ACE) inhibitors Antiarrhythmics Anticoagulants Valvuloplasty Valve replacement	*Activity Intolerance* *Decreased Cardiac Output*
Aortic stenosis	None Angina Murmur Syncope Orthopnea Exertional dyspnea	ECG Chest x-ray Serial echocardiograms Stress (exercise) test Computed tomography (CT) scan	HF	Valve replacement: surgical or transcatheter	*Activity Intolerance* *Decreased Cardiac Output*

Continued

Table 23.1

Cardiac Valvular Disorders Summary—cont'd

Valve Disorder	Signs and Symptoms	Diagnostic Tests	Complications	Therapeutic Measures	Priority Nursing Diagnoses
	Fatigue HF	MRI Cardiac catheterization			
Aortic regurgitation	None Forceful pulse Murmur Chest pain Palpitations Fatigue Exertional dyspnea Corrigan pulse Diaphoresis	ECG Chest x-ray Echocardiogram Cardiac catheterization	HF Life-threatening arrhythmia Symptoms of shock	Digitalis Diuretics Vasodilators Valve replacement	*Activity Intolerance* *Decreased Cardiac Output*

A two-dimensional echocardiogram with Doppler can show valve abnormalities and identify mitral regurgitation from MVP. For more severe cases, cardiac catheterization can show the bulging flaps of the mitral valve on a coronary angiogram.

Therapeutic Measures

MVP is a benign disorder. No treatment is needed unless it becomes severe with symptoms. A healthy lifestyle, including a good diet, exercise, stress management, and avoidance of stimulants such as caffeine, can help prevent symptoms. Treatment depends on severity of symptoms and may include beta blockers to reduce the heart rate and perhaps relieve chest pain, aspirin or anticoagulants to help prevent formation of blood clots on the valve, and antiarrhythmics (also known as antidysrhythmics) for an arrhythmia. Surgical repair or replacement of the valve can be done for severe cases of MVP. (See surgical interventions discussion later in the chapter.)

CRITICAL THINKING

Mrs. Tepley, age 32, has mitral valve prolapse and reports palpitations whenever she experiences stress. She drinks three cups of coffee daily.

1. What might you hear when auscultating Mrs. Tepley's heart sounds?
2. Why does Mrs. Tepley experience palpitations? Would experiencing palpitations make you fearful?
3. What patient-centered information does Mrs. Tepley need to manage her mitral valve prolapse?

Suggested answers are at the end of the chapter.

Mitral Stenosis

Pathophysiology and Etiology

Mitral stenosis (MS) results from thickening of the mitral valve flaps and shortening of the chordae tendineae, causing narrowing of the mitral valve opening. Older patients with MS usually have calcification and fibrosis of the mitral valve flaps. This obstructs blood flow from the left atrium into the left ventricle. The left atrium enlarges to hold the extra blood volume caused by the obstruction. Because of the increased blood volume, pressure rises in the left atrium; in turn, pressure rises in the pulmonary circulation and the right ventricle. The right ventricle dilates to handle the increased volume. Eventually, the right ventricle fails from excessive workload, reducing blood volume delivered to the left ventricle and decreasing cardiac output.

Rheumatic fever is the major cause of MS, which is seen in older adults who had rheumatic fever as children or in those in underdeveloped countries. Even though rheumatic fever is rare in developed nations, when it does occur, the resultant rheumatic heart disease may not appear for two to four decades after the rheumatic fever is resolved. Less common causes of MS include congenital defects of the mitral valve, tumors, rheumatoid arthritis, systemic lupus erythematosus, and calcium deposits.

Signs and Symptoms

Patients can be asymptomatic with MS (see Table 23.1). A click or low-pitched murmur might be heard as a rumbling sound over the heart apex during diastole. The click or murmur is more pronounced right before systole. Chest pain and pulmonary symptoms such as exertional dyspnea, cough, hemoptysis (bloody sputum), and respiratory infections can occur. Fatigue, intolerance to activity, dizziness, or syncope result from decreased cardiac output. Edema of ankles and feet may be present. Palpitations from atrial flutter or fibrillation caused by atrial enlargement and chest pain from decreased cardiac output may occur.

Complications
Emboli can form from the stasis of blood in the left atrium that may cause stroke. If the right ventricle fails, symptoms of HF and pulmonary edema can be seen (see Chapter 26).

Diagnostic Tests
MS is diagnosed with the patient history, physical examination, and diagnostic tests findings. The ECG shows enlargement of the left atrium and right ventricle and changes in the P waveform (see Fig. 25.1). Atrial flutter or fibrillation may be seen (see Chapter 25). A chest x-ray examination confirms enlargement of the affected heart chambers. Transthoracic two-dimensional color flow Doppler echocardiogram and Doppler ultrasound are the noninvasive gold standard tests for evaluation of valvular disease. They show the narrowed mitral valve opening and decreased motion of the valve. Computed tomography (CT) scan and magnetic resonance imaging (MRI) may be done.

Therapeutic Measures
When the patient is asymptomatic, no treatment is needed. Anticoagulants might be given to prevent emboli from stasis of blood in the atrium. Atrial fibrillation, an irregular heart rhythm, or HF may develop and require treatment (see Chapter 26).

If invasive treatment is needed, percutaneous balloon **valvuloplasty** (a balloon dilates the stenosed heart valve) is done in the cardiac catheterization lab (Fig. 23.2). Surgical treatment can include valvular repair (valvuloplasty), but mitral valve replacement is typically needed (Fig. 23.3).

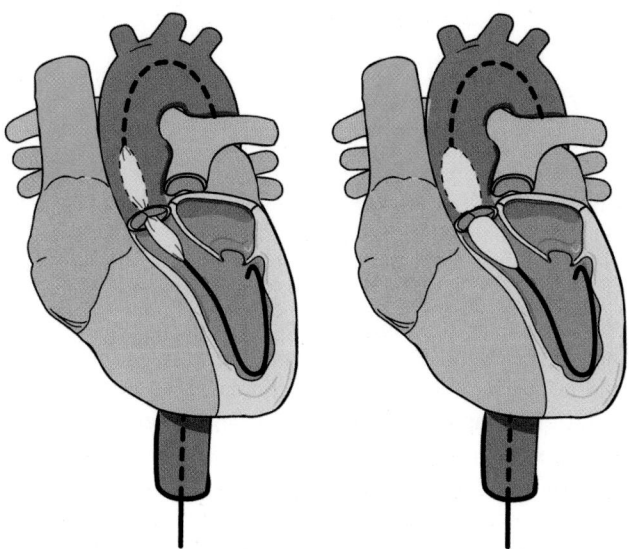

FIGURE 23.2 Percutaneous balloon valvuloplasty.

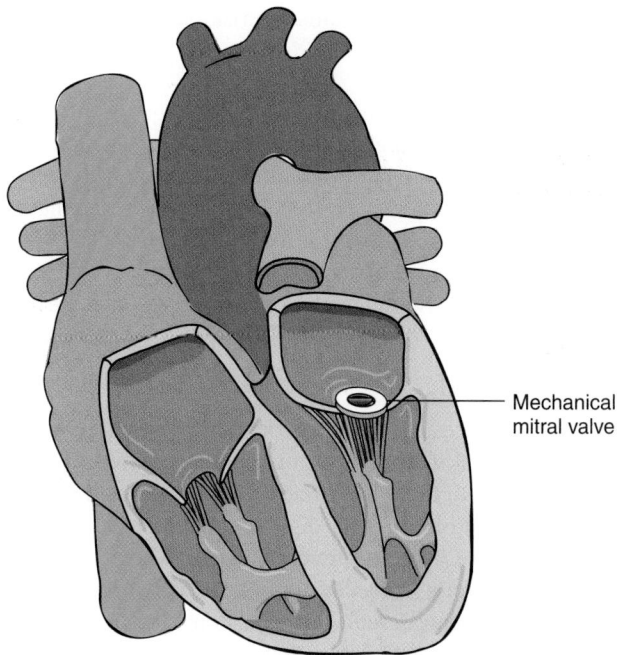

Mechanical mitral valve

FIGURE 23.3 Mitral valve replacement with mechanical valve.

Mitral Regurgitation
Pathophysiology and Etiology
Mitral regurgitation (MR), or insufficiency, is the incomplete closure of the mitral valve leaflets. It allows backflow of blood into the left atrium with each contraction of the left ventricle. This blood is then extra volume that is added to the incoming blood from the lungs. With chronic MR, the increase in blood volume dilates and increases pressure in the left atrium. In response to the extra blood volume delivered by the left atrium, the left ventricle compensates by dilating. If the compensatory mechanism of dilation is inadequate, pressure rises in the pulmonary circulation and then in the right ventricle as blood volume backs up from the left atrium. The left ventricle and eventually the right ventricle may fail from this increased strain.

Causes of MR include rheumatic heart disease, endocarditis, rupture or dysfunction of the chordae tendineae or papillary muscle, MVP, hypertension, myocardial infarction (MI), cardiomyopathy, annulus calcification, aging, or congenital defects.

Signs and Symptoms
Patients with MR are usually asymptomatic. A murmur may be heard. It begins with S_1 (first heart sound) and continues during systole up to S_2 (second heart sound). With severe MR, HF symptoms can develop as the left ventricle fails (see Table 23.1). Exertional dyspnea, fatigue, syncope, cough, hemoptysis, and edema may occur. If acute MR develops, as in papillary muscle rupture following MI, pulmonary edema and shock symptoms will be exhibited.

Complications
Palpitations due to atrial fibrillation may result as the left atrium enlarges. Pulmonary hypertension or HF may occur

(see Chapter 26). Endocarditis is a risk due to the damaged valve.

Diagnostic Tests

The ECG shows enlargement of the left atrium and left ventricle and changes in the P waveform (see Fig. 25.1). Atrial flutter or fibrillation may be seen. A chest x-ray examination confirms hypertrophy of the affected heart chambers. Two-dimensional echocardiogram with Doppler or transesophageal echocardiogram shows left atrial enlargement and regurgitation of blood.

Therapeutic Measures

Without the presence of symptoms and depending on the cause, medical treatment is not usually required. If atrial fibrillation with rapid heart rate develops, calcium channel blockers, beta blockers, or digitalis may be ordered; anticoagulants are used to prevent emboli. When symptoms develop, surgery is needed for severe MR, or acute MR mitral valve repair or replacement is done. For those unable to have surgery, vasodilators may be used.

Aortic Stenosis
Pathophysiology and Etiology

In aortic stenosis (AS), blood flow from the left ventricle into the aorta is obstructed through the stenosed aortic valve. The opening of the aortic valve may be narrowed from thickening, scarring, calcification, or fusing of the valve's flaps. To compensate for the difficulty in ejecting blood into the aorta, the left ventricle contracts more forcefully. In chronic AS, the left ventricle hypertrophies to maintain normal cardiac output. As narrowing increases, the compensatory mechanisms are unable to continue. The left ventricle fails to move blood forward, resulting in decreased cardiac output and HF.

The major causes of AS are congenital defects or rheumatic heart disease. Calcification of the aortic valve may be age related and occurs after age 60.

Signs and Symptoms

Many years may pass before signs or symptoms of AS are observed (see Table 23.1). Early symptoms include dizziness, syncope, exertional dyspnea, or activity intolerance. Late symptoms are angina pectoris (chest pain) from a lack of oxygen to the myocardium or HF signs and symptoms. A systolic murmur can develop, beginning just after systole with increasing intensity until midsystole. The murmur then decreases and ends right before the second heart sound.

Complications

Life-threatening arrhythmias, sudden cardiac death, endocarditis, emboli, or HF can occur.

Diagnostic Tests

The ECG usually shows enlargement of the left ventricle and left atrium. Two-dimensional and Doppler echocardiogram show thickening of the left ventricular wall, impaired

movement of the aortic valve, and the severity of the disease. Cardiac catheterization will show elevated left ventricular pressure and decreased cardiac output. Cardiac MRI, CT scan, or positron emission tomography (PET) scan can also be used.

Therapeutic Measures

Aortic valve replacement is the only effective treatment for AS. For those considered high risk for traditional open-heart surgery, a transcatheter aortic valve replacement (TAVR) can be done (see the section on heart valve replacement). **Valvotomy** (expansion of a balloon to open the mitral valve) is used only for those who are unable to have valve replacement.

If symptoms of HF are present, they are treated. Medications that reduce the contractility of the heart and, subsequently, cardiac output are avoided to prevent further HF.

CRITICAL THINKING

Mrs. Pryor, age 48, has aortic stenosis and is admitted to the hospital with angina. She had an episode of syncope 2 days ago. She reports that she tires easily.

1. Mrs. Pryor asks what aortic stenosis is. What should the nurse tell her, and how should it be documented?
2. Why might Mrs. Pryor be experiencing angina?
3. What nursing care related to safety needs is important to include in Mrs. Pryor's plan of care? Think of how you would feel knowing you will continue to have episodes of syncope and fatigue. What concerns would you have regarding completing your activities of daily living?
4. What nursing diagnoses and care are relevant for Mrs. Pryor's report of being tired?
5. Digoxin (Lanoxin) 0.25 mg has been prescribed for Mrs. Pryor. Digoxin is available in 0.125-mg tablets. How many tablets will the nurse give?

Suggested answers are at the end of the chapter.

Aortic Regurgitation
Pathophysiology and Etiology

In chronic aortic regurgitation (AR), the aortic valve cusps may become scarred, thickened, or shortened. Chronic AR may slowly develop over many years or decades. A backflow of blood from the aorta into the left ventricle occurs if the aortic valve cusps do not close completely. The left ventricle's blood volume increases with this backflow of blood; this is in addition to the normal flow of blood from the left atrium. To handle the increased volume, the left ventricle compensates with dilation and hypertrophy to deliver a stronger contraction ejecting more blood volume to maintain cardiac output. Over time, the heart's contraction weakens and the left ventricle fails, causing cardiac output to drop.

Congenital defects, aging, rheumatic heart disease, syphilis, severe hypertension, and ankylosing spondylitis can cause AR. An acute cause of AR may be endocarditis or aortic dissection.

Signs and Symptoms

Symptoms may not become apparent for many years with chronic AR (see Table 23.1). Initially, the patient may report feeling a forceful heartbeat that is more pronounced when lying down. Palpitations and pounding in the head may also be experienced. Next, exertional dyspnea, fatigue, and worsening levels of dyspnea (e.g., orthopnea, paroxysmal nocturnal dyspnea) occur after years of progressive valvular dysfunction. A murmur is heard during diastolic after the second heart sound. The palpated pulse is forceful and then quickly collapses (Corrigan pulse). The diastolic blood pressure decreases to widen the pulse pressure. This compensates for an increase in systolic blood pressure. Later in the disease, atypical angina pectoris may occur. This often happens at rest or at night, along with diaphoresis, when a lower pulse rate results in delivery of less oxygen to the myocardium. Eventually, symptoms of HF develop if the left ventricle fails. In acute aortic dysfunction, profound symptoms of pulmonary distress, chest pain, and cardiogenic shock symptoms occur and require immediate treatment.

Diagnostic Tests

The ECG shows left ventricle hypertrophy, ST-segment depression (see Fig. 25.8), and T-wave inversion (see Fig. 25.6) in some leads. A chest x-ray confirms hypertrophy of the left ventricle and aorta. With severe AR, left atrial enlargement may also be seen. An echocardiogram, Doppler echocardiogram, or transesophageal echocardiogram show an enlarged left ventricle and severity of the AR. Cardiovascular CT scan or cardiac MRI provide accurate disease severity assessment and effect on ventricular function. Cardiac catheterization reveals elevated left ventricular diastolic pressure and, with contrast injection, shows the regurgitation of blood into the left ventricle.

Therapeutic Measures

Treatment with vasodilators, digitalis, or diuretics may be useful for some patients to reduce systolic blood pressure and, subsequently, cardiac workload until surgery is needed. Occasionally, surgical valve repair can be done, but valve replacement is typically needed when symptoms develop.

Nursing Process for the Patient With a Cardiac Valvular Disorder

Data Collection

A history is obtained that includes information presented in Table 23.2. Vital signs are measured, heart sounds are auscultated to detect murmurs, and any signs and symptoms of HF are noted and reported (see Chapter 26).

Nursing Diagnoses, Planning, Implementation, and Evaluation

The major nursing diagnoses for all valvular disorders are the same. They include those for HF as well, if symptoms of HF are present. See "Nursing Care Plan for the Patient With a Cardiac Valvular Disorder."

Nursing Care Plan for the Patient With a Cardiac Valvular Disorder

Nursing Diagnosis: *Decreased Cardiac Output* related to valvular stenosis or insufficiency or heart failure
Expected Outcome: The patient will have adequate cardiac output as evidenced by vital signs within normal limits (WNL), less dyspnea, and minimal fatigue.
Evaluation of Outcome: Are the patient's vital signs WNL with less dyspnea or fatigue?

Intervention	Rationale	Evaluation
Monitor vital signs, oxygen saturation, chest pain, and edema.	*These are indicators of cardiac output decline.*	Are vital signs WNL with no chest pain or peripheral edema noted?
Administer oxygen as ordered.	*Supplemental oxygen provides more oxygen to the heart by increasing the oxygen saturation in the blood.*	Is oxygen saturation WNL?
Elevate head of bed 45 degrees.	*Venous return to heart is reduced and chest expansion improved, which increases the amount of oxygen coming into the lungs.*	Is there use of accessory muscles of respiration? Does patient report dyspnea?

(nursing care plan continues on page 380)

Nursing Care Plan for the Patient With a Cardiac Valvular Disorder—cont'd

Intervention	Rationale	Evaluation
Geriatric		
Review cardiac medications and presence of side effects, and teach patient side effects to report.	*Toxic side effects are more common, owing to altered metabolism and excretion of medications in the older adult.*	Are side effects present for medications patient is taking? Does patient understand side effects to report?

Nursing Diagnosis: *Activity Intolerance* related to decreased oxygen delivery from decreased cardiac output
Expected Outcome: The patient will exhibit normal changes in vital signs and less fatigue in response to activity.
Evaluation of Outcome: Does the patient have normal changes in vital signs with activity? Does the patient report less fatigue with activity?

Intervention	Rationale	Evaluation
Assist as needed with activities of daily living (ADLs).	*Conserve energy with ADL assistance.*	Are all ADLs completed? Are vital signs WNL with activity?
Provide rest between activities.	*Cardiac workload and oxygen needs are reduced with rest.*	Is patient able to perform activities when allowed extra time?
Geriatric		
Slow pace of care and allow patient extra time to perform activities.	*Patients can often perform activities if allowed time to slowly perform them and rest at intervals.*	Does blood pressure remain WNL when changing position?
Ensure safety when mobilizing older patient.	*Orthostatic hypertension is common in the older adult.*	Does patient ambulate without injury?

Table 23.2

Data Collection for Patients With Cardiac Valvular Disorders

Data Collection	Subjective Data Questions
Health History	Infections (rheumatic fever, endocarditis, streptococcal or staphylococcal, syphilis)? Congenital defects? Cardiac disease (myocardial infarction, cardiomyopathy)?
Respiratory	Dyspnea at rest, on exertion, when lying, or that awakens patient? How many pillows are you accustomed to sleeping on? Cough or hemoptysis?
Cardiovascular	Chest pain, qualities—when does it occur? Loss of consciousness? Edema? Palpitations, dizziness, fatigue, activity intolerance?
Medications	What medications are you taking?
Knowledge of Condition	What is the reason that you are here today? Have you ever been diagnosed with any type of heart disease?

Table 23.2

Data Collection for Patients With Cardiac Valvular Disorders—cont'd

Coping Skills	How do you normally cope with stressors? Support system? What, if anything, seems to help alleviate symptoms? Have there been any adaptations in lifestyle and/or environment?
Objective Data	
Respiratory	Crackles, wheezes, tachypnea, use of accessory muscles
Cardiovascular	Murmurs, extra heart sounds, arrhythmias, edema, jugular venous distention, Corrigan pulse, increased or decreased pulse pressure or blood pressure
Integumentary	Clubbing; cyanosis; diaphoresis; cold, clammy skin; pallor
Diagnostic Test Findings	Review test results.

Patient Education

Education should include caregivers and focus on understanding of the nature of the disorder, health maintenance including medications, prevention of complications, and early recognition of symptoms so that medical care can be sought. For patients on warfarin (Coumadin), a medical ID should be used, and international normalized ratio should be regularly monitored. For high-risk patients, the health care provider (HCP) should explain the American Heart Association guidelines for prophylactic antibiotics to prevent IE (see the prevention section for IE later in this chapter).

Cardiac Valve Repairs

A **commissurotomy** repairs a stenosed valve, which is most commonly the mitral valve. The valve flaps that have adhered to each other—and thus closed the opening between them, known as the *commissure*—are separated to enlarge the valve opening. The patient is placed on cardiopulmonary bypass (CPB; see Chapter 21). An atriotomy (incision into the atrium) is made to expose the valve. The valve cusps are either incised with a knife or broken apart with a dilator. The atrium is sewn closed. CPB is discontinued. Surgery continues as described in Chapter 21.

Annuloplasty is the repair or reconstruction of the valve flaps or annulus. Sutures or a prosthetic ring may be placed in the valve annulus to improve closure of the leaflets. The mitral valve is the most common valve repaired in this way. Similar procedures are used on the tricuspid valve; however, the aortic valve is not readily repaired in this manner.

Heart Valve Replacement

Valves used for cardiac valve replacement may be either mechanical or biological (tissue). Research is ongoing to develop tissue engineered heart valves. Tissue valves (**bioprosthesis**) come from **xenograft** (porcine [pig] and bovine [cow]; also known as a **heterograft**) or **allograft** (a human cadaveric or living donor; also known as a **homograft**) ("Cultural Considerations"). Allografts are available in limited numbers because they rely on donors. An **autograft** (self-donor) in the Ross procedure uses the patient's own pulmonary valve to replace the removed aortic valve; an allograft (human donor) pulmonary valve then replaces the patient's pulmonary valve. Visit www.lifenethealth.org for more information on allografts.

Cultural Considerations

Cardiac Valves

Adherents to the Jewish and Islam religions may not consume pork products. These patients should be asked whether they would prefer bovine, mechanical, or human valves. In the Hindu religion, the cow is considered sacred. Adherents to the Hindu religion should be asked whether they would prefer porcine, mechanical, or human valves.

For mitral valve replacement, a left atriotomy is made after the patient is on CPB. For an aortic valve replacement, an incision is made above the right coronary artery in the aorta. Then, in either valvular procedure, the diseased

• WORD • BUILDING •
commissurotomy: commissura—joining together + tome—incision
annuloplasty: annulus—ring + plasty—formed

valve is excised and the new valve sutured in place. The incision is closed. Surgery then continues as described in Chapter 21.

TAVR is a minimally invasive procedure available for intermediate- to high-risk patients. This procedure replaces the valve without the need to remove the old defective valve. A balloon catheter is introduced via the femoral artery. Then, it is inserted through the diseased valve and inflated to open the stenosed valve leaflets (visit www.corevalve.com to view this procedure). For mitral valve valvoplasty, after the balloon catheter is inserted into the right atrium, it is threaded through a small hole pierced into the right atrial septum that emerges into the left atrium. The catheter is passed through the mitral valve. Inflating the balloon within the mitral valve opens the stenosed valve flaps. Complications may include arrhythmias, emboli, hemorrhage, and cardiac tamponade. A balloon valvuloplasty results in fewer complications than traditional open-heart surgery.

Complications of Valve Replacement

Tissue valves have a low incidence of thrombus formation. They do not require lifelong anticoagulant therapy. However, they do not last as long as mechanical valves because of degenerative changes and calcification. Mechanical valves are durable (lasting 20 to 30 years). However, they create turbulent blood flow, requiring lifelong anticoagulant therapy to prevent blood clots. Anemia from hemolysis of red blood cells as they come in contact with mechanical valve structures can occur. Also, IE can occur due to microorganisms growing on the valve leaflets or the sewing ring of mechanical valves. These growths can make valves incompetent or break off to become emboli.

Nursing Process for the Preoperative Cardiac Surgery Patient

DATA COLLECTION. Baseline data collection is important for postoperative comparison and to begin discharge planning. Pain management, circulatory status, and results of diagnostic tests are all significant. Typing and crossmatching for ordered units of blood is done.

NURSING DIAGNOSES, PLANNING, IMPLEMENTATION, AND EVALUATION. See the "Nursing Process for Preoperative Patients" in Chapter 12.

Nursing Process for the Postoperative Cardiac Surgery Patient

After cardiac surgery, the patient goes to a cardiac universal bed unit (CUB) or an intensive care unit (ICU) to be monitored for 1 to 2 days. In the CUB unit, the patient recovers in the same room until discharge. This avoids transfers to other units and increases continuity of care. In the ICU, as recovery progresses, the patient is transferred to a step-down or general surgical unit for continued cardiac monitoring.

DATA COLLECTION. The patient is accompanied to ICU/CUB by the anesthesiologist. The anesthesiologist gives the nurse a report of the procedure, complications, and hemodynamic and ventilatory management of the patient. The patient remains on a cardiac monitor and mechanical ventilator for up to 24 hours.

A head-to-toe assessment of the patient is performed. This includes dressings, tubes (chest tube, nasogastric tube, urinary catheter), and intravenous (IV) lines. Of importance are signs of awakening, pain, lung and heart sounds, and palpation of the entire chest and neck to detect crepitus (air in the subcutaneous tissue from opening the chest). Trends in cardiac output are monitored. Body temperature is continuously monitored if warming measures such as a warming blanket are used. Warming is discontinued when the core body temperature nears 98.6°F (37°C). Warming should occur slowly to avoid peripheral vasodilation, which can result in shock. While being rewarmed, patients are monitored for shivering. Shivering may be felt as a fine vibration at the mandibular angle of the jaw. Shivering greatly increases cardiac oxygen needs. As ordered, paralyzing agents given with narcotics eliminate shivering. Complete blood count (CBC), electrolytes, coagulation studies, and arterial blood gases (ABGs) are monitored.

After the initial transfer assessment, vital signs, oxygen saturation, and cardiac pressures are monitored. They are recorded every 15 to 30 minutes, with decreasing frequency as the patient stabilizes. Intake and output is measured. A 12-lead ECG is done to detect perioperative MI. A chest x-ray is done to check central line and endotracheal tube placement and to detect a pneumothorax or hemothorax, diaphragm elevation, or mediastinal widening from bleeding.

Awakening with many questions, strange auditory and tactile sensations, and the inability to speak are frightening and frustrating to the patient. Give explanations regarding procedures in simple terms. Keeping eye contact with the patient and using touch appropriately can be soothing to the patient. Communicating with the intubated patient is done with simple closed-ended questions for yes and no answering, nonverbal gestures, communication boards, or magic slates. The family will need a great deal of support during this time.

After cardiac surgery, pain is monitored in relation to the patient's preoperative anginal or MI-associated pain. Chest pain after surgery can be frightening. Knowing that chest pain can occur from the surgical incision rather than from anginal or MI pain is comforting to the patient.

NURSING DIAGNOSES, PLANNING, IMPLEMENTATION, AND EVALUATION. Nursing diagnoses for postoperative cardiac surgery are discussed in the "Nursing Care Plan for the Postoperative Patient Undergoing Cardiac Surgery" and in Chapter 12.

Nursing Care Plan for the Postoperative Patient Undergoing Cardiac Surgery

Nursing Diagnosis: *Acute Pain* related to sternotomy or pericarditis
Expected Outcomes: The patient will state that pain is relieved or tolerable within 30 minutes of report of pain. Patient will be able to rest and perform respiratory treatments.
Evaluation of Outcomes: Does the patient state pain is within acceptable levels? Is the patient able to rest and perform respiratory therapies?

Intervention	Rationale	Evaluation
Ask location and characteristics of pain with each report of pain. Explain pain scale, with 0 being no pain and 10 being the worst pain imaginable.	*A thorough description is needed to determine cause and plan actions.*	Does patient describe pain using scale of 0 to 10?
Splint chest incision with all movement, including coughing and deep breathing.	*Stabilizes sternum and incision to increase comfort.*	Can patient splint chest incision independently?
Turn and reposition every 2 hours.	*Relieves skin pressure points and changes muscle position, relieving stiffness.*	Does patient report comfort without stiffness?
Offer back rubs frequently.	*Relaxes tense muscles retracted during operation.*	Does patient report resting comfortably?
Instruct patient to take a deep breath before movement and exhale slowly during movement.	*Keeps muscles relaxed, minimizing tension with guarding and pain.*	Can patient perform deep-breathing techniques as instructed?

Nursing Diagnosis: *Decreased Cardiac Output* related to myocardial depression, hypothermia, bleeding, unstable arrhythmias, or hypoxemia
Expected Outcomes: The patient will maintain normal sinus rhythm, maintain vital signs within normal limits (WNL), and have palpable peripheral pulses and urine output greater than 30 mL/hr.
Evaluation of Outcomes: Is rhythm normal sinus? Are vital signs WNL and pulses palpable? Is urine output greater than 30 mL/hr?

Intervention	Rationale	Evaluation
Monitor vital signs trends.	*Trends can identify problems.*	Are vital signs WNL?
Monitor peripheral circulation.	*Mottling or weak pulses may indicate poor cardiac output (CO).*	Do peripheral pulses remain strong with normal skin color, temperature, and capillary refill?
Monitor intake and output.	*Fluid deficit or excess can alter CO.*	Does total intake equal output?
Listen to lung sounds and note character of sputum.	*Wet lung sounds may indicate heart failure or pulmonary edema.*	Are lungs clear with no sputum?
Monitor temperature closely while rewarming the patient.	*Febrile state increases heart rate and myocardial oxygen consumption.*	Does temperature remain less than or equal to 98.6°F (37°C)?
Monitor for shivering.	*Shivering increases the blood pressure, decreasing CO and increasing risk for bleeding.*	Is patient's shivering controlled?
Monitor chest tube drainage for increase or sudden decrease.	*Drainage greater than 200 mL/hr may lead to hypovolemia and decreased CO.*	Is patient free from cardiac tamponade and hypovolemia?

(nursing care plan continues on page 384)

Nursing Care Plan for the Postoperative Patient Undergoing Cardiac Surgery—cont'd

Intervention	Rationale	Evaluation
Monitor electrocardiogram.	*Premature ventricular contractions and atrial fibrillation decrease CO.*	Does patient remain in normal sinus rhythm or a controlled arrhythmia?
Monitor electrolytes.	*Low calcium and magnesium and high potassium decrease contractility and CO.*	Are electrolytes WNL?
Monitor arterial blood gases (ABGs).	*Acidosis decreases heart function, and a low CO may lead to further acidosis.*	Are ABGs WNL?

Nursing Diagnosis: *Risk for Infection* related to inadequate primary defenses from surgical wound
Expected Outcome: The patient will remain free from infection.
Evaluation of Outcome: Does the patient remain free from infection?

Intervention	Rationale	Evaluation
Observe incision for signs and symptoms of infection. These include redness, warmth, fever, and/or edema.	*Redness, warmth, fever, and swelling indicate the body's response to an invading pathogen.*	Are signs and symptoms of infection present?
Monitor patency of drains and drainage.	*Drains remove fluid from the surgical site to prevent infection.*	Are drains functioning with amount and color of drainage as expected for procedure?
Monitor and report abnormal findings for temperature, lung sounds, sputum, and urine consistency.	*Low-grade (immunosuppressed) or high-grade fever, crackles, yellow-green sputum color, or cloudy urine can indicate infection.*	Is the patient's temperature WNL, and are lung sounds, sputum, and urine clear?
Practice excellent hand hygiene, and cleanse stethoscope with ethanol-based cleanser or alcohol between patients and with each hand hygiene.	*Hands and stethoscopes can carry and transfer infectious agents.*	Are infectious preventive techniques used? Does patient remain free from infection?

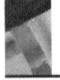

INFLAMMATORY AND INFECTIOUS CARDIAC DISORDERS

The layers of the heart are the endocardium, pericardium, and myocardium (Fig. 23.4). They can become inflamed or infected, leading to endocarditis, pericarditis, and myocarditis, respectively.

Infective Endocarditis

Infective endocarditis, or IE, is an infection of the endocardium that mostly occurs in hearts with artificial or damaged valves or pacemakers. Men develop IE more often than women, as do older adults compared with younger.

Pathophysiology and Etiology

Cardiac defects result in turbulent blood flow that erodes the normally infection-resistant endocardium. IE begins when the invading organism (most commonly bacteria but possibly a fungi or other organism) attaches to eroded endocardium where platelets and fibrin deposits have formed a vegetative lesion. Then, more platelets and fibrin cover the multiplying organism. This covering protects the microbes, reducing the ability to destroy them. Damage to valve leaflets occurs as the vegetations grow. As blood flows through the heart, these vegetations may break off and become emboli.

Damaged valves from conditions such as MVP with regurgitation, rheumatic heart disease, congenital defects, and valve replacements are especially prone to bacterial invasion. The mitral valve is the valve most commonly infected, with the aortic valve being second. HF may result from valve damage, especially of the aortic valve.

Risk factors include the following:

• Compromised immune system
• Artificial heart valve

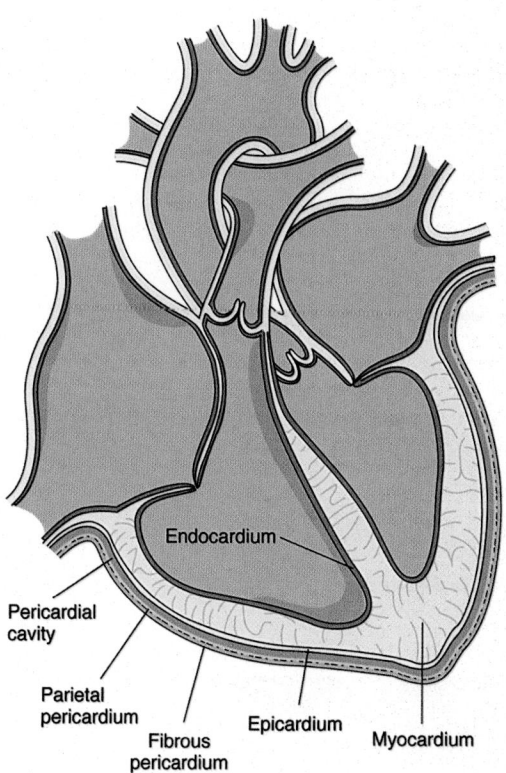

FIGURE 23.4 Layers of the heart.

- Congenital or valvular heart disease
- History of endocarditis
- IV drug use
- Gingival gum disease

Prevention

Dental disease may be a contributing factor to IE. Therefore, daily tooth brushing and flossing along with regular dental care is important. Antibiotic prophylaxis guidelines have been updated by the American Heart Association (Nishimura et al., 2017). The guidelines recommend prophylactic antibiotics before dental procedures for only the highest risk individuals who have an artificial heart valve or a valve repaired with artificial material, a history of IE, a heart transplant with abnormal valve function, or certain congenital heart defects.

Signs and Symptoms

The onset of symptoms can be rapid or slow. Fever (99°F to 103°F [37.2°C to 39.4°C]) is a common sign, although the older adult may be afebrile (Table 23.3). Chills, aching muscles and joints, fatigue, dyspnea, cough, edema, and hematuria may occur. A new or different murmur is heard with valvular damage. Splinter hemorrhages may be seen in the distal nailbed (black or red-brown longitudinal short lines). **Petechiae** (tiny red or purple flat spots) resulting from microembolization of the vegetation may occur on mucous membranes, conjunctivae, or skin (Fig. 23.5). Janeway lesions (small, painless red-blue lesions on palms

and soles) are an acute finding. Osler nodes (small, painful nodes on fingers and toes) from cardiac emboli are a late finding (Fig. 23.6). Roth spots can also occur. These are hemorrhages in the retina that have a white center.

Complications

Vegetative emboli can be a major complication of IE. If organ embolization occurs, signs and symptoms that reflect the organ that was affected by the emboli are seen. Brain emboli may produce changes in level of consciousness or stroke. Kidney emboli cause pain in the flank area, hematuria, or renal failure. Pulmonary emboli result in sudden dyspnea, cough, and chest pain. Spleen emboli cause abdominal pain. Emboli in the small blood vessels can impair circulation in the extremities.

Heart structures can be damaged or destroyed by IE, leading to MI or arrhythmias. Stenosis (narrowing) or regurgitation (leakage) of a heart valve may also result. As the infection progresses and causes more damage to heart structures, HF may occur. Abscesses may also develop in the heart or other parts of the body.

Diagnostic Tests

Table 23.3 lists diagnostic tests for IE. Positive blood cultures identify the causative organism. Echocardiogram shows cardiac vegetation and effects. Chest x-ray, CT scan, or MRI may be used to identify other areas of infection.

Therapeutic Measures

Initial treatment begins with hospitalization and high doses of intravenous antibiotics. The specific pathogen will be identified by blood cultures. The length of therapy is dependent on the type of pathogen; however, treatment is prolonged to penetrate vegetations and kill all microbes. A combination of two antibiotics has proven to be effective. Rest and supportive symptom care are also used. When afebrile without complications after about 1 week, the patient is discharged to continue IV antibiotic therapy at home. Monitoring is continued by the home health care nurse and laboratory testing.

Surgical replacement or repair of valves is needed for severely damaged heart valves, prosthetic valve infection, multiple emboli from damaged valves, or HF. Surgery may be needed for infections that do not resolve.

Nursing Process for the Patient With Infectious Endocarditis

DATA COLLECTION. A patient history is obtained that includes risk factors for IE and recent infections or invasive procedures (Table 23.4). Vital signs are recorded, and heart sounds are auscultated for murmurs. Signs of HF and emboli are noted. The HCP should be notified immediately if circulatory impairment (e.g., cold skin, decreased capillary refill, cyanosis, or absent peripheral pulses in an extremity) or symptoms of organ-related emboli are detected.

• WORD • BUILDING •
petechiae: petecchia—skin spot

Table 23.3

Infective Endocarditis Summary

Signs and Symptoms	Dyspnea, cough Fatigue, weakness Fever, chills, aching muscles Heart murmur Janeway lesions, Osler nodes, Roth spots Nailbed splinter hemorrhages Petechiae Weight loss
Diagnostic Tests	Blood cultures Complete blood count (CBC) Echocardiogram or transesophageal echocardiogram Chest x-ray Electrocardiogram (ECG)
Therapeutic Measures	*Acute therapy:* Prolonged intravenous antimicrobial medications such as penicillin, vancomycin, amphotericin B Antipyretics Rest Valve replacement or repair Prophylactic antibiotic therapy per high-risk infective endocarditis criteria
Complications	Emboli Heart failure Abscesses
Priority Nursing Diagnoses	*Decreased Cardiac Output* related to impaired valvular function or heart failure *Activity Intolerance* related to reduced oxygen delivery from decreased cardiac output

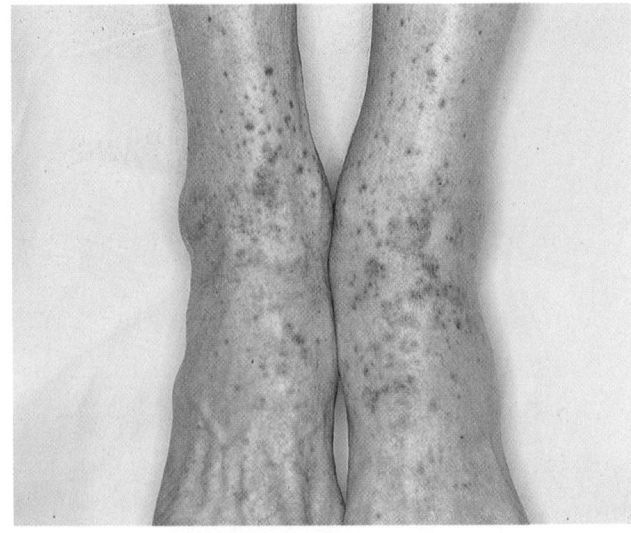

FIGURE 23.5 Petechiae.

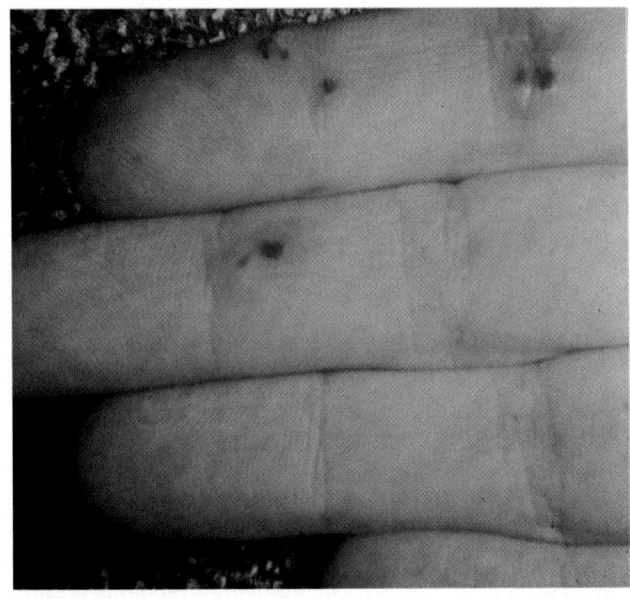

FIGURE 23.6 Osler nodes.

Table 23.4

Data Collection for Patients With Infective Endocarditis

Data Collection	Subjective Data Questions
Health History	Infections (rheumatic fever, scarlet fever, previous endocarditis, streptococcal or staphylococcal, syphilis)? Cardiac disease (valvular surgery, congenital)? Childbirth? Invasive procedures (surgery, dental, catheterization, intravenous [IV] therapy, cystoscopy, gynecological)? Illicit drug use?

Table 23.4

Data Collection for Patients With Infective Endocarditis—cont'd

Gastrointestinal	Malaise? Anorexia? Weight loss?
Respiratory	Dyspnea on exertion or orthopnea (when lying down)? Cough?
Cardiovascular	Palpitations, chest pain, fatigue, activity intolerance?
Musculoskeletal	Weakness, arthralgia, myalgia?
Medications	Steroids, immunosuppressants, prolonged antibiotic therapy? IV drug use?
Knowledge of Condition	What is your understanding of this condition?
Objective Data	
Body Temperature	Fever, diaphoresis
Respiratory	Crackles, tachypnea
Cardiovascular	Murmurs, tachycardia, arrhythmias, edema
Integumentary	Nailbed splinter hemorrhages; petechiae on lips, mouth, conjunctivae, feet, or antecubital area; paleness
Renal	Hematuria
Diagnostic Test Findings	Positive blood cultures, anemia, elevated white blood cell count, elevated erythrocyte sedimentation rate (ESR), electrocardiogram (ECG) showing conduction problems, echocardiogram showing valvular dysfunction and vegetations, chest x-ray exam showing heart enlargement (cardiomegaly) and lung congestion

NURSING DIAGNOSES, PLANNING, IMPLEMENTATION, AND EVALUATION. See "Nursing Care Plan for the Patient With Infective Endocarditis." Teaching provides patients and families with the ability to provide IV antibiotics at home and maintain health to prevent future IE. Good hygiene including brushing with a soft-bristle toothbrush (to prevent gum trauma) twice a day, flossing daily, and having biannual dental cleaning is important. Good skin care includes bathing, proper hand-washing technique, avoiding nail biting, not popping pimples or lancing boils, and cleansing and applying antibiotic ointment to cuts. Recognition of symptoms (e.g., fever, chills, sweats), seeking prompt medical care, and a statement of patient's understanding along with printed material for home reference promote health maintenance.

Nursing Care Plan for the Patient With Infective Endocarditis

Nursing Diagnosis: *Decreased Cardiac Output* related to impaired valvular function or heart failure as manifested by activity intolerance
Expected Outcome: The patient will have adequate cardiac output as evidenced by vital signs within normal limits (WNL), no dyspnea, and minimal fatigue in response to activity.
Evaluation of Outcome: Are the patient's vital signs WNL with less dyspnea and fatigue? Can the patient participate in desired activities?

Intervention	Rationale	Evaluation
Monitor vital signs, murmurs, dyspnea, and fatigue.	*Abnormal vital signs, dyspnea, and fatigue are indicators of cardiac output decline.*	Are vital signs WNL with less dyspnea or fatigue?

(nursing care plan continues on page 388)

Nursing Care Plan for the Patient With Infective Endocarditis—cont'd

Intervention	Rationale	Evaluation
Administer oxygen as ordered and measure saturation.	*Supplemental oxygen will increase oxygen level in the blood.*	Is oxygen saturation WNL?
Elevate head of bed 45 degrees.	*Venous return to heart is reduced and chest expansion improved.*	Is dyspnea reported or use of accessory respiratory muscles seen?
Assist with activities of daily living (ADLs) and provide rest periods as ordered.	*Cardiac workload and oxygen needs are reduced with rest.*	Are ADLs completed and level of fatigue reduced?

Nursing Diagnosis: *Decreased Diversional Activity* related to restricted mobility from prolonged intravenous (IV) therapy
Expected Outcome: The patient will state diversional activities are satisfying.
Evaluation of Outcome: Does the patient participate in diversional activities? Does the patient state satisfaction with activities?

Intervention	Rationale	Evaluation
Identify patient's preferred activities and hobbies.	*Activity preference should be known to plan satisfactory diversional activities.*	Are patient's preferred activities known?
Plan patient's schedule around relaxing and fun activities, using the patient's input.	*Self-esteem is fostered with increased patient control.*	Does patient offer input into scheduled care? Is input followed?
Explore pet therapy.	*Individuals who interact with pets live longer and are healthier.*	Does patient state enjoyment of pet therapy?

CRITICAL THINKING

Mrs. Jones, age 28, is admitted to the hospital with a fever of 100°F (37°C), chills, fatigue, anorexia, and pain in her joints. A physical exam reveals splinter hemorrhages in the left index finger nailbed and petechiae on her chest. She is diagnosed with a heart murmur and infective endocarditis.

1. Why is a heart murmur heard with endocarditis?
2. What do splinter hemorrhages look like?
3. What do petechiae indicate?
4. How would Mrs. Jones's data collection findings be documented?
5. What type of medication would the nurse expect to be ordered to treat the infection?
6. Why does Mrs. Jones have chills if her temperature is elevated?
7. What signs and symptoms might occur if the complications of heart failure develop?
8. Acetaminophen (Tylenol) 650 mg every 6 hours for pain is ordered. It comes as 325-mg tablets. How many tablets would be given for each dose?

Suggested answers are at the end of the chapter.

Pericarditis
Pathophysiology and Etiology

Pericarditis is an acute or chronic inflammation of the pericardium (the sac surrounding the heart for protection and to reduce friction). The inflammation creates a problem for the heart as it tries to expand and fill. As a result, ventricular filling is reduced, which then decreases cardiac output and blood pressure. Acute pericarditis usually resolves in less than 6 weeks but can reoccur. It can be caused by a variety of factors, including:

• Infections (e.g., viruses, bacteria, fungi, or Lyme disease)
• **Dressler syndrome** (autoimmune response)
• Medications
• Neoplastic disease
• Postpericardiotomy (e.g., after cardiac surgery)
• Postmyocardial infarction
• Renal disease or uremia
• Rheumatic disorders (e.g., systemic lupus erythematosus, rheumatoid arthritis)
• Trauma from chest injury or invasive thoracic procedures

There are several forms of chronic pericarditis. It is the result of fibrous scarring of the pericardium. The heart becomes surrounded by a thickened, stiff sac that limits the stretching ability of the heart's chambers for filling. This may result in HF. Chronic constrictive pericarditis results from neoplastic disease and metastasis, radiation, or tuberculosis.

Signs and Symptoms

Chest pain is the most common symptom of acute pericarditis (Table 23.5). The pain is located substernally and over the heart. It may radiate to the clavicle, neck, and left scapula. Typically, there is an intense, sharp, creaky, grating pain that increases with deep inspiration, coughing, moving of the trunk, or lying flat. For some, the pain is not as intense and is instead a dull ache. The pain may be relieved by sitting up and leaning forward. Other symptoms depend on the cause of the pericarditis. They may include orthopnea, low-grade fever, fatigue, cough, and edema.

A **pericardial friction rub** is a grating, scratchy, high-pitched sound that is the result of friction from the inflamed pericardial and epicardial layers rubbing together as the heart fills and contracts. Depending on the severity of the pericarditis,

the rub may be faint when auscultated or loud enough to be audible without auscultation. It may be heard intermittently or continuously. It is usually heard over the lower left sternal border of the chest during each heartbeat. However, this occurs in only about 50% of those with pericarditis.

Chronic constrictive pericarditis produces dyspnea and signs and symptoms of right-sided HF. It may also cause atrial fibrillation.

> **LEARNING TIP**
>
> To simulate the sound of a pericardial friction rub, hold the diaphragm of a stethoscope against the palm of one hand; listen through the stethoscope as you rub the index finger of the opposite hand over the knuckles of the hand holding the diaphragm. This sound is similar to a pericardial friction rub.

Diagnostic Tests

Table 23.5 lists diagnostic tests for pericarditis. The ECG reveals ST-T wave elevation in all leads (see Fig. 25.8). Echocardiogram results show a **pericardial effusion** (buildup of fluid in pericardial space). C-reactive protein (CRP) is elevated from inflammation and can be monitored to show therapy effects. In chronic constrictive pericarditis, a CT scan or MRI may show a thickened pericardium.

Therapeutic Measures

Mild acute cases may resolve without treatment. The cause is determined for appropriate treatment such as antibiotics for bacterial infections. Bedrest is advised to reduce the heart's workload during acute symptoms. Nonsteroidal anti-inflammatory drugs (NSAIDs) or aspirin are given along with colchicine (Colsalide) to resolve inflammation and reduce pain. Corticosteroids are used if initial treatment is not effective. Hemodialysis is used to treat uremic pericarditis. If the patient is unstable, prompt intervention is required, such as an emergency pericardiocentesis.

Chronic effusive pericarditis can be treated with a pericardial window. It is a surgical opening to remove a portion of the outer pericardial layer, allowing continuous drainage of pericardial fluid into the pleural space. Chronic constrictive pericarditis is treated with **pericardiectomy.** This is the surgical removal of the entire tough, calcified pericardium, relieving constriction of the heart and allowing normal filling of the ventricles.

Complications

A pericardial effusion is the most common complication of pericarditis. A rapidly developing effusion, such as one occurring from trauma, can produce symptoms with smaller amounts of fluid than slowly developing effusions, such as pericarditis from tuberculosis, with larger amounts of fluid. The increasing fluid presses on nearby tissue, such as lung tissue producing dyspnea, cough, and tachypnea. The heartbeat sounds distant.

Table 23.5

Pericarditis Summary

Signs and Symptoms	Chest pain
	Cough
	Dyspnea, orthopnea
	Edema
	Low-grade fever
	Palpitations
	Pericardial friction rub
	Weakness
Diagnostic Tests	Complete blood count (CBC)
	Blood chemistry
	Chest x-ray
	Electrocardiogram (ECG)
	Echocardiogram
	Magnetic resonance imaging (MRI)
	Computed tomography (CT) scan
Therapeutic Measures	Treat underlying cause
	Anti-inflammatory medication
	Corticosteroids
	Pericardiocentesis
	Pericardial window
	Pericardiectomy
Complications	Pericardial effusion
	Cardiac tamponade
Priority Nursing Diagnoses	*Acute Pain* related to inflammation of pericardium
	Anxiety related to disease process
	Decreased Cardiac Output related to cardiac constriction

As the fluid accumulation grows, **cardiac tamponade,** another complication of pericarditis, can occur. Cardiac tamponade is a life-threatening compression of the heart by fluid accumulated in the pericardial sac. Cardiac output drops. To compensate, the heart rate increases. Then, blood pressure falls as compensatory mechanisms fail. Symptoms of decreased cardiac output, such as restlessness, confusion, tachycardia, and tachypnea, occur. Jugular venous distention is present from increased venous pressure, and heart sounds are distant.

Cardiac tamponade requires emergency treatment with **pericardiocentesis.** The pericardium is punctured with a needle, and excess fluid in the pericardial sac is removed (Fig. 23.7). Fluid obtained during pericardiocentesis can be examined to diagnose the cause. Complications include bleeding, infection, pneumothorax, or heart damage from laceration of a coronary artery or the myocardium.

Nursing Care

Nursing care focuses on relieving the patient's pain and anxiety and maintaining normal cardiac function. Pain is rated and treated as ordered. Allowing the patient to assume a position of comfort by sitting up and leaning forward also relieves pain. Teaching the patient about pericarditis and its treatment

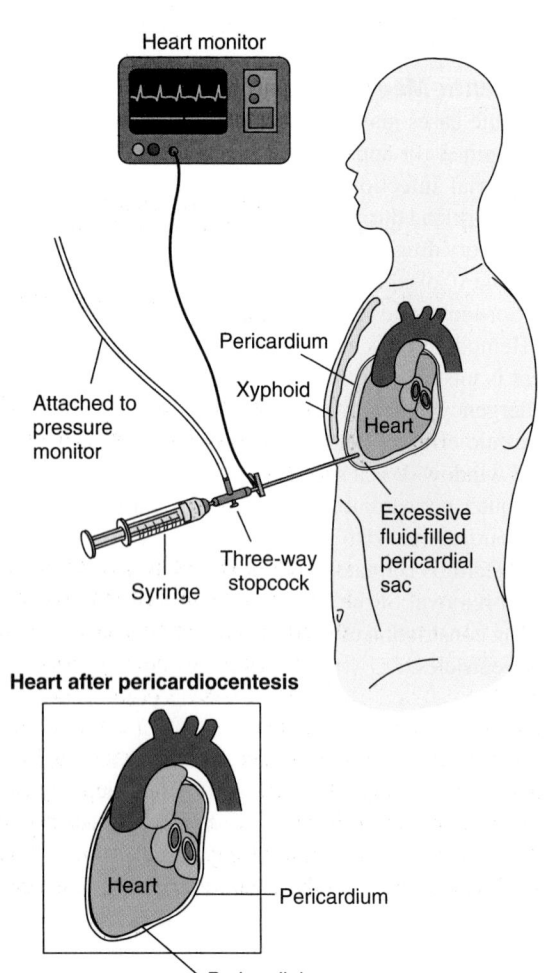

FIGURE 23.7 Pericardiocentesis.

relieves anxiety, giving a feeling of control by allowing the patient to make knowledgeable health care decisions.

Myocarditis

Pathophysiology and Etiology

Myocarditis is inflammation of the myocardium. The amount of muscle destroyed with myocarditis determines the extent of damage to the heart. The heart may enlarge in response to the damaged muscle fibers. However, most cases of myocarditis are benign, with few signs or symptoms.

Myocarditis is a rare condition that most commonly develops after a viral infection. Other causes are bacteria, parasites, fungi, rickettsiae, spirochetes, medications, lead toxicity, autoimmune factors, HIV, rheumatic fever, systemic lupus erythematosus, pericarditis, IE, or cardiac transplant rejection.

Signs and Symptoms

Signs and symptoms of myocarditis vary from none to severe cardiac manifestations. Fatigue, fever, pharyngitis, malaise, dyspnea, palpitations, muscle aches, gastrointestinal discomfort, and enlarged lymph nodes may occur early from a viral infection. Cardiac manifestations such as chest pain or tachycardia may occur about 2 weeks after a viral infection. Occasionally, sudden death may occur.

Diagnostic Tests

An endomyocardial biopsy during cardiac catheterization can be used to diagnose myocarditis. Chest x-ray, echocardiogram, and MRI are helpful to show heart structure and function. An ECG shows arrhythmias, commonly sinus tachycardia. Blood tests are done, including CBC, viral antibodies, and enzyme levels that look for heart damage.

Therapeutic Measures

Treatment is aimed at the cause, if known. Interventions to reduce the heart's workload during recovery are essential. These include bedrest and limited activity. Exercise increases myocardial inflammation and mortality. It should be avoided until symptoms improve and inflammation is gone. The use of alcohol and tobacco should be avoided. Symptoms of HF are treated with medications such as angiotensin-converting enzyme (ACE) inhibitors, angiotensin II receptor blockers (ARBs), beta blockers, or diuretics to reduce the heart's workload. Severe myocarditis may require inotropic medications to vasodilate and strengthen contraction or heart transplantation.

Nursing Care

Nursing care is aimed at maintaining normal cardiac function by monitoring vital signs and symptoms, and administering medications as ordered. Interventions to reduce fatigue

• WORD • BUILDING •

cardiac tamponade: kardia—heart + tamponade—plug
pericardiocentesis: peri—around + kardia—heart + centesis—puncture
myocarditis: myo—muscle + kardia—heart + itis—inflammation

include providing assistance as needed, allowing for frequent rest periods, and teaching energy conservation methods. Determining diversional activities with the patient when activity is restricted further reduces patient anxiety.

Cardiac Trauma

Two types of cardiac trauma can occur: nonpenetrating and penetrating. Nonpenetrating injuries, or contusions, occur from blunt trauma such as motor vehicle accidents or contact sports in which direct compression or force is applied to the upper torso. Contusions may vary from small bruises to hemorrhage.

There may be few or no external injuries indicating cardiac injury. The patient may be asymptomatic or exhibit signs and symptoms identical to a MI. In severe contusions, laboratory results may show elevated creatine kinase MB (CK-MB, an enzyme) or troponin I (a protein).

If bleeding into the pericardial sac occurs, cardiac tamponade can occur. If signs of shock are present, a pericardiocentesis must be performed. With its own pressure, the tamponade may seal the area of bleeding, so no cardiac decompensation occurs. In this case, only bedrest and observation are required. There are no long-term effects with most contusions. With severe contusions, however, scarring and necrosis of the myocardium may decrease cardiac output and increase the risk for cardiac rupture.

Penetrating traumas include an external injury to the chest, such as a stab or gunshot wound, or an internal injury, such as invasive lines that penetrate the cardiac muscle. Complications vary depending on the size, location, and cause of injury. Tamponade occurs from bleeding into the pericardial sac if the pericardium is sealed off by clot formation. A hemothorax develops if blood drains into the pleural space in the chest. A pneumothorax occurs if air collects in the pleural space. Signs and symptoms of hemorrhage and myocardial ischemia can be noted. Surgical repair may be indicated.

Cardiomyopathy

Cardiomyopathy is abnormality and enlargement of the heart muscle that leads to ineffective pumping of the blood. There are three types of cardiac structure and function abnormalities in cardiomyopathy: dilated, hypertrophic, and restrictive (Fig. 23.8). A consequence of each type of cardiomyopathy can be HF, myocardial ischemia, or MI due to reduced cardiac output. There is no cure. The greatest advancement for the cardiomyopathies has been in genetic research, which has identified genetic mutations that cause these diseases.

Dilated Cardiomyopathy

In dilated cardiomyopathy, the size of the heart chambers increases and the walls of the heart become thin. Since the heart is weakened, cardiac output is reduced. Blood moves more slowly from the left ventricle. This often results in blood clot formation. Dilated cardiomyopathy is the most frequent type of cardiomyopathy and one of the most frequent causes of HF. The left ventricle is most often affected. Dilated cardiomyopathy may be caused by genetics (family testing may be recommended), infectious myocarditis, hypertension, heart valve disorders, MI, chronic alcohol or

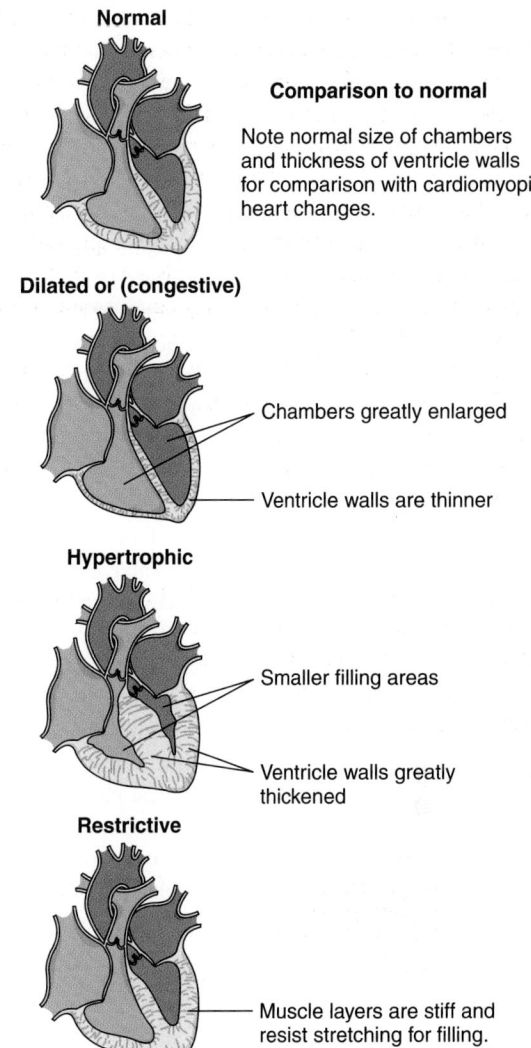

Normal

Comparison to normal

Note normal size of chambers and thickness of ventricle walls for comparison with cardiomyopic heart changes.

Dilated or (congestive)

Chambers greatly enlarged

Ventricle walls are thinner

Hypertrophic

Smaller filling areas

Ventricle walls greatly thickened

Restrictive

Muscle layers are stiff and resist stretching for filling.

FIGURE 23.8 Comparison of the normal heart structure with each type of cardiomyopic heart structure.

cocaine use, metals such as lead, elevated iron levels, HIV, thiamine or zinc deficiencies, cardiac infections, chemotherapy, or neuromuscular disorders.

Hypertrophic Cardiomyopathy

Hypertrophic cardiomyopathy is a hereditary disorder that is transmitted as an autosomal dominant trait (family testing with ECG and echocardiogram is recommended). Prognosis and life span are very good as symptoms often do not develop to restrict lifestyle. Thickening (hypertrophy) of the cardiac muscle wall, often of the upper ventricular septum and left ventricle during adolescence, occurs. The hypertrophy may occur asymmetrically. Hypertrophic cardiomyopathy causes the ventricular wall to be rigid. Therefore, it does not relax to allow normal ventricular filling. If the mitral valve is affected and, along with the enlarged septum, obstructs the

• WORD • BUILDING •

cardiomyopathy: kardia—heart + myo—muscle + pathy—disease

outflow of blood through the aortic valve, it is known as obstructive hypertrophic cardiomyopathy. Occasionally, sudden death can occur, primarily in those who are young.

Restrictive Cardiomyopathy

Restrictive cardiomyopathy impairs ventricular stretch limiting ventricular filling. Cardiac muscle stiffness is present with no ventricular dilation, although systolic emptying of the ventricle is normal. Restrictive cardiomyopathy is the rarest form of cardiomyopathy. It may be caused by infiltrative diseases such as amyloidosis that deposit the protein amyloid within the myocardial cells. This makes the muscle stiff and resistant to stretching for easy ventricular filling. Treating the underlying cause may help reduce heart damage.

Signs and Symptoms

Manifestations of cardiomyopathy depend on the type of abnormality, with varying degrees of HF (Table 23.6). Often there are no early symptoms, and it can occur abruptly. With dilated cardiomyopathy, left ventricular and then right-sided HF with a poor prognosis are seen. Dyspnea on exertion, orthopnea, extreme fatigue, and sometimes atrial fibrillation occur. With hypertrophic cardiomyopathy, if symptoms develop, middle to older age is the most common time. These symptoms can include exertional dyspnea, fatigue, chest pain, syncope, dizziness, and palpitations related to obstruction of cardiac output through the aortic valve. With restrictive cardiomyopathy, HF symptoms result from the ventricles' inability to fill during diastole. Syncope, arrhythmias, and thrombi may occur.

Diagnostic Tests

Cardiomegaly is visible on a chest x-ray. Echocardiogram shows muscle thickness and chamber size to differentiate between the types of cardiomyopathy. Changes related to enlarged chamber size, tachycardia, and arrhythmias can be seen on the ECG. Cardiac catheterization and biopsy as well as cardiovascular MRI may be useful. An endomyocardial biopsy may be done for restrictive cardiomyopathy. Blood tests may be done to identify HF (brain natriuretic peptide [BNP]), infections, or elevated metal or iron levels. For those with hypertrophic cardiomyopathy, a stress (exercise) test may identify exertional problems due to obstruction.

Therapeutic Measures

Treatment for both dilated and restrictive cardiomyopathies is palliative, focusing on the underlying cause, if known, and managing HF (see Chapter 26). For dilated cardiomyopathy, treatment focuses on the symptoms of HF. ACE inhibitors, ARBs, beta blockers, diuretics, aldosterone antagonists, and digoxin (Lanoxin) may be given. Biventricular pacing and implantable defibrillators may be used. For severe HF, primarily in those with dilated cardiomyopathy, a heart transplant may be done. A ventricular assist device along with extracorporeal membrane oxygenation (ECMO) may be used until a donor is found (see Chapter 26).

Therapy is not very useful for restrictive cardiomyopathy. Diuretics or nitrates may be used to relieve venous congestion that occurs because of HF. However, a fine balance is needed when using these drugs so that preload is not reduced too greatly, which would worsen symptoms. With atrial fibrillation, anticoagulants are given to prevent emboli formation. Antiarrhythmics or cardioversion is used for arrhythmias.

Treatment is not required for most people with hypertrophic cardiomyopathy as symptoms do not usually develop. For obstructive hypertrophic cardiomyopathy, beta blockers and calcium channel blockers are given to slow the heart rate to allow more filling time and lessen the strength of the heart's contraction. An antiarrhythmic agent might be used. Adequate hydration is vital, helping to maintain cardiac output. Digoxin and vasodilators are avoided because they can increase the obstruction. Strenuous exercise and athletic sports are restricted to prevent sudden death. Lower levels of exercise may be allowed. For patients in whom medical therapy is not effective, dual chamber pacemakers, implantable automatic defibrillators, or invasive procedures are considered. For those without obstruction, fewer treatment options exist. Diuretics are used to reduce elevated pressures along with beta blockers and calcium channel blockers.

When medical therapy is not successful, surgery can be done for the hypertrophied muscle to remove part of the ventricular septum (**myectomy**). This allows greater outflow of blood. For those not candidates for surgery, a septal ablation delivers alcohol via a catheter to necrose and reduce septal heart wall thickness over time.

Nursing Care

Nursing care focuses on maintaining normal cardiac function, increasing activity tolerance, and relieving anxiety. Careful monitoring is done to detect complications, such as HF, emboli, or arrhythmias. The HCP is immediately notified of problems. Maintenance of normal cardiac function includes increasing activity tolerance, planning rest periods, scheduling activities in small amounts, avoiding tiring activities, and providing small meals that require less energy to digest than large meals. Patient and caregiver education is vital due to the chronic nature of the disease and emotional needs. Education increases the sense of control, decreases anxiety, and aids informed decision making (Box 23.1). Home health care may assist in maintaining functional ability and reduce hospitalizations.

VENOUS DISORDERS

Thrombophlebitis

Thrombophlebitis is the formation of a clot, followed by inflammation within a vein. It is the most common disorder of veins. It can occur in any superficial or deep vein in the

---

• WORD • BUILDING •

cardiomegaly: kardia—heart + mega—large
myectomy: myo—muscle + ectomy—cutting out
thrombophlebitis: thromb—lump (clot) + phleb—vein + itis—
    inflammation

Table 23.6
Cardiomyopathy Summary

Signs and Symptoms	Angina Arrhythmias Dyspnea Edema Fatigue Syncope
Diagnostic Tests	Brain natriuretic peptide (BNP) Electrocardiogram (ECG) Chest x-ray Cardiac catheterization Cardiac magnetic resonance imaging (MRI) Echocardiogram
Therapeutic Measures	Anticoagulants Antihypertensives Diuretics Corticosteroids Antiarrhythmics *Dilated cardiomyopathy:* vasodilators, cardiac glycosides, cardiac resynchronization, implantable cardioverter device, heart transplant *Hypertrophic cardiomyopathy:* beta blockers, calcium channel blockers, myectomy, septal ablation *Restrictive cardiomyopathy:* vasodilators, heart transplant
Complications	Heart failure
Priority Nursing Diagnoses	*Activity Intolerance* related to cardiac insufficiency *Anxiety* related to disease process *Decreased Cardiac Output* related to impaired myocardial function

body. Most commonly, it occurs in the legs, thighs, or pelvis. Deep vein thrombosis (DVT) is the most serious form because pulmonary emboli can result if the thrombus detaches (see Chapter 31). Venous thromboembolism (VTE) disease includes DVT and pulmonary emboli. VTE can be fatal. It occurs most often in hospitalized patients due to immobility or after surgery.

Pathophysiology and Etiology

A venous thrombus is made up of platelets, red blood cells, white blood cells, and fibrin. Platelets attach to a vein wall. Then, a tail forms as more blood cells and fibrin collect. As the tail grows, it drifts in the blood flowing past it. The turbulence of blood flow can cause parts of the drifting thrombus to break off, becoming emboli that travel to the lungs.

Box 23.1
Patient Education

Cardiomyopathy
Patients and families should understand the importance of the following:
- Adherence to medication regimen to prevent heart failure
- Having emergency contact numbers readily available
- Cardiopulmonary resuscitation (CPR) training for family members
- The availability of hospice care and emotional support for families during the grieving process

Three factors are involved in the formation of a thrombus: stasis of blood flow, damage to the lining of the vein wall, and increased blood coagulation (Table 23.7). They are referred to collectively as *Virchow's triad*.

Prevention

Identification of risk factors for thrombosis (see Table 23.7) and patient education promote the use of interventions (discussed later) to prevent thrombosis ("Evidence-Based Practice"). Dehydration should be avoided to reduce thrombus risk. (Visit the Centers for Disease Control and Prevention Stop the Clot campaign page at www.cdc.gov/features/blood-clot-awareness/index.html for further information.)

Evidence-Based Practice

Clinical Question
Is combined intermittent pneumatic compression (IPC) of the legs and pharmacological prophylaxis more effective than single modalities in preventing venous thromboembolism in hospitalized surgical or trauma patients?

Evidence
A systematic review of 22 trials (with 9,137 participants and including 15 randomized control trials) revealed moderate evidence that combined IPC and pharmacological prophylaxis was more effective in decreasing deep vein thrombosis (DVT) than IPC alone and in decreasing pulmonary embolism (PE) more than with anticoagulation alone (Kakkos et al., 2016).

Implications for Nursing Practice
Recognize and teach patients the need for combined therapy to reduce DVT and PE.

Reference
Kakkos, S. K., Caprini, J. A., Geroulakos, G., Nicolaides, A. N., Stansby, G., Reddy, D. J., & Ntouvas, I. (2016). Combined intermittent pneumatic leg compression and pharmacological prophylaxis for prevention of venous thromboembolism. *Cochrane Database of Systematic Reviews, 2016*(9). CD005258. doi:10.1002/14651858.CD005258.pub3

Table 23.7

Predisposing Conditions for Thrombophlebitis (Virchow's Triad)

Condition	*Example*
Venous stasis	
• Reduction of blood flow	Shock, heart failure, myocardial infarction, atrial fibrillation
• Dilated veins	Vasodilators
• Decreased muscle contractions	Sitting for long periods (e.g., traveling) Immobility due to fractured hip, paralysis, anesthesia, surgery, obesity, advanced age
• Faulty valves	Varicose veins, venous insufficiency
Venous wall injury	Venipuncture, venous cannulation at same site for more than 48 hours, venous catheterization, surgery, trauma, burns, fractures, dislocation, intravenous (IV) medications (potassium, chemotherapy drugs, antibiotics, IV hypertonic solutions), IV contrast agents, diabetes, cerebrovascular disease
Increased coagulation of blood	Anemia, malignancy, antithrombin III deficiency, oral contraceptives, estrogen therapy, smoking, discontinuance of anticoagulant therapy, dehydration, malnutrition, polycythemia, leukocytosis, thrombocytosis, sepsis, pregnancy

---

BE SAFE!

For prevention of thrombophlebitis:

• Teach and encourage leg exercises if patient is immobilized in bed.
• Ambulate as early as possible.
• Change intravenous sites every 48 to 72 hours.

IMMOBILITY. People traveling long distances (e.g., in cars, airplanes) or with sedentary jobs that require extended periods of sitting or standing should change positions, perform knee and ankle flexion exercises, or walk at regular intervals to prevent stasis of blood. Patients on bedrest should have legs elevated above the level of the heart, if possible, and turn every 2 hours to prevent pooling of blood. Postoperatively or in times of bedrest, active or passive range-of-motion exercises should be done to increase blood flow. Ambulation should begin as soon as the patient's condition allows. Pain should be controlled to facilitate movement. Deep-breathing aids improve blood flow in the large thoracic veins. Smoking should be avoided because nicotine causes vasoconstriction.

PROPHYLACTIC ANTIEMBOLISM DEVICES. Patients with peripheral venous disease, those on bedrest, and those who have had surgery or trauma may use antiembolism devices to improve blood flow. Knee- or thigh-length elastic compression stockings apply pressure to the leg. They must be applied correctly to avoid a tourniquet effect. Older patients with decreased manual dexterity may need assistance. Stockings should be removed for skin inspection, cleansing, and moisturizing daily. Intermittent pneumatic compression (IPC) devices fill intermittently with air to move venous blood in the legs by simulating contraction of the leg muscles. They may be used in combination with elastic compression stockings. Research has shown that the lowest incidence of DVT in surgical patients occurs with elastic compression stockings and IPC devices used together.

PROPHYLACTIC MEDICATION. Low molecular weight heparin (LMWH) can be given postoperatively to prevent thrombosis (Table 23.8). Anticoagulation monitoring is not required with LMWH because of the predictability of its dose-related response. Subcutaneous heparin may also be used postoperatively to prevent thrombosis. Platelet counts must be monitored with either LMWH or heparin to detect heparin-induced thrombocytopenia.

Oral anticoagulants such as warfarin (Coumadin) can be used in the high-risk patient to decrease thrombosis. The **international normalized ratio** (INR) measures the effectiveness of warfarin therapy using a standardized testing reagent. Therefore, INR can be used around the world with no variation in results as occurs with prothrombin time (PT). INR is the preferred monitoring value but PT is also reported ("Learning Tip").

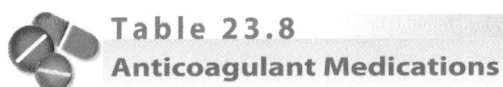

Table 23.8
Anticoagulant Medications

Medication Class/Action

Coumarin

Inhibits liver synthesis of vitamin K dependent clotting factors: II, XII, IX, X.

Examples	**Nursing Implications**
warfarin (Coumadin)	Monitor international normalized ratio (INR) regularly.
	Monitor for bleeding, and teach patient to report bleeding.
	Acetaminophen (Tylenol) for analgesia used instead of aspirin during therapy (can continue aspirin for heart disease).
	Antidote: Vitamin K.

Direct Thrombin Inhibitors

Examples	**Nursing Implications**
dabigatran (Pradaxa)	Monitor for bleeding.

Heparin

Binds to antithrombin III, which then inhibits fibrin formation.

Examples	**Nursing Implications**
heparin sodium	Do not give intramuscularly as can cause pain and hematoma.
	Monitor heparin antifactor Xa or partial thromboplastin time: 1.5 to 2 times control.
	Monitor platelet count for decrease.
	Monitor for bleeding.
	Teach:
	Report bleeding.
	Antidote: Protamine sulfate.

Factor Xa Inhibitors

Bind with antithrombin III, inhibiting making of factor Xa and the formation of thrombin.

Examples	**Nursing Implications**
apixaban (Eliquis)	Bleeding rare.
dalteparin sodium (Fragmin)	Contraindicated with kidney disease due to increased bleeding risk.
enoxaparin (Lovenox)	Compliance is key for efficacy.
fondaparinux (Arixtra)	*Teach:*
rivaroxaban (Xarelto)	Give injection subcutaneously (with a prefilled syringe;
edoxaban (Savaysa)	the air bubble is not to be removed).

Thrombolytics

Promote fibrinolysis to break down fibrin in blood clot.

Examples	**Nursing Implications**
reteplase; rPA (Retavase)	Minimize blood draws for 24 hours. Monitor for bleeding.
tenecteplase; TNK (TNKase)	Avoid acetylsalicylic acid, nonsteroidal anti-inflammatory drugs.
tissue plasminogen activator; tPA (Alteplase)	

LEARNING TIP

Before administering the anticoagulant warfarin (Coumadin), laboratory values must be checked to ensure patient safety:

• Normal and desired therapeutic international normalized ratio (INR) values for the patient's disorder are provided on the laboratory report. These INR values do not require calculation of a therapeutic range because the values are given on the report.

• Compare the patient's INR value with the desired INR value to determine whether it is safe to give warfarin.

• Although INR is the preferred test for warfarin effectiveness, you might still want to know how to calculate a therapeutic range for prothrombin time (PT) if it is also reported. PT is measured in seconds. The normal value range gives the seconds required for a fibrin clot to form during the test. If a patient is on warfarin, the purpose is to increase the time (seconds) it takes the blood to clot.

• Because a *therapy*, warfarin, is being given, a PT range that safely considers the expected effects of the warfarin is needed. This is called the therapeutic range (i.e., a low and a high value). Warfarin's therapeutic range is 1.5 to 2 times the normal PT range. To monitor the patient's therapeutic PT, compare the patient's result with the therapeutic range that you calculate.

• Example:
  Normal PT range: 9 to 12 seconds
  To calculate therapeutic range, multiply:

$$
\begin{array}{ccc}
9 & & 12 \\
\underline{\times\,1.5} & & \underline{\times\,2} \\
13.5 & \text{to} & 24 \text{ seconds (Therapeutic range)}
\end{array}
$$

  Patient's value on warfarin: 16 seconds

Compare the patient's value of 16 seconds with the therapeutic range of 13.5 to 24 seconds to determine that the patient's PT value is indeed safely within the therapeutic range. So, it is safe to give warfarin.

IV THERAPY. Monitoring of IV sites should be performed according to institutional policy in order to detect signs of thrombophlebitis. Venous cannula sites should be changed regularly per institutional guidelines (e.g., every 48 to 72 hours) to prevent thrombus formation.

Signs and Symptoms

Symptoms vary according to the size and location of a thrombus. In some cases, the thrombus becomes an embolus (Table 23.9).

SUPERFICIAL VEINS. Thrombophlebitis in a superficial vein may produce redness, warmth, swelling, and tenderness in the area. The vein feels like a firm cord. This is referred to as *induration*. The saphenous vein is the most commonly affected vein in the leg. Varicosity of the vein is usually the cause. In the arm, IV therapy is the most common cause.

Table 23.9

Thrombophlebitis Summary

Signs and Symptoms	*Superficial veins:* redness, warmth, swelling, tenderness, induration *Deep veins:* swelling, pain, warmth, venous distention, edema and tenderness
Diagnostic Tests	D-dimer (small protein fragment in blood as a blood clot dissolves) Compression ultrasonography Contrast venography Magnetic resonance imaging (MRI) or computed tomography (CT) scan
Therapeutic Measures	*Superficial veins:* warm, moist heat; analgesics; nonsteroidal anti-inflammatory drugs (NSAIDs); compression stockings *Deep veins:* anticoagulants; warm, moist heat; leg extremity elevation above heart level; compression stockings; thrombolytic therapy; thrombectomy; early ambulation
Complications	Pulmonary embolism Chronic venous insufficiency Recurrent deep vein thrombosis
Priority Nursing Diagnoses	*Acute Pain* related to inflammation of vein *Impaired Skin Integrity* related to venous stasis *Anxiety* related to uncertain prognosis of disease

DEEP VEINS. Up to 50% of patients have no symptoms with thrombophlebitis in the legs. With a DVT in a femoral vein, swelling, pain, warmth, venous distention, edema, and tenderness of the calf may be present in the affected leg. Obstruction of blood flow from the leg back to the heart causes the edema. An elevated temperature can be present. Cyanosis and edema may occur if the large veins (vena cava) are involved.

Complications

The most serious complication is pulmonary embolism (PE), which is a life-threatening emergency (see Chapter 31). Chronic venous insufficiency, results from damage to the valves in the vein and results in venous stasis. Signs and symptoms that may appear years after a thrombus include edema, pain, brownish discoloration and ulceration of the medial ankle, venous distention, and dependent cyanosis of the leg. Postthrombotic syndrome (PTS) is a symptomatic chronic venous insufficiency after a DVT that occurs in about

50% of DVT patients within 2 years. It occurs from damage to the vein valves that normally prevent backflow of blood within the leg veins. PTS results in pain, swelling, and sometimes leg ulcers, which can reduce quality of life. The routine use of compression stockings is no longer recommended to prevent PTS (Kearon et al., 2016).

Diagnostic Tests

Diagnostic tests guide treatment needs (see Table 23.9). Compression ultrasonography is a reliable, rapid bedside test to diagnosis a suspected DVT, allowing quick initiation of treatment.

Therapeutic Measures

The goals of treatment are to relieve pain and to prevent pulmonary emboli, thrombus enlargement, or development of another thrombus. Superficial thrombophlebitis is treated at home with warm, moist heat; analgesics; NSAIDs; and, for the leg, elastic compression stockings and leg elevation for symptom relief. Anticoagulants are not typically needed since the risk of PE is low. A proximal DVT may be treated at home if there is no PE. Traditionally, bedrest has been recommended for DVT care. However, increasing evidence has not shown an increased risk for PE and DVT deaths with early ambulation, after pain and swelling subside, which has many benefits (Liu et al., 2015).

Traditional medical care for some DVTs involves a hospital stay of about 5 days. Interventions may include warm, moist heat; elevation of the leg above heart level for swelling; elastic compression stockings; and anticoagulants. Additional classes of anticoagulants that do not require ongoing lab monitoring have provided options to the traditional anticoagulant therapy of heparin and warfarin (see Table 23.8). Typically, anticoagulants are initially prescribed for 3 months. Then, the patient is evaluated for further need for them.

Other approaches are surgical treatment to prevent pulmonary emboli or chronic venous insufficiency when anticoagulant therapy cannot be used or the risk of pulmonary emboli is great. Venous thrombectomy removes the clot through a venous incision. In some cases, a vena cava filter is placed into the vena cava through the femoral or right internal jugular vein (Fig. 23.9). Once in place, it is opened and attaches to the vein wall. The filter traps clots traveling toward the lungs without hindering blood flow. An inferior vena cava filter is not recommended for those with acute DVT or PE when taking anticoagulants (Kearon et al., 2016).

Nursing Process for the Patient With Thrombophlebitis

DATA COLLECTION. A patient history is obtained that includes questions regarding recent IV therapy or use of contrast media, surgery, extremity trauma, childbirth, bedrest, recent long trips, cardiac disease, recent infections, and current medications that can put the patient at high risk of thrombus. Data are gathered for pain, fever, peripheral pulses, sensation, tenderness, redness, warmth, edema, and a firm, cordlike vein in the affected extremity. Daily extremity circumference measurements are taken and documented (bilateral thighs and calves for leg DVT) and recorded to monitor edema. Coagulation tests are monitored. Signs and symptoms of a pulmonary embolism must be immediately reported to the HCP (see Chapter 31).

NURSING DIAGNOSES, PLANNING, IMPLEMENTATION, AND EVALUATION. For the patient identified as being at risk for blood clots, the nursing diagnosis *Risk for Venous Thromboembolism* applies. Interventions would include the preventive measures previously discussed. See "Nursing Care Plan for the Patient With Thrombophlebitis" for specific nursing interventions. Teaching the patient about the disease and treatment is important to reduce anxiety about complications and to enhance adherence to treatment to prevent complications (see Patient Teaching Guidelines for this chapter on Davis Edge).

Nursing Care Plan for the Patient With Thrombophlebitis

Nursing Diagnosis: *Acute Pain* related to inflammation of vein
Expected Outcome: The patient will report satisfactory pain relief within 30 minutes of pain report.
Evaluation of Outcome: Does the patient report satisfactory pain relief?

Intervention	Rationale	Evaluation
Monitor pain using rating scale, such as 0 to 10.	*Self-report is the most reliable indicator of pain.*	Does patient report pain using scale?
Provide analgesics and nonsteroidal anti-inflammatory drugs (NSAIDs) as ordered.	*Pain is reduced when inflammation is decreased.*	Is patient's rating of pain lower after medication?
Apply warm, moist compresses as ordered.	*Moist heat penetrates deeply to relieve pain and increase circulation to aid comfort.*	Does patient report increased comfort with warm, moist compresses?

(nursing care plan continues on page 398)

Nursing Care Plan for the Patient With Thrombophlebitis—cont'd

Nursing Diagnosis: *Impaired Skin Integrity* related to venous stasis
Expected Outcome: The patient's skin will remain intact.
Evaluation of Outcome: Does the patient's skin remain intact?

Intervention	Rationale	Evaluation
Observe skin for edema, skin color changes, and ulcers. Measure both extremities' circumference at the same site in each extremity daily or as ordered.	*Monitoring will detect signs of skin integrity impairment. Edematous skin breaks down more easily.*	Is there a change in edema or skin integrity?
Elevate feet above heart level.	*Elevation decreases swelling by increasing blood flow to heart.*	Is swelling reduced?
Fit and apply elastic compression stockings after edema is reduced, as ordered.	*Elastic compression stockings are fitted after edema is reduced to avoid constriction. The compression of elastic stockings increases blood flow to reduce swelling.*	Is swelling reduced?
Teach patient to avoid crossing legs or wearing constricting clothes.	*Crossing legs and constrictive clothes impair venous return.*	Does patient demonstrate understanding of teaching?

Home Health Hints

• The caregiver often answers the door. When the patient is alone, a note can be placed on the door with instructions; however, the instructions should not convey that the patient is alone.

• On admission, measure the patient's midcalf area for a baseline size. Reassess measurements at every visit. Slight changes in size can indicate a problem.

• Observe if pressure is being applied on the popliteal area or calf muscle when a patient with venous circulation problems is sitting in a recliner with the leg rest in the up position. A small, flat pillow can be placed underneath the knees and lower legs to open the angle and relieve the pressure.

• Encourage the patient to move often because immobility can contribute to thrombophlebitis and other complications.

• Assist patients to develop energy-conserving techniques by being observant of their environment. Things that the patient uses frequently can be placed in trays and baskets close to the patient's chair. A carrying pouch on the front bar of a walker can carry items such as a portable phone or tissues. Chairs for resting can be placed at the top and bottom of stairs.

• If the patient is bedbound and the health care provider is in agreement, instruct both the patient and caregiver on simple active and passive range-of-motion exercises.

If necessary, consider involving occupational and physical therapists to work collaboratively, planning an appropriate activity program.

• Teach patients to report the signs and symptoms of thrombophlebitis, pulmonary emboli, incisional infection, or pneumonia.

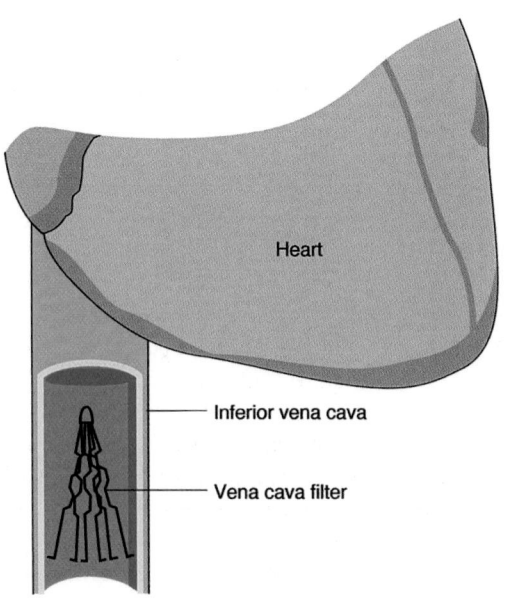

Heart

Inferior vena cava

Vena cava filter

FIGURE 23.9 Vena cava filter placed in the inferior vena cava to prevent emboli from reaching the lungs.

SUGGESTED ANSWERS TO CRITICAL THINKING

Mrs. Tepley

1. You might hear a murmur.
2. Stress and caffeine increase the occurrence of palpitations.
3. She needs education regarding mitral valve prolapse, stress management techniques, and reduction of caffeine intake (e.g., drink decaffeinated coffee).

Mrs. Pryor

1. In aortic stenosis, the aortic valve is narrowed, making it more difficult for blood to leave the left ventricle and go into the aorta, resulting in less blood flow to the body. This is most likely why Mrs. Pryor is feeling tired. Documentation of subjective data: "What is aortic stenosis?" Documentation of objective data: Listened attentively during explanation of aortic stenosis and its effects. Expressed interest in learning more about diagnosis.
2. Angina results if the heart is not getting enough oxygen-rich blood.
3. Nursing care should include fall precautions due to syncope and fatigue. Teaching should be based on Mrs. Pryor's need for safety at home, assistance with activities of daily living (ADLs), and answering her questions and concerns.
4. Nursing diagnoses and care include *Self-Care Deficit* related to fatigue (plan for these ADL needs) and *Activity Intolerance* related to fatigue (plan rest periods between activities, include energy-conserving techniques, and monitor vital signs with activity).
5. You should give two tablets. Unit analysis method solution:

$$\frac{0.25 \text{ mg}}{} \left| \frac{1 \text{ tablet}}{0.125 \text{ mg}} \right. = 2 \text{ tablets}$$

Mrs. Jones

1. A heart murmur is heard from damaged heart valves.
2. Splinter hemorrhages appear as black or red-brown lines in the distal nailbed.
3. Petechiae indicate that tiny pieces of a lesion on the endocardium or valves have broken off and become microemboli.
4. Subjective data may include statements such as, "I have pain in my joints and am chilled" or "I am fatigued and have no appetite." Objective findings may include fever of 100°F (37°C), splinter hemorrhages in the nailbed, petechiae on chest.
5. Expected medications include intravenous antibiotics.
6. Shivering is muscular work that raises the body's temperature. Raising the body's temperature is part of the inflammatory process. It is the body's attempt at developing an unfavorable environment for the pathogen. Removing blankets to decrease fever results in chills and shivering. This further increases body temperature and adds to cardiac workload from muscular activity during shivering. Therefore, Mrs. Jones should be kept covered to prevent chills.
7. For left-sided heart failure, crackles or wheezes may be auscultated cough or dyspnea might be noted. In right-sided hear failure, peripheral edema or jugular venous distention may be present.
8. Two tablets.

$$\frac{650 \text{ mg}}{} \left| \frac{1 \text{ tablet}}{325 \text{ mg}} \right. = 2 \text{ tablets}$$

Review Questions

1. The nurse is caring for a group of patients. After completing morning rounds, which of the following patients require priority care?
   1. A patient who is 2 days postsurgery reporting severe constipation
   2. A patient with a deep vein thrombosis who has peripheral edema
   3. A patient with aortic stenosis who is reporting chest pain
   4. A patient with mitral valve prolapse who has lost 2 pounds of weight this morning

2. The nurse is evaluating patient teaching for mitral valve prolapse. The patient shows understanding of the prognosis by stating which of the following?
   1. "The prognosis is poor."
   2. "Heart failure often occurs."
   3. "There are often no symptoms."
   4. "Symptoms quickly progress."

3. The nurse is evaluating a patient's preoperative teaching for a commissurotomy. The patient shows understanding of the purpose of this procedure by stating which of the following?
   1. "Fused valve flaps are separated to enlarge the valve opening."
   2. "A mechanical valve is inserted to replace a valve."
   3. "The valve flaps are repaired or reconstructed."
   4. "A biological valve is inserted to replace a valve."

4. The nurse is evaluating understanding after a teaching session for mechanical cardiac valve replacement surgery. Which statement by the patient indicates understanding of teaching?
   1. "I will need anticoagulants for the first month after surgery."
   2. "I will need anticoagulant therapy for life."
   3. "I will need anticoagulant therapy for the first year after valve replacement."
   4. "I will not need to be on anticoagulant therapy."

5. The nurse evaluates the patient as understanding how to prevent rheumatic fever if the patient identifies that rheumatic fever can be prevented by treating streptococcal infections with which of the following?
   1. Cortisone
   2. Cyclosporine
   3. Penicillin
   4. Prednisone

6. The nurse is caring for a patient with cardiomyopathy. Which of the following symptoms, if reported by the patient, require priority action by the nurse? **Select all that apply.**
   1. Decreased appetite
   2. Dyspnea
   3. Fatigue
   4. Headache
   5. Left great toe pain

7. The nurse is collecting data on a patient who had surgery. Which of the following signs and symptoms indicate to the nurse the possible presence of a deep vein thrombosis in the patient's leg that should be reported to the health care provider? **Select all that apply.**
   1. Calf swelling
   2. Crackles
   3. Jugular venous distention
   4. Fever
   5. Warmth
   6. Redness

8. After the nurse reviews medication orders and patient allergies to give warfarin (Coumadin), which of the following actions should the nurse take first?
   1. Obtain a glass of water.
   2. Prepare the medication for administration.
   3. Review international normalized ratio result.
   4. Document the medication administration.

Answer rationales available in your online resources.

ANSWERS 1. 3; 2. 3; 3. 1; 4. 2; 5. 3; 6. 2, 3; 7. 1, 4, 5, 6; 8. 3

Key Points

Find the chapter key points in your online resources available through Davis Edge.

Additional Resources

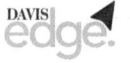 Use the scratch off code on the inside front cover of your book to access online quizzes that will help you to improve your scores on course exams and prepare for NCLEX-PN®.

 Study Guide

CHAPTER 24

Nursing Care of Patients With Occlusive Cardiovascular Disorders

Maureen McDonald

KEY TERMS

acute coronary syndrome (ah-KYOOT KOR-uh-nare-ee sin-DROHM)

anastomosed (an-AST-tah-most)

aneurysm (AN-yur-izm)

angina pectoris (an-JY-nah PEK-tuh-ris)

arteriosclerosis (ar-TEER-ee-oh-skleh-ROH-sis)

atherosclerosis (ATH-er-oh-skleh-ROH-sis)

collateral circulation (kuh-LAH-tur-al SIR-kew-LAY-shun)

coronary artery disease (KOR-uh-nar-ee AR-ter-ee dih-ZEEZ)

embolism (EM-buh-lizm)

endarterectomy (en-DAR-ter-eck-toe-mee)

high-density lipoprotein (HY DEN-sih-tee LIH-poh-PROH-teen)

hyperlipidemia (HY-per-LIH-pih-DEE-mee-ah)

intermittent claudication (IN-tur-MIT-tent KLAW-dih-KAY-shun)

ischemia (is-KEY-me-ah)

low-density lipoprotein (LOH DEN-sih-tee LIH-poh-PROH-teen)

lymphangitis (lim-FAN-jee-EYE-tis)

myocardial infarction (MY-oh-KAR-dee-yuhl in-FARK-shun)

peripheral arterial disease (puh-RIFF-uh-ruhl ar-TEER-ee-uhl dih-ZEEZ)

plaque (PLAK)

Raynaud disease (rah-NOH dih-ZEEZ)

thrombosis (throm-BOH-sis)

varicose veins (VAR-ih-kohz VAINS)

venous stasis ulcers (VEE-nus STAY-sis UL-sers)

CHAPTER CONCEPT

Perfusion

LEARNING OUTCOMES

1. Explain the etiologies, signs, symptoms, and therapeutic measures of coronary artery disease, angina pectoris, and myocardial infarction.
2. List data to collect for patients with coronary artery disease, angina pectoris, or myocardial infarction.
3. Describe therapeutic measures used to treat coronary artery disease, angina pectoris, and myocardial infarction.
4. Explain the etiologies, signs, and symptoms for each of the peripheral vascular disorders.
5. Identify therapeutic measures used to treat peripheral vascular disorders.
6. Plan nursing care for patients with a peripheral vascular disorder.

Cardiovascular disease (CVD) is the leading cause of disability and death in the United States. Diseases of the heart and peripheral vessels can affect quality of life and alter the ability of the individual to perform tasks of everyday living. Many factors leading to CVD can be controlled or modified. Education is important in preventing and treating occlusive CVD.

An estimated 92.1 million American adults have one or more types of CVD. CVD accounts for more than 800,000 deaths annually in the United States. More than 2,200 Americans die every day of CVD (Benjamin et al., 2017). As of 2015, the prevalence of CVD was 7.8% among men and 4.6% among women. CVD occurs on average about 10 years later in women than in men. However, the age gap narrows with advancing age. The average age in 2015 for a person having a first **myocardial infarction** (MI; heart attack) was 65.3 years for men and 71.8 years for women. Smoking lowers the age of having a first heart attack for both genders, but even more so for women. Women who smoke and use oral contraceptives have a higher risk of MI. Women are more likely to die of a heart attack within the first few weeks after one occurs (Benjamin et al., 2017).

ARTERIOSCLEROSIS

Arteriosclerosis is the thickening, loss of elasticity, and calcification of arterial walls. It is part of the aging process. The intimal lining of the artery wall losses elasticity and weakens due to the high pressure within the arteries.

ATHEROSCLEROSIS

Atherosclerosis is the formation of plaque in the arteries. Arteriosclerosis and atherosclerosis are both conditions that may begin in early childhood and progress without symptoms through adulthood. Atherosclerosis causes coronary heart disease (CHD), also known as **coronary artery disease** (CAD).

Pathophysiology

Atherosclerosis is a multistep process that affects the inner lining of the artery (Fig. 24.1). First, injury to the endothelial cells that line the walls of the arteries occurs, causing inflammation and immune responses. Damage to the endothelium stimulates the growth of smooth muscle cells. These cells secrete collagen and fibrous proteins. Lipids, platelets, and other clotting factors accumulate. Scar tissue replaces some of the arterial wall.

An early indication of injury is a fatty streak on the lining of the artery. This buildup of fatty deposits is known as **plaque.** It is composed of smooth muscle cells, fibrous proteins, and cholesterol-laden foam cells. Plaque has irregular,

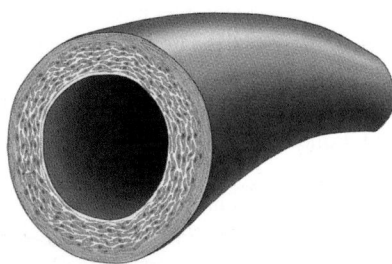

Normal artery

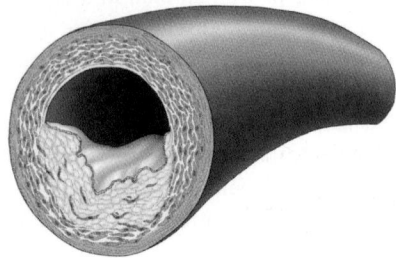

Atherosclerotic artery

FIGURE 24.1 (*Top*) Cross section of normal coronary artery. (*Bottom*) Coronary artery with atherosclerosis narrowing the lumen.

jagged edges that allow blood cells and other material to adhere to the wall of the artery. The portion of the plaque that faces the bloodstream develops a fibrous cap (a firm shell that often contains calcium). Over time, this buildup becomes calcified and hardened, causing turbulence that damages cells and increases the buildup within the vessel. Sometimes the plaque's fibrous cap tears or ruptures, and a blood clot forms. This blood clot can completely block the coronary artery, or it may break loose and lodge within a smaller artery leading to the heart. The vessel may also become stenosed (narrowed) by plaque buildup. This buildup of plaque may cause partial or total occlusion of the artery, resulting in reduced blood flow. The area distal to the occlusion may become ischemic as a result.

Etiology

Risk factors for atherosclerosis can be divided into two categories: those that can be modified and those that cannot (Table 24.1).

Diagnostic Tests

Total cholesterol levels above 200 mg/dL increase risk of CAD and MI (Table 24.2). Elevated **low-density lipoproteins** (LDLs) and low levels of **high-density lipoproteins** (HDLs) are associated with increased risk of CAD. A risk factor for premature CAD is a high level of Lp(a) cholesterol (a genetic variation of plasma LDL). An excellent predictor of MI risk is the LDL particle number. It is measured directly or indirectly as apolipoprotein B, the protein particle in each LDL. A high LDL particle number with a low LDL still creates a high risk for MI. (The amount of cholesterol contained in each LDL particle varies.) Apolipoprotein B particles in LDL-type cholesterol are able to infiltrate the arterial wall, rapidly causing damage. A new way to measure one function of HDL, cholesterol efflux capacity (CEC) and its relationship to CAD, is being researched. This HDL function promotes the efflux of cholesterol from macrophages for biliary excretion, which may be a better indicator of CAD risk than HDL level. C-reactive protein (CRP) can indicate low-grade inflammation in blood vessels and an increased CAD risk. Elevated blood glucose levels can increase the risk for atherosclerosis. Radiological studies of the arteries can be performed to show narrowed or occluded vessels (see Chapter 21).

Therapeutic Measures

A healthy lifestyle, reducing risk factors, medications, and medical examinations are helpful in controlling atherosclerosis.

Diet

Because the formation of plaque within arteries is primarily caused by fatty deposits, an adherence to a heart-healthy diet is recommended by the American Heart Association (AHA; "Nutrition Notes").

• WORD • BUILDING •

arteriosclerosis: arterio—artery + sklerosis—hardness

Nutrition Notes

Controlling Blood Cholesterol With Diet. Two-thirds of the body's cholesterol is produced by the liver and intestines. Most, but not all, people produce less cholesterol or increase its excretion in response to high levels of dietary cholesterol. To reduce cholesterol and overall cardiovascular disease risk, the American Heart Association set a 2020 Impact Goal and developed seven factors for health, Life's Simple 7, that include lifestyle and diet recommendations (visit https://playbook.heart.org/index.php/lifes-simple-7). More information for some of these factors can be found at:

- The Dietary Approaches to Stop Hypertension (DASH) eating plan (www.nhlbi.nih.gov/files/docs/public/heart/new_dash.pdf)
- U.S. Department of Agriculture Food Patterns (https://health.gov/dietaryguidelines/2015/guidelines/appendix-3)
- American Heart Association Diet (click on the Healthy Eating tab at https://healthyforgood.heart.org)

   Recommendations include the following:

- Consuming fruits, vegetables, and whole grains; low-fat dairy; poultry and fish; legumes; nontropical vegetable oils; and nuts
- Avoiding trans fats
- Reducing saturated fats (no more than 6% of calories)
- Limiting sugar (e.g., sweets, sugar-sweetened beverages)
- Reducing sodium to 2,300 mg/day (a reduction to 1,500 mg/day is even more beneficial to reduce blood pressure but difficult to attain for many individuals)

   Eating foods approved by the U.S. Food and Drug Administration (2013) to reduce cholesterol can be beneficial. These foods include the following:

- Marine omega-3 fatty acids (e.g., herring, mackerel, rainbow trout, salmon, sardines, swordfish, tuna)
- Soluble fiber (Kellogg's Bran Buds, barley, oatmeal)
- Soy
- Plant sterols (e.g., found in butter and margarine spreads, juices, salad dressings, soy milk) that interfere with intestinal absorption of cholesterol

Reference

U.S. Food and Drug Administration. (2013). Guidance for industry: Food labeling guide. Retrieved from www.fda.gov/Food/GuidanceRegulation/GuidanceDocumentsRegulatory Information/LabelingNutrition/ucm2006828.htm

Table 24.1

Risk Factors for Atherosclerosis/Coronary Artery Disease

Risk Factors That Cannot Be Changed	
Age	Men have increased incidence after age 50. Women have increased incidence after menopause.
Ethnicity	African Americans have a higher incidence of atherosclerosis.
Gender	Men have more risk factors and higher incidence of coronary artery disease (CAD).
Genetics	CAD risk factors such as hyperlipidemia can run in families.

Risk Factors That Can Be Changed or Controlled	
Diabetes mellitus	Increases the risk of hypertension, obesity, and elevated blood lipids.
Hypertension	Vasoconstriction increases myocardial oxygen demand.
Elevated serum cholesterol	Level above 200 mg/dL increases the risk of developing CAD.
Elevated low-density lipoprotein (LDL) particle number or apolipoprotein B	Infiltrates arterial wall, rapidly causing damage.
Elevated serum homocysteine	Increases CAD risk. Foods that contain folic acid (e.g., fruits, green leafy vegetables) reduce homocysteine level.

Continued

Table 24.1

Risk Factors for Atherosclerosis/Coronary Artery Disease—cont'd

Excessive alcohol use	Raises blood pressure, increases triglycerides, and causes irregular heartbeats.
Obesity	Increases heart workload and risk of hypertension, diabetes, glucose intolerance, and hyperlipidemia.
Sedentary lifestyle	Increases obesity, hypertension, and hyperlipidemia.
Emotional stress	Increases heart workload and risk for hypertension.
Tobacco use, including secondhand smoke	Causes vasoconstriction and increases myocardial oxygen demand. Decreases high-density lipoproteins (HDLs).

Table 24.2

Atherosclerosis Summary

Diagnostic Tests	Cholesterol Low-density lipoprotein (LDL) particle number Triglycerides Arteriogram
Therapeutic Measures	Low-fat, low-cholesterol diet Smoking cessation Exercise
Priority Nursing Diagnoses	*Acute Pain* *Deficient Knowledge*

Smoking

The risk of developing CAD is greater in cigarette smokers than in nonsmokers. Risk is proportionate to the number of cigarettes smoked. Smoking contributes to a loss of HDL. HDL is the best cholesterol to decrease the risk of any CVD. Smoking also causes vasoconstriction, which leads to angina pectoris and cardiac arrhythmias. The benefits of smoking cessation are dramatic and almost immediate. Education about the risks of smoking and effects of exposure to secondhand and thirdhand smoke should be presented to patients and their families. Thirdhand smoke is residual nicotine and toxic chemicals left on surfaces (e.g., skin, hair, clothing, bedding, carpets, floors, furniture, walls) by tobacco smoke. The American Cancer Society has many programs to help people quit smoking (visit www.cancer.org/healthy/stay-away-from-tobacco.html).

Exercise

Increased activity raises HDL levels. Increasing physical activity may also lower insulin resistance and facilitate weight loss. Over time, exercise also leads to the development of **collateral circulation,** which allows blood to flow around occluded sites. Before an exercise program is begun, the patient's health care provider (HCP) should be consulted.

Medications

Lowering lipid levels is the primary therapy for atherosclerosis. If dietary control is not effective, medication is also used (Table 24.3). It may take 4 to 6 weeks before lipid levels respond to drug therapy ("Evidence-Based Practice"). If one drug does not lower lipids, another drug can be added.

Evidence-Based Practice

Clinical Question

What interventions help increase compliance with lipid-lowering medications?

Evidence

Within a systematic review of 35 randomized studies of 925,171 subjects on lipid-lowering therapy, 11 studies that focused on intensive interventions to increase medication compliance were included in a meta-analysis. Subjects in the intervention group, which consisted of electronic reminders, pharmacist involvement, and education by health care team members, complied better with their medication regimen than did those who did not receive intervention. Total cholesterol and low-density lipoprotein (LDL) levels also decreased in the intervention group (van Driel et al., 2016).

Implications for Nursing Practice

Interventions provided by health care team members to help people remember to take prescribed medications result in lower cholesterol levels. Nurses should include medication education in the patient's plan of care.

References

van Driel, M. L., Morledge, M. D., Ulep, R., Shaffer, J. P., Davies, P., & Deichmann, R. (2016). Interventions to improve adherence to lipid-lowering medication. *Cochrane Database of Systematic Reviews, 2016*(12). CD004371. doi:10.1002/14651858.CD004371.pub4

Table 24.3
Medications Used to Lower Lipid Levels

Medication Class/Action

Statins

First-line drugs to reduce low-density lipoprotein (LDL) by reducing cholesterol synthesis.

Examples	**Nursing Implications**
atorvastatin (Lipitor)	Monitor liver function studies. Monitor for rhabdomyolysis (lethal breakdown of
fluvastatin (Lescol XL)	skeletal muscle).
lovastatin (Mevacor)	*Teach:*
pravastatin (Pravachol)	Take medication in evening when cholesterol synthesis is highest.
rosuvastatin (Crestor)	Report muscle pain to health care provider.
simvastatin (Zocor)	

Fibrates

Reduce triglycerides.

Examples	**Nursing Implications**
clofibrate (Atromid-S)	*Teach:*
fenofibrate (TriCor)	Take 30 minutes before morning and evening meal.
gemfibrozil (Lopid)	May increase the effects of anticoagulants and hypoglycemia.

Bile Acid Sequestrants

Lower cholesterol by binding bile acids, so stored cholesterol is used to make more bile acids.

Examples	**Nursing Implications**
cholestyramine (Questran)	*Teach:*
colesevelam hydrochloride	Add fruits and vegetables high in fiber to diet to reduce constipation and other
(Welchol, Sankyo)	gastrointestinal associated effects.
colestipol (Colestid)	Can interfere with absorption of digoxin, thiazides, and beta blockers.

Niacin

Prevents conversion of fats into very low LDLs. Rarely used because of flushing.

Examples	**Nursing Implications**
niacin (Nicotinic acid)	*Teach:*
extended-release niacin	Take aspirin 30 minutes before taking medication to reduce flushing.
(Niaspan)	

Cholesterol Absorption Inhibitor

Inhibits the absorption of cholesterol. Decreases LDLs and increases high-density lipoproteins (HDLs).

Examples	**Nursing Implications**
ezetimibe (Zetia)	*Teach:*
	Take with liquids and meals.
	Take other medications 1 hour before or 4 hours after.

Combination Agent

See each agent.

Examples	**Nursing Implications**
Vytorin = ezetimibe (Zetia) +	See each agent.
simvastatin (Zocor)	

CORONARY ARTERY DISEASE

CAD is the obstruction of blood flow through the coronary arteries to the heart muscle cells, typically from atherosclerosis. Blood flow reduction resulting from CAD can cause angina, MI, or sudden death if blood flow is not restored.

Prevention

Risk factors for CAD are listed in Table 24.1. The risk factors that can be changed should be modified following the AHA's guidelines (see the therapeutic measures discussion for atherosclerosis). Low-dose aspirin may be recommended for certain patients by their HCP to prevent the formation of a thrombus.

Angina Pectoris

Angina pectoris is chest pain due to **ischemia** resulting from a reduction in coronary artery blood flow and oxygen delivery to the heart muscle. Angina is a symptom, not a disease. It usually occurs as a result of narrowed arteries caused by CAD.

Types of Angina

STABLE ANGINA. Stable angina occurs with moderate exertion in a pattern that is familiar to the patient. The pain is predictable and lasts only a few minutes. It can usually be relieved by resting and using nitroglycerin (NTG).

UNSTABLE ANGINA. Unstable angina is angina that increases unpredictably in frequency or that occurs with less exertion, at rest, or during sleep. It is not relieved by rest or medication as stable angina may be. Blood clots that form in response to injury to the artery from atherosclerosis cause a reduction in blood flow leading to unstable angina. This is a serious condition that can lead to an MI. See the discussion on acute coronary syndrome.

VARIANT OR VASOSPASTIC ANGINA (PRINZMETAL ANGINA). This type of angina is caused by coronary artery spasms and is serious. The pattern of occurrence is often cyclical, with the pain happening about the same time each day. The pain lasts longer than stable angina, can occur with exercise or at rest, and often occurs at night.

MICROVASCULAR ANGINA. Spasms in the walls of the tiniest arteries of the heart reduce coronary blood flow and result in microvascular angina. Compared with other types of anginal pain, this pain might be more severe and last longer.

Signs and Symptoms

Patients (especially men) often describe anginal chest pain as discomfort, burning, fullness, heaviness, pressure, or squeezing (Fig. 24.2). The pain can radiate down one or both arms (left arm is common) or into the shoulder, neck, jaw, or back. Patients may also describe heaviness in their arms or a feeling of impending doom. During the episode of pain, the patient may be pale, diaphoretic, or dyspneic.

Women might experience chest pain, jaw pain, or heartburn with angina but often have atypical symptoms. These include shortness of breath, fatigue, nausea, or pain that is less severe. Atypical symptoms should not be ignored and treatment sought. (See the "Women and Heart Health" section.)

Diagnostic Tests

Common tests used to diagnose CAD or the causes of angina include electrocardiogram (ECG), exercise stress test, echocardiography, chemical stress testing, cardiac computed tomography (CT) scan, cardiac magnetic resonance imaging (MRI)/magnetic resonance angiogram (MRA), radioisotope imaging, and coronary angiography.

Therapeutic Measures

Risk factors identified for the patient determine treatment to prevent anginal attacks and MI. Weight reduction, a heart-healthy diet, and emotional stress reduction may help slow disease progression. The three major groups of medication used for relieving angina are vasodilators (nitrates), calcium channel blockers, and beta blockers (Table 24.4).

VASODILATORS. NTG, a nitrate, is the drug of choice for acute anginal attacks. Nitrates dilate coronary arteries to increase oxygen to the myocardium and dilate peripheral vessels so the heart does not have to work so hard to pump blood into them. NTG can be administered sublingually, orally, transdermally, intravenously (IV), or as a lingual spray. When administered sublingually, NTG may relieve chest pain within 1 to 2 minutes (Box 24.1).

> **BE SAFE!**
> **Sublingual nitroglycerin (NTG):** After one tablet, call 911 after 5 minutes have elapsed if pain is unrelieved or worsens, especially with symptoms of a myocardial infarction. Take two more doses, 5 minutes apart, as needed while waiting.
> **Transdermal NTG:** Wear gloves to protect yourself from hypotension from touching the ointment or patch medication. Always remove the previous ointment or patch before applying a new one to prevent overdose.

Long-acting nitrates are used to prevent chest pain rather than to treat acute pain. They can be given orally, in ointment, or by transdermal patches. To prevent development of tolerance, the patch or ointment is usually removed at bedtime and reapplied in the morning. This gives the patient an 8- to 12-hour nitrate-free period. Headaches may be experienced when nitrates are first begun and can be relieved with aspirin. This side effect usually subsides after a week or two.

• WORD • BUILDING •
angina pectoris: angina—to choke + pectora—chest

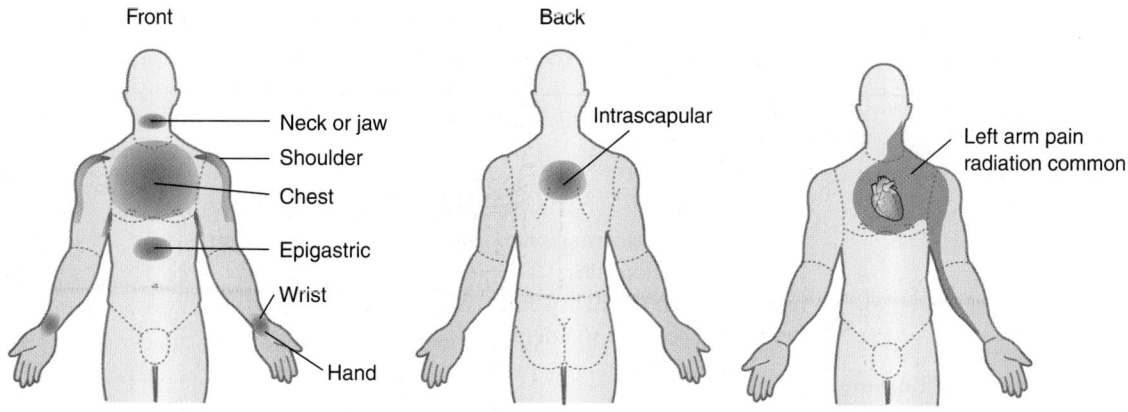

FIGURE 24.2 Common locations of anginal pain, which may vary in combination and intensity.

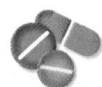

Table 24.4

Medications Used to Treat Angina Pectoris

Medication Class/Action

Antiplatelets

Inhibit platelet activation, adhesion, or procoagulant activity.

Examples	**Nursing Implications**
aspirin	Enteric-coated aspirin beneficial for daily use.
clopidogrel (Plavix)	Monitor for bleeding.
ticagrelor (Brilinta)	

Statins

See Table 24.3.

Nitrates

Vasodilate to reduce preload and afterload. Reduce oxygen consumption of myocardium.

Examples	**Nursing Implications**
nitroglycerin (Nitrostat, NitroQuick)	Document onset, type, radiation, location, and duration of chest pain.
nitroglycerin sublingual spray (Nitrolingual Pumpspray)	Take apical pulse and blood pressure (BP) pre- and postadministration.
isosorbide dinitrate (Isordil)	Place sublingual (SL) tablet in buccal pouch to lessen burning sensation under tongue.
isosorbide mononitrate (Imdur, ISMO)	Do not shake aerosol canister before administration of lingual spray.
	Remove patch before magnetic resonance imaging or defibrillation.
	Teach:
	Explain need to rise slowly, especially with SL spray.
	If chest pain is not relieved, call 911.
	Tablets should be replaced every 3 to 6 months.
	Keep tablets in original bottle as they become inactive when exposed to light, air, heat, and moisture.
	Burning or tingling sensation may be felt under the tongue with SL nitroglycerin.
	Use of erectile dysfunction medications is contraindicated because they can cause a drop in blood pressure.
	Avoid alcohol.

Continued

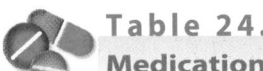

Table 24.4

Medications Used to Treat Angina Pectoris—cont'd

Medication Class/Action

nitroglycerin (Transderm Nitro, Nitro-Bid) nitroglycerin patch (Nitro-Dur, Nitrek)	*Teach:* (Transdermal) Remove old transdermal patch before applying new patch. Rotate application sites. Apply patch to clean, dry, hairless area. Remove at bedtime so tolerance does not develop.

Angiotensin-Converting Enzyme (ACE) Inhibitors

Block production of angiotensin II, a potent vasoconstrictor. Vasodilate and improve cardiac output and exercise tolerance.

Examples	**Nursing Implications**
captopril (Capoten) enalapril (Vasotec) lisinopril (Prinivil, Zestril) ramipril (Altace)	If pulse is less than 60 beats per minute (bpm) or systolic BP less than 90 mm Hg, notify health care provider (HCP) before administering medication. Give 1 hour before meals. Give captopril on empty stomach. *Teach:* Take first dose at night to adjust to lower BP. Rise slowly. Check BP weekly. Report development of dry cough or other side effects.

Calcium Channel Blockers

Dilate peripheral arteries, decrease myocardial contractility, depress conduction system, and decrease workload of the heart. In variant angina, reduce coronary artery spasm.

Examples	**Nursing Implications**
amlodipine (Norvasc) diltiazem (Cardizem, Dilacor XR) felodipine (Plendil) nicardipine (Cardene)	If pulse is less than 60 bpm or systolic BP less than 90 mm Hg, notify HCP before administering medication.

Beta Blockers

Decrease pulse, BP, and cardiac output, and suppress renin activity. Decrease the risk of sudden death.

Examples	**Nursing Implications**
atenolol (Tenormin) metoprolol (Lopressor, Toprol XL)	Beta blockers contraindicated in asthma, heart block, and bronchoconstriction. If pulse is less than 60 bpm or systolic BP less than 90 mm Hg, notify HCP before administering medication. *Teach:* Explain need to rise slowly. Abrupt withdrawal may result in diaphoresis, palpitations, headache, and tremors.

Anti-Ischemic Agent

Antianginal agent used as combination therapy for those not responding to other antianginal medication.

Examples	**Nursing Implications**
ranolazine (Ranexa)	May not be as effective in women. Prolongs QT interval on electrocardiogram.

CALCIUM CHANNEL BLOCKERS. Calcium is required for electrical excitability of cardiac cells and contraction of the myocardium and vascular smooth muscle. Calcium channel blockers relax vascular smooth muscle. This leads to decreased peripheral vascular resistance (afterload) and decreased myocardial oxygen demand. These drugs dilate main coronary arteries, increasing the myocardial oxygen supply. Calcium channel blockers are also used to decrease systolic and diastolic blood pressures and to slow the heart rate. Because these drugs are slow acting, they are ineffective in relieving acute anginal attacks.

Box 24.1

Key Points for Using Sublingual Nitroglycerin

- Carry nitroglycerin (NTG) tablets at all times.
- Keep NTG tablets tightly sealed in the original container and protected from heat, light, and moisture.
- Replace NTG prescription at least every 6 months for maximum effect or every 3 to 4 months if carried in a pocket next to body heat.
- Take NTG tablet before an activity known to cause chest pain.
- Sit or lie down when taking NTG tablets, if possible.
- Take one NTG tablet. If the symptoms are not worsening but not completely relieved, your health care provider may tell you to repeat a tablet every 5 minutes up to a total of three tablets. If pain is not relieved after three tablets, call 911.
- If pain is unrelieved after one NTG tablet and other symptoms of myocardial infarction are present, call 911 for emergency medical care.
- Tingling should be felt under the tongue when NTG tablets are used.
- NTG may cause a headache initially. Aspirin may relieve it.
- NTG may cause light-headedness. Rise slowly to prevent falls.

BE SAFE!

Patients who take nitrates should not use drugs for erectile dysfunction, such as sildenafil (Viagra), tadalafil (Cialis), or vardenafil (Levitra). These types of drugs dilate blood vessels and may cause a significant drop in blood pressure if used with nitrates.

BETA BLOCKERS. Beta blockers decrease heart rate, lower blood pressure, and prevent release of renin. This reduces the workload of the heart to help prevent anginal attacks. Because of these decreased effects, beta blockers should be used with caution in patients with any degree of heart failure because it may make heart failure worse. There are nonselective and selective types of beta-adrenergic blockers. People with asthma or chronic obstructive pulmonary disease (COPD; including emphysema, bronchitis, and bronchiectasis) should avoid nonselective beta-adrenergic blockers because they cause bronchoconstriction. Metoprolol (Lopressor) and atenolol (Tenormin) are cardioselective. They can be used in patients with asthma and COPD. Beta blockers are not effective for coronary artery spasms. They should not be used for variant (Prinzmetal) angina.

LEARNING TIP

To help you identify beta blockers, remember that their generic names end with -olol.

ANGIOTENSIN-CONVERTING ENZYME INHIBITORS. Angiotensin-converting enzyme (ACE) inhibitors block production of angiotensin II, which is a potent vasoconstrictor. This action reduces peripheral arterial resistance (vasodilation), which lowers blood pressure. ACE inhibitors may cause retention of potassium in some patients. If a patient taking an ACE inhibitor develops a dry cough, inform the HCP so the medication can be changed.

STATINS. Cholesterol and inflammation in artery walls are involved in atherosclerosis development. Statins lower cholesterol levels by reducing cholesterol production in the liver (see Table 24.3). They also reduce inflammation and CRP levels, which improves patient outcomes in CAD. Statins are used to prevent and treat atherosclerosis.

ANTIPLATELETS. Aspirin and clopidogrel (Plavix) are commonly used antiplatelets that help prevent cardiovascular events.

Nursing Process for the Patient With Coronary Artery Disease and Angina
Data Collection
Record height, weight, allergies, over-the-counter and prescription medications, use of herbs, and typical diet. Identify the patient's nonmodifiable and modifiable risks for atherosclerosis and CAD. Obtain vital signs and oxygen saturation. Note dyspnea, labored respirations, diaphoresis, nausea, skin color, and temperature.

A history of chest pain, fatigue, or activity intolerance is noted. Document patient's description of anginal pain (e.g., type, location, pain radiation to other areas of the body). Note any factors that may make the pain worse or better. This will provide information to determine improvement or lack of improvement in pain. Ask how long the patient has had angina, what are triggering activities, and how the pain has been relieved in the past.

Nursing Diagnoses, Planning, and Implementation

Acute Pain related to reduced coronary artery blood flow

EXPECTED OUTCOME: The patient will report an absence or acceptable level of pain within 30 minutes of reporting pain.

- Ask patient to use a rating scale (such as 0 to 10) to identify pain level *to provide consistency in pain reporting.*
- Administer oxygen as ordered via nasal cannula *to increase oxygen availability to myocardium.*
- Administer NTG (sublingual, spray) as prescribed *to provide pain relief.*
- Notify HCP if pain is unrelieved after three doses of NTG or as prescribed, or if vital signs change. *Chest pain unrelieved by nitrates (sublingual, spray) may represent unstable angina or MI and need for IV nitrates.*
- Administer aspirin as prescribed *to decrease platelet aggregation.*

- Administer analgesic (such as morphine) as prescribed and recheck pain level frequently *to provide pain relief.*
- Remain with patient and provide emotional support. *A patient who has chest pain should never be left alone.*

Deficient Knowledge related to ineffective management of regimen for coronary artery disease

EXPECTED OUTCOME: The patient will report understanding and management of atherosclerosis and CAD.

- Collect data on patient's readiness to learn, desired learning needs, and feelings about incorporating lifestyle changes into daily routine *to prioritize teaching topics.*
- Include significant other as appropriate *to support patient during learning.*
- Use appropriate teaching tools written in patient's native language and an interpreter as needed *to meet individual learning needs.*
- Collect data on patient's present understanding of atherosclerosis and CAD *to determine baseline knowledge.*
- Explain pathophysiology of atherosclerosis and CAD, control of risk factors, and management of CAD symptoms *to promote understanding.*
- Explain action, side effects, and importance of taking medications as prescribed *to relieve pain and prevent complications.*
- Provide information about community resources *that can assist in making lifestyle changes, such as weight loss, smoking cessation, emotional stress management, and exercise.*
- Teach patient to monitor blood pressure and heart rate as appropriate and to report chest pain or dyspnea, *which may point to the presence of complications from CAD.*
- Encourage questions and allow patient the opportunity to verbalize new information and skills *to enhance learning.*
- Document teaching and evaluation of patient knowledge *to validate understanding.*

Evaluation

Interventions are successful if the patient is pain-free, demonstrates an increased understanding of atherosclerosis and CAD and their management, and states that risk factors of CAD will be modified.

 ACUTE CORONARY SYNDROME

The term **acute coronary syndrome** (ACS) includes the conditions of unstable angina pectoris and MI. ACS is caused by a sequence of inflammatory processes. This can lead to thrombus formation and reduced blood flow (unstable angina) or to partial or complete coronary artery occlusion (MI).

Silent Ischemia

Silent ischemia occurs without pain. It can carry great risk since the ischemia goes undetected. Older adults and those with hypertension or diabetes most often have silent ischemia.

Sudden Cardiac Death

Sudden cardiac death is cardiac arrest triggered by lethal ventricular arrhythmias or asystole from an abrupt occlusion of a coronary artery (see Chapter 25). Prompt treatment is required to attempt to prevent death.

Myocardial Infarction

An MI results in the death of heart muscle. It occurs from a sudden partial or complete blockage of a coronary artery. The cells of the heart in the area that is supplied by the blocked coronary artery do not receive blood and die. The extent of the cardiac damage varies depending on the location and amount of blockage in the coronary artery. The ability of the heart to contract, relax, and propel blood throughout the body requires healthy cardiac muscle. Cellular death may not occur with timely and effective reperfusion.

MI is identified by the type of changes seen on the ECG. Non–ST-segment elevation MI (NSTEMI) is caused by a partial artery blockage. ST-segment elevation MI (STEMI) is the deadliest type because it is caused by a complete blockage of the artery. (See Chapter 25 for ST-segment definition.)

Pathophysiology

MI does not happen immediately. Ischemic injury evolves over several hours before complete necrosis and infarction take place. The ischemic process affects the subendocardial layer, which is most sensitive to hypoxia. This process leads to depressed myocardial contractility. The body's attempt to compensate for decreased cardiac function triggers the sympathetic nervous system to increase the heart rate. The change in heart rate increases myocardial oxygen demand, further depressing the myocardium.

Prolonged ischemia can produce severe cellular damage and necrosis of cardiac muscle. Once necrosis takes place, the contractile function of the muscle is permanently lost. The heart has a zone of ischemia and injury around the necrotic area (Fig. 24.3). The zone of injury is next to the necrotic area. It is susceptible to becoming necrosed. If treatment is initiated within the first hour of symptoms of the MI and restores the blood supply from the blocked artery, the area of damage can be minimized. Around the injury zone is an area of ischemia and viable tissue. If the heart responds to treatment, this area can rebuild and develop collateral circulation. If prolonged ischemia takes place, the size of the infarction can be quite large.

The area affected by an MI depends on the coronary artery (Fig. 24.4). Being familiar with the anatomy of the heart and the area of the MI helps the nurse anticipate arrhythmias, conduction disturbances, and heart failure. All of these are the major complications of MIs (Table 24.5).

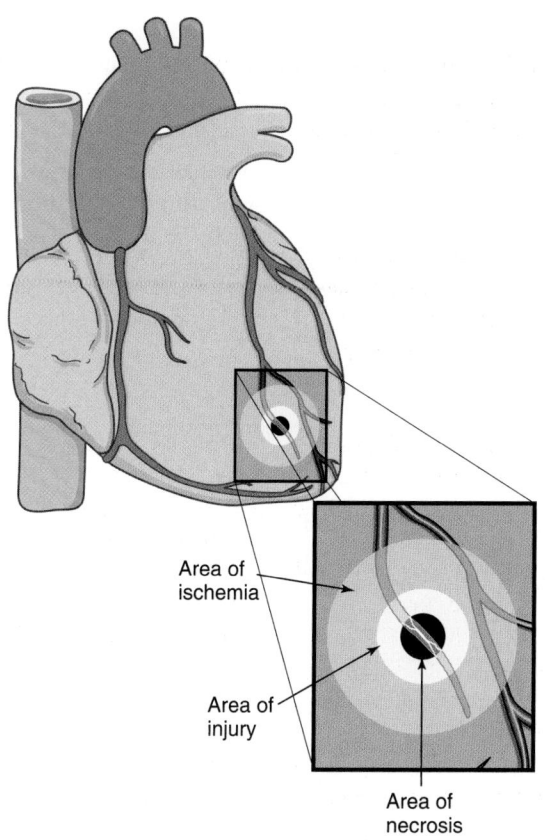

Area of ischemia

Area of injury

Area of necrosis

FIGURE 24.3 Myocardial infarction. Areas of ischemia, injury, and necrosis caused by a blockage in the left anterior coronary artery.

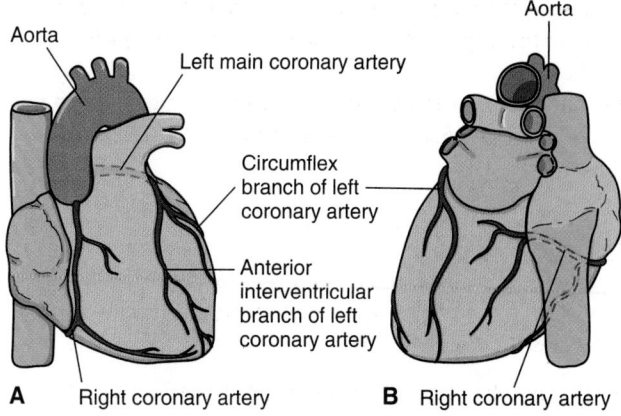

FIGURE 24.4 Coronary arteries. (A) Anterior view. (B) Posterior view.

The left coronary artery supplies the anterior wall of the heart, which also includes most of the left ventricle. An occlusion in this area causes an anterior wall MI. When the left ventricle is affected, there can be severe loss of left ventricular function. This leads to severe changes in the hemodynamic status of the patient.

The right coronary artery supplies the heart's inferior wall and parts of the atrioventricular node and the sino-atrial node. An occlusion of the right coronary artery leads to an inferior MI and abnormalities in cardiac conduction.

Table 24.5

Complications of Myocardial Infarction

Complication	Types or Symptoms	Interventions
Arrhythmias	Premature ventricular contractions, ventricular tachycardia, ventricular fibrillation, heart block	Continuous cardiac monitoring Protocol treatment of arrhythmias (see Chapter 25)
Cardiogenic shock	Decreased blood pressure; increased heart rate; diaphoresis; cold, clammy, gray skin	Immediate initiation of treatment to decrease infarct size, control pain and arrhythmias Intra-aortic balloon pump Thrombolytic therapy Dopamine, dobutamine
Heart failure/ pulmonary edema	Dizziness, orthopnea, weight gain, edema, enlarged liver, jugular venous distention, crackles	Correct underlying cause Relieve symptoms Increase cardiac contractility Administer diuretics as ordered
Emboli	Dependent on location of emboli	Anticoagulants to prevent clots Supportive symptom treatment
Rupture of muscles or valves of the heart, septal rupture	Signs of cardiogenic shock, death	Immediate treatment of myocardial infarction to limit extent of damage
Pericarditis (inflammation of the pericardium)	Chest pain, increased with movement, deep inspiration, or cough; pericardial friction rub (fine grating sound)	Position upright, leaning forward Anti-inflammatory medications

Serious arrhythmias can occur early in an inferior MI that may be life threatening.

The left circumflex coronary artery supplies the heart's lateral wall and part of the posterior wall. A blockage in this artery causes a lateral wall infarction of the left ventricle.

LEARNING TIP

To remember which coronary artery occlusion results in a specific myocardial infarction (MI) location, use U.S. location initials that match the first initials of coronary artery and MI location, such as those given below. You can personalize the locations with initials of places familiar to you.

Location	Coronary Artery	Resulting MI Location
Los Angeles	Left anterior descending	Anterior
Cedar Point	Circumflex	Posterior
Rhode Island	Right	Inferior

Signs and Symptoms

Chest pain is a classic symptom of an MI. The pain begins suddenly and is not relieved by rest or administration of NTG. Pain occurring in the center of the chest is usually described as crushing or viselike or as if an elephant is standing on the chest. Pain can radiate to the back, one or both arms and shoulders, neck, or jaw. The pain can imitate indigestion or a gallbladder attack with abdominal pain and vomiting. Other classic MI symptoms include shortness of breath, dizziness, nausea, and sweating (Table 24.6). The heart rate may be rapid and the heart's rhythm irregular. An extra heart sound (S_3 or S_4) may be present, which is a sign the myocardium is failing. When listening to lung sounds, crackles or wheezing may be heard with heart failure.

TIMELY SYMPTOM TREATMENT. Individuals, especially women, often deny or fail to recognize that an MI is occurring because they experience atypical MI symptoms or their symptoms are similar to other mild conditions such as indigestion ("Gerontological Issues"). Patients have reported that the symptoms of an MI they experienced were not what they expected. If people expect to have the dramatic heart attack symptoms as seen on television shows (which are usually not the same as those in real life) and they do not, they are likely to wait to seek treatment. Waiting 2 to 24 hours before seeking medical care is common, yet the first hour after symptom onset is crucial for administering reperfusion treatments that restore blood flow, minimize tissue damage, and save lives. Individuals should not drive themselves or let someone else drive them to the hospital when having chest pain. Calling for emergency medical care (911 or local emergency services) allows timely lifesaving treatment

---

Table 24.6

Myocardial Infarction Summary

Signs and Symptoms	**Classic**
	Crushing, viselike chest pain with radiation to arm, shoulder, neck, jaw, or back
	Shortness of breath
	Dizziness
	Nausea
	Sweating
	Atypical
	Absence of chest pain
	Fatigue
	Cramping in chest
	Anxiety
	Feeling of impending doom
	Falling
	More Common in Women
	Epigastric or abdominal pain
	Chest discomfort, pressure, or burning
	Arm, shoulder, neck, jaw, or back pain
	Discomfort/pain between shoulder blades
	Shortness of breath
	Fatigue
	Indigestion or gas pain
	Nausea or vomiting
Diagnostic Tests	Electrocardiogram (ECG)
	Serum cardiac troponin I or T
	Serum myoglobin
	Serum creatine kinase-MB (CK-MB)
	Complete blood count (CBC)
	Serum magnesium and potassium
	Vital signs, oxygen saturation
	Intake and output
Therapeutic Measures	Oxygen
	Angiotensin-converting enzyme (ACE) inhibitors
	Anticoagulants
	Antiarrhythmics
	Antiplatelets (e.g., aspirin)
	Beta blockers
	Morphine sulfate
	Nitrates
	Statins
	Thrombolytics
	Vasodilators
	Percutaneous coronary interventions and stents
	Myocardial revascularization (coronary artery bypass grafting)

Table 24.6
Myocardial Infarction Summary—cont'd

	Daily weight
	Bedrest with use of bedside commode/bathroom
	Low-sodium diet advanced to diet as tolerated; no caffeine
	Cardiac rehabilitation
Complications	Arrhythmias
	Heart failure
	Cardiogenic shock
	Valvular insufficiency
Priority Nursing Diagnoses	*Acute Pain*
	Decreased Cardiac Output
	Fear

to begin. Individuals, especially women, need to be educated that "time is muscle." As time passes during an MI, more muscle is lost.

For more information and an animation, visit:

- www.nhlbi.nih.gov/health/health-topics/topics/heartattack/names
- www.womenshealth.gov/heart-health-stroke/heart-disease-stroke-prevention/index.html
- www.heart.org

Gerontological Issues

Myocardial Infarction. With age, the heart has decreased elasticity and decreased ability to respond to changes in pressure. This increases resistance to its pumping action and increases the workload of the myocardium. Older patients should be taught never to neglect symptoms of shortness of breath, fatigue, fast or slow heartbeats, or chest discomfort. For older patients, the following is common with myocardial infarction (MI):

- When pain is not present, the only symptom may be a sudden onset of shortness of breath or fainting, restlessness, or a fall.
- Atypical presentation of MI symptoms is normal in older people, especially those older than age 85. Because the older adult has had more time to develop collateral circulation than younger people, they often do not have as many complications with an MI.
- In the older adult, reperfusion therapies such as angioplasty and bypass surgery seem to be superior in improving quality of life without increasing mortality risk.

Women and Heart Health

Heart disease remains the leading cause of death in women in the United States. Heart disease kills more women over the age of 65 than all cancers combined. African American women are more likely than Caucasian women to develop heart disease. Compared with men, women tend to have acute MIs at an older age, with a higher mortality rate and more complications, such as ventricular fibrillation and heart failure.

Women may have classic chest pain, but they are also likely to have other symptoms as well that men do not typically have. Research is ongoing to understand women and cardiac disease. Atypical symptoms reported by women may include extreme fatigue, epigastric pain, jaw pain, indigestion, nausea and vomiting, dyspnea, shortness of breath, or cramping in the chest. Many women noted prodromal symptoms a month before an acute MI. These symptoms include unusual fatigue, sleep disturbances, and shortness of breath.

Diagnostic Tests

Patients with a strong familial history of MI should be considered at risk until an MI is ruled out. Indicators of an MI are patient history, ECG, and levels of serum cardiac troponin I or T, myoglobin, and creatine kinase (CK)-MB (see Chapter 21). The ECG usually shows the area that has infarcted as well as the ischemic areas of the heart. Myocardial damage can be seen as ST-segment elevation, the presence of a Q-wave, or T-wave abnormalities (Fig. 24.5). Serial ECGs monitor changes indicating damage or ischemia. Magnesium and potassium levels are checked. Both are essential for normal cardiac function, especially for those on diuretic therapy.

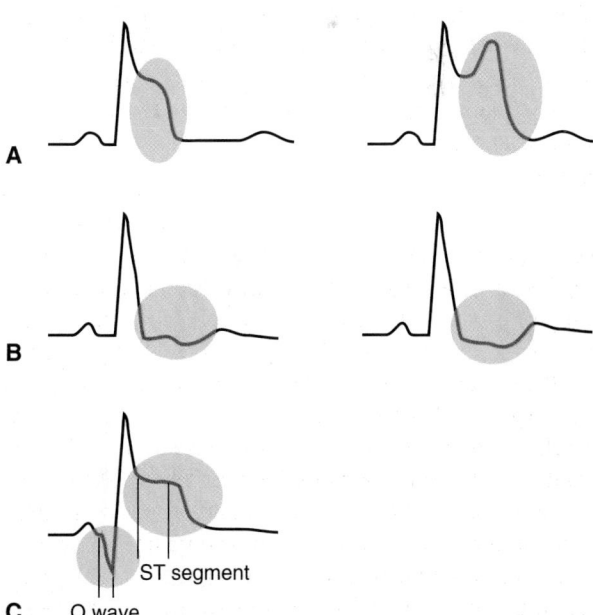

FIGURE 24.5 Electrocardiogram changes during STEMI myocardial infarction. (A) Injury: ST-segment elevation. (B) Ischemia: ST-segment inversion. (C) Necrosis: large Q-wave and ST-segment elevation.

Therapeutic Measures

Medical treatment should be sought within 5 minutes for unrelieved chest pain. The AHA recommends chewing one uncoated adult aspirin at the onset of chest pain as directed by an HCP. Time until intervention is directly related to mortality (Box 24.2). The goal is to restore blood flow to the heart muscle within 90 minutes or less of the patient's arrival at the emergency department door.

PERCUTANEOUS CORONARY INTERVENTION. Percutaneous coronary intervention (PCI), also called coronary angioplasty, uses a small balloon to increase blood flow and oxygen to the myocardium. Emergency PCI is used frequently in the management of acute MI. PCI should be initiated within 90 minutes of arrival in the emergency department.

In a cardiac catheterization laboratory, a catheter with a balloon tip is inserted, usually via the femoral or radial artery. It is advanced into the heart to open the blocked coronary artery (Fig. 24.6). Once the blocked artery is entered, the balloon on the catheter is inflated and the atherosclerotic plaque is compressed. The dilated vessel is able to deliver more oxygen-rich blood to the myocardium. Angioplasty can be done with or without the placement of stents.

Coronary Artery Stent. A coronary artery stent, placed during angioplasty, is used to prevent closure of a coronary artery from an atherosclerotic lesion. A stent is an expandable metal mesh tube that is implanted at the site of blockage in the coronary artery (Fig. 24.7). A stent provides support to a coronary artery wall at the area of stenosis to keep blood flowing through the artery. Complications associated with stent placement include **thrombosis** (formation of a blood clot inside a blood vessel), bleeding from anticoagulation, stent occlusion, or coronary artery dissection. Drug-eluting stents are coated with immunosuppressant medication that can be released at the implantation site to reduce the risk of restenosis. The medication is released over months to inhibit smooth muscle cell proliferation to reduce risk of restenosis. Antiplatelet medications are recommended after stent placement to help prevent clot formation.

THROMBOLYTIC THERAPY. Thrombolytic medications may be used to dissolve a blood clot that is occluding a coronary artery. (PCI has greatly reduced the use of thrombolytics.) Thrombolytic therapy must be started within a specified time range from the onset of symptoms, usually within 1 to 6 hours, before necrosis results. The goal is to

---

Box 24.2

Preventing Delays in Myocardial Infarction Treatment

- Understand symptoms, the "time is muscle" principle, and that a delay in calling for help results in untoward effects.
- Develop an action plan and rehearse it.
- Understand normal emotional responses of anxiety, denial, or embarrassment.
- Educate family to follow action plan.
- Establish protocols in workplaces for employees experiencing myocardial infarction.
- Establish emergency room policies that reduce delays, such as having equipment and medication readily available.

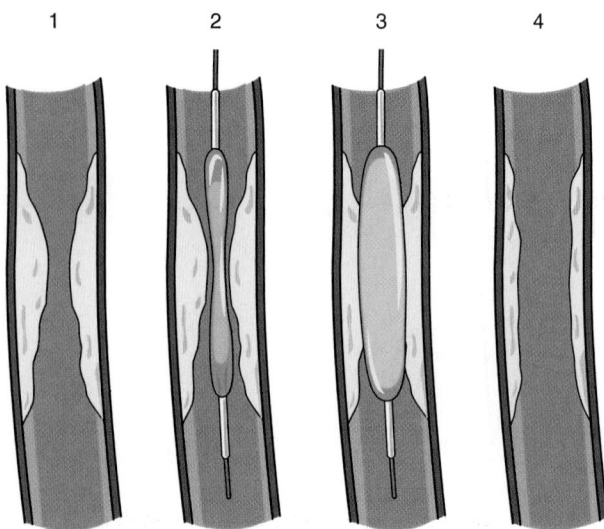

FIGURE 24.6 Percutaneous coronary intervention: Balloon angioplasty opens narrowed coronary arteries.

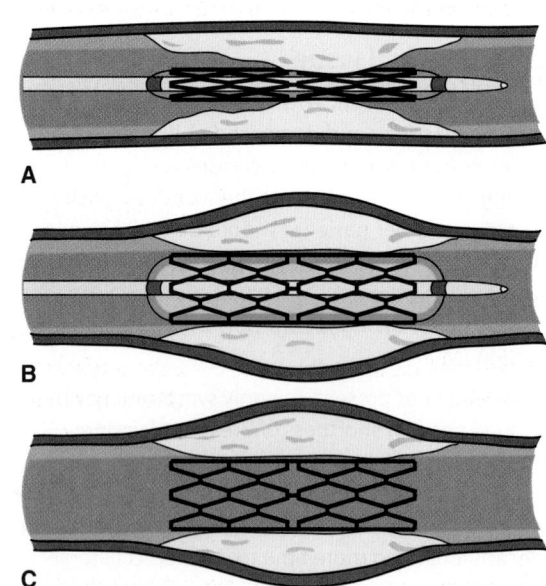

FIGURE 24.7 Insertion of a coronary artery stent: (A) A balloon catheter with a collapsed stent is advanced to the location of a coronary artery lesion. (B) The balloon is inflated, which expands the stent and compresses the lesion to increase the artery opening. (C) The balloon is then deflated and removed, leaving the expanded stent in place to prevent the artery from closing.

give thrombolytics within 30 minutes of arrival in the emergency department.

MEDICATIONS. For those with unstable angina, taking antiplatelets, statins, ACE inhibitors, and beta blockers can be beneficial. A drug from each of these drug classes should be considered. When taken together, these drugs have a synergistic effect in fighting plaque. This means they have a greater positive result for the patient.

Table 24.7 summarizes pharmacological treatment of MI. **MONA** is a mnemonic to remember medications for treating MI patients: morphine, oxygen, nitroglycerin, and aspirin.

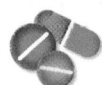

Table 24.7
Medications Used to Treat Myocardial Infarction

Medication Class/Action

Analgesics

Opioid relieves pain, reduces preload and afterload, decreases anxiety. Reduce preload and afterload. Decrease anxiety.

Examples	Nursing Implications
morphine sulfate	Monitor vital signs and sedation level before and after administration.

Angiotensin-Converting Enzyme (ACE) Inhibitors

See Table 24.4.

Anticoagulants

Heparin: *Inhibits conversion of prothrombin to thrombin to prevent thrombus formation.*

Examples	Nursing Implications
heparin sodium	Do not give if bleeding risk.
	Dose regulated by heparin antifactor Xa or activated partial thromboplastin time (aPTT).
	aPTT Goal: 1.5 to 2.5 times control.
	Monitor for bleeding.

Low Molecular Weight Heparin (LMWH): *Antithrombotic. Prophylaxis of ischemic complications in unstable angina or non-ST-elevation myocardial infarction with aspirin therapy.*

Examples	Nursing Implications
dalteparin (Fragmin)	Do not remove prefilled syringe air bubble.
enoxaparin (Lovenox)	Give deep subcutaneously: Hold fold of skin while giving injection.
fondaparinux (Arixtra)	Rotate sites.
	Teach:
	Monitor for bleeding.

Antiarrhythmics

Inhibit ventricular arrhythmias.

Examples	Nursing Implications
amiodarone (Cordarone, Pacerone)	Contraindicated in atrioventricular block or pregnancy.
	Obtain baseline vital signs and electrocardiogram (ECG).
	Monitor for lung toxicity.
	Teach:
	Avoid grapefruit juice with oral form.

Antiplatelets

Inhibit platelet activation, adhesion, or procoagulant activity.

Examples	Nursing Implications
aspirin	*Teach:*
clopidogrel (Plavix)	Chew aspirin when acute coronary syndrome (ACS) or myocardial infarction (MI) suspected.
prasugrel (Effient)	Report bleeding or bruising.
ticagrelor (Brilinta)	
vorapaxar (Zontivity)	

Continued

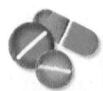

Table 24.7
Medications Used to Treat Myocardial Infarction—cont'd

Medication Class/Action

Glycoprotein IIb/IIIa Inhibitors

Inhibit platelet aggregation.

Examples	Nursing Implications
abciximab (ReoPro) bivalirudin (Angiomax) eptifibatide (Integrilin) tirofiban (Aggrastat)	Given via intravenous route only during percutaneous coronary intervention. Prevent injury for bleeding risk. Monitor vital signs and ECG. *Teach:* Report bleeding or bruising.

Beta Blockers

See Table 24.4.

Nitrates

Vasodilate to reduce preload and afterload. Reduce myocardial oxygen consumption. See Table 24.4 for other forms.

Examples	Nursing Implications
nitroglycerin	Document onset, type, radiation, location, and duration of chest pain. Monitor apical pulse and blood pressure. *Teach:* Headache may occur but will resolve over time. Change position slowly to avoid orthostatic hypotension and fall risk.

Statins

See Table 24.3.

Thrombolytics

Dissolve blood clots in blood vessels or catheters, such as dialysis catheters.

Examples	Nursing Implications

alteplase; tissue plasminogen
  activator [t-PA] (Activase)
reteplase; rPA (Retavase)
tenecteplase; TNK (TNKase)
	Most effective when given within 6 hours of coronary event. Goal is 90 minutes
	  from arrival in emergency department.
	Baseline international normalized ratio (INR), activated partial thromboplastin time
	  (aPTT), platelet count, and fibrinogen levels checked.
	Avoid venipunctures for 24 hours after administration.

Additional Medications as Needed

Specific for drugs given.

Examples	Nursing Implications
antiemetics anxiolytics antacids stool softeners	Control nausea, vomiting, anxiety, gastric upset, and straining/constipation.

ANALGESICS. Analgesics are given for relief of chest pain. Morphine sulfate is the most commonly used narcotic. It is usually given in increments of 2 to 8 mg IV every 5 to 15 minutes until pain is relieved. The patient should be monitored for hypotension, respiratory depression, oversedation, and morphine sensitivity. In addition to pain relief, morphine helps decrease anxiety, opens bronchioles, and increases peripheral blood pooling to decrease preload (blood returning to heart) and afterload (pressure within the aorta). This can help increase blood supply and oxygen to the myocardium.

OXYGEN. Oxygen is administered, usually at 2 L/min via nasal cannula. Oxygen therapy may be limited to the first 6 hours in stable patients. Too much oxygen can lead to systemic vasoconstriction. This may increase myocardial workload. Arterial blood gases (ABGs) guide the patient's oxygen needs. Oxygen saturation should be monitored and stay above 94%. Oxygen can be administered via mask if higher concentrations are needed. Mechanical ventilation can be provided when indicated by ABGs.

VASODILATORS. NTG sublingually, topically, or by IV drip can be administered for vasodilation to supply more blood to the myocardium to reduce pain and the workload of the heart. In the acute phase, the IV route is usually used. Nitrates should not be given if the patient has a systolic blood pressure of less than 90 millimeters of mercury (mm Hg) or of 30 mm Hg or more below baseline, has severe bradycardia less than 50 beats per minute, or has taken a phosphodiesterase inhibitor for erectile dysfunction. Catastrophic hypotension may result.

ANTIPLATELETS. Antiplatelet medication is given to reduce platelets from forming clots. Antiplatelet examples include aspirin, clopidogrel (Plavix), ticagrelor (Brilinta), and prasugrel (Effient). Antiplatelet therapy may be given long term after an MI.

ACTIVITY. Initially, patients are kept on bedrest to decrease myocardial oxygen demand. A bedside commode for bowel movements is usually ordered to reduce straining on a bedpan. Activity is advanced gradually as tolerated.

INTRA-AORTIC BALLOON PUMP. To support an ischemic heart, an intra-aortic balloon pump (IABP) may be used to increase circulation to the coronary arteries and reduce the work of the heart (see Chapter 26). While the heart is relaxed (diastole), the balloon is inflated, sending more blood into the coronary arteries. Just before the heart contracts (systole), the balloon deflates, creating a suction effect that allows blood to flow past it with less resistance (decreased afterload) into the aorta.

DIET AND WEIGHT LOSS. Initially, a low-sodium, clear liquid diet is ordered as tolerated, which helps reduce the risk of vomiting. Then, small, easily digested, heart-healthy meals are served. Caffeine is restricted because it increases heart rate and causes vasoconstriction. Fluids may be restricted if the patient is in heart failure as well. If the patient is obese, weight loss can reduce cardiac workload. A dietitian can help the patient and family to devise a weight-loss diet for the patient.

TOBACCO USE. Patients are instructed on the hazards of smoking and/or exposure to secondhand and thirdhand smoke. Referral to a tobacco cessation program can be made. The nurse can help patients work toward making lifestyle changes.

Coronary Artery Bypass Graft

AHA guidelines help determine which type of procedure would benefit the patient: PCI or coronary artery bypass graft (CABG). During bypass surgery, the saphenous vein from the leg or an internal mammary artery from the chest wall is used to reroute blood around a segment of a coronary artery that is narrowed by atherosclerosis (Fig. 24.8). One or more vessels can be bypassed ("Patient Perspective"). There are two types of bypass procedures: arrested heart surgery and beating heart surgery.

Patient Perspective

Keith. When I was 72, a heart catheterization showed significant coronary artery blockage, so I had five coronary artery bypass grafts performed. It was a long surgery. I felt disoriented for several days afterward, mostly while I was in the intensive care unit.

I was provided excellent care at home after discharge from the hospital. I had a capable visiting nurse, physical therapist, or occupational therapist almost every day. Physical therapy was difficult at first but shortly became routine and easy. I have had a strange sensation in my legs at the incision sites ever since surgery but no pain. I have not experienced depression, although I hear post-op depression is common.

My experience during cardiac rehab of three sessions per week for 12 weeks was outstanding. I enjoyed the association with others in the same situation. We even staged a graduation when we finished. I wore a tuxedo jacket with my gym shorts!

Since completing my rehab, I have maintained a minimum 40-minute exercise schedule three times per week. I am trying to be more conscious of my diet. I do this because I want to stay healthy for a long time.

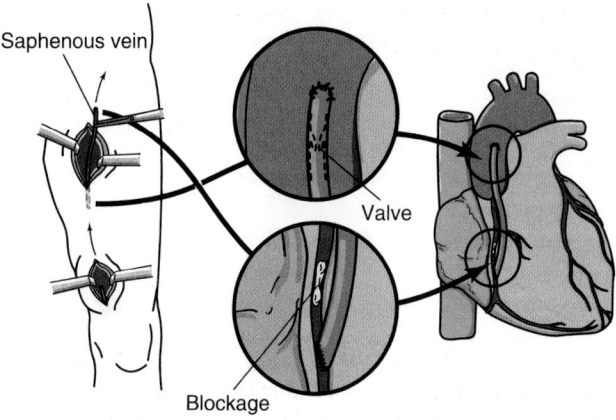

FIGURE 24.8 Myocardial reperfusion by coronary artery bypass graft surgery.

ARRESTED HEART SURGERY. Most bypasses are done while the heart is stopped with a cardiopulmonary bypass machine (on pump) in use (see Chapter 21). While the median sternotomy is made, the vein graft is being removed from the body. The graft is flushed with a heparinized solution to check for leaks and then set aside for use during the surgery. After the patient is placed on cardiopulmonary bypass and the heart is stopped, one end of the graft is **anastomosed** (joined) to the coronary artery distal to the occlusion while the proximal end of the graft is anastomosed, often to the ascending aorta.

BEATING HEART SURGERY. This surgery is done with the heart beating and does not use the heart-lung machine (off pump). A device is used to stabilize a vessel while the surgeon works on it. Either traditional median sternotomy or minimally invasive surgery can be used.

MINIMALLY INVASIVE SURGERY. Less invasive approaches include the minimally invasive coronary artery bypass grafting (MICS CABG), which is done off pump, and totally endoscopic coronary artery bypass surgery (TECAB), which can be done on or off pump. MICS CABG is done through a small fifth intercostal incision. TECAB uses three or four chest holes for insertion of robotic arms and a camera that a surgeon then views to control the robotic arms.

CRITICAL THINKING

Mr. Jones is transferred to the critical care unit after a quadruple coronary artery bypass grafting. Preoperative vital signs were blood pressure 144/84 mm Hg, apical pulse 62 beats per minute (regular), respiratory rate 18 breaths per minute, and temperature 98.4°F (36.9°C). Data collection findings are blood pressure 100/56 mm Hg, apical pulse 105 beats per minute, respiratory rate 28 breaths per minute (irregular and shallow), temperature 99.8°F (37.7°C), lung sounds diminished with crackles in bilateral bases, pedal pulses weak bilaterally, and chest and leg dressings dry and intact.

1. Which findings may indicate pulmonary problems?
2. List four nursing interventions for the altered pulmonary status.
3. List three reasons why the apical pulse could be elevated.
4. Name two reasons why the blood pressure could be low.
5. With which health care team members will the nurse collaborate?

Suggested answers are at the end of the chapter.

Nursing Process for the Patient Experiencing Myocardial Infarction

DATA COLLECTION. A thorough history is obtained to identify risk factors that may contribute to an MI. All patients admitted with chest pain are treated as having a possible MI until it has been ruled out. Continuous cardiac monitoring, serial ECGs, and laboratory values help identify life-threatening arrhythmias and determine the degree of cardiac damage. Controlling chest pain immediately helps diminish anxiety and the negative physiological effects pain has on the body. Screening for depression after an MI is important to make appropriate treatment referrals.

NURSING CARE TIP

When caring for a patient after a coronary artery bypass grafting (CABG), be sure to use infection-control procedures at all times to prevent surgical site infection. Surgical site infection following CABG (mediastinitis) is a "Never Event." This means that Medicare will not pay the hospital for care required for this condition.

NURSING DIAGNOSES, PLANNING, IMPLEMENTATION, AND EVALUATION. See "Nursing Care Plan for the Patient With Myocardial Infarction." Also see "Nursing Care Plan for the Patient Undergoing Cardiac Surgery" for additional nursing care.

Patient Education

Teaching about the therapeutic regimen includes information about the disease, medications, diet, activity, and rehabilitation needs that may require lifestyle changes. Diet, emotional stress reduction, a regular exercise program, smoking cessation (if necessary), and following a medication schedule require extensive patient and family teaching. This disease can affect all aspects of a patient's lifestyle including family and job roles.

Patients recovering from cardiac disorders are often anxious about resuming sexual activity but are embarrassed to discuss it. This is an area that is often overlooked when caring for patients. Sexual counseling should be offered to patients and their partners. Patients often have misconceptions that are unfounded but interfere with resuming sexual activity. If patients have angina, NTG can be taken prophylactically before sexual activity. After an MI, sexual activity can be resumed in 1 to 2 months or when the patient can climb two flights of stairs without symptoms, as approved by the HCP. Patients are given information to make an informed decision on when they are ready to resume this physical activity. Referral to a sexuality counselor for information on ways to cope with sexual issues in relation to the illness can be helpful to the patient.

Cardiac Rehabilitation and Exercise

Cardiac rehabilitation begins when the patient's acute symptoms are relieved to improve cardiac function and quality of life. Phase 1 of rehabilitation occurs in the hospital. Activities

Nursing Care Plan for the Patient With Myocardial Infarction

Nursing Diagnosis: *Acute Pain* related to decreased coronary blood flow causing myocardial ischemia
Expected Outcomes: The patient will report an absence or acceptable level of pain within 30 minutes of reporting pain.
Evaluation of Outcomes: Does the patient state that pain is reduced?

Intervention	Rationale	Evaluation
Monitor location, duration, intensity, and radiation of pain; use a pain rating scale.	*Identifies type and severity of pain.*	What is pain level, location, duration, intensity, and radiation?
Monitor blood pressure, pulse, and respiration.	*Vital signs may change with episodes of pain.*	Are vital signs within normal limits (WNL)?
Administer oxygen as ordered.	*Oxygen administration helps decrease hypoxia and pain.*	Is oxygen saturation greater than 94%? Are arterial blood gases WNL?
Administer analgesics as prescribed, and recheck pain level frequently to provide pain relief.	*Relieves pain.*	Is pain relieved?
Assist with alternative pain relief measures (e.g., positioning, encouraging rest, relaxation techniques, diversional activities).	*These measures help decrease oxygen demand because patient is restful and relaxed.*	Does patient express pain relief and decreased emotional stress?

Geriatric

Monitor and ensure that older patient's pain is relieved.	*Pain is not an expected part of the aging process as may be believed.*	Does patient report pain is relieved?

Nursing Diagnosis: *Decreased Cardiac Output* related to ischemia or infarction, changes in heart rate and rhythm, and decreased contractility
Expected Outcomes: The patient will maintain adequate cardiac output and tissue perfusion.
Evaluation of Outcomes: Does the patient have vital signs and urine output within normal limits?

Intervention	Rationale	Evaluation
Monitor blood pressure, heart rate, and urine output, and report abnormalities.	*These are indirect indicators of cardiac output.*	Are indicators WNL?
Monitor electrocardiogram (ECG), and report abnormalities.	*Identifies arrhythmias that reduce cardiac output.*	Is patient's ECG WNL?
Monitor peripheral circulation, pulses, capillary refill, edema, color, and temperature.	*These are indicators of adequate tissue perfusion.*	Does patient have strong peripheral pulses, capillary refill less than 3 seconds, no edema, warm skin, and pink nailbeds?
Administer cardiac medications as ordered by health care provider.	*Helps improve cardiac output and tissue perfusion.*	Does patient show signs of improved contractility, increased cardiac output, and tissue perfusion?
Promote quiet environment and rest in semi-Fowler position.	*Decreases cardiac workload.*	Is patient relaxed?

(nursing care plan continues on page 420)

Nursing Care Plan for the Patient With Myocardial Infarction—cont'd

Intervention	Rationale	Evaluation
Geriatric		
Observe for atypical pain, such as jaw pain, or no pain with dyspnea or fatigue.	*In acute myocardial infarction (MI), older adults may not have typical chest pain or may have a silent MI.*	Does patient have atypical symptoms of MI?
Monitor for medication side effects.	*Older patients may have more medication toxicity due to reduced renal and hepatic function.*	Does patient exhibit side effects of medications?

Nursing Diagnosis: *Fear* related to threat of death, changes in lifestyle, chest pain, and procedures
Expected Outcomes: The patient will verbalize reduced fear and demonstrate effective coping mechanisms.
Evaluation of Outcomes: Does the patient verbalize reduced fear?

Intervention	Rationale	Evaluation
Identify level of fear and allow patient to verbalize fear of dying.	*Verbalization helps identify and reduce fear.*	Is patient able to verbalize fears?
Ask about patient's usual coping pattern.	*This allows building on patient's coping strengths.*	What are patient's coping techniques?
Assure patient heart's function is being closely monitored and explain equipment in use.	*Assurance of detection for prompt treatment of any complications will reduce fear.*	Does patient state less fear due to continuous monitoring?
Offer family support and allow them to be with the patient and involved in the care.	*Significant others often ignore their own needs and experience anxiety so supporting them allows them to support the patient.*	Does family verbalize ability to support patient without anxiety?
Geriatric		
Provide protective, safe environment with consistent caregivers.	*Older adults adapt to change with more difficulty during illness than younger adults.*	Is continuity of care provided? Does patient report less fear?

Nursing Diagnosis: *Activity Intolerance* related to imbalance between oxygen supply and demand, weakness, and fatigue
Expected Outcome: The patient will tolerate progressive activity as evidenced by heart rate, blood pressure, pulse oximetry, and respiratory rate WNL.
Evaluation of Outcome: Is the patient's heart rate, blood pressure, pulse oximetry, and respiratory rate WNL with progressive activity?

Intervention	Rationale	Evaluation
Obtain patient's vital signs before activity.	*Identifies baseline data comparison with activity.*	Are vital signs WNL?
Observe and document patient response during and after activity. Stop activity and report abnormal responses, including heart rate over 120 beats per minute or 20 beats over resting rate, systolic blood pressure increased	*Observation allows detection of abnormal responses to stop activity.*	Are vital signs WNL and activity tolerated without symptoms?

Nursing Care Plan for the Patient With Myocardial Infarction—cont'd

Intervention	Rationale	Evaluation
over 20 mm Hg, chest pain, dizziness, skin color changes, diaphoresis, dyspnea, arrhythmias, excessive fatigue, and ST-segment changes on ECG.		
Maintain progression of ordered activities as tolerated. *Initial activities:* activities of daily living, dangling feet at bedside for 15 minutes, using commode with assistance. *Progressive activities:* Out of bed to chair for 30 to 60 minutes, partial bath, range-of-motion exercises.	*Patient should have increasing activity to condition the myocardium.*	Is patient able to progress activity?
Geriatric		
Refer patient to cardiac rehabilitation as able.	*Older adults benefit comparably to younger persons from exercise programs.*	Does patient participate in cardiac rehab?
Slow the pace of care but allow independence as able.	*Allow patient extra time to complete activity to reduce cardiac demand and fatigue.*	Is patient able to complete care without symptoms or fatigue?

Nursing Care Plan for the Patient Undergoing Cardiac Surgery

Nursing Diagnosis: *Acute Pain* related to sternotomy, leg incisions, internal mammary artery resection, or pericarditis
Expected Outcomes: The patient will state pain is relieved or tolerable within 30 minutes of report of pain, be able to rest, and perform respiratory treatments.
Evaluation of Outcomes: Does the patient state pain is within acceptable levels? Is the patient able to rest and perform respiratory therapies?

Intervention	Rationale	Evaluation
Have patient use a pain rating scale and describe characteristics of pain.	*A thorough description is needed to determine cause and plan actions.*	Does patient rate pain using a rating scale and describe the pain's characteristics?
Administer analgesics as prescribed, and recheck pain level in 30 minutes to provide pain relief.	*Relieves pain.*	Is pain relieved?
Turn and reposition every 2 hours.	*Turning changes muscle position, relieving stiffness.*	Is patient comfortable without stiffness?
Offer back rubs frequently.	*Relaxes tense muscles retracted during operation.*	Is patient able to rest comfortably?

(nursing care plan continues on page 422)

Nursing Care Plan for the Patient Undergoing Cardiac Surgery—cont'd

Intervention	Rationale	Evaluation
Teach patient "sternal precautions": no pushing or pulling with arms; hug pillow for all movement, coughing, and deep breathing; do not use arms to rise out of a chair; no lifting more than 5 to 10 lb; do not raise elbows higher than shoulders; and bend elbows and lower head for grooming.	*Stabilizes sternum and incision to increase comfort.*	Does patient understand sternal precautions and use them?
Instruct patient to take a deep breath before movement and exhale slowly during movement.	*Keeps muscles relaxed, minimizing tension with guarding and pain.*	Can patient perform deep-breathing techniques as instructed?

Nursing Diagnosis: *Decreased Cardiac Output* related to myocardial depression, hypothermia, bleeding, unstable arrhythmias, or hypoxemia
Expected Outcomes: The patient will maintain vital signs within normal limits (WNL), palpable peripheral pulses, urine output greater than 30 mL/hr, and normal sinus rhythm.
Evaluation of Outcomes: Is the patient free of major side effects? Are vital signs WNL?

Intervention	Rationale	Evaluation
Monitor vital signs and electrocardiogram (ECG) and report abnormalities.	*Abnormal trends reflect problems.*	Are vital signs and ECG WNL (see Chapter 25)?
Monitor peripheral circulation and report abnormalities.	*Mottling or weak pulses may indicate poor cardiac output (CO).*	Do peripheral pulses remain strong with normal skin color, temperature, and capillary refill?
Listen to lung sounds and report crackles or wheezes.	*Crackles and wheezes may indicate heart failure or pulmonary edema.*	Are lungs clear?
Report intake and output imbalances.	*Fluid deficit or excess can alter CO.*	Does intake equal output?
Report chest tube drainage excessive increases.	*Drainage more than 200 mL/hr may lead to hypovolemia and a decrease in CO.*	Is patient free from hypovolemia?
Report electrolyte and arterial blood gas abnormalities.	*Low calcium and magnesium and abnormal potassium levels decrease contractility and CO. Acidosis decreases heart function.*	Are electrolytes and arterial blood gases WNL?

Nursing Diagnosis: *Risk for Infection* related to inadequate primary defenses from surgical wound
Expected Outcome: The patient will remain free from infection.
Evaluation of Outcome: Does the patient remain free from infection?

Intervention	Rationale	Evaluation
Monitor incision, temperature, drains, and drainage for signs and symptoms of infection to report.	*Redness, warmth, fever, and swelling of incision and foul drainage odor indicate infection.*	Are signs and symptoms of infection present and reported?
Maintain sterile technique for dressing changes.	*Sterile technique reduces infection development.*	Does incision remain free of signs and symptoms of infection?

for each hospital day, such as types and amounts of self-care and activity, are specified in protocols. Phase 2 occurs 4 to 6 weeks after discharge in an outpatient program. It focuses on returning the patient to previous levels of activity and function. Phase 3 follows, during which patients are encouraged to maintain optimal physical fitness and continue healthy lifestyles that include exercising and losing weight to maintain an ideal body weight.

CRITICAL THINKING

Mrs. Sims, age 43, is admitted to the intensive care unit with a diagnosis of atypical chest pain that radiates to her left shoulder and down her left arm. She has a history of midsternal chest cramping. Her pain increases with activity and decreases with rest. She smokes one and a half packs of cigarettes per day and is 50 pounds overweight. The cardiac monitor shows normal sinus rhythm without arrhythmias. She has nitroglycerin sublingual ordered as needed for chest pain.

One hour after admission, Mrs. Sims reports acute midsternal chest pain radiating to her left neck and jaw. The cardiac monitor shows sinus tachycardia with occasional premature ventricular contractions. Her blood pressure is 100/70 mm Hg, respirations are 20 breaths per minute and unlabored, and skin is warm and dry.

1. What actions should you take?
2. What is happening to Mrs. Sims?
3. How is angina differentiated from a myocardial infarction (MI)?
4. What are four indicators of an MI?
5. What medical interventions can be used for an MI?
6. What patient-centered education is indicated for Mrs. Sims?

Suggested answers are at the end of the chapter.

 PERIPHERAL VASCULAR SYSTEM

Peripheral vascular disease (PVD) may be either arterial or venous in origin. PVD is common in older people and people with diabetes. It is important to understand whether the origin of the problem is arterial or venous to prevent serious complications from occurring.

Arterial Thrombosis and Embolism
Pathophysiology

Acute arterial occlusions are often sudden and dramatic. Occlusions are most common in the lower extremity but may occur in the upper extremity. A thrombus (blood clot) adheres to the vessel wall. Acute arterial thrombi occur where there is injury to an arterial wall, sluggish flow, or plaque formation secondary to atherosclerotic changes. Other causes of arterial thrombosis are polycythemia, dehydration, and repeated arterial needlesticks. If a thrombus breaks off and travels, it

becomes an **embolism** that occludes an arterial vessel that is too small to allow it to pass. Some of the causes of an arterial embolism are arrhythmias, prosthetic heart valves, MI, and rheumatic heart disease.

Signs and Symptoms

Usually there is an abrupt onset of symptoms with acute arterial occlusion, unless collateral circulation has developed that is able to supply some blood to the occluded area. Symptoms depend on the artery occluded, the tissue supplied by that artery, and whether collateral circulation is present.

The clinical signs of acute arterial occlusion are known as the "six Ps": **p**ain, **p**allor, **p**ulselessness, **p**aresthesia (numbness), **p**aralysis, and **p**oikilothermia (assumes environmental temperature). There is decreased movement in the affected extremity. The extremity is pale, mottled, and without pulses distal to the occlusion. The extremity will feel cold because blood provides warmth.

Therapeutic Measures

Immediate treatment is necessary to save the affected limb. Anticoagulant therapy, usually with IV unfractionated heparin (UFH), is started immediately to prevent further clotting. UFH has no effect on existing clots. The patient remains on UFH therapy for several days. UFH levels are monitored with activated partial thromboplastin time (aPTT) or anti-factor Xa. After 3 to 7 days, an oral anticoagulant such as warfarin (Coumadin) or a low molecular weight heparin (LMWH) is started. Warfarin takes 3 to 5 days to reach therapeutic levels. UFH is continued until a therapeutic warfarin level is reached, unless LMWH injections are used for bridging therapy. Warfarin levels are monitored by international normalized ratios (INRs). Daily adjustments in warfarin doses are made to reach therapeutic levels. Examples of LMWHs include enoxaparin (Lovenox), dalteparin (Fragmin), and tinzaparin (Innohep). These often require no laboratory monitoring. Other types of anticoagulants may also be used.

For patients with severe occlusions, especially if the risk of limb loss is imminent, surgery or thrombolytic agents are used to save the extremity. During an emergency embolectomy or thrombectomy, the artery is cut open, the emboli or thrombus is removed, and the vessel is sutured closed. Thrombolytic agents dissolve a thrombus or embolus.

Peripheral Arterial Disease

Peripheral arterial disease (PAD) is a disorder of the arterial circulation usually caused by chronic, progressive narrowing of arterial vessels that leads to obstruction or occlusion. PAD usually affects the lower extremities. PAD is sometimes referred to as lower extremity arterial disease (LEAD). Atherosclerosis is the leading cause of occlusive disease. PAD can be described as organic or functional. Organic disease is caused by structural changes from plaque or inflammation in the blood vessels. Functional disease is a short-term localized spasm in the blood vessel as occurs in Raynaud disease.

Pathophysiology

The purpose of the arterial system is to deliver oxygen-rich blood to the vascular beds. Anything that impedes this flow causes an imbalance in supply and demand for oxygen. Decreased nutrition, cellular waste accumulation, and the development of ischemia occur at the area distal to the obstruction. With the increased debris and sluggish flow, thrombosis and embolism can become major problems.

The body has several mechanisms that attempt to compensate for reduced blood flow. These include peripheral vasodilation, anaerobic metabolism, and development of collateral circulation. However, these mechanisms are not intended to meet the ongoing blood supply needs of the body. It takes time for collateral circulation to develop. Blood vessels eventually reach their limit of dilation, and anaerobic metabolism is only a very short-term compensatory mechanism. Eventually, a lack of blood supply produces signs of ischemia. If not corrected, this results in ulceration, gangrene, and necrosis of the extremity; amputation of the limb may then become necessary.

CRITICAL THINKING

Mrs. May is admitted with severe rheumatoid arthritis. It has left her relatively immobile for 7 months. She is returning to her room following physical therapy when she suddenly reports severe pain in her left groin.

1. What is your first action?
2. After data collection for Mrs. May, what action should you take next?
3. What are the possible causes of this sudden symptom?
4. How would you document Mrs. May's signs and symptom?
5. What immediate interventions are necessary?
6. What medical interventions do you anticipate?
7. What surgical procedure may need to be done if the risk of losing the limb is imminent?

Suggested answers are at the end of the chapter.

Signs and Symptoms

Many people with PAD, especially women, have no symptoms. Symptoms often occur late in the course of PAD when diminished blood flow begins to produce changes in the extremities. Pain in the calves associated with activity or exercise is called **intermittent claudication.** This is a common symptom of arterial occlusive disease. When blood supply to the muscles is decreased, the muscles are unable to receive adequate oxygen. Ischemia develops. As ischemia increases, the muscle develops a cramping-type pain that usually subsides when the activity is stopped. As PAD progresses, the pain is present even at rest, thus indicating severe arterial occlusion.

Skin color changes are associated with decreased blood supply. The extremity is pale when the leg is elevated. If the leg is in a dependent position, it becomes reddish-purple or cyanotic. The extremity is cool to touch even in warm environments. There may be hair loss on the lower calf, ankle, and foot. Other findings include dry, flaky, scaly, pale, or mottled skin. The toenails may be thickened. As occlusion of the arteries progresses, arterial pulses become diminished or absent.

Diagnostic Tests

The ankle-brachial index (ABI) is used to compare blood pressures in the upper and lower extremities. Normally, blood pressure readings in the thigh and calf are higher than those in the upper extremities. With the presence of arterial disease, thigh and calf blood pressures are lower than the brachial blood pressure. Normally, the ankle blood pressure is equal to or greater than the brachial blood pressure. When an occlusion occurs in the lower extremities, the blood pressures between the upper and lower extremities become unequal. After treadmill exercise, the ABI decreases in arterial insufficiency. A duplex ultrasound measures the velocity of the blood flow. MRI and CT scan can give definitive images of blood vessels and degrees of arterial closure. Plethysmography and angiography can also be used to evaluate arterial flow in lower extremities (see Chapter 21).

Therapeutic Measures

Conservative treatment is initiated with mild to moderate occlusive disease. This includes patients who experience pain on activity that ceases with rest. This type of patient usually receives medication for vasodilation and diet management if necessary. Surgical intervention is used for the patient who experiences pain at rest or who has leg ulcers that do not heal. Surgical treatment includes endarterectomy to remove atherosclerotic lesions, balloon angioplasty with stents, or grafting to bypass the occluded area. (See the discussion of vascular surgery later in this chapter.)

DIET. Teaching the patient to eat a healthy diet to control atherosclerosis development is important.

MEDICATIONS. Statins used to decrease cholesterol and lipid levels in atherosclerosis are also used for occlusive disease. Antiplatelet agents such as aspirin and clopidogrel (Plavix) prevent blood clots. Cilostazol (Pletal), an antiplatelet drug, treats claudication to improve walking ability.

INVASIVE THERAPIES. Percutaneous transluminal angioplasty can be used to dilate a narrowed peripheral vessel. However, it does not provide long-term results. It is similar to PCI, which was discussed earlier. Peripheral atherectomy is another invasive procedure used to remove plaque from atherosclerotic arteries. Intravascular stents can also be used to maintain patency of the artery. After stent placement, patients are given platelet aggregation inhibitors to prevent blood clots.

Raynaud Disease

Raynaud disease (also called syndrome or phenomenon) is a local overreaction by the blood vessels that results in vasospasm, primarily in the digits, when exposed to cold or emotional stress. The abnormal vasoconstriction in the small arteries in the digits reduces arterial blood flow. It also can affect the ears, lips, or the nose. Primary Raynaud disease does not occur due to another disorder. Secondary Raynaud disease may be seen with collagen diseases such as rheumatoid arthritis, scleroderma, systemic lupus erythematosus, and endocrine disorders.

Women who live in cold climates are more often affected. With exposure to cold (e.g., opening the refrigerator/freezer, touching cold water) or emotional stress, the affected skin area exhibits obvious skin color changes that can vary. The affected area of skin may turn white and then blue, with reports of coldness and numbness. With warming, pain, tingling, and redness (hyperemia) occurs. Normal blood flow returns in about 15 minutes.

Initial therapy goals are to improve the quality of life and prevent injury to the tissue from ischemia. Education on cold avoidance, keeping warm, and emotional stress management is essential for patients with Raynaud disease. To protect the hands from cold, gloves should be worn when going outside, cleaning a refrigerator, or preparing cold foods. Patients are instructed in the importance of protecting the hands from injury. They must also avoid vasoconstrictors such as smoking, alcohol, caffeine, and emotional stress. Immersing the hands in warm water may decrease vasospasm. Calcium channel blockers may be prescribed if preventive measures do not effectively prevent vasoconstriction. Other therapies may be used if initial therapy is not effective.

Thromboangiitis Obliterans (Buerger Disease)

Thromboangiitis obliterans, or Buerger disease, is a rare recurring inflammation and thrombosis of small and medium arteries and veins in the limbs. The cause is unknown but may be autoimmune. It is associated with all types of tobacco use. To stop its progression, all use of tobacco must be avoided. Periodontal disease may be a factor in the development of the disease. Symptoms include intermittent pain with activity, vein inflammation, numbness, and pale digits with cold exposure. Distal extremity ischemia can lead to ulceration, gangrene, and even amputation. There is no cure so there is urgency in helping the patient to cease smoking. Treatments such as platelet inhibitors and vasodilators may be tried with less effect. The goal of nursing care for Buerger disease is to reduce complications of ulceration, gangrene, and amputation.

Nursing Process for the Patient With a Peripheral Arterial Disorder

DATA COLLECTION. Careful assessment of extremity pulses, capillary refill, temperature, color, and presence of edema helps identify patients at risk for complications. Absent pulses are reported immediately to prevent limb loss. Skin that is shiny and hairless points to chronic diminished blood flow to the extremity. A serum glucose and lipid panel identifies diabetes and **hyperlipidemia,** which are significant risk factors for PAD. Skin lesions and ulcerations are photographed.

NURSING DIAGNOSES, PLANNING, IMPLEMENTATION, AND EVALUATION. See "Nursing Care Plan for the Patient With a Peripheral Arterial Occlusive Disorder."

Aneurysms

An **aneurysm** is a bulging, ballooning, or dilation at a weakened point of an arterial wall. The artery diameter is often increased by 50%. Atherosclerosis, hypertension, smoking, trauma, and congenital abnormalities are risk factors for an aneurysm. Heredity may also play a role. Aneurysms can occur in any artery in the body but are common in the abdominal aorta, which is the focus of the rest of this discussion.

An abdominal aortic aneurysm (AAA) is often silent if it is less than 4 cm. The incidence of AAA increases with age. Medicare covers a one-time screening ultrasound for those with a family history of AAA or men aged 65 to 75 with a smoking history of 100 or more cigarettes. Men older than age 50 are at the highest risk of death from rupture and bleeding of an AAA. The mortality rate is high with a ruptured aneurysm. Survival improves with elective repair.

Types of Aneurysms

The various types of aneurysms are shown in Figure 24.9. A fusiform aneurysm is the dilation of the entire circumference of the artery. A saccular aneurysm is one that bulges on only one side of the artery wall. A dissecting aneurysm occurs when a cavity is formed from a tear in the artery wall, usually the intimal (inner) layer. The layers of the artery wall separate as blood is pumped into the tear with each heartbeat, expanding the cavity, which then becomes prone to rupturing.

Signs and Symptoms

An AAA usually exhibits few if any symptoms until it grows (Table 24.8). Back or flank pain is the classic symptom; the pain is caused by the aneurysm pressing against nerves of the vertebrae. Depending on the location and size of the aneurysm, there may be reports of abdominal pain, a feeling of fullness, or nausea caused by pressure on the intestines. Changing positions may temporarily relieve the symptoms. Because the symptoms are vague, they are often not associated with an AAA. There may be a pulsating mass in the abdomen caused by an AAA that is discovered during routine physical or x-ray examination.

Severe, sudden back, flank, or abdominal pain and a pulsating abdominal mass can indicate that the aneurysm may be about to rupture. With rupture and bleeding, signs of shock may develop. Immediate surgery is needed for a ruptured AAA.

• WORD • BUILDING •

hyperlipidemia: hyper—above + lipos—fat + emia—blood

Nursing Care Plan for the Patient With a Peripheral Arterial Occlusive Disorder

Nursing Diagnosis: *Acute Pain* related to impaired circulation to extremities, causing intermittent or continuous pain
Expected Outcome: The patient will report an absence or acceptable level of pain within 30 minutes of reporting pain.
Evaluation of Outcome: Does the patient report relief from pain by nonpharmacological or pharmacological methods?

Intervention	Rationale	Evaluation
Monitor for intermittent claudication or pain at rest.	*Helps determine degree of occlusive disease. Pain at rest is an indicator that the arterial occlusion is becoming worse.*	Does patient have pain during activity or at rest?
Administer medication as ordered (e.g., analgesics, vasodilators, calcium channel blockers).	*Relieves chronic or acute pain. Increases blood flow to extremities. Decreases vasospastic episodes.*	Does patient show signs of increased circulation and relief of pain following administration of medications?
Encourage rest if pain is present.	*Rest decreases muscle contraction and helps prevent further ischemia in extremities.*	Is patient able to rest?

Nursing Diagnosis: *Ineffective Peripheral Tissue Perfusion* related to interruption of arterial flow in arms and legs
Expected Outcome: The patient will show signs of increased arterial blood flow and tissue perfusion.
Evaluation of Outcome: Does the patient have strong peripheral pulses, capillary refill less than 3 seconds, warm skin, pink nailbeds, and absence of edema?

Intervention	Rationale	Evaluation
Check extremity peripheral pulses, capillary refill, color, temperature, and presence of edema every 4 hours, and report abnormal findings.	*These are indications of adequate tissue perfusion.*	Are peripheral pulses strong, nailbeds pink, and capillary refill of 3 seconds or less with no edema noted?
Check skin for intactness, healed areas, and signs of ulceration or infection.	*Chronic arterial occlusion leads to decreased blood flow, resulting in tissue damage and poor wound healing.*	Is skin intact?
Place extremities lower than heart, feet on floor in sitting position, or head of bed elevated on blocks.	*Dependent position increases blood flow to the legs and feet.*	Does patient have adequate tissue perfusion signs?
Avoid bending knees, pillows under knees, prolonged sitting, or crossing legs.	*These activities impede blood flow to extremities.*	Does patient exhibit understanding of ways to improve peripheral blood flow?
Encourage wearing of shoes that fit well.	*Prevents irritation and tissue breakdown leading to ulcer.*	Does patient verbalize that shoes fit well?

Nursing Diagnosis: *Activity Intolerance* related to activity pain and diminished blood flow
Expected Outcome: The patient will report that pain is relieved during desired activities.
Evaluation of Outcome: Does patient participate in activities without pain?

Intervention	Rationale	Evaluation
Refer to progressive activity program.	*Gradual progressive exercise promotes collateral circulation.*	Does patient participate in exercise program?

Nursing Care Plan for the Patient With a Peripheral Arterial Occlusive Disorder—cont'd

Nursing Diagnosis: *Readiness for Enhanced Health Literacy* related to complications, medications, or postoperative care
Expected Outcome: The patient and family will verbalize self-care measures to control disease and prevent complications.
Evaluation of Outcome: Are the patient and family able to verbalize an understanding of teaching?

Intervention	Rationale	Evaluation
Determine patient's and family's health literacy for the physiology of the disease, and treatment and preventive techniques.	*Health literacy level determines the ability to learn.*	Does patient's and family's health literacy promote understanding of peripheral artery disease (PAD)?
Describe PAD, symptoms, diagnosis, treatment, and complications to patient and family.	*The patient should understand PAD to help control it.*	Do patient and family verbalize understanding of PAD?
Teach healthy lifestyle and risk factor control (e.g., smoking cessation, healthy diet, walking programs, hyperlipidemia, and diabetes and hypertension control).	*Healthy lifestyle promotes circulation and decreases functional impairment and pain.*	Is patient willing and able to incorporate healthy lifestyle into daily routine?
Explain daily foot care: Inspect feet for ingrown toenails, redness, sores, or blisters; wash feet with warm soap and water; dry with gentle patting; lubricate skin to prevent cracking; wear clean socks; do not walk barefoot; and inspect inside of footwear for foreign objects before inserting foot.	*Daily foot care and reporting problems promptly can help prevent complications of PAD.*	Does patient verbalize understanding and state will perform daily foot care?
Explain prescribed drug treatment protocols.	*Medication explanation can help patient comply with therapy.*	Does patient verbalize understanding of medications?

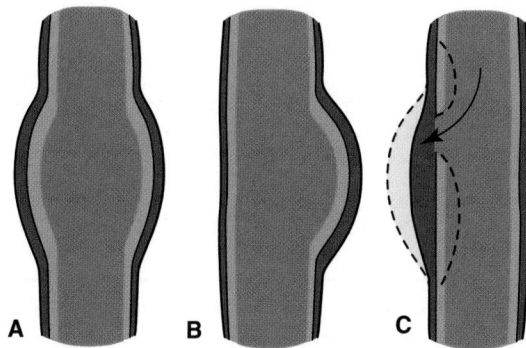

FIGURE 24.9 Types of aneurysms. (A) Fusiform: The entire circumference of the artery is dilated. (B) Saccular: One side of the artery is dilated. (C) Dissecting: A tear in the inner layer causes a cavity to form between the layers of the artery and fill with blood. The cavity expands with each heartbeat.

Diagnostic Tests

Abdominal ultrasound, CT scan, MRI, or aortography diagnose an AAA. Small aneurysms, less than 4 cm, are monitored for enlargement with ultrasound about every 6 to 12 months.

Therapeutic Measures

Medical treatment includes smoking cessation, gentle exercise such as walking and bike riding, avoiding the lifting of heavy objects, blood pressure control to prevent arterial wall rupture, and beta blockers to slow AAA enlargement. Surgical repair (a bypass graft) is performed for pain, signs of circulatory compromise, and an aneurysm that is larger than 5.5 cm or rapidly enlarging.

An open surgical repair or an endovascular stent graft may be done to repair an AAA. Open repair is done under anesthesia. The dilated aorta section is removed and replaced

Table 24.8

Aneurysm Summary

Signs and Symptoms	Back pain
	Flank pain
	Abdominal fullness
	Nausea
	Pulsating mass in abdomen
	Severe sudden back pain with rupture
Diagnostic Tests	Ultrasound
	Computed tomography (CT) scan
	Aortography
Therapeutic Measures	Observe for growth of aneurysm
	Maintain blood pressure
	Surgical repair and graft
Complications	Rupture
	Shock
	Hemorrhage
Priority Nursing Diagnoses	*Acute Pain*
	Risk for Deficient Fluid Volume
	Risk for Ineffective Peripheral Tissue Perfusion

with a synthetic graft that is sutured in place. Endovascular grafting involves the placement (through the femoral artery) of a stent graft at the site of the AAA. Dye is used to guide a balloon catheter that positions and opens the graft against the aorta wall. Blood flows through the stent graft to reduce pressure on the aneurysm, which will shrink over time. A fenestrated (perforated) endograft is used when the AAA is near other arteries, such as the renal arteries, to maintain their blood flow. Endovascular surgery requires less hospitalization time (2 to 3 days) and a quicker recovery. Monitoring of the endograft is necessary.

Nursing Process for the Patient With an Abdominal Aortic Aneurysm

DATA COLLECTION. Careful monitoring of a patient with an AAA is necessary. Emotional stress may be a risk factor that should be addressed. Patient understanding must be determined so patients understand their medication regimen and the importance of taking antihypertensives as prescribed. The patient is cared for in the intensive care unit after surgery.

NURSING DIAGNOSES, PLANNING, IMPLEMENTATION, AND EVALUATION. See "Nursing Care Plan for the Patient After Vascular Surgery."

Nursing Care Plan for the Patient After Vascular Surgery

Nursing Diagnosis: *Acute Pain* related to surgical incision and reperfusion of tissue
Expected Outcomes: The patient will report an absence or acceptable level of pain within 30 minutes of reporting pain. The patient will rest comfortably, perform respiratory treatments as necessary, and perform activities of daily living (ADLs).
Evaluation of Outcomes: Does the patient state that pain is relieved or acceptable? Is the patient able to rest and participate in respiratory treatments and ADLs?

Intervention	Rationale	Evaluation
Have patient rate using pain scale and describe characteristics of pain, including severity of pain.	*Peripheral vascular surgery pain is usually mild; severe pain may indicate reocclusion. Major vascular surgery pain is severe.*	Does patient state that pain is at a tolerable level with a patent vessel?
Administer analgesics as prescribed, and recheck pain level in 30 minutes to provide pain relief.	*Relieves pain.*	Is pain relieved?
Geriatric		
Notify health care provider if pain is unrelieved.	*Pain is not a normal part of aging, and older patients need and are entitled to adequate pain relief. This may require trials of various analgesics.*	Does patient rate pain as none or at a tolerable level using a pain scale?
Use opioid pain medications cautiously. Consider reducing frail older patients' first opioid dose by 25% to 50%, and then increase if safe as ordered.	*Older patients are more susceptible to peak effects and duration of analgesia of opioids.*	Are patient's vital signs and sedation levels within normal limits?

Nursing Care Plan for the Patient After Vascular Surgery—cont'd

Nursing Diagnosis: *Ineffective Peripheral Tissue Perfusion* related to hypotension, hypothermia, emboli, vascular spasm, or reocclusion
Expected Outcomes: The patient will have palpable peripheral pulses, adequate capillary refill, and normal color, temperature, motor, and sensory function of extremities. The patient will have reactive pupils and baseline cognitive function.
Evaluation of Outcomes: Is the patient's circulatory status within normal limits? Does the patient have reactive pupils and baseline cognitive function intact?

Intervention	Rationale	Evaluation
Monitor circulation, movement, and sensation in extremities every 1 to 4 hours.	*Early detection of spasm or reocclusion minimizes risk of ischemia and necrosis.*	Does graft or vessel remain patent?
Perform neurologic checks every 2 to 4 hours (carotid).	*Allows early detection of complications.*	Are major neurologic or circulatory problems detected?
Measure abdominal girth every shift (abdominal aortic surgery).	*Increasing girth may indicate bleeding into abdomen.*	Does abdominal girth remain unchanged?
Take temperature every 4 hours as ordered.	*May indicate hypothermia with need for further warming or an infection.*	Does patient remain normothermic?
Monitor complete blood count (CBC) as ordered.	*Red blood cell count, hemoglobin, and hematocrit decrease with insidious bleeding into abdomen or significant hematoma formations.*	Is CBC within normal limits?
Avoid constricting measures on affected extremity (e.g., knee gatch of bed, adhesive tape, tight dressings).	*Prevent further decrease in blood flow to compromised extremity.*	Is blood flow to affected extremity maintained?

Varicose Veins

Varicose veins are elongated, tortuous, dilated veins. Primary varicosities are likely caused by a structural defect in the vessel wall. Along with the defect, the dilation of the vessel can lead to incompetent venous valves. Valves normally help prevent blood from refluxing. If reflux occurs, it can cause further dilation of the vessel and blood pooling in the lower extremities. Superficial veins are most often involved in primary varicosities.

Secondary varicosities are caused by an acquired or congenital pathological condition of the deep venous system. This produces dilation of collateral and superficial veins. As a result, there is an interference of blood return to the heart. This leads to stasis, or pooling, of the blood in the deep venous system. This increases the pressure within the system, pushing blood into the collateral vessels and producing varicosities in the superficial veins.

Etiology

Wall defects have been identified as a familial tendency. Any factor that contributes to increasing hydrostatic pressure within the leg, such as prolonged standing, pregnancy, and obesity, can promote venous dilation.

Signs and Symptoms

The appearance of telangiectasias (spider veins) indicates minor chronic venous disease. With more advanced disease, there can be dull pain, cramping, edema, and feelings of heaviness in the lower extremities, especially after prolonged standing. This can usually be relieved by walking or elevating the extremity. With secondary varicosities, pain and disfigurement can be more severe. Edema or ulceration can develop if venous return is severely compromised.

Therapeutic Measures

To help prevent varicose veins during your nursing career, consider wearing compression stockings. The primary goals for varicose vein therapy are to improve circulation, relieve pain, and avoid complications. Conservative treatment is exercise, leg elevation, and compression therapy (e.g., compression stockings, intermittent pneumatic compression pump, or compression bandages) as ordered. Injection sclerotherapy to collapse the vein and laser or light therapy can treat superficial varicosities. Minimally invasive ablation to seal the vein includes radiofrequency or laser ablation. These procedures can be done in the HCP's office with local anesthesia. Traditional vein stripping is done in surgery although rarely anymore.

Venous Insufficiency

Venous insufficiency is a chronic condition. Damaged or aging valves within the veins interfere with blood return to the heart, causing pooling of blood in the lower extremities. Chronic venous insufficiency can lead to venous stasis ulcers.

Venous Stasis Ulcers

PATHOPHYSIOLOGY. **Venous stasis ulcers** are the end result of chronic venous insufficiency. Dysfunctional valves in the venous system prevent or reduce venous blood return. As venous pressure increases, venous stasis occurs. Over time, the congestion and decreased venous circulation lead to changes in the lower extremities. There may be edema and a brownish discoloration of the leg and foot, with the surrounding skin hardened and leathery in appearance. The brown color occurs when veins rupture, releasing red blood cells into the tissues; the red blood cells then break down and stain the tissue brown.

Stasis ulcers develop from the increased pressure and rupture of small veins. Signs of skin breakdown are most commonly seen at the medial malleolus of the ankle. Stasis ulcers are a serious complication of venous insufficiency that are difficult to cure and can affect the patient's quality of life.

THERAPEUTIC MEASURES. The focus of treatment is to decrease edema and heal skin ulcerations. Compression wraps such as elastic stockings or bandage wraps are necessary to decrease edema. Bedrest and elevation of legs and feet above the heart are important to assist with venous drainage of lower extremities. Patients are advised not to keep legs dependent and to avoid long periods of standing or sitting to prevent increased pressure and pain. The foot of the bed should be elevated 5 to 6 inches. Additionally, patients should be encouraged to exercise and walk often during nonacute episodes. Patients should be taught not to cross their legs or wear constrictive clothing that would decrease venous blood return to the heart.

Skin ulcers are usually cultured and treated with topical antibiotics if needed. Wound care can be chronic and challenging (see Chapter 54). An Unna Boot is a gauze dressing coated with zinc oxide, calamine, and glycerine. It may be used to promote healing in severe ulcers. Zinc promotes wound healing and can be soothing. The Unna Boot is applied snugly and provides compression therapy as well. It is changed every 2 to 7 days. Skin grafting may be necessary if ulcerations are severe or do not heal.

Nursing Process for the Patient with a Venous Disorder.

DATA COLLECTION. Risk factors and knowledge of contributing factors for venous disorders are identified for teaching plans. Symptoms and concerns about body image are noted. Leg appearance, presence of edema, and ulcerations are noted. Patient-coping skills are identified to cope with chronic ulcers that may affect quality of life.

NURSING DIAGNOSES, PLANNING, AND IMPLEMENTATION.

Acute Pain related to edema in extremities

EXPECTED OUTCOME: The patient will report an absence or acceptable level of pain within 30 minutes of reporting pain.

- Ask patient to use rating scale (such as 0 to 10) to identify pain level *to provide consistency in pain reporting.*
- Elevate legs above heart level and avoid long periods of sitting or standing *to reduce impaired venous return or pooling of fluid.*
- Utilize compression therapy as ordered *to promote drainage and reduce edema.*
- Administer analgesics as prescribed and recheck pain level in 30 minutes *to provide pain relief.*

Impaired Tissue Integrity related to chronic venous congestion

EXPECTED OUTCOME: The patient will have intact tissue integrity.

- Note and document size, shape, and depth of wound *to evaluate healing of wound over time.*
- Provide a comprehensive plan for wound care including pressure relief, treatments, and nutrition as ordered *to ensure that quality wound care is provided.*
- Provide wound care as ordered *to aid in wound healing.*

Ineffective Health Maintenance related to deficient knowledge of venous disorder

EXPECTED OUTCOME: The patient will report understanding of how to manage venous disorder.

- Identify patient's understanding of the venous disorder *to determine baseline knowledge.*
- Explain venous disorder pathophysiology, signs and symptoms, prevention, and therapeutic regimen *to empower patient to manage disorder.*
- Explain that tight-fitting clothes at tops of legs or waist should not be worn *to prevent venous occlusion.*
- Explain how to control risk factors and prevent varicose veins (e.g., weight reduction, elevation of the extremities, walking, exercise, and compression therapy) *to assist blood flow return to the heart.*
- Document teaching and evaluation of patient knowledge *to communicate patient progress toward goal attainment.*

See also the "Nursing Care Plan for the Patient After Vascular Surgery."

EVALUATION. Interventions are successful if the patient reports pain is at an acceptable level and verbalizes an understanding of venous disease and prevention.

Vascular Surgery

Vascular impairments requiring surgery may be acute or chronic. They may involve arteries, veins, or lymphatic vessels. When intermittent claudication becomes severe or disabling or when the limb is at risk for amputation, then surgical vascular grafting may be done.

Nursing Process for the Patient Undergoing Preoperative Vascular Surgery

DATA COLLECTION. Circulatory status and pain control needs are monitored. Laboratory test results, including complete blood count (CBC), INR, partial thromboplastin time (PTT), and bleeding time, are reviewed.

NURSING DIAGNOSES. The nursing diagnoses for preoperative vascular surgery may include the following:

• *Acute* or *Chronic Pain* related to ischemia of tissue distal to occlusion or aneurysm
• *Anxiety* related to unknown outcome, pain, powerlessness, or threat of death
• *Deficient Knowledge,* preoperative and postoperative procedures, related to unfamiliar process

See Chapter 12 for further preoperative nursing process information.

Embolectomy and Thrombectomy

When an artery becomes completely occluded by an embolus or thrombus, it is considered a surgical emergency. Surgical removal to restore blood flow and oxygenation to the tissue distal to the occlusion is imperative to decrease ischemia and necrosis.

Vascular Bypasses and Grafts

Vascular bypass surgery involves the use of either autografts, such as the patient's own saphenous vein, or a synthetic graft material. The graft is anastomosed to the artery proximal to the occlusion and tunneled past the occlusion. There, the distal end of the graft is anastomosed to the artery (Fig. 24.10). The graft is assessed for hemostasis and function. The wound is then sutured closed.

Endarterectomy

Arteriosclerotic plaques are dissected from the lining of the arterial wall and removed in a procedure called an **endarterectomy.** This is most commonly performed on the carotid artery but may be done on peripheral arterial vessels as well. To control blood flow, the artery is clamped on both

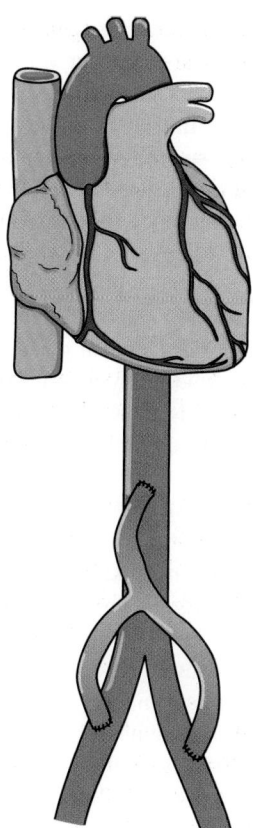

FIGURE 24.10 Aortofemoral bypass.

sides of the occlusion. An incision is made into the artery. The plaque within the artery is removed with forceps. The artery is irrigated to remove any further debris and then closed with sutures. The clamps are removed, and the skin incision is closed. A drain may be placed to help prevent hematoma formation.

Angioplasty

Minimally invasive techniques can also be used to open plaque-blocked arteries. These techniques include balloon or laser angioplasty. A flexible laser-tipped catheter is inserted into an artery and advanced to the site of the blockage. The laser sends out pulsating beams of light, which vaporize the plaque. This procedure is used for patients with smaller occlusions in the distal superficial femoral, proximal popliteal, and common iliac arteries.

Stents

Stents are placed inside an artery to provide support to the artery walls to keep them open. See the PCI discussion earlier.

• WORD • BUILDING •

endarterectomy: end—inside + arter—artery + ectomy—excision

Complications of Vascular Surgery

Bleeding and hemorrhage can occur with any vascular surgery. If hemorrhage occurs, manual pressure is applied to the site of bleeding, and the HCP is notified immediately. Drainage may cause swelling and hematoma formation. Drains can be placed to help prevent this. Extensive surgeries may result in significant blood loss, leading to fluid volume deficit or shock.

Reocclusion is possible with any vascular surgery. If thrombi or emboli develop and block blood flow, a surgical emergency results. Loss of a pedal pulse may signify reocclusion and must be immediately reported to the HCP. Blood flow needs to be reestablished within 4 to 6 hours to prevent risk of amputation of the extremity.

Nursing Process for the Patient After Vascular Surgery

DATA COLLECTION. Upon transfer postoperatively to either the intensive care or surgical unit, the patient is positioned comfortably. Head-to-toe data collection is obtained and documented. A patent airway is ensured, and vital signs are monitored. The patient's pain level is rated with a pain scale. All IVs and drains are monitored. Measurement of intake and output is done hourly, then every 4 to 8 hours. CBC, INR, PTT, and electrolytes are monitored. Increasing abdominal girth measurements (for AAA repair) can indicate hemorrhage. Abnormal findings are reported immediately to the HCP.

Initially, neurovascular checks are ordered every 15 minutes for the first 2 hours, then every 30 minutes for 1 to 3 hours, and then hourly for aortic or extremity vascular surgery. Neurovascular checks include extremity movement and sensation, presence of numbness or tingling, pulses, temperature, color, and capillary refill (less than 3 seconds normally). Peripheral pulses are palpated or checked with Doppler ultrasound if not palpable. Then, they are compared with the unaffected extremity to detect deficits. If a pulse is absent or weak or the extremity is cool or dusky, the HCP is notified immediately.

NURSING DIAGNOSES, PLANNING, IMPLEMENTATION, AND EVALUATION. See "Nursing Care Plan for the Patient After Vascular Surgery."

NURSING CARE TIP

Neurovascular checks refer to the assessment of an extremity. (Neurologic checks refer to assessment of the central nervous system.) The following are areas to examine on an extremity when doing neurovascular checks:

NEURO	VASCULAR
Movement	Pulses
Sensation	Capillary refill
Numbness	Color (nailbed or skin)
Tingling	Temperature

 ## LYMPHATIC SYSTEM

The lymphatic system returns fluid from other tissues in the body to the bloodstream. It is a pumpless system with one-way valves that return the fluid to the heart. Any interruption in the flow of lymph results in edema.

Lymphangitis

Lymphangitis is inflammation of the lymphatic channels due to an infection. The infection can occur in the arms or legs. It is most commonly caused by *Streptococcus* bacteria. *Staphylococcus* bacteria and other organisms may also cause it. It is a serious infection that can cause sepsis and be fatal. Symptoms include painful red streaks in the extremity. Fever and chills may be present. Lymph nodes in the area of infection can be enlarged and painful. Therapy is initiated with an appropriate antimicrobial agent. Moist heat and elevation help reduce pain and swelling.

Nursing Process for the Patient With Lymphangitis

DATA COLLECTION. The affected area is monitored for size changes, edema, and skin breakdown to prevent complications. Pain level and fever occurrence are monitored. Abnormal changes are reported to the HCP.

NURSING DIAGNOSES, PLANNING, AND IMPLEMENTATION.

Acute Pain related to tissue damage and edema from infection

EXPECTED OUTCOME: The patient will report an absence or acceptable level of pain within 30 minutes of reporting pain.

- Administer analgesics as prescribed, and recheck pain level in 30 minutes *to provide pain relief.*
- Position extremity *for comfort,* and elevate *to reduce edema, which can cause pressure and pain.*

Excess Fluid Volume related to congested lymph nodes from infection

EXPECTED OUTCOME: The patient will exhibit no evidence of edema.

• Apply moist, heat on the extremity as ordered *to increase circulation and reduce edema.*

• Elevate extremity *to help improve circulation and prevent edema.*

EVALUATION. Interventions are successful if the patient reports pain is at an acceptable level and no edema is present.

Home Health Hints

Cardiac

• After open-heart surgery, many patients suffer from depression. Utilize a depression screening tool and follow up with the health care provider (HCP). Interventions that might be appropriate include antidepressants, support groups, and social work referrals.

• Chest pain from esophageal reflux can mimic cardiovascular symptoms. Ask if the pain is related to consuming large meals, lying down, or bending over, or if it is relieved with antacids or food. Inform the HCP of these findings.

• The agency's social worker can help the patient and family adjust to lifestyle changes. The social worker can also reduce caregiver strain by facilitating the use of resources available within the family or community, such as respite care or housekeeping services.

• Teach the caregiver stress management techniques to use. This can include deep-breathing exercises, reading a book, meditation, massage therapy, guided imagery, exercise, socializing with friends, and/or working on a favorite hobby.

Vascular

• Monitor peripheral pulses and capillary refill to ensure adequate tissue perfusion. Report absent pulses or sluggish capillary refill to the patient's HCP.

• Teach the patient to report changes in skin color, insect bites, and/or rashes to the HCP. Patients with peripheral vascular disorders are at a high risk for developing lower extremity wounds that are often slow to heal.

• Teach the patient to stop and rest if pain develops in the lower extremities during exercise.

SUGGESTED ANSWERS TO CRITICAL THINKING

Mr. Jones

1. Irregular, respiratory rate 28 breaths per minute and shallow, lung sounds diminished with crackles in bilateral bases.
2. Pain control, coughing and deep breathing, and incentive spirometer.
3. Pain, compensation for respiratory status, and elevated temperature.
4. Hemorrhage and reduced cardiac output.
5. Health care provider (HCP) for orders, pharmacist for medication orders, and respiratory therapist for pulmonary concerns.

Mrs. Sims

1. Place patient on bedrest, administer oxygen via nasal cannula at 2 L/min, obtain blood pressure and pulse, administer nitroglycerin (NTG) sublingual as ordered, obtain electrocardiogram (ECG), and notify HCP.
2. She may be having an anginal attack versus acute myocardial infarction (MI).
3. NTG usually stops chest pain associated with angina. Rest may also alleviate chest pain. Neither NTG nor rest will relieve the pain of an acute MI.
4. Indicators of an MI include patient history, ECG changes with or without ST-segment elevation, elevated troponin I, and creatine kinase (CK)-MB elevation.
5. Medical interventions may include oxygen, NTG drip, morphine, anticoagulant therapy (heparin), and thrombolytic agents to dissolve the clot. A cardiac catheterization can determine which coronary artery is blocked. Percutaneous coronary intervention or a coronary artery bypass graft can reperfuse the heart.
6. Educate Mrs. Sims about the risks of smoking and being overweight.

Mrs. May

1. Monitor the patient's left leg for color, temperature, capillary refill, and pulses (femoral, popliteal, dorsalis pedis, and posterior tibial). Compare findings with findings in the right leg.
2. If unable to palpate pulses, use a Doppler ultrasound that enhances sound to locate pulses.

Continued

SUGGESTED ANSWERS TO CRITICAL THINKING—cont'd

3. The patient's signs and symptom could be caused by an embolism above the left femoral artery.
4. To document findings, you would collect more data. A sample of **SOAP** (Subjective, Objective, Analysis, Plan) charting for your additional findings is given: **S:** "I have severe pain in my left groin that just started. It is at 9 on a scale of 0 to 10."; **O:** Grimacing, moaning, and holding left upper leg. Left leg cool, color pale, nailbeds pale, capillary refill 8 seconds, unable to palpate pulses. Faint femoral and popliteal pulse, no dorsalis pedis or posterior tibial pulse heard with Doppler. Right leg warm, pink, capillary refill 3 seconds, with all pulses palpable.; **A:** Ineffective tissue perfusion.; **P:** Notify HCP immediately.
5. Immediate interventions include complete bedrest, protecting the leg, and notifying the HCP.
6. Medical interventions could include medication for pain and use of an anticoagulant, such as heparin. If no pulses are present, a thrombolytic agent may be ordered. Surgery is possible.
7. Thrombectomy or embolectomy may be necessary to save the limb.

Mr. Janeway

1. Priority areas for data collection include respiratory status, circulatory status of right leg and foot, vital signs, and pain level.
2. A medical history should include Mr. Janeway's usual blood glucose values and medications, ambulation aids, gait, knowledge base regarding his various disease processes, and what led to this hospitalization.
3. Priority nursing diagnoses include (1) *Acute Pain* related to surgery of right lower leg; (2) *Ineffective Peripheral Tissue Perfusion* related to embolectomy of right lower leg and renal insufficiency; and (3) *Risk for Injury* related to leg surgery, diabetes, and obesity.
4. Outcomes include (1) verbalizes relief of pain; (2) maintains adequate tissue perfusion as evidenced by palpable peripheral (pedal) pulses and warm and dry skin; and (3) remains free from injury.
5. Nursing interventions include the following: (1) Position (especially right leg) for comfort; keep the right leg slightly elevated; educate the patient regarding the need to ask for pain medication before pain is too severe; educate the patient regarding the need to take pain medication to minimize the negative physiological effects of pain; monitor pain on a pain scale; evaluate the effectiveness of medication using the same pain scale; report ineffective pain measures. (2) Check pedal pulses, surgical dressing, pedal sensation and movement, and color initially and every hour; report changes; check capillary refill; monitor for pain in extremities; monitor for edema in extremities; keep leg elevated slightly. (3) Make sure the nursing call light is within reach; provide assistance with ambulation; use walking aids.

Review Questions

1. The nurse would evaluate the patient as understanding teaching for prevention of coronary artery disease if the patient stated that which of the following is a risk factor for coronary artery disease that can be controlled?
    1. "Family history of cardiovascular disease."
    2. "Hypertension."
    3. "Ethnicity."
    4. "Family history of diabetes mellitus."

2. The licensed practical nurse is assisting with collecting data on a female patient. Which of these findings should be reported to the registered nurse that could be possible symptoms of a myocardial infarction in the absence of chest pain? **Select all that apply.**
    1. Fatigue
    2. Dizziness
    3. Nausea
    4. Pain between shoulder blades
    5. Sweating
    6. Shortness of breath

3. The nurse would evaluate the patient as understanding teaching on the purpose of coronary artery bypass graft surgery if the patient made which of the following statements?
    1. "It cures coronary artery disease."
    2. "It is done to increase blood flow to the myocardium."
    3. "It prevents spasms of the coronary arteries."
    4. "It will decrease blood flow to the coronary arteries."

4. The nurse is reinforcing teaching for a patient prescribed sublingual nitroglycerin tablets. The nurse should instruct the patient to use this medication in which of the following ways?
    1. Take one tablet and lie down for 1 hour, and repeat if pain unrelieved.
    2. Place two tablets under the tongue daily to prevent angina.
    3. Swallow one tablet, wait 10 minutes; swallow two tablets if pain persists; swallow three tablets if pain remains after 15 minutes.
    4. With angina and symptoms of myocardial infarction, place one tablet under the tongue and if, after 5 minutes has elapsed, the pain is unchanged or worse, call 911.

5. What actions can the nurse take to reduce the anxiety of a patient who is experiencing chest pain? **Select all that apply.**
   1. Remain with the patient at all times.
   2. Dim lights, close door, and leave patient to sleep.
   3. Explain heart's function is being monitored.
   4. Explain procedures and actions taken.
   5. Turn television on for distraction.
   6. Allow family to be involved in care.

6. The nurse would evaluate the patient as understanding teaching for peripheral arterial occlusive disease if the patient stated that which of the following is the classic symptom?
   1. Angina
   2. Edema
   3. Intermittent claudication
   4. Stasis ulcers

7. The nurse is caring for a patient who has peripheral arterial disease. Which of the following statements by the patient indicates understanding of how to manage the pain of peripheral arterial disease?
   1. "I will sit with my legs down."
   2. "I will use a reclining chair."
   3. "I will lie down frequently."
   4. "I will do knee flexion exercises."

8. The nurse is teaching a patient about medications used to treat peripheral arterial disease and claudication. Which of these would the nurse include in the teaching plan? **Select all that apply.**
   1. Aspirin
   2. Cholestyramine (Questran)
   3. Cilostazol (Pletal)
   4. Clopidogrel (Plavix)
   5. Enoxaparin (Lovenox)
   6. Ranolazine (Ranexa)

Answer rationales available in your online resources.

ANSWERS 1. 2; 2. 1, 3, 4, 6; 3. 2; 4. 4; 5. 1, 3, 4, 6; 6. 3; 7. 1; 8. 1, 3, 4

Key Points

Find the chapter key points in your online resources available through Davis Edge.

Additional Resources

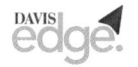

Use the scratch off code on the inside front cover of your book to access online quizzes that will help you to improve your scores on course exams and prepare for NCLEX-PN®.

Study Guide

CHAPTER 25

Nursing Care of Patients With Cardiac Arrhythmias

Michele Dickson, Linda S. Williams

KEY TERMS

ablation (uh-BLAY-shun)

arrhythmia (uh-RITH-mee-ah)

atrial depolarization (AY-tree-uhl DEE-poh-lur-ih-ZAY-shun)

atrial systole (AY-tree-uhl SIS-tuh-lee)

atrioventricular node (AY-tree-oh-ven-TRIK-yoo-lur NOHD)

bigeminy (by-JEM-ih-nee)

bradycardia (BRAY-dih-KAR-dee-ah)

bundle of His (BUN-duhl of HIS)

cardioversion (KAR-dee-oh-VER-zhun)

defibrillation (dee-FIB-ri-lay-shun)

dysrhythmia (dis-RITH-mee-ah)

electrocardiogram (ee-LEK-troh-KAR-dee-oh-GRAM)

fluoroscopy (fluh-RAHS-kuh-pee)

hyperkalemia (HY-per-kuh-LEE-mee-ah)

hypomagnesemia (HY-poh-MAG-nuh-ZEE-mee-ah)

isoelectric line (EYE-so-ee-LEK-trik LINE)

multifocal (MUHL-tee-FOH-kuhl)

quadrigeminy (kwa-drih-JEM-ih-nee)

sinoatrial node (SY-noh-AY-tree-al NOHD)

trigeminy (try-JEM-ih-nee)

unifocal (YOO-ni-FOH- kuhl)

ventricular diastole (ven-TRIK-yoo-lar dye-AS-tuh-lee)

ventricular repolarization (ven-TRIK-yoo-lar RE-pol-lahr-i-ZAY-shun)

ventricular systole (ven-TRIK-yoo-lar SIS-tuh-lee)

ventricular tachycardia (ven-TRIK-yoo-lar TAK-ee-KAR-dee-ah)

CHAPTER CONCEPT

Perfusion

LEARNING OUTCOMES

1. Describe how electrical activity flows through the heart.
2. List the six steps used for arrhythmia interpretation.
3. Explain current medical treatments for cardiac arrhythmias.
4. Discuss cardiac pacemakers and implantable cardioverter defibrillators and their uses.
5. Plan nursing care for patients with an arrhythmia.
6. Plan nursing care for patients with an implanted device.

CARDIAC CONDUCTION SYSTEM

The heart's electrical conduction system initiates an impulse. Its purpose is to stimulate the mechanical cells of the heart to contract (see Fig. 21.3). Electrical activity can be seen on a cardiac monitor or recorded on an **electrocardiogram** (ECG) tracing. Activity seen on an ECG is not proof that the mechanical cells of the heart have contracted in response to the electrical impulse seen. So how can you verify that the heart muscle contracted and perfusion occurs? With physical data collection! Obtain the patient's blood pressure and apical and peripheral pulses. This is the evidence that cardiac contraction and perfusion occurred.

Do you recall what part of the conduction system is called the normal pacemaker of the heart? It is the **sinoatrial** (SA) **node.** The SA node is the primary pacemaker of the heart. This is because its inherent (built-in) rate is faster than those of other conduction sites located in the **atrioventricular** (AV) **node** or ventricles. The SA node normally fires at a rate of 60 to 100 beats per minute (bpm).

If the SA node slows or fails, other areas of the heart can initiate impulses to keep the heart beating. This protective mechanism is referred to as *escape*. The AV node has an inherent rate of 40 to 60 bpm. Body functions are usually adequate at this rate. If the AV node is unable to initiate an impulse, the ventricles can take over at 20 to 40 bpm. However, the ventricular rate of 20 to 40 bpm is not enough to meet the body's oxygen needs. At this rate, the patient will begin to show signs of inadequate cardiac output (decompensation). These signs include dyspnea, abnormal vital signs, and changes in level of consciousness. Treatment is needed to reestablish a normal heart rate immediately.

After the SA node fires, the impulse spreads through the atria conduction system to the AV node. This stimulates the atria to contract. This is known as **atrial systole.** The atrial contraction propels blood out of the atria and into the relaxed ventricles during **ventricular diastole.** At the AV node, the impulse is briefly delayed. Next, the impulse travels down the **bundle of His,** which divides into right and left bundle branches through the Purkinje fibers. This stimulates both ventricles to contract upward from the apex of the heart. Blood is pushed toward the arteries. This contraction is known as **ventricular systole.**

Cardiac Cycle

A cardiac cycle is the period from the beginning of one heartbeat to the beginning of the next. The cardiac cycle is the electrical representation of the impulse that stimulates depolarization (contraction) and repolarization (relaxation) of the atria and ventricles. Within the normal cardiac cycle, there is a P wave, a QRS complex, and a T wave (Fig. 25.1).

ELECTROCARDIOGRAM

The electrical activity of the heart can be seen with either an ECG or continuous cardiac monitoring. An ECG test shows electrical activity at the moment when the ECG is obtained. Electrodes placed on the patient's skin allow various views of the heart's electrical activity to be seen. Each view of the heart is referred to as a *lead.* A 12-lead ECG provides 12 different views of the heart's electrical activity. An 18-lead ECG shows 18 views. For continuous monitoring, one lead or two leads are viewed. Continuous 12-lead monitoring can also be done.

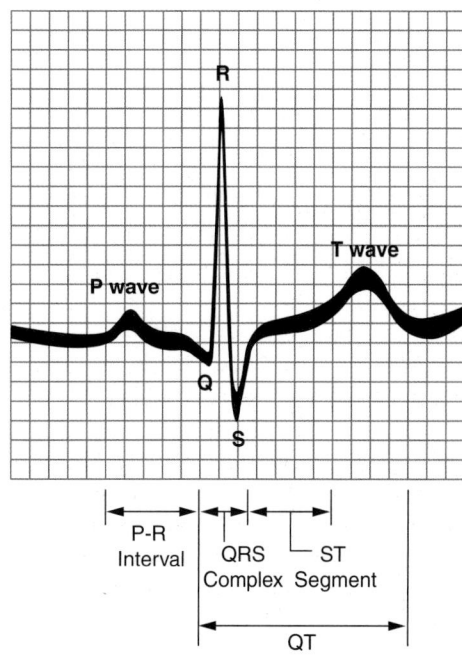

FIGURE 25.1 Components of the cardiac cycle.

Specialized training, usually obtained by physicians, is required to interpret ECGs for normal and abnormal heart rhythms. By learning the characteristics of a normal heart rhythm and rules for common **arrhythmias,** you will be able to report rhythm changes to your supervisor or the health care provider (HCP).

LEARNING TIP
Think of a 12- or 18-lead electrocardiogram (ECG) as if you had a camera that you were using to take pictures (views) of an object such as an apple. To obtain views that showed you all of the areas of the apple (front, side, back, side), you would take a picture and then move the camera a little to get the view next to the one you had just taken. You would continue moving the camera until you had gone around the entire apple. This would then give you a view of the entire apple. This is what a 12- or 18-lead ECG does to allow viewing of the entire conduction system of the heart.

Electrocardiogram Graph Paper

Intervals of each of the components of a cardiac cycle are measured in seconds of time on the ECG graph paper. The graph paper is calibrated within a grid. Small squares are divided into heavy lined blocks of 25 that are five squares wide and five squares high (Fig. 25.2). Each small square is 0.04 seconds wide. One-half of a square is 0.02 seconds wide. Nothing smaller than one-half of a square is used. There are five small squares horizontally between two heavy, vertical black lines. The waveforms are measured horizontally from left to right on the graph paper. The height of the waveforms (amplitude) is measured vertically.

You have probably seen a heart monitor, perhaps on television, with a straight line displayed on it. This straight line is called the **isoelectric line** (baseline). It occurs when there is no electrical current (e.g., when the ECG machine is turned on but not attached to a person). It also occurs when the positive and negative electrical activity is equal. So, it is seen when there are no positive (upward) or negative (downward) electrical wave deflections present.

COMPONENTS OF A CARDIAC CYCLE

P Wave

The P wave is the first wave of the cardiac cycle. It represents **atrial depolarization.** When the SA node fires, the electrical impulse spreads from the right to left atrium. The normal P wave appears rounded. When compared with other waveforms, it looks like a small hill. Disorders that change atrial size cause alterations in P-wave shape and size.

• WORD • BUILDING •
arrhythmia: an—without or away + rhythm—rhythm + ia— condition

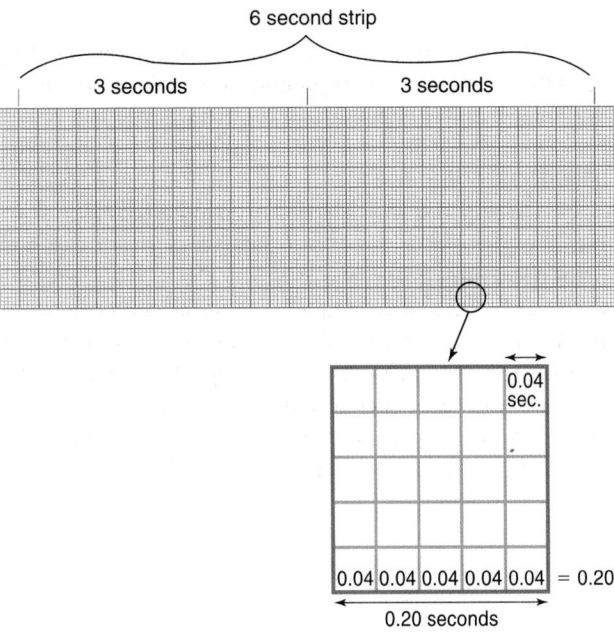

FIGURE 25.2 Electrocardiogram recording paper time intervals.

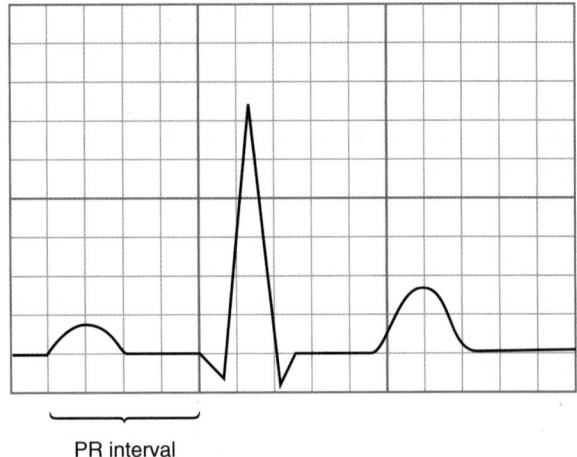

FIGURE 25.3 PR interval. This PR interval covers four squares. Each square is 0.04 seconds: 4 × 0.04 = 0.16 seconds.

PR Interval

The PR interval (PRI) represents the time it takes for the electrical impulse to travel from the SA node to the AV node. The PRI starts at the beginning of the P wave and ends at the beginning of the QRS complex. Count the number of small squares horizontally that the interval covers. Then multiply by 0.04 to identify the length of the PRI (Fig. 25.3). The normal PRI is 0.12 to 0.20 seconds (three to five small horizontal squares).

QRS Complex

The QRS complex represents ventricular depolarization. It is composed of three waves: Q, R, and S. The Q wave is the first downward deflection after the P wave. The R wave is the first upward deflection after the P wave. The S wave is the first negative deflection after the R wave (see Fig. 25.1). The S wave ends when it returns to the isoelectric line. (This is why locating the isoelectric line is helpful when first learning to identify waves.) It is important to note that all three waves are not always present in every QRS complex. Even with absent waves, it is still referred to as the QRS complex and can be considered normal (Fig. 25.4). The QRS complex is larger than the P wave. This is because the ventricles are larger because of more muscle mass. This makes the QRS complex look like a mountain when compared with the size of other waveforms.

QRS Interval

The QRS interval (duration) represents the time it takes for the electrical impulse to travel from the AV node rapidly through the ventricles. To measure the QRS interval, count the number of squares from the wave that starts the QRS complex to the end of the wave that completes the QRS complex. For example, when a Q, R, and S are present, measure

> ### LEARNING TIP
>
> To make measuring waves easier:
>
> • Identify the isoelectric line as you measure waveform tracings to help you determine the presence and type of wave. Place a straight edge along the isoelectric line so that it lays below the line; next, note any positive waves occurring above the line. Then, lay the straight edge above the line and note any waveforms that are below the line.
> • Find a wave that begins on a vertical line, if possible, to make it visually easier to double-check the caliper measurement (see Fig. 25.3).

> ### LEARNING TIP
>
> To remember the normal PR interval (PRI), use the "R" to recall normal respiratory rate and then add a decimal before each number. A normal respiratory rate is 12 to 20 breaths per minute, and a normal PRI is 0.12 to 0.20 seconds.

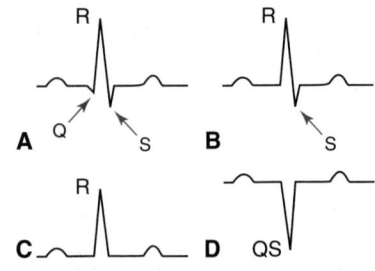

FIGURE 25.4 (A) QRS complex with a Q wave. (B) QRS complex without a Q wave. (C) QRS complex without a Q or an S wave. (D) QRS complex with no R wave. The wave present is called a QS because it is not known whether it is a Q or an S.

from the beginning of the Q wave to the end of the S wave (Fig. 25.5). If there is an R and an S present, measure from the beginning of the R to the end of the S. But if there is only an R present, measure from the beginning of the R to the end of the R. The normal QRS interval is 0.06 to 0.10 seconds (1.5 to 2.5 boxes).

T Wave

The T wave represents **ventricular repolarization,** which is the resting state of the heart when the ventricles are filling with blood and preparing to receive the next impulse. The T wave is a rounded wave. In size comparison with the other waves, it is a medium-sized hill. In most leads, the T wave is an upward (positive) deflection. It follows the QRS complex (remember depolarization must occur first!). The T wave ends with a return to the isoelectric line. An inverted (downward) T wave can indicate cardiac ischemia (Fig. 25.6).

QT Interval

The QT interval measures the time from the start of the Q wave to the end of the T wave (see Fig. 25.1). This represents the time for ventricular depolarization and repolarization. Normal ranges are 0.34 to 0.43 seconds. These vary based on gender, heart rate, and age. A QT chart for identifying normal values is used. Prolonged or shortened QT intervals can lead to ventricular arrhythmias. Abnormal intervals may be due to genetic causes, heart conditions, electrolyte imbalances, or medications that can prolong the QT interval.

U Wave

The U wave is small and often not seen. It occurs shortly after the T wave. It is most prominent in patients with hypokalemia (low serum potassium level; Fig. 25.7).

ST Segment

The ST segment reflects the time from completion of a contraction (depolarization) to recovery (repolarization) of myocardial muscle for the next impulse. The ST segment starts at the end of the QRS complex. It ends at the beginning of the T wave (Fig. 25.8A). The ST segment is checked when patients experience chest pain. If a patient has nontransmural ischemia, the ST segment can become inverted or depressed (Fig. 25.8B). With transmural ischemia, the ST segment can elevate from the isoelectric line (Fig. 25.8C).

INTERPRETATION OF CARDIAC RHYTHMS

Six-Step Process for Arrhythmia Interpretation

An orderly, systematic method for interpreting ECG rhythms should be used. This will increase understanding of the items to examine and ensure nothing is overlooked. Six steps are used (Table 25.1). The findings of the first five steps identify the ECG rhythm according to the five rules for each arrhythmia. Then, the QT interval is measured in the sixth step. A 6-second ECG tracing is used when interpreting rhythms (see Fig. 25.2).

Step 1. Regularity of the Rhythm

The regularity of the rhythm can be determined by looking at the R-to-R spacing on the ECG tracing (Fig. 25.9). The same spacing between each R to R, with a rare variation of

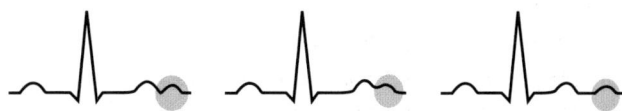

FIGURE 25.7 Various locations where U waves may appear.

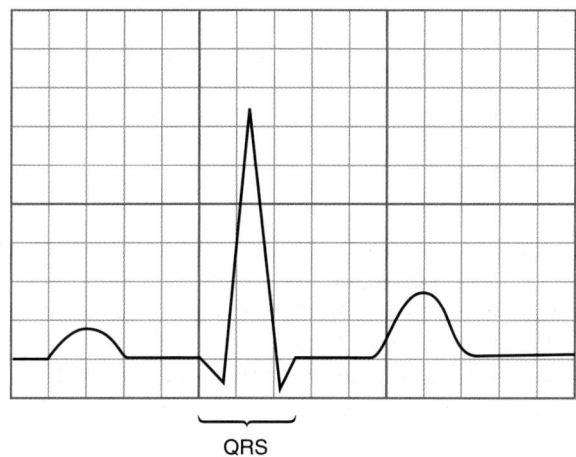

FIGURE 25.5 QRS interval. This QRS interval covers two and a half squares. Each square is 0.04 seconds. One-half square is 0.02 seconds: 2.5 × 0.04 = 0.10 seconds.

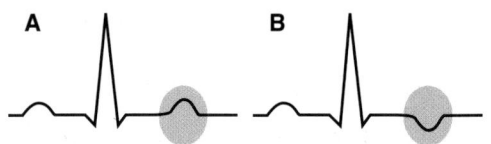

FIGURE 25.6 (A) T wave with positive deflection. (B) T wave with inverted, negative deflection, indicating ischemia.

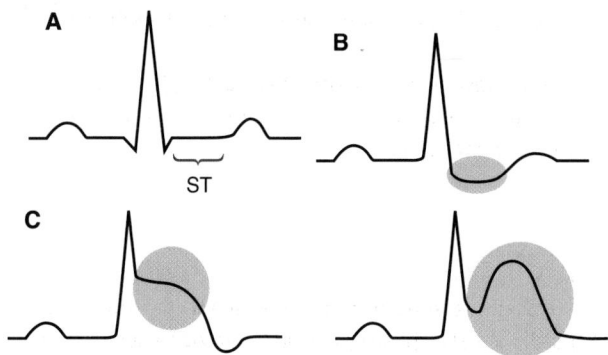

FIGURE 25.8 (A) ST segment. (B) ST segment inverted or depressed. (C) ST segment elevated.

Table 25.1

Six-Step Process for Arrhythmia Interpretation

After answering these questions with the patient's electrocardiogram (ECG) data, you can name the patient's arrhythmia.

Step	Questions
Step 1: Regularity of the rhythm	Is the rhythm regular? Irregular? Is there a pattern to the irregularity?
Step 2: Heart rate	What is the heart rate?
Step 3: P waves	Is there one P wave in front of every QRS complex? Is the atrial rate the same as the ventricular rate? Are the P waves smooth, rounded, and upright?
Step 4: PR interval	Is the PR interval normal and constant? Does the PR interval vary?
Step 5: QRS interval	Is the QRS duration normal and constant? Do the QRS complexes all look alike?
Step 6: QT interval	Is the QT interval normal?

no greater than two small squares, is seen in a normal rhythm. To determine the regularity of a rhythm, count the number of small squares between each R wave. They should normally be the same. A caliper (a two-sided, movable metal instrument with sharp points) can also be used to measure the R-to-R spacing.

To use a caliper for measuring R waves, place one metal point on an R wave. Place the other point in the same location on the next R wave. Next, stabilize the caliper. Without changing the distance between the caliper points, move the caliper from R wave to R wave across the ECG tracing (also known as an *ECG strip*) to see if R waves are regularly (evenly) spaced. If the distance is always the same, the rhythm is regular. If the distance varies, the rhythm is irregular. An irregular rhythm can be regularly irregular or irregularly irregular. *Regularly irregular* means it has a predictable pattern of irregularity. *Irregularly irregular* means it has no pattern to the occurrence of the irregularity.

LEARNING TIP

If a caliper is not available, a piece of paper can be placed on the electrocardiogram tracing. A mark can be made on the paper at the peak of one R wave and another mark made at the peak of the next R wave. The marks on the paper can then be moved along the R-to-R intervals on the tracing (just as caliper points would be) to determine the rhythm regularity.

Step 2. Heart Rate

After rhythm regularity is determined, a 1-minute heart rate is calculated. One of the two following methods is used:

1. Count the number of small (0.04-second) squares between two R waves. Divide that number into 1,500. This gives the bpm, because 1,500 small squares equal 1 minute (Fig. 25.10). This method is used only for regular rhythms. It is very accurate. A *rate meter* is a visual paper copy of this mathematical calculation for an entire 6-second ECG tracing. The nurse views it to calculate the 1-minute heart rate.
2. The 6-second method is used for irregular rhythms. It may also be used when a rapid estimate of a regular rhythm is needed. However, it is not the most accurate method for regular rhythms. At the top of ECG graph paper are vertical marks at 3-second intervals (see Fig. 25.2). Count the number of R waves in a 6-second strip (three vertical marks) and multiply the total by 10 (the number of 6-second time periods in a minute) to obtain the bpm (6 seconds × 10 = 60 seconds or 1 minute; Fig. 25.11).

Step 3. P Waves

The P waves on the ECG tracing are examined to see whether (1) there is one P wave in front of every QRS, (2) the P waves are regularly occurring, and (3) the P waves all look alike (see Fig. 25.9). If all of the P waves meet these criteria, they are considered normal. If they do not, further examination of the tracing is necessary to determine the arrhythmia.

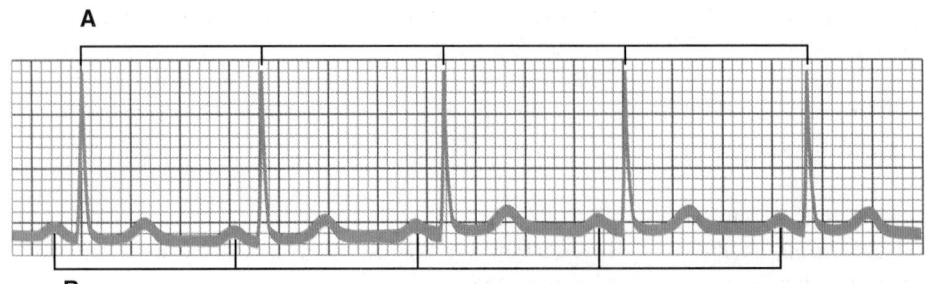

FIGURE 25.9 Normal cardiac waves are equal distances apart. (A) R to R waves. (B) P to P waves.

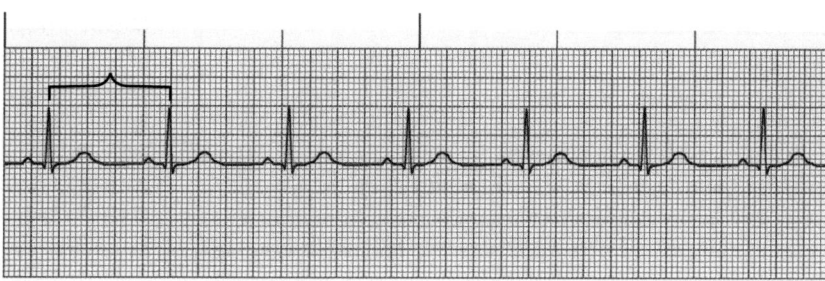

FIGURE 25.10 Normal sinus rhythm, rhythm regular: Count the small squares between two of the R waves and divide into 1,500: 1,500/22 = 68 bpm. Modified from Jones, S. A. (2008). *ECG success: Exercises in ECG interpretation*. Philadelphia, PA: F.A. Davis.

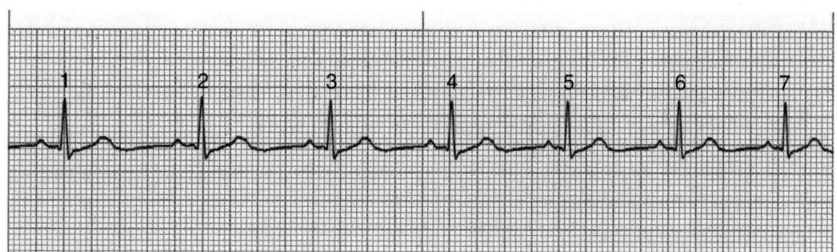

FIGURE 25.11 Rhythm irregular: Counting R waves in a 6-second strip. There are seven R waves in this 6-second strip, and 7 × 10 = 70 bpm.

Step 4. PR Interval

All PRIs are measured to determine whether they are normal (0.12 to 0.20 seconds) and constant. If the PRI is found to vary, it is important to note whether there is a pattern to the variation.

Step 5. QRS Interval

The QRS complexes are measured to determine whether they are all within normal range (0.06 to 0.10 seconds). Abnormal QRS complexes require further examination.

Step 6. QT Interval

Finally, the QT interval is measured to ensure that it is not shortened or prolonged. This can lead to arrhythmias. Abnormal QT intervals should be reported to the HCP.

 NORMAL SINUS RHYTHM

Normal sinus rhythm (NSR) is the heart's normal rhythm (see Fig. 25.10). It originates in the SA node. NSR has complete, regular cardiac cycles at 60 to 100 bpm.

Normal Sinus Rhythm Rules
1. Rhythm: regular
2. Heart rate: 60 to 100 bpm
3. P waves: rounded, upright, precede each QRS complex, alike
4. PRI: 0.12 to 0.20 seconds
5. QRS interval: less than or equal to 0.10 seconds

 ARRHYTHMIAS

An arrhythmia, which is also called a **dysrhythmia,** is an abnormal rhythm of the heart.

Several mechanisms can cause an arrhythmia. Examples of these mechanisms are disturbances in the formation of an impulse or in the conduction of the impulse. When impulse formation is disturbed, an impulse may arise from the atria, the AV node, or the ventricles instead of the SA node. This disturbance can result in an increased or decreased heart rate, early or late beats, or atrial or ventricular fibrillation. With a disturbance in conduction, the impulse becomes blocked within the electrical conduction system (as in heart blocks or right or left bundle branch block). Check out the American Heart Association (AHA) Guidelines for Cardiopulmonary Resuscitation [CPR] and Emergency Cardiovascular Care [ECC] at www.heart.org.

Arrhythmias Originating in the Sinoatrial Node

Rhythms arising from the SA node are referred to as *sinus rhythms*. Disturbances in conduction from the SA node can cause irregular rhythms or abnormal heart rates. Arrhythmias arising from the SA node are rarely dangerous. Patients, especially those with heart, lung, or kidney disease, who cannot tolerate a rapid or slow heart rate can require treatment.

LEARNING TIP

The origin and the type of a problem are used to name an arrhythmia. Let's name a slow arrhythmia that originates in the sinoatrial (SA) node. The origin is sinus, and the type of problem (slow rate) is bradycardia. So, the arrhythmia is sinus bradycardia. The term *normal* is not used because there is an abnormality! So, what would a fast arrhythmia originating in the SA node be called? It is sinus tachycardia. It is easy to understand what is happening in the arrhythmia when you look at what the name is telling you.

• WORD • BUILDING •

dysrhythmia: dys—difficult or abnormal + rhythm—rhythm + ia—condition

Sinus Bradycardia

Bradycardia is a rate slower than 60 bpm. It can be asymptomatic or symptomatic (usually when below 50 bpm). Sinus bradycardia has the same cardiac cycle components as NSR. The only difference between the two is a slower rate. This is caused by fewer impulses originating from the SA node (Fig. 25.12). Do you see that the name *sinus bradycardia* tells you this difference? The name says the impulse is coming from the sinus node (sinus) but at a slower rate than normal (bradycardia).

ETIOLOGY. Medications such as digoxin (Lanoxin), myocardial infarction (MI), and electrolyte imbalances can cause bradycardia. Well-conditioned athletes can also have slower heart rates. This is because their hearts work so efficiently.

SINUS BRADYCARDIA RULES.
1. Rhythm: regular
2. Heart rate: less than 60 bpm
3. P waves: rounded, upright, precede each QRS complex, alike
4. PRI: 0.12 to 0.20 seconds
5. QRS interval: less than or equal to 0.10 seconds

SIGNS AND SYMPTOMS. With symptomatic bradycardia, decreased blood pressure, respiratory distress, diminished or absent peripheral pulses, fatigue, or syncope can occur.

THERAPEUTIC MEASURES. Asymptomatic bradycardia does not require treatment. Observe the patient for symptom development. The underlying cause must be identified for correction. For the symptomatic patient, begin treatment while the cause is corrected. Treatment can include intravenous (IV) atropine or infusions of dopamine or epinephrine. Transcutaneous pacing is used if atropine is ineffective (Table 25.2). Transvenous pacing can also be considered.

Sinus Tachycardia

Tachycardia is defined as a heart rate greater than 100 bpm. It originates from the SA node. Sinus tachycardia has the same components as NSR except the rate is faster (Fig. 25.13).

ETIOLOGY. Sinus tachycardia causes include physical activity; hemorrhage; shock; medications such as epinephrine, atropine, or nitrates; dehydration; fever; MI; electrolyte imbalance; fear; and anxiety. Tachycardia occurs as a compensatory mechanism for hypoxia. It helps produce additional cardiac output to deliver oxygen to tissues.

SINUS TACHYCARDIA RULES.
1. Rhythm: regular
2. Heart rate: 101 to 180 bpm
3. P waves: rounded, upright, precede each QRS complex, alike
4. PRI: 0.12 to 0.20 seconds
5. QRS interval: less than or equal to 0.10 seconds

SIGNS AND SYMPTOMS. Sinus tachycardia can be asymptomatic. A very rapid rate (usually greater than 150 bpm) that is sustained for long periods may cause symptoms. The patient may have angina, dyspnea, syncope, or tachypnea. Older patients can become symptomatic more rapidly than younger patients ("Gerontological Issues"). Patients with MI may not tolerate a rapid heart rate. They may have more severe symptoms because cardiac workload is increased.

Gerontological Issues

Arrhythmia Risk. The main factors that increase the risk of arrhythmias in older adults include the following:

- Digitalis toxicity (most common)
- Hypokalemia
- Angina
- Coronary insufficiency or cardiomyopathy (exercise, stress)
- Sleep apnea
- Hypothyroidism or hyperthyroidism

Arrhythmias that occur most often in older adults include the following:

- Atrial fibrillation (atria beating 400 to 700 times per minute)
- Sick sinus syndrome (alternating episodes of bradycardia, normal sinus rhythm, tachycardia, and periods of long sinus pause)
- Heart blocks (delayed or blocked impulses to the atria or ventricles)

Some of the common age-related effects of arrhythmias include the following:

• Bradycardia	• Fatigue
• Confusion	• Hypotension
• Dizziness	• Palpitations
• Dyspnea or shortness of breath	• Syncope
	• Weakness

Older adults have less ability to adapt to sudden changes or stressors. They may not be able to tolerate tachycardia for very long. Any new-onset tachycardia in an older patient should be reported promptly.

THERAPEUTIC MEASURES. If the patient is stable, obtain an ECG and treat the cause. Medications such as adenosine (Adenocard), beta blockers, or calcium channel blockers are considered to slow the heart rate (when equal to or greater than 150 bpm; see Table 25.2). The treatment goal is to decrease the heart's workload and correct the cause. This

• WORD • BUILDING •
bradycardia: bradys—slow + kardia—heart

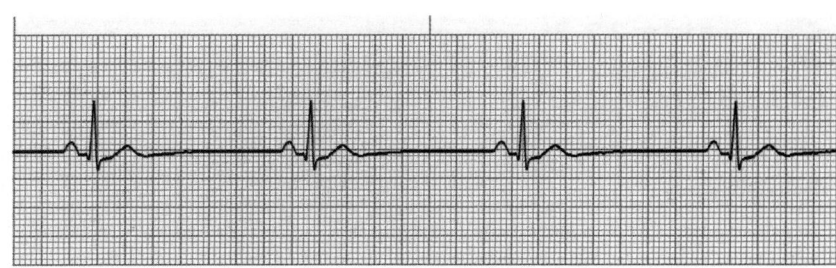

FIGURE 25.12 Sinus bradycardia. Heart rate is 38.

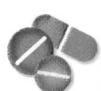

Table 25.2
Medications Used in Treatment of Arrhythmias

Medication Class/Action

Anticoagulant (Oral)
Increases clotting time.

Examples	Nursing Implications
Reduces risk of blood clots in atrial fibrillation (AF). warfarin (Coumadin)	Monitor international normalized ratio regularly. Monitor for bruising and bleeding. Acetaminophen (Tylenol) should be used rather than aspirin for analgesia during therapy. Reversal agent is vitamin K.
Reduces risk of blood clots in nonvalvular AF. apixaban (Eliquis) dabigatran (Pradaxa) edoxaban (Savaysa, Lixiana) rivaroxaban (Xarelto)	No regular monitoring needed. No specific reversal agent available.

Antidysrhythmics

Examples	Nursing Implications
In supraventricular tachycardia, slows conduction through AV node to restore normal sinus rhythm. adenosine (Adenocard)	Inform health care provider (HCP) if female pregnant or nursing. Record rhythm strip during administration. Given via intravenous (IV) push fast (1 to 3 seconds), followed by normal saline flush fast. Contraindicated in atrioventricular (AV) block or pregnancy.
Inhibits AF, atrial flutter, and ventricular arrhythmias. amiodarone (intravenous: Nexterone; by mouth: Cordarone, Pacerone)	Obtain baseline vital signs and electrocardiogram. Monitor for toxicity. Monitor heart rate and rhythm.
Inhibits ventricular tachycardia. lidocaine (Xylocaine)	

Anticholinergic
Increases heart rate to treat symptomatic bradycardia and asystole.

Examples	Nursing Implications
atropine sulfate	Contraindicated in angle closure glaucoma.

Continued

Table 25.2
Medications Used in Treatment of Arrhythmias—cont'd

Medication Class/Action

Beta Blockers

Decrease myocardial contractility. Control rate in sinus tachycardia, premature atrial contraction, atrial flutter, AF, and premature ventricular contractions.

Examples	Nursing Implications
atenolol (Tenormin)	Check apical pulse and blood pressure (BP) before giving.
esmolol (Brevibloc)	If pulse is less than 60 bpm and BP less than 100 mm Hg systolic, notify HCP.
metoprolol succinate (Lopressor, Toprol XL)	*Teach:*
	Change positions slowly and to not stop drug abruptly.

Calcium Channel Blocker

Decreases myocardial contractility and depresses conduction system. Controls rate in sinus tachycardia, atrial flutter, and AF.

Examples	Nursing Implications
diltiazem (Cardizem)	IV route used for symptomatic arrhythmias.
verapamil (Calan, Isoptin, Verelan)	Monitor for bradycardia and hypotension.

Inotrope—Cardiac Glycoside (Positive Inotrope and Negative Chronotrope)

Slows heart rate. Maintains sinus rhythm for sinus tachycardia, atrial flutter, and AF.

Examples	Nursing Implications
digoxin (Lanoxicaps, Lanoxin)	Take apical pulse for 1 minute; if less than 60 bpm, notify HCP.
	Therapeutic digoxin levels: 0.5 to 2 mg/mL.
	Monitor drug level and electrolytes as hypokalemia, hypomagnesemia, and hypercalcemia increase toxicity.

Vasopressors

Examples	Nursing Implications
For cardiac stimulation, vasoconstriction, and bronchodilation. Treats asystole, ventricular tachycardia, ventricular fibrillation, and symptomatic bradycardia.	Contraindicated with nonselective beta blockers.
epinephrine/adrenalin	
Increases cardiac output and blood pressure; treats bradycardia.	Monitor blood pressure and heart rate.
dopamine	

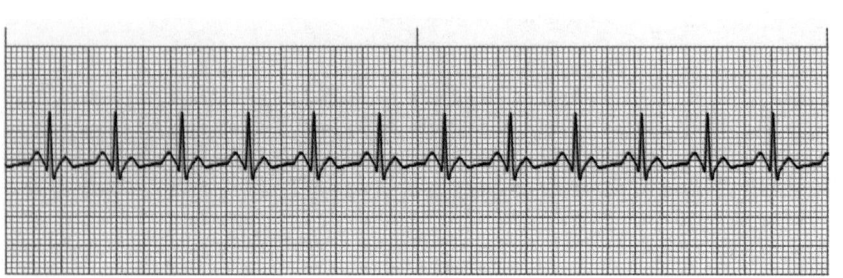

FIGURE 25.13 Sinus tachycardia. Heart rate is 125.

usually resolves the tachycardia. For example, if the patient is hemorrhaging, immediate intervention is needed to stop the bleeding and restore normal blood volume. Once normal blood volume is restored, the heart rate should return to normal.

LEARNING TIP

Tachycardia is often the first sign of hemorrhage. It is a compensatory mechanism to maintain cardiac output. If a patient develops sudden tachycardia, consider whether hemorrhage could be the cause. This could occur in postoperative patients, patients with gastrointestinal bleeding or cancer, or trauma patients. The bleeding may be external. It could be internal and, therefore, not visible. Apply pressure to the site if bleeding is seen. Report the tachycardia and any bleeding promptly for treatment.

Arrhythmias Originating in the Atria

As discussed, all areas of the heart can initiate an impulse. The SA node is the primary pacemaker. But if the atria begin to initiate impulses faster than the SA node, they become the primary pacemaker. Atrial rhythms are usually faster than 100 bpm. They can exceed 200 bpm. When an impulse originates outside the SA node, the P waves produced look different (flatter, notched, or peaked) from the rounded P waves from the SA node. This indicates that the SA node is not controlling the heart rate. The atrial impulses travel to the ventricles. They initiate a normal-shaped QRS complex after each P wave.

LEARNING TIP

If a QRS complex measures less than or equal to 0.10 seconds and an arrhythmia is present, the problem originated above the ventricles. This is known as a *supraventricular* (above the ventricle) *arrhythmia*.

Ventricular-originating arrhythmias produce wide QRS complexes that are greater than 0.10 seconds.

Premature Atrial Contractions

The term *premature* refers to an "early" beat. When the atria fire an impulse before the SA node fires, a premature beat results. If the underlying rhythm is NSR, the distance between R waves is the same except where the early beat occurs. When looking at the ECG strip, a shortened R-to-R interval

is seen where the premature beat occurs. The R wave preceding the premature atrial contraction (PAC) and the PAC's R wave are close together, followed by a pause, with the next beat being regular (Fig. 25.14).

ETIOLOGY. Causes of PACs include hypoxia, cigarette smoking, stress, myocardial ischemia, enlarged atria in valvular disorders, medications (such as digoxin), electrolyte imbalances, atrial fibrillation onset, and heart failure.

PREMATURE ATRIAL CONTRACTIONS RULES.
1. Rhythm: premature beat interrupts underlying rhythm where it occurs
2. Heart rate: depends on the underlying rhythm; if NSR, 60 to 100 bpm
3. P waves: early beat is abnormally shaped
4. PRI: usually appears normal, but premature beat could have shortened or prolonged PRI
5. QRS interval: less than or equal to 0.10 seconds (indicates normal conduction to ventricles)

SIGNS AND SYMPTOMS. PACs can occur in healthy individuals and those with a diseased heart. No symptoms are usually present. If several PACs occur in succession, the patient may report feeling palpitations.

THERAPEUTIC MEASURES. PACs are usually not serious. Often no treatment is required other than correcting the cause. Frequent PACs indicate atrial irritability. This can worsen into other atrial arrhythmias. Beta blockers can be given for frequent PACs to slow the heart rate (see Table 25.2).

Atrial Flutter

In atrial flutter, the atria contract, or flutter, at a rate of 250 to 350 bpm. The very rapid P waves appear as *flutter*, or F waves, on the ECG. They appear in a sawtooth pattern. Some of the impulses get through the AV node and reach the ventricles. This results in normal QRS complexes. There can be from two to four F waves between QRS complexes. If impulses pass through the AV node at a consistent rate, the rhythm is regular (Fig. 25.15). The classic characteristics of atrial flutter are more than one P wave before a QRS complex, a sawtooth pattern of P waves, and an atrial rate of 250 to 350 bpm.

ETIOLOGY. Causes of atrial flutter include rheumatic or ischemic heart diseases, congestive heart failure, hypertension, pericarditis, pulmonary embolism, and postoperative coronary artery bypass surgery. Many medications can also cause this arrhythmia.

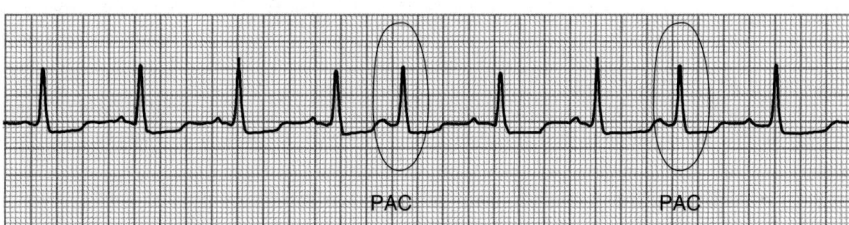

FIGURE 25.14 Premature atrial contractions.

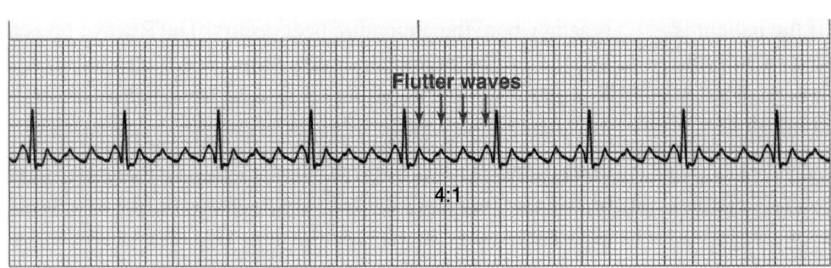

FIGURE 25.15 Atrial flutter.

ATRIAL FLUTTER RULES.
1. Rhythm: atrial rhythm regular; ventricular rhythm regular or irregular depending on consistency of AV conduction of impulses
2. Heart rate: ventricular rate varies
3. P waves: flutter or F waves with sawtooth pattern
4. PRI: none measurable
5. QRS interval: less than or equal to 0.10 seconds

SIGNS AND SYMPTOMS. The presence of symptoms in atrial flutter depends on the ventricular rate. If the ventricular rate is normal, usually no symptoms are present. If the rate is rapid, the patient may experience palpitations, angina, or dyspnea.

THERAPEUTIC MEASURES. The ventricular rate and adequacy of cardiac output guide treatment. The goal is to control the ventricular rate with conversion to NSR. For an unstable patient with a rapid ventricular rate, synchronized **cardioversion** (electrical shock) is used. Medications such as calcium channel blockers can be used to control the ventricular rate (see Table 25.2). Antiarrhythmic medications are used to convert atrial flutter. To terminate the atrial flutter in symptomatic patients, catheter **ablation** (usually in the right atrium) may be done.

Atrial Fibrillation
In atrial fibrillation (AF), the atrial rate is extremely rapid and chaotic. An atrial rate of 350 to 600 bpm can occur. However, the AV node blocks most of the impulses. So, the ventricular rate is much lower than the atrial rate. There are no definable P waves. The atria are fibrillating, or quivering, rather than beating effectively. No P waves can be seen or measured. A wavy pattern is produced on the ECG. Because the atrial rate is so irregular and only a few of the atrial impulses are allowed to pass through the AV node, the R waves are irregular. The ventricular rate varies from normal to rapid.

AF can be self-limiting, persistent, or permanent, which doubles the risk of death. Stroke risk is increased with AF. This is due to the risk of thrombus formation in the atria from blood stasis caused by poor emptying of blood from the quivering atria (Fig. 25.16).

ETIOLOGY. AF increases with age (65 and above), especially in those with heart disease. Causes include cardiac surgery, heart failure, hypertension, heart valve disease, MI, hyperthyroidism, emphysema, sleep apnea, and some medications. Sometimes the cause is unknown.

ATRIAL FIBRILLATION RULES.
1. Rhythm: irregularly irregular
2. Heart rate: atrial rate not measurable; ventricular rate under 100 bpm is controlled response; greater than 100 bpm is rapid ventricular response
3. P waves: no identifiable P waves
4. PRI: none can be measured because no P waves are seen
5. QRS interval: less than or equal to 0.10 seconds

> **LEARNING TIP**
> Atrial fibrillation is easy to identify based on its two classic characteristics on an electrocardiogram (ECG) strip: a lack of identifiable P waves and an irregularly irregular rhythm (R waves).

SIGNS AND SYMPTOMS. With AF, most patients feel the irregular rhythm. Many describe it as palpitations, a racing heart, or a skipping heartbeat. They may feel short of breath, be dizzy, or have chest discomfort. A patient's radial pulse may be faint because of a decreased stroke volume (volume of blood ejected with each contraction). If the ventricular rhythm is rapid and sustained, the patient can go into left-sided heart failure.

THERAPEUTIC MEASURES. The focus of AF treatment is to control rate, prevent thromboembolism, and restore normal rhythm. If the patient is unstable, synchronized cardioversion is done immediately to try to return the heart to NSR. For the patient who is stable, medications to control the ventricular rate are used. These include beta blockers, calcium channel blockers, or digoxin (see Table 25.2). Anticoagulant therapy is given to reduce thrombi and stroke risk. Pharmacological or electrical cardioversion may be used to convert the rhythm to NSR. It should be done after sufficient anticoagulation (3 to 4 weeks) to stabilize or resolve any existing blood clots in the atria. This prevents them from being dislodged and causing a stroke. Rhythm control medications such as sodium or potassium channel blockers are used to restore and maintain NSR. If known, the underlying cause of AF is treated. For patients with AF who do not respond to medications or electrical cardioversion, other therapies can be used.

• WORD • BUILDING •
ablation: ab—away from + lat—carry

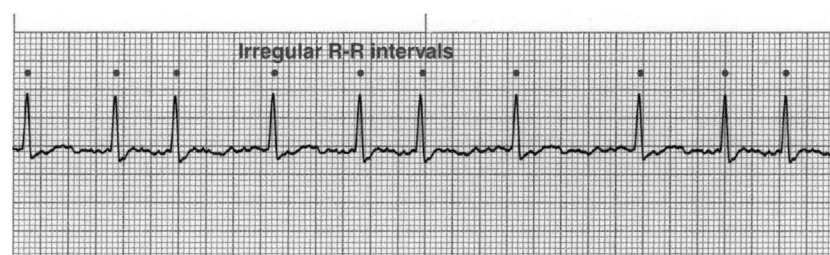

FIGURE 25.16 Atrial fibrillation.

Catheter Ablation. To isolate impulses coming from the pulmonary veins (most AF impulses arise from pulmonary veins) or AV node, catheter ablation may be used to cure AF. Intracardiac echocardiography maps the area of the heart requiring treatment. Then, released energy, such as cryothermy or radiofrequency energy, creates lesions either on all four pulmonary veins or near the AV node. The lesions heal and scar. This blocks those pathways to future impulses. Postprocedural care is similar to postangioplasty or postcardiac catheterization care (see Chapter 21).

Surgery. The maze procedure is often done as minimally invasive robotic-guided surgery. Incisions are made in the atria that create a "maze," or route, for electrical impulses to travel to the AV node. These impulses cannot go off course because scar tissue surrounds the incision sites.

Third-Degree Atrioventricular Block

In third-degree AV block, SA node impulses are blocked and do not reach the ventricles to stimulate them to contract (Fig. 25.17). This is also known as *complete heart block* (CHB) or *third-degree heart block*. The escape pacemakers for the heart (junctional [AV node] or ventricular) must produce electrical impulses to cause the ventricles to contract or else cardiac arrest will occur. Depending on the origin of the escape beat, the QRS complex will either be narrow (junctional) or wide (ventricular) on the ECG. Normal P waves march across the ECG strip at a constant P-to-P interval without any relationship to the regularly occurring but slower QRS complexes.

ETIOLOGY. Cardiac ischemia or infarction, **hyperkalemia** (elevated serum potassium), infection, antiarrhythmic medications, or digoxin toxicity are some common causes of CHB.

SIGNS AND SYMPTOMS. With narrow QRS complex escape rhythms, there are fewer symptoms such as dizziness, chest pain, and fatigue. Typically, severe symptoms are seen, including when wide QRS complex escape rhythms occur. These include confusion, dyspnea, severe chest pain, hypotension, or syncope.

THIRD-DEGREE ATRIOVENTRICULAR BLOCK RULES.
1. Rhythm: P-to-P interval regular; R-to-R interval regular; atria and ventricles controlled by separate electrical impulses from foci that are firing regularly
2. Heart rate: atrial 60 to 100 bpm; ventricular rate slower: 40 to 60 bpm is junctional foci; 20 to 40 bpm is ventricular foci

3. P waves: rounded, upright, alike; more P waves than QRS complexes; may occur within a QRS complex or upon a T wave
4. PRI: no P waves conducted to the ventricles, so no relationship to the QRS complexes; therefore, there is no actual PRI (may appear as if the PRI varies)
5. QRS interval: less than or equal to 0.10 (junctional origin); greater than 0.10 (ventricular origin)

THERAPEUTIC MEASURES. CHB is a medical emergency. Oxygen is given. If the patient is symptomatic, transcutaneous pacing is needed immediately. Atropine might be carefully considered, if the patient is not symptomatic. Depending on the cause, a permanent pacemaker may be required for the rest of the patient's life. A temporary pacemaker may be used until the permanent pacemaker can be implanted. If medication toxicity is the cause, the CHB may be gone after the toxicity is resolved. A temporary pacemaker may be needed until this occurs.

Ventricular Arrhythmias

Premature ventricular contractions (PVCs) originate in the ventricles from an ectopic focus (a site other than the SA node). The irritable ventricles fire prematurely, before the SA node does. When the ventricles fire first, the impulses are not conducted normally through the electrical pathway. This results in a wide (greater than 0.10 seconds), bizarre QRS complex on an ECG (Fig. 25.18).

PVCs can occur in different shapes. **Unifocal** (one focus) PVCs all look the same. This is because they come from the same irritable ventricular area. **Multifocal** (multiple foci) PVCs do not all look the same because they are originating from several irritable areas in the ventricle.

There can be several repetitive cycles or patterns of PVCs:

- **Bigeminy** occurs every other beat (a normal beat and then a PVC; Fig. 25.19).
- **Trigeminy** occurs every third beat (two normal beats and then a PVC).
- **Quadrigeminy** occurs every fourth beat (three normal beats and then a PVC).
- When two PVCs occur together, they are referred to as a couplet (pair).

• WORD • BUILDING •

hyperkalemia: hyper—above + kalium—potassium + emia—blood

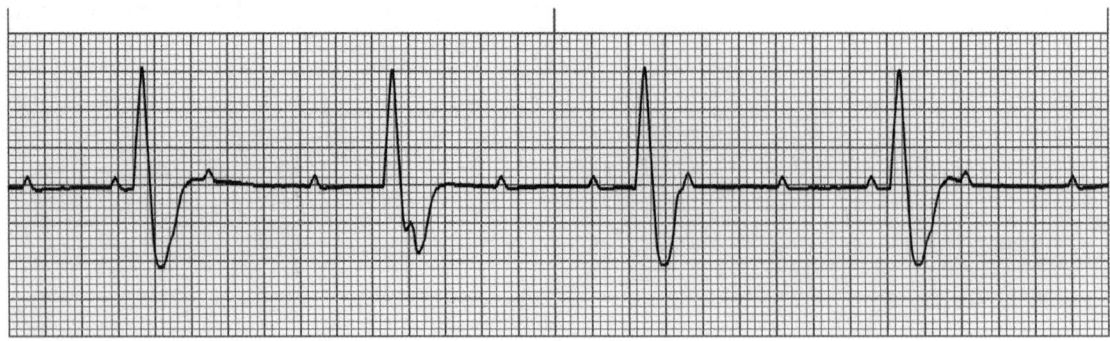

FIGURE 25.17 Third-degree atrioventricular block.

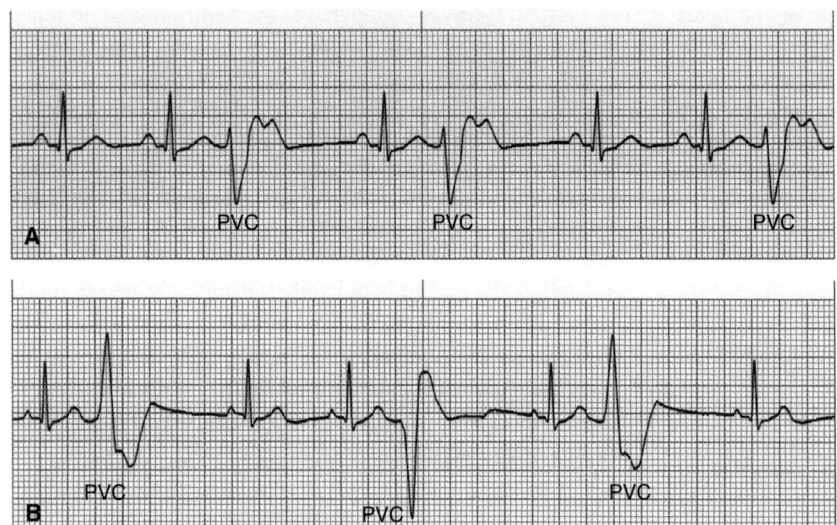

FIGURE 25.18 Premature ventricular contractions. (A) Unifocal PVCs arise from one foci (area) and look the same. (B) Multifocal PVCs arise from different foci and may look different.

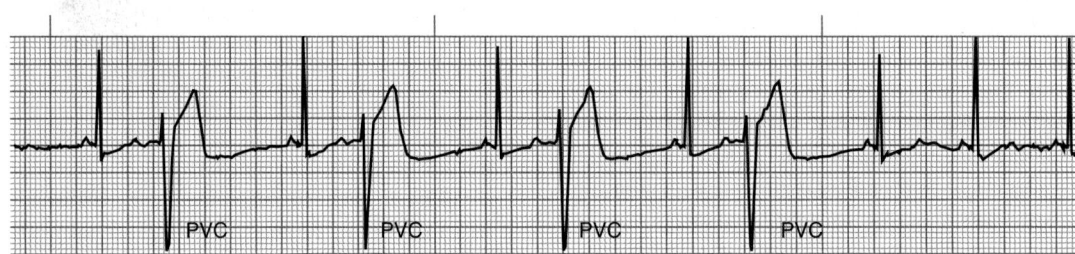

FIGURE 25.19 Bigeminal premature ventricular contractions.

• If three or more PVCs occur in a row, it is referred to as a run of PVCs or ventricular tachycardia.

ETIOLOGY. Use of caffeine or alcohol, anxiety, hypokalemia, cardiomyopathy, ischemia, and MI are common causes of PVCs.

PREMATURE VENTRICULAR CONTRACTION RULES.
1. Rhythm: depends on the underlying rhythm; PVC usually interrupts rhythm
2. Heart rate: depends on underlying rhythm
3. P waves: absent before PVC QRS complex
4. PRI: none for PVC
5. QRS interval: if PVC, is greater than 0.10 seconds; T wave is in the opposite direction of QRS complex (i.e., QRS upright, T downward; or QRS downward, T upright).

SIGNS AND SYMPTOMS. PVCs may be felt by the patient. They are described as a skipped beat or palpitations. With frequent PVCs, cardiac output can be decreased. This leads to fatigue, dizziness, or more severe arrhythmias.

THERAPEUTIC MEASURES. Treatment depends on the type and number of PVCs and whether symptoms are produced. Occasional PVCs do not usually require treatment. However, if the PVCs are more than six per minute, regularly occurring, multifocal, falling on the T wave (known as *R-on-T phenomenon,* which can trigger life-threatening arrhythmias), or caused by an acute MI, they can be dangerous. Antidysrhythmic drugs such as lidocaine (Xylocaine) and beta blockers that depress myocardial activity are used to treat PVCs (see Table 25.2).

CRITICAL THINKING

Mrs. Mae, age 70, is 5 days postmyocardial infarction without complications. You assist her back to bed after she ambulates at 1400 hours. Her oxygen is on at 2 L/min via nasal cannula. Her vital signs are blood pressure 126/78 mm Hg, apical pulse 82 bpm, and respiratory rate 18 breaths per minute. She has no pain and says she feels good after walking. The cardiac monitor shows normal sinus rhythm. Five minutes later, you see that the monitor shows sinus rhythm with premature ventricular contractions of less than six per minute. Her vital signs are now blood pressure 132/84 mm Hg, apical pulse 92 bpm (regularly irregular), and respiratory rate 22 breaths per minute. She reports no pain but says, "I can feel my heart skipping. It takes my breath away." You call the registered nurse while staying with the patient to provide reassurance.

1. What should you do first?
2. What should you do regarding the arrhythmia?
3. What might be some causes for this arrhythmia?
4. What symptoms, if any, would you expect to be present?
5. What would you do if symptoms were present?
6. With which health care team members might you collaborate?
7. What type of orders would you anticipate from the health care provider?
8. How would you document your findings?

Suggested answers are at the end of the chapter.

Ventricular Tachycardia

The occurrence of three or more PVCs in a row is referred to as **ventricular tachycardia** (VT) (Fig. 25.20). VT results from the continuous firing of an ectopic ventricular focus. During VT, the ventricles rather than the SA node become the pacemaker of the heart. The pathway of the ventricular impulses is different from normal conduction, producing a wide (greater than 0.10 seconds), bizarre QRS complex.

ETIOLOGY. Myocardial irritability, MI, and cardiomyopathy are common causes of VT. Respiratory acidosis, hypokalemia, digoxin toxicity, cardiac catheters, and pacing wires can also produce VT.

VENTRICULAR TACHYCARDIA RULES.

1. Rhythm: usually regular, may have some irregularity
2. Heart rate: 150 to 250 ventricular bpm; slow VT is below 150 bpm
3. P waves: absent
4. PRI: none
5. QRS interval: greater than 0.10 seconds

SIGNS AND SYMPTOMS. Patients are aware of a sudden onset of rapid heart rate. They can experience dyspnea, palpitations, and light-headedness. Angina commonly occurs. The seriousness of VT is determined by the duration of the arrhythmia. Sustained VT compromises cardiac output. It can become pulseless VT.

THERAPEUTIC MEASURES. For a patient who is stable, antidysrhythmic medications are used. If the patient is pulseless or not breathing, cardiopulmonary resuscitation (CPR) and immediate **defibrillation** are required ("Evidence-Based Practice"). Advanced cardiac life support (ACLS) protocols for pulseless VT treatment are used. Medications may include epinephrine, and lidocaine or amiodarone (see Table 25.2).

Evidence-Based Practice

Clinical Question

What is the best method for bystander cardiopulmonary resuscitation (CPR) on an adult?

Evidence

A systematic review of three randomized and quasi-randomized studies for bystander-provided CPR revealed high-quality evidence. When bystanders used chest compressions during CPR, guided by telephone instruction from emergency personnel, there was an increase in those who survived to hospital discharge when compared with conventional interrupted chest compression CPR with rescue breathing (Zhan, Yang, Huang, He, & Liu, 2017).

Implications for Nursing Practice

Encourage patients and their families to become certified in basic life support to be able to respond to an emergency.

Reference

Zhan, L., Yang, L. J., Huang, Y., He, Q., & Liu, G. J. (2017). Continuous chest compression versus interrupted chest compression for cardiopulmonary resuscitation of non-asphyxial out-of-hospital cardiac arrest. *Cochrane Database of Systematic Reviews, 2017*(3). CD010134. doi:10.1002/14651858.CD010134.pub2

CRITICAL THINKING

Mrs. Parker, age 76, is admitted to the long-term care unit where you are working. She has been transferred from the hospital after treatment for a recent myocardial infarction and several episodes of ventricular tachycardia (VT). At 1600 hours, you find her unresponsive, with no palpable pulses and shallow respirations. Vital signs are blood pressure 80/40 mm Hg, apical pulse 150 bpm, and respiratory rate 6 breaths per minute.

1. Why are there no palpable pulses?
2. What is happening to the heart when VT is occurring?
3. What action should you take?
4. How will you document your findings?

Suggested answers are at the end of the chapter.

• **WORD · BUILDING** •
defibrillation: de—from + fibrillation—quivering fibers

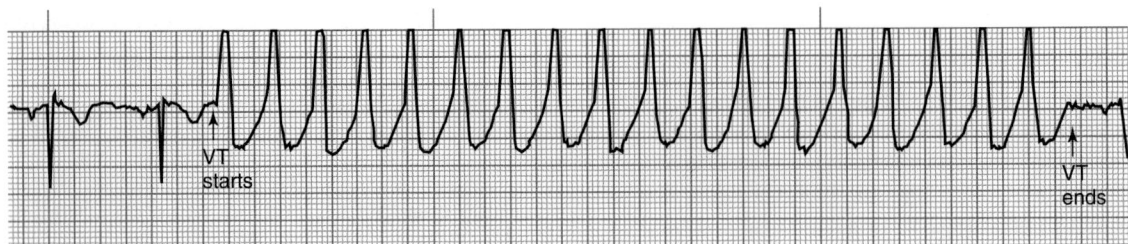

FIGURE 25.20 Ventricular tachycardia.

Ventricular Fibrillation

Ventricular fibrillation (VF) occurs when many ectopic ventricular foci fire at the same time. Ventricular activity is chaotic. There are no discernible waves (Fig. 25.21). The ventricle quivers. It is unable to initiate a contraction. There is a complete loss of cardiac output. If this rhythm is not corrected immediately, death occurs.

ETIOLOGY. Hyperkalemia, **hypomagnesemia** (low serum magnesium), electrocution, coronary artery disease, and MI are all possible causes of VF. Placement of intracardiac catheters and cardiac pacing wires can also lead to ventricular irritability and then VF.

VENTRICULAR FIBRILLATION RULES.
1. Rhythm: chaotic and extremely irregular
2. Heart rate: not measurable
3. P waves: none
4. PRI: none
5. QRS complex: none

SIGNS AND SYMPTOMS. Patients experiencing VF lose consciousness immediately. There are no heart sounds, peripheral pulses, or blood pressure readings. These are all indicative of circulatory collapse. Respiratory arrest, cyanosis, and pupil dilation occur.

THERAPEUTIC MEASURES. Immediate defibrillation is the best treatment for terminating VF. Each minute that passes without defibrillation reduces survival. CPR is started until the defibrillator is available. Automatic external defibrillators provide quick access to easily used technology for defibrillation (see "Defibrillation" section). Endotracheal intubation with oxygen supports respiratory function. Medications are given according to ACLS protocols. They include epinephrine, and amiodarone or lidocaine (see Table 25.2).

Asystole

Asystole (the silent heart) is the absence of electrical activity within the cardiac muscle. It is referred to as cardiac arrest. A straight line appears on an ECG strip (Fig. 25.22).

ETIOLOGY. Hyperkalemia, VF, or a loss of a majority of functional cardiac muscle due to an MI are common causes of asystole. VF usually precedes asystole. VF must be reversed immediately to help prevent asystole.

ASYSTOLE RULES.
1. Rhythm: none
2. Heart rate: none
3. P waves: none
4. PRI: none
5. QRS interval: none

SIGNS AND SYMPTOMS. Patients in asystole are unconscious and unresponsive. There are no heart sounds, peripheral pulses, blood pressure readings, or respirations.

THERAPEUTIC MEASURES. CPR is started immediately. Endotracheal intubation and oxygen supports respirations. Epinephrine is administered per ACLS protocols (see Table 25.2). Reversible causes are treated.

CARDIAC PACEMAKERS

Pacemakers are used to generate an electrical impulse when there is a problem with the heart's conduction system. Permanent pacemakers are used for symptomatic bradycardia and third-degree AV block (complete dissociation between atrial and ventricular activity). Pacemakers can be temporary (epicardial, transcutaneous, transvenous) or permanent (Fig. 25.23). The newest advance in pacemaker technology is the leadless pacemaker.

Temporary pacemakers treat bradycardia or tachycardia (overdrive pacing) that does not respond to medications or synchronized cardioversion. They may also be used after an MI to allow the heart time to heal. The temporary pacemaker becomes the electrical conduction system. It stimulates the atria and ventricles to contract. This maintains cardiac output. Temporary pacemakers can be inserted during valve or open heart surgery (epicardial). They can also be used in the cardiac catheterization lab or critical care unit (CCU; transvenous) for emergency treatment. They are kept in place until surgery can be scheduled to implant a permanent pacemaker. Transcutaneous pacemakers are used in emergency situations. They are quick and easy to apply. Impulses are delivered from the external generator via electrodes on the skin to the heart. The electrodes are placed on the chest and back.

• WORD • BUILDING •
hypomagnesemia: hypo—below + magnes—magnesium + emia—blood

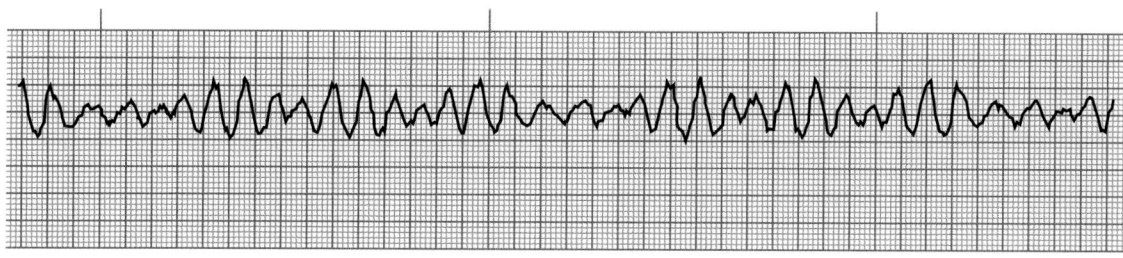

FIGURE 25.21 Ventricular fibrillation.

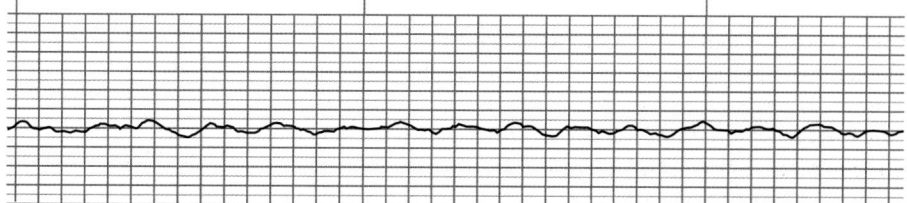

FIGURE 25.22 Asystole.

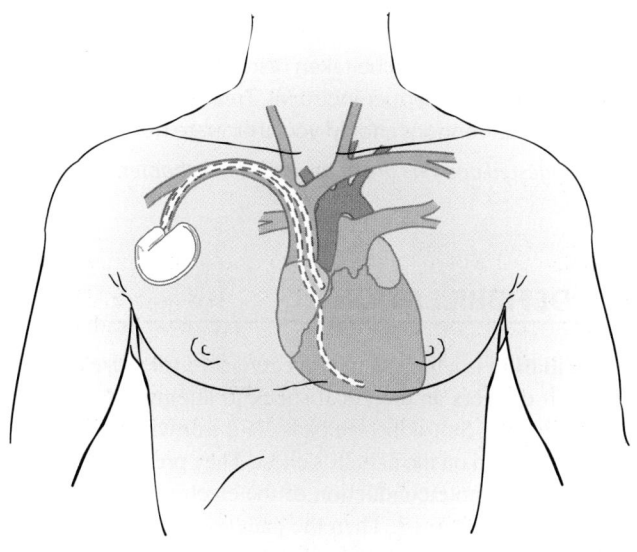

FIGURE 25.23 Dual-chamber permanent pacemaker.

Permanent Pacemaker

Permanent pacemaker implantation is a procedure in which **fluoroscopy,** a screen that shows an image similar to a radiograph, is used. The pacemaker generator is implanted subcutaneously. It is attached to leads (insulated conducting wires) that are inserted via a vein into the heart. The lead then delivers an impulse directly to the heart wall. A single-lead pacemaker paces either the right atrium or right ventricle into which it is placed. Dual-chamber pacemakers have two leads. One is in the right atrium, and the other is in the right ventricle. This allows pacing of both chambers. Activity-responsive pacemakers provide a rate range (e.g., 60 to 115 bpm). They allow rate changes in response to a person's activity level. This provides the patient with greater flexibility for increasing cardiac output when needed, such as during exercise.

Leadless Pacemaker

The first leadless pacemaker was approved by the U.S. Food and Drug Administration in 2016 (visit www.medtronic.com). It is implanted into the right ventricle, with no leads. Everything is contained within the pacemaker. It is inserted via a leg vein so no chest incision is needed. It is about the size of a vitamin capsule. The battery lasts about 12 years. Currently, it is only available for single-chamber right ventricular pacing. Traditional pacemakers will continue to be used until additional types of leadless pacemakers are developed.

Pacemaker Activity

When a patient is in a paced rhythm, a small spike (vertical line) is seen on the ECG at the start of the paced beat. This spike is the electrical stimulus. It can precede the P wave, QRS complex, or both depending on what is being paced (Fig. 25.24). Patients may have 100% paced beats, a mixture of their own beats and paced beats, or 100% their own beats. Pacemakers should not fire during a patients' own beat.

Problems that can occur with pacemakers include the following:

- Failure to sense a patient's own beat
- Failure to pace because of a malfunction of the pulse generator
- Failure to capture, which is the heart's lack of depolarization

Nursing Care for Patients With Pacemakers

Patients' heart rhythm, apical pulse, and incision are monitored after implantation of a pacemaker. Irregular heart rhythms or a rate slower than the pacemaker's set rate can indicate pacemaker malfunction. Any change in heart rhythm, reports of

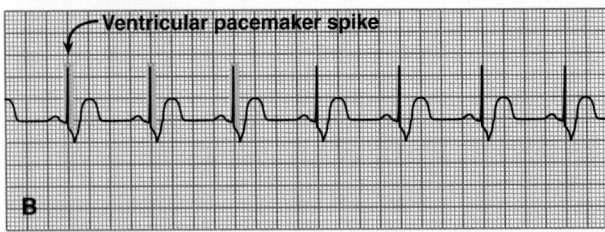

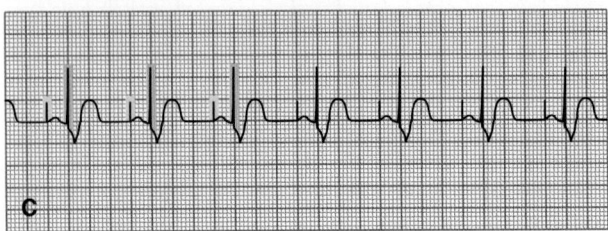

FIGURE 25.24 ECG tracings. (A) Atrial-only pacemaker (yellow spike before P wave). (B) Ventricular-only pacemaker (green spike before QRS). (C) Dual-chamber pacemaker that paces both atrial and ventricular chambers (yellow spike before P and green spike before QRS).

chest pain, or changes in vital signs are reported immediately. The patient may have outpatient surgery or remain in the hospital overnight.

Pacemaker teaching before discharge includes:

- Care for incision as instructed (e.g., dressing removal, keeping it clean and dry, resuming showers).
- Maintain ordered activity restrictions (e.g., limit raising arm on pacemaker side, driving, returning to work).
- Be aware of devices:
  - Safe devices: microwaves, cell phones less than 3 watts, Bluetooth headset, most common household devices.
  - Caution to be used with devices: security metal detectors (avoid having a hand wand passed over the pacemaker), antitheft systems, MP3 player headphones (keep 3 cm away), extracorporeal shock-wave lithotripsy.
  - Devices with risk: strong electromagnetic fields such as from magnetic resonance imaging (MRI; unless your system is one that has been designed for use with MRI, such as the complete Revo MRI SureScan pacing system), welders above 130 amps, radio towers, or touching running car engines (information is available on pacemaker manufacturer and the AHA Web sites regarding various devices).
  - If you become light-headed or dizzy near an electromagnetic device, move away from it.
- Carry a pacemaker identification card to show to HCPs, airport security, or other security staff. Pacemaker metal

may set off alarms, but the device is not harmed if one walks normally through the security device.

- Report chest pain, dizziness, fainting, irregular heartbeats, palpitations, muscle twitching, or hiccups to the HCP.
- Report signs of incision infection (e.g., redness, swelling, warmth, pain, fever, discharge) to the HCP.
- Keep scheduled appointments with the HCP. Periodic pacemaker checks will be done by the HCP or remotely from home. The HCP can reprogram the pacemaker if needed.

CRITICAL THINKING

Mr. Treacher, age 58, underwent pacemaker placement 6 days ago and has a 100% paced rhythm. You are making patient rounds. You find his vital signs are blood pressure 138/72 mm Hg and apical pulse 72 bpm. Thirty minutes later, he says that he feels weak and tired. His vital signs are now blood pressure 100/60 mm Hg and apical pulse 60 bpm and irregular.

1. What is your first action?
2. What actions should be taken next?
3. What might be happening to Mr. Treacher?
4. What interventions should you anticipate next?

Suggested answers are at the end of the chapter.

 DEFIBRILLATION

Defibrillation is a lifesaving procedure used for pulseless VT or VF. It delivers an electrical shock to attempt to reset the heart's rhythm. Self-adhesive pads (saline or with conductive jelly) are placed on the patient's chest. They prevent electrical burns and promote conduction of the electrical charge. The defibrillator is charged. Then the paddles are pressed firmly and evenly against the chest wall to prevent burns or electrical arcing (Fig. 25.25). For safety, the person who is defibrillating must announce "Clear." The phrase "One. I'm clear. Two. You're clear. Three. All clear" is suggested. No one, including the person defibrillating, should touch the bed or patient during this time to avoid also being shocked. ACLS protocols specify the guidelines for resuscitation.

After successful defibrillation, the patient is assessed for a pulse and adequate tissue perfusion. The patient is treated in the CCU after successful resuscitation.

Emotional support for an alert patient who experienced cardiac arrest and defibrillation is an important aspect of nursing care. This can be an extremely frightening event for the patient. It is important to explain to the patient what happened. Then listen and allow him or her to express concerns. The patient is reassured that continuous cardiac monitoring is done in the CCU. Families also require emotional support during resuscitation of a loved one. They may be present during the resuscitation per agency policy.

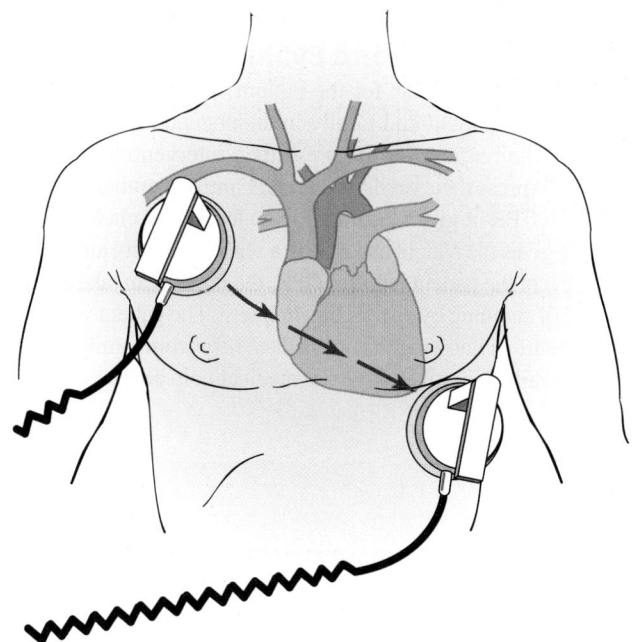

FIGURE 25.25 Placement of defibrillator paddles on chest.

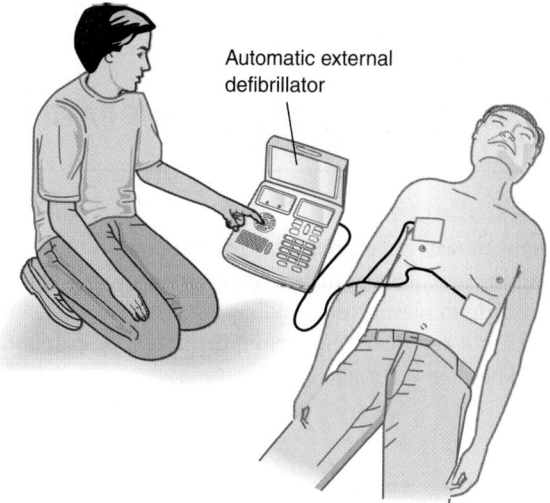

Automatic external defibrillator

FIGURE 25.26 Automatic external defibrillator.

 CARDIOVERSION

Cardioversion is performed with a defibrillator set in the synchronized mode. In the synchronized mode, a mark is highlighted on the patient's R waves. The R wave must be recognized for a shock to be delivered. When the discharge button is pressed, the shock is released when the machine senses it is safe to do so. The number of joules delivered with each shock usually ranges from 25 to 50. The procedure for delivering the shock safely is the same as for defibrillation.

Synchronized cardioversion is used for VT with a pulse. Elective synchronized cardioversion is used for arrhythmias that are not responsive to drug therapy. These include AF, atrial flutter, and supraventricular tachycardia. The patient is given a sedative and monitored by anesthesia professionals during the procedure.

If cardioversion is successful, there should be a return to NSR. If the rhythm does not immediately convert, additional cardioversion attempts can be made by the HCP. After the procedure, the patient is monitored for skin burns, rhythm disturbances and changes in the ST segment, vital sign changes and hypotension, and respiratory problems.

 OTHER METHODS TO CORRECT ARRHYTHMIAS

Automatic External Defibrillators

An automatic external defibrillator (AED) is an external device that automatically analyzes rhythms. For VF or VT, it will either automatically deliver or prompt the operator to deliver an electrical shock for a shockable rhythm (Fig. 25.26).

Minimally trained laypersons or hospital and rescue personnel can use these devices with little risk of injury to the patient because the AED analyzes the rhythm rather than the operator. The patient is connected to the AED with adhesive sternal-apex pads attached to cables coming from the device. This connection allows hands-free defibrillation.

AEDs are found in public places such as shopping malls, airports, stadiums, casinos, golf courses, and airplanes for immediate access. Defibrillation attempts must occur within minutes of cardiac arrest to increase chance of survival. AEDs are available for home use. They are recommended for people at high risk of sudden cardiac arrest. They are helpful for those at risk with rescue access that will take longer than 4 minutes, such as people living in rural areas, gated communities, or secured-access buildings.

Implantable Cardioverter Defibrillator

An implantable cardioverter defibrillator (ICD) or a combination pacemaker/ICD is placed into the chest of a patient who experiences life-threatening arrhythmias or is at risk for sudden cardiac death. ICDs have decreased the number of deaths from these arrhythmias by analyzing and treating these heart rhythms. When a life-threatening rhythm is detected that could cause death (VF), the ICD automatically delivers an electrical shock. If the arrhythmia does not convert on the initial shock, more shocks are delivered sequentially.

If the device detects VT, it cardioverts the rhythm with lower energy. ICDs also have antitachycardia pacing ability if a tachycardia rhythm is detected. Battery life depends on usage. When battery life is getting low, the entire unit needs to be changed within a few months.

Patients with ICDs can be extremely anxious about receiving shocks from the ICD. Defibrillator or cardioversion shocks may feel like a kick in the chest. Reinforcement of patient and family education is important. To prevent problems, those with ICDs should take the same precautions as discussed earlier for those with pacemakers. Provide emotional support and answer questions.

 NURSING PROCESS FOR THE PATIENT WITH ARRHYTHMIAS

Data Collection

Patients at risk for arrhythmias require careful monitoring. Obtaining apical and radial pulses at frequent intervals helps detect arrhythmias. Most arrhythmias are not life-threatening. A patient's report of chest pain, dizziness, or palpitations should be reported to the HCP.

Nursing Diagnoses, Planning, Implementation, and Evaluation

See "Nursing Care Plan for the Patient With Arrhythmias."

Assist the patient and family in understanding the plan of care and the reasons for the prescribed interventions. Allow them to express their needs and fears. Family members should be taught CPR or given information on local CPR classes. This training gives the patient and family a sense of control and hope. In the event the patient requires CPR, the family can take action instead of standing by and feeling helpless. The patient will feel more secure in knowing that immediate help from family members is available until emergency medical help arrives.

Nursing Care Plan for the Patient With Arrhythmias

Nursing Diagnosis: *Decreased Cardiac Output* related to arrhythmias
Expected Outcomes: The patient's cardiac status will be stabilized. Patient will be able to perform activities of daily living (ADLs).
Evaluation of Outcomes: There is an absence of arrhythmias. The patient performs ADLs without tachycardia, chest pain, or weakness.

Intervention	Rationale	Evaluation
Take apical and radial pulses with frequency based on stability. Monitor blood pressure and urinary output.	*Monitors for arrhythmias, impending cardiac arrest, or shock. Blood pressure, pulse, and urinary output are indicators of cardiac output.*	Is patient free of arrhythmias with vital signs within normal limits?
Monitor mental status every 2 to 4 hours.	*Dizziness, confusion, and restlessness may indicate decreased cerebral blood flow.*	Does patient show signs of decreased cerebral perfusion, such as confusion?
Listen to lung sounds every 2 to 4 hours.	*Arrhythmias can cause heart failure.*	Are lungs clear with no report of dyspnea?
Administer oxygen as ordered.	*Increases oxygenation to the heart and brain.*	Is patient free of chest pain, confusion, and light-headedness?
Ensure that patient gets adequate rest and does not exceed activity tolerance.	*Reduces dyspnea and decreases oxygen demand on the myocardium.*	Does patient rest and tolerate activity without dyspnea or chest pain?

Geriatric

Administer medications as ordered, and observe for adverse reactions.	*Older patients may have decreased kidney and liver function that may lead to rapid development of toxicity.*	Does patient have signs of toxicity?

Nursing Diagnosis: *Anxiety* related to situational crisis
Expected Outcomes: The patient will be able to effectively manage anxiety. The patient will report decreased anxiety.
Evaluation of Outcomes: The patient uses effective coping mechanisms to manage anxiety. Patient expresses decreased anxiety.

Intervention	Rationale	Evaluation
Ask about level of anxiety.	*Establishes a baseline.*	What is patient's level of anxiety?
Encourage patient and family to verbalize fears.	*Helps correct and clarify their concerns.*	What are patient's feelings or fears?

Nursing Care Plan for the Patient With Arrhythmias—cont'd

Intervention	Rationale	Evaluation
Explain procedures to patient and family.	*Lack of knowledge increases anxiety. This knowledge will help with compliance of therapy.*	Does patient express understanding of therapy with decreased anxiety?
Identify and reduce as many environmental stressors as possible.	*Anxiety often results from lack of trust in the environment.*	Can patient describe two situations that increase tension?
Teach patient relaxation techniques to be performed every 4 to 6 hours, such as guided imagery, muscle relaxation, and meditation.	*These measures can restore psychological and physical equilibrium and help decrease anxiety.*	Is patient successful in demonstrating relaxation methods?
Medicate with antianxiety agents as ordered.	*Aids the patient in decreasing anxiety.*	Does patient show decreased anxiety?

Home Health Hints

• The home health care nurse should have a pocket mask for cardiopulmonary resuscitation (CPR) available at all times.
• If the patient reports straining, request a laxative or stool softener order from the health care provider (HCP). Patients prone to arrhythmias should avoid straining with bowel movements.
• Visual disturbances can occur from digitalis toxicity. If the patient sees halos around lights or red-green tinting on everything, report this to the HCP.

• Teach patients on beta blockers and inotropic agents (e.g., digoxin) how to take their radial pulse, because bradycardia is a major side effect. For a pulse below 50 bpm, call the HCP.
• Teach patients who are leaving home for the weekend or holidays to refill medicines ahead of time. The HCP might write a prescription for patients to have while away for emergencies.
• Teach patients with a new pacemaker to wear loose tops. Women may want to wear a small pad over the pacemaker to protect it from the bra strap.

SUGGESTED ANSWERS TO CRITICAL THINKING

Mrs. Mae

1. Assess the patient's vital signs and heart sounds, note symptoms, and obtain an electrocardiogram (ECG) per agency protocol.
2. Report the patient findings to the registered nurse (RN) or health care provider (HCP).
3. Possible causes include hypokalemia or ischemia leading to irritability of the heart.
4. Symptoms might include light-headedness, feeling of heart skipping, chest pain, or fatigue.
5. To alleviate symptoms, elevate the head of bed for comfort, monitor vital signs, and maintain oxygen at 2 L/min via nasal cannula per agency protocol. Remain with the patient to help alleviate anxiety. Notify the RN.

6. RN, respiratory therapist, HCP.
7. Orders might include ECG, oxygen, potassium, or electrolytes.
8. Documentation should include the following:
   • 1400: Ambulated 20 feet with one assist. Vital signs stable. Stated: "Feel good. Pain zero."
   • Tolerated well. Assisted to bed. Oxygen at 2 L/min via nasal cannula.
   • 1405: see ECG strip with intermittent PVCs. Vital signs: BP 132/84 mm Hg; apical 92 bpm, irregular; R 22 breaths per minute.
   • "Pain zero. I can feel my heart skipping, it takes my breath away." RN notified.

Continued

SUGGESTED ANSWERS TO CRITICAL THINKING—cont'd

Mrs. Parker

1. A heart in ventricular tachycardia (VT) has an ectopic focus that is initiating impulses. The heart is unable to maintain adequate cardiac output with such a rapid heart rate. The rapid and irregular heart rhythm does not allow the heart chambers time to adequately fill and empty, thereby reducing the blood volume with each beat. This in turn affects the peripheral circulation, causing the absence of palpable pulses.

2. In VT, one or more sites in the ventricle may be initiating impulses. The rapid rate of VT overrides the normal pacemaker of the heart. The rhythm can be regular or irregular. The inability of the heart to conduct impulses along normal pathways prevents the chambers from emptying and filling properly. This leads to a decreased cardiac output and can lead to cardiac arrest if the rhythm is not converted.

3. Understand advance directive status. Begin cardiopulmonary resuscitation (CPR), if applicable. Call for assistance and have 911 called.

4. Documentation should include the following: 1600: Patient found in bed unresponsive to verbal and tactile stimuli. Respirations shallow. No palpable pulses. BP 80/40 mm Hg, P 150 bpm, R 6 breaths per minute. CPR started. Assistance arrived at 1602 and 911 called.

Mr. Treacher

1. Your first actions should be to obtain an ECG per agency protocol and to notify the RN or HCP. The emergency number 911 may need to be called.

2. You should keep the head of the bed elevated and administer oxygen at 2 L/min via nasal cannula per protocol. Turn the patient onto his side because this may help float the pacemaker wire to the chamber wall for better contact. Monitor the patient's vital signs and symptoms, and remain with patient to provide emotional support.

3. Mr. Treacher could be experiencing pacemaker malfunction.

4. Interventions may include transfer to a hospital emergency department for assessment and reprogramming of the pacemaker or a return to surgery for manipulation or replacement of the pacemaker wires.

Review Questions

1. Place the following in the correct sequence for normal electrical impulse movement through the cardiac conduction system.
   1. Atrioventricular node
   2. Bundle of His
   3. Internodal tracts
   4. Purkinje fibers
   5. Sinoatrial node

2. The nurse prepares to document an electrocardiogram rhythm. The nurse uses a systematic method for analyzing the electrocardiogram tracing for which of the following reasons?
   1. To prevent abnormalities from being missed
   2. To save time
   3. To develop a routine for examining tracings
   4. To increase memory of the analysis steps

3. The nurse responds to a call for assistance with a patient in pulseless ventricular tachycardia. The nurse should prepare for what first-line treatment for this rhythm?
   1. Antiarrhythmic medication
   2. Defibrillation
   3. Pacemaker
   4. Synchronized cardioversion

4. The nurse is reinforcing teaching to a patient after insertion of a pacemaker. Which of the following instructions should the nurse give the patient regarding pacemaker care? **Select all that apply.**
   1. "Avoid microwaves."
   2. "All types of pacemakers are compatible with magnetic resonance imaging."
   3. "Avoid strong electromagnetic devices."
   4. "You will need to be on bedrest for 48 hours."
   5. "MP3 player headphones should be kept 3 centimeters from the pacemaker."
   6. "Take pulse daily and report rates 5 beats under or over set rate."

5. The nurse is ambulating a patient who is recovering from a myocardial infarction when the patient develops chest pain with an irregular pulse. Which of these is the safest way for the nurse to return the patient to bed?
   1. Ambulation to room with one assistant
   2. With assistance by gurney
   3. With assistance by a wheelchair
   4. After completion of ambulation

6. A patient has a radial pulse of 58 beats per minute. Which of the following should the nurse use to document this finding?
   1. Normal
   2. Asystole
   3. Bradycardia
   4. Tachycardia

7. The nurse is to give a patient amiodarone 800 mg/day by mouth in two divided doses. The nurse has available 200-mg tablets. How many tablets should the nurse give for each dose? **Fill in the blank.**
   Answer: _____ tablets

Answer rationales available in your online resources.

ANSWERS 1. 5, 3, 1, 2, 4, 2. 1; 3. 2; 4. 3, 5, 6; 5. 2; 6. 3; 7. 2

Key Points

Find the chapter key points in your online resources available through Davis Edge.

Additional Resources

DAVIS **edge.**   Use the scratch off code on the inside front cover of your book to access online quizzes that will help you to improve your scores on course exams and prepare for NCLEX-PN®.

Study Guide

CHAPTER 26

Nursing Care of Patients With Heart Failure

Kathy Berchem

KEY TERMS

afterload (AF-ter-lohd)
cor pulmonale (KOR PUL-mah-NAH-lee)
cyanosis (SIGH-an-NOH-siss)
hepatomegaly (HEP-ah-toh-MEH-gah-lee)
orthopnea (or-THOP-nee-ah)
paroxysmal nocturnal dyspnea (PEAR-ox-IS-mul knock-TURN-al DISP-nee-ah)
perfusion (pur-FEW-shun)
peripheral vascular resistance (puh-RIFF-uh-ruhl VAS-kyoo-lar ree-ZIS-tense)
preload (PREE-lohd)
pulmonary edema (PULL-muh-NARE-ee eh-DEE-muh)
splenomegaly (SPLEE-noh-MEG-ah-lee)

CHAPTER CONCEPT

Perfusion

LEARNING OUTCOMES

1. Describe the pathophysiology of left- and right-sided heart failure.
2. Define acute heart failure.
3. List causes of acute and chronic heart failure.
4. Identify signs and symptoms of acute and chronic heart failure.
5. Plan nursing care for patients undergoing diagnostic tests for heart failure.
6. Explain medical treatments used for acute and chronic heart failure.
7. Plan nursing care for acute and chronic heart failure.
8. Plan teaching for patients with heart failure and their families.

OVERVIEW OF HEART FAILURE

Heart failure (HF) is a clinical syndrome that affects **perfusion.** It occurs from the inability of the ventricle(s) to fill or pump enough blood to meet the body's oxygen and nutrient needs. It may cause dyspnea, fatigue, and fluid volume overload. It can reduce quality and length of life. Causes of HF are varied. They can include coronary artery disease (most often), myocardial infarction, cardiomyopathy, heart valve problems, and hypertension (HTN). Any heart problem can potentially lead to HF. In the older adult, the most common cause of HF is cardiac ischemia. HF may develop rapidly (acute), as with cardiogenic shock and **pulmonary edema.** It can also occur over time (chronic) as a result of another disorder. This could include HTN or pulmonary disease.

Incidences of HF are growing. This is due to an increasing older adult population and treatment advances with better survival rates. According to the American Heart Association (AHA), an estimated 6.5 million people have HF. There are 960,000 new cases each year. A total of 3.6 million women have HF. Black females have the highest incidence of HF. In 2014, 1 in 8 deaths had HF as a contributing cause (Benjamin et al., 2017). HF is also the most common reason for hospital admission in the older adult. Readmission rates to hospitals soon after discharge for HF treatment are high and pose a challenge for health care providers (HCPs).

Congestive Heart Failure

Congestive HF is an older term for HF. It is still used by some for HF. The term HF is used because volume overload ("congestion") either in the lungs or periphery (extremities) is not present in everyone with HF.

• WORD • BUILDING •
perfusion: per—throughout + fundere—pour

Pathophysiology

The heart is divided into two separate pumping systems: the right side of the heart and the left side of the heart. Proper cardiac functioning requires each ventricle to pump out equal amounts of blood over time. If the amount of blood returned to the heart becomes more than either ventricle can handle, the heart can no longer function effectively as a pump.

HF can be the result of systolic (contractile) dysfunction, diastolic (relaxation) dysfunction, or a mixed systolic and diastolic dysfunction. Systolic dysfunction is a contractile problem in which the ventricle is unable to generate enough force to pump blood from the ventricle. Diastolic dysfunction is a problem with the ventricle's ability to relax and fill. Mixed systolic and diastolic dysfunction is a combination of the two defects.

LEARNING TIP

To understand heart failure (HF), compare it to a dam in a river:

• In a river without a dam, water flows freely; in the normal circulatory system, blood flows freely.

• In a river with a dam, the water is blocked by the dam and builds up behind it; in HF, the failing ventricle acts like a dam in the river, causing blood to back up behind it.

• When too much water builds up behind the dam, the riverbanks are flooded; in HF, if too much blood builds up behind the failing ventricle, the lungs (pulmonary edema) or peripheral tissues (peripheral edema) are flooded.

Conditions causing HF can affect one or both of the heart's pumping systems. Therefore, HF can be classified as right-sided HF, left-sided HF, or biventricular HF. The left ventricle typically weakens first. This is because it has the greatest workload. It must eject blood against the resistance in the aorta. The right and left sides of the heart's pumping system work together in a closed system. So, failure of one side will lead to failure of the other side.

LEARNING TIP

To understand and see the effects of heart failure (HF), trace the flow of blood backward from each ventricle. Along the backward path from the failing ventricle, congestion develops. This produces the signs and symptoms seen in HF. Understanding the backward path of congestion can help you identify the signs and symptoms of either right- or left-sided HF.

Left-Sided Heart Failure

The left ventricle must generate a certain amount of force during a contraction to eject blood into the aorta through the aortic valve. This force is referred to as **afterload.** The pressure within the aorta and arteries acts as resistance. This influences the force needed to open the aortic valve to pump blood into the aorta. This pressure is called **peripheral vascular resistance.**

HTN is a major cause of left-sided HF. It increases the pressure within arteries. This makes the left ventricle work harder to pump blood into the aorta. Over time, the strain caused by the increased workload causes the left ventricle to weaken and fail as an effective pump. See Table 26.1 for other causes of left-sided HF.

With left-sided HF, blood first backs up from the left ventricle into the left atrium. Then it backs up into the four pulmonary veins and lungs (Fig. 26.1). This increases pulmonary pressure. The pressure causes fluid to move into the interstitium and then into the alveoli. Alveolar edema is serious. It reduces gas exchange across the alveolar capillary membrane. This causes shortness of breath and cyanosis from decreased oxygenation of the blood. If the fluid buildup is severe, acute pulmonary edema occurs. This requires immediate medical treatment.

Right-Sided Heart Failure

Conditions causing right-sided HF increase the work of the right ventricle. They either increase the amount of contractile force needed or require pumping of excess blood volume (**preload**). Causes of right-sided HF are described in Table 26.2. The major cause of right-sided HF is left-sided HF. When the left side fails, fluid backs up into the lungs. Pulmonary pressure is increased. The right ventricle must continually pump blood against this increased fluid and pressure. Over time, this strain causes it to weaken and fail

---

T a b l e 26.1

Causes of Left-Sided Heart Failure

Cause	*Primary Effect on Left Ventricular Workload*
Aortic stenosis	Increased volume to pump from restricted blood outflow
Cardiomyopathy	Increased workload from impaired contractility
Coarctation of the aorta	Restricted outflow and increased resistance from narrowing of aorta
Hypertension	Resistance increased from elevated pressure
Heart muscle infection	Increased workload from damaged myocardium
Myocardial infarction	Increased workload from impaired contractility
Mitral regurgitation	Increased volume to pump from backward blood flow

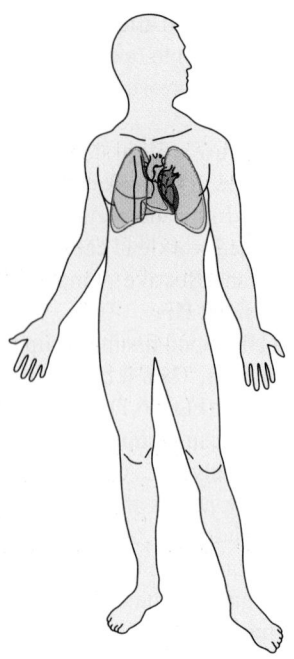

FIGURE 26.1 Left-sided heart failure. Shaded areas indicate areas of congestion from blood backup caused by the failing left side of the heart.

Table 26.2
Causes of Right-Sided Heart Failure

Cause	Primary Effect on Right Ventricular Workload
Atrial septal defect	Left atrial blood flow into right atrium increases right ventricular volume to pump
Cor pulmonale	Resistance increased from elevated pressure
Left-sided heart failure	Resistance increased from backup of fluid and elevated pressures
Pulmonary hypertension	Resistance increased from elevated pressure
Pulmonary valve stenosis	Increased volume to pump from restricted right ventricular blood outflow

as a pump. When the right ventricle hypertrophies (increases muscle mass) or fails from disorders of the lung, it is called **cor pulmonale.**

When the right ventricle fails, it does not empty normally. There is a backward buildup of blood in the systemic blood vessels. With the blood backed up from the right ventricle, right atrial and systemic venous blood volume increases. This causes the jugular veins to become distended. Normally, they are not visible. But with the patient in a 45-degree upright position, the jugular vein distension can be seen. Edema may occur in the peripheral tissues. The abdominal organs can become distended (Fig. 26.2). Fluid congestion causes upset in the gastrointestinal (GI) tract. Anorexia, abdominal pain, and nausea can occur. As the right-sided failure progresses, blood pools in the hepatic veins. The liver becomes congested (**hepatomegaly**). Liver function is impaired. Pain occurs in the right upper quadrant of the abdomen. Systemic venous congestion also leads to distension of the spleen (**splenomegaly**).

LEARNING TIP

To understand the signs and symptoms of left-sided versus right-sided heart failure, remember that left-sided signs and symptoms are found in the lungs. "Left" begins with L, as does "lung" (Left = Lungs = L). Any signs and symptoms not related to the lungs are caused by right-sided failure.

COMPENSATORY MECHANISMS TO MAINTAIN CARDIAC OUTPUT

Compensatory mechanisms help ensure that enough blood is being pumped out of the heart. Although these mechanisms are designed to maintain cardiac output, they contribute to a cycle that, instead of being helpful, leads to further HF. Let's see how that occurs.

When the sympathetic nervous system detects low cardiac output, it releases epinephrine and norepinephrine. This speeds up the heart rate (cardiac output = heart rate × stroke volume). Normally, this is helpful to maintain an adequate cardiac output. However, whenever the heart beats faster, the heart itself also requires more oxygen. The failing heart finds it difficult to supply this additional oxygen, thus worsening HF.

With a low cardiac output, blood flow to the kidneys is reduced. So, the kidneys activate the renin-angiotensin-aldosterone system to save water. Antidiuretic hormone is also released from the pituitary gland to conserve water. Urine output decreases. This adds further fluid to the fluid retention problem already occurring in HF.

Over time, the heart responds to its increased workload by enlarging its chambers (dilation) and increasing its muscle mass (hypertrophy). This is known as *remodeling*. In dilation, the heart muscle fibers stretch. This increases the force of myocardial contractions. This stretch is known as the *Frank–Starling phenomenon*. In hypertrophy, the muscle mass of the heart increases, also creating more contractile force. Both

---

• **WORD** • **BUILDING** •

cor pulmonale: cor—heart + pulm—lung
hepatomegaly: hep—liver + mega—large
splenomegaly: splen—spleen + mega—large

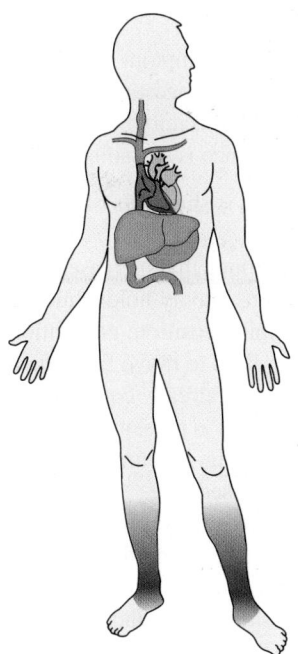

FIGURE 26.2 Right-sided heart failure. Shaded areas indicate areas of congestion from blood backup due to the failing right side of the heart.

compensatory mechanisms temporarily improve patient symptoms. However, they also increase the heart's oxygen needs. As you now know, this further contributes to HF. Additionally, the heart walls stiffen. This further reduces the heart's pumping ability.

PULMONARY EDEMA (ACUTE HEART FAILURE)

Pulmonary edema (acute HF) is sudden, severe fluid congestion within the lung alveoli. It is life-threatening. Pulmonary edema can occur with an acute event such as a myocardial infarction. It can also happen when the heart is severely stressed, causing the left ventricle to fail. Complications of pulmonary edema include arrhythmias and cardiac arrest.

Pathophysiology

First, pressure rises in the lung's venous blood vessels as blood builds up. This causes fluid to move into the interstitial spaces. Then, with continued pressure increases, fluid containing red blood cells leaks into the alveoli. Finally, the alveoli and airways become filled with fluid. This reduces gas exchange and oxygen levels.

Signs and Symptoms

Signs and symptoms of pulmonary edema are listed in Table 26.3. Pink, frothy sputum is the classic symptom of pulmonary edema. It is caused by the lung congestion and increased pressure that cause leaking of fluid and red blood cells into the alveoli. Compensatory mechanisms increase

Table 26.3	
Acute Heart Failure Summary	
Signs and Symptoms	Anxiety and restlessness
	Clammy, cold skin
	Coughing
	Crackles and wheezes
	Pale skin and mucous membranes
	Pink, frothy sputum
	Rapid respirations with accessory muscle use
	Severe dyspnea and orthopnea
Diagnostic Tests	Arterial blood gases (ABGs)
	Chest x-ray examination
	Electrocardiogram (ECG)
	Hemodynamic monitoring
Therapeutic Measures	Oxygen via cannula, mask, or mechanical ventilation
	Positioning in Fowler or semi-Fowler position
	Bedrest
	Intravenous drugs (e.g., morphine, diuretics, inotropic agents, vasodilators)
	Frequent vital signs and urinary output
	Pulmonary pressures
	Daily weights
	Treatment of underlying cause
Priority Nursing Diagnoses	*Impaired Gas Exchange*
	Decreased Cardiac Output
	Excess Fluid Volume

the heart rate and blood pressure. But as pulmonary edema worsens, the blood pressure may fall.

Diagnostic Tests

Diagnostic studies are listed in Table 26.3. X-rays show the congestion in the pulmonary system. Arterial blood gases (ABGs) show a decrease in partial pressure of oxygen (Pao_2). This continues to drop as the edema worsens. Partial pressure of carbon dioxide ($Paco_2$) is increased. This causes respiratory acidosis. The pulmonary artery catheter shows elevated pulmonary pressures and a decreased cardiac output.

Therapeutic Measures

Immediate treatment is needed to prevent acute respiratory distress (see Table 26.3). The goal of therapy is to reduce the workload of the left ventricle. This will improve cardiac output and reduce the patient's anxiety. Place the patient in a semi-Fowler or Fowler position based on comfort. This reduces venous return. It also allows the lungs to expand more easily. Give oxygen as ordered. A mask is used to provide higher concentrations. Endotracheal intubation and mechanical ventilation may be necessary for severe cases.

Medications are given intravenously. They are ordered to reduce anxiety, relax airways, and increase peripheral blood pooling (decreases preload). Medications can also reduce fluid congestion, strengthen heart contractions, reduce arterial pressure (afterload), and reduce sodium and water retention to relieve dyspnea.

Nursing Care

The patient is typically critically ill and is treated in an intensive care unit. Psychosocial care is important because the patient, if alert, will be anxious.

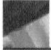 ## CHRONIC HEART FAILURE

Signs and Symptoms

Chronic HF is a progressive disorder. Signs and symptoms worsen over time (Table 26.4).

Fatigue and Weakness

Fatigue and weakness are the earliest symptoms of chronic HF. They occur from reduced oxygen reaching the tissues. During the day, the fatigue worsens, especially with activity ("Evidence-Based Practice").

Evidence-Based Practice

Clinical Question

What are the challenges for patients living with heart failure (HF)?

Evidence

A systematic review of qualitative literature included five studies and the voices of 32 men and 29 women (Schjoedt, Sommer, & Bjerrum, 2016). The results revealed that persons living with HF experience three types of fatigue: decreased physical capacity, unpredictability of fatigue, and fluctuating intensity of fatigue. Persons living with HF experienced changes in everyday activities, such as the ability to complete household chores; social activities, such as going out for lunch; and personal well-being, such as loss of self-esteem and identity as well as alterations in intellectual function.

Implications for Nursing Practice

Nurses should recognize that patients with HF experience different types of fatigue. They should consider this as they help patients set goals and plan self-care.

Reference

Schjoedt, I., Sommer, I., & Bjerrum, M. B. (2016). Experiences and management of fatigue in everyday life among adult patients living with heart failure: A systematic review of qualitative evidence. *JBI Database of Systematic Reviews and Implementation Reports, 14*(3), 68–115. doi:10.11124/JBISRIR-2016-2441

Dyspnea

Dyspnea is a common symptom of left-sided chronic HF. It occurs from pulmonary congestion that impairs gas exchange. Dyspnea triggers compensatory mechanisms. Short, rapid respirations result. Dyspnea is classified in several ways:

- *Exertional dyspnea* is shortness of breath that increases with activity.
- **Orthopnea** is dyspnea that increases when lying flat. In an upright position, gravity holds fluid in the lower extremities. In a supine position, gravitational forces are removed, allowing fluid to move from the legs to the heart. This overwhelms the already congested pulmonary system. When orthopnea is present, two or more pillows are often used for sleeping. Documentation should state the number of pillows used (e.g., "three-pillow orthopnea").
- **Paroxysmal nocturnal dyspnea** is a sudden shortness of breath that occurs after lying flat for a time. It results from excess fluid in the lungs. The sleeping person awakens with feelings of suffocation and anxiety. Relief is obtained by sitting upright for a short time, reducing the amount of fluid returning to the heart.

Cough

A chronic, dry cough is common in chronic HF. Coughing increases when lying down from increased irritation of the lung mucosa. This irritation is due to increased pulmonary congestion that occurs when gravity releases fluid in the legs. This extra fluid then returns to the heart and lungs.

Crackles and Wheezes

Pulmonary congestion causes abnormal breath sounds. These include crackles and wheezes. Crackles are the sound of the fluid buildup in the alveoli. Wheezes occur from bronchiolar constriction from increased fluid.

Tachycardia

As discussed earlier, low cardiac output triggers the sympathetic nervous system to increase the heart rate.

LEARNING TIP

To simulate the sound of crackles heard with a stethoscope, open a piece of Velcro or rub hair together next to your ear.

Chest Pain

Chest pain may occur from ischemia. Several factors cause ischemia. A low cardiac output does not deliver adequate oxygen to the heart muscle. Tachycardia raises the heart's

• WORD • BUILDING •
orthopnea: orth—straight + pnea—to breathe

Table 26.4
Chronic Heart Failure Summary

	Right-Sided Heart Failure	*Left-Sided Heart Failure*
Signs and Symptoms	Ascites Dependent peripheral edema Fatigue, weakness Gastrointestinal (e.g., anorexia, nausea, pain) Hepatomegaly Jugular vein distention Nocturia Splenomegaly Tachycardia Weight gain	Cheyne–Stokes respiration Crackles, wheezing Cyanosis Dry hacking cough, especially when supine Dyspnea on exertion Nocturia Orthopnea Paroxysmal nocturnal dyspnea Tachypnea, tachycardia
Diagnostic Tests	Arterial blood gases (ABGs) Cardiac catheterization Cardiac magnetic resonance imaging (MRI) Chest x-ray Coronary angiography Echocardiography, two-dimensional with Doppler Electrocardiogram (ECG) Exercise stress test Hemodynamic monitoring Laboratory tests: complete blood count (CBC), serum B-type natriuretic peptide (BNP), electrolytes, blood urea nitrogen (BUN), creatinine, liver function tests, thyroid-stimulating hormone, fasting blood glucose, lipid profile, ferritin Nuclear imaging studies Sleep studies Urinalysis	
Complications	Cardiogenic shock Hepatomegaly Left ventricular thrombus and emboli Pleural effusion Splenomegaly	
	Noninvasive	*Invasive*
Therapeutic Measures	Treatment of underlying cause Oxygen by cannula or mask Drug therapy (see Table 26.5) Individualized activity plan Dietary sodium restriction Fluid restriction Daily weights	Pacemaker Resynchronization therapy Implantable cardioverter defibrillator (ICD) Intra-aortic balloon pump (IABP) Left ventricular assist device Total artificial heart Surgery: coronary artery bypass graft (CABG), valvuloplasty, heart valve replacement, cardiac transplant
Priority Nursing Diagnoses	*Impaired Gas Exchange* *Decreased Cardiac Output* *Excess Fluid Volume*	

oxygen needs. Increased preload also increases the heart's workload and oxygen needs. Ischemic pain results. Pain also increases oxygen requirements. These factors all contribute to the vicious cycle of HF.

Cheyne–Stokes Respiration

Cheyne–Stokes breathing is a pattern of shallow respirations building to deep breaths followed by a period of apnea. The period of apnea occurs because deep breathing causes carbon dioxide (CO_2) levels to drop. Low CO_2 levels do not stimulate the respiratory center. The apnea may last up to 30 seconds. Then, the Cheyne–Stokes breathing pattern begins again.

Edema

Edema occurs in chronic HF. It is the result of systemic blood vessel congestion and, as previously discussed, compensatory mechanisms that save water. Systemic edema or pulmonary edema (also discussed earlier) can occur. Systemic edema is seen with jugular vein distension, swelling of the legs and feet, sacral edema in the supine patient, and increased abdominal cavity fluid (ascites).

Anemia

Many patients with HF are anemic. This is due to hemodilution from fluid overload and decreased angiotensin-converting enzyme (ACE) action. The reduced ACE action decreases erythropoietin release. This results in decreased production of red blood cells.

Nocturia

Nocturia is an increase in urine output at night during sleep. After lying down, fluid in the lower legs returns to the circulatory system. Renal blood flow and filtration are increased, resulting in greater urine production and the need to urinate frequently during the night. Nocturia may occur up to six times per night, contributing to the patient's fatigue from lack of sleep.

NURSING CARE TIP

Patients will often void shortly after going to bed as a result of fluid in the legs returning to the heart and then the kidneys for filtering after they lie down. To help patients get as much undisturbed rest as possible, teach them to recline with their legs at or above heart level for at least 30 minutes before going to bed. Then, they can void before going to bed, instead of soon after.

Cyanosis

The skin, nailbeds, or mucous membranes may appear blue, or cyanotic, from decreased oxygenation of the blood. **Cyanosis** is a late sign of chronic HF and occurs primarily with left-sided HF.

Altered Mental Status

Reduced cardiac output decreases the amount of oxygen delivered to the brain. As a result, restlessness, insomnia, confusion, decreased level of consciousness, and impaired memory may occur.

Malnutrition

Several factors contribute to malnutrition for those with chronic HF. Altered mental status, dyspnea, and fatigue affect eating. GI upset, anorexia, and malabsorption occur from excess fluid pressing on the GI structures (ascites).

CRITICAL THINKING

Part 1: Mr. Shepard, age 66, has a family history of cardiac disease. He has been hypertensive for 10 years and takes captopril (Capoten) daily. His baseline vital signs are blood pressure 122/78 mm Hg, pulse 80 beats per minute (bpm), respirations 18 breaths per minute, height 66 inches, and weight 170 lb. During a visit to his health care provider (HCP), Mr. Shepard states that he has been short of breath during his daily 2-mile walk and has been using two pillows at night for sleep. As he talks, his HCP notes that he has an intermittent dry cough. His physical examination shows blood pressure 140/86 mm Hg, pulse 106 bpm, respiration 24 breaths per minute, weight 178 lb, and bilateral crackles in the lung bases.

1. What signs and symptoms of heart failure (HF) does Mr. Shepard display?
2. Do the signs and symptoms reflect right- or left-sided HF?
3. Why are each of the signs and symptoms occurring?
4. Why is Mr. Shepard using two pillows for sleeping? What is the medical term for this?
5. What health care team members might collaborate on Mr. Shepard's care during the course of his HF?

Suggested answers are at the end of the chapter.

Complications of Heart Failure

Complications of chronic HF are listed in Table 26.4. The liver and spleen enlarge from the fluid congestion. This causes impaired function, cellular death, and scarring. The elevated pressures in the capillaries of the lung can cause a pleural effusion. This is a leakage of fluid from the capillaries of the lung into the pleural space. Thrombosis and emboli can occur as a result of poor emptying of the ventricles. This leads to stasis of blood. Aspirin or anticoagulants are often prescribed. They prevent thrombus formation in patients with HF. Cardiogenic shock is often caused by a myocardial infarction that damages the left ventricle. It occurs when the left ventricle is unable to supply the tissues with enough oxygen and nutrients to meet their needs. Cardiogenic shock is a life-threatening condition that requires immediate treatment (see Chapter 9).

Diagnostic Tests

Diagnostic tests are done to identify the cause of chronic HF and identify the degree of failure present (see Table 26.4):

- Serum laboratory tests can evaluate contributing factors for HF. These include elevated serum blood urea nitrogen (BUN) and serum creatinine from renal failure, elevated liver enzymes from liver damage, elevated ferritin with hemochromatosis (iron overload), and thyroid function tests.
- A serum B-type natriuretic peptide (BNP) or N-terminal proBNP (NT-proBNP) level is obtained. Elevated levels indicate HF and severity; higher levels of this cardiac biomarker correlate with a worse prognosis. BNP is made by the heart to regulate blood volume to reduce cardiac workload. When the heart has to work harder over time, it releases more BNP.
- Elevated serum cystatin C (a protein produced by all nucleated cells) is a risk factor for HF.
- A chest x-ray examination shows the size, shape, and any enlargement of the heart as well as congestion in the pulmonary vessels.
- Cardiac arrhythmias that precipitate and contribute to HF are diagnosed with an electrocardiogram (see Chapters 21 and 25).
- Echocardiography may measure ventricular size, wall thickness, motion, and ejection fraction and assess valvular function.
- Exercise stress testing and nuclear imaging studies show activity tolerance, which is usually limited in HF.
- Cardiac magnetic resonance imaging (MRI) shows both moving and still pictures of the heart and major blood vessels. Cardiac structure and function are analyzed to determine treatment for cardiac disease.
- Cardiac catheterization and angiography are used to detect underlying heart disease that may be the cause of HF.
- Sleep studies may be done because sleep apnea or breathing disorders can contribute to HF.
- Measurement of the pressure in the heart and lungs is done with hemodynamic monitoring to guide medical therapy.

CRITICAL THINKING

Part 2: Mr. Shepard's chest x-ray examination shows an enlarged heart (cardiomegaly).

1. Why is Mr. Shepard's heart enlarged?
2. What is the significance of an enlarged heart?

Suggested answers are at the end of the chapter.

Therapeutic Measures

The goal of treatment for chronic HF is to improve the heart's pumping ability and decrease the heart's oxygen demands. Treatment of HF focuses on (1) identifying and correcting the underlying cause, (2) increasing the strength of the heart's contraction, (3) maintaining optimal water and sodium balance, and (4) decreasing the heart's workload. HF management requires a team approach that may involve HCPs, case managers, nurses, dietitians, physical therapists, occupational therapists, pharmacists, social workers, and clergy. HF pathways guide treatment. HF clinics ensure quality-based outcomes while reducing treatment costs.

The severity of HF determines the patient-centered therapy selected. Noninvasive approaches are usually tried first. Then, as needed, invasive treatments are used. Often, multiple therapies are used for better patient outcomes.

Oxygen Therapy

One of the major problems caused by HF is a reduction in oxygen delivered to the tissues. The signs and symptoms of this are fatigue, dyspnea, altered mental status, and cyanosis. Oxygen therapy may assist in supplying tissue oxygen needs. In mild HF, oxygen may be delivered by nasal cannula. For severe cases, ABG values guide oxygen delivery. Masks that provide high concentrations of oxygen or mechanical ventilation are used.

Activity

Activity tolerance is dependent on the severity of HF signs and symptoms. Severe symptoms may require bedrest until treatment reduces the symptoms. For stable HF, a regular exercise program can improve cardiac function. Patients are encouraged to stay as active as possible. An activity plan is developed with the health care team. A referral to a cardiac rehabilitation program can be made. A walking program that increases activity over time is often prescribed. Patients are educated on how to exercise safely. They are taught how to identify symptoms to prevent overexertion.

Sodium Restriction and Weight Control

Dietary sodium is restricted to decrease fluid retention. Salt substitutes often use potassium in place of sodium. The patient and HCP should discuss their use. A healthy weight range should be maintained. A dietitian can develop a plan for a low-sodium diet and weight reduction, if needed.

> **BE SAFE!**
> In severe HF, when abdominal discomfort is present, malnutrition is a concern. The patient can be anorexic. But the weight gain that occurs with fluid retention can mask the weight loss occurring from the anorexia. Monitor food intake. Ensure that weight gain from fluid retention does not allow malnutrition to go undetected.

Medication Therapy

There is no cure for chronic HF. Medications, however, can improve symptoms and quality of life. The American College of Cardiology Foundation/American Heart Association/Heart

Failure Society of America 2016 guidelines recommend medication classes (Table 26.5) with qualifiers for the following stages of HF development (Yancy et al., 2016):

- Stage A: Those at high risk of HF
- Stage B: Those who have no HF symptoms but do have structural heart disease
- Stage C: Those with HF with reduced ejection fraction and symptoms
- Stage D: Those with refractory HF, requiring extraordinary support or hospice care

Generally, medication categories are used as follows:

- First, ACE inhibitors or angiotensin II receptor blockers (ARBs) are used to control HTN, if present in Stage A.
- Next, beta blockers (bisoprolol, carvedilol, metoprolol succinate SR) are added along with the ACE inhibitors or ARBs for Stage B.
- Then, ACE inhibitors or ARBs are replaced with valsartan/sacubitril (Entresto), an angiotensin receptor neprilysin inhibitor (ARNi); diuretics are added for fluid retention; and aldosterone antagonists, nitrates, digitalis,

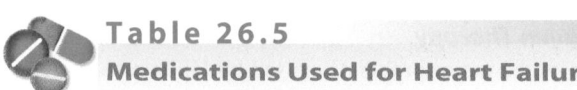

Table 26.5
Medications Used for Heart Failure

Medication Class/Action

Angiotensin-Converting Enzyme (ACE) Inhibitors

First-line therapy to decrease afterload to prevent hypertension (HTN). Decrease cardiac hypertrophy.

Examples	Nursing Implications
captopril (Capoten) benazepril (Lotensin) enalapril (Vasotec) fosinopril (Monopril) lisinopril (Prinivil, Zestril) moexipril (Univasc) quinapril (Accupril) perindopril (Aceon) ramipril (Altace) trandolapril (Mavik)	Check apical pulse and blood pressure (BP). If pulse is less than 60 bpm or systolic BP less than 100 mm Hg, notify health care provider (HCP). Give 1 hour before meals. *Teach:* Take first doses at night to adjust to lower BP. Rise slowly. Check BP weekly. Report if persistent cough or other side effects develop.

Angiotensin II Receptor Blockers (ARBs)

Block angiotensin II receptor to reduce extracellular fluid and cause vasodilation. May be used if ACE inhibitor not tolerated.

Examples	Nursing Implications
candesartan (Atacand) irbesartan (Avapro) losartan (Cozaar) valsartan (Diovan)	Check apical pulse and BP. If pulse is below 60 bpm or systolic BP below 100 mm Hg, notify HCP. *Teach:* Rise slowly. Report rash, sore throat/mouth, fever, swelling, difficulty breathing, chest pain, or irregular heartbeat.

Angiotensin Receptor Neprilysin Inhibitors (ARNis)

Reduce blood volume and vasodilate to reduce cardiac workload.

Example	Nursing Implications
valsartan/sacubitril (Entresto)	Contraindicated with ACE inhibitors or history of angioedema. Check apical pulse and BP. If pulse is below 60 bpm or systolic BP below 100 mm Hg, notify HCP. Monitor for hyperkalemia, kidney problems and angioedema (swelling of lips/face). *Teach:* Rise slowly. Report cough. Seek emergency care for swelling of lips/face.

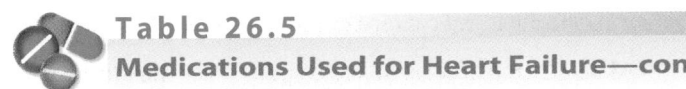

Table 26.5
Medications Used for Heart Failure—cont'd

Medication Class/Action

Beta-Adrenergic Blockers (Beta Blockers)

Reduce sympathetic nervous system input and cardiac remodeling; improve cardiac output to reduce symptoms; reduce disease progression and sudden death.

Examples	**Nursing Implications**
bisoprolol (Zebeta)	Check apical pulse and BP. If pulse is below 60 bpm or systolic BP below
carvedilol (Coreg)	100 mm Hg, notify HCP.
metoprolol succinate (Toprol XL)	*Teach:*
	Take pulse daily and notify HCP if below 60.
	Take BP biweekly.
	Rise slowly.

Loop Diuretics

Decrease fluid overload

Potassium-Wasting

Examples	**Nursing Implications**
bumetanide (Bumex)	Check BP and pulse before giving.
furosemide (Lasix)	Monitor electrolyte levels (especially potassium and in those on digitalis) and
torsemide (Demadex)	fluid status (daily weight, intake and output, thirst, dry mouth, weakness,
	oliguria) throughout therapy.
	Administer per patient lifestyle (usually in the morning) to avoid nocturia.

Potassium-Sparing

Example	**Nursing Implications**
spironolactone (Aldactone)	Do not give a potassium-sparing diuretic if patient is hyperkalemic.
	Teach:
	Report signs of hyperkalemia (e.g., weakness, fatigue, confusion,
	dyspnea, arrhythmias, confusion)

Thiazide Diuretics

Decrease fluid overload; potassium-wasting.

Examples	**Nursing Implications**
chlorothiazide (Diuril)	Monitor potassium.
hydrochlorothiazide (HydroDIURIL,	*Teach:*
HCTZ, Microzide)	Do not give a potassium-wasting diuretic if patient is hypokalemic.
metolazone (Zaroxolyn)	Administer potassium supplements as ordered; if on digitalis, increased risk of
	toxicity with hypokalemia.
	Monitor weight daily, and report 2- to 3-pound change over 1 to 2 days.

Inotropes: Cardiac Glycoside (Positive Inotrope and Negative Chronotrope)

Increase force and contraction of myocardium, which increases cardiac output. Slow heart rate to reduce workload of heart and control atrial fibrillation, if present.

Examples	**Nursing Implications**
digoxin (Lanoxin)	Take apical pulse for 1 minute; if below 60 bpm, notify HCP.
	Older patients are more susceptible to toxicity. Periodically monitor drug level
	and electrolytes (hypokalemia, hypomagnesemia, and hypercalcemia make
	patient more susceptible to toxicity).

Continued

Table 26.5
Medications Used for Heart Failure—cont'd

Medication Class/Action

Teach:

Take medication exactly as directed, at the same time each day.

Take pulse before taking medication; if below 60 bpm, hold and contact HCP.

Report signs of digitalis toxicity: abdominal pain, anorexia, nausea, vomiting, visual changes (blurred, yellow-green halos, photophobia, diplopia), bradycardia, arrhythmias.

Vasodilators

Decrease afterload to prevent HTN; used for patients who cannot take ACE inhibitors.

Examples	**Nursing Implications**
isosorbide dinitrate (Isorbid, Isordil)	Take blood pressure and pulse before giving. Notify HCP if not within normal limits.
hydralazine (Apresoline)	*Teach:*
nitroglycerin	Rise slowly.
	Headache common initially, treated with aspirin.

and hydralazine (Apresoline) are considered for Stage C. Sinoatrial heart rate reduction therapy with ivabradine (Corlanor) is considered.

- Finally, anticoagulants are used on an individual basis for risk of blood clots.

ANGIOTENSIN-CONVERTING ENZYME INHIBITORS. ACE inhibitors are considered the first-choice drug. They are used for their vasodilation effect. This lowers blood pressure and reduces workload on the heart. They also prevent cardiac remodeling. This remodeling leads to progressive cardiac deterioration.

LEARNING TIP

To help you identify angiotensin-converting enzyme, or ACE, inhibitors, remember that their generic names end with *-pril*.

ANGIOTENSIN II RECEPTOR BLOCKERS. ARBs are an alternative to ACE inhibitors. They inhibit the renin-angiotensin-aldosterone system. This lowers blood pressure and workload on the heart. ARBs do not produce a cough as much as ACE inhibitors do.

ANGIOTENSIN RECEPTOR NEPRILYSIN INHIBITORS. The new medication class of ARNis has been found to reduce hospitalizations and deaths from chronic HF and reduced ejection fraction. Entresto, a combination drug of valsartan/sacubitril, is often used with beta blockers and diuretics. A serious side effect is angioedema (swelling of lips/face) that can be life-threatening. ACE inhibitors increase the risk of angioedema. They must be stopped with a 36-hour wash-out period before Entresto is started.

BETA-ADRENERGIC BLOCKERS. The sympathetic nervous system acts to compensate for HF. Long-term sympathetic nervous system effects, however, are not helpful. Beta-adrenergic blockers, or beta blockers, help avoid these adverse effects. They improve cardiac output, reduce symptoms, reduce disease progression, and reduce sudden death.

DIURETICS. Diuretics act on various areas of the kidneys. They reduce fluid volume and increase urine output. This reduces pulmonary venous pressure. In turn, cardiac workload decreases. Diuretics are given to help prevent edema. However, edema does not need to be present for their use. A combination of diuretics may be ordered. Potassium supplements may be given with potassium-wasting diuretics. Electrolytes (especially potassium levels to prevent hypokalemia) and fluid balance (to prevent dehydration) should be carefully monitored.

ALDOSTERONE ANTAGONISTS. Spironolactone (Aldactone) blocks the effects of aldosterone, which causes the retention of sodium and fluid. Potassium must be monitored carefully, because spironolactone is a potassium-sparing agent. The risk of hyperkalemia increases if ACE inhibitors or ARBs are also used.

BE SAFE!

Always check serum potassium levels before giving a potassium-wasting diuretic (e.g., loop diuretics furosemide [Lasix], bumetanide [Bumex], and torsemide [Demadex]) or before giving a potassium supplement. Do not give a diuretic if the potassium level is low or a potassium supplement if the potassium level is high.

INOTROPIC AGENTS. Inotropic drugs strengthen ventricular contraction. This increases cardiac output. Inotropic agents include digitalis (e.g., digoxin), sympathomimetics (e.g., dobutamine), and phosphodiesterase inhibitors (e.g., milrinone). The sympathomimetics and phosphodiesterase inhibitors are usually used short term.

CRITICAL THINKING

Part 3: Mr. Shepard visits his health care provider. He is told to continue the angiotensin-converting enzyme (ACE) inhibitor, the diuretic, and a 2-g sodium diet.

1. Why is the ACE inhibitor continued?
2. Will the ACE inhibitor affect preload or afterload?
3. Why is the diuretic ordered?
4. What laboratory test result is checked before administering diuretics?
5. Why is a 2-g sodium diet ordered?
6. What is the overall goal of the ordered treatment?

Suggested answers are at the end of the chapter.

Pacemakers and Implantable Cardioverter Defibrillator

Pacemakers and implantable cardioverter defibrillators (ICDs) are used along with medication therapy for patients at risk of sudden death. Pacemakers pace the heart rate and abnormal rhythm. ICDs deliver an electric countershock if a shockable life-threatening rhythm occurs.

Cardiac Resynchronization Therapy

With HF, the ventricles do not always beat in normal synchrony with each other. This dyssynchrony results in less effective pumping by the ventricles. It reduces stroke volume. Cardiac resynchronization therapy restores normal timing of ventricular contraction. It reduces symptoms and improves quality of life. A biventricular cardiac pacing system is used. It synchronizes ventricle contraction to atrial pacing when three-chamber pacing is used. Left ventricular filling and, thus, contraction is then improved. Cardiac resynchronization therapy is also available with an ICD. For more information and pictures of cardiac resynchronization devices, visit www.medtronic.com.

Mechanical Assistive Devices

Mechanical cardiopulmonary support provides temporary function to patients with impaired cardiac function or who are experiencing cardiogenic shock. Assistive devices can act as a bridge to recovery or transplantation, to destination therapy (a long-term solution when other options are not available for the failing heart), or as heart replacement. These devices include extracorporeal membrane oxygenation (ECMO), the intra-aortic balloon pump (IABP), ventricular assist devices, total artificial heart, and implantable replacement heart. Technology in this area is continually changing.

ECMO is a portable bedside device that uses extrathoracic cannulation to perform respiratory (oxygenation and carbon dioxide removal) and circulatory support (somewhat similar to cardiopulmonary bypass used during cardiac surgery).

INTRA-AORTIC BALLOON PUMP. For acute care, an IABP increases circulation to the coronary arteries and reduces the work of the heart. The pump catheter is inserted into the femoral artery and positioned in the descending aortic arch (Fig. 26.3). It is attached to a computer that senses ventricular contraction. This controls the balloon. While the heart is relaxed (diastole), the balloon is inflated. This sends more blood into the coronary arteries. Just before the heart contracts (systole), the balloon deflates. This allows blood to flow past it. The deflation of the balloon creates a suction effect. The blood then flows past it with less resistance (decreased afterload) into the aorta. The IABP is inserted in a cardiac catheterization laboratory, critical care unit, or surgical suite. It is used short term for several days.

VENTRICULAR ASSIST DEVICES. Ventricular assist devices can be transcutaneous (pump located outside the body), which may be used short term after cardiac surgery or implanted mechanical devices. They assist cardiac pumping to maintain cardiac output (Fig. 26.4). They allow the failing ventricle to rest. Ventricular assist devices are used temporarily. They can be a bridge to transplantation (for patients awaiting a donor heart), a bridge to recovery (for patients whose hearts may recover), or as a destination therapy (a long-term therapy) for

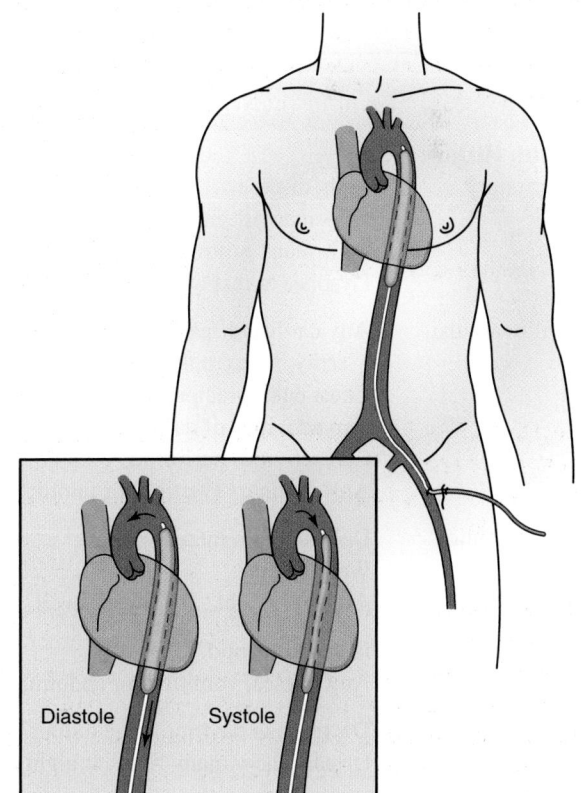

Diastole   Systole

FIGURE 26.3 Intra-aortic balloon pump.

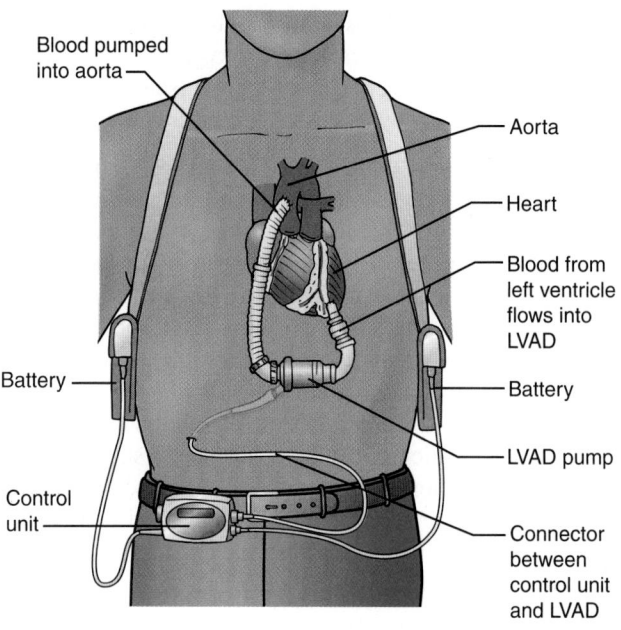

Blood pumped into aorta

Aorta

Heart

Blood from left ventricle flows into LVAD

Battery

Battery

LVAD pump

Control unit

Connector between control unit and LVAD

FIGURE 26.4 Schematic of a left ventricular assist device.

those who are not candidates for heart transplant. They are referred to as left ventricular assist devices if only used in the left ventricle, right ventricular assist devices if only used in the right ventricle, or biventricular assist devices if used in both ventricles. Two devices are used for biventricular failure.

Surgical Management

The causes of HF may be treated surgically (see Chapters 23 and 24). HF symptoms may resolve after these conditions are corrected. Surgical ventricular reconstruction reduces left ventricular volume. It might be done along with coronary artery bypass surgery. Reconstruction can reduce left ventricle end-systolic volume more than coronary artery bypass grafting (CABG) alone. However, this does not translate into better cardiovascular morbidity or mortality. Based on these results, *routine* surgical ventricular reconstruction at the time of CABG is not recommended (Velazquez, Kumbhani, & Bhatt, 2017).

Nursing Process for the Patient With Chronic Heart Failure
Data Collection

While obtaining data for the patient with chronic HF, focus on areas that might indicate the presence of HF (Table 26.6).

Nursing Diagnoses, Planning, Implementation, and Evaluation

See "Nursing Care Plan for the Patient With Chronic Heart Failure" for common nursing diagnoses. The major focus of nursing care for chronic HF patients is to improve oxygenation. This can be done by decreasing the body's need for oxygen with rest, positioning, medications, fluid balance, and oxygen consumption control.

Table 26.6
Nursing Data Collection for the Patient With Chronic Heart Failure

Subjective Data	
Health History	
Respiratory	Lung disease? How many flights of stairs can be climbed without dyspnea? How many pillows used for sleeping? Dyspnea at rest or that awakens from sleeping?
Cardiovascular	Any cardiac disease history: hypertension, myocardial infarction, valvular problem, anemia, arrhythmias, palpitations? Chest pain: precipitating factors, severity, relieving factors? Can activities of daily living be performed? Can activities performed 6 months, 4 months, 2 months, 2 weeks ago still be done? Any dizziness (vertigo) or fainting (syncope)?
Fluid retention	Daily sodium intake? Weight gain? Are shoes tight? Do ankles swell?
Gastrointestinal	Is appetite good? Any nausea, vomiting, or abdominal pain?
Urinary	Decrease in daytime urine output? Urinates how many times at night (nocturia)?

T a b l e   26.6

Nursing Data Collection for the Patient With Chronic Heart Failure—cont'd

Subjective Data	
Neurologic	Any change in behavior?
Knowledge of Condition	What are you being treated for? What questions do you have?
Coping Skills	What coping techniques do you usually use? Are they effective? Who is a part of your support system?
Medications	What are all of the medications that you take?
Objective Data	
Respiratory	Tachypnea, crackles, wheezing, respiratory effort, dyspnea with exertion
Cardiovascular	Tachycardia, arrhythmias, jugular vein distention, peripheral edema (degree of pitting)
Gastrointestinal	Abdominal distention, ascites, hepatomegaly, splenomegaly
Neurologic	Confusion, decreased level of consciousness, restlessness, impaired memory
Integumentary	Cold, clammy skin; pallor; cyanosis
General	Weight
Diagnostic Tests	Review findings.

Nursing Care Plan for the Patient With Chronic Heart Failure

Nursing Diagnosis: *Decreased Cardiac Output* related to the heart's inability to effectively pump adequate blood
Expected Outcome: The patient will demonstrate vital signs within normal limits (WNL).
Evaluation of Outcome: Are vital signs WNL without dyspnea or chest pain?

Intervention	Rationale	Evaluation
Monitor for primary signs of heart failure (HF): dyspnea, orthopnea, paroxysmal nocturnal dyspnea, fatigue, edema and secondary signs of weight gain, jugular vein distension, lung crackles, oliguria, coughing, and clammy skin with color changes.	*These signs were identified as being either primary or secondary in HF.*	Does patient exhibit any of these signs of HF?
Monitor daily weight after voiding with the same clothing, at the same time each day, and on the same scales. Report weight gains.	*Daily weights show fluid gain when fluid is being retained.*	Does daily weight remain the same?

(nursing care plan continues on page 472)

Nursing Care Plan for the Patient With Chronic Heart Failure—cont'd

Intervention	Rationale	Evaluation
Maintain bedrest with head of bed elevated for breathing ease for an acute episode.	*Bedrest with the head of the bed elevated reduces the workload of the heart and eases breathing.*	Does bedrest with head of the bed elevated relieve HF signs and symptoms?

Geriatric

Monitor for fatigue and depression.	*Fatigue and depression can be signs of HF in the older adult.*	Are fatigue or depression present?

Nursing Diagnosis: *Activity Intolerance* related to oxygen imbalance
Expected Outcome: The patient will demonstrate increased activity tolerance with vital signs WNL in response to activity.
Evaluation of Outcome: Does the patient participate in activities and maintain vital signs WNL?

Intervention	Rationale	Evaluation
Provide rest, space activities, and conserve energy.	*Myocardial oxygen need is decreased with rest and energy conservation.*	Does patient participate in activity with minimal pulse rate or electrocardiogram changes?
Assist patient as needed with activities of daily living (ADLs).	*Conserve energy by assisting with ADLs.*	Are patient's ADLs met?
Teach use of assistive devices and lifestyle changes.	*Assistive devices can overcome limitations to increase activity.*	Does patient incorporate assistive devices into lifestyle changes?

Geriatric

Increase time allowed to complete activities.	*Independence and participation are increased if extra time is allowed for tasks.*	Does patient report greater ability to complete activities with fewer symptoms?

Nursing Diagnosis: *Excess Fluid Volume* related to HF and the secondary reduction in renal blood flow for filtration
Expected Outcomes: The patient will remain free from edema and dyspnea, have clear lung sounds, and maintain baseline weight at all times.
Evaluation of Outcomes: Does the patient have clear lung sounds with baseline weight maintained?

Intervention	Rationale	Evaluation
Monitor for edema, weight gain, jugular vein distention, and lung crackles.	*Excess fluid is indicated by edema, daily weight gain, jugular vein distension, and crackles in the lungs.*	Are edema, weight gain, jugular vein distension, or crackles present? Are they worsening or improving?
Monitor intake and output (I&O).	*I&O will show fluid imbalances.*	Are I&O balanced for 24 hours?
Decrease sodium intake as ordered.	*Sodium retains fluid.*	Does patient restrict sodium intake?
Maintain fluid restriction as ordered.	*Excess fluid intake contributes to edema.*	Does patient restrict fluid intake?

Nursing Care Plan for the Patient With Chronic Heart Failure—cont'd

Nursing Diagnosis: *Disturbed Sleep Pattern* related to nocturia and inability to lie down and sleep comfortably
Expected Outcome: The patient will awaken refreshed and be less fatigued during the day.
Evaluation of Outcome: Does the patient wake up less frequently during the night and feel more refreshed with less fatigue during the day?

Intervention	Rationale	Evaluation
Identify and discuss barriers to sleep.	*Anxiety, nocturia, diuretics, orthopnea, or paroxysmal nocturnal dyspnea can make sleep difficult.*	Does patient identify sleep barriers?
Encourage patient to recline for 30 to 60 minutes before bedtime.	*Reclining before bedtime redistributes fluid to the kidneys so that the patient can void before going to sleep instead of soon afterward.*	Are there less instances of nocturia?
Geriatric		
Encourage patient to take diuretics in early hours. If patient sleeps during nighttime hours, then recommend taking diuretics early in the day. If patient sleeps during daytime hours, then recommend taking medications after rising.	*Nocturia is reduced if diuretics are taken earlier in time frame when awake.*	Does patient take diuretics early in time frame when awake and report less nocturia?

OXYGEN. Oxygen therapy is ordered by the HCP. It is guided by blood gas analysis and patient medical history and symptoms. It requires careful monitoring. For chronic HF, oxygen may be administered at 2 to 6 L/min via nasal cannula.

REST AND ACTIVITY. Reduction of the body's oxygen demands decreases the workload of the heart. A balance of rest and activity without signs or symptoms of oxygen deprivation is essential. The activity level of the patient is determined by the severity of the HF. During times of exertion, monitor the patient's vital signs and respiratory effort. Look for signs of oxygen deprivation. If activity intolerance develops, stop the activity.

POSITIONING. Semi-Fowler or high-Fowler position makes breathing easier. In upright positions, the lungs can expand more fully. Gravity decreases the amount of fluid returned to the heart. This reduces the heart's workload.

FLUID RETENTION. Daily weights identify fluid weight gain. It is important to detect fluid retention in this way. Edema is usually not observed until 5 to 10 pounds of extra fluid are present. A baseline weight is obtained when HF is diagnosed. Daily weights should be measured on the same scale, at the same time of day, and with the same type of clothing worn for accuracy. A good time to obtain a daily weight is in the morning after the bladder is emptied. Document daily weights. Include the date and time of the weight, the scale used, the clothing worn, and the weight measurement. The patient can keep a weight journal. Teach the patient to report weight gains of 2 to 3 pounds over 1 to 2 days.

OXYGEN CONSUMPTION. Activities that increase oxygen consumption by the heart should be avoided. Sustained tachycardia increases the oxygen needs of the heart. It should be reported promptly to the HCP for treatment. Older patients are especially vulnerable to the effects of tachycardia. This is due to their decreased cardiac reserves. Constipation should be prevented. Straining during defecation (Valsalva maneuver) increases the heart's workload by increasing venous return to the heart. Stool softeners can prevent straining.

To reduce fatigue, patients should be taught to alternate activity with periods of rest. This will save energy while performing activities of daily living. The occupational therapist and physical therapist can be helpful. They will develop ways to help the patient save energy during self-care. Suggestions for conserving energy include putting frequently used objects at waist level to avoid reaching overhead, planning bathing activities to include rest periods, and using Velcro fasteners to make dressing easier.

MEDICATIONS. HF is a progressive, chronic condition. Patients may require lifetime medication. Combination drug therapy is often needed. Taking multiple pills daily can be challenging. Financial resources, adherence to therapy regimen, and ongoing monitoring must be considered.

Diuretics. Diuretics require monitoring of the patient's potassium levels and blood pressure. To prevent hypokalemia, potassium supplements may be prescribed. Also, a diet with high-potassium foods is encouraged. If too much fluid is removed, the patient may become hypotensive. Orthostatic hypotension can develop. This causes dizziness and a risk of falling. Caution the patient to change positions slowly. They should dangle their legs at the bedside before standing. This will help prevent falls.

Digitalis. Before giving a digitalis drug, the patient's apical pulse should be counted for 1 minute. This drug slows the heart rate. If the pulse is below 60 bpm, notify the HCP. Some patients are given digitalis with heart rates between 50 and 60 bpm. This would occur if the heart's conduction system is normal or if the rate is due to other medications such as a beta blocker. When giving digitalis, be aware that hypokalemia increases the heart's sensitivity to digitalis. This can lead to toxicity with a normal dose of digitalis when hypokalemia is present. It is important to know this because many people on digitalis also take diuretics. Some diuretics lower potassium levels. Monitoring for signs and symptoms of digitalis toxicity should be done routinely. Early signs and symptoms of digitalis toxicity are anorexia, nausea, and vomiting; bradycardia or other arrhythmias; visual problems; and mental changes. Older adults are especially prone to the toxic effects of this drug. They may exhibit confusion when levels are elevated.

Vasodilators. Medications with vasodilating effects reduce the heart's workload by decreasing vascular pressure. Blood pressure is monitored when giving vasodilators.

Medication Teaching. Patients and their families are taught the purpose, side effects, and precautions for prescribed medications. Patients should understand the importance of taking their medication as prescribed, even if they do not have symptoms. A schedule should be developed so patients remember to take their medications. Teach them to report side effects to the HCP. If dizziness occurs from drugs that reduce blood pressure, the drugs can be staggered so that they are not all taken at the same time. Patients taking digitalis or a beta blocker should be taught to take their pulse. They should be informed to notify their HCP if it is below 60 bpm or below the lower limit heart rate set by their HCP. Patients on diuretics should be taught the following:

- Take the drug during the day before 1600 to decrease being awakened at night to void.
- Have a readily available and obstacle-free bathroom or commode to prevent incontinence and falls.
- Eat high-potassium foods if taking a potassium-wasting diuretic.
- Weigh oneself daily, and report weight gains of 2 to 3 pounds over 1 to 2 days.

LOW-SODIUM DIET AND WEIGHT CONTROL. A dietitian consult helps the patient and family understand the need for following a special diet. Menus that are appealing and easy to use are discussed. Eating should remain pleasurable for the patient to avoid malnutrition. Discuss foods the patient likes

and can still have. Do not talk only about foods they cannot have. Patients are taught to read food labels to determine which foods are high and low in sodium content. Salt substitutes may contain potassium. With this knowledge, patients can help design a daily meal plan using low-sodium foods that are appealing. Food preparers are taught not to salt food during cooking. Table salt should be eliminated. Spices, herbs, and lemon juice may be used to flavor unsalted foods.

For overweight patients, weight reduction may help eliminate the underlying cause of HF. Diet counseling and support should be given to obese patients to encourage weight loss. The body mass index and waist-to-hip ratio should guide weight loss.

If anorexia occurs in the later stages of HF, the patient's intake should be evaluated. Several small meals rather than three large meals will decrease the heart's workload. If the patient's nutritional needs are not being met, the HCP should offer a referral to a dietitian.

EDUCATION. Chronic management of HF requires patient and family understanding of the disease process, management of home oxygen therapy, diet and weight control, and the need for immunizations, such as the annual flu shot, and medications ("Home Health Hints"). The patient and family must recognize the importance of all of these factors to foster quality of life for the patient with chronic HF. A discussion of HF and signs and symptoms to report to the HCP using simple terms should be included in the teaching plan (Box 26.1).

COPING. Living with a chronic illness can be frustrating for both patients and their families. An assessment of coping skills used by patients and their families can be used to develop a plan for coping with this current illness. Available support systems are explained to patients. Referrals to social workers, sex counselors, and nurse-managed clinics can be helpful in providing resources that may make living with HF easier.

Understanding the chronic nature of HF is important for patients, families, and caregivers. This helps them positively deal with the emotions and feelings that can result. Nurse-managed HF clinics decrease hospitalization rates. They also increase effective management of the therapeutic regimen.

Box 26.1

Patient and Family Education

Heart Failure Signs and Symptoms to Report to the Health Care Provider

- Ankle or foot edema
- Anorexia
- Dry cough
- Episodes of sudden awakening with shortness of breath (paroxysmal nocturnal dyspnea)
- Fatigue
- Nocturia
- Shortness of breath
- Shortness of breath when lying down (orthopnea)
- Weight gain of 2 to 3 pounds over 1 to 2 days

Home Health Hints

- A telehealth unit in the home can alert the agency to signs of exacerbation such as a weight gain of 2 pounds in 24 hours. Interventions such as medication changes can then be ordered to prevent hospital admissions.
- Blood drawn for potassium level needs to be transported to the laboratory within 1 hour. Ice should not be put directly on the blood-draw tube because this can cause destruction of the cells and a false elevation in the potassium level.
- Observe for signs of oxygen deprivation and hypoxia, such as confusion, combativeness, or unusual expressions of anger.
- Measure for edema using a tape measure in centimeters on the abdominal girth, thigh, calf, and ankle. Measure at the same place each time (e.g., girth of calf at specified distance above medial malleolus). Edema can be present if the patient reports jewelry, waistband, or shoes and socks feel tighter.
- The sacrum, back, and sides of a bedridden patient should be observed for edema. These are dependent areas in the bedridden patient, so fluid accumulates in these areas instead of the ankles.
- Observe the contents of medicine bottles. If pills have been cut in half, question the patient because this is often an attempt by the patient to "stretch" the medicine to decrease expenses. Refer to the social worker for financial assistance.
- Adjust medication times to fit the patient's lifestyle. A dose of diuretic too late in the day may cause frequent awakenings during the night to void. This may lead to a lack of adherence and then rehospitalization.
- For the patient on a low-sodium diet, an effective diet-teaching technique is to have the patient name the foods highest in sodium. Asking the patient to rename the list on each visit helps knowledge retention and adherence to the diet.
- Teach patients on sodium-restricted diets to use no-salt-added canned vegetables or to pour off the liquid and rinse the vegetables. Herbs and spices can make them flavorful.
- Teach patients that long oxygen tubing allows movement around the home. For safety, caution about keeping the tubing out of the way and advise them not to kink the tubing.
- Teach patients and caregivers about the explosive nature of oxygen and the danger of an open flame or smoking in its presence.
- Teach patients with orthopnea that a foam wedge can be obtained from a medical equipment company to use under the head instead of pillows when sleeping.
- Teach patients self-management skills to reduce the odds of hospital readmission (e.g., sodium restrictions, daily weights, and warning signs of exacerbation to report).
- If an ambulance is called, teach caregivers to turn on an outside light and clear a pathway to enable the emergency technicians to get to the patient more easily.

Should the patient's condition worsen irreversibly, a discussion regarding the possibility of organ donation could be considered. Such a discussion would require a team approach involving other members of the health care team, such as the HCP, social worker, and clergy.

> **NURSING CARE TIP**
>
> Provide written discharge instructions to all patients with HF and their caregivers. Instructions should focus on medications (stressing adherence to following the medication regimen), diet, activity level, follow-up appointments, and daily weights. Instructions should also tell patients and caregivers to report or seek medical care for symptoms that worsen.

 ## CARDIAC TRANSPLANTATION

Cardiac transplantation is reserved for patients with end-stage cardiac disease. Transplant centers use selection guidelines for donors and recipients to improve survival.

> **CRITICAL THINKING**
>
> **Part 4: Mr. Shepard** talks with the nurse after his health care provider orders a continued angiotensin-converting enzyme (ACE) inhibitor, a diuretic, and a 2-g sodium diet.
>
> 1. What patient-centered information should the nurse teach Mr. Shepard based on the prescribed treatment?
> 2. What types of foods should be included in Mr. Shepard's diet?
> 3. Why does the nurse instruct Mr. Shepard to weigh himself daily?
> 4. Why does the nurse tell Mr. Shepard to weigh himself at the same time of day, on the same scale, and wearing the same type of clothing?
> 5. What guidelines does the nurse teach Mr. Shepard to follow in reporting of weight gain?
>
> *Suggested answers are at the end of the chapter.*

Preoperative teaching is started after the recipient is accepted into the transplant program. For more information on heart transplantation, visit www.nhlbi.nih.gov/health-topics/heart-transplant.

To increase the number of organs for transplant, a transport device has been developed. It keeps the heart beating and nourished with the donor's blood for up to 12 hours. The Organ Care System (Heart in a Box) is used in Europe. It is in trials in the United States.

Surgical Procedure

Once a donor heart is found, the recipient is notified, admitted to the hospital, and prepared for surgery. The general procedures for this surgery are similar to those described in Chapter 21. Two types of cardiac transplant procedures are performed: orthotopic and heterotopic. In the orthotopic procedure, once the patient is on cardiopulmonary bypass, the recipient's diseased heart is removed, leaving the posterior wall of the atria, superior and inferior vena cava, and pulmonary vein (Fig. 26.5). The donor's atria, aorta, and pulmonary artery are then anastomosed to the recipient's atria, aorta, and pulmonary artery. The heterotopic procedure joins the donor heart and vessels to the recipient's heart and vessels without removing the recipient's heart. So the donor heart rests in the right side of the chest.

Immunosuppressive therapy is required to prevent rejection of the transplanted heart. Medications such as cyclosporine (Neoral, Sandimmune), mycophenolate mofetil (CellCept), tacrolimus (Prograf), sirolimus (Rapamune), and prednisone are used ("Nutrition Notes"). A high loading dose of one of these medications begins preoperatively. The risk for rejection is highest immediately after surgery. Over time, it decreases but never goes away. Dosages of immunosuppressive medication are also highest initially after surgery and decrease with time. Lifelong antirejection therapy is required and involves the combination of drugs to allow lower doses. This helps to reduce side effects.

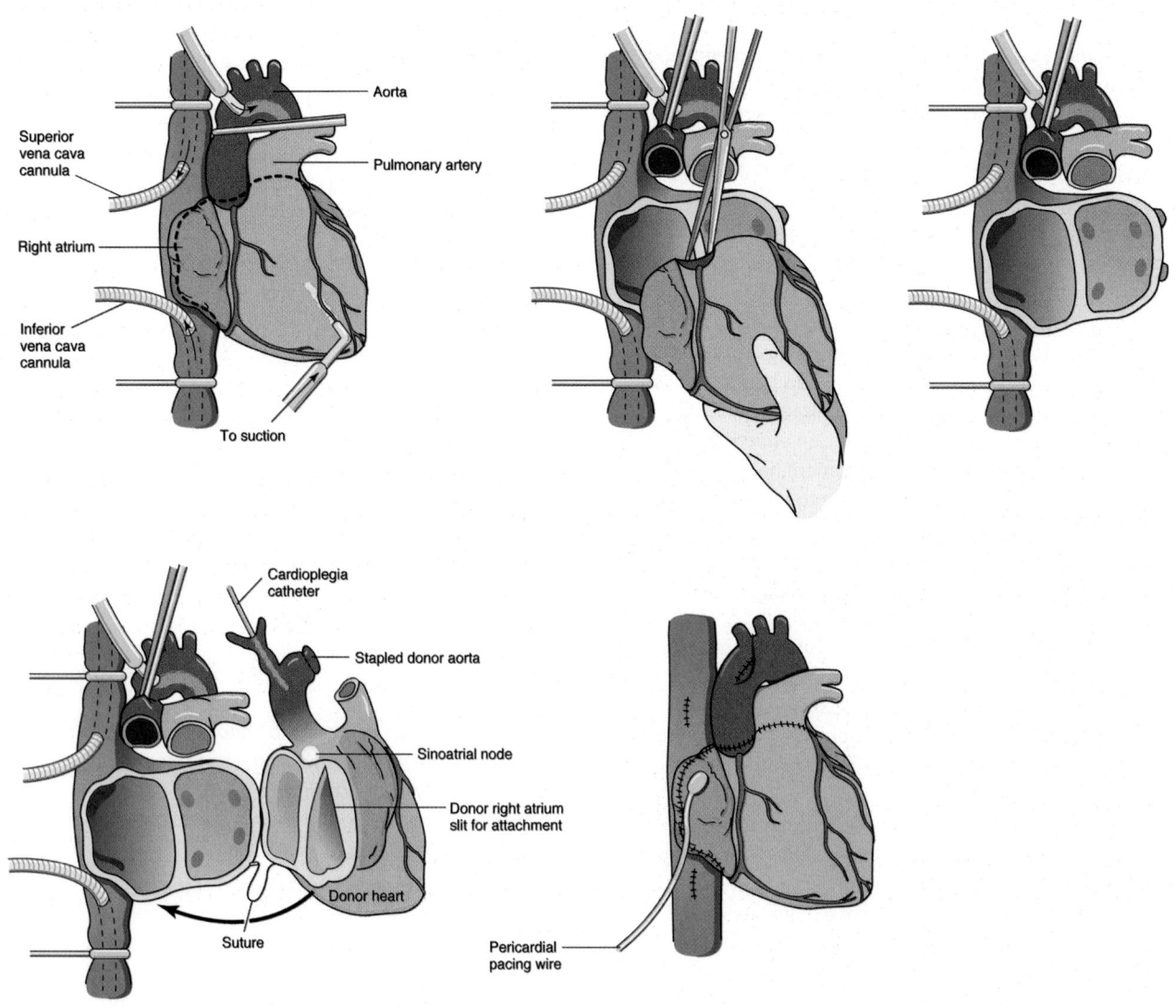

FIGURE 26.5 Heart transplantation.

Nutrition Notes

Cyclosporine, an immunosuppressant used to prevent transplant rejection, is metabolized by intestinal CYP3A4. Taking cyclosporine with grapefruit juice may cause elevated blood levels of the drug. St. John's wort, sold as a dietary supplement, has interacted with cyclosporine (through both CYP3A4 and P-glycoprotein mechanisms) sufficiently to cause organ rejection.

Complications

Heart transplantation complications may include those associated with cardiac surgery. Heart rejection, which is the major cause of death within the first year, is another complication. To detect rejection, frequent biopsies of cardiac muscle or a newer blood test to detect activation of rejection genesis is done during the first year. If a biopsy shows damaged cells, indicating rejection, antirejection drug therapy may be changed.

Due to immunosuppressive therapy, infection and cancer may occur. The medications used for immunosuppressive therapy also may cause adverse reactions. They include increased cataracts, high cholesterol, diabetes, kidney disease, and osteoporosis.

Therapeutic Measures

After cardiopulmonary bypass is stopped, the patient receives a diuretic to aid in excretion of excessive circulating fluid. Intake and output are monitored hourly. The patient is observed for fluid overload. Lung sounds are assessed for crackles. Weight and electrolyte levels are checked daily.

Postcardiotomy syndrome may occur from days 2 to 5 after surgery and last a few weeks. Patients may rouse normally and be oriented but exhibit mild confusion or psychosis. Pupillary reaction and motor response are assessed. The safety of the patient is maintained with side rails up, bed in low position, and nursing call light within reach. The patient is given as much rest and as little sensory stimulation as possible.

Sleeping is difficult. This is because of postoperative pain and the continuous level of activity in the intensive care unit. Sleep is promoted in 90-minute intervals. The lights are dimmed. Decreasing all sensory stimulation near the patient is important. Additionally, listening to a favorite soothing type of music with earphones or the use of ordered narcotics for pain may also help sedate and relax the patient to allow for healing.

Temperature is monitored every 4 hours. Complete blood cell count and white blood cell results are monitored for indications of infection. If oral thrush (white patches) develops, an antifungal agent is ordered. A urine culture to diagnose a urinary tract infection is ordered if cloudy urine or urinary tract burning occurs.

Nursing Process for the Preoperative Cardiac Transplant Patient

General preoperative and postoperative surgical care is discussed in Chapter 12. Postoperative needs for the patient undergoing cardiac surgery are discussed next.

Nursing Process for the Postoperative Cardiac Transplant Patient
Data Collection

The patient is accompanied to the intensive care unit by the anesthesiologist. The HCP gives the nurse a report of the procedure. In addition, complications as well as hemodynamic and ventilatory management of the patient are reported. The patient is connected to a cardiac monitor and a mechanical ventilator for 4 to 24 hours. A temporary pacemaker is connected to the epicardial pacing wires if they were placed during surgery as a precaution to treat bradycardia and other arrhythmias. The patient is placed under a forced-air warming device, such as a blanket. The chest tubes are monitored. The nasogastric tube is placed to suction. The urinary catheter is placed for gravity drainage.

A head-to-toe assessment of the patient, including dressings, tubes, and intravenous lines, is performed. Of importance are signs of awakening, shivering, pain, lung and heart sounds, and palpation of the entire chest and neck to detect crepitus (air in the subcutaneous tissue from opening the chest). Complete blood count, electrolytes, coagulation studies, and ABGs are monitored. Cardiac transplant patients may be in isolation for their own protection, depending on the agency's policy.

After the initial transfer assessment, vital signs, oxygen saturation, and cardiac pressures are monitored and recorded every 15 to 30 minutes. An electrocardiogram is done to detect perioperative myocardial infarction. A chest x-ray examination is done to check central line and endotracheal tube placement. An x-ray can also detect a pneumothorax or hemothorax, diaphragm elevation, or mediastinal widening from bleeding. At this point, the family may see the patient. Patient care is explained.

Nursing Diagnoses, Planning, Implementation, and Evaluation

Nursing diagnoses for postoperative cardiac surgery or transplant are discussed in "Nursing Care Plan for the Postoperative Patient Undergoing Cardiac or Transplant Surgery."

Nursing Care Plan for the Postoperative Patient Undergoing Cardiac or Transplant Surgery

Nursing Diagnosis: *Acute Pain* related to sternotomy, leg incisions, internal mammary artery resection, or pericarditis
Expected Outcomes: The patient will state pain is relieved or tolerable within 30 minutes of report of pain. The patient will be able to rest and perform respiratory treatments.
Evaluation of Outcomes: Does the patient state pain is within acceptable levels? Is the patient able to rest and perform respiratory treatments?

Intervention	Rationale	Evaluation
Obtain report of characteristics of pain with each episode.	*A thorough description is needed to determine cause and plan actions.*	Does patient describe pain on scale of 0 to 10?
Splint chest incision with all movement and coughing and deep breathing.	*Stabilizes sternum and incision to increase comfort.*	Can patient splint chest incision independently?
Encourage patient to report pain even when pain is mild.	*Mild pain is easier to control.*	Does patient report pain when mild?
Turn, reposition every 2 hours, and offer back rub.	*Changes muscle position, relieving stiffness and tense muscles.*	Is patient comfortable without stiffness?
Instruct patient to take a deep breath before movement and exhale slowly during movement.	*Keeps muscles relaxed, minimizing tension with guarding and pain.*	Can patient perform coughing and deep-breathing techniques as instructed?
Explain that chest pain can occur from the surgical incision rather than the heart.	*Chest pain after surgery can be frightening. Patients may not associate surgical chest pain with the incision. They may instead think the pain is anginal or infarction pain.*	Does patient state understanding of pain sources?

Nursing Diagnosis: *Decreased Cardiac Output* related to myocardial depression, hypothermia, bleeding, unstable arrhythmias, or hypoxemia
Expected Outcomes: The patient will remain free of major side effects of pharmacological support. The patient will maintain vital signs within normal limits (WNL), palpable peripheral pulses, urine output greater than 0.5 to 1 mL/kg/hr, and normal sinus rhythm post-transplant.
Evaluation of Outcomes: Is the patient free of major side effects? Are vital signs WNL?

Intervention	Rationale	Evaluation
Monitor vital signs. Observe temperature closely while rewarming the patient.	*Trends reflect problems. Febrile state increases heart rate and myocardial oxygen consumption.*	Are vital signs WNL? Is temperature less than or equal to 98.6°F (37°C)?
Monitor peripheral circulation.	*Mottling or weak pulses may indicate poor cardiac output (CO).*	Do peripheral pulses remain strong with normal skin color, temperature, and capillary refill?
Monitor intake and output.	*Fluid deficit or excess can alter CO.*	Does total intake equal output?
Listen to lung sounds and note character of sputum.	*Crackles may indicate heart failure (HF) or pulmonary edema.*	Are lungs clear?
Monitor chest tube drainage for increase or sudden decrease.	*Drainage of 200 mL/hr may lead to hypovolemia and a decrease in CO.*	Is patient free from cardiac tamponade and hypovolemia?
Monitor echocardiogram.	*Premature ventricular contractions and atrial fibrillation decrease CO.*	Does patient remain in normal sinus rhythm or controlled arrhythmia?

Nursing Care Plan for the Postoperative Patient Undergoing Cardiac or Transplant Surgery—cont'd

Intervention	Rationale	Evaluation
Monitor electrolytes.	*Low calcium and magnesium and high potassium decrease contractility and CO.*	Are electrolytes WNL?
Monitor arterial blood gases (ABGs).	*Acidosis decreases heart function. A low CO may lead to further acidosis.*	Are ABGs WNL?

Nursing Diagnosis: *Risk for Infection* related to inadequate primary defenses from surgical wound or immunosuppression (transplants)
Expected Outcome: The patient will remain free from infection post-transplant.
Evaluation of Outcome: Does the patient remain free from infection?

Intervention	Rationale	Evaluation
Monitor and report abnormal findings for temperature, lung sounds, sputum, and urine consistency.	*Low-grade (immunosuppressed) or high-grade fever, crackles, yellow-green sputum color, or cloudy urine can indicate infection.*	Is patient's temperature WNL? Are lung sounds, sputum, and urine clear?
Encourage coughing, deep breathing, and incentive spirometer use.	*Lung infections can be prevented with lung expansion and secretion removal.*	Does patient perform coughing and deep breathing and use incentive spirometer?
Observe incision for signs and symptoms of infection.	*Erythema (redness), warmth, fever, and swelling indicate infection.*	Are signs and symptoms of infection present?
Monitor drainage and maintain drains.	*Drains remove fluid from the surgical site to prevent infection development.*	Are drainage amount and color normal for procedure? Are drains functioning?
Maintain sterile technique for dressing changes.	*Sterile technique reduces infection development.*	Is incision free of signs and symptoms of infection?

Nursing Diagnosis: *Deficient Knowledge* related to lack of prior experience with transplant
Expected Outcome: The patient will demonstrate understanding of posttransplant care before discharge.
Evaluation of Outcome: Does the patient verbalize understanding and ability to carry out post-transplant care?

Intervention	Rationale	Evaluation
Give information in small increments, and use written and video materials.	*Cardiac transplant patients commonly have memory deficits, cognitive dysfunction, and short attention spans resulting from long-term decreased cerebral perfusion.*	Does patient verbalize understanding of information?
Include families in teaching sessions, and encourage them to promote self-care by the patient.	*Family involvement promotes understanding and retention.*	Does the family participate and verbalize understanding of teaching sessions?
Address or refer sexual functioning questions with patients and their partners.	*Patients usually have questions regarding sexual functioning. Referrals can be made to sex counselors.*	Does patient verbalize that questions have been addressed?
Discharge teaching includes treatment, complications, activity, medications, and enhancing quality of life.	*Patients need comprehensive information to comply with posttransplant care.*	Does patient verbalize understanding of discharge care?

Coping With Cardiac Transplant

Cardiac transplant patients may have feelings of sadness and grief for the donor and his family while also experiencing great elation, relief, and hope after a long wait for the transplant. Patients should be told that these feelings are normal. They should be allowed to express their feelings when they are ready. Emotional support may be needed.

Transplant rejection can occur. Patient education is very important. Instructions for medications and testing must be followed. This is vital to prevent or detect rejection.

After a cardiac transplant, patients work out in an exercise rehabilitation program. Their activity is closely monitored for signs of activity intolerance. Most patients can reach an activity level to play some recreational sports.

CRITICAL THINKING

Mrs. Eden, age 45 and a single mother of two, is transferred to a surgical unit 5 days after a cardiac transplant. She is withdrawn and has a poor appetite. Her vital signs are stable. When ambulating to the bathroom, she is very weak, requiring two nurses to help her. Her respiratory rate increases from 20 to 32 breaths per minute and is slightly labored. Her apical pulse increases from 88 to 103 mm Hg.

1. Is Mrs. Eden tolerating this activity? Why or why not?
2. List four reasons why Mrs. Eden has a poor appetite.
3. Give four patient-centered nursing interventions for Mrs. Eden's poor appetite.
4. Give three reasons why Mrs. Eden is withdrawn.
5. What health care team members might collaborate in Mrs. Eden's care?

Suggested answers are at the end of the chapter.

SUGGESTED ANSWERS TO CRITICAL THINKING

Part 1: Mr. Shepard

1. Signs and symptoms of heart failure (HF) include shortness of breath, two-pillow orthopnea, dry cough, tachycardia (pulse 106 bpm), tachypnea (respiration 24 breaths per minute), and bilateral crackles.
2. Left-sided HF is indicated by the findings.
3. *Shortness of breath:* fluid in the lungs impairs gas exchange; *orthopnea:* lying flat increases fluid accumulation in the lungs, causing dyspnea; *dry cough:* fluid in the lungs irritates the mucosal lining of the lungs; *tachycardia:* sympathetic compensation to increase cardiac output; *tachypnea:* sympathetic compensation to increase blood oxygenation; *bilateral crackles:* fluid trapped in the lungs.
4. The two pillows help prevent orthopnea by using a more upright position, which allows gravity to decrease fluid accumulation in the lungs.
5. The health care provider (HCP; e.g., physician, physician's assistant, nurse practitioner), case manager, nurses, dietitian, physical therapist, occupational therapist, pharmacist, social worker, and clergy.

Part 2: Mr. Shepard

1. Mr. Shepard's heart is enlarged to compensate for the strain caused by increased peripheral vascular resistance from hypertension to maintain an adequate cardiac output.
2. An enlarged heart requires more oxygen, which often cannot be supplied in HF.

Part 3: Mr. Shepard

1. The angiotensin-converting enzyme (ACE) inhibitor is needed for vasodilation to reduce peripheral vascular resistance and decrease the heart's workload. This in turn prevents cardiac remodeling and improves cardiac output.
2. The ACE inhibitor will affect afterload.
3. The diuretic is ordered to decrease fluid volume, which reduces preload and decreases the heart's workload.
4. Potassium needs to be monitored because diuretics can be either potassium-wasting or potassium-sparing.
5. The low-sodium diet is ordered to reduce water retention, which reduces preload and decreases the heart's workload.
6. The goal is to (a) decrease the heart's workload and increase its efficiency by reducing preload and peripheral vascular resistance, and (b) decrease progression of chronic HF and improve survival.

Part 4: Mr. Shepard

1. After determining Mr. Shepard's knowledge base, medication teaching should be given on the ACE inhibitor and diuretic, including their purpose, side effects, and precautions. A schedule for taking the medications can be planned. Explain the purpose of a low-sodium diet and menu planning based on Mr. Shepard's likes and dislikes.
2. Low-sodium foods should be selected to prevent fluid retention. High-potassium foods should be included to prevent hypokalemia from the diuretic, if appropriate. Encourage Mr. Shepard to read food labels. Low-sodium foods include puffed rice, wheat cereals, fruits, chicken, beef, eggs, and potatoes. High-sodium foods include tomato juice, sauerkraut, softened water, buttermilk, cheese, smoked meats, canned tuna, canned soup, pickles, instant rice, and instant potatoes. High-potassium foods include salt substitutes, bran products, avocado, bananas, prunes, oranges, baked potato, sweet potato, spinach (cooked), chocolate, nuts, and molasses.
3. Daily weighing is necessary to detect a rapid weight gain that indicates fluid retention (2 pounds in 24 hours) and to measure weight loss resulting from the diuretic.

SUGGESTED ANSWERS TO CRITICAL THINKING—cont'd

4. These instructions ensure accuracy of the weight so that comparison to the baseline weight detects a weight gain or loss.
5. The guideline for reporting a weight increase is an increase of 2 to 3 pounds in 1 to 2 days.

Mrs. Eden

1. No, Mrs. Eden is not tolerating this activity, as evidenced by her increased respiratory rate and apical rate.
2. Steroids, immunosuppressive therapy, depression, and fatigue could be causing her poor appetite.
3. Nursing interventions related to Mrs. Eden's poor appetite could include the following: offer small, frequent meals; have her family bring favorite foods from home; allow the patient to rest before meals; provide oral hygiene before meals; administer antiemetics before meals; and give a high-calorie meal at peak appetite.
4. Mrs. Eden could be withdrawn because of changes in her lifestyle as a result of her transplant, extreme fatigue, concerns regarding how she will raise her children, grieving for the donor, and fear that she will reject her new heart.
5. HCP (e.g., surgeon, physician's assistant, nurse practitioner), case manager, nurses, dietitian, physical therapist, occupational therapist, pharmacist, social worker, and clergy.

Review Questions

1. The nurse is providing patient education. The patient asks the nurse what heart failure is. Which of the following is the nurse's best response?
   1. "The heart pumps too much blood into the pulmonary veins."
   2. "The heart is unable to pump enough blood for the body's oxygen needs."
   3. "Heart failure is a buildup of blood in the aorta from the heart's left ventricle."
   4. "With a failing heart, the heart stops beating, so blood is not pumped out."

2. The nurse is to administer bumetanide (Bumex) to a patient but first reviews laboratory results. Which of these results requires action by the nurse?
   1. Potassium 3.0 meq/dL
   2. Sodium 135 meq/dL
   3. International normalized ratio 0.8
   4. Partial thromboplastin time 36 seconds

3. A patient who has been treated for heart failure is being prescribed 20 mg furosemide (Lasix) daily upon discharge from the hospital. Which of the following statements by the patient would indicate to the nurse the need for further teaching for this medication? **Select all that apply.**
   1. "I will take the Lasix in the morning."
   2. "I will take the Lasix at bedtime."
   3. "I will drink lots of fluids with the Lasix."
   4. "I will take it with each meal."
   5. "I will count my pulse for 2 minutes."
   6. "I will eat more bananas."

4. The nurse is caring for a patient receiving bumetanide (Bumex) to reduce preload for heart failure. While collecting data, the nurse sees the patient has less ankle edema and jugular vein distention than earlier. The next dose of bumetanide is scheduled in 1 hour. Which of the following actions should the nurse take?
   1. Notify the physician.
   2. Hold the bumetanide.
   3. Give the bumetanide as scheduled.
   4. Give the bumetanide early.

5. The nurse is reinforcing teaching for a patient with chronic heart failure. Which of the following weight assessments should the nurse teach the patient to perform to monitor fluid status at home?
   1. Weigh daily.
   2. Weigh weekly.
   3. Weigh biweekly.
   4. Weigh monthly.

6. A 160-pound patient is to receive cyclosporine (Neoral) 12.5 mg/kg daily in two divided doses. How many milligrams will the patient receive with each dose? Fill in the blank.
   Answer: _____ mg

Answer rationales available in your online resources.

ANSWERS 1. 2; 2. 1; 3. 2, 3, 4, 5; 4. 3; 5. 1; 6. 454.5 mg per dose (160/2.2 = 72.72 × 12.5 = 909/2 = 454.5)

Key Points

Find the chapter key points in your online resources
available through Davis Edge.

Additional Resources

Use the scratch off code on the inside front
cover of your book to access online quizzes
that will help you to improve your scores
on course exams and prepare for the NCLEX-PN®.

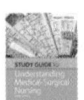 Study Guide

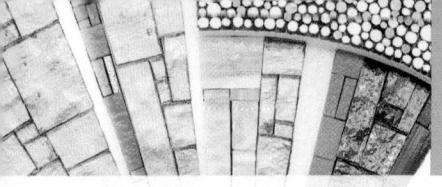
CHAPTER 27

Hematologic and Lymphatic System Function, Assessment, and Therapeutic Measures

Jennifer Mitchell, Janice L. Bradford, Lucy L. Colo

KEY TERMS

ecchymoses (EK-ih-MOH-sis)
hemolysis (hee-MAHL-ih-sis)
lymphedema (LIMPF-uh-DEE-mah)
petechiae (puh-TEE-kee-eye)
purpura (PURR-purr-uh)

CHAPTER CONCEPTS

Hematologic Regulation
Infection

LEARNING OUTCOMES

1. List the components of blood.
2. List the components of the lymphatic system.
3. Describe how changes in the blood or lymph systems can manifest as disease processes.
4. Describe the sequence of events in the process of blood clotting.
5. Identify data to collect when caring for a patient with a disorder of the hematologic or lymphatic system.
6. Identify laboratory and diagnostic studies that are used when evaluating the hematologic and lymphatic systems.
7. Plan nursing care for patients undergoing diagnostic tests of the hematologic or lymphatic systems.
8. List common therapeutic measures used for patients with hematologic and lymphatic disorders.
9. Discuss the role of the licensed practical nurse/licensed vocational nurse in administering blood products.

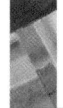

NORMAL HEMATOLOGIC AND LYMPHATIC SYSTEM ANATOMY AND PHYSIOLOGY

The hematologic system includes the bone marrow, blood, and blood components. The lymphatic system includes lymph nodes; nodules, which filter pathogens for destruction; and lymph vessels, which return lymph to the blood.

Blood

The general functions of blood are transport of substances; regulation of body temperature, pH, and fluid balance; and transport of cells that offer the body protection.

The human body contains 4 to 6 L of blood. Approximately 45% is formed elements. The remainder is plasma (Fig. 27.1). All formed elements are produced from stem cells in the red bone marrow (hematopoietic tissue) found in flat bones, irregular bones, and the epiphyses of long bones (Fig. 27.2). T-lymphocyte maturation and differentiation occur in the thymus. Table 27.1 shows normal blood cell counts.

Plasma

Plasma, the transporting medium, is about 91% water. Plasma proteins are synthesized by the liver. They include clotting factors, albumin, and globulins. Clotting factors such as prothrombin and fibrinogen circulate until activated for coagulation. Albumin helps maintain blood volume and pressure by pulling tissue fluid into the venous ends of the capillary networks. Alpha and beta globulins are carrier molecules for substances such as fats. Gamma globulins are antibodies produced by lymphocytes.

Plasma is also important in maintaining body temperature. The water of plasma is warmed by passage through active organs, such as the liver or skeletal muscles; then blood distributes this heat throughout the body. The flush of fever or vigorous exercise is caused by vasodilation in the dermis, allowing blood to circulate near the body surface, resulting in heat loss. A person in a cold environment may appear pale. This is because vasoconstriction in the dermis shunts blood toward the core of the body for heat retention.

The normal pH range of blood is 7.35 to 7.45. Buffer systems in the blood moderate acid–base changes to maintain homeostasis.

Plasma is the clear, extracellular matrix of this liquid connective tissue. It accounts for 55% of blood.

The main component of plasma is water; however, plasma also contains proteins (the main one being **albumin**), nutrients, electrolytes, hormones, and gases. Plasma proteins play roles in blood clotting, the immune system, and the regulation of fluid volume. Plasma without the clotting proteins (which occurs when blood is allowed to clot and the solid portion is removed) is called **serum**.

WBCs and platelets form a narrow buff-colored band just underneath the plasma. Called the *buffy coat*, these cells constitute 1% or less of the blood volume.

Formed elements—which include cells and cell fragments—make up 45% of blood. Specific blood cells include **erythrocytes** (red blood cells, or RBCs), **leukocytes** (white blood cells, or WBCs), and **platelets**.

RBCs are the heaviest of the formed elements and sink to the bottom of the sample. They account for most of the formed elements. This value—the percentage of cells in a sample of blood—is called the **hematocrit**.

FIGURE 27.1 Components of blood.

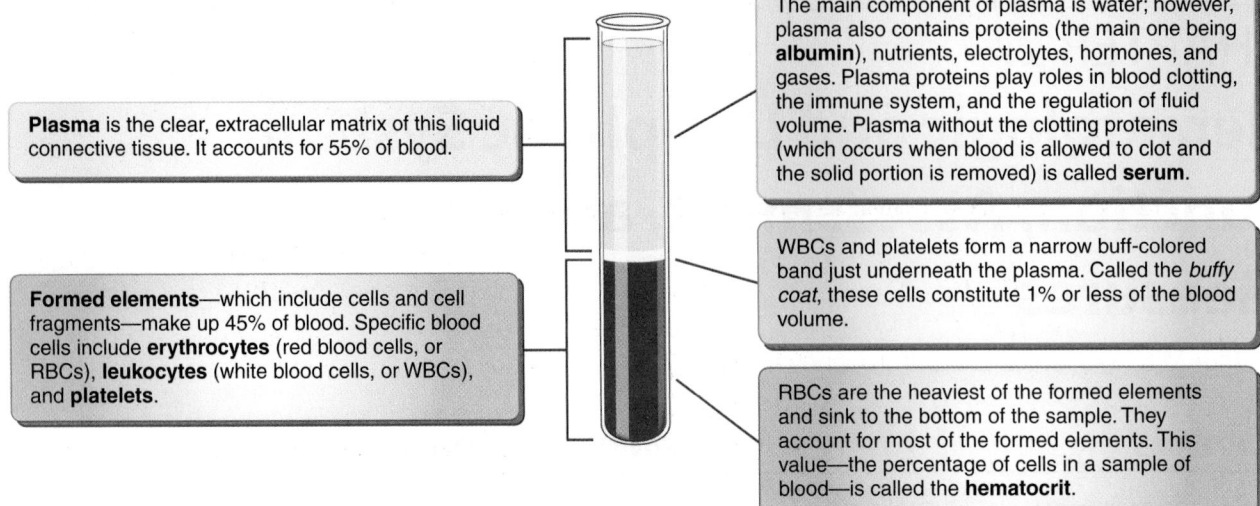

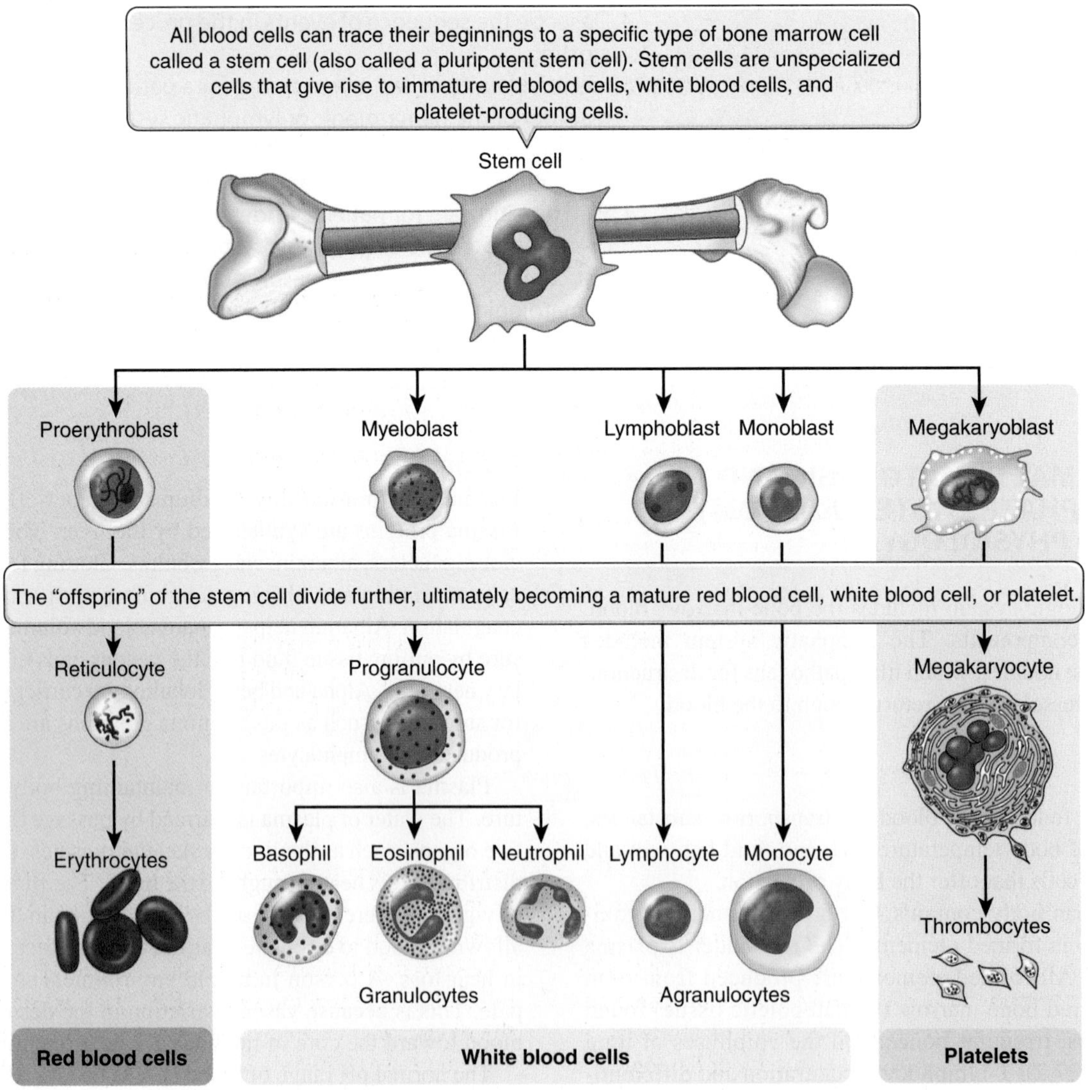

All blood cells can trace their beginnings to a specific type of bone marrow cell called a stem cell (also called a pluripotent stem cell). Stem cells are unspecialized cells that give rise to immature red blood cells, white blood cells, and platelet-producing cells.

Stem cell

Proerythroblast   Myeloblast   Lymphoblast   Monoblast   Megakaryoblast

The "offspring" of the stem cell divide further, ultimately becoming a mature red blood cell, white blood cell, or platelet.

Reticulocyte   Progranulocyte   Megakaryocyte

Erythrocytes   Basophil   Eosinophil   Neutrophil   Lymphocyte   Monocyte   Thrombocytes

Granulocytes   Agranulocytes

Red blood cells   **White blood cells**   **Platelets**

FIGURE 27.2 Blood cell formation.

Table 27.1

Review of Blood Cell Values and Disorders

Test	*Normal Value*	*Significance of Abnormal Findings*
Red Blood Cells (RBCs)		
Increased RBCs is called polycythemia; decreased RBCs is called anemia.		
RBCs	*Male:* 4.71–5.14 million/mm³ *Female:* 4.2–4.87 million/mm³	Increased in chronic hypoxia Decreased in anemia or blood loss
Hematocrit (Hct; cellular portion of blood)	*Male:* 43%–49% *Female:* 38%–44%	Increased in dehydration or chronic hypoxia Decreased in anemia or blood loss
Hemoglobin (Hgb; reflects oxygen-carrying capacity of blood)	*Male:* 13.2–17.3 g/100 mL *Female:* 11.7–15.5 g/100 mL	Increased in chronic hypoxia Decreased in blood loss or anemia
Reticulocytes (number of circulating immature RBCs)	1.5%–2.5%	Increased in hypoxia or anemia Decreased in RBC maturation defect
White Blood Cells (WBCs)		
Increased WBCs is called leukocytosis; decreased WBCs is called leukopenia.		
WBCs	4,500–11,000/mm³	Increased in infection
Neutrophils (Bands) (Segments)	59% (3%) (56%)	Increased in infection
Eosinophils	2.7%	Increased in allergic response, some leukemias
Basophils	0.5%	Increased in hyperthyroidism, some bone marrow disorders, ulcerative colitis
Lymphocytes	34%	Increased in viral infections, chronic bacterial infection, some leukemias
Monocytes	4%	Increased in chronic inflammatory disorders, some leukemias
Platelets		
Increased platelets is called thrombocytosis; decreased platelets is called thrombocytopenia.		
Thrombocytes/platelets	150,000–450,000/mm³	Increased from trauma Decreased with blood disorders Increased risk of bleeding with low platelet count

Red Blood Cells

Mature red blood cells (RBCs) are biconcave disks without nuclei; they carry oxygen bonded to the iron in hemoglobin. *Oxyhemoglobin* is formed in the pulmonary capillaries when oxygen bonds to the iron in hemoglobin. Once hemoglobin gives up its oxygen to the cells of the body, it becomes *reduced hemoglobin*. The amount of hemoglobin in RBCs, the amount of iron in that hemoglobin, and the number of RBCs determine the amount of oxygen the blood can carry. Reduced oxygen-carrying capacity causes anemia. This results in symptoms such as shortness of breath and fatigue.

Hypoxia stimulates the kidneys to secrete erythropoietin. This increases the rate of RBC production and, thus, the oxygen-carrying capacity of the blood. A *reticulocyte* (immature RBC) becomes a mature RBC when it ejects its nucleus. This causes the characteristic biconcave disk shape. The presence of large numbers of reticulocytes in peripheral blood indicates an insufficient number of mature RBCs to meet the oxygen demands of the body.

Sufficient dietary intake of protein and iron to synthesize hemoglobin is required for normal production of RBCs. The vitamins folic acid and vitamin B_{12} are needed for DNA synthesis in the stem cells of the red bone marrow; mitosis is dependent on the ability to produce new sets of chromosomes. Vitamin B_{12} is called *extrinsic factor* because it comes from an extrinsic source: food. The parietal cells of the stomach lining produce *intrinsic factor*. This is a chemical that combines with vitamin B_{12} to promote its absorption in the small intestine.

RBCs live for about 120 days. After that, they become fragile and are phagocytized by fixed macrophages in the liver, spleen, and red bone marrow (Fig. 27.3). Diseases such as malaria and sickle cell anemia cause an accelerated destruction of RBCs (**hemolysis**). The resulting release of excess hemoglobin can cause the blood level of bilirubin to rise. Elevated bilirubin levels discolor the sclerae, skin, and mucous membranes to a yellowish orange hue; this condition is known as jaundice.

Each person has an inherited blood type. Blood type is determined by the antigens present on the RBCs. The two most important type categories are the ABO group and the Rh factor. The ABO type (A, B, O, or AB) indicates the antigens present (or not present, as in type O) on the RBCs. The plasma contains antibodies for antigens that are not present in the blood. These antibodies can interact with antigens in transfused blood if the donor's blood does not match the recipient's blood (Table 27.2). To be Rh-positive means that the D antigen is present on the RBCs; Rh-negative means that the antigen is not present. Rh-negative people do not have natural antibodies to the D antigen but will produce them if given Rh-positive blood.

White Blood Cells

White blood cells (WBCs) are larger than RBCs. They have nuclei when mature. The granular WBCs (neutrophils, eosinophils, and basophils) and the agranular WBCs (lymphocytes and monocytes) are produced in the red bone marrow; the T lymphocytes complete their development in the thymus. The T lymphocytes and B lymphocytes become activated, proliferate, and differentiate in the lymph nodes, spleen, and lymphatic nodules. Table 27.1 shows normal values and percentages for each type of WBC in a differential count. WBCs function within tissue fluid and blood. All are involved in the immune or inflammatory response to injury.

Monocytes become macrophages in tissues, which phagocytize pathogens and viral-infected cells. Neutrophils are more numerous and phagocytize foreign materials. Eosinophils combat the effects of histamine, detoxify foreign proteins during allergic reactions, and respond to parasitic infections. Basophils release heparin and histamine as part of inflammatory reactions. There are two groups of lymphocytes: T cells and B cells. T cells may be helper, suppressor, killer, or memory T cells. B cells become memory cells and plasma cells; plasma cells produce antibodies to foreign antigens.

Platelets

Platelets are formed in the red bone marrow. They are fragments of large cells called megakaryocytes. Platelets are involved in all mechanisms of hemostasis: vascular spasm, platelet plugs, and chemical clotting.

After a platelet plug is formed, one of two pathways initiates a cascade of events to bring about coagulation. When a blood vessel or surrounding tissues *outside* the blood are damaged, the extrinsic pathway begins. Conversely, when platelets adhere to damaged endothelium and release clotting factors, this initiates the *intrinsic* pathway. Either way, the end result is a fibrin clot (Fig. 27.4).

Excessive clotting in the vascular system is prevented in several ways. The smooth endothelial lining of blood vessels repels platelets so that they do not stick to intact vessel walls. Heparin produced by mast cells inhibits the clotting mechanism. Antithrombin inactivates excess thrombin to prevent the clotting mechanism from becoming a vicious cycle.

Lymphatic System

The lymphatic system consists of lymph, lymph vessels, lymph nodes and nodules, the spleen, and the thymus (Fig. 27.5). Functions of the lymph system include the return of tissue fluid to maintain blood volume and protecting the body against pathogens and other foreign material. (Immunity is covered in Unit 4.)

Lymphatic Vessels

Lymph is tissue fluid that has entered lymph capillaries. Lymph must be returned to the blood to maintain blood volume and blood pressure. Lymph capillaries are found in most tissue spaces. They anastomose, forming larger and larger lymph vessels, which have valves to prevent backflow. Lymph from areas below the diaphragm and the upper left half of the body enters the thoracic duct. It is returned to the blood in the left subclavian vein. Lymph from the upper right body enters the right lymphatic duct. It is returned to the blood in the right subclavian vein.

Lymph Nodes and Nodules

Lymph *nodes* are masses of lymphatic tissue along the pathways of the lymph vessels. They house activated lymphocytes and macrophages. Nodes are scattered throughout the body. They are concentrated in the cervical, axillary, and

• **WORD** • **BUILDING** •
hemolysis: heme—blood + lysis—dissolution

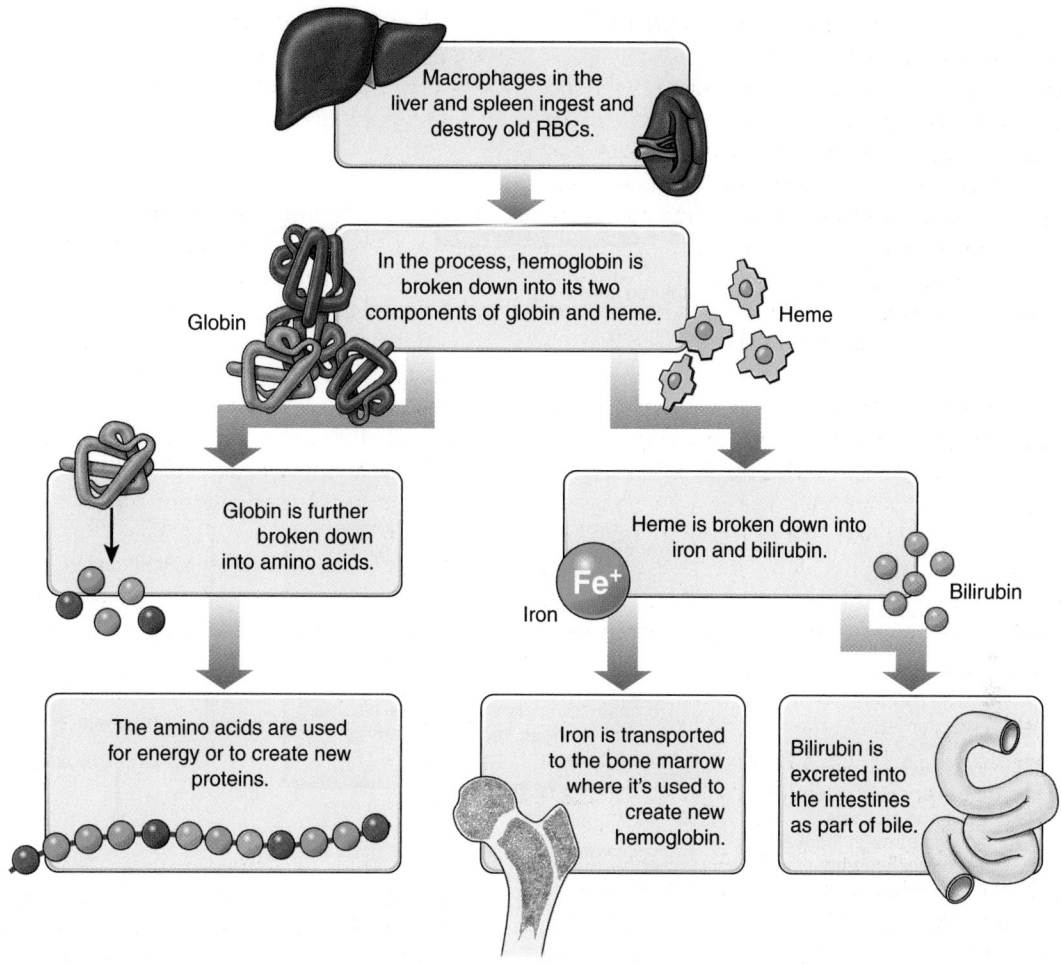

FIGURE 27.3 Breakdown of red blood cells.

Table 27.2

ABO Blood Types

Type	Antigens Present on Red Blood Cells	Antibodies Present in Plasma
A	A	Anti-B
B	B	Anti-A
AB	Both A and B	Neither anti-A nor anti-B
O	Neither A nor B	Both anti-A and anti-B

inguinal regions, where they are well situated to remove pathogens before the lymph is returned to the blood. Foreign materials are phagocytized by fixed macrophages; lymphocytes form immune responses.

Lymph *nodules* (or mucosa-associated lymphatic tissue) are small masses of lymphatic tissue found just beneath the epithelium of all mucous membranes. Mucosal-lined tracts

(respiratory, digestive, urinary, and reproductive) have openings to the external environment. Any natural body opening is a potential portal of entry for pathogens. Microbes that penetrate the epithelium are usually destroyed by the macrophages in the lymph nodules. The tonsils, which protect the oral and nasal portions of the pharynx, are familiar examples of lymph nodules.

Spleen

The spleen is located in the upper left quadrant of the abdominal cavity, just below the diaphragm and behind the stomach. The lower rib cage protects the spleen from mechanical injury. In the fetus, the spleen produces RBCs, a function assumed by the bone marrow after birth.

The spleen has several functions after birth. It contains B cells and T cells, which conduct immune responses. It also contains fixed macrophages that phagocytize pathogens and worn or defective blood cells and platelets. The heme unit from RBC destruction forms bilirubin. Bilirubin is sent to the liver by way of portal circulation for excretion in the bile. The spleen stores up to one-third of the body's platelets.

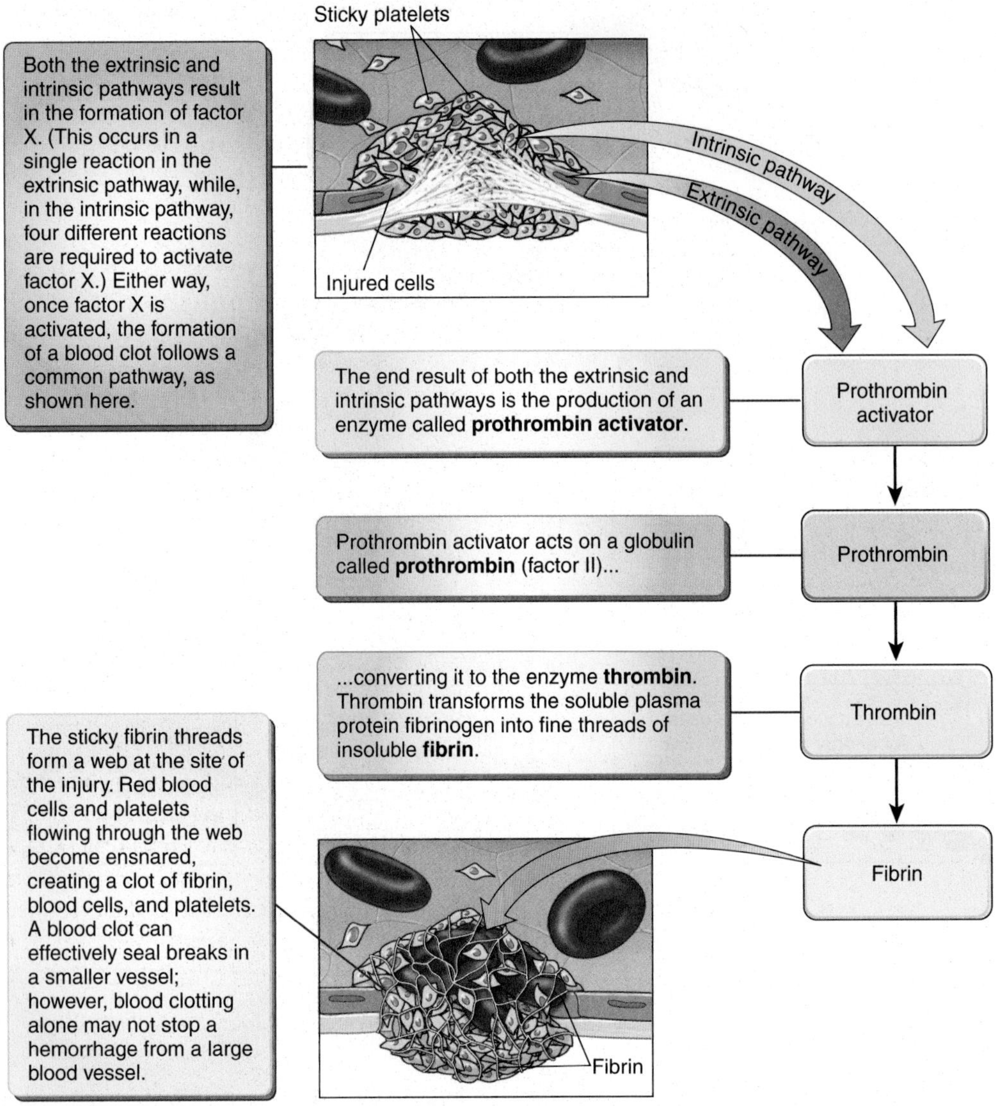

Sticky platelets

Both the extrinsic and intrinsic pathways result in the formation of factor X. (This occurs in a single reaction in the extrinsic pathway, while, in the intrinsic pathway, four different reactions are required to activate factor X.) Either way, once factor X is activated, the formation of a blood clot follows a common pathway, as shown here.

Injured cells

Intrinsic pathway

Extrinsic pathway

The end result of both the extrinsic and intrinsic pathways is the production of an enzyme called **prothrombin activator**.

Prothrombin activator acts on a globulin called **prothrombin** (factor II)...

...converting it to the enzyme **thrombin**. Thrombin transforms the soluble plasma protein fibrinogen into fine threads of insoluble **fibrin**.

The sticky fibrin threads form a web at the site of the injury. Red blood cells and platelets flowing through the web become ensnared, creating a clot of fibrin, blood cells, and platelets. A blood clot can effectively seal breaks in a smaller vessel; however, blood clotting alone may not stop a hemorrhage from a large blood vessel.

Fibrin

Prothrombin activator

Prothrombin

Thrombin

Fibrin

FIGURE 27.4 Formation of a blood clot.

The spleen is not considered a vital organ because other organs compensate for its functions if it must be removed. The liver and red bone marrow also remove worn RBCs from circulation. The many lymph nodes and nodules produce lymphocytes and macrophages for protection. However, a person without a spleen is somewhat more susceptible to certain bacterial infections, such as pneumonia and meningitis.

Thymus

The thymus is located in the mediastinum, anterior to the trachea. As we age, the thymus atrophies, so relatively little thymic tissue is found in adults. The thymus contains T lymphocytes (T cells) that mature and proliferate. Thymic hormones contribute to the maturation of the T cells. (Immunity is covered in Unit 4.)

Aging and the Hematologic and Lymphatic Systems

Older adults undergo a number of changes in the hematologic and lymphatic systems (Fig. 27.6).

NURSING ASSESSMENT OF HEMATOLOGIC AND LYMPHATIC SYSTEMS

Health History

A thorough nursing assessment starts with an in-depth patient history (Table 27.3). Specific problems that might be seen in patients with hematologic disorders include abnormal bleeding, **petechiae** (small purplish hemorrhagic spots under the skin), **ecchymoses** (larger areas of discoloration

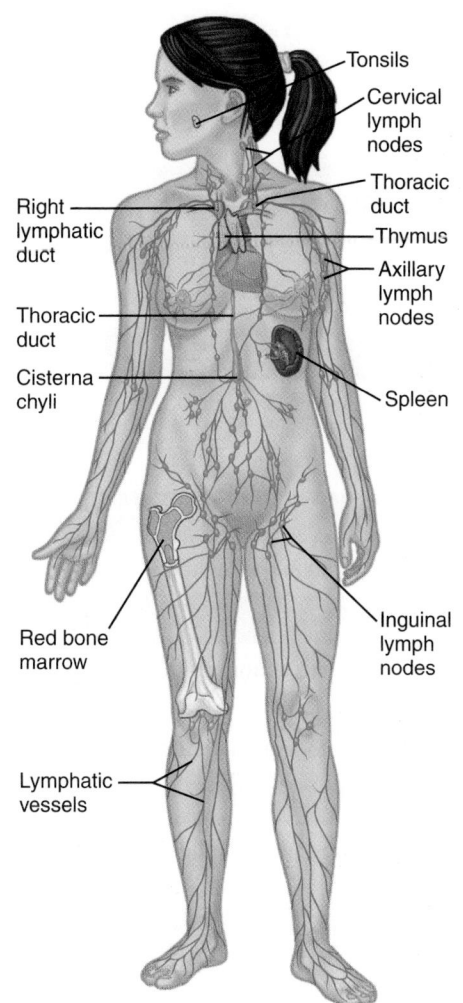

Tonsils
Cervical lymph nodes
Thoracic duct
Right lymphatic duct
Thymus
Axillary lymph nodes
Thoracic duct
Cisterna chyli
Spleen
Red bone marrow
Inguinal lymph nodes
Lymphatic vessels

FIGURE 27.5 The lymphatic system.

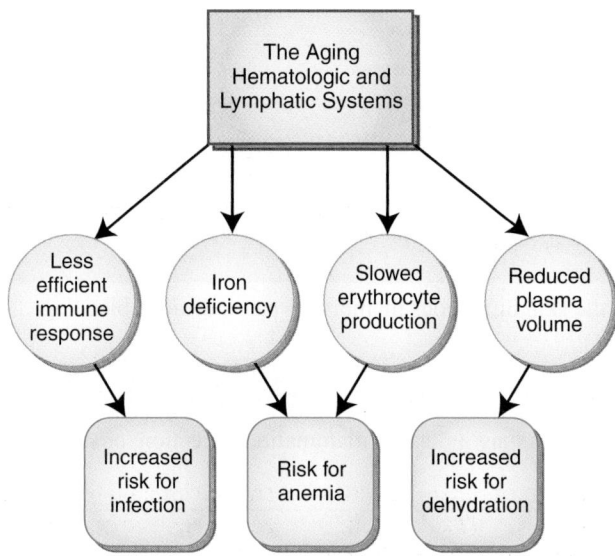
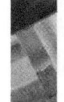

The Aging Hematologic and Lymphatic Systems

Less efficient immune response

Iron deficiency

Slowed erythrocyte production

Reduced plasma volume

Increased risk for infection

Risk for anemia

Increased risk for dehydration

FIGURE 27.6 Effects of aging on the hematologic and lymphatic systems.

from hemorrhage under the skin), and **purpura** (hemorrhage into the skin, mucous membranes, and organs). Additional symptoms include fatigue, weakness, shortness of breath, and fever. Fatigue, malaise, and weight loss can accompany cancers of the lymphatic system.

Begin by obtaining the patient's biographical data, marital status, occupation, religion, age, sex, and ethnic background. This information can give you valuable clues to risk factors. For example, even though hemophilia almost always occurs in males, females can carry the gene. Sickle cell anemia occurs mostly in African Americans but also affects people of Mediterranean or Asian ancestry. Pernicious anemia occurs most often in people of northern European ancestry. By carefully collecting this information, you can obtain important clues that will help pinpoint a patient's problem. Finally, focus on collecting data about symptoms by using the *WHAT'S UP?* format presented in Chapter 1.

A complete review of past illnesses and family history is always indicated and can provide valuable information. A social history is also useful. After developing good rapport with the patient, explore dietary and alcohol intake habits, any drug use or abuse, and sexual habits, all of which can cause changes in the hematologic system.

An occupational review can reveal exposure to hazardous substances that can cause bone marrow dysfunction. Certain occupations, such as working in a paint factory, tool and dye processing, and even dry cleaning, can be related to the formation of some hematologic cancers. Military history can also reveal sources of exposure that can help during the diagnostic phase for hematologic and lymphatic disorders.

Physical Examination

Hematologic and lymphatic disorders can involve almost every body system, so each system must be assessed. Signs and symptoms of hematologic and lymphatic disorders can be vague, such as shortness of breath or fatigue. A careful assessment will guide nursing care but may also uncover important data that should be reported to the primary care provider. Table 27.4 reviews objective data that should be collected and possible interpretations of findings.

DIAGNOSTIC TESTS FOR THE HEMATOLOGIC AND LYMPHATIC SYSTEMS

Blood Tests

Examples of laboratory studies routinely done for patients with hematologic disorders include complete blood count (CBC), total hemoglobin (Hgb) concentration, hematocrit (Hct) level, and platelet level. See normal values in Table 27.1.

Coagulation Tests

Coagulation tests are shown in Table 27.5. Agglutination tests include ABO blood typing, Rh typing, crossmatching

Table 27.3

Subjective Data Collection for the Hematologic and Lymphatic Systems

Questions to Ask During the Health History	*Rationale/Significance*
Reason for Seeking Health Care	
Why are you seeking health care?	Signs and symptoms of hematologic/lymphatic disorders may be nonspecific. Any body system can be involved.
Family History	
How is the health of your blood relatives? Does anyone in your family have any blood-related diseases?	Some blood and immune disorders are hereditary.
Diet History	
Describe your usual diet.	Dietary deficiencies can lead to anemia or altered immune responses.
Medications/Supplements	
What medications do you take? What herbs or alternative therapies do you use?	Herbs and drugs can cause adverse reactions in the blood and immune systems.
How much alcohol do you drink each day?	Excess alcohol intake can lead to folic acid–deficiency anemia.
Occupational/Exposure History	
What is your occupational history? What is your military history?	Exposure to certain hazardous substances can lead to anemias, leukemias, or other cancers.
Fatigue	
Have you noticed any change in your energy level?	Anemia and many cancers are associated with fatigue.
Bleeding Tendency	
Have you experienced nosebleeds or any other unusual bleeding? Have you had bloody or black bowel movements?	Bleeding may indicate low platelet levels or a clotting factor deficiency.
Respiratory	
Do you experience shortness of breath or faintness?	Red blood cells (RBCs) carry oxygen, so a reduced RBC count can cause dyspnea.
Integumentary	
Have you noticed any changes in your skin?	Bleeding into the skin or mucous membranes can indicate a bleeding disorder.
Lymphadenopathy	
Have you noticed swelling in your neck, armpits, or groin?	Swollen lymph nodes may indicate inflammation, infection, or some cancers.

T a b l e 2 7 . 4
Objective Data Collection for the Hematologic and Lymphatic Systems

Abnormal Findings	*Possible Hematologic/Lymphatic Causes*
Vital Signs	
Fever	Poor immune function, infection
Subnormal temperature	Possible overwhelming Gram-negative infection
Elevated heart rate	Blood loss
Elevated respiratory rate	Anemia, decreased oxygen supply
Level of Consciousness	
Decreased level	Hypoxia, fever, intracranial bleeding
Skin, Mucous Membranes	
Pallor	Anemia
Cyanosis	Poor oxygenation of red blood cells
Jaundice (yellow color)	Hemolysis, liver involvement
Inflammation, redness, swelling, drainage	Poor immune function, infection
Purpura, ecchymoses, petechiae	Bleeding disorder
Dry or coarse skin	Some anemias
Itching	Blood or lymph disorders, jaundice, liver involvement
Fingernails	
Striations	Anemia
Spoon-shaped nails	Anemia
Clubbed fingers	Long-term hypoxia, anemia
Abdomen	
High-pitched, tinkling bowel sounds	Intestinal obstruction
Increasing abdominal girth	Ascites, bleeding
Neck, Axillae	
Lymph nodes greater than 1 cm in size or tender nodes	**Lymphedema,** inflammation, some cancers
Sternum	
Tenderness	Bone marrow packed with abnormal cells

of blood samples, and direct antiglobulin tests (also known as the Coombs test).

Bone Marrow Biopsy
Biopsy information can be obtained through removal of a small amount of bone marrow with a needle. Aspiration of marrow is done to obtain a specimen that can be viewed under the microscope. Purposes of this test include the diagnosis of hematologic disorders; monitoring the course of

· WORD · BUILDING ·

lymphedema: lymph—fluid found in lymphatic vessels + edema—swelling

CRITICAL THINKING

Mrs. Brown is on warfarin (Coumadin) therapy because of a blood clot in her leg. She has an international normalized ratio (INR) done at her health care provider's (HCP) office. The result is 4. Will the HCP most likely increase Mrs. Brown's daily dose of warfarin, decrease it, or leave it the same? (Use Table 27.5 to figure out the answer.)

Suggested answers are at the end of the chapter.

LEARNING TIP

When a patient has a bacterial infection, the neutrophils, which are the most numerous of the white blood cells (WBCs), rise in number to help fight it. There are two forms of neutrophils: segmented (mature) and bands (immature). Initially, the number of segmented neutrophils rises. Then, as the infection becomes more severe, the number of immature bands will rise.

An easy way to remember this is that the WBCs are part of the body's defenses, just like the military is part of a country's defenses. When needed, sergeants who are fully trained or mature are called to assess the battle first. If they are unable to fight off the invading enemy, new recruits being trained in boot camp are called in to help.

Segmented neutrophils (called **s**egs) are like the **s**ergeants, fully mature and ready to fight. The **b**ands are like **b**oot camp recruits, immature and not fully trained. However, in an acute infection, bands are needed to keep the body from being overwhelmed by the infection and losing the battle.

As you look at the differential WBC count, if the segs are elevated but the bands are normal, the infection is probably new. If the bands are also elevated, the infection is worsening. The more elevated they are, the more severe the infection.

Lymphocytes fight viral infections and are elevated during a virus. A common pattern in the WBCs is produced for either a bacterial or viral infection. If the infection is acute bacterial:

Segs ↑ Bands ↑ Lymphocytes ↓
If the infection is viral:
Segs ↓ Bands ↓ Lymphocytes ↑

The bone marrow produces the cells most needed during the time of viral infection and reduces production of those cells least needed. When the infection is resolved, all of the cells should return to their normal production levels.

---

treatment; discovery of other disorders, such as primary and metastatic tumors, infectious diseases, and certain granulomas; and isolation of bacteria and other pathogens by culture.

An accurate bone marrow specimen in an adult can be obtained from the sternum, the spinous processes of the vertebrae, or the anterior or posterior iliac crest. Bone marrow biopsy is considered a minor surgical procedure. It is carried out under aseptic conditions. For iliac crest aspiration, the patient is placed comfortably on the side with the back slightly flexed. The posterior iliac crest is cleansed and covered with antiseptic solution. The skin, subcutaneous tissue, and periosteum are anesthetized using 1% or 2% lidocaine (Xylocaine). A 2- to 3-mm incision is made to facilitate penetration with a 14-gauge, 2- to 4-cm-long bone marrow needle. The incision is made to avoid introducing a skin plug into the marrow cavity, which can cause infection.

The nurse's role in bone marrow biopsy is multifaceted. You may need to help coordinate between the laboratory and the health care provider (HCP), establish a time to do the procedure, and determine who obtains the supplies, such as the disposable bone marrow aspiration tray and specialized needles. Be sure to obtain an order for an analgesic and to administer it before the procedure. Assist with positioning the patient before and during the procedure. Afterward, observe the aspiration site for bleeding and infection. Provide emotional support to the patient before, during, and after the procedure.

BE SAFE!

Make sure that the correct surgery is done on the correct patient and at the correct place on the patient's body. (Joint Commission's 2018 National Patient Safety Goals, © The Joint Commission, 2018. Reprinted with permission.)

Lymphangiography

Problems in the lymph system, such as lymphoma or metastatic cancers, can be evaluated using lymphangiography. This procedure involves injection of a dye into the lymphatic vessels of the hand or foot. X-ray views are then taken to determine lymph flow or blockages. X-ray examinations are repeated in 24 hours to assess lymph node involvement.

Following the procedure, the HCP may order a pressure dressing and immobilization of the injected limb to prevent bleeding at the site. Continue to monitor the limb for swelling, circulatory status, and changes in sensation. Warn the patient that the skin, urine, or feces may be tinged blue from the dye for about 2 days.

Lymph Node Biopsy

If a lymph node is enlarged, it may be biopsied to determine whether the cause is infection or malignancy. A biopsy is done with a needle aspiration or surgical incision. A small dressing or bandage is applied to the site. Following the procedure, review signs of bleeding and infection with the patient that should be reported to the HCP.

Table 27.5
Coagulation Studies

Test	Normal Value	Significance of Abnormal Findings
Prothrombin time (PT; affected by activity of clotting factors V, VII, and X; prothrombin; and fibrinogen)	*Male:* 9.6–11.8 seconds *Female:* 9.5–11.3 seconds *Therapeutic range:* 1.5–2.0 times normal for patient on warfarin (Coumadin) therapy	Abnormalities in these values when the patient is not receiving anticoagulant therapy can indicate liver malfunction and bleeding tendency.
International normalized ratio (INR; standardized test adopted by World Health Organization)	Less than 1.3 *Therapeutic range:* 2.0–3.0 for patient on warfarin (Coumadin); 3.0–4.5 for recurrent problems	When receiving anticoagulant therapy, indicates if dosage needs to be increased or decreased.
Activated partial thromboplastin time (aPTT; evaluates factors I, II, V, VIII, IX, X, XI, and XII)	25–39 seconds *Therapeutic range:* 1.5–2.0 times normal for patient on heparin therapy	When receiving anticoagulant therapy, indicates if dosage needs to be increased or decreased.
Bleeding time (measures time for small puncture wound to stop bleeding)	2.5–9.5 minutes	Prolonged bleeding time indicates a platelet disorder.
Capillary fragility test (tests ability of capillaries to resist rupture under pressure)	Fewer than 10 petechiae appearing in a 2-inch circle after application of a blood pressure cuff at 100 mm Hg for 5 minutes	More than 10 petechiae could be related to fragile capillaries or thrombocytopenia.

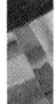

THERAPEUTIC MEASURES FOR THE HEMATOLOGIC AND LYMPHATIC SYSTEMS

Blood Administration

Blood may be administered by a registered nurse (RN) or licensed practical nurse/licensed vocational nurse (LPN/LVN), depending on the state in which you practice. As an LPN/LVN, you may be called on to assist with proper identification procedures and monitoring of vital signs during the transfusion.

Table 27.6 lists blood components that may be ordered. The main goals are to administer them safely and to avoid mistakes. Make sure to use proper identifying information to ensure that the right patient is receiving the right blood products. In addition, most institutions require a special transfusion consent form to be completed and present in the patient's chart.

> **BE SAFE!**
>
> **BE VIGILANT!** Use at least two ways to identify patients. For example, use the patient's name *and* date of birth. This is done to make sure that each patient gets the correct medicine and treatment.
>
> Make sure that the correct patient gets the correct blood when they get a blood transfusion. (Joint Commission's 2018 National Patient Safety Goals, © The Joint Commission, 2018. Reprinted with permission.)

Table 27.6
Blood Products

Product	Use
Packed red blood cells (RBCs)	Severe anemia or blood loss
Frozen RBCs	Autotransfusion (blood taken from patient and saved for future surgery), prevention of febrile reactions
Platelets	Bleeding caused by thrombocytopenia
Albumin	Hypovolemia caused by hypoalbuminemia
Fresh frozen plasma	Provides clotting factors for bleeding disorders; occasionally used for volume replacement
Cryoprecipitates	Bleeding caused by specific missing clotting factors

Special Precautions

FLUID COMPATIBILITY. Make sure to use only normal saline solution to help dilute the blood and to flush the intravenous (IV) lines before and after the transfusions. Solutions that contain dextrose can cause RBCs to lyse (i.e., destroy their cell membranes). Solutions with calcium can cause the blood product to clump, clot, or not infuse at all.

TIMING. Transfuse each unit of packed cells over 2 hours. If it must transfuse more slowly because of the patient's condition, make sure the unit does not hang longer than 4 hours to prevent deterioration and bacterial growth.

FILTERING. Filters are used with blood administration tubing to prevent potentially harmful particles from entering the patient. Most often, the filter that comes with the transfusion tubing is sufficient for each unit of packed RBCs. In some situations, special filters may be needed to remove leukocytes or micro-aggregates. The blood bank can advise in these situations.

WASHED OR LEUKOCYTE-DEPLETED BLOOD. In some instances, packed RBCs are ordered as "washed." They arrive from the blood bank in a special bag. The washing process removes almost all of the plasma. This can decrease the risk or severity of a febrile reaction. In addition, leukocyte filters may be used to completely remove all WBCs. This removal process is used in cases in which many transfusions are anticipated, in order to decrease the risk of antigen sensitization. It can also reduce transmission of certain viruses, such as cytomegalovirus.

WARMED BLOOD. If the patient has had severe bleeding and is receiving multiple rapid transfusions, the HCP may consider a blood warmer. It works just as the name implies, warming the cold blood from the blood bank to the standard body temperature of 98.6°F (37.0°C). This warming helps prevent hypothermia, which can cause heart arrhythmias. It also prevents shivering, which can destroy blood cells and platelets.

Monitoring

Whether or not you actually administer the blood, you will likely participate in monitoring to prevent complications or to detect and treat them quickly if they occur. Stay with the patient for the first 15 minutes of the blood transfusion to assess for any immediate reactions. The 15 minutes begins when the blood enters the vein. If saline solution is in the tubing, it may take several minutes before the blood reaches the patient. Check and document vital signs before starting the transfusion, after the blood has begun to infuse, and after the infusion is complete. Always follow institution guidelines for vital sign monitoring. During the transfusion, assess the patient for signs and symptoms of complications.

Complications

Quick detection of complications can be lifesaving. It is easy to think of transfusing blood components as a routine procedure because it is a common activity. Do not be fooled. *It is a serious procedure that can be life threatening if errors occur.* Complications include febrile reactions, hypersensitivities, hemolytic reactions, anaphylaxis, circulatory overload, and even death. Regular monitoring according to

institution policy can help detect complications early when treatment is most effective.

FEBRILE REACTION. By far, the most common reaction is fever (febrile reaction). It occurs up to 2% of the time. Make sure that blood never transfuses for more than 4 hours. The risk of a febrile reaction goes up with each unit of blood product given to the patient. Many times, febrile reactions occur after the transfusion is completed, but they can occur at any time. This is the reason for obtaining a set of baseline vital signs, including the patient's temperature. Once a febrile reaction begins, the most common signs are an increase in temperature and shaking chills, which can be severe. Other symptoms include headache and back pain. If febrile symptoms occur, stop the transfusion and notify the HCP. Acetaminophen may be ordered. If a hemolytic reaction is not suspected, the HCP may order the transfusion to continue once the patient is more comfortable. Administering leukocyte-depleted blood can usually prevent future febrile reactions.

URTICARIAL REACTION. Urticarial (hive) reactions are considered to be minor allergic reactions. They are usually associated with antigens in the plasma accompanying the transfusion. There may be a fever, but the cardinal sign is the appearance of urticaria, a hive-like rash. On discovery of this reaction, stop the transfusion and notify the HCP immediately. Expect that the patient will be given a dose of an antihistamine, such as diphenhydramine (Benadryl). If the transfusion is restarted, continue to monitor the patient closely. Make sure the 4-hour administration rule is not violated.

HEMOLYTIC REACTION. The deadliest and, fortunately, rarest of the reactions is an acute hemolytic reaction. The cause of this reaction is transfusion of incompatible blood. The result is hemolysis (destruction) of RBCs. This serious reaction is usually noticed within minutes of starting the transfusion. The patient may report back pain, chest pain, chills, fever, shortness of breath, nausea, vomiting, or a feeling of impending doom. As the reaction progresses, the patient begins to show signs of shock, hypotension, oliguria, and decreased consciousness. Late signs and symptoms include those associated with disseminated intravascular coagulation (e.g., uncontrollable bleeding from many different sites at the same time, usually causing death).

At the first sign of this type of reaction, immediately stop the transfusion and stay with the patient. Institute emergency procedures to notify the supervisor, the HCP, and the blood bank. Keep the vein open with normal saline using a new tubing set (ensuring that no more incompatible blood is administered) so that emergency drugs can be administered. High volumes of fluids are administered to decrease shock and hypotension. High doses of diuretics are given to promote urine flow because the kidneys are the most likely organs to be damaged.

ANAPHYLACTIC REACTION. Anaphylactic reactions are not common but may be seen more often in patients who have received many transfusions or have had many pregnancies.

Usually, the source of the anaphylaxis is sensitization to immunoglobulins passed from the donor blood product. In this type of reaction, the very first milliliters of blood containing the allergens to pass into the patient's system may be enough to cause the patient to develop respiratory or cardiovascular collapse. Other more common symptoms include severe gastrointestinal cramping, vomiting, and uncontrollable diarrhea.

If the patient exhibits these signs and symptoms, stop the transfusion at once and stay with the patient. Have someone else notify the RN and the HCP, using institutional emergency procedures. Emergency resuscitation measures, including cardiopulmonary resuscitation (CPR) if necessary, must be instituted until the rapid response or code team arrives. Expect the patient to be intubated and receive oxygen, steroids, and other drugs as needed for life support. After the emergency has passed, this patient will likely need to receive transfusions from frozen, deglycerolized blood cells.

CIRCULATORY OVERLOAD. Circulatory overload is caused by rapid transfusion in a short period, particularly in older and debilitated patients. Usual signs and symptoms include chest pain, cough, frothy sputum, distended neck veins, crackles and wheezes in the lung fields, and increased heart rate. If symptoms occur, stop the transfusion and notify the HCP. Anticipate administration of diuretics, which help get rid of the excess fluid. The transfusion may be restarted later at a slower rate ("Gerontological Issues").

Gerontological Issues

Monitoring for Fluid Excess. Older patients have less cardiac and renal ability to adapt to changes in blood volume, so they have a much higher risk of fluid overload when receiving intravenous infusions or blood transfusions. Carefully monitor lung sounds and vital signs both before, during, and after a blood transfusion. New onset of dyspnea, crackles, hypertension, or bounding pulse during any infusion should be reported to the registered nurse or health care provider immediately. If an older adult requires more than one unit of blood, a diuretic may be ordered between units.

SUGGESTED ANSWERS TO CRITICAL THINKING

Mrs. Brown

The health care provider will most likely decrease Mrs. Brown's warfarin (Coumadin) dose. Note in Table 27.5 that the international normalized ratio (INR) for a patient on warfarin should be 2 to 3. A value of 4 means her blood is taking too long to clot, and she needs a lower dose to avoid bleeding.

Review Questions

1. Which of the following actions should the nurse prioritize when taking care of a patient with a platelet count of 23,000/mm³?
   1. Request an order for an anticoagulant.
   2. Protect the patient from injury.
   3. Encourage the patient to drink plenty of fluids.
   4. No action is necessary. This is a normal level.

2. A nurse is assessing a patient and finds small red-purple dots over most skin surfaces. The patient denies noticing them before. Which action should the nurse take first?
   1. Report the findings immediately to the registered nurse or health care provider.
   2. Document the findings objectively in the medical record.
   3. Assist the patient to apply lotion.
   4. Administer an antihistamine as needed.

3. A nurse is preparing a patient for lymphangiography. Which statement by the patient shows that more teaching is needed?
   1. "My skin might turn a bluish color."
   2. "I will need a sandbag on my groin to prevent bleeding."
   3. "My nurse will be checking my circulation routinely after the procedure."
   4. "I will need more x-rays tomorrow."

4. Which of the following activities should be carried out to keep the patient safe before starting a blood transfusion? **Select all that apply.**
   1. Match the blood to the order.
   2. Match the patient to the blood.
   3. Match the room number to the order.
   4. Check the patient's vital signs.
   5. Check the temperature of the blood.
   6. Check the patient's weight.

5. A nurse is monitoring a patient during a blood transfusion. After the blood has been hanging for 30 minutes,
   the patient's temperature rises from 98.6°F (37.0°C)
   at baseline to 101.0°F (38.3°C). The patient also
   experiences severe chills. Which action should the
   nurse take first?
   1. Document the vital signs in the medical record.
   2. Administer acetaminophen for the fever.
   3. Notify the health care provider of the change.
   4. Stop the transfusion and hang normal saline solution.

Answer rationales available in your online resources.

ANSWERS 1. 2; 2. 1; 3. 2; 4. 1; 4. 5. 4

Key Points

Find the chapter key points in your online resources
available through Davis Edge.

Additional Resources

DAVIS
edge. ◀ Use the scratch off code on the inside front
cover of your book to access online quizzes
that will help you to improve your scores
on course exams and prepare for the NCLEX-PN®.

 Study Guide

CHAPTER 28

Nursing Care of Patients With Hematologic and Lymphatic Disorders

Jennifer Mitchell, Lucy L. Colo

KEY TERMS

anemia (uh-NEE-mee-ah)
aplastic (ay-PLAS-tik)
disseminated intravascular coagulation
   (dis-SEM-ih-NAY-ted IN-trah-VAS-kyoo-lar
   koh-AG-yoo-LAY-shun)
glossitis (gloss-SY-tis)
hemarthrosis (HEE-mar-THROH-sis)
hemolysis (hee-MAHL-ih-sis)
hemolytic (HEE-moh-LIT-ik)
hemophilia (HEE-moh-FIL-ee-ah)
idiopathic thrombocytopenic purpura
   (ID-ee-uh-PATH-ik THROM-boh-SY-toh-PEE-nik
   PURR-purr-uh)
leukemia (loo-KEE-mee-ah)
lymphoma (lim-FOH-mah)
pancytopenia (PAN-sy-toh-PEE-nee-ah)
panmyelosis (PAN-my-eh-LOH-sis)
pathological fracture (PATH-uh-LAW-jik-uhl
   FRAK-chur)
phlebotomy (fleh-BAW-tuh-mee)
polycythemia (PAW-lee-sy-THEE-mee-ah)
splenectomy (spleh-NEK-tuh-mee)
splenomegaly (SPLEE-noh-MEG-ah-lee)
thrombocytopenia (THROM-boh-SY-toh-
   PEE-nee-ah)

CHAPTER CONCEPTS

Cellular Regulation
Hematologic Regulation
Infection
Safety

LEARNING OUTCOMES

1. Explain the pathophysiology of each of the hematologic and lymphatic disorders discussed in this chapter.
2. Describe the etiologies, signs, and symptoms of each disorder.
3. Identify tests used to diagnose each of the disorders.
4. Describe current therapeutic measures for each disorder.
5. List data you should collect when caring for patients with disorders of the hematologic or lymphatic systems.
6. Plan nursing care for patients with hematologic disorders.
7. Plan nursing care for patients with lymphatic disorders.
8. Explain how you will know whether your nursing interventions have been effective.
9. Describe precautions you should institute to prevent bleeding in patients with clotting disorders.
10. Identify nursing care and teaching you will provide for patients undergoing a splenectomy.

HEMATOLOGIC DISORDERS

Patients with hematologic disorders have problems related to their blood. What do you suppose happens when there are too many blood cells, or too few, or the cells are defective?

• When red blood cells (RBCs) are affected, oxygen transport is also affected, causing symptoms related to poor oxygenation.
• When white blood cells (WBCs) are affected, the patient is unable to effectively fight infections.
• If platelets or clotting factors are affected, bleeding disorders occur.

DISORDERS OF RED BLOOD CELLS

Anemias

The term **anemia** describes a condition in which there is a deficiency of RBCs, hemoglobin (Hgb), or both, in the circulating blood. Because Hgb carries oxygen, this results in a reduced capacity to deliver oxygen

• WORD • BUILDING •
anemia: a—not + emia—blood

497

to the tissues. Symptoms such as weakness and shortness of breath occur, which lead the patient to seek medical help.

Pathophysiology

A decrease in the number of RBCs can be traced to three conditions: (1) impaired production of RBCs, as in aplastic anemia and nutrition deficiencies; (2) increased destruction of RBCs, as in hemolytic or sickle cell anemia; or (3) massive or chronic blood loss. Some anemias are related to genetic problems in certain cultures ("Cultural Considerations"). It is important to remember that the general term *anemia* refers to a symptom or condition secondary to another problem and is not a diagnosis. Different types of anemia are discussed later in this chapter.

Cultural Considerations

A gender-linked genetic disease common in parts of China is an enzyme deficiency affecting the person's red blood cells that results in anemia. Deficiency of this enzyme, Mediterranean-type glucose-6-phosphate dehydrogenase (G6PD), is common worldwide, causing a hemolytic crisis when fava beans are eaten, when aspirin or certain other drugs are taken, or in acidotic or hypoxemic states. Mediterranean-type G6PD deficiency is an inherited disorder in males, although some females are carriers.

Among Asian Indians, sickle cell disease is highly prevalent: The gene is detected in 16.5% of selected populations. Sickle cell anemia is the most common genetic disorder among African American populations. Sickle cell anemia is also found in individuals who live in areas where malaria is endemic, such as the Caribbean, the Middle East, the Mediterranean region, and Asia.

Etiology

DIETARY DEFICIENCIES. Iron, folic acid, and vitamin B_{12} are all essential to the production of healthy RBCs. A deficiency of any of these nutrients can cause anemia. *Pernicious anemia* is associated with a lack of intrinsic factor in stomach secretions, which is necessary for absorption of vitamin B_{12}. See "Nutrition Notes" for more information.

Nutrition Notes

Understanding Common Nutritional Anemias. Nutritional deficiencies can produce some forms of anemia. Nutrients vital to the synthesis of red blood cells (RBCs) include iron, folic acid, and vitamin B_{12}. Even if the cause of the anemia is dietary, other therapies may be used in addition to nutritional interventions.

Microcytic Anemia. Iron-deficiency anemia is characterized by smaller-than-normal RBCs. Poor intake of iron,

excessive blood loss, dialysis treatments, ingestion of lead, gastrointestinal surgeries (including gastric bypass), or lack of stomach acid can lead to iron-deficiency anemia. Those at greatest risk of iron deficiency are women of childbearing age and young children. Even before obvious anemia is seen, cognitive abilities can be impaired.

Good sources of iron include meat, fish, and poultry, which contain 50% to 60% heme iron that is absorbed intact. Plant sources and the other 40% of iron in meat, fish, and poultry must be reduced by stomach acids to an absorbable form. Vitamin C helps in this conversion of iron.

If iron supplements are given to treat iron deficiency, they should be continued for several months after hemoglobin (Hgb) and hematocrit (Hct) levels return to normal to enable the body to rebuild iron stores.

Macrocytic Anemia. Folic acid or vitamin B_{12} deficiencies produce anemias characterized by larger-than-normal RBCs. Folic acid aids in the formation of DNA and heme, the iron-containing portion of Hgb. It is particularly necessary for rapidly growing cells, including those in the gastrointestinal tract, blood, and fetal tissue. Many drugs, including alcohol, anticonvulsants, and aspirin, interfere with the use of folic acid and can lead to anemia.

Good food sources of folic acid include fortified flours, grains, cereals, and wheat germ; liver and eggs; green leafy vegetables; legumes; and bananas and oranges. Because folic acid markedly decreases the occurrence of fetal neural tube defects such as spina bifida, women capable of becoming pregnant should consume 400 mcg of synthetic folic acid daily from fortified foods or supplements in addition to the folate furnished by a balanced diet.

Vitamin B_{12} is essential for the manufacture of DNA and RBCs and for synthesis and maintenance of myelin, the fatty covering on nerves. Vitamin B_{12} requires a highly specific protein-binding factor called *intrinsic factor,* secreted by glands in the stomach. The intrinsic factor protects vitamin B_{12} from digestive enzymes and intestinal bacteria until it reaches the ileum, where the vitamin is absorbed.

Vitamin B_{12} is found in meat, fish, shellfish, poultry, and eggs; dairy products (milk, cheese, yogurt); and vitamin B_{12}-fortified foods such as soy milk, tofu, and breakfast cereals. A healthy person eating these foods regularly is not at risk of vitamin B_{12} deficiency. Strict vegetarians may be at risk and can pass that risk to their breastfed infants. Pregnant and lactating vegan women's diets should be evaluated carefully for deficiency of vitamin B_{12}. Continued lack of vitamin B_{12} can cause irreparable nerve damage and should be considered in a person being evaluated for dementia.

Reference
National Institute of Health National Heart, Lung, and Blood Institute. (2016). Anemia. Retrieved from www.nhlbi.nih.gov/health/health-topics/topics/anemia

HEMOLYSIS. **Hemolysis** is the destruction, or lysis, of RBCs. Destruction of RBCs leads to a type of anemia called **hemolytic** anemia. This may be a congenital disorder, or it may be caused by exposure to certain toxins.

OTHER CAUSES. Thalassemia anemia is a hereditary anemia found in persons from Southeast Asia, Africa, the Middle East, Italy, and the Mediterranean islands. People with thalassemia do not synthesize Hgb normally. People with chronic disease also develop anemia ("Gerontological Issues"). Additional causes of anemia are discussed under the separate headings of "Aplastic Anemia" and "Sickle Cell Anemia."

Gerontological Issues

Anemia. Hemoglobin (Hgb) and hematocrit (Hct) levels should remain unchanged in healthy older adults. Anemia is usually brought on by an underlying medical condition that causes altered iron metabolism, deficiency of erythropoietin, or shortened life span of red blood cells. Anemia of chronic disease is often mistaken for iron-deficiency anemia; nutritional deficiencies and blood loss are common causes of iron-deficiency anemia.

Signs and Symptoms

Symptoms of anemia include paleness (pallor), tachycardia, tachypnea, fatigue, and shortness of breath (Table 28.1). These symptoms occur because of the reduced number of functioning RBCs with reduced ability to carry oxygen to tissues. In addition to these symptoms, the patient with pernicious (vitamin B_{12}) anemia may experience numbness of the hands or feet and weakness. This is because vitamin B_{12} is needed for normal neurologic function. Pernicious anemia is also associated with a sore, beefy red tongue. Patients with iron deficiency may have fissures at the corners of the mouth, an inflamed tongue (**glossitis**), and spoon-shaped fingernails.

Diagnostic Tests

A complete blood count (CBC) is done to determine the number of RBCs and WBCs per cubic millimeter. The size, color, and shape of the blood cells are determined by microscopic examination. Hgb and hematocrit (Hct) levels are below normal in anemia. Serum iron, ferritin, and total iron-binding capacity (TIBC) measurements are done to diagnose iron-deficiency anemia. Serum folate is measured if folic acid deficiency is suspected. A bone marrow biopsy and analysis may also be done.

Patients with pernicious anemia have low gastric acid levels. Many patients have antibodies to intrinsic factor. Both abnormalities are associated with poor absorption of vitamin B_{12}. If blood loss is suspected, additional tests are done to determine the source of bleeding.

Therapeutic Measures

Treatment begins with elimination of causes. Intake of the deficient nutrient can be increased in the diet or administered as a supplement (see "Nutrition Notes"). Changing cooking habits, decreasing alcohol intake, and controlling chronic diarrhea can help correct folic acid deficiency. If symptoms of anemia are acute, a blood transfusion may be needed.

Nursing Process for the Patient With Anemia

DATA COLLECTION. Monitor Hgb and Hct levels and other laboratory studies ordered. Report any downward trend. Monitor responses to therapy, the patient's fatigue level, and the patient's ability to ambulate safely and perform activities of daily living (ADLs). Monitor dyspnea and oxygen saturation, but be aware that, at lower Hgb levels, oxygen saturation values may not be accurate. Assess for pallor in the skin and conjunctivae.

NURSING DIAGNOSES, PLANNING, AND IMPLEMENTATION. Possible nursing diagnoses are listed next along with outcomes and interventions.

Activity Intolerance related to tissue hypoxia and dyspnea

EXPECTED OUTCOME: The patient will be able to tolerate activity as evidenced by ability to complete ADLs with minimal assistance. The patient will have knowledge about conserving energy as evidenced by a verbal statement.

- Monitor vital signs before and after activity. *The patient experiencing activity intolerance may have tachycardia, increased respiratory rate, and decreased blood pressure with activity.*
- If the pulse or respiratory rate increases more than 20% from baseline during activity, reduce the activity level. *This is evidence that the activity is too strenuous and can result in hypoxia and dyspnea.*
- Plan care to conserve energy after periods of activity. *Balancing activities and rest periods helps the patient conserve energy.*
- Assist the patient with self-care activities as needed. *Assisting with ADLs helps to decrease the amount of energy expended by the patient.*
- Encourage the patient to limit visitors, telephone calls, and unnecessary interruptions *to conserve energy.*
- Administer oxygen as ordered to relieve dyspnea. *The patient with anemia does not have enough Hgb to carry oxygen to vital organs.*
- Assist with blood transfusion as ordered. *A blood transfusion is a quick way to raise Hgb levels and to correct severe symptoms.*

• WORD • BUILDING •

hemolysis: heme—blood + lysis—dissolution
hemolytic: heme—blood + lytic—break down
glossitis: glos—tongue + itis—inflammation

Table 28.1

Clinical Manifestations of Anemia

Body System	Mild (Hgb 10 to 14 g/dL)	Moderate (Hgb 6 to 10 g/dL)	Severe (Hgb less than 6 g/dL)
Skin	None	None	Pallor, jaundice, pruritus
Eyes	None	None	Jaundiced conjunctivae and sclerae, retinal hemorrhages, blurred vision
Mouth	None	None	Glossitis, smooth tongue
Cardiovascular	Palpitations	Increased palpitations	Tachycardia, increased pulse pressure, systolic murmurs, angina, congestive heart failure, myocardial infarction
Lungs	Exertional dyspnea	Significant dyspnea	Tachypnea, orthopnea, dyspnea at rest
Neurologic	None	None	Headache, vertigo, irritability, depression, impaired thought processes
Gastrointestinal	None	None	Anorexia, hepatomegaly, splenomegaly
Musculoskeletal	None	None	Bone pain
General	None	Fatigue	Sensitivity to cold, weight loss, lethargy

Imbalanced Nutrition: Less Than Body Requirements related to disease, treatment, or lack of knowledge about adequate nutrition

EXPECTED OUTCOME: The patient will (1) have improved nutrition as evidenced by stable weight, Hgb level, and Hct level; and (2) will be able to appropriately select foods to meet nutritional requirements.

• Consult a dietitian *to provide diet instruction if the anemia is caused by a dietary deficiency.*
• Teach the patient with folic acid deficiency to include foods from each food group at every meal. *A balanced diet includes adequate amounts of folic acid.*
• Instruct the patient to take supplements as ordered by the health care provider (HCP). *The patient should not stop taking the supplements until the HCP advises him or her to do so.*
• Instruct the patient with pernicious anemia that vitamin B_{12} injections are given for life *because pernicious anemia is a chronic disease.*
• Instruct the patient with iron deficiency about high-iron foods and correct use of an iron supplement. *An iron supplement should be taken with vitamin C to enhance absorption.*
• Instruct the patient to notify the HCP of any side effects related to iron supplements *such as nausea, diarrhea, constipation, and dark stools.*
• Administer intramuscular iron injections by the Z-track method *to avoid staining the injection site.*

• Administer oral iron 1 hour before or 2 hours after meals *to enhance absorption.*
• Administer liquid supplements with a drinking straw *to avoid staining the teeth.*

Impaired Oral Mucous Membrane Integrity related to altered dietary status

EXPECTED OUTCOME: The patient will have intact oral mucous membranes.

• Monitor condition of oral mucous membranes *to detect changes.*
• Provide good oral hygiene *to keep the oral cavity clean and prevent infection.*
• Encourage soft, bland foods, *which are more tolerable until healing can occur.*
• Instruct the patient to use a soft toothbrush for oral care *because it is gentler until healing can occur.*

EVALUATION. When successfully treated, patients should be able to tolerate their usual level of activity without shortness of breath or excess fatigue. The patient should be able to explain the treatment plan and therapeutic measures for long-term prevention of problems, including dietary choices, supplements, and self-care measures. The oral mucosa will be intact.

Aplastic Anemia

PATHOPHYSIOLOGY. **Aplastic** anemia differs from other types of anemia in that the bone marrow becomes fatty and unable to produce enough RBCs. It is also called *hypoplastic* anemia. The cells that are produced are normal in size and shape, but there are not enough of them to sustain life. The result is **pancytopenia.** This is reduced numbers of all cells from the bone marrow, including RBCs, platelets, and WBCs. Left untreated, aplastic anemia is almost always fatal.

ETIOLOGY. Aplastic anemia may be congenital—that is, the person is born with bone marrow incapable of producing the correct number of cells. It also may be due to exposure to toxic substances, such as industrial chemicals (e.g., benzenes and insecticides) or chemotherapy medications, or from use of cardiopulmonary bypass during surgery. Other causes include certain bacterial and viral infections, such as tuberculosis and hepatitis, or autoimmune disease.

SIGNS AND SYMPTOMS. The clinical features of aplastic anemia vary with the severity of bone marrow failure. As with other anemias, early symptoms include progressive weakness, fatigue, pallor, shortness of breath, and headaches. As the disease progresses and the pancytopenia worsens, other symptoms, such as tachycardia and heart failure, may appear. Ecchymoses (Fig. 28.1) and petechiae (Fig. 28.2) appear on the skin surface because of reduced platelet count. Blood may ooze from mucous membranes. Injection sites may progress from oozing to frank bleeding. There is often bleeding into vital organs. Infection occurs because of reduced WBCs. Without treatment, most patients die of infection or bleeding.

DIAGNOSTIC TESTS. The diagnosis of aplastic anemia begins with a CBC. Usually, all values are very low, with the occasional exception of the RBC count, in part because of the longer life span of RBCs. Eventually, the RBCs are also depleted. If the patient has bleeding internally or externally, the RBC level can drop rapidly and dramatically. The most definitive test is a bone marrow biopsy. Because the bone

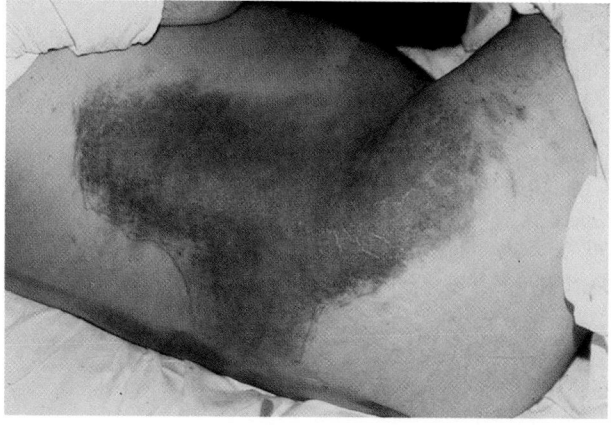

FIGURE 28.1 Ecchymoses. Extensive hemorrhage into the skin (in disseminated intravascular coagulation). Note how the area is outlined in pen so the nurse can assess if the area is spreading.

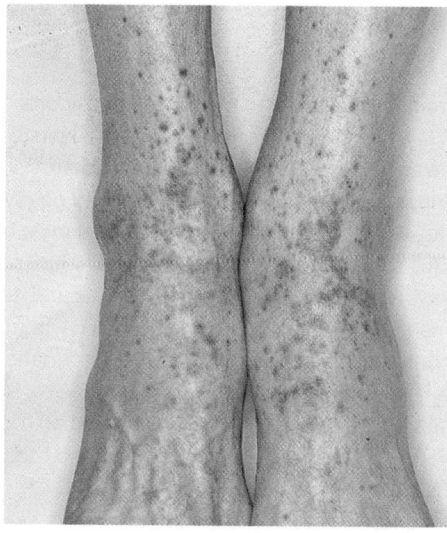

FIGURE 28.2 Petechiae on the skin (from thrombocytopenia).

marrow is essentially dead, the result is often described as a "dry tap," in which pale, fatty, yellow, fibrous bone marrow is extracted instead of the red, gelatinous bone marrow normally seen. Other diagnostic tests include TIBC and serum iron level. It is common to find both of these levels elevated because the RBCs are not being produced and are not using up the stores of iron in the production of Hgb.

THERAPEUTIC MEASURES. Early identification of the cause of aplastic anemia and correction of the underlying problem are important to survival. Unfortunately, it is often difficult to determine the cause. There is no way to reverse the damage. Aggressive supportive measures may be the only treatment. Most of these measures are aimed at prevention of infection and bleeding. Transfusions may be administered to replace deficient cells.

Steroids may be administered to stimulate production of cells in the weakened bone marrow. Immunosuppressant agents may be given if an autoimmune disorder is the underlying cause. Occasionally, the administration of hormones may work to increase the viability of the marrow. The most effective treatment for aplastic anemia is bone marrow transplantation ("Patient Perspective").

In many treatment institutions, limited success is being obtained with the use of colony-stimulating factors, natural elements that can now be produced synthetically. (You can read more about these medications in Chapter 11.) For example, epoetin alfa, a form of erythropoietin (Epogen), stimulates production of RBCs, and filgrastim (a granulocyte colony stimulator; Neupogen) stimulates production of WBCs. The major drawback to this type of therapy is cost. Many of the

• **WORD** • **BUILDING** •

aplastic: a—not + plastic—develop

pancytopenia: pan—all + cyto—cell + penia—poverty

Patient Perspective

Janet. I took my daughter to the doctor for a sports physical. Later that day, I received a call telling me to take her to the university hospital immediately because she had a serious life-threatening illness. I kept telling myself and my husband that our small-town hospital must have made some sort of error. As it turned out, they had not. My daughter was diagnosed with aplastic anemia and needed a bone marrow transplant. I became obsessed with the illness, poring over every tidbit of medical information I could find. Sometimes I found myself out in the car unable to remember where I was going; sometimes I had to pull over because my eyes were filled with tears and I could no longer see.

My daughter was 16 at the time of her illness, yet it is the parents who sign consent forms and make the choices in care. When the chemotherapy was started and was running through the intravenous tubing, I felt like grabbing the tubing and pinching it off, yelling, "I need more time to think about this decision," but time was running out. Without a bone marrow transplant, she had about 8 months to live.

After transplantation, my daughter was in an isolation room for a month. I stayed with her every day, and at night I stayed at the inn that was attached to the hospital. If I was needed, I wanted to be no more than a minute away. I was one of the luckier parents because I had the financial means to manage this process. I thought about how horrible it would be if I had other children at home. Sometimes I would have such an urge to run away and escape from it all. I attended support groups that were held on the hospital unit. I got to know a lot of other parents with sick kids, and it became very upsetting to me at times. One day parents told me how well their child was doing; the next day I saw the child's room empty and thought he must have gone home, only to find out later that he had died during the night. I wondered if my daughter would be next.

I look at my daughter now, 4 years later, alive and perfectly healthy, and I tell myself that I made the right choices for her. But she tells me that if it happens again, she will not go through chemotherapy. I wonder, is chemo worse than death?

pharmaceutical manufacturers have patient access programs that help reduce the costs of these medications.

NURSING MANAGEMENT. Nursing care of patients with symptoms related to reduced RBCs was presented earlier in the "Nursing Process for the Patient With Anemia" section. If the patient's platelet count is low (usually less than 20,000), the patient is placed on bleeding precautions (Box 28.1). If the WBC count is low, the patient must be protected from infection (Box 28.2).

Box 28.1

Interventions to Prevent Bleeding

- Use an electric razor instead of a safety razor for shaving.
- Use a soft toothbrush or gauze to clean the teeth. Avoid flossing.
- Avoid invasive procedures as much as possible, including enemas, douches, suppositories, and rectal temperatures.
- Avoid intramuscular injections.
- To avoid injury when checking blood pressure, pump cuff up only until pulse is obliterated.
- Avoid blood draws whenever possible. Use established access sites or group specimen collections into once-daily draws.
- Maintain pressure on intravenous, blood draw, and other puncture sites for 5 minutes.
- Encourage use of shoes or slippers when out of bed.
- Keep area clutter-free to prevent bumps and bruises.
- Avoid use of drugs that interfere with platelet function, such as aspirin products and nonsteroidal anti-inflammatory drugs (NSAIDs; e.g., aspirin, ibuprofen, naproxen).
- Administer stool softeners as ordered to prevent straining to have a bowel movement.
- Move and turn patient gently to avoid bruising.
- Instruct patient to blow nose very gently and only when necessary.
- Advise patient to consult with health care provider about whether sexual intercourse is safe.

Box 28.2

Interventions for the Patient at Risk for Infection

- Place the patient in a private room.
- Ensure that all staff and visitors wash hands before entering the room.
- Teach the patient to wash hands before and after using the toilet and before and after eating.
- Teach the patient and family to wash hands before touching each other.
- Prevent staff or visitors with known infections from entering the patient's room.
- Teach the patient not to handle flowers or plants brought into the room.
- Teach the patient to avoid unwashed fruits and vegetables.
- Avoid use of indwelling urinary catheters and other invasive devices.
- Use strict aseptic technique if invasive procedures are needed.
- Use acetaminophen (Tylenol) if an antipyretic is needed; aspirin can induce bleeding.

BE SAFE!

BE VIGILANT! Watch carefully for even subtle signs of bleeding, such as early skin changes or pink-tinged urine. Report findings before bleeding worsens.

Sickle Cell Anemia

PATHOPHYSIOLOGY. Sickle cell anemia is an inherited anemia in which the RBCs have a specific mutation that makes the Hgb very sensitive to oxygen changes. Any time a decrease in the oxygen tension is sensed, the cells begin an observable physical change from their usual spherical shape to a sickle or crescent shape (Fig. 28.3). Sickled cells are very rigid and easily cracked and broken. The abnormal shape also causes the cells to become tangled in the blood vessels and organs. The result is congestion, clumping, and clotting.

As RBCs are broken, the cellular contents spill out into the general circulation. The resulting increase in the bilirubin level causes jaundice. Gallstones (cholelithiasis) may develop because of the increased amounts of bile pigments. The spleen and liver may enlarge because of the increase in retained cells and cellular materials.

Because the cells are fragile, their life span is significantly decreased. Normal RBCs live about 120 days. Sickled cells survive only about 10 to 20 days, an 80% to 90% decrease in cell survival.

ETIOLOGY. Sickle cell disease (SCD) is an autosomal recessive hereditary disorder. This means that, if both parents pass on the abnormal Hgb, the child will have the disease.

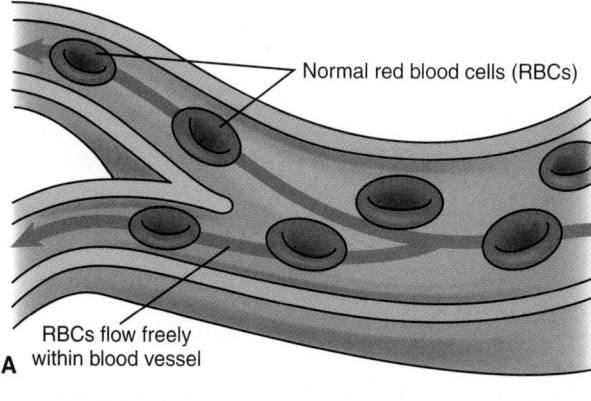

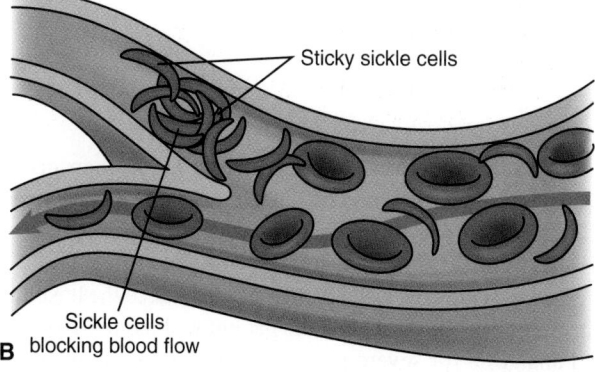

FIGURE 28.3 (A) Normal red blood cells (RBCs) flowing freely in a blood vessel. The inset image shows a cross-section of a normal RBC with normal hemoglobin (Hgb). (B) Abnormal, sickled RBCs blocking blood flow in a blood vessel. The inset image shows a cross-section of a sickle cell with abnormal (sickle) Hgb forming abnormal strands.

If only one parent passes on the abnormal Hgb, the child will have the sickle cell trait and will be able to pass the trait (or the disease if the other parent is also affected) on to his or her child.

In the United States, sickle cell anemia is most often found in those of African or Eastern Mediterranean heritage. Worldwide, many persons residing in Asia, the Caribbean, the Middle East, and Central America are affected. Nearly 10% of African Americans have the sickle cell trait; one out of every 365 African American infants born has inherited the two sets of abnormal genes needed to have the disease (Centers for Disease Control and Prevention, 2016). Symptoms do not appear in infants until after the age of 4 or 5 months. This is because, up to that age, the infant is using Hgb manufactured during fetal life, which is not affected by the sickling process.

SIGNS AND SYMPTOMS. The sickling changes happen on a daily basis. The rapid return of the oxygen level to normal usually returns the cells to their normal shape.

Occasionally, the sickling process cannot be reversed. This sudden and severe sickling is called a *sickle cell crisis.* As more and more sickling occurs, the blood flow becomes sluggish. It tends to collect in the capillaries and veins of the joints, chest, and abdominal organs, which can cause infarction with resulting tissue necrosis (death) from lack of blood supply. Tissue necrosis causes pain, fever, and swelling. Clotting in the cerebral blood vessels can lead to stroke. Refer to Chapter 49 for detailed information on stroke.

Any condition that leads to decreased oxygenation can contribute to the development of a sickle cell crisis. Some examples include pneumonia, exposure to cold, diabetic acidosis, and severe infection. Sickle cell anemia presents problems for the patient who needs surgery. Anesthesia and blood loss during surgery and postoperative dehydration can trigger a crisis.

Common symptoms produced during sickle cell crises include severe pain and swelling in the joints, especially of the elbows and knees, as the sickled cells impede circulation. Abdominal pain is common with swelling of the spleen and engorgement of the vital organs. Hypoxia occurs as fever and pain increase, causing the patient to breathe rapidly. A male patient may have a continuous, painful erection (priapism) from impaired blood flow through the penis. Symptoms of kidney failure are common as circulation is slowed and the kidneys become clogged with cellular debris.

Repeated crises and infarctions lead to chronic manifestations such as hand-foot syndrome, an unequal growth of fingers and toes from infarction of the small bones in the hands and feet (Fig. 28.4). Additional manifestations of SCD are shown in Figure 28.5.

The patient with sickle cell anemia has impaired quality of life. Strenuous exercise may be impossible because of the risk of crisis. Crises may occur without any apparent cause. In general, crises last from 4 to 6 days. They may occur in cycles close together for a time and then become dormant for

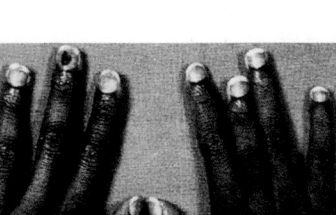
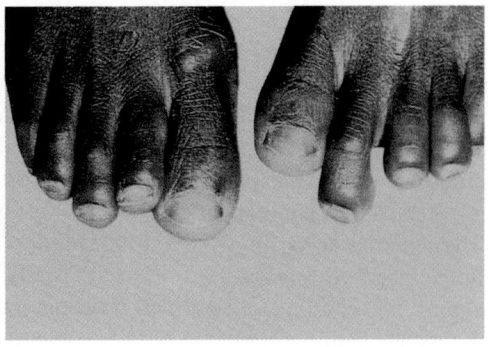

FIGURE 28.4 Hand-foot syndrome. Note different lengths of fingers and toes.

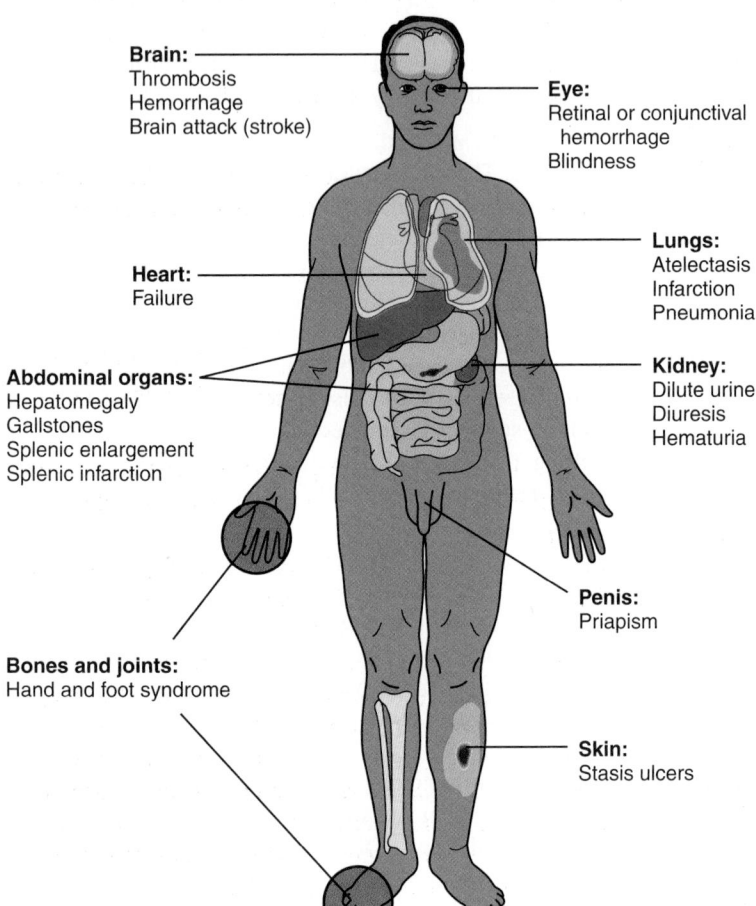

Brain:
Thrombosis
Hemorrhage
Brain attack (stroke)

Eye:
Retinal or conjunctival
 hemorrhage
Blindness

Heart:
Failure

Lungs:
Atelectasis
Infarction
Pneumonia

Abdominal organs:
Hepatomegaly
Gallstones
Splenic enlargement
Splenic infarction

Kidney:
Dilute urine
Diuresis
Hematuria

Penis:
Priapism

Bones and joints:
Hand and foot syndrome

Skin:
Stasis ulcers

FIGURE 28.5 Clinical manifestations of sickle cell anemia.

months to years. The cause of death in patients with sickle cell anemia is usually infection, stroke, or organ failure.

DIAGNOSTIC TESTS. The Sickledex test is a screening test that shows sickling of RBCs when oxygen tension is low. Hgb electrophoresis is a test used to determine the presence of Hgb S, the abnormal form of Hgb. There is also a decreased amount of Hgb, a lowered RBC count, an elevated WBC count, and a decreased erythrocyte sedimentation rate (ESR).

THERAPEUTIC MEASURES. Treatment depends on the severity of the disease. All patients should receive education on how to prevent crises and supportive care when crises occur. Some patients may be placed on low-dose oral penicillin to help prevent infections, decreasing the risk of crises.

During acute crises, the patient is admitted to the hospital. The nurse can anticipate that the patient will require sedation and analgesia for severe pain and blood transfusions to replace the sickled red cells. Oxygen therapy decreases dyspnea caused by the anemia. Large amounts of oral and intravenous (IV) fluids are given to flush the kidneys of the by-products of the broken cells' debris. Antibiotics are used to treat infection that may have triggered the crisis.

Frequent blood transfusions, often monthly, can help supply normal blood cells. However, they can cause high levels of iron to build up in the body. Deferasirox (Exjade) is a medication that may be given to decrease the excess iron levels. Corticosteroids can reduce the need for analgesics and oxygen. Hydroxyurea (Droxia) is a drug that has been shown to decrease crises, but it can cause life-threatening side effects; it should also be used with caution in women of childbearing years because of the risk of birth defects. Patients may not adhere to hydroxyurea therapy because they don't feel different; it may take months to years to make a difference in outcomes.

Bone marrow transplantation has shown promise in the treatment of SCD, although it is not without risk. In 2015, data were reviewed from several transplant centers of 22 adults who received bone marrow transplants for treatment of SCD. From 2012 to 2015, the patients were matched either by a sibling (17 patients) or unrelated donor (5 patients). Four patients experienced a severe adverse reaction and one patient died, but there were no incidents of transplant failure or recurrence of SCD post–bone marrow transplant (Krishnamurti et. al, 2015). This pilot study reported excellent outcomes in the adult population; more research is needed for the pediatric population.

NURSING PROCESS FOR THE PATIENT WITH SICKLE CELL ANEMIA.

Data Collection. In the patient in crisis, assess circulation in the extremities every 2 hours, including pulse oximetry, capillary refill, peripheral pulses, and temperature. Monitor neurological status. Frequent pain assessment is also essential.

Nursing Diagnoses, Planning, and Implementation.

Risk for Ineffective Cerebral/Peripheral Tissue Perfusion related to sickled cells and infarction

EXPECTED OUTCOME: The patient will have adequate cerebral/peripheral tissue perfusion as evidenced by the presence of peripheral pulses, absence of neurological changes, warm extremities, urine output within normal limits, and a capillary refill time of less than 3 seconds.

- Monitor neurological status (level of consciousness, orientation, bilateral muscle strength, pupil size, speech) *to identify any changes due to cerebrovascular thrombosis from cell debris.*
- Encourage oral fluids, and assist the registered nurse (RN) to monitor IV fluids *to dilute and aid in elimination of cell debris.*
- Apply warm compresses as ordered to the painful areas, cover the patient with a blanket, and keep the room temperature above 72°F (22°C) *to reduce the vasoconstrictive effects of cold.*
- Avoid cold compresses *because they decrease circulation and increase the number of sickled cells caught in a painful area.*

- Avoid restrictive clothing and raising the knee gatch (the adjustable joint in the hospital bed, which allows for the patient's knee to be flexed and the legs supported). *These can restrict circulation.*

Acute Pain related to tissue infarction

EXPECTED OUTCOME: The patient will state pain is at an acceptable level at all times.

- Administer opioid analgesics such as morphine as ordered *for acute pain.* (Analgesics may be given via IV route or by use of patient-controlled analgesia [PCA].)
- Administer acetaminophen (Tylenol) *to control fever.*
- Avoid giving aspirin *because it may increase acidosis, which can worsen the crisis.*
- Encourage bedrest during the acute phase of the crisis *to reduce oxygen demand.*

Evaluation. If nursing care has been effective, the patient will state that he or she is comfortable and will not have signs of poor circulation.

Ineffective Health Maintenance

EXPECTED OUTCOME: The patient will state reasons why treatment is important and follow therapeutic regimen as prescribed.

- Assess the patient and family's readiness to learn. *Readiness to learn affects ability to adhere to a prescribed therapeutic regimen.*
- Assess the patient and family's understanding of rationale for treatment and expected effects. *Assessment of knowledge base should guide teaching.*
- Assess the patient's ability to obtain medication, including ability to make trips to the laboratory and pharmacy. *A trial intervention performed in 2016 showed that community health workers teaching parents regarding treatment with hydroxyurea for their children improved adherence to the regimen as compared with a control group with no intervention (18.1% deviation from regimen vs. -42.6%) (Green et al., 2016).*
- Refer the patient and family for in-depth education as needed about treatment regimen. *Patients must understand therapy in order to adhere to it.*
- Refer the patient and family to a support group with others who have sickle cell anemia. *Support groups are a venue for sharing stories about personal experiences with the disease and to encourage each other to stay adherent to the medication.*

Evaluation. If interventions have been effective, the patient will state that he is comfortable, have evidence of adequate circulation, state understanding of the importance of adhering to treatment plan, and have fewer crises.

PATIENT EDUCATION. During remission, teach the patient and caregiver how to prevent acute episodes. Advise the patient to avoid tight-fitting clothing that restricts circulation. Urge the patient to avoid strenuous exercise, which increases oxygen demand. Instruct the patient to avoid cold temperatures and smoking, which cause vasoconstriction. Alcoholic beverages can also trigger a crisis and should be avoided. Patients should never fly in an unpressurized aircraft or undertake mountain climbing or other sports that can cause hypoxia. Encourage patients to get a pneumococcal vaccine and yearly flu vaccine. Encourage fluids to maintain hydration and reduce blood viscosity. Genetic counseling is important to prevent passing on the trait or disease to children. For more information, visit www.sicklecelldisease.org.

Polycythemia
Pathophysiology and Etiology
Polycythemia includes two separate disorders that are easily recognizable by similar characteristic changes in the RBC count. In both forms of polycythemia, the blood becomes so thick with too many RBCs that it resembles sludge. This thickness does not allow the blood to circulate easily.

Polycythemia vera (PV) is known as *primary polycythemia.* Most people with PV have a specific genetic mutation. In PV, the RBCs, platelets, and WBCs are all overproduced, and the bone marrow becomes packed with too many cells. As this overabundance of cells spills out into the general circulation, the organs become congested with cells and the tissues become packed with blood. The thick blood and excess platelets can cause thrombosis and occlusion of vessels. PV is usually found in patients over age 50.

In contrast, secondary polycythemia is the result of long-term hypoxia. Common coexisting conditions that may predispose a patient to secondary polycythemia include pulmonary diseases such as chronic obstructive pulmonary disease (COPD), cardiovascular problems such as chronic heart failure, living in high altitudes, and smoking. The body makes more RBCs in response to the low oxygenation associated with these conditions. Secondary polycythemia is a compensatory mechanism rather than an actual disorder.

Signs and Symptoms
A patient with PV commonly presents with hypertension, vision changes, headache, vertigo, dizziness, and ringing in the ears (tinnitus). Laboratory results show an increased level of all bone marrow components (RBCs, WBCs, platelets), which is called **panmyelosis.** Patients may also be at risk for developing a bleeding disorder called *acquired von Willebrand syndrome,* in which the platelets don't clump together well. The patient may have nosebleeds and bleeding gums, retinal hemorrhages, exertional dyspnea, and chest pain due to increased pressure exerted by the excess cells. The patient usually has a dark, flushed complexion from build-up of red cells. Intense itching is related to excess mast cells (and, therefore, histamine) in the skin. Abdominal pain with an early feeling of fullness with meals occurs because of the enlarged liver and spleen. Nearly all of the symptoms in PV are due to the major problems of hypervolemia, hyperviscosity, and engorgement of capillary beds. Without treatment, patients with PV die of thrombosis or hemorrhage.

Diagnostic Tests
Diagnosis of PV is made based on a CBC and bone marrow aspiration. Laboratory tests show a Hgb level greater than 18 mg/dL, an RBC mass greater than 6 million, and a Hct level of greater than 55%. A low level of erythropoietin is present, caused by negative feedback to the kidneys, where erythropoietin is made. The bone marrow or blood may show a genetic mutation known as *janus kinase 2* (JAK2).

Therapeutic Measures
Treatment of PV takes place in two stages. The first stage is to decrease the hyperviscosity problem. The most common first-line treatment is therapeutic **phlebotomy.** Phlebotomy involves withdrawal of blood, which is then discarded. From 350 to 500 mL of blood are removed once or twice a week, with the goal being a Hct level of about 45%. This reduces the RBC level. The patient usually feels more comfortable quickly. Repeated phlebotomies eventually cause iron-deficiency anemia. This in turn stabilizes RBC production; phlebotomies can then be reduced to every 2 to 3 months. Low-dose aspirin reduces the risk of blood clots.

The problem that remains is the increased WBC and platelet counts because phlebotomy does little to correct these overloads. Chemotherapeutic agents or radiation therapy, including radioactive phosphorus or interferon-alpha, may be used to suppress production of blood cells in some patients. Leukemia is a side effect of this therapy, so it is used only if the benefits outweigh the risks.

Nursing Management
Explain the phlebotomy procedure and reassure the patient that the treatment will relieve the most distressing symptoms. The procedure is the same as that used for donating blood. The patient should remain active and ambulatory to help prevent thrombus formation. If bedrest is needed, passive and active range-of-motion exercises should be implemented. Monitor the patient for complications such as hypovolemia and bleeding.

If the patient has more advanced manifestations, such as an enlarged liver or spleen, offer several small meals each day so the patient will be more comfortable while still receiving adequate nutrition. A dietitian can be consulted to discuss ways to maintain good nutrition. If the patient is on drug therapy, monitor CBC and platelet counts.

Patient Education
Instruct the patient to drink at least 3 L of water daily to reduce blood viscosity. Encourage smoking cessation, avoidance of tight or restrictive clothing, and elevation of feet when resting to promote good circulation. Use of support

• WORD • BUILDING •
polycythemia: poly—many + cyt—cells + emia—in the blood

hose when active also promotes circulation. If anticoagulant or antiplatelet agents are ordered, instruct the patient about side effects to watch for and the importance of routine laboratory tests. Routine bleeding precautions are implemented (see Box 28.1). Warn the patient to stop activities at the first sign of chest pain. Instruct the patient to report chest pain, increased joint pain, decreased activity tolerance, fever, and signs of iron-deficiency anemia, such as pallor, weight loss, and dyspnea. Advise the patient to report any signs or symptoms of bleeding or thrombosis immediately.

HEMORRHAGIC DISORDERS

Disseminated Intravascular Coagulation

Pathophysiology

Disseminated intravascular coagulation (DIC) involves a series of events that results in severe hemorrhage. DIC is a catastrophic, overwhelming state of accelerated clotting throughout the peripheral blood vessels. In a short period, all of the clotting factors and platelet supplies are exhausted, and clots can no longer be formed. This results in bleeding from nearly every bodily route possible. DIC is not a disease; it is a syndrome that develops secondary to another severe physical problem. Once this deadly syndrome develops, the progression of symptoms is rapid.

Massive clotting in blood vessels leads to organ and limb necrosis. Organs most often affected include the kidneys and the brain. Other blood-engorged organs, such as the lungs, the pituitary and adrenal glands, and the gastrointestinal (GI) mucosa, are also commonly involved. DIC is usually acute in onset, although in some patients it becomes a chronic condition. The prognosis depends on early diagnosis and intervention as well as the severity of the hemorrhaging. DIC has a very high mortality rate.

Etiology

DIC can develop after any condition in which the body has sustained major trauma. The sources of trauma are varied and can include an overwhelming infection; obstetric complications such as abruptio placentae, amniotic fluid embolism, or a retained dead fetus; or cancer-related causes such as acute leukemia or lung cancer. Massive tissue necrosis found in severe crush or burn injuries can increase the risk of DIC. Tissue necrosis secondary to extensive abdominal surgery with leakage of the intestinal contents can also be related to DIC onset.

Signs and Symptoms

Abnormal bleeding without a history of a serious hemorrhagic disorder is a cardinal sign of DIC. Early signs of bleeding include ecchymoses (see Fig. 28.1), petechiae (see Fig. 28.2), and bleeding from venipuncture sites. Bleeding may progress to IV sites, skin tears, surgical sites, incisions, and the GI tract and oral mucosa. Joints become painful and enlarged if bleeding into the joints occurs. All of these signs and symptoms may occur at the same time. Massive bleeding may also be accompanied by nausea, vomiting, dyspnea, oliguria, convulsions, coma, shock, major organ system failure, and severe muscle, back, and abdominal pain.

Diagnostic Tests

Initial laboratory findings in DIC include a prolonged prothrombin time (PT) and partial thromboplastin time (PTT), decreased platelet count, and increased evidence of fibrin degradation products (Table 28.2). A decrease in Hgb is the result of spilled Hgb from the increased numbers of broken RBCs. Blood urea nitrogen (BUN) and serum creatinine levels may also be increased.

Therapeutic Measures

Effective treatment of DIC depends on early recognition of the condition. Treatment is first aimed at correcting the underlying cause. Additional treatment consists of supportive interventions, including administration of blood, fresh frozen plasma, platelets, vitamin K, and the infusion of cryoprecipitate (which provides clotting factors) to support hemostasis. IV heparin may be used to help prevent the initial microembolization. It may also be used for chronic DIC cases. Additional therapies are being investigated.

Nursing Management

Care of the patient with DIC is a nursing challenge. Early intervention requires vigilance in recognizing and reporting

Table 28.2

Laboratory Abnormalities in Disseminated Intravascular Coagulation

Screening Test	Finding
Prothrombin time (PT)	Prolonged
Partial thromboplastin time (PTT)	Prolonged
Activated partial thromboplastin time (APTT)	Prolonged
Thrombin time (TT)	Prolonged
Fibrinogen	Reduced
Platelets	Reduced
Fibrin split products (FSP; also known as *fibrin degradation products* [FDP])	Elevated
Protamine sulfate	Strongly positive
Dimers (cross-linked fibrin fragments)	Elevated
Antithrombin III	Reduced
Factor assays (V, VII, VIII, X, and XIII)	Reduced

signs of bleeding. In addition to supportive care, focus on the prevention of further bleeding episodes. Care should be taken to avoid any trauma that might cause bleeding. Be careful not to dislodge clots from any site because another clot may not form and the patient will hemorrhage. See Box 28.1 for bleeding precautions.

Patient Education

Because a patient with DIC is often cared for in the intensive care unit, there are many opportunities for patient and family teaching. Explain all diagnostic tests to the patient and family. A large part of family education is preparing the family for what the patient may look like in terms of bleeding and bruising as well as specific equipment that may be in place, such as IV lines, a nasogastric (NG) tube, and an indwelling urinary catheter. It may be helpful to enlist the aid of social workers, chaplains, and other members of the health care team to help support the family.

CRITICAL THINKING

Mrs. Johns is admitted to your unit with disseminated intravascular coagulation (DIC) following the difficult delivery of her new baby.

1. What data will you collect as you care for Mrs. Johns?
2. What treatment do you anticipate?
3. What concerns is Mrs. Johns likely to have?
4. Mrs. Johns is to receive 300 mL of intravenous (IV) fresh frozen plasma over 30 minutes. How many milliliters per hour should be set on the IV controller?
5. With which members of the health care team should you anticipate collaborating?

Suggested answers are at the end of the chapter.

Idiopathic Thrombocytopenic Purpura
Pathophysiology and Etiology

Acute **idiopathic thrombocytopenic purpura** (ITP) results from increased platelet destruction by the immune system. Any time platelet numbers are reduced, the risk for bleeding increases. Acute ITP usually affects children between ages 2 and 6, whereas chronic ITP mainly affects adults over age 60.

Acute ITP usually occurs after an acute viral illness such as rubella or chickenpox. Hepatitis C virus and HIV can also be triggers. It may be drug-induced or associated with pregnancy. ITP is believed to be related to an immune system dysfunction. Antibodies responsible for platelet destruction have been found in nearly all diagnosed patients.

Signs and Symptoms

ITP produces clinical changes that are common to all forms of **thrombocytopenia**: petechiae, ecchymoses, and bleeding from the mouth, nose, or GI tract. Bleeding may occur in vital organs, such as the brain, which may prove fatal. In the acute type, onset may be sudden and without warning, causing easy bruising, nosebleeds, and bleeding gums. Onset of chronic ITP is usually insidious.

Diagnostic Tests

A platelet count of less than 20,000/mm^3 and a prolonged bleeding time suggest ITP. The greatly decreased platelet level places the patient at serious risk for hemorrhage. Examination of platelets under the microscope shows them to be small and immature. Anemia may be present if there has been a bleeding episode. If a bone marrow aspiration is performed, the results show an adequate number of megakaryocytes, the precursor cells for platelets. However, instead of the 7- to 10-day life span that platelets usually have, these immature platelets have a life span of just a few hours.

Therapeutic Measures

The goal of treatment is to have an adequate platelet count and no bleeding. Most cases of acute ITP resolve spontaneously without treatment. Initial treatment, if needed, often involves the administration of steroids. The purpose of the steroids is to prolong the life of the platelets by decreasing immune activity. In acute situations, immunoglobulin may be given to quickly increase the blood count. Some patients receive chemotherapeutic drugs. The spleen may be removed because it is the primary site of platelet destruction. Often the patient undergoing splenectomy has tried all other courses of treatment unsuccessfully and may be having bleeding episodes. Acute bleeding episodes are treated with transfusions of blood, platelets, and vitamin K.

Nursing Care

Care for the patient with ITP is the same as any patient with a bleeding disorder. See Box 28.1 for bleeding precautions. Teach the patient to watch for and report signs and symptoms of bruising and bleeding (Box 28.3). The patient should avoid trauma and restrict activity during severe episodes.

Hemophilia

Hemophilia is a group of hereditary bleeding disorders that result from a severe lack of specific clotting factors. The two most common are hemophilia A (classic hemophilia) and hemophilia B (Christmas disease). Von Willebrand disease is another related bleeding disorder, but it represents a minority of cases and is not discussed in this chapter.

Pathophysiology

Recall that many different clotting factors make up the clotting mechanism. Hemophilia A accounts for 80% of all types

• WORD • BUILDING •
idiopathic thrombocytopenic purpura: idio—unknown + pathic—disease + thrombo—clot + cyto—cell + penic—lack + purpura—hemorrhage in the skin
thrombocytopenia: thrombocyte—platelet + penia—lack
hemophilia: hemo—blood + philia—to love

Patient Education

Signs and Symptoms of Bleeding
Notify your health care provider if the following occur:
- Easy bruising of skin
- Petechiae (small red spots on skin)
- Blood in urine
- Black tarry stools
- Bleeding from nose or gums
- Increase in vaginal bleeding
- New onset of painful joints

of hemophilia. It results from a deficiency of factor VIII. Hemophilia B is a factor IX deficiency; about 15% of people with hemophilia have this type. The severity and prognosis of hemophilia depend on the degree of deficiency of the clotting factors. Mild hemophilia has the best prognosis because it does not cause spontaneous bleeding and joint deformities like severe hemophilia can.

After an injury, the person with hemophilia forms a platelet plug (which differs from a clot) at the site of an injury as would normally be expected. However, the clotting factor deficiency keeps the patient from forming a stable fibrin clot. Continued bleeding washes away the platelet plug that initially formed. Contrary to popular myth, people with hemophilia do not bleed faster and are not at risk from small scratches.

Etiology
Hemophilia A and B are inherited as X-linked recessive traits. This means that the female carrier (daughter of an affected father) has a 50% chance of transmitting the gene to each son or daughter. Daughters who receive the gene are carriers, and sons who receive the gene are born with hemophilia. It is technically possible for daughters to be affected with hemophilia, although it is rare.

Signs and Symptoms
Bleeding occurs as a result of injury or, in severe cases, spontaneously (unprovoked by injury). Bleeding into the muscles and joints (**hemarthrosis**) is common and can cause acute pain. Severe and repeated episodes of joint hemorrhage cause joint deformities, especially in the elbows, knees, and ankles. This decreases the patient's range of motion and ability to walk.

In mild hemophilia, excessive bleeding is usually associated only with surgery or significant trauma. However, once a person with mild hemophilia begins to bleed, the bleeding can be just as serious as that of the patient with a more severe form.

Spontaneous bleeding can occur with more severe hemophilia. It is possible for a patient to bleed into the joints or brain without any precipitating trauma. Severe episodes can produce large subcutaneous and deep intramuscular hematomas. Major trauma can cause bleeding so severe that it becomes life threatening.

Another unfortunate problem related to hemophilia treatment is the frequent need to replace clotting factors and other blood products. Before 1986, blood banks did not routinely test for HIV antibodies. Depending on the patient's age and frequency of treatment, many patients may have been exposed to HIV or hepatitis. Blood banks and pharmacies have checked their blood supplies for the presence of HIV since 1986. Today, plasma proteins are artificially created or thoroughly cleansed to prevent transmission of disease.

Diagnostic Tests
In some cases of mild hemophilia, a surgical procedure or trauma is the first time a bleeding problem is noticed. Laboratory data reveal a prolonged PTT. The various clotting factor levels are measured to determine which is missing. Once the missing factor is identified, the type of hemophilia is determined, and necessary treatments can be implemented.

Therapeutic Measures
Hemophilia is not curable. However, treatment advances have improved outcomes. Many patients can now live a normal life span. Treatment is aimed at preventing crippling deformities and increasing life expectancy. This involves stopping bleeding episodes by administering the missing clotting factors. Mild hemophilia A may be treated with injection or nasal inhalation of desmopressin (antidiuretic hormone; DDAVP). Desmopressin stimulates the body to release more clotting factors. It can be administered before dental procedures or sports. More severe hemophilia A is treated with factor VIII; hemophilia B is treated with factor IX. Each is available in a freeze-dried powder that is reconstituted with water and administered via IV route. The newest treatment employs factors made using recombinant DNA technology without the use of any human blood products. Blood transfusions are uncommon but may be necessary after severe trauma or surgery.

Complications occur when therapy is started too late. Minor trauma typically needs to be treated with at least 72 hours of added clotting factors; major traumas and surgeries may require up to 14 days of added factors to prevent sudden bleeding. Health care workers should pay careful attention to the patient who says that bleeding is starting even when no outward signs are evident. The patient usually knows from experience whether bleeding is starting. If treatment is delayed at this time, the results can be disastrous. Some patients with severe disease are treated prophylactically to prevent bleeding.

Nursing Process for the Patient With Hemophilia
DATA COLLECTION. Assess the patient and family for knowledge of the disease and its treatment and understanding of how to prevent bleeding episodes. Most patients care for themselves at home, starting their own IVs and administering

• WORD • BUILDING •

hemarthrosis: hem—bleeding + arthr—joint + osis—condition

treatment independently. Hospitalization is needed only for surgery or major trauma. During an acute episode of bleeding, monitor Hgb and Hct levels carefully. Monitor factor VIII or IX levels to determine whether factor replacement has reached adequate levels. Monitor vital signs for falling blood pressure and rising pulse rate, which are signs of hypovolemic shock. Assess all body systems for signs of bleeding (see Box 28.3). Perform a pain assessment using the *WHAT'S UP?* format.

NURSING DIAGNOSES, PLANNING, AND IMPLEMENTATION.

Acute Pain related to bleeding into tissues

EXPECTED OUTCOME: The patient's pain will be controlled as evidenced by verbalization that pain is relieved to a satisfactory level within a specified time frame depending on medication and route of intervention.

- Have the patient report the location, intensity, and quality of the pain. *Assessment provides the caregiver with data that can be used to develop a treatment plan.*
- Administer opioids as prescribed, including PCA. *Analgesics are the primary way to manage moderate to severe pain.*
- Avoid the administration of intramuscular injections *because of the risk of bleeding into the muscle.*
- Reassess the level of pain after administration of analgesia *to determine the effectiveness of the treatment ordered. IV medications will work almost immediately; oral medications may take 30 to 60 minutes.*
- Monitor sedation and respiratory status of the patient receiving opioids for pain. *Opioids depress the respiratory center of the brain.*

Risk for Bleeding related to factor deficiencies

EXPECTED OUTCOME: The patient will experience no signs or symptoms of bleeding. The patient will verbalize understanding of bleeding precautions.

- Instruct the patient on bleeding precautions and signs and symptoms of bleeding (see Boxes 28.1 and 28.3). *Identification of signs of bleeding will promote early intervention and prevent injury.*
- Assist with administration of factor concentrates, fresh frozen plasma, cryoprecipitate, blood, or a combination of these as ordered *to treat acute episodes of bleeding.* See Chapter 27 for transfusion of blood products.
- Apply ice or pressure on bleeding sites *to help slow bleeding.*
- Avoid intramuscular, subcutaneous, or rectal medications. *These routes can cause bleeding into tissues.*
- Instruct the patient that preventive care will be needed if surgery or dental procedures are needed. *These invasive procedures can be life-threatening events for the patient with hemophilia.*
- Instruct the patient to obtain emergency care in the event that bleeding occurs. *Intervention is critical for survival of an acute bleeding episode.*

- Instruct the patient and families on community services and hemophilia treatment centers available to the patient. *These centers are nationwide and coordinate care for patients with hemophilia.*

EVALUATION. If interventions have been effective, the patient will be comfortable. Bleeding will be prevented or complications minimized. The patient and family will be able to state appropriate measures to prevent and treat bleeding episodes. The patient will be knowledgeable about the resources available to cope with the diagnosis of hemophilia.

 DISORDERS OF WHITE BLOOD CELLS

Leukemia

The term **leukemia** literally means "white blood." It was first identified in 1845 when the blood of patients was examined and found to have an excess of "colorless" cells.

Pathophysiology

Leukemia is a malignant disease of the WBCs that affects all age-groups. The immature WBCs (blast cells) generate in an explosive fashion in the bone marrow, lymph tissue, and spleen. The cells are abnormal and unable to effectively fight infection. So many abnormal cells develop and are dumped into the peripheral circulation that they tend to collect in the body tissues and organs, especially where circulation is sluggish. Areas especially prone to infiltration with immature WBCs are the oral mucosa, anus, sinuses, and lungs. At the time of diagnosis, these areas are often inflamed, painful, and infected. It is common for patients to be diagnosed only after experiencing an infection that does not clear up easily with treatment.

As the disease progresses, the bone marrow continues to produce large numbers of the useless cells. The peripheral circulation is filled with them. The bone marrow is packed with blast cells. Because so many of the blood stem cells are being used to make defective WBCs, production of most other normal cells is impossible. The patient becomes anemic because of the lack of RBC production. Bleeding becomes a problem, as fewer and fewer platelets are manufactured. Most important, even though the WBC count is very high, there are few normal, mature, and active WBCs with which to fight infection. Thus, the patient often develops severe infections that do not respond to antibiotics. Without treatment, leukemia leaves the patient unable to fight infection, unable to control bleeding, and with increasing fatigue and anorexia. Untreated leukemia is almost always fatal.

Classifications

Leukemias are classified as either (1) acute or chronic and either (2) lymphoid or myeloid. Symptoms of the acute leukemias begin suddenly, and the patient is very sick. Chronic leukemias develop slowly, and patients can be surprised by the diagnosis because they feel well. Lymphoid leukemias affect the lymphocytes. Myeloid leukemias originate in the stem cells of the bone marrow that develop into monocytes, granulocytes, erythrocytes, and platelets. The most common leukemias are discussed next.

ACUTE LEUKEMIAS. Acute lymphocytic leukemia (ALL) is the most common cancer in children. ALL involves abnormal growth of the lymphocyte precursors (lymphoblasts). Acute myelogenous (myeloblastic) leukemia (AML) usually affects people over age 60. AML has a poor prognosis.

The patient with acute leukemia may present with sudden onset of high fever, abnormal bleeding from the mucous membranes, petechiae, ecchymoses, and easy bruising after minor trauma. Death usually results from infection.

CHRONIC LEUKEMIAS. Chronic lymphocytic leukemia (CLL) predominantly affects the B and T lymphocytes. CLL usually occurs in adults. Chronic myelogenous leukemia (CML) is characterized by the Philadelphia chromosome. CML occurs most often in older adults.

Chronic leukemia usually develops in a three-phase process. The first insidious phase is characterized by anemia and mild bleeding abnormalities. During this phase, the patient often feels well and is not even aware of being sick. After a time, generally years, the disease progresses to the accelerated and acute phases, in which the scenarios are similar to the events seen in acute leukemias. Chronic leukemia is almost always fatal; the average survival time is 3 to 5 years after onset of the chronic phase and 3 to 6 months after onset of the acute phase. With advances in treatments, however, it is not uncommon to encounter patients who have been living with chronic leukemia for 10 years or more.

Etiology

There is no single clear-cut cause for the development of leukemia. Risk factors are thought to include certain viruses because remnants of viruses have been found in leukemic cells. Genetic and immunological factors are often involved. For example, persons with Down syndrome are more likely to develop leukemia. Exposure to radiation is believed to be a factor, in part because radiologists have been found to have a higher than average development of leukemia. Some patients have developed leukemia after being treated for another unrelated malignancy using radiation or chemotherapy. Researchers have noted the higher occurrence rate of leukemia in persons who lived through the Hiroshima and Nagasaki atomic bombings during World War II. Water polluted with benzene and other chemicals may be a factor.

Signs and Symptoms

Symptoms are similar for all types of leukemia. They include low-grade fever caused by infection, pallor, weakness, lethargy, shortness of breath, and malaise caused by anemia. These symptoms may be present weeks or months before the appearance of other symptoms. The patient also may have fatigue, tachycardia, palpitations, and abdominal pain. Sternal pain and rib tenderness may result from crowding of bone marrow. If the leukemia has invaded the central nervous system, the patient may experience confusion, headaches, and personality changes. During the acute phase, the patient may have high fevers from infection. Ecchymosis or petechiae may result from thrombocytopenia.

Diagnostic Tests

Although a simple CBC often points toward the diagnosis, only bone marrow aspiration can show the degree of proliferation of the malignant WBCs and confirm the diagnosis of leukemia. The CBC may also show a decrease in the numbers of platelets, RBCs, and mature WBCs. A lumbar puncture helps determine whether the central nervous system is involved. Genetic analysis of the peripheral blood and bone marrow components may show the presence of the Philadelphia chromosome in patients with CML.

Therapeutic Measures

CHEMOTHERAPY. Systemic chemotherapy aims to eradicate the leukemic cells and induce a remission. Remission means that the bone marrow is free to produce normally occurring cells in normal proportions without production of the immature WBCs. The type of chemotherapy used varies with the type of leukemia and the level of involvement. Occasionally, partial remission is achieved when everything looks good except for an occasional leukemic cell seen in the bone marrow. Remission is not the same as cure.

There are four phases to the treatment of leukemia: induction, intensification, consolidation, and maintenance. Induction is the period in which an attempt is made to get the patient into remission. This first phase is difficult because chemotherapy is given in very high doses and on an aggressive timetable. Often, the patient becomes quite ill from the treatment. The patient may become depressed because the treatment seems worse than the disease at this stage. The nurse must help the patient deal with anemia, thrombocytopenia, and leukopenia as well as other side effects (Table 28.3; also see Box 28.2 and Chapter 11).

If the first remission is accomplished, the other phases of treatment are begun. Intensification is similar to the initial induction phase, using the same drugs at even higher doses. The next phase, consolidation, is used to ensure that all leukemic cells have been eradicated from the body. Finally, the patient graduates to maintenance therapy, in which the patient is kept free of leukemic cells and in remission for a period of years (and hopefully a lifetime). This requires years of continued chemotherapy treatments, often on a monthly basis.

RADIATION THERAPY. Radiation therapy is sometimes used in addition to chemotherapy for initial treatment of leukemia. It may be directed at the entire body or at specific areas where leukemic cells are collecting.

BONE MARROW TRANSPLANT. Bone marrow transplant is sometimes used to treat leukemia. Preparation includes high-dose chemotherapy and/or total body irradiation. The goal is

Table 28.3
Leukemia Summary

Signs and Symptoms	Fever (related to infection)
	Pallor
	Weakness, malaise
	Tachycardia
	Dyspnea
	Bone pain
	Headaches, confusion
Diagnostic Tests	Complete blood count (CBC)
	Bone marrow aspiration
	Lumbar puncture
Therapeutic Measures	Chemotherapy
	Radiation therapy
	Bone marrow transplant
Priority Nursing Diagnoses	*Risk for Injury* (infection, bleeding) related to pancytopenia
	Fatigue related to decreased tissue oxygenation
	Impaired Oral Mucous Membrane Integrity related to chemotherapy and pancytopenia

to destroy all of the patient's malignant bone marrow and then, at the last possible moment, replace it with a donor's clean and healthy bone marrow (allogenic transplant). Another type of bone marrow transplant is known as an autologous transplant. It uses the patient's own diseased bone marrow, which is harvested, chemically treated and cleaned, stored, and later reinfused. Transplanted bone marrow is given to the patient like a blood transfusion, typically through a central line placed in the chest. Once infused into the bloodstream, the new marrow travels to the bones, where it is hoped that it will begin to grow and function normally. Bone marrow transplants are being performed at more and more centers across the United States.

A new and promising treatment for leukemia is peripheral blood stem cell transplantation. Hematopoietic stem cells can be collected from the patient during remission and then reinfused at a later time. Donor stem cells are also sometimes used if a good match can be found.

OTHER THERAPIES. Biological therapies may be used to boost the patient's immune system. They may be used to help the body attack cancer cells or to control side effects by boosting RBC or WBC production. Kinase inhibitors (the most common is imatinib [Gleevec], an oral agent) may be used to inhibit abnormal proteins in leukemic cells in CML. By targeting just the cancer cells, the incidence of side effects is reduced.

Nursing Process for the Patient With Leukemia

The patient with leukemia is at risk for many problems, including fatigue, bleeding, infection, and other complications of the disease and its treatment. The patient must understand the disease process and treatment regimen to participate in self-care. See "Nursing Care Plan for the Patient With Leukemia" for interventions to deal with these problems. Additional diagnoses include *Deficient Knowledge* and *Anxiety*. The following websites provide resources for patients and families with leukemia:

- American Cancer Society, www.cancer.org
- Leukemia & Lymphoma Society, www.lls.org
- National Cancer Institute, www.cancer.gov

Also see Chapter 11 for general care of the patient with cancer.

Nursing Care Plan for the Patient With Leukemia

Nursing Diagnosis: *Risk for Injury* (infection, bleeding) related to pancytopenia
Expected Outcomes: The patient will be free from injury and infection as evidenced by temperature within normal limits and no signs or symptoms of bleeding. Signs and symptoms of infection or bleeding will be reported promptly.
Evaluation of Outcomes: Is the patient free from infection and bleeding, or are problems reported so that quick intervention can prevent further complications?

Intervention	Rationale	Evaluation
Monitor vital signs every 4 hours and as needed.	*Elevated temperature is a sign of infection. Falling blood pressure and elevated pulse rate may indicate sepsis or blood loss.*	Are vital signs stable?
Monitor patient for swelling, redness, or purulent drainage.	*These are signs of infection and should be reported promptly.*	Are signs of infection present?

Nursing Care Plan for the Patient With Leukemia—cont'd

Intervention	Rationale	Evaluation
Protect patient from sources of infection (see Box 28.2).	*Patient is at risk for infection because of ineffective white blood cells.*	Are precautions being observed to prevent infection?
Observe for tarry stools, petechiae, and ecchymoses (see Box 28.3).	*These are signs of bleeding and should be reported promptly.*	Are signs of bleeding present?
Protect patient from injury that could cause bleeding (see Box 28.1).	*Patient is at risk for bleeding because of reduced platelet count.*	Are precautions being observed to prevent injury and bleeding?

Nursing Diagnosis: *Fatigue* related to decreased red blood cell count and oxygenation and effects of treatments as evidenced by patient statement of lack of energy and inability to participate in desired activities
Expected Outcome: The patient's fatigue will be controlled at a level that is acceptable to the patient as evidenced by ability to participate in activities that are important to the patient.
Evaluation of Outcome: Is the patient able to identify and participate in activities as desired?

Intervention	Rationale	Evaluation
Assess fatigue using the *WHAT'S UP?* format.	*A good assessment establishes a baseline and aids in planning.*	Is fatigue present? To what degree?
Help patient identify activities that are important (e.g., activities of daily living [ADLs], attending a child's wedding, taking a trip). Assist in setting goals to work toward the desired activity.	*If the patient cannot do everything the patient wishes, it may help to focus on the most important things.*	Can patient identify important activities? What are they? How can you assist the patient to reach activity goals?
Encourage a balanced diet. Contact dietitian as needed.	*Poor nutrition contributes to fatigue.*	Is patient eating a balanced diet? Is weight stable?
Allow periods of rest between activities.	*Any activity (e.g., ADLs, getting x-rays, even talking) can increase fatigue.*	Is patient able to rest?
Ensure adequate sleep. Obtain order for sleeping aid if indicated.	*Lack of sleep worsens fatigue.*	Does patient state feeling rested on awakening? Is medication needed?
Provide for ADLs when patient is unable to do so independently.	*Extreme fatigue may prevent the patient from participating in self-care.*	Does patient need total assistance?

Nursing Diagnosis: *Impaired Oral Mucous Membrane Integrity* related to chemotherapy and pancytopenia as evidenced by bleeding, ulcerations, statement of pain, and difficulty eating
Expected Outcomes: The patient's oral mucous membranes will remain intact as evidenced by pink, moist, smooth tissue without ulceration. The patient will be able to eat a balanced diet.
Evaluation of Outcomes: Are oral mucous membranes intact without lesions? Is patient eating a balanced diet?

Intervention	Rationale	Evaluation
Assess mouth daily for redness, edema, and lesions.	*Routine assessment helps identify problems early so treatment can be implemented.*	Are mucous membranes intact?
Encourage adequate nutrition and fluids.	*Poor nutrition and dehydration increase the risk of oral lesions.*	Is patient eating and drinking?

(nursing care plan continues on page 514)

Nursing Care Plan for the Patient With Leukemia—cont'd

Intervention	Rationale	Evaluation
Encourage patient to brush teeth after meals with a soft toothbrush. If irritation is severe or if the patient is at risk for bleeding, use swabs or sponge Toothettes instead of a toothbrush.	*Brushing the teeth controls tooth and gum disease; a toothbrush may be too harsh if the patient is at risk for bleeding.*	Is mouth care being provided after meals? Is mouth care irritating? Are alternative methods needed?
Avoid use of lemon-glycerin swabs for mouth care.	*Lemon-glycerin swabs are drying to oral mucosa.*	Are products used appropriate?
Obtain an order for a mouthwash containing diphenhydramine (Benadryl). Obtain an order for a topical anesthetic if mouth is very inflamed and painful.	*Diphenhydramine reduces inflammation; anesthetics reduce pain.*	Does mouthwash soothe pain?
Encourage patient to avoid smoking, alcohol, acidic food or drinks, extremely hot or cold foods and drinks, and commercial mouthwash.	*These things can be irritating to the mucosa.*	Does patient state understanding of things to avoid?
Geriatric		
Advise patient to remove dentures for cleaning and at bedtime.	*Dentures left in for long periods can impair circulation and increase risk of lesions.*	Are oral mucous membranes intact?

BE SAFE!

BE VIGILANT! Monitor the patient carefully for subtle signs of infection. With inadequate or immature white blood cells, symptoms may not be obvious. Any redness, swelling, or even slight increase in temperature should be reported.

CRITICAL THINKING

Mr. Washington is on your unit and undergoing initial treatment for leukemia. You enter his room and find it full of visitors.

1. What concerns do you have?
2. What do you do?
3. How can you promote patient-centered care during Mr. Washington's treatment?

Suggested answers are at the end of the chapter.

MULTIPLE MYELOMA

Multiple myeloma is a deadly cancer of the plasma cells in the bone marrow. When the disease is caught in its early stages, treatment can prolong life by 3 to 5 years. More important, early detection can decrease the amount of pain and disability due to bony destruction and **pathological fractures.** Unfortunately, many patients die within 2 years of diagnosis. Multiple myeloma currently has a 47% survival rate at 5 years (American Society of Clinical Oncology, 2016). Multiple myeloma most often affects men aged 50 to 70.

Pathophysiology

In this disorder, cancerous plasma cells in the bone marrow begin reproducing uncontrollably. These cells infiltrate bone tissue all over the body. This produces hundreds of tumors that begin to devour the bone tissue. X-ray examination may show holes in the bones forming a Swiss-cheese pattern (Fig. 28.6). As more and more holes form, the integrity of the bone is compromised and weakened. Multiple myeloma usually affects the bones of the skull, pelvis, ribs, and vertebrae.

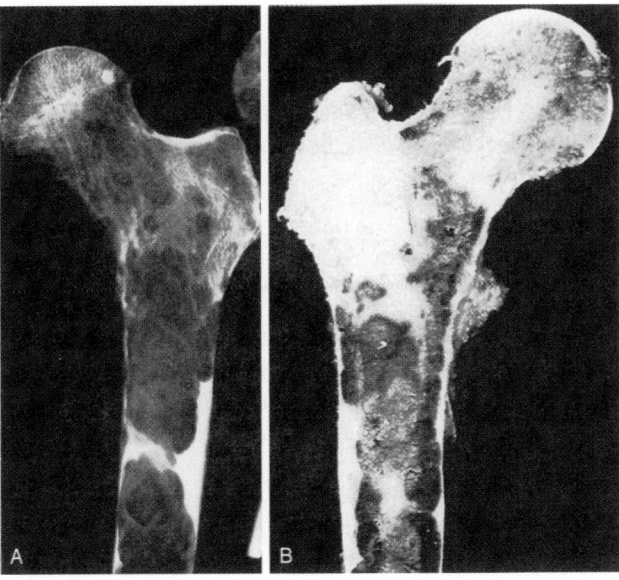

FIGURE 28.6 X-ray of bone destruction in multiple myeloma.

As the disease progresses, plasma cells infiltrate the major organs, including the liver, spleen, lymph nodes, lungs, adrenal glands, kidneys, skin, and GI tract. Because the diagnosis is usually made only after widespread invasion of the bones is well under way, the prognosis for patients with this disease is poor. Although the overall result of the disease is the devastating destruction of the bone and widespread osteoporosis, death is often from sepsis.

Etiology

The cause of multiple myeloma is unknown. Research suggests genetics may be one factor. People who work in rubber, leather, farming, and petroleum industries are more likely to develop multiple myeloma. Obesity, exposure to radiation, and long-term exposure to hair dyes also increase risk.

Signs and Symptoms

Skeletal pain is the most common complaint. The patient may describe the pain as constant severe back pain that increases with exercise or movement or as pain in the ribs. Other signs and symptoms include achiness of the long bones, joint swelling and tenderness, low-grade fever, and general malaise. Sometimes, there is evidence of early peripheral neuropathy secondary to vertebral collapse and spinal cord compression. The patient may be unable to feel the true temperature of bath water and be burned. In addition, the patient may be unable to feel wounds and infections on the feet. In more severe cases of cord compression, the patient may lose control of bladder and bowels. This is a true oncological emergency. Prompt emergency treatment is needed to keep the patient from becoming paralyzed.

Patients may have pathological fractures of the long bones. These are fractures that occur with no trauma (e.g., the patient breaks a leg turning over in bed or breaks a rib while sneezing). In advanced disease, the patient experiences anemia, weight loss, thoracic spinal deformities from multiple rib destruction, and a loss of height because of pathological fractures and compacting of the vertebrae.

Because calcium is mobilized from the bones and into the blood, the patient is at risk for hypercalcemia. Signs and symptoms of hypercalcemia include anorexia, nausea, vomiting, mental changes (especially confusion), seizures, weakness, and fatigue. Kidney stones may result as the excess calcium passes through the kidneys.

Patients are susceptible to infection because of compromised immune function. Pneumonia is a common finding in patients with multiple myeloma. They may develop anemia because of bone marrow dysfunction and reduced erythropoietin formation by diseased kidneys. Risk for bruising and bleeding occurs due to thrombocytopenia.

Patients often develop kidney failure because the filtering capacity of the kidney becomes blocked by calcium. Other factors include recurrent infections and deposits of myeloma cells in the kidneys.

Diagnostic Tests

A CBC shows moderate to severe anemia. The WBC count may show an increase in the number of WBCs secondary to infection. Blood and urine studies are positive for M-type globulins (called *Bence–Jones proteins* when found in the urine) in 40% of patients. X-ray examinations or magnetic resonance imaging (MRI) may show changes in the lungs and diffuse osteoporosis in bones not already riddled with holes. Bone marrow biopsy is done to confirm the diagnosis and determine the stage of the disease.

Blood chemistries often show an increased amount of calcium in the blood. Hypercalciuria results when the calcium released out of the bones is flushed out in the urine. An IV pyelogram may be done to see how much calcium is collecting in the kidneys. A 24-hour urine collection is done to evaluate protein excretion.

C-reactive protein (CRP) is elevated in multiple myeloma; it is believed that the CRP actually promotes the cancer cells' proliferation and protects them from the effects of chemotherapy agents. Measurement of CRP helps determine prognosis. Elevated CRP levels are also associated with increased fatigue.

Therapeutic Measures

Long-term treatment of multiple myeloma consists of a two-pronged approach: (1) managing the disease, and (2) managing the symptoms. To manage the disease, corticosteroids (prednisone or dexamethasone) and oral or IV chemotherapy agents are given. Thalidomide (Thalomid) may be given to slow the progression of the disease. Lenalidomide (Revlimid) is chemically similar to thalidomide but has fewer side effects. The goal of drug therapy is to suppress plasma cell proliferation. This helps decrease the amount and speed of bone destruction.

Another medication for multiple myeloma is bortezomib (Velcade). Bortezomib is a proteasome inhibitor that inhibits enzymes to disrupt cancer cell growth and survival.

Another option is high-dose chemotherapy combined with stem cell transplantation. Donor stem cells can be used, or a patient's own peripheral stem cells can be removed and re-infused in a process called *immunotherapy*. These stem cells can then differentiate into new, healthy cells. Additional treatment options are being researched.

The second approach is control of symptoms. The patient is monitored for signs and symptoms of hypercalcemia, hyperuricemia, dehydration, respiratory infection, renal problems, and pain. The HCP may order the administration of IV bisphosphonate agents such as pamidronate (Aredia). This class of drugs inhibits bone resorption. It is used to help keep serum calcium levels controlled. Oral compounds are also available to help keep the calcium within normal limits. The goal is to get the serum calcium level below 10 mg/dL. If hypercalcemia occurs, the HCP will order an IV infusion of normal saline solution at a high rate, followed by regular administration of diuretics.

External beam irradiation may be given to especially painful areas of bone involvement. Fortunately, this treatment is quite effective, usually decreasing pain intensity in just a few days. The patient can expect to have a daily (or perhaps a twice-daily) treatment over a course of 10 to 14 days that is delivered directly to the painful bony areas. Vigorous attention to administering pain medications during the early course of treatment greatly reduces the patient's pain levels.

The patient may need spinal surgery if vertebral collapse occurs. Because of demineralization of the bone, with resulting large amounts of calcium in the blood and urine, surgery for kidney stones and eventual dialysis for acute or chronic kidney failure may be needed.

Nursing Process for the Patient With Multiple Myeloma

The patient with multiple myeloma is at risk for many problems. In addition to the following, the diagnoses in "Nursing Care Plan for the Patient With Leukemia" are appropriate.

Data Collection

Assess for fever or malaise, which can signal the onset of infection. Other conditions to be alert for include anemia, hypercalcemia, fractures, and kidney complications. Monitor intake and output, and strain urine for stones. Elevated BUN and creatinine levels will alert you to possible kidney failure. Report back pain, leg weakness, sensory loss, or loss of bowel or bladder function because these can indicate spinal cord compression. Monitor the patient for elevated CRP and low Hgb, which are associated with increased fatigue.

Nursing Diagnoses, Planning, and Implementation

Risk for Infection related to compromised immune function

EXPECTED OUTCOME: The patient will remain free from infection as evidenced by temperature within normal limits and no signs or symptoms of infection.

• Intervene as appropriate *to reduce the risk of infection* (see Box 28.2).

• Encourage deep breathing, and keep patient active *to decrease the risk of respiratory complications.*

Risk for Injury (fracture) related to weakened bones, complications of immobility, and complications due to hypercalcemia

EXPECTED OUTCOME: The patient will remain free from injury as evidenced by no fracture and no complications related to immobility or hypercalcemia.

• Keep the patient mobile. Consult physical and occupational therapy as needed. Bones in use are strongest, so the patient should remain up and moving as much as possible *to help stimulate calcium resorption and decrease demineralization.*
• Assist the patient with walking *to reduce the risk of pathological fractures of the long bones.*
• If the patient is unsteady, use a walker or a support belt *to reduce the risk of falls.*
• If the patient is bedridden, reposition every 2 hours *to prevent complications related to immobility.*
• Use a lift sheet to move the patient gently in bed *to decrease the risk of skin damage and pathological fractures.*
• Provide passive range-of-motion exercises *to maintain mobility if the patient is unable to be independently mobile.*
• Administer fluids so that daily output is never less than 1,500 mL *to flush kidneys and reduce the risk of kidney stones.*
• Teach the patient the importance of good hydration at all times *to minimize complications of hypercalcemia.* Depending on time of year and the type and level of patient activities, the patient may need to have an intake of more than 4 L daily.

Evaluation

If nursing care has been effective, the patient will be free of infection or infection will be recognized and treated promptly. The patient will avoid injury, with no fracture, skin breakdown, or complications related to hypercalcemia. See "Home Health Hints" at the end of this chapter for additional suggestions for patients being cared for at home.

 LYMPHATIC DISORDERS

Lymphatic disorders include Hodgkin disease and the non-Hodgkin lymphomas.

Hodgkin Disease

Despite its name, Hodgkin disease is a **lymphoma,** which is a cancer of the lymph system. Its distinguishing feature is the presence of Reed–Sternberg cells. This makes it different

• WORD • BUILDING •
lymphoma: lymph—fluid found in lymphatic vessels + oma—tumor

from all the other forms of lymphoma. Hodgkin disease is more prevalent in men than in women. It occurs most often from ages 15 to 40. After a decrease in incidence in persons aged 40 to 55, the incidence peaks again in adults older than age 55. Of all the lymphomas, Hodgkin disease is the most curable type, even when the disease is widespread at the time of diagnosis.

Pathophysiology

Lymph nodes are made of tightly bound fibers and cells that serve as filtering devices for the body's immune system. Most often, Hodgkin disease begins as a single changed lymph node, usually one of the cervical lymph nodes of the neck. As the disease progresses, the cancer invades the lymph node chains node by node. The cancer infiltration usually follows the path of lymph fluid flow. Left untreated, other lymphoid tissues such as the spleen become infiltrated with Hodgkin disease. The major organs eventually become involved. Common reports of patients with organ involvement include shortness of breath, a feeling of fullness, weakness, and malaise. These organ-related symptoms usually motivate the patient to seek medical help.

A tentative diagnosis of Hodgkin disease is based on one or more painlessly enlarged nodes in the cervical, axillary, or inguinal areas. A biopsy of several of the enlarged nodes is performed to search for the presence of Reed–Sternberg cells, which confirms the diagnosis.

Etiology

The exact cause of Hodgkin disease is unknown. A possible viral origin has been proposed; it is more common in people who have had mononucleosis. Sometimes, it occurs in families, suggesting a genetic link. Patients with impaired immune function are also at higher risk, such as those with AIDS or taking immunosuppressant drugs.

Signs and Symptoms

Painless swelling in one or more of the common lymph node chains is a usual presentation (Fig. 28.7). Swelling can range from barely perceptible to the size of a softball, occasionally even larger. The patient may report generalized pruritus. One other curious event, alcohol-induced pain, is occasionally present. With just a few sips of any type of alcohol-containing beverage (beer, wine, or liquor), the patient may describe intense pain at the site of disease. Because the lymph nodes in the upper chest and neck are often involved, the patient may have symptoms of obstruction, such as cough, dysphagia, or stridor.

Other common symptoms include persistent low-grade fever, night sweats, fatigue, weight loss, and malaise. When these additional symptoms are present, the prognosis is worse. In older adults, enlarged lymph nodes might not be visible, so these secondary symptoms may be the only presenting symptoms. Other symptoms associated with late-stage disease include edema of the neck and face, jaundice, nerve pain, enlargement of the retroperitoneal nodes, and infiltration of the spleen; liver and bones may also be involved.

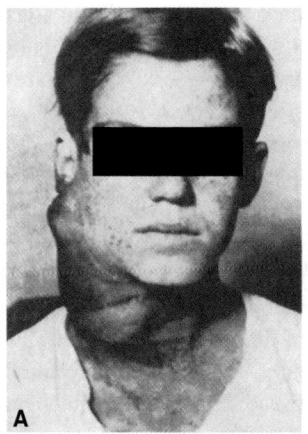

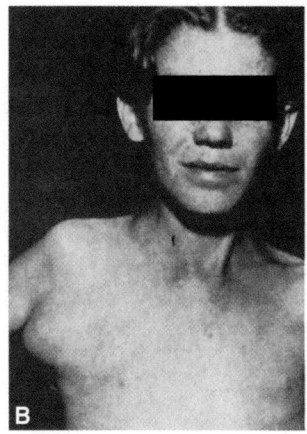
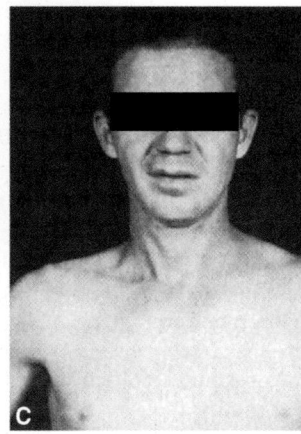

FIGURE 28.7 Cervical Hodgkin disease. (A) Young boy with extensive cervical Hodgkin disease. (B) Appearance several years later, when axillary manifestation developed. (C) Appearance 23 years after initial treatment with radiation.

Diagnostic Tests and Staging

Diagnosis usually begins with a lymph node biopsy of the easiest lymph node to access. Lymph node biopsies are done to check for abnormal histiocytic proliferation, nodular fibrosis, and necrosis. Other tests include bone marrow biopsy and aspiration, liver and spleen biopsies, routine chest x-ray examination, abdominal computed tomography (CT) scan to check for disease in the liver and spleen, lung scan, and bone scan. Lymphangiography may be performed to view the flow of lymph in the lymph network. A gallium scan can also be done to view lymph tissue.

Hematologic tests (e.g., CBC) may show wide variability of RBCs, indicating mild to severe anemia. The WBC count is often abnormal and extreme (either very high or very low) because of bone marrow infiltration by disease. These same tests are used for staging the disease into one of four stages:

- Stage I disease is limited to a single lymph node or site or a single organ.
- Stage II disease occurs when two or more nodes are involved on the same side of the diaphragm.
- Stage III disease affects nodes on both sides of the diaphragm.

• Stage IV, the most serious form of the disease and the least curable, includes widely disseminated disease in both lymph nodes and other organs, such as bone marrow or liver.

Therapeutic Measures

Appropriate therapy includes the use of radiation and chemotherapy. It depends on the stage of the disease. Radiation therapy is administered on an outpatient basis over a 4- to 6-week period. It can cure most patients with stage I or stage II disease. Combinations of chemotherapy and radiation therapy are used for patients with stage III and stage IV disease. Results vary depending on the location and the stage of disease. If the disease recurs after initial treatment, bone marrow or stem cell transplant may be considered.

Nursing Management

Most nursing interventions are aimed at symptom management. If the patient is experiencing pruritus or night sweats, nursing interventions are aimed at alleviation of discomfort. These may include changing the gown and bed linens several times a night and helping the patient remain clean and dry. Keeping the patient and family involved in the plan of care may relieve anxiety.

Later, nursing interventions are tailored to alleviate problems that arise secondary to chemotherapy and radiation therapy. See Chapter 11 for nursing interventions for these problems. Also see "Nursing Care Plan for the Patient With Lymphoma." See Box 28.2 and Chapter 11 for additional interventions for patients with cancer.

Nursing Care Plan for the Patient With Lymphoma

Nursing Diagnosis: *Activity Intolerance* related to fatigue and anemia as evidenced by inability to carry out activities of daily living (ADLs) without excessive fatigue or dyspnea
Expected Outcome: The patient will have ADL needs met by self or caregiver as evidenced by patient statement of met needs.
Evaluation of Outcome: Are ADL needs met?

Intervention	Rationale	Evaluation
Assess amount of activity that causes fatigue or dyspnea.	*Assessment helps guide plan of care.*	How much can patient do before becoming fatigued or dyspneic?
Assist patient with activities as needed.	*Patient may need assistance with ADLs if fatigue is extreme.*	Does assistance help reduce fatigue?
Provide oxygen therapy as ordered.	*Oxygen therapy can increase oxygen levels and activity tolerance.*	Does patient tolerate activity better with oxygen therapy?
Instruct patient to space rest with activities.	*Rest periods decrease oxygen needs and allow patient to conserve energy for next activity.*	Is patient able to tolerate activity better after a rest period?

Nursing Diagnosis: *Risk for Infection* related to bone marrow involvement and side effects of treatment as evidenced by elevated temperature, redness, swelling, or other signs and symptoms based on infection site
Expected Outcome: The patient will remain infection-free as evidenced by temperature within normal limits and no signs or symptoms of infection.
Evaluation of Outcome: Are signs and symptoms of infection absent? Is temperature within normal limits?

Intervention	Rationale	Evaluation
Assess patient for risk factors for infection.	*The white blood cell count may be very high or very low, placing the patient at risk for infection.*	Is patient at risk? Are additional interventions indicated?
Monitor patient for signs and symptoms of infection, such as cough, fever, malaise, erythema, pain, or drainage. Report immediately.	*Early detection and treatment of infection provide the best results.*	Are signs and symptoms of infection present?

Patient Education

In addition to the teaching needs outlined, make sure that the patient and the family know about local chapters of the American Cancer Society (www.cancer.org) and the Leukemia & Lymphoma Society (www.lls.org). Both organizations provide information, financial assistance, and counseling referral sources, which most patients find valuable.

CRITICAL THINKING

Jeanie is a 60-year-old nurse diagnosed with stage II Hodgkin disease. She wishes to continue working at her job on a respiratory unit at the local hospital while she undergoes treatment. What concerns do you have about this?

Suggested answers are at the end of the chapter.

Non-Hodgkin Lymphomas

All of the other types of lymphomas are clumped into a diverse classification known as the *non-Hodgkin lymphomas* (NHLs). It is possible to sort these other types of lymphomas into different categories based on the degree of malignancy. NHLs arise in the lymphoid tissues of the body, just as Hodgkin disease does, but they differ in several ways (Table 28.4).

Pathophysiology

The most distinguishing difference is the absence of the Reed–Sternberg cells in an NHL. Instead, many of these lymphomas arise from the B cells and T cells. The B cells are involved in recognizing and destroying specific antigens. Cells specifically involved include the memory B cells and the plasma cells. The T cells also are involved in registering

Table 28.4

Hodgkin Disease versus Non-Hodgkin Lymphoma

	Hodgkin Disease	*Non-Hodgkin Lymphomas*
Age	15 to 40 and over 55 years	Usually over 50 years
Incidence	Less common	More common
Prognosis	Good	Poorer
Reed–Sternberg cells	Present	Absent
Alcohol-induced pain	May be present	Absent

antigens, but there are many kinds of T cells. An abnormality in any of the T cells can result in a type of NHL. Cancerous cells are found most commonly in the lymph nodes, but they can also be found in other lymph tissues such as the tonsils, thymus, or bone marrow.

Etiology

The cause of an NHL is unclear. However, some viruses, such as the Epstein-Barr and herpes viruses, are thought to play a role in their development. *Helicobacter pylori,* the bacterium that causes ulcers, has been associated with NHLs. Genetics play a role, as do immune problems such as AIDS. People working in farming, printing, medicine, electronics, and leather also have a higher risk for developing an NHL.

Signs and Symptoms

Clinical features of malignant NHLs include enlarged, painless, rubbery nodes in the cervical and supraclavicular areas, axillae, and groin; enlarged tonsils and adenoids; and occasional symptoms of dyspnea and cough. As the disease progresses, the patient may report fatigue, malaise, weight loss, and night sweats similar to Hodgkin disease. NHLs usually progress more rapidly than Hodgkin disease.

Diagnostic Tests

Diagnosis is confirmed by histological evaluation of biopsied lymph nodes, tonsils, bone marrow, liver, bowel, skin, or other affected tissues. Other relevant tests include bone scans, chest x-rays, lymphangiography, liver and spleen scans, CT of the abdomen, MRI, positron emission tomography (PET) scan, and IV pyelogram to determine the extent of the disease. Laboratory tests include a CBC (which often indicates anemia), serum uric acid level, and liver function studies. Serum calcium level may be elevated if bone lesions are present.

Therapeutic Measures

Treatment usually involves multimodal therapy, including the use of chemotherapy and radiation therapy in combination. Radiation therapy is given to affected areas in advanced stages of NHL. Stem cell transplant may be tried in patients with advanced disease. Newer therapies include the use of monoclonal antibodies to target and destroy cancer cells and interferon therapy to help boost the immune system to fight the cancer.

Nursing Management

You can provide emotional support by keeping the patient and family informed during the testing phase. Symptoms such as night sweats can be managed with frequent linen and gown changes. Help the patient maintain nutrition with attractively prepared meals. Spend time listening to the patient's concerns; involve the hospital chaplain in the patient's care if the patient desires. See Table 28.5 and "Nursing Care Plan for the Patient With Lymphoma" for more information.

Table 28.5
Lymphoma Summary

Signs and Symptoms	Swollen lymph nodes Fatigue Low-grade fever Night sweats
Diagnostic Tests	Complete blood count (CBC) Lymph node biopsy Lymphangiography Computed tomography (CT) scan
Therapeutic Measures	Chemotherapy Radiation Bone marrow or stem cell transplant
Priority Nursing Diagnoses	*Activity Intolerance* *Risk for Infection*

 SPLENIC DISORDERS

The spleen is involved in a number of disorders, including cancers of the blood, lymph, and bone marrow; hereditary conditions such as SCD; and acquired problems such as idiopathic thrombocytopenia. Under normal circumstances, the spleen is not paid much attention; it generally performs its functions without much fanfare.

If the spleen enlarges markedly, the condition is referred to as **splenomegaly.** Other times, the spleen may or may not be enlarged, but the function is out of control so that too many RBCs and platelets are removed from the peripheral circulation. Sometimes, the spleen is not able to perform its job because of bleeding into the pulp of the organ, which makes it useless. Bleeding into the spleen can occur from various illnesses or from trauma. Regardless of the nature of the malfunction, one treatment option may be splenectomy.

Splenectomy

Splenectomy is the surgical removal of the spleen. This is used to treat selective hematologic disorders. It is also used to determine the stage of lymphomas. It may be done with traditional, open surgery or laparoscopically. Splenectomy is performed fairly often in the United States. However, like any surgery, it is not without risk. Some patients have splenic autotransplantation. This involves implantation of some of the removed tissue, usually in the peritoneal cavity. This allows for return of some splenic function.

Patient Education

Explain to patients that this surgery removes the spleen, usually under general anesthesia. Inform patients that they can live a normal life after the surgery. However, tell them that they may be more prone to infection and should receive vaccines against pneumonia, meningococci, and *Haemophilus influenzae* disease, as well as a yearly influenza vaccine.

Preoperative Care

Before the surgery, ensure that the CBC and coagulation profile are completed and reported to the HCP. Blood transfusion may be ordered to correct underlying anemia and to prepare for the loss of a great deal of blood stored in the spleen. Vitamin K is often ordered to correct clotting factor deficiencies.

Check the patient's vital signs, and perform a baseline respiratory assessment. Note any signs of respiratory infections such as fever, chills, crackles, wheezes, or cough. If any of these are noted, make sure that the surgeon is aware of them because surgery may need to be delayed. Teach the patient routine coughing and deep-breathing techniques to help prevent postoperative respiratory complications.

Postoperative Care

During the early postoperative period, watch carefully for bleeding, either external or internal. Be prepared to administer opioids for pain, usually on an around-the-clock schedule so the patient is comfortable enough to deep breathe, cough, and ambulate. After opioid administration, be sure to observe for side effects. These may include incomplete pain relief or hypoventilation. Monitor for fever every 4 hours, and expect a mild, low-grade, transient fever postoperatively. A persistent fever may indicate abscess or hematoma formation.

If the surgery was performed to decrease the numbers of cells being removed from the peripheral circulation, monitor the platelet count. Often the count begins to rise in just a few days, but it may take up to 2 weeks for the platelets to normalize.

Complications

A splenectomy can lead to complications such as bleeding, pneumonia, and atelectasis (collapsed alveoli). Respiratory problems occur because of the spleen's position close to the diaphragm and the need for a high surgical incision that is very painful. Often, the patient tries to restrict lung expansion after surgery to keep from hurting. However, this splinting behavior may leave the patient at risk for pneumonia and respiratory problems. In addition, splenectomy patients are usually more vulnerable to infection, especially influenza. This is because the spleen's role in the immune response is no longer filled.

Another possible complication of splenectomy includes the development of pancreatitis. This is because the tail of the pancreas is close to the spleen, and irritation can occur.

• WORD • BUILDING •
splenomegaly: splen—spleen + megaly—large
splenectomy: splen—spleen + ectomy—excision

Another serious complication is overwhelming post-splenectomy infection (OPSI). The causative agents in OPSI include streptococci, *Neisseria* spp., and influenza bacteria (as opposed to a flu virus). OPSI can occur at any time from 1 week to 20 years after the splenectomy. Patients most at risk are those with poor immune function.

Early symptoms of OPSI include fever and malaise that seem unremarkable. However, the infection may progress within a few hours to sepsis and death. Unfortunately, OPSI can have a mortality rate as high as 70%. Be sure to include the signs and symptoms of OPSI in presplenectomy patient education. Also, stress the need to promptly obtain medical attention for the patient at the first signs and symptoms of OPSI. The patient should be directed to continue to receive lifetime vaccinations against these bacteria.

Home Health Hints

- Patients who are at risk for infection can place a sign on the front door of their homes to limit visitors or ask persons with colds to come back when they are well. The patient may appreciate the home health nurse giving permission to be assertive in such circumstances.

- Teach patients with infection risk to wear gloves when gardening, avoid manicures and pedicures, avoid hot tubs or Jacuzzis, and wash hands after contact with pets, fresh flowers, or plants.
- To prevent bruising, have the patient cut the feet off long, white sport socks and wear them on the arms. They can be hidden under long-sleeve shirts and blouses. They provide a cushion when doing housework.
- Teach patients with thrombocytopenia to avoid contact sports and to consult with their health care provider (HCP) about whether sexual intercourse is safe.
- Teach patients with thrombocytopenia to avoid over-the-counter medications unless approved by the HCP. Many such agents contain aspirin or nonsteroidal anti-inflammatory drugs (NSAIDs).
- Patients with sickle cell anemia usually have a lower blood pressure. It is important to report even mild hypertension in these patients.
- Provide a high-calorie/-protein nutritional supplement between meals. If fatigue or nausea causes poor appetite, discuss eating smaller, more frequent meals. Ask the HCP for an antiemetic order if needed.

SUGGESTED ANSWERS TO CRITICAL THINKING

Mrs. Johns

1. Monitor Mrs. Johns's vital signs and report falling blood pressure and rising pulse immediately. Inspect her skin for petechiae and ecchymoses. Outline ecchymotic areas with a marker to see whether the area is increasing in size. Monitor urine for signs of blood. Test stools for occult blood. Monitor vaginal discharge for increasing bleeding. Report any changes promptly.
2. Anticipate assisting the registered nurse (RN) with administration of blood or blood products. Instruct Mrs. Johns in the importance of preventing injury that could cause further bleeding. Other care will be supportive.
3. Mrs. Johns will be concerned for her new baby, who is most likely on another unit or already discharged home. Allow Mrs. Johns to talk about her concerns. Arrange visits with her family and baby if permitted by her condition and her health care provider.

4.

$$\frac{300 \text{ mL}}{30 \text{ min}} \left| \frac{60 \text{ min}}{1 \text{ hour}} \right. = 600 \text{ mL per hour}$$

5. Collaborate with the RN, internist, obstetrician, hematologist, neonatal nurse, husband, family, and social worker to provide holistic, patient-centered care for this new mother.

Mr. Washington

1. Because of his leukemia and treatment, Mr. Washington is at risk for infection. If he develops an infection, he will have great difficulty getting over it. With so many visitors in the room, it is likely that one or more has a cold or virus. They may not be aware of the risk this poses to Mr. Washington. Mr. Washington is probably also fatigued because of his disease and treatment, and visiting requires energy.
2. You should kindly explain that although family visits are important, Mr. Washington is very susceptible to catching colds or other illnesses and that it would be best to limit visitors to one or two at a time. Point out that persons with symptoms of colds or flu should not enter the room at all. Visits should also be brief to prevent overtiring the patient.
3. Ask Mr. Washington about his preferences, and attempt to honor them if possible. He may choose one or two (healthy!) visitors to come regularly, or choose a time of day when he is less fatigued to have visitors. As his nurse, you can help enforce visiting limitations so Mr. Washington does not have to feel ungracious toward his visitors.

Continued

SUGGESTED ANSWERS TO CRITICAL THINKING—cont'd

Jeanie

Jeanie will probably be fatigued from her disease, and fatigue may increase further as a side effect of treatment. Staff nursing jobs can be tiring even for healthy nurses. In addition, she will be around patients with respiratory diseases, many of whom are contagious. Because of the risk of infection secondary to the disease process and the treatment regimen, Jeanie might want to take a leave of absence during treatment or ask to be reassigned to an area that is less demanding and away from direct patient care until her treatments have been completed.

Review Questions

1. The nurse is caring for a patient admitted with pancytopenia with complaints of dyspnea upon exertion. For which condition should the nurse assess further?
   1. Pain
   2. Thrombocytopenia
   3. Anemia
   4. Neutropenia

2. A nurse is teaching a patient with sickle cell anemia about activities to avoid. Which of the following activities the patient plans to do shows that more teaching is needed?
   1. Going to the beach
   2. Taking a long car trip
   3. Running in a marathon
   4. Listening to a concert

3. The family of a patient with disseminated intravascular coagulation has questions about the bleeding that is occurring. Which statement by the nurse is the best response to explain why the patient is bleeding?
   1. "Bleeding is caused by a lack of red blood cells."
   2. "Bleeding is caused by depleted white blood cells."
   3. "Extremely high blood pressure forces blood from mucous membranes."
   4. "Bleeding happens when the body's clotting factors have all been used up."

4. The nurse is teaching the parent of a child with hemophilia. Which of the following statements by the parent demonstrates understanding about preventing bleeding episodes?
   1. "My son will have to avoid contact sports."
   2. "My son will have to avoid irritating foods in his diet."
   3. "My son will have to grow a beard."
   4. "My son will always have to live near a major hospital."

5. Which family member should be restricted from visiting a patient with newly diagnosed leukemia?
   1. The one who has a new baby at home
   2. The one who has a history of asthma
   3. The one who has received recent radiation treatment for cancer
   4. The one who has a runny nose

6. Which of the following nursing interventions is a priority for the patient with multiple myeloma found in the ribs and femur?
   1. Implement safety measures to prevent falls.
   2. Assist with all activities of daily living.
   3. Provide a high-protein, low-sodium diet.
   4. Institute infection precautions.

7. Which of the following nursing interventions are appropriate for a patient with thrombocytopenia? **Select all that apply.**
   1. Avoid intramuscular injections.
   2. Keep visitors who are ill away from the patient.
   3. Encourage 4 liters of fluid daily.
   4. Avoid use of aspirin and nonsteroidal anti-inflammatory drugs.
   5. Allow rest between activities.
   6. Encourage use of shoes or slippers.

8. A patient with hypercalcemia needs to drink at least 3 liters of fluid per day. Today, the patient has had 1 measuring cup of coffee, 1 liter of water, a can of soda that says it has 355 milliliters, and a half cup of juice. How many milliliters has he had so far today? Fill in the blank.
   Answer: _____ mL

9. What assessment data will best help the nurse determine whether interventions for neutropenia have been effective?
   1. Temperature
   2. Fatigue level
   3. Oxygen saturation
   4. Hemoglobin level

10. Which circumstance places the patient at most risk for
postoperative pneumonia following a splenectomy?
1. Disturbance of clotting factors
2. Nothing by mouth status
3. Need for frequent dressing changes
4. Location of surgical incision

Answer rationales available in your online resources.

Key Points

Find the chapter key points in your online resources
available through Davis Edge.

Additional Resources

DAVIS
edge. ◀ Use the scratch off code on the inside front
cover of your book to access online quizzes
that will help you to improve your scores
on course exams and prepare for NCLEX-PN®.

 Study Guide

CHAPTER 29

Respiratory System Function, Assessment, and Therapeutic Measures

Paula D. Hopper, Janice L. Bradford

KEY TERMS

adventitious (ad-ven-TISH-us)
apnea (AP-nee-ah)
crepitus (KREP-ih-tus)
cyanosis (SY-uh-NOH-sis)
dyspnea (DISP-nee-ah)
respiratory excursion (RES-per-uh-TOR-ee eks-KUR-shun)
retraction (rih-TRAK-shun)
thoracentesis (THOR-uh-sen-TEE-sis)
tidaling (TY-dah-ling)
tracheostomy (TRAY-key-AH-stuh-mee)
tracheotomy (TRAY-key-AH-tuh-mee)

CHAPTER CONCEPTS

Acid–Base Balance
Evidence-Based Practice
Oxygenation
Safety

LEARNING OUTCOMES

1. Describe the normal structures and functions of the respiratory system.
2. Identify how aging affects the respiratory system.
3. List data to collect when caring for a patient with a respiratory disorder.
4. Recognize expected findings when inspecting, palpating, percussing, and auscultating the chest.
5. Identify common diagnostic tests performed to diagnose disorders of the respiratory system.
6. Plan nursing care for patients undergoing each of the diagnostic tests.
7. Discuss therapeutic measures used to help patients with respiratory disorders.

NORMAL RESPIRATORY SYSTEM ANATOMY AND PHYSIOLOGY

The respiratory system is basically a tract, divided into upper and lower respiratory portions. The upper tract is above the thoracic cavity. The lower portion is within the thoracic cavity. The alveoli of the lungs are the site of gas exchange between the air and the blood of pulmonary circulation; the rest of the system moves air into and out of the lungs. Together with the cardiovascular system, the respiratory system supplies the body with oxygen and eliminates carbon dioxide.

Nose and Nasal Cavities

The nose is made mostly of bone and cartilage covered with muscle and epithelium. Hairs inside the nostrils block the entry of dust and other particles. The nasal cavities are separated at midline by the nasal septum, which is made of bone and cartilage. The nasal mucosa is highly vascular, ciliated epithelium that warms and moistens inhaled air. Dust and microorganisms become trapped on mucus produced by goblet cells and then are swept back into the pharynx by the cilia. Table 29.1 provides a summary of protective mechanisms in the respiratory system.

The paranasal sinuses are air cavities in the maxillary, frontal, sphenoid, and ethmoid bones that open into the nasal cavities, releasing mucus. The sinuses lessen the weight of the skull and provide resonance for the voice.

Pharynx

The pharynx is posterior to the nasal and oral cavities. It has three regions (Fig. 29.1). The soft palate and uvula rise to block the nasopharynx during swallowing. The lingual tonsils, the adenoid (pharyngeal tonsil), and the palatine tonsils form a ring of lymphatic tissue around the pharynx and destroy pathogens that penetrate the mucosa.

Table 29.1

Protective Mechanisms in the Respiratory System

Nasal hairs and turbinates	Trap dust and microorganisms.
Mucous membranes	Warm and moisten inhaled air; trap inhaled particles.
Cilia	Move particles toward pharynx to be swallowed or coughed out.
Irritant receptors in nose and airways	Trigger sneeze and cough to remove foreign debris.
Alveolar macrophages	Phagocytize foreign particles and bacteria.

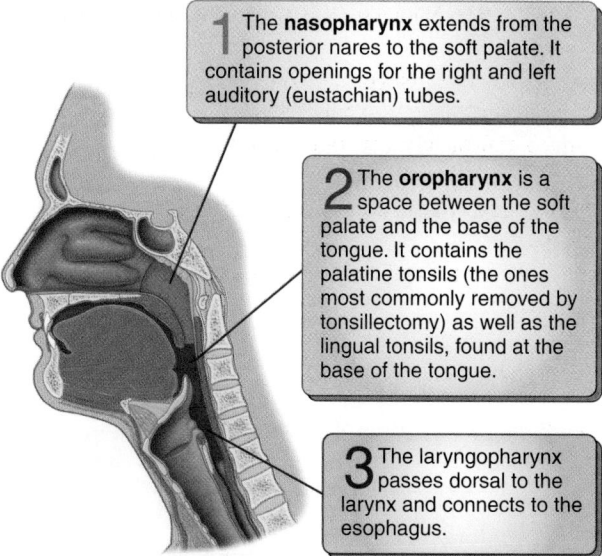

1 The **nasopharynx** extends from the posterior nares to the soft palate. It contains openings for the right and left auditory (eustachian) tubes.

2 The **oropharynx** is a space between the soft palate and the base of the tongue. It contains the palatine tonsils (the ones most commonly removed by tonsillectomy) as well as the lingual tonsils, found at the base of the tongue.

3 The laryngopharynx passes dorsal to the larynx and connects to the esophagus.

FIGURE 29.1 Pharynx.

Larynx

The larynx is the airway between the pharynx and trachea. It houses the vocal cords and produces sound that can be formed into speech. The epiglottis at the top of the larynx prevents ingested materials from entering the trachea (Fig. 29.2). The cartilaginous walls are lined with ciliated epithelium. The vagus and accessory cranial nerves innervate the larynx.

Trachea and Bronchial Tree

The trachea descends from the larynx to the primary bronchi (Fig. 29.3). The mucosa is ciliated epithelium. Mucus with trapped dust and microorganisms is swept upward toward the pharynx and is swallowed.

Deeper into the bronchial tree, cartilage diminishes, and smooth muscle in the walls increases. The bronchioles have

no cartilage in the walls to maintain patency. Therefore, they can be closed completely by bronchoconstriction.

Lungs and Pleural Membranes

The lungs occupy the thoracic cavity on each side of the heart, extending from the clavicles to the diaphragm. They are protected by the ribs (costae). On the medial (mediastinal) surface of each lung is an indentation called the hilus. This is where the primary bronchus and the pulmonary vessels enter the lung (Fig. 29.4). A thin layer of fluid between the visceral and parietal pleural membranes provides lubrication to reduce friction during lung expansion.

The functional units of the lungs are the millions of alveoli, the air sacs where gas exchange occurs. Both the alveoli and the surrounding alveolar capillaries are made of simple squamous epithelium—that is, their walls are only one cell in thickness to permit diffusion of gases (Fig. 29.5).

Each alveolus is lined with a thin layer of tissue fluid that is essential for the diffusion of gases. However, the surface tension of the fluid tends to make the walls of an alveolus stick together internally. Alveolar cells secrete *surfactant*, a lipoprotein that mixes with the tissue fluid and decreases surface tension to permit inflation.

Between clusters of alveoli is elastic connective tissue that can stretch during inhalation and recoil during exhalation. The recoil of this tissue allows passive exhalation without the expenditure of energy.

Mechanism of Breathing

Ventilation is the term for the movement of air into and out of the alveoli. The primary respiratory muscles are the diaphragm, inferior to the lungs, and the external intercostal muscles, between the ribs. Accessory muscles of respiration are used during exercise and times of respiratory distress. These include muscles for deep inspiration (sternocleidomastoid, scalene, pectoralis minor) and for forced expiration (internal intercostal muscles and abdominal musculature; Fig. 29.6). Respiratory centers of the brain, located in the medulla oblongata and pons, innervate muscles of respiration via the intercostal and phrenic nerves. A normal respiratory rate is 12 to 20 breaths/minute.

Ventilation is accomplished by respiratory muscle contractions, causing changes in lung volumes. Movement of air follows Boyle's law, which states that in a closed container of gases, volume and pressure are inversely related. Air moves from high-pressure to low-pressure areas.

Inhalation

Inhalation, also called inspiration, occurs when motor impulses from the medulla cause contraction of the respiratory muscles. Impulses travel along the phrenic nerves and cause the dome-shaped diaphragm to contract and flatten inferiorly. Intercostal nerves cause the external intercostal muscles to expand the thoracic cavity in the anteroposterior dimension. These movements then expand the pleural membranes and, therefore, the lungs as a result of adhesion from serous fluid. As the lungs

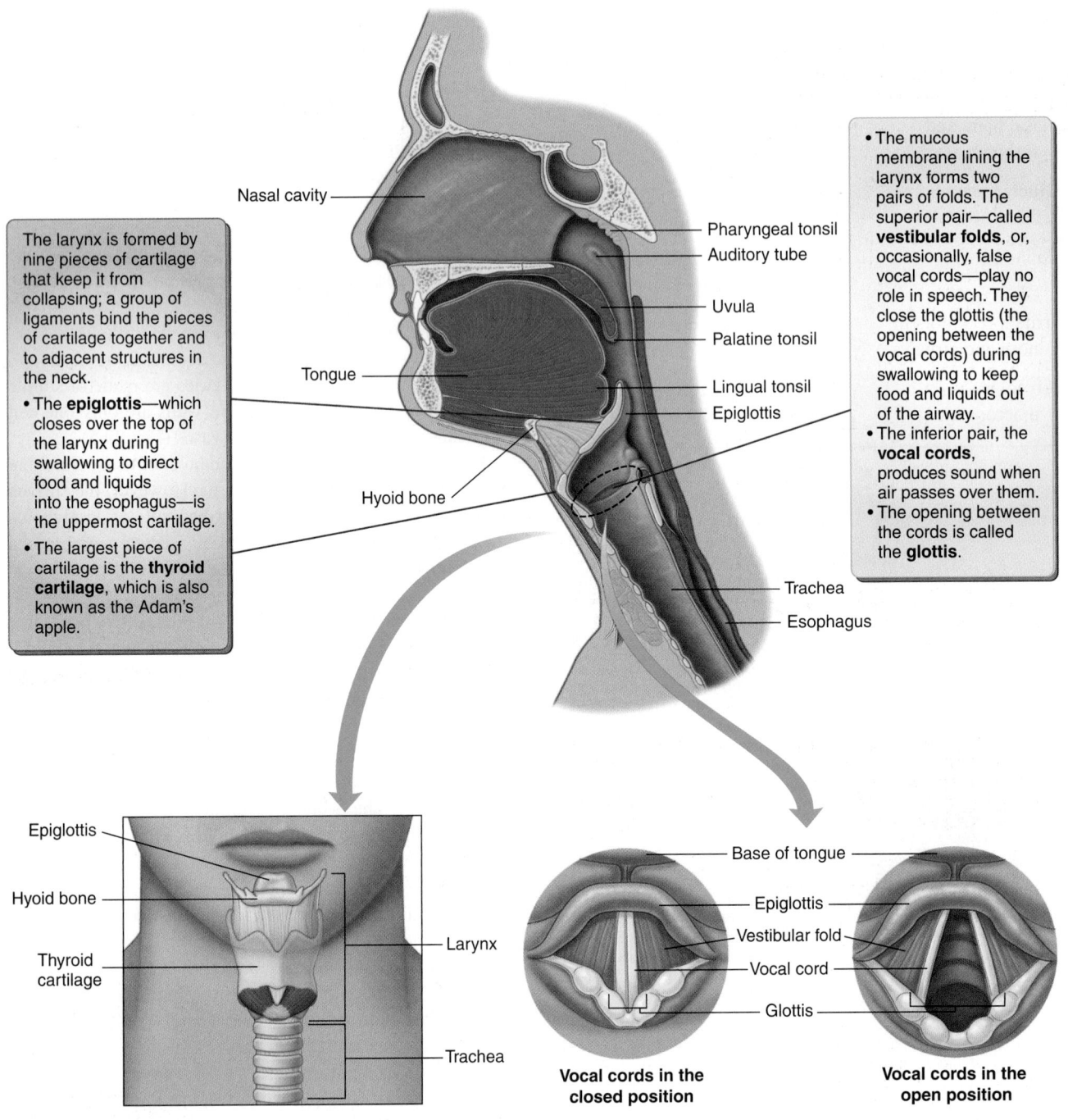

The larynx is formed by nine pieces of cartilage that keep it from collapsing; a group of ligaments bind the pieces of cartilage together and to adjacent structures in the neck.

- The **epiglottis**—which closes over the top of the larynx during swallowing to direct food and liquids into the esophagus—is the uppermost cartilage.
- The largest piece of cartilage is the **thyroid cartilage**, which is also known as the Adam's apple.

- The mucous membrane lining the larynx forms two pairs of folds. The superior pair—called **vestibular folds**, or, occasionally, false vocal cords—play no role in speech. They close the glottis (the opening between the vocal cords) during swallowing to keep food and liquids out of the airway.
- The inferior pair, the **vocal cords**, produces sound when air passes over them.
- The opening between the cords is called the **glottis**.

Nasal cavity

Pharyngeal tonsil
Auditory tube
Uvula
Palatine tonsil
Tongue
Lingual tonsil
Epiglottis
Hyoid bone
Trachea
Esophagus

Epiglottis
Hyoid bone
Thyroid cartilage
Larynx
Trachea

Base of tongue
Epiglottis
Vestibular fold
Vocal cord
Glottis

Vocal cords in the closed position

Vocal cords in the open position

FIGURE 29.2 Larynx.

expand, alveolar pressure falls below atmospheric pressure, and air enters the nose and respiratory passages. A deeper inhalation requires a more forceful contraction of the respiratory muscles (including accessory inspiratory muscles) to expand the thoracic cavity and lungs even further. Ease of thoracic and lung expansion is called *compliance*.

Exhalation

Normal exhalation is a passive process. The lungs are compressed as the thoracic cavity reduces volume and the recoil of the elastic lung tissue compresses the alveoli. Alveolar

pressure rises above atmospheric pressure, and air is forced out of the lungs. At rest, energy is not used in exhalation because no muscle contraction is required. Forced exhalation is an active process, requiring contraction of the internal intercostal muscles compressing the thorax and abdominal muscles that force the diaphragm superiorly, increasing compression of the lungs.

● Transport of Gases in the Blood

A total of 98.5% of oxygen is carried in the blood, bound to iron of hemoglobin (Hgb) in red blood cells (RBCs).

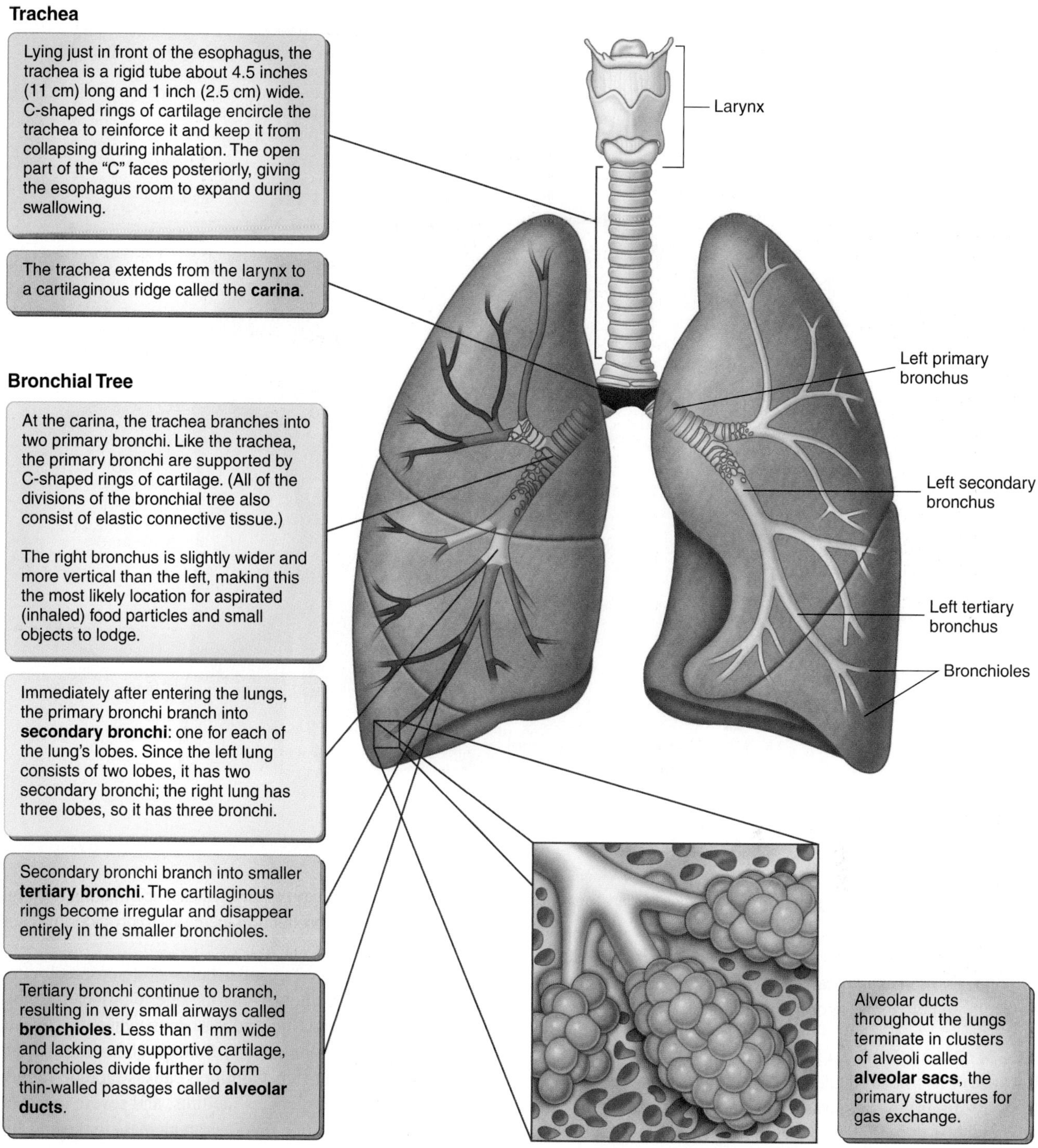

Trachea

Lying just in front of the esophagus, the trachea is a rigid tube about 4.5 inches (11 cm) long and 1 inch (2.5 cm) wide. C-shaped rings of cartilage encircle the trachea to reinforce it and keep it from collapsing during inhalation. The open part of the "C" faces posteriorly, giving the esophagus room to expand during swallowing.

The trachea extends from the larynx to a cartilaginous ridge called the **carina**.

Bronchial Tree

At the carina, the trachea branches into two primary bronchi. Like the trachea, the primary bronchi are supported by C-shaped rings of cartilage. (All of the divisions of the bronchial tree also consist of elastic connective tissue.)

The right bronchus is slightly wider and more vertical than the left, making this the most likely location for aspirated (inhaled) food particles and small objects to lodge.

Immediately after entering the lungs, the primary bronchi branch into **secondary bronchi**: one for each of the lung's lobes. Since the left lung consists of two lobes, it has two secondary bronchi; the right lung has three lobes, so it has three bronchi.

Secondary bronchi branch into smaller **tertiary bronchi**. The cartilaginous rings become irregular and disappear entirely in the smaller bronchioles.

Tertiary bronchi continue to branch, resulting in very small airways called **bronchioles**. Less than 1 mm wide and lacking any supportive cartilage, bronchioles divide further to form thin-walled passages called **alveolar ducts**.

Larynx

Left primary bronchus

Left secondary bronchus

Left tertiary bronchus

Bronchioles

Alveolar ducts throughout the lungs terminate in clusters of alveoli called **alveolar sacs**, the primary structures for gas exchange.

FIGURE 29.3 Trachea and bronchial tree.

Oxyhemoglobin is formed in the lungs, where the partial pressure of oxygen (Pa_{O_2}) is high. In tissues where the Pa_{O_2} is low, Hgb releases much of its oxygen. The remaining oxygen is dissolved in the plasma.

Most carbon dioxide (70%) is carried as bicarbonate ion in the blood plasma. These ions form when carbon dioxide enters RBCs and is converted to carbonic acid (H_2CO_3). H_2CO_3 ionizes into bicarbonate ions (HCO_3^-) and hydrogen ions (H+). The bicarbonate ions leave the RBCs for the plasma. The remaining hydrogen ions are buffered by the Hgb in the RBCs. When the blood reaches the lungs, an area of lower partial pressure of carbon dioxide (Pa_{CO_2}), these reactions are reversed: Carbon dioxide is reformed and diffuses into the alveoli to be exhaled. Carbon dioxide is also transported as carbaminohemoglobin (23%) and dissolved in plasma (7%).

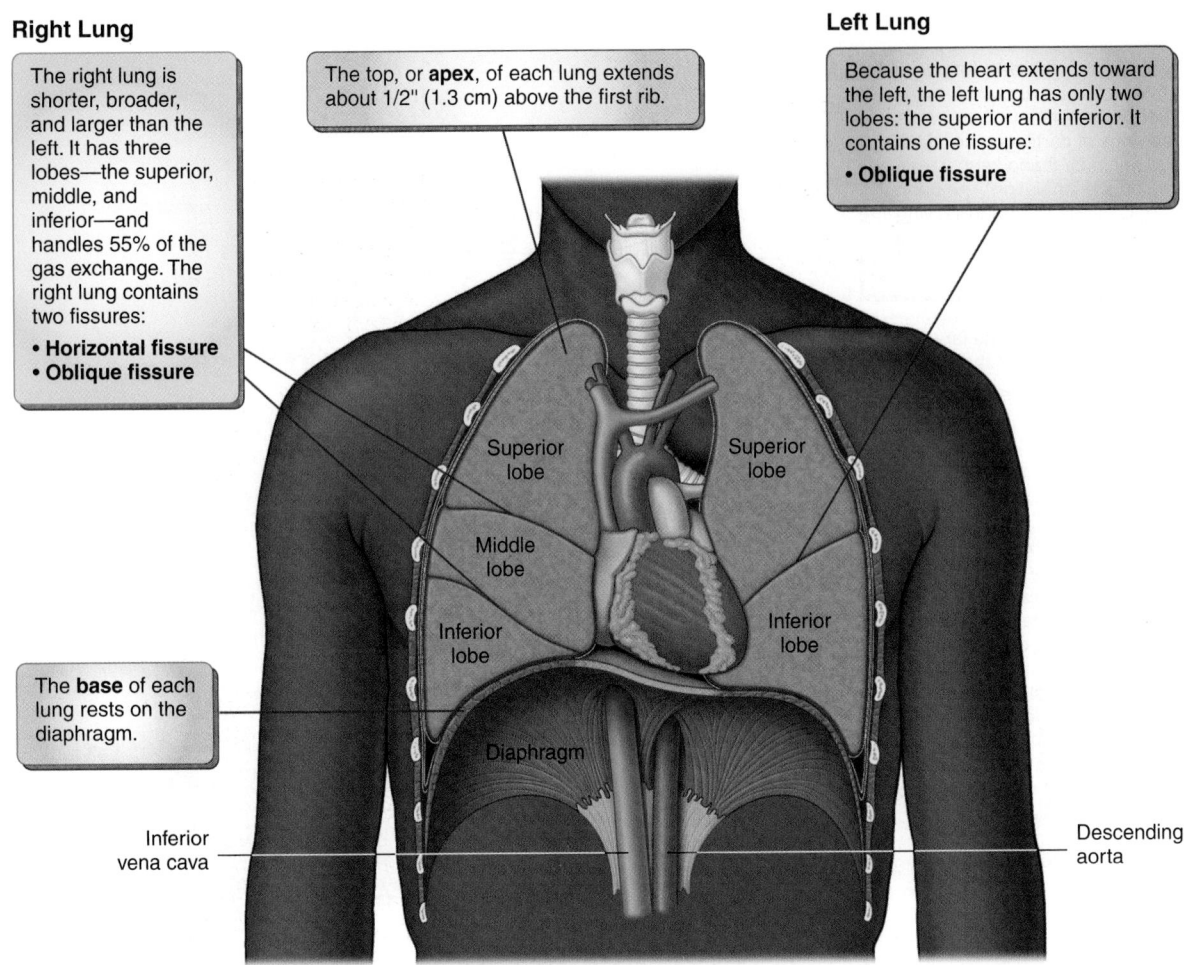

Right Lung

The right lung is shorter, broader, and larger than the left. It has three lobes—the superior, middle, and inferior—and handles 55% of the gas exchange. The right lung contains two fissures:
• **Horizontal fissure**
• **Oblique fissure**

The top, or **apex**, of each lung extends about 1/2" (1.3 cm) above the first rib.

Left Lung

Because the heart extends toward the left, the left lung has only two lobes: the superior and inferior. It contains one fissure:
• **Oblique fissure**

Superior lobe

Superior lobe

Middle lobe

Inferior lobe

Inferior lobe

The **base** of each lung rests on the diaphragm.

Diaphragm

Inferior vena cava

Descending aorta

FIGURE 29.4 Lungs.

Chemical Regulation and Respiration

Chemoreceptors (in the carotid and aortic bodies) monitor blood levels of oxygen, carbon dioxide, and pH. The medulla responds by increasing heart and respiratory rates during hypoxemia, hypercapnia, and/or acidemia.

Respiration and Acid–Base Balance

Because of its role in regulating the amount of carbon dioxide in body fluids, the respiratory system is important in the maintenance of acid–base balance, measured by blood pH. Any decrease in the rate or efficiency of respiration permits excess carbon dioxide to accumulate in the blood. The resulting accumulation of excess hydrogen ions lowers pH. This is called *respiratory acidosis*. It can occur as a consequence of pulmonary disease or any impairment of gas exchange in the lungs.

Respiratory alkalosis occurs when the rate of respiration increases, eliminating exhaled carbon dioxide rapidly. Less carbon dioxide in the blood means fewer hydrogen ions are formed and the pH rises. Although it is not a common condition, respiratory alkalosis may occur during states of hyperventilation caused by anxiety or hypoxemia, or when acclimating to a high altitude, before RBC production increases to provide sufficient oxygenation of tissues.

The respiratory system also helps compensate for pH changes that are metabolic—that is, due to any cause other than respiratory. Metabolic acidosis occurs when the concentration of hydrogen ions in body fluids is above normal due to lowered HCO_3^- buffer. Common causes include kidney disease, uncontrolled diabetes mellitus, and severe diarrhea. Respiratory compensation involves an increase in the rate and depth of respiration to exhale more carbon dioxide. This decreases hydrogen ion formation and raises the pH toward normal. Metabolic alkalosis can be caused by overingestion of antacid medications or by vomiting acidic gastric contents. Respiratory compensation involves a decrease in the breathing rate to retain carbon dioxide in the body, increasing the formation of hydrogen ions. This lowers the pH toward normal. Respiratory compensation occurs very quickly, within moments.

Respiratory compensation for an ongoing metabolic pH imbalance (such as kidney failure) cannot be complete

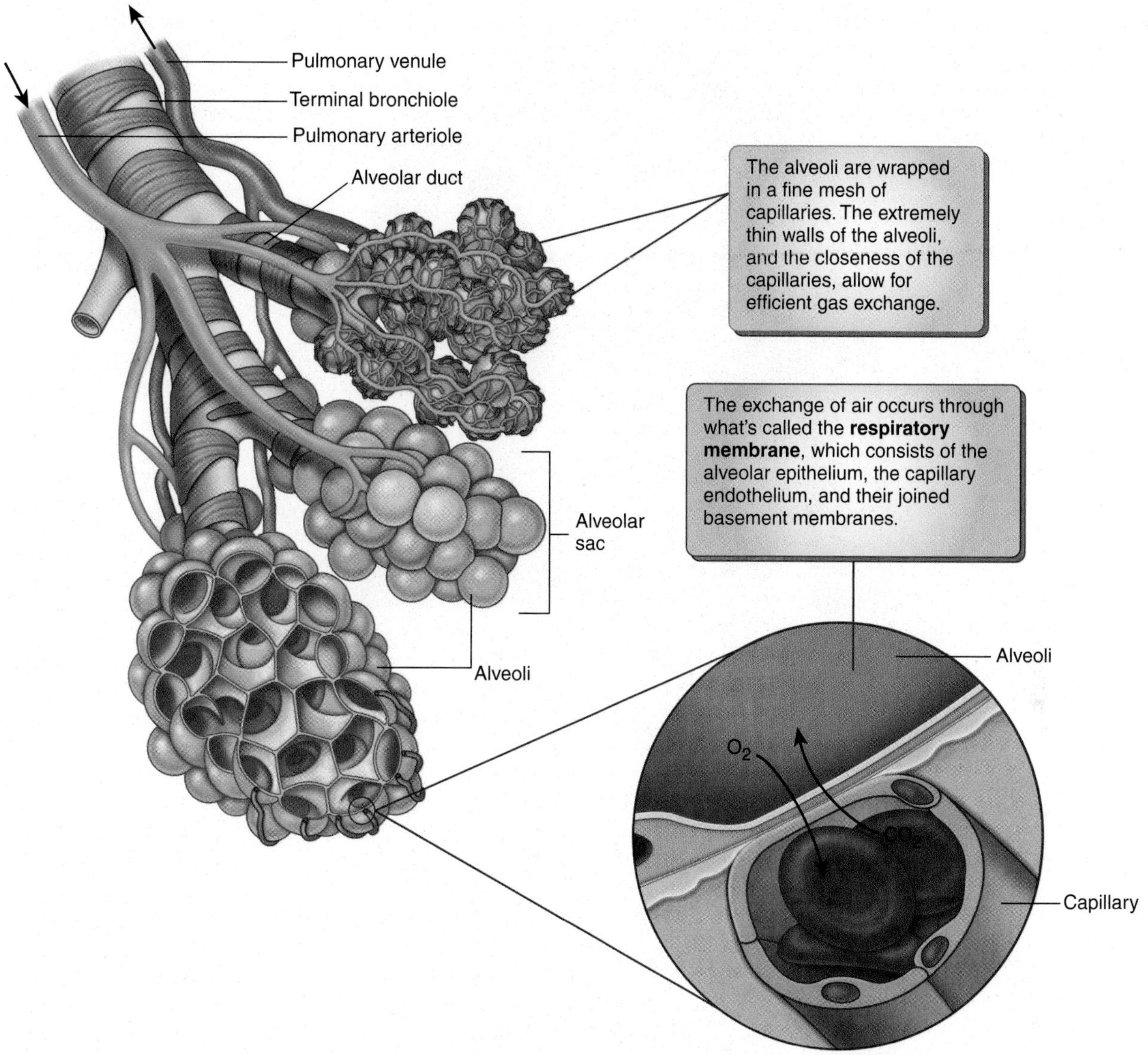

Pulmonary venule

Terminal bronchiole

Pulmonary arteriole

Alveolar duct

> The alveoli are wrapped in a fine mesh of capillaries. The extremely thin walls of the alveoli, and the closeness of the capillaries, allow for efficient gas exchange.

> The exchange of air occurs through what's called the **respiratory membrane**, which consists of the alveolar epithelium, the capillary endothelium, and their joined basement membranes.

Alveolar sac

Alveoli

Alveoli

O_2

CO_2

Capillary

FIGURE 29.5 Alveoli.

because the amount of carbon dioxide that may be exhaled or retained is limited. At most, respiratory compensation is only about 75% effective.

Acid–base balance is discussed further in Chapter 6.

Effects of Aging on the Respiratory System

See Figure 29.7 for the effects of aging on respiration.

NURSING ASSESSMENT OF THE RESPIRATORY SYSTEM

Health History

Many factors in a patient's personal and family history affect respiratory function. Questions to ask while assessing the patient with a history of respiratory problems are

presented in Table 29.2. If at any time while you are taking the history the patient relates a specific symptom, use the *WHAT'S UP?* format to gather additional data. For example, if the patient reports shortness of breath, respond with the following questions:

- **W**here is it? (Doesn't apply to shortness of breath, so it may be skipped.)
- **H**ow does it feel? Does your breathing feel tight, gasping, painful, suffocating?
- **A**ggravating and alleviating factors? How much activity causes your shortness of breath? Does anything else aggravate it? What do you do to relieve your shortness of breath?
- **T**iming? When did you first experience shortness of breath? Does it happen at any particular time of day or year?

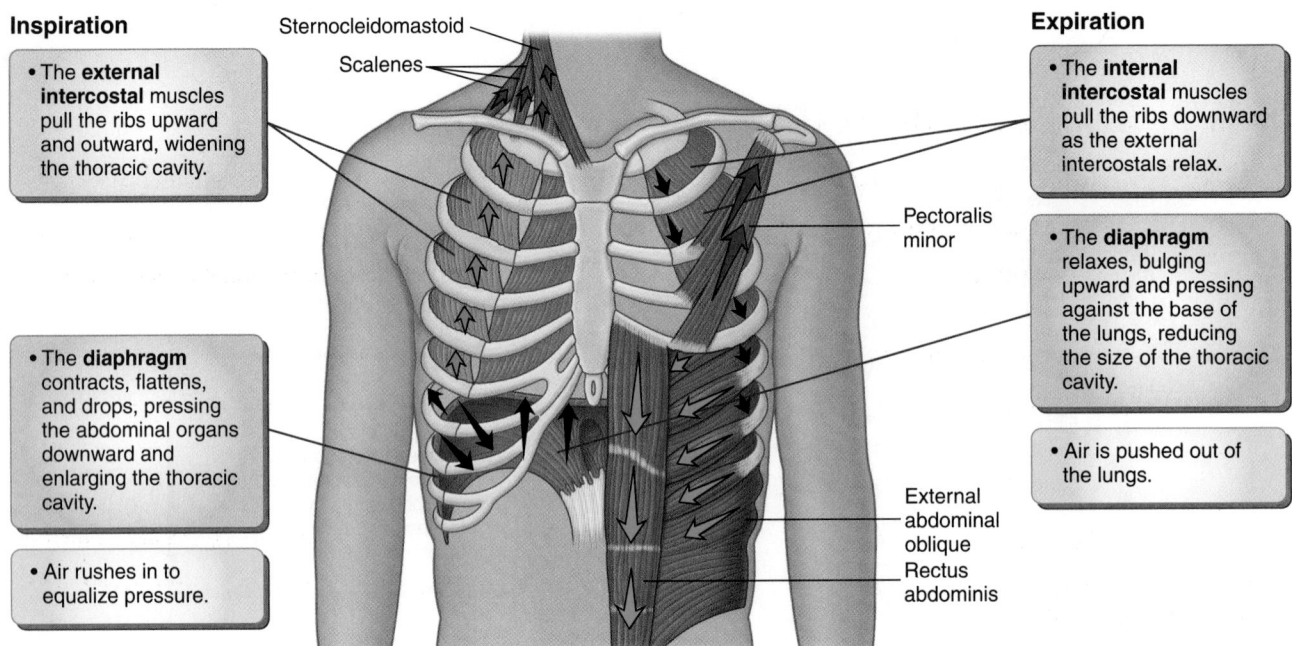

Inspiration

Sternocleidomastoid
Scalenes

- The **external intercostal** muscles pull the ribs upward and outward, widening the thoracic cavity.

- The **diaphragm** contracts, flattens, and drops, pressing the abdominal organs downward and enlarging the thoracic cavity.

- Air rushes in to equalize pressure.

Expiration

- The **internal intercostal** muscles pull the ribs downward as the external intercostals relax.

- The **diaphragm** relaxes, bulging upward and pressing against the base of the lungs, reducing the size of the thoracic cavity.

- Air is pushed out of the lungs.

Pectoralis minor

External abdominal oblique
Rectus abdominis

FIGURE 29.6 Respiratory muscles.

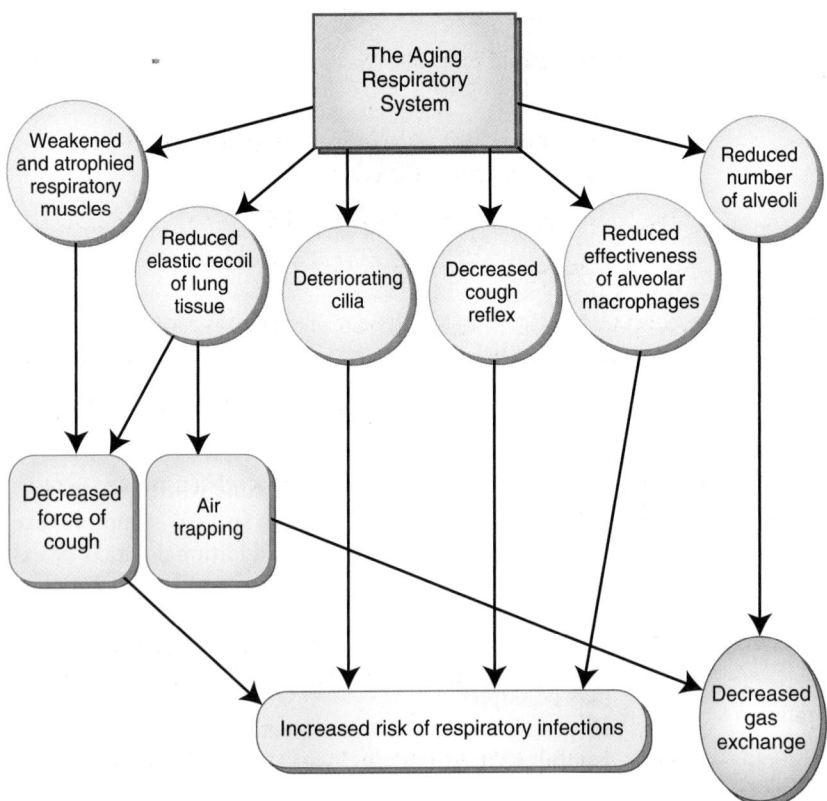

The Aging Respiratory System

Weakened and atrophied respiratory muscles

Reduced elastic recoil of lung tissue

Deteriorating cilia

Decreased cough reflex

Reduced effectiveness of alveolar macrophages

Reduced number of alveoli

Decreased force of cough

Air trapping

Increased risk of respiratory infections

Decreased gas exchange

FIGURE 29.7 Effects of aging on respiration.

- **S**everity? Rate your shortness of breath on a scale of 0 to 10, with 0 being easy breathing and 10 being the worst shortness of breath you can imagine.
- **U**seful other data? Do you have any other symptoms that occur along with the shortness of breath?

- **P**atient's perception? What do you think is causing your shortness of breath?

Because smoking is such a major risk factor for many types of lung disease, it is essential to ask about smoking history and

Table 29.2

Table 29.2
Subjective Data Collection for the Respiratory System

Questions to Ask During the Health History	*Rationale/Significance*
Upper Respiratory Tract	
Do you often have headaches or sinus tenderness?	These may indicate sinusitis.
Do you often experience nosebleeds?	A history of nosebleeds may indicate an abnormality that can predispose to future nosebleeds.
Do you snore? Are you sleepy during the day?	These may be symptoms of sleep apnea.
Has your voice changed?	A voice change may indicate a variety of disorders of the nose or throat, including cancer.
Lower Respiratory Tract	
Do you have chest pain?	Chest pain can indicate a variety of respiratory or cardiac problems.
Do you ever feel short of breath, as though you can't get enough air?	Many respiratory and cardiac problems result in shortness of breath.
Do you have a cough? Is it productive?	A cough indicates respiratory irritation or excessive secretions.
What does the sputum look like?	Yellow, tan, or green sputum may accompany an infection. Blood in the sputum is usually serious; it can occur with pneumonia, tuberculosis, pulmonary embolism, or cancer.
Have you recently experienced night sweats, chills, or fever?	These are symptoms of tuberculosis.
Do you ever feel confused, light-headed, or restless?	These symptoms might indicate a low partial pressure of oxygen (Pao_2), reducing oxygen to the brain.
Have you had any chest surgeries?	This may reveal problem areas the patient has not yet mentioned.
Exposures	
Do you have any allergies that cause respiratory symptoms? How do you treat them?	The patient may take over-the-counter medications for allergies that affect respiratory function or interact with prescribed medications.
Do you smoke? How many packs per day? For how many years?	Many respiratory disorders are caused or aggravated by exposure to tobacco smoke.
Are you exposed to environmental smoke? Have you been exposed to airborne pollutants at home or work?	Pollutants such as asbestos, radon, coal dust, or chemicals can cause lung disease.
Treatments	
Do you take any medications or use inhalers (prescribed or over-the-counter) for your respiratory problems?	Information about medications gives further information about disorders, severity, and treatment. Also consider drug interactions and side effects.
Do you use home oxygen or other home respiratory treatments?	This helps determine the severity of disease and the treatment.
Family History	
Do any of your blood relatives have respiratory problems such as emphysema, asthma, or tuberculosis?	Some respiratory disorders have a hereditary tendency. Tuberculosis is contagious.

encourage the patient to quit (see the discussion of smoking cessation later in this chapter). Document the patient's smoking history in terms of pack-years. For example, if a patient has smoked two packs of cigarettes per day for 20 years, he has a 40 pack-year smoking history (2 × 20 = 40 pack-years). It is also important to be aware of cultural influences on the patient's respiratory health ("Cultural Considerations").

Cultural Considerations

Pulmonary diseases associated with people from Japan include asthma, possibly related to dust mites in straw mats that commonly cover floors in Japanese homes and air pollution from living in urban areas.

Patients from Poland, Ireland, or other countries where mining is a primary occupation may have an increased incidence of respiratory disease. It is essential for health care providers (HCPs) to carefully screen patients from these countries for respiratory conditions.

HCPs also should be aware of variations among ethnic persons of color when assessing for cyanosis. Cyanosis and decreased blood hemoglobin levels in darker-skinned individuals give the skin an ashen color instead of the bluish color seen in light-skinned people. Thus, the nurse must examine the sclerae, conjunctivae, buccal mucosa, tongue, lips, nailbeds, and palms and soles of the feet to assess for cyanosis.

Physical Examination
Inspection
Inspection begins during the nursing history and continues during the physical assessment. Start with the nose, observing for symmetry, swelling, or other abnormalities. Note whether the patient is short of breath while speaking or moving. If the patient feels very breathless, he or she may speak in short sentences.

Observe the patient for use of accessory muscles of breathing (Fig. 29.8). Use of the sternocleidomastoid muscles causes the shoulders to rise during labored inspiration. During forced expiration, the abdominal and intercostal muscles contract. The use of accessory muscles for breathing indicates respiratory distress. **Retraction** of the chest wall between the ribs occurs when airways are obstructed. This can indicate serious distress. When the patient inhales and air cannot easily flow into the lungs, negative pressure in the chest pulls the soft tissue between the ribs inward.

Note the color of the skin, lips, mucous membranes, and nailbeds. A bluish color is called **cyanosis.** This is a late sign of oxygen deprivation. Observe the trachea and chest for symmetry. Count the number of respirations per minute, noting depth and rhythm. Irregular respirations, or periods of **apnea** (absence of respirations), can indicate a pathological condition. These are described in Figure 29.9. Observe the shape

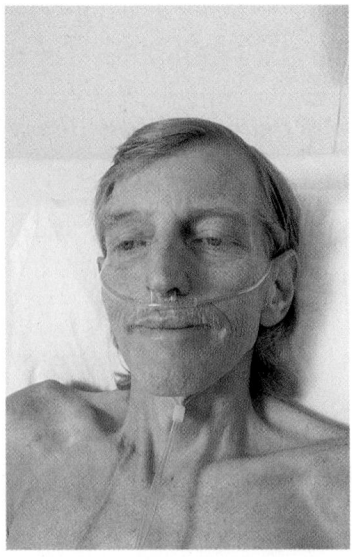

FIGURE 29.8 Accessory muscles of breathing. Note the prominent sternocleidomastoid muscles.

of the chest. Normally, the chest is about twice as wide (side to side) as it is deep (front to back). If it is more rounded, it is called a *barrel chest,* which is associated with trapped air in the lungs. See Table 29.3 for a summary of objective data.

Palpation
Palpate the frontal and maxillary sinuses if sinus inflammation is suspected (Fig. 29.10). Use your thumbs to palpate gently below the eyebrows and below each cheekbone. Tenderness may indicate sinus inflammation or infection.

Respiratory excursion can also be palpated. This is a rough measurement of chest expansion on inspiration. Figure 29.11 illustrates how to palpate for respiratory excursion. You can palpate for **crepitus** (also called *subcutaneous emphysema*) if indicated. Crepitus feels like Rice Krispies under the skin when felt with the fingers. It occurs when air leaks into subcutaneous tissues because of pneumothorax or a leaking chest tube site. Palpation is not done routinely but only when indicated by other assessment findings.

Percussion
Percussion is typically done by the experienced nurse. It involves tapping on the anterior and posterior chest, in each intercostal space, and comparing sounds from side to side. A normal chest sounds resonant and is the same bilaterally, except over the heart. If other percussion notes are heard, they can indicate a pathological condition and should be reported.

· WORD · BUILDING ·
cyanosis: cyan—dark blue + osis—condition
apnea: a—not + pnea—breath

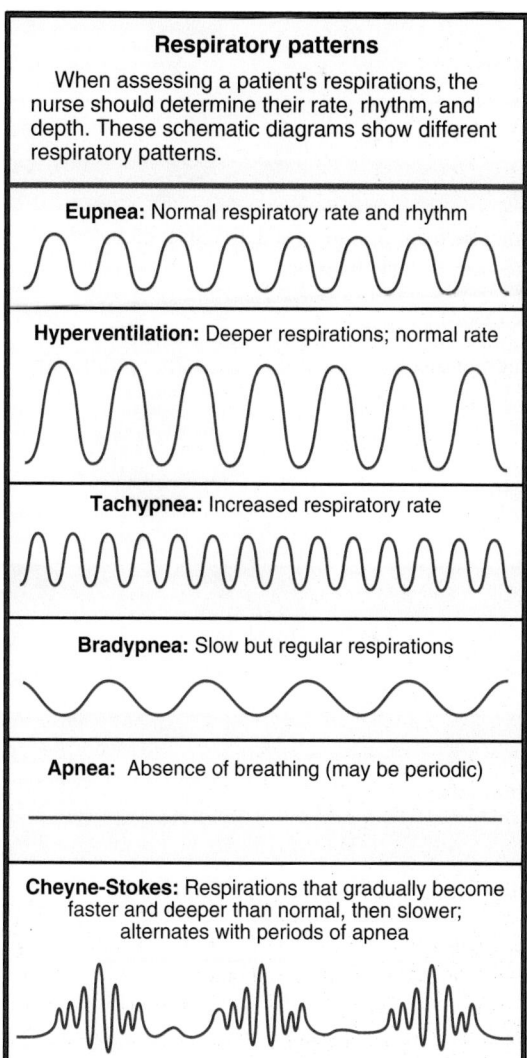

Respiratory patterns

When assessing a patient's respirations, the nurse should determine their rate, rhythm, and depth. These schematic diagrams show different respiratory patterns.

Eupnea: Normal respiratory rate and rhythm

Hyperventilation: Deeper respirations; normal rate

Tachypnea: Increased respiratory rate

Bradypnea: Slow but regular respirations

Apnea: Absence of breathing (may be periodic)

Cheyne-Stokes: Respirations that gradually become faster and deeper than normal, then slower; alternates with periods of apnea

Kussmaul's: Faster and deeper respirations without pauses

FIGURE 29.9 Abnormal respiratory patterns.

Auscultation

Auscultation provides valuable information about respiratory status. Use the diaphragm of your stethoscope to listen to the anterior, lateral, and posterior chest during an entire inspiration and expiration at each interspace (Fig. 29.12). Auscultation of the posterior chest is easiest if the patient is sitting. However, if necessary, it may be done with the patient in a side-lying position. Ask the patient to breathe deeply through the mouth to help enhance the sounds. Allow the patient to rest at intervals to prevent hyperventilation. Regular and frequent practice helps you learn to distinguish normal from abnormal breath sounds. Abnormal extra sounds (another term is **adventitious**) indicate a pathological condition. These are described in Table 29.4.

 DIAGNOSTIC TESTS FOR THE RESPIRATORY SYSTEM

Laboratory Tests

For normal values for the following laboratory tests, see Appendix B.

Blood Tests
Complete Blood Count (CBC)

Measurement of RBCs and Hgb can give information about the oxygen-carrying capacity of the blood. **Dyspnea** (shortness of breath) can be caused by a reduction in RBCs or Hgb. Elevated white blood cells (WBCs) indicate infection.

Arterial Blood Gas Analysis

Arterial blood gases (ABGs) are measured to determine the effectiveness of gas exchange. See Table 29.5 for a basic interpretation of ABGs. The blood sample is usually taken from the radial artery in the wrist by a specially trained respiratory therapist (RT) or laboratory technician. This can be painful for the patient. Place pressure on the site after the test until bleeding stops; this may take 5 minutes or more.

• WORD • BUILDING •
dyspnea: dys—bad + pnea—breathing

Table 29.3
Objective Data Collection for the Respiratory System

Abnormal Findings	Possible Causes
Respiratory	
Respiratory rate less than 12 or greater than 20 per minute	Respiratory depression may be from opioid or sedative use; elevated respiratory rate indicates respiratory distress
Use of accessory muscles	Restrictive or obstructive disorders
Barrel chest	Air trapping from obstructive disorder (chronic obstructive pulmonary disorder)
Adventitious sounds	*See Table 29.4.*
Cough	Airway irritation or secretions
Sputum	*See Table 29.2*
Integumentary	
Cyanosis	Tissue hypoxia
Nail clubbing	Chronic tissue hypoxia
Neurologic	
Confusion	Lack of oxygen to the brain
Gastrointestinal	
Weight loss	Dyspnea interfering with eating; use of excessive calories for breathing

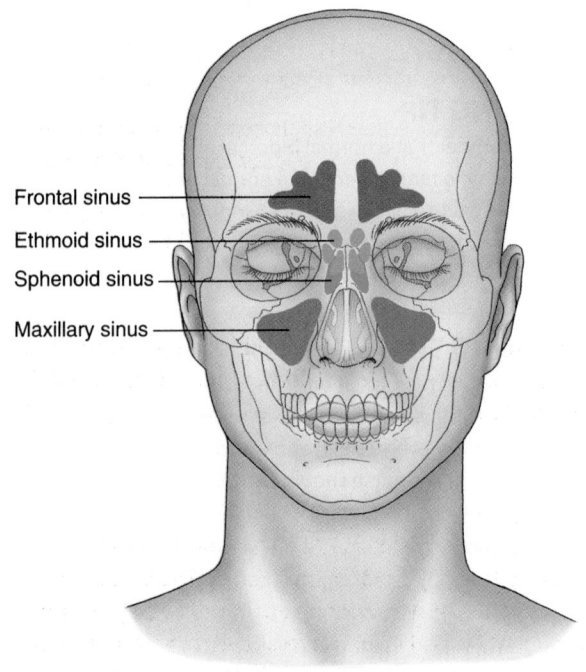

FIGURE 29.10 Paranasal sinuses.

Frontal sinus
Ethmoid sinus
Sphenoid sinus
Maxillary sinus

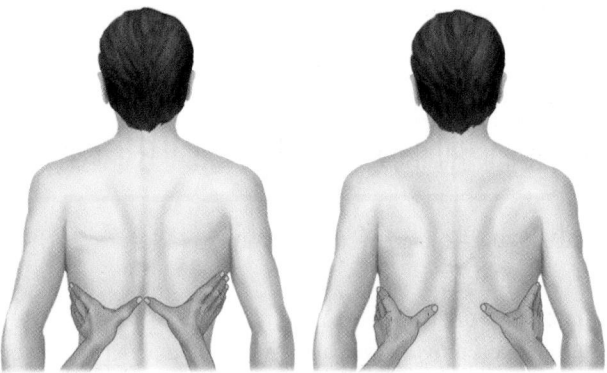

FIGURE 29.11 Palpation of respiratory excursion. Left: during exhalation. Right: after inhalation.

D-Dimer
This blood test measures fibrin degradation products. These are present if there is a blood clot in the body. It helps diagnose the presence of a blood clot in a pulmonary artery.

Sputum Culture and Sensitivity
A sputum culture identifies pathogens present in the sputum. The sensitivity test determines which antibiotics will be

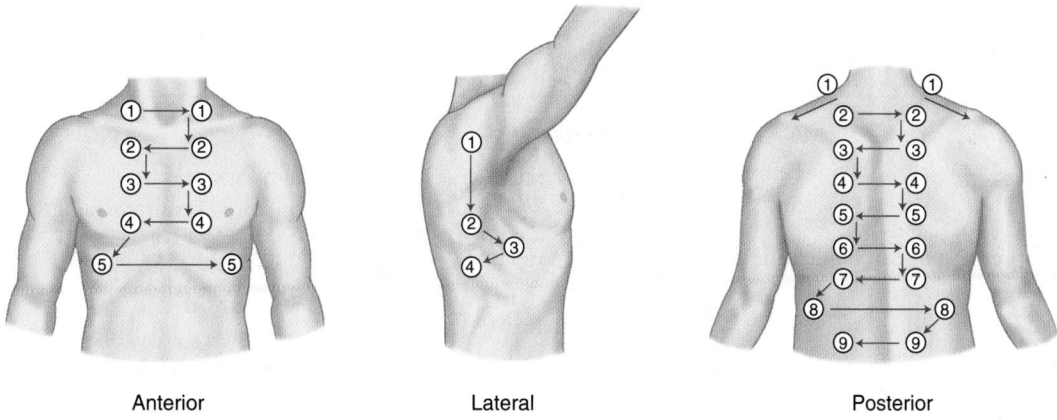

Anterior   Lateral   Posterior

FIGURE 29.12 Auscultation of the chest. Use a systematic approach to auscultate the chest, comparing sounds from side to side.

Table 29.4
Abnormal Lung Sounds

Abnormal (Adventitious) Sound	Cause of Sound	Description	Associated Disorders
Coarse crackles (sometimes called rales)	Fluid or secretions in airways	Moist bubbling sound, heard on inspiration or expiration	Pulmonary edema, bronchitis, pneumonia
Fine crackles (rales)	Alveoli popping open on inspiration	Velcro being torn apart, heard at end of inspiration	Heart failure, atelectasis
Wheezes	Narrowed airways	Fine high-pitched violin sound, mostly on expiration	Asthma
Stridor	Airway obstruction	Loud crowing noise heard without stethoscope	Obstruction from tumor or foreign body
Pleural friction rub	Inflamed pleura rubbing together	Sound of leather rubbing together; grating sound	Pleurisy, lung cancer, pneumonia, pleural irritation
Diminished	Decreased air movement	Faint lung sounds	Emphysema, hypoventilation, obesity, muscular chest wall
Absent	No air movement	No sounds heard	Pneumothorax, pneumonectomy, pleural effusion

effective against those pathogens. To obtain a sputum specimen, first check the order and obtain a sterile container. Some institutions have special containers for sputum that help prevent transmission of infection to the HCP (Fig. 29.13). Instruct the patient to take several deep breaths and then cough sputum into the container. It is important that the patient not simply spit saliva or sinus drainage into the cup. The specimen must come from the lungs. It may be easiest to obtain a specimen first thing in the morning (after mouth care) because secretions build up during the night. Send the specimen to the laboratory immediately. If the patient is unable to cough up sputum, extra fluids or a bedside humidifier may help. An RT may be able

to help obtain a specimen with a nebulized mist treatment or with a special suction catheter with a sputum trap. The HCP's order may be needed for these procedures.

BE SAFE!

If the health care provider orders a "sputum for AFB," tuberculosis is suspected, which is caused by an acid-fast bacillus (AFB). Ask whether the patient should be placed in isolation while waiting for test results. *Always* practice standard precautions when handling laboratory specimens.

Table 29.5

Arterial Blood Gas Analysis

	Normal Values	*Interpretation*
Pa_{O_2} (partial pressure of oxygen)	75–100 mm Hg	↑ in hyperventilation ↓ in impaired respiratory function
Pa_{CO_2} (partial pressure of carbon dioxide)	35–45 mm Hg	↑ in impaired gas exchange ↓ in hyperventilation
pH	7.35–7.45	↑ in respiratory alkalosis with low Pa_{CO_2} ↓ in respiratory acidosis with high Pa_{CO_2}
HCO_3^- (bicarbonate ions)	22–26 mEq/L	↑ to buffer Pa_{CO_2} in acidosis ↓ to buffer Pa_{CO_2} in alkalosis
Oxygen saturation	95%–100%	↓ in impaired respiratory function

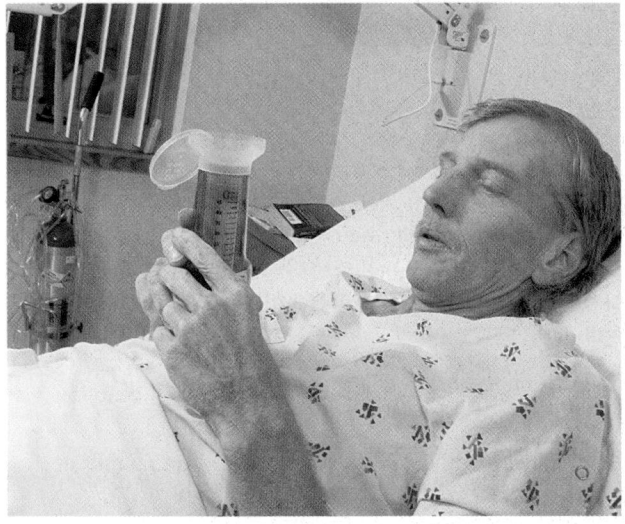

FIGURE 29.13 A special container that helps prevent transmission of infection is often used to collect sputum for culture.

Throat Culture

A throat culture is done to determine the presence of viral or bacterial pathogens in the pharynx. Use a swab to reach into the posterior pharynx behind the uvula (without touching the patient's mouth) and swab the red area or lesions. Use a tongue blade to help hold the tongue down while obtaining the culture. Warn the patient that a gag reflex may be triggered. Once the culture has been obtained, place it in a sterile tube with culture medium, according to package instructions. Send it to the laboratory immediately for analysis.

Nasal Samples

A nasopharyngeal swab or a nasal wash can be used to identify flu or other respiratory viruses. To be accurate, it must be done in the first few days a person has symptoms. The sample may be obtained by swabbing the nasal passages or pharynx or by using a small amount of saline to wash out the nose, depending on the type of test ordered.

Oxygen Saturation

The oxygen saturation test (also called pulse oximetry, O_2 sat, or Sp_{O_2}) is a simple and noninvasive way to measure arterial oxygenation. A sensor is placed on the patient's finger or ear. The sensor measures the percentage of Hgb that is saturated with oxygen. Oxygen saturation can be measured at rest or while the patient is walking to determine the patient's exercise tolerance. It is also often done with and without supplemental oxygen to determine the patient's need for oxygen supplementation at home. See Table 29.5 for normal values. Collaborate with the HCP for an appropriate Sp_{O_2} level for your patient. Although 95% or greater is considered normal, some patients with chronic lung disease may be maintained at 90% to 92%. If the Sp_{O_2} is less than 75%, prepare for emergency intervention.

Oxygen saturation measurement may be inaccurate in patients with low blood flow or decreased perfusion, patients who are moving, and patients who have smoke inhalation injury or carbon monoxide poisoning. Dark-skinned patients may have falsely high readings. Acrylic nails may need to be removed for accurate readings. Always correlate Sp_{O_2} results with other patient assessment findings.

Capnography

The process of measuring a person's exhaled carbon dioxide level is called capnography. It provides a continuous measurement of the patient's ventilation status. It is most often used when patients are intubated. A special sensor is placed between the endotracheal (ET) tube and the ventilator to measure the exhaled carbon dioxide. Special nasal cannulas with sensors are also available. Results are displayed on a special monitor.

Other Tests

For explanations of the following diagnostic tests, see Appendix A.

Chest X-Ray Examination

A chest x-ray examination may be ordered to help diagnose a variety of pulmonary disorders. Usually, posterior–anterior

(PA) and side views (lateral) are taken. If a hospitalized patient is too ill to go to the radiology department, a portable chest x-ray machine can be used at the bedside to obtain a PA view.

Computed Tomography

A computed tomography (CT) scan can show cancers, pneumonia, emphysema, and more. It may be used to obtain additional information after an abnormal chest x-ray. A spiral CT scan can be useful for evaluating trauma or blood vessel abnormalities in the chest.

Ventilation-Perfusion Scan

During a ventilation-perfusion scan (also called a lung scan or VQ scan), a radioactive substance is injected via intravenous (IV) route. A scan is then done to view blood flow to the lungs (perfusion). Another radioactive substance is inhaled. Scanning then shows how well gas is distributed in the lungs (ventilation). If an area of the lungs is well ventilated but has no blood supply, a pulmonary embolism is suspected. Chronic lung disease may cause poor ventilation and perfusion.

Pulmonary Function Studies

Pulmonary function studies are a series of tests done to determine lung volume, capacity, and flow rates. These are commonly used to help diagnose and monitor restrictive or obstructive lung disease. The patient is asked to use a special mouthpiece to blow into a cylinder that is connected to a computer. A computer printout is generated to show the results. Table 29.6 lists normal values. Some patients use handheld peak expiratory flow rate (PEFR) meters at home to monitor asthma symptoms. They might notice changes in

PEFR before symptoms occur, allowing them to begin treatment before the problem becomes more serious.

Pulmonary Angiography

Pulmonary angiography involves an x-ray examination of the pulmonary vessels after IV administration of a radiopaque dye. Pulmonary angiography is used to help diagnose pulmonary embolism or other pulmonary vessel disorders. See Appendix A for pre- and postprocedure care.

Bronchoscopy

Bronchoscopy involves the use of a flexible endoscope to examine the larynx, trachea, and bronchial tree. Bronchoscopy can be used diagnostically for visualization or to obtain a biopsy specimen for examination. It can also be used therapeutically to remove an obstruction, foreign body, or thick secretions. See Appendix A for pre- and postprocedure care.

 ## THERAPEUTIC MEASURES FOR THE RESPIRATORY SYSTEM

Smoking Cessation

Probably the *most* important intervention for preventing and treating respiratory disease is smoking cessation. Many respiratory disorders are caused or aggravated by smoking. Stopping can prevent disease from occurring or slow its progression significantly. Table 29.7 lists interventions to help patients stop smoking. Remind patients that if they have tried quitting before and failed, that does not mean that they will never be able to quit ("Evidence-Based Practice"). Many patients try several times before quitting successfully.

Table 29.6
Normal Values for Pulmonary Function Studies

Test	Definition	Normal Values*
Tidal volume (V$_T$)	Air inspired and expired in one breath	400–600 mL at rest
Residual volume (RV)	Air remaining in lungs after maximum exhalation	1,000–1,500 mL
Functional residual capacity (FRC)	Air remaining in lungs after normal expiration	1,800–2,300 mL
Inspiratory reserve	Amount of air beyond V$_T$ that can be taken in with the deepest possible inhalation	2,000–3,000 mL
Expiratory reserve	Amount of air beyond V$_T$ in the most forceful exhalation	1,000–1,500 mL
Forced vital capacity (FVC)	Maximum amount of air expired forcefully after maximum inspiration	3,000–5,000 mL
Forced expiratory volume (FEV) 1% (FEV$_1$/FVC)	Amount of air expired in first second of forced exhalation divided by FVC	65%–85% of the FVC
Peak expiratory flow rate (PEFR)	Maximum flow of air expired during FVC (this is a rate rather than a volume)	450 L/min

*Normal values are approximate. They are individualized based on patient's sex, height, and age.

Table 29.7
Interventions to Stop Smoking

Intervention	Rationale
Behavior modification	If the patient can identify situations associated with smoking, such as eating a meal or experiencing stress, then other healthier behaviors can be substituted, such as going for a walk.
Counseling	Counseling by a health care worker alone or in combination with other methods can greatly increase success.
Setting a quit date	The "cold turkey" (all-at-once) method is more effective than slow tapering, although the patient may choose to taper before the quit date.
Nicotine replacement therapy	Nicotine gum, patches, nasal sprays, lozenges, and inhalers can reduce withdrawal symptoms.
Drug therapy (bupropion [Zyban], varenicline [Chantix], nortriptyline [Pamelor])	Bupropion and nortriptyline interfere with smoking's effect on brain neurotransmitters. Varenicline attaches to nicotine receptors in the brain to block nicotine and reduce its pleasurable effects.
Hypnosis	Hypnosis is believed to help the person be open to the suggestion that smoking is undesirable.
Physical activity	Physical activity reduces cravings and post-cessation weight gain.
Electronic cigarettes (e-cigarettes)	Nicotine-containing e-cigarettes may help promote smoking cessation, although more research needs to be done.

Many Internet sites have information to help people stop smoking. Simply type "smoking cessation" into any search engine. Alternatively, individuals can call 800-QUIT NOW to speak with a representative who will assist with cessation strategies.

Evidence-Based Practice

Clinical Question
Can nurses make a difference in helping patients stop smoking?

Evidence
Thirty-one randomized trials comparing targeted nursing interventions to controls (usual care interventions) found that nursing intervention significantly increased the likelihood of patients quitting smoking (Rice & Stead, 2008). Nursing interventions were more effective in hospital settings but less effective in outpatient settings.

Implications for Nursing Practice
Advice and support from nursing staff can increase people's success in quitting smoking, especially in a hospital setting.

Reference
Rice, V. H., & Stead, L. F. (2008). Nursing interventions for smoking cessation. *Cochrane Database of Systematic Reviews, 2008*(1). CD001188. doi:10.1002/14651858. CD001188.pub3

Deep Breathing and Coughing
Effective coughing can keep the airways clear of secretions. An ineffective cough is exhausting and fails to bring up secretions. Instruct the patient to take two or three deep breaths, using the diaphragm. This helps get the air behind the secretions. After the third deep inhalation, have the patient hold the breath for a few seconds and then cough forcefully. This is repeated as necessary, usually every 1 to 2 hours. Good hydration can facilitate mucous removal.

Huff Coughing
Patients with chronic obstructive pulmonary disease (COPD) typically have a weak cough and airways that collapse easily. *Huff* coughing may work better for them. Instruct the patient to deep breath and cough, as just described. Instead of closing the glottis to generate a forceful cough, the patient should keep the glottis and mouth open, and use the abdominal muscles to create a series of forced expirations, moving air and mucus up the bronchial tree. This creates "huff" sounds. A short "huff" helps clear larger airways, and a longer "huff" held out for several seconds helps open and clear smaller airways. Finally, the patient should take one more controlled inhalation and a final huff cough to expel the mucus.

Autogenic Drainage
Autogenic drainage is a variation on deep breathing and coughing that may be more effective for patients with thick

secretions that are difficult to raise, such as those with cystic fibrosis or severe COPD. It is also gentler and less likely to cause declines in oxygen saturation or uncontrolled coughing than other methods. The patient is taught to sit upright and breathe in more deeply than usual, slowly through the nose, and then hold the breath for 2 to 4 seconds. When holding the breath, the patient should keep the glottis open, to prevent airway collapse. Exhaling is done as a quiet sigh, as if trying to steam up a mirror.

Using these breathing techniques, the patient is taught three phases:

1. *Unstick.* The patient breathes out completely, then takes a slow breath, and exhales fully several times, suppressing the urge to cough. This loosens mucus in the lower airways.
2. *Collect.* The patient takes 10 to 20 slightly deeper breaths, exhaling normally, still suppressing the urge to cough. This helps move mucus up to the middle airways.
3. *Evacuate.* The patient takes 10 to 20 breaths and huff coughs to move the mucus up and out.

During the *unstick* and *collect* phases, airflow should be high enough to produce a rattle if secretions are present. This is a complex process that is typically taught by an RT.

Breathing Exercises

Breathing exercises are essential for patients with chronic lung disease. Diaphragmatic and pursed-lip breathing increase the effectiveness of breathing and help reduce panic when dyspnea occurs.

Diaphragmatic Breathing

The diaphragm is the major muscle of breathing. However, patients often use less-efficient accessory muscles when they are short of breath. Conscious use of the diaphragm during breathing can be relaxing and conserve energy. Teach the patient to do the following:

1. Place one hand on the abdomen and the other on the chest.
2. Concentrate on pushing out the abdomen during inspiration and relaxing the abdomen on expiration. The chest should move very little.

Pursed-Lip Breathing

The pursed-lip breathing technique can be used any time the patient feels short of breath. It helps keep airways open during exhalation, which promotes carbon dioxide excretion. It should be done with diaphragmatic breathing. Counting during breathing also distracts the patient, reducing panic. Teach the patient to do the following:

1. Inhale slowly through the nose to the count of two (using diaphragmatic breathing).
2. Exhale slowly through pursed lips to the count of four.

> **NURSING CARE TIP**
> When teaching patients to do pursed-lip breathing, try teaching them to "smell the roses" while inhaling slowly through the nose and "blow out the candle" while exhaling. If you remind them not to let the wax splatter, then they'll blow slowly and gently!

Positioning

The patient who is short of breath should be positioned to conserve energy while allowing for maximum lung expansion. Most respiratory patients do not tolerate lying flat. The patient in bed can use Fowler or semi-Fowler position to keep abdominal contents from crowding the lungs. Some patients prefer to sit in a chair while leaning forward and placing their elbows on their knees or an over-the-bed table (tripod position; Fig. 29.14).

Patients with unilateral (one-sided) lung disease can benefit from the "good lung down" lateral position. This is a side-lying position with the good lung in the dependent position. Gravity causes greater blood flow to the dependent, "good" lung, thereby increasing oxygen saturation. Some patients may also benefit from prone positioning.

> **NURSING CARE TIP**
> Patients at home may choose to sleep in a recliner or La-Z-Boy–type chair to keep their head elevated. Others may use a wedge under their mattress or a hospital bed.

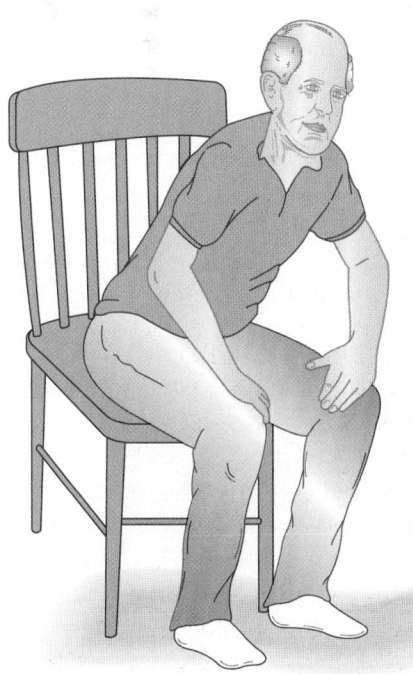

FIGURE 29.14 The tripod position may help reduce dyspnea.

Oxygen Therapy

Oxygen therapy is ordered by the HCP when the patient is unable to maintain oxygenation. Patients are typically placed on supplemental oxygen when their oxygen saturation is less than 90% on room air. The HCP's order should include the method of administration and the flow rate. A variety of delivery methods are described next.

The role of the licensed practical nurse/licensed vocational nurse (LPN/LVN) in oxygen therapy includes monitoring the flow rate, ensuring that the cannula and tubing or other device remain properly placed, and monitoring the patient's response to treatment. If the patient becomes short of breath while on oxygen therapy, notify the RT, registered nurse (RN), or HCP. Instruct the patient to avoid smoking, using electrical equipment, and performing other activities that can cause fire in the presence of oxygen. The RT is knowledgeable about oxygen therapy and is an excellent resource when questions arise.

> **NURSING CARE TIP**
>
> If a patient suddenly becomes confused, check the oxygen saturation (SpO_2) and oxygen delivery system. The patient may have taken off the cannula or the tubing may be kinked or disconnected, resulting in hypoxia and confusion.

Low-Flow Devices

NASAL CANNULA. The nasal cannula is the most common method of oxygen administration. Oxygen is delivered through a flexible catheter that has two short nasal prongs (Fig. 29.15). For the nasal cannula to be most effective, the patient must breathe through his or her nose. The cannula allows the patient to eat and talk. It is generally more comfortable than other methods of administration. If the nasal mucous membranes become dry, a water source can be placed on the system to humidify the oxygen. Oxygen can be delivered at 1 to 6 L/min via a nasal cannula; special high-flow cannulas can deliver much higher rates. Patients with COPD may benefit from a special cannula with a reservoir. Oxygen is stored in the reservoir during exhalation and delivered during inhalation. Patients, therefore, receive a higher concentration of oxygen.

Masks. Masks are used when a higher oxygen concentration is needed (Fig. 29.16). A disadvantage of masks is that they make some patients feel claustrophobic. Also, a mask must be replaced by a cannula while the patient eats.

- *Simple face mask.* A rate of 5 to 10 L/min can deliver oxygen concentrations from 40% to 60% with a simple face mask.
- *Partial rebreather mask.* A partial rebreather mask uses a reservoir bag to store oxygen. Vents on the sides of the

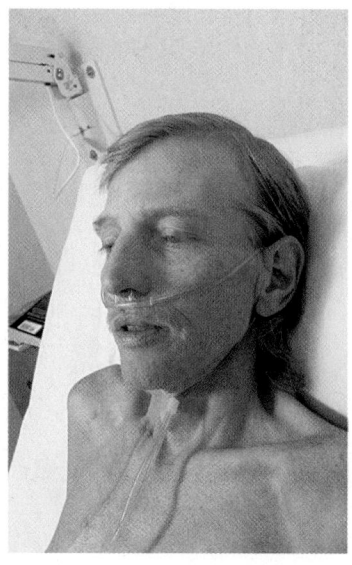

FIGURE 29.15 Nasal cannula for oxygen delivery.

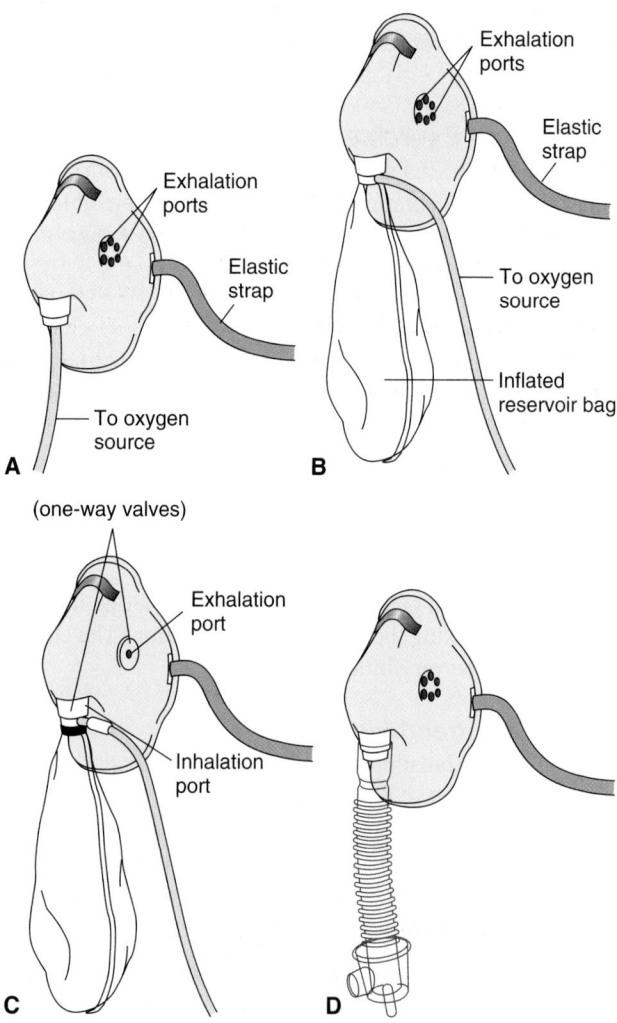

FIGURE 29.16 Oxygen masks. (A) Simple mask. (B) Partial rebreather mask. (C) Nonrebreather mask. (D) Venturi mask.

mask allow room air to mix with oxygen. It can deliver oxygen concentrations of 50% or greater.

- *Nonrebreather mask.* A nonrebreather mask has one or both side vents closed to limit the mixing of room air with oxygen. The vents open to allow exhalation but remain closed on inhalation. The reservoir bag has a valve to store oxygen for inhalation but does not allow entry of exhaled air. It is used to deliver oxygen concentrations of 70% to 100%.

> ### NURSING CARE TIP
> When a patient is using a partial rebreather or nonrebreather mask, make sure that the reservoir bag is never allowed to collapse to less than two-thirds full.

High-Flow Devices

VENTURI MASK. A Venturi mask is used for the patient who requires precise percentages of oxygen, such as the patient with chronic lung disease with CO_2 retention. A combination of entrainment ports and specified flow rates delivers exactly the right concentration of oxygen.

Transtracheal Catheter

A transtracheal catheter is a small tube that is surgically placed through the base of the neck directly into the trachea to deliver oxygen (Fig. 29.17). This is an attractive alternative for some patients who are on long-term oxygen therapy at home because it does not obstruct the nose or mouth. In addition, it can be easily covered with a loose scarf or collar. The patient is taught to remove and clean the catheter two or three times a day to prevent mucus obstruction. Check institution policy and procedure for specific care instructions.

Risks of Oxygen Therapy

In the past, health care professionals believed that patients with COPD should never receive oxygen at rates greater than 2 L per minute. This is because higher rates might depress breathing. Now, with pulse oximetry technology, oxygen administration rates are adjusted based on the SpO_2 level. Oxygen is administered at the flow rate needed to achieve 88% to 89% saturation, depending on the HCP order.

In addition, any patient can suffer lung damage from high oxygen concentrations (greater than 50%) delivered for more than 24 hours. If a patient exhibits symptoms of dry cough, chest pain, numbness in the extremities, lethargy, or nausea, the HCP should be contacted. A PaO_2 greater than 100 mm Hg should also be reported.

Nebulized Mist Treatments

Nebulized mist treatments (NMTs) use a nebulizer to mist medication directly into the lungs (Fig. 29.18). Such topical use of medication reduces systemic side effects. Bronchodilators such as albuterol (Proventil, ProAir HFA), mixed with normal saline solution and sometimes with supplemental oxygen, are most commonly administered. Medications such as corticosteroids, mucolytics, and antibiotics may also be given. An RT or a specially trained nurse administers the NMT. The patient uses a handheld reservoir with tubing and a mouthpiece to breathe in the medication. Some patients are taught to administer their own NMTs at home.

Inhalers

Inhalers are another way to administer topical medication directly into the lungs, minimizing systemic side effects. Corticosteroids and bronchodilators are often administered by inhaler. Metered-dose inhalers (MDIs) use propellants to deliver medication. Figure 29.19 shows use of a traditional MDI. Use of a spacer can increase the amount of medication that gets to the lungs (Fig. 29.20). Dry-powder inhalers (DPIs) deliver medication without the use of propellant. With so many different types of inhalers, it is important to carefully read the instructions for use before assisting a patient.

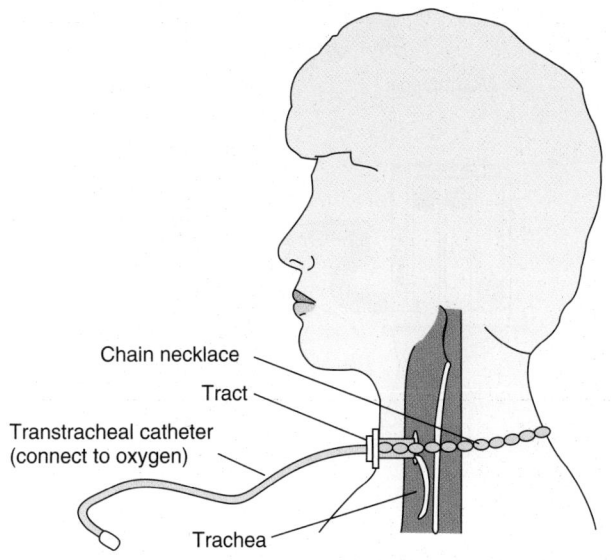

Chain necklace

Tract

Transtracheal catheter (connect to oxygen)

Trachea

FIGURE 29.17 Transtracheal oxygen catheter.

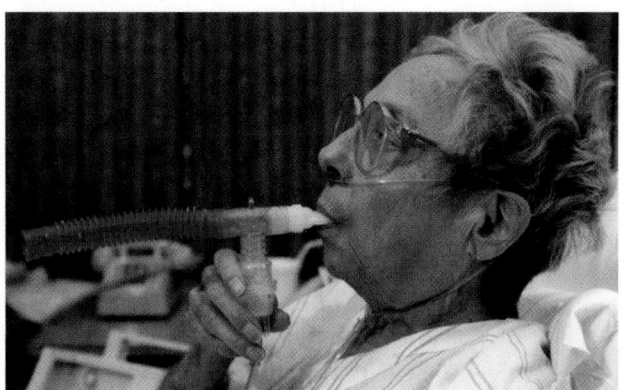

FIGURE 29.18 Patient receiving nebulized mist treatment.

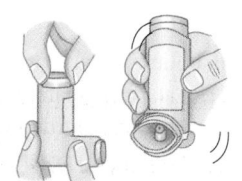

1. Gently twist the canister into the inhaler unit. Shake the inhaler and remove the cap.

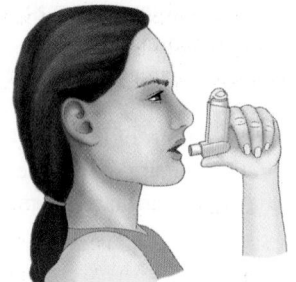

2. Exhale.

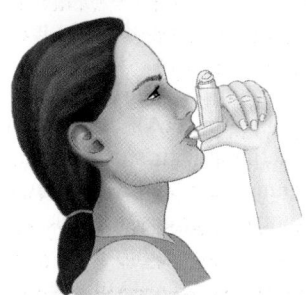

3. Place the inhaler mouthpiece in your mouth.

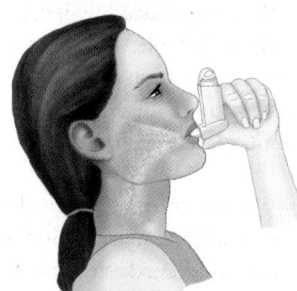

4. Press the canister down to actuate a dose of medication. As you do so, breathe in slowly and deeply. Time the dose and breath so the medication goes into the lungs and not onto the tongue.

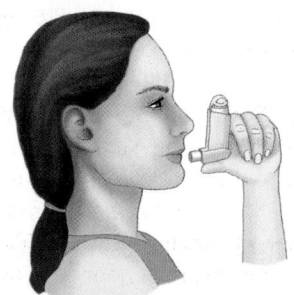

5. Hold your breath for 5–10 seconds. Repeat steps 2–4 if two puffs are ordered.

FIGURE 29.19 Instructions for use of a metered-dose inhaler. See package inserts for specific instructions because many types of inhalers are available.

The RT or nurse must carefully instruct the patient because improper use can reduce the effectiveness of the medication. It is also important to teach the patient to avoid overuse of adrenergic bronchodilator inhalers. Adrenergic bronchodilators can cause severe rebound bronchoconstriction and even death when used more often than prescribed.

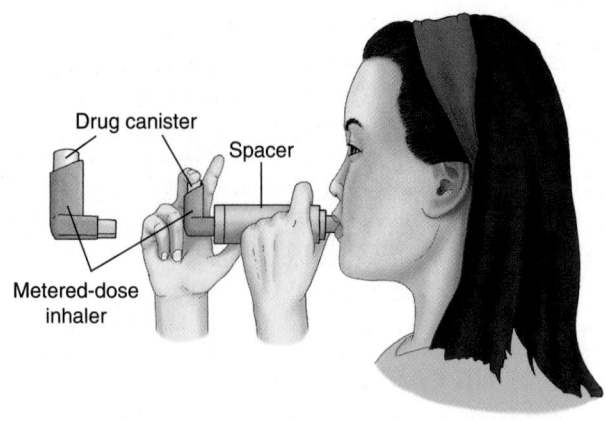

Drug canister
Spacer
Metered-dose inhaler

FIGURE 29.20 Use of a spacer increases the amount of medication that gets to the lungs.

Incentive Spirometry

Incentive spirometers (Fig. 29.21) are used to encourage deep breathing in patients at risk for collapse of lung tissue, a condition called *atelectasis*. These devices are commonly ordered for postoperative patients. Patients are instructed to use the spirometer 10 times each hour they are awake. Because a variety of spirometers are available, consult with an RT and read package inserts for specific directions for use.

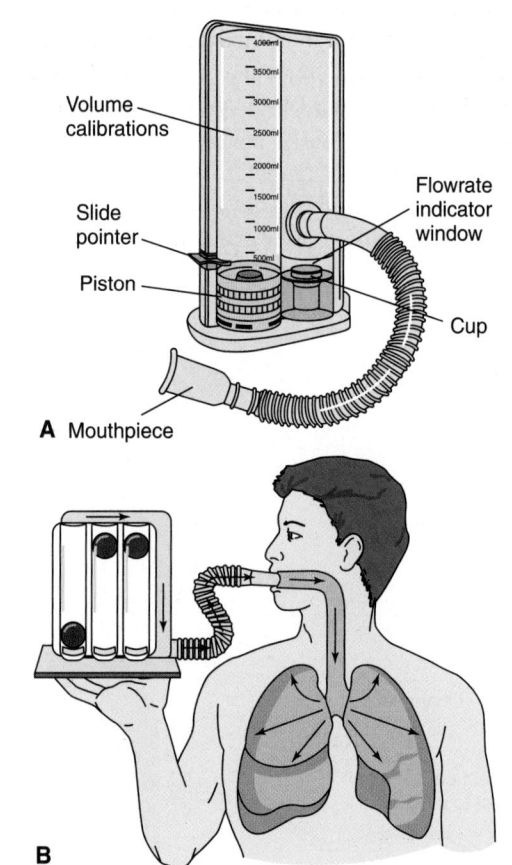

Volume calibrations
Flowrate indicator window
Slide pointer
Piston
Cup
A Mouthpiece

B

FIGURE 29.21 Incentive spirometers. (A) Voldyne volumetric deep-breathing exerciser. (B) TriFlo II incentive breathing exerciser.

Chest Physiotherapy

Chest physiotherapy (CPT) includes postural drainage, percussion, and vibration. It helps move secretions out from deep inside the lungs (Fig. 29.22). It is indicated for the patient who has a weak or ineffective cough and is at risk for retaining secretions. Patients with retained secretions due to conditions such as COPD, cystic fibrosis, or bronchiectasis and patients on ventilators benefit from CPT.

CPT is performed by an RT, physical therapist, or specially trained nurse. For postural drainage, the patient is placed in various positions (head down to help drain secretions) and turned periodically during the treatment so all lobes of the lungs are drained. The therapist uses cupped hands to strike the chest repeatedly (percussion), producing sound waves that are transmitted through the chest, loosening secretions. The therapist may also apply vibration to the patient's chest, using the hands or a vibrator, to loosen secretions. An NMT should be given before CPT to humidify secretions. The patient is instructed to deep breathe and cough at intervals during and after the treatment.

High-Frequency Chest Wall Oscillation Vest

The high-frequency chest wall oscillation vest (sometimes called vest therapy) is an alternative to CPT. Because it does not require the presence of an RT, it is less expensive over time. An inflatable vest is placed on the patient. A compressor generates pulses of air into the vest to vibrate the patient's chest. Like CPT, this helps loosen secretions so they can be expectorated. The patient must cough during and after the therapy for it to be effective. It can easily be used at home.

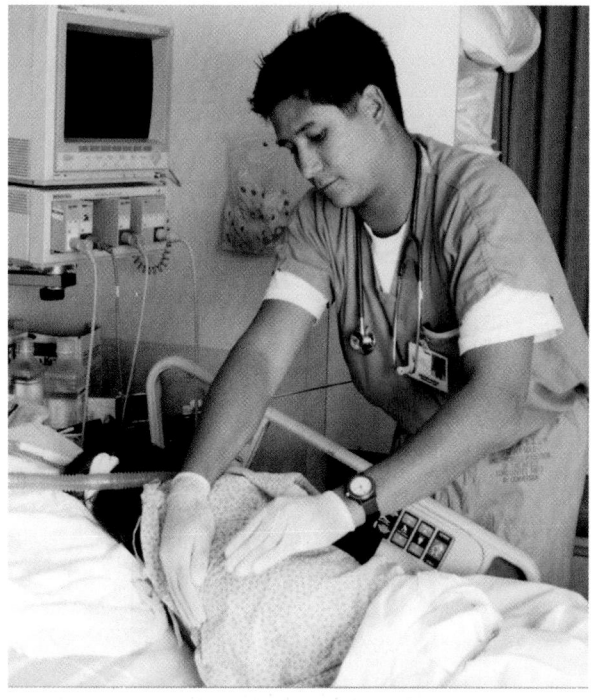

FIGURE 29.22 Patient receiving chest physiotherapy.

Vibratory Positive Expiratory Pressure Device

Another alternative to CPT is a small handheld device called a vibratory positive expiratory pressure (PEP) device. One brand is the Flutter mucus clearance device (Fig. 29.23). When the patient blows into the mouthpiece, it makes a heavy steel ball inside bounce around in its chamber, which then sends vibrations back into the airways to help loosen mucus. Blowing into the device also creates positive pressure, which opens airways.

Thoracentesis

Thoracentesis involves the insertion of a needle into the pleural space. It is commonly done to aspirate fluid trapped in the pleural space (pleural effusion; see Chapter 31). The procedure may be diagnostic to determine the source of fluid or therapeutic to remove fluid and reduce respiratory distress. It may also be performed to aspirate blood or air or to inject medication.

You may be asked to assist an HCP with a thoracentesis. First, verify that the patient understands the procedure and that written consent has been obtained if required by institution policy. Have the patient void before the procedure. The patient should be aware that a sensation of pressure may be felt but that severe pain is rare. Administer an analgesic, if ordered, before the procedure. Obtain a special procedure tray that has the equipment needed by the HCP. Place the patient in a sitting position, bending over a bedside table, or in a side-lying position if unable to sit. You can position yourself in front of the patient and encourage relaxation during the procedure. If you are asked to hand equipment to the HCP, be sure to keep everything sterile.

The HCP uses a local anesthetic before inserting a needle into the patient's back through the desired interspace. Specimens are withdrawn through the needle, labeled, and sent to the laboratory. A sterile container is used to collect the remaining fluid. As much as 2 L can be removed, sometimes more. The patient will usually report immediate reduction of dyspnea.

After the procedure, the HCP may apply a petroleum jelly dressing to prevent air leakage into the wound. Assess vital signs, breath sounds, and the puncture site according to the HCP's orders (e.g., every 15 minutes times two, every 30 minutes times two, then every 4 hours for 24 hours). The patient is usually maintained on bedrest for 1 hour after the procedure. Label and send specimens to the laboratory as ordered. The HCP may order a postprocedure x-ray examination to ensure that the lung was not punctured, causing a pneumothorax.

Chest Drainage

Continuous chest drainage involves insertion of one or two chest tubes by the HCP into the pleural space to drain fluid

• WORD • BUILDING •

thoracentesis: thoraco—chest + centesis—puncture

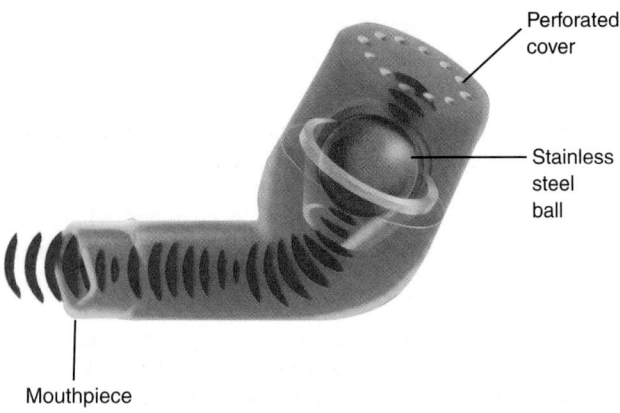

FIGURE 29.23 Flutter mucus clearance device.

Labels for Figure 29.23:
- Perforated cover
- Stainless steel ball
- Mouthpiece

or air. The tubes are connected to a chest drainage system that collects the fluid or allows escape of air.

Indications

Chest tubes and a chest drainage system are used when fluid or air has collected in the pleural space. This can occur with a collapsed lung (pneumothorax), pleural effusion, penetrating chest injury, or during chest surgery. These conditions are covered in Chapter 31.

Chest Tube Insertion

The HCP inserts drainage tubes through the chest wall into the pleural space either in surgery or at the bedside. If removal of air from around a collapsed lung is the goal, the tube is inserted into the upper anterior chest, in the second to fourth intercostal space. If removal of fluid or blood is the goal, such as after an injury, the tube is inserted in the lower lateral chest, in the eighth or ninth intercostal space. If a patient has both air and fluid to drain, two tubes are inserted and may be joined with a Y connector before connecting to tubing that leads to a drainage system.

You can assist the HCP by obtaining a chest tube insertion tray and chest drainage system. Prepare it according to the manufacturer's directions. Ensure that the patient understands the procedure and that written consent has been obtained according to institutional policy. Administer an analgesic as ordered. Help position the patient as directed by the HCP. Chest tube insertion is often an emergency intervention. This necessitates preparing the patient quickly.

Once the tube has been inserted and the system is in place, ensure that each connection is securely taped to prevent a break in the system. Sterile petroleum jelly gauze and an occlusive dressing are applied over the insertion site to prevent air leakage. If the dressing becomes soiled, do not change it; reinforce it with additional dressings, and notify the RN or HCP. Some nurses may change chest tube dressings with special training.

Obtain two padded clamps to keep at the bedside. These are used for clamping the chest tube if the chest drainage system becomes accidentally disconnected from the tubing, for

changing the drainage system, or for a trial period before chest tube removal. The tubes are never clamped for more than a few seconds, however, because this prevents air escape and can cause a buildup of air in the pleural space. This can create a tension pneumothorax, which is a life-threatening emergency (see Chapter 31).

Chest Drainage System

The drainage system has evolved from a set of glass bottles to a one-piece molded plastic system with chambers that correspond to the bottles. Studying the bottle system will help you understand the one-piece system (Fig. 29.24). One, two, or three bottles can be used. Study Figure 29.24 as you read the following sections.

WATER SEAL BOTTLE OR CHAMBER. Each time the patient exhales, trapped air also escapes the pleural space and travels through the chest tube to the water seal bottle or chamber, under the water, and then bubbles up and out of the bottle. The water acts as a seal, allowing air to escape from the pleural space but preventing air from getting back in during the negative pressure of inspiration. When the system is initiated, bubbling will occur on each exhalation until the lung is reexpanded. Once most of the pneumothorax is resolved, water in the tube fluctuates up with each inspiration and down with each expiration, as much as 5 to 10 cm. This is called **tidaling.** When the lung is fully reinflated, tidaling stops. If tidaling stops before the lung is reinflated, the tubing should be checked for a kink or occlusion. If constant bubbling occurs

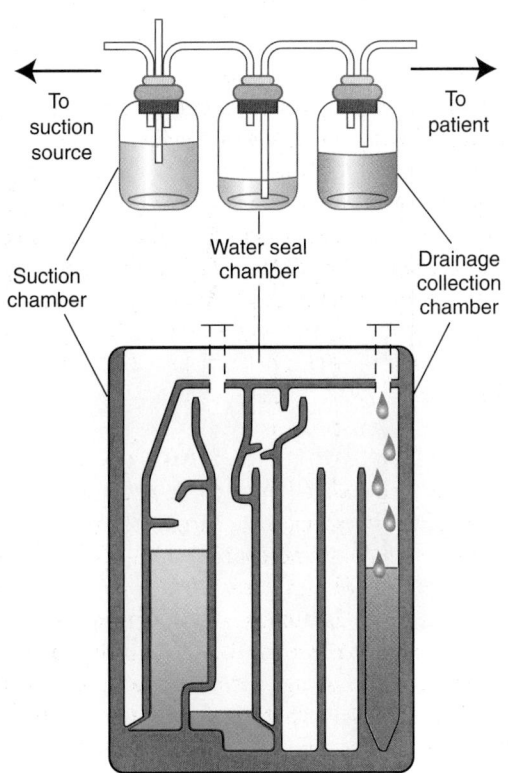

Labels for Figure 29.24:
- To suction source
- To patient
- Suction chamber
- Water seal chamber
- Drainage collection chamber

FIGURE 29.24 Pleur-evac chest drainage system.

in the water seal chamber, the system should be checked immediately for leaks.

> ## LEARNING TIP
> Do you remember blowing bubbles through a straw into a glass of water as a child? The air could escape through the water, but you could not suck the air back through the water after it escaped. A water seal chamber operates under the same principle.

SUCTION BOTTLE OR CHAMBER. Sometimes, a suction source is used to speed lung reinflation. A separate bottle with tubing attached to suction is used. The amount of suction depends on the level of water in the bottle, not the amount of suction set on the machine. As shown in Figure 29.24, some air is being suctioned from the atmosphere from the center straw, and some is being suctioned from the patient. The farther the straw is immersed in the water, the harder it will be for the suction to draw air from the atmosphere, creating more suction to the patient. The suction level is ordered by the HCP. It is almost always negative 20 cm of water. The suction source should be turned on far enough to cause gentle bubbling in the suction bottle or chamber. Vigorous bubbling causes water evaporation, which alters the amount of suction. If water evaporates, more must be added to maintain the correct amount of suction. Some newer one-piece systems use special suction control valves to eliminate the need for water.

DRAINAGE BOTTLE OR CHAMBER. Sometimes a third bottle is needed to catch fluid drained from the pleural space. Drainage may be from pleural effusion, chest trauma, or surgery. Sometimes, a small amount of drainage occurs because of the insertion of the chest tube. The drainage chamber is not emptied to measure drainage. Rather, the drainage level in the bottle or chamber is marked and timed each shift to monitor the amount. It is documented as output on the intake and output record. If drainage suddenly increases or becomes very bloody, notify the HCP. If the drainage chamber fills up, either the chamber or the entire unit will need to be changed, depending on the type of system used.

Nursing Care for the Patient With a Chest Tube

Nursing care for a patient with a chest tube involves regular assessment of the patient and the drainage system. See Box 29.1 for specific assessment and care. If permitted by the HCP, patients can be free to move around with the chest tube and drainage system. The drainage system must always be kept upright and below the level of the chest. If the patient must be transported, the drainage system is transported with the patient. Ask the HCP whether the patient can be safely transported without suction. If the answer is yes, the suction control chamber is then left open to allow air to escape. Do not clamp tubing for transport.

> ## Box 29.1
> ### Care of the Patient With a Chest Drainage System
>
> Assess the patient according to institution policy. Start with the patient and move toward the drainage system.
>
> #### Patient
> 1. Observe respiratory rate, effort, and symmetry.
> 2. Assess shortness of breath, pain, anxiety, or other discomforts.
> 3. Auscultate lung sounds (lung sounds may initially be muffled or absent on the side of a collapsed lung but should gradually return to normal as the lung reinflates).
> 4. Confirm that dressing is intact; observe for drainage. If necessary, reinforce the dressing and notify the health care provider (HCP). Do not change the dressing unless specifically ordered to and trained to do so.
> 5. Palpate around insertion sites for crepitus, a sign that air is leaking into the tissues.
>
> #### Tubing
> 6. Check all tubing for kinks, breaks, or broken connections. Verify that all connections are securely taped.
> 7. Ensure that there are no dependent loops of tubing. Excess tubing should be coiled on the bed.
>
> #### Draining System
> 8. Verify that drainage system is below level of patient's chest at all times.
> 9. Check drainage system for cracks or leaks.
> 10. Check water seal chamber for correct water level and for tidaling (unless lung is reinflated). Add sterile water if evaporation has decreased level. If continuous bubbling is present, check entire system for leaks and notify registered nurse (RN) or HCP.
> 11. Check suction control chamber for gentle bubbling (or open to air). Confirm correct amount of water as ordered. Add water if needed.
> 12. Check and mark amount of drainage in collection chamber every 8 hours and as needed or as ordered. Report any marked increase in bloody drainage. Record drainage as output.
> 13. Document findings.
>   *Notify RN or HCP if any of the following occur:*
> - *The patient suddenly reports increasing dyspnea.*
> - *There is a change in the patient's assessment findings.*
> - *The drainage chamber is full and needs to be changed.*

If a chest tube is accidentally pulled out before the pneumothorax is resolved, air can re-enter the pleural space. Contact the RN or HCP immediately if this occurs.

Stripping and Milking

You may hear about stripping or milking tubing to dislodge clots and maintain patency. Stripping is done by holding the proximal end of the tubing and using the other hand to squeeze the tubing between two fingers while sliding the fingers toward the drainage system. This is repeated on small sections of tubing until all have been stripped. It is now known, however, that this process can create negative pressure at the openings in the tubing that are within the pleural space. This can suck lung tissue in and cause damage. Stripping should not be done.

Milking is done by gently squeezing portions of tubing from the patient to the system without any sliding motion. This is somewhat safer for the patient but is still not done routinely. If tubing appears to be occluded, consult with the HCP for specific orders.

CRITICAL THINKING

Miss Israel has a chest tube in place for a spontaneous pneumothorax.

1. You note that the water seal chamber is bubbling vigorously. What could cause this? What should you do?
2. You are totaling intake and output for your 8-hour shift. There is 240 mL of serous fluid in the drainage chamber of the drainage system at 2200. At 1400, there was 190 mL. How much output should you record?

Suggested answers are at the end of the chapter.

Removal of Chest Tube

When the reason for the chest tube is resolved, the HCP removes it and places petroleum jelly gauze and a sterile occlusive dressing over the site. Continue to watch for development of crepitus. Monitor the patient's respiratory status and dressing site.

Tracheostomy

A **tracheotomy** is a surgical opening through the base of the neck into the trachea. It is called a **tracheostomy** when it is more permanent and has a tube inserted into the opening to maintain patency (Fig. 29.25). The patient breathes through this opening, bypassing the upper airways. A tracheostomy is performed for a variety of reasons, such as in patients who have had a cancerous larynx removed, patients with airway obstruction caused by trauma or a tumor, patients who have difficulty clearing secretions from the airway, or patients who need prolonged mechanical ventilation.

The tracheostomy tube consists of three parts: an outer cannula, an inner cannula, and an obturator (Fig. 29.26A and B). The obturator is a guide that is used only during insertion of the tube. After insertion, the obturator is immediately removed and kept at the bedside (commonly in a plastic bag taped to the wall above the bed) for emergency use if the tracheostomy tube is accidentally removed. The outer cannula remains in place at all times and is secured by ties or a Velcro strap to prevent dislodging. The inner cannula is removed at intervals, usually every 8 hours and as needed for cleaning. Some newer tracheostomy tubes eliminate the need for an inner cannula.

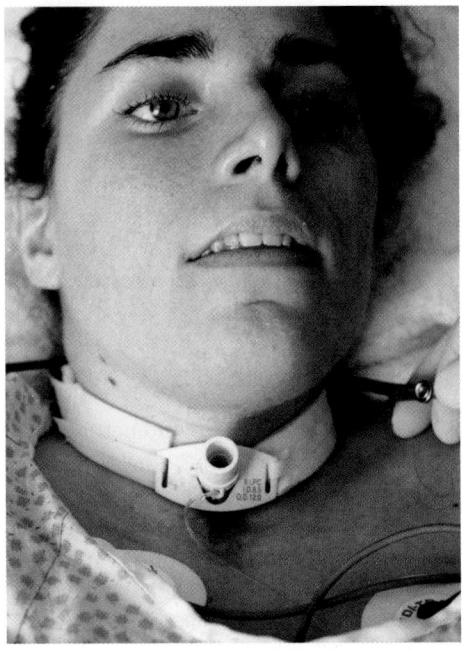

FIGURE 29.25 Patient with tracheostomy.

The tube may be metal or plastic. Plastic tubes typically have disposable inner cannulas, which can be replaced rather than cleaned. Plastic tubes also may have balloon-like cuffs that are inflated to prevent air escape during mechanical ventilation. You know that the cuff is inflated if the small pilot balloon on the tubing used to inject air is inflated (see Fig. 29.26B and C). Cuffs are deflated routinely to prevent tissue damage. See "Performing Tracheostomy Care" on Davis Edge for steps required for a routine tracheostomy cleaning.

Communication is problematic for the patient with a tracheostomy tube because air is diverted out the tube rather than past the vocal cords and out the mouth. Fenestrated tubes are tubes with openings (fenestra) in the cannula to allow air to flow up into the larynx for speaking (see Fig. 29.26C). The patient can be taught to plug the opening of the tube while speaking to divert air through the fenestra. Another option is a valve such as the Passy Muir tracheostomy speaking valve (Fig. 29.27). This is a special valve that allows air to flow into the tracheostomy during inspiration. It then closes and redirects air up around the tracheostomy tube, through the vocal cords, and out the nose and mouth on expiration, allowing the patient to speak. Use of the valve eliminates the need for the patient to use a finger over the opening to speak. For the valve to be used safely and effectively, the tracheostomy tube must be small enough for air to flow around it or it must be fenestrated to allow air to flow up through the vocal cords. If cuffed, the cuff must be completely deflated.

• WORD • BUILDING •
tracheotomy: trach—trachea + otomy—incision
tracheostomy: trach—trachea + ostomy—opening or mouth

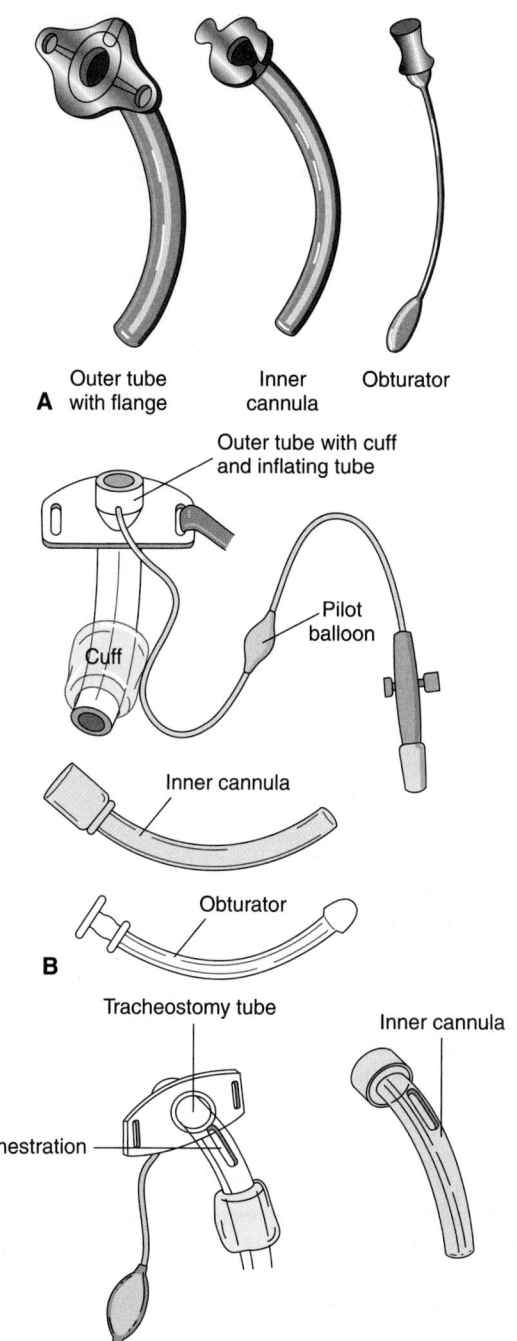

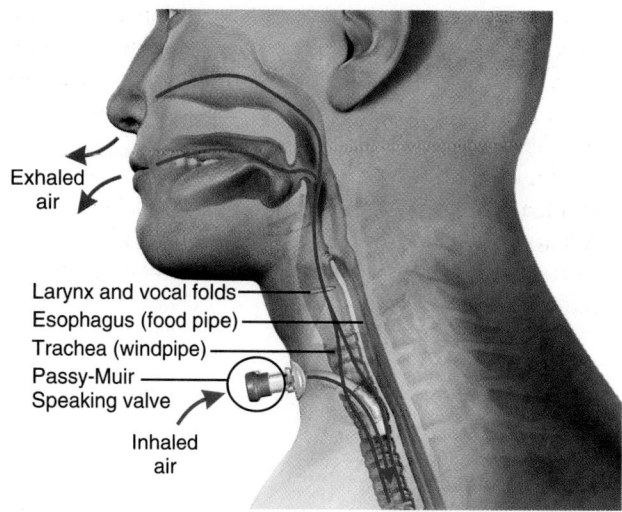

FIGURE 29.27 The Passy Muir tracheostomy speaking valve.

FIGURE 29.26 Tracheostomy tube. (A) Metal tube. (B) Cuffed plastic tube. (C) Fenestrated tube.

BE SAFE!

A patient with a tracheostomy tube in place as a result of laryngectomy surgery will not have vocal cords, and the trachea will no longer connect to the nose and mouth. The patient will not be able to plug the tube or use a valve to talk; plugging a laryngectomy tube would cause suffocation. Laryngectomy is covered in Chapter 30.

Some tracheostomies are permanent. However, some patients can be weaned from the tracheostomy tube when their condition has improved enough to allow breathing without it. The HCP may replace the tube with a smaller tube to prepare the patient for its removal. This allows a plug to be inserted into the tracheostomy tube at intervals to force the patient to breathe around the tube through the nose and mouth. When the tracheostomy tube has been removed, the opening may be taped shut and covered with gauze until it is healed. The gauze often becomes saturated with secretions and is changed as needed.

CRITICAL THINKING

Mr. Smith has a plastic, cuffed tracheostomy tube that is small enough to allow airflow around it for talking when the cuff is deflated. A friend stops by for a chat and helps Mr. Smith to plug his tracheostomy so he can talk. Mr. Smith's face turns dark red, and he gets panicky. His friend calls for help.

1. What happened? What should you do right away?
2. How can you help prevent this in the future?
3. How will you document this occurrence?

   Suggested answers are at the end of the chapter.

Nursing Process for the Patient With a Tracheostomy

See "Nursing Care Plan for the Patient With a Tracheostomy."

Suctioning

Suctioning involves the use of a sterile flexible catheter inserted into the tracheostomy tube to remove secretions from a patient who is unable to cough effectively. This may be

Nursing Care Plan for the Patient With a Tracheostomy

Nursing Diagnosis: *Ineffective Airway Clearance* related to excessive secretions
Expected Outcome: The patient's airway will be free of secretions as evidenced by no audible crackles or wheezes in airway and a clear cannula.
Evaluation of Outcome: Is airway free of secretions?

Intervention	Rationale	Evaluation
Assess lung sounds every 4 hours and as needed (prn).	*Coarse crackles or wheezes may indicate secretions in airways.*	Are coarse crackles or wheezes present?
Monitor oxygen saturation every 4 hours and prn.	*Secretions may reduce gas exchange.*	Is oxygen saturation less than 90% to 95%, indicating a problem?
Encourage patient to deep breathe and cough as able.	*Patient may be able to clear own secretions without suctioning.*	Is patient able to cough up secretions effectively?
Encourage fluids if not contraindicated.	*Fluids help hydrate secretions, making them easier to cough up.*	Is patient taking adequate fluids? Are secretions thin?
Provide humidified oxygen or a room humidifier.	*Humidification helps prevent drying of mucosa and secretions.*	Are mucosa moist and secretions easily removed?
Encourage ambulation as able, or turn every 2 hours.	*Movement helps mobilize secretions.*	Is patient mobilized as much as possible?
Clean tracheostomy according to agency policy.	*Cleaning helps remove excess mucus and keeps airway clear.*	Does cleaning help maintain an open airway?
Suction patient using sterile technique, only when needed.	*Suctioning clears secretions from airways. Unnecessary suctioning irritates airways.*	Is suction necessary? Is airway free of secretions after suctioning?
Monitor and document amount, color, and character of secretions. Report change in secretions accompanied by fever.	*Purulent sputum accompanied by fever can indicate pneumonia.*	Is sputum clear or white and scant in amount? Is purulent sputum reported?

Nursing Diagnosis: *Risk for Infection* related to bypass of normal respiratory defense mechanisms and increased aspiration risk
Expected Outcome: The patient will be free of infection, as evidenced by vital signs within normal limits and clear secretions.
Evaluation of Outcome: Is patient free from symptoms of infection?

Intervention	Rationale	Evaluation
Monitor and report signs and symptoms of infection (e.g., fever, increased respiratory rate, purulent sputum, elevated white blood cell count).	*Early recognition and treatment of infection improves outcome.*	Are signs of infection present?
Use good hand hygiene practice.	*Hand hygiene is important in preventing infection.*	Do all caregivers use good hand hygiene technique?
Protect tracheostomy opening from foreign material, such as food, sprays, and powders.	*Foreign materials in the tracheostomy can cause pneumonia.*	Is the tracheostomy adequately protected?

Nursing Care Plan for the Patient With a Tracheostomy—cont'd

Intervention	Rationale	Evaluation
Use meticulous sterile technique for all tracheostomy care and suctioning.	*Use of nonsterile technique may introduce microorganisms into the respiratory tract.*	Is sterile technique used by all caregivers?
Encourage a well-balanced diet. Consult dietitian prn.	*A well-balanced diet enhances immune function.*	Is patient eating a balanced diet or receiving adequate supplementation?
Keep head of bed elevated 30 to 45 degrees.	*Elevation helps reduce aspiration of gastric contents, which can lead to pneumonia.*	Is the head of bed elevated?
Consult with speech therapist and health care provider (HCP) about whether to have cuff inflated or deflated on cuffed tube.	*An inflated cuff can impair swallowing in some patients.*	Is the cuff properly inflated or deflated according to specific orders?

Nursing Diagnosis: *Impaired Verbal Communication* related to presence of tracheostomy tube
Expected Outcomes: The patient will use alternate methods of communication effectively. The patient will express satisfaction with ability to communicate needs.
Evaluation of Outcomes: Is the patient able to use alternative methods to express needs?

Intervention	Rationale	Evaluation
Take time to allow patient to communicate needs.	*Patient may become frustrated if hurried.*	Does patient feel adequate time is given for communication of needs?
Watch for patient's nonverbal cues.	*Gestures and facial expression can provide valuable cues.*	Are nonverbal cues recognized?
Offer pen and paper or magic slate (if patient is literate).	*Patient may be able to write out his or her needs/concerns.*	Is patient able to communicate in writing?
Use a picture board (available from speech therapy department).	*The patient can point to a picture (water, toileting) that indicates need.*	Is patient able to point appropriately to needs?
Teach patient with fenestrated or small tracheostomy tube how to cover opening with a plug or clean finger to talk, or to use Passy Muir valve, according to HCP or speech therapy recommendations.	*Covering the opening or using a valve diverts air into larynx and allows speech.*	Is patient able to communicate in this manner?
Consult with speech therapist.	*Speech therapist may have additional methods for communicating with patient.*	Are alternative methods effective?

Nursing Diagnosis: *Disturbed Body Image* related to presence of tracheostomy
Expected Outcomes: The patient will demonstrate adaptation to changes in appearance due to tracheostomy. The patient will be willing to participate in tracheostomy care.
Evaluation of Outcomes: Does the patient look at and talk about tracheostomy? Does the patient participate in learning to care for tracheostomy?

Intervention	Rationale	Evaluation
Assess patient's and family members' feelings about tracheostomy.	*Assessment provides basis for care.*	Are patient's feelings within an expected range for such a change in body image? Are family members accepting?

(nursing care plan continues on page 550)

Nursing Care Plan for the Patient With a Tracheostomy—cont'd

Intervention	Rationale	Evaluation
Approach patient with an accepting attitude.	*Patient will be aware of the nurse's nonverbal body language.*	Does patient indicate a feeling of acceptance from the nurse?
Allow patient opportunity to share concerns about tracheostomy.	*Sharing concerns helps patient to sort out feelings and problem solve.*	Does patient share feelings as needed? (*Note:* Some patients do not wish to share feelings and should not be forced to do so.)
Refer patient to support group if available.	*Patient may benefit from communicating with others with tracheostomies.*	Is patient receptive to a support group referral?
Assist patient in finding attractive ways to conceal tracheostomy if desired.	*Loose scarves or collars can help conceal and protect the tracheostomy.*	Is patient satisfied with appearance of tracheostomy?

Nursing Diagnosis: *Deficient Knowledge* related to care of new tracheostomy
Expected Outcomes: The patient and significant other will verbalize understanding of self-care, demonstrate tracheostomy self-care procedures, and state resources for help after discharge.
Evaluation of Outcomes: Are the patient and significant other able to verbalize self-care and correctly demonstrate care procedures? Is the patient able to state how to obtain help after discharge?

Intervention	Rationale	Evaluation
Assess patient's and significant other's baseline knowledge of self-care.	*Teaching should only be initiated if a knowledge deficit exists.*	Does patient exhibit knowledge of self-care?
Instruct patient and significant other in tracheostomy cleaning, deep breathing and coughing, suctioning, prevention of infection and symptoms to report to the HCP, and protection of tracheostomy from pollutants and water (no swimming, careful showering).	*Patient will need to care for self after discharge.*	Does patient verbalize understanding of self-care and demonstrate all procedures correctly?
Provide follow-up with the home health nurse after discharge.	*A home health nurse can provide reinforcement of instruction at home.*	Is patient receptive to having a home health nurse assist?

a patient with overwhelming secretions or a patient with a tracheostomy or ET tube who is unable to clear the tube with coughing.

The procedures for suctioning are found on Davis Edge. Consult a procedure manual for more detailed instruction. Remember that suctioning is both frightening and uncomfortable for a patient. Patients sometimes feel as though oxygen is being "vacuumed" from their lungs. Suctioning can cause hypoxia, vagal stimulation with resulting bradycardia, and even cardiac arrest. Only suction when necessary rather than on a routine basis. Coughing is the most effective way to clear secretions and should be encouraged if the patient is capable. Signs that suctioning is needed include crackles or wheezes heard with or without a stethoscope or a dropping oxygen saturation value. Explain each step to the patient during suctioning even if he or she is unresponsive.

Intubation

Some patients are intubated with a special ET tube through the nose or mouth and into the trachea (Fig. 29.28). Cardiopulmonary arrest, general anesthesia during surgery, and respiratory failure are examples of situations that may require intubation. Most intubated patients are also mechanically ventilated. Some patients have advance directives that indicate they do not wish to be intubated. You should be familiar with the patient's wishes and bring them to the attention of the HCP if necessary.

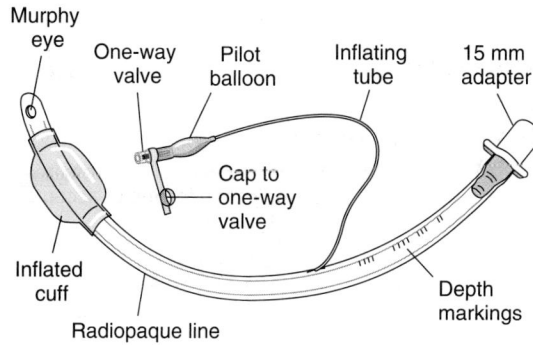

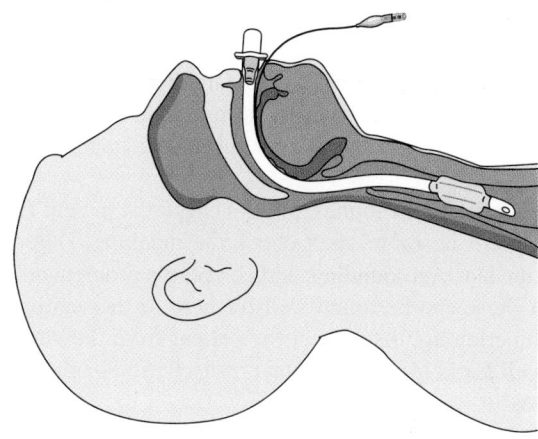

Placement of tube in airway

FIGURE 29.28 Endotracheal tube.

Because intubation can damage the vocal cords and surrounding tissues, it is usually a short-term intervention. Patients who need long-term ventilatory support have a tracheostomy tube placed.

Nursing Care for the Intubated Patient

Nursing care for the intubated patient includes regular assessment of the patient's respiratory status and tube placement. Auscultate lung sounds bilaterally to ensure that the tube has not been displaced into one bronchus. Carefully secure the tube with tape or a Velcro holder to avoid dislodging. Reposition and secure oral tubes to the opposite side of the mouth every 24 hours or according to institution policy to prevent tissue damage. Apply an adhesive skin barrier under the tape to protect the skin. If alert, instruct the patient to be careful not to pull on the tube. You may need to obtain an order for soft wrist restraints if absolutely necessary for the confused patient. Restraints can be avoided if a family member is available to sit with the patient. Many nursing interventions for the patient with a tracheostomy are also appropriate for the intubated patient. (See "Nursing Care Plan for the Patient With a Tracheostomy.")

Like tracheostomy tubes, ET tubes have a cuff (balloon-like area around the tube) to help maintain proper placement

and to prevent leakage of air around the tube. Consult the RT to help monitor the cuff pressure.

Patients will need suctioning because they are unable to cough effectively with an ET tube. Visible secretions in the tube, crackles or wheezes heard with or without the stethoscope, or a drop in SpO_2 without another obvious cause are signs that suctioning is necessary. The ET tube suctioning procedure is sterile. It is the same as suctioning a tracheostomy tube. Most institutions have in-line suctioning devices, which are connected to the ET tube within a sterile sleeve. This maintains sterility, protects the nurse, and simplifies the suctioning procedure. Oral suction may also be necessary to keep the mouth free of secretions.

The intubated patient is often extremely anxious, especially if she or he is alert. Explain the purpose of all care activities. Suctioning is a particularly anxiety-producing activity. It should be explained carefully even if the patient is unresponsive.

Intubated patients are at risk of developing ventilator-associated pneumonia (VAP) because normal respiratory defense mechanisms are bypassed. Good hand hygiene and frequent mouth care to reduce risk of aspirating oral microorganisms can help prevent VAP. The head of the bed should also be kept elevated 30 to 45 degrees at all times.

Because the ET tube passes between the vocal cords, the patient is unable to speak. Provide paper and pencil or a picture board for communication. Yes/no questions can be answered by a nod or shake of the head.

Monitor ABG and oxygen saturation values and notify the HCP of changes. If oxygen values drop or the patient becomes confused or agitated, immediately assess the patient for a disconnected oxygen source or excessive secretions.

If the HCP determines that the patient can breathe effectively without the tube, the tube will be removed. The patient will be slowly weaned from the ventilator first. Before tube removal, the patient's mouth and tube are suctioned, and the cuff is deflated. After removal, the patient is observed closely for laryngeal edema or respiratory distress. The patient is maintained in high Fowler position to maximize chest expansion.

Mechanical Ventilation

Ventilators are devices that provide ventilation (respirations) for patients who are unable to breathe effectively on their own (Fig. 29.29). Ventilators use positive pressure to push oxygenated air via a cuffed ET or tracheostomy tube into the lungs at preset intervals. Patients may need mechanical ventilation after some surgeries, after cardiac or respiratory arrest, for declining ABGs related to worsening respiratory disease, or for neuromuscular disease or injury that affects the muscles of respiration.

Ventilator Modes

Ventilators can control ventilation or assist the patient's own respirations. See Table 29.8 for terms related to ventilator

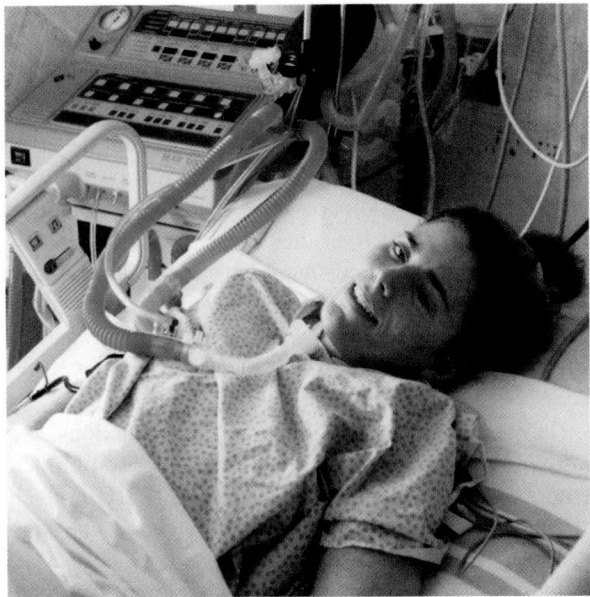

FIGURE 29.29 Patient on ventilator.

function. There are many types and models of ventilators. Consult with the respiratory care department for an explanation of a patient's ventilator and how to troubleshoot alarms.

Ventilator Alarms

Several types of alarms are found on ventilators. Low-pressure alarms sound if the ventilator senses reduced pressure in the system. Low pressure can be caused by disconnected tubing, leaks in tubing or around the ET tube, or an underinflated cuff.

A low-pressure alarm may also sound if the patient has attempted to remove the tube.

High-pressure alarms sound for higher-than-normal resistance to airflow. This might occur if the patient needs to be suctioned; if the patient is biting on the tube, coughing, or trying to talk; if tubing is kinked or otherwise obstructed; or if worsening respiratory disease causes decreased lung compliance. In addition, the high-pressure alarm may be triggered if the patient is anxious and unable to time his or her breaths with those of the ventilator. Water in the tubing might also cause a high-pressure alarm. Consult with the respiratory care department for guidance in draining the tubing.

A loss-of-power alarm may signal a power failure or a disconnected plug. Be aware of emergency power sources and be prepared to ventilate the patient manually if necessary. Volume and frequency alarms sound when tidal volume or number of breaths per minute fall outside preset parameters.

When an alarm sounds, always check the patient first. If the patient is stable, then check the machine. Determine why the alarm is sounding, and correct the problem quickly. If no cause can be found, call for help. If the ventilator is not functioning, disconnect the patient from the ventilator and call for help. Use a manual resuscitation bag until help arrives.

Nursing Care

Before initiating mechanical ventilation, it is important for the health care team to be aware of advance directives and consult with the patient and family, because some patients do not wish to be intubated or mechanically ventilated. Some

Table 29.8
Ventilator Terminology

Fraction of inspired oxygen (FIO_2)	Range: 21%–100%.
Tidal volume (V_T)	Amount of air delivered with each breath. Range: 6–8 mL/kg of ideal body weight.
Rate	Frequency of breaths delivered.
Assist control mode (AC; also called continuous mechanical ventilation, or CMV)	Does all the work of breathing for the patient. Ventilator delivers a breath each time patient begins to inspire. If patient does not breathe, the machine continues to deliver a preset number of breaths per minute.
Synchronized intermittent mandatory ventilation (SIMV)	Allows patient to breathe independently but delivers a minimum number of ventilations per minute as necessary. Synchronized to patient's own respiratory pattern.
Pressure support (PS)	Provides positive pressure on inspiration to decrease the work of breathing.
Continuous positive airway pressure (CPAP)	Provides positive pressure on inspiration and expiration to keep alveoli open in a spontaneously breathing patient.
Positive end-expiratory pressure (PEEP)	Provides positive pressure on expiration to help keep small airways open.

patients accept mechanical ventilation if it is a temporary measure but not if it might be a permanent intervention.

In the past, ventilators were used only in intensive care units. Now, ventilators are seen on medical-surgical units, in nursing homes, and even in patients' homes. It is important to use a team approach when caring for a patient who is mechanically ventilated. The social worker; RT; physical, occupational, and speech therapist(s); dietitian; nurse; and HCP all work together to provide the comprehensive care needed by the patient. RTs usually take responsibility for routine monitoring and equipment maintenance.

The nurse is responsible for monitoring the patient, ensuring that ventilator settings are maintained as prescribed, providing initial response to alarms, keeping tubing free from water accumulation, and keeping the patient's airway free from secretions. In addition, keep a manual resuscitation bag at the bedside for emergencies. Good nursing care is essential for preventing ventilator-associated complications, especially pneumonia. Keep the head of the bed at a 30- to 45-degree angle to reduce the risk of aspiration and pneumonia (Wang et al., 2016). Oral care with chlorhexidine mouthwash can reduce the incidence of VAP (Hua et al., 2016). Keep the airway clear with suctioning as needed. Good nutrition is also essential and can increase the success of eventual weaning.

Patients who are mechanically ventilated are unable to talk and can become very uncomfortable and anxious if there is no easy way to communicate. Box 29.2 provides tips for making ventilated patients feel more secure.

Noninvasive Positive-Pressure Ventilation

Noninvasive positive-pressure ventilation (NIPPV) is an alternative to intubation and mechanical ventilation for patients who are able to breathe on their own but are unable to maintain normal ABGs. Patients with severe respiratory disease, sleep apnea, or neuromuscular diseases such as amyotrophic lateral sclerosis (ALS) that weaken respiratory muscles can benefit from this treatment. Instead of the invasive ET or tracheostomy tube, NIPPV uses an external masklike device that fits over the nose or mouth and nose (Fig. 29.30). It can be successful in patients who are alert, able to cooperate, do not have excessive secretions, and are able to breathe on their own for periods of time. It can be used with or without supplemental oxygen. In an acutely ill patient, oxygen saturation is monitored.

Two basic types of NIPPV are available: continuous positive airway pressure (CPAP) and bilevel positive airway pressure (BiPAP). With CPAP, the same amount of positive pressure is maintained throughout inspiration and expiration to prevent airway collapse. In BiPAP, a higher level of positive pressure is used on inspiration, and a lower level on expiration.

Nursing Care

Monitor patients receiving NIPPV for skin irritation from the mask and gastric distention from swallowing air. Apply an adhesive skin barrier to the areas that come in contact with the mask to prevent irritation. To prevent gastric distention,

---

Box 29.2

Tips for Caring for Patients Who Are Mechanically Ventilated

- Mechanically ventilated patients report feeling panicky but less so if relatives or nursing staff are present:
  - Speak to the patient each time you enter the room and explain everything you do.
  - Encourage family to visit.
  - Answer the patient's call light and attend to ventilator alarms promptly.
  - Use restraints only as a last resort.
- Patients may have difficulty relaxing and sleeping while on a ventilator:
  - Administer sedatives or antianxiety drugs as ordered. Request an order if necessary.
  - Allow uninterrupted blocks of time for sleep.
- Patients with endotracheal tubes report pain and discomfort:
  - Assess for comfort and reposition at regular intervals.
  - Be careful not to pull on the ventilator tubing.
  - Administer analgesics as ordered.
  - Provide good oral care, moistening the lips with a cool washcloth and water-based lubricant.
- Suctioning is painful and frightening for patients:
  - Suction quickly and smoothly, and avoid inserting the catheter too deeply.
  - Avoid the use of saline with suctioning, which can reduce oxygen saturation.
  - Allow the patient to suction him or herself if possible (with health care provider order and appropriate instruction).
- Communication is very difficult for the patient:
  - Be patient when trying to understand communication efforts.
  - Provide a pencil and paper, but be aware that even writing can be exhausting.
  - Ask yes/no questions when possible. Establish a response system with the patient such as blinking (once for no, twice for yes), hand squeezes, or nodding.
  - Validate patient expressions and body language; don't assume that a patient is sad or wants to be left alone based on facial expression.
  - Make sure the call light is within reach at all times.

Source: Modified from Jablonski, R. A. S. (1995). If ventilator patients could talk. *RN, 58*(2), 32.

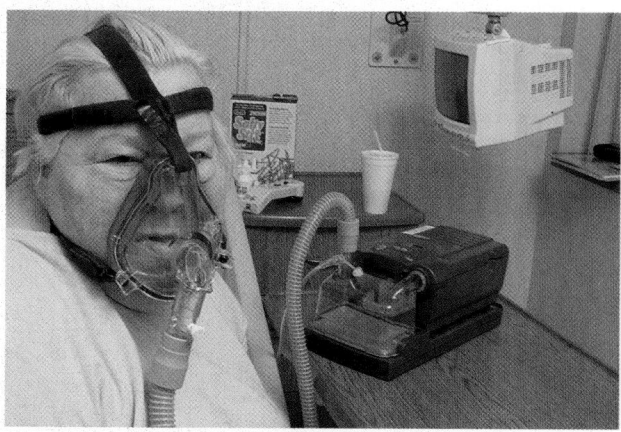

FIGURE 29.30 Noninvasive positive-pressure ventilation. Note round face from steroid use.

place the patient in semi-Fowler position. Consult with the RT to adjust air delivery pressure if necessary. A special humidifier on the machine can reduce nose and mouth dryness. An air leak around the mask can cause air to blow in the patient's eyes, which can be irritating. If this happens, remove the mask and reposition it. Many patients do not like the tight mask covering their nose or mouth. Be patient in explaining the reason for this treatment. Check the patient frequently to help control anxiety. Be sure to assess the patient's goals for therapy. Some patients may choose not to use NIPPV, but they must be fully aware of possible consequences.

Patients can use NIPPV nearly continuously, removing it to eat or use the bathroom. Other patients who are able to breathe effectively on their own during the day use it only when they are sleeping. Some use it for a few days until an acute exacerbation of disease is resolved. Others continue its use indefinitely at home.

SUGGESTED ANSWERS TO CRITICAL THINKING

Miss Israel

1. Bubbling in the water seal chamber indicates a leak in the system. Vigorous bubbling may indicate a large leak. The health care provider should be contacted immediately. After checking the patient, check the entire system for cracks or leaks and correct any problems discovered.
2. 50 mL.

Mr. Smith

1. Mr. Smith plugged his tracheostomy while the cuff was still inflated, so no air could get to his lungs. If the plug is not removed immediately, he will be totally unable to breathe. *Immediately* remove the plug!

2. To prevent this from happening in the future, teach Mr. Smith how his tracheostomy tube works and how to care for it. Show him how to check the pilot balloon if he is unsure.
3. "Answered call for help at 12:30, found patient dark red in color, unable to breathe, trach plugged. Trach unplugged, respirations restored, vital signs stable. Patient stated he plugged trach so he could talk to his friend. Function of trach cuff explained to patient and friend. Both verbalize understanding to only plug trach when cuff is deflated or to call for nurse if unsure."

Review Questions

1. How should the nurse record smoking history for a patient who has smoked 2.5 packs of cigarettes per day for 10 years?
   1. Patient has smoked cigarettes for 10 years.
   2. Patient smokes 2.5 packs of cigarettes per day.
   3. Patient has a 12.5 pack-year smoking history.
   4. Patient has a 25 pack-year smoking history.

2. Which term should be used to document the musical sounds generated by airflow through narrowed airways?
   1. Crackles
   2. Wheezes
   3. Friction rub
   4. Stridor

3. Which laboratory result should alert the nurse to perform further assessment on a patient admitted with respiratory distress?
   1. Partial pressure of carbon dioxide ($Paco_2$) less than 50 mm Hg
   2. Bicarbonate ions (HCO_3^-) less than 27 mEq/L
   3. Partial pressure of oxygen (Pao_2) less than 90 mm Hg
   4. Oxygen saturation (Spo_2) less than 90%

4. Place the following steps in the correct sequential order for obtaining a sputum specimen for culture.
   1. Have the patient cough deeply from the lungs.
   2. Teach the patient to inhale deeply several times.
   3. Check the order for the test.
   4. Send the specimen immediately to the laboratory.
   5. Obtain the appropriate container.

5. Which instruction is correct when teaching a patient how to use a traditional metered-dose inhaler?
   1. "Inhale deeply, place canister in mouth, depress top of canister, exhale."
   2. "Exhale, place canister in mouth, inhale while depressing canister."
   3. "Cough, place canister in mouth, inhale deeply, cough again."
   4. "Exhale, depress canister, place in mouth, inhale deeply."

6. Which nursing interventions can improve comfort in a
patient with a continuous positive airway pressure mask?
Select all that apply.
   1. Use an adhesive barrier to protect skin from the mask.
   2. Remove the mask for sleeping.
   3. Use a humidifier to reduce dryness.
   4. Tape the patient's eyes closed.
   5. Maintain patient in semi-Fowler position.

Answer rationales available in your online resources.

ANSWERS 1. 4; 2. 3; 3. 4; 4. 3, 5, 2, 1, 4; 5. 2; 6. 1, 3, 5

Key Points

Find the chapter key points in your online resources
available through Davis Edge.

Additional Resources

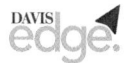 Use the scratch off code on the inside front
cover of your book to access online quizzes
that will help you to improve your scores
on course exams and prepare for NCLEX-PN®.

 Study Guide

CHAPTER 30
Nursing Care of Patients With Upper Respiratory Tract Disorders

Paula D. Hopper

KEY TERMS

dysphagia (dis-FAY-jee-ah)
epistaxis (EP-uh-STAX-is)
exudate (EKS-yoo-date)
laryngectomee (lare-in-JEK-tuh-mee)
laryngitis (lare-in-JY-tis)
myalgia (my-AL-jyah)
nasoseptoplasty (NAY-zoh-SEP-toh-plas-tee)
pharyngitis (fair-in-JY-tis)
rhinitis (ry-NY-tis)
rhinoplasty (RY-noh-plas-tee)
sinusitis (SY-nuh-SY-tis)

CHAPTER CONCEPTS

Comfort
Grief and Loss
Infection
Oxygenation

LEARNING OUTCOMES

1. Explain the pathophysiologies of disorders of the upper respiratory tract.
2. Describe etiologies, signs, and symptoms of disorders of the upper respiratory tract.
3. Describe current therapeutic measures for disorders of the upper respiratory tract.
4. Plan nursing care for the patient with an upper respiratory disorder.
5. Discuss how you will know whether your care has been effective.
6. Identify the special needs of the patient who has undergone a laryngectomy.

Disorders of the upper respiratory tract include problems occurring in the nose, sinuses, pharynx, larynx, and trachea. Many of these problems are minor illnesses that can be cared for at home. Others can become serious if they are not recognized and treated in a timely manner.

 DISORDERS OF THE NOSE AND SINUSES

Epistaxis
Pathophysiology
Epistaxis is more commonly known as a nosebleed. The nose can bleed either from the anterior or posterior region. Anterior bleeds are much more common and originate from a group of vessels called the Kiesselbach plexus. Anterior bleeds are easier to locate and treat than posterior bleeds. The blood vessels of the posterior nose are larger, and bleeding can be severe and difficult to control.

Etiology
The most common cause of epistaxis is dry, cracked mucous membranes. Trauma, forceful nose blowing, nose picking, and tumors are also factors. Anything that reduces the blood's ability to clot, such as hemophilia or leukemia, regular aspirin use, anticoagulant therapy, or chemotherapy, can predispose a patient to nosebleeds. Cocaine use can also cause epistaxis. High blood pressure can prolong a nosebleed but is not usually the cause.

Therapeutic Measures
Instruct a patient with a nosebleed to sit in a chair and lean forward slightly to avoid aspirating or swallowing blood. If the patient swallows blood, it will be difficult to assess the extent of bleeding. Also, it might cause nausea and vomiting. Be sure to wear gloves and follow standard precautions. Place pressure on the nares for 5 to 10 minutes to stop bleeding. However, avoid placing pressure on the nose if a fracture is

suspected to avoid further trauma. Ice packs to the nose and eye area may be used to constrict the bleeding vessels.

If first aid measures are ineffective in stopping bleeding, the health care provider (HCP) may attempt more invasive treatment. Local application of a vasoconstrictive agent such as phenylephrine (Neo-Synephrine) might be used to constrict the bleeding vessels. If the bleeding vessel can be located, the HCP may cauterize it by use of an electrical cauterizing device or by application of silver nitrate.

Gauze may be used to pack the anterior nasal cavity. The cavity is packed firmly but gently, usually with half-inch petroleum or iodoform gauze. Placement and removal of packing can be uncomfortable for the patient. If there is time, administer an analgesic before the procedure. Petroleum jelly on the packing helps prevent gauze from adhering to the nasal mucosa. If the packing is to remain in place for several days, it is coated with an antibiotic ointment to reduce the risk of infection. Oral antibiotics may be ordered.

Commercial products such as compressed sponges and nasal tampons are available to pack the nose. For anterior and posterior bleeds, balloon catheters such as the Rapid Rhino device can be inserted and inflated near the bleeding vessels in the nasal cavity (Fig. 30.1). The inflated balloon places pressure on the vessels to stop the bleeding. A small Foley catheter can also be used for this procedure. If these measures are not effective,

materials such as a gelatin sponge or a tiny coil can be inserted into the bleeding artery. Patients who are treated for posterior bleeding are typically hospitalized until they are stable.

If the patient has lost a significant amount of blood, intravenous (IV) fluid replacement or a transfusion may be needed. Nosebleeds rarely cause death because blood loss lowers blood pressure, which in turn slows the bleeding. Ultimately, the cause of the epistaxis is determined and corrected if possible. Rarely, surgical correction may be necessary for repeat episodes of epistaxis.

Nursing Care for the Patient With Epistaxis

Monitor bleeding, noting the amount and color of drainage. Monitor vital signs and hemoglobin level for signs of excessive blood loss. If the patient swallows repeatedly, inspect the back of the throat for bleeding. If bleeding does not stop within 10 to 15 minutes or if it worsens, notify a registered nurse (RN) or HCP immediately.

If posterior packing has been used, monitor the patient for airway obstruction from a slipped device. Know how to remove the device in case of emergency. Institute comfort measures, and maintain the placement of the external portion of the device. The HCP will remove the packing or catheter. Once bleeding is controlled, caution the patient not to blow the nose for up to 48 hours and to avoid nose picking. The patient should also avoid bending over, which can increase pressure in the nose. If the cause of the bleeding is dryness, teach the patient to use nasal saline spray or a room humidifier.

CRITICAL THINKING

Mr. Jondahl is brought to the emergency room with a nosebleed. His vital signs are blood pressure 140/90 mm Hg, pulse 92 beats per minute, and respirations 20 breaths per minute. He states that he has never had a nosebleed before. He denies any history of coagulation disorders. His current medications include captopril (Capoten), furosemide (Lasix), and ibuprofen (Motrin). What are two areas you should assess further in trying to determine a cause? (Hint: If you are not familiar with Mr. Jondahl's medications, look them up.)

Suggested answers are at the end of the chapter.

Nasal Polyps
Pathophysiology and Etiology

Polyps are grapelike clusters of mucosa in the nasal passages. They are usually benign, but they can obstruct the nasal passages and are sometimes complicated by sinus infections. Although the exact cause is unknown, they are related to chronic inflammation, and people with allergies are prone to developing them. They are also associated with cystic fibrosis. Some patients with nasal polyps also have asthma and are allergic to aspirin. This is called *aspirin-exacerbated respiratory disease (AERD)*. People with AERD produce high levels of leukotrienes, which promote inflammation.

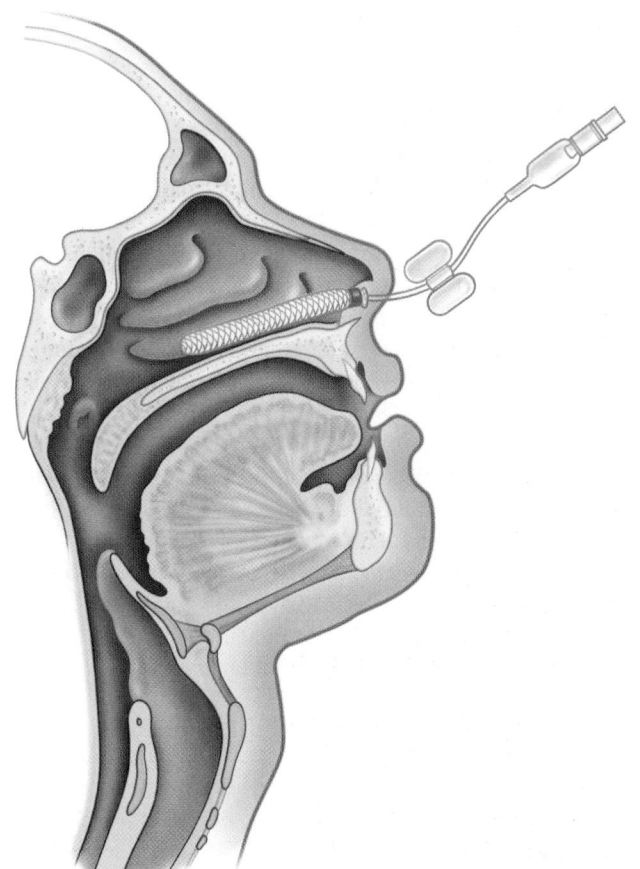

FIGURE 30.1 Rapid Rhino. Courtesy of ArthroCare, Inc., Austin, TX.

Therapeutic Measures

Control of allergy symptoms may help control polyp development. Oral antihistamines, leukotriene antagonists, or nasal corticosteroid sprays can help control symptoms. Some patients may benefit from aspirin desensitization and treatment. Antibiotics are used if there is a related sinus infection. If polyps obstruct breathing, they can be removed. This is done as an outpatient procedure under local anesthesia, using laser or endoscopic surgery. Patients are taught to avoid aspirin products after surgery because they increase the risk of postoperative bleeding and recurrence of the polyps.

Deviated Septum

Pathophysiology and Etiology

The septum dividing the nasal passages is slightly deviated in most adults. This may result from nasal trauma but often has no cause. Some septa may be so deviated that they block sinus drainage or interfere with breathing.

Signs and Symptoms

The patient may report a chronically stuffy nose or discomfort from blocked sinus drainage. Some patients have headaches, sinus infections, or nosebleeds.

Therapeutic Measures

Symptoms may be treated with decongestants, antihistamines, or intranasal cortisone sprays to reduce inflammation. However, if the deviated septum is causing chronic problems, a **nasoseptoplasty** can be done. This surgery involves revising or removing the deviated portion of the septum. Nasal packing is then placed to reduce bleeding. This is typically done as an outpatient surgical procedure under local anesthesia.

Nursing Care for the Patient After Nasoseptoplasty

After surgery, monitor vital signs and bleeding until the patient is stable. Excessive swallowing should alert you to check for blood running down the back of the throat. The patient will have nasal packing and a "mustache dressing" of folded gauze under the nose to catch drainage.

Most patients are discharged home once they are stable, so teaching is important. Box 30.1 details additional care and teaching following nasal surgery.

Rhinoplasty

Rhinoplasty is the surgical reconstruction of the nose, usually for cosmetic purposes. It may also be done to correct deformity caused by trauma. Nursing care is similar to that for the patient after nasoseptoplasty.

Sinusitis

Pathophysiology and Etiology

Sinusitis is inflammation of the mucosa of one or more sinuses. It can be either acute or chronic. Chronic sinusitis is diagnosed if symptoms have existed for more than 3 months and are unresponsive to treatment. The maxillary and ethmoid sinuses are the most commonly affected. The inflammation is

---

Box 30.1

Patient Education

Nasal Surgery

1. Your nose will feel stuffy and may drain. Change the moustache dressing as often as needed. Do *not* blow your nose. If you must sneeze, do so with your mouth open.
2. Avoid strenuous exercise, including swimming, for several weeks.
3. Drink plenty of fluids unless your health care provider (HCP) advises otherwise.
4. Use a cool mist vaporizer to humidify air and prevent nasal drying.
5. Keep your head elevated on two pillows or sleep in a recliner chair.
6. Expect some bruising around your eyes.
7. Use an ice pack on your face to help reduce swelling and bruising.
8. Take pain medication as prescribed. Antibiotics may be prescribed if packing is in place.
9. Avoid aspirin because it can increase bleeding.
10. Request a stool softener if needed to avoid straining to have a bowel movement.
11. Call your HCP if you experience bleeding that doesn't stop, excessive swelling, or a fever.
12. Avoid alcohol and smoking. Alcohol can increase congestion; smoking can delay healing.
13. Return to see your HCP for removal of packing as directed. Check hospital or surgeon policy for specific instructions.

---

often the result of a bacterial infection. It may follow a cold or other viral upper respiratory illness. Because the mucous lining of the nose and sinuses is continuous, nasal organisms easily travel to the sinuses. When the infected mucous lining of the sinuses swells, drainage is blocked. Bacteria that normally reside in the sinuses multiply in the retained secretions. The most common infecting organisms are *Streptococcus pneumoniae* and *Haemophilus influenzae*. Other causes of sinusitis include swelling caused by allergies, nasal polyps, fungal infection, or intubation with a nasotracheal or nasogastric tube.

Signs and Symptoms

The patient usually has pain over the region of the affected sinuses and purulent nasal discharge. If a maxillary sinus is affected, the patient will have pain over the cheek and upper teeth. In ethmoid sinusitis, pain occurs between and behind the eyes. Pain in the forehead typically indicates frontal sinusitis. Fever may be present in acute infection, with or without generalized fatigue and foul breath.

• WORD • BUILDING •

nasoseptoplasty: naso—nose + septo—septum + plasty—to mold, as in plastic surgery

rhinoplasty: rhin—nose + plasty—to mold, as in plastic surgery

sinusitis: sinu—sinus + itis—inflammation

Complications

The patient who has received inadequate treatment or who has not complied with treatment is at risk for complications. Uncontrolled sinusitis may spread to surrounding areas, causing osteomyelitis, cellulitis of the orbit (infection of the soft tissues around the eye), abscess, or meningitis. Sinusitis can also trigger asthma symptoms.

Diagnostic Tests

Uncomplicated sinusitis may be diagnosed based on symptoms alone. If repeated episodes occur, x-ray examination, nasal endoscopy, computed tomography (CT) scan, or magnetic resonance imaging (MRI) may be done to confirm the diagnosis and determine the cause. Nasal discharge may be cultured to determine appropriate antibiotic therapy.

Therapeutic Measures

Treatment is aimed at relieving pain and promoting sinus drainage. Nasal irrigation with normal saline solution helps some sufferers of chronic sinusitis. Corticosteroids, usually via a nasal spray (such as fluticasone [Flonase]), reduce inflammation. Adrenergic nasal sprays, such as oxymetazoline (Afrin), constrict blood vessels and, therefore, reduce swelling. However, they should be used cautiously by patients with heart disease or hypertension because vasoconstriction increases blood pressure. Adrenergic sprays may be used for up to 3 days; longer use may cause rebound congestion. Warm, moist packs over the affected sinus for 1 to 2 hours twice a day may help decrease inflammation. Acetaminophen or ibuprofen is given for pain and fever. Oral fluids and a room humidifier can help loosen secretions. Antihistamines dry and thicken secretions and usually are avoided. Antibiotics are not recommended for most sinus infections. If conservative treatment does not relieve symptoms, the HCP may surgically drain the affected sinus and irrigate it with normal saline or an antibiotic solution.

One such drainage procedure is the Caldwell-Luc procedure. The surgeon enters the maxillary sinus above the upper teeth, under the upper lip. The infected mucosa and bone are removed, and a new, larger opening is made to drain the sinus. Newer procedures, now more common, use nasal endoscopy to open and drain a chronically infected sinus.

Nursing Care for the Patient With Sinusitis

Patients with uncomplicated sinusitis are cared for at home. Instruct the patient to increase water intake to 8 to 10 glasses per day unless contraindicated. Excess water might be contraindicated in patients with fluid overload, such as those with cardiovascular or kidney disease. Pressure may be relieved if the patient maintains a semi-Fowler position, as in a reclining chair. Explain the use of warm and moist packs, analgesics, and prescribed medications. If antibiotics are ordered, instruct the patient to finish the antibiotic prescription even if he or she is feeling better before it is completed. Advise the patient to call the HCP if pain becomes severe or if signs of complications, such as a change in level of consciousness, occur.

Sleep Apnea
Pathophysiology and Etiology

The patient with obstructive sleep apnea (OSA) has periods of apnea during sleep. This most often occurs when sleeping supine. The muscles of the throat relax, and the tongue and soft tissues fall back to obstruct the airway (Fig. 30.2). The resulting hypoxemia sends a signal to take a breath, causing a sudden, loud inhalation. This can occur up to 100 times an hour throughout the night. Men are affected more often

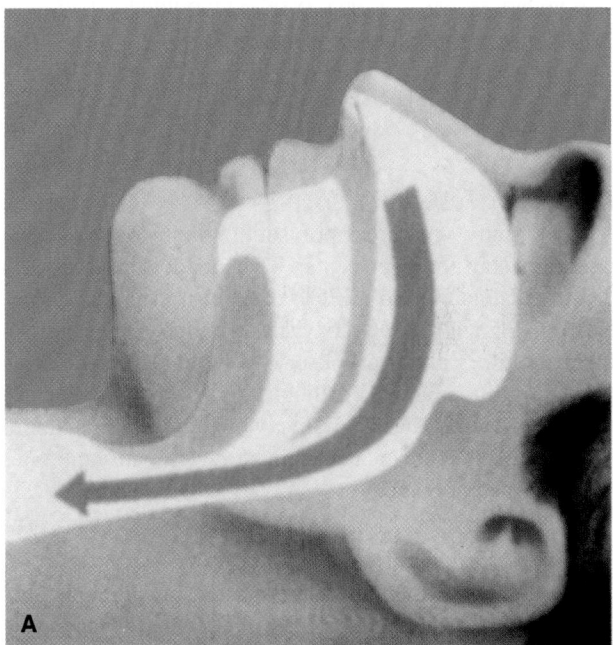

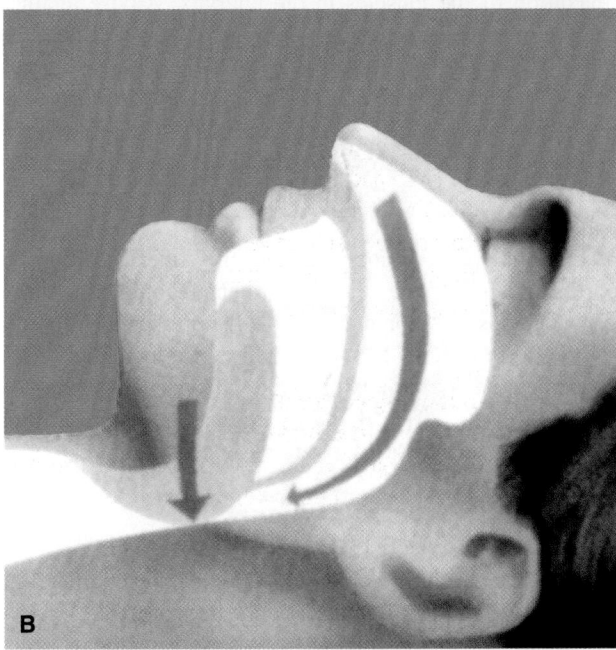

FIGURE 30.2 Obstructive sleep apnea (OSA). (A) Normal open airway. (B) Obstructed airway in OSA. Courtesy of Philips Respironics, Murrysville, PA.

than women, as are those who are overweight, are smokers, or have high arched palates or receding jawlines. OSA is associated with increased risk for heart disease, high blood pressure, stroke, and diabetes.

Signs and Symptoms

Ask the sleeping partner of someone with sleep apnea, and he or she will tell you that sleep apnea is noisy. When the tongue falls back and obstructs the airway, the result is total silence. When breathing resumes, it is like a very loud snore. Spouses often find themselves lying awake waiting for the next breath. Because the quality of sleep is impaired, the sufferer may awaken feeling unrested and with a headache, be sleepy throughout the day, and may have difficulty with memory and attention. Sudden sleepiness can make driving dangerous.

Diagnostic Tests

A sleep study (nocturnal polysomnography) involves an overnight stay at a sleep center. The patient is hooked up to electroencephalogram (EEG), electrocardiogram (ECG), electromyography (EMG), oxygen saturation, and eye movement monitors and then observed while sleeping. Many people find it somewhat difficult to fall asleep hooked up to so many wires, but a sedative would alter the results of the test. A less sophisticated form of the test can sometimes be performed at home.

Therapeutic Measures

Teach patients self-care measures such as avoiding alcohol or sedatives at bedtime; these can worsen apnea by increasing relaxation of the muscles in the pharynx. Advise against sleeping on the back, and encourage smoking cessation. Weight loss may help reduce sleep apnea and is also a good idea for reducing cardiovascular and diabetes risks. A newer treatment involves nasal patches (such as Provent) that have valves that impede airflow on exhalation, causing increased pressure in the airway. This holds the airway open during exhalation.

Evidence-based guidelines from the American College of Physicians provide three treatment recommendations: (1) weight loss, (2) noninvasive positive-pressure ventilation (NIPPV; see Chapter 29), and (3) use of a mandibular advancement device (a mouthpiece to advance the mandible) (Qaseem et al., 2013). If all other measures have failed, surgery may be necessary to remove excess tissue.

NURSING CARE TIP

If your patients have trouble avoiding sleeping on their back, have them sew a pocket on the back of an old tee shirt and put a tennis ball in it. As soon as patients roll over onto the ball, they will quickly be back on their side!

 ### INFECTIOUS DISORDERS

Viral Rhinitis/Common Cold
Pathophysiology and Etiology

Rhinitis (also called coryza) is inflammation of the nasal mucous membranes. The release of histamine and other substances causes vasodilation and edema. It may occur as a reaction to allergens (sometimes called hay fever) such as pollen, dust, molds, or some foods. It may also be caused by viral or bacterial infection. Viral rhinitis is another name for the common cold. The most common cold virus is the rhinovirus, which is contagious.

Signs and Symptoms

Common symptoms include nasal congestion, localized itching, sneezing, sore throat, and nasal discharge. Viral or bacterial rhinitis may also be accompanied by fever and malaise. Sometimes it is difficult to differentiate between a cold and influenza (flu). Table 30.1 lists signs and symptoms of each.

Diagnostic Tests

A throat culture or rapid flu test can help identify whether symptoms are caused by the flu virus.

Prevention

Staying away from others who are ill and good hand hygiene are the best preventive measures.

Therapeutic Measures

Treatment of viral rhinitis is symptomatic. Because colds are caused by viruses, antibiotics are not effective. Inappropriate use of antibiotics can lead to antibiotic-resistant infections. Explain to the patient that taking antibiotics for a viral infection is not only ineffective but also potentially dangerous.

Acetaminophen can be used for generalized discomfort. Decongestants cause vasoconstriction, which reduces swelling and congestion. Any drugs that cause vasoconstriction should be used cautiously in patients with heart disease or hypertension. Cough syrups and cold medicines should be used with caution. They do not treat the underlying cause of the cold and often contain several drugs, many of which are not really needed. Teach the patient that rest and fluids are the most effective treatment (see "Nursing Care Plan for the Patient With an Upper Respiratory Infection"). Echinacea, vitamin C, and zinc are alternative remedies that might help reduce the severity or length of symptoms by supporting the immune system. However, there is not enough evidence to be sure at this time.

• WORD · BUILDING ·
rhinitis: rhin—nose + itis—inflammation

Table 30.1

Differentiating Respiratory Tract Infections

Signs and Symptoms	Cold	Influenza	Bacterial Infection
Onset	Slow	Sudden	Usually slow
Fever	None or low grade	Common, may exceed 101°F (38.3°C)	Common, may exceed 101°F (38.3°C)
Headache	Rare	Common	Less common
Muscle aches	Less common	Common, may be severe	Less common
Cough	Present	Present, usually dry	Present, may be dry or productive
Chest pain	Absent	Common	Common
Fatigue	Slight	Common, prolonged, may be severe	Common
Runny nose	Common	Less common	Less common
Sore throat	Common	Less common	Less common
Complications	Rare	Pneumonia	Pneumonia
Treatment	Rest and fluids	Rest and fluids, antiviral agents in some cases	Antibiotics

Evidence-Based Practice

Clinical Question
Are antibiotics useful for the common cold or purulent rhinitis?

Evidence
Eleven research studies were reviewed. Researchers found that patients receiving antibiotics did not do better than those receiving placebos and had higher risk for adverse effects (Kenealy & Arroll, 2013).

Implications for Nursing Practice
Routine use of antibiotics for the common cold or purulent rhinitis is not recommended.

Reference
Kenealy, T., & Arroll, B. (2013). Antibiotics for the common cold and acute purulent rhinitis. *Cochrane Database of Systematic Reviews, 2013*(6). CD000247. doi:10.1002/14651858.CD000247.pub3

Pharyngitis
Pathophysiology and Etiology

Pharyngitis, or inflammation of the pharynx, is usually related to bacterial or viral infection. It may also occur as a result of trauma to the tissues. From 5% to 15% of pharyngitis cases are caused by beta-hemolytic streptococci, commonly referred to as strep throat. If strep throat is not treated with antibiotics, it can lead to rheumatic fever, glomerulonephritis, or other serious complications.

Signs and Symptoms
The most common symptom of pharyngitis is a sore throat. Some patients may also experience **dysphagia** (difficulty swallowing). The throat appears red and swollen, and **exudate** (drainage or pus) may be present. Exudate usually signifies bacterial infection and may be accompanied by fever, chills, headache, and generalized malaise.

Diagnostic Tests
The HCP may order a rapid streptococcal antigen test or a throat culture and sensitivity test (explained in Chapter 29) to identify the causative organism and determine which antibiotic will be effective.

Therapeutic Measures
If the pharyngitis is bacterial, antibiotics are ordered. Penicillin is commonly used for streptococcal infection. Acetaminophen or throat lozenges may be used to relieve discomfort. Saltwater gargles (one-quarter teaspoon of salt in a glass of warm water) or honey and lemon mixed with warm water help soothe

· WORD · BUILDING ·
pharyngitis: pharyng—pharynx + itis—inflammation
dysphagia: dys—bad + phagia—to swallow
exudate: to sweat out

Nursing Care Plan for the Patient With an Upper Respiratory Infection

Nursing Diagnosis: *Impaired Comfort* related to infectious process
Expected Outcomes: The patient will be comfortable as evidenced by statement of increased comfort and ability to swallow and sleep at night.
Evaluation of Outcomes: Does the patient express comfort? Is the patient able to sleep?

Intervention	Rationale	Evaluation
Assess for cause of discomfort (e.g., malaise, muscle aches, fever, sore throat).	*Knowing the cause of discomfort helps guide intervention.*	Can interventions be directed toward specific symptoms?
Offer acetaminophen or nonsteroidal anti-inflammatory drugs (NSAIDs) as ordered.	*Analgesics relieve pain. Antipyretics relieve fever, which may contribute to discomfort.*	Do analgesics/antipyretics relieve symptoms?
Offer throat lozenges, saltwater, or honey and lemon gargles as ordered for irritated throat.	*Lozenges or gargles soothe irritated mucous membranes.*	Do measures relieve throat irritation?
Encourage rest.	*Physical stress increases need for sleep. Rest boosts immune function.*	Is patient resting comfortably?

Nursing Diagnosis: *Hyperthermia* related to infectious process
Expected Outcomes: The patient will have a temperature lower than 103°F (39.4°C) and show no signs/symptoms of dehydration.
Evaluation of Outcomes: Is the patient's fever controlled at a safe level? Is the patient well hydrated?

Intervention	Rationale	Evaluation
Monitor temperature daily; every 4 hours if fever present.	*Screening helps detect temperature changes early.*	Is patient febrile?
If patient begins chilling, recheck temperature when chilling subsides.	*Chilling indicates rising temperature.*	Is chilling present? Should temperature be checked more often?
Monitor for signs of dehydration (e.g., dry skin and mucous membranes, thirst, weakness, hypotension).	*Fever causes loss of body fluids.*	Are signs of dehydration present?
Encourage oral fluids if not contraindicated.	*Fluids prevent or treat dehydration.*	Is patient taking fluids well?
Administer antipyretic such as acetaminophen if fever is higher than 102°F (39°C) or for discomfort.	*Antipyretics reduce fever. Fever enhances immune function and so should be treated only if high, if patient has a history of febrile seizures, or if patient is uncomfortable.*	Is fever higher than 102°F (39°C)? Are antipyretics indicated? Are they effective?
If fever rises above 103°F (39.4°C) in an adult, contact health care provider (HCP).	*A fever above 103°F (39.4°C) can indicate more serious infection and may require treatment.*	Is fever above 103°F? Has HCP been contacted? (*Note:* Ask pediatrician about fever in a child.)

Nursing Care Plan for the Patient With an Upper Respiratory Infection—cont'd

Nursing Diagnosis: *Risk for Infection* (transmission to others) related to presence of infectious disease
Expected Outcomes: Risk for infection of others will be reduced, as evidenced by the patient stating measures to prevent transmission and the patient taking precautions against spread.
Evaluation of Outcomes: Is transmission to others prevented?

Intervention	Rationale	Evaluation
Assess patient's understanding of infection transmission.	*Understanding of mode of transmission is essential to prevention.*	Does patient understand how infection is transmitted?
Based on patient's previous knowledge, teach patient and all caregivers the importance of good hand hygiene after contact with patient or patient's belongings, to cover nose and mouth when coughing or sneezing, and to not share eating or drinking utensils. See cough etiquette guidelines in Chapter 8.	*Hand hygiene prevents spread of infection. Covering nose and mouth prevents spread of infectious droplets. Many infections are transmitted via contaminated objects.*	Does patient take precautions to prevent spread of infection?

inflamed tissues. Encourage fluids (if not contraindicated) and rest. (See "Nursing Care Plan for the Patient With an Upper Respiratory Infection.")

Laryngitis
Pathophysiology and Etiology
Laryngitis is an inflammation of the mucous membrane lining the larynx (voice box). It can be caused by irritation from smoking, alcohol, chemical exposure, gastroesophageal reflux disease (GERD), or a viral, fungal, or bacterial infection. It often follows an upper respiratory infection. Laryngeal cancer can also cause symptoms of laryngitis.

Signs and Symptoms
The most common symptom is hoarseness. Cough, dysphagia, or fever may also be present.

Diagnostic Tests
The HCP may use a tiny mirror to view the larynx. If hoarseness persists for more than 2 weeks, a laryngoscopy and biopsy may be done to rule out cancer of the larynx.

Therapeutic Measures
Treatment includes rest, fluids, humidified air, and aspirin (adults only) or acetaminophen. Antibiotics are used if bacterial infection is present. Medication to control acid reflux is used if GERD is the cause. Encourage the patient to rest the voice. Advise the patient that whispering strains the voice even more than normal speech. Use paper and pen to help the

patient communicate. Throat lozenges may help increase comfort. Help the patient to identify and avoid causative factors. (See "Nursing Care Plan for the Patient With an Upper Respiratory Infection.")

Tonsillitis/Adenoiditis
Pathophysiology and Etiology
The tonsils are masses of lymphoid tissue that lie on each side of the oropharynx. They filter microorganisms to protect the lungs from infection. Tonsillitis occurs when the filtering function becomes overwhelmed with a virus or bacteria and infection results. The adenoids, a mass of lymphoid tissue located at the back of the nasopharynx, can also become involved. Tonsillitis is more common in children but is more serious when it occurs in adults. Tonsillitis is usually viral, but bacteria that are commonly associated with tonsillitis include *Streptococcus* species, *Staphylococcus aureus, H. influenzae,* and *Pneumococcus* species.

Signs and Symptoms
Tonsillitis usually begins suddenly with a sore throat, fever, chills, and pain on swallowing. Generalized symptoms include headache, malaise, and **myalgia.** On examination, the tonsils appear red and swollen and may have yellow or white

• WORD • BUILDING •
laryngitis: laryng—larynx + itis—inflammation
myalgia: myo—muscle + algia—pain

exudate on them. If the adenoids are involved, the patient may experience snoring, a nasal obstruction, and a nasal tone to the voice.

Diagnostic Tests

A throat culture is done to discover the causative organism and determine effective treatment. A white blood cell count and differential can also help identify whether the infection is viral or bacterial. A chest x-ray may be done if respiratory symptoms are present.

Therapeutic Measures

Antibiotics are prescribed for bacterial infection. Acetaminophen, lozenges, and saline gargles help promote comfort. For care of the patient who is not having a tonsillectomy, see "Nursing Care Plan for the Patient With an Upper Respiratory Infection."

If tonsillitis becomes chronic or if breathing or swallowing is affected, a tonsillectomy may be considered, although this is not a common procedure in an adult. An adenoidectomy may be performed at the same time. After the tonsillectomy, the patient is maintained in a semi-Fowler position to reduce swelling and promote drainage. Monitor the patient for bleeding and airway patency, and provide comfort measures. Encourage fluids for hydration; cold fluids may help reduce pain and bleeding. Red-colored drinks are avoided because they interfere with observation for bleeding. A room humidifier helps prevent drying. Keep suction equipment available for emergencies.

CRITICAL THINKING

Mrs. Hiler is recovering after a tonsillectomy. She is sleeping, but you notice that she swallows every few seconds. She has an intravenous (IV) line of normal saline solution running at 100 mL per hour.

1. How do you respond?
2. What should you be vigilant for?
3. At how many drops per minute should her IV run if the tubing has a drop factor of 15?

   Suggested answers are at the end of the chapter.

Influenza
Pathophysiology and Etiology

Influenza, commonly called the *flu,* is a viral infection of the respiratory tract. Many different flu viruses have been identified, and new strains appear each year. Influenza is the cause of millions of lost workdays each year. Young children, chronically ill patients, and older adults are at increased risk for complications and even death from influenza because of compromised immune function.

Influenza is easily transmitted via droplets from coughs and sneezes of infected people. It may be transmitted by physical contact with a person or object that harbors the virus. The incubation period from time of exposure to onset of symptoms is 1 to 3 days.

Prevention

According to Healthy People 2020, influenza leads to more than 200,000 hospitalizations and 36,000 deaths each year. One of the Healthy People 2020 goals is to reduce, eliminate, or maintain elimination of cases of vaccine-preventable diseases (Office of Disease Prevention and Health Promotion, 2017). The Centers for Disease Control and Prevention (2017) recommends a yearly flu vaccine for anyone older than 6 months of age. Although Medicare covers the cost of a flu shot, many older adults do not get one. Emphasize to older people that they will not get the flu from the shot because it does not contain a live virus. Once the shot has been administered, it takes about 2 weeks for antibodies to develop; it is then effective for about 4 months. Other important preventive measures include hand hygiene and avoidance of people with influenza. Visit www.cdc.gov/flu for more information.

BE SAFE!

Use hand cleaning guidelines from the Centers for Disease Control and Prevention or the World Health Organization. Set goals for improving hand cleaning. (Joint Commission's 2018 National Patient Safety Goals, © The Joint Commission, 2018. Reprinted with permission.)

BE SAFE!

Patients who have had severe reactions to eggs should receive the flu vaccine in a setting where reactions can be treated. Flu vaccines contain small amounts of egg protein. While rare, reactions can be deadly.

Signs and Symptoms

Symptoms of flu include abrupt onset of fever, chills, myalgia, sore throat, cough, general malaise, and headache. Flu can last for 2 to 5 days, with malaise lasting up to several weeks.

Complications

The most common complication of influenza is pneumonia, which may be caused by the same virus as the flu or by a secondary bacterial infection. This should be suspected if the patient has persistent fever and shortness of breath or if the lungs develop crackles or wheezes.

Diagnostic Tests

Viral cultures of throat or nasal swabbing can be done to identify influenza, but results may take 3 to 10 days.

Rapid tests can identify the presence of flu virus in less than 15 minutes in an office setting but are less reliable than cultures. Cultures may also be done to rule out bacterial infection. Once influenza has been identified in a geographical area, HCPs will test less often and treat based on symptoms.

Therapeutic Measures

Treatment is primarily symptomatic. Acetaminophen is given for fever, headache, and myalgia. Aspirin is avoided in children because it increases the risk of Reye syndrome. Rest and fluids are essential. Antibiotics are used only if a secondary bacterial infection is present.

Antiviral medications, such as zanamivir (Relenza, an inhaled agent) and oseltamivir (Tamiflu, an oral medication), may reduce the severity and duration of symptoms if given within 48 hours of becoming ill. Antiviral agents may also be given prophylactically to high-risk people who have not been immunized or to control outbreaks in high-risk situations, such as in long-term care facilities.

Nursing Care for the Patient With Influenza

Older adults or other high-risk patients may be hospitalized for treatment of influenza. These patients are closely monitored for complications. Assess lung sounds and vital signs every 4 hours and monitor for dehydration. Report changes to an RN or HCP. Encourage rest and fluids (if not contraindicated), and provide comfort measures. Teach patients and families not to give aspirin to treat influenza symptoms in children aged under 18 years because of the risk of Reye syndrome. (See "Nursing Care Plan for the Patient With an Upper Respiratory Infection.")

CRITICAL THINKING

Mrs. Murdock is a 97-year-old resident of a long-term care facility who develops flu symptoms. She is lethargic, confused, and feverish. Because of her mental status changes, you want to send her to the hospital, but her son asks you to please keep her where she is. She has a history of chronic obstructive pulmonary disease (COPD) and diabetes.

1. How could Mrs. Murdock have caught the flu?
2. How could it have been prevented?
3. What can be done now to prevent her from developing complications that could lead to pneumonia or even death?
4. What other concerns do you have?
5. What other team members should you involve in her care?

Suggested answers are at the end of the chapter.

Other Respiratory Viruses

West Nile virus is less deadly than some flu viruses but can still cause serious complications. West Nile virus is transmitted from birds to humans by mosquitoes. It causes either no symptoms or flu-like symptoms. However, in a few people, especially older adults, it can progress to encephalitis (inflammation of the brain) and meningitis (inflammation of the covering of the brain and spinal cord). Teach patients to prevent exposure by using mosquito repellent and to eliminate standing water where mosquitoes lay eggs. There is no specific treatment for West Nile virus. Patients who develop complications are hospitalized for supportive care.

Other viruses that have caused concern in recent years include avian influenza (bird flu), severe acute respiratory syndrome (SARS), and H1N1 (swine flu).

 ## MALIGNANT DISORDERS

Cancer of the Larynx
Pathophysiology

Cancer of the larynx (the voice box) usually develops in the squamous cells of the mucosal epithelium. It is evaluated based on the tumor-node-metastasis (TNM) staging system described in Chapter 11. It is most often a primary cancer and can spread to the lungs, liver, or lymph nodes. The prognosis for a patient with laryngeal cancer is good with early diagnosis but is poor when diagnosis and treatment are delayed.

Etiology

Risk factors for cancer of the larynx include a history of alcohol and tobacco use. Exposure to industrial chemicals or hardwood dust, chronic overuse of the voice, and a diet low in fruits and vegetables are also factors. Men are more likely to be affected than women.

Prevention

Prevention begins with education. You can help educate patients about the relationship between cancer of the larynx and use of alcohol and tobacco. It is also important to teach patients to seek help when symptoms first occur because a delayed diagnosis may mean metastasis of the cancer and a poor prognosis. Teach that any hoarseness that lasts longer than 2 weeks should be investigated by a HCP.

Signs and Symptoms

The most common symptom is persistent hoarseness because the vocal cords are located in the larynx (Table 30.2). The patient may also have throat or ear pain, shortness of breath, a chronic cough, and difficulty swallowing. Stridor may indicate a tumor obstructing the airway. Late signs include weight loss and halitosis (foul breath).

Diagnostic Tests

Laryngoscopic examination and biopsy are used to diagnose and determine the stage of laryngeal cancer. CT scan, MRI,

Table 30.2
Laryngeal Cancer Summary

Signs and Symptoms	Hoarse voice Pain Cough Shortness of breath Difficulty swallowing Weight loss Foul breath
Diagnostic Tests	Examination with laryngeal mirror Laryngoscopy with biopsy Additional blood and radiographic studies to detect metastasis
Therapeutic Measures	Radiation therapy Chemotherapy (adjunct to radiation or surgery) Endoscopic laser surgery to destroy tumor Partial laryngectomy (preserves some voice) Radical neck dissection with total laryngectomy (loss of voice)
Priority Nursing Diagnoses	*Ineffective Airway Clearance* *Acute Pain* *Impaired Verbal Communication* *Risk for Imbalanced Nutrition: Less Than Body Requirements* *Impaired Swallowing* *Grieving* *Disturbed Body Image*

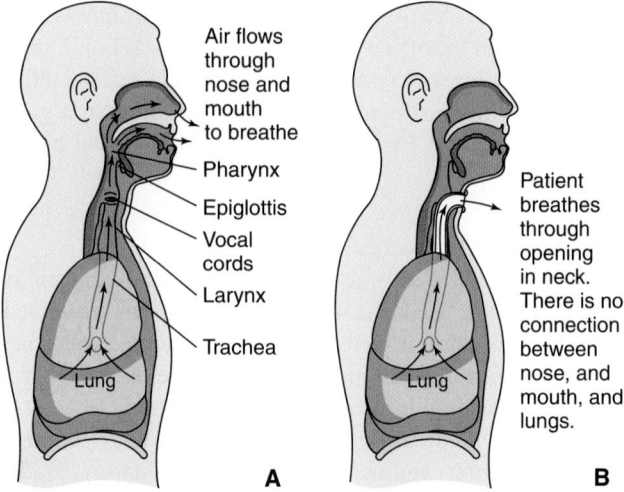

FIGURE 30.3 (A) Before laryngectomy. (B) After laryngectomy.

Several alternatives for speech exist:

- Esophageal speech involves swallowing air and forming words as the air is regurgitated back up the esophagus.
- Electronic devices are available, which the patient places next to the neck or mouth. These devices use sound vibrations to help the patient form words. UltraVoice is an electronic device that is placed inside an upper denture or retainer, and the patient speaks into a small microphone (Fig. 30.4A).
- Another alternative is a tracheoesophageal puncture (TEP), such as the Blom-Singer voice prosthesis, which uses a surgically implanted voice prosthesis that creates a valve between the trachea and esophagus. If the patient holds a finger over the laryngectomy, air is diverted into the esophagus and the patient forms words as the air exits the mouth (Fig. 30.4B).

All of these devices take time to adjust to, and the patient will need support after discharge to continue to develop communication skills.

LEARNING TIP

Did you ever "burp the ABCs" as a child? If not, ask most any child to demonstrate! This uses the same idea as esophageal speech.

---

or other diagnostic tests may be done to determine the presence or extent of metastasis.

Therapeutic Measures

If laryngeal cancer is diagnosed early in the disease, it may be treatable with radiation therapy; this treatment can preserve the patient's voice. Chemotherapy may be used with radiation or surgery, but it is not usually used alone. New targeted chemotherapy attacks only certain cells in the body. Surgery may be done at any stage of the disease. The larynx will be either partially or completely removed (Fig. 30.3). If cancer has spread beyond the larynx, a radical neck dissection, which removes adjacent muscle, lymph nodes, and tissue, may be done. Surgery can be done using laser technology, endoscopy, or traditional methods.

After a partial laryngectomy, the patient may have a permanently hoarse voice. If a total laryngectomy is done, the patient will have a permanent tracheostomy (in this case, called a laryngectomy) tube in place and no voice. The patient will need to learn alternative methods of communication. A person who has had a total laryngectomy is sometimes referred to as a **laryngectomee.**

Nursing Process for the Patient Undergoing Total Laryngectomy

PREOPERATIVE CARE. In addition to routine preoperative teaching, the patient undergoing a total laryngectomy surgery must be prepared for the loss of ability to breathe through the mouth and nose and loss of ability to speak.

· WORD · BUILDING ·

laryngectomee: laryng—larynx + ectome—excision (person who has undergone laryngectomy)

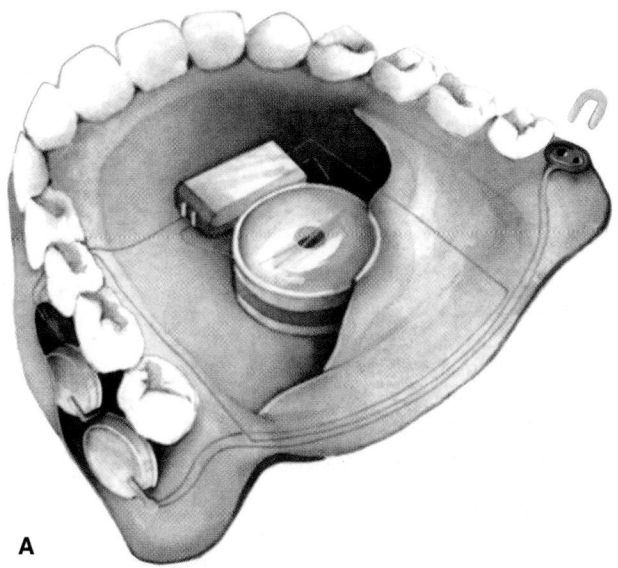

A

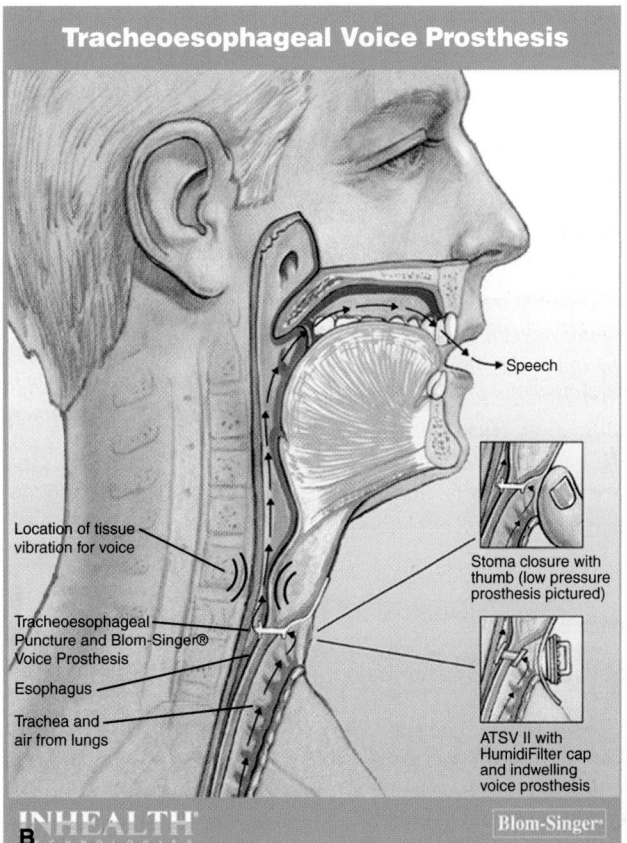

Tracheoesophageal Voice Prosthesis

Speech

Location of tissue vibration for voice

Tracheoesophageal Puncture and Blom-Singer® Voice Prosthesis

Esophagus

Trachea and air from lungs

Stoma closure with thumb (low pressure prosthesis pictured)

ATSV II with HumidiFilter cap and indwelling voice prosthesis

INHEALTH TECHNOLOGIES

B

Blom-Singer® voice restoration systems

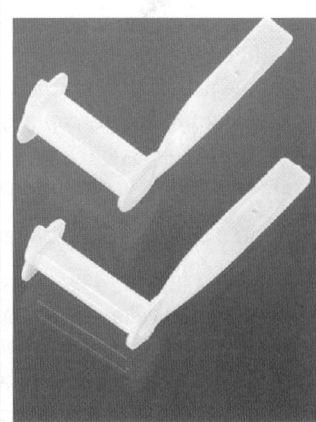

FIGURE 30.4 Devices to aid speech in the laryngectomy patient. (A) UltraVoice is an electronic device placed inside a denture or retainer; the patient speaks into a small microphone. Courtesy of UltraVoice Ltd., Newtown Square, PA. (B) The Blom-Singer voice prosthesis diverts air into the esophagus and out the mouth to form tracheoesophageal speech. Courtesy of InHealth Technologies, Carpinteria, CA.

Initial instruction in communication techniques should take place before surgery to prevent the patient from feeling panicky after surgery when he or she cannot speak. A variety of techniques and devices are available. Consult a speech therapist before surgery to provide a picture board, magic slate, or paper and pencil (see Chapter 49). Instruct the patient to point to the picture that corresponds with the need or to write out his or her concern. A dietary consult is also important before surgery if the patient has been undernourished.

POSTOPERATIVE CARE.

Data Collection. Collecting data about the patient's physical and psychosocial status, comfort, nutritional status, and ability to swallow is important both before and after surgery. After surgery, assessment of airway patency and respiratory function takes priority. Monitor lung sounds, oxygen saturation, and arterial blood gases. In addition, be sure to assess the patient's understanding of the disease process and self-care needs after surgery. It is important to evaluate the patient's support systems and ability to cope with the partial or total loss of voice after surgery.

Nursing Diagnoses, Planning, and Implementation.

Ineffective Airway Clearance *related to excessive secretions and new tracheostomy/laryngectomy*

EXPECTED OUTCOME: The patient will maintain a clear airway as evidenced by clear lung sounds and ability to cough up secretions.

- Monitor and record amount, color, and consistency of secretions; vital signs; oxygen saturation; lung sounds; and signs of respiratory distress. *Visible secretions from the stoma, a drop in oxygen saturation (SpO$_2$), or an increase in crackles may indicate airway compromise and a need for suctioning. A change in amount or color of secretions, increased temperature, or presence of adventitious sounds can indicate infection and should be reported to the HCP immediately.*
- Provide tracheostomy care and suctioning according to agency policy (see Chapter 29) *to keep the airway clear.*
- Maintain strict sterile technique with tracheostomy care and suctioning. *Prevention of infection is essential, because the airway no longer has the protection of normal upper airway defense mechanisms.*
- Place the patient in semi-Fowler position *to allow for lung expansion and more effective coughing.*
- Encourage the patient to deep breathe and cough every hour *to keep airway free of secretions.*
- Administer oxygen as ordered. A special tracheostomy collar should be used. *Supplemental oxygen helps maintain oxygenation. The oxygen must be applied to the stoma because there is no connection between the nose and lungs.*
- Provide room or oxygen humidification. *Humidification can help keep secretions mobile.*
- Avoid use of powders, sprays, or other airborne materials near the patient. *These can cause irritation or infection if they enter the laryngectomy.*

Acute Pain *related to surgical procedure*

EXPECTED OUTCOME: The patient will state his or her pain level is acceptable.

- Assess pain level every 4 hours and as needed. *A good assessment must guide treatment.*
- Assess sedation and respiratory status often. Opioids are given carefully *because they may reduce respiratory rate and cough reflex, which is vital to clearing the airway.*
- Include nonpharmacological pain control interventions (see Chapter 10). *Interventions such as distraction and relaxation may help with pain control and reduce (not eliminate) the need for opioids.*
- Administer analgesics as ordered, on an around-the-clock basis or via patient-controlled pump, for the first few days after surgery. If the liver has been damaged from previous alcohol use, dosages are adjusted by the HCP. *The patient who is comfortable will be better able to participate in care and take measures to prevent complications, such as coughing and ambulating.*

Impaired Verbal Communication *related to loss of vocal cords*

EXPECTED OUTCOME: The patient will be able to communicate his or her needs.

- Use a picture board or paper and pencil *so the patient can communicate without speaking.*
- Make sure the patient has a call light or bell nearby at all times. *Patients can become panicky if they have a need and no way to summon a nurse.*
- Work with the speech therapist and HCP to provide the patient with a method of communication that best fits his or her needs (see Fig. 30.4). *Different patients prefer different long-term communication methods.*

Risk for Imbalanced Nutrition: Less Than Body Requirements *related to absence of oral feeding immediately following surgery and possible previous alcohol use or abuse*

EXPECTED OUTCOME: The patient's weight will be within normal limits for height and age.

- Monitor weight. *Underweight or weight loss reflects inadequate nutrition.*
- Monitor parenteral nutrition or tube feedings after surgery until the neck has begun to heal and swallowing can be evaluated. *Nutrition must be maintained to support healing.*
- Consult a dietitian for nutrition guidance. If the patient has a history of alcohol abuse, he or she may have been undernourished before surgery. *You may need to advocate for the patient and ensure that he or she is receiving adequate calories for healing. A dietitian can assist with specific recommendations.*

Impaired Swallowing *related to edema or presence of laryngectomy tube*

EXPECTED OUTCOME: The patient will be able to swallow safely.

- Consult a speech therapist to assist with a swallowing assessment and recommendations. *Speech therapists are trained to assess and treat swallowing disorders.*
- Assure the patient that aspiration will not occur *because there is no longer a connection between the mouth and the lungs.*
- Place the patient in high-Fowler position *to make swallowing easier.*
- Stay with the patient during the first attempts *to eat to help alleviate anxiety.*

Grieving *related to loss of voice*

EXPECTED OUTCOME: The patient will express feelings of loss and begin to plan for the future.

- Assess the patient's feelings of loss. *Inability to speak is a loss that cannot be overemphasized. The patient may also be facing a career change if job-related exposure contributed to the disease or if loss of voice prevents return to a previously held job.*

- Actively listen to the patient's communication of feelings *to show your support and validate feelings.*
- Assess and involve support systems. *Family support is important to the patient's long-term adjustment to a laryngectomy.*
- Contact the patient's clergy if patient wishes. *A religious counselor can help with grief and spiritual distress.*

Disturbed Body Image related to change in body structure and function

EXPECTED OUTCOME: The patient will verbalize acceptance of new laryngectomy and participate in self-care.

- Portray an accepting attitude. *Patients are very aware of nurses' nonverbal behavior, and looks of distaste can be disturbing.*
- Allow the patient to share feelings if he or she indicates a need to do so. *This may help the patient to work through feelings about the changes to his or her body image.*
- With the patient's permission, contact a local support group that may have names of people who have had similar experiences who are willing to visit with the patient. *Such visitors can provide firsthand information and support.*
- Assist the patient to find ways to camouflage the change, such as scarves or necklines that conceal but do not obstruct the airway. *Camouflage can help the patient feel less conspicuous while protecting the airway.*

Evaluation. When evaluating the patient's progress toward goals, ask the following questions:

- Is the airway clear, without signs of infection or obstruction?
- Does the patient verbalize an acceptable level of comfort?
- Do the patient and significant others demonstrate understanding of self-care at home or have referrals to continue learning self-care at home?

- Does the patient indicate satisfaction with the level and quality of communication?
- Is the patient's weight stable?
- Is the patient able to swallow if taking oral nutrition?
- Is the patient able to grieve appropriately?
- Does the patient have someone to talk to if he or she wishes to do so?
- Does the patient show acceptance of the laryngectomy by learning to care for it?

Note that many of these evaluative criteria are long-term and may not be seen while the patient is hospitalized, so follow-up by a home health nurse is essential.

Patient Education. After assessing the patient's readiness to learn, teach the patient self-care measures for the laryngectomy, including how to perform cleaning and suctioning (see Chapter 29). Teach the patient to protect the laryngectomy from water and debris. Lightweight scarves or purchased products can protect the stoma. Involve the significant other or family whenever possible.

The patient must also be instructed to perform gentle range-of-motion exercises of the neck. Some patients may avoid extending the neck because of the location of the incision, causing muscle contracture.

Referral to a home health care agency after discharge will provide assessment of the home environment as well as follow-up instruction. A social service referral may be made for financial or psychosocial concerns if needed. Consult with the HCP or check the local phone directory for laryngectomee support groups, and refer the patient to them if appropriate. The local branch of the American Cancer Society may also be able to provide information. Assist the patient in finding resources to support alcohol and smoking cessation. Continued alcohol and tobacco use will increase the patient's risk of cancer recurrence.

To find additional information for laryngectomees, visit the National Cancer Institute website at www.cancer.gov.

SUGGESTED ANSWERS TO CRITICAL THINKING

Mr. Jondahl
Explore the amount of ibuprofen being taken daily because nonsteroidal anti-inflammatory drugs (NSDAIDs) can interfere with platelet aggregation. In addition, high blood pressure can aggravate the bleeding.

Mrs. Hiler
1. Mrs. Hiler may be swallowing blood. Examine the back of her throat with a flashlight. Check vital signs for evidence of impending shock. Notify a health care provider (HCP) if bleeding is confirmed.
2. Continue to be vigilant for signs of bleeding (e.g., frequent swallowing or bright red blood from the mouth). Monitor for changes in vital signs and report even small changes to the registered nurse (RN) or HCP.

3. Use this formula to determine drops per minute:

$$\frac{100 \text{ mL}}{1 \text{ hour}} \cdot \frac{1 \text{ hour}}{60 \text{ minutes}} \cdot \frac{15 \text{ gtt}}{1 \text{ mL}} = 25 \text{ gtt per minute}$$

Mrs. Murdock
1. Mrs. Murdock may have contracted the flu from a visitor or a staff person at the long-term care facility. Most health care facilities require flu vaccines of all employees. She is susceptible because of her age and comorbid conditions (i.e., chronic obstructive pulmonary disease [COPD], diabetes).
2. Mrs. Murdock's flu could probably have been prevented with a flu vaccination, but her son refused it because he

Continued

SUGGESTED ANSWERS TO CRITICAL THINKING—cont'd

believed it could cause her to get the flu. Good hand hygiene by staff and urging visitors not to visit when ill will also help.

3. If it is within 48 hours of symptom onset, an HCP may prescribe an antiviral agent to help reduce her symptoms and shorten the course of her illness. In addition, you can provide fluids, acetaminophen, and comfort measures. You should also monitor her closely for evidence of bacterial infection or pneumonia and report signs or symptoms immediately to the HCP.

4. A major concern is that Mrs. Murdock could transmit the flu to other residents or staff, although they should all have been vaccinated. In addition, you must decide whether to send Mrs. Murdock to the hospital. Check her advance directives and talk to her son about goals for her care. If needed, educate him about differences in long-term care and hospital care.

5. Involve the RN, supervisor or director, and infection control nurse. Collaborate to determine not only how to manage Mrs. Murdock but also ways to protect other residents.

Review Questions

1. Which is the best explanation to a patient by a nurse for why a health care provider does not prescribe antibiotics for influenza?
   1. "Most cases of influenza are caused by antibiotic-resistant bacteria."
   2. "Influenza is caused by viruses."
   3. "Antibiotics have too many serious side effects."
   4. "Antibiotics can interact with other medications used for influenza."

2. After a laryngectomy, which of the following assessments takes priority?
   1. Airway patency
   2. Nutritional status
   3. Lung sounds
   4. Patient acceptance of surgery

3. Which of the following responses is correct when a patient asks why the health care provider did not order a new antiviral drug for flu symptoms that started 3 days ago?
   1. "Antiviral drugs are for acquired immunodeficiency syndrome, not the flu."
   2. "The side effects of the antiviral drugs are worse than having the flu."
   3. "Antiviral drugs are only prescribed for children."
   4. "Antivirals work best if you start them within 48 hours after flu symptoms begin."

4. Which of the following positions is recommended for a patient experiencing a nosebleed?
   1. Lying down with feet elevated
   2. Sitting up with neck fully extended
   3. Lying down with a small pillow under the head
   4. Sitting up leaning slightly forward

5. The nurse knows that the patient understands teaching related to prevention of influenza transmission when the patient demonstrates which behaviors? **Select all that apply.**
   1. Washing hands frequently
   2. Covering the nose and mouth during coughing or sneezing
   3. Taking acetaminophen as ordered
   4. Drinking extra fluids
   5. Avoiding sharing eating utensils with others
   6. Taking antibiotics until the entire prescription is finished

6. Which of the following communication methods is inappropriate for the patient with a total laryngectomy?
   1. Placing a finger over the stoma
   2. Providing a special valve that diverts air into the esophagus
   3. Obtaining a picture board
   4. Teaching the patient esophageal speech

Answer rationales available in your online resources.

ANSWERS 1. 2. 1; 3. 4. 4; 5. 1, 2, 5; 6. 1

Key Points

Find the chapter key points in your online resources available through Davis Edge.

Additional Resources

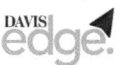 Use the scratch off code on the inside front cover of your book to access online quizzes that will help you to improve your scores on course exams and prepare for the NCLEX-PN®.

 Study Guide

CHAPTER 31

Nursing Care of Patients With Lower Respiratory Tract Disorders

Paula D. Hopper

KEY TERMS

anergic (AN-ur-jik)
antitussive (AN-tee-TUS-iv)
atelectasis (AT-eh-LEK-tah-sis)
atypical (ay-TIP-ih-kuhl)
blebs (BLEBS)
bronchiectasis (BRONG-key-EK-tah-sis)
bronchitis (brong-KY-tis)
bronchodilator (BRONG-koh-DY-lay-ter)
bronchospasm (BRONG-koh-spazm)
bullae (BUL-ah)
ectopic (ek-TOP-ik)
emphysema (EM-fih-SEE-mah)
empyema (EM-pye-EE-mah)
exacerbation (egg-ZAS-ur-BAY-shun)
expectorant (eks-PEK-tah-rant)
exudate (EKS-yoo-dayt)
hemoptysis (hee-MOP-tih-sis)
hemothorax (HEE-moh-THOR-aks)
induration (IN-doo-RAY-shun)
lobectomy (loh-BEK-tuh-mee)
mucolytic (MYOO-koh-LIT-ik)
paradoxical respiration (PEAR-uh-DOK-sih-kuhl
    RES-per-AY-shun)
pleurodesis (PLOO-roh-DEE-sis)
pneumonectomy (NOO-moh-NEK-tuh-mee)
pneumothorax (NOO-moh-THOR-aks)
polycythemia (PAW-lee-sy-THEE-mee-ah)
status asthmaticus (STAT-us az-MAT-ih-kus)
tachypnea (TAK-ip-NEE-uh)
thoracotomy (THOR-ah-KOT-ah-mee)

CHAPTER CONCEPTS

Acid–Base Balance
Infection
Oxygenation
Perfusion

LEARNING OUTCOMES

1. Explain the pathophysiology of each of the disorders of the lower respiratory tract.
2. Describe the etiologies, signs, and symptoms of each of the disorders.
3. Identify tests that are used to diagnose lower respiratory disorders.
4. Describe therapeutic measures used for disorders of the lower respiratory tract.
5. List data to collect when caring for patients with disorders of the lower respiratory tract.
6. Plan nursing care for patients with disorders of the lower respiratory tract.
7. Identify interventions for patients experiencing impaired gas exchange, ineffective airway clearance, or ineffective breathing pattern.
8. Explain how you will know whether your nursing interventions have been effective.

Disorders of the lower respiratory tract include problems of the lower portion of the trachea, bronchi, bronchioles, and alveoli. These disorders may be related to infection, noninfectious alterations in function, neoplasm (cancer), or trauma. Any pathological condition of the lower respiratory tract can seriously impair carbon dioxide and oxygen exchange.

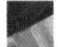 INFECTIOUS DISORDERS

Acute Bronchitis

Bronchitis is an inflammation of the bronchial tree. The bronchial tree includes the right and left bronchi, secondary bronchi, and bronchioles. When the mucous membranes lining the bronchial tree become irritated and inflamed, excessive mucus is produced. The result is congested airways. Acute bronchitis is usually an isolated episode, caused by a virus. If bronchitis occurs more than 3 months out of the year for two consecutive years, chronic bronchitis is

• WORD • BUILDING •
bronchitis: bronch—airway + itis—inflammation

diagnosed. See the discussion of chronic bronchitis later in this chapter for more information that applies to both the acute and chronic forms.

Bronchiectasis
Pathophysiology
Bronchiectasis is a dilation of the bronchial airways (Fig. 31.1). The dilated areas become flabby and scarred. Bronchiectasis can remain localized or spread throughout the lungs. Secretions pool in these areas and are difficult to cough up. This creates an environment where bacteria can flourish, and infection is common.

Etiology
Bronchiectasis usually occurs secondary to another chronic respiratory disorder, such as cystic fibrosis, asthma, tuberculosis, bronchitis, or exposure to a toxin. Airway obstruction from a tumor or foreign body can also be a predisposing factor. Infection and inflammation of the airways in these underlying disorders weaken the bronchial walls and reduce ciliary function. Airway obstruction from excessive secretions then predisposes the patient to development of bronchiectasis. Vitamin D deficiency may play a role in bronchiectasis (Bekir et al., 2016).

Signs and Symptoms
The patient with bronchiectasis experiences recurrent lower respiratory infections. Sputum is copious and purulent. The accompanying cough can produce as much as 200 mL of thick, foul-smelling sputum in a single episode of coughing. Extreme airway inflammation may cause sputum to be bloody. If bronchiectasis is widespread throughout the lungs, the patient may experience dyspnea even with minimal exertion. Wheezes and crackles may be auscultated. Fever is present during active infection. Cor pulmonale (right-sided heart failure; covered in Chapter 26) and clubbing of the fingers may develop with chronic disease.

Diagnostic Tests
A chest x-ray examination is done, but it may not show early disease. A computed tomography (CT) scan provides a better view of the dilated airways. Bronchoscopy may be done, if needed. Sputum cultures determine infecting organisms and guide antibiotic therapy. Additional testing may be done to determine the cause of bronchiectasis.

Therapeutic Measures
Treatment is aimed at keeping the airways clear of secretions, controlling infection, and correcting the underlying problem, if possible. Antibiotics may be used intermittently or for prolonged periods. Azithromycin (Zithromax) may reduce **exacerbations** (acute worsening of symptoms). Measures to prevent infection, including vaccinations for flu and pneumonia, should be implemented. **Bronchodilators** relax smooth muscle in the airways to reduce obstruction. **Mucolytic** agents and **expectorants** help loosen and mobilize secretions so they can be coughed up. Bronchitol, a form of mannitol, is an inhaled mucolytic that promotes mucus clearance. It is a sugar that draws fluid into the airways to help liquefy mucus. Anti-inflammatory agents such as corticosteroids or leukotriene inhibitors reduce airway inflammation.

Chest physiotherapy (CPT) or a high-frequency chest wall oscillation vest can help mobilize secretions. Noninvasive positive-pressure ventilation (NIPPV; see Chapter 29) can help maintain oxygenation. Oxygen is used if hypoxemia is present. Oral fluids are encouraged. If the affected area of the lung is localized and symptoms are severe, surgery may be considered to remove the diseased area. Lung transplant may be considered in severe cases. Nursing care is found in "Nursing Care Plan for the Patient With a Lower Respiratory Tract Disorder."

> **NURSING CARE TIP**
> If your patient is coughing up a lot of sputum, line an emesis basin with a white tissue. This makes it easier to assess the color of the sputum and simplifies cleaning out the basin!

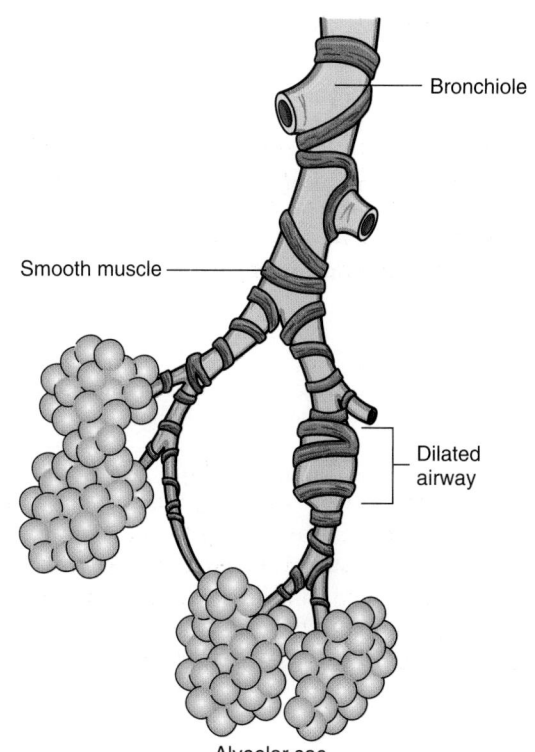

FIGURE 31.1 Bronchiectasis. Note dilated airway.

Labels: Bronchiole, Smooth muscle, Dilated airway, Alveolar sac

• **WORD** • **BUILDING** •
bronchiectasis: bronch—airway + ectasis—dilation or expansion
bronchodilator: broncho—airway + dilator—to expand
mucolytic: muco—mucus + lytic—break up
expectorant: ex—out of + pec—chest

Nursing Care Plan for the Patient With a Lower Respiratory Tract Disorder

Note: The most commonly used nursing diagnoses related to respiratory disorders are presented in the following care plan. This is not a care plan for any one respiratory disorder. Rather, use it as a reference when one of the nursing diagnoses applies to the patient, based on a thorough respiratory assessment.

Nursing Diagnosis: *Impaired Gas Exchange* related to decreased ventilation or perfusion as evidenced by partial pressure of oxygen (Pao_2) less than 80 mm Hg, partial pressure of carbon dioxide ($Paco_2$) greater than 45 mm Hg, or peripheral capillary oxygen saturation (Spo_2) less than 90%, statement of dyspnea

Expected Outcomes: The patient will experience improved gas exchange, as evidenced by improving arterial blood gases (ABGs) or pulse oximetry and statement of acceptable level of dyspnea.

Evaluation of Outcomes: Are the patient's ABGs or Spo_2 improving? Does the patient state that dyspnea is resolved or controlled at an acceptable level?

Intervention	Rationale	Evaluation
Monitor ABG values and pulse oximetry as ordered.	*Pao_2 less than 80 mm Hg, $Paco_2$ greater than 45 mm Hg, or Spo_2 less than 90% indicate impaired gas exchange.*	Are values within patient's baseline values?
Assess degree of dyspnea on a scale of 0 to 10, with 0 being dyspnea and 10 being worst dyspnea.	*The patient's subjective report is the best measure of dyspnea; dyspnea indicates impaired gas exchange.*	Is patient's degree of dyspnea within parameters that are acceptable to patient?
Assess lung sounds, respiratory rate and effort, use of accessory muscles.	*Respiratory rate less than 12 per minute or more than 24 per minute or use of accessory muscles indicates distress. Diminished or adventitious lung sounds can indicate risk factors for impaired gas exchange.*	Are lung sounds clear and audible? Is respiratory rate 12 to 20 per minute and unlabored?
Observe skin and mucous membranes for cyanosis.	*Cyanosis indicates poor oxygenation. Oral mucous membrane cyanosis indicates serious hypoxia.*	Are skin and mucous membranes cyanotic?
Monitor for confusion or changes in mental status.	*Changes in mental status can signal impaired gas exchange.*	Is patient alert and oriented? If not, could poor gas exchange be the reason?
Elevate head of bed or help patient to lean on over-bed table.	*Upright positioning promotes lung expansion.*	Did change of position relieve some distress?
Position with good lung dependent ("good lung down").	*This position allows the healthier lung to be better perfused and increases gas exchange.*	Is Spo_2 improved in this position?
Administer supplemental oxygen as ordered.	*Supplemental oxygen decreases hypoxemia.*	Is oxygen placed properly on patient? Does it provide relief from dyspnea?
Place a fan in patient's room or provide a handheld fan.	*The handheld fan directed toward the face reduces feelings of breathlessness.*	Is a fan available to patient, and does it help?
Teach patient relaxation exercises.	*Relaxation exercises decrease perceived dyspnea.*	Does patient use relaxation effectively?
For chronic disease, teach patient diaphragmatic and pursed-lip breathing. (See Chapter 29.)	*Breathing exercises promote relaxation and increase CO_2 excretion.*	Does patient use breathing exercises correctly? Do they help?
Encourage patient to stop smoking if patient is a current smoker.	*Smoking is damaging to lungs and respiratory function.*	Is patient receptive to smoking cessation? Are resources available?

Nursing Care Plan for the Patient With a Lower Respiratory Tract Disorder—cont'd

Intervention	Rationale	Evaluation
For severe dyspnea, ask health care provider (HCP) about an order for intravenous (IV) morphine sulfate.	*Low doses of IV morphine reduce anxiety and cause peripheral vasodilation, which helps relieve pulmonary edema.*	Does morphine provide relief from dyspnea?

Nursing Diagnosis: *Ineffective Airway Clearance* related to excessive secretions as evidenced by crackles or wheezes, and ineffective cough
Expected Outcome: The patient will have improved airway clearance as evidenced by clear breath sounds and ability to cough up secretions.
Evaluation of Outcome: Are the patient's breath sounds clear? Is the patient able to effectively cough up and expectorate secretions?

Intervention	Rationale	Evaluation
Assess lung sounds every 4 hours and as needed (prn).	*Crackles and wheezes may indicate excess secretions in airways.*	Do lung sounds indicate retained secretions?
Monitor amount, color, and consistency of sputum.	*Thick, purulent sputum indicates infection and should be reported to the HCP.*	Does sputum indicate infection?
Turn patient every 2 hours or encourage ambulating if able.	*Movement mobilizes secretions.*	Is patient mobile?
Encourage oral fluids; use cool steam room humidifier.	*Hydration decreases viscosity of secretions and aids expectoration.*	Is patient able to take oral fluids? Are secretions thin and easily expectorated?
Encourage patient to cough and deep breathe every hour and prn.	*Controlled coughing following deep breaths is more effective in clearing the airway.*	Does patient cough and deep breathe effectively?
Administer expectorants or mucolytics as ordered.	*Expectorants help liquefy secretions and trigger the cough reflex.*	Are expectorants effective?
If patient is unable to cough up secretions, suction per institution policy.	*Suctioning is necessary to remove secretions when patient is unable to cough effectively.*	Is suctioning necessary? Does it help remove secretions?
Obtain order for chest physiotherapy (CPT) or vibratory positive expiratory pressure (PEP) device, if indicated.	*CPT and PEP help mobilize secretions.*	Is CPT (or PEP) effective and well tolerated by patient?

Nursing Diagnosis: *Ineffective Breathing Pattern* related to anxiety or pain as evidenced by respiratory rate less than 12 per minute or greater than 24 per minute, labored or shallow respirations, and abnormal ABGs and Spo$_2$ values.
Expected Outcomes: The patient will maintain an effective breathing pattern as evidenced by a respiratory rate between 12 and 20 per minute that is even and unlabored, and ABG and oxygen saturation results within the patient's normal range.
Evaluation of Outcomes: Is the patient's respiratory rate within normal limits and unlabored? Does the patient's breathing pattern support normal ABG and Spo$_2$ values?

Intervention	Rationale	Evaluation
Assess respiratory rate, depth, and effort every 4 hours and prn.	*Respirations less than 12 per minute or more than 20 per minute may indicate an ineffective pattern.*	Is respiratory pattern ineffective?
Monitor ABG and oxygen saturation values	*An ineffective breathing pattern will not maintain oxygenation.*	Is breathing pattern adversely affecting oxygenation?

(nursing care plan continues on page 576)

Nursing Care Plan for the Patient With a Lower Respiratory Tract Disorder—cont'd

Intervention	Rationale	Evaluation
Determine and treat the cause of ineffective breathing pattern.	*Pain or anxiety can cause a patient to change the breathing pattern.*	Is a contributing factor identifiable and correctable?
Place patient in Fowler or semi-Fowler position.	*This allows for maximum chest expansion.*	Is patient in a comfortable position that enables adequate expansion?
Teach patient to use diaphragmatic breathing, with a regular 2-second in, 4-second out pattern.	*Breathing exercises promote relaxation and increase CO_2 excretion.*	Is patient able to demonstrate an effective breathing pattern?

Nursing Diagnosis: *Activity Intolerance* related to imbalance between oxygen supply and demand as evidenced by dyspnea or drop in Spo_2 with routine activity
Expected Outcomes: The patient will tolerate increasing activity level as appropriate based on prognosis, as evidenced by stable respiratory rate and Spo_2 with activity. The patient will receive assistance with self-care until he or she is able to carry out own activities of daily living (ADLs).
Evaluation of Outcomes: Are the patient's care needs met by self or caregiver?

Intervention	Rationale	Evaluation
Assess amount of activity patient can tolerate without becoming short of breath (SOB).	*Patients should be encouraged to do as much as they can for themselves to avoid becoming deconditioned.*	What is patient able to do?
Monitor vital signs and oxygen saturation with activities.	*Respiratory and heart rates will rise and Spo_2 will drop if activity is not tolerated.*	Are vital signs and Spo_2 stable?
Allow patient to rest between activities. Bedrest may be needed during acute dyspnea.	*Even talking or eating can be exhausting to a patient who is dyspneic.*	Is patient able to catch his or her breath between activities?
Obtain bedside commode, shower chair, and handheld showerhead, if needed.	*Assistive devices can help patient conserve energy.*	Do assistive devices allow patient more independence?
Obtain portable oxygen if patient is able to ambulate.	*Portable oxygen may enable patient to ambulate and prevent deconditioning.*	Is patient able to ambulate and maintain Spo_2 within normal limits with portable oxygen?
Allow uninterrupted rest at night as much as possible.	*Lack of sleep can contribute to activity intolerance.*	Is patient able to sleep uninterrupted? Can interferences be delayed until morning?
Slowly increase activity as able.	*Increasing activity helps maintain muscle tone and endurance.*	Is patient able to increase a little each day? Is this a realistic goal for patient?
Refer patient with chronic lung disease to a pulmonary rehabilitation program.	*Pulmonary rehabilitation programs can help patient increase exercise tolerance.*	Is patient willing to participate in a rehabilitation program?

Pneumonia

Pneumonia is the cause of many hospital admissions each year and is a common cause of death from infection. Persons at risk for pneumonia are the very young, adults over age 65, smokers, those with chronic disease, and people with compromised immune systems, such as those with AIDS, alcoholism, or who take medications that reduce immune function. Pneumonia is categorized according to where it is acquired. For example, hospital-acquired pneumonia (HAP) is defined as pneumonia that develops at least 48 hours after a hospital admission. One type of HAP is ventilator-associated pneumonia (VAP). Healthcare-associated pneumonia (HCAP) is pneumonia that develops in outpatient settings or nursing homes. Community-acquired pneumonia (CAP) develops in the community and is usually less serious than other forms. Each type of pneumonia may be caused by different organisms.

Pathophysiology

Pneumonia is an acute inflammation and/or infection of the lungs that occurs when an infectious agent enters and multiplies in the lungs of a susceptible person. Infectious particles can be transmitted by the cough of an infected individual, from contaminated respiratory therapy equipment, from infections in other parts of the body, or from aspiration of bacteria from the mouth, pharynx, or stomach. Organisms from the mouth and pharynx may be related to poor oral hygiene or may be present because of a cold or influenza virus. When pathogens enter the body of a healthy person, normal respiratory defense mechanisms and the immune system prevent the development of infection. In a person who is immunocompromised, however, even microorganisms that are normally present in the oropharynx can cause an infection.

When the microorganisms multiply, they release toxins that induce inflammation in the lung tissue, causing damage to mucous and alveolar membranes. This leads to the development of edema and **exudate,** which fills the alveoli and reduces the surface area available for exchange of carbon dioxide and oxygen. Some bacteria also cause necrosis of lung tissue.

Pneumonia may be confined to one lobe (lobar pneumonia), or it may be scattered throughout the lungs (bronchopneumonia). Bronchopneumonia occurs more often as HAP or in the very young or old, and can be quite serious. Patients may use terms such as *walking pneumonia* or *double pneumonia.* These are not medical terms, but it is helpful to understand them. *Walking pneumonia* refers to a mild infection that may not even keep the patient from working (or walking); *double* is a lay term for "bilateral."

Etiology

BACTERIAL PNEUMONIA. The most common cause of community-acquired bacterial pneumonias is *Streptococcus pneumoniae,* also called pneumococcal pneumonia. Other community-acquired infections are caused by *Staphylococcus aureus, Chlamydia trachomatis,* and *Mycoplasma pneumoniae.* HAPs are often antibiotic resistant and tend to be much more serious than CAPs. HAPs can be caused by *Escherichia coli, Haemophilus influenzae,* and *Klebsiella pneumoniae,* among others. Methicillin-resistant *Staphylococcus aureus* (MRSA), *Pseudomonas aeruginosa,* and other antibiotic-resistant pneumonias are especially difficult to treat.

VIRAL PNEUMONIA. Influenza viruses are the most common cause of viral pneumonia. The presence of viral pneumonia increases the patient's susceptibility to a secondary bacterial pneumonia. Generally, patients are less ill with viral pneumonia than with bacterial pneumonia, but they may be ill for a longer period because antibiotics are ineffective against viruses.

FUNGAL PNEUMONIA. *Candida* and *Aspergillus* are two types of fungi that can cause pneumonia. *Pneumocystis jiroveci* pneumonia (PJP) is caused by a fungus and typically causes pneumonia in patients with AIDS.

ASPIRATION PNEUMONIA. Some pneumonias are caused by aspiration of foreign substances. This most often occurs in patients with decreased levels of consciousness or an impaired cough or gag reflex. These conditions can occur with alcohol ingestion, stroke, general anesthesia, seizures, gastrointestinal reflux disease (GERD), or other serious illness. Aspiration pneumonia increases the risk for subsequent bacterial pneumonia.

VENTILATOR-ASSOCIATED PNEUMONIA. VAP is a type of aspiration pneumonia that develops in patients who are intubated and mechanically ventilated. The endotracheal (ET) tube keeps the glottis open, so secretions can be easily aspirated into the lungs.

CHEMICAL PNEUMONIA. Inhalation of toxic chemicals can cause inflammation and tissue damage, which can lead to chemical pneumonia. This increases the risk for subsequent bacterial infection.

Prevention

Both flu and pneumonia vaccination are essential to preventing pneumonia. All individuals age 6 months and older should receive the yearly flu vaccine. Check the Centers for Disease Control and Prevention (CDC; www.cdc.gov) web site for flu and pneumonia vaccine recommendations, which change frequently ("Gerontological Issues: Respiratory Infections in Advanced Age").

Nursing care plays an important role in the prevention of HAP. Regular coughing, deep breathing, and position changes for patients on bedrest or after surgery, prevention

---

• WORD • BUILDING •
exudate: to sweat out

Gerontological Issues

Respiratory Infections in Advanced Age. Advanced age is a significant risk factor for serious complications from respiratory infections such as influenza, pneumococcal pneumonia, and aspiration pneumonia. Therefore, it is recommended that people over age 65 and people with chronic disease have yearly influenza vaccines and two pneumococcal vaccines (a dose of pneumococcal conjugate vaccine [PCV13] first, followed by a dose of pneumococcal polysaccharide vaccine [PPSV23]). Consistent oral care and twice-yearly dental cleanings are important to help prevent morbidity and mortality from aspiration pneumonia.

of aspiration for patients at risk, and good hand hygiene practices by both patients and health care personnel can help prevent many cases.

The risk of VAP can be reduced with frequent mouth care using chlorhexidine and use of a special ET tube that allows continuous suctioning of secretions above the inflated cuff. All patients should be positioned with the head of the bed elevated 30 to 45 degrees to help prevent aspiration. Medication to reduce gastric acid secretion and stress ulcers may help reduce aspiration but may also increase bacterial growth.

CRITICAL THINKING

Mr. Smith is an 86-year-old man who was watching television when he couldn't sleep one night. After seeing a commercial for toilet cleaner, he decided his own toilet could use some attention. He used bleach and ammonia "to get it really clean." The combination created toxic fumes, which caused a severe chemical pneumonia. He was brought to the emergency room in acute respiratory distress.

1. As his nurse, what questions might you ask as you further assess the cause of his pneumonia?
2. What can you teach Mr. Smith related to prevention of similar episodes in the future?
3. How can you be vigilant in preventing complications in Mr. Smith?

Suggested answers are at the end of the chapter.

Signs and Symptoms

Patients with pneumonia present with fever, shaking, chills, chest pain, dyspnea, fatigue, and a productive cough. Sputum is purulent or may be rust-colored or blood-tinged. Crackles and wheezes may be heard on lung auscultation because of the exudate in the alveoli and airways.

Some bacterial and many viral pneumonias cause **atypical** symptoms. The patient may experience fatigue, sore throat, dry cough, or nausea and vomiting.

Older adult patients may not exhibit expected symptoms of pneumonia. New-onset confusion or lethargy in an older patient can indicate reduced oxygenation. This should alert you to look for other symptoms or request evaluation by the health care provider (HCP). New onset of fever or dyspnea should also cause suspicion of pneumonia in older adults.

BE SAFE!

Use the hand cleaning guidelines from the Centers for Disease Control and Prevention or the World Health Organization. Set goals for improving hand cleaning. Use the goals to improve hand cleaning. (The Joint Commission's 2018 National Patient Safety Goals, © The Joint Commission, 2018. Reprinted with permission.).

Complications

Complications from pneumonia most commonly occur in patients with other underlying chronic diseases. Pleurisy and pleural effusion (discussed later in this chapter) are two of the most common complications and generally resolve within 1 to 2 weeks. **Atelectasis** (collapsed alveoli) can occur as a result of trapped secretions. It may be resolved by efforts to keep the airways clear, such as use of an incentive spirometer. Other complications result from spread of infection to other parts of the body, causing septicemia, meningitis, septic arthritis, pericarditis, or endocarditis. Treatment for each of these is antibiotics. Although antibiotics can greatly reduce the incidence of death related to pneumonia, it is still a common cause of death in older people.

Diagnostic Tests

A chest x-ray examination is done to identify the presence of pulmonary infiltrate, which is fluid leakage into the alveoli from inflammation (Fig. 31.2). In addition, sputum and blood cultures are obtained to identify the organism causing the pneumonia and determine appropriate treatment. If the patient is unable to produce a sputum specimen, a nebulized mist treatment (NMT) may be ordered to promote sputum expectoration. Nasotracheal suctioning or a bronchoscopy can be done to obtain a specimen from a very ill patient.

NURSING CARE TIP

Obtain culture specimens before antibiotics are started to avoid altering culture results. The best time to obtain a specimen is first thing in the morning, before breakfast. If the patient has eaten, be sure he or she has rinsed the mouth to keep food particles out of the specimen.

• WORD • BUILDING •
atypical: a—not + typical—usual
atelectasis: atel—imperfect + ectasis—expansion

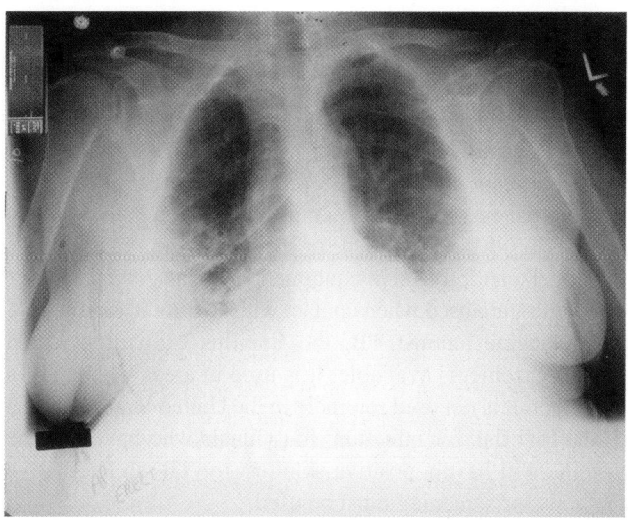

FIGURE 31.2 Chest x-ray examination showing infiltrates in pneumonia.

Therapeutic Measures

Broad-spectrum antibiotics are initiated as soon as cultures are sent to the lab, even if results are not completed. Once the culture and sensitivity (C&S) report is available, antibiotic orders may change to more narrow-spectrum agents. Many patients can be treated with oral antibiotics as outpatients. However, hospitalization and intravenous (IV) therapy may be necessary in older adults or in individuals who are chronically or acutely ill. If the pneumonia is caused by a virus, rest and fluids are recommended. Occasionally, antiviral medications are used.

Evidence-Based Practice

Clinical Question

What are nursing care activities that can help prevent ventilator-associated pneumonia (VAP)?

Evidence

In a systematic review, 18 studies provided high-quality evidence that chlorhexidine antiseptic mouth rinse or gel as part of oral hygiene care reduces risk of VAP from 25% to 19% (Hua et al., 2016).

Implications for Nursing Practice

Follow institution policy for oral hygiene care in ventilated patients. If chlorhexidine is not part of routine care, discuss its benefits with the registered nurse or health care provider.

Reference

Hua, F., Xie, H., Worthington, H. V., Furness, S., Zhang, Q., & Li, C. (2016). Oral hygiene care for critically ill patients to prevent ventilator-associated pneumonia. *Cochrane Database of Systematic Reviews, 2016*(10). CD008367. doi:10.1002/14651858.CD008367.pub3

Expectorants, bronchodilators, and analgesics may be given for comfort and symptom relief. NMTs or metered-dose inhalers (MDIs) may be used to deliver bronchodilators. Supplemental oxygen via nasal cannula or mask is used as needed. Nursing care is found in "Nursing Care Plan for the Patient With a Lower Respiratory Tract Disorder." (See "Evidence-Based Practice" and Table 31.1 for a pneumonia summary.)

Nursing Process for the Patient With Pneumonia

Nursing diagnoses for pneumonia include *Impaired Gas Exchange, Ineffective Airway Clearance,* and *Activity Intolerance.* These are found in "Nursing Care Plan for the Patient With a Lower Respiratory Tract Disorder."

Tuberculosis

Pathophysiology and Etiology

Tuberculosis (TB) is an infectious disease caused by the bacterium *Mycobacterium tuberculosis.* TB primarily affects the lungs, but the kidneys, liver, brain, and bone may be affected as well. *M. tuberculosis* is an acid-fast bacillus (AFB): When it is stained in the laboratory and then washed with an acid, the stain remains, or stays, "fast." *M. tuberculosis* can live in dark places in dried sputum for months but is killed in a few hours of direct sunlight. It is spread by inhalation of the TB bacilli from respiratory droplets (droplet nuclei) of an infected person.

Once the bacilli enter the lungs, they multiply and begin to disseminate to the lymph nodes and then to other parts of

Table 31.1

Pneumonia Summary

Signs and Symptoms	Fever, chills Chest pain Dyspnea Productive cough Crackles and wheezes
Diagnostic Tests	Chest x-ray Sputum cultures
Therapeutic Measures	Antibiotics Supplemental oxygen Bronchodilators Expectorants Rest, fluids
Complications	Pleurisy Pleural effusion Atelectasis
Priority Nursing Diagnoses	*Impaired Gas Exchange* *Ineffective Airway Clearance* *Activity Intolerance*

the body. The patient is then infected but may or may not go on to develop clinical (active) disease. TB infection without disease is called *latent TB infection* (LTBI). During this time the body develops immunity, which keeps the infection under control. If the lungs are involved, the immune system surrounds the infected area in the lung with neutrophils and alveolar macrophages. This process creates a lesion called a *tubercle,* which seals off the bacteria and prevents spread. Similar processes take place in other affected areas of the body. The bacteria within the tubercle die or become dormant, and the patient is no longer infectious. If the patient's immune system becomes compromised, however, some of the dormant bacteria can become active, causing active disease. Only 5% to 10% of infected people in the United States actually develop the disease. Even then, it may not occur for many years ("Gerontological Issues: Aging and Tuberculosis").

Gerontological Issues

Aging and Tuberculosis. The age-related decline in immune system function can decrease the effectiveness of the tuberculosis (TB) antibodies in someone who previously had latent infection. The TB bacilli can be activated, causing active disease. Because of the risk of false-negative tuberculin test results, a two-step test is recommended, with the second test done 1 to 3 weeks after the first. Decline in immune system function can also have an impact on clinical manifestations of TB. Patients may exhibit fewer symptoms, making recognition difficult.

Risk Factors

Crowded or poorly ventilated living conditions place people at risk for becoming infected with TB. Although TB can infect any age group, older people are especially at risk. While they may have contracted the disease many years before, it can reactivate as the aging process reduces immune function. AIDS, chronic drug or alcohol abuse, and certain drugs (e.g., chemotherapy and some drugs used for rheumatoid arthritis, Crohn disease, or psoriasis) can also compromise immune function and increase risk of activation. In the United States, TB is also prevalent among the urban poor and minority groups.

Before 1985, the incidence of TB in the United States was steadily decreasing. At that time, it began to increase in incidence, in part because of the prevalence of AIDS, the development of antibiotic-resistant strains of the TB bacillus, and ineffective treatment programs. Now it is again on the downswing.

Prevention

Clean, well-ventilated living areas are essential to the health of all people. If a hospitalized patient is known or suspected to have TB, he or she is placed in respiratory isolation to prevent spread to staff or other patients. Special negative-pressure isolation rooms are ventilated to the outside. Staff should wear special high-efficiency filtration masks when in the room of a patient with TB; a regular surgical mask is not effective against TB. Verify with the institution's infection control department that the masks provided are effective for use with TB patients. If the patient must travel through the hallway for tests or other activities, he or she must wear a mask. Additional personal protective equipment, such as gowns, gloves, or goggles, are used when contact with sputum is likely.

A vaccine against TB, the Bacillus Calmette–Guérin (BCG) vaccine, is available. It is used in areas where TB is prevalent. It is not used routinely in the United States because of the low risk for infection. Individuals who have had the vaccine will have a positive skin test for TB, so alternative methods for screening must be used.

Ultimately, prevention will come from adequate treatment of patients with TB. A current concern is the development of antibiotic-resistant strains of the TB bacillus, which can develop when patients are noncompliant with drug therapy. When antibiotics are taken intermittently or discontinued early, the more virulent (stronger) bacteria survive and multiply and become resistant to the drugs being used. This multidrug-resistant TB (MDR-TB) can then be passed on to someone else. Some strains are resistant to nearly all antibiotics. These strains are called extensively drug resistant TB (XDR-TB). It is, therefore, vital to teach all patients the importance of strict adherence to drug therapy. Patients who are at risk for nonadherence to drug therapy must have a visiting nurse or other health professional observe each dose of antibiotic taken. This is called directly observed therapy, or DOT. DOT transfers responsibility for making sure the drugs are taken from the patient to the health care worker. The World Health Organization reports the highest treatment success rates with DOT.

Because TB is much more prevalent in other countries, especially in Asia and Africa, Healthy People 2020 has developed a goal of reducing the case rate for foreign-born people living in the United States (Office of Disease Prevention and Health Promotion, 2017). This is essential to protecting both foreign-born and U.S.-born people.

Signs and Symptoms

Active pulmonary TB is characterized by a chronic productive cough, blood-tinged sputum, and drenching night sweats. Chest pain, fatigue, poor appetite, weight loss, and a low-grade fever are common. If effective treatment is not initiated, a downhill course occurs, with pulmonary fibrosis, **hemoptysis,** and progressive weight loss.

Complications

Spread of the TB bacilli throughout the body can result in pleuritis, pericarditis, peritonitis, meningitis, bone and joint

---

• WORD • BUILDING •

hemoptysis: hem—blood + ptysis—to spit

infections, genitourinary or gastrointestinal (GI) infection, or infection of many other organs.

Diagnostic Tests

Routine screening for TB infection is usually done with a purified protein derivative (PPD) skin test. The PPD is injected intradermally. The test is considered positive if a raised area of **induration** occurs within 48 to 72 hours. If a red area appears around the induration, this is not measured. The size of induration that indicates a positive test varies based on the individual's history (Table 31.2). If a person is **anergic** (has limited ability to react to the test due to immune dysfunction), a smaller area of induration would be considered a positive result. A red area without induration is considered a negative result. A positive result indicates that a person has been exposed to TB; it does not mean that active TB disease is present.

Some health care institutions use a two-step process for baseline testing of employees and residents. If an individual has a negative PPD test, he or she is retested in 1 to 3 weeks. This is because someone who was exposed many years ago may not react to the first test. The first test acts as a reminder to the immune system to react. The second test will then be positive in the person with a past TB infection.

> ### NURSING CARE TIP
> You have probably had a purified protein derivative (PPD) skin test so you can do your clinical practice for school. When you have it checked, the clinician should touch your arm. Just looking at it is not adequate to judge whether there is a raised area of induration.

The QuantiFERON-TB (QFT-TB) and T-SPOT tests are blood tests that detect the cell-mediated immune response to TB bacteria in blood. Unlike the PPD skin test, these are simple blood tests and are valid in individuals who have been vaccinated against TB.

A chest x-ray examination is used as a screening tool in someone with a known positive test. Final diagnosis is made based on sputum culture results.

> ### BE SAFE!
> While awaiting culture results on a hospitalized patient, ask the health care provider whether the patient should be isolated to protect staff and other patients.

Therapeutic Measures

Treatment consists of specific antibiotic therapy. First-line drugs have the fewest adverse effects:

- Isoniazid
- Rifampin

Table 31.2

Classifying a Tuberculin Skin Test Reaction

Size of Induration	Considered Positive for:
5 mm or more	People infected with HIV Recent contacts of infectious tuberculosis (TB) cases Persons with fibrotic changes on chest radiograph consistent with prior TB Organ transplant recipients Those who are immunosuppressed for other reasons (e.g., taking immune suppressing drugs)
10 mm or more	Recent immigrants (within last 5 years) from high-prevalence countries Injection drug users Residents or employees of high-risk congregate settings Mycobacteriology laboratory personnel Persons with clinical conditions that place them at high risk Children younger than age 4 Infants, children, or adolescents exposed to adults in high-risk categories
15 mm or more	People with no risk factors for TB

Source: Centers for Disease Control and Prevention. (2016). Tuberculosis skin testing. Retrieved from www.cdc.gov/tb/publications/factsheets/testing/skintesting.htm

- Ethambutol
- Pyrazinamide

However, they can still be toxic to the liver and nervous system and have other side effects. Other, more toxic antibiotics are reserved for cases that do not respond to first-line drug therapy. Generally, two or three antibiotics are given simultaneously to allow lower doses of each individual drug, reducing the incidence of serious side effects as well as the risk of developing resistant bacteria. Drugs must be taken for 6 to 9 months or up to 2 years for MDR-TB. Because of the length of therapy and the incidence of side effects, adherence to therapy is often a problem.

Additional treatment is supportive. Rest and good nutrition are important for helping the patient's own immune system

• WORD • BUILDING •
induration: in—in + durus—hard

to work. Patients must be isolated until their sputum no longer contains TB bacteria. Typically, after about 2 weeks on antibiotic therapy, the patient is no longer contagious, but a sputum culture must be done to confirm this. Teach the patient to avoid being around others and to use proper hand hygiene during this time period.

Patients with LTBI do not need to be treated, but some health departments recommend treatment to reduce the risk of progression to active disease and subsequent spread to others. LTBI is easier to treat than active TB.

The CDC provides information about TB at www.cdc.gov; simply type "tuberculosis" into the search window.

Nursing Process for the Patient With Tuberculosis

DATA COLLECTION. Perform a thorough history and head-to-toe physical examination, because TB can affect many systems. Focus on respiratory and psychosocial assessments. The severity of the disease determines the impact on the patient's lifestyle. It is also important to determine the patient's knowledge of the disease and treatment and adherence to drug treatment.

NURSING DIAGNOSES, PLANNING, AND IMPLEMENTATION. Nursing interventions for *Impaired Gas Exchange, Ineffective Airway Clearance,* and *Activity Intolerance* are found in "Nursing Care Plan for the Patient With a Lower Respiratory Tract Disorder." Additional nursing diagnoses for the patient with TB follow.

Ineffective Health Management related to deficient knowledge and length of treatment

EXPECTED OUTCOME: The patient will follow treatment regimen and infection will be resolved, as evidenced by negative cultures.

• Assess the patient's and family's ability and intent to follow treatment regimen. *It is essential for patients to be diligent about taking their drugs to eradicate the infection and to prevent spread to others.*
• Teach the patient and family that drugs must be taken as scheduled for the entire course (6 months or longer) or a drug-resistant form of disease may develop. *Patients may be more willing to adhere to treatment if they understand the rationale for taking their medications.*
• Forewarn the patient that rifampin turns urine and other body fluids red. *This might frighten the patient and prevent adherence to treatment.*
• Teach patient to report side effects of medications. *If side effects can be managed, the patient is more likely to adhere to therapy.*
• Request an order for a home health nurse. *A nurse can monitor adherence to therapy. DOT has been found to increase adherence to medication therapy.*
• Teach the patient and family how to avoid spreading the disease to others. *TB is contagious.*
  • Stay home and away from others for a few weeks until sputum cultures are negative.

• Have patient wear a mask when around others.
• Use a tissue to cover the mouth and nose when coughing or sneezing, and flush tissue down toilet or discard in a sealed bag.
• Use good hand-washing technique.
• Keep home and room well ventilated.

EVALUATION. If nursing care has been effective, the patient will understand his or her disease and the importance of taking care of himself or herself. The patient will take medications and receive follow-up care as ordered. He or she will take measures to protect others from catching TB.

CRITICAL THINKING

Mr. Woo is being tested for tuberculosis. You check his skin test and find that the purified protein derivative (PPD) test in his forearm has a 13-mm area of induration.

1. How do you document these results?
2. How do you interpret them?

   Suggested answers are at the end of the chapter.

 RESTRICTIVE DISORDERS

Restrictive disorders are those problems that limit the ability of the patient to expand his or her lungs and, therefore, inhale air. Restrictive disorders can be intrinsic, involving lung tissue (such as pulmonary fibrosis), or extrinsic, involving structures outside the lungs (such as pleural effusion). Restrictive disorders covered next include pleurisy, pleural effusion, empyema, pulmonary fibrosis, and atelectasis.

Pleurisy (Pleuritis)
Pathophysiology
Recall that the visceral and parietal pleurae are the membranes that surround the lungs. Between these membranes is a small amount of serous fluid that prevents friction as the pleurae slide over each other during inhalation and exhalation. If the membranes become inflamed for any reason, they do not slide as easily. Instead of sliding, one membrane may "catch" on the other, causing it to stretch as the patient attempts to take a breath. This causes the characteristic sharp pain on inspiration. The irritation causes an increase in the formation of pleural fluid. This, in turn, reduces friction and decreases pain.

Etiology
Pleurisy is usually related to another underlying respiratory disorder, such as pneumonia, TB, a tumor, or trauma. Nonrespiratory disorders such as pancreatitis or certain autoimmune disorders can also result in pleurisy.

Signs and Symptoms
Pleurisy causes a sharp pain in the chest on inspiration. Pain also occurs during coughing or sneezing. Breathing may be

shallow and rapid because deep breathing increases pain. The patient may also exhibit fever, chills, and an elevated white blood cell (WBC) count if the cause is infectious. A pleural friction rub is heard on auscultation.

Complications

As pleural membranes become more inflamed, serous fluid production increases, which may result in pleural effusion (see next section). If pleuritic pain is not controlled, patients have difficulty breathing deeply and coughing, which may lead to atelectasis. If infection goes untreated, empyema can result.

Diagnostic Tests

Diagnosis is based on signs and symptoms, including auscultation of a pleural friction rub. A chest x-ray examination, CT scan, or ultrasound and complete blood count (CBC) may be done. FVC (forced vital capacity) is reduced more than FEV_1 (forced expiratory volume in 1 second) because expansion is limited by the restrictive disorder; airways and FEV_1 may be normal. Additional testing is done to determine the underlying cause.

Therapeutic Measures

Treatment is aimed at correcting the underlying cause. Non-steroidal anti-inflammatory drugs (NSAIDs) or opioids are given to control pain and facilitate deep breathing and coughing. The physician may perform a nerve block by injecting anesthetic near the intercostal nerves to block pain transmission. Patients may also experience some pain relief when lying on their affected side.

Pleural Effusion
Pathophysiology

When excess fluid collects in the pleural space, it is called a pleural effusion. Fluid normally enters the pleural space from surrounding capillaries and is then reabsorbed by the lymphatic system. When a pathological condition causes an increase in fluid production or inadequate reabsorption of fluid, excess fluid collects. A normal amount of pleural fluid around each lung is 1 to 15 mL. More than 25 mL of fluid is considered abnormal; in pleural effusion, as much as several liters of fluid can collect at one time. The effusion can be either *transudative,* forming a watery fluid from the capillaries, or *exudative,* with fluid containing WBCs and protein from an inflammatory or infectious process.

Etiology

Like pleurisy, pleural effusion is generally caused by another lung disorder. It is a symptom rather than a disease. Transudative effusion may result from heart failure, liver disorders, or kidney disorders. Exudative effusion more commonly occurs with lung cancer, infection, or inflammation.

Signs and Symptoms

Symptoms depend on the amount of fluid in the pleural space. The patient may or may not experience pleuritic pain.

Increasing shortness of breath occurs because of the decreasing space for lung expansion. Cough and **tachypnea** may be present. A dull sound is heard when the affected area is percussed. Lung sounds are decreased or absent over the effusion, and a friction rub may be auscultated.

Diagnostic Tests

A chest x-ray or CT scan is done to determine whether pleural effusion is present. If a thoracentesis is done, fluid samples are sent to the laboratory for C&S and cytological examination. Further tests are done to determine the cause of the effusion.

Therapeutic Measures

Bedrest is recommended to enhance spontaneous resolution of the effusion. If symptoms are severe, a therapeutic thoracentesis is done to remove the excess fluid from the pleural space and relieve the patient of dyspnea. (Chapter 29 discusses how to assist with a thoracentesis.) Patients usually experience immediate improvement in dyspnea following thoracentesis. The HCP will use x-ray examinations and percussion or sometimes ultrasound to determine where to insert the needle to obtain the fluid. If the fluid accumulation is large or recurring, a chest tube might be placed to continuously drain the pleural space. Occasionally, talc or another irritating agent will be instilled via the chest tube to cause the pleural membranes to adhere to each other (this is called **pleurodesis**), eliminating the pleural space and preventing future episodes of pleural effusion. Treatment of the underlying cause of the effusion is necessary to prevent recurrence.

Empyema

Empyema is the collection of pus in the pleural space. It is a pleural effusion that is infected. Empyema is usually a complication of pneumonia, TB, or lung abscess. Symptoms, diagnosis, therapeutic measures, and nursing care are the same as the care of the patient with a pleural effusion, with an added emphasis on identifying and resolving the infection. A chest tube or surgery may be necessary to drain the area.

Pulmonary Fibrosis
Pathophysiology

Pulmonary fibrosis (PF), sometimes called interstitial lung disease, is a group of disorders that cause scarring and fibrosis of lung tissue. PF may evolve from injury to the alveoli, causing chronic inflammation; inflamed tissues are gradually replaced by fibrous connective tissue. Alveoli become thick and scarred, and gas exchange becomes difficult.

• WORD • BUILDING •

tachypnea: tachy—rapid + pnea—breathing
pleurodesis: pleur—pleural membrane + desis—binding

Etiology

Various factors are linked with PF, including heredity, exposure to certain viral illnesses, wood and metal dust exposure, medications, radiation therapy, and smoking. It may also be associated with some autoimmune disorders such as lupus erythematosus or rheumatoid arthritis. Chronic GERD may play a role. Often PF is called idiopathic PF because no specific cause can be found.

Signs and Symptoms

Patients with PF experience progressive shortness of breath. Inspiratory crackles and chronic cough are present. Some experience flu-like symptoms. Fatigue is common, and clubbing of fingers may be present. Patients usually follow a downhill course.

Diagnostic Tests

A chest x-ray may show lung infiltrates. A CT scan may be done. Spirometry is done to verify that the condition is restrictive. Arterial blood gases (ABGs) may show reduced partial pressure of oxygen (Pao_2). A bronchoscopy and lung biopsy can help rule out other causes of the patient's symptoms. They can also show inflammation and fibrosis. A blood test (antinuclear antibodies [ANA] titer) shows whether an autoimmune process is involved.

Therapeutic Measures

Two new antifibrotic drugs, pirfenidone (Esbriet) and nintedanib (Ofev), can reduce disease progression and preserve lung function. Patients should be encouraged to stop smoking and to avoid secondhand smoke. Oxygen is used if needed to maintain oxygenation. Patients should receive flu and pneumococcal vaccines. Younger patients may be considered for a lung transplant. Pulmonary rehabilitation helps patients maintain optimum activity tolerance.

Atelectasis

Atelectasis is the collapse of alveoli. It most commonly occurs in postsurgical patients who do not cough and deep breathe effectively. However, it can be caused by anything that causes hypoventilation. Areas of the lungs that are not well aerated become plugged with mucus, which prevents inflation of alveoli. As a result, alveoli collapse. Compression of lung tissue from effusion or a tumor can also cause atelectasis. The focus of nursing care is on prevention. Patients should be taught the importance of coughing and deep breathing or the use of an incentive spirometer whenever the risk for hypoventilation is present. Frequent position changes and ambulation are also helpful.

Nursing Process for the Patient With a Restrictive Disorder

Data Collection

Perform a routine respiratory assessment. Monitor lung sounds for friction rub or decreasing breath sounds in any of the lobes. Assess pain level and vital signs. Be vigilant for an increase in dyspnea or tachypnea, changes in vital signs or pulse oximetry, or an increased WBC count or temperature.

Nursing Diagnoses, Planning, and Implementation

Priority nursing diagnoses are similar to those for other respiratory disorders and are addressed in "Nursing Care Plan for the Patient With a Lower Respiratory Tract Disorder." In addition, it is essential to address pain (discussed next), because pain can prevent the patient from breathing effectively.

Ineffective Breathing Pattern related to acute pain

EXPECTED OUTCOME: The patient will be comfortable enough to breathe deeply and cough effectively and will have a respiratory rate of 12 to 20 per minute.

- Monitor respiratory rate and depth as well as pain location and level. *Some types of pain can cause shallow respirations, especially pleuritic pain.*
- Position the patient for comfort. *Sometimes, lying on the affected side for short periods will help reduce chest wall movement and pain.*
- Administer pain medication as ordered, preferably around the clock, to prevent pain from becoming severe. *Pain must be controlled so the patient can breathe deeply and prevent further complications. Acetaminophen or NSAIDs are usually tried first because they will not suppress cough and respirations.*
- If opioids are required to control pain, carefully monitor respirations and cough. *Opioids can suppress respirations and cough, which can further complicate the underlying disorder.*
- Teach the patient the importance of effective deep breathing and coughing (see Chapter 29). *This can help prevent further complications. If opioids have suppressed cough reflex, the patient will need to purposefully deep breath and cough.*
- Request an order for an incentive spirometer. *Incentive spirometry can help encourage the patient to breathe deeply.*

Evaluation

If interventions have been effective, the patient should report a decrease in dyspnea and anxiety. Pain will be controlled so that the patient is able to take deep breaths and cough effectively. Breath sounds will be clear and equal bilaterally, and the patient will be free of signs and symptoms of infection.

OBSTRUCTIVE DISORDERS

Obstructive disorders are characterized by air trapping and difficulty getting air out of the lungs. Obstructive disorders covered in this chapter include chronic obstructive pulmonary disease, emphysema, chronic bronchitis, asthma, and cystic fibrosis.

Chronic Obstructive Pulmonary Disease/Chronic Airflow Limitation

According to the National Heart, Lung, and Blood Institute (NHLBI), 16 million adults in the United States have been diagnosed with chronic obstructive pulmonary disease (COPD). In addition, many more likely have it but have not yet been diagnosed (NHLBI, 2017). Death rates in men have fallen slightly in recent years, but death rates in women are steady, due to more women smoking.

Pathophysiology

COPD is a group of pulmonary disorders characterized by difficulty exhaling. In COPD, airways are narrowed or blocked by inflammation and mucus, and there is loss of elasticity in the alveoli. Both conditions make it difficult for air to be removed from the alveoli, leading to trapping of air. More effort is required for weakened alveoli to push air out through obstructed airways (Fig. 31.3). Emphysema, chronic bronchitis, and asthma are disorders that limit airflow. A patient with COPD may have some degree of both emphysema and chronic bronchitis. Asthma may also be present, but it differs somewhat because the airway limitation in asthma is usually reversible. A patient with unremitting asthma is treated as having COPD. Airflow limitation in emphysema and bronchitis is progressive and minimally reversible (Fig. 31.4).

COPD may also be referred to as chronic airflow limitation (CAL) or chronic obstructive lung disease (COLD). COPD develops slowly and may be present for many years before symptoms become evident, and it may be advanced by the time the patient seeks treatment. It is characterized by periods of relative stability and exacerbations, which may be triggered by respiratory infection or other stressors. (See Table 31.3 for a COPD summary.)

> ## LEARNING TIP
> **R**estrictive disorders cause difficulty with inhalation or air ente**R**ing the lungs. **O**bstructive disorders are associated with difficulty exhaling or getting air **O**ut.

CHRONIC BRONCHITIS PATHOPHYSIOLOGY. Chronic bronchitis is similar to acute bronchitis, with symptoms occurring for at least 3 months of the year for two consecutive years. Patients may have multiple exacerbations, each lasting 2 weeks or more. The bronchial tree becomes inflamed from inhaled irritants. Impaired ciliary function reduces the ability to remove the irritants. The mucus-producing glands in the airways become hypertrophied, producing excessive thick, tenacious mucus, which obstructs airways and traps air (Fig. 31.5). These changes lead to chronic low-grade infection.

EMPHYSEMA PATHOPHYSIOLOGY. **Emphysema** affects the respiratory bronchioles and alveoli distal to the terminal bronchioles, causing destruction of the alveolar walls and loss of elastic recoil (see Fig. 31.5). This also causes damage to adjacent pulmonary capillaries. Because of the loss of elastic recoil, passive exhalation is impaired and air is trapped in the alveoli. The combination of damaged alveoli and capillaries causes reduced surface area for gas exchange.

Etiology

Smoking is the single most important risk factor for COPD. Other factors include passive (secondhand and possibly third-hand) smoking, indoor and outdoor air pollution, and exposure to industrial chemicals. Some familial predisposition to chronic bronchitis has been demonstrated. A small number of individuals have an inherited deficiency of the enzyme alpha-1 antitrypsin (α_1AT), which causes a predisposition to the development of emphysema. Patients with this inherited tendency who also smoke have a very high risk of developing the disease. Children of smoking parents are at higher risk because of smoke exposure.

AIR TRAPPING IN CHRONIC AIRFLOW LIMITATION

Air trapping from excess mucus

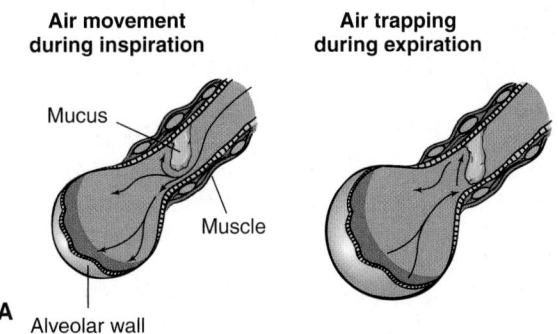

Air movement during inspiration   **Air trapping during expiration**

Mucus

Muscle

A Alveolar wall

Air trapping from decreased elastic recoil and narrowed airways

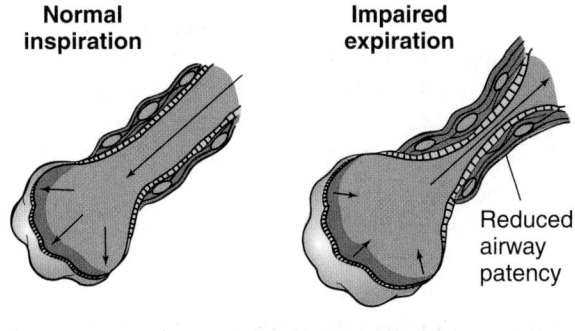

Normal inspiration   **Impaired expiration**

Reduced airway patency

B

Air trapped due to decreased elastic recoil of alveolus and collapsed airway

FIGURE 31.3 Air trapping in COPD.

• WORD • BUILDING •
emphysema: to inflate

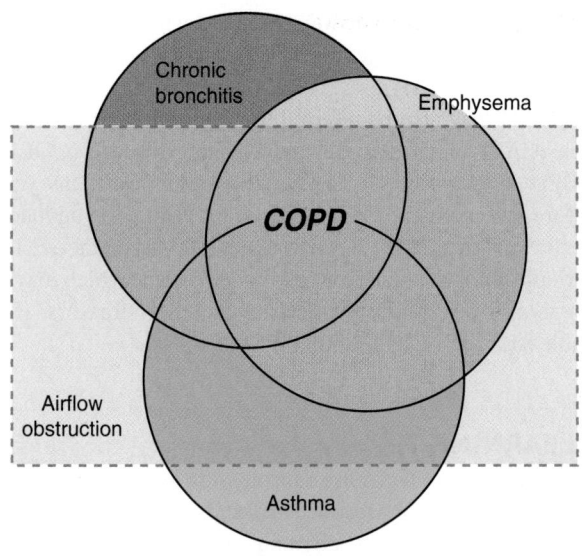

FIGURE 31.4 Chronic bronchitis and emphysema are the primary underlying disorders in COPD. Asthma also may play a role.

Table 31.3
COPD Summary

Signs and Symptoms	Cough
	Chronic sputum production
	Dyspnea that occurs every day, worsens with exercise
	Activity intolerance
	Crackles, wheezes, diminished breath sounds
	Barrel chest
	Use of accessory muscles
Diagnostic Tests	Chest x-ray examination, computed tomography (CT) scan
	Arterial blood gas (ABG) analysis
	Complete blood count (CBC)
	Sputum analysis
	Spirometry
	Alpha-1 antitrypsin (α_1AT) level if hereditary deficiency suspected
Therapeutic Measures	Smoking cessation
	Bronchodilators: per os, or by mouth (PO), nebulized mist treatment (NMT), metered-dose inhaler (MDI)
	Corticosteroids, expectorants
	Flu and pneumonia vaccinations
	Supplemental oxygen
	Breathing exercises
	Chest physiotherapy (CPT)
	Pulmonary rehabilitation
Priority Nursing Diagnoses	*Impaired Gas Exchange*
	Ineffective Airway Clearance
	Activity Intolerance

Prevention

Prevention is important because no cure for COPD is currently available. Avoidance of smoking and other inhaled irritants is vital, especially in those individuals with parents or siblings with COPD.

NURSING CARE TIP

This is a self-care tip. If you are a smoker, now is a good time to quit. COPD is deadly. Check Chapter 29 for ways to quit smoking or visit www.tobaccofreenurses.org. You **can** do it! Good luck!

Signs and Symptoms

Classic symptoms of COPD are chronic cough, with or without sputum production, and progressive dyspnea on exertion. Patients exhibit prolonged exhalation because of obstructed air passages and reduced elastic recoil. Air trapping causes the lungs to become hyperinflated, which in turn leads to the classic barrel-shaped chest.

The patient with chronic bronchitis has a chronic productive cough, shortness of breath, and activity intolerance. Symptoms may initially be worse in the winter months. Crackles and wheezing are often noted on auscultation and may improve after coughing.

The most characteristic symptom of emphysema is progressive shortness of breath, accompanied by activity intolerance. Use of accessory muscles to breathe is evident. Auscultation reveals diminished breath sounds. Remember that many patients have symptoms of both chronic bronchitis and emphysema.

ABGs may be checked during an acute exacerbation of COPD and show an increase in partial pressure of carbon dioxide ($PaCO_2$) and a low PaO_2. The patient develops **polycythemia** in response to chronic hypoxemia, which results in a ruddy skin color. Cyanosis may also be present.

In late stages of COPD, patients may lose weight and become malnourished. They have difficulty eating because of severe dyspnea, and the increased work of breathing expends more calories. Chronic hypoxemia causes release of certain chemicals that may also lead to weight loss. Patients use accessory muscles to breathe and tend to assume the classic tripod position to aid breathing.

Complications

Some patients with emphysema develop a large air spaces within the lung tissue (**bullae**) or adjacent to the pleurae (**blebs**). These are like blisters that can rupture and cause the lung to collapse. Right-sided heart failure may develop because the heart has to work harder to pump blood to the diseased lungs. (See the section on cor pulmonale in Chapter 26.) Death usually results from respiratory infection or respiratory failure.

• WORD • BUILDING •

polycythemia: poly—many + cyt—cells + emia—in the blood

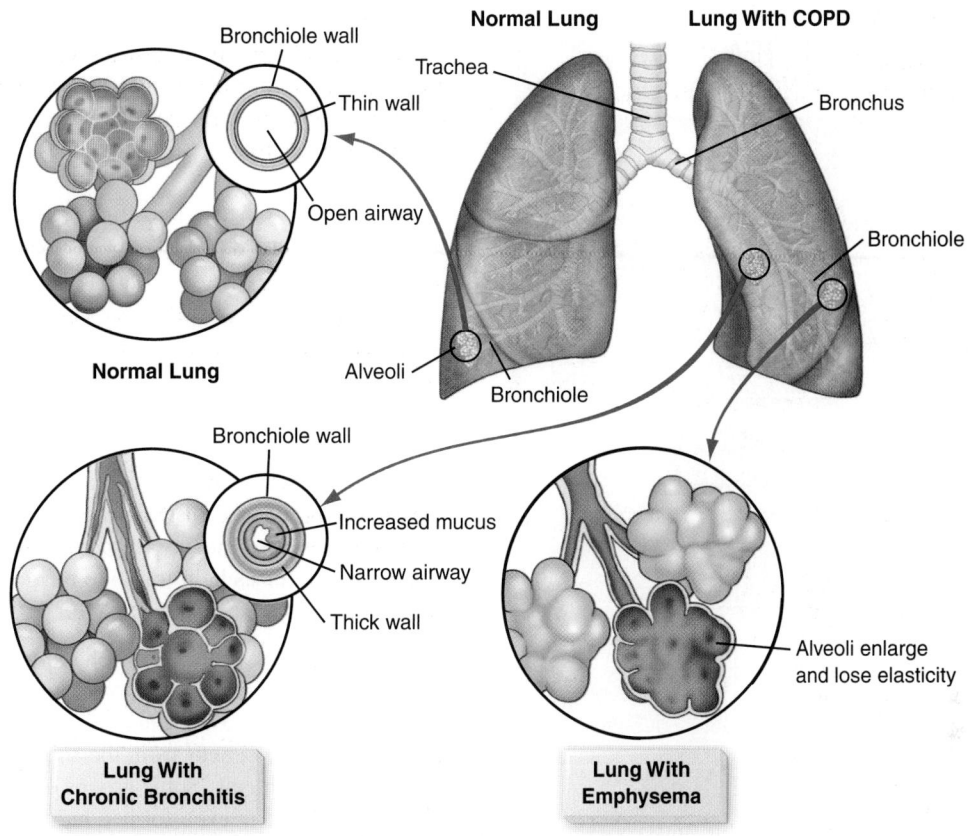

FIGURE 31.5 Normal lung versus lung with COPD.

Diagnostic Tests

Information from spirometry is correlated with the history and physical examination to diagnose COPD. Spirometry is essential for diagnosis. Normally, the FEV_1 is about 70% to 80% of the FVC. In COPD, the FEV_1 following bronchodilator use is less than 70%. This is because the patient with airflow limitation is unable to forcefully exhale as much air in the first second as would normally be expected.

If lung function improves after administration of a bronchodilator, asthma is suspected rather than COPD. An $\alpha_1 AT$ level is checked if deficiency is suspected, especially in patients with a family history of COPD. CBC, electrolytes, and sputum culture may also be assessed during exacerbations.

COPD is classified according to spirometry results into four grades, from GOLD 1 (mild airflow limitation) to GOLD 4 (very severe airflow limitation), and into four categories (A, B, C, D) based on symptoms (Global Initiative for Chronic Obstructive Lung Disease [GOLD], 2017). So 1A would be very mild, and 4D would indicate severe disease.

Therapeutic Measures

The goals of COPD treatment, according to the GOLD guidelines, are to reduce symptoms and reduce risk of exacerbations (GOLD, 2017). In addition, cessation of cigarette smoking should be included as a goal throughout any management program.

SMOKING CESSATION. Even late in the disease process, stopping smoking can slow disease progression and prolong life.

Exposure to other respiratory contaminants should also be minimized. Hair spray, other household aerosols, and body powder should be avoided. Fig. 31.6 shows the benefits of smoking cessation. "Patient Perspective" provides a personal account from one woman who understood too late the importance of smoking cessation. See Chapter 29 for more information on smoking cessation.

Patient Perspective

Sarah. At age 17, I started the habit that would change my life. I started to smoke.

At first it was just a few cigarettes, but as time passed I smoked more and more until I reached two packs a day. This habit continued for 42 years. I disregarded all the warnings about what could happen. I was sure this would never happen to me.

Now at age 75, I must do three breathing treatments a day and carry an inhaler with me at all times. I have a cough that cannot be controlled. I can no longer ride a bike with my grandchildren, play badminton, or even bowl. My lungs won't let me. Going shopping is no longer fun—it's a chore. I have to walk slowly or I can't breathe.

All the things I enjoyed most I've given up because for 42 years I was a slave to cigarettes. If any of you smoke, stop now. Smell the coffee and roses without coughing.

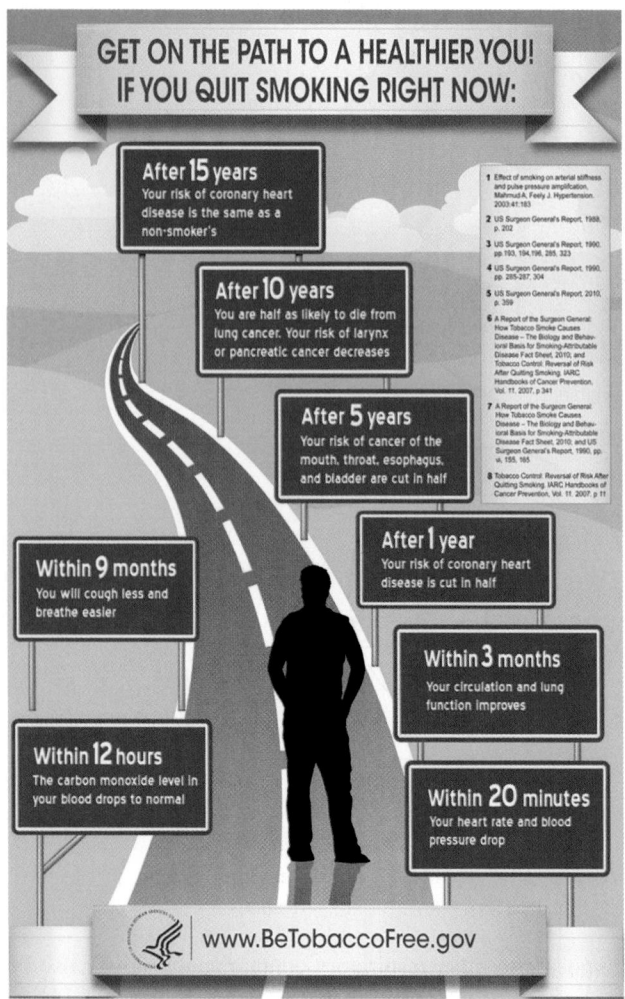

GET ON THE PATH TO A HEALTHIER YOU!
IF YOU QUIT SMOKING RIGHT NOW:

After 15 years
Your risk of coronary heart disease is the same as a non-smoker's

After 10 years
You are half as likely to die from lung cancer. Your risk of larynx or pancreatic cancer decreases

After 5 years
Your risk of cancer of the mouth, throat, esophagus, and bladder are cut in half

After 1 year
Your risk of coronary heart disease is cut in half

Within 9 months
You will cough less and breathe easier

Within 3 months
Your circulation and lung function improves

Within 12 hours
The carbon monoxide level in your blood drops to normal

Within 20 minutes
Your heart rate and blood pressure drop

www.BeTobaccoFree.gov

FIGURE 31.6 Benefits of smoking cessation.

OXYGEN. Oxygen therapy is used in patients with chronic oxygen saturation levels of 88% or less. Oxygen flow rate is titrated (adjusted) to achieve oxygen saturation between 88% and 92%. If the patient tends to retain CO_2, having a much higher saturation could reduce the respiratory drive. But remember that our brains need oxygen! Always aim for 88% to 92% in patients with COPD, and watch your patients closely. If they become drowsy or their respiratory rate falls too low, call the registered nurse (RN) or HCP.

MEDICATIONS. Medications commonly used include adrenergic and anticholinergic MDIs or NMTs to open airways, corticosteroid inhalers to control inflammation, and, intermittently when needed, antibiotics. **Antitussive** agents should be avoided in patients with COPD because they need to be able to cough up secretions.

Oral theophylline bronchodilators are sometimes used but have significant side effects so are avoided if possible. Oral or IV corticosteroids are used for acute exacerbations. Replacement of 1AT may be used in emphysema patients who are deficient. See Table 31.4 for a more detailed list of medications used in the treatment of COPD.

Patients with COPD should also be assessed for depression. Depression is common with chronic illness and often goes undiagnosed. Patients may not report feeling depressed but may experience more physical symptoms. Antidepressant medications, if indicated, can increase quality of life for COPD patients.

Morphine or other opioids may be effective in reducing acute dyspnea and anxiety. They are reserved for end-stage disease.

SUPPORTIVE CARE. Pneumococcal and yearly influenza vaccinations are recommended to reduce the risk of respiratory infection. Avoidance of crowds and exposure to people with respiratory infections is advised.

Good hydration and a cool mist humidifier help keep secretions loose. A dietitian consultation is helpful for the patient who is unable to maintain a desirable weight. Typically, a high-protein, high-fat, low-carbohydrate diet is prescribed. Breathing exercises help improve oxygenation and reduce anxiety (see Chapter 29).

REHABILITATION. Pulmonary rehabilitation programs can help patients increase exercise tolerance and maintain a sense of well-being (Fig. 31.7). Patients exercise in a monitored environment and benefit from the support of other patients with similar problems. Some groups of pulmonary rehabilitation patients have even formed harmonica clubs! Playing their harmonicas mimics pursed-lip breathing and may strengthen the diaphragm, the major muscle of breathing.

SURGERY. Surgical removal of emphysematous lung tissue (called *lung volume reduction surgery,* or LVRS) increases the space available for good lung tissue to expand, reducing dyspnea and increasing exercise tolerance. This is a high-risk procedure, but it has allowed some patients to return to a more normal activity level and improved quality of life. Surgery may also be performed to remove blebs in an attempt to prevent pneumothorax. Lung transplant may be an option in select patients.

ENDOBRONCHIAL VALVE. A newer treatment is similar to lung reduction surgery, but without the surgery. It is placement of a tiny one-way valve, called an endobronchial valve, via bronchoscopy into an area of emphysematous lung, which causes the diseased area to collapse. This then allows the healthy lung tissue more space to expand. This can increase FEV_1 and exercise tolerance.

MECHANICAL VENTILATION. If ABGs worsen despite treatment, intubation and mechanical ventilation may be considered, depending on the patient's advance directive. Unfortunately, mechanical ventilation will not make a patient's disease better, and weaning may be difficult or impossible once it is initiated. Use of NIPPV (see Chapter 29) may be a good alternative for many patients.

• WORD • BUILDING •
antitussive: anti—against + tussive—cough

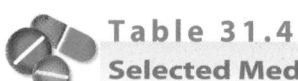

Table 31.4
Selected Medications Used for Lower Respiratory Tract Disorders

Medication Class/Action

Adrenergic Bronchodilators

Stimulate beta receptors to dilate bronchioles.

Examples	**Nursing Implications**
albuterol (Ventolin, Proventil, ProAir)	Use with care in patients with cardiac disease.
metaproterenol (Alupent)	Overuse can cause rebound bronchospasm.
pirbuterol (Maxair)	Short acting; used as rescue inhalers.

Anticholinergic Agents

Block parasympathetic response, causing bronchodilation.

Examples	**Nursing Implications**
ipratropium (Atrovent)	Should be avoided with narrow-angle glaucoma and prostatic
tiotropium (Spiriva)	hypertrophy.
umeclidinium (Incruse Ellipta)	
aclidinium (Tudorza Pressair)	

Corticosteroids

Reduce inflammation in airways.

Examples	**Nursing Implications**
methylprednisolone (Medrol, Solu-Medrol)	Must be used regularly to prevent symptoms.
prednisone	Never discontinue abruptly; must be tapered.
triamcinolone acetonide (Azmacort)	Monitor blood glucose while on high doses.
beclomethasone (Beclovent, QVAR)	*Teach:*
fluticasone (Flovent)	Rinse mouth after inhaler use to prevent local infection
budesonide (Pulmicort)	(candidiasis).
Mometasone (Asmanex)	If using glucocorticoid and adrenergic metered-dose inhalers
	together, use adrenergic inhaler first to open airways.
Combination agents:	See individual agents.
albuterol and ipratropium (Combivent)	Salmeterol and formoterol are long-acting beta agonists that
fluticasone and salmeterol (Advair)	are unsafe for use alone but appear to be safer when used
budesonide and formoterol (Symbicort)	with inhaled corticosteroids.
fluticasone and vilanterol (Breo Ellipta)	Use only as directed.
	Not for use as rescue inhalers.

Phosphodiesterase-4 Inhibitor

Reduces COPD exacerbations.

Examples	**Nursing Implications**
roflumilast (Daliresp)	*Not* effective for acute symptoms. Used prophylactically to reduce exacerbations.

Expectorants

Liquefy secretions and stimulate cough.

Examples	**Nursing Implications**
guaifenesin (Robitussin, Mucinex)	Encourage fluids.

Continued

Table 31.4
Selected Medications Used for Lower Respiratory Tract Disorders—cont'd

Medication Class/Action

Antileukotrienes

Inhibit leukotriene synthesis or activity, a mediator of inflammation in asthma.

Examples
zafirlukast (Accolate)
montelukast (Singulair)
zileuton (Zyflo)

Nursing Implications
Must be taken regularly to prevent symptoms.
Monitor for elevation of liver enzymes.

Antitussives

Suppress cough reflex.

Examples
codeine
dextromethorphan (DM suffix in cough preparations)

Nursing Implications
Avoid giving to patient who has secretions that need to be expectorated.

Note: This table is an overview. A drug guide should be consulted for complete administration guidelines.

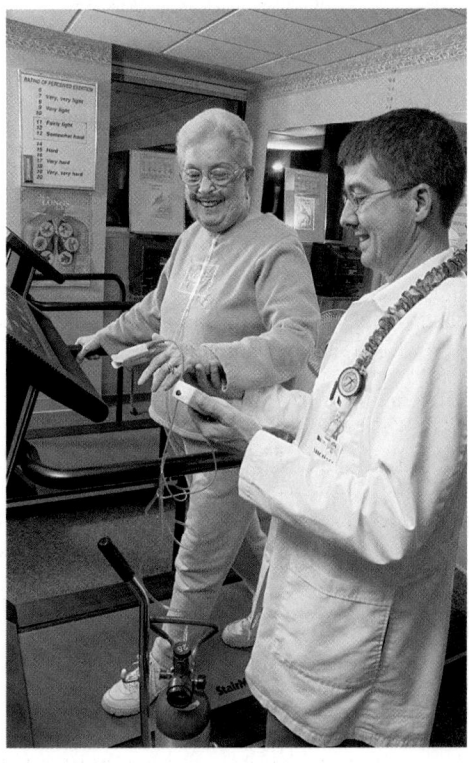

FIGURE 31.7 Patients build exercise tolerance in pulmonary rehabilitation programs. Note therapist monitoring oxygen saturation.

END-OF-LIFE PLANNING. It is important to assess whether the patient has a living will or durable power of attorney for health care (see Chapter 17). COPD is a progressive disease, and patients can increase the quality of their life and death by making decisions in advance. Patients should make decisions about whether they would want to be intubated and mechanically ventilated, or have cardiopulmonary resuscitation (CPR) in event of a cardiac arrest. CPR is rarely successful in a patient with end-stage disease. Patients should be made aware of palliative care options and assured that they will be kept as comfortable as possible.

Nursing Process for the Patient With COPD

See "Nursing Process for the Patient With an Obstructive Disorder" and "Nursing Care Plan for the Patient With a Lower Respiratory Tract Disorder." Priority nursing diagnoses for the patient with COPD include *Impaired Gas Exchange, Ineffective Airway Clearance,* and *Activity Intolerance.*

Asthma

Asthma affects more than 300 million people worldwide (Global Initiative for Asthma [GINA], 2017) and 24.6 million in the United States (CDC, 2017a). Asthma can lead to disability and even death. With careful monitoring and treatment, however, patients with asthma can manage their symptoms and lead normal lives.

Pathophysiology

Asthma is characterized by chronic inflammation of the airways and hyperresponsiveness of the bronchial smooth muscles (**bronchospasm**). This causes narrowed airways and air trapping, which is why it is considered an obstructive disorder. Inflammation occurs in part because things that trigger asthma (asthma triggers) cause the release of inflammatory substances such as histamine and leukotrienes. Symptoms are intermittent and generally reversible, with

• WORD • BUILDING •
bronchospasm: broncho—airway + spasm—convulsion, involuntary narrowing

periods of normal airway function. Some people develop permanent changes in their airways, called remodeling; this leads to a progressive loss of lung function.

Many patients develop the disorder in childhood, and some outgrow it. However, a significant number develop symptoms again later in life. Children with asthma should be counseled that smoking can increase the risk of recurrence in adulthood. Asthma may also complicate chronic bronchitis or emphysema. Asthma is classified as mild, moderate, or severe based on the amount and type of medication required to control it (GINA, 2017).

Etiology

The tendency to develop asthma is inherited. The most common predisposing factor is the genetic tendency to be allergic to airborne allergens such as pollen or mold. Viral respiratory infections are also a contributing factor to asthma diagnosis and exacerbation. Tobacco smoke, air pollution, early use of antibiotics, and sensitization to house-dust mites and cockroaches have also been linked to asthma development.

Asthma Triggers

Once asthma develops, a number of triggers can cause an acute attack. Exposure to allergens such as dust mites, cockroaches, cat and dog dander, or pollen can trigger an attack. Other possible triggers include viral infection, emotional upset, exercise, stress, and certain medications (e.g., aspirin, beta blockers).

Prevention

Although asthma cannot be prevented at this time, research is ongoing to determine factors associated with its development. Current research recommendations include (1) avoidance of environmental tobacco smoke during pregnancy and a child's first year of life, (2) vaginal delivery (exposing baby to mother's vaginal flora may be beneficial), and (3) avoidance of acetaminophen and broad-spectrum antibiotics during the first year of life (GINA, 2017). Appropriate control of childhood asthma may prevent more serious asthma in later years. Avoidance of smoking may reduce the risk of recurrence of asthma that started in childhood. To prevent acute attacks, it is important that the patient identify triggers of asthma symptoms and avoid them whenever possible. Monitoring of symptoms and compliance with prophylactic and maintenance therapy is also important.

Signs and Symptoms

Asthma symptoms are intermittent and are often referred to as attacks. Attacks may last from minutes to days. Patients report wheezing, chest tightness, dyspnea, coughing, and difficulty moving air in and out of the lungs. Symptoms are often worse at night. Some patients experience coughing but no wheezing. Once initial symptoms are controlled, airways may remain hypersensitive and prone to asthma symptoms for many weeks.

On examination, you will note an increased respiratory rate as the patient attempts to compensate for narrowed airways. Inspiratory and expiratory wheezing is heard because of turbulent airflow through swollen airways with thick secretions; wheezing may sometimes be audible even without a stethoscope. Air is trapped in the lungs, and expiration is prolonged. A cough is common and may produce thick, clear sputum. Use of accessory muscles to breathe is a sign that the attack is severe and warrants immediate attention.

Be aware that an absence of audible wheezing may not signal open airways but rather may be an ominous sign that the patient is not moving enough air to make any sound. If wheezing is not heard, use of accessory muscles and peak expiratory flow rate (PEFR) values must be carefully evaluated. Once treatment begins to open the airways, wheezing may become audible.

Complications

Status asthmaticus occurs if bronchospasm is not controlled and symptoms are prolonged. As the patient increases the respiratory rate to compensate for narrowed airways, a lot of carbon dioxide is blown off and respiratory alkalosis occurs. If the attack is not resolved and the patient begins to tire, the patient will no longer be able to compensate. $Paco_2$ will rise, resulting in respiratory acidosis. This can lead to respiratory failure and death if untreated.

Diagnostic Tests

Diagnosis is based on the patient's report of symptoms, physical examination, and spirometry results. PEFR and FEV_1 are reduced, especially during symptomatic periods. Asthma can be differentiated from COPD during spirometry testing by administering an adrenergic agonist (such as an albuterol inhaler) and then retesting. Asthma symptoms can generally be reversed with the medication, but COPD cannot. Allergy skin testing and increased serum immunoglobulin E and eosinophil levels indicate allergic involvement and may help determine appropriate treatment. ABGs may be evaluated during an acute severe attack.

On a long-term basis, asthma control can be evaluated using FEV_1 or PEFR measurements, frequency and severity of exacerbations and nighttime awakenings, and frequency of short-acting beta-agonist use.

CRITICAL THINKING

Timothy is a 16-year-old whose mother brought him to the emergency room because of an asthma attack. He says he feels short of breath, but when you listen to his lungs, you hear no wheezing.

1. Does Timothy really need to be in the emergency room?
2. What should you do?
3. What do you think could be happening?
4. What other team members can you collaborate with as you care for Timothy?

Suggested answers are at the end of the chapter.

Therapeutic Measures

Patients must learn to manage asthma at home. If they can monitor and manage their symptoms, acute episodes and hospitalizations can be avoided.

SELF-MONITORING. All patients benefit from learning to monitor their asthma symptoms and make treatment decisions accordingly. This can be done by carefully monitoring symptoms or by monitoring of the peak expiratory flow rate, or PEFR (Fig. 31.8). PEFR is a measurement in liters per minute of the amount of air a patient can blow into a peak flowmeter from fully inflated lungs. The patient determines his or her baseline PEFR during symptom-free times. Readings can be charted to keep track of progress (Fig. 31.9). If symptoms worsen or PEFR begins to fall below the patient's baseline, the patient should begin self-treatment according to an asthma action plan (Fig. 31.10). If treatment does not improve PEFR to the expected degree, the patient is advised to go to the emergency room. PEFR results may indicate the onset of asthma before the patient experiences any obvious symptoms.

AVOIDANCE OF TRIGGERS. The patient is instructed to identify and avoid asthma triggers. If triggers cannot be avoided, the patient can use a bronchodilator as prescribed before exposure. Inhalers can be especially useful before exercise. Animal dander and foods that cause symptoms are best avoided when possible. Eliminating carpets and curtains in bedrooms, using vinyl mattress and pillow covers, and installing a portable or central air filter can reduce dust mite exposure. Maintenance of indoor humidity between 40% and 50% can reduce mold growth. If cold air triggers symptoms, the patient should keep the nose and mouth covered when outside in cold weather. Smoking and exposure to secondhand smoke are strongly discouraged.

Aspirin and NSAIDs can cause asthma symptoms in some individuals. Beta-blocking medications (e.g., propranolol, metoprolol), used commonly for hypertension, block beta receptors in the lungs, preventing the sympathetic nervous system from promoting bronchodilation. These drugs should be avoided if they make symptoms worse.

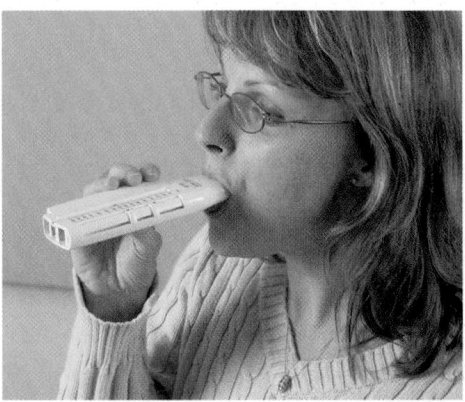

FIGURE 31.8 Patient with asthma using a peak flowmeter to monitor peak expiratory flow rate.

MEDICATIONS. Medications for asthma treatment may be used intermittently or continuously, depending on the persistence of symptoms. Inhaled medications are preferred because they cause fewer adverse effects than oral or injected medications. See Table 31.4 for a summary of medications used in the treatment of lower respiratory disorders.

For patients with intermittent symptoms, short-acting beta agonists (SABAs) such as albuterol are used to dilate bronchioles. They are administered via an MDI when symptoms occur and are often called *rescue inhalers*. They can also be administered preventively before exercise or other events that trigger asthma.

If the patient needs to use a rescue inhaler more than two times a week for symptoms, maintenance medications to prevent symptoms will likely be started. Inhaled corticosteroids such as fluticasone (Flovent) or budesonide (Pulmicort) are generally added first to control inflammation. Instruct the patient that corticosteroids must be used regularly to prevent symptoms and that they do not provide immediate symptom relief during an acute attack.

Long-acting beta-agonist (LABA) bronchodilators such as salmeterol (Serevent) or formoterol (Foradil) can also help prevent symptoms by keeping airways dilated for up to 12 hours or more. Research in recent years, however, has questioned their safety, and they are no longer recommended to be used alone. If they are used, they should be used in combination with inhaled corticosteroids (fluticasone and salmeterol [Advair], budesonide and formoterol [Symbicort]).

If inhaled medications do not control symptoms or if the patient has nocturnal symptoms, oral antileukotrienes may be added. Immunotherapy (allergy shots) may be used for some patients with allergic asthma.

An acute asthma attack may be treated with an inhaler (MDI or NMT) or SABA (bronchodilator). IV or oral corticosteroids (e.g., methylprednisolone, prednisone) are potent anti-inflammatory agents that are useful in an acute episode but are avoided for long-term therapy if possible because of significant side effects. Long-term corticosteroids must be tapered before discontinuing to prevent withdrawal symptoms. (See the section on addisonian crisis in Chapter 39.)

It is important for patients to understand the difference between long-acting maintenance medications and rescue medications and to use them appropriately. Oxygen is generally not necessary because many patients hyperventilate during an acute attack. If the attack is prolonged and the patient becomes cyanotic or Pao_2 levels begin to fall, oxygen therapy will be used.

> **NURSING CARE TIP**
> Instruct the patient to contact the health care provider if using more than one adrenergic metered-dose inhaler canister per month. This has been associated with an increased risk of death.

Name															
Green zone _____			Yellow zone _____				Red zone _____								
Date															
	AM	PM	AM	PM	AM	PM	AM	PM	AM	PM	AM	PM	AM	PM
800															
750															
700															
650															
600															
550															
500															
450															
400															
350															
300															
250															
200															
150															
100															
Notes															

FIGURE 31.9 Peak flow chart. The green zone is 80% to 100% of the patient's normal peak flow rate. The yellow zone is 50% to 80% of normal. The red zone is less than 50% of normal. The patient works with the health care provider to determine which actions to take when readings fall in the yellow or red zones.

Asthma Action Plan for _____ Doctor's Name _____ Date _____

Doctor's Phone Number _____ Hospital/ Emergency Room Phone Number _____

GREEN ZONE: Doing Well

- No cough, wheeze, chest tightness, or shortness of breath during the day or night
- Can do usual activities

And, if a peak flow meter is used,

Peak flow: more than _____
(80% or more of my best peak flow)

My best peak flow is: _____

Take These Long-Term-Control Medicines Each Day (include an anti-inflammatory)

Medicine	How much to take	When to take it

Before exercise ☐ _____ ☐ 2 or ☐ 4 puffs 5 to 60 minutes before exercise

YELLOW ZONE: Asthma Is Getting Worse

- Cough, wheeze, chest tightness, or shortness of breath, or
- Waking at night due to asthma, or
- Can do some, but not all, usual activities

-Or-

Peak flow: _____ to _____
(50% – 80% of my best peak flow)

First **Add: Quick-Relief Medicine – and keep taking your GREEN ZONE medicine**

_____ (short-acting beta$_2$-antagonist) ☐ 2 or ☐ 4 puffs, every 20 minutes up to 1 hour
☐ Nebulizer, once

Second **If your symptoms (and peak flow, if used) return to GREEN ZONE after 1 hour of above treatment**

☐ Take the quick-relief medicine every 4 hours for 1 to 2 days
☐ Double the dose of your inhaled steroid for _____ (7–10) days
-Or-
If your symptoms (and peak flow, if used) do not return to GREEN ZONE after 1 hour of above treatment
☐ Take: _____ (short-acting beta$_2$-antagonist) ☐ 2 or ☐ 4 puffs or ☐ Nebulizer
☐ Add: _____ (oral steroid) _____ mg/day For _____ (3–10) days
☐ Call the doctor before/ ☐ within _____ hours after taking the oral steroid.

RED ZONE: Medical Alert!

- Very short of breath, or
- Quick-relief medicines have not helped, or
- Cannot do usual activities, or
- Symptoms are same or get worse after 24 hours in Yellow Zone

-Or-
Peak flow: less than _____
(50% of my best peak flow)

Take this Medicine

☐ _____ (short-acting beta$_2$-antagonist) ☐ 4 or ☐ 6 puffs or ☐ Nebulizer
☐ _____ (oral steroid) _____ mg

Then call your doctor NOW. Go to the hospital or call for an ambulance if:
✔ You are still in the red zone after 15 minutes AND
✔ You have not reached your doctor

DANGER SIGNS
- **Trouble walking and talking due to shortness of breath**
- **Lips or fingernails are blue**

✔ Take ☐ 4 or ☐ 6 puffs of your quick-relief medicine AND
✔ Go to the hospital or call for an ambulance (_____) NOW!

WHITE – PATIENT COPY   YELLOW – WORK/SCHOOL COPY   PINK – PROVIDER COPY

FIGURE 31.10 Asthma action plan.

Nursing Process for the Patient With Asthma

See "Nursing Process for the Patient With an Obstructive Disorder" section, following the section on cystic fibrosis in this chapter. Primary nursing diagnoses include *Impaired Gas Exchange, Ineffective Airway Clearance,* and *Anxiety.* See Table 31.5 for an asthma summary.

Cystic Fibrosis

In the past, cystic fibrosis (CF) was thought to be just a childhood disease because most affected children did not survive past puberty. However, with new treatments, patients with CF are living longer and more productive lives. Some CF patients now live into their 60s.

Pathophysiology

CF is a disorder of the exocrine glands that affects primarily the lungs, GI tract, and sweat glands. Abnormal sodium and chloride transport across cell membranes, causing thick, tenacious secretions, is responsible for many of the characteristic symptoms. Thick, sticky respiratory secretions are difficult to remove and cause airway obstruction, resulting in air trapping and frequent respiratory infections.

Similar abnormalities in the pancreas cause blocked ducts and retained digestive enzymes. These retained enzymes digest and destroy the exocrine pancreas. The absence of digestive enzymes in the intestines causes malabsorption of essential nutrients; frequent foul-smelling, fatty stools; and excess flatus.

Patients with CF secrete sweat that is high in sodium and chloride because these electrolytes are not reabsorbed as they pass through the sweat ducts.

Etiology

CF is a genetic disorder. Both parents must be carriers of the defective gene for CF to be present in a child. Patients with CF who marry are counseled on the risk of potential offspring having the disease.

Signs and Symptoms

Symptoms usually first appear in infancy or childhood, although a few individuals are not diagnosed until adulthood. Respiratory symptoms are often the first visible manifestation of the disease and range from chronic sinusitis to production of thick, tenacious sputum. Finger clubbing is common. Over time, bouts of infection become more frequent, with eventual loss of lung function and respiratory failure.

Frequent foul-smelling stools, poor appetite, bowel obstruction, cirrhosis, cholecystitis, and cholelithiasis are associated findings. Chronic disease causes delayed sexual maturation in both males and females, and infertility is common. Death is usually the result of pulmonary complications, especially antibiotic-resistant infection.

Diagnostic Tests

Diagnostic tests begin with genetic testing. A blood test for immunoreactive trypsinogen may show high levels in CF. A sweat chloride test determines whether sweat is high in sodium and chloride. You may recall public health campaigns that advise parents to kiss their babies and report any salty taste to their HCPs. Chest x-ray, spirometry, and GI tests also may be done.

Therapeutic Measures

Because there is no cure for CF, treatment is aimed at controlling infection and relieving symptoms. Removal of thick sputum is promoted with hydration, use of a vibratory positive expiratory pressure (PEP) device, CPT, or a high-frequency chest wall oscillation vest (see Chapter 29). All forms of smoke should be avoided. NMTs using normal or hypertonic saline or mucolytic medications may be used before CPT. An inhaled medication called dornase alfa (Pulmozyme) is an enzyme that breaks up and loosens mucus; it has been shown to reduce lung infections and improve lung function. Bronchitol, mentioned earlier in the section on bronchiectasis, is also being studied for CF. Inhaled beta-agonist bronchodilators help keep airways open. Ivacaftor (Kalydeco) is a new oral medication that is being studied to improve the function of a protein that is defective in patients with CF. It is the first drug that will target the underlying cause of CF rather than treat symptoms. High doses of ibuprofen (Motrin) may slow lung deterioration. Lung transplant is a potentially promising treatment. Pulmonary rehabilitation programs help patients maintain activity tolerance.

Patients should receive a yearly flu vaccination. Antibiotics must be administered as soon as signs of infection occur. Antibiotic-resistant infections are a deadly threat to the patient with CF. Patients must be vigilant in avoiding others with infections.

Table 31.5
Asthma Summary

Signs and Symptoms	Chest tightness, dyspnea, cough Wheezing
Diagnostic Tests	Spirometry, before and after bronchodilator Arterial blood gas (ABG) analysis in acute attack
Therapeutic Measures	Identification and avoidance of triggers Inhaled corticosteroids Inhaled bronchodilators Oral bronchodilators and steroids if inhaled ineffective
Complications	Status asthmaticus
Priority Nursing Diagnoses	*Impaired Gas Exchange* *Ineffective Airway Clearance* *Anxiety*

Pancreatic enzyme replacement (pancrelipase; Pancrease, Viokase) helps reduce symptoms related to malabsorption and improve nutritional status. An increase in calorie requirements necessitates a high-calorie, nutrient-dense diet. For more information, visit the Cystic Fibrosis Foundation at www.cff.org.

Nursing Process for the Patient With Cystic Fibrosis

See "Nursing Process for the Patient With an Obstructive Disorder" section next. *Ineffective Airway Clearance* is the priority nursing diagnosis. Also, be sure to remember the special needs of the adolescent patient with this chronic, debilitating disease. Not only are normal physical growth and development delayed, but psychosocial development is also affected by repeated hospitalizations and the necessity of routine daily medication and treatments.

CRITICAL THINKING

Mr. Jenkins is a 36-year-old accountant with bronchiectasis secondary to cystic fibrosis. You enter his room during an episode of uncontrollable coughing and offer him support. You observe his sputum as you dispose of it—a whole Styrofoam coffee cup full of thick, bright yellow sputum; the smell makes you nauseated. Even after coughing, his lungs sound congested from retained secretions. You offer him mouth care before you leave his room.

1. What questions can you ask Mr. Jenkins to assess his cough?
2. What nursing diagnosis is most appropriate for Mr. Jenkins?
3. What nursing care can you provide to enhance secretion removal?
4. How would you document this episode of coughing?
5. What other team members can you collaborate with to provide the best care for Mr. Jenkins?

   Suggested answers are at the end of the chapter.

Nursing Process for the Patient With an Obstructive Disorder
Data Collection

Perform a complete respiratory assessment as presented in Chapter 29. Frequency of assessment is dictated by the severity of the patient's condition. Note orientation and level of consciousness; poor gas exchange can cause confusion and lethargy. Assess respiratory rate and effort. Observe skin and mucous membranes for cyanosis. Auscultate lungs for adventitious sounds. Monitor cough and the color, viscosity, odor, and amount of sputum. Note exercise tolerance and have the patient report degree of dyspnea on a scale of 0 to 10. Monitor vital signs, oxygen saturation, and ABGs if ordered. Careful documentation of findings allows you to be vigilant for trends in the patient's progress.

Nursing Diagnoses, Planning, and Implementation

A number of nursing diagnoses are appropriate for the patient with an obstructive disorder. As always, choose diagnoses based on defining characteristics and the patient's individual assessment findings.

Priority nursing diagnoses for most chronic respiratory patients include *Impaired Gas Exchange, Ineffective Airway Clearance, Ineffective Breathing Pattern,* and *Activity Intolerance.* Interventions for these diagnoses are presented in "Nursing Care Plan for the Patient With a Lower Respiratory Tract Disorder." Related diagnoses are discussed next.

Imbalanced Nutrition: Less Than Body Requirements related to poor appetite and increased calorie expenditure as evidenced by weight loss or low weight for height

EXPECTED OUTCOME: The patient's weight will be stable at desired weight for height.

- Monitor food intake and weekly weight. *Regular monitoring can help identify nutrition problems before they are severe.*
- If the patient is too dyspneic to eat, schedule rest periods and bronchodilator treatments before meals. *Eating takes a lot of energy, and resting can help conserve energy before a meal. Bronchodilators can reduce dyspnea while eating.*
- Create a pleasant eating environment. *Unpleasant views or odors can spoil an appetite.*
- Provide smaller, more frequent meals of the patient's favorite foods. *Eating a lot at one time can fill up the stomach and reduce room for lung expansion.*
- Encourage family members to bring favorite foods from home for the hospitalized patient. *A large tray of unappetizing food may be more than a patient can handle and may spoil the appetite. Be sure to note sodium or other restrictions; although the patient with end-stage disease may be allowed a more lenient diet, excess sodium can cause fluid retention and increase dyspnea.*
- Consult a dietitian for liquid supplement recommendations. *A specialized supplement such as Pulmocare provides less carbon dioxide than other supplements when metabolized and may be used for patients with chronic respiratory disease.*
- See also "Nutrition Notes."

Nutrition Notes

Optimizing Nutrition in Patients With Respiratory Disease. Caloric requirements commonly are increased in patients with respiratory disease. When caloric intake is inadequate, the body begins to break down muscle stores, including the respiratory and gastrointestinal (GI) muscles, which only worsens the problem.

Causes of inadequate food intake can include the following:

• Anorexia
• Shortness of breath
• Fatigue (too tired to eat)
• Pressure from the GI tract impinging on the chest
• Medication side effects

Many patients with COPD have carbon dioxide retention and oxygen depletion. Because fat calories produce less carbon dioxide when metabolized than carbohydrate calories, diets with increased fat and decreased carbohydrate may help. Special supplements for pulmonary patients are available. Energy and protein needs may be increased for normal maintenance of nutritional status. Nevertheless, it is important not to overfeed the patient. Excess intake can raise the demand for oxygen and the production of carbon dioxide beyond the patient's capacity to manage them.

The American Lung Association recommends the following dietary strategies:

• Offer small, frequent feedings. Eat more food earlier in the morning if more fatigued later in the day. Rest prior to eating.
• Consume a diet composed of complex carbohydrates (20 to 30 g of fiber per day), limiting simple carbohydrates; adequate, high-quality protein; and monounsaturated and polyunsaturated fats.
• Limit sodium in diet.
• Drink adequate fluids.
• Consult health care provider regarding a multivitamin.
• Avoid foods that cause gas or bloating (these may include carbonated beverages, legumes, and cruciferous vegetables).
• Drink liquids between meals if drinking with meals causes early fullness.
• Add a nutrition supplement, especially a low-carbohydrate supplement such as Pulmocare, at night to help improve nutrition.

Reference
American Lung Association: Lung Health and Diseases. (2016, November). Nutrition. Retrieved from http:// www.lung.org/lung-health-and-diseases/lung-disease-lookup/copd/living-with-copd/nutrition.html

Anxiety related to acute dyspnea as evidenced by statement of anxiety, tense appearance, and tremors

EXPECTED OUTCOME: The patient will state that anxiety is controlled; appearance of tension and tremors will be absent. The patient will use techniques to control dyspnea and anxiety when they occur.

• Stay with a patient who is acutely dyspneic and anxious. *Feeling alone during episodes of dyspnea can increase anxiety.*

• Calmly remind the patient to breathe slowly in through the nose and out through pursed lips. *During acute episodes of dyspnea, the patient may forget that breathing exercises can help.*
• Teach relaxation exercises during times when anxiety is minimal, and remind the patient to use them during acute anxiety. *Relaxation exercises can help reduce muscle tension and distract the patient.*
• Administer antianxiety medications as ordered. *Medications can reduce anxiety but can also depress respirations, so should be used with caution.*
• Administer IV morphine as ordered (or contact RN to do so). *Morphine helps acute dyspnea and anxiety in patients with end-stage disease.*

Evaluation

If interventions have been effective, the patient will learn techniques to make breathing as comfortable as possible and will be able to cough up secretions and maintain a clear airway. The patient will be able to manage anxiety symptoms and complete activities of daily living or other desired activity without dyspnea. The patient's intake should be adequate to maintain a stable weight. If any of the patient's goals have not been met, the plan of care should be revised.

Patient Education

The patient must be aware of the contributing factors to the disease and eliminate them if at all possible. The patient who is a smoker should not simply be told to quit smoking but referred to a smoking cessation program and provided with medication, nicotine patches, or other resources and support as necessary to quit (see Chapter 29). Techniques for effective breathing and anxiety control should also be taught. A formal pulmonary rehabilitation program is an excellent resource for patient education.

CRITICAL THINKING

Mr. Franklin is admitted to the respiratory unit with exacerbated COPD. He has a history of emphysema and now has an acute infection complicating his disease. His lung sounds are very diminished, and he is short of breath at rest, even on 2 L of oxygen per nasal cannula. You walk into his room to respond to his call light and find him sitting on the bedside commode with a look of panic in his eyes. He is gasping for breath, his color is gray, and his respiratory rate is 36 per minute.

1. What do you do first? What assessment is appropriate? Whom can you call for assistance?
2. What can you teach Mr. Franklin to prevent an acute dyspneic episode in the future?
3. How will you document this episode?

Suggested answers are at the end of the chapter.

PULMONARY VASCULAR DISORDERS

Pulmonary Embolism

Pathophysiology

An embolism is a foreign object that travels through the bloodstream. It may be a blood clot, air, or fat. A pulmonary embolism (PE), sometimes called a pulmonary thromboembolism (PTE), is usually a blood clot that has traveled into a pulmonary artery (Fig. 31.11). Resulting obstruction of blood flow causes a ventilation-perfusion mismatch. In this case, it means that an area of the lung is well ventilated with air but has no blood flow, or perfusion. Because reduced or no blood supply is available to pick up the oxygen in the affected portion of the lung, it becomes pulmonary "dead space," causing seriously impaired gas exchange.

Occasionally, damage occurs to a portion of the lung because of lack of oxygen. This is called lung infarction. It is not common because oxygen is delivered to lung tissue not only from the pulmonary arteries but also via the bronchial arteries and the airways.

Etiology

Most pulmonary emboli originate in the deep veins of the lower extremities (deep vein thrombosis [DVT]). Therefore, every effort should be made to avoid risk factors for DVT

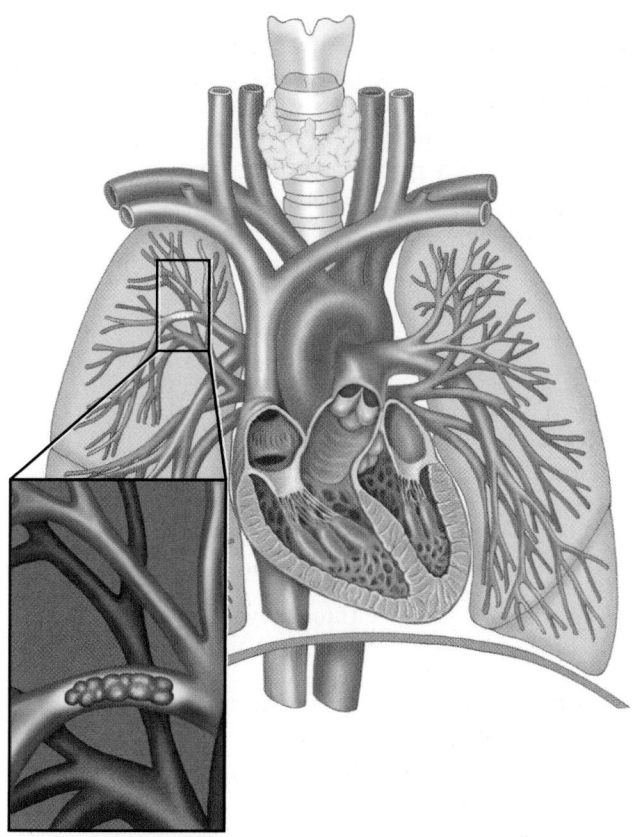

Pulmonary embolism

FIGURE 31.11 Pulmonary embolism.

(see Chapter 23). Less common causes of PE include fat emboli from compound fractures, amniotic fluid embolism during labor and delivery, and air embolism from entry of air into the bloodstream.

Prevention

Prevention of thrombi in the deep veins of the legs is the most important factor in the prevention of a PE. Regular ambulation is advised if the patient is able. If a patient is at risk for DVT or PE, such as following surgery or during times of immobility, anticoagulant medications may be ordered. Intermittent compression stockings may also be used. If a DVT is diagnosed, prompt treatment is essential to prevent PE.

Signs and Symptoms

The most common symptom of PE is a sudden onset of dyspnea for no apparent reason. The patient may be gasping for breath and appear anxious. Tachycardia, tachypnea, cough, and pleuritic chest pain may be present. Auscultation may reveal crackles or a friction rub. If lung infarction has occurred, hemoptysis may also be present. Some patients have no symptoms at all. Be vigilant for the presence of risk factors, and obtain immediate assistance if the cause of dyspnea might be PE. Death can occur if treatment is not fast and effective.

Complications

High blood pressure within the pulmonary circulation (pulmonary hypertension) may result from arterial occlusion and lead to right ventricular failure. This occurs because the right ventricle is unable to push blood into the occluded artery. As a result, the contraction becomes weak, cardiac output falls, and the patient becomes hypotensive.

Diagnostic Tests

A D-dimer blood test can be helpful to rule out PE. Results can be obtained in less than an hour. D-dimer is a fibrin fragment that is found in the blood after any thrombus formation. It can be present in a number of disorders, but if it is negative, PE can be eliminated as a possible cause of the patient's symptoms.

A spiral CT scan with contrast dye is noninvasive and can diagnose PE quickly. If this is not available, a lung scan (ventilation-perfusion scan) is done to assess the degree of ventilation of lung tissue and the areas of blood perfusion. If an area is well ventilated but poorly perfused (i.e., a mismatch), PE is suspected.

A pulmonary angiogram is an invasive test that can outline the pulmonary vessels with a radiopaque dye injected via a cardiac catheter. It can show where blood flow is diminished or absent, suggesting an embolism.

Chest x-ray examination, electrocardiogram (ECG), ABG analysis, or magnetic resonance imaging (MRI) may also be done. However, many of these show changes only in the presence of a very large embolism or infarction.

Therapeutic Measures

Thrombolytic agents such as alteplase (Activase) or reteplase (Retavase) may be used in life-threatening emergencies to dissolve the clot; heparin or another anticoagulant is used to prevent new clots from forming. Thrombolytics must be administered within 4 to 6 hours of the clot's occurrence and are associated with risk for hemorrhage.

In patients who cannot tolerate a thrombolytic agent, the clot may be removed with a cardiac catheter, or a surgical embolectomy can be performed. The latter is a rare procedure that is reserved for emergency situations.

Oxygen is administered even if peripheral capillary oxygen saturation (SpO_2) is normal, because it may help dilate pulmonary vessels. Intubation and mechanical ventilation may be required in some cases.

Long-term use of anticoagulants follows initial treatment to prevent formation of additional clots. Drugs such as heparin or rivaroxaban (Xarelto) may be used. Clotting studies must be monitored for patients receiving heparin. Sometimes heparin therapy is initiated even before a diagnosis of PE is made. It is believed that it is safer to begin therapy and then stop if PE is ruled out than to wait until all test results are available.

An oral anticoagulant is used for at least 3 to 6 months after PE to prevent recurrence. It can also be used for long-term prevention of repeated clots in patients who have risk factors that cannot be resolved. Oral therapy can begin 2 to 3 days after the heparin therapy begins. Because it has a slow onset of action, it may take several days for the full anticoagulant effect to occur. See Chapter 23 for nursing care of patients on anticoagulant therapy.

If clots are a recurring problem, a filter may be placed into the inferior vena cava via the jugular or femoral vein to filter out clots traveling from the lower extremities toward the heart and lungs.

Nursing Process for the Patient With a Pulmonary Embolism

DATA COLLECTION. Assess the patient for respiratory distress, including respiratory rate and effort, cyanosis, confusion, chest pain, and subjective feelings of dyspnea and anxiety. Auscultate lung sounds. Note sputum color and amount, watching especially for hemoptysis. Monitor ABGs and oxygen saturation. Monitor heart sounds and peripheral edema for signs of heart failure. Contributing factors, such as calf pain, should be noted. Remember, any sudden onset of dyspnea should be taken seriously and reported quickly.

NURSING DIAGNOSES, PLANNING, AND IMPLEMENTATION. The priority nursing diagnosis for a patient with a PE is *Impaired Gas Exchange* (see "Nursing Care Plan for the Patient With a Lower Respiratory Tract Disorder"). Because of the impaired perfusion of the affected area of the lung, oxygen and carbon dioxide exchange are limited. *Anxiety* occurs related to dyspnea. *Risk for Bleeding* related to anticoagulant therapy is a concern once treatment is initiated (also see Chapter 23).

Risk for Bleeding related to anticoagulant therapy

EXPECTED OUTCOME: The patient will remain safe as evidenced by absence of bleeding. The patient will verbalize understanding of self-care measures.

- Monitor coagulation studies and report results to the HCP. *Anticoagulant therapy may be adjusted as often as every 6 hours on the basis of laboratory results.*
- Protect the patient from injury *so that excessive bleeding does not occur.*
- Encourage the patient to wear shoes or slippers when ambulating *to protect from injury.*
- Teach the patient to use a soft toothbrush and an electric razor *to prevent injury.*
- Avoid use of intramuscular (IM) injections. *An IM injection can result in hematoma in an anticoagulated patient.*
- Instruct the patient to report any signs of bleeding, such as hematuria or easy bruising. *Bleeding may be associated with excessively prolonged clotting and may require a change in anticoagulant dosing or administration of an antidote.*

EVALUATION. The patient should state that dyspnea and anxiety are resolved and verbalize understanding of anticoagulant therapy and precautions. (See Table 31.6 for a PE summary.)

Table 31.6
Pulmonary Embolism Summary

Signs and Symptoms	Sudden-onset dyspnea, tachypnea Chest pain Tachycardia Hemoptysis Crackles History of blood clot
Diagnostic Tests	D-dimer Computed tomography (CT) scan Ventilation-perfusion lung scan Angiogram
Therapeutic Measures	Thrombolytic therapy Anticoagulants Oxygen
Complications	Pulmonary hypertension
Priority Nursing Diagnoses	*Impaired Gas Exchange* *Anxiety* *Risk for Bleeding* due to anticoagulant therapy

CHEST TRAUMA

Pneumothorax

The term **pneumothorax** literally means "air in the chest." It is used to describe conditions in which air has entered the space between the visceral and parietal pleurae. If the pneumothorax occurs without an associated injury, it is called a spontaneous pneumothorax. A secondary spontaneous pneumothorax may occur due to underlying lung disease. A traumatic pneumothorax results from a penetrating chest injury. An iatrogenic (caused by medical treatment) pneumothorax results from complications of hospital procedures, such as central line insertion, pleural biopsy, or positive pressure ventilation.

Pathophysiology and Etiology

Recall that the lungs are surrounded by the visceral and parietal pleurae. These membranes are normally separated only by a thin layer of pleural fluid. Each time a breath is taken in, the diaphragm descends, creating negative pressure in the thorax. This negative pressure pulls air into the lungs via the nose and mouth. If either the visceral pleura or the chest wall and parietal pleura are perforated, air will enter the pleural space, negative pressure will be lost, and the lung on the affected side will collapse (Fig. 31.12). Each time the patient takes a breath, the resulting increase in negative pressure will draw more air into the pleural space via the perforation. During exhalation, air may or may not be able to escape through the perforation.

SPONTANEOUS PNEUMOTHORAX. If no injury is present, the pneumothorax is considered spontaneous. This occurs mostly in tall, thin individuals and in smokers. Patients who have had one spontaneous pneumothorax are at greater risk for a recurrence. Patients with underlying lung disease (especially emphysema) may have blister-like defects in lung tissue (called bullae or blebs) that can rupture, allowing air into the pleural space. Weakened lung tissue from lung cancer can also lead to pneumothorax.

TRAUMATIC PNEUMOTHORAX. Penetrating trauma to the chest wall and parietal pleura allows air to enter the pleural space. This can occur as a result of a knife or gunshot wound or from protruding broken ribs.

OPEN PNEUMOTHORAX. If air can enter and escape through the opening in the pleural space, it is considered an open pneumothorax.

CLOSED PNEUMOTHORAX. If air collects in the space and is unable to escape, a closed pneumothorax exists.

TENSION PNEUMOTHORAX. In a closed pneumothorax, air, and, therefore, tension, builds up in the pleural space and is unable to escape. As tension increases, pressure is placed on the heart and great vessels, pushing them away from the affected side of the chest. This is called a mediastinal shift. When the heart and vessels are compressed, venous return to

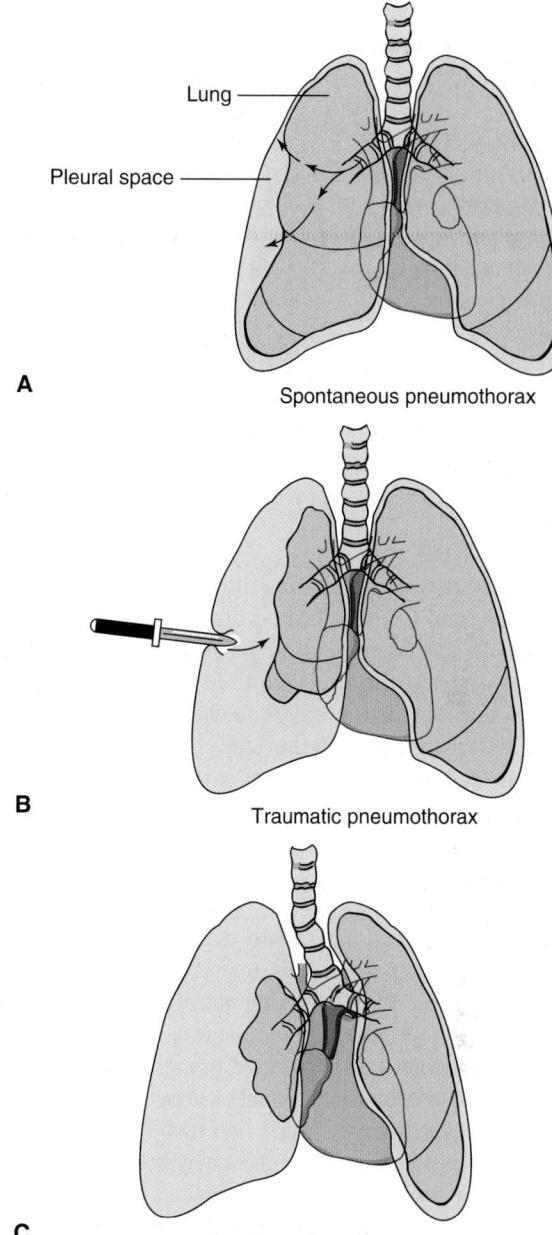

FIGURE 31.12 Types of pneumothorax. (A) Spontaneous pneumothorax. (B) Traumatic pneumothorax. (C) Tension pneumothorax with mediastinal shift.

the heart is impaired, resulting in reduced cardiac output and symptoms of shock. A tension pneumothorax is often related to the high pressures present with mechanical ventilation. It is a life-threatening emergency.

HEMOTHORAX. The term **hemothorax** refers to the presence of blood in the pleural space. This can occur with or without an accompanying pneumothorax (when they occur together

---

• WORD • BUILDING •
pneumothorax: pneumo—air + thorax—chest
hemothorax: hem—blood + thorax—chest

it is called a hemopneumothorax). It is often the result of traumatic injury. Other causes include lung cancer, PE, and anticoagulant use.

Signs and Symptoms

Sudden dyspnea, chest pain, tachypnea, tachycardia, restlessness, and anxiety occur with pneumothorax. On examination, asymmetrical chest expansion on inhalation may be noted. Breath sounds may be absent or diminished on the affected side. In a "sucking" chest wound, air can be heard as it enters and leaves the wound.

If a tension pneumothorax develops, the patient becomes hypoxemic and hypotensive as well. The trachea may deviate to the unaffected side. Heart sounds may be muffled. Bradycardia and shock occur if emergency intervention is not provided.

Diagnostic Tests

History, physical examination, ultrasound, chest x-ray examination, and CT scan can be used to diagnose pneumothorax. In the emergency department, bedside ultrasound can shorten the time required for diagnosis and intervention and avoid the wait for a chest x-ray to be completed. Chest x-ray examination may be done to monitor the resolution of the pneumothorax after treatment. ABGs and oxygen saturation are monitored as needed throughout the course of treatment.

Therapeutic Measures

A small pneumothorax may absorb with no treatment other than rest or high-flow oxygen or the trapped air can be removed with a small-bore needle inserted into the pleural space. Chest tubes connected to a water seal drainage system are used to remove larger amounts of air or blood from the pleural space. See Chapter 29 for complete information about chest drainage. Smaller devices that have special one-way valves to allow air to escape but not re-enter the chest may be used for some patients who are treated at home. Some injuries require surgical repair before the pneumothorax can be resolved. Oxygen and positioning help maintain oxygenation.

If the pneumothorax is recurrent, other treatments can be used to prevent additional episodes. Sterile talc or tetracycline can be injected into the pleural space via thoracentesis, irritating the pleural membranes and making them stick together. This is called *pleurodesis,* or *sclerosis,* and prevents recurrent pneumothorax. Pleurodesis is painful; prepare the patient with an analgesic before the procedure.

Nursing Care of the Patient With a Pneumothorax

Nursing care of the hospitalized patient with a pneumothorax involves close monitoring of the condition. Frequent and thorough assessments should be done, including level of consciousness, skin and mucous membrane color, vital signs, oxygen saturation, respiratory rate and depth, and presence of dyspnea, chest pain, restlessness, or anxiety. Regular auscultation of lung sounds provides information

about reinflation of the affected lung. Be especially vigilant for signs of increasing or tension pneumothorax, and report them to the HCP immediately. Nursing diagnoses to consider include *Impaired Gas Exchange, Acute Pain,* and *Anxiety.* See Chapter 29 for care of the patient with a chest tube and water seal drainage system. See Table 31.7 for a pneumothorax summary.

Rib Fractures

Etiology and Signs and Symptoms

Chest trauma is often accompanied by fractured ribs. Uncontrolled coughing, especially in the presence of osteoporosis or cancer, can also fracture ribs. Falls are a common cause of broken ribs in older people. The fourth through ninth ribs are the most commonly affected. Broken ribs can be painful and often prevent the patient from breathing deeply or coughing effectively, which can result in atelectasis or pneumonia. Displaced ribs can also damage abdominal organs or lung tissue, causing pneumothorax.

Therapeutic Measures

In the past, elastic rib belts were used to stabilize the ribs while healing took place. These are no longer used because it restricts deep breathing. Pain control is the most important treatment. Keeping the patient comfortable allows coughing and deep breathing, which in turn prevents complications such as pneumonia and atelectasis. If traditional pain control measures such as NSAIDs or opioids are ineffective, intercostal nerve blocks may be used. Ribs generally heal in about 6 weeks.

Table 31.7

Pneumothorax Summary

Signs and Symptoms	Sudden-onset dyspnea, chest pain, tachypnea Asymmetrical chest expansion Diminished or absent breath sounds on affected side
Diagnostic Tests	Ultrasound Chest x-ray, computed tomography (CT) scan Arterial blood gas (ABG) analysis
Therapeutic Measures	Chest tube and water seal drainage Pleurodesis for recurrent pneumothorax
Complications	Tension pneumothorax Shock
Priority Nursing Diagnoses	*Impaired Gas Exchange* *Acute Pain* *Anxiety*

Flail Chest
Pathophysiology and Etiology
When multiple ribs are fractured, the structural support of the chest is impaired. As a result, the affected part of the chest collapses with the negative pressure of inhalation and bulges with exhalation. This is called **paradoxical respiration,** which may be ineffective in ventilating the lungs and result in hypoxia.

Signs and Symptoms
The patient with a flail chest exhibits chest movement that is opposite to that usually seen with respiration. The patient is dyspneic and anxious and may also be tachypneic and tachycardic.

Therapeutic Measures
Treatment includes supplemental oxygen and analgesics. Intubation and mechanical ventilation may be necessary but are avoided if possible because of related risk for infection. If lung damage has occurred, treatment for a pneumothorax may be needed. Surgical stabilization of the ribs may be done in some cases.

Nursing Process for the Patient With Chest Trauma
The following nursing process is based on the stabilized patient. For emergency care of the trauma patient, see Chapter 13.

Data Collection
When caring for the patient following chest trauma, it is important to monitor respiratory status continuously. Be vigilant for any sign of worsening status, such as a change in vital signs, oxygen saturation, or lung sounds; change in respiratory rate; increase in dyspnea, chest pain, pallor, or cyanosis; development of tracheal deviation; or new onset of anxiety or restlessness. Report changes to the RN or HCP immediately. Monitor pain and condition of the chest wound, if present. Additional assessment may be necessary depending on the type of injury sustained.

Nursing Diagnoses, Planning, and Implementation
Priority nursing diagnoses for the patient with chest trauma include *Impaired Gas Exchange, Ineffective Breathing Pattern,* and *Acute Pain.* Additional diagnoses may be appropriate depending on the individual patient's assessment. See "Nursing Care Plan for the Patient With a Lower Respiratory Tract Disorder" for interventions for *Impaired Gas Exchange* and *Ineffective Breathing Pattern.*

Acute Pain related to chest trauma as evidenced by pain rating

EXPECTED OUTCOME: The patient will state pain is controlled and will be able to cough and deep breathe effectively.

• Administer NSAIDs or opioids as ordered. *Pain must be controlled so that the patient is able to breathe deeply and prevent atelectasis and pneumonia.*

• If opioids are used, monitor for depressed respirations and reduced cough reflex. *Depressed respirations and cough increase the risk of atelectasis and pneumonia.*

• Teach the patient to splint the chest with a pillow for coughing. *This may help reduce chest movement and pain during coughing.*

Evaluation
Are pain, anxiety, and dyspnea controlled? Are respiratory rate and SpO_2 within normal limits? Are vital signs stable? Frequent evaluation is essential, so that failure to progress can be quickly reported.

 # RESPIRATORY FAILURE

Acute Respiratory Failure
Pathophysiology
Acute respiratory failure is diagnosed when the patient is unable to maintain adequate blood gas values. Hypoxemia may result from inadequate ventilation (air movement in and out of lungs) or poor oxygenation (adequate ventilation but inability to get the oxygen into the blood and, therefore, the cells), or both. Hypercapnia and respiratory acidosis occur when the diseased lungs are unable to effectively eliminate carbon dioxide.

Etiology
An acute respiratory infection in a patient with chronic obstructive disease is often the precipitating factor in acute respiratory failure. Other causes include central nervous system (CNS) disorders that affect the muscles of breathing, such as a stroke, spinal cord injury, or myasthenia gravis; inhalation of toxic substances; opioid overdose; and aspiration.

Prevention
Avoidance of respiratory infections in patients with chronic respiratory disease is important. Instruct patients to notify their HCP immediately if sputum becomes purulent so treatment can be initiated.

Sedatives and narcotics should be used carefully or avoided in patients with chronic respiratory disease because these are respiratory depressants and can precipitate failure. Careful monitoring and early intervention are essential in patients at risk for respiratory failure.

Signs and Symptoms
The patient with impending respiratory failure may become restless, confused, agitated, or sleepy. ABGs show decreasing PaO_2 and pH and increasing $PaCO_2$, which lead to respiratory acidosis. The patient is cyanotic and dyspneic. Respirations become rapid and deep in an effort to blow off excess CO_2.

Diagnostic Tests
Respiratory failure is diagnosed when PaO_2 falls below 60 mm Hg or $PaCO_2$ is elevated above 50 mm Hg. Some patients with chronic respiratory disease have adapted to

impaired gas exchange. In these patients, a drop in Pao_2 of 10 to 15 mm Hg is considered acute failure. Sputum cultures or chest x-ray examinations may be used to identify underlying respiratory problems. Additional tests may be done to determine nonpulmonary causes and guide treatment. Pulse oximetry is used to continuously monitor oxygen saturation. Patients cared for in intensive care units (ICUs) may have additional monitoring, including capnography (Chapter 29).

Therapeutic Measures

Carefully observe the patient, and report significant findings to the HCP immediately. It is easy to mistakenly treat symptoms of agitation or confusion with sedatives. However, this will speed the onset of respiratory failure. Oxygen therapy via nasal cannula or mask is provided. Oxygen saturation should be maintained at 88% to 92%. Higher levels could depress the stimulus to breathe, worsening the situation.

Antibiotics or other treatments are ordered to correct the underlying cause of the failure. Bronchodilators promote ventilation and secretion removal. Interventions for ineffective airway clearance and impaired gas exchange are initiated. Suctioning is indicated if the patient is unable to cough effectively.

Acute Respiratory Distress Syndrome/Acute Lung Injury

Acute respiratory distress syndrome (ARDS) is a group of disorders that has diverse causes but similar pathophysiology, symptoms, and treatment.

Pathophysiology and Etiology

ARDS occurs because of acute lung injury (ALI). The most common cause of injury is widespread sepsis. Other causes include pneumonia, trauma, shock, narcotic overdose, inhalation of irritants, burns, pancreatitis, and aspiration. Each of these causes begins a chain of events leading to alveolocapillary damage and noncardiogenic pulmonary edema (pulmonary edema that is not caused by heart failure). ARDS usually affects patients without a previous history of lung disease.

Tired respiratory muscles, in combination with edema and atelectasis, reduce gas exchange and result in hypoxia. As the condition progresses, atelectasis and edema worsen, and the lungs may hemorrhage. A chest x-ray examination appears white because of the excessive fluid in the lungs. These changes explain some of the older names for what is now known as ARDS (e.g., wet lung, white lung, shock lung, and stiff lung).

Prevention

Early recognition and treatment of underlying disorders are important in the prevention of ARDS. Good nursing care can help reduce aspiration and some types of pneumonia.

Signs and Symptoms

The patient presents with dyspnea, tachypnea, and cyanosis. Initial respiratory alkalosis (from tachypnea) develops into acidosis as the patient tires. Fine inspiratory crackles are auscultated. The patient is often confused and lethargic. If ARDS is not reversed, eventually hypoxemia leads to decreased cardiac output, shock, and death.

Complications

Complications that can result from ARDS include heart failure, a pneumothorax related to mechanical ventilation, infection, and disseminated intravascular coagulation (DIC). The death rate for ARDS in the past was 100%. With newer treatments, it is now closer to 40%. Most patients who survive ARDS recover completely.

Diagnostic Tests

Diagnosis is made based on history of a causative injury, physical examination, chest x-ray examination, CT scan, and ABG analysis. An ECG is done to rule out a cardiac-related cause.

Therapeutic Measures

The patient with ARDS is cared for in the ICU. Treatment is supportive and aimed at the underlying cause. Oxygen therapy is adjusted on the basis of repeated ABG results. NIPPV or intubation and mechanical ventilation are necessary in most cases, with the use of positive end-expiratory pressure (PEEP) to keep the airways open. Diuretics may be used to reduce pulmonary edema, but care must be taken to prevent fluid depletion. IV fluids are administered if blood pressure or urine output is low. A pulmonary artery catheter may be used to monitor hemodynamic status. If infection or sepsis is the underlying cause, antibiotics are administered. Tube feeding or parenteral nutrition maintain nutritional status while the patient is acutely ill. Positioning the patient with the less involved lung in the dependent position ("good lung down") allows the better lung to be well perfused with blood and may increase Pao_2. Prone positioning has also been shown to increase oxygenation and reduce death rate in patients with ARDS.

Nursing Process for the Patient Experiencing Respiratory Failure
Data Collection

Assess the patient's degree of dyspnea on a scale of 0 to 10 if the patient is able to participate. Monitor respiratory rate and effort, use of accessory muscles, ABGs, and oxygen saturation values. Note the presence of cyanosis.

Monitor mental status, including restlessness, confusion, and level of consciousness, because reduced oxygenation can produce CNS symptoms. Monitor symptoms of the underlying cause of respiratory failure. If the cause is infectious, monitor temperature and WBC counts; if the infection is respiratory in origin, monitor cough and sputum.

All assessment findings should be compared with earlier data. Even subtle changes in the assessment findings can be significant and should be reported.

Nursing Diagnoses, Planning, and Implementation

Priority nursing diagnoses include *Impaired Gas Exchange, Ineffective Airway Clearance,* and *Ineffective Breathing*

Pattern (see "Nursing Care Plan for the Patient With a Lower Respiratory Tract Disorder"). Related diagnoses include *Activity Intolerance, Anxiety, Risk for Acute Confusion, and Self-Care Deficit.*

Evaluation

If interventions have been effective, the patient will state that dyspnea is controlled. Mental status will be at baseline for the patient. Airways will be kept clear at all times, and SpO_2 and respiratory rate will be within normal limits.

> **NURSING CARE TIP**
>
> The "good lung down" position can help increase oxygenation in patients with lung disease. Gravity results in more blood in the dependent lung, where it can receive oxygen from the healthier lung tissue. If both lungs are diseased, the right lung down position may be beneficial because the right lung has a larger surface area (Yeaw, 1992).

LUNG CANCER

Lung cancer is the leading cause of cancer death in the United States for both men and women. In 2014, the most recent year for which statistics are available, 113,326 men and 102,625 women were diagnosed with lung cancer, an increase from 2009; in addition, 84,859 men and 70,667 women died from lung cancer (CDC, 2017b).

Pathophysiology

Lung cancers originate in the respiratory tract epithelium; most originate in the lining of the bronchi (Fig. 31.13). The four major types of lung cancer are identified by the type of cells that are affected: small cell lung cancer (SCLC), large cell carcinoma, adenocarcinoma, and squamous cell carcinoma. The latter three types are classified as non–small cell lung cancer (NSCLC).

About 10% to 15% of lung cancers are SCLC. SCLC grows rapidly and often has metastasized by the time of diagnosis. It is usually caused by smoking and is most often found centrally, near the bronchi. The patient with SCLC has a poor prognosis, with survival time averaging less than 1 year.

The remaining lung cancers are NSCLC. Large cell carcinoma is a rapidly growing cancer that can occur anywhere in the lungs. It metastasizes early in the disease, so these patients also have a poor prognosis.

Adenocarcinoma occurs more often in women, and most often in the peripheral lung fields. It is slow growing but often is not diagnosed until metastasis has occurred. It is less closely linked with smoking.

Squamous cell carcinoma is the most common form of NSCLC. It usually originates in the lining of the bronchi and metastasizes late in the disease. It is associated with a history of smoking. The prognosis for individuals with squamous cell carcinoma may be better than for some other lung cancers.

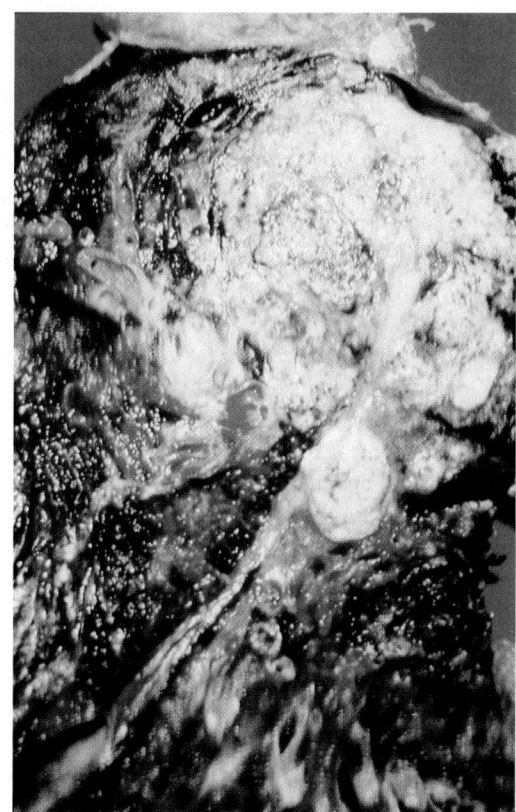

FIGURE 31.13 Cross section of a human lung. The white area in the upper lobe is cancer; the black areas indicate the patient was a smoker.

Etiology

Tobacco smoke causes 80% to 90% of lung cancers. Cigarettes contain chemicals that cause DNA to mutate, creating changes in cells and development of tumors. If a patient stops smoking, the risk of lung cancer decreases significantly. Unfortunately, even with all this information, 15% of adults in the United States continue to smoke (CDC, 2017c).

Living with a smoker increases a nonsmoker's risk of lung cancer by 20% to 30% (National Cancer Institute, 2017). Secondhand smoke may also be related to breast cancer, nose and throat cancers, leukemia, lymphoma, and brain tumors in children. Other factors that contribute to increased lung cancer risk are exposure to asbestos, radon, arsenic, air pollution, diesel exhaust, and radiation. Genetic predisposition and a diet poor in fruits and vegetables may also be factors.

> **NURSING CARE TIP**
>
> Exposure to radon gas, which can be found in homes, is a significant risk factor for lung cancer. Check out www.epa.gov/radon for more information and to find out if radon is a concern in your area. Many local health departments and hardware stores have inexpensive radon test kits available for purchase.

Prevention

The single most important way to prevent lung cancer is to stop smoking. Many programs educate school children about the dangers of smoking. Smoking cessation programs are available for people who desire to quit. Contact your local American Cancer Society chapter (www.cancer.org) for smoking cessation programs that can be recommended to patients.

Signs and Symptoms

Manifestations of lung cancer depend on the location of the tumor. Commonly, patients exhibit a persistent cough with sputum production. The patient may ignore these symptoms because they are also associated with smoking and other chronic respiratory disorders. Repeated respiratory infections may occur, producing thick, purulent sputum. Sputum may become bloody (hemoptysis). The patient may experience dyspnea. If the airway becomes obstructed by the tumor, wheezing or stridor may be heard. Late signs include chest pain, weight loss, anemia, and anorexia.

Complications
Pleural Effusion

Pleural fluid collects in the pleural space as a result of irritation or obstruction of lymphatic or venous drainage by the tumor (see earlier "Pleural Effusion" section).

Superior Vena Cava Syndrome

If the tumor obstructs the superior vena cava, blood flow is interrupted, causing distention of the jugular veins and swelling of the chest, face, and neck. Diuretics may help relieve the fluid buildup. Radiation may be used to shrink the obstruction.

Ectopic Hormone Production

Some lung cancers produce **ectopic** hormones that mimic the body's own hormones. Ectopic production of antidiuretic hormone (ADH) can produce syndrome of inappropriate ADH (SIADH) production, with resulting fluid retention. Ectopic production of adrenocorticotropic hormone (ACTH) can cause Cushing syndrome. High calcium levels can be caused by ectopic secretion of a parathyroid-like hormone. These disorders are discussed in Chapter 39.

Atelectasis and Pneumonia

Atelectasis occurs when tumor growth prevents ventilation of areas of the lung. Patients with lung cancer also have a greater risk for pneumonia. (See earlier sections on both of these disorders.)

Metastasis

Common sites of lung cancer metastasis include the brain, bones, opposite lung, liver, adrenal gland, and lymph nodes.

Diagnostic Tests

A complete medical history and physical examination are done to look for symptoms and risk factors for lung cancer. A chest x-ray examination is done to identify a mass. However, all tumors may not show up on x-ray. A CT or positron emission tomography (PET) scan or MRI may be done to provide more specific information about the size and location of a tumor. Sputum is analyzed for abnormal cells. Brain and bone scans are done to find metastatic lesions.

Diagnosis is confirmed with a biopsy of the lesion. A biopsy specimen may be obtained via bronchoscopy, percutaneous biopsy (a needle through the skin guided by radiograph), or mediastinoscopy (placement of an endoscope into the mediastinum to look for changes in mediastinal lymph nodes).

Therapeutic Measures

Tumors are staged based on the tumor-node-metastasis (TNM) staging system. Staging helps determine appropriate treatment (Table 31.8). If NSCLC is localized and in an early stage, it may be cured with surgical removal of the tumor. This can be accomplished with a segmental or wedge resection, which removes only the affected lung segment. A **lobectomy** (removal of a lobe) or removal of an entire lung may be done in more advanced cases (Fig. 31.14).

Chemotherapy or radiation may be done alone or in addition to surgery. Patients with Stage IV cancer may opt for using experimental drugs in clinical research trials. Palliative surgery may make a patient more comfortable.

Chemotherapy is the treatment of choice in SCLC, because usually it has metastasized by the time of diagnosis. Radiation may be used in combination with chemotherapy. Surgery is not usually indicated in SCLC; the goal of treatment may be palliation of symptoms rather than cure.

Newer therapies for lung cancer include targeted therapies, such as monoclonal antibodies, antiangiogenesis agents, and growth factor inhibitors. Targeted therapies attack the cancer cells and spare normal cells from damage. Vaccines and gene therapy are also being studied to treat lung cancer.

For more information about cancer treatment and nursing care, see Chapter 11. For more on lung cancer, visit the American Cancer Society at www.cancer.org.

Nursing Process for the Patient With Lung Cancer
Data Collection

Perform a complete biopsychosocial assessment of the patient with lung cancer. Assess and document respiratory rate and depth, skin and mucous membrane color, lung sounds,

• WORD • BUILDING •
ectopic: displaced
lobectomy: lobe—lobe (of lung) + ectomy—excision

Table 31.8

Stages of Lung Cancer

Stage	Characteristics
Non–Small Cell Lung Cancer	
I	Cancer in lung with no spread to lymph nodes
II	Cancer in lung and nearby lymph nodes
III	Cancer in in lung, lymph nodes, and mediastinum
IV	Cancer is in both lungs and pleurae or in distant areas
Small Cell Lung Cancer	
Limited	Cancer is limited to one side of the chest
Extensive	Cancer cells are found outside one side of the chest or in distant sites

oxygen saturation, cough, and sputum amount and character. Ask the patient to rate the degree of pain and dyspnea on appropriate scales. Ask about appetite and weight loss as well as symptoms of other complications. Note activity tolerance and fatigue.

The patient will likely be grieving about the illness and prognosis. Assessment of the patient's coping strategies and support systems will help you plan care for psychosocial needs. The presence of a living will or durable power of attorney and the desire for assistance with end-of-life planning should be noted (see Chapter 17).

Nursing Diagnoses, Planning, and Implementation

Possible diagnoses that may be experienced by the patient with lung cancer include *Impaired Gas Exchange, Ineffective Airway Clearance, Imbalanced Nutrition: Less Than Body Requirements, Pain, Constipation* related to opioid use, *Grieving,* and *Activity Intolerance.* See "Nursing Care Plan for the Patient With a Lower Respiratory Tract Disorder" for care of patients with respiratory diagnoses. See Chapter 11 for interventions related to cancer diagnoses.

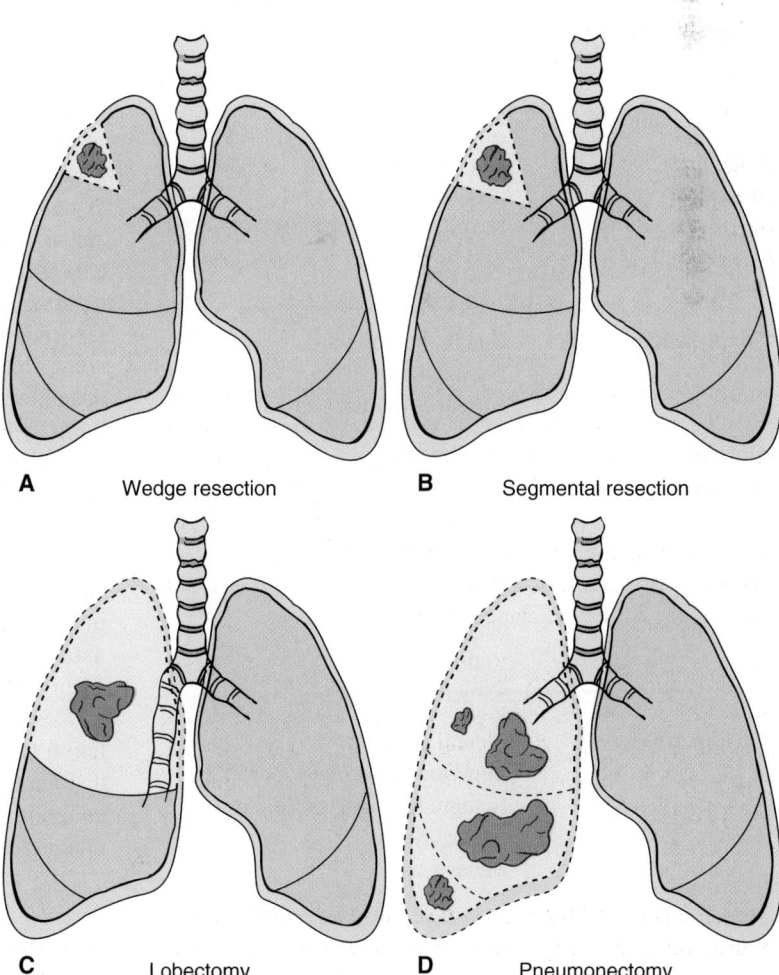

A   Wedge resection

B   Segmental resection

C   Lobectomy

D   Pneumonectomy

FIGURE 31.14 Types of surgeries for lung cancer. (A) Wedge resection. (B) Segmental resection. (C) Lobectomy. (D) Pneumonectomy.

Evaluation

Carefully consider the patient's individual goals when evaluating care. Is the patient comfortable and free from unnecessary dyspnea? Is the airway clear and is nutrition being maintained? Are medication side effects manageable? Have patients with terminal conditions come to terms with their impending death, and have they been able to do those things most important to them before their death? See Table 31.9 for a lung cancer summary.

 ## THORACIC SURGERY

A surgical incision made into the chest wall is called a **thoracotomy.** A thoracotomy may be performed for a number of reasons, including biopsy; removal of tumors, lesions, or foreign objects; to repair trauma following penetrating or crushing injuries; or to repair or revise structural problems.

Pneumonectomy

A **pneumonectomy** is the surgical removal of a lung. This is usually done to treat lung cancer. It may also be used to treat severe cases of TB, bronchiectasis, or lung abscesses. Chest drainage is not usually used following a pneumonectomy. This is because, once the lung is removed, the air in the thoracic cavity is absorbed, and the cavity fills with serosanguineous fluid. At about 6 months after surgery, the fluid is coagulated, and the thoracic cavity is stabilized.

Lobectomy

Lobectomy is the surgical removal of one lobe. This may be done for lung cancer, TB, or another localized problem.

Resection

Resection refers to removal of a smaller amount of lung tissue—that is, less than one lobe. A segmental resection is the removal of one segment of a lobe; a wedge resection is removal of a small wedge of lung tissue (see Fig. 31.14).

Video-Assisted Thoracoscopic Surgery

Video-assisted thoracoscopic surgery (VATS) is a newer technique that uses a specialized endoscope to perform surgery. It can be done with two or three small incisions, so it is much less invasive than a traditional thoracotomy, which requires opening the chest. It can be used for biopsy, staging, or treatment of tumors.

Lung Transplantation

Lung transplant can benefit patients with a variety of serious pulmonary disorders, including pulmonary hypertension, emphysema, CF, and bronchiectasis. Either a single lung, both lungs, or heart and lungs have been successfully transplanted. Better criteria for selecting patients and donors as well as advancements in surgical techniques have improved outcomes for transplant patients.

Nursing Process for the Patient Undergoing Thoracic Surgery

Preoperative Nursing Care

Work with the RN to perform a thorough assessment before surgery, with a focus on the respiratory system. This gives a baseline against which to judge changes postoperatively. Routine preoperative teaching is done by the nurse in collaboration with the health team. The patient should understand that he or she will wake up in the ICU. If at all possible, it is helpful to have the patient and family tour the ICU before the surgery to decrease anxiety postoperatively. Prepare the patient for waking up after surgery with an ET tube connected to a ventilator, oxygen, chest tubes, IV fluids, cardiac monitor, Foley catheter, and possibly an epidural catheter for pain control. Let the patient know he or she will not be able to talk while the ET tube is in. Explain the use of the call light, picture board, or alternate communication techniques. Consult the surgeon for specific plans.

Advise the patient that position changes and early ambulation help prevent complications following surgery. Also instruct the patient in the use of an incentive spirometer and coughing and deep-breathing techniques for after the ET tube is removed.

Table 31.9
Lung Cancer Summary

Signs and Symptom	Cough, hemoptysis Dyspnea, wheezing Repeat respiratory infections
Diagnostic Tests	Chest x-ray Computed tomography (CT) scan Biopsy
Therapeutic Measures	Surgery Chemotherapy Radiation Targeted therapies
Complications	Pleural effusion Superior vena cava syndrome Ectopic hormone production Atelectasis Metastasis
Priority Nursing Diagnoses	*Impaired Gas Exchange* *Ineffective Airway Clearance* *Activity Intolerance*

• WORD • BUILDING •
thoracotomy: thora—chest + otomy—incision
pneumonectomy: pneum—lung + ectomy—excision

Postoperative Nursing Care

DATA COLLECTION. Frequent assessment of vital signs and hemodynamic stability; respiratory rate, depth, and effort; and lung sounds is performed. Remember that lung sounds are absent on the side of a pneumonectomy. An increase in pulse rate or a falling blood pressure may indicate internal bleeding and should be reported immediately. Oxygen saturation is monitored continuously. Often, patients report an immediate improvement in breathing because the pulmonary blood supply is no longer being routed to diseased lung tissue.

Assessment for tracheal deviation alerts you to the possible complication of mediastinal shift. The trachea is normally positioned straight above the sternal notch. If the trachea deviates from the midline position, the surgeon should be notified immediately. Secretions are monitored and reported to the HCP if they become thick, yellow or green, or foul smelling. ABGs are monitored closely. Chest tubes are usually present (except following pneumonectomy) and are monitored as explained in Chapter 29. Pain is assessed using a pain rating scale. Incision sites are monitored for redness, edema, or drainage. If the patient is mechanically ventilated, additional assessment of the ET tube and ventilator settings will be needed.

NURSING DIAGNOSES, PLANNING, AND IMPLEMENTATION. See "Nursing Care Plan for the Patient With a Lower Respiratory Tract Disorder" for basic interventions. Following are some additional interventions specific to the patient following thoracic surgery.

Ineffective Airway Clearance related to presence of ventilator, inability to cough, and sedation, as evidenced by presence of crackles and wheezes, and high-pressure ventilator alarm

EXPECTED OUTCOME: The patient will have a clear airway as evidenced by clear lung sounds and by absence of airway noise and high-pressure ventilator alarms.

• Suction according to agency policy. *The airway must remain free of secretions to prevent VAP and dyspnea.*
• Once extubated, remind the patient to cough and deep breathe regularly. *This helps clear the airway.*
• Administer analgesics as ordered. *Postoperative pain must be controlled for the patient to be able to cough effectively.*

Impaired Gas Exchange related to surgical intervention, opioid use, and removal of lung tissue, as evidenced by ABGs and by Spo$_2$ not within normal limits

EXPECTED OUTCOME: The patient's gas exchange will be within acceptable limits as evidenced by Spo$_2$ of 90% or above.

• Monitor Spo$_2$. *Interventions should maintain Spo$_2$ at 90% or above.*
• Reposition patient every 1 to 2 hours. Consult surgeon for specific positioning orders. *Some surgeons want patients positioned with the operative side up, and others with the operative side down. Fowler position allows room for lung expansion and helps prevent aspiration.*
• Encourage use of an incentive spirometer as ordered following extubation *to encourage the patient to deep breathe and maximize oxygenation.*
• Monitor chest tube and water seal drainage system, if used. *This helps re-expand the lung and must remain intact at all times.*
• Administer oxygen and bronchodilators as ordered *to maintain oxygenation.*

Acute Pain related to surgical procedure as evidenced by pain rating

EXPECTED OUTCOME: The patient will be comfortable as evidenced by statement or indication that pain is controlled. If unable to communicate, objective signs of acute pain (e.g., increase in vital signs, restlessness) will be absent.

• Administer analgesics as ordered, around the clock. *Pain control is important for the patient to be able to ambulate and deep breathe and cough effectively.*
• Monitor respiratory rate and effort if not mechanically ventilated. *Opioids depress respirations.*
• Teach the patient to splint the incision while coughing. *This can stabilize the site and reduce pain, increasing the likelihood of effective coughing.*

Impaired Physical Mobility related to discomfort at surgical site as evidenced by inability or unwillingness to move

EXPECTED OUTCOME: The patient will maintain mobility as evidenced by ability to move arm and shoulder through range-of-motion exercises.

• Perform range-of-motion exercises, passively at first, then actively when the patient is able. *This helps prevent contracture of the arm and shoulder on the affected side.*
• Assist the patient to ambulate as tolerated on first or second postoperative day as ordered. *Ambulation helps maintain mobility and prevent postoperative complications.*

Risk for Infection related to intubation, Foley catheterization, surgical incision, and major surgery

EXPECTED OUTCOME: The patient will be free of signs of infection as evidenced by clean and dry incision, temperature and WBC count within normal limits, clear sputum, and clear urine.

• Monitor temperature, WBC count, incision, sputum, and urine for signs of infection *so infection can be identified and treated quickly.*

• Use standard infection control precautions, including careful hand hygiene, *because the patient is at increased risk for infection.*

• Use meticulous sterile technique for all invasive procedures (e.g., suctioning, dressing changes, catheter insertion). *This prevents introduction of pathogens.*

• Monitor nutritional intake. Consult dietitian for recommendations. *Adequate nutrients are essential for wound healing and immune function.*

• Maintain head of bed at a minimum 30-degree elevation *to help prevent aspiration of gastric contents.*

• Provide frequent oral care *to reduce risk of aspiration of oral bacteria.*

• Assist with ventilator weaning and extubation as soon as possible. *Mechanical ventilation is associated with increased risk of pneumonia.*

• Request order to remove Foley catheter as soon as possible. *Foley catheter insertion is associated with risk of urinary tract infection (UTI).*

EVALUATION. The patient's airway should remain clear, and secretions should be easily coughed up. The patient should report an acceptable comfort level and be able to cough, deep breathe, and ambulate without excessive discomfort. The patient's breathing should be unlabored, with a respiratory rate of 12 to 20 per minute. The patient's affected arm and shoulder should maintain full range of motion. Urine should be clear. Signs of infection should be absent.

Home Health Hints

• If the patient with chronic obstructive pulmonary disease (COPD) is tempted to adjust his or her own oxygen flow rate, equipment suppliers can put on a locking flowmeter. Increasing the flow rate can reduce hypoxic drive and cause hypoventilation if the Spo_2 is too high.

• Teach the patient with COPD to conserve energy. The patient should be encouraged to sit on a stool when cooking at the stove or doing dishes. A shower stool can be obtained from a medical supply store. Personal care activities should be spaced throughout the day.

• When a patient is using oxygen by nasal cannula, the area around the ears can become irritated or excoriated. A small sponge-type hair roller can be placed around the tubing to protect the ears. Avoid using gauze for this purpose. It can be abrasive and worsen the problem.

• Teach the patient how to use inhalers properly and have the patient do a return demonstration.

• When a patient requires more than one metered-dose inhaler, number the canisters in the order they are to be used.

• Teach the patient or caregiver to clean nebulizer parts at least three times a week, using warm water and a common home disinfectant solution for 30 minutes.

• Observe the caregiver for signs of role strain. Discuss options available and consider having a social worker consulted to assist with counseling and community resources. Contact the health care provider to discuss your concerns and ideas.

SUGGESTED ANSWERS TO CRITICAL THINKING

Mr. Smith

1. A complete respiratory history is taken as described in Chapter 29. An open-ended question such as, "What happened to bring you to the hospital?" elicits information about the incident. In addition, questions to determine mental status and ability to make decisions and function safely on his own are appropriate. If any concerns arise, a social service consultation will be helpful for discharge planning.

2. Mr. Smith should be instructed to always read label warnings before using any cleaning products in the future and to never mix bleach and ammonia!

3. Monitor Mr. Smith closely for signs or symptoms of bacterial pneumonia. Assist with good mouth care, and maintain careful hand-washing and infection-control practices. Discourage ill visitors.

Mr. Woo

1. Document exactly what you see: "13 mm induration at test site." Date and time your entry, and sign.

2. Mr. Woo's test is positive. The induration has occurred because Mr. Woo's immune system has responded to the injected antigen. Mr. Woo will need a chest x-ray and a sputum culture to confirm his diagnosis.

Mr. Jenkins

1. Ask questions based on the *WHAT'S UP?* format:
   • *Where* (not applicable)
   • *How* does it feel? Does the coughing cause chest pain? Are you short of breath?
   • *Aggravating and alleviating factors.* What makes the cough worse? What seems to help? Do you use any techniques at home that are helpful?
   • *Timing.* How often do you cough during a day? Is it interfering with sleep and rest?
   • *Severity.* How bad is it on a scale of 0 to 10? How much sputum are you coughing up? Is it usually this color?
   • *Useful other data.* Are you experiencing any other symptoms with your cough (such as shortness of breath, nausea, loss of appetite)?
   • *Patient's perception.* Is it better or worse than usual today? How can I help? (The patient with long-standing disease often knows what will help but is hesitant to ask.)

2. The most appropriate nursing diagnosis is *Ineffective Airway Clearance* related to excessive secretions and ineffective cough.

3. Provide hydration with oral liquids and a room humidifier to liquefy secretions. Administer expectorants as ordered.

SUGGESTED ANSWERS TO CRITICAL THINKING—cont'd

Instruct the patient in coughing and deep-breathing exercises such as autogenic drainage to increase the effectiveness of his cough. Provide good oral care following expectoration of sputum to freshen the patient's mouth. Obtain an order for chest physiotherapy (CPT) or a vibratory positive expiratory pressure (PEP) device (Chapter 29) to help loosen and drain secretions.

4. "Patient expectorated 200 mL of bright yellow, foul-smelling sputum. Lungs have scattered crackles and wheezes throughout after coughing episode. Expectorant given; fluids encouraged. Mouth care provided."

5. Respiratory therapy should be involved with nebulized mist treatments (NMTs) and assistance with airway clearance interventions. Occupational or physical therapy can help with mobilization and increasing exercise tolerance. Discharge planning may be needed to help set up home therapies or pulmonary rehabilitation. Social work or pastoral care can help with emotional distress related to having a chronic disease.

Timothy

1. There is no way to know whether Timothy needs to be in the emergency room without further assessment. Remember that shortness of breath is very subjective and must be evaluated before discharge.

2. Collect further data. Have Timothy rate his shortness of breath. Look at his color and use of accessory muscles. Check his vital signs, peak expiratory flow rate, and oxygen saturation.

3. If Timothy is having an asthma attack, one explanation for the absence of wheezing on auscultation is that he is not moving enough air to generate the wheezing sound. If his airways are extremely tight, breath sounds may be so diminished that wheezing is not heard. This is a bad sign rather than a good one.

4. If Timothy's assessment findings are abnormal, call for help. The health care provider (HCP) may want to begin treatment quickly before further evaluation is done. A respiratory therapist (RT) can be helpful with both

further assessment and treatment. Collaborate with the registered nurse (RN) to determine the cause of Timothy's problems and provide appropriate education to prevent repeat episodes.

Mr. Franklin

1. You need to do several things at once. Begin by speaking in a calm voice and trying to help Mr. Franklin to calm himself by doing pursed-lip breathing. Assure him that you will help him and won't leave. At the same time, check his oxygen to make sure it is on the ordered number of liters and that his tubing is not kinked or disconnected. Grab the bedside table for him to lean on. Call for someone to page an RT to do an NMT if ordered. Have someone bring a pulse oximeter to check his oxygen saturation. Also call for the RN to administer intravenous morphine if ordered. All this should take about 1 minute! Once Mr. Franklin is a bit calmer, you can find out what happened. Did the exertion of moving to the bedside commode cause his dyspnea? Check his vital signs and lung sounds, and work with the RN to determine whether this represents a change in Mr. Franklin's condition that should be reported to the HCP.

2. Teach Mr. Franklin that he should probably stay on bedrest until his acute exacerbation is resolved. Once he is able to start moving around, he should call for help to get up. Review his controlled breathing exercises, which he can use during movement, and encourage rest between activities.

3. "3:00: Patient up on bedside commode (BSC), respiratory rate (RR) 36 per minute and labored, color gray, appeared very apprehensive. O_2 on at 2 L per min per nasal cannula (NC), assisted to lean on over-bed table. Encouraged pursed-lip breathing. Vital signs (VS) blood pressure 146/64 mm Hg, pulse 102 beats per minute, respirations 36 breaths per minute, SpO_2 82%. RT paged; administered as needed (prn) NMT. Breath sounds diminished, no cough. At 3:15, patient appears much calmer, RR 24 per minute and less labored, SpO_2 90%."

Review Questions

1. A patient asks the nurse why he doesn't feel sick even though the tuberculosis test is positive. The nurse knows the patient has been diagnosed with latent tuberculosis infection. Which explanation is best to provide the patient?
   1. "Tuberculosis often does not make people feel sick, but it is contagious nevertheless."
   2. "You have latent disease, which just stays in your system but won't ever make you sick."
   3. "You have tuberculosis infection but not active disease. As long as your immune system stays strong, it can keep the infection from making you sick."
   4. "Even though you do not feel sick, the positive test shows that you have the disease and must be treated with antibiotics."

2. Which of the following assessment findings does the nurse expect in the patient with emphysema?
   1. Purulent sputum
   2. Diminished breath sounds
   3. Generalized edema
   4. Dull chest pain

3. A patient with shortness of breath is being tested for lung cancer. Which diagnostic test will be most conclusive?
   1. Chest x-ray
   2. Magnetic resonance imaging
   3. Sputum culture
   4. Biopsy

4. A patient with recurrent pneumothorax is scheduled to have pleurodesis done in 1 hour. Which nursing intervention should take priority at this time?
   1. Encourage fluids.
   2. Encourage coughing and deep breathing.
   3. Administer an analgesic as needed as ordered.
   4. Administer a bronchodilator as needed as ordered.

5. Which of the following assessment findings in the patient with pneumonia most indicates a need to remind the patient to cough and deep breathe?
   1. The patient reports chest pain.
   2. The patient has removed the oxygen cannula.
   3. The patient develops coarse wheezes and crackles.
   4. The patient has a fever of 101°F (38.3°C).

6. A patient is admitted to the hospital with shortness of breath. The nurse notes increasing confusion and combativeness during the past hour. Which of the following actions is appropriate first?
   1. Assess peripheral capillary oxygen saturation and apply oxygen per protocol if indicated.
   2. Page the physician stat.
   3. Put up the patient's side rails and apply soft restraints.
   4. Administer a dose of sedative as needed.

7. Which of the following interventions is most appropriate for the patient with an ineffective breathing pattern?
   1. Encourage the patient to cough and deep breathe.
   2. Teach the patient controlled diaphragmatic breathing.
   3. Encourage oral fluids.
   4. Allow the patient to rest between activities.

8. A patient with end-stage obstructive pulmonary disease has a nursing diagnosis of *Impaired Gas Exchange*. Which assessment finding shows that interventions have been effective?
   1. The patient's peripheral capillary oxygen saturation is 92% on 2 liters of oxygen.
   2. The patient appears comfortable.
   3. The patient is coughing up copious white sputum.
   4. The patient is able to move in bed without difficulty.

Answer rationales available in your online resources.

ANSWERS 1. 3; 2. 2; 3. 4; 4. 3; 5. 3; 6. 1; 7. 2; 8. 1

Key Points

Find the chapter key points in your online resources available through Davis Edge.

Additional Resources

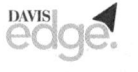 Use the scratch off code on the inside front cover of your book to access online quizzes that will help you to improve your scores on course exams and prepare for the NCLEX-PN®.

 Study Guide

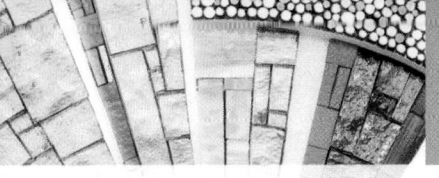
CHAPTER 32

Gastrointestinal, Hepatobiliary, and Pancreatic Systems Function, Assessment, and Therapeutic Measures

Linda S. Williams, Janice L. Bradford

KEY TERMS

basal cell secretion test (BAY-zuhl SELL seh-KREE-shun TEST)

caput medusae (KAP-ut meh-DOO-see)

colonoscopy (KOH-lun-AW-skuh-pee)

endoscopy (EN-daw-skuh-pee)

enteral nutrition (EN-ter-uhl new-TRISH-un)

esophagogastroduodenoscopy (ee-SOFF-ah-go-GAS-troh-doo-AW-den-AW-skuh-pee)

esophagoscopy (ee-SOFF-ah-GAW-skuh-pee)

fluoroscope (FLOOR-oh-skope)

gastric acid stimulation test (GAS-trik AS-id STIM-yoo-LAY-shun TEST)

gastric analysis (GAS-trik ah-NAL-ih-sis)

gastroscopy (gas-STRAW-skuh-pee)

gastrostomy (gas-STRAW-stoh-mee)

gavage (gah-VAZH)

icterus (ICK-ter-us)

impaction (im-PAK-shun)

jaundice (JAWN-dis)

lavage (lah-VAZH)

occult blood (oh-KULT BLUHD)

parenteral nutrition (par-EN-ter-uhl new-TRISH-un)

peristalsis (pear-ih-STALL-sis)

proctosigmoidoscopy (PROK-toh-SIG-moy-DAWS-kuh-pee)

retrograde cholangiopancreatography (RET-roh-grade koh-LAN-jee-oh-PAN-kree-ah-TOG-rah-fee)

spider angioma (SPY-der AN-jee-OH-mah)

steatorrhea (STEE-ah-toh-REE-ah)

striae (STREYE-ee)

CHAPTER CONCEPTS

Elimination
Nutrition

LEARNING OUTCOMES

1. List the structures of the gastrointestinal tract and of the accessory glands: liver, gallbladder, and pancreas.
2. Describe the functions of each organ of the gastrointestinal tract and of the accessory glands: liver, gallbladder, and pancreas.
3. Discuss how age affects the gastrointestinal tract and accessory glands.
4. List data to collect when caring for a patient with a disorder of the gastrointestinal system, liver, gallbladder, or pancreas.
5. Differentiate normal and abnormal data collection findings.
6. Explain techniques used to conduct a physical examination of the abdomen.
7. Plan nursing care for patients having diagnostic tests of the gastrointestinal tract.
8. Explain types of nasogastric tubes and their uses.
9. Plan nursing care for insertion and maintenance of nasogastric tubes.
10. Describe therapeutic measures used for patients with gastrointestinal diseases.

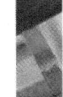

NORMAL GASTROINTESTINAL, HEPATOBILIARY, AND PANCREATIC SYSTEMS ANATOMY AND PHYSIOLOGY

The gastrointestinal (GI) tract (or alimentary tract) is part of the digestive system (Fig. 32.1). Digestion begins in the oral cavity and continues in the stomach and small intestine. Most absorption of nutrients takes place in the small intestine. The large intestine is where the majority of water is reabsorbed. Indigestible material, mainly cellulose, is then eliminated from the large intestine. Accessory organs include teeth, tongue, salivary glands, liver, gallbladder, and pancreas.

Oral Cavity and Pharynx

The boundaries of the oral cavity are the hard and soft palates superiorly, the cheeks laterally, and the floor of the mouth inferiorly. Within the oral cavity are the teeth, tongue, and the openings of the ducts of the salivary glands.

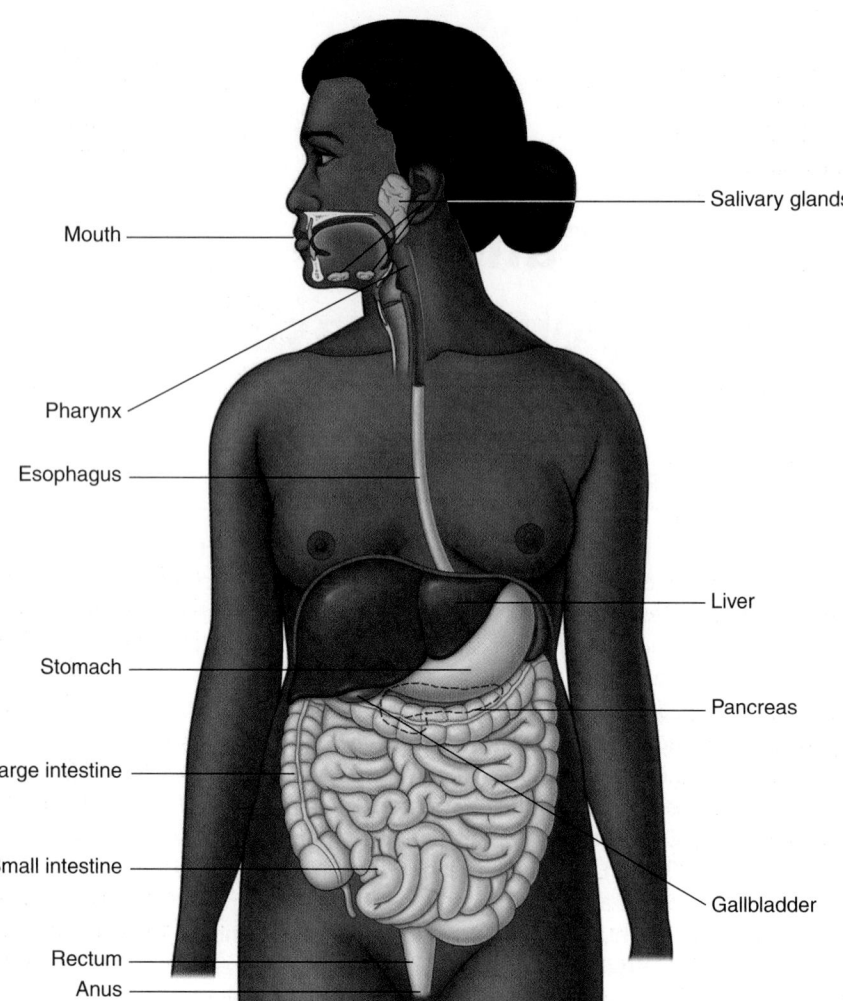

Mouth

Pharynx

Esophagus

Stomach

Large intestine

Small intestine

Rectum
Anus

Salivary glands

Liver

Pancreas

Gallbladder

FIGURE 32.1 Digestive system.

The teeth begin mechanical digestion to create more sur-face area for the chemical digestion regulated by enzymes. The roots of the teeth are in sockets in the mandible and max-illae. The tongue is made of skeletal muscle innervated by the hypoglossal nerve. Taste buds surround the base of each papilla. Innervation for tasting is by the facial, glossopharyn-geal, and vagus nerves. Elevation of the tongue is the first step in swallowing.

The three pairs of salivary glands are the parotid, sub-mandibular, and sublingual glands. Their ducts secrete saliva to the oral cavity. Salivation is a parasympathetic response mediated by the facial and glossopharyngeal nerves. Saliva is mostly water. It is used to dissolve food for gustation and moisten the food for swallowing. The only digestive enzyme in saliva that functions in the mouth is amylase, which digests starch to maltose. However, food does not remain in the mouth long enough for significant starch digestion. There is also lingual lipase. When activated by acidic pH, it begins its action in the stomach.

The pharynx is a muscular tube connecting the oral cavity to the esophagus. When a mass of food is pushed posteriorly by the tongue, the smooth muscles of the pharynx contract as part of the swallowing reflex. This reflex is regulated by the medulla and pons. The uvula closes off the nasopharynx while the epiglottis closes the opening to the larynx.

Esophagus

The esophagus is about 10 inches long. It carries ingested items from the pharynx to the stomach. No digestion takes place in the esophagus. **Peristalsis** of the muscle layer in the wall of the esophagus propels food inferiorly to the stomach. At the junction with the stomach, the lumen of the esophagus is surrounded by the lower esophageal sphincter (LES; also cardiac sphincter, gastroesophageal sphincter, or esophageal sphincter). It is a circular, smooth muscle. The LES relaxes to permit food to enter the stom-ach and then contracts to prevent the backflow of stomach contents. The esophagus penetrates the diaphragm at the esophageal hiatus. The remainder of the digestive system is within the abdominopelvic cavity.

• **WORD** • **BUILDING** •
peristalsis: peri—around + stellein—to place

Stomach

The stomach is in the upper left abdominal quadrant, to the left of the liver and in front of the spleen. It is a J-shaped, sac-like organ that extends from the esophagus to the duodenum of the small intestine. Some digestion takes place in the stomach; it serves mainly as a reservoir for food so that digestion may take place gradually.

The four regions of the stomach are the cardia, fundus, body, and pylorus (Fig. 32.2). The pylorus is divided into an antrum and canal. It narrows at the pyloric sphincter, which guards entry to the duodenum.

When the stomach is empty, the mucosa (inner lining) has folds called rugae that permit expansion of the lining. The mucosa contains gastric pits with glands of the stomach that produce gastric juice.

Gastric juice begins secretion at the sight or smell of food; this is a parasympathetic response. The presence of food in the stomach stimulates the secretion of the hormone gastrin by the gastric mucosa. Gastrin increases the secretion of gastric juice.

The three layers of smooth muscle in the stomach wall achieve efficient mechanical digestion, changing ingested food to a thick liquid called *chyme.* The pyloric sphincter contracts when the stomach is churning food and relaxes at intervals to allow small amounts of chyme to pass into the duodenum. Carbohydrates are most readily digested by the stomach, followed by proteins and fats.

Small Intestine

The small intestine is about 1 inch in diameter and approximately 10 feet long. Within the peritoneal cavity, the coils of the small intestine are encircled by the colon. The small intestine extends from the stomach to the cecum of the colon. The duodenum is the first 10 inches and contains

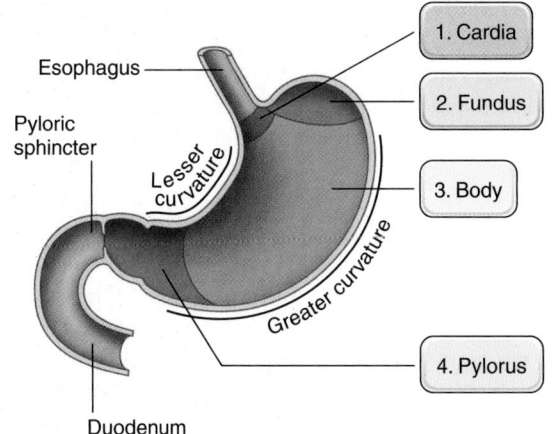

FIGURE 32.2 Parts of the stomach.

the hepatopancreatic ampulla (ampulla of Vater), the entrance of the common bile duct and the pancreatic duct. The jejunum is about 3 feet long; the ileum is about 6 feet in length.

Digestion is completed in the small intestine. The end products of digestion are absorbed into the blood and lymph. Bile from the liver and enzymes from the pancreas function in the small intestine (Table 32.1). When chyme enters the duodenum, the intestinal mucosa produces the enzymes sucrase, maltase, and lactase, which complete the digestion of disaccharides to monosaccharides; the peptidases, which complete the digestion of proteins to amino acids; and the nucleosidases and phosphatases, completing nucleotide digestion.

The absorption of nutrients requires a large surface area; the small intestine has extensive folds for this purpose. Macroscopic circular folds and microscopic villi with apical

Table 32.1

Digestive Secretions

Organ	Enzyme or Other Secretion	Function	Site of Action
Salivary glands	Amylase	Converts starch to maltose	Oral cavity
Stomach	Pepsin Hydrochloric acid	Converts proteins to polypeptides Changes pepsinogen to pepsin Maintains pH of 1–2 Destroys pathogens	Stomach
Liver	Bile salts	Emulsify fats	Small intestine
Pancreas	Amylase Lipase Trypsin	Converts starch to maltose Converts emulsified fats to fatty acids and glycerol Converts polypeptides to peptides	Small intestine
Small intestine	Peptidases Sucrase, maltase, lactase	Convert peptides to amino acids Convert disaccharides to monosaccharides	Small intestine

border microvilli greatly expand the absorptive surface. Water-soluble nutrients (monosaccharides, amino acids, minerals, water-soluble vitamins) are absorbed into the blood in the capillary networks. Fat-soluble vitamins and fatty acids and glycerol are absorbed into the chyle of the lacteals.

Large Intestine

The large intestine extends from the ileum of the small intestine to the anus. It is about 5 feet long and 2.5 inches in diameter. The ileocecal valve prevents backup of fecal material from the large intestine into the small intestine. No further digestion takes place in the colon; it temporarily stores and then eliminates indigestible material. The mucosa absorbs significant amounts of water and minerals as well as the vitamins produced by the normal bacterial flora.

Elimination of feces is accomplished by involuntary and voluntary actions. Parasympathetic control initiates the defecation reflex from centers in the sacral region of the spinal cord. Baroreceptor input produces returning motor impulses. This causes contraction of the smooth muscle of the rectum and relaxation of the internal anal sphincter. Defecation is voluntarily controlled via actions of the external anal sphincter.

Liver

The liver occupies the right side and center of the upper abdominal cavity just below the diaphragm. Its right lobe is larger than the left lobe.

The blood supply of the liver differs from that of other organs. The liver receives oxygenated blood by way of the hepatic artery. By way of the hepatic portal vein, blood from the abdominal digestive organs and the spleen is brought to the liver before being returned to the heart. This special pathway is called hepatic portal circulation. It permits the liver to regulate blood levels of nutrients or to remove potentially toxic substances such as alcohol from the blood before the blood circulates to the rest of the body. All blood leaving the liver exits via the hepatic vein.

The only digestive function of the liver is the production of bile by the hepatocytes. Bile flows to the duodenum via ducts from either the liver or gallbladder (Fig. 32.3).

Bile is mostly water and bile salts. Its excretory function is to carry bilirubin and excess cholesterol to the intestines for elimination in feces. The digestive function of bile is accomplished via bile salts, which emulsify fats in the small intestine. Emulsification is a type of mechanical digestion in which large fat globules are broken into smaller globules, producing greater surface area for chemical catabolism. Secretion of bile is stimulated by the hormone secretin. Ejection of bile from the gallbladder is stimulated by cholecystokinin.

Functions of the Liver

The liver is involved in a variety of functions, most of which involve organic molecule metabolism. These functions can be grouped into categories.

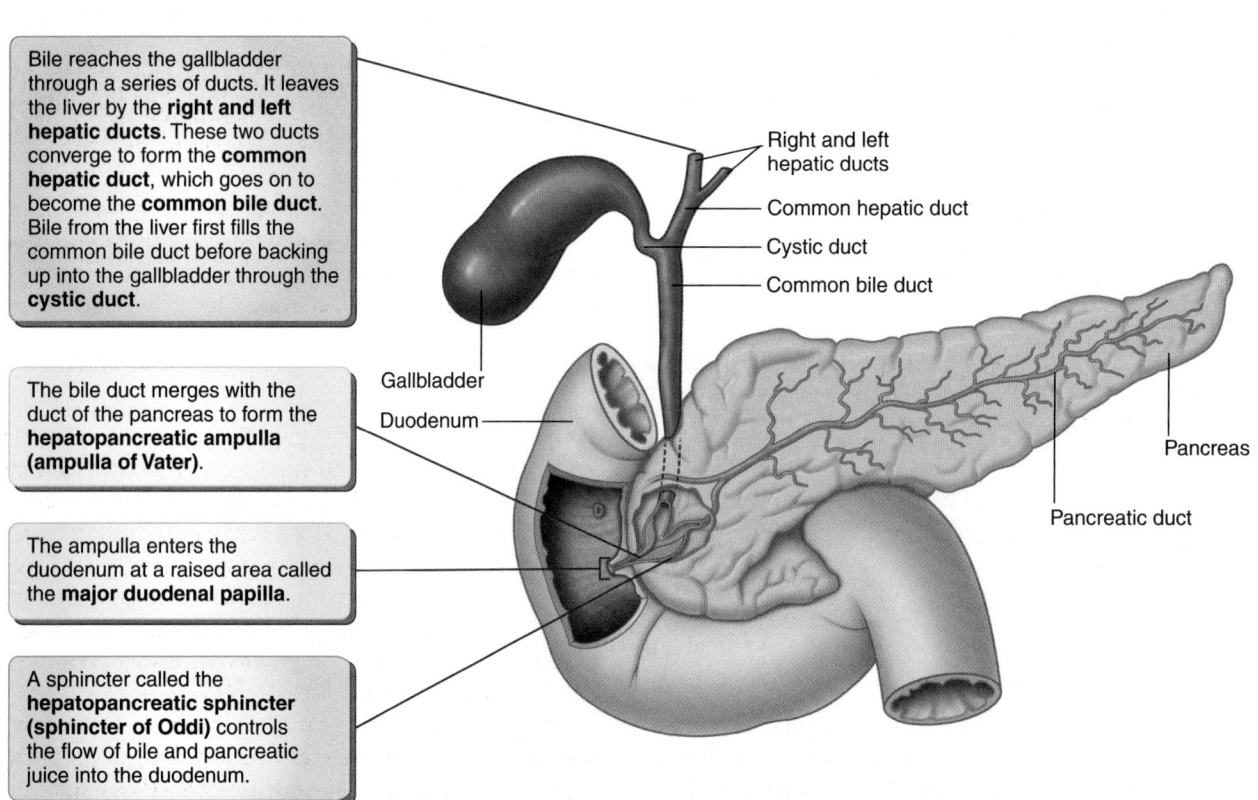

Bile reaches the gallbladder through a series of ducts. It leaves the liver by the **right and left hepatic ducts**. These two ducts converge to form the **common hepatic duct**, which goes on to become the **common bile duct**. Bile from the liver first fills the common bile duct before backing up into the gallbladder through the **cystic duct**.

The bile duct merges with the duct of the pancreas to form the **hepatopancreatic ampulla (ampulla of Vater)**.

The ampulla enters the duodenum at a raised area called the **major duodenal papilla**.

A sphincter called the **hepatopancreatic sphincter (sphincter of Oddi)** controls the flow of bile and pancreatic juice into the duodenum.

Right and left hepatic ducts

Common hepatic duct

Cystic duct

Common bile duct

Gallbladder

Duodenum

Pancreas

Pancreatic duct

FIGURE 32.3 Gallbladder and pancreas.

CARBOHYDRATE METABOLISM. The liver regulates the blood glucose level by storing excess glucose as glycogen and performing glycogenolysis when the blood glucose level is low. The liver also changes other monosaccharides to glucose, which is more readily used by cells for energy production.

AMINO ACID METABOLISM. The liver regulates the blood levels of amino acids based on tissue needs for protein synthesis. Of the 20 amino acids needed for the production of human proteins, the liver is able to synthesize 12, called the nonessential amino acids, by the process of transamination. The other eight amino acids, which the liver cannot synthesize, are called the essential amino acids. Essential amino acids are required in the diet.

Excess amino acids (those not needed for protein synthesis) undergo the process of deamination in the liver; the amino group is removed, and the remaining carbon chain is converted to a simple carbohydrate that is used for energy production or converted to fat for energy storage. The amino groups are converted to urea, a nitrogenous waste product that is removed from the blood by the kidneys and excreted in urine.

LIPID METABOLISM. The liver forms lipoproteins for the transport of lipids in the blood to other tissues. The liver also synthesizes cholesterol and excretes excess cholesterol into bile to be eliminated in feces.

Beta oxidation is another task of the liver, in which fatty acid molecules are split into two-carbon acetyl groups. These acetyl groups may be used by the liver to produce energy, or they may be combined to form ketones to be transported to other cells for energy production.

SYNTHESIS OF PLASMA PROTEINS. The liver synthesizes albumin, clotting factors, and globulins. Albumin is the most abundant plasma protein; it maintains osmotic balance. Clotting factors produced by the liver include prothrombin and fibrinogen, which circulate in the blood until needed for coagulation. Globulin functions include becoming part of lipoproteins, acting as carriers, and acting as antibodies.

PHAGOCYTOSIS BY KUPFFER CELLS. The fixed macrophages of the liver (named Kupffer cells or stellate reticuloendothelial cells) phagocytize worn formed elements and pathogens.

FORMATION OF BILIRUBIN. Hepatocytes form bilirubin from the *heme* portion of hemoglobin removed from worn erythrocytes and collect bilirubin from the spleen. Bilirubin is excreted as a part of bile to be eliminated in feces.

STORAGE. The liver stores the minerals iron and copper; the fat-soluble vitamins A, D, E, and K; and the water-soluble vitamin B_{12}.

DETOXIFICATION. The liver synthesizes enzymes that convert harmful substances to less harmful ones. Alcohol and medications are examples of potentially toxic chemicals. The liver also converts ammonia from protein metabolism to urea, a less toxic substance.

ACTIVATION OF VITAMIN D. The skin, kidneys, and liver each perform a role in providing the body with activated vitamin D.

Gallbladder

The gallbladder is a muscular sac approximately 4 inches long located on the undersurface of the liver. Bile in the common hepatic duct from the liver flows through the cystic duct into the gallbladder. The gallbladder stores bile until it is needed in the small intestine (see Fig. 32.3). The gallbladder concentrates bile by absorbing water.

When fatty foods or partially digested proteins enter the duodenum, the duodenal mucosa secretes the hormone cholecystokinin. One function of cholecystokinin is to stimulate contraction of the smooth muscle of the wall of the gallbladder. Contraction of the gallbladder forces bile into the cystic duct and then into the common bile duct, which empties into the duodenum.

Pancreas

The pancreas is about 6 inches long. It is located posterior to the greater curvature of the stomach. Digestive secretions enter the duodenum either via the pancreatic duct or the alternate accessory duct (see Fig. 32.3).

The pancreatic digestive enzymes are involved in the digestion of all four of the organic molecule categories. The enzyme pancreatic amylase digests starch to maltose. Pancreatic lipase converts emulsified fats to fatty acids and monoglycerides. Trypsinogen is an inactive enzyme that is changed to active trypsin in the duodenum. Trypsin digests polypeptides to shorter chains of amino acids. Pancreatic juice also contains proteolytic enzymes: chymotrypsin, carboxypeptidase, and elastase. Ribonuclease and deoxyribonuclease, for the digestion of RNA and DNA, respectively, are contributed by the pancreas as well.

Secretion of pancreatic juice is stimulated by the hormones of the duodenal mucosa. Secretin stimulates the production of bicarbonate pancreatic juice. Cholecystokinin stimulates secretion of the pancreatic enzyme juice.

Aging and the Gastrointestinal, Hepatobiliary, and Pancreatic Systems

Many changes occur in the aging GI system (Fig. 32.4). The sense of taste is less acute. If teeth have been lost, chewing may be difficult. Periodontal disease and oral cancer increase. Secretions throughout the GI tract are reduced. Effective peristalsis diminishes because of loss of muscle elasticity and slowed motility. Indigestion episodes may increase, especially with loss of tone of the LES. Peptic ulcers are more common. In the colon, diverticula may form. Hemorrhoids and constipation may be problems. Colon cancer risk also increases with age.

The liver and pancreas usually continue to function well into old age. Liver damage can occur from pathogens such as hepatitis viruses or toxins such as alcohol ("Gerontological Issues"). Gallstone formation increases. Acute pancreatitis of unknown cause is more common.

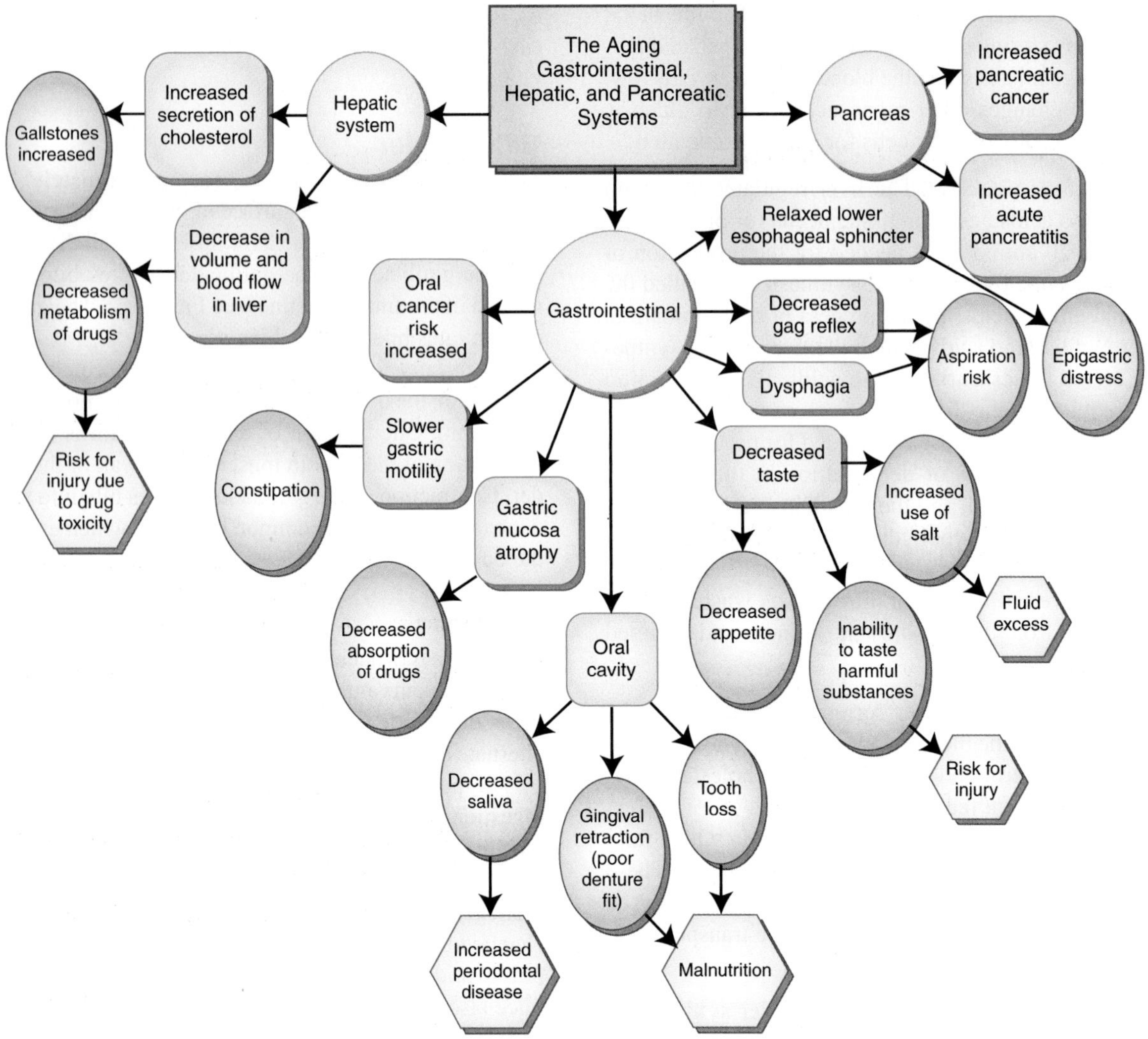

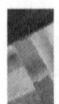

FIGURE 32.4 The effects of aging on the gastrointestinal, hepatic, and pancreatic systems are shown on this concept map.

Gerontological Issues

Medication Metabolism. With aging, the liver decreases in mass, volume, and blood flow. The liver metabolizes many drugs, and, with impaired liver function, toxic levels of a drug can occur. Check liver function tests and review medications that are metabolized by the liver. The older adult may require a lower dosage of these medications.

NURSING ASSESSMENT OF THE GASTROINTESTINAL, HEPATOBILIARY, AND PANCREATIC SYSTEMS

Health History

Data collection includes asking the *WHAT'S UP?* questions (see Chapter 1) (Table 32.2). Demographic data are obtained, including travel history to help diagnose the cause of GI symptoms such as diarrhea and work history for potential exposure to liver toxic chemicals.

Medications

Ask the patient about all medications, including acetaminophen, antacids, aspirin, nonsteroidal anti-inflammatory drugs (NSAIDs), and laxatives. NSAIDs or aspirin can cause irritation and bleeding in the GI tract. Acetaminophen can be hepatotoxic. Older adults may use these medications for arthritis pain control (see "Gerontological Issues"). Older adults may use laxatives regularly and become dependent on them. Teaching may be needed on normal bowel patterns and laxative use.

CLOSTRIDIUM DIFFICILE. Ask the patient about recent hospitalizations, antibiotic use, or uncontrolled diarrhea. Recent hospitalizations and antibiotic use is a risk factor for *Clostridium difficile* (see Chapter 8). If risk factors are present, monitor patients closely for indicators of *C. difficile* infection (e.g., diarrhea, nausea, anorexia, abdominal tenderness or

Table 32.2

Subjective Data Collection for the Gastrointestinal, Hepatobiliary, and Pancreatic Systems

Questions to Ask During the Health History	*Rationale/Significance*
Gastrointestinal	
Do you have any history of gastrointestinal (GI) illnesses or surgeries?	Patient may have a recurring problem.
Nausea, vomiting, bloating, excess gas?	Can be associated with GI disorders.
Do you smoke?	Nicotine can irritate the GI mucosa. Smoking is related to esophagitis, ulcers, and GI cancers such as esophagus and mouth cancer.
What are your bowel patterns and frequency? Any changes? Stool color, consistency? Diarrhea or constipation? Bowel incontinence? Ostomy?	Changes in bowel habits could indicate new disease process. Black stools: bleeding; clay-colored stools: liver or gallbladder disease; fatty stools: pancreatic disease. Constipation may result from dehydration.
Have you had any blood in your stool or on the toilet tissue?	Blood in stool may indicate hemorrhoids, sign of cancer, or inflammatory diseases such as ulcerative colitis.
Gallbladder, Liver, and Pancreas	
Do you have abdominal pain? Do any foods cause pain?	Pain can be associated with disease of the liver, gallbladder, or pancreas. Fatty foods can cause pain in gallbladder disease.
Does your abdomen feel distended or full?	Fluid in the abdomen, or ascites, occurs with liver disease.
Do you bruise or bleed easily?	Bleeding is associated with liver disease, because clotting factors are made in the liver.
How much alcohol do you drink each day?	Excess alcohol intake is associated with liver disease and pancreatitis.
Have you had any recent blood transfusions or blood products, dental procedures, body piercing or tattooing, or intravenous injection with a potentially contaminated needle?	Breaks in skin may be the route of entry for hepatitis (type B or C) or other pathogens.
Medications	
What prescription, over-the-counter, or herbal remedies do you take?	Provides baseline information. Many drugs and herbs are toxic to the liver.
Have you recently taken any nonsteroidal anti-inflammatory drugs (NSAIDs), aspirin, anticoagulants, or steroids?	These medications can cause gastric upset and/or bleeding.
Do you routinely take laxatives or use fiber?	Patient may have dependency on laxatives.
Are you taking or have you recently taken antibiotics?	Diarrhea due to *Clostridium difficile* can be caused by recent antibiotic use.

Continued

Table 32.2

Subjective Data Collection for the Gastrointestinal, Hepatobiliary, and Pancreatic Systems—cont'd

Questions to Ask During the Health History	*Rationale/Significance*
Nutrition	
Describe your usual diet. Tell me what you ate yesterday for the entire day. Do you use nutritional supplements or vitamins?	Provides information about adequacy of nutritional status. Older adults may be on a fixed income and unable to afford adequate nutrition.
Do you have any food allergies?	These may interfere with proper nutrition.
Do you have indigestion, dysphagia, heartburn, nausea, or vomiting? Have you had a change in appetite? Have you had a change in weight—gain or loss? Are there any foods that you cannot eat?	Use *WHAT'S UP?* format for further details.
Family History	
Do you have a family history of alcoholism or GI, liver, gallbladder, or pancreatic diseases?	Certain diseases are hereditary.

pain). Report these signs and symptoms to the health care provider (HCP) promptly. *C. difficile* infection can be fatal.

CRITICAL THINKING

Mrs. Todd, age 74, has arthritis and takes eight aspirin daily for pain control. She is scheduled for an esophagogastroduodenoscopy (EGD) for anemia due to suspected gastrointestinal (GI) bleeding.

1. What is a likely cause of Mrs. Todd's GI bleeding?
2. What could you do to help prevent future bleeding episodes for Mrs. Todd?
3. What nursing care is required before and after the test?

   Suggested answers are at the end of the chapter.

Nutritional History

Ask about patterns of gastric acid reflux, heartburn, indigestion, nausea, vomiting, diarrhea, constipation, flatulence, and bowel incontinence. These conditions may interfere with proper nutrition. Acid reflux can be identified by asking patients if they experience a bile taste or awaken with an unpleasant taste in their mouth.

Cultural Influences

Respecting and assisting the patient to maintain desired cultural food practices is important for nutritional maintenance (Box 32.1).

Physical Examination

Table 32.3 summarizes findings from the objective assessment of the GI, hepatobiliary, and pancreatic systems, discussed next.

Height, Weight, and Body Mass Index

The patient's height and weight are obtained for planning care. Excess waist circumferences (for women, more than 35 inches; for men, more than 40 inches) place people at greater risk for diabetes and cardiovascular disease. Body mass index (BMI) is calculated to measure body fat and used along with waist-to-hip ratio measurements to determine the patient's health risk factors (Table 32.4).

Oral Cavity

Oral health is very important to a person's overall health and well-being. The ability of the patient to perform oral care is noted. The lips are examined for lesions, abnormal color, and symmetry. With a penlight and tongue blade, the oral cavity is inspected for inflammation, tenderness, ulcers, swelling,

Box 32.1

Cultural Nutritional Assessment

Questions to ask when performing a cultural nutritional assessment:
- What types of foods are common in your culture or community?
- What are your preferred foods?
- Which foods do you most commonly consume?
- How and where are your foods chosen and purchased?
- Who prepares the food in your household?
- Who purchases the food in your household?
- How is your food stored for future use?
- How is your food prepared before being eaten?
- What foods do you eat or avoid to maintain your health?
- What foods do you eat or avoid when you are ill?

Table 32.3

Objective Data Collection for the Gastrointestinal, Hepatobiliary, and Pancreatic Systems

Normal Physical Examination Findings	*Possible Abnormal Findings/Causes*
Height, Weight, and Body Mass Index (BMI)	
Normal height, weight, and BMI	Decreases in height, weight, and BMI could indicate inadequate nutrition or malabsorption problems. Current weight loss could indicate cancer.
Oral Cavity	
Moist, pink oral mucosa, without lesions, inflammation, tenderness, or discolorations	Foul odor may indicate infection or poor oral hygiene.
Pink, rough-surfaced tongue	A dry tongue with cracks or furrows indicates dehydration, possibly due to vomiting or diarrhea.
Intact teeth; properly fitting dentures	Broken teeth or ill-fitting dentures can contribute to inadequate nutrition.
Abdominal	
Inspection	
Abdomen contour flat, rounded, or convex; shape symmetrical	Irregularities in contour and symmetry such as bulging or masses may be due to distention, tumors, hernia, abdominal aortic aneurysm, or previous surgeries.
Skin color consistent with skin tone	Jaundice color may indicate liver or gallbladder disease. Bruising could be related to injury or altered liver function.
No scars, stomas, or discolorations	Scars, dressings, stoma, and ostomy appliance are noted. Striae are present if the skin has been stretched (i.e., with pregnancy or weight gain). Note any spider angiomas or caput medusae.
Auscultation	
Bowel sounds present	Absent due to ileus or obstruction.
Circulatory sounds absent	Humming sound may be heard over liver with cirrhosis, indicating overloaded liver venous circulation.
Percussion	
Completed by health care provider	Fluid, air, and masses may be in abdomen.
Palpation (Light)	
Abdomen is soft, with no pain, muscle tension, rigidity, or masses felt	Muscle tension, rigidity, or pain may occur in many abdominal disorders.
Abdominal girth should be appropriate for patient without increasing over time	Ascites from liver disease may increase girth that increases as the disease worsens.
Anus	
No lumps, rashes, scars, erythema, bleeding, fissures, or hemorrhoids	Hemorrhoids may be present. Diarrhea may cause skin breakdown or rash.

Table 32.4

Calculating Body Mass Index and Waist-to-Hip Ratio Measurement

To calculate body mass index (BMI)	*Formulas:* *Pounds and inches:* weight (lb) / [height (in.)]^2 × 703 Step 1. Multiply height (in inches) by height. Step 2. Divide weight (in pounds) by Step 1 answer. Step 3. Multiply Step 2 answer by 703. *Kilograms and meters:* weight (kg) / [height (m)]^2 Step 1. Multiply height (in meters) by height. Step 2. Divide weight (in kilograms) by Step 1 answer.
BMI findings	• Below 18.5: underweight • 18.5–24.9: normal • 25–29.9: overweight • 30 and over: obese
To obtain waist-to-hip ratio measurement	Step 1. Stand. Place measuring tape around bare waist at top of hip bones. Step 2. Pull snugly around the waist. Step 3. Read measurement after exhale. Step 4. Place measuring tape around hip at widest part and read measurement. Step 5. Waist measurement is divided by hip measurement.
Waist-to-hip ratio findings/risk for health complications	Female: 0.8 = low risk; 0.85 or greater = high risk Male: 0.95 = low risk; 1.0 or greater = high risk

bleeding, discoloration, and foul breath odor. The tongue should be pink with a rough texture with no signs of dehydration, such as dryness, cracks, or furrows. The patient's gums should be pink without swelling, redness, or irregularities. Loose, broken, or absent teeth and problems with the fit of dentures are noted. Loose teeth can become dislodged and aspirated into the airway. Broken teeth can be a source of pain and contribute to poor nutritional intake. Ill-fitting dentures can affect the patient's nutritional intake and obstruct the airway

Abdomen

Instead of following the usual inspect-palpate-percuss-auscultate (IPPA) format, abdominal examination starts with inspection, then auscultation, percussion, and palpation. This prevents palpation from altering other data collection findings.

INSPECTION. To inspect the abdomen, patients are placed in a supine position with their arms at their sides. Wounds, tubes, or ostomy devices, including type and location, are noted.

Inspect the patient's skin for bruising, **caput medusae** (bluish purple, swollen vein pattern extending out from the navel), **jaundice** (also called **icterus**; a yellowing of the skin and the sclerae of the eyes), petechiae, scars, **striae**

(commonly called stretch marks; light silver-colored or thin red lines on the abdomen), and **spider angiomas** (thin, reddish purple vein lines close to the skin surface). Observe for visible masses, visible movement, or peristalsis.

Jaundice is a symptom of liver or gallbladder disease and red blood cell disorders. Old red blood cells are cleared from the circulatory system by phagocytes in the spleen, liver, lymph nodes, and bone marrow. In the process, the compound heme (part of hemoglobin) is split into iron and another substance that is metabolized to bilirubin. The liver is then responsible for converting bilirubin to a water-soluble compound that can be excreted in bile. If the liver is unable to convert or conjugate bilirubin to a water-soluble compound or if bile drainage is obstructed, serum bilirubin is elevated and pigments are deposited in body tissues.

When serum bilirubin levels elevate, the patient's skin color changes to yellow. The yellow color varies from pale yellow to a striking golden orange. The color intensity is directly related to the amount of elevation of the serum bilirubin. Jaundice can be seen in body tissue and fluid

• WORD • BUILDING •

caput medusae: caput—head + medusae—Medusa's snaky locks
jaundice: jaune—yellow

where there is any amount of albumin ("Cultural Considerations"). Pigment may occasionally be seen in cerebrospinal fluid or joint fluid. Pigment is not seen in saliva or tears. Urine becomes dark. If bile flow to the bowel is obstructed, stools will be a light clay color.

Cultural Considerations

To observe for jaundice in a patient with dark skin, look at the sclerae, conjunctivae, palms of hands, soles of feet, and in the buccal mucosa for patches of yellow bilirubin pigment.

The perianal and anal areas are inspected for color, rashes, scars, fissures, external hemorrhoids, and skin breakdown.

Observe the patient's stool for evidence of bacteria (e.g., a foul smell), fat (e.g., stool floats on the water surface and appears greasy), pus, blood, mucus, and color. With liver or gallbladder disease, stools may be pale or clay colored.

AUSCULTATION. Bowel sounds are soft clicks and gurgles that vary normally in frequency and rate. To listen for bowel sounds, the stethoscope is pressed lightly on the abdomen (Fig. 32.5). Bowel sounds can be categorized as normal, hyperactive, hypoactive, or absent. With a bowel obstruction, a high-pitched tinkling sound that is proximal to the obstruction and absent distal to the obstruction may be heard.

Research has shown that there is great variability in how bowel sounds are auscultated. Therefore, the value of listening to bowel sounds has been questioned. Further research is needed to determine if there is value in listening to bowel sounds and to standardize the method for auscultating.

PERCUSSION. Percussion produces a sound that identifies the density of the organs beneath the area being percussed. It is performed by the HCP. Percussion detects fluid, air, and masses in the abdomen. It also identifies size and location of abdominal organs (especially the liver and spleen). Tympanic high-pitched sounds indicate the presence of air. Dull thuds indicate fluid or solid organs.

PALPATION. Light palpation of the abdomen concludes the physical assessment. If the patient is having pain, palpate that area last. Lightly depress the abdomen no more than 0.5 to 1.0 inch during the palpation using the finger pads. Note any muscle tension, rigidity, masses, or expressions of pain.

Deep palpation of the abdomen is done only by the HCP. Rebound tenderness is determined by pressing down on the abdomen a few inches and quickly releasing the pressure. If the patient feels a sharp pain during this procedure, appendicitis may be indicated.

Abdominal girth is measured by placing a tape measure around the patient's abdomen at the iliac crest. A mark is made at the measurement site so measurements are made at the same location for comparison. Abdominal girth is increased in patients with distention or conditions such as ascites (accumulation of fluid in the peritoneal cavity). When abdominal girth is abnormal, daily measurements should be monitored for changes.

DIAGNOSTIC TESTS FOR THE GASTROINTESTINAL, HEPATOBILIARY, AND PANCREATIC SYSTEMS

See Appendix B for general information on common diagnostic tests. See Tables 32.5 and 32.6 for summary of laboratory tests and Table 32.7 for a summary of diagnostic procedures.

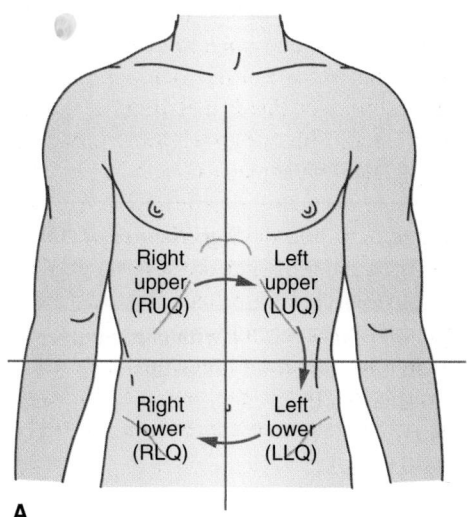

A

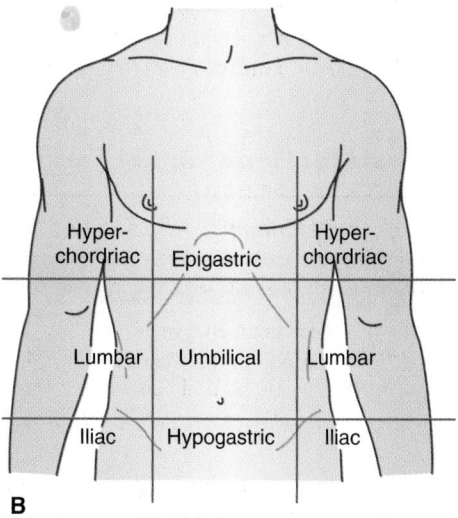

B

FIGURE 32.5 (A) Abdominal quadrants. Auscultation may begin from the right upper quadrant in a clockwise manner. (B) Nine abdominal regions.

Table 32.5
Laboratory Tests for Gastrointestinal System

Test	Definition	Normal Range	Significance of Abnormal Findings
Carcinoembryonic antigen (CEA)	Blood test to detect glycoproteins produced during rapid multiplication of epithelial cells.	Nonsmoker: Less than 2.5 ng/mL Smoker: Less than 5 ng/mL	Identifies stage of colorectal cancer. Tests for recurrence or metastasis of colon or liver cancer. Monitors response to liver and gastrointestinal (GI) cancer therapy. Elevated: benign tumors, cirrhosis, GI cancer, inflammatory bowel disease, pancreatitis.
Fecal Analysis			
Stool for occult blood	Stool sample tested for presence of blood.	Negative	Blood presence may indicate peptic ulcer, colorectal cancer, ulcerative colitis.
Stool cultures	Stool sample tested for pathogenic bacteria.	No pathogen growth	Bacterial infection, botulism.
Stool for fat (lipids)	Test measuring fat content in stool. Used to confirm diagnosis of steatorrhea.	Adult: 2–7 g per 24 hours	Increased: Crohn disease, malabsorption syndrome, malnutrition, pancreatic disease, peptic ulcer disease.
Stool for immunochemical test	Stool sample tested for presence of hidden blood	Negative	Blood presence can be early sign of colorectal cancer requiring further testing.
Stool for multitarget DNA	Stool sample tested for 10 biomarkers for pre-cancerous lesions and colorectal cancer	Negative	Pre-cancerous lesions or colorectal cancer
Stool for ova and parasites	Stool sample tested for parasites	No parasites, ova, or larvae	Parasitic infection

Table 32.6
Laboratory Tests for Hepatobiliary and Pancreatic Systems

Test	Definition	Normal Range	Significance of Abnormal Findings
Blood			
Alanine aminotransferase (ALT)	ALT is an enzyme made in the liver.	*13 months to 60 years:* Male 19–36 units/L; Female 24–36 units/L *61 to 90 years:* Male 13–40 units/L; Female 10–28 units/L *Older than 90:* Male 6–38 units/L; Female 5–24 units/L	↑ with chronic liver damage and hepatitis

Table 32.6

Laboratory Tests for Hepatobiliary and Pancreatic Systems—cont'd

Test	Definition	Normal Range	Significance of Abnormal Findings
Albumin	The body protein in the greatest concentration. Evaluates liver, kidney, and nutritional status.	*20 to 40 years:* 3.7–5.1 g/dL *41 to 60 years:* 3.4–4.8 g/dL *61 to 90 years:* 3.2–4.6 g/dL *Older than 90:* 2.9–4.5 g/dL	↓ in acute and chronic liver disease, kidney disease, and malnutrition
Ammonia	A by-product of protein catabolism.	15–60 mcg/dL	↑ in cirrhosis and hepatitis
Amylase	Detects and evaluates treatment for pancreatitis.	100–300 units/L	↑ in biliary tract disease, common bile duct obstruction or stones, pancreatitis, pancreatic ascites, cancer, cyst, or tumor ↓ in hepatic disease, pancreatectomy, and pancreatic insufficiency
Aspartate aminotransferase (AST); also called serum glutamic-oxaloacetic transaminase (SGOT)	Enzyme found in large amounts in the liver and smaller amounts in the pancreas that is released into bloodstream with tissue damage. Levels reflect degree of damage.	*20 to 49 years:* Male 20–40 units/L; Female: 15–30 units/L *Male older than 50 years or Female older than 45 years:* 10–35 units/L	Greatly ↑ acute hepatitis, especially viral, and acute pancreatitis Moderately ↑ biliary tract obstruction, cirrhosis, chronic hepatitis, and liver tumors
Bilirubin			
• Total serum bilirubin	Evaluates liver function. Sum of conjugated, unconjugated, and delta bilirubin.	Less than 1.2 mg/dL	↑ in excessive red blood cell destruction, liver damage, and bile duct obstruction
• Conjugated (direct) bilirubin	Bilirubin that is conjugated in the liver (joined with glucuronic acid).	Less than 0.3 mg/dL	↑ with gallstones and gallbladder obstruction
• Delta	Irreversibly binds to albumin. Remains elevated the longest during recovery, likely causing the persistent jaundice.	Less than 0.2 mg/dL	↑ with gallstones and gallbladder obstruction
• Unconjugated (indirect) bilirubin	Bilirubin in the bloodstream that has not yet passed through the liver.	Less than 1.1 mg/dL	↑ with excessive red blood cell destruction or liver damage, hepatitis, or cirrhosis

Continued

Table 32.6

Laboratory Tests for Hepatobiliary and Pancreatic Systems—cont'd

Test	Definition	Normal Range	Significance of Abnormal Findings
Calcium, total	Identifies serum calcium level, which is involved in almost all of the body's essential processes.	*Adult:* 8.2–10.2 mg/dL *Older than 90 years:* 8.2–9.6 mg/dL	↓ with acute pancreatitis, cirrhosis, malabsorption, and malnutrition
Cholesterol	Identifies 12-hour fasting serum cholesterol level.	Greater than 200 mg/dL	↑ in pancreatitis and gallbladder disease ↓ may indicate severe liver disease
Lactic dehydrogenase (LDH)	Determines level of this intracellular enzyme, which is released with injury or disease. LDH_3 fraction elevates with liver damage.	*15 to 43 years:* 90–156 units/L *Older than 43 years:* 90–176 units/L LDH_3: 20% to 26%	↑ in cirrhosis, liver cancer, pancreatitis, obstructive jaundice, and viral hepatitis
Lipase	Digestive enzymes mainly secreted by the pancreas. Released into bloodstream with damage to pancreatic acinar cells. Serum levels diagnose pancreatic disease.	0–60 units/L	↑ in pancreatic diseases, especially pancreatitis and acute cholecystitis
Prothrombin time (PT)	Prothrombin is a vitamin K–dependent protein produced by the liver. PT is a coagulation test measuring time for a fibrin clot to form.	10–13 seconds	↑ in biliary obstruction, cirrhosis, and vitamin K deficiency
Urine			
Urine bilirubin	Detects liver disorders.	Negative	Present in cirrhosis, hepatitis, and biliary obstruction
Urobilinogen	Detects liver disorders.	Up to 1 mg/dL	↑ with hepatitis, cirrhosis, and bile duct obstruction

Table 32.7

Diagnostic Procedures for the Gastrointestinal, Hepatobiliary, and Pancreatic Systems

Procedure	Definition/Normal Findings	Significance of Abnormal Findings	Nursing Management
Noninvasive			
Barium swallow	X-ray examination of esophagus, stomach, duodenum, and jejunum using oral barium. Fluoroscope outlines organs. Normal findings: normal organ structures.	Hiatal hernias, motility problems, polyps, strictures, tumors, and ulcers	*Pretest:* Nothing by mouth (NPO) for 6 hours before test. Encourage no smoking morning of procedure. *Posttest:* Increase fluids. Laxatives may be ordered. Monitor for constipation.
Barium enema	Colon filled with barium. X-rays visualize position, movement, and filling of colon. Normal findings: colon structures normal.	Diverticula, inflammation, obstructions, polyps, stenosis, tumors, and ulcerative colitis	*Pretest:* Low-residue diet several days before test; clear liquids 24 hours before test; NPO 8 hours before test. Laxative and enema the evening before the test; enema the morning of test as needed. *Posttest:* Encourage fluids. Laxatives may be ordered. Monitor for constipation.
Computed tomography colonography	X-ray examination of interior of colon using CT scanner Normal findings: colon structures normal	Colorectal cancer, polyps	Pretest: Clear liquids only 24 hours before test with water hourly as directed; NPO on day of test. Laxatives as instructed the day before and the morning of test. Posttest: May expel instilled air and feel bloated for several hours.
Invasive			
Nuclear scanning: cholescintigraphy, diisopropyl iminodiacetic acid (DISIDA) scintigraphy, hepatobiliary iminodiacetic acid (HIDA) scan, or iminodiacetic acid (IDA) scan	Injection of small amount of intravenous radioactive isotope. Serial images of gallbladder, bile duct, and duodenum are recorded. Normal findings: normal structures and function.	Cholecystitis, biliary ejection problem, or obstruction	*Pretest:* NPO 4–6 hours before test. *Posttest:* Discard urine in first 24 hours. Wash gloved hands and then wash ungloved hands. *Teach:* Increase fluids to flush isotope. Flush toilet immediately and wash hands well for 24 hours.
Esophagogastro-duodenoscopy (EGD)	Endoscopy allowing visualization of esophagus, stomach, and upper duodenum. Biopsy or cytology specimens can be obtained. Normal findings: normal structures.	Inflammation, cancer, bleeding, injury, or infection	*Pretest:* Laxative and enema the evening before the test; enema the morning of test as needed. NPO 6 hours before test. *Posttest:* Monitor vital signs. Keep NPO until swallow and gag reflex present. Monitor for pain, bleeding, fever, and dysphagia.

Continued

Table 32.7

Diagnostic Procedures for the Gastrointestinal, Hepatobiliary, and Pancreatic Systems—cont'd

Procedure	Definition/Normal Findings	Significance of Abnormal Findings	Nursing Management
Endoscopic retrograde cholangiopan-creatography (ERCP)	Endoscopy allowing visualization of pancreatic and biliary ducts, and x-rays with contrast media. Normal findings: normal structures without obstruction.	Gallstones, bile duct or pancreatic disease	*Pretest:* See EGD. *Teach:* Fast 6 hours, restrict clear fluids 2 hours before exam, and avoid anticoagulants as ordered. *Posttest:* Keep NPO until swallow and gag reflex returns, then eat lightly for 24 hours. Monitor vital signs, contrast reaction signs, and intake and output. *Teach:* Throat will be sore with hoarseness.
Proctosigmoidoscopy	Examination of distal sigmoid colon, rectum, and anal canal using a rigid or flexible endoscope (sigmoidoscope). Normal findings: normal mucosa.	Ulcerations, punctures, lacerations, tumors, hemorrhoids, polyps, fissures, fistulas, early malignancies, and abscesses	*Pretest:* Low-residue diet for 3 days before test; clear liquids evening before test; NPO 8 hours before test. Laxative and enema the evening before the test; enema morning of test as needed. *Posttest:* Monitor vital signs and for rectal bleeding.
Colonoscopy	Visualization of lining of the lower colon through a flexible endoscope. Biopsy specimen may be obtained or polyps removed. Normal findings: normal mucosa.	Colon cancer, polyps, or inflammation	*Pretest:* Low-residue diet for several days before test; clear liquids evening before test; fast for 6 hours and restrict fluids 2 hours before test. Laxative and enema the evening before the test; enema morning of test as needed. *Posttest:* Monitor vital signs and for rectal bleeding.
Percutaneous liver biopsy	Needle inserted through skin into liver to obtain a small tissue sample. Normal findings: normal liver tissue.	Liver cancer, cirrhosis, or hepatitis	*Pretest:* Consent signed. Complete blood count (CBC) and coagulation studies reviewed. *Posttest:* Monitor vital signs and biopsy site for bleeding. Give analgesics as ordered.

Laboratory Tests

The complete blood count (CBC) reveals if anemia or infection is present. Anemia may occur with GI bleeding or cancer. Electrolyte imbalances often occur with GI illness as a result of vomiting, diarrhea, malabsorption, or use of GI suction. Genetic testing can be done to identify family members at risk of developing serious conditions such as the polyps associated with colon cancer.

Stool Tests

Stool samples can be tested for **occult blood** (blood not seen by the naked eye). A series of three tests is usually done to increase the chances of detecting blood. False-positive occult blood results can occur with bleeding gums following a dental procedure; ingestion of red meat within 3 days before testing; ingestion of fish, turnips, or horse-radish; and use of drugs, including anticoagulants, aspirin, colchicine, iron preparations in large doses, NSAIDs, and steroids.

Stool is collected to detect intestinal infections caused by parasites and their ova (eggs). The test usually requires a series of three stool specimens collected every second or third day. The stool specimen is collected using a tongue blade, placed in a container with a preservative, and taken immediately to the laboratory. The stool must be examined within 30 minutes of collection. False-negative results can occur as a result of urine in the specimen or if the specimen is not fresh.

Stool cultures (via sterile collection technique) are done to determine the presence of pathogenic organisms in the GI tract. Stool can also be examined for lipids (fat). Excessive secretion of fecal fats (**steatorrhea**) may occur in various digestive and absorptive disorders. The stools are collected for 72 hours and stored on ice if necessary before being sent to the laboratory.

Stool tests for colorectal screening beginning at age 45 until age 75 include an annual guaiac-based occult blood test or immunochemical test or a multitarget DNA test every three years.

Radiographic Tests
Barium Swallow
A barium swallow is an x-ray examination of the esophagus, stomach, duodenum, and jejunum using an oral liquid radiopaque contrast medium (barium) and a **fluoroscope** (an x-ray source and fluorescent screen between which the patient is placed) to outline the contours of the organs. A barium swallow detects strictures, ulcers, tumors, polyps, hiatal hernias, and motility problems.

The patient usually receives nothing by mouth (NPO) for 6 hours before the procedure. Because smoking can stimulate gastric motility, the patient is discouraged from smoking the morning of the procedure. Patient teaching includes information about being NPO and increasing fluids after the procedure, the barium ingestion, and the white appearance of stools 2 to 3 days afterward. During the procedure, the patient drinks thick, chalky barium while standing in front of a fluoroscopic tube. X-ray films are taken in various positions and at specific intervals to visualize the outline of the organs. The passage of the barium through the GI tract is viewed.

A laxative is usually ordered after the procedure to expel the barium and prevent constipation or a barium **impaction** (impassable mass of stone-like feces). The patient is asked to increase fluid intake to expel barium. The abdomen is checked for distention. Stool color is monitored to determine whether the barium has been completely eliminated. Constipation with distention indicates a barium impaction.

Barium Enema
A barium enema is performed to visualize the position, movements, and filling of the colon. Tumors, diverticula, stenosis, obstructions, inflammation, ulcerative colitis, and polyps can be detected. If the patient has active inflammatory disease of the colon or suspected perforation or obstruction, a barium enema is contraindicated. Active GI bleeding may prohibit the use of laxatives and enemas.

The patient eats a low-residue diet for several days before the test to empty the bowel. Clear liquids only should be consumed 24 hours before the test. The patient is NPO 8 hours before the test. Laxatives, bowel-cleansing solutions, and enemas may be administered the day before the test with cleansing enemas the morning of the examination. Bowel preparation is necessary for adequate visualization during the procedure. Inadequate bowel preparation may result in poor test results or test cancellation (Fig. 32.6). The area around the rectum should be clean when the patient is sent for the procedure.

During the procedure, barium is instilled through a rectal tube with an inflated balloon or through a colostomy (with special prep and colostomy irrigation first). Fluoroscopy shows the barium's movement in the colon. The procedure takes about 15 minutes. After the test, most of the barium is removed with the rectal tube; an x-ray confirms this. The patient is allowed to use the bathroom after the procedure to expel the remaining barium.

The patient's stool color is monitored after the procedure to note if all the barium is passed. The patient is encouraged to increase fluids to help remove the barium. Laxatives may be ordered to help clear the barium from the colon. The patient is told to report any abdominal pain, bloating, or absence of stool (any of these could indicate constipation or bowel obstruction) as well as any rectal bleeding.

CRITICAL THINKING

Mrs. Pearl is a 95-year-old woman undergoing a barium enema for abdominal pain. What concerns might you, as her nurse, have for Mrs. Pearl as she undergoes this test? How can you address them?

Computed Tomography Colonography
Computed tomography colonography (CTC) is a CT scan that looks at the colon. It is an option to screen for colorectal cancer every 5 years. Bowel preparation is needed.

Nuclear Scanning
Hepatobiliary scanning primarily determines patency of the cystic and common bile ducts. It can also show hepatic and gallbladder function or gallstones. A small amount of radioactive isotope is injected. The scan is called cholescintigraphy, diisopropyl iminodiacetic acid (DISIDA) scintigraphy, hepatobiliary iminodiacetic acid (HIDA) scan, or iminodiacetic acid (IDA) scan, depending on the radioactive isotope and exact procedure that is used. Cholecystitis, biliary disease,

· **WORD · BUILDING ·**

steatorrhea: steato—fat + rrhea—flow
fluoroscope: fluor—a flowing + skopeîn—to look at

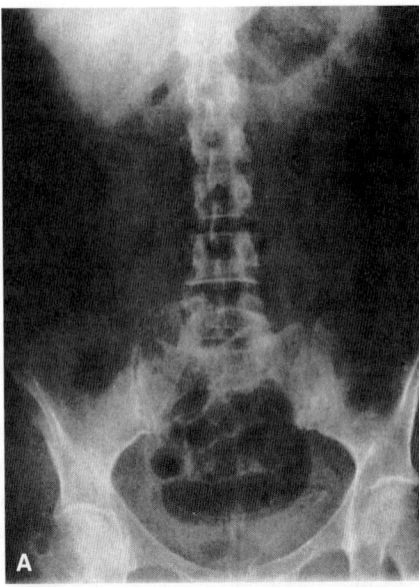

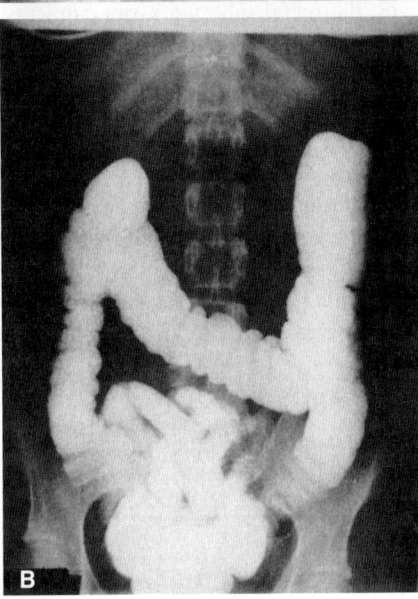

FIGURE 32.6 (A) An image of a patient who was poorly prepared for a barium enema. (B) An image of a patient who was adequately prepared for a barium enema.

ejection problem, or obstruction can be confirmed with this examination.

Liver Scan

A liver scan involves injecting a slightly radioactive medium that is taken up by the liver. An instrument is passed over the liver that records the amount of material taken up by the liver and forms a composite picture of the liver. It may show tumors, masses, and abnormal size and patterns of blood vessels.

Endoscopy

Esophagogastroduodenoscopy

Esophagogastroduodenoscopy (EGD) visualizes the esophagus (**esophagoscopy**), the stomach (**gastroscopy;** Fig. 32.7), and the upper duodenum. Sedation is used to relax and ease

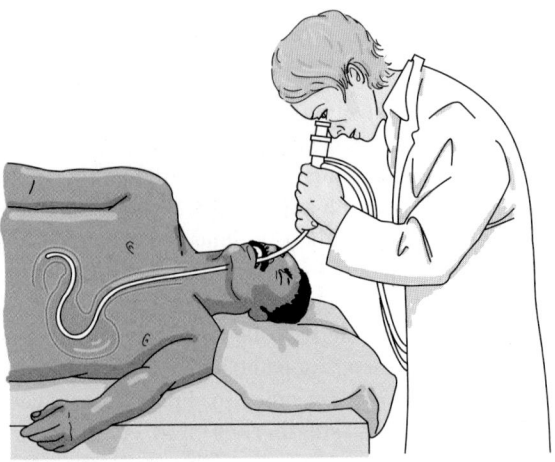

FIGURE 32.7 Gastroscopy.

pain during the procedure. The oropharynx is sprayed or swabbed with a local anesthetic, which may inhibit the swallow and gag reflex. Abnormalities such as inflammation, cancer, bleeding, injury, and infection can be seen. Biopsy or cytology specimens can be obtained.

After the procedure, vital signs are monitored. If a local anesthetic in the oropharynx was used, keep the patient NPO. Check for swallow and gag reflex return before allowing fluids or food (usually within 4 hours). Patients are monitored for signs of perforation (e.g., bleeding, fever, dysphagia). Mid-esophageal perforation can cause referred substernal or epigastric pain. Blood loss secondary to perforation can lead to hematoma formation, which in turn can result in cyanosis and referred back pain. Distal esophageal perforation may result in shoulder pain, dyspnea, or symptoms similar to those of a perforated ulcer. The patient may have a sore throat for a few days.

Capsule **endoscopy** makes use of a capsule with a microchip in it that is swallowed. As the capsule moves through the GI tract, pictures are taken of the stomach and small intestine to diagnose conditions such as bleeding, tumors, or Crohn disease. It is most helpful in the small intestine, which is difficult to scope because of its length and twists.

Endoscopic Retrograde Cholangiopancreatography

Endoscopic **retrograde cholangiopancreatography** (ERCP) shows the pancreatic and biliary ducts (Fig. 32.8). The procedure allows direct viewing, x-rays with contrast media, and intervention if needed, such as biopsy, stone or tumor removal, stricture balloon dilation, or bile duct stent placement. An endoscope is passed through the esophagus to the duodenum, where dye is injected that outlines the pancreatic and bile ducts.

The patient is prepared for an ERCP the same as for an EGD. The patient fasts 6 hours before the procedure and stops clear liquids 2 hours before the test. Allergies to contrast agents are identified and reported. Ensure that ordered laboratory studies have been done before the procedure and

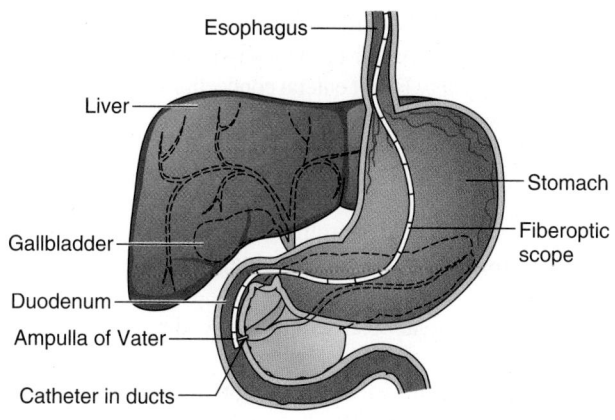

Esophagus

Liver

Gallbladder

Duodenum

Ampulla of Vater

Catheter in ducts

Stomach

Fiberoptic scope

FIGURE 32.8 Endoscopic retrograde cholangiopancreatography.

that the patient has removed dentures. Postprocedure pancreatitis can develop. A pancreatic stent may be placed to help prevent this. Follow-up care is similar to that for an EGD. Teach the patient to report increased right upper quadrant pain, fever, or chills, which may indicate infection. Teach also to report hypotension, tachycardia or rapid heart rate, increasing right upper quadrant pain, nausea, or vomiting, which may indicate perforation or the onset of pancreatitis.

Lower Gastrointestinal Endoscopy

PROCTOSIGMOIDOSCOPY. **Proctosigmoidoscopy** is the examination of the distal sigmoid colon, the rectum, and the anal canal using a flexible endoscope (sigmoidoscope). Ulcerations, punctures, lacerations, tumors, hemorrhoids, polyps, fissures, fistulas, and abscesses can be detected. Malignancies at an early stage can be detected, so an examination for patients age 45 and older is recommended every 5 years until age 75.

Proctosigmoidoscopy requires the lower bowel to be cleaned out. The patient eats a low-residue diet for 3 days before the test, clear liquids the evening before the test, and is NPO 8 hours before the test. A laxative and enema the night before the test and an enema the morning of the procedure may be given. Bowel preparation may not be ordered for patients with bleeding or severe diarrhea.

The patient is positioned in a left lateral knee-to-chest position. This allows the sigmoid colon to straighten by gravity. A rigid proctoscope is used to visualize the rectum. A flexible scope is then used to permit visualization above the rectosigmoid junction. Patients are told they may feel pressure as though they are going to have a bowel movement. During the procedure, one or more small pieces of intestinal tissue may be removed (biopsy specimens). Rectal or sigmoid polyps are removed with a snare. An electrocoagulating current is used to cauterize sites to prevent or stop bleeding. Specimens are labeled and sent to the pathology laboratory immediately for examination.

After the procedure, the patient is allowed to rest for a few minutes in the supine position to avoid orthostatic hypotension when standing. Pain and flatus may occur from instilled air.

The patient is observed for signs of perforation, such as heavy bleeding, pain, and fever.

COLONOSCOPY. **Colonoscopy** provides visualization of the lining of the lower colon to identify abnormalities through a flexible endoscope, which is inserted rectally. During the colonoscopy, biopsy and fluid specimens may be obtained, polyps removed, and bleeding controlled with a laser. Examination for patients age 45 and older is recommended every 10 years until age 75.

The patient eats a low-residue diet for several days before the test and fasts 6 hours before the procedure. Fluids are restricted 2 hours before the test. A laxative and enema the evening before the test and enema the morning of the test are used as needed.

> **BE SAFE!**
>
> Older patients may experience fatigue and weakness during bowel preparation and may be unable to complete it. Monitor the patient for distress. Consult the health care provider if you note any patient distress during bowel preparation. Observe the patient frequently because defecation urgency, especially in unfamiliar surroundings, may create a fall risk.

Procedural sedation and analgesia are used. The patient is positioned on the left side. Air is instilled into the colon to help the HCP visualize the bowel. The air causes pressure and may be uncomfortable for the patient. The patient is encouraged to relax and take slow deep breaths through the nose and out the mouth. Vital signs are monitored throughout the procedure to watch for a vasovagal response, which can lead to hypotension and bradycardia.

After the procedure, the patient is monitored until stable. Hemorrhage or severe pain are immediately reported. When giving the patient discharge instructions, explain that flatus and cramping may occur for several hours after the test, that blood may be present in the stool if a biopsy specimen was taken, and to report problems to the HCP.

Gastric Analysis

Gastric analysis measures the secretions in the stomach. Diagnoses of duodenal ulcer, gastric carcinoma, pyloric or duodenal obstruction, and pernicious anemia are made with this test. A diagnosis of pernicious anemia is ruled out with the finding of acid. A diagnosis of gastric carcinoma may be made by the presence of cancer cells in the gastric secretions. The two gastric analysis tests performed are the basal cell secretion test and the gastric acid stimulation test.

Before the **basal cell secretion test,** the patient should avoid taking any drugs that could interfere with gastric acid secretion, such as anticholinergics and antacids. The patient is NPO after midnight the night before the test. For the procedure, a nasogastric (NG) tube is inserted, and the contents of the stomach are suctioned out through the tube using a syringe. The NG tube is connected to wall suction. Stomach contents are collected every 15 minutes for 1 hour. The specimens are labeled according to the time they were collected and the order in which they were obtained. The gastric acid is tested for pH using indicator paper or a pH meter. The amount of gastric acid is also measured. Too much hydrochloric acid may indicate a peptic ulcer; too little could be a sign of cancer or pernicious anemia.

The **gastric acid stimulation test** measures the amount of gastric acid for 1 hour after subcutaneous injection of a histamine drug. If abnormal results occur, radiographic tests or endoscopy can be done to determine the cause.

Percutaneous Liver Biopsy

If less invasive tests do not aid in diagnosis of liver disease, a needle biopsy for analysis can be done. This type of biopsy can identify cancer, cirrhosis, hepatitis, or other causes of liver disease. After a local anesthetic, the HCP makes a small incision over the liver. Ultrasound may be used to guide the insertion of the hollow needle through the skin and into the liver. Tissue samples are withdrawn for examination. This procedure places the patient at risk for bleeding because the liver is highly vascular and because many patients with liver disease have reduced clotting ability.

During the procedure, the nurse assists the patient onto his or her back or left side and instructs the patient to hold very still. The patient is instructed to exhale and hold the breath while the needle is being inserted. After the needle is removed, pressure is applied on the site up to 5 minutes, followed by application of a pressure dressing.

After the biopsy, the patient lies on the right side for 2 hours to prevent bleeding. Vital signs are monitored as well as the site for signs of bleeding for several hours. The patient is advised to avoid coughing or straining and to avoid exercise and heavy lifting for one week. Analgesics are offered for comfort as ordered.

CRITICAL THINKING

Mr. Wozynski is admitted with cirrhosis and jaundice. What specific laboratory value can you expect to be elevated related to his jaundice? Mr. Wozynski's health care provider orders a liver biopsy. Why is it important for you to check Mr. Wozynski's laboratory reports before the procedure?

Suggested answers are at the end of the chapter.

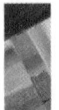

THERAPEUTIC MEASURES FOR THE GASTROINTESTINAL, HEPATOBILIARY, AND PANCREATIC SYSTEMS

Gastrointestinal Intubation

GI intubation is the placement of a tube within the GI tract for therapeutic or diagnostic purposes (Fig. 32.9). When the GI tube is inserted orally into the stomach, it is an orogastric tube. When it goes from the nares into the stomach, it is a nasogastric,

or NG, tube. A variety of tubes are available with specific purposes (Table 32.8). An all-in-one NG system has been developed, with the safety ENFit enteral connection, that can perform multiple functions. Orogastric tubes reduce sinus infection risk because they do not block normal drainage of the sinuses, as can nasal tubes. GI intubation is done for a variety of reasons:

- To remove gas and fluids from the stomach (decompression)
- To diagnose GI motility and to obtain gastric secretions for analysis
- To relieve and treat obstructions or bleeding within the GI tract
- To provide a means for nutrition (**gavage** feeding), hydration, and medication when the oral route is not possible or is contraindicated
- To promote healing after esophageal, gastric, or intestinal surgery by preventing distention of the GI tract and strain on the suture lines
- To remove toxic substances (**lavage**) that have been ingested either accidentally or intentionally and to provide for irrigation

Feeding tubes include NG, esophagostomy, **gastrostomy,** or jejunostomy tubes (see Fig. 32.9). A new type of small bore feeding tube has a camera for viewing landmarks during insertion. NG tubes are usually temporary and short term. Esophagostomy, gastrostomy, or jejunostomy tubes are generally used for longer-term nutrition delivery.

Provide emotional support and explanations to the patient and significant others to facilitate the process of tube insertion and maintenance. Verifying tube placement is essential to prevent complications or death from incorrect tube placement. NG tube placement must be verified after insertion and then intermittently to ensure the tube is in the correct position and not in the lungs, esophagus, pleural space, or brain. A device can be placed on an NG tube to detect CO_2 to identify lung placement. (See Davis Edge for procedures on the insertion and maintenance of NG tubes.)

Gastrostomy or jejunostomy tube placement is verified by comparing current exposed length with documented exposed length at insertion. The tube may not be in the desired position if the current and insertion exposed tube lengths are different, so the HCP should be consulted before using the tube.

Enteral Nutrition

Enteral nutrition (EN) provides patients with supplemental or total nutrition when oral intake is not possible. Enteral feedings are delivered directly into the stomach, duodenum, or proximal jejunum. Sometimes, the esophagus and stomach may need to be bypassed due to inability to swallow, severe burns or trauma to the face or jaw, debilitation, and oropharyngeal or esophageal paralysis. Complications associated with EN are presented in Table 32.9.

Enteral Nutrition Formulas

EN formulas are prescribed by the HCP based on the patient's nutritional needs, the consistency of the formula, the size and location of the tube, the method of delivery, and

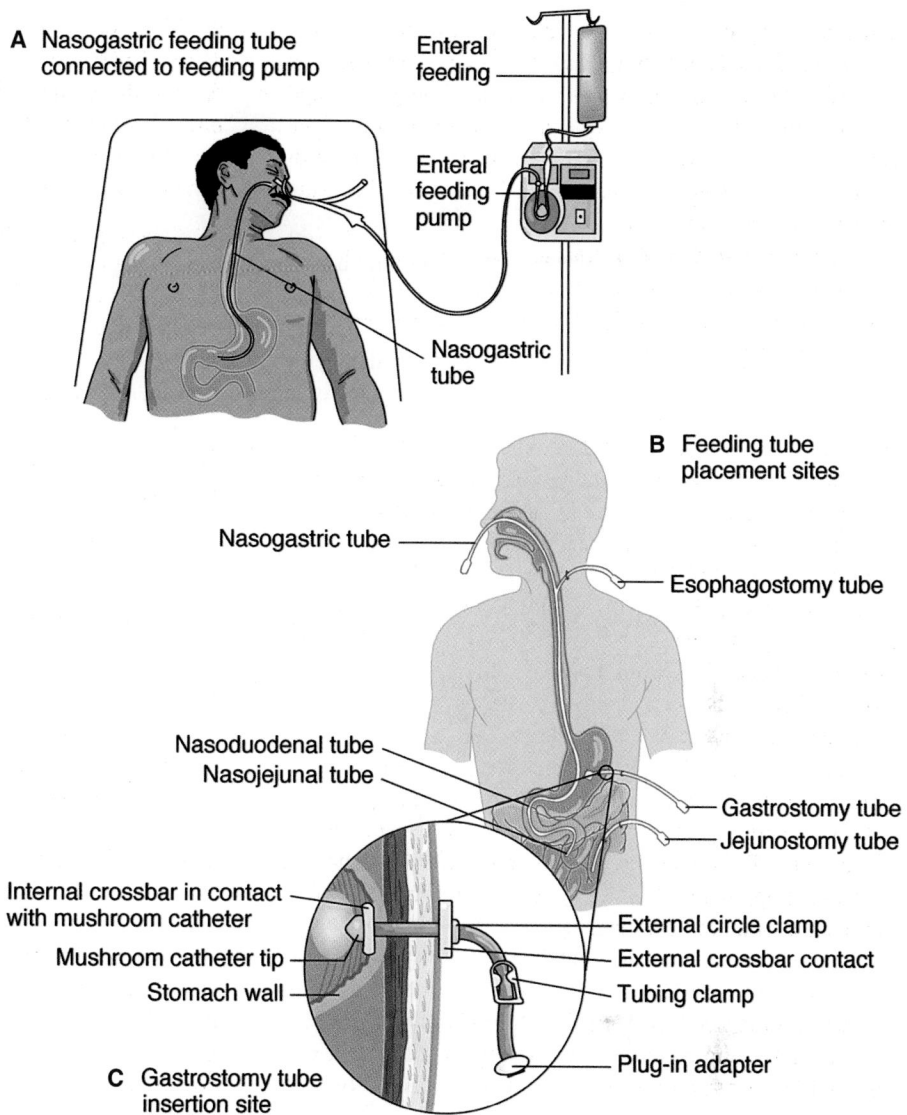

A Nasogastric feeding tube connected to feeding pump

Enteral feeding

Enteral feeding pump

Nasogastric tube

B Feeding tube placement sites

Nasogastric tube

Esophagostomy tube

Nasoduodenal tube

Nasojejunal tube

Gastrostomy tube

Jejunostomy tube

Internal crossbar in contact with mushroom catheter

Mushroom catheter tip

Stomach wall

External circle clamp

External crossbar contact

Tubing clamp

Plug-in adapter

C Gastrostomy tube insertion site

FIGURE 32.9 Feeding tubes. (A) Nasogastric tube connected to feeding tube pump. (B) Feeding tube placement sites (esophagostomy, nasointestinal, gastrostomy, and jejunostomy). (C) Gastrostomy tube insertion site.

Table 32.8

Gastric Tube Examples

Tube	Uses and Description	Nursing Considerations
Levin tube	Single lumen. May be used for gastric decompression, irrigation, lavage, and feeding.	Tube is not vented. Avoid use with continuous suction to prevent injury to stomach lining.
Sump tube	Double lumen with one lumen; an air vent prevents tube adherence to the stomach lining. Used for decompression, irrigation, lavage, and medication administration.	May be used with continuous suction because of air vent. Air vent must not be plugged off. Can remain in place for 30 days.
Weighted or nonweighted, flexible feeding tube, with or without stylets	Small-bore tube for enteral feeding only. Less injury. Can remain in place for extended periods.	Suction collapses tube. Use 10-mL syringe or greater because smaller syringe creates too much pressure, leading to possible rupture of tube. Inject 30 mL of air with a 60-mL syringe immediately before withdrawing fluid to make it easier to withdraw.

Table 32.9

Common Mechanical, Gastrointestinal, and Metabolic Complications of Tube-Fed Patients and Prevention Strategies

Complication	Prevention Strategies
Mechanical	
Tube irritation	Consider oral tubes and avoid nasal tubes due to sinus infection risk. Oral tubes also help prevent ventilator-associated pneumonia (VAP). Consider using a smaller or softer tube. Lubricate tube before insertion. Make sure tube is secured in place.
Tube obstruction	Flush tube with water after each use, and before and after medication administration. Do not mix medications with tube-feeding formula. Use liquid medications, if available. Crush nonliquid medications thoroughly (if crushing not contraindicated). Use infusion pump to maintain constant flow (see Fig. 32.9).
Aspiration and regurgitation	Feeding should not be started until tube placement is radiographically confirmed. Elevate head of patient's bed 30 degrees or more at all times. Discontinue feeding at least 30 to 60 minutes before treatments requiring head to be lowered (e.g., chest percussion). If patient has an endotracheal tube in place, keep cuff inflated during feeding. Avoid use of blue dye to detect aspiration because it has not been shown predictive, and dye can be absorbed in critically ill patients, who then turn blue and can die.
Tube displacement	Place a black mark at the point where the tube, when properly placed, exits the nostril. Measure exposed length for future placement verification. If available, place CO_2 monitoring device on tube to detect displacement. For dislodgement, replace tube and obtain health care provider's order to confirm with x-ray imaging.
Gastrointestinal	
Cramping, distention, bloating, gas pains, nausea, vomiting, diarrhea*	Practice excellent personal hygiene when handling any feeding product. Keep formula at room temperature before feeding. Initiate and increase amount of formula gradually. Change to a lactose-free formula. Decrease fat content of formula. Administer drug therapy as ordered. Change to formula with a lower osmolality. Change to formula with a different fiber content. Evaluate medications for diarrhea side effect (e.g., antibiotics, digoxin).
Metabolic	
Dehydration	Note patient's recommended fluid requirements. Provide adequate daily water. Monitor hydration status.
Overhydration	Note patient's recommended fluid requirements. Monitor hydration status.
Hyperglycemia	Initiate feeding at a slow rate. Monitor blood glucose. Use hyperglycemic medication if needed. Select a low-carbohydrate formula.

Table 32.9

Common Mechanical, Gastrointestinal, and Metabolic Complications of Tube-Fed Patients and Prevention Strategies—cont'd

Complication	Prevention Strategies
Hypernatremia	Note patient's fluid and electrolyte status. Provide adequate fluids as ordered.
Hyponatremia	Note patient's fluid and electrolyte status. Restrict fluids as ordered. Supplement feeding with rehydration solution and saline as ordered.
Hypophosphatemia	Monitor serum level. Replenish phosphorus before refeeding as ordered.
Hypercapnia	Low-carbohydrate, high-fat formula is helpful.
Hypokalemia	Monitor potassium level. Supplement feeding with potassium as ordered.
Hyperkalemia	Reduce potassium intake as ordered. Monitor potassium level.

Source: Modified from Lutz, C. A., Mazur, E. E., & Przytulski, K. R. (2014). *Nutrition & diet therapy* (6th ed.). Philadelphia, PA: F.A. Davis.
  *The most commonly cited complication of enteral feeding is diarrhea.

the convenience for the patient at home. Commercially prepared formulas are composed of protein, carbohydrates, and fats. Full-strength formula can be used. When patients receive EN, their daily water needs in addition to any water supplied by the feeding should be considered. Dietitians can help calculate the patient's free water needs. Water is the best fluid to use to flush the tube at intervals and before and after administration of medications to prevent clogging. Sterile water may be desired to prevent infection due to contaminated tap water. Use 30 mL every 4 hours to routinely flush the tube. This can count toward the patient's daily total water needs. Dehydration can occur if the patient's daily water needs are not met.

Method of Enteral Feeding Delivery

Feedings are administered either by gravity or by a controller pump that delivers continuous volume through the feeding tube. Gravity feedings are placed above the level of the stomach and dripped in by gravity slowly. Intermittent feedings are defined as either being delivered by a pump that runs continuously throughout the day and is discontinued each night or as a 4- to 6-hour volume of feeding given over 20 to 30 minutes. A continuous feeding administered 24 hours a day through a pump allows for small amounts to be given over a long period. Pumps are set at the specified rate to control the feeding being delivered to the patient.

When feedings are administered, patients must be positioned with the head of the bed at 30 to 45 degrees to reduce the risk of aspiration. Monitoring for the risk of aspiration is essential. Ensure proper labeling of the formula and correct feeding tube connection. Monitor the ordered beginning rate

and advancement rate of the feeding to ensure nutritional needs are being met.

Watch for signs that the feeding is not being tolerated. Vomiting, abdominal distention, patient report of a feeling of fullness or discomfort, limited flatus or stool, diarrhea, and abnormal abdominal x-rays are indicators that the feeding is not being tolerated. Research has shown that residual volumes do not reflect gastric emptying and may not be a good reflection of aspiration risk. It was found that eliminating residual volume checks did not decrease patient safety. It did result in better delivery of the feeding to meet the patient's nutritional needs. Residual checks can result in clogged tubes, increased interruption of feeding, stoppage of a tolerated feeding in the absence of other intolerance indicators, and reduced feeding volume delivered to the patient, resulting in malnutrition. If residual checks are used, consideration can be given to raising feeding cut-off limits when other signs of intolerance are not present. Be aware of current evidence-based guidelines. Follow your agency's policy when administering enteral feedings.

If medications are administered via a feeding tube, ensure that the medication is made for the GI route. *Never* interchange the routes of a medication to prevent serious effects or even death. Obtain a new medication order if needed for the correct route form of the medication. Also understand possible drug–nutrient interactions. Some medications cannot be given with certain substances and may require feedings to be interrupted. Other medications, such as enteric-coated or sustained-release medications, *cannot* be crushed. Liquid medications should be used when possible to reduce clogging of the tube. Pharmacists and dietitians should be consulted for special considerations.

BE SAFE!

Incorrect connection of enteral feeding equipment is a hazard to patient safety. An enteral feeding incorrectly connected and administered through a nonenteral system (such as an intravenous [IV] line, peritoneal dialysis catheter, oxygen tubing, or tracheostomy tube cuff) can result in patient injury or death. Worldwide equipment redesigns have been made to prevent tubing misconnections. Nurses must be vigilant to ensure that they understand the appropriate use of the equipment and all tubing connections being made to prevent harmful errors:

- Avoid rigging connections that may impair designed safety features.
- Package together all parts needed for enteral feeding within the agency to avoid improper equipment being selected and connected.
- Label or color-code feeding tubes and connectors within the institution.
- Verify the solution's label.
- Label enteral bags with large words such as "ALERT! For Enteral Use Only."
- Use adequate room lighting when working with equipment.
- Route tubes/catheters with different purposes in standardized directions (IV lines routed toward the patient's head; enteric lines routed toward the feet).
- If disconnection occurs, only staff familiar with the equipment should make a reconnection.
- During a reconnection, always trace the lines back to their origins and then ensure that they are secure.
- During the handoff process, trace all tubes to their origin and check connections.

CRITICAL THINKING

Mrs. Wood is receiving enteral nutrition because of dysphagia, the cause of which is being investigated. She is not receiving any medications. You note that Mrs. Wood's tongue is bright red with deep furrows. She states her mouth is very dry. Her skin remains tented when skin turgor is checked.

1. What do Mrs. Wood's data collection findings indicate?
2. How would you document your findings?
3. What other data should you gather?
4. Why might Mrs. Wood be exhibiting this condition?
5. What actions can you take for this condition?
6. How would you record the total of Mrs. Wood's 8-hour intake: enteral feeding at 50 mL per hour?

   Suggested answers are at the end of the chapter.

Gastrointestinal Decompression

GI decompression may be necessary when the stomach or small intestine becomes filled with air or fluid. Swallowed air and GI secretions enter the stomach and intestines and collect there if they are not propelled through the GI tract by peristalsis. Accumulating air or fluid causes distention, a feeling of fullness, and possibly pain in the abdomen. Gastric distention

may occur after major abdominal surgery. Ambulating or turning the patient frequently can help prevent this. However, when GI decompression is necessary, a NG tube or rarely a nasointestinal tube may be inserted and suction applied. Nasointestinal tubes are more difficult and slower to place and may be uncomfortable, so they are not used often. The tube remains in place until full peristaltic activity (passage of flatus, bowel movement, no distention, bloating or cramps) has returned.

Parenteral Nutrition

Parenteral nutrition (PN) supplies complete nutrition via a central or peripheral intravenous route (see Chapter 7). It is given to improve the patient's nutritional status, achieve weight gain, or enhance the healing process.

LEARNING TIP

- Patients may respond to the glucose in parenteral nutrition (PN) with an elevated serum glucose level. After PN is discontinued, the serum glucose levels should return to baseline levels.
- Regular insulin is ordered to control hyperglycemia during PN therapy. It can be given as an additive to the PN solution or subcutaneously per a sliding scale based on specified blood glucose monitoring results, such as every 6 hours, or both.
- The insulin type that is given for sliding scale coverage is always *regular* insulin. Can you figure out why? Because regular insulin is rapid acting, it reduces the *current* blood glucose level.

Home Health Hints

- Observe the patient's food preparation facilities to ensure that the patient's nutritional needs can be met. Some older patients may have outdated or spoiled food in their refrigerators or cupboards because they are unable to see dates or mold growing on foods.
- Observe and ensure that patients can use appliances to heat food safely. Patients with limited vision may not see gas flames and can ignite their clothing. Confused patients might try to heat foods in cardboard containers. If the patient can obtain and learn to use a microwave, it may be a safer cooking appliance than a stove.
- Share community nutritional support services with patients, such as Women, Infants, and Children (WIC) programs, nutrition sites for older adults, Meals on Wheels, school food programs, and government surplus food programs.
- Prevent a feeding tube from kinking by slipping a split straw lengthwise around the area that tends to kink and then lightly taping over the split in the straw.
- Use wire coat hangers that are bent to hang over doors or closet bars for enteral feeding solution bags.
- Teach patients to notify the home health nurse for a clogged feeding tube and not to unclog it with items such as meat tenderizer or carbonated beverages.

SUGGESTED ANSWERS TO CRITICAL THINKING

Mrs. Todd

1. Daily aspirin use is the most likely cause of her bleeding.
2. Medication teaching including side effects can help Mrs. Todd prevent future bleeding episodes. Mrs. Todd should be instructed to take aspirin with food to minimize gastrointestinal upset and help prevent formation of ulcers. Identifying pain relief needs and consultation with the health care provider (HCP) will also help.
3. See Table 32.7.

Mrs. Pearl

Mrs. Pearl is at risk for dehydration and electrolyte loss as a result of the laxative and enema preparation and NPO (nothing by mouth) status. This risk is increased because of her age. Her fluid and electrolyte status should be monitored closely.

Mrs. Pearl will likely have a concern about "making it" to the bathroom during the preparation and should have a bedside commode placed within easy reach. Her call light should be answered promptly. If enemas are ordered "until clear," Mrs. Pearl will be at greater risk for fluid and electrolyte loss. If more than two or three enemas are required, the HCP should be notified.

Older patients can become very fatigued during testing and test preparation. Mrs. Pearl should be allowed plenty of rest before and after the test. She may also have a concern about being able to hold the barium in her bowel during the test without having an "accident." She should be assured that the barium is held in with a balloon that is on the end of the enema catheter and that bathrooms are nearby.

Mr. Wozynski

You can expect to find that Mr. Wozynski's serum bilirubin is elevated because his liver is unable to convert or conjugate bilirubin into a water-soluble compound that can be eliminated in the feces. Mr. Wozynski is at risk for bleeding because the liver is highly vascular and prone to bleed when a biopsy specimen is taken. In addition, he may not be manufacturing the necessary amount of prothrombin needed for blood clotting and may bleed after the biopsy has been performed. It will be especially important to check his coagulation studies and report any elevations to the HCP before the biopsy.

Mrs. Wood

1. Dehydration.
2. Document as follows: "0800 'Mouth very dry.' Tongue bright red with deep furrows, tented turgor. Enteral feeding infusing (include solution and rate). HCP notified. K. Ohno, LVN."
3. Monitor Mrs. Wood's vital signs to look for changes such as increased heart rate, decreased blood pressure, and possibly mildly elevated temperature. Review current lab work if available for indications of dehydration such as elevated blood urea nitrogen (BUN) and elevated hematocrit (see Chapter 6).
4. Mrs. Wood's daily water needs are not being met. She is not receiving medications that would incidentally provide water during their administration.
5. Consult a dietitian and/or HCP to review Mrs. Wood's daily water needs. Divide the water needs over 24 hours, and ensure that water is administered. Ensure tubing is flushed per agency policy, and calculate water used toward daily water needs. Monitor intake and output. Continue assessing Mrs. Wood's signs and symptoms, and report abnormal findings.

6. 50 mL × 8 hours = 400 mL.

Review Questions

1. The nurse is contributing to the plan of care for a 78-year-old patient's elimination needs. Which of the following interventions should the nurse recommend to reduce complications due to the aging change of slowed motility? **Select all that apply.**
   1. Decrease ambulation.
   2. Decrease fluid intake.
   3. Increase dairy products.
   4. Increase dietary fiber.
   5. Increase activity level.

2. The nurse is to collect data on a patient who reports diarrhea. What data should the nurse collect? **Select all that apply.**
   1. Bruising
   2. Consistency of stools
   3. Color of stools
   4. Frequency of stools
   5. Antibiotic use
   6. Body piercings

3. The nurse is to palpate the patient's abdomen during data collection. Which of the following techniques should the nurse use?
   1. Firmly place hands on abdomen, depressing tissues 1 to 2 inches.
   2. Lightly depress the abdomen 0.5 to 1 inch.
   3. Randomly feel the patient's abdomen with fingertips.
   4. Light palpation must be completed by an experienced practitioner.

4. The nurse is caring for a patient who had a barium enema. Which of the following actions should the nurse implement? **Select all that apply.**
   1. Have patient cough and deep breathe hourly while awake.
   2. Encourage fluids.
   3. Monitor for return of swallow and gag reflex.
   4. Maintain the patient in semi-Fowler position.
   5. Keep NPO, or nothing by mouth.
   6. Provide ordered laxative.

5. A patient is admitted with an order for a nasogastric sump tube. The nurse knows this tube is used for which of the following purposes? **Select all that apply.**
   1. Supplemental feeding
   2. Decompression
   3. Irrigation
   4. Lavage
   5. Gavage
   6. Parenteral nutrition

6. The nurse assisted with inserting a flexible feeding tube into a patient. Which of the following actions should the nurse take to confirm tube placement?
   1. Aspirate gastric contents to observe for green-colored fluid.
   2. Measure the pH of secretions from tube.
   3. Obtain ordered chest x-ray results.
   4. Look in the back of the mouth for coiling of the tube.

7. The nurse is caring for a patient who is receiving a parenteral nutrition infusion. The nurse performs blood glucose monitoring every 6 hours to detect which complication?
   1. Hypocalcemia
   2. Hyponatremia
   3. Hyperglycemia
   4. Hyperkalemia

Answer rationales available in your online resources.

ANSWERS 1. 4, 5; 2. 2, 3, 4, 5; 3. 2; 4. 2, 6; 5. 2, 3, 4; 6. 3; 7. 3

Key Points

Find the chapter key points in your online resources available through Davis Edge.

Additional Resources

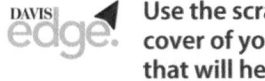 Use the scratch off code on the inside front cover of your book to access online quizzes that will help you to improve your scores on course exams and prepare for the NCLEX-PN®.

 Study Guide

CHAPTER 33
Nursing Care of Patients With Upper Gastrointestinal Disorders

Lazette V. Nowicki

KEY TERMS

anorexia (AN-uh-REK-see-ah)
aphthous stomatitis (AF-thus STOH-mah-TY-tis)
bariatric (BEAR-ee-AT-trik)
gastrectomy (gas-TREK-tuh-mee)
gastritis (gas-TRY-tis)
gastroduodenostomy (GAS-troh-DOO-oh-den-AW-stuh-mee)
gastrojejunostomy (GAS-troh-JAY-joo-NAW-stuh-mee)
Helicobacter pylori (HEH-lih-koh-back-tur PIE-lore-ee)
hiatal hernia (hy-YAY-tuhl HER-nee-ah)
obesity (oh-BEE-sih-tee)
peptic ulcer disease (PEP-tik UL-sir dih-ZEEZ)
Roux-en-Y (roo-ehn-WHY)
steatorrhea (STEE-ah-toh-REE-ah)

CHAPTER CONCEPT

Nutrition

LEARNING OUTCOMES

1. Explain anorexia, nausea, and vomiting.
2. Describe therapeutic measures and nursing care for anorexia, nausea, and vomiting.
3. Describe medical, surgical, and nursing management for obesity.
4. Plan nursing care for patients with acute or chronic gastritis.
5. Explain the pathophysiology, signs and symptoms, and diagnostic testing for hiatal hernia, peptic ulcer disease, gastric bleeding, and gastric cancer.
6. List current pharmacological treatments used for peptic ulcer disease.
7. Plan nursing care for patients with hiatal hernia, peptic ulcer disease, gastric bleeding, and gastric cancer.

 ## ANOREXIA

Anorexia is a lack of appetite. It is a common symptom of many diseases. Causes include noxious food odors, certain drugs (intentional or as a side effect), emotional stress, fear, psychological problems, and infections. Prolonged anorexia can lead to serious electrolyte imbalances. These imbalances can lead to cardiac arrhythmias. Eating is the preferred method for gaining weight but other measures such as enteral feedings and intravenous (IV) infusion can be used. Ask patients what causes loss of appetite and what improves it to plan their care. Nursing actions for the patient with anorexia include documenting accurate intake and output (I&O); monitoring vital signs, electrolytes, and electrocardiograms (ECGs); and monitoring the rate of an IV infusion or enteral feeding.

 ## NAUSEA AND VOMITING

Nausea is the subjective feeling of the urge to vomit. Vomiting is the act of expelling stomach contents from the body through the esophagus and mouth. It is a protective function to rid the body of harmful substances from the gastrointestinal (GI) tract. This reflex is controlled by the vomiting center of the brain. Stimuli and conditions that are either directly related to the GI tract or independent of it can trigger nausea and vomiting. Viral GI infection and other infections, motion sickness, stress, pregnancy, medications, myocardial infarction, uremia, and other conditions may cause nausea and vomiting. Emesis that looks like coffee grounds (dark brown) occurs from bleeding in the stomach and requires further investigation. If vomiting is prolonged, dehydration and electrolyte imbalances can occur. The loss of hydrochloric acid from the stomach can result in metabolic alkalosis.

Therapeutic Measures

Nausea and vomiting may be self-limited and require no intervention. If the cause of vomiting is known, it is treated. Antiemetics may be given. Ginger used with antiemetic medications may help ease nausea. For severe or prolonged vomiting, IV fluids and possibly nutrition need to be provided. Occasionally, an orogastric or nasogastric (NG) tube with suction may be ordered to decompress the stomach. After the vomiting is resolved, clear liquids are started, with water preferred. If liquids are tolerated, crackers or dry toast may be tolerated as well.

> **BE SAFE!**
> Protection of the airway during vomiting is a priority to prevent aspiration. Those at risk of aspiration are persons who are unconscious, have a gag reflex impairment, or are older and frail. Place these types of persons on their side when they begin to vomit. This allows the gastric contents to be expelled from the mouth rather than pooling at the back of the throat and being aspirated.

Nursing Process for the Patient With Nausea and Vomiting

Data Collection

The characteristics of the episodes of nausea and vomiting are noted. Medical conditions, medications, and treatments are documented to aid in diagnosing the cause. With continued vomiting, monitor to report signs of early fluid deficit, such as weakness, headache, muscle cramps, restlessness, inability to concentrate, and postural hypotension.

Nursing Diagnoses, Planning, and Implementation

Nausea related to various causes

EXPECTED OUTCOME: The patient will report relief from nausea within 30 minutes of reporting nausea.

- Provide a quiet, odor-free, visually clean environment *to avoid triggering stimuli.*
- Give antiemetics as ordered *to relieve nausea.*
- Provide frequent oral care *to remove taste of emesis.*
- Teach patient to avoid triggering fluids or foods *to prevent nausea and vomiting.*

Risk for Aspiration related to decreased gag reflex or unconsciousness with vomiting

EXPECTED OUTCOME: The patient's airway and lung sounds will remain clear at all times.

- Identify patients who are nauseated and at risk of aspiration *to plan preventive care.*
- Turn patient onto side if nauseated and vomiting *to protect airway and prevent aspiration.*

Evaluation

The patient's goals are met if nausea is not present and lung sounds remain clear.

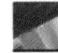 ## OBESITY

Several methods can be used to diagnose a patient as overweight or obese. Factors such as gender, age, body frame size, and being an athlete with larger muscle mass can influence these measurements:

- *Ideal height-weight chart:* Weight 10% to 20% above ideal body weight is overweight; 20% or more above ideal body weight is obese.
- *Waist circumference:* Obesity for women is greater than 35 inches and for men greater than 40 inches.
- *Body mass index (BMI):* Calculated using height-to-weight ratios (Fig. 33.1).

Obesity is caused by a caloric intake that exceeds energy expenditure. Having a large waist results in an apple-shaped body. This is associated with greater health risks, especially for heart disease and cancer. This type of fat is referred to as *visceral* fat, which is metabolically more active. The metabolic activity increases substances such as triglycerides, low-density lipoprotein (LDL) cholesterol, and serum glucose that contribute to health risks.

Only a small percentage of obesity is associated with a metabolic or endocrine abnormality. Obesity that interferes with activities of daily living, such as breathing or walking, is known as morbid obesity. Morbid obesity refers to people whose BMI is above 40, which is about 100 pounds overweight for men and about 80 pounds overweight for women. Surgery can be an option for people whose BMI is above 40 or for people whose BMI is between 35 and 40 and who have life-threatening obesity-related diseases such as severe sleep apnea or heart disease. Diseases associated with being overweight or obese are called *comorbidities.* These can include atherosclerosis, gallbladder disease, heart disease, hypertension, osteoarthritis, sleep apnea, type 2 diabetes mellitus, decreased mobility, lack of self-esteem, and depression. For more information, visit the Centers for Disease Control and Prevention (CDC) at www.cdc.gov/obesity/index.html or the Obesity Society at www.obesity.org.

Therapeutic Measures

Initial treatment for obesity is weight loss through education regarding a healthy and balanced diet, exercise, and calorie restriction. Support groups, such as Take Off Pounds Sensibly (www.tops.org) and Weight Watchers (www.weightwatchers.com), can help patients be successful. Many helpful free apps are available for mobile devices such as MyFitnessPal, Lose It, and Weight Watchers. Short-term use of medications that suppress appetite or block fat absorption may also be suggested.

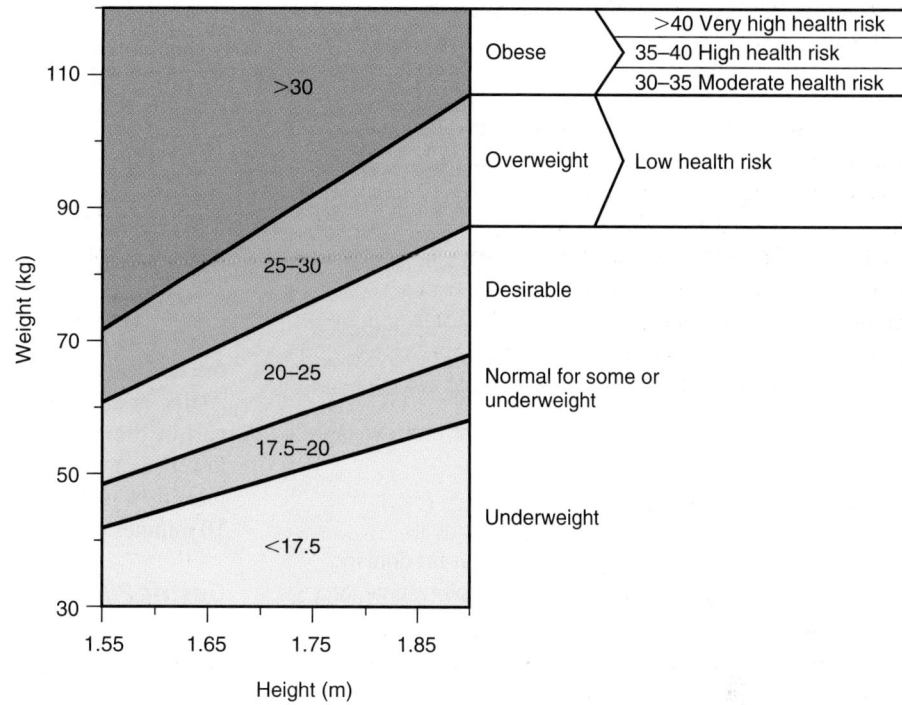

FIGURE 33.1 Body mass index ranges and associated level of health risk with obesity.

Bariatric Surgery

Patients who do not respond to medical methods of weight loss, weigh 100 pounds over ideal body weight, have a BMI over 40, have a BMI over 35 with severe health effects or type 2 diabetes mellitus, or have ineffectively controlled type 2 diabetes mellitus with a BMI of 30 to 35 might be candidates for surgical weight loss ("Patient Perspective"). Additional screening for psychiatric and social stability is required.

Weight loss surgery is called **bariatric** surgery (from Greek *baros* meaning "weight") or metabolic surgery by the American Diabetes Association when referring to its use to treat type 2 diabetes mellitus. Surgical techniques produce weight loss by limiting how much the stomach can hold and/or decreased calorie and nutrient absorption ("Nutrition Notes"). For a list of surgical weight loss centers and surgical procedures, visit the American Society for Metabolic and Bariatric Surgery (https://asmbs.org) web site.

Patient Perspective

Curtis. By the time I was in high school, I weighed 250 pounds, and the weight just kept building from there. I had tried many weight control programs. At age 38, I began to consider weight loss surgery. I had spoken to many people who had bariatric surgery. They pointed out the psychological aspect of how differently people treated you after weight loss and how some couples ended up divorcing. This was a very scary aspect to me.

However, after much research and reaching a weight of 380 pounds, I had surgery at a bariatric surgery facility. I felt very comfortable through the presurgical testing and psychological evaluation and counseling. One of the nice features was that the facility itself was patient-friendly, with large chairs and other amenities for larger people. When I had the surgery, the first 24 hours in the critical care unit was rough. The nursing staff was very professional and understanding. The care was responsive to my needs. I think that understanding the medical field you are working in is important to promoting patient comfort. Several of my nurses had gone through the procedure themselves. This really helped them to know what I was experiencing.

I lost 120 pounds. My health has improved a good deal. I would do it again, even though, at about day 21, I would have said, "Never again."

As nursing professionals, it is very important to treat all patients with respect, regardless of their socioeconomic status or medical needs. I believe it is not only kind but helps in the healing and recovery processes as well. I was treated with a great deal of kindness and respect during my procedure, and I greatly appreciated this. Thanks to all the professional nurses out there who do a great job!

Nutrition Notes

Supplying Nutrition in Upper Gastrointestinal Conditions

Bariatric Surgery. Candidates for bariatric surgery are counseled that the procedure is a tool to assist with weight control, along with behavioral changes, diet, and exercise. If the patient overeats, the small pouch that was created can be stretched and weight regained.

The type and amount of food intake are strictly controlled after surgery and during about 12 weeks of recovery. Long-term dietary strategies include the following:

• Choosing foods that are high protein, low fat, and low sugar
• Eating six small meals daily
• Chewing thoroughly and eating slowly
• Drinking sufficient fluids, mostly between meals
• Avoiding carbonated beverages and straws for drinking, as this introduces excess air into the gastrointestinal tract
• Taking vitamin and mineral supplements as prescribed

Common micronutrient deficiencies after gastric bypass include thiamin, vitamin B_{12}, vitamin D, iron, and copper. Intake of less than recommended amounts of calcium, magnesium, and phosphorus also occurs.

Gastroesophageal Reflux Disease (GERD) and Hiatal Hernia. Guidelines to help control symptoms of GERD and hiatal hernia include the following:

• Maintaining ideal body weight
• Chewing food completely
• Avoiding high-fat, spicy, or trigger foods that cause symptoms (individualized), such as citrus or tomato products.
• Avoiding alcohol, chocolate, coffee, peppermint, and spearmint
• Avoiding food within 3 hours of bedtime

Dumping Syndrome. Ways to decrease dumping syndrome include the following:

• Eating six small meals per day
• Eating meals that include high-protein, high-fiber complex carbohydrates, and no simple sugars
• Thickening foods with guar gum and pectin
• Avoiding fluids with meals
• Lying down for 30 to 60 minutes after meals

Gastric Cancer. If a patient has a poor prognosis after a total gastrectomy for cancer, dietary interventions should focus on symptoms the patient wishes to control. An overly restricted diet may cause the patient discomfort or distress.

Adjustable Gastric Banding

Laparoscopic adjustable gastric banding is done with an inflatable silicone band placed around the upper portion of the stomach (Fig. 33.2). This creates a small pouch to limit the amount of food the patient eats. The band is adjustable with a saline solution injected into the band through a port in the skin, making a larger or smaller pouch. The procedure is reversible.

Gastric Bypass

The **Roux-en-Y** gastric bypass is a successful weight loss surgery that reduces stomach size and bypasses some of the small intestine, which reduces absorption of calories, causing weight loss (see Fig. 33.2). It is mostly done laparoscopically but can be done as open surgery. First, a small stomach pouch the size of a thumb is created. This small pouch causes a quick satisfactory feeling of fullness during a meal, which is the key to the success of this procedure. Next, the small intestine is divided, and the pouch is connected to the lower part of the cut small intestine to allow food to bypass the lower stomach, duodenum, and part of the jejunum. Digestive juice flow is maintained, and food enters the jejunum within 10 minutes of eating.

Gastric Plication

Laparoscopic gastric plication folds the stomach inwardly, and then sutures hold the folds in place. This reduces the stomach's volume and limits the food that can be ingested at one time. It can be reversed. It is investigational.

Sleeve Gastrectomy

Laparoscopic sleeve **gastrectomy** removes about 75% of the stomach, leaving a slim narrow tube (gastric sleeve). This reduces the stomach's volume and limits food intake at one time. It decreases the hormone ghrelin produced by the stomach that causes hunger.

Biliopancreatic Diversion With Duodenal Switch

Like the sleeve gastrectomy, a small tubular pouch is created. Then, most of the small intestine is bypassed, so that, with the connection of a piece of the distal small intestine to the pouch, the food goes directly to the end portion of the small intestine. The end of the bypassed small intestine is reconnected to this end portion of the small intestine so that digestive juices are not lost and can mix with the food.

Complications of Bariatric Surgery

Complications of bariatric surgery are nausea and vomiting caused by overeating or by not chewing food well, bloating, heartburn, staple disruption, obstruction, dumping syndrome, gout, gallstones, kidney stones, and osteoporosis. Protein, vitamin, and mineral deficiencies can result. Band slippage or intestinal leakage can occur.

Postoperative Care

Patients who have had bariatric surgery require care similar to that for most types of gastric surgeries. (See "Nursing Process for the Patient Having Gastric Surgery.") The bariatric diet, however, is very different and requires individualized

• WORD • BUILDING •
gastrectomy: gastr—stomach + ectomy—to remove

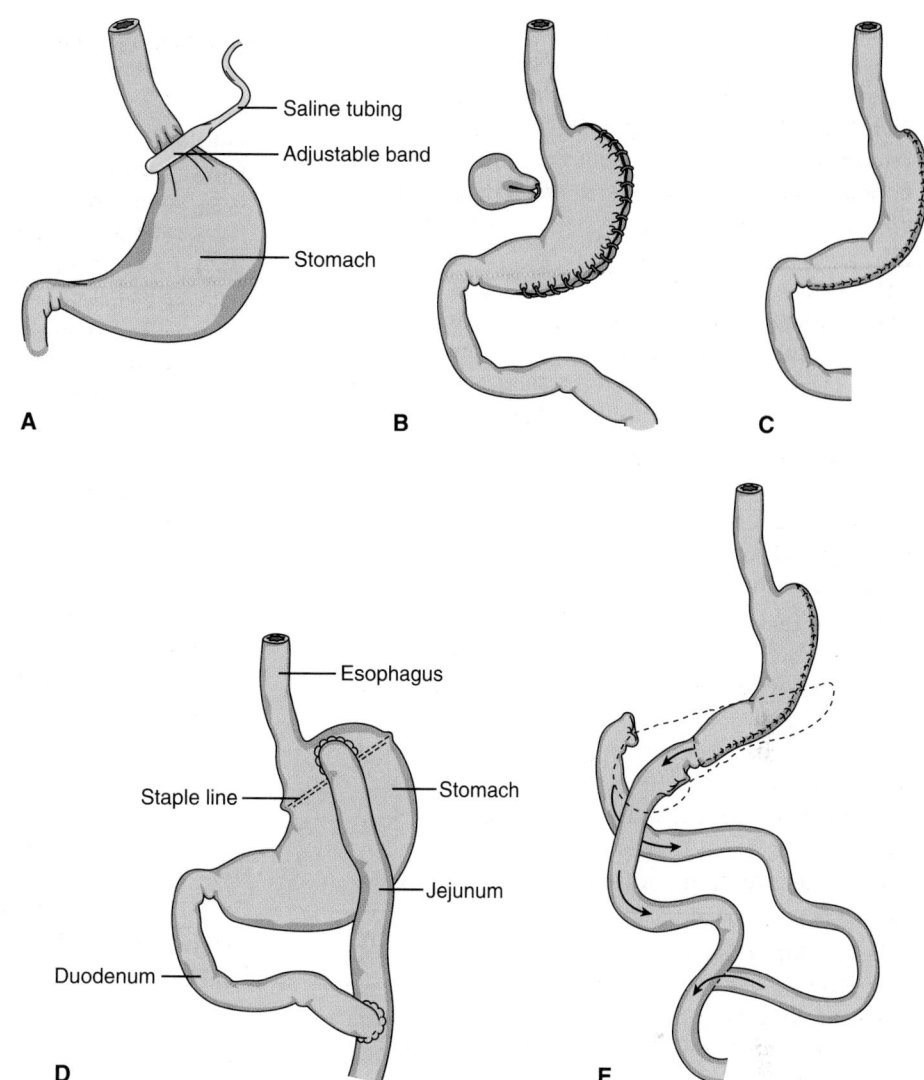

FIGURE 33.2 (A) Adjustable gastric band. (B) Gastric plication. (C) Sleeve gastrectomy. (D) Roux-en-Y gastric bypass. (E) Biliopancreatic diversion with duodenal switch.

dietary education. Some patients will have an NG tube placed during surgery. It is important to keep the head of the bed elevated to ensure adequate lung expansion. Patients are started on a clear liquid diet because of the small stomach pouch that has been created. Only a small amount of fluid, 30 mL, is allowed at a time. Then, the diet progresses to full liquids, pureed foods, and, finally, at about 6 weeks after surgery, regular foods, as tolerated. Patients will need to be taught to restrict the amount of food ingested at one time. Long-term follow-up is needed. Many patients experience significant weight loss by 6 to 8 months after surgery. This can lead to a large amount of flabby skin. It is recommended that patients wait at least 1 full year before having reconstructive surgery to remove the excess skin.

Nursing Process for the Patient Who Is Obese
Data Collection
Data collection for the patient with obesity should include measurements of height, weight, and BMI and physical examination. Information about eating patterns and exercise patterns

is obtained. The nurse determines if any problems exist for the patient related to excess weight, such as physical limitations, social interaction issues, and personal issues (e.g., changes in sexuality or financial status). People who are overweight have an increased risk for other diseases, which should be explored.

Nursing Diagnoses, Planning, and Implementation

Obesity related to caloric intake greater than metabolic needs and/or decreased activity level

EXPECTED OUTCOME: The patient will achieve and maintain weight loss to specified weight.

• Establish desired weight goal and monitor weight *to track progress toward goal.*
• In collaboration with a dietitian, modify eating habits and patterns *to lose weight and then maintain weight loss.*
• Establish and maintain increased activity pattern *to lose weight and then maintain weight loss.*
• Discuss realistic weight loss goals of about 1 to 2 lb (0.5 to 1 kg) per week *to achieve lasting weight loss effects.*

- Discuss emotions, events, and patterns of eating *to help patient identify when the patient is eating to satisfy an emotional need versus a physiological hunger.*
- Provide preoperative instructions if surgical interventions are planned *to help patient understand the procedure.*

Evaluation

The patient's goals are met if the patient maintains progressive weight loss to a specified weight goal and safely progresses through the perioperative period if a surgical intervention is completed.

NURSING CARE TIP

Special bariatric equipment for providing patient-centered care includes the following:

- Larger hospital bed, wheelchair, or walker
- Patient lifting devices
- Extra pillows to ease breathing
- Larger hospital gowns
- Larger blood pressure cuff

 ## ORAL HEALTH AND DENTAL CARE

Good oral health care is important to overall health. Nutrition can be affected if oral problems interfere with eating and drinking. Respiratory illness and cardiac disease are associated with pathogens in the mouth. Regular mechanical oral hygiene is needed to remove plaque and prevent infections. Functional limitations may interfere with self-care for oral hygiene, especially for older adults ("Gerontological Issues"). Suction toothbrushes are available for those patients who are unable to control secretions (see Fig. 2.2). During data collection, the nurse should note any signs of oral inflammation or infection requiring prompt treatment. Regular dental care is also important in the prevention of infections (Box 33.1).

Gerontological Issues

Oral Hygiene. Nurses can have a positive impact on older patients' outcomes by providing mechanical oral hygiene. Studies have shown that, because mechanical oral care removes plaque, it helped to prevent pneumonia and pneumonia-related death in older patients who were either hospitalized or in a long-term care facility.

 ## ORAL INFLAMMATORY DISORDERS

Aphthous Stomatitis (Canker Sores)

Aphthous stomatitis (oral inflammation) appears as small, white, painful ulcers on the inner cheeks, lips, tongue, gums, palate, or pharynx. It typically lasts for several days to 2 weeks. Triggers may include injury to the mouth from biting the cheeks or dental work; a vitamin B_{12}, zinc, folate, or iron deficiency; toothpaste with sodium lauryl sulfate; stress; menstruation; *Helicobacter pylori;* or exposure to irritating foods. Application of topical tetracycline several times a day usually shortens the healing time. A topical anesthetic such as benzocaine or lidocaine provides pain relief and makes it possible to eat with minimal pain.

Herpes Simplex Virus Type 1 Infection

Herpes simplex virus type 1 (HSV-1) infection may appear as painful cold sores or fever blisters on the face, lips, perioral area, cheeks, nose, or conjunctivae. These lesions recur over time but last only for a few days each time. The onset can be provoked by fever or stress, among other things. Acyclovir ointment can be used to ease the pain, but it does not cure the lesions. Oral acyclovir may reduce recurrences. These lesions are infectious, and standard precautions should be used when ointment is applied or oral care is given.

 ## ORAL CANCER

Pathophysiology and Etiology

Oral cancer can occur anywhere in the mouth or throat. If detected early enough, it is curable. Oral cancer is found most commonly in patients who use alcohol or any form of tobacco. The highest incidence of oral cancer is found in the pharynx (throat), with the lowest incidence being on the lips.

Signs and Symptoms

Any oral sore that does not heal in 2 weeks should be assessed by the patient's health care provider (HCP). Cancerous ulcers are often painless but may become tender as the cancer progresses. In the later stages, the patient may report difficulty chewing, swallowing, or speaking or have swollen cervical lymph glands.

Diagnostic Tests

Biopsy specimens are taken to identify the presence of cancer.

Therapeutic Measures

Oral cancer treatment varies depending on the individualized diagnosis. Radiation, chemotherapy, and surgery are used alone or in combination to treat oral cancer. Radical or modified neck dissection is often performed because this type of

• WORD • BUILDING •

stomatitis: stoma—mouth + itis—inflammation

Box 33.1

Common Concerns in Oral Health and Dental Care

Daily and ongoing oral care is important throughout life and has been found to have a link to cardiac health.

Angular Cheilosis. A condition known as angular cheilosis (red, raw corners of the mouth) develops more often in older adults. It may be from infection, deficiency of riboflavin (vitamin B$_2$), or loss of facial profile caused by worn-down or damaged dentures or the patient not wearing his or her dentures. It is treated with anti-infective medications, vitamins, or new dentures.

Antibiotic Prophylaxis. People who have artificial joints or certain heart conditions may need to take prophylactic antibiotics before certain dental procedures. This is to prevent bacteria from entering the circulation and causing bacterial endocarditis. The patient's health care provider identifies the length of time after a joint replacement (e.g., for 1 or 2 years, or for life) that antibiotics are required. The dentist is informed of the patient's history to prescribe appropriate antibiotics.

Dental Implants. An implant is an artificial root placed in the jawbone. The implant is usually tubular and made of titanium. Implants can be used to replace one tooth, multiple teeth, or an entire arch. They can also be used to stabilize a complete denture.

Dentures. It is helpful to have the dentist place a small identity tag in the acrylic of the denture with the person's name on it to avoid lost or mixed-up dentures, especially when the person lives in a long-term care facility.

Those with complete dentures still need to be routinely screened by a dentist or dental hygienist for proper denture fit, sore areas, oral fungal infections, and oral cancer detection.

Gingival Recession. As people age, it is not unusual for their gingivae (gums) to recede or shrink, exposing the root surfaces of the teeth. This can lead to root sensitivity, tooth decay, or both. To protect the teeth from tooth decay as a result of dry mouth or gingival recession, a fluoride gel (Gel-Kam), rinse (ACT), or a prescription toothpaste with high fluoride is strongly recommended.

Gingivitis. As people get older, the gingivae have a greater tendency to bleed, a condition known as gingivitis. If the supporting tissues in the sockets of the teeth become inflamed, bone loss occurs, resulting in a condition known as periodontitis (pyorrhea). Periodontitis can lead to tooth mobility or loss.

Good oral hygiene habits cannot be overemphasized in the prevention of gum disease. Flossing every day is very important. If the patient is unable to floss because of arthritis or other conditions, an electric toothbrush or a Waterpik device is helpful in providing oral hygiene.

Thrush (Candida albicans Fungus). Older adults are susceptible to oral yeast infections (caused by *Candida albicans*) caused by certain medications, systemic conditions, or chemotherapy. Nystatin oral rinse treats this infection.

Xerostomia (Dry Mouth). As people age, it is not unusual for them to experience a condition known as xerostomia (dry mouth). Some medications and radiation treatment of the head and neck can cause it. Xerostomia can lead to rampant tooth decay in older adults, putting their dentition at risk. Before any radiation therapy of the head or neck area, a thorough oral examination and any needed restorative dental procedures should be completed.

Although water is used as a common substitute for saliva, it does not contain the necessary compounds, such as lubricants, to protect the teeth. There are many products available for dry mouth, such as Biotene gel, ACT rinse, and sprays to help with the discomfort of dry mouth. Brushing with a high fluoride toothpaste that is available by prescription is also recommended.

Source: Dr. Ralph Kluk and Dr. Cheryl Kluk, Jackson, MI.

cancer frequently has metastasized to cervical lymph nodes by the time it is diagnosed (Fig. 33.3). The tumor is removed along with lymph nodes, muscles, blood vessels, glands, and part of the thyroid, depending on the extent of the cancer. Drains are usually inserted into the incision to prevent fluid accumulation. A tracheostomy may also be performed to protect the airway and prevent obstruction.

Nursing Care

See "Nursing Process for the Patient With Oral or Esophageal Cancer."

 ESOPHAGEAL CANCER

Pathophysiology and Etiology

Esophageal cancer is usually detected in advanced stages because of its location near many lymph nodes that allows it to metastasize. As the cancer progresses, obstruction of the esophagus can occur, with possible perforation or fistula development that may cause aspiration. Risk factors for esophageal cancer are use of tobacco or alcohol, being overweight or obese, and Barrett's esophagus, a precancerous condition discussed later.

Signs and Symptoms

Signs and symptoms may include progressive dysphagia (difficulty swallowing), a feeling of fullness, pain in the chest after eating, foul breath, or regurgitation of foods if there is an obstruction.

Diagnostic Tests

Diagnosis of esophageal cancer can be made by barium swallow studies, biopsy, or endoscopy procedures such as esophagogastroduodenoscopy (EGD) or mediastinoscopy (endoscopic examination of mediastinum). Mediastinoscopy is used to determine whether the cancer has spread to the lymph nodes and surrounding structures.

Therapeutic Measures

Treatment for esophageal cancer includes surgery (most common), radiation, chemotherapy, laser therapy, and

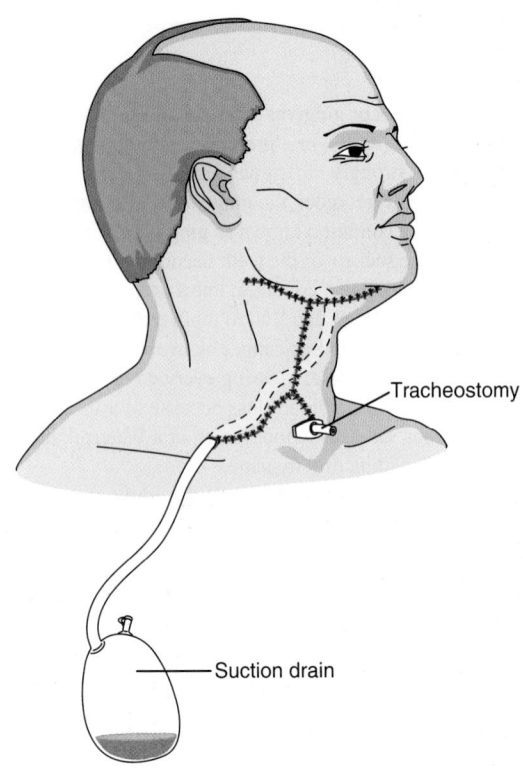

—Tracheostomy

—Suction drain

FIGURE 33.3 Radical neck dissection with tracheostomy tube and drains inserted.

electrocoagulation. These therapies may be used alone or in combination. Surgical procedures include esophageal resection (esophagectomy), resection of the esophagus and anastomosis to the remaining part of the stomach (esophagogastrostomy), Dacron esophageal replacement, or use of a section of colon to replace the esophagus (esophagoenterostomy). If the tumor is inoperable, esophageal dilation or stent placement can be done to relieve dysphagia and allow food to pass through the esophagus.

Nursing Process for the Patient With Oral or Esophageal Cancer

The patient with oral or esophageal cancer may undergo various forms of treatment, including chemotherapy, radiation,

or surgery. Nursing care is provided based on the effects from these therapies (see Chapters 11 and 12). Preoperatively, the use of alcohol or tobacco is discussed and referrals to cessation programs and support groups offered as desired. Postoperatively, major concerns are airway patency, pain management, swallowing ability, and fluid and nutritional needs. The airway must be monitored, and secretions controlled to prevent aspiration. Tracheostomy care is discussed in Chapter 29. Preoperative teaching includes communication methods if a tracheostomy is to be placed. Pain is monitored, and analgesics given as needed. A speech pathologist may perform a swallowing evaluation to develop a plan of care for nutritional needs. Swallowing ability is monitored. IV fluids and parenteral nutrition or enteral feedings (see Chapter 32) are given to meet the patient's hydration and nutritional needs while swallowing is difficult.

■ HIATAL HERNIA

Pathophysiology

The esophagus passes through an opening in the diaphragm called the hiatus. A **hiatal hernia** is a condition in which the stomach slides up through the hiatus of the diaphragm into the thorax (Fig. 33.4). A sliding hiatal hernia is the most common type, in which the junction of the stomach and esophagus slides up into the thoracic cavity when a patient is supine and then usually goes back into the abdominal cavity when the patient stands upright. A paraesophageal hernia is rarer but serious, as part of the stomach squeezes through the hiatus and is at risk for strangulation (blood supply is cut off). Hiatal hernia occurs most commonly in smokers and in those who are older than age 50, obese, or pregnant. People with hiatal hernia often have gastroesophageal reflux disease (GERD) as well (discussed later).

Signs and Symptoms

A small hernia may not produce any discomfort or require treatment. However, a large hernia can cause pain, heartburn, a feeling of fullness, or reflux, which can injure the esophagus with possible ulceration and bleeding.

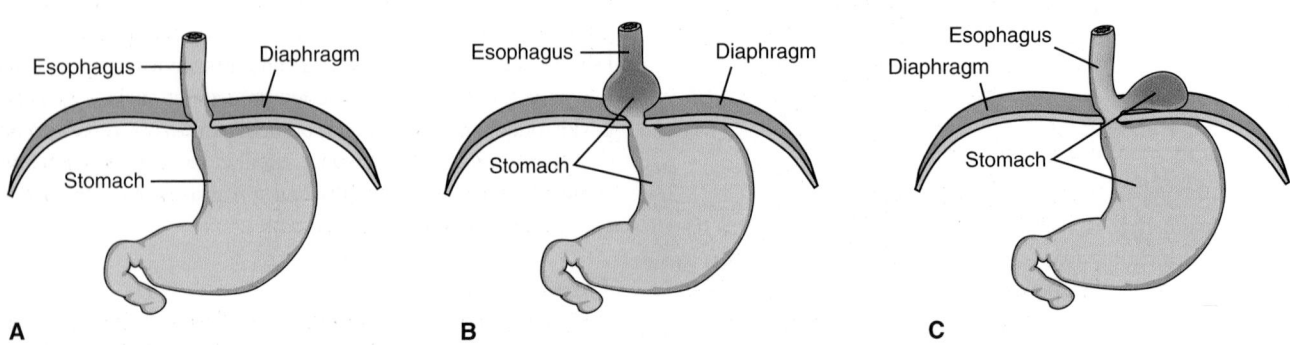

FIGURE 33.4 Hiatal hernia. (A) Normal esophagus and stomach. (B) Sliding hiatal hernia. (C) Rolling hiatal hernia.

Diagnostic Tests

Hiatal hernias are diagnosed by x-ray studies and fluoroscopy.

Therapeutic Measures

Lifestyle changes for symptomatic hiatal hernia include not smoking and elevating the head of the bed 6 to 12 inches to prevent reflux, in addition to dietary interventions in "Nutrition Notes."

Surgical Management

Surgery is done for symptomatic hiatal hernia when GERD, strangulation, or obstruction is present. Fundoplication, in which the stomach fundus is wrapped around the lower part of the esophagus, is the most common surgical procedure performed (Fig. 33.5).

Nursing Care

The patient is taught lifestyle interventions to reduce the symptoms of hiatal hernia. If the patient undergoes surgery, general postoperative nursing care is provided. In addition, following fundoplication, patients are monitored for dysphagia during their first postoperative meal. If dysphagia occurs, the physician should be notified because the repair may be too tight, causing obstruction of the passage of food.

 ## GASTROESOPHAGEAL REFLUX DISEASE

Pathophysiology

GERD is a condition in which gastric secretions reflux into the esophagus. The esophagus can be damaged by acidic gastric secretions and exposure to digestive enzymes. GERD is caused primarily by conditions that affect the ability of the lower esophageal sphincter to close tightly, such as hiatal hernia.

Signs and Symptoms

Signs and symptoms of GERD include heartburn two to three times a week, regurgitation, sour taste in the mouth, or dysphagia (Table 33.1).

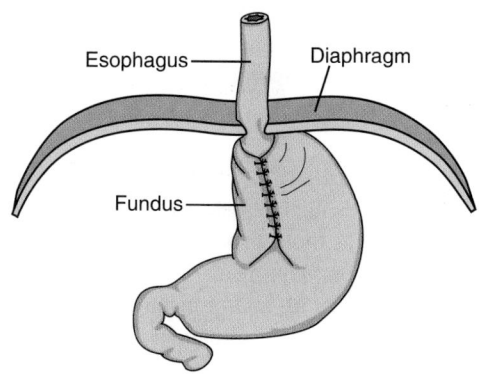

FIGURE 33.5 Hiatal hernia repair. Nissen fundoplication wraps the stomach fundus around the esophagus and then sutures it onto itself to hold it in place.

Table 33.1
GERD Summary

Signs and Symptoms	Heartburn two to three times weekly Regurgitation Dysphagia Hoarseness Sore throat
Diagnosis	Symptoms Response to treatment Endoscopy 24-hour esophageal pH study
Therapeutic Measures	Avoid smoking Raise head of bed on 4- to 6-inch blocks For mild symptoms: antacids, histamine 2 (H2)-receptor antagonists For moderate to severe symptoms: proton pump inhibitors (PPIs) Also see "Nutrition Notes"
Complications	Esophagitis Barrett's esophagus Respiratory symptoms
Priority Nursing Diagnoses	*Acute Pain* *Deficient Knowledge*

Diagnostic Tests

Diagnostic tests include a barium swallow, esophagoscopy (an endoscopic procedure), or pH monitoring of the normally alkaline esophagus.

Complications

Respiratory complications such as asthma, aspiration pneumonia, bronchospasm, laryngospasm, and chronic bronchitis can occur due to aspiration of gastric contents.

Barrett's esophagus

GERD can result in esophagitis (inflammation of the esophagus) due to acid reflux. Over time, this can change the epithelium of the esophagus and lead to Barrett's esophagus. This is a precancerous lesion that puts the patient at risk of developing esophageal cancer. Barrett's tissue can be removed during a 30-minute outpatient endoscopic procedure using radiofrequency ablation (the Barrx system). Normal tissue returns, and the risk of cancer is reduced.

Therapeutic Measures

Lifestyle changes are recommended first and then medications if needed (see "Nutrition Notes" and Table 33.1). If medications are not effective, a fundoplication or endoscopic procedure can be done. A minimally invasive procedure called transoral incisionless fundoplication (TIF) is performed through the mouth without incisions. It employs the EsophyX device to create an esophagogastric fundoplication that is up to 270 degrees and 2 to 3 cm in length. EsophyX uses an endoscope to tighten the lower esophageal sphincter. This aids in improving or eliminating GERD with good success (for more information, visit www.endogastricsolutions.com/tif-procedure/tif-vs-antireflux-surgery). What do you think the benefit of this procedure is over fundoplication surgery? If you think that it's minimally invasive and, therefore, has a speedier recovery, you would be correct. Other endoscopic procedures that use radiofrequency waves, such as the Stretta, can be done. The radiofrequency waves are injected into the lower esophageal sphincter muscle to form collagen contraction, which leads to a barrier against reflux.

Nursing Process for the Patient With GERD
Data Collection
Data collection for the patient with GERD includes evaluation of heartburn episodes. The onset, duration, characteristics, and precipitating or relieving factors are noted.

Nursing Diagnoses, Planning, and Implementation

Acute Pain related to inflammation of esophageal tissues

EXPECTED OUTCOME: The patient will state a reduction of pain to an acceptable level or total relief of pain within 30 minutes of report of pain.

- Identify characteristics of heartburn and factors that trigger pain *to develop teaching plan.*
- Instruct the patient in lifestyle changes, including maintaining ideal weight and avoiding smoking, caffeine, peppermint, and alcohol *because they decrease functioning of the lower esophageal sphincter.*
- Instruct the patient to avoid trigger foods *to avoid pain.*
- Instruct the patient to sleep with head of bed elevated 4 to 6 inches and avoid eating 3 hours before bedtime *to prevent reflux of gastric contents into esophagus.*
- Teach the patient about medications *to ensure appropriate use.*

Evaluation
The goal is met if the patient's pain is controlled and symptoms are relieved.

MALLORY-WEISS TEAR

A Mallory-Weiss tear (MWT) is a longitudinal tear in the mucous membrane of the esophagus at the stomach junction (gastric cardia). It occurs from a sudden powerful or prolonged force due to coughing, vomiting, seizures, prolapse of the stomach into the esophagus, or cardiopulmonary resuscitation (CPR). Up to 15% of GI bleeding is caused by MWTs. It occurs most in men. Alcohol use should be avoided. Up to 75% of those with MWTs use alcohol

excessively. Symptoms include bright red, bloody emesis or bloody or tarry stools. The tear can be diagnosed with an EGD. Hemoglobin and hematocrit are monitored.

The tear usually self-heals without intervention in several days, and bleeding stops within a few hours. It is rare to have it happen again. A proton pump inhibitor (PPI) and an antiemetic may be given. Bleeding is treated with an injection of epinephrine to constrict the blood vessel. During endoscopy, endoclips can be placed to stop the bleeding. Rarely, excessive bleeding may occur, resulting in shock and/or the need for a blood transfusion.

The focus of nursing care is to monitor the patient for signs of bleeding and report them. Patient teaching includes medications and the avoidance of alcohol use. See the section on gastric bleeding later in the chapter for more information.

ESOPHAGEAL VARICES

Esophageal varices are dilated blood vessels in the esophagus (see Chapter 35). Their rupture can precipitate a life-threatening event.

GASTRITIS

Gastritis is inflammation of the stomach mucosa and can be acute or chronic. Causes are listed in Box 33.2.

Acute Gastritis
Pathophysiology
Gastritis results when the protective mucosal barrier is broken down and allows autodigestion from hydrochloric acid and pepsin to occur. Inflammation results in edema of the tissue and possible hemorrhage. With severe gastritis, the gastric mucosa can become gangrenous and perforate, which can lead to peritonitis (infection of the peritoneum). Scarring may also occur, resulting in pyloric obstruction.

Signs and Symptoms
The major symptom of gastritis is abdominal pain, which is often accompanied by nausea and anorexia. The patient may also experience abdominal tenderness, a feeling of fullness, reflux, belching, and hematemesis. If the cause of the gastritis is contaminated food, symptoms, including diarrhea, usually start within 5 to 6 hours.

Therapeutic Measures
Treatment of gastritis includes avoiding alcohol; avoiding irritating foods such as those that are acidic, greasy, or spicy; and eating smaller frequent meals. Antiemetics are given to control vomiting. Antacids and/or histamine 2 (H2)-receptor antagonists are given to control pain.

• WORD • BUILDING •
gastritis: gastr—stomach + itis—inflammation

Causes of Gastritis

- Alcohol use
- Endoscopic procedures
- Microorganisms (e.g., *Helicobacter pylori, Salmonella*)
- Medications (e.g., aspirin, nonsteroidal anti-inflammatory drugs [NSAIDs], corticosteroids, digitalis, chemotherapy agents)
- Nasogastric suctioning
- Radiation
- Reflux of bile
- Smoking
- Stress (emotional, physiological)
- Trauma

Chronic Gastritis

Chronic gastritis occurs over time and is classified as type A or type B.

Type A

Type A chronic gastritis is often referred to as autoimmune gastritis. It occurs in the fundus (body of stomach), usually with no symptoms. It is diagnosed by endoscopy, upper GI x-ray examination, and gastric aspirate analysis (see Chapter 32). In those with this condition, there is usually not enough intrinsic factor secreted from their stomach cells. As a result, there is difficulty absorbing vitamin B_{12}, which leads to pernicious anemia (discussed later; Carabotti et al., 2017).

Type B

Type B chronic gastritis affects the antrum and pylorus (lower end of the stomach near the duodenum). It is associated with *H. pylori* bacterial infection. Type B is the most common type of chronic gastritis. Signs and symptoms include poor appetite, heartburn after eating, belching, a sour taste in the mouth, and nausea and vomiting. Type B chronic gastritis can also be diagnosed by endoscopy, upper GI x-ray examination, and gastric aspirate analysis. *H. pylori* infection is treated with antibiotics.

Stress-Induced Gastritis

A small number of patients who are critically ill may develop GI mucosal damage from ischemia. The stress response to the illness causes reduced blood flow to the stomach and small intestine, resulting in ischemia and damage to the mucosa. The damaged mucous barrier then allows acid secretions to create ulcerations. Preventive treatment has dramatically reduced stress ulceration, which can have a high mortality rate because of the multiple bleeding ulcer sites. This treatment includes trauma care that quickly restores oxygen to the stomach as well as early feeding within 24 hours of the trauma and prophylactic sucralfate (which forms a gel that binds to the base of an ulcer), antacids, or histamine blockers.

PEPTIC ULCER DISEASE

Pathophysiology

Peptic ulcer disease (PUD) is a condition in which the lining of the stomach, pylorus, duodenum, or the esophagus is eroded, usually from infection with *H. pylori*. The erosion may extend into the muscular layers or the peritoneum. Peptic ulcers occur in the portions of the GI tract that are exposed to hydrochloric acid and pepsin. The erosion is due to an increase in the concentration or activity of hydrochloric acid and pepsin. The damaged mucosa is unable to secrete enough mucus to act as a barrier against the hydrochloric acid. Some individuals have more rapid gastric emptying. When combined with hypersecretion of acid, this creates a large amount of acid moving into the duodenum. As a result, peptic ulcers occur more often in the duodenum. Ulcers are named by their location: gastric or duodenal. Duodenal ulcers are more common than gastric ulcers.

Etiology

Until 1982, the cause of peptic ulcers was poorly understood and thought to be related to stress, diet, and alcohol or caffeine ingestion. It is now known that PUD is primarily caused by the gram-negative bacterium *H. pylori*. About half of all people worldwide are infected with *H. pylori*. North America has a low prevalence. The discovery of *H. pylori* has led to changes in treating and curing peptic ulcers. Nonsteroidal anti-inflammatory drug (NSAID) use and smoking also increase the risk for PUD.

Signs and Symptoms

Symptoms vary with the location of the ulcer (Table 33.2). Symptoms may not be experienced until complications such as hemorrhage, obstruction, or perforation develop. If pain does occur with gastric ulcer, it is a burning and gnawing pain in the high-left epigastric region that may increase with food ingestion or 1 to 2 hours after a meal. Duodenal ulcers produce cramping or burning pain in the mid-epigastric or upper abdominal area, which occurs 2 to 4 hours after meals or in the middle of the night. This intermittent pain may be relieved by the ingestion of food or antacids. Anorexia and nausea and vomiting may also occur with either ulcer location. Bleeding may occur with massive hemorrhaging or slow oozing. Patients often have low hematocrit and hemoglobin levels. Gastric or fecal occult blood may be found, depending on where the ulcers are located.

Complications

Bleeding, perforation of stomach or duodenum wall, and obstruction can occur. Bleeding can occur in varying degrees, from occult blood in stool and emesis to massive bright red bleeding. Hemorrhage tends to occur more often with gastric ulcers in older adults. Treatment includes stopping the bleeding and replacing fluid and electrolytes.

Table 33.2

Peptic Ulcer Disease Summary

Signs and Symptoms	
Gastric ulcer	Intermittent high-left epigastric or upper abdominal burning or gnawing pain, increased 1 to 2 hours after meals or with food Variable pain pattern possibly made worse by food Antacids ineffective Possible malnourishment Hematemesis more common than melena
Duodenal ulcer	Intermittent mid-epigastric or upper abdominal burning or cramping pain, increased 2 to 4 hours after meals or in the middle of the night Relieved by food or antacids Patient usually well nourished Melena more common than hematemesis Anorexia Nausea and vomiting Bleeding (stomach secretions or stool positive for occult blood)

Diagnostic Tests	
Helicobacter pylori	Urea breath test Immunoglobulin G antibody detection test for *H. pylori* Biopsy Culture
Peptic ulcer	Upper gastrointestinal series (barium swallow) Esophagogastroduodenoscopy (EGD)

Therapeutic Measures	
H. Pylori	Antibiotics Bismuth subsalicylate
Peptic ulcer	Avoid smoking, caffeine, alcohol, trigger foods Antacids Histamine 2 (H2)-receptor antagonists Proton pump inhibitors (PPIs) Sucralfate (Carafate)

Complications	
	Bleeding Perforation Obstruction

Priority Nursing Diagnoses	
	Acute Pain *Risk for Injury* *Deficient Knowledge*

Diagnostic Tests

H. pylori can be diagnosed with several tests. The urea breath test is performed by having the patient drink carbon-labeled urea. The urea is metabolized rapidly if *H. pylori* is present, allowing the carbon to be absorbed and measured in exhaled carbon dioxide. An immunoglobulin G antibody detection test for *H. pylori* identifies whether the patient is infected with *H. pylori*. These are both noninvasive detection tests. Biopsy specimens for the *Campylobacter*-like organism (CLO) biopsy urease test and a histological examination can be obtained during EGD. Biopsy is the most conclusive test for *H. pylori*. Cultures of the biopsy specimen may also be done to determine antimicrobial susceptibility.

Peptic ulcers are diagnosed on the basis of symptoms, upper GI series (barium swallow), and EGD. Endoscopy allows direct visualization of the ulcer and mucosal tissues.

Therapeutic Measures

Several treatment options are used to cure *H. pylori* without recurrence (Table 33.3). For better effectiveness, triple therapy with two antibiotics to decrease resistance of the bacteria and a PPI or H2-receptor antagonist is used. Sequential treatment lasting 14 days has better eradication rates than 10-day treatments (Liou et al., 2016). Bismuth subsalicylate (e.g., in Pepto-Bismol) may also be used for its antibacterial effects.

PPIs are powerful agents that stop the final step of gastric acid secretion to reduce mucosa erosion and aid in healing ulcers (Table 33.4). H2-receptor antagonists block H2 receptors to decrease acid secretion, although they are not as powerful as gastric acid pump inhibitors. Alcohol and foods known to

Table 33.3
Medication Regimen Examples for *H. Pylori* Infection

Type of Therapy	Included in Therapy	Examples of Therapy Options
Triple therapy	Two antibiotics + proton pump inhibitor (PPI)	Amoxicillin (Amoxil) + clarithromycin (Biaxin) + omeprazole (Prilosec) Amoxicillin (Amoxil) + clarithromycin (Biaxin) + lansoprazole (Prevacid) (available as Prevpac, combined for convenience)
Other therapy	Two antibiotics + bismuth subsalicylate Add histamine 2 (H2)-receptor antagonist	metronidazole (Flagyl) + tetracycline + bismuth subsalicylate (Pepto-Bismol) + H2-receptor antagonist

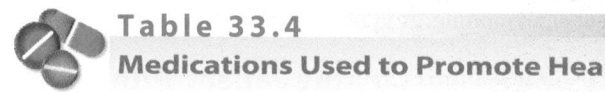

Table 33.4
Medications Used to Promote Healing of Peptic Ulcers

Medication Class/Action

Antisecretory Agents

Histamine 2 (H2)-Receptor Antagonist
Inhibit gastric acid secretion by blocking H2-receptors on gastric parietal cells.

Examples	Nursing Indications
cimetidine (Tagamet) famotidine (Pepcid) nizatidine (Axid) ranitidine (Zantac)	If giving an antacid, give it at least 1 hour before or 2 hours after an H2-receptor antagonist because absorption may be reduced. Can be given in single bedtime dose or, if given twice a day, one dose in morning and one at bedtime.

Proton Pump Inhibitors (PPIs)
Bind to an enzyme in the presence of acidic gastric pH, preventing final transport of hydrogen ions into the gastric lumen.

Examples	Nursing Indications
dexlansoprazole (Dexilant) esomeprazole (Nexium) lansoprazole (Prevacid) omeprazole (Prilosec) pantoprazole (Protonix) rabeprazole (Aciphex)	Delayed release. Capsule swallowed whole. Give before morning meal. Notify health care provider of bleeding, diarrhea, headache, or abdominal pain.

Continued

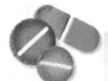

Table 33.4

Medications Used to Promote Healing of Peptic Ulcers—cont'd

Medication Class/Action

Antacids	
Increase gastric pH to reduce pepsin activity; strengthen gastric mucosal barrier and esophageal sphincter tone.	
Examples	**Nursing Indications**
aluminum-magnesium combinations (Riopan, Maalox, Mylanta, Gelusil) calcium carbonate (Tums, Titralac)	Do not give to patients with kidney disease. Give at least 1 hour before or 2 hours after an H2-receptor antagonist, tetracycline, or enteric-coated tablets because absorption may be reduced. Do not give with milk. Monitor bowel movements and for signs of hypermagnesemia or hypercalcemia.

Mucosal Barrier Fortifiers	
In presence of mild acid condition, form viscid and sticky gel and adhere to ulcer surface, forming a protective barrier.	
Examples	**Nursing Indications**
sucralfate (Carafate)	Take on an empty stomach, 1 hour before meals and at bedtime. Monitor for constipation.

cause discomfort to the patient, such as spicy foods, carbonated drinks, and caffeine, should be avoided until the ulcer heals.

A perforated ulcer is a medical emergency and may require surgery. Gastroduodenal contents escape through the perforation into the peritoneal cavity. This can result in peritonitis and hypovolemic shock. Perforation most often occurs with duodenal ulcers and presents with an acute onset of sharp, severe pain. An NG tube is inserted, and IV fluids are given. Surgical treatment includes cleaning the peritoneal cavity and closing the perforation.

Obstruction may be due to scar tissue because of repeated ulcerations and healing in a patient with long-standing PUD. Obstruction frequently occurs at the pylorus, causing pain at night and vomiting. A pyloroplasty corrects the problem.

CRITICAL THINKING

Mr. Smith, a patient on your medical unit, has a duodenal ulcer. His wife runs to the nursing station and says that you need to help her husband because he is in terrible pain. As you enter the room, you see Mr. Smith curled up in a knee-to-chest position on the bed. He is moaning and says he has excruciating abdominal pain.

1. What additional data would you gather?
2. What nursing actions would you complete to provide patient-centered care?
3. What emotional support would you offer to Mrs. Smith?
4. What complication do you suspect Mr. Smith is experiencing?
5. What member(s) of the health care team would you anticipate collaborating with?
6. What nursing actions will you anticipate implementing after receiving orders from the health care provider?

Suggested answers are at the end of the chapter.

Nursing Process for the Patient With Peptic Ulcer Disease
Data Collection
Data are collected about the patient's PUD history and factors that trigger or relieve symptoms. The primary focus of nursing care for PUD is educating patients on the importance of diagnosing this condition because ulcers may be caused by an infection that can be cured with antibiotics.

Nursing Diagnoses, Planning, Implementation, and Evaluation
See "Nursing Care Plan for the Patient With Peptic Ulcer Disease."

 GASTRIC BLEEDING

Gastric bleeding may be caused by ulcer perforation, tumors, gastric surgery, or other conditions. Bleeding peptic ulcers are the most common cause of blood loss into the stomach or intestine. Blood loss can be hidden (occult) blood in the stool, observable vomited blood (hematemesis), or black tarry stools (melena). When blood mixes with hydrochloric acid and enzymes in the stomach, a dark, granular material resembling

Nursing Care Plan for the Patient With Peptic Ulcer Disease

Nursing Diagnosis: *Acute Pain* related to gastric mucosal erosion
Expected Outcome: The patient's pain will be relieved as evidenced by no report of pain within 30 minutes of report of pain.
Evaluation of Outcome: Is pain relieved to patient's satisfaction?

Intervention	Rationale	Evaluation
Ask about factors precipitating and relieving pain.	*Peptic ulcer pain may be relieved by food, antacids, or other interventions.*	Is patient able to state precipitating and relieving pain factors?
Ask patient to rate pain level every 3 hours and as needed. Note location, onset, intensity, characteristics of pain, and nonverbal pain cues.	*Prompt assessment can lead to timely intervention and relief of pain.*	Does patient rate pain using scale and describe pain?
Administer medications as ordered.	*Acid suppressing medications help heal ulcer and relieve pain.*	Do medications reduce patient's symptoms?
Provide small, frequent meals four to six times a day.	*Small, frequent meals dilute and neutralize gastric acid.*	Does patient report relief of gastric pain between meals?

Nursing Diagnosis: *Risk for Injury* related to complications of peptic ulcer activity such as hemorrhage and perforation
Expected Outcomes: The patient's vital signs will be maintained within normal limits, and bleeding or hemorrhage will be promptly detected.
Evaluation of Outcomes: Are patient's vital signs within normal limits?

Intervention	Rationale	Evaluation
Monitor for signs and symptoms of hemorrhage, such as hematemesis (vomiting blood) and melena (blood in the stool).	*Rapid assessment can lead to prompt intervention.*	Does patient have any bleeding?
Monitor vital signs (e.g., blood pressure, pulse, respirations, temperature) and report abnormalities.	*Severe blood loss of more than 1 L per 24 hours may cause evidence of shock, such as hypotension; weak, thready pulse; chills; palpitations; and diaphoresis.*	Are vital signs normal?
Maintain intravenous infusion as ordered	*Normal fluid balance prevents hypovolemia and shock due to hemorrhage.*	Are intake and output balanced?

coffee grounds is produced. This material can be vomited or passed through the GI system and mixed with stools. Melena occurs from slow bleeding in an upper GI area.

Signs and Symptoms

With mild bleeding, the patient may experience only slight weakness or diaphoresis (Table 33.5). Severe blood loss (more than 1 L in 24 hours) may result in hypovolemic shock, with signs and symptoms such as hypotension; a weak, thready pulse; chills; palpitations; and diaphoresis.

Therapeutic Measures

The goal of treatment for a massive GI bleed is to prevent or treat hypovolemic shock and prevent dehydration,

electrolyte imbalance, and further bleeding. The following steps are taken:

• The patient is kept on nothing by mouth (NPO) status.
• An IV line is started to replace lost fluids and administer blood if necessary.
• A complete blood count (CBC) is obtained to determine the amount of blood lost.
• A urinary catheter may be inserted to monitor output.
• An NG tube is inserted to assess the rate of bleeding, decompress the stomach, monitor the pH of gastric secretions, and administer saline lavage if ordered.
• Oxygen therapy may be required if the patient has lost a large amount of blood.

Table 33.5

Gastric Bleeding Summary

Signs and Symptoms	Occult blood in stool Hematemesis Melena Hypovolemic shock
Diagnostic Tests	Endoscopy Decreased hemoglobin and hematocrit
Therapeutic Measures	Hypovolemic shock: NPO (nothing by mouth), intravenous fluids, oxygen therapy, nasogastric tube Removal or ligation of bleeding area Acid suppressing medications
Complications	Hypovolemic shock
Priority Nursing Diagnoses	*Deficient Fluid Volume*

- To prevent aspiration with vomiting, the patient is turned to the left side and elevating the head of the bed is considered.
- The HCP may perform endoscopy to help control the bleeding and instill medications.
- For severe cases, surgery may be needed to remove the bleeding area or ligate bleeding vessels.
- Acid suppression medications are given to decrease the secretion of gastric acid.

Nursing Process for the Patient With Gastric Bleeding

Data Collecton

The nurse monitors at-risk patients for signs and symptoms of bleeding. If bleeding occurs, monitor for signs of hypovolemic shock, including hypotension, tachycardia, tachypnea, chills, palpitations, and diaphoresis. Also monitor changes in level of consciousness, confusion, dry mucous membranes, fatigue, and thirst, which could indicate a decrease in circulating blood volume.

Nursing Diagnoses, Planning, and Implementation

Deficient Fluid Volume related to bleeding from GI tract via vomiting or diarrhea

EXPECTED OUTCOME: The patient's vital signs will remain within normal limits and I&O will be balanced over 24 hours.

- Monitor color, amount, and frequency of fluid loss *to determine fluid balance changes.*
- Monitor vital signs and level of consciousness to report abnormal findings *for prompt treatment.*
- Monitor hematocrit and hemoglobin levels as ordered *to detect a decrease in circulating blood volume.*

- Obtain daily weights and monitor mucous membranes and skin turgor *to detect changes in fluid volume.*
- Offer oral fluids or monitor IV infusions as ordered *to ensure adequate intake.*

Evaluation

If interventions have been effective, vital signs are within the normal range and the patient has a balanced I&O over 24 hours.

GASTRIC CANCER

Gastric cancer refers to malignant lesions found in the stomach. It is more common in men than in women. *H. pylori* bacteria can play a role in gastric cancer development. The antioxidants in fruits and vegetables can protect these cells. Other factors that may be associated with gastric cancer development include pernicious anemia; exposure to occupational substances such as lead dust, grain dust, glycol ethers, or leaded gasoline; and a diet high in smoked fish or meats. A poor prognosis is often associated with gastric cancer because most patients have metastasis at the time of diagnosis (see "Nutrition Notes").

Signs and Symptoms

Gastric cancer is rarely diagnosed in its early stages because symptoms do not appear until late in the disease (Table 33.6). In the early stages, there may not be any symptoms at all, and metastasis to another organ, such as the liver, may have already occurred. The symptoms of gastric cancer are often mistaken for PUD; these include indigestion, anorexia, pain relieved by antacids, weight loss, and nausea and vomiting. Anemia from blood loss commonly occurs, and occult blood may be present in the stool.

Diagnostic Tests

Diagnosis of gastric cancer is made by upper GI x-ray examination, gastroscopy, gastric fluid analysis, and measurement of serum gastrin levels.

Therapeutic Measures

There is little effective medical treatment available for gastric cancer. Surgical removal of the cancer is the most effective treatment. Typically, the cancer has already metastasized, and surgery is performed only to relieve symptoms. Chemotherapy and radiation are sometimes used in conjunction with surgery. Biological therapies with natural substances to boost the immune system might also be tried.

GASTRIC SURGERY

Two types of surgical interventions are typically used to treat upper GI diseases: subtotal gastrectomy (partial removal of the stomach) and total gastrectomy (total removal of the stomach). There are two types of subtotal gastrectomy. It is used to treat cancer or, rarely, PUD that does not respond to

Table 33.6
Gastric Cancer Summary

Signs and Symptoms	Rarely detected during early stages Symptoms often mistaken for peptic ulcer disease (e.g., indigestion, anorexia, pain, weight loss, nausea, vomiting, anemia) Late symptoms include involvement of other organs such as the liver
Diagnostic Tests	X-ray studies Gastroscopy Gastric fluid analysis Serum gastrin levels
Therapeutic Measures	Medical treatment not very effective Surgical treatment: subtotal or total gastrectomy
Complications	Related to disease and surgery (e.g., hemorrhage, acute gastric distention, nutritional problems)
Priority Nursing Diagnoses	*Acute Pain* *Fear*

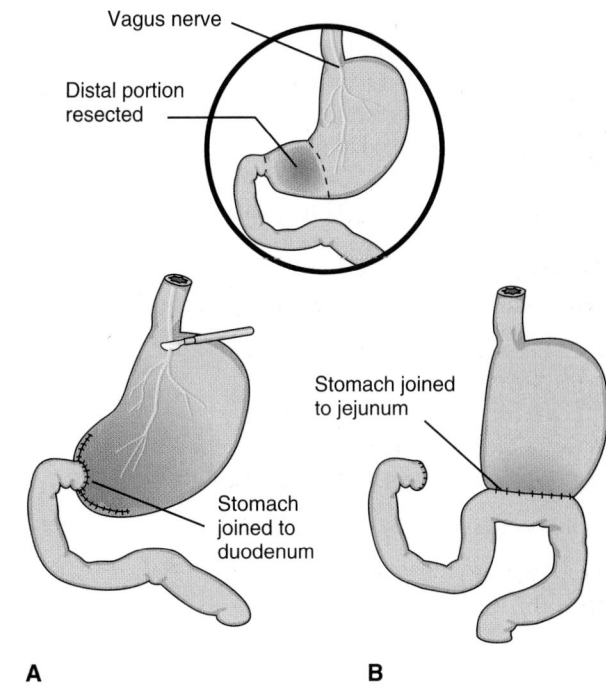

FIGURE 33.6 Subtotal gastrectomy involves removing the distal portion of the stomach. The remaining portion of the stomach is then sutured (A) to the duodenum (Billroth I procedure) or (B) to the proximal jejunum (Billroth II procedure).

therapy. For a **gastroduodenostomy** (Billroth I), the distal portion of the stomach is removed, and the remainder of the stomach is anastomosed (surgically attached) to the duodenum (Fig. 33.6). A **gastrojejunostomy** (Billroth II) involves removal of a larger amount of the distal stomach and reanastomosis of the proximal remnant of the stomach to the proximal jejunum (see Fig. 33.6). Because it results in bypassing of the duodenum, the Billroth II procedure is used to treat duodenal ulcers. Pancreatic secretions and bile are necessary for digestion and continue to be secreted from the common bile duct even after partial gastrectomy. Total gastrectomy is the treatment for extensive gastric cancer. This surgery involves total removal of the stomach, with anastomosis of the esophagus to the jejunum (Fig. 33.7). Rarely, a vagotomy may also be performed.

Nursing Process for the Patient Having Gastric Surgery
Data Collection
Preoperatively, identify the patient's fears or concerns to allow the provision of information on postoperative care and discharge instructions. Postoperatively, the patient's vital signs are monitored as ordered. Respiratory status is carefully observed because the high location of the surgical incision may cause pain, which interferes with deep breathing and coughing. Atelectasis or pneumonia can develop as a result of guarding and shallow breathing. The patient's pain is

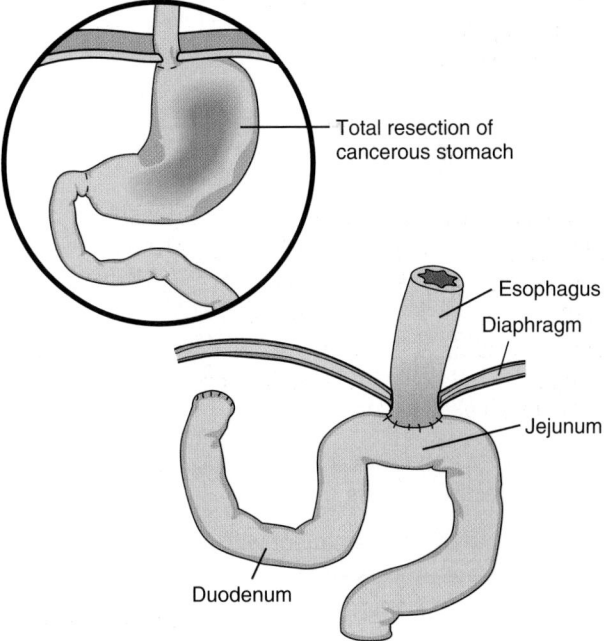

FIGURE 33.7 Total gastrectomy.

• WORD • BUILDING •

gastroduodenostomy: gastro—stomach + duoden—duodenum + ostomy—mouth or opening

gastrojejunostomy: gastro—stomach + jejeun—jejunum + ostomy—mouth or opening

identified and relieved, which also helps the patient's ability to deep breathe or cough. The patient's IV site and infusion are monitored, and I&O are recorded. The incisional site and dressings are observed for drainage and bleeding. Early ambulation is encouraged to promote a quicker recovery by improving respiratory and GI function.

Patients may have an NG tube inserted during surgery. The drainage from the NG tube is monitored for color and amount. If bleeding or excessive amounts of drainage or abdominal distention are noted, they are reported to the HCP.

BE SAFE!
After gastric surgery, do not irrigate or reposition a nasogastric tube to prevent damaging the suture line.

Nursing Diagnoses, Planning, and Implementation

Acute Pain related to postoperative status

EXPECTED OUTCOME: The patient will report pain is relieved or tolerable within 30 minutes of report of pain.

- Evaluate pain regularly, noting characteristics, location, and intensity on a pain rating scale *to provide information regarding patient's pain level and effectiveness of interventions.*
- Provide comfort measures such as positioning every 2 hours and back rub *to improve circulation and reduce tension associated with pain.*
- Use relaxation techniques with the patient such as deep breathing, guided imagery, music, and distraction therapy *to enhance relaxation and improve pain relief.*
- Administer medications as ordered on a routine schedule for 24 to 48 hours *to control postoperative pain and prevent pain from becoming unbearable for patient.*
- Ensure functioning of NG tube (usually low intermittent suction) *to prevent distention and increased pain.*
- Notify HCP if pain control measures are unsuccessful *to allow revision of treatment plan.*

Fear related to body image changes, treatment, and life-threatening illness

EXPECTED OUTCOME: The patient will understand and discuss disease process and treatment options and possible outcomes of treatment before surgical procedure.

- Use open communication and convey acceptance of the patient's fears *to help patient cope with fears.*
- Explain disease process and treatment options, and reinforce as needed *to decrease the patient's fear of the unknown.*
- Explain all postoperative procedures and interventions (such as medications, NG tube, drains) *to help decrease the patient's fear.*

Evaluation

If interventions have been effective, the patient will report relief or reduction of pain to a tolerable level and report that fear is reduced because of an understanding of the disease process, treatment options, and possible outcomes of treatment.

Complications of Gastric Surgery
Hemorrhage

The incidence of hemorrhage after gastric surgery is very low and most often caused by a dislodged clot at the surgical site or slippage of a suture. The patient experiencing hemorrhage exhibits restlessness, cold skin, increased pulse and respirations, and decreased temperature and blood pressure. The patient may have a change in level of consciousness and become confused. In addition, the patient may vomit bright red blood.

The abdominal dressing is monitored for drainage or bleeding. Following gastric surgery, patients usually have an NG tube that has been inserted in the operating room. The drainage from the tube should be monitored for color and amount. A small amount of pink or light red drainage may be expected for the first 12 hours, but moderate or excessive bleeding should be immediately reported to the HCP.

Gastric Distention

Symptoms of gastric distention include an enlarged abdomen, epigastric pain, tachycardia, and hypotension. The patient may report feeling full and hiccup or gag repeatedly. These symptoms must be reported to the HCP.

The HCP usually inserts the NG tube during surgery so that the suture line is not damaged. If suction is desired, an order is required. Irrigating or repositioning the NG tube is not performed by the nurse to prevent harm to the suture line. Any problems with distention or an improperly functioning NG tube are reported to the surgeon who may need to reposition the NG tube to correct the problem. The patient's vital signs should be monitored until the patient's distention is relieved and the patient is stable.

CRITICAL THINKING

Mr. Wong had gastric surgery today. He has an intravenous (IV) infusion of 1,000 mL dextrose 5% in 0.45 normal saline over 8 hours and a nasogastric tube set to low intermittent suction. Mr. Wong is restless and reporting pain. His abdomen is distended. The suction canister contains no gastric output.

1. What nursing interventions, in order of priority, are needed to help Mr. Wong?
2. What equipment do you need to provide patient-centered care for Mr. Wong?
3. As you monitor the IV, it is set for how many drops per minute with a 10-drop factor IV set?

Suggested answers are at the end of the chapter.

Dumping Syndrome

Dumping syndrome is one of the most common complications of gastric surgery. It occurs with the rapid entry of food into the jejunum without proper mixing of the food with digestive juices. On entering the jejunum, the hyperosmolar food draws extracellular fluid into the bowel from the circulating blood volume to dilute the high concentration of electrolytes and sugars. This rapid shift of fluids decreases the circulating blood volume and produces symptoms. The symptoms occur 5 to 30 minutes after eating. They include dizziness, tachycardia, fainting, sweating, nausea, diarrhea, a feeling of fullness, and abdominal cramping. Additionally, the blood sugar rises, and excessive insulin is excreted in response. This release of insulin causes the patient to have symptoms of hypoglycemia about 2 hours later. Symptoms include weakness, sweating, anxiety, shakiness, confusion, and tachycardia. The patient should immediately eat some candy or drink juice containing sugar to relieve the symptoms. See "Nutrition Notes" for ways to reduce dumping syndrome. Inform the patient that these symptoms may last for up to 6 months after gastric surgery but usually slowly subside over time.

Nutritional Problems

Nutritional problems that commonly occur after removal of part or all of the stomach include vitamin B_{12} and folic acid deficiency as well as reduced absorption of calcium and vitamin D. Also, rapid entry of food into the bowel often results in inadequate absorption of food.

Following gastric surgery, patients may be NPO. IV fluid provides hydration. If patients are to be NPO for any length of time, they will need an alternate form of nutrition to meet their caloric and nutritional needs. After removal of the NG tube, clear fluids may be ordered with progression to full liquids, and then soft foods as the patient tolerates them. Foods and fluids should be introduced into the diet gradually following gastric surgery. If the patient eats too much or too fast, regurgitation may result.

PERNICIOUS ANEMIA. Vitamin B_{12} deficiency may occur after some or all of the stomach is removed because intrinsic factor secretion is reduced or absent. Normally, vitamin B_{12} combines with intrinsic factor to prevent its digestion in the stomach and promote its absorption in the intestines. Lifelong replacement of vitamin B_{12} is required to prevent the development of pernicious anemia. Patients must be taught the importance of complying with this treatment. Traditionally after gastric surgery, it is given by the parenteral route. However, other routes such as oral tablets or nasal gel might be effectively used. Vitamin B_{12} injections are given daily initially, then weekly, and then monthly for life. Symptoms of pernicious anemia include anemia, weakness, sore tongue, numbness and tingling, and GI upset.

Steatorrhea

Steatorrhea is the presence of excessive fat in the stools. It is the result of rapid gastric emptying, which prevents adequate mixing of fat with pancreatic and biliary secretions. In most cases, steatorrhea can be controlled by reducing the intake of fat in the diet.

Pyloric Obstruction

Pyloric obstruction can occur after gastric surgery as a result of scarring, edema, inflammation, or a combination of these. The signs and symptoms are vomiting, a feeling of fullness, gastric distention, nausea after eating, loss of appetite, and weight loss. As the obstruction increases, it gradually becomes more difficult for the stomach to empty, and symptoms worsen. Conservative methods are used first, such as replacing fluids and electrolytes through IV fluids and decompressing the distended stomach using an NG tube. Surgery may be necessary if conservative measures do not relieve the signs and symptoms. Pyloroplasty widens the exit of the pylorus to improve emptying of the stomach.

SUGGESTED ANSWERS TO CRITICAL THINKING

Mr. Smith

1. Data include vital signs (looking for signs of shock); checking Mr. Smith's abdomen (looking for location of pain, tenderness, rigidity); noting vomiting and characteristics of emesis, including blood; and verifying patency of intravenous (IV) site access.
2. Assist Mr. Smith to a comfortable position and stay with him. Call for help. Inform the registered nurse (RN) so the health care provider (HCP) can be notified immediately and provide data regarding Mr. Smith's change in condition. Administer oxygen, monitor IV fluids, and continue to monitor vital signs. Medicate for pain as ordered.
3. Explain that you will stay with Mr. Smith as you gather data and take vital signs. Explain that you have informed the RN, who will assess Mr. Smith and report findings to the HCP. Explain that treatments ordered by the HCP will be started, including oxygen, IV fluids, and pain medication. Inform Mrs. Smith you will explain Mr. Smith's care. Invite questions and have a nursing assistant provide Mrs. Smith with comfort needs, such as a beverage, tissues, and a chair.
4. You suspect a perforated duodenal ulcer, which is a medical-surgical emergency.
5. RN, HCP.

Continued

SUGGESTED ANSWERS TO CRITICAL THINKING—cont'd

6. Prepare Mr. Smith for surgery by maintaining NPO (nothing by mouth) status, ensure IV access is present, verify consent is signed, obtain labs (may include complete blood count, chemistry panel, type, and cross-match for blood), and administer antibiotics as ordered.

Mr. Wong

1. Prioritize the nursing interventions:
   a. Take Mr. Wong's vital signs to determine whether he is stable. Gastric distention can cause pain, and once the distention is relieved, the pain caused by distention subsides.
   b. Check placement of Mr. Wong's nasogastric (NG) tube by comparing the insertion length with the current length and, if ordered by the HCP, by aspirating gastric contents and verifying the pH of the contents. It is important to check for abdominal placement of Mr. Wong's NG tube to make sure it is not misplaced in the lungs. After abdominal placement is determined, if ordered, the NG tube can be connected to suction equipment. Do not reposition an NG tube in a patient who has had gastric surgery, as it could damage the surgical suture line.
   c. Next, check the suction equipment for ordered settings and to ensure that it is turned on. The suction

setting normally is ordered to be on low. A whistling sound is heard when the tube is disconnected from the suction setup. The seals should be tight on the suction canister. When the tubing is hooked to suction, gastric contents should start flowing into the suction canister.
   d. Check the NG tube for clogging only if the physician orders aspiration or irrigation to be done. If ordered, the tube is gently aspirated with a 60-mL catheter-tipped syringe. If the tube remains clogged, it is gently flushed as ordered with 10 to 20 mL of sterile normal saline.
   e. After the gastric distention has been relieved, Mr. Wong's pain level is reevaluated to determine whether he needs pain medication. Considering that he is less than 1 day postoperative, he probably does.

2. Necessary equipment includes stethoscope, 60-mL catheter-tipped syringe, gloves, goggles, and normal saline for irrigation.

3.
$$\frac{1{,}000 \text{ mL}}{480 \text{ min}} \times \frac{10 \text{ gtt}}{\text{mL}} = \frac{10{,}000 \text{ drops}}{480 \text{ min}} = 21 \text{ drops/min}$$

Review Questions

1. To deliver 1,000 mL of 5% dextrose in 0.45 normal saline at 150 mL per hour using 10 drop tubing, the nurse would monitor the intravenous infusion at how many drops per minute? Fill in the blank.
   Answer: _____ drops per minute

2. The nurse is planning care for a team of patients. To provide patient-centered care safely, for which patients should the nurse use specialized mobility equipment designed for the patient who is obese? **Select all that apply.**
   1. A woman with body weight 22% above ideal body weight
   2. A man with body weight 30% above ideal body weight
   3. A man with body mass index of 31
   4. A woman with a body mass index of 24
   5. A woman with waist measurement of 36 inches
   6. A man with waist measurement of 44 inches

3. The nurse is caring for a patient with gastritis. Which intervention should the nurse implement for a patient with acute gastritis?
   1. Monitor patient for bloody diarrhea.
   2. Explain that aspirin rarely causes gastritis.
   3. Administer phenothiazine to control vomiting.
   4. Encourage a regular diet during the acute phase of gastritis.

4. The nurse is planning a teaching session for a patient with a peptic ulcer. Which of these would the nurse include in the teaching plan as the primary cause of peptic ulcers?
   1. Eating spicy foods
   2. A stressful life
   3. A bacterial infection
   4. Excessive caffeine intake

5. The nurse provides teaching for a patient with a peptic ulcer. Which patient statement would the nurse evaluate as indicating understanding of the purpose of histamine 2 (H2)-receptor antagonists?
   1. "H2-receptor antagonists neutralize gastric acid."
   2. "H2-receptor antagonists form a protective paste."
   3. "H2-receptor antagonists determine gastric pH levels."
   4. "H2-receptor antagonists inhibit secretion of gastric acid."

6. A patient who has just returned from surgery after a total gastrectomy begins to vomit bright red blood. What is the priority action for the nurse to take?
   1. Increase the intravenous rate.
   2. Take blood pressure.
   3. Place patient onto side.
   4. Administer oxygen.

7. The nurse is teaching a patient with dumping syndrome about food choices. Which of these foods would the nurse instruct the patient to avoid?
   1. Spinach and avocado salad
   2. Coffee and glazed doughnut
   3. Sausage and liver
   4. Creamed chipped beef

Answer rationales available in your online resources.

ANSWERS 1. 25; 2. 2, 3, 5, 6; 3. 1; 4. 3; 5. 4; 6. 3; 7. 2

Key Points

Find the chapter key points in your online resources available through Davis Edge.

Additional Resources

DAVIS
edge.

Use the scratch off code on the inside front cover of your book to access online quizzes that will help you to improve your scores on course exams and prepare for the NCLEX-PN®.

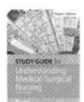 Study Guide

CHAPTER 34

Nursing Care of Patients With Lower Gastrointestinal Disorders

Linda S. Williams

KEY TERMS

appendicitis (uh-PEN-dih-SY-tis)
colectomy (koh-LEK-tuh-me)
colitis (koh-LY-tis)
colostomy (kuh-LAW-stuh-mee)
constipation (KON-stih-PAY-shun)
diarrhea (DY-uh-REE-ah)
diverticulitis (DY-ver-tik-yoo-LY-tis)
diverticulosis (DY-ver-tik-yoo-LOH-sis)
enteritis (en-tur-EYE-tis)
fissures (FISH-ers)
fistulas (FIST-yoo-lahs)
hematochezia (HEM-uh-toh-KEE-zee-uh)
hemorrhoids (HEM-uh-royds)
hernia (HER-nee-uh)
ileostomy (IL-ee-AW-stuh-mee)
impaction (im-PAK-shun)
intussusception (IN-tuh-suh-SEP-shun)
megacolon (MEG-ah-KOH-lun)
melena (muh-LEE-nah)
obstipation (OB-stih-PAY-shun)
peristomal (PEAR-ih-STOH-muhl)
peritonitis (pear-ih-toh-NY-tis)
stoma (STOH-mah)
volvulus (VOL-view-lus)

CHAPTER CONCEPT

Elimination

LEARNING OUTCOMES

1. List data to collect when caring for patients with lower gastrointestinal disorders.
2. Identify the causes, signs and symptoms, and therapeutic measures of constipation and diarrhea.
3. Plan nursing care and teaching for patients with constipation or diarrhea.
4. Describe pathophysiology, therapeutic measures, nursing care, and teaching for patients with inflammatory and infectious disorders of the lower gastrointestinal tract.
5. Describe pathophysiology, therapeutic measures, nursing care, and teaching for inflammatory bowel disease.
6. Plan nursing care for an abdominal hernia.
7. Plan nursing care and teaching for patients with absorption disorders.
8. Describe causes, signs and symptoms, therapeutic measures, and nursing care for intestinal obstruction.
9. Plan nursing care for anorectal problems.
10. Describe causes, signs and symptoms, therapeutic measures, and nursing care for lower gastrointestinal bleeding.
11. Describe the causes, signs and symptoms, therapeutic measures, and nursing care for colon cancer.
12. Plan nursing care and teaching for a patient with an ostomy.
13. Discuss evaluation of nursing care for various lower gastrointestinal disorders.

The lower gastrointestinal (GI) system includes the small and large intestines, rectum, and anus.

 ## PROBLEMS OF ELIMINATION

Constipation
Pathophysiology
Constipation occurs when the fecal mass is held in the rectal cavity for a period of time that is unusual for the patient or less than three times per week. When the feces are held for a prolonged time in the rectum, more water is absorbed. This makes the feces smaller, drier, harder, and more difficult and, sometimes, painful to pass.

If a patient repeatedly ignores the urge to have a bowel movement (laxation), the musculature and rectal mucous membrane become insensitive to the presence of feces. Eventually, a stronger stimulus is needed to produce the peristaltic rush required for defecation. Prolonged constipation is called **obstipation.**

Etiology

There are many causes of constipation. Medications such as narcotics, tranquilizers, and antacids with aluminum decrease motility of the large intestine and may contribute to constipation. Rectal or anal conditions such as hemorrhoids or fissures may lead to a delay in defecation because of the associated pain. Metabolic or neurologic conditions such as diabetes mellitus, multiple sclerosis, systemic lupus erythematosus, or scleroderma may interfere with normal bowel innervation and function. Colon cancer may cause an obstruction that prevents normal bowel function and leads to constipation. Low intake of dietary fiber and fluids decreases the bulk of the feces and causes constipation. Decreased mobility, weakness, and fatigue, especially in the older adult, reduce the strength of the muscles used for defecation, increasing the likelihood of constipation.

Signs and Symptoms

Abdominal pain and distention, indigestion, rectal pressure, a sensation of incomplete emptying, and intestinal rumbling are indications of constipation (Table 34.1). The patient may also report headache, fatigue, decreased appetite, straining at stool, and elimination of hard, dry stool.

Table 34.1
Constipation Summary

Signs and Symptoms	Abdominal pain and distention Indigestion Intestinal rumbling Rectal pressure Sensation of incomplete emptying Straining at stool Hard, dry stool
Diagnostic Tests	History Physical with rectal examination
Therapeutic Measures	High-fiber diet 2–3 L fluid daily Strengthening of abdominal muscles Exercise Bulk-forming agents Stool softeners Laxatives
Priority Nursing Diagnoses	*Constipation* *Deficient Knowledge*

Complications

A variety of problems can result from constipation. Fecal **impaction** may result when the fecal mass is so dry it cannot be passed. Pressure on the colon mucosa from a mass of stool may cause ulcers to develop. Often, small amounts of liquid stool ooze around the fecal mass and cause incontinence of liquid stools. The incontinence may be treated with an antidiarrheal medication. This will worsen the constipation if a thorough assessment is not performed to rule out impaction. Straining to have a bowel movement (Valsalva maneuver) can result in cardiac, neurologic, and respiratory complications. If the patient has a history of heart failure, hypertension, or recent myocardial infarction, straining can lead to cardiac rupture and death. Grossly dilated loops of the colon, known as **megacolon,** can occur proximal to the dry fecal mass and obstruct the colon. Abdominal distention occurs. In severe cases, loops of bowel can be palpated through the abdominal wall.

Diagnostic Tests

Constipation is usually self-diagnosed or diagnosed by history and physical with rectal examination. If complications are suspected, a radiographic examination, sigmoidoscopy, or colonoscopy may be needed.

Therapeutic Measures

Treatment of constipation depends on the cause. Fiber intake and physical activity should be increased, and exercises to strengthen abdominal muscles performed. Behavior changes, such as appropriately responding to the urge to defecate and drinking 8 oz of warm water or a caffeine beverage in the morning and 2 to 3 L of water every day, if not contraindicated for other reasons, can help establish a more normal bowel pattern. Bulk-forming agents such as psyllium (Metamucil) or stool softeners such as docusate sodium (Colace) can be tried instead of other laxatives. Laxatives for severe constipation include lubiprostone (Amitiza) and linaclotide (Linzess). Enemas and rectal suppositories are used only for severe cases and are discontinued when an acute episode is resolved. Medications such as methylnaltrexone (Relistor) or naloxegol (Movantik) are available for opioid-induced constipation, which usually requires intervention.

Nursing Process for the Patient With Constipation

DATA COLLECTION. The patient may feel self-conscious or embarrassed when interviewed about bowel habits and history. Consideration should be given to the patient's feelings by establishing rapport first. Provide privacy to gather data. Include the onset and duration of constipation, past elimination pattern, current elimination pattern, occupation, lifestyle (stress, exercise, nutrition), history of laxative or enema use, medical-surgical history, and current medications being taken. Color, consistency, and any odor of the stool as well as any intestinal symptoms are noted.

• WORD • BUILDING •
megacolon: mega—large + colon—colon

Evidence-Based Practice

Clinical Question
What is the most effective way to treat functional constipation?

Evidence
A systematic review of 58 studies (41 clinical trials, 8 observational studies, and 9 systematic reviews or meta-analysis) examined the use of polyethylene glycol (PEG), with or without electrolytes, compared with other treatments such as milk of magnesia, paraffin oil or sodium phosphate, lactulose, and psyllium in the management of functional constipation and the treatment of fecal impaction. Results showed that PEGs are the most efficacious and safest osmotic laxatives (more than lactulose), and they have a low incidence of side effects.

Implications for Nursing Practice
Negative health effects are associated with constipation, including discomfort and intestinal obstruction that can lead to increased morbidity–mortality. Using PEG has been shown to be the most effective, safe, and well-tolerated method for treating functional constipation.

Reference
Minguez, M., Higueras, A., & Judez, J. (2016). Use of polyethylene glycol in functional constipation and fecal impaction. *Revista Española de Enfermedades Digestivas, 108*(12), 790–806.

After the interview, the patient's abdomen is inspected and palpated for distention and symmetry. Inspection of the perianal area may reveal fissures, external hemorrhoids, or irritation.

NURSING DIAGNOSES, PLANNING, AND IMPLEMENTATION.

Constipation related to irregular defecation habits

EXPECTED OUTCOME: The patient will maintain passage of soft, formed stool every 1 to 3 days without straining.

- Identify normal pattern of defecation, diet and fluid intake, medications, surgeries, and use of laxatives *to help identify factors contributing to constipation.*
- Explain the physiology of defecation and the importance of responding to the urge to defecate when it occurs *to help prevent constipation.*
- Determine the patient's access to the bathroom and ability to use the toilet *to ensure barriers to safe toileting, such as unsafe obstructing furniture arrangements or clutter, are removed.*
- Set a specific time for defecation, such as after a meal when bowels are most active, *to facilitate the urge reflex.*
- Use a footstool *to promote flexion of the hips, which promotes defecation.*
- Encourage a high-fiber, high-residue diet *to decrease constipation* ("Nutrition Notes: Treating Constipation With Food Choices").

- Teach to increase fluid, if not contraindicated, to 2 to 3 L per day *to soften feces.*
- Teach to increase activity through a daily walking program and abdominal exercises designed to improve the muscle tone *to improve peristalsis and promote more spontaneous defecation.*

EVALUATION. The plan has been effective if the patient has established a regular bowel function pattern (Box 34.1) and expresses satisfaction with the outcomes.

Nutrition Notes

Treating Constipation With Food Choices. Achieving the recommended fiber intake of 19 to 38 grams per day (depending on gender and age) is a matter of prudent choices at every meal. Listed here are examples of higher fiber foods in the column on the left and examples of foods in the same category but with less fiber in the column on the right.

Higher Fiber Foods	Grams of Fiber	Lower Fiber Foods	Grams of Fiber
Breakfast			
All-bran buds, 1/3 cup	13	Corn flakes, 1 cup	1
Orange sections, 1 cup	4	Orange juice reconstituted from frozen concentrate, 1 cup	0
Lunch			
Chili, 1 cup	5	Chicken noodle soup, 1 cup	2
Raw apple with skin, 2¾" diameter	4	Raw apple peeled, 2¾" diameter	2
Dinner			
Whole wheat spaghetti, 1 cup cooked	6	Spaghetti, 1 cup cooked	3
Banana, 1 cup sliced	4	Watermelon, 1 cup diced	1
Totals	**36**		**9**

Other foods contribute to fiber intake. They can be evaluated via nutrition labels or at https://ndb.nal.usda.gov/ndb or http://nutritiondata.self.com. Individuals who wish to correct constipation without medications should determine their present fiber intake and increase it gradually to the U.S. Department of Agriculture recommended dietary allowance while also drinking sufficient water.

Criteria for Regular Bowel Function

- A regular time for defecation is planned.
- Fluid intake is 2 to 3 L per day.
- High-fiber and high-residue foods are added to the diet.
- A regular exercise program is followed.
- Laxative use is limited or avoided.
- Outcome is frequency of stools every 1 to 3 days and consistency of stools reported is soft and formed.

CRITICAL THINKING

Mrs. Burns is a 93-year-old resident in an assisted living facility. The nurse notes that she has not had a bowel movement in 5 days. What action should the nurse take to provide patient-centered care?

Suggested answers are at the end of the chapter.

Diarrhea

Diarrhea occurs when fecal matter passes through the intestine rapidly, resulting in decreased absorption of water, electrolytes, and nutrients and causing frequent, watery stools. It is more than three loose or watery stools in 24 hours. Severe diarrhea can result in over 20 bowel movements per day. Acute diarrhea usually resolves in several days. Chronic diarrhea lasts more than 14 days.

Pathophysiology and Etiology

The most common cause of acute diarrhea is infection from contaminated food or water. The infection can be viral or bacterial. Food intolerance or allergies can also cause diarrhea. Foods that most commonly cause diarrhea are milk products, if lactose intolerant; wheat, if gluten intolerant; sugar substitutes, due to sugar alcohols; excessive caffeine; excessive fat substitute Olestra; or high-fat and fried foods. Antibiotics have diarrhea as a side effect. Inflammatory diseases such as Crohn disease or ulcerative colitis (discussed later) may impair absorption, resulting in frequent, watery stools. An irritable bowel or a neurologic disorder may cause increased motility problems. Radiation therapy for cancer also may induce a malabsorption syndrome. Enteral feedings can result in diarrhea, especially when malnutrition has caused edema in the gut wall, which decreases absorption.

Prevention

To prevent diarrhea, proper handling, storage, and refrigeration of all fresh foods helps to minimize contact with infectious agents. Milk and milk products must be kept refrigerated and protected. Hand hygiene and cleaning of the kitchen as well as food preparation and serving items are extremely important. Also, enteral feedings should be given using full-strength formula rather than diluting the formula. This reduces the risk of contaminating the formula.

Signs and Symptoms

Initial diarrhea stools may be foul smelling and have undigested food particles and mucus (Table 34.2). The stools could contain blood or pus. Diarrhea resulting from food poisoning usually has an explosive onset and may be accompanied by nausea and vomiting. Abdominal cramping, intestinal rumbling, and thirst are common. Fever indicates an infection. Weakness and dehydration from fluid loss may occur ("Gerontological Issues: Dehydration and Hypokalemia").

Gerontological Issues

Dehydration and Hypokalemia. Diarrhea can cause older people to quickly become dehydrated and hypokalemic because both fluid and potassium are lost in stools. The signs and symptoms of hypokalemia include muscle weakness, hypotension, anorexia, paresthesia, and drowsiness. It can also cause cardiac arrhythmias, such as atrial and ventricular tachycardia, premature ventricular contraction, and ventricular fibrillation, which can be fatal.

If the older person has decreased mobility, quick access to the bathroom is important. Because of poor muscle control, older patients may be incontinent. This might embarrass patients or cause them to hurry, which increases chances of patients falling and causing other problems such as fracture, dislocation, or hematoma. Also, because older patients' skin is more sensitive as a result of poor turgor and a reduction in subcutaneous fat layers, perirectal skin excoriation can occur secondary to the acidity and digestive enzyme content of diarrheal stools.

Diagnostic Tests

The diagnosis of diarrhea is determined by the onset and progression of the condition, presence of fever, laboratory examinations, and visual inspection of the stool for bacteria, pus, or blood. Stool mixed with red blood cells (RBCs) and mucus is associated with cholera, typhoid, typhus, large-bowel cancer, or amebiasis. Stool mixed with white blood cells (WBCs) and mucus is associated with shigellosis, intestinal tuberculosis, salmonellosis, regional **enteritis,** or ulcerative colitis. Bulky, frothy stool is seen in celiac disease. Pasty stools usually have a high fat content and may be associated with common bile duct obstruction and celiac disease.

Therapeutic Measures

Most people with diarrhea do not require treatment ("Nutrition Notes: Deciding When an Adult With Diarrhea Should Seek Medical Care"). Replacing fluids and electrolytes is important. Intravenous (IV) fluid replacement may be necessary for dehydration, especially in the very young or very old. For three or more watery stools per day, motility of the intestines can

• WORD • BUILDING •

diarrhea: dia—through + rhea—to flow
enteritis: entero—intestine + itis—inflammation

Table 34.2
Diarrhea Summary

Signs and Symptoms	Frequent, watery stools Abdominal cramping Distention Anorexia Intestinal rumbling
Causes	Inflammatory diseases, such as Crohn disease and ulcerative colitis Infectious organisms Recent antibiotic use Surgical procedures such as bowel resection Laxatives Enteral feedings Radiation therapy
Diagnostic Tests	History Laboratory examinations of stool
Therapeutic Measures	Replacement of fluids and electrolytes Antidiarrheal medications Antimicrobials Probiotic (Lactinex) Fecal transplant
Priority Nursing Diagnoses	*Diarrhea* *Risk for Deficient Fluid Volume* *Deficient Knowledge*

Nutrition Notes

Deciding When an Adult With Diarrhea Should Seek Medical Care. Most instances of diarrhea in healthy adults are self-limiting and resolve without treatment. Indications for medical care include the following:

- Lasts for more than 3 days
- Causes severe pain in the abdomen or rectum
- Fever of 102°F or higher
- Produces blood in the stool or black, tarry stools
- Is accompanied by signs of dehydration
- Occurs in a person with medical conditions for which fasting, dehydration, or infectious disease is a hazard

Maintaining adequate hydration is important and individuals should be encouraged to drink water and electrolyte-replacing beverages. Educate the person to progress to clear liquids, then to full liquids, progressing to a low-residue diet (one limited in high-fiber foods), and, finally, to a regular diet as tolerated.

be decreased with the use of medications, such as diphenoxylate (Lomotil), difenoxin hydrochloride (Motofen), and loperamide (Imodium). Antimicrobial agents are prescribed for some infections. If diarrhea is thought to be caused by antibiotics that change the normal flora of the bowel, a *Lactobacillus* granule probiotic supplement (Lactinex) may be used to help restore the normal flora. Fecal transplant can restore the normal intestinal flora in those who are ill (see Chapter 32).

Nursing Process for the Patient With Diarrhea

DATA COLLECTION. Ask the patient whether there is a known cause for the diarrhea, what the signs and symptoms are, and when they began. The patient's usual dietary habits and any changes or recent exposure to contaminated food or water are noted. Identify whether medications, such as antibiotics or laxatives, may be contributing to the diarrhea. If the patient has traveled recently, determine the geographic location and whether exposure to an infected person or someone with similar symptoms occurred. Document stool consistency, color, odor, and frequency.

Observe for symptoms of dehydration, such as tachycardia, hypotension, decreased skin turgor, weakness, thready pulse, dry mucous membranes, and oliguria. Obtain the patient's height and weight to establish a baseline. Abnormal laboratory studies that may indicate dehydration include increased serum osmolality, increased specific gravity of urine, and increased hematocrit. Decreased serum potassium may result from intestinal loss of potassium.

NURSING DIAGNOSES, PLANNING, AND IMPLEMENTATION.

Diarrhea related to infection or possible ingestion of irritating foods

EXPECTED OUTCOME: The patient will maintain formed, soft stool every 1 to 3 days.

- Obtain patient history, including medications, about diarrhea *to help identify cause.*
- Monitor and record stool characteristics, amount, and frequency *to plan care.*
- Promote hand hygiene by patient, family, and health care staff *to prevent the spread of infection.*
- Identify potentially infected persons or contaminated foods *to prevent the spread of infection.*
- Utilize transmission precautions and consider a private patient room *to prevent infection transmission.*
- Give antidiarrheal medications as ordered *to control diarrhea.*
- Keep skin clean, dry, and protected with a moisture barrier, such as petrolatum or medicated ointment, after each bowel movement or use a fecal incontinence appliance *to protect perianal skin from contact with liquid stools and their enzymes.*
- Limit caffeine intake *because it stimulates intestinal motility.*
- Teach the patient hand hygiene *to prevent spread of infection.*

Risk for Deficient Fluid Volume related to frequent passage of stools and insufficient fluid intake

EXPECTED OUTCOME: The patient will maintain a stable weight and vital signs, and urine output will remain within normal limits at all times.

• Weigh the patient daily and record intake and output (I&O; including diarrheal stools) *to determine fluid balance.*
• Maintain IV fluid replacement as ordered *to maintain fluid balance if output is greater than intake.*
• Encourage oral intake *to prevent dehydration from diarrhea.*
• Teach the patient signs and symptoms of dehydration to report *to allow prompt treatment.*

EVALUATION. Goals have been met if frequency of diarrheal stools is decreased and balance of fluids is achieved.

 ## INFLAMMATORY AND INFECTIOUS DISORDERS

Many diseases of the lower GI tract are a result of inflammation in the bowel. Sometimes the inflamed areas become infected, resulting in a worsening of symptoms.

Appendicitis
Pathophysiology
Appendicitis is the inflammation of the appendix, the small, finger-like appendage attached to the cecum of the large intestine (see Fig. 32.1). Because of the small size of the appendix, obstruction may occur, causing inflammation and making it susceptible to infection.

Signs and Symptoms
Signs and symptoms of appendicitis include fever, increased WBCs, and generalized pain in the upper abdomen. Within hours of onset, the pain usually becomes localized to the right lower quadrant at the McBurney's point, midway between the umbilicus and the right iliac crest (Fig. 34.1). This is one of the classic symptoms of appendicitis. Nausea, vomiting, and anorexia are also usually present.

Physical examination reveals slight abdominal muscular rigidity (guarding), normal bowel sounds, and local rebound tenderness (intensification of pain when pressure is released after palpation) in the right lower quadrant of the abdomen. Sometimes there is pain in the right lower quadrant when the left lower quadrant is palpated (Rovsing's sign). The patient might keep the right leg flexed for comfort and experience increased pain if the leg is straightened.

Diagnostic Tests
A complete blood count (CBC) reveals elevated leukocyte (WBC) and neutrophil counts. An ultrasound, computed tomography (CT) scan, or magnetic resonance imaging (MRI) reveals an enlargement in the area of the cecum.

Therapeutic Measures
The patient is NPO (nothing by mouth), and, after diagnosis, surgery is performed immediately unless there is evidence of perforation or peritonitis. Applying ice to the site of pain and placing the patient in a semi-Fowler position may help reduce pain while the diagnosis is being made. The use of a heating pad on the abdomen is avoided because the warmth may increase inflammation and risk of rupture. Laxatives and enemas are avoided because they may cause or complicate a rupture. After surgery, the diet is advanced as ordered and tolerated.

If the appendix has ruptured, IV fluids and antibiotic therapy are started to treat infection and peritonitis. Surgery may or may not be done right away. The patient may have an orogastric or nasogastric (NG) tube to decompress the stomach. If infection is present, a drain may be inserted into the abdomen by a radiologist. Surgery may then be delayed for up to several weeks while the infection is resolved.

Complications
In addition to peritonitis, an abscess of the appendix can occur. An abscess is a localized collection of pus separated from the peritoneal cavity by the omentum or small bowel. This is usually treated with IV antibiotics and surgical drainage. An appendectomy is done about 6 weeks later.

Peritonitis
Peritonitis is inflammation of the peritoneum that occurs from a variety of causes. It is a serious condition that can be life threatening.

Pathophysiology and Etiology
Trauma, ischemia, or perforation in an abdominal organ causes leakage of the organ's contents into the peritoneal cavity, causing inflammation and infection. The tissues become edematous and begin leaking fluid containing increasing

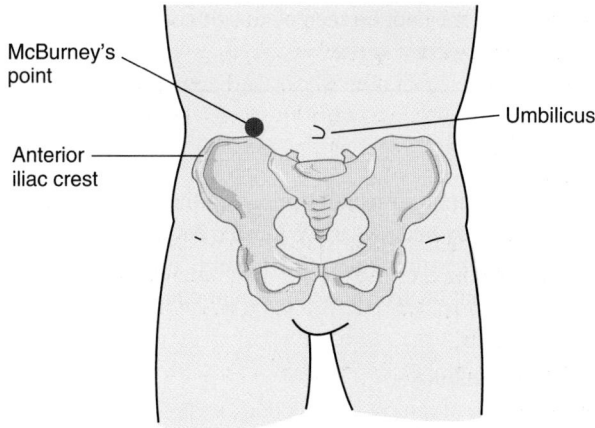

FIGURE 34.1 Pain at McBurney's point is a symptom of appendicitis.

• WORD • BUILDING •

peritonitis: periton—pertaining to peritoneum + itis—inflammation

amounts of blood, protein, cellular debris, and WBCs. Initially, the intestinal tract responds with hypermotility, but this is soon followed by paralysis (paralytic ileus).

Common causes of peritonitis that permit GI bacteria to enter the peritoneum are a ruptured appendix, peptic ulcer, gangrenous gallbladder or perforated colon, pancreatitis, peritoneal dialysis, diverticulitis, incarcerated hernia, or gangrenous small bowel. It may also be a spontaneous complication of cirrhosis due to ascites.

Signs and Symptoms

Generalized abdominal pain evolves into localized pain at the site of the perforation or leakage. The area of the abdomen that is affected is extremely tender and aggravated by movement. Rebound tenderness and abdominal rigidity (board-like) are present. Decreased peristalsis results in bloating, full feeling, anorexia, nausea and vomiting, and no bowel movement or flatus. Infection causes fever, increased WBCs, and an elevated pulse. Dehydration signs can be present. Peritonitis can cause sepsis and be life threatening, so medical care should be sought.

Diagnostic Tests

Tests include WBCs to identify elevation, an abdominal x-ray or CT scan to show distention or perforation, paracentesis and laboratory analysis to identify a causative organism, or exploratory surgery to identify the cause.

Therapeutic Measures

The patient is NPO because of impaired peristalsis. Fluid and electrolyte replacement is crucial to correct hypovolemia and prevent or treat shock. Antibiotics are used to treat or prevent sepsis. Abdominal distention is relieved through insertion of an orogastric (or NG) tube with low intermittent suction. Depending on the cause of the peritonitis, surgery may be performed to excise, drain, or repair the cause. An ostomy may be formed to divert stool, allowing resolution of the infection. After surgery, the patient usually has a wound drain, an NG tube, and a urinary catheter. Pain control is essential to overall recovery. A nutritional plan will be developed to meet the patient's nutritional needs.

Complications

Complications of peritonitis are intestinal obstruction (discussed later), hypovolemia caused by the shift of fluid into the abdomen, and septicemia from bacteria entering the bloodstream. Shock and ultimately death may result.

Diverticulosis and Diverticulitis
Pathophysiology

A diverticulum (singular) is a small outpouching of the bowel mucous membrane through areas of weakness in the wall of the colon. **Diverticulosis** is when multiple diverticula (plural) are present without evidence of inflammation (Fig. 34.2). Many people have diverticulosis without knowing it. With

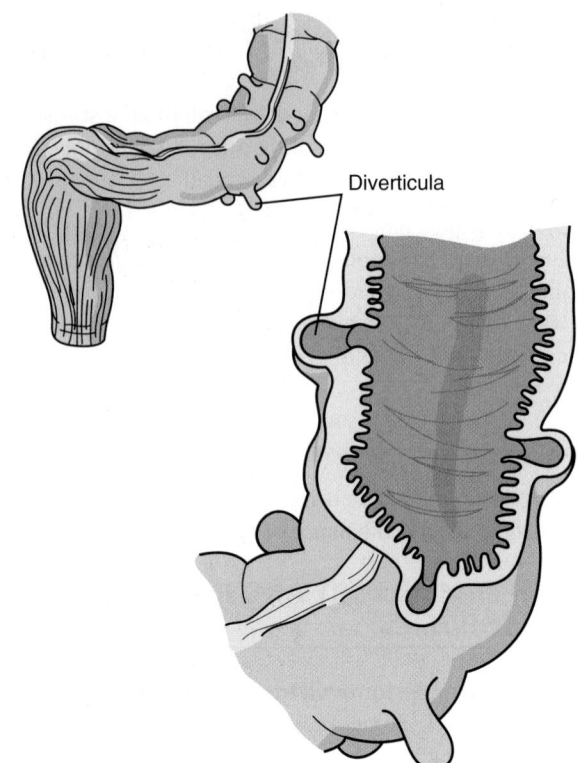

FIGURE 34.2 The presence of diverticula in diverticulosis.

increased pressure within the colon or stool trapped in a diverticulum, a tear can occur, and inflammation and infection can develop. This is called **diverticulitis.** If an abscess develops, the diverticulum may rupture, leading to peritonitis ("Gerontological Issues: Diverticulitis").

Gerontological Issues

Diverticulitis. With aging, the incidence of diverticular disease increases as a result of chronic constipation, obesity, hiatal hernia, or atrophy of the intestinal walls. Symptoms are often not reported early because patients fear it may be cancer. Blood in the stool, which can be an indication of diverticulitis, may not be seen by the older adult because of impaired vision.

Etiology

Chronic constipation usually precedes the development of diverticulosis by many years. When the patient is chronically constipated, pressure within the bowel is increased, leading to development of diverticula. A major cause of the disease

· WORD · BUILDING ·

diverticulosis: diverticul—blind pouch + osis—condition
diverticulitis: diverticul—blind pouch + itis—inflammation

is a decreased intake of dietary fiber. Diverticulosis is most common in the sigmoid colon. A small percentage of patients with diverticulosis develop diverticulitis.

Risk Factors

People older than age 60 most commonly experience diverticulitis. A diet low in fiber and high in animal fats, obesity, sedentary lifestyle, and smoking may increase risk for diverticulitis. Medications such as nonsteroidal anti-inflammatory drugs (NSAIDs), opioids, and steroids can increase risk. Some health care providers (HCPs) recommend avoiding nuts and seeds that can get caught in diverticula, such as in tomatoes and raspberries. However, this has not been shown to prevent diverticulitis.

Signs and Symptoms

Most people with diverticulosis never experience symptoms. When diverticulitis is present, the patient experiences constipation and possibly diarrhea (Table 34.3). Steady or crampy pain in the left lower quadrant of the abdomen is the most common symptom. Bleeding may occur, along with fever and fatigue. Abdominal tenderness may be present.

Diagnostic Tests

Diverticulosis is typically found with flexible sigmoidoscopy (proctosigmoidoscopy) or colonoscopy. Diverticulitis is confirmed with a CT scan, especially if complications such as an abscess are suspected. WBCs are checked for infection. A stool specimen can show infection or occult blood.

Therapeutic Measures

Severity of an attack guides treatment. Home treatment is possible for mild cases. It includes over-the-counter analgesics such as acetaminophen (Tylenol), an antibiotic, and a liquid diet. With severe diverticulitis, the patient is hospitalized for pain control, administration of IV antibiotics and fluids while being NPO, and drainage of any abscesses. When the acute period is over, a progressive diet is started.

Surgery may be considered, especially for perforation, abscess, or bowel obstruction. A bowel resection to remove the diseased area of the colon with anastomosis (reconnection) may be done. For increased inflammation, a temporary colostomy (discussed later) may be created to allow the inflammation to subside and the diseased portion of the colon to rest. Later, the colostomy can be reversed and the colon reconnected.

Nursing Process for the Patient With an Inflammatory or Infectious Disorder
Data Collection

Identifying pain is essential for patients experiencing inflammation or infection. Monitor the patient closely, and notify the HCP immediately if pain increases, especially if associated with abdominal rigidity. Increased pain may indicate that the bowel has ruptured and peritonitis is developing. Abdominal distention is recorded and reported. Vital signs are monitored for fever and other signs of sepsis. Reduced urinary output, dropping blood pressure, and rising pulse rate reflect fluid volume imbalance.

Nursing Diagnoses, Planning, and Implementation

Acute Pain related to inflammatory process

EXPECTED OUTCOME: The patient will report pain is relieved or at an acceptable level within 30 minutes of report of pain.

- Have the patient rate pain using a rating scale such as 0 to 10 *to determine pain level.*

Table 34.3
Symptoms Associated With Diverticulitis

W—Where is the pain?	Usually in the left lower quadrant
H—How does it feel? (Describe quality)	Tender, crampy
A—Aggravating and alleviating factors	Constipation and low-fiber diet may aggravate; treatment of constipation may alleviate
T—Timing (onset, duration, frequency)	Gradual onset and intermittent, gradual increase in frequency of pain events
S—Severity (0–10)	Usually 5 to 7
U—Useful other data/associated symptoms	Intermittent rectal bleeding; straining at stool; constipation alternating with diarrhea; elevated white blood cells and sedimentation rate; elevated temperature and pulse rate; and pus, mucus, and blood in stool
P—Patient's perception	Fear of cancer diagnosis

• Give analgesics or antispasmodic drugs as ordered *to relieve pain.*
• Use position changes, diversion, and relaxation exercises to help relieve pain. *Semi-Fowler position may reduce tension on the abdomen.*
• Provide frequent mouth care if an NG tube is in place *to increase comfort.*

Risk for Deficient Fluid Volume related to diarrhea or fluid shifting from the circulation to the peritoneal cavity

EXPECTED OUTCOME: The patient will maintain vital signs and urine output within normal limits at all times.

• Record I&O *to determine fluid balance.*
• Weigh patient daily *to determine fluid loss.*
• Monitor vital signs and urine output and report changes *to detect change from normal limits.*
• Maintain IV fluid replacement as ordered *to maintain fluid balance if output is greater than intake.*

    For constipation related to a low-fiber diet, see the earlier section on constipation.

Evaluation

The goals are met if the patient reports that pain is controlled, vital signs and urinary output remain stable, and the patient has regular, comfortable bowel elimination.

INFLAMMATORY BOWEL DISEASE

Crohn Disease
Pathophysiology

Crohn disease is an autoimmune inflammatory bowel disease (IBD) that can involve any part of the GI tract. It most commonly affects the terminal portion of the ileum, or first part of the large intestine. The inflamed areas from Crohn disease can alternate with areas of healthy tissue, so the inflamed areas are referred to as "skip lesions" (as they are not continuous lesions along the intestine). As the disease progresses, obstruction occurs because the intestinal lumen narrows with inflamed mucosa and scar tissue.

    The inflammation extends through the intestinal mucosa. This leads to the formation of abscesses, **fistulas** (abnormal connections between structures), and **fissures** (unnatural tracts or ulcers). Fistulas may include enterovaginal (small bowel to vagina), enterovesicular (small bowel to bladder), enterocutaneous (small bowel to skin), entero-entero (small bowel to small bowel), or enterocolonic (small bowel to colon) (Fig. 34.3). Fistulas communicating with organs that then drain externally can cause tremendous skin irritation as well as increased risk of developing infections.

Etiology

Although the exact cause of Crohn disease has not been identified, it tends to occur within families. Infections or environmental agents can trigger the immune system's attack on the GI tract. Crohn disease is most often diagnosed between the ages of 15 and 30. It occurs more often in women than men. Smoking increases the risk for Crohn disease.

Signs and Symptoms

Crampy abdominal pains (unrelieved by defecation), diarrhea with blood possible, weight loss, fatigue, fever, and mouth sores are the most common symptoms. They can be mild to severe. Because the crampy pains occur after eating, the patient often does not eat to avoid the pain. A lack of eating and poor absorption of nutrients result in weight loss and malnutrition.

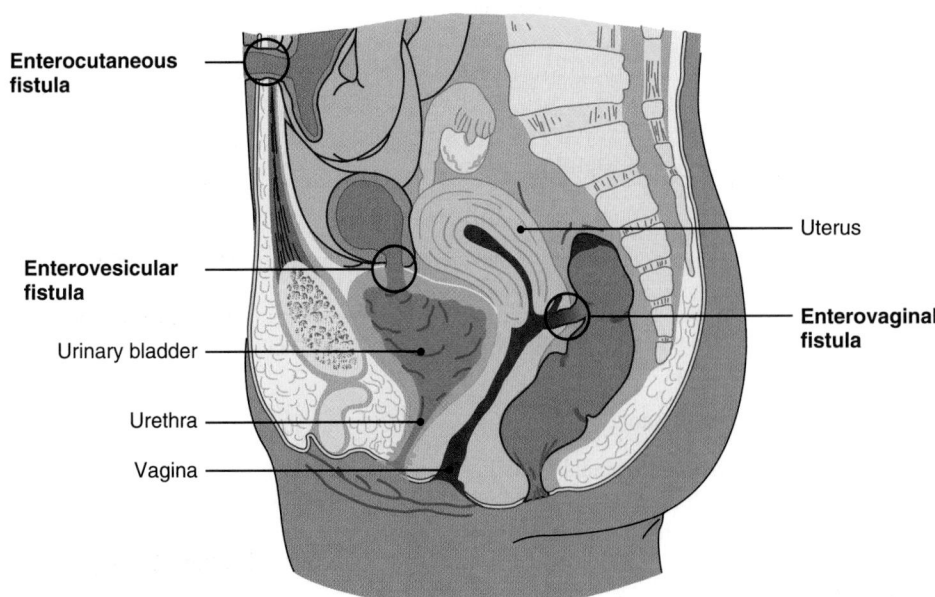

Enterocutaneous fistula

Enterovesicular fistula

Urinary bladder

Urethra

Vagina

Uterus

Enterovaginal fistula

FIGURE 34.3 Fistulas are a common complication of Crohn disease.

Chronic diarrhea contributes to fluid deficit and electrolyte imbalance. There can also be inflammatory symptoms outside the GI tract of the eyes, liver, bile ducts, skin, and joints. Periods of remission and exacerbations occur. Physical or psychological stress may trigger exacerbations ("Cultural Considerations").

Cultural Considerations

Crohn disease and ulcerative colitis are more common in Caucasians, people of Eastern European Jewish descent, and urban populations. The incidence of Crohn disease is increasing in blacks who live in the United Kingdom and North America. These findings support possible hereditary or environmental risk factors for inflammatory bowel disease.

Diagnostic Tests

Laboratory testing looks for anemia, infection, liver function, low albumin due to poor absorption of protein, and stool infections or occult blood. Endoscopy (colonoscopy and sigmoidoscopy), with multiple biopsies of the diseased colon and terminal ileum, is used to diagnose Crohn disease. Other endoscopic tests include capsule endoscopy (swallowed camera the size of a pill), ultrasound to identify fistulas and areas of bleeding, and double balloon enteroscopy, which provides views of the inside of tissue folds. Crohn disease is confirmed by granulomas in the biopsy specimen. Imaging tests include multiphase CT enterography and magnetic resonance enterography (MRE), which provide detailed images of the intestines.

Therapeutic Measures

There is no cure for Crohn disease. Management is aimed at achieving and maintaining remission. Treatment is individualized. Symptoms are controlled by reducing the intestinal inflammation that is the underlying cause of the symptoms. Classes of medications used to achieve these goals are 5-aminosalicylates, corticosteroids, biologic response modifiers, immunomodulators, and antibiotics (Table 34.4). To reduce inflammation, 5-aminosalicylates are used; however, they do not prevent acute episodes and are not used as much as in the past. Corticosteroids are used during acute inflammation, then tapered and discontinued. Biologic

Table 34.4
Medications for Crohn Disease and/or Ulcerative Colitis

Medication/Action

5-Aminosalicylates

Decrease intestinal inflammation.

Examples	**Nursing Implications**
mesalamine (Asacol, Canasa, Pentasa, Rowasa)	Monitor for signs of reduced kidney function.
olsalazine (Dipentum)	Take with food.
balsalazide (Colazal)	Take with food.
sulfasalazine (Azulfidine)	Contraindicated in sulfa allergy.

Biologic Response Modifiers

Selectively target inflammatory agents to interfere with inflammatory response.

Examples	**Nursing Implications**
adalimumab (Humira)	Tuberculosis test must be done before therapy begins and annually.
certolizumab pegol (Cimzia)	
infliximab (Remicade)	Monitor for infections, bone marrow suppression, and central nervous system disorder.
ustekinumab (Stelara)	
vedolizumab (Entyvio)	

Corticosteroids

Decrease inflammation and suppress immune system.

Examples	**Nursing Implications**
prednisone (Deltasone)	Teach patient not to stop taking medication abruptly.
methylprednisolone (Medrol, Solu-Medrol)	

Continued

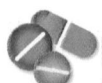

Table 34.4
Medications for Crohn Disease and/or Ulcerative Colitis—cont'd

Medication/Action

Anti-Inflammatory Synthetic Corticosteroid

Reduce inflammation locally for Crohn disease.

Examples	**Nursing Implications**
budesonide (Entocort EC)	*Teach:* Grapefruit and grapefruit juice should be avoided. Take in morning. Swallow whole.

Immunomodulators

Most commonly used in immunosuppression to reduce inflammation.

Examples	**Nursing Implications**
azathioprine (Imuran) 6-mercaptopurine (6-MP, Purinethol) Methotrexate (Trexall)	Report symptoms of infection when taking an immunomodulator. Monitor for infections. Monitor for side effects. *Teach:* Grapefruit and grapefruit juice should be avoided. Take in morning. Swallow whole.

response modifiers selectively target agents in the inflammatory process to block their action and effects. Immunomodulators modify the immune system to decrease inflammation. They may be used with steroids to treat acute episodes because they have a longer onset of action. Antibiotics are used to reduce bacterial counts in the intestine that may be contributing to the inflammation.

Antidiarrheal medications such as diphenoxylate with atropine (Lomotil) or loperamide (Imodium) are used. Bulk-forming laxatives may help reduce loose stools and, subsequently, skin irritation.

As complications develop, surgery may be indicated for obstruction, stricture, fistula, abscess, excessive bleeding, perforation, toxic megacolon (loss of muscle tone and dilation in colon), or symptoms that do not respond to treatment. Surgery does not cure Crohn disease because it can recur elsewhere in the GI tract. Surgical procedures include strictureplasty to widen areas of stricture, resection of an affected area with anastomosis, **colectomy** with ileorectal anastomosis, or proctocolectomy (rectum and colon) with ileostomy. See details regarding intestinal ostomies later in this chapter. A Kock pouch is not recommended for those with Crohn disease because the disease may affect the pouch.

A healthy diet is important in overall health, but there is no special diet for Crohn disease. A dietitian referral is important for nutritional support. Adequate fluid intake is essential to prevent dehydration if diarrhea is present. Malnutrition is a concern if the small intestine is affected and nutrients are not absorbed properly. Multivitamin and mineral supplements may be needed. Foods that increase symptoms, such as dairy products, fatty food, and fresh fruits and vegetables, should be limited.

Nursing Process for the Patient With Crohn Disease
Because of the similarities between Crohn disease and ulcerative colitis, the nursing processes for both are discussed together in the "Nursing Process for the Patient With Inflammatory Bowel Disease" section that follows.

Ulcerative Colitis
Pathophysiology
Ulcerative **colitis** is similar to Crohn disease. Crohn disease, however, can occur anywhere in the GI system, whereas ulcerative colitis occurs in the large intestine and rectum. Multiple ulcerations and diffuse inflammation occur in the superficial mucosa and submucosa of the colon. The lesions spread in a continuous pattern.

• WORD • BUILDING •

colectomy: col—pertaining to colon + ectomy—surgical excision

colitis: col—pertaining to colon + itis—inflammation

Etiology

Infection, allergy, and autoimmune response are possible causes of ulcerative colitis, although an exact cause is unknown. Environmental agents such as pesticides, tobacco, radiation, and food additives may precipitate an exacerbation. Ulcerative colitis usually begins between ages 15 and 30. Heredity may play a role for about a quarter of those with ulcerative colitis.

Signs and Symptoms

Diarrhea with blood or pus, abdominal and rectal pain, rectal bleeding, and fecal urgency with straining are common symptoms of ulcerative colitis (Table 34.5). Anorexia, weight loss, cramping, vomiting, fever, fatigue, and severe dehydration associated with passing 5 to 10 or more liquid stools a day may also occur. Along with the potential for fluid and electrolyte imbalance, calcium is lost. Anemia often develops as a result of rectal bleeding. Symptoms are usually intermittent, with remissions lasting from weeks to years. Diet or psychological stress may trigger or worsen an attack of symptoms.

Complications

Malnutrition occurs less often with ulcerative colitis than with Crohn disease. As discussed with Crohn disease, other inflammatory disorders can occur. Additional complications include hemorrhage, toxic megacolon, perforation, peritonitis, osteoporosis, and increased risk for colorectal cancer.

Diagnostic Tests

A history and physical examination with laboratory tests are used to diagnose ulcerative colitis. Anemia is often present because of blood loss. Examination of stool specimens is done to rule out the presence of bacterial or amoeba organisms. The stool is positive for blood in the presence of ulcerative colitis. Electrolytes may be depleted from chronic diarrhea. There is protein loss because of liver dysfunction and malabsorption. A colonoscopy to see the whole colon or a flexible sigmoidoscopy to view the lower colon is done. Biopsy specimens show inflamed cells. Barium enema, ultrasound, CT scan, and MRI are also used. Leukocyte scintigraphy, a noninvasive imaging test, uses the patient's WBCs tagged with a radioactive material to detect infection and inflammation in the colon.

Therapeutic Measures

Diet, lifestyle changes, medications, and surgery are used for treatment. Many of the medication classes used with Crohn disease are used for ulcerative colitis (see Table 34.4). Foods that cause gas or diarrhea should be avoided. Because the offending foods may be different for each patient, foods are tried in small amounts and eliminated if they are thought to cause symptoms. In general, high-fiber foods, caffeine, spicy foods, and milk products are avoided. Diarrhea may increase the need for fluids to prevent dehydration.

Surgery is considered for excessive bleeding, severe symptoms, perforation, or toxic megacolon. Because ulcerative colitis usually involves the entire large intestine, the entire colon and rectum are removed for a proctocolectomy with ileostomy (discussed later). This procedure is curative. The anal sphincter of the rectum can be preserved for an ileoanal pouch (restorative proctocolectomy) procedure. This is not curative, as the disease can return in the preserved rectum.

An ileoanal pouch does not require an ostomy pouch to be worn and is the more common surgery performed. Because the anus and sphincter are saved, stool still passes through the anus. The rectum and colon are removed. The end of the ileum, which is made into a J-shaped pouch, is attached to the anus. A temporary ileostomy is created to allow the pouch to heal. After about 12 weeks, the ileostomy is closed. Several bowel movements per day occur. The stool is of soft consistency. Surgical complications can include a bowel obstruction or an inflammation of the pouch (pouchitis), which is treated with antibiotics.

Nursing Process for the Patient With Inflammatory Bowel Disease
Data Collection

A history obtained from the patient includes symptoms, including their onset, duration, frequency, and severity. Ask whether there has been any correlation between exacerbations

Table 34.5
Inflammatory Bowel Disease Summary

Signs and Symptoms	Diarrhea Abdominal and rectal pain or cramping Rectal bleeding Fecal urgency with straining Weight loss Fluid and electrolyte imbalance Fissures, fistulas, and abscesses Arthritis and skin lesions Inflammatory eye disorders Inflammatory liver disease
Diagnostic Tests	Stool examination Endoscopy with biopsy Barium enema, ultrasound, computed tomography (CT) scan, magnetic resonance imaging (MRI) Leukocyte scintigraphy
Therapeutic Measures	Medications: see Table 34.4 Surgery if necessary Avoidance of offending foods Elemental formula or parenteral nutrition (PN) if required
Priority Nursing Diagnoses	*Constipation* *Diarrhea* *Risk for Deficient Fluid Volume* *Deficient Knowledge*

of symptoms and dietary changes or stress. Determine the presence of any food allergies or intolerances that may increase diarrhea. Also, note the daily and weekly intake of caffeine, nicotine, and alcohol because all these stimulate the bowel and can cause cramping and diarrhea.

Identify the patient's nutritional status and signs of dehydration. Ten to 20 pounds can be lost in a 2-month period. Perianal skin should be observed for irritation and excoriation.

Identification of emotional status, coping skills, and verbal and nonverbal behaviors is essential. The patient may withdraw from family and friends because of frequent bowel movements. Anxiety, sleep disturbances, depression, and denial can be problems. If surgery involving an ileostomy is planned, the patient is at risk for altered body image.

Nursing Diagnoses, Planning, and Implementation

Acute Pain related to increased peristalsis and cramping

EXPECTED OUTCOME: The patient will state pain is relieved or at an acceptable level within 30 minutes of report of pain.

- Ask patient to rate pain on a scale such as 0 to 10 *to determine pain level.*
- Document the character of the pain (e.g., dull, cramping, burning) and ask whether the pain is associated with meals or other activities *to plan care.*
- Give analgesics and medications *to relieve cramping, as prescribed.*

Diarrhea related to the inflammatory process

EXPECTED OUTCOME: The patient will maintain formed, soft stool every 1 to 3 days.

- Document characteristics of stools, including color, consistency, amount, frequency, and odor *to plan care.*
- Ensure the patient has quick access to the bathroom or provide a bedside commode *to prevent incontinence.*
- Administer antidiarrheal medication as prescribed. *Controlling diarrhea controls comfort and fluid balance.*
- Encourage bedrest *to decrease peristalsis during exacerbations.*
- Keep the environment clean and odor free *to help promote comfort.*
- Teach the patient to avoid dairy products and high-fiber foods such as whole grains and raw fruits and vegetables as well as caffeine, alcohol, and nicotine *because they stimulate intestinal motility.*

Risk for Deficient Fluid Volume related to diarrhea and insufficient fluid intake

EXPECTED OUTCOME: The patient will maintain vital signs and urine output within normal limits at all times.

- Weigh patient daily *to determine fluid loss.*
- Record I&O (including diarrhea stools) *to determine fluid balance.*

- Document and report signs of deficient fluid volume to the HCP *to allow treatment.*
- Maintain IV fluids as ordered *to maintain fluid balance.*
- Encourage fluids when acute diarrhea subsides *to maintain fluid balance.*
- Teach the patient signs and symptoms of dehydration to report *to allow prompt treatment.*

Anxiety related to symptoms and frequency of stools and treatment

EXPECTED OUTCOME: The patient will report that anxiety is reduced.

- Answer questions; talk in a calm, confident manner; and actively listen to the patient *to reduce anxiety, which aggravates symptoms of IBD.*

Impaired Skin Integrity related to frequent loose stools

EXPECTED OUTCOME: The patient's skin will remain intact at all times.

- Keep perianal skin clean, dry, and protected with a moisture barrier, such as petrolatum or medicated ointment, after each bowel movement *to protect perianal skin from contact with liquid stools and their enzymes.*
- Provide sitz baths, which may be comforting and helpful in keeping skin clean, *to prevent excoriation.*

Imbalanced Nutrition: Less Than Body Requirements related to malabsorption

EXPECTED OUTCOME: The patient will maintain weight within normal range for height and age.

- Weigh weekly *to detect weight loss.*
- Give special liquid (elemental) formula that is absorbed in the upper bowel as ordered *to allow the colon to rest.*
- Maintain parenteral nutrition (PN) as ordered to provide nourishment *if the patient is unable to tolerate oral intake.*

See "Nursing Care Plan for the Patient With Inflammatory Bowel Disease."

Evaluation

Goals have been met if pain is relieved, frequency of diarrhea stools is decreased, fluid and electrolyte balance is achieved, anxiety is reduced, skin is intact, and weight is within normal range for height and age.

 IRRITABLE BOWEL SYNDROME

Pathophysiology

Irritable bowel syndrome (IBS) is not a disease but rather a functional problem. The colon mucosa is not damaged by the condition, and there is no increased risk of colorectal cancer. IBS is a disorder of altered intestinal motility in which the

Nursing Care Plan for the Patient With Inflammatory Bowel Disease

Nursing Diagnosis: *Ineffective Coping* related to inflammatory bowel disease
Expected Outcome: The patient will identify strategies that promote effective coping.
Evaluation of Outcome: Is the patient able to state strategies for effective coping?

Intervention	Rationale	Evaluation
Identify patient's knowledge of the disease.	*Many people have little knowledge of a disease, and accurate information is essential.*	Does patient verbalize information about the disease and its effects on the body?
Encourage patient to express feelings about the disease and how it is affecting his or her life.	*Expressing feelings about the disease and its perceived effect enables patient to talk about concerns. Once identified, the health care team can then address these concerns.*	Does patient talk about feelings regarding the potential impact of the disease on his or her life?
Determine whether patient would like to speak with a person of similar age from the Crohn's & Colitis Foundation.	*Speaking with someone close in age with the same disease lets the patient know that he or she is not the only person coping with this disorder. It can also help the patient learn some strategies for effectively coping with the disease.*	Does patient show an interest in speaking with someone with the same disease?
Identify strategies for effective coping that are acceptable to patient.	*Talking about concerns and possible solutions is a positive step. Coping strategies identified with the patient are more likely to be implemented.*	Is patient able to identify strategies for effective coping that he or she believes will work?

CRITICAL THINKING

Judy Moore is an 18-year-old college student who has just been diagnosed with Crohn disease.

1. What questions should the nurse ask Judy to identify her symptoms?
2. What nursing diagnoses would be relevant for Judy's condition?
3. What patient-centered care can help Judy adapt to this disease?
4. If Judy's condition were to worsen, what manifestations would be exhibited?
5. With which members of the health care team might the nurse collaborate?

Suggested answers are at the end of the chapter.

colon muscle contracts more easily. It contracts in a disorderly way that can be violent and last for a long time, or, at times, it may not contract at all. The abnormal contractions lead to changes in bowel patterns. Thus, the disorder may be classified as IBS with diarrhea, IBS with constipation, or IBS with mixed diarrhea and constipation. Mucus may be seen in the stool, although this is not abnormal.

Etiology

The cause is unknown. There is a hereditary tendency for IBS. IBS is more common in women than men and in those who are young to middle aged. Intestinal muscle contractions, nerve conduction abnormalities, immune response, and the microbiome are influencing factors in the disorder. The nerves in the bowel are overly sensitive in people with IBS. At times of stress in daily living or with food intolerances, abnormal contractions may result. Flare-ups can be caused by infections or the menstrual cycle.

Signs and Symptoms

Patients experience abdominal pain, bloating, gas, or constipation or diarrhea, which can alternate. Other symptoms include feeling of incomplete evacuation, depression, and anxiety.

Diagnostic Tests

Diagnosis of IBS is made based on history and physical examination along with stool examination, colonoscopy, flexible sigmoidoscopy, CT scan, or lower GI series to rule out other disorders, including lactose intolerance or celiac disease if diarrhea occurs. IBSchek is a new antibody test that identifies IBS cases that have developed two antibodies in response to exposure to a bacterial toxin found in food poisoning that results in watery diarrhea.

Therapeutic Measures

IBS is a chronic condition, but symptoms can generally be controlled with diet, lifestyle, and stress management and medication. Treatment varies based on the bowel pattern. In general, adequate hydration, exercise, rest, and avoiding food triggers, especially those that cause gas and contain gluten or FODMAPs (fermentable oligosaccharides, disaccharides, monosaccharides, and polyols), are important ("Nutrition Notes: Low FODMAP Diet"). A high-fiber and high-bran diet and fiber supplements (psyllium [Metamucil] or methylcellulose [Citrucel]) may help to form softer, larger stools to relieve constipation. Eating smaller, frequent meals can be helpful in reducing bowel contractions. Patients can keep a diary of foods eaten, stressors, and symptoms. This can help the HCP identify flare-up triggers. Stress management and behavioral therapy (e.g., biofeedback, hypnosis, psychotherapy) are helpful in relaxing the bowel as well as contributing to overall health.

Nutrition Notes

Low FODMAP Diet. The Low FODMAP diet restricts certain carbohydrates that are known to cause symptoms in patients with IBS because of their poor absorption, osmotic activity, and rapid fermentation. FODMAP stands for Fermentable Oligosaccharides, Disaccharides, Monosaccharides, And Polyols. The Low FODMAP Diet has been shown to reduce IBS symptoms and is the primary diet therapy used internationally (St. Charles & O'Brien, 2015).

High FODMAP foods include fermentable:

- Oligosaccharides: fructans (e.g., agave, wheat, onions, garlic, leeks, artichokes, asparagus, jicama) and galactans (GOSs; e.g., legumes [soybeans, beans, chickpeas, lentils]; cabbage, Brussels sprouts, wheat, rye, onions, garlic, inulin, artichokes, leeks, asparagus, broccoli)
- Disaccharides (lactose): milk, dairy products
- Monosaccharides (fructose): honey, apples, dates, mangoes, papaya, pears, prunes, watermelon, high-fructose corn syrup
- Polyols (sugar alcohols, i.e., sorbitol, mannitol, maltitol, xylitol, ismalt): low-calorie food products, sugar-free mints/gums/beverages

Not all FODMAPs will trigger symptoms for all patients. Only those that are malabsorbed are likely to be clinically significant. Fructans and GOSs are always malabsorbed and fermented by intestinal bacteria, resulting in gas production and associated flatulence even in healthy people.

The remaining FODMAP carbohydrates will only induce symptoms in the patients with IBS that malabsorb them. Identification of susceptible patients can be achieved by breath tests after ingestion of lactose or fructose or by eliminating all FODMAP foods and relating their reintroduction to returning symptoms.

Individualizing the diet is important, particularly for vegetarians who may depend on legumes for protein intake, as it may show patients that they can cope with garlic as a minor ingredient or wheat products occasionally, which would expand the nutritional composition of their diet. The low FODMAP diet requires a registered dietitian's expertise both to maximize compliance with instigating the complete list of FODMAP sources and to avoid an overly restrictive approach unnecessarily. The latter is of great import in the event the diet is successful and likely to be followed long term.

Reference

St. Charles, A., & O'Brien, M. (2015). *Irritable bowel syndrome and inflammatory gastrointestinal disorders* (3rd ed.). Concord, CA: Institute for Natural Resources Health Update.

Medications taken depend on the type of IBS. Laxatives or antidiarrheal medication are used as appropriate. Antidepressants help to relieve pain. For IBS with constipation, selective serotonin reuptake inhibitors (SSRIs), such as paroxetine hydrochloride (Paxil) or fluoxetine (Prozac, Sarafem), are given. Low-dose tricyclic antidepressants, such as desipramine (Norpramin), imipramine (Tofranil), or nortriptyline (Pamelor), are used for IBS with diarrhea because they slow movement through the intestines. Antispasmodics, such as hyoscyamine (Levbid) or dicyclomine (Bentyl), are used in IBS for diarrhea to relieve painful bowel spasms. Rifaximin (Xifaxan), an antibiotic, treats IBS with diarrhea. Medications that increase fluid secretion in the intestine to help pass stool and reduce constipation include linaclotide (Linzess), which is for those who do not respond to other treatments. For women for whom treatment for IBS with constipation has not been successful, lubiprostone (Amitiza) is used.

Nursing Process for the Patient With Irritable Bowel Syndrome
Data Collection

Height, weight, and symptoms, including pain that the patient experiences, are documented. Timing of the symptoms, food and fluid intake, elimination patterns, effects on self-esteem, and socialization are explored. Personal and family roles are identified because IBS is a significant cause of missed work and school. It also causes social withdrawal and feelings of embarrassment. Patient knowledge of the disorder and readiness for managing the syndrome is determined to plan care.

Nursing Diagnoses, Planning, and Implementation

Constipation related to irregular motility of GI tract

EXPECTED OUTCOME: The patient will maintain passage of soft, formed stool every 1 to 3 days without straining.

- Identify normal bowel pattern, diet and fluid intake, and medications *to help identify factors contributing to constipation for planning care.*
- Increase fluid intake, if not contraindicated, to 2 to 3 L per day *to prevent hard stools.*
- Teach the patient about the benefits of increasing fiber and bran in the diet *to promote soft, larger stools that are easier to pass.*
- Give medication as ordered *to prevent constipation.*

Diarrhea related to irregular motility of GI tract

EXPECTED OUTCOME: The patient will maintain formed, soft stool every 1 to 3 days.

- Obtain history and medications taken for diarrhea episodes *to help identify cause.*
- Monitor and record stool characteristics, amount, and frequency *to plan care.*
- Give antidiarrheal medications as ordered. *Controlling diarrhea controls comfort and fluid balance.*
- Limit caffeine intake *because it stimulates intestinal motility.*
- Keep skin clean, dry, and protected with a moisture barrier, such as petrolatum or medicated ointment, after each bowel movement *to protect perianal skin from contact with liquid stools and their enzymes.*

Readiness for Enhanced Health Management related to desire to manage symptoms of IBS

EXPECTED OUTCOME: The patient will state understanding and ability to carry out preventive measures to control symptoms before discharge.

- Explain IBS, including symptoms, aggravating factors, and treatments, *to promote understanding, which will aid ability to follow therapeutic regimen.*

- Consult a registered dietitian *to develop meal plan to prevent symptoms.*
- Encourage use of food diary documenting foods eaten and timing of symptom occurrence *to identify food triggers for symptoms including lactose intolerance.*

Evaluation

The plan has been effective if the patient has regular bowel function pattern, verbalizes understanding of self-care measures, and expresses satisfaction with the outcomes.

ABDOMINAL HERNIAS

Pathophysiology and Etiology

A **hernia** is an abnormal protrusion of an organ or structure through a weakness or tear in the wall of the cavity normally containing it, such as the abdominal wall. A hernial sac is formed by the peritoneum protruding through the weakened muscle wall. Hernias occur from increased intra-abdominal pressure, such as the pressure from coughing, straining, or heavy lifting. Contents in the hernia sac can be the small or large intestine or the omentum.

Figure 34.4 illustrates the various types of hernias. Umbilical hernias are seen most often in obesity, ascites, peritoneal dialysis, or multiple pregnancies. Inguinal hernias (direct or indirect) are located in the groin where the spermatic cord in males or the round ligament in females emerges from the abdominal wall. Femoral hernias occur in the groin below the inguinal ligament and are not common. Ventral (incisional) hernias usually result from a weakness in the abdominal wall after abdominal surgery, especially in the obese patient, if a drainage system was used, if the patient experienced poor wound healing, or if the patient received inadequate nutrition.

Prevention

Congenital defects cannot be prevented. However, reducing strain on abdominal muscles is helpful. Those who do heavy lifting, tugging, or pushing should wear a support binder or avoid the lifting. A healthy lifestyle of maintaining normal weight, not smoking, and eating high-fiber foods is recommended.

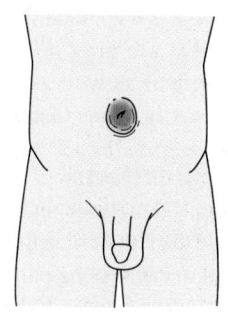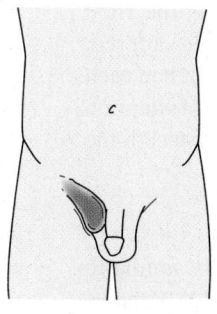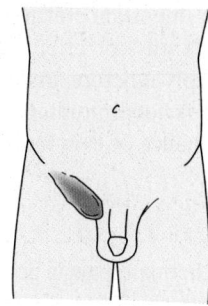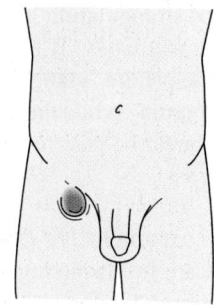

Umbilical hernia   Direct inguinal hernia   Indirect inguinal hernia   Femoral hernia

FIGURE 34.4 Types of hernias.

Signs and Symptoms

Unless complications occur, few symptoms are associated with hernias. An abnormal bulging can be seen in the affected area of the abdomen, especially when straining or coughing. The patient may have some discomfort due to tension on tissues around the hernia. The herniation may disappear when the patient lies down. If the intestinal mass easily returns to the abdominal cavity or can be manually placed back in the abdominal cavity, it is called a reducible hernia. When adhesions or edema occur between the sac and its contents, the hernia becomes irreducible or incarcerated.

Complications

An incarcerated hernia may become strangulated if the blood and intestinal flow are completely cut off in the trapped loop of bowel. Strangulated hernias do not develop in adults very often. Incarceration leads to an intestinal obstruction and possibly gangrene and bowel perforation. Symptoms are pain at the site of the strangulation, nausea and vomiting, and colicky abdominal pain.

Therapeutic Measures

Hernias are diagnosed by physical examination. Treatment options include no treatment, observing the hernia, using short-term support devices, or surgery to repair the hernia. A supportive truss or brief applies pressure to keep the reduced hernia in place. Emergency surgery is needed for strangulation or the threat of bowel obstruction. Surgical repair is recommended for inguinal hernias. Surgical procedures are most often done laparoscopically and include hernioplasty (open or laparoscopically) or herniorrhaphy (open hernia repair). Herniorrhaphy involves making an incision in the abdominal wall, replacing the contents of the hernial sac, sewing the weakened tissue, and closing the opening. Hernioplasty involves replacing the hernia into the abdomen and reinforcing the weakened muscle wall with wire, fascia, or mesh. Bowel resection or a temporary colostomy may be necessary if the hernia is strangulated.

Nursing Care

The patient is instructed to avoid activities that increase intra-abdominal pressure, such as lifting heavy objects or coughing. The patient is taught to recognize signs of incarceration or strangulation and the importance of notifying the HCP immediately. If a support truss or brief has been ordered, the patient is taught to apply it before arising from bed each morning while the hernia is not protruding. Special attention should be paid to maintenance of skin integrity beneath the truss.

Postoperative Care

Care following inguinal hernia repair is generally similar to any abdominal postoperative care (see Chapter 12). Patients can perform deep breathing to keep lungs clear postoperatively but should avoid coughing. Coughing increases abdominal pressure and could affect the hernia repair. The male patient may experience swelling of the scrotum. Ice packs and elevation of the scrotum may be ordered to reduce the swelling. Because most patients are discharged the same day of surgery, they are taught to change the dressing and report difficulty urinating, bleeding, and signs and symptoms of infection, such as redness, incisional drainage, fever, or severe pain. The patient is also instructed to avoid lifting, driving, or sexual activities for 2 to 6 weeks as specified by the HCP. Most patients can return to nonstrenuous work within 2 weeks.

 ## ABSORPTION DISORDERS

The process of digestion reduces nutrients to a liquid form that can be absorbed through intestinal mucosa into the portal bloodstream. More than 8,000 mL of liquid with nutrients and electrolytes is absorbed daily, mostly proximal to the ileocecal valve.

Pathophysiology and Etiology

Malabsorption occurs when the GI system is unable to absorb one or more of the major nutrients (carbohydrates, fats, or proteins). Some causes of malabsorption are ileal dysfunction, jejunal diverticula, parasitic disease, celiac disease, enzyme deficiency, and IBD such as Crohn disease and ulcerative colitis. The primary malabsorption disorders are celiac disease and lactose intolerance.

In celiac disease, a sensitivity to gluten is thought to cause malabsorption of protein. Gluten is a protein found in wheat, barley, and rye. Oats may become contaminated with gluten in the milling process of these other grains ("Nutrition Notes: Treating Celiac Disease").

A deficiency in lactase, an enzyme that breaks down lactose (milk sugar), causes lactose intolerance. When lactose is not digested, a high concentration of it occurs in the intestines, causing an osmotic retention of water in the colon and watery stools.

Signs and Symptoms

Weight loss, fatigue, and general malaise resulting from malnutrition are associated with malabsorption disorders. Lactose intolerance causes abdominal cramping, excessive gas, and loose stools after eating milk products. Celiac disease symptoms can range from none to many in various body systems (visit www.csaceliacs.org). Frequent loose, bulky, foul stools that are gray in color with an increased fat content (steatorrhea) as well as gas, bloating, and abdominal pain may occur in celiac disease.

Complications

Vitamin K deficiency and resulting hypoprothrombinemia can increase the risk of bleeding. Calcium deficiency can be severe enough to cause bone pain and neuromuscular hyperirritability, including tetany. Folic acid, vitamin B_{12}, and iron deficiencies can result in glossitis, stomatitis, anemia, and dry, rough skin. In celiac disease, dermatitis herpetiformis occurs, which is a skin rash with severe pruritus and blistering.

Nutrition Notes

Treating Celiac Disease. Celiac disease, or gluten-sensitive enteropathy, has a multifactorial etiology involving a combination of

- genetic predisposition,
- ingestion of gluten, and
- an autoimmune response that produces chronic inflammation of the small intestine.

Definitive diagnosis is made with a biopsy of the small intestine. The Celiac Disease Foundation (http://celiac.org) estimates that it affects 1 in 10 people worldwide. Treatment requires permanent elimination of wheat, rye, and barley from the diet. Gluten-free grains, such as oats, can be cross-contaminated with gluten during milling. An individual must look for a "gluten-free" claim on food packaging to ensure a food is, in fact, gluten free. This is a voluntary U.S. Food and Drug Administration (FDA) labeling rule, which, if used, guarantees less than 20 parts per million (ppm) of gluten in the product. Products that don't contain other ingredients and are normally gluten free (e.g., frozen vegetables) are not required to be labeled as gluten free (www.fda.gov/Food/GuidanceRegulation/GuidanceDocumentsRegulatoryInformation/Allergens). If someone with celiac disease ingests gluten, the intestinal villi are damaged even in the absence of symptoms. This frequently causes nutritional deficiencies of iron, calcium, magnesium, zinc, folate, niacin, riboflavin, vitamin B_{12}, and vitamin D. Absence of gluten allows the healing of the villi, causing symptoms to resolve. Because dietary restriction is permanent, instruction from and follow-up by a registered dietitian are indicated to ensure adequate nutritional intake despite the many dietary limitations.

Table 34.6
Diagnostic Tests for Disorders of Malabsorption

Diagnostic Test	Test Result and Associated Malabsorption Syndrome
Hematocrit	Decreased if anemia is present.
Mean corpuscular volume	Decreased values are found with malabsorption of vitamin B_{12}.
Upper gastrointestinal series	Thickening of the intestinal mucosa, narrowed mucosa of the terminal ileum, or a change in fecal transit time are indicative of malabsorption syndrome.
D-xylose absorption test	Decreased excretion of xylose after 5 hours is indicative of malabsorption.
Sudan stain for fecal fat	Malabsorption can be distinguished from maldigestion if this test shows abnormally large numbers of fat droplets.
72-hour stool collection for fat	Stool fat greater than 5 g per 24 hours after ingestion of 80 g of fat in 2 days implies a fat digestion disorder.
Biopsy	Shows flattened mucosa and loss of villi with celiac disease.

Diagnostic Tests

See Table 34.6 for diagnostic studies used to identify malabsorption diseases. It is important to be tested before making diet changes.

Therapeutic Measures
Celiac Disease

A consultation with a dietitian is essential to plan a gluten-free diet to relieve symptoms, promote intestinal healing, and improve nutritional status. However, because gluten is used as a filler or binder in many products, even in those labeled "wheat free," diligence in identifying potentially offending foods is essential. The dietitian can assist with choosing safe foods.

Lactose Intolerance

Lactose intolerance is treated by having very small servings of foods that contain lactose, such as milk and milk products. Whole milk and some dairy products, such as hard cheeses (cheddar, Swiss) and yogurt, may be better tolerated. Lactase enzyme drops or tablets (e.g., Lactaid or Dairy Ease) digest about 70% of lactose in foods. They can be added to milk in liquid form or taken as a tablet before eating foods containing lactose. Vitamin D supplements may be needed.

Nursing Care

Nursing care involves monitoring fluid and electrolyte balance, nutritional status, and skin integrity. Recording daily weight and I&O helps determine whether fluid loss is occurring. Intake of electrolyte-rich fluids is encouraged to replace losses. Diet teaching is reinforced. Perianal skin is kept clean and dry, and barrier ointments are used as needed to protect the skin from excoriation.

 INTESTINAL OBSTRUCTION

Intestinal obstructions occur when the flow of intestinal contents is blocked. The two types of intestinal obstruction are mechanical and nonmechanical, both of which can be either partial or complete.

Mechanical obstruction is when a blockage occurs within the intestine from conditions causing pressure on the intestinal walls. Nonmechanical obstruction occurs when peristalsis is impaired and the intestinal contents cannot be propelled through the bowel. The severity of the obstruction depends on the area of bowel affected, the amount of occlusion within the lumen, and the amount of disturbance in the blood flow to the bowel

Small-Bowel Obstruction
Pathophysiology
When obstruction occurs in the small bowel, a collection of intestinal contents, gas, and fluid occurs proximal to the obstruction. The distention that results stimulates gastric secretion but decreases the absorption of fluids. As distention worsens, the intraluminal pressure causes a decrease in venous and arterial capillary pressure, resulting in edema, necrosis, and eventually perforation of the intestinal wall.

Etiology
There are a variety of mechanical obstruction causes. Following abdominal surgery, loops of intestine may adhere to areas in the abdomen that are not healed. This may cause a kink in the bowel that occludes the intestinal flow. These adhesions, or bands of scar tissue, are the most common cause of small-bowel obstruction. They are usually acquired from previous abdominal surgery or inflammation. Hernias and neoplasms are the next most common causes, followed by IBD, foreign bodies, strictures, volvulus, and intussusception. A **volvulus** occurs when the bowel twists, occluding the lumen of the intestine. **Intussusception** occurs when peristalsis causes the intestine to telescope into itself (Fig. 34.5).

Paralytic, or adynamic, ileus is a nonmechanical obstruction that occurs when the intestinal peristalsis decreases or stops because of a neuromuscular condition. Causes of

nonmechanical obstructions include abdominal surgery, hypokalemia, myocardial infarction, peritonitis, pneumonia, spinal injuries, trauma, and vascular insufficiency.

Signs and Symptoms
The patient initially reports wavelike abdominal pain and vomiting. Initially, flatus and feces that are already near the end of the colon and blood and mucus may be passed, but this stops as the obstruction worsens (Table 34.7). As the obstruction becomes more extreme, peristaltic waves may occur to attempt to relieve the obstruction and propel the intestinal contents into the stomach. This can eventually lead to fecal vomiting. Pain and abdominal distention are present. Pain that is sharp and sustained may indicate perforation. In mechanical obstructions, high-pitched, tinkling bowel sounds are heard proximal to the obstruction and are absent distal to it. If the obstruction is nonmechanical, there is an absence of bowel sounds.

Loss of fluid and electrolytes can lead to dehydration, with its associated symptoms of extreme thirst, drowsiness, aching, and general malaise. The lower in the GI tract the obstruction is, the greater the abdominal distention. An uncorrected obstruction can lead to shock and possibly death.

Diagnostic Tests
Dilated loops of bowel are evident in radiographic studies and CT scans. If strangulation or perforation occurs, leukocytosis is evident. Hematocrit levels are elevated if the patient is dehydrated and serum electrolyte levels are decreased.

Therapeutic Measures
In most cases, the patient is NPO. The bowel is decompressed using an NG tube to suction, which relieves symptoms and may allow the obstruction to resolve on its own. An IV solution with electrolytes is initiated to correct the fluid and electrolyte imbalance. Complete mechanical obstruction requires surgical intervention, such as removal of tumors, release of adhesions, or a bowel resection with anastomosis.

Large-Bowel Obstruction
Pathophysiology
Obstruction in the large bowel is less common and not usually as dramatic as small-bowel obstruction. Radiological examination reveals a distended colon. Dehydration occurs more slowly because of the colon's ability to absorb fluid and distend well beyond its normal full capacity. If the blood supply to the colon is cut off, the patient's life is in jeopardy because of bowel strangulation and necrosis.

Etiology
Most large-bowel obstructions occur in the sigmoid colon and are caused by carcinoma, IBD, diverticulitis, or benign tumors. Impaction of stool may also cause obstruction.

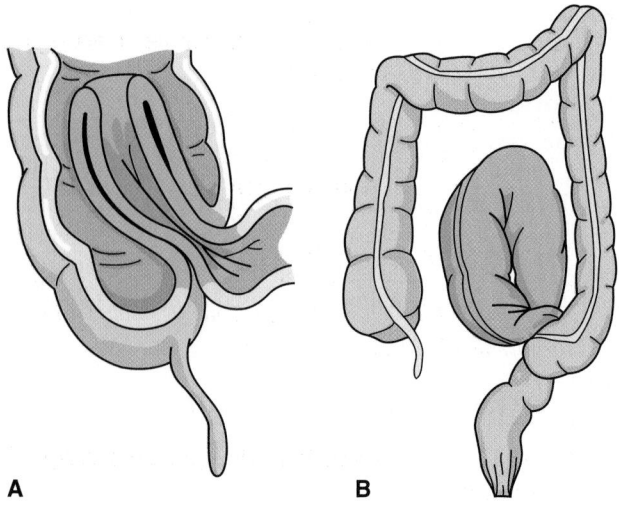

A   **B**

FIGURE 34.5 Mechanical bowel obstructions. (A) Intussusception. (B) Volvulus.

• WORD • BUILDING •
intussusception: intus—within + suscept—to receive

Table 34.7
Bowel Obstruction Summary

Signs and Symptoms	Wavelike abdominal pain Vomiting Possible fecal vomiting Blood and mucus from rectum Flatus and feces cease Bowel sounds high pitched, tinkling, or absent Abdominal distention
Diagnostic Tests	Abdominal x-ray examination Computed tomography (CT) scan Complete blood count (CBC) and electrolytes
Therapeutic Measures	Nothing by mouth (NPO) status Nasogastric tube Fluid and electrolyte replacement Parenteral nutrition (PN) as needed Medications (antibiotics, antiemetics, analgesics) Surgery
Priority Nursing Diagnoses	*Acute Pain* *Risk for Deficient Fluid Volume* *Risk for Electrolyte Imbalance* *Risk for Dysfunctional Gastrointestinal Motility*

Signs and Symptoms

Symptoms of large-bowel obstruction develop slowly and depend on the location of the obstruction. If the obstruction is in the rectum or sigmoid, the only symptom may be constipation. As the loops of bowel distend, the patient may report crampy lower abdominal pain and abdominal distention. Vomiting, if it occurs, is a late sign and may be fecal. High-pitched, tinkling bowel sounds may be heard. A localized tender area and mass may be felt on palpation. Large-bowel obstructions, if not diagnosed and treated, can lead to gangrene, perforation, and peritonitis.

Therapeutic Measures

If impaction is present, enemas and manual disimpaction may be effective. Other mechanical blockages may require surgical resection of the obstructed colon. A temporary colostomy may be indicated to allow the bowel to rest and heal. Sometimes, an ileoanal anastomosis is done. A stent may be placed to expand the colon to facilitate fecal movement if surgery cannot be done immediately. A patient who is a poor surgical risk may have a cecostomy (an opening from the cecum to the abdominal wall) to allow diversion of stool. A consult with the nutrition support team to evaluate for PN should be made.

Nursing Process for the Patient With a Bowel Obstruction
Data Collection

Each quadrant of the abdomen is auscultated for bowel sounds to identify the location of the obstruction. The abdomen is palpated for distention, firmness, and tenderness. The amount and character of stool, if any, are documented. Pain is monitored using the institution's pain scale and described according to location and character, such as crampy or wavelike. Vital signs are monitored for signs of infection or shock. Daily weight and I&O are monitored. Skin turgor is assessed for fluid deficit. The amount, color, and character of NG drainage are documented.

Nursing Diagnoses, Planning, and Implementation

Acute Pain related to abdominal distention

EXPECTED OUTCOME: The patient will state pain is relieved or at an acceptable level within 30 minutes of report of pain.

- Monitor pain level using rating scale *to consistently communicate pain level.*
- Give medications ordered for pain cautiously *because they may mask symptoms of perforation and decrease intestinal motility.*
- Position patient in semi-Fowler position *to reduce tension on the abdomen.*

Risk for Deficient Fluid Volume related to vomiting

EXPECTED OUTCOME: The patient will maintain vital signs and urine output within normal limits at all times.

- Accurately monitor I&O and report abnormal trends *to identify fluid deficit.*
- Maintain fluid replacement as ordered *to prevent dehydration.*

Risk for Electrolyte Imbalance related to suctioning

EXPECTED OUTCOME: The patient will maintain electrolytes within normal limits at all times.

- Monitor electrolyte values *to identify imbalances.*
- Monitor vital signs and watch for signs of electrolyte imbalances such as weakness accompanied by low potassium levels *to identify imbalances for prompt treatment.*
- Give ice chips sparingly if ordered by the HCP. *Melted ice increases electrolyte and hydrochloric acid removal when suctioned from the stomach, and electrolyte imbalance and metabolic alkalosis occur.*

Risk for Dysfunctional Gastrointestinal Motility

EXPECTED OUTCOME: The patient will maintain passage of flatus and stool.

- Monitor GI function for presence of flatus and bowel movements *to detect problems.*

- Maintain orogastric or NG tube on low intermittent suction as ordered *to relieve discomfort from distention.*
- Maintain NPO status *to rest the bowel and promote comfort.*

Evaluation

Goals are met if the patient states that pain is controlled, fluid is balanced, electrolytes are within normal limits, and GI motility is normal.

CRITICAL THINKING

Mrs. Loos is admitted for abdominal pain. She has a history of abdominal surgery. Her abdomen is distended, firm, and tender to touch. She states that she feels nauseous.

1. How would you know if Mrs. Loos might be developing a small-bowel obstruction?
2. Is she at risk for developing an obstruction?
3. If she is at risk, what data should be collected?
4. What findings would be normal?
5. How would you recognize that an obstruction is developing?
6. What should you do if the patient's data collection findings have changed?
7. How will you document the findings?
8. After treatment is started, how will you know the patient is improving, getting worse, or developing complications as a result of a bowel obstruction?

Suggested answers are at the end of the chapter.

 ## ANORECTAL PROBLEMS

Hemorrhoids

Hemorrhoids are enlarged veins within the anal tissue. They are caused by an increase in pressure in the veins, often from increased intra-abdominal pressure. Internal hemorrhoids occur above the internal sphincter, and external hemorrhoids occur below the external sphincter. Most hemorrhoids are caused by straining during bowel movements. They are common during pregnancy. Prolonged sitting or standing, obesity, and chronic constipation also contribute to hemorrhoids. Portal hypertension related to liver disease may also be a contributing factor.

Internal hemorrhoids are usually not painful unless they prolapse. They may bleed during bowel movements. External hemorrhoids cause itching and pain when inflamed and filled with blood (thrombosed). Inflammation and edema occur with thrombosis, causing severe pain and possibly infarction of the skin and mucosa over the hemorrhoid.

Treatment is aimed at preventing constipation, avoiding straining during defecation, maintaining good personal hygiene, and making lifestyle changes to relieve hemorrhoid symptoms and discomfort. Prolonged standing and sitting are avoided. Increased fluid intake and stool softeners can be used to reduce the need for straining. Daily sitz baths increase circulation to the area and aid in comfort and healing. Astringents, such as witch hazel, can be used for symptom relief. Anti-inflammatory medications may be tried, such as steroid creams or suppositories. Alternating ice and heat helps relieve edema and pain for thrombosed hemorrhoids. The blood clot is removed by a HCP.

If surgery is required for internal hemorrhoids, methods include rubber-band ligation using a rubber band around the hemorrhoid that cuts off the blood supply, causing the hemorrhoid to slough off into the stool; infrared coagulation that burns off the hemorrhoid; sclerotherapy that shrinks the hemorrhoid with a chemical solution; and hemorrhoidectomy to surgically remove the hemorrhoid.

If the patient has surgery, analgesics are given as needed because the many nerve endings in the anal canal can cause severe pain. Comfort measures such as a side-lying position and fresh ice packs can be used to relieve pain. After the first postoperative day, sitz baths may be ordered. Unfortunately, a side effect of opioid analgesics is constipation, which needs to be avoided, especially in the immediate postoperative period. Because the first bowel movement can be painful and anxiety provoking, stool softeners are given and analgesics administered before the first bowel movement.

Patient education includes prevention and self-care. The patient should be instructed to consume a high-fiber diet and 2 to 3 L of fluid a day to promote regular bowel movements. The effects and side effects, proper dosage, and frequency of local or topical medications should be explained.

Anal Fissures

Anal fissures are cracks or ulcers in the lining of the anal canal. They are most commonly associated with constipation and stretching of the anus with passage of hard stool, although Crohn disease or other factors may also play a role. The patient may experience bright red bleeding. Pain may be so severe that the patient delays defecation, leading to further constipation and worsening symptoms. Treatment of anal fissures involves measures to ensure soft stools to allow fissures time to heal. Sitz baths may be used to promote circulation to the area to aid in healing. Anesthetic suppositories and nonopioid analgesics may be ordered for comfort. If conservative measures are not helpful, surgical excision of the fissure may be needed.

Anorectal Abscess

An anorectal abscess is a collection of pus in the rectal area. Common causative organisms include *Escherichia coli, Proteus* spp., staphylococci, and streptococci. Symptoms include pain, redness and swelling, fever, and sometimes drainage. Abscesses are treated with antibiotics and surgical incision and drainage of pus. The area may be left open to drain, with gauze packing placed to assist with drainage and healing.

Nursing care includes dressing or packing changes as ordered. Sitz baths are used to keep the area clean and promote healing, especially after bowel movements. The patient is instructed in the importance of keeping the area clean and dry. Postoperative care is similar to care following hemorrhoidectomy.

 LOWER GASTROINTESTINAL BLEEDING

Etiology
Major causes of lower GI bleeding are diverticulitis, polyps (growths in the colon), anal fissures, hemorrhoids, IBD, and cancer.

Signs and Symptoms
Bleeding from the GI tract is seen in the stool. When blood has been in the GI tract for more than 8 hours and has come in contact with hydrochloric acid, it causes **melena,** or black and tarry stools. The presence of melena indicates bleeding above or in the small bowel. Bleeding from the colon or rectum is usually bright red (**hematochezia**).

Significant blood loss causes hypotension, light-headedness, nausea, and diaphoresis. The patient may be pale and have cool skin. The onset of tachycardia and worsening hypotension indicate hypovolemic shock and should be reported to the HCP immediately.

Diagnostic Tests
A thorough history is necessary to determine underlying disorders that may be causing the bleeding. Decreased hemoglobin and hematocrit levels result from blood loss. Blood urea nitrogen (BUN) may be elevated as a result of breakdown of proteins in the blood by the GI tract. Stool can be tested for occult blood if it is not evident on inspection. Digital examination, colonoscopy, or sigmoidoscopy may be done by the HCP.

Therapeutic Measures
Treatment involves correction of the cause of the bleeding. Surgery to correct diverticulosis, correct IBD, or resect cancer may be considered.

Nursing Care
Stools are checked for the presence and amount of blood. Vital signs are monitored for signs of shock. Decreasing blood pressure and rising heart rate are reported to the HCP immediately. The patient is prepared for diagnostic tests, and nursing care for the underlying disorder is provided.

 COLORECTAL CANCER

Pathophysiology and Etiology
Colorectal cancer is one of the most common types of internal cancer in the United States. It originates in the epithelial lining of the colon or rectum and can occur anywhere in the large intestine. People with a personal or family history of ulcerative colitis, colon cancer, or polyps of the rectum or large intestine are at higher risk for developing cancer. Colorectal cancer has also been linked with previous gallbladder removal and dietary carcinogens. A major causative factor is lack of fiber in the diet, which prolongs fecal transit time and in turn prolongs exposure to possible carcinogens. Also, bacterial flora is believed to be altered by excess fat, which converts steroids into compounds having carcinogenic properties. Lifestyle factors such as obesity, smoking, alcohol intake, and a large amount of red meat in the diet increase the risk of colon cancer.

Healthy People 2020 has a target goal to reduce incidence of colorectal cancer deaths per 100,000 population from 17.1 (as of 2007) to 14.5 in 2020. Data show that as of 2015 the goal has been exceeded at 14.3 (Office of Disease Prevention and Health Promotion, 2018).

Signs and Symptoms
Manifestations of colorectal cancer vary according to the type of tumor and the location. A change in bowel habits is the most common symptom (Table 34.8). Blood or mucus in stools may occur. All tumors cause varying degrees of obstruction. Tumors in the descending colon and rectum generally do not cause nausea or vomiting, anemia, or weight loss.

Diagnostic Tests
Screening for colorectal cancer in those over age 45 at average risk is the best prevention, but screening rates could be higher. Screening guidelines can be found in Chapter 11 or at the American Cancer Society web site at www.cancer.org.

Home screening for blood in the stool can be done with a home colon cancer test kit. Immunological tests look for small amounts of blood. If blood is found, an HCP is contacted for follow-up. Most colorectal cancers are identified by biopsy done at the time of endoscopy (proctosigmoidoscopy, sigmoidoscopy, or colonoscopy). A CT scan can perform a virtual colonoscopy to view the inside of the colon. The carcinoembryonic antigen (CEA) blood test is used to assess response to treatment of GI cancer. CEA is present when epithelial cells rapidly divide and provides an early warning that the cancer has returned.

Therapeutic Measures
Small, localized tumors may be excised and treated during endoscopy or laparoscopy. These procedures can also be used as palliative care for patients with advanced tumors who cannot tolerate major surgery. If a tumor is causing obstruction, a stent can be placed to keep the colon open for bowel function until surgery.

Surgery is performed either to resect larger tumors and anastomose the remaining bowel or to create a fecal diversion by forming an ostomy. A variety of surgical procedures can be done depending on the location and extent of the cancer (Table 34.9 and Fig. 34.6). Medical management can include radiation therapy, chemotherapy, and monoclonal antibody therapy. When used along with surgery, increased survival rates have been demonstrated.

• **WORD • BUILDING** •

hematochezia: hemat—blood + chezia—in stool

Table 34.8

Colon Cancer Summary

Signs and Symptoms	Change in bowel habits Blood or mucus in stools
Diagnostic Tests	Colonoscopy with biopsy Sigmoidoscopy with biopsy Proctosigmoidoscopy Barium enema Abdominal and rectal examination Fecal occult blood
Therapeutic Measures	Surgery, possibly colostomy Radiation Chemotherapy and/or radiation Medications (analgesics) Parenteral nutrition (PN) as needed Support and education
Priority Nursing Diagnoses	*Acute Pain* *Fear* *Imbalanced Nutrition: Less Than Body Requirements*

Monoclonal antibody therapy uses antibodies that are made in a laboratory and work like normal antibodies do for advanced colon cancer. They can enhance immune system function, interfere with the cancer cell's growth, or even carry treatment such as drugs or radiation to cancer cells. The antibody is designed to attach to cancer cells to flag them for the immune system so they can be destroyed. Bevacizumab (Avastin) blocks the making of new blood vessels to deprive cancer cells of nourishment. Cetuximab (Erbitux) blocks the cell's growth signal to stop it from growing. Additional medications used are panitumumab (Vectibix), regorafenib (Stivarga), ramucirumab (Cyramza), and ziv-aflibercept (Zaltrap).

Complications

Complications include bleeding, complete obstruction of the colon, perforation, anastomosis leaking leading to peritonitis, and extension of the tumor to adjacent organs. Colorectal cancer can metastasize to the lymphatic system and liver.

If the patient has an anastomotic leak, the location of the leak determines the effects that are seen. The patient may need to be NPO for up to 4 weeks to rest the GI tract and prevent more leakage as well as to receive high-dose antibiotic therapy such as ciprofloxacin (Cipro) or metronidazole

Table 34.9

Intestinal Surgeries

Types of Intestinal Surgery	Definition	Effect on Stool Elimination
Colectomy	Affected part of colon and nearby lymph nodes removed with laparoscope through smaller incisions.	Anastomosed ends. Stool is passed via rectum and anus.
Open colectomy	Affected part of colon and nearby lymph nodes removed through traditional incision.	Anastomosed ends. Stool is passed via rectum and anus.
Ileocolectomy	Right side of colon and diseased portion of ileum removed.	Anastomosed ends. Stool is passed via rectum and anus.
Hemicolectomy	Right or left side of colon removed.	Right: Colon attached to small intestine. Left: Anastomosed ends. Stool is passed via rectum and anus.
Total colectomy	Entire colon removed; rectum and anus remain.	Ileorectal anastomosis. Stool is passed via rectum and anus.
Total proctocolectomy	Entire colon, rectum, and sometimes anus removed.	Ileostomy. If anus left, ileal pouch-anal anastomosis and stool is passed via anus.

Table 34.9
Intestinal Surgeries—cont'd

Types of Intestinal Surgery	Definition	Effect on Stool Elimination
Rectal Cancer		
Local transanal resection: cancer in lower area of rectum Transanal endoscopic microsurgery: cancer higher in rectum	No incision. Rectal cancer removed through anus.	Anastomosed ends. Stool is passed via anus.
Lower anterior resection: cancer in upper two-thirds of rectum	Affected part of colon and nearby lymph nodes removed through traditional incision.	Anastomosed ends. Stool is passed via rectum and anus.
Abdominoperineal resection: cancer in lower one-third of rectum	Sigmoid colon, rectum, and anus removed.	Colostomy ends. Stool passed via ostomy.
Proctectomy: cancer in lower two-thirds of rectum	Rectum removed.	Coloanal anastomosis. Stool passed via anus.

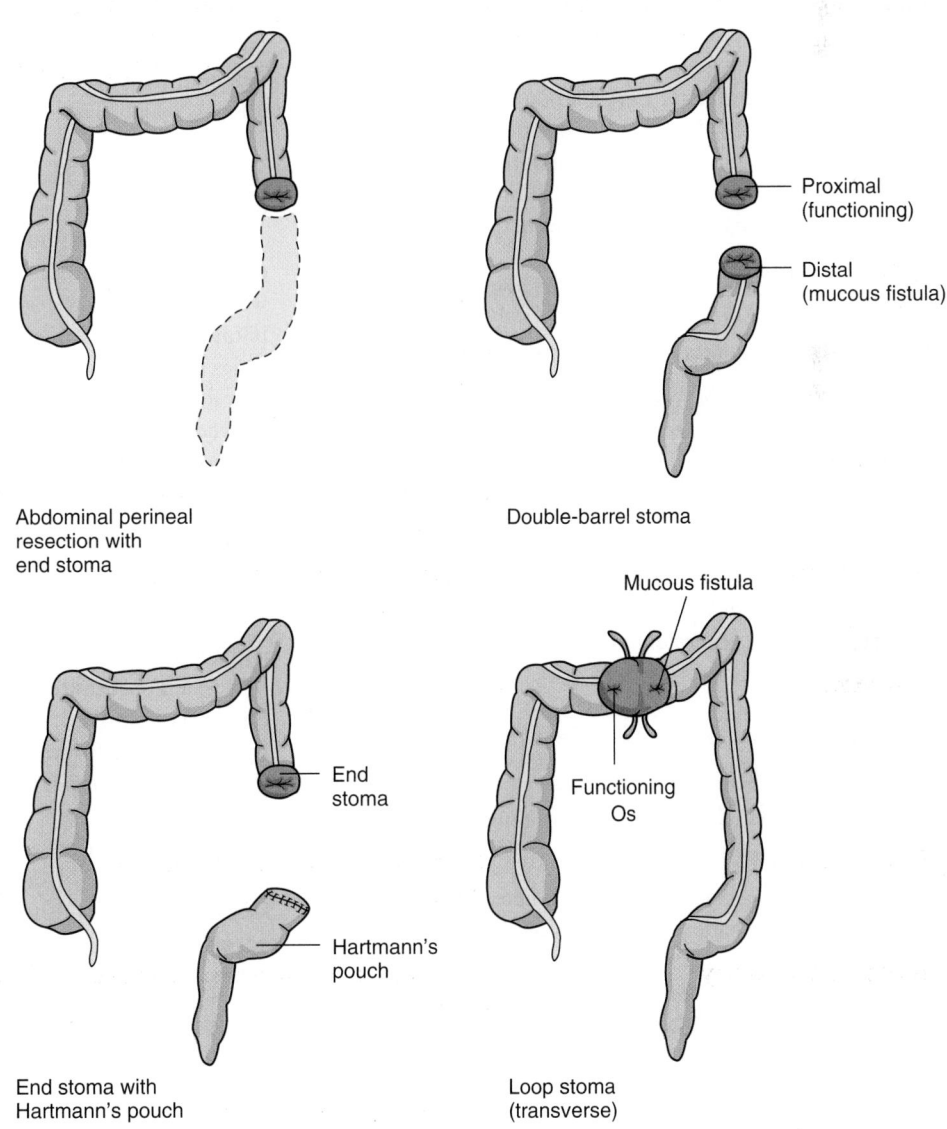

Abdominal perineal resection with end stoma

Double-barrel stoma

Proximal (functioning)

Distal (mucous fistula)

End stoma

Hartmann's pouch

End stoma with Hartmann's pouch

Mucous fistula

Functioning Os

Loop stoma (transverse)

FIGURE 34.6 Types of stomas.

(Flagyl). Ongoing monitoring includes WBCs, sedimentation rate, and fever. The patient will likely go home with special home care needs. A peripherally inserted central catheter line is placed to continue the antibiotic therapy.

Nursing Process for the Patient With Colorectal Cancer

Data Collection

Risk factors for colorectal cancer are identified by asking questions about the patient's personal and family histories: Is there a history of IBD? What are the patient's dietary habits? What foods ae usually eaten, and how much fluid is usually consumed? Prior to diagnosis, did the patient experience constipation or diarrhea? Has there been a change in bowel habits? Has mucus or blood been noted in the stools? Is there pain? What social habits does the patient have? Does the patient smoke, drink alcoholic beverages, exercise? Has there been a recent weight loss? If so, how much and over what period of time? Does the patient have unusual fatigue or insomnia? Stool is checked for mucus or blood.

If the patient has surgery, postoperative monitoring includes vital signs, pain, and the return of flatus and bowel movements. Lung sounds are monitored for response to coughing and deep breathing and early ambulation. Dressings are observed for drainage. Large amounts of drainage or bleeding are reported. If a drain is inserted in the perineal wound, moderate amounts of serosanguineous (light pink) drainage are expected. If the patient has an ostomy, it is monitored (see the ostomy section later in the chapter).

Nursing Diagnoses, Planning, and Implementation

Fear related to serious threat to well-being

EXPECTED OUTCOME: The patient will state fear is reduced after information is given related to patient's condition.

• Assist patient in identifying fears *to develop plan for reducing fears.*
• Set aside time to allow the patient who so desires to talk, cry, or ask questions about the diagnosis and planned surgery *to help reduce fear.*
• Answer questions accurately *to provide a trusting relationship.*

Imbalanced Nutrition: Less Than Body Requirements related to nausea and anorexia

EXPECTED OUTCOME: The patient will maintain normal weight for height and age.

• Give antiemetics as ordered *to relieve nausea.*
• Identify foods the patient likes and provide them *to stimulate appetite.*
• Monitor PN as ordered *to provide nutrients.*
• Provide the patient with a high-protein, high-calorie diet, as ordered, that is low in residue *to decrease excessive peristalsis and minimize cramping.*

Evaluation

Expected outcomes are that the patient verbalizes less fear and attains an optimum level of nutrition.

OSTOMY AND CONTINENT OSTOMY MANAGEMENT

An ostomy is a surgically created opening (traditional abdominal incision or laparoscopic) that diverts stool (or urine) to the outside of the body through an opening on the abdomen called a **stoma.** A stoma is the portion of bowel that is sutured onto the abdomen. A continent ostomy uses an internal reservoir to collect stool. The types of abdominal ostomies include ileostomy, colostomy, and urostomy. (Urinary ostomies are discussed in Chapter 37.) The stomas can be end, loop, or double barrel (see Fig. 34.6).

Ileostomy

An **ileostomy** is an end stoma formed by bringing the terminal ileum out to the abdominal wall following a total proctocolectomy. Two types of ileostomies can be formed: a conventional ileostomy and a continent ileostomy, such as a Kock pouch (sometimes called a Koch pouch) or Barnett continent internal reservoir, which is a modification of a Kock pouch (Fig. 34.7). A conventional ileostomy has a small stoma in the right lower quadrant that requires a pouch at all times because of the continuous flow of liquid effluent.

Continent ileostomies are formed by taking a portion of the terminal ileum to construct an internal reservoir with a nipple valve. A stoma is created, and the patient is taught to insert a catheter into the stoma three or four times a day to empty the reservoir. A continent ileostomy surgical procedure takes longer and requires additional instruction for the patient to be able to do self-care. It is important for the patient to empty the pouch routinely to prevent pouch rupture. Complications can occur, especially for the Kock pouch, such as valve slippage or leaking, pouch rupture, or pouchitis. Corrective surgery may be required.

An ileoanal anastomosis connects the ileum to the anus and avoids the need for a stoma (Fig. 34.8). This is usually a two-step procedure. During the first surgery, the diseased bowel is removed. A reservoir (named by its shape, J pouch) is then formed from part of the ileum and connected to the anus. A temporary ileostomy is also formed to divert stool while the reservoir heals. After about 3 months, the temporary ileostomy is reversed and the patient can have bowel movements from the anus. Problems with perianal skin irritation resulting from frequent liquid stools may occur.

• WORD • BUILDING •

ileostomy: ileo—pertaining to ileum + stoma—mouth or opening

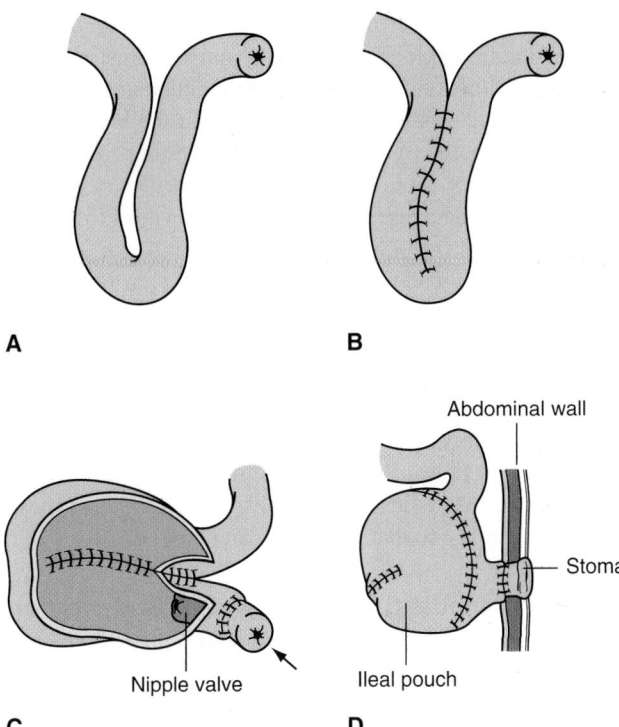

FIGURE 34.7 Surgical formation of continent ileostomy (Kock pouch). (A) Loop of terminal ileum. (B) Both limbs of ileum are brought together and sutured into a U shape. (C) Pouch created with nipple valve. (D) Pouch sutured to abdominal wall.

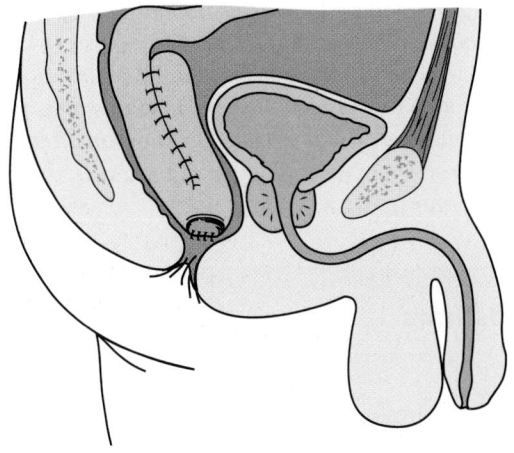

FIGURE 34.8 Ileal J pouch-anal anastomosis. The two-loop ileal pouch is simple to construct, provides adequate storage capacity, and is evacuated spontaneously and fully.

LEARNING TIP

As stool travels through the colon, water is absorbed and the stool becomes firmer. Therefore, an ileostomy produces the most liquid effluent, followed by an ascending colostomy. A descending or sigmoid colostomy produces the firmest stool. Those with an ileostomy are at increased risk for dehydration because of greater water loss.

Colostomy

A colostomy is named according to where in the bowel it is formed; it may be an ascending, transverse, descending, or sigmoid colostomy. The type of effluent is dependent on the location of the bowel used (Table 34.10).

End Stoma

An end stoma is formed when the proximal end of the bowel is brought to the outside abdominal wall. If an abdominoperineal (AP) resection is done, the rectum is removed, and the proximal sigmoid or descending colon is brought out as a stoma. Another procedure that may be done involves removing the segment of diseased or injured bowel and using the proximal portion to form the stoma. The remaining limb of bowel is sutured closed and left in the peritoneal cavity so that the rectum is intact. This is called a Hartmann's pouch, or mucous fistula, and may be permanent or temporary depending on the diagnosis. Because the rectum is intact, the patient may feel the urge to defecate. This is normal because the colon continues to produce mucus. As the rectal stump fills with mucus, the sphincter is triggered and alerts the patient as though stool were present.

Loop Stoma

To create a loop stoma, a loop of bowel, usually the transverse colon, is pulled to the outside abdominal wall and a bridge is slipped under the loop to hold it in place. An incisional slit is made in the top of the exposed colon to allow stool to exit. The entire loop of bowel is not cut through.

Double-Barrel Stoma

With a double-barrel stoma, the bowel is completely dissected. Both ends of the colon are brought to the outside abdominal wall to form two separate stomas. The proximal stoma is the functioning stoma that expels stool. The distal stoma is called a mucous fistula because mucus produced by the bowel passes from it. A double-barrel stoma is often temporary, allowing the bowel to rest during healing after trauma or surgery.

Preoperative Care

A wound, ostomy, and continence nurse (WOCN) should be consulted before surgery. The WOCN can help prepare the patient both emotionally and physically for the surgery. In addition, the WOCN has expertise in selecting the stoma site for the surgeon to ensure that it is easy to sit with it, care for it, and wear clothing over it. This involves observing the abdomen as the patient assumes various positions to note how clothing is worn, such as where a belt rests. The site for the stoma can then be chosen so it is visible to the patient for self-care, avoids skin or fat folds, and is placed where clothing will not interfere with the appliance. Properly planned

• WORD • BUILDING •

colostomy: colo—pertaining to colon + stoma—mouth or opening

Table 34.10
Location of Stomas and Type of Effluent

Location of Stoma	Type of Effluent
Ileostomy	Liquid to mushy
Cecostomy, ascending colostomy	Liquid to mushy, foul odor
Right transverse colostomy	Mushy to semiformed
Left transverse colostomy	Semiformed, soft
Descending or sigmoid colostomy	Soft to hard formed

stoma placement can prevent discomfort when sitting, inability to perform self-care, and uncomfortable, leaking, or poorly fitting appliances postoperatively.

Routine preoperative instruction, including the importance of coughing and deep breathing, splinting, and early ambulation, is provided. Orders for cleansing of the bowel are performed to reduce the risk for infection following surgery. Unless the patient has chronic diarrhea related to IBD, an oral agent to cleanse the bowel is given.

Nursing Process for the Patient With a New or Established Ostomy or Continent Ostomy
Data Collection

For a patient with a new ostomy, in addition to routine postoperative assessment, a stoma should be inspected at least every 8 hours. The stoma should be pink to red, moist (similar to the inside of the mouth), and well attached to the surrounding skin (Fig. 34.9). A bluish stoma indicates inadequate blood supply; a black stoma indicates necrosis. Either complication should be reported to the HCP immediately for treatment, which may require that the patient return to surgery. Note edema of the stoma. The stoma size will gradually decrease over the first few weeks following surgery.

For both new and established ostomies, skin is assessed for irritation around the pouch and under the pouch each time it is changed. Ostomy discharge (effluent) is monitored and documented. Unexpected changes, such as liquid stool from a descending ostomy, are reported. For the patient with a continent ostomy pouch, monitoring that regular emptying of the pouch is done is important to prevent rupture and leakage. The characteristics of the stool are noted for any type of continent ostomy so that problems can be reported.

Nursing Diagnoses, Planning, and Implementation
See "Nursing Care Plan for the Patient With an Intestinal Ostomy" and Table 34.11.

Deficient Knowledge related to ostomy

EXPECTED OUTCOME: The patient will demonstrate how to care for ostomy.

- Determine patient readiness and ability to learn and perform self-care. *The patient experiencing pain, nausea, or vomiting is not likely to be ready to look at the ostomy or learn about ostomy care.*
- Include the caregiver in teaching if the patient is not ready or able to learn. *With short hospital stays, time for teaching is limited and must begin soon after surgery.*

Nursing Care Plan for the Patient With an Intestinal Ostomy

Nursing Diagnosis: *Disturbed Body Image* related to new ostomy
Expected Outcome: The patient will verbalize acceptance of intestinal ostomy before discharge.
Evaluation of Outcome: Does the patient verbalize acceptance of the ostomy?

Intervention	Rationale	Evaluation
Identify knowledge of self-care of ostomies and feelings about the stoma.	*Identification of misconceptions and "hearsay" knowledge is important to clarify or correct.*	Does patient verbalize appropriate knowledge of ostomy care and express feelings?
Explain the normal characteristics of the stoma before patient's first look.	*Helping patient understand what to expect will help relieve anxiety.*	Does patient look at the stoma without hesitation?
Demonstrate ostomy appliance change and daily care, and encourage patient participation.	*When patient observes and participates in self-care, self-concept improves.*	Is patient participating in self-care? Has patient performed return demonstration of appliance change and emptying of pouch?

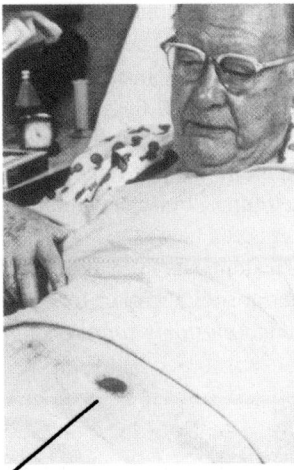

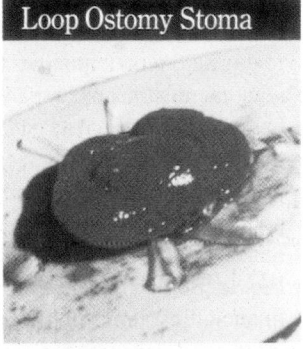

Loop Ostomy Stoma

Colostomy Stoma

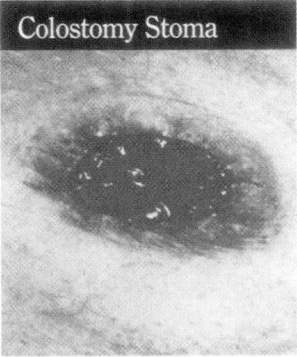

Man above has a descending or "dry" colostomy.

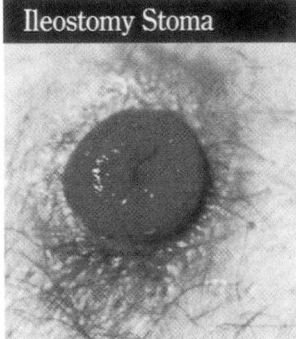

Ileostomy Stoma

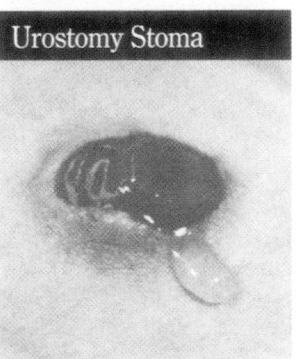

Urostomy Stoma

FIGURE 34.9 Images of stomas. Note moist, pink to red appearance of healthy stoma. Reproduced with permission of Hollister Inc., Libertyville, IL.

- Consult a WOCN or ostomy equipment supplier if needed *to identify appliances suited to individual patient's needs.* Figure 34.10 shows types of appliances.
- Ensure referral to a home health nurse is made *to continue teaching in the patient's home.*
- Provide special instructions or a specific type of ostomy appliance for patients with special needs, such as blindness, deafness, language barrier, severe arthritis, or other physical conditions that limit ability to perform self-care, *so they will be able to perform self-care.*
- Explain how to change appliance (Fig. 34.11) *to promote self-care.*
- Demonstrate how to apply appliance using moldable or traditional skin barrier to promote self-care. *A moldable (able to change shape) skin barrier does not require measuring a pattern or cutting and does not leave a gap around the stoma.*

- For the traditional skin barrier:
  - Measure stoma with a stoma-sizing guide initially with each appliance change *because the stoma will shrink for up to 6 months.*
  - Trace the stoma pattern on the cut-to-fit skin barrier and cut to fit, if using a nonmoldable barrier, *to teach the patient proper size and shape because most stomas are not round.*
  - Apply a moldable barrier ring or strips to the skin barrier as needed to fill in gaps or fit convex shapes *to protect the skin and prevent leakage.*
  - Fit the traditional skin barrier over the stoma on the skin with no gaps around the base of the stoma *to prevent skin contact with stool.*
- Change appliance first thing in the morning every 3 days or every 10 to 14 days depending on the type of appliance *to reduce skin shearing from frequent removal.*
- Change appliance immediately if leakage occurs *to avoid **peristomal** skin irritation.*
- Use an open-ended or drainable pouch for all colostomies or ileostomies, especially during the first 8 weeks after surgery *to facilitate emptying and comfort.*
  - Explain to the patient who has a left-sided (descending or sigmoid) colostomy that the bowel can be regulated either by diet or regular irrigation of the stoma. After bowel regulation has been achieved, the patient may use a closed-end pouch or a stoma cap.
- Explain daily care and hygiene:
  - Empty pouch when it is one-third to one-half full. The amount of effluent and the frequency of emptying depend on the location of the stoma in the bowel. *If the pouch is allowed to become more than half full of stool, the weight of the effluent will pull on the pouch and weaken the seal of the skin barrier.*
  - Empty the pouch and then clean inside of the tail of the pouch before the self-seal or clamp is replaced *to help control odor.*
  - Place deodorants in the pouch *to control odor.*
  - Bathe or shower with the appliance in place but check seal and retape or change it if it is loosening. *Water will not harm stoma or leak into stoma.*
- Explain diet considerations ("Nutrition Notes: Dietary Management of Ostomies").

Readiness for Enhanced Health Management related to difficulty carrying out self-care measures

EXPECTED OUTCOME: The patient will demonstrate ability to perform self-care measures.

- Identify financial ability *to obtain supplies.* The cost and availability of ostomy supplies is problematic for many patients. Most insurers, including Medicare, pay for ostomy supplies, although some limit the type of appliance and number allowed per month. Each state-funded

• WORD • BUILDING •
peristomal: peri—surrounding + stoma—mouth or opening

Nutrition Notes

Dietary Management of Ostomies. Ostomy patients receive a soft diet initially, progressing to a general diet as the health care provider prescribes and is tolerated. Stringy, high-fiber foods are initially avoided. Then, they are best tried in small amounts, one at a time, until tolerance has been demonstrated. They include the following:

- Cabbage (including coleslaw and sauerkraut), corn, peas, and spinach
- Coconut, dried fruit, pineapple, and membranes on citrus fruits
- Popcorn, nuts, seeds, and skins of fruits and vegetables

Legumes, cruciferous vegetables (broccoli, Brussels sprouts), eggs, fish, beer, and carbonated beverages might be avoided because they produce excessive flatus and subsequent odor.

Low-fiber foods may be more easily tolerated:

- Applesauce and bananas
- Cheese
- Creamy peanut butter
- Pasta, white bread, and white rice

Patients with ostomies should be encouraged to:

- Drink adequate amounts of fluid.
- Eat at regular intervals.
- Chew food completely to avoid blockage of the stoma.
- Avoid foods that produce excessive gas, loose stools, offensive odors, and undesirable bulk.
- Avoid excessive weight gain.

Medicaid system is different. The type of appliance needed to eliminate leakage may not always be covered, requiring the patient either to pay the difference or wear what the insurance company will provide. If the patient has no insurance, costs can be high. Some patients find they have to choose whether to purchase ostomy appliances or prescriptions with their limited funds. Fortunately, the pouches in most two-piece systems can be washed out and reused to save money ("Home Health Hints").

- Provide referral to case manager or social worker for financial resources *in order to obtain ostomy supplies.*

Home Health Hints

- Some ostomy supplies may be covered by insurance. Record product numbers for ease of reordering. Most companies will deliver supplies to the patient's home.
- If the patient requires a stool for occult blood test, deliver a collection device (hat) to assist with obtaining the specimen before your visit. Plan to deliver the specimen to the laboratory the day it is collected.
- Teach patients about their diet and provide written instructions.

Sexual Dysfunction related to body image change or erectile dysfunction

EXPECTED OUTCOME: The patient will discuss satisfying acceptable sexual practices for self and partner.

- Identify if a male patient who had an AP resection is experiencing erectile dysfunction. *This impotence may be*

Table 34.11

Summary of Recovery from Intestinal Surgery

Intestinal Surgery	Elimination Needs	Discharge Teaching Needs	Possible Psychological Needs
Total colectomy	Normal or continent anal passage	Continent ostomy care. Soft diet until first doctor visit. Monitor for constipation and report.	Chronic sorrow related to inflammatory bowel disease (IBD)
Hemicolectomy (right or left) or ileocolectomy	Normal, no appliance needed	Avoid stress to abdomen: heavy lifting, sit-ups. Soft diet until first doctor visit. Monitor for constipation and report.	Fear of cancer Chronic sorrow related to IBD
Partial colectomy	Normal, no appliance needed	Monitor for constipation.	Fear of cancer

Table 34.11

Summary of Recovery from Intestinal Surgery—cont'd

Intestinal Surgery	Elimination Needs	Discharge Teaching Needs	Possible Psychological Needs
Abdominoperineal resection	Pouch	Ostomy care.	Fear of cancer Body image changes
Proctosigmoidectomy	Normal, no appliance needed	Soft diet until first doctor visit. Monitor for constipation and report.	Fear of cancer
Total proctocolectomy	Continent anal passage or pouch	Continent ostomy care. Soft diet until first doctor visit. Monitor for constipation and report.	Chronic sorrow related to IBD

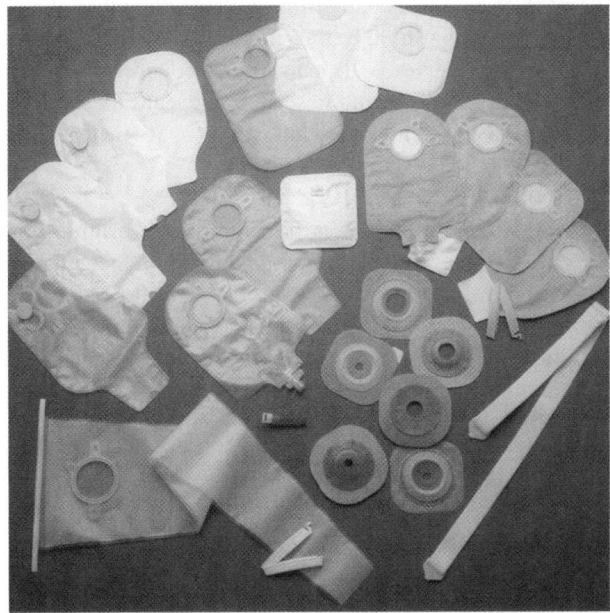

FIGURE 34.10 Appliances used for ostomies. The long sleeve at the lower left of the photograph is used to drain the bowel following irrigation. Reproduced with permission of Hollister Inc., Libertyville, IL.

transient, depending on the severity of nerve damage or edema associated with the surgery.
• Ensure consultation with urologist is made *to treat erectile dysfunction if present.*
• Encourage the patient to discuss concerns regarding sexuality with his or her sexual partner. *This may help them work through any fears or embarrassment.*
• Explain that attractive pouch covers can be purchased and worn *to help disguise the pouch and its contents.*
• Encourage personal hygiene and emptying ostomy pouch before sexual encounters *to decrease odors and enhance experience.*

Risk for Injury related to skin and stomal complications

EXPECTED OUTCOME: The patient will remain free from injury with intact skin; red, moist stoma; and functioning ostomy.

• Consult WOCN for complications associated with care of the ostomy. *A WOCN has had specialized instruction in caring for the stoma and peristomal skin.*
• Identify allergies *to prevent allergic dermatitis from sensitivity to the adhesive from developing.*
• Use a protective skin paste *to prevent skin breakdown from leakage.*
• Apply a stoma powder to absorb moisture from broken skin around the stoma *to allow the skin to heal.*
• Remove tape and adhesive only when necessary *to prevent skin shearing from frequent removal.*
• Leave pouches on for several days unless leakage occurs *to prevent skin shearing from frequent removal.*
• Monitor for peristomal hernia *to detect hernias that may develop around the stoma as a result of weakened abdominal muscles and cause leakage by the change in body contours associated with the hernia.*
• Use a more flexible ostomy appliance if peristomal hernia is present *to fit body contours better.*
• Monitor for and report stomal prolapse, especially in older adults. *Weakened abdominal muscles contribute to the falling down (or out) of the intestinal mucosa, which can make pouching difficult.*
• Monitor stoma color and immediately report dusky or blue color, *which occurs when there is circulatory compromise.* This may arise as a result of vascular collapse, blockage in the mesentery of the intestines, or edema in the intestine from obstruction proximal to the stoma. Usually, necrotic tissue occurs only at the very end of the stoma and will eventually slough off, revealing viable mucosa.

Preparation of the Stomahesive Wafer with Sur-Fit Flange

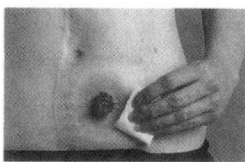

1. Cleanse the peristomal area with water and pat thoroughly dry. Measure your stoma size with the measuring guide provided and trace the proper opening on the white paper backing of the Stomahesive® disc.

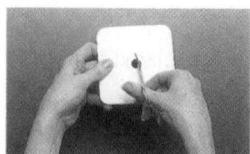

2. Leaving the white paper backing of the wafer in place, cut a hole in the wafer to the same shape and size as the base of the stoma. The best result is usually obtained by cutting from the reverse side of the wafer, using curved, short-bladed scissors.

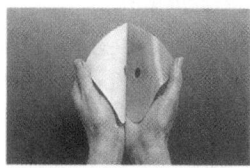

3. Peel the white paper backing from the wafer just prior to application.

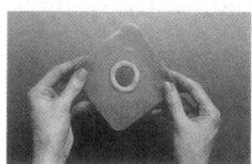

4. Gaps between the wafer and the base of the stoma may be further protected by applying Stomahesive® Paste to the wafer.

Application of the Stomahesive Wafer with Sur-Fit Flange

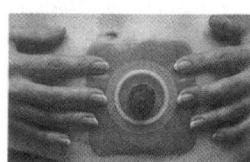

5. Center the enlarged hole over the stoma, place on abdomen, and apply light pressure.

FIGURE 34.11 Preparation to apply an ostomy appliance. Courtesy ConvaTec, a Bristol-Myers Squibb Company, Princeton, NJ, with permission.

- Explain signs and symptoms of an ileostomy blockage (e.g., absent stool, abdominal cramping, edematous stoma, and stoma color that is pale or dusky) *to allow it to be treated.*
- Have the patient recall what was eaten in the past 24 hours if intestinal blockage occurs *because certain foods are considered to cause stomal blockage.*
- Have the patient get into a tub of warm water (not too hot or cold), get into a knee-to-chest position, and sip on warm liquid, such as coffee, tea, bouillon, broth, or hot chocolate, for an ileostomy blockage. *If the blockage is partial, relief will occur fairly soon after these measures are taken.*
- Explain to the patient that if no relief from an intestinal blockage is obtained, medical treatment should be sought. *For a complete blockage, an ileostomy lavage must be performed by a HCP or WOCN.*

Evaluation

The plan of care has been effective if the patient is able to accept the change in body image, competently care for the ostomy (or caregiver will), carry out self-care, is satisfied with sexual practices, and describes self-care measures to prevent injury or treat complications.

Rehabilitative Needs

Ensuring that the patient is becoming comfortable with self-care, is able to perform the ostomy appliance change, and is able to return to work or social activities as before are the goals of care. The patient can generally perform any activity he or she was able to do before the ostomy including swimming.

SUGGESTED ANSWERS TO CRITICAL THINKING

Mrs. Burns

Collect data about the situation before intervening. First, ask Mrs. Burns or her caregivers whether she had a bowel movement that was inadvertently not charted. Next, ask Mrs. Burns whether she feels constipated or whether she has abdominal discomfort. Check Mrs. Burns's abdomen for distention and presence or absence of bowel sounds. A digital examination may be necessary to determine whether a fecal impaction is present. If simple constipation appears to be the problem, the medical record should be checked for as-needed laxative or enema orders. Once Mrs. Burns has had a bowel movement, laxatives should be discontinued and preventive measures such as regular fluids, fiber, and exercise should be instituted.

Judy Moore

1. Ask about characteristics of pain (e.g., location, quality, intensity, precipitating factors, relieving factors), characteristics of bowel elimination (frequency, characteristic of stool, amount, color, consistency), nutritional status (weight loss, appetite, daily food intake, food likes/dislikes, irritating foods, fluid intake), and anxiety and coping skills (support systems, usual coping methods).
2. Appropriate nursing diagnoses include: *Acute Pain* related to increased peristalsis and cramping; *Diarrhea* related to inflammatory process; *Risk for Deficient Fluid Volume* related to diarrhea and insufficient fluid intake; *Anxiety* related to symptoms and frequency of stools and treatment; *Impaired Skin Integrity* related to frequent loose stools; *Imbalanced Nutrition, Less Than Body Requirements* related to malabsorption; and *Ineffective Coping* related to frequency of stools.
3. Further explore how Judy perceives that Crohn disease will affect her lifestyle. What does she know about Crohn disease? What is she concerned about? How has Crohn disease affected her ability to sleep, what she eats, her participation in sports, and her relationships with other people? Convey a caring attitude to Judy by being accepting of her, listening actively to her concerns, and helping her to find acceptable ways of resolving them. Provide her with information that she needs about Crohn disease. Arrange to have a Crohn's & Colitis Foundation representative, one who has adapted well to an ostomy and who is approximately Judy's age, meet with her to share coping strategies with her.
4. Increased frequency of stools leading to fluid volume deficit and possibly shock symptoms; bleeding leading to anemia and hypovolemia and possibly shock symptoms.
5. Health care provider (HCP), dietitian, psychologist, registered nurse.

Mrs. Loos

1. The first consideration is to be aware of whether the patient is at risk for a small-bowel obstruction. After abdominal surgery, loops of intestine may adhere to areas in the abdomen that are not healed, causing a kink in the bowel that occludes the intestinal flow.
2. Yes, due to her history of abdominal surgery, she is at risk of adhesion development that can cause obstruction. If data collection findings confirm this possibility, the HCP should be contacted. Because of the nausea and the potential obstruction, withhold food and oral fluids until the HCP is consulted.
3. Begin by asking the *WHAT'S UP?* questions, including exactly where the pain is occurring, how it feels, whether there is anything that aggravates or alleviates the pain, when it started, how bad it is on a scale of 0 to 10, whether there are associated symptoms, and whether Mrs. Loos has some insight regarding the cause of her problem. Then, in this order, inspect, auscultate, and palpate; doing the examination in this order prevents palpation from changing other assessment findings. Inspect her abdomen to note distention. Listen for bowel sounds in each quadrant. Lightly palpate her abdomen, noting tenderness or rigidity. Ask when her last bowel movement was.
4. Bowel sounds normal in all quadrants, abdomen flat, soft with no tenderness, flatus present.
5. Abnormal bowel sounds, absent for a nonmechanical obstruction or a mechanical obstruction; high-pitched, tinkling bowel sounds proximal to the obstruction and absent distal to it; pain; abdominal distention.
6. Findings should be discussed with the registered nurse or HCP. New orders such as a nasogastric tube, NPO (nothing by mouth) status, and pain management should be anticipated.
7. When documenting, answer what, why, when, where, how, and who (either explicitly or implicitly by professional knowledge, in narrative or flow sheet format) for completeness:

   What = Patient is experiencing large, firm, tender to touch abdomen with nausea (additional assessment data should be included).

   Why = Unknown, HCP notified

   When = Current date and time

   Where = Abdomen

   How = Unknown

   Who = S. Snyder, LPN
8. If improving, symptoms will be resolving: no nausea, abdomen soft, bowel sounds present in all quadrants, flatus present, and bowel movements normal. If condition is worsening or complications are developing, symptoms will not improve, and fecal vomiting and shock may occur.

Review Questions

1. The nurse is collecting data on a patient admitted with a history of severe diarrhea. Findings include cool, pale skin, and red tongue with furrows. Vitals signs are blood pressure 102/74 mm Hg, pulse 106 beats per minute, respirations 20 breaths per minute, and temperature 99.9°F (37.7°C). Which action should the nurse take now?
   1. Apply warm blankets.
   2. Give acetaminophen (Tylenol) as ordered.
   3. Obtain bedside commode.
   4. Report findings to registered nurse.

2. The nurse is caring for a patient after an appendectomy. Which of the following interventions should the nurse include in the patient's plan of care to prevent respiratory complications? **Select all that apply.**
   1. Pain control
   2. Early ambulation
   3. Bedrest
   4. Coughing and deep breathing
   5. Incentive spirometer

3. The nurse is reinforcing patient teaching. Which of the following foods would the nurse reinforce that the patient with ulcerative colitis is to avoid?
   1. Fresh fruits
   2. White bread
   3. Sweet dessert
   4. Meat

4. The nurse participated in a patient's teaching session for care to prevent respiratory complications after a hernia repair. Which statement by the patient would indicate to the nurse that the patient understood the teaching?
   1. "I will cough every hour while awake."
   2. "I will deep breathe four times daily."
   3. "I will cough and deep breathe every hour."
   4. "I will deep breathe every hour while awake."

5. The nurse would evaluate the patient as understanding diet teaching for celiac disease if the patient selected which of the following breakfast foods to eat? **Select all that apply.**
   1. Fresh fruit and oatmeal with milk
   2. Tomato juice and waffles
   3. Hard-boiled egg, bacon, and blueberries
   4. Banana, cream of wheat cereal, and coffee
   5. Scrambled eggs and orange juice
   6. Protein smoothie with carrots and spinach

6. The nurse is caring for a patient with a small-bowel obstruction who is NPO (nothing by mouth) with an orogastric tube on low intermittent suction. Which of the following ongoing data would be a priority for the nurse to monitor and collect? **Select all that apply.**
   1. Intake and output
   2. Pain level
   3. Temperature
   4. Pulse rate
   5. Edema
   6. Firmness of abdomen or distention

7. The nurse is caring for a patient who has a sudden onset of diarrhea with black tarry stools. Which action should the nurse take?
   1. Obtain vital signs.
   2. Monitor output.
   3. Ask about a history of food allergies.
   4. Place the patient on nothing by mouth status.

8. Which of these patient's dietary habits does the nurse understand may increase the risk for development of colon cancer?
   1. Low meat and protein intake
   2. High intake of milk and milk products
   3. High-fat, low-fiber intake
   4. Low-fat, high-carbohydrate intake

9. The nurse is caring for a 1-day postoperative patient who has a new end colostomy that is a dusky color. Which action is the priority for the nurse to take?
   1. Check the stoma drainage in 1 hour.
   2. Monitor the stoma color in 4 hours.
   3. Place a new ostomy appliance over the stoma.
   4. Report this finding to the health care provider now.

10. A patient with Crohn disease is to receive sulfasalazine (Azulfidine) 500 mg oral suspension four times daily. The oral suspension is available as 250 mg/5 mL. How many milliliters should the nurse give for the 0800 dose?
   1. 5 mL
   2. 10 mL
   3. 20 mL
   4. 50 mL

Answer rationales available in your online resources.

ANSWERS 1. 4; 2. 1, 2, 4, 5; 3. 1; 4. 4; 5. 3, 5, 6; 6. 1, 2, 3, 4, 6; 7. 1; 8. 3; 9. 4; 10. 2

Key Points

Find the chapter key points in your online resources
available through Davis Edge.

Additional Resources

Use the scratch off code on the inside front
cover of your book to access online quizzes
that will help you to improve your scores
on course exams and prepare for the NCLEX-PN®.

 Study Guide

CHAPTER 35
Nursing Care of Patients With Liver, Pancreatic, and Gallbladder Disorders

Linda S. Williams

KEY TERMS

ascites (ah-SY-teez)
asterixis (AS-tur-IK-sis)
cholecystitis (KOH-lee-sis-TY-tis)
choledocholithiasis (koh-LED-oh-koh-lih-THIGH-ah-sis)
cholelithiasis (KOH-lee-lih-THIGH-ah-sis)
cirrhosis (sih-ROH-sis)
colic (KAW-lick)
encephalopathy (en-SEF-uh-LAW-pah-thee)
extracorporeal shock-wave lithotripsy (EKS-trah-kor-POR-ee-uhl SHAWK-WAYV LITH-oh-TRIP-see)
fetor hepaticus (FEE-tur heh-PAT-tih-kus)
hepatitis (HEP-uh-TY-tis)
hepatorenal syndrome (heh-PAT-oh-REE-nuhl SIN-drohm)
laparoscopy (LAP-uh-ROS-kuh-pee)
pancreatectomy (PAN-kree-uh-TEK-tuh-mee)
pancreatitis (PAN-cree-uh-TY-tis)
portal hypertension (POR-tuhl HY-per-TEN-shun)
transjugular intrahepatic portosystemic shunt (TRANZ-jug-yoo-lur in-trah-heh-PAT-tik por-toe-sis-TEM-ik SHUNT)
varices (VAR-i-seez)

LEARNING OUTCOMES

1. Explain the causes, risk factors, and pathophysiology of the various types of liver disease.
2. Describe therapeutic measures used for patients with liver disease.
3. Plan nursing care for the patient experiencing a liver disorder.
4. Explain the causes, risk factors, and pathophysiology of the various pancreatic disorders.
5. Describe therapeutic measures used for patients with pancreatic disorders.
6. Plan nursing care for a patient with a pancreatic disorder.
7. Explain the causes, risk factors, and pathophysiology of gallbladder disorders.
8. Describe therapeutic measures used for patients with gallbladder disorders.
9. Plan nursing care for the patient with a gallbladder disorder.

CHAPTER CONCEPTS

Cognition
Infection
Inflammation
Nutrition

 ## DISORDERS OF THE LIVER

Hepatitis

Hepatitis is inflammation of the liver resulting from viral or bacterial infection; drugs, alcohol, or chemicals toxic to the liver; and metabolic or vascular disorders. Symptoms of hepatitis range from no symptoms to life-threatening symptoms due to death of liver tissue. Viral hepatitis, which is common, is discussed here.

Pathophysiology and Etiology
Viral hepatitis is caused by one of five viruses:

• Hepatitis A virus (HAV)
• Hepatitis B virus (HBV)
• Hepatitis C virus (HCV)
• Hepatitis D virus (HDV)
• Hepatitis E virus (HEV)

The viral agents vary by mode of transmission, incubation period, symptoms, diagnostic tests, vaccines, and postexposure prophylaxis (Table 35.1). The infecting organism causes inflammation of the liver, with resulting damage to liver cells and liver function. If damage involves the bile canaliculi (thin tubes that collect secreted bile), obstructive jaundice will occur. If complications do not

• WORD • BUILDING •
hepatitis: hepat—liver + itis—inflammation

Table 35.1

Viral Hepatitis Infections

	Hepatitis A (HAV)	Hepatitis B (HBV)	Hepatitis C (HCV)	Hepatitis D (HDV)	Hepatitis E (HEV)
Mode of transmission	Fecal–oral route: fecal contact; fecal-contaminated food, water, or raw shellfish from poor hand hygiene by infected person or inadequate sanitation.	Blood or body fluids such as saliva, semen, menstrual or vaginal fluid; equipment contaminated by infected blood.	Blood transfusions, IV drug use. Rarer: unprotected sex.	Blood or body fluids. Co-infection with HBV required for HDV replication.	Water contaminated with human feces or raw or undercooked pork or venison.
Incubation period	14–28 days	30–180 days	2 weeks to 6 months	30–180 days	15–60 days
Signs/symptoms, if they occur	Prodromal: anorexia, fatigue, malaise, nausea, vomiting. Icteric: jaundice, pale stools, pruritus, dark urine, RUQ pain.	Most asymptomatic. Prodromal: 1–2 months of fatigue, malaise, anorexia, fever, nausea, headache, RUQ pain, myalgia. Icteric: jaundice, rashes.	Many asymptomatic. Same as HBV, but usually less severe.	Most asymptomatic. Same as HBV with coinfection but more severe.	Prodromal: anorexia, dehydration, myalgia, nausea, RUQ pain, vomiting, fever. Icteric: jaundice, pale stools, pruritus, dark urine.
Diagnostic tests	**Anti-HAV IgM** Acute infection. **Anti-HAV IgG** Recovery and immunity to virus.	**HBsAg** Surface antigen of virus. Appears 1–10 weeks postexposure. Disappears 4–6 months after recovery. Continued presence indicates chronic infection. **Anti-HBs IgM** Antibody to surface antigen that attacks HBV. Provides immunity to HBV.	**Anti-HCV** Antibody to virus made after exposure/infection at unknown time. Does not provide future immunity. **HCV-RNA** Presence of replicating virus indicates current infection; done when antibody test positive.	**HDV-RNA** Presence of replicating virus. **HDAg** Acute infection.	**Anti-HEV** Acute infection.

Continued

Table 35.1

Viral Hepatitis Infections—cont'd

	Hepatitis A (HAV)	Hepatitis B (HBV)	Hepatitis C (HCV)	Hepatitis D (HDV)	Hepatitis E (HEV)
		Anti-HBc IgM Antibody to core antigen. Present during acute illness and up to 6 months after recovery. **HBeAg** High HBV replication. **Anti-HBe** Slowed viral replication. Lower infectivity.	**HCV Viral Load** Monitors amount of viral RNA present at diagnosis and during treatment. **HCV genotype (1–6)** Identifies virus strain to guide treatment.		
Vaccines	Hepatitis A vaccine.	Hepatitis B vaccine.	None.	Hepatitis B vaccine conveys protection if not already HBV infected.	Hepatitis E vaccine currently available in China only.
Postexposure prophylaxis (when not already immune from vaccination)	Within 2 weeks after exposure: 12 months to 40 years, hepatitis A vaccine; over 40 years or immunocompromised or with chronic liver disease, IG.[1]	Hepatitis B IG (HBIG) within 7 days of exposure, and vaccination.[2]	None, due to the virus's rapid mutation rate. Follow-up with testing for HCV infection.[3]	Prevented with hepatitis B prophylaxis.	None available.
High-risk groups/ activities	Travelers without vaccination to endemic areas.	Workers at risk of blood exposure, including health care workers and correctional staff; those with multiple sexual partners; men who have sex with men; people receiving	Similar to HBV; rarely through monogamous heterosexual sex.	Same as HBV and for chronic HBV carriers.	Travelers to endemic areas.

Table 35.1

Viral Hepatitis Infections—cont'd

	Hepatitis A (HAV)	Hepatitis B (HBV)	Hepatitis C (HCV)	Hepatitis D (HDV)	Hepatitis E (HEV)
		hemodialysis; those with HIV; sharing needles/equipment; sharing toothbrushes, nail clippers, and razors.			
Prognosis	Acute onset with short illness. Rarely fatal.	Acute: asymptomatic or ill for several weeks; Chronic: developed by some, leading to potentially fatal complications of cirrhosis or hepatocellular carcinoma.	High cure rate with medication.	Co-infection with HBV: mild to severe illness with recovery. Superinfection with chronic HBV: progression to more severe disease.	Self-limiting infection. Rarely fatal but increases for pregnant women.

Anti = antibody; ALT = alanine aminotransferase; IG = immunoglobulin; IV = intravenous; RUQ = right upper quadrant.

Sources: [1]Centers for Disease Control and Prevention. (2017). Hepatitis A questions and answers for health professionals. Retrieved from www.cdc.gov/hepatitis/hav/havfaq.htm - protection. [2]Schillie, M. D., Murphy, T. V., Sawyer, M., Ly, K., Huges, E., Jiles, R., ... Ward, J. W. (2013). CDC guidance for evaluating health care personnel for hepatitis B virus protection and for administering postexposure management. *Morbidity and Mortality Weekly Report, 62*(RR10), 1–19. [3]Centers for Disease Control and Prevention. (2017). Information for healthcare personnel potentially exposed to hepatitis C virus (HCV). Retrieved from www.cdc.gov/hepatitis/pdfs/testing-followup-exposed-hc-personnel.pdf

occur, cells regenerate and normal liver function eventually resumes.

HAV, HBC, and HCV are the most common types of viral hepatitis in the United States (Centers for Disease Control and Prevention, 2016). The virus causing the highest number of new hepatitis infections each year as well as chronic hepatitis is HCV.

HEPATITIS C VIRUS. Many people who are infected with HCV, especially baby boomers (people born from 1945 to 1965), are not aware of it and can live for 20 years without symptoms. Those infected can develop chronic infection, chronic liver disease, cirrhosis, or liver cancer. Risk factors for becoming infected with HCV include sharing needles or other equipment to inject drugs or working in health care. Before 1992, when widespread screening of the blood supply began in the United States, HCV was also commonly spread through blood transfusions and organ transplants. It is recommended by the Centers for Disease Control and Prevention

(2016) that all baby boomers be tested for HCV. Healthy People 2020 has a target goal to increase those who are aware that they have a HCV to 60%. Data show awareness increased to 54% in 2014. Healthy People 2020 also has a target goal to reduce new cases of HCV to 0.25 per 100,000 population. However, the data from 2007 to 2014 show an increase in cases to 0.74 (Office of Disease Prevention and Health Promotion, 2018).

Prevention

The hepatitis viruses are very resistant to a wide range of anti-infective measures, such as drying, heat, ultraviolet light exposure, freezing, and bleach and other disinfectants. At least 30 minutes in boiling water is required to destroy them. Infection control precautions should reflect the usual mode of transmission of the specific hepatitis virus. The best methods for preventing the transmission of the hepatitis viruses are careful attention to hygiene, not sharing personal hygiene items, use of sterile needles for tattoos or body piercings, use of condoms for higher risk sex, not sharing drug needles or equipment, getting available vaccinations, and/or the use of immunoglobulin (IG) after an exposure (see Table 35.1).

IGs are plasma donor antibodies that circulate in the recipient's blood for up to 3 months. They do not stimulate the recipient's immune system to develop its own antibodies, so they only provide short-term passive protection. In the United States, vaccines for HAV and HBV are available that provide permanent, active immunity since stimulation of the immune system results in development of a person's own antibodies. The active immunity is to the specific virus to which the body developed antibodies. Health care workers and those in high-risk groups should be vaccinated for HBV.

Public health measures such as health education programs, licensing and supervision of public facilities, screening of blood donors and organs for transplant, and screening of food handlers are general measures to prevent the transmission of hepatitis viruses.

Signs and Symptoms

People can be asymptomatic with viral hepatitis. Because of this, many people do not know they are infected. An acute infection of hepatitis with symptom appearance often shows a typical pattern of decreased liver function, which generally occurs in three stages:

1. The prodromal (preicteric [prejaundice]) stage occurs about 2 weeks after exposure to the hepatitis virus and lasts until jaundice occurs (see Table 35.1).
2. With the appearance of jaundice (see Chapter 32), the icteric stage begins (Fig. 35.1). It occurs about 5 to 10 days after the prodromal stage and lasts 2 to 6 weeks. The patient continues to have prodromal symptoms.
3. The convalescent stage (posticteric) begins when the patient starts feeling better. It can last from 2 to 6 weeks. Recovery varies and depends on the type of hepatitis. Full recovery is measured by the return to normal of all liver function tests. This may take as long as 1 year. The effects of hepatitis can be considered reversible if the patient adheres to a medical regimen of adequate rest, proper nutrition, and abstinence from alcohol and other liver-toxic agents for at least 1 year after liver function laboratory values return to normal.

Complications

Hepatitis may lead to fulminant (sudden and severe), acute, or chronic liver failure. Chronic infection can develop in those with HBV, HCV, and, rarely, HDV. Some people can become asymptomatic carriers of HBV or HCV and never have an active illness. However, they can infect others. They have a greater risk of developing cancer of the liver.

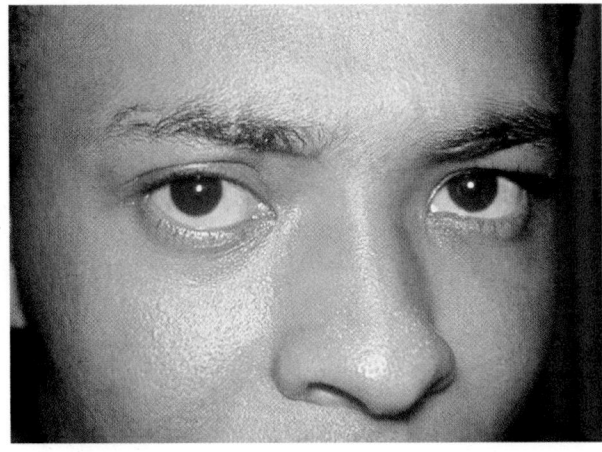

FIGURE 35.1 Jaundice of the conjunctivae and facial skin.

Diagnostic Tests

Serological tests can determine the specific virus causing the hepatitis via viral antigens. They can also identify the presence of antibodies to the virus (see Table 35.1). Serum liver enzymes are elevated and possibly bilirubin (Table 35.2). In patients with severe hepatitis, prothrombin time (PT) may be prolonged. An abdominal x-ray may show an enlarged liver. Liver function tests or biopsy may be done to determine liver damage and healing.

Therapeutic Measures

Treatment goals are to identify the cause of hepatitis, monitor liver status, provide symptom relief, and prevent cirrhosis development. Adequate fluid and nutrition intake are important due to nausea and vomiting. Extreme exertion should be avoided. Alcohol or drugs known to be toxic to the liver should not be used (Box 35.1). Treatment for HAV and HEV infection is supportive care based on signs and symptoms. Coinfection of HBV and HDV is treated with pegylated interferon therapy, although it is not very effective in reducing HDV RNA replication.

Acute HBV infection may resolve over time and require no treatment. If treatment is needed for chronic hepatitis B, potent antivirals that reduce viral resistance are used, such as entecavir (Baraclude) and tenofovir (Vemlidy, Viread). Pegylated interferon-alfa therapy (peginterferon alfa-2b [PEG-Intron] or peginterferon alfa-2a [Pegasys]) may be used for a few patients. Liver transplantation may be needed.

Management of HCV infection continues to evolve as new therapies are developed. The newer direct-acting antiviral (DAA) oral medications have a high cure rate and are safe with few side effects. Various combination medication regimens are available for each HCV genotype. Examples of DAA combination medications are elbasvir plus grazoprevir, sofosbuvir plus ledipasvir (Harvoni), sofosbuvir plus velpatasvir (Epclusa), and ombitasvir plus paritaprevir plus ritonavir plus dasabuvir (Viekira Pak).

Table 35.2

Laboratory Tests for Liver Function in Hepatitis and Cirrhosis

Test	Normal Value	Significance of Abnormal Findings
Indicates Liver Damage		
Alanine aminotransferase (ALT)	**13 months to 60 years** *Male:* 19–36 units/L *Female:* 24–36 units/L **61 to 90 years** *Male:* 13–40 units/L *Female:* 10–28 units/L **Over 90 years** *Male:* 6–38 units/L *Female:* 5–24 units/L	Most specific enzyme for liver damage. Can elevate 50 times normal with death of liver cells.
Aspartate aminotransferase (AST)	**20 to 49 years** *Male:* 20–40 units/L *Female:* 15–30 units/L **Male over 50 years** 10–35 units/L **Female over 45 years** 10–35 units/L	Enzyme found in liver and heart. Over 500 units/L seen with acute hepatitis.
Alkaline phosphatase (ALP)	**21 years and older** *Male:* 35–142 units/L *Female:* 25–125 units/L **Older adults** Slightly elevated	Enzyme found in liver and other areas; released and elevates greatly with severe liver damage.
Measures Functioning of Liver		
Albumin	**20 to 40 years** 3.7–5.1 g/dL **41 to 60 years** 3.4–4.8 g/dL **61 to 90 years** 3.2–4.6 g/dL **Over 90 years** 2.9–4.5 g/dL	Decreased because of impaired liver protein synthesis. Maintains plasma oncotic pressure, so low levels can cause edema and ascites.
Ammonia	**25 months to adult** 15–60 mcg/dL	Increased because liver cannot metabolize this protein end product; contributes to hepatic encephalopathy.
Total bilirubin	**Adults** Less than 1.2 mg/dL	Increased because the liver is unable to use it to produce bile.
Prothrombin time (PT)	10–13 seconds	Value prolonged. Liver can no longer make prothrombin; patient bleeds more easily.

Nursing Process for the Patient With Hepatitis

DATA COLLECTION. Identify subjective data such as malaise, fatigue, pruritus (itching), nausea, anorexia, and right upper quadrant (RUQ) abdominal pain. Objective data, such as baseline weight, vomiting, pale stools, dark-colored (tea-colored) urine, and jaundice, are recorded. The patient's vital signs are obtained. Fever or abnormal bruising or bleeding is reported immediately. Ask the patient about knowledge of the disease and how to prevent its spread ("Evidence-Based Practice").

Evidence-Based Practice

Clinical Question
What do people experience when living with hepatitis C virus (HCV)?

Evidence
Forty-six studies that looked at the experience of living with hepatitis C virus were included in this systematic review. The research showed that those living with HCV faced reduced quality of life due to physical symptoms, discrimination, stigma, lack of disease information, feeling unsupported, and not being a partner in health care decision making.

Implications for Nursing Practice
Nurses can be more compassionate, provide patient-centered care, and increase education to enhance the lives of those living with HCV.

Reference
Dowsett, L. D., Coward, S., Lorenzetti, D. L., MacKean, G., & Clement, F. (2017). Living with hepatitis C virus: A systematic review and narrative synthesis of qualitative literature. *Canadian Journal of Gastroenterology and Hepatology, 2017*, 3268650. doi:10.1155/2017/3268650

NURSING DIAGNOSES, PLANNING, AND IMPLEMENTATION.

Acute Pain related to inflammation and enlargement of the liver

EXPECTED OUTCOME: The patient will state that pain level is acceptable.

- Monitor pain level using pain rating scale (e.g., 0 to 10) and ask *WHAT'S UP?* questions *to determine treatment needs.*
- Give analgesics as ordered, around the clock and as needed (prn) for intermittent breakthrough pain, recognizing that lower doses might be needed with liver dysfunction, *to control pain and prevent toxicity.*
- Avoid use of acetaminophen (Tylenol) and combination drugs containing acetaminophen *due to risk of liver toxicity.*
- Encourage nondrug pain relief, such as distraction, imagery, and relaxation *to supplement and possibly decrease need for analgesics.*

Imbalanced Nutrition, Less Than Body Requirements related to anorexia, nausea, or vomiting

EXPECTED OUTCOME: The patient's weight will be stable and appropriate for height.

- Make dietitian referral *for development of a nutritional plan.*
- Monitor weight and nutritional intake, recording percentage of food eaten, *to determine ongoing treatment needs.*

Box 35.1

Common Causes of Hepatic Inflammation

Medications
- Acetaminophen (Tylenol)
- Acetylsalicylic acid (aspirin)
- Allopurinol (Zyloprim)
- Captopril (Capoten)
- Carbamazepine (Tegretol)
- Diazepam (Valium)
- Erythromycin estolate (Ilosone)
- Estrogen
- Halothane (Fluothane)
- Isoniazid (INH)
- Methotrexate (Trexall)
- Methyldopa (Aldomet)
- Oral contraceptives
- Phenobarbital (Luminal)
- Phenytoin (Dilantin)
- Sulfonamides
- Tetracycline (Sumycin)

Metabolic Disorders
- Alpha-1 antitrypsin deficiency
- Hemochromatosis (iron buildup)
- Wilson disease (copper buildup)

Toxins
- Carbon tetrachloride
- Cholecystographic dyes
- Ethyl alcohol
- Kava-containing products (herb)
- Poisonous wild mushrooms
- Toluene
- Trichloroethylene

Vascular Disorders
- Budd–Chiari syndrome (hepatic vein occlusion)
- Heart failure
- Shock

Viruses
- Cytomegalovirus
- Epstein-Barr virus
- Hepatitis A, B, C, D, E
- Herpes simplex virus
- Yellow fever

- Administer antiemetic drugs as ordered *to reduce nausea and increase appetite.*
- Provide frequent, smaller meals *because these may be better tolerated than larger meals.*
- Teach the patient to avoid alcohol, herbal supplements, and vitamin supplements unless specifically prescribed by the HCP *to prevent further liver damage, as these can be toxic to the liver.*

Risk for Impaired Liver Function related to viral infection

- Monitor liver function tests and signs of liver dysfunction, including ascites, mental changes (check ammonia levels), and bleeding (check coagulation studies), *to detect liver infection.*
- Review medications for hepatotoxicity and administer medications carefully *to protect liver function.*
- Calculate total acetaminophen 24-hour dosage for all medications that contain it so daily limit of 2,000 mg or less is not exceeded in presence of hepatitis *to protect liver function.*
- Refer to alcohol cessation program if applicable *to preserve liver function.*

Risk for Impaired Skin Integrity related to pruritus secondary to bilirubin pigment deposits in skin

EXPECTED OUTCOME: The patient's skin will remain intact and free from secondary infection.

- Administer antihistamine such as diphenhydramine (Benadryl) as ordered *to decrease itching.*
- Encourage the patient not to scratch skin but to press firmly on the itchy area. *Scratching can damage skin and increase risk for infection.*
- Encourage the patient to keep fingernails trimmed short *so that vigorous scratching does not tear the skin.*

Ineffective Health Management related to lack of knowledge of hepatitis and its transmission and treatment

EXPECTED OUTCOME: The patient will state how to self-manage the treatment regimen for viral hepatitis and how to prevent spread of the disease.

- Determine the patient's knowledge of hepatitis *to plan teaching.*
- Teach the patient how hepatitis affects the body and the importance of taking medications as prescribed, adequate rest, and proper nutrition *to promote recovery.*
- Teach the importance of avoiding alcohol and other liver-toxic drugs *to prevent further damage to liver.*
- Teach the patient and family how to prevent the spreading of the hepatitis virus, including vaccination as appropriate for family; hand washing after toileting; using soap and hot water to clean eating utensils, cookware, and food preparation surfaces; practicing safer sex (abstinence, condoms, monogamy); and not sharing needles, *because hepatitis is contagious* (see "Home Health Hints").

EVALUATION. Management of the patient with hepatitis has been successful if the patient reports pain is satisfactorily relieved; body weight is maintained within 2 pounds of pre-illness weight; skin has no breaks, cuts, or tears or secondary infections; the patient can define the disease; and the patient and family understand and follow the treatment plan and transmission precautions.

Home Health Hints

Abdominal Ascites
- A hospital bed at home may be needed so the patient can be positioned to aid in breathing. A health care provider's order must be obtained for insurance coverage.
- Measure and document abdominal girth at each visit.
- Teach the patient to obtain weight on the same scale first thing in the morning and to record the weight so the nurse can document the findings.

Hepatitis
- Teach the caregiver to wear disposable gloves when cleaning the patient's bathroom. If possible, the patient should have a separate bedroom and bathroom. Advise the family to use liquid soap instead of bar soap.
- Teach the patient and caregiver to wash contaminated linens separately from household laundry and to use detergent and hot water. Presoak in cold water if soiled with blood. Rubber gloves should be worn to handle the patient's laundry.

CRITICAL THINKING

Carl Young, 23, has returned from a missionary trip in Africa. He reports that during his time there, he sustained a serious laceration that required sutures. Carl also mentions his fondness for seafood, and that since his return, he has had several "feasts" that have included raw oysters. Carl states that since his return, he has lost nearly 8 pounds, is nauseated, has frequent headaches, tires easily, and is very irritable.

1. What information might lead you to suspect hepatitis A infection? Hepatitis B infection?
2. What precautions should be instituted for Carl until a diagnosis is made?
3. What additional health care team members will be beneficial to Carl's care?
4. What patient-centered care actions might you implement to help Carl improve his nutrition?
5. What classes of medications should Carl avoid?
6. What information should be included in a teaching plan related to hepatitis for Carl?

Suggested answers are at the end of the chapter.

Acute Liver Failure

Acute liver failure is a rare but serious condition that can develop rapidly, sometimes in just 2 days. When the liver is severely damaged, its many functions are impaired. The outcome of the disease may be decided within 48 to 72 hours of diagnosis. Possible outcomes are liver recovery, need for liver transplantation, or death. See Box 35.1 for causes.

Box 35.2 teaches patients ways to prevent liver damage and possible liver failure.

Acetaminophen Toxicity

Acetaminophen (Tylenol) overdose is the most common cause of acute liver failure. Acetaminophen intake should not exceed 3,000 mg in a 24-hour period in a person with no liver disease. Prescription drugs containing more than 325 mg of acetaminophen should not be prescribed or taken per U.S. Food and Drug Administration (FDA) guidelines. To prevent excessive dosage, visit www.knowyourdose.org, an acetaminophen awareness program, for more information and a list of more than 600 medications containing acetaminophen.

For overdose of acetaminophen, activated charcoal is given to absorb acetaminophen if it is within 1 hour of ingestion and the patient is alert with an intact or protected airway. N-acetylcysteine is the antidote for acetaminophen. It is effective in preventing hepatotoxicity if given within 8 hours of ingestion.

BE SAFE!

Understand how to monitor the 24-hour dosage of acetaminophen taken by a patient. Look back at the previous 24-hour time frame from the current time and add up the dosage of any acetaminophen taken alone and in combination drugs. This is a floating 24-hour period, not shift times or a calendar day. The acetaminophen dose should not exceed 3,000 mg in a 24-hour period for the patient who does not have liver disease. Teach the patient how to monitor this, too.

Signs and Symptoms

Initial symptoms of liver failure, including fatigue, gastrointestinal (GI) upset, and diarrhea, are vague and make detection difficult. As the condition worsens, symptoms become more severe; these include jaundice, hepatic **encephalopathy** (HE), bleeding, and abdominal distention. The patient may suddenly lapse into an extremely serious illness, starting with confusion and progressing to hepatic coma. In a matter of hours, on x-ray, the liver shows a rapid reduction in size, a typical sign of onset of acute liver failure. In addition, there is a sudden elevation of liver enzymes, alanine aminotransferase (ALT), aspartate aminotransferase (AST), and bilirubin. PT is elevated, with marked elevation being an ominous sign. Potassium and blood glucose levels drop.

Therapeutic Measures

Treatment is directed toward stopping and reversing the damage to the liver. Dialysis may be ordered if the liver damage results from an overdose of a hepatotoxic substance to filter the substance from the blood. The patient needs intensive amounts of supportive care. Maintaining the airway (head elevated 30 degrees, NPO [nothing by mouth], nasogastric

---

Box 35.2

Patient Education

Liver Failure Prevention

To avoid causes of liver failure:
- Wash hands after using the bathroom and before handling food.
- Do not share personal grooming items (especially toothbrushes or razors).
- Obtain hepatitis A and B vaccines.
- Eat a balanced diet.
- Do not exceed 3,000 mg of acetaminophen in a 24-hour period or a prescribed drug with more than a 325-mg dose of acetaminophen in it.
- Review prescribed and over-the-counter medications to know which are combination drugs that contain acetaminophen to prevent excessive dosage. There are more than 600 drugs containing acetaminophen, such as Norco, NyQuil, Percocet, Vicodin, Tylenol with Codeine, or Tylox.
- Know how to read medicine labels and dosage found in the active ingredient list on the label. Visit www.knowyourdose.org to interactively read a drug label.
- Avoid alcohol or drink it only in moderation. Do not drink alcohol when taking acetaminophen.
- Avoid exposure to blood.
- Use condoms for safer sex.
- Ensure sanitary conditions and equipment when obtaining a body piercing or tattoo.
- Do not share intravenous needles.

[NG] tube, endotracheal intubation) is important if HE develops. An attempt is made to put the liver completely at rest. The patient is often on bedrest. Stimulation is avoided. Most medications are discontinued because they are metabolized by the liver. Nutrition may be provided via enteral or parenteral nutrition. Medications may be given to decrease ammonia levels (see later section on HE).

Nursing Process for the Patient With Acute Liver Failure

Nursing care of the patient with acute liver failure is the same as it is for the patient with cirrhosis, which is discussed next.

Chronic Liver Disease and Cirrhosis

In 2015, 3.9 million adults had chronic liver disease and cirrhosis (Blackwell & Villarroel, 2016). **Cirrhosis** is the progressive replacement of healthy liver tissue with scar tissue. It results from a chronic liver disease. There are a variety of causes of chronic liver disease (see Box 35.1). Cirrhosis is usually irreversible unless the cause is identified and treated early. Common causes of cirrhosis are chronic alcohol use, chronic hepatitis B and C, or nonalcoholic steatohepatitis (NASH). NASH is also known as fatty liver disease due to

---

• WORD • BUILDING •

encephalopathy: encephalo—brain + pathy—disease
cirrhosis: cirrh—orange yellow + osis—condition

the buildup of fat in the liver. It is common in those with diabetes, obesity, heart disease, or elevated cholesterol levels.

> ## BE SAFE!
> Many consequences of alcohol abuse, such as cirrhosis, can take years to develop, but not acute alcohol toxicity! Ingesting a large quantity of ethanol (or a smaller quantity of alcohol not intended for beverages) in a short time can be fatal within a few hours. Alcohol poisoning is especially heartbreaking when, through ignorance or fear of retribution, a young person dies because he or she was left to "sleep it off." Education on the effects of alcohol use is an important health teaching topic for nurses.

Pathophysiology

Healthy liver cells exposed to toxins become inflamed. Then, the liver cells are infiltrated with fat and white blood cells (WBCs) and are replaced by fibrotic tissue. As the liver makes repairs, scar tissue forms. If the damage continues over years, and more and more scar tissue is created, cirrhosis can develop. Liver regeneration continues abnormally, disrupting the lobes of the liver and creating nodules. The liver becomes enlarged and hardened and lumpy instead of soft. Blood flow through the liver becomes impaired due to the nodules, resulting in portal venous hypertension. Later, the liver shrinks and is covered with gray connective tissue. As the disease progresses, liver function is impaired. After many years, cirrhosis can lead to liver failure.

Signs and Symptoms

Initially, symptoms often do not occur with cirrhosis. As liver function becomes impaired, many signs and symptoms are possible (Table 35.3). The liver may be enlarged, firm, and tender upon palpation. Laboratory values reflect progressive loss of liver function. As cirrhosis progresses, signs and symptoms of increasing loss of liver function and complications related to the increasing loss of function develop (Fig. 35.2).

Complications

Complications of cirrhosis include blood clotting defects, portal hypertension, ascites, HE, and hepatorenal syndrome.

CLOTTING DEFECTS. Blood clotting defects develop because of impaired prothrombin and fibrinogen production in the liver. Furthermore, the absence of bile salts prevents the absorption of fat-soluble vitamin K, which is essential to make certain blood-clotting factors. As a result, bruising, disseminated intravascular coagulation, or hemorrhage can occur.

PORTAL HYPERTENSION. **Portal hypertension** is persistent elevated blood pressure in the portal vein. Liver scarring obstructs blood flow in the portal vein. This causes blood to back up into surrounding blood vessels. The increased

Table 35.3
Cirrhosis Summary

Signs and Symptoms	Anorexia, nausea, weight loss Ascites Bruising Cramping Dull right upper quadrant pain Gastrointestinal bleeding Itching (from bile products deposited in skin) Jaundice Telangiectasias (group of small, dilated veins)
Diagnostic Tests	Elevated alanine aminotransferase (ALT), alkaline phosphatase (ALP), aspartate aminotransferase (AST), ammonia, bilirubin, prothrombin time (PT) Liver biopsy
Therapeutic Measures	Prevent disease progression Treat complications
Complications	Remember the pneumonic **CHEAP** (see Learning Tip)
Priority Nursing Diagnoses	*Acute Pain* *Excess Fluid Volume* *Imbalanced Nutrition: Less Than Body Requirements*

pressure causes the abdominal veins around the umbilicus to become enlarged and visible (called *caput medusae*) as well as rectal hemorrhoids, spleen enlargement (splenomegaly), and esophageal **varices** (dilated veins; Fig. 35.3).

The most serious result of portal hypertension is bleeding esophageal varices. Varices usually develop from the fundus of the stomach upward and may extend into the upper esophagus. The blood-filled, thin-walled varices may tear easily, causing severe bleeding from sudden excessive pressure, such as from coughing, lifting, or straining.

ASCITES. **Ascites** is an accumulation of serous fluid in the peritoneal (abdominal) cavity from portal hypertension. Low production of the protein albumin by the failing liver can also allow fluid to leak from the blood vessels into the peritoneal cavity. The kidneys respond to the decreased circulating blood volume by releasing aldosterone to save sodium and thus water. Accumulated fluid in the peritoneal cavity causes a markedly enlarged abdomen. The fluid may cause severe respiratory distress as a result of elevation of the diaphragm.

HEPATIC ENCEPHALOPATHY. HE is caused by elevated ammonia, a by-product of protein metabolism, which disrupts

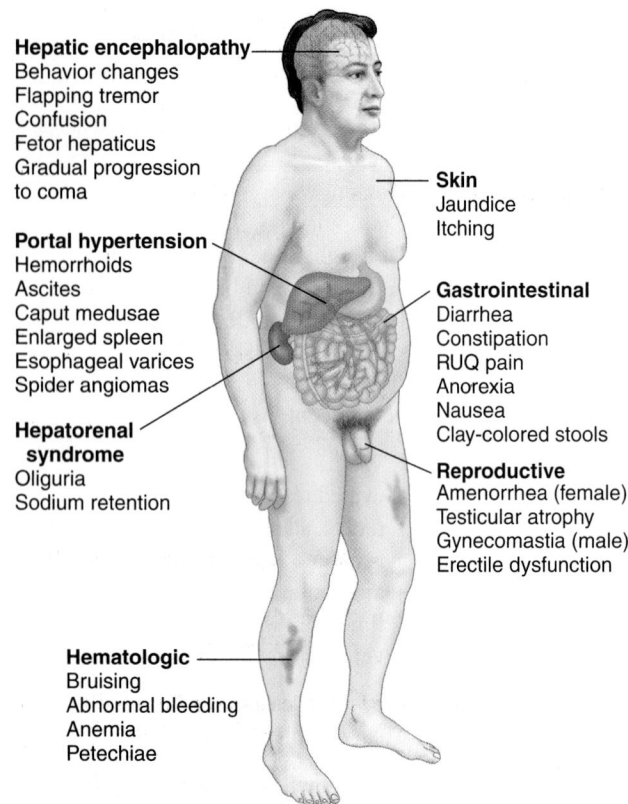

Hepatic encephalopathy
Behavior changes
Flapping tremor
Confusion
Fetor hepaticus
Gradual progression
to coma

Portal hypertension
Hemorrhoids
Ascites
Caput medusae
Enlarged spleen
Esophageal varices
Spider angiomas

**Hepatorenal
syndrome**
Oliguria
Sodium retention

Skin
Jaundice
Itching

Gastrointestinal
Diarrhea
Constipation
RUQ pain
Anorexia
Nausea
Clay-colored stools

Reproductive
Amenorrhea (female)
Testicular atrophy
Gynecomastia (male)
Erectile dysfunction

Hematologic
Bruising
Abnormal bleeding
Anemia
Petechiae

FIGURE 35.2 Signs and symptoms of cirrhosis.

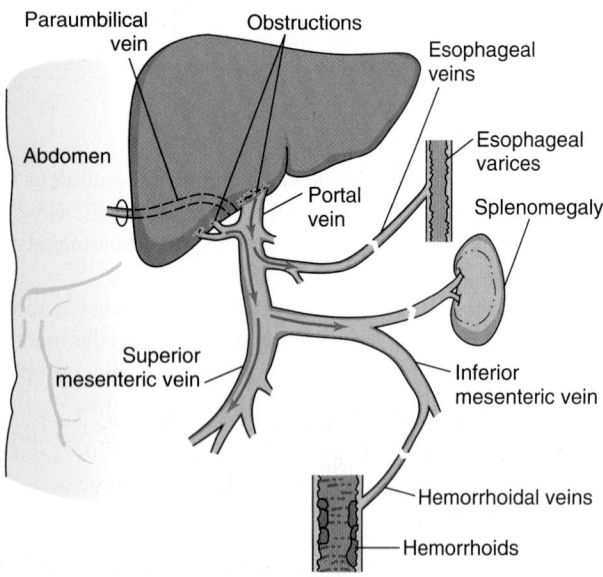

Paraumbilical vein
Obstructions
Esophageal veins
Esophageal varices
Abdomen
Portal vein
Splenomegaly
Superior mesenteric vein
Inferior mesenteric vein
Hemorrhoidal veins
Hemorrhoids

FIGURE 35.3 Portal hypertension.

mental status. The damaged liver is unable to convert the ammonia to urea for excretion in the urine. Signs and symptoms of HE include progressive confusion, **asterixis** (flapping tremors in the hands caused by toxins at peripheral nerves), and **fetor hepaticus** (foul breath caused by metabolic end products related to sulfur).

Stages of HE and signs and symptoms of the stages are as follows:

- *Early:* The patient exhibits subtle changes in personality, fatigue, drowsiness, and changes in handwriting (the best assessment for the early stage).
- *Stupor and confusion:* The patient is often belligerent and irritable and develops asterixis, muscle twitching, hyperventilation, and marked confusion.
- *Comatose:* The patient gradually loses consciousness and becomes comatose.

With treatment, as ammonia levels decrease, the patient usually gradually regains consciousness. HE represents end-stage liver failure and has a high mortality rate once coma begins.

HEPATORENAL SYNDROME. Hepatorenal syndrome is a secondary failure of the kidneys from cirrhosis. The impaired liver circulation reduces renal blood flow. Symptoms of hepatorenal syndrome include oliguria without detectable kidney damage, reduced glomerular filtration rate (GFR) with essentially no urine output or less than 200 mL per day, and nearly total sodium retention. Albumin and fresh frozen plasma to increase intravascular volume and blood flow can be given. Liver transplant may be necessary.

LEARNING TIP

For complications of cirrhosis, remember the pneumonic **CHEAP:**

C: Clotting defects
H: Hepatorenal syndrome
E: Encephalopathy
A: Ascites
P: Portal hypertension

WERNICKE–KORSAKOFF SYNDROME. Wernicke–Korsakoff syndrome may be a complication of alcoholic liver disease. It is a brain disorder caused by thiamine (B_1) deficiency. Wernicke encephalopathy and Korsakoff psychosis often occur together. They are primarily diagnosed in those who abuse alcohol and occasionally in malnourished patients with no history of alcohol abuse.

Wernicke encephalopathy is an acute condition resulting in confusion, delirium, visual disturbances, and ataxia. When caused by dietary deficiency, this encephalopathy can usually be successfully treated with oral or subcutaneous thiamine. Korsakoff psychosis is the result of permanent damage to the

---

· WORD · BUILDING ·

asterixis: a—not + sterixis—fixed position

fetor hepaticus: fetor—offensive odor + hepat—liver + icas—related to

hepatorenal syndrome: hepato—liver + renal—kidneys + syndrome—group of symptoms

brain tissue. Administration of thiamine will not reverse this brain damage. Patients with Korsakoff psychosis display an abnormal mental state in which memory and learning are affected in an otherwise alert and responsive patient.

Diagnostic Tests

Tests that show liver damage and functioning of the liver are shown in Table 35.2. Abdominal x-rays of patients with cirrhosis may show ascites and enlargement of the liver. An abdominal ultrasound may show liver enlargement early in cirrhosis or a small liver later in the disease. An esophagogastroduodenoscopy (EGD) detects esophageal varices and bleeding (discussed later in the chapter). A liver biopsy may be done to determine the extent and nature of the liver damage (see Chapter 32).

> **NURSING CARE TIP**
>
> Patients with cirrhosis undergoing a liver biopsy need careful observation for bleeding after the procedure because of possible impaired clotting.

Therapeutic Measures

Interventions for cirrhosis are to prevent advancement of the disease and treat complications. A liver transplant may be considered if cirrhosis cannot be treated.

ASCITES. Ascites is treated with diuretics such as spironolactone (Aldactone) or furosemide (Lasix), sodium and fluid restriction (800 to 1,000 mL/day), and albumin infusions for severe ascites. Paracentesis can be done to remove accumulated fluid from the peritoneal cavity when the fluid is compromising the patient's breathing, causing abdominal discomfort, or posing a threat of ruptured umbilical hernia. If large amounts of fluid are removed, albumin may be given to replace lost proteins to prevent further fluid shifting.

Ascites may be treated by the nonsurgical placement of a shunt, called a **transjugular intrahepatic portosystemic shunt** (TIPS), under fluoroscopy (Fig. 35.4). A stent is placed via the jugular vein to connect the portal vein to the hepatic vein, in the middle of the liver. This reduces portal pressure by allowing blood to bypass the liver and be carried to the heart. It reduces fluid accumulation and aids in reducing the risk of bleeding. Complications can develop with TIPS.

ESOPHAGEAL VARICES. Bleeding varices are a medical emergency, and 911 should be called. Large amounts of blood can be lost, and death can result, so screening for the presence of varices should be done. For bleeding prevention, the beta blockers propranolol (Inderal) and nadolol (Corgard) as well as endoscopic variceal ligation using rubber bands are used.

Bleeding from esophageal varices must be stopped immediately. Bleeding varices can be treated with a vasoconstrictor such as octreotide (Sandostatin) and variceal ligation (Fig. 35.5). TIPS is another procedure that may be recommended to reduce the pressure in the portal vein and stop the

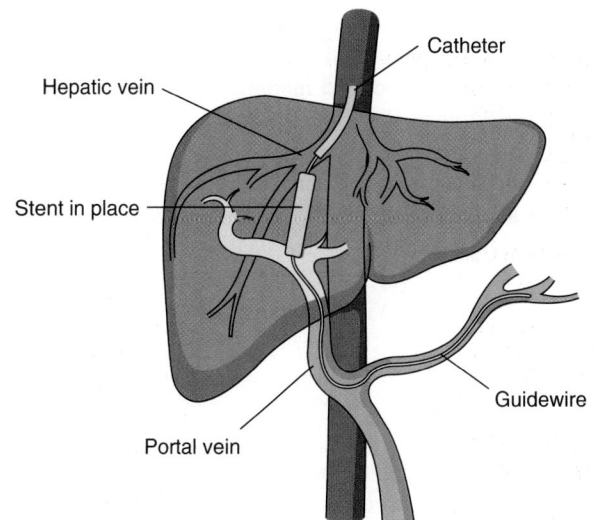

FIGURE 35.4 Transjugular intrahepatic portosystemic shunt (TIPS).

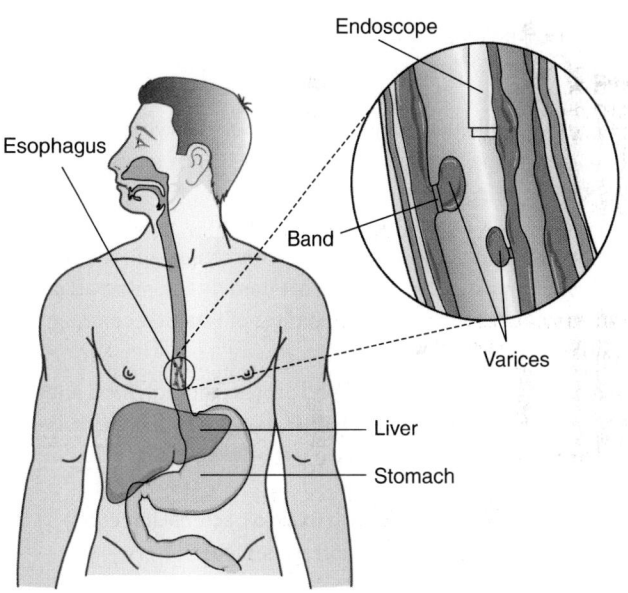

FIGURE 35.5 Variceal banding.

bleeding varices. A blood transfusion may be needed for lost blood volume. Antibiotic prophylaxis is given with hemorrhage because infection is a risk and can be a precursor to rebleeding varices.

HEPATIC ENCEPHALOPATHY. To reduce serum ammonia levels to prevent or treat HE, the osmotic disaccharide laxative lactulose is given by mouth, NG tube, or enema (depending

• **WORD** • **BUILDING** •

transjugular intrahepatic portosystemic shunt: trans— across + jugular—jugular vein + intra—within + hepatic— liver + porto—portal (liver circulation) + systemic—systemic (circulation) + shunt—to divert

on how alert the patient is). It lowers the pH of the colon, inhibiting ammonia from moving into the blood so that it can be excreted in the stool and inhibiting ammonia-producing bacteria. Lactulose also causes water to be drawn into the colon, which increases ammonia's transport from the body. Antibiotics may also be given to reduce bacteria in the gut that produce ammonia. Rifaximin (Xifaxan) is commonly used. Neomycin (Neo-Fradin), an intestinal antibiotic, or other antibiotics have also been used ("Nutrition Notes: Supplying Nutrients to Patients With Liver Disease").

Nutrition Notes

Supplying Nutrients to Patients With Liver Disease.
A registered dietitian consultation is needed to assess nutritional status, help diagnose malnutrition, and make diet recommendations to improve nutrient intake.

Nutritional Care for Hepatitis Patients
A well-balanced diet is recommended following the principles of the 2015–2020 Dietary Guidelines for Americans (https://health.gov/dietaryguidelines/2015/guidelines). Herbal supplements and alcohol should be avoided, and vitamin/mineral supplements should be taken only under health care provider supervision.

Nutritional Care for Cirrhosis Patients
Patients with cirrhosis may have a decreased appetite and be malnourished. Absorption of vitamins and minerals can be impaired. The National Institutes of Health recommends that patients:

- Obtain adequate calories and protein through food and nutritional supplements (either orally or by feeding tube)
- Monitor vitamin status and use appropriate supplementation
- Avoid alcohol and shellfish (due to bacterial infection)
- Restrict sodium based upon ascites level

Branched-chain amino acids (isoleucine, leucine, and valine) can improve hepatic encephalopathy. Branched-chain amino acids do not require oxidation by the liver and are available for direct use by other tissues. A special formula for oral or enteral feeding is Hepatic-Aid II.

Nursing Process for the Patient With Acute Liver Failure, Chronic Liver Disease, or Cirrhosis

Data Collection
A complete history and physical assessment are done. Be alert to subjective symptoms of liver dysfunction, such as abdominal pain, anorexia, nausea, severe itching, and dull, aching RUQ pain. Note objective evidence of liver problems, such as jaundice, light-colored stools, ascites, ecchymosis (bruising) of the skin, GI bleeding, and any evidence of alterations in thought processes, such as confusion, disorientation, or inability to make decisions.

Nursing Diagnoses, Planning, and Implementation
Common nursing diagnoses for the patient with acute liver failure, chronic liver disease, or cirrhosis include the following:

Excess Fluid Volume related to portal hypertension and ascites

EXPECTED OUTCOME: Fluid volume will be controlled as evidenced by stable weight and abdominal girth within normal limits for the patient.

- Obtain baseline weight and then weigh daily *to reveal fluid retention.*
- Measure the patient's abdominal girth (circumference) daily at the same marked location *to monitor ascites.*
- Measure intake and output *to accurately monitor fluid volume changes.*
- Monitor the patient's vital signs and lung sounds and report changes or difficulty breathing or changes in mental status promptly *to detect fluid overload and obtain prompt treatment.*
- Report weight gain or increase in girth promptly *so treatment can be ordered and complications minimized.*
- Maintain a low-sodium diet and fluid restrictions *to reduce fluid retention.*
- Administer ordered diuretics as scheduled *to reduce fluid overload.*

Imbalanced Nutrition: Less Than Body Requirements related to anorexia and impaired metabolism of needed nutrients

EXPECTED OUTCOME: The patient's nutritional needs will be maintained within normal limits.

- Obtain dietitian referral *to assess for malnutrition and then develop nutritional plan.*
- Offer frequent mouth care *to increase comfort and make food more palatable.*
- Make sure that odors and other unpleasant stimuli are eliminated *to reduce anorexia.*
- Offer the patient frequent, small, high-calorie meals *to reduce feeling of fullness that can occur with larger meals.*

Acute Pain related to abdominal pressure

EXPECTED OUTCOME: The patient will state pain level is acceptable.

- Monitor pain level using pain rating scale (e.g., 0 to 10) and ask **WHAT'S UP?** questions *to guide treatment.*
- Give analgesics as ordered to control pain. *Lower doses may be needed for the patient with liver dysfunction.*
- Encourage nondrug pain relief activities, such as distraction, imagery, and relaxation *to possibly decrease the need for analgesics.*

Acute Confusion related to elevated ammonia levels

EXPECTED OUTCOME: The patient will remain alert and oriented to person, place, and time.

- Monitor the patient's level of consciousness and orientation often *to allow prompt treatment.*
- Monitor neuromuscular function by asking the patient to hold arms steady and straight out in front. *If asterixis, or liver flap, is present, the patient's hands will unwillingly dip and return to the horizontal position in a flapping motion due to elevated ammonia.*
- Give medications such as lactulose as scheduled *to decrease serum ammonia levels.*
- Recognize that lactulose causes loose stools but do not withhold the medication when the patient has the desired two soft or loose stools per day; report severe diarrhea. *Loose stools are a sign that the medication is working, not a reason to withhold it when treating ammonia levels.*
- Question giving medications such as sedatives, opioids, and tranquilizers *because these can precipitate HE.*
- Reorient the patient to time and place if needed *to reinforce reality.*
- Give simple, clear explanations of care and give the patient time to understand the explanation *because short, simple explanations are easier to process.*
- Provide a safe environment for the confused or unsteady patient *to prevent injury.*

Ineffective Breathing Pattern related to excess fluid in the abdomen

EXPECTED OUTCOME: The patient's respirations will be even and unlabored, 16 to 20 per minute.

- Monitor the patient's respiratory rate, rhythm, chest movement, skin color, and oxygen saturation frequently *to determine breathing pattern and its effectiveness.*
- Assist the patient to use an incentive spirometer *to encourage deep breathing and keep airways clear.*
- Elevate the head of the patient's bed *so that the patient's lungs have maximum room for expansion.*
- Administer analgesics carefully, as ordered, if pain is causing shallow respirations. *Reducing painful breathing allows for a more effective breathing pattern.*
- Reposition the patient at least every 2 hours *to ventilate all areas of the lungs.*

Risk for Deficient Fluid Volume related to bleeding esophageal varices or GI bleeding secondary to clotting disorder

EXPECTED OUTCOME: Fluid volume will remain within normal limits as evidenced by no signs of bleeding, and vital signs, weight, and fluid balance within normal limits for the patient.

- Monitor gastric secretions, stool, and urine at least every 8 hours, and report any signs of bleeding *for prompt treatment.*

- Monitor blood clotting laboratory studies such as PT and report any abnormal values *to identify risk for bleeding.*
- Caution the patient to use a soft-bristle toothbrush and an electric rather than straight razor *to avoid injury and bleeding.*
- Avoid suctioning the patient if possible *because suctioning can cause esophageal varices to bleed.*
- Use a small-gauge needle for injections and apply direct pressure to all puncture sites *to prevent bleeding.*
- Teach the patient to avoid forceful coughing or nose blowing, straining, vomiting, or gagging if at all possible. Administer medications as ordered to prevent their occurrence. *These can increase pressure and risk of bleeding varices.*

Evaluation

Nursing care has been effective if the patient is alert and oriented and has no signs of fluid retention, a stable weight appropriate for height, no abdominal pain or pain reported as tolerable using pain rating scale, a respiratory rate between 16 and 20 respirations per minute with no cyanosis or changes in level of consciousness, no bleeding, no injuries, and an accurate knowledge of acute liver failure, chronic liver disease, or cirrhosis and proper disease management requirements.

Patient Education

Teach patients how acute liver failure, chronic liver disease, or cirrhosis affects their bodies and health. In particular, patients need to know about portal system hypertension and HE. In addition, teach patient to do the following:

- Avoid alcohol.
- Obtain adequate rest and avoid strenuous activity.
- Use opioids, sedatives, and tranquilizers cautiously due to potential mental function impairment.
- Report bleeding; confusion, tremors, or personality changes; signs of low potassium, such as muscle cramps, nausea, or vomiting caused by diuretics; changes in weight; or other symptoms promptly.
- Maintain adequate nutrition (see "Nutrition Notes: Supplying Nutrients to Patients With Liver Disease").

CRITICAL THINKING

Mrs. Conner, a 76-year-old retired businesswoman, has lived alone for the past 20 years since the death of her husband. She has a history of poor nutritional habits but does not consume alcohol. She is admitted with cirrhosis.

1. What risk factors does Mrs. Conner have for cirrhosis?
2. What symptoms would you expect Mrs. Conner to exhibit with early cirrhosis?
3. What values do you expect to see for serum albumin? Prothrombin time?
4. What are the two greatest concerns with portal hypertension?
5. What is the usual treatment for ascites?

Suggested answers are at the end of the chapter.

Liver Transplantation

The patient with end-stage liver failure from cirrhosis, hepatitis, biliary disease, metabolic disorders, or hepatic vein obstruction may be considered for a liver transplant. The American Association for the Study of Liver Diseases and the American Society of Transplantation have guidelines for liver transplantation and evaluation of potential patients for liver transplantation (Martin, DiMartini, Feng, Brown, & Fallon, 2014). The patient will be evaluated for emotional and physical stability as well as acceptance of the need for daily medications for life ("Cultural Considerations: Organ Donation").

Cultural Considerations

Organ Donation. Certain considerations may need to be made for potential donor recipients who adhere to Judaism. Jewish law addresses organ transplantation from the perspectives of the recipient, the living donor, the cadaver donor, and the dying donor. If a recipient's life can be prolonged without considerable risk, transplant is ordained. For a living donor to be approved, the risk to the life of the donor must be considered. One is not obligated to donate a part of himself or herself unless the risk is small. The use of a cadaver for transplant is usually approved if it is saving a life. A rabbi can be helpful when making decisions regarding organ donation or transplantation.

After the surgical implantation of a donor liver, the patient is closely observed for evidence of donor organ rejection. The patient will be placed on drugs to suppress immune system responses and prevent tissue rejection. The patient is observed for the following signs of impending rejection:

- Pulse greater than 100 beats per minute
- Temperature greater than 101°F (38°C)
- Reports of RUQ pain
- Increased jaundice
- Decrease in bile from the T-tube or a change in bile color

In addition, laboratory studies may show increased serum transaminases (ALT and AST), serum bilirubin, alkaline phosphatase (ALP), and PT. Symptoms of acute tissue rejection usually develop between the fourth and tenth postoperative days. The patient who has received an organ transplant needs extended medical follow-up. Teach the patient to promptly report to the HCP symptoms of infection, bleeding episodes, or RUQ pain.

As a short-term bridge to liver transplant, bioartificial livers with filtering membranes have been used. Hepatocyte transplantation via a splenic artery catheter for longer-term support is being researched.

Cancer of the Liver

Cancer of the liver usually results from metastasis from a primary cancer at a distant location. The liver is a likely area of involvement for cancers that originated in the esophagus, lungs, breast, stomach, colon, pancreas, kidney, bladder, or skin. For some patients, the primary tumor site is the liver. Patients with a history of chronic HBV or HCV, nutritional deficiencies, heavy alcohol use or smoking, and exposure to hepatotoxins have an increased risk for cancer of the liver.

Symptoms of cancer of the liver include encephalopathy, abnormal bleeding, jaundice, and ascites. Laboratory tests show elevated serum ALP. Radiologic examinations may include abdominal radiographs or radioisotope scans, which show tumor growth. Liver cancer is definitively diagnosed with a positive needle biopsy combined with an ultrasound examination of the liver.

Liver cancer is staged upon diagnosis. If found early, surgery can be curative. However, it is rarely found early. Postoperative care is similar to care for other abdominal surgeries. If surgery is not an option, the patient may receive chemotherapeutic drugs by injection directly into the affected lobe of the liver or into the hepatic artery; sorafenib (Nexavar), which slows the multiplication of cancer cells; or radiation therapy. The overall survival rate for liver cancer is low. (See Chapter 11 for care of patients with cancer.)

DISORDERS OF THE PANCREAS

Pancreatitis

Pancreatitis, inflammation of the pancreas, may be either acute or chronic. The two forms of pancreatitis have different courses and are considered two different disorders.

Acute Pancreatitis
Pathophysiology

Inflammation of the pancreas appears to be caused by a process called autodigestion. Recall that the pancreas normally secretes digestive enzymes. For reasons not fully understood, pancreatic enzymes can be activated while they are still in the pancreas and begin to digest the pancreas. In addition, large amounts of enzymes are released by inflamed cells. As the pancreas digests itself, chemical cascades occur. Trypsin destroys pancreatic tissue and causes vasodilation. As capillary permeability increases, fluid is lost to the retroperitoneal space, causing shock. In addition, trypsin appears to set off another chain of events that causes the conversion of prothrombin to thrombin, so that clots form. The patient may develop disseminated intravascular coagulation (see Chapter 28).

Etiology

Acute pancreatitis (AP) is most commonly associated with heavy alcohol consumption or cholelithiasis (gallstones). Alcohol appears to act directly on the acinar cells of the pancreas and the pancreatic ducts to irritate and inflame the structures. Gallstones may plug the pancreatic duct and cause inflammation from excessive fluid pressure on sensitive ducts. The irritant effect of bile itself may cause inflammation. Elevated triglycerides, endoscopic retrograde cholangiopancreatography (ERCP)-induced pancreatitis, pancreatic tumors, or, rarely, medications can cause pancreatitis. Sometimes, the cause is unknown and referred to as idiopathic.

Prevention
Caution patients who drink alcohol to stop. People with biliary disease should seek medical treatment so that pancreatitis does not develop as a complication.

Signs and Symptoms
Patients with AP may present with severe pain, guarding, a rigid (boardlike) abdomen, hypotension or shock, and respiratory distress from accumulation of fluid in the retroperitoneal space (Table 35.4). Pain is located in the epigastric area or left upper quadrant (LUQ), with radiation to the chest, back, and flanks. Respirations are likely to be shallow as the patient attempts to splint the painful areas. The patient may have a low-grade fever, dry mucous membranes, and tachycardia. If the primary cause is biliary, the patient may report nausea and vomiting, and jaundice may be evident.

Complications
It may be useful to think of severe AP as a chemical burn to the organ. As with severe burns, death is likely to occur from organ failure. From the onset of symptoms, cardiovascular, pulmonary (including acute respiratory distress syndrome), and acute kidney injury are the most likely causes of death. Electrolyte imbalance, hemorrhage, peripheral vascular collapse, and infection are also major concerns. The presence of Chvostek sign (twitching of facial muscles with tapping in front of ear over facial nerve) indicates neuromuscular irritability and decreased calcium levels. A purplish discoloration of the flanks (Turner sign) or a purplish discoloration around the umbilicus (Cullen sign) may occur with extensive hemorrhagic destruction of the pancreas.

Diagnostic Tests
Diagnosis of AP is made when two of these are present: abdominal pain, serum amylase (normal: 100 to 300 units/L), and/or serum lipase (normal: 0 to 60 units/L) more than three times normal. Also, abdominal imaging may indicate it. Serum amylase rises quickly and then returns to normal in 3 to 5 days in most patients. Serum lipase is most specific for AP; it elevates and stays elevated for a longer period of time. Ultrasonography may show pleural effusion from local inflammatory reaction to pancreatic enzymes or a change in the size of the pancreas. Computed tomography (CT) scan and magnetic resonance imaging (MRI) can confirm AP.

Therapeutic Measures
Early aggressive intravenous (IV) hydration during the first 24 hours for hypovolemia treatment is recommended. In asymptomatic, mild AP, oral nutrition is given ("Nutrition Notes: Nourishing the Patient With Pancreatitis"). In severe cases, enteral feeding is begun. Pain relief is essential, especially for severe pain. Antibiotics are given if sepsis is present. Minimally invasive debriding of necrotic tissue may be considered for some symptomatic patients.

Table 35.4
Pancreatitis Summary

Signs and Symptoms	Epigastric or lower upper quadrant abdominal pain Low-grade fever Nausea and vomiting
Diagnostic Tests	Elevated serum amylase and lipase
Therapeutic Measures	Aggressive intravenous fluid hydration Pain control Mild acute pancreatitis: oral feeding Severe acute pancreatitis: enteral feeding
Complications	Hemorrhage, shock, sepsis, organ failure
Priority Nursing Diagnoses	*Pain* *Imbalanced Nutrition: Less Than Body Requirements* *Ineffective Breathing Pattern*

Nutrition Notes

Nourishing the Patient With Pancreatitis. Nutritionally, acute pancreatitis (AP) is treated with the following:

- Aggressive hydration with intravenous fluids
- Clear liquids or low-fat diet as tolerated after pain and nausea and vomiting are controlled
- Total abstinence from alcohol

If the disease progresses to severe AP, enteral pump-assisted feedings are started and should:

- Begin as early as possible
- Consist of a high-protein, low-fat, semielemental formula
- Start slowly (10 to 40 mL/hour, advancing every 8 to 12 hours by 10 to 20 mL/hour, as tolerated), until the goal rate is met

General dietary management principles for chronic pancreatitis depend on the stage of disease and include the following:

- Total abstinence from alcohol and smoking
- Adequate hydration, limiting caffeinated beverages
- Small, frequent, low-fat, and nutritionally balanced meals
- Vitamin–mineral supplements as appropriate
- Medium-chain triglycerides, a dietary fat in oil form, for easily digested calories
- Pancreatic enzyme supplements, which reduce pain

CRITICAL THINKING

Mrs. Samuels, an 85-year-old retired librarian, is admitted to the nursing unit from the emergency department with severe mid-epigastric pain that radiates to her back. On admission, she is noted to have guarding of the abdomen, and her abdomen is distended and rigid. Her medical record documents that she had an endoscopic retrograde cholangiopancreatography (ERCP) 2 days ago for recurrent episodes of right upper quadrant abdominal pain. She has no history of excessive alcohol intake.

1. What is the most common cause of acute pancreatitis (AP)? Does Mrs. Samuels fit the description?
2. Why might Mrs. Samuels have difficulty breathing?
3. Why is Mrs. Samuels at risk for hemorrhage?
4. What laboratory test is most likely to be abnormal in early AP?
5. Why are opioids commonly ordered for AP?
6. What nutrition orders will likely be given for Mrs. Samuels?

Suggested answers are at the end of the chapter.

Chronic Pancreatitis
Pathophysiology

Chronic pancreatitis (CP) is a progressive fibro-inflammatory disease in which functioning pancreatic tissue is replaced with fibrotic tissue because of inflammation. Pancreatic ducts become obstructed, dilated, and, finally, atrophied. The acinar, or enzyme-producing, cells of the pancreas ulcerate in response to inflammation. The ulceration causes further tissue damage and tissue death. It also may cause cystic sacs filled with pancreatic enzymes to form on the surface of the pancreas. The pancreas becomes smaller and hardened. Progressively smaller amounts of pancreatic enzymes are produced (exocrine insufficiency). Later, islet tissue is lost, causing diabetes mellitus (endocrine insufficiency).

Etiology

The usual age when CP develops is between 43 and 62 years. It occurs in men more than women and predominately in Caucasians (Conwell et al., 2017). Causes of CP include alcohol abuse (most common), obstructive biliary disease, and hyperlipidemia. Causes may also be idiopathic, genetic, and autoimmune related. Cigarette smoking and repeated attacks of AP are risk factors.

Signs and Symptoms

CP may by asymptomatic. If signs and symptoms occur, they are less severe than for AP. The patient will report epigastric or LUQ pain that worsens after eating, nausea and vomiting, weight loss, steatorrhea (greasy, foul-smelling, loose stools), and intolerance of fatty foods. The patient's history will show a pattern of exacerbations and remissions.

Complications

A variety of complications can result from CP. Abscesses and fistulas may develop when cysts filled with pancreatic enzymes burst into the abdominal cavity, causing severe inflammation and tissue necrosis. Pleural effusion may develop from inflammation just under the diaphragm. Pancreatic enzymes are essential for normal absorption of nutrients from the intestines. Fat intolerance and malabsorption syndrome with fatty stools and diarrhea may develop in response to the limited amount of pancreatic enzymes produced. In addition, biliary obstruction may further complicate fat absorption. As the terminal third of the pancreas becomes involved and the islets of Langerhans are destroyed, diabetes mellitus results (discussed in Chapter 40). CP is a risk factor for pancreatic cancer.

Diagnostic Tests

CT scan is the preferred initial radiologic test. If inconclusive, then MRI with IV secretin, endoscopic ultrasound, and pancreas function tests would be indicated. CT and ultrasonography best show late characteristic pancreatic structural changes, such as masses, calcification of ducts, cysts, and change in pancreatic size. Serum amylase and serum lipase levels will be normal or low. Fecal fat analysis shows higher than normal amounts of fat but are helpful only in late CP to identify the degree of exocrine insufficiency. ERCP can locate specific obstructions and detect ductal leaks for intervention.

Therapeutic Measures

Treatment is aimed at promoting comfort, maintaining adequate pancreatic function and nutrition, and treating complications (see "Nutrition Notes: Nourishing the Patient With Pancreatitis"). Alcohol abstinence is crucial to reduce pain. Other interventions to relieve pain include small low-fat meals, nonsteroidal anti-inflammatory drugs (NSAIDs) and analgesic, nerve block, or pancreatic enzyme supplements (Table 35.5). Procedures can be done to stent the pancreatic ducts or remove ductal stones (**extracorporeal shock-wave lithotripsy**). Surgery may be necessary to treat biliary disease, repair fistulas, drain cysts, or remove part of the pancreas.

Nursing Process for the Patient With Pancreatitis

See "Nursing Care Plan for the Patient With Acute and Chronic Pancreatitis."

Cancer of the Pancreas

Pancreatic cancer is the third-leading cause of cancer deaths in the United States, killing more than 43,000 people each year. The incidence of pancreatic cancer is rising. More than 55,000 new cases of cancer of the pancreas are projected to be diagnosed in 2018 (American Cancer Society, 2016).

• WORD • BUILDING •
extracorporeal shock-wave lithotripsy: extra—outside + tripsy—rub or crush

Nursing Care Plan for the Patient With Acute and Chronic Pancreatitis

Nursing Diagnosis: *Acute Pain* related to edema and inflammation
Expected Outcome: The patient will state pain level is tolerable within 30 minutes of pain report.
Evaluation of Outcome: Does the patient state pain level is tolerable?

Intervention	Rationale	Evaluation
Monitor patient for pain every 2 hours by asking patient to rate pain (such as with scale of 0 to 10).	*Intense pain is likely to occur with acute pancreatitis. A pain scale allows for a consistent and individual evaluation of pain.*	Does patient state that pain is tolerable?
Administer analgesics as ordered, before pain becomes severe.	*Analgesics are most effective if given before pain becomes too great.*	Are analgesics effective?
Assist patient to a position of comfort, usually high Fowler or leaning forward slightly.	*An upright position keeps abdominal organs from pressing against the inflamed pancreas.*	Does positioning promote comfort?
Keep the environment free from excessive stimuli.	*A quiet, restful, anxiety-free atmosphere permits patient to relax and may decrease pain perception.*	Does patient state atmosphere is relaxing?
Teach patient alternative pain control strategies, such as guided imagery and relaxation techniques.	*Successful use of pain control strategies may decrease the amount of analgesics needed and give patient a greater sense of control.*	Are alternative strategies effective?

Nursing Diagnosis: *Imbalanced Nutrition: Less Than Body Requirements* related to pain, anorexia, and treatment
Expected Outcome: The patient will experience improved nutrition as evidenced by stable weight.
Evaluation of Outcome: Is weight stable?

Intervention	Rationale	Evaluation
Observe for diarrhea, bloating, or steatorrhea (fatty stools). Report steatorrhea immediately.	Diarrhea, bloating, or fatty stools may indicate malabsorption syndrome. Steatorrhea may indicate that the enzyme replacement doses are not meeting the patient's needs.	Are stools normal?
Weigh patient every other day.	A loss of 1 lb of body weight occurs when the body uses 3,500 calories more than is taken in.	Has patient lost less than 5% of total baseline body weight?
Administer pancreatic enzymes and nutritional supplements as ordered.	Aids digestion and provides adequate nutrition.	Does patient take supplements?
Teach patient to avoid alcohol and provide alcohol cessation resources.	Alcohol may trigger another episode of pancreatitis.	Does patient verbalize understanding of importance of avoiding alcohol and use of resources?
Teach patient and family to self-monitor for symptoms of malabsorption syndrome, such as fatty stools, weight loss, dry skin, or bleeding.	Absence of pancreatic enzymes causes problems with digestion of fats, carbohydrates, and proteins.	Does patient verbalize understanding of symptoms of malabsorption to report?
Teach patient and family the signs and symptoms of diabetes mellitus.	Patients with pancreatitis are at great risk for developing diabetes mellitus.	Does patient verbalize signs and symptoms of diabetes to report?

(nursing care plan continues on page 710)

Nursing Care Plan for the Patient With Acute and Chronic Pancreatitis—cont'd

Nursing Diagnosis: *Ineffective Breathing Pattern* related to abdominal pressure and pain
Expected Outcome: The patient will have an effective breathing pattern as evidenced by unlabored respirations, 16 to 20 per minute and oxygen saturation (Sao$_2$) 95% or greater at all times.
Evaluation of Outcome: Are respirations unlabored and 16 to 20 per minute, and is Sao$_2$ 95% or greater?

Intervention	Rationale	Evaluation
Observe patient's breathing pattern, including respiration depth, regularity, rate, effort, and distress, such as use of accessory muscles or intercostal muscles or Sao$_2$ less than 95%.	*Abdominal pressure from inflammation and tissue damage under the diaphragm may cause patient to take shallow, rapid respirations, which can tire the patient.*	Are patient's respirations 16 to 20 per minute, unlabored, and regular?
Administer oxygen as ordered.	*Oxygen increases the Sao$_2$.*	Is Sao$_2$ 95% or greater?
Place patient in an upright or slightly forward-leaning position.	*Relieves pressure on the diaphragm.*	Is positioning effective?

Nursing Diagnosis: *Risk for Injury* related to hemorrhage or fluid and electrolyte imbalances
Expected Outcome: The patient will experience no injury during illness.
Evaluation of Outcome: Is there evidence of injury? Are signs and symptoms of impending injury recognized and reported early?

Intervention	Rationale	Evaluation
Monitor sodium, potassium, calcium, and magnesium levels daily.	*Electrolyte levels can become imbalanced in pancreatitis.*	Are laboratory values within normal range?
Observe for nausea and vomiting and give antiemetics as ordered.	*Vomiting can contribute to fluid loss.*	Is nausea controlled to prevent vomiting?
Monitor patient's hematocrit level, hemoglobin level, and blood clotting times frequently.	*Destruction of the pancreas can result in hemorrhage.*	Does patient have any abnormal bruising, bleeding gums, or pink urine?
Observe abdomen and flanks for Cullen and Turner signs.	*These are signs of hemorrhage.*	Are signs of hemorrhage present?
Weigh the patient daily.	*Weight accurately monitors fluid balance.*	Is weight stable?
Measure and record intake and output.	*Monitors and reflects fluid balance.*	Is urinary output greater than 30 mL/hr?
Teach patient to report weakness or muscle twitching.	*May indicate electrolyte imbalance.*	Does patient verbalize understanding of signs and symptoms of electrolyte imbalance to report?

Pathophysiology

Most primary tumors of the pancreas are ductal adenocarcinomas. They occur in the exocrine (digestive secretion) parts of the pancreas. Exocrine tumors will be discussed in this section because neuroendocrine pancreatic tumors are less common. The tumors in the head and body of the pancreas tend to be large. Cancer of the pancreas spreads rapidly by direct extension to the stomach, gallbladder, and duodenum. Cancer located in the body of the pancreas usually spreads farther and more rapidly than do masses in the head. Cancer of the pancreas may spread by the lymphatic and vascular systems to distant organs and lymph nodes.

Etiology

The cause of pancreatic cancer is associated most commonly with smoking followed by dietary factors (obesity, especially during early adulthood; possibly consumption of red meat and processed meat), work place exposure to chemicals used

Table 35.5

Medications Used for Pancreatic and Gallbladder Disorders

Medication Class/Action

Antiemetics

Reduce nausea.

Examples	Nursing Implications
prochlorperazine (Compazine)	Contraindicated in glaucoma or prostatic hypertrophy. Give antacids 2 hours before or after.
metoclopramide (Reglan)	Monitor for extrapyramidal symptoms. Administer 30 minutes before meals.
promethazine (Phenergan)	May be additive when used with opioids. Monitor intake and output, sedation, and urine retention.
ondansetron (Zofran)	Monitor for hypersensitivity.

Bile Acid Sequestrants

Bind with circulating bile acids for excretion in the stool to relieve itching.

Examples	Nursing Implications
cholestyramine (Questran, LoCholest) colestipol (Colestid)	Give 4 to 6 hours before or 1 hour after other medications.

Bile Acid Dissolution Agents

Prevent or dissolve (noncalcified) cholesterol gallstones.

Examples	Nursing Implications
ursodiol (Actigall) chenodiol (Chenix)	Give with a full glass of water. Aluminum antacids may reduce absorption.

Pancreatic Supplements

Replace pancreatic digestive enzymes (lipase, protease, amylase).

Examples	Nursing Implications
pancrelipase (Cotazym, Creon, Ultrase, Viokase)	Give with meals. Teach not to hold medication in mouth because it may irritate inside of mouth.

in dry cleaning and metal industries, diabetes mellitus, chronic pancreatitis, cirrhosis, *Helicobacter pylori* infection, and heredity. African American males have the highest rate of pancreatic cancer. Prevention may be provided with high-folate and lycopene fruits and vegetables.

Signs and Symptoms

The patient with early pancreatic cancer often does not experience signs or symptoms. When signs or symptoms appear, the cancer may have already metastasized. Epigastric or back pain, anorexia, nausea, fatigue, and malaise are early symptoms. Weight loss is the classic sign of pancreatic cancer. The patient may report abdominal pain that is worse at night. The pain is described as gnawing or boring, and it radiates to the back. The pain may be lessened by a side-lying position with the knees drawn up to the chest or by bending over when walking. The pain becomes increasingly severe and unrelenting as the cancer grows. Depression may be experienced. The patient may report a bloated feeling or fullness after eating. If the cancer obstructs the bile duct, the patient may have jaundice, pruritus, dark urine, and light-colored stools. The patient's health history may include a recent diagnosis of diabetes mellitus.

Complications

Complications may occur before or after surgical treatment. Preoperative complications include malnutrition, spread of the cancer, and gastric or duodenal obstruction. Postoperative complications include infection, breakdown of the surgical site, fistula formation, diabetes mellitus, and malabsorption syndrome.

Thrombophlebitis is a common complication of cancer of the pancreas. As the tumor grows, by-products of the tumor growth appear to increase the levels of thromboplastic (clotting) factors in the blood, making clotting easier. The potential for thrombophlebitis increases if the patient is on bedrest or has surgery.

Diagnostic Tests

Serum ALP, glucose, and bilirubin levels may be elevated. Amylase and lipase levels are elevated if the cancer has caused secondary pancreatitis. Blood coagulation tests, such as clotting time, are done. Carcinoembryonic antigen (CEA) is ordered to confirm the presence of cancer (normal: less than 5 ng/mL).

Abdominal x-rays determine the size of the pancreas and the presence of masses. CT scan, MRI, or ultrasonography are done to precisely locate masses in the pancreas. ERCP can be used to visualize the common ducts and to take tissue samples for microscopic analysis. Pancreatic biopsy is necessary for definitive diagnosis of pancreatic cancer. A tissue sample may be obtained by needle aspiration during ultrasonography. Staging of the cancer with **laparoscopy** and biopsy can be done to guide treatment options.

Therapeutic Measures

The prognosis for pancreatic cancer can be poor because most cases are diagnosed after the cancer has already spread. If diagnosed early enough, surgical treatment may provide a cure. The HCP can develop a survivorship care plan for tests and follow-up appointments, healthy lifestyle choices, and things to report to the HCP. If the patient's cancer has progressed to distant involvement of other organ structures and lymph nodes, treatment is directed at easing symptoms and making the patient more comfortable.

Curative (if all of the cancer can be removed) or palliative focused surgery can be used. When the tumor is located at the head of the pancreas, there is the greatest possibility for cure. The Whipple procedure (pancreatoduodenectomy), a very complex surgery, is the most commonly used surgery for exocrine pancreatic cancer. This surgery removes the head and sometimes the body of the pancreas, lymph nodes nearby, the lower portion of the common bile duct, the gallbladder, most of the duodenum, and possibly parts of the stomach nearby (Fig. 35.6). This can be done as an open or laparoscopic surgery. Potential postoperative problems after the Whipple procedure include failure of the suture lines to hold, causing leakage of pancreatic enzymes and bile into the abdomen; pneumonia or atelectasis from shallow breathing because the incision line is directly under the diaphragm; paralytic ileus; gastric retention or ulceration; wound infection; fistula formation; unstable diabetes mellitus; and kidney failure.

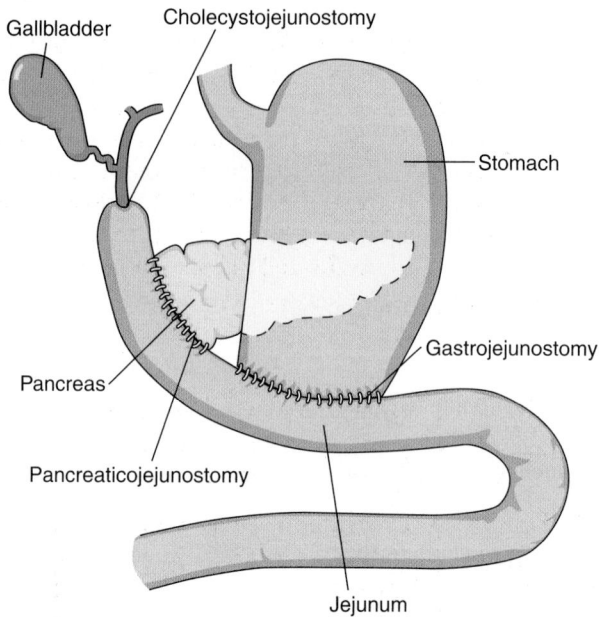

FIGURE 35.6 Pancreatoduodenectomy (Whipple procedure) for cancer of the head of the pancreas.

Rarely, for tumors in the tail of the pancreas, a distal **pancreatectomy** along with spleen removal is done, in which the tail or the tail and some of the pancreas body is removed. Relief of biliary obstruction can sometimes be accomplished by implanting a stent or plastic tube in the common bile duct during an endoscopic procedure. Pain can be reduced by surgical removal of a portion of the greater splanchnic nerve. Also less common is a total pancreatectomy with removal of the gallbladder, a portion of the stomach, small intestine, and the spleen. However, there are more side effects, and insulin and digestive enzymes must be used for life.

Palliative surgery such as stent placement or bypass surgery for a blocked bile duct is used to promote comfort. Chemotherapy and/or radiation therapy can be used to shrink or destroy the tumor, treat or prevent metastasis, or provide relief of symptoms if the cancer has become too widespread for surgery. (See Chapter 11 for care of the patient undergoing radiation or chemotherapy.)

Nursing Process for the Patient With Pancreatic Cancer

DATA COLLECTION. Observe the patient with cancer of the pancreas for evidence of malnutrition and fluid imbalance, including weight loss, inelastic skin turgor, nausea and vomiting, and fatty stools. Review laboratory tests, especially blood glucose, liver function studies, and clotting studies. Monitor the patient for pain. Observe the skin for bruising, scaling, and yellowing, and ask about itching. Evaluate the patient's mental status for evidence of depression.

• WORD • BUILDING •
laparoscopy: laparo—pertaining to flank + scopy—to examine
pancreatectomy: pancreat—pancreas + ectomy—excision

NURSING DIAGNOSES, PLANNING, AND IMPLEMENTATION. The patient with cancer of the pancreas will have numerous problems. Interventions for the nursing diagnoses *Imbalanced Nutrition: Less Than Body Requirements* (related to inability to digest food, anorexia, nausea, and vomiting) and *Acute Pain* (related to pancreatic tumor or surgical incision) are the same as for patients with pancreatitis (see "Nursing Care Plan for the Patient With Acute and Chronic Pancreatitis"). Additional care is listed next. Interventions for patients with cancer, including psychosocial interventions, can be found in Chapter 11.

Risk for Deficient Fluid Volume related to nausea and vomiting

EXPECTED OUTCOME: The patient will have adequate fluid volume as evidenced by stable vital signs, elastic skin turgor, and moist mucous membranes.

• Monitor the patient's intake and output accurately. *Low intake increases risk of deficient fluid volume; low output is a sign of deficient fluid.*
• Monitor vital signs and report abnormal findings. *Tachycardia, tachypnea, and low blood pressure may indicate excessive fluid loss.*
• Monitor laboratory values and report abnormal values, especially serum electrolytes. *If electrolyte values are low, the HCP may order IV replacement solutions.*

Risk for Impaired Tissue Integrity related to itching

EXPECTED OUTCOME: The patient's skin will remain intact.

• Monitor the patient for reports of itching *because scratching can cause a break in the skin.*
• Help the patient keep fingernails short *to reduce damage to skin with scratching.*
• Provide frequent skin care with products free of soap or alcohol *to prevent further dryness and itching.*
• Apply products such as calamine lotion as ordered *to decrease itching.*

EVALUATION. The plan of care for the patient with pancreatic cancer is successful if the patient maintains body weight within 5% of normal body weight and experiences no nausea or vomiting; states that pain remains tolerable; and has urinary output greater than 30 mL/hr, elastic skin turgor, moist mucous membranes, and pulse and blood pressure within 10% of patient's baseline.

PATIENT EDUCATION. Teach the patient and family self-care measures such as blood glucose monitoring, insulin administration, signs and symptoms of hyperglycemia and hypoglycemia (see Chapter 40), and the regimen for pancreatic enzyme replacement. Instruct the patient on how to manage dressing changes if he or she is to be discharged with tubes or drains after surgery. The patient and family should know the signs and symptoms of complications to report. A patient being cared for at home should have a referral for hospice care or home health nursing. For more information, visit the National Pancreas Foundation at www.pancreasfoundation.org.

DISORDERS OF THE GALLBLADDER

Cholecystitis, Cholelithiasis, and Choledocholithiasis

Gallstones and inflammations of the gallbladder and common bile duct are the most common disorders of the biliary system.

Pathophysiology

Cholecystitis is inflammation of the gallbladder. Acute cholecystitis is a serious response to obstruction of the common bile duct by a stone, resulting in edema and inflammation. Urgent medical treatment is required with surgery to prevent gallbladder rupture. Chronic cholecystitis may be the result of repeated attacks of acute cholecystitis or chronic irritation from gallstones. The gallbladder then becomes fibrotic and thickened, and does not empty easily or completely.

Cholelithiasis is the formation of gallstones in the gallbladder. The most common composition of gallstones in the United States is cholesterol. **Choledocholithiasis** refers to gallstones within the common bile duct. Gallstones form when bile becomes supersaturated with a substance such as cholesterol. The substance then crystallizes, forming sludge, with continued enlargement to form stones. Another type of gallstone is a pigment stone, which is composed of calcium bilirubinate that forms when free bilirubin combines with calcium.

Etiology and Incidence

CHOLELITHIASIS. Causes of gallstones include aging, heredity ("Cultural Considerations: Gallbladder Disease"), obesity, stasis of bile, frequent fasting, diabetes mellitus, cirrhosis, pregnancy, estrogen, and other medications. They occur mostly in women. Stasis may be caused by a decreased gallbladder-emptying rate, a partial obstruction in the common duct, or pregnancy. Excessive cholesterol intake combined with a sedentary lifestyle is linked to an increased incidence of cholelithiasis, as are hemolytic blood disorders such as sickle cell disease and bowel disorders such as Crohn disease.

CHOLECYSTITIS. Cholelithiasis is responsible for most cases of cholecystitis, or inflammation of the gallbladder.

Cultural Considerations

Gallbladder Disease. Gallbladder disease is common among Mexican Americans. Native Americans have an increased incidence of pancreatic disease and gallbladder disease. The nurse can positively affect the nutritional status of at-risk patients by teaching food preparation practices that use less fat.

• WORD • BUILDING •

cholecystitis: chole—bile + cyst—bladder + itis—inflammation
cholelithiasis: chole—bile + lith—stone + iasis—condition
choledocholithiasis: chole—bile + docho—duct + lith—stone + iasis—condition

Signs and Symptoms

Gallstones are asymptomatic (silent stones) and require no treatment in most people. Signs and symptoms of cholecystitis and cholelithiasis are similar. Signs include evidence of inflammation such as an elevated temperature, pulse, and respirations as well as vomiting. The patient may have a positive Murphy sign, which is the inability to take a deep breath when an examiner's fingers are pressed below the liver margin.

CHOLELITHIASIS. The epigastric pain caused by cholelithiasis may also be called biliary **colic**. The pain is a steady, aching, severe pain in the epigastrium and RUQ that may radiate back to behind the right scapula or to the right shoulder. The pain usually begins suddenly after a fatty meal and lasts for 1 to 3 hours. If the pain is caused by a stone in the common bile duct (choledocholithiasis), the pain may last until the stone has passed into the duodenum. Jaundice is more commonly present with acute choledocholithiasis because the common bile duct is blocked or inflamed.

CHOLECYSTITIS. The biliary colic caused by cholecystitis typically lasts 4 to 6 hours. The pain is made worse with movement such as breathing. The patient usually has nausea, vomiting, and a low-grade fever with the pain. Heartburn, indigestion, and flatulence are more common with chronic cholecystitis. Patients often report repeated attacks of acute cholecystitis symptoms (Table 35.6).

CRITICAL THINKING

Donna Stewart, a 48-year-old woman, is suspected of having acute cholecystitis. She is 5 feet, 4 inches tall and weighs 188 pounds. After testing, the health care provider (HCP) recommends surgery.

1. What risk factors does Donna have for cholecystitis?
2. What diagnostic tests might be ordered to confirm Donna's diagnosis of cholecystitis?
3. What medication can you anticipate that the HCP will order for Donna?
4. If the diagnosis of cholecystitis is confirmed, what type of surgical treatment might be ordered?
5. What type of diet will Donna need to eat after discharge?

Suggested answers are at the end of the chapter.

Complications

Complications of cholecystitis include acute cholangitis (inflammation of the bile ducts), necrosis or perforation of the gallbladder, empyema (a collection of purulent drainage in the gallbladder), fistulas, and adenocarcinoma of the gallbladder. A major complication of choledocholithiasis is AP if the pancreatic duct is obstructed.

Diagnostic Tests

An ultrasound of the gallbladder is the classic test done to detect stones, inflamed walls of the gallbladder, and dilated ducts. An endoscopic ultrasound can provide more detailed images of the gallbladder and bile ducts. A CT scan may also

---

Nutrition Notes

Modifying the Diet for Patients With Gallbladder Disease

- During an acute attack of cholecystitis, depending on severity and treatment, the patient's prescribed diet may range from nothing by mouth (NPO) to a low-fat diet.
- For treatment of chronic cholecystitis, caused by gallstones, the patient is taught to:
  - Lose weight gradually, if needed, and then maintain an ideal body weight.
  - Eat a high-fiber diet with complex carbohydrates (whole grains, fruits, and vegetables), and limit simple carbohydrates (white bread, white rice, sugars).
  - Eat healthy fats, such as low-fat dairy products, lean meats, healthy monounsaturated fats (avocado and nuts), and polyunsaturated fats (vegetable oils and fish).
- After a cholecystectomy, the patient may initially be NPO or have a clear liquid diet. The diet is advanced as tolerated. Later, balanced low-fat meals are often well tolerated because bile enters the duodenum continuously to digest fat.

Reference

National Institute of Health, National Institute of Diabetes and Digestive and Kidney Diseases. (2017). Dieting and gallstones. Retrieved from www.niddk.nih.gov/health-information/digestive-diseases/gallstones/dieting

---

be done. Tests to view the bile ducts include magnetic resonance cholangiopancreatography (MRCP), ERCP that directly visualizes the pancreatic ducts and bile ducts for the presence of stones to then remove them, and a hepatobiliary iminodiacetic acid (HIDA) scan in which the patient is given an IV injection of a radioactive isotope that is metabolized by the liver and excreted in the bile. The scanning camera then traces the path of the isotope as it travels through the bile ducts, gallbladder, and intestines to identify blockages.

The patient may have an elevated WBC count (normal: 5,000 to 10,000 cells/mm³). If direct bilirubin is elevated (normal: less than 0.3 mg/dL), its cause is likely obstruction in the biliary or liver areas. Liver enzymes can rise from hepatic inflammation. Serum amylase and lipase levels may be elevated if the pancreas is involved or if there is a stone in the common duct.

Therapeutic Measures

Treatment of an acute episode of cholecystitis centers on pain control with analgesics, prevention of infection, and maintenance of fluid and electrolyte balance. For itching relief with jaundice from bile acid deposits in the skin, colestipol (Colestid) or cholestyramine (Questran, LoCholest) is given (see Table 35.5). These drugs bind with the circulating bile acids for excretion in the stool. If the patient has nausea and vomiting, an antiemetic may be ordered (see Table 35.5). See "Nutrition Notes: Modifying the Diet for Patients With Gallbladder Disease."

· WORD · BUILDING ·

colic: colic—spasm

Table 35.6

Symptoms of Gallbladder Disorders

	Acute Cholecystitis	*Chronic Cholecystitis*	*Cholelithiasis and Choledocholithiasis*
Biliary colic	Lasts 4–6 hours Worse with movement	Only during acute attack	Sudden onset
Jaundice	Present (if common bile duct is inflamed or blocked)	Present	Lasts 1–3 hours Radiates to right scapula or shoulder
Low-grade fever	Present	Present	Present
Nausea, vomiting	Present	Only during acute attack	Present
Repeated attacks	Do not occur	Occur	Do not occur
Heartburn, indigestion, and flatulence	Not present	Present	Not present
Complications	Cholangitis Necrosis or perforation Fistulas	Empyema Fistulas Adenocarcinoma	Acute pancreatitis

SURGERY. Treatment for cholelithiasis typically involves cholecystectomy (surgical removal of gallbladder) via laparoscopy. A laparoscopic cholecystectomy is done with a laparoscope through four small puncture wounds in the abdomen. Choledochoscopy (using endoscope) may also be used to view the common bile duct to prevent retained stones there. Patients are usually discharged in 24 hours or less, and recovery time is reduced with laparoscopic surgery.

For large stones or an infected gallbladder, a traditional open cholecystectomy may be required. A T-tube may be inserted into the common duct to ensure that bile drainage is not obstructed (Fig. 35.7). T-tube drainage ranges from 500 to 1,000 mL the first day and decreases to 200 mL by the third day. The patient with a traditional cholecystectomy has incisional pain that creates difficulty with coughing and deep breathing postoperatively. This is because deep breathing causes the diaphragm to press on the operative site. Patients are hospitalized for 2 to 3 days with a traditional cholecystectomy.

MEDICATION. Dissolution of small noncalcified (primarily cholesterol) stones (less than 1.5 cm) with a bile acid dissolution agent (see Table 35.5) is used for those who are not surgical candidates. Treatment with a dissolution drug may take up to 2 years and stones often return.

Nursing Process for the Patient With a Gallbladder Disorder

DATA COLLECTION. Monitor the patient frequently for pain, using the *WHAT'S UP?* questions. Take the patient's vital signs, particularly the temperature, frequently to monitor for signs of infection. Evaluate laboratory studies for elevation in the WBC count or abnormalities in electrolytes or serum bilirubin levels. Weigh the patient and inspect mucous membranes, skin turgor, and urinary output for signs of dehydration. Measure intake and output, including any emesis or drainage from T-tubes. Observe stools and urine for color and consistency. Obstruction of bile flow may result in stools that are clay-colored or have a foul, greasy appearance, or urine that is dark amber or tea colored. Report these findings immediately.

NURSING DIAGNOSES, PLANNING, AND IMPLEMENTATION. Common nursing diagnoses for the patient with cholecystitis include *Acute Pain* and *Risk for Deficient Fluid Volume*.

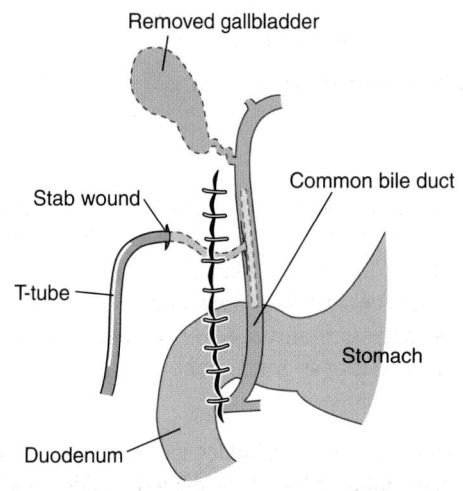

FIGURE 35.7 T-tube to drain bile after a cholecystectomy until swelling of the duct subsides.

Additional nursing diagnoses for the patient with cholelithiasis who has a surgical procedure include *Risk for Impaired Skin Integrity* related to surgical incision and T-tube drainage and *Ineffective Breathing Pattern* related to abdominal incision.

Acute Pain related to biliary colic

EXPECTED OUTCOME: The patient will rate pain as 2 or less on a 0 to 10 pain scale.

• Monitor the patient frequently for pain *to guide treatment.*
• Administer analgesics as ordered *to reduce pain.*
• Administer antispasmodics or anticholinergics as ordered *for biliary colic.*
• Assist patient with positioning *to assume the position that provides the most comfort.*

Risk for Deficient Fluid Volume related to nausea, vomiting, or excessive tube drainage

EXPECTED OUTCOME: The patient will have adequate fluid volume as evidenced by stable vital signs, elastic skin turgor, and moist mucous membranes at all times.

• Monitor intake and output, daily weights, and skin turgor, and report changes *to monitor fluid balance.*
• Monitor T-tube drainage. Carefully observe the T-tube drainage unit to prevent kinking of the tubing. *Pressure in the biliary drainage system from poor drainage may greatly increase the patient's pain and the risk for infection.*
• Give antiemetics as ordered *to control nausea and vomiting.*
• Assist with administration of IV fluids and electrolytes as ordered if the patient is on restricted oral intake *to maintain hydration.*

Risk for Impaired Skin Integrity related to pruritic from jaundice, surgical incision, and T-tube drainage

EXPECTED OUTCOME: The patient's skin will remain intact at all times.

• Inspect the patient's skin and the sclerae of the eyes for jaundice, and report jaundice or pruritus *to provide treatment to reduce itching injury to skin.*
• Inspect the cholecystectomy incision for infection signs such as redness, edema, warmth, or drainage, *which can irritate and break down skin.*
• Keep dressings dry *to protect the skin around the incision site from irritating drainage.*

Ineffective Breathing Pattern related to abdominal incision

EXPECTED OUTCOME: The patient will have effective breathing pattern that has a respiratory rate of 16 to 20 per minute, is even and unlabored, and has depth within normal limits at all times.

• Monitor respiratory rate, depth, and effort, and ability to cough effectively. *The high abdominal incision can cause pain with deep breathing and coughing.*

• Monitor pain and provide analgesics as ordered *to allow the patient to cough without pain.*
• Encourage the patient to cough and deep breathe as taught before surgery hourly while awake. *Deep breathing and coughing after any surgical procedure helps prevent atelectasis and respiratory tract infections.*
• Assist the patient with splinting the abdomen when coughing *to make coughing less painful.*
• Encourage early ambulation as soon as possible *to help mobilize secretions.*

EVALUATION. The plan of care for a patient with cholecystitis or cholelithiasis is successful if the patient reports tolerable pain not greater than 2 on a pain scale of 0 to 10, no weight loss, no excessive thirst, and urinary output greater than 30 mL/hour; has moist mucous membranes, elastic skin turgor, and intact skin with no warmth, redness, swelling, or purulent drainage at the wound site; no jaundice or itching; clear breath sounds; and a normal WBC count (Table 35.7).

PATIENT EDUCATION. Discharge education focuses on a high-protein, low-fat diet. Obese patients are encouraged to lose weight. After a cholecystectomy, fat should be slowly reintroduced into the diet. Once the duodenum becomes accustomed to a constant infusion of bile, the patient's individual tolerance for fat intake guides food choices.

Table 35.7
Cholecystitis Summary

Signs and Symptoms	Biliary colic: Epigastric/right upper quadrant pain, especially after a fatty meal Elevated temperature, pulse, respirations Jaundice if common bile duct blocked
Diagnostic Tests	Ultrasound, endoscopic ultrasound Computed tomography (CT) Scan Magnetic resonance cholangiopancreatography (MRCP) Endoscopic retrograde cholangiopancreatography (ERCP) Hepatobiliary iminodiacetic acid (HIDA) scan White blood cell count elevated
Therapeutic Measures	Pain control Laparoscopic or open cholecystectomy Medications (see Table 35.5) Low-fat diet
Priority Nursing Diagnoses	*Acute Pain* *Ineffective Breathing Pattern* *Risk for Impaired Skin Integrity*

SUGGESTED ANSWERS TO CRITICAL THINKING

Carl Young

1. Foreign travel within the past 2 months, eating raw oysters, fatigue, nausea, and irritability suggest hepatitis A virus infection. Recent possible exposure to materials contaminated with blood or body fluids and fatigue, headache, and nausea suggest hepatitis B virus infection.
2. Careful hand hygiene and standard precautions when handling any body fluids or feces should be instituted.
3. Infectious disease health care provider (HCP), dietitian for nutritional needs, social worker for financial information during recovery period.
4. Plan to give an antiemetic if Carl is nauseated. The nurse should also ensure that the environment is free of noxious stimulants such as unpleasant odors. The diet should be high calorie, high protein, high carbohydrate, and low fat.
5. Any medication that is known to be hepatotoxic, such as acetaminophen, aspirin, and diazepam (Valium), should be avoided.
6. Carl should be taught that cleanliness, especially with food preparation, is essential; that he should avoid eating raw oysters or raw or undercooked shellfish; that frequent hand washing is crucial; and that alcohol and other liver-toxic substances should be avoided.

Mrs. Conner

1. Mrs. Conner has a history of poor nutrition that puts her at risk, as does her age.
2. Mrs. Conner may report that she has malaise, nausea, weight loss, a change in bowel habits, and dull, aching right upper quadrant pain.
3. Serum albumin level may be less than 3.2 g/dL. Her prothrombin time will probably be prolonged and greater than 25 seconds.
4. Esophageal varices and ascites are the two greatest concerns for the patient with portal hypertension.
5. The HCP will usually order diuretics, a sodium-restricted diet, and possibly intravenous albumin infusions.

Mrs. Samuels

1. The most common cause of acute pancreatitis (AP) is heavy alcohol intake. Mrs. Samuels reports no alcohol consumption, but she does have the risk factor of having had a recent endoscopic retrograde cholangiopancreatography (ERCP), which may have dislodged a gallstone or irritated the pancreatic duct.
2. Respiratory distress may result from excess fluid accumulation in the retroperitoneal space and from shallow respirations that seek to decrease pressure from the diaphragm on the inflamed pancreas and surrounding tissues.
3. Pancreatitis is similar to a chemical burn and may cause erosion of major blood vessels in surrounding tissue.
4. Serum amylase rises quickly and then returns to normal in 3 to 5 days. Serum lipase is thought to be more specific for AP, and elevates and stays elevated for a longer period of time.
5. Opioids are ordered because pain is intense, and pain with anxiety stimulates the autonomic nervous system, which may stimulate greater production of pancreatic enzymes.
6. Enteral nutrition until symptoms (pain) are resolved, then oral nutrition.

Donna Stewart

1. Aging and obesity.
2. Donna's HCP might order a white blood cell count, which will be elevated if she has cholecystitis. In addition, the HCP may order an ultrasound or radionuclide scan to visualize the gallbladder and its contents and the common bile duct.
3. You can anticipate that the HCP will order analgesics.
4. If the diagnosis is confirmed, Donna will probably have a laparoscopic cholecystectomy unless her HCP decides that she needs a traditional cholecystectomy.
5. Donna will need to eat a low-fat diet after discharge. Eventually she may be able to add more fats to her diet as her body adjusts to the loss of the gallbladder.

Review Questions

1. The nurse is planning care for a patient with cirrhosis. For which condition would the nurse place the patient on bleeding precautions?
   1. Encephalopathy
   2. Low vitamin K
   3. Elevated liver enzymes
   4. Hepatorenal syndrome

2. The nurse is caring for a patient with cirrhosis. The nurse would cautiously use sedatives for the patient due to which of the following?
   1. The liver's ability to synthesize protein is altered.
   2. Sedatives may increase the risk of jaundice.
   3. Sedatives are potentially toxic to the cirrhosis patient.
   4. Sedatives promote the conversion of ammonia to ammonium ion.

3. The nurse is collecting data for a patient with suspected acute hepatitis A infection. Which clinical manifestations would the nurse expect the patient to report? **Select all that apply.**
   1. Headache
   2. Flu-like symptoms
   3. Light-colored stools
   4. Nausea
   5. Abdominal pain
   6. Brown-colored urine

4. The nurse is caring for a patient with chronic pancreatitis. While reviewing laboratory data, the nurse would expect an elevation in which serum laboratory value?
   1. Albumin
   2. Amylase
   3. Bilirubin
   4. Calcium

5. The nurse is planning care for a newly admitted patient with acute pancreatitis. Which patient outcome should receive the highest priority in the plan of care?
   1. Patient increases activity tolerance.
   2. Patient maintains normal bowel function.
   3. Patient verbalizes understanding of medications at discharge.
   4. Patient expresses satisfaction with pain control.

6. The nurse is collecting data for a patient who develops jaundice and dark-colored urine. The nurse recognizes that which of the following is most likely the cause of these clinical manifestations?
   1. Encephalopathy
   2. Pancreatitis
   3. Bile duct obstruction
   4. Cholecystitis

7. The nurse reinforces teaching for a patient after a cholecystectomy who is on a low-fat diet. The nurse will know that the patient understands the diet if which menu items are selected?
   1. Roast chicken, rice, gelatin dessert
   2. Cream of chicken soup, milk, gelatin dessert
   3. Meat loaf, mashed potatoes with small amount of gravy, green beans
   4. Turkey and cheese sandwich on whole-grain bread, apple, milk

8. The nurse is caring for a patient who had an open cholecystectomy 24 hours ago. Which actions should the nurse take to assist the patient to maintain an effective breathing pattern? **Select all that apply.**
   1. Place in a supine position.
   2. Provide analgesics for pain relief.
   3. Encourage coughing and deep breathing.
   4. Monitor bowel sounds.
   5. Assist with splinting during coughing.
   6. Maintain bedrest for 48 hours after surgery.

9. The nurse is to administer promethazine 12.5 mg intramuscularly and has 50 mg/mL on hand. How many milliliters should be drawn up? Fill in the blank.
   Answer: _____ mL

Answer rationales available in your online resources.

ANSWERS 1. 2; 2. 3; 3. 1, 2, 4, 5, 4; 6. 3; 7. 1; 8. 2, 3, 5; 9. 0.25

Key Points

Find the chapter key points in your online resources available through Davis Edge.

Additional Resources

DAVIS
edge. ◀ Use the scratch off code on the inside front cover of your book to access online quizzes that will help you to improve your scores on course exams and prepare for the NCLEX-PN®.

 Study Guide

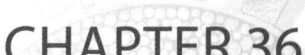

CHAPTER 36

Urinary System Function, Assessment, and Therapeutic Measures

Maureen McDonald, Janice L. Bradford

KEY TERMS

azotemia (AY-zoh-TEE-me-ah)
cystoscopy (sis-TAW-skuh-pee)
dysuria (dis-YOO-ree-ah)
hematuria (HEE-muh-TOOR-ee-ah)
incontinence (in-CON-tin-ense)
nephrotoxic (NEF-row-TOK-sik)
nocturia (knock-TOO-ree-ah)
percutaneously (PURR-kyoo-TAY-nee-us-lee)
polyuria (pa-lee-YOO-ree-ah)
pyelogram (PIE-eh-loh-gram)

LEARNING OUTCOMES

1. Identify the normal anatomy of the urinary system.
2. Describe the normal function of the urinary system.
3. Discuss the effects of aging on the urinary system.
4. Explain data to collect when caring for a patient with a disorder of the urinary system.
5. Plan preparation and postprocedure care for patients undergoing diagnostic tests of the urinary system.
6. Plan nursing care for patients with incontinence.
7. Discuss nursing actions to decrease the risk of infection in urinary catheterized patients.

CHAPTER CONCEPT

Elimination

NORMAL URINARY SYSTEM ANATOMY AND PHYSIOLOGY

The urinary system consists of two kidneys and two ureters, the urinary bladder, and the urethra. The kidneys form urine, and the rest of the system eliminates urine. The purpose of urine formation is the removal of potentially toxic waste products from the blood; however, the kidneys have other equally important functions as well:

- Regulation of blood pressure, volume, and composition by the excretion or conservation of water
- Regulation of the electrolyte balance of the blood by the excretion or conservation of minerals
- Regulation of the acid–base balance of the blood by the excretion or conservation of ions such as hydrogen or bicarbonate
- Production of erythropoietin, which then stimulates erythrocyte production in the bone marrow
- Activation of vitamin D, which maintains bone health

The process of urine formation thus helps maintain the normal composition, volume, and pH of blood and tissue fluid.

Kidneys

The bilateral kidneys are located against the posterior wall of the abdominal cavity. They are retroperitoneal. The superior portions of both kidneys rest on the inferior surface of the diaphragm; these portions are protected by the lower rib cage. The kidneys are cushioned by surrounding adipose tissue. This tissue, in turn, is covered by a fibrous connective membrane called the renal fascia. On the medial surface of each kidney is an indentation called the hilus, where the renal artery enters and the renal vein and ureter emerge. The ureter carries urine from the kidney to the urinary bladder.

Internal Structure of the Kidney

A frontal section of the kidney shows three distinct areas: the cortex, medulla, and pelvis (Fig. 36.1).

Blood Vessels of the Kidney

The pathway of blood flow through the kidney is an essential part of the process of urine formation. Blood enters the kidney from the renal artery and exits through the renal vein. Extensive branching within the kidney eventually leads arterial blood to each afferent arteriole. This vessel

719

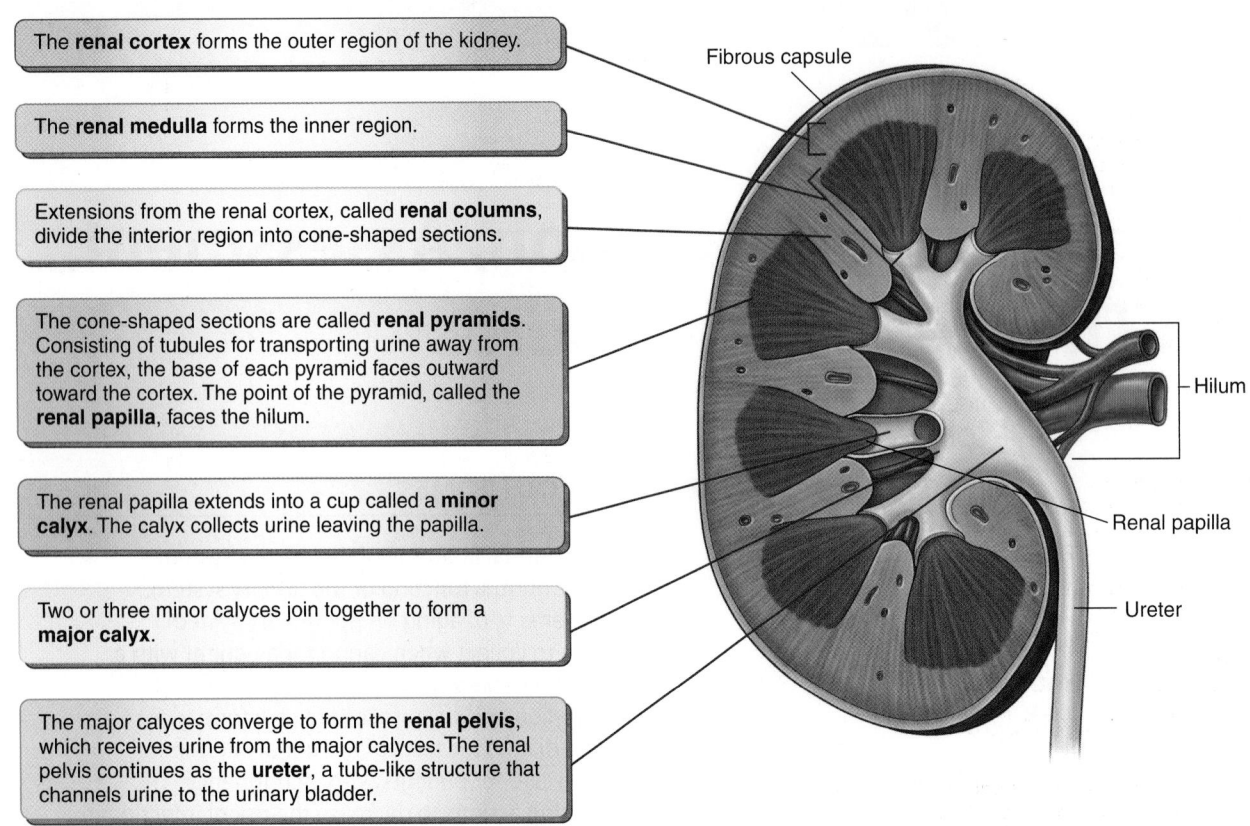

The **renal cortex** forms the outer region of the kidney.

The **renal medulla** forms the inner region.

Extensions from the renal cortex, called **renal columns**, divide the interior region into cone-shaped sections.

The cone-shaped sections are called **renal pyramids**. Consisting of tubules for transporting urine away from the cortex, the base of each pyramid faces outward toward the cortex. The point of the pyramid, called the **renal papilla**, faces the hilum.

The renal papilla extends into a cup called a **minor calyx**. The calyx collects urine leaving the papilla.

Two or three minor calyces join together to form a **major calyx**.

The major calyces converge to form the **renal pelvis**, which receives urine from the major calyces. The renal pelvis continues as the **ureter**, a tube-like structure that channels urine to the urinary bladder.

Fibrous capsule

Hilum

Renal papilla

Ureter

FIGURE 36.1 Interior of the kidney.

begins the microcirculation at the *nephron,* the functional unit of the kidney. The exchanges that take place in the capillaries of the nephrons form urine from blood plasma.

Nephron

Urine is formed in the approximately 1 million nephrons per kidney. The two major parts of a nephron are the renal corpuscle with glomerulus and the renal tubule with peritubular capillaries (Fig. 36.2). These are the two sites of exchange between blood plasma and urinary filtrate within the nephron. All parts of the renal tubule are surrounded by the peritubular capillaries. The capillaries arise from the efferent arteriole and receive the materials reabsorbed by the renal tubules.

Formation of Urine

The formation of urine involves three major processes: glomerular filtration, tubular reabsorption, and tubular secretion.

Glomerular Filtration

In glomerular filtration, blood pressure forces water and small solutes out of the glomeruli and into Bowman capsules. This fluid is then called renal filtrate (Fig. 36.3).

Tubular Reabsorption and Secretion

Exiting the glomerular capsule, renal filtrate then enters the renal tubules. Tubular reabsorption is the recovery of useful materials from the renal filtrate and their return to the blood in the peritubular capillaries (Table 36.1). In tubular secretion, substances are actively secreted from the blood in the peritubular capillaries into the filtrate in the renal tubules.

The Kidneys and Acid–Base Balance

Other than exhalation of carbon dioxide by the respiratory system, the kidneys are the organs most responsible for maintaining the normal pH range of blood and tissue fluid. They compensate for the pH changes that are part of normal body metabolism or the result of disease. In acidosis, the kidneys secrete more hydrogen ions into the renal filtrate and return more bicarbonate ions back to the blood. When body fluids become too alkaline, the kidneys return hydrogen ions to the blood and excrete bicarbonate ions in urine.

Elimination of Urine

The ureters, urinary bladder, and urethra do not change the composition or volume of urine but are responsible for its elimination.

Ureters

The ureters are behind the peritoneum of the dorsal abdominal cavity. Each ureter extends from the hilus of a kidney to the lower, posterior side of the urinary bladder. The smooth muscle in the wall of the ureter contracts in peristaltic waves to propel urine toward the urinary bladder. As the bladder fills, it expands and compresses the lower ends of the ureters to prevent backflow of urine.

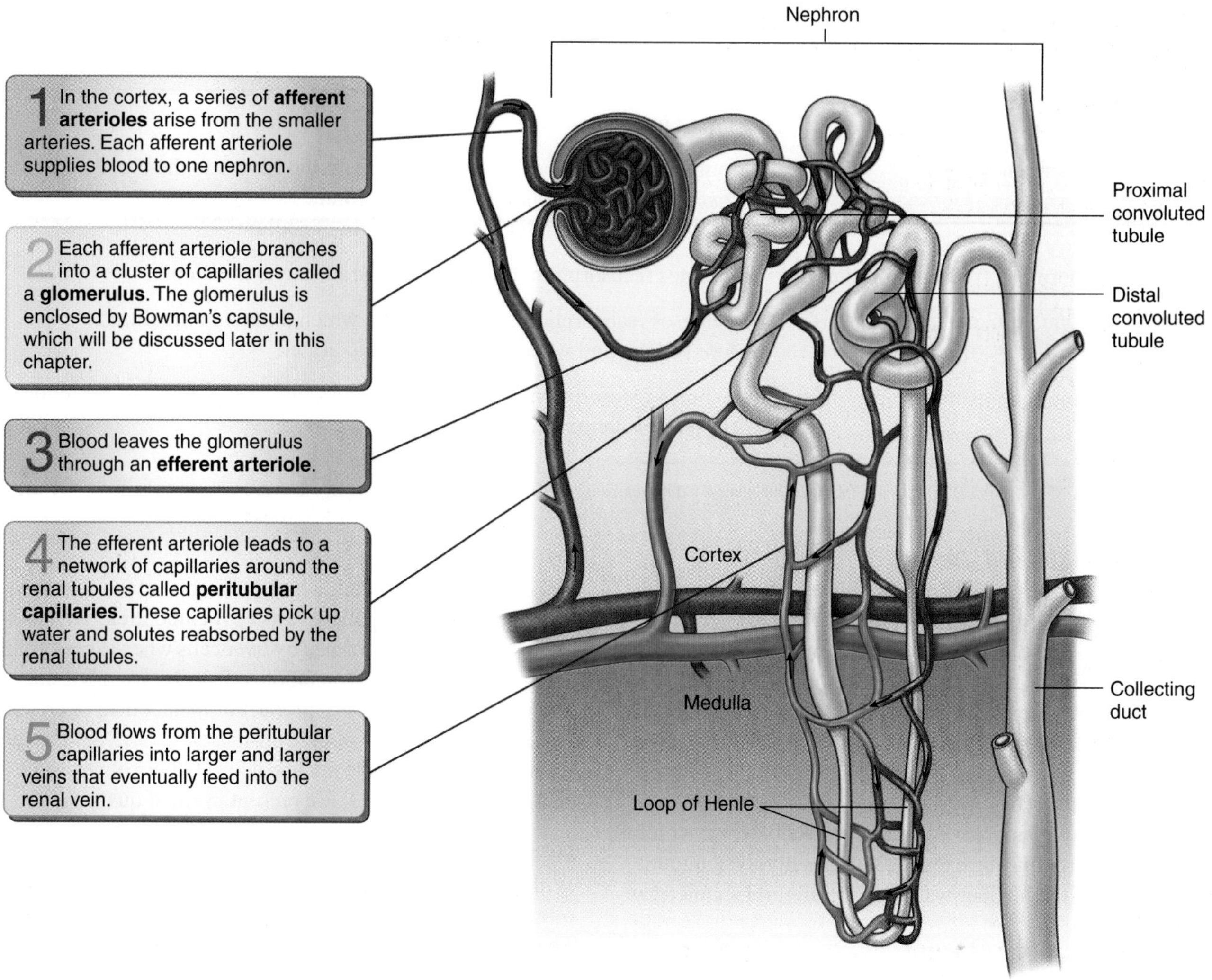

Nephron

1 In the cortex, a series of **afferent arterioles** arise from the smaller arteries. Each afferent arteriole supplies blood to one nephron.

2 Each afferent arteriole branches into a cluster of capillaries called a **glomerulus**. The glomerulus is enclosed by Bowman's capsule, which will be discussed later in this chapter.

3 Blood leaves the glomerulus through an **efferent arteriole**.

4 The efferent arteriole leads to a network of capillaries around the renal tubules called **peritubular capillaries**. These capillaries pick up water and solutes reabsorbed by the renal tubules.

5 Blood flows from the peritubular capillaries into larger and larger veins that eventually feed into the renal vein.

Proximal convoluted tubule

Distal convoluted tubule

Cortex

Medulla

Collecting duct

Loop of Henle

FIGURE 36.2 Nephron.

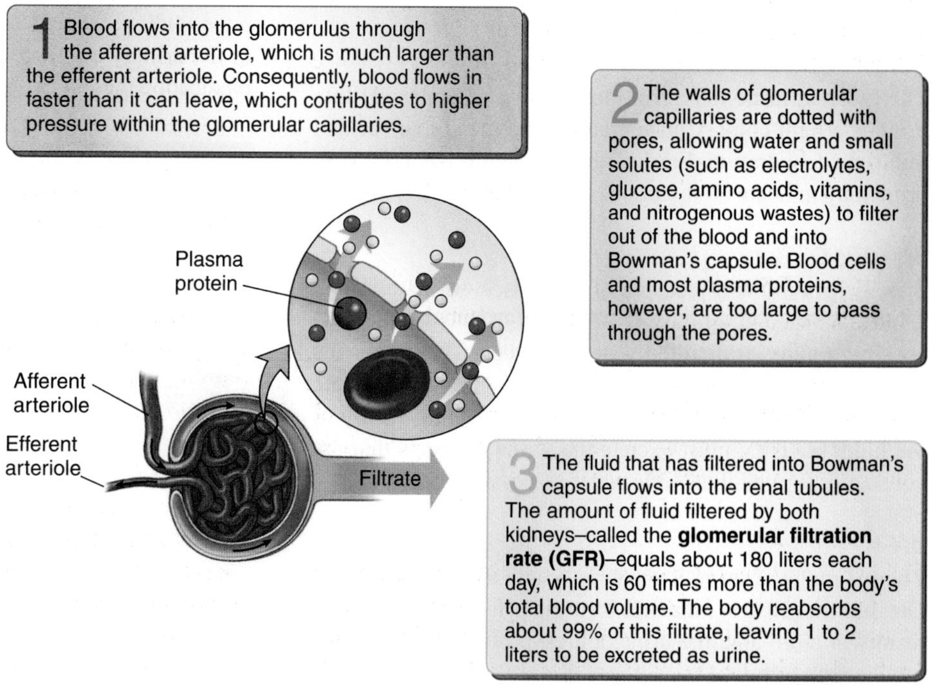

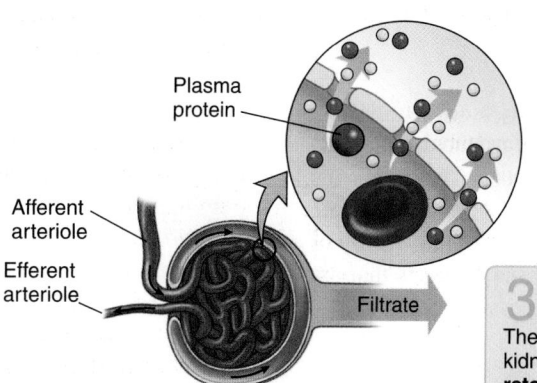

1 Blood flows into the glomerulus through the afferent arteriole, which is much larger than the efferent arteriole. Consequently, blood flows in faster than it can leave, which contributes to higher pressure within the glomerular capillaries.

2 The walls of glomerular capillaries are dotted with pores, allowing water and small solutes (such as electrolytes, glucose, amino acids, vitamins, and nitrogenous wastes) to filter out of the blood and into Bowman's capsule. Blood cells and most plasma proteins, however, are too large to pass through the pores.

Plasma protein

Afferent arteriole

Efferent arteriole

Filtrate

3 The fluid that has filtered into Bowman's capsule flows into the renal tubules. The amount of fluid filtered by both kidneys—called the **glomerular filtration rate (GFR)**—equals about 180 liters each day, which is 60 times more than the body's total blood volume. The body reabsorbs about 99% of this filtrate, leaving 1 to 2 liters to be excreted as urine.

FIGURE 36.3 Glomerular filtration.

Table 36.1

Effects of Hormones on the Kidneys

Hormone (Gland)	Function
Aldosterone (adrenal cortex)	Promotes reabsorption of sodium ions from the filtrate to the blood and excretion of potassium ions into the filtrate. Water is reabsorbed after the reabsorption of sodium.
Antidiuretic hormone (posterior pituitary)	Promotes reabsorption of water from the filtrate to the blood.
Atrial natriuretic hormone (atria of heart)	Decreases reabsorption of sodium ions, which remain in the filtrate. More sodium and water are eliminated in urine.
Parathyroid hormone (parathyroid glands)	Promotes reabsorption of calcium ions from filtrate to blood and excretion of phosphate ions into filtrate.

Source: Scanlon, V. C., & Sanders, T. (2019). *Essentials of anatomy and physiology* (8th ed.). Philadelphia, PA: F.A. Davis.

Urinary Bladder and Urethra

The urinary bladder is a muscular sac inside the peritoneum just posterior to the pubic symphysis. In women, the bladder is anterior and inferior to the uterus; in men, the bladder is superior to the prostate gland. The functions of the bladder are the temporary storage of urine and its elimination. Urethra anatomy differs between men and women.

Urination Reflex

Urination (micturition) is a spinal cord reflex over which voluntary control may be exerted. Muscles involved include the detrusor of the bladder wall and two urethral sphincters.

Characteristics of Urine

Amount

Normal urinary output is 1,000 to 2,000 mL per 24 hours. Any changes in fluid intake or other fluid output (such as sweating) affect this volume.

Color

The color of urine is referred to as straw or amber. Dilute urine is a light color. Concentrated urine is dark amber and indicates dehydration. Freshly voided urine is clear. Cloudy urine may indicate an infection.

Specific Gravity

Specific gravity is a measure of the dissolved materials in urine. The specific gravity of urine is 1.005 to 1.030. (The specific gravity of distilled water is 1.000.) The higher the specific gravity, the more dissolved material present. Specific gravity of urine is a measure of the concentrating ability of the kidneys. They must excrete the waste products that are constantly formed in as little water as possible.

pH

The pH range of urine is 4.6 to 8.0, with an average of 6.0. Diet has the greatest influence on urine pH. A vegetarian diet results in more alkaline urine; a high-protein diet results in more acidic urine.

Constituents

Urine is about 95% water, which is the solvent for waste products and salts. Nitrogenous wastes include urea, creatinine, and uric acid. Urea is formed by liver cells when excess amino acids are deaminated (metabolized) to be used for energy production. Creatinine is a product of metabolism of creatine phosphate, an energy source in muscles. Uric acid results from the metabolism of nucleic acids. Other solutes, such as enzymes and hormones, are present in small quantities.

Aging and the Urinary System

With age, the number of nephrons in the kidneys decreases, often to half the original number by age 70 or 80 (Fig. 36.4). The glomerular filtration rate (GFR) also decreases. This results in part from arteriosclerosis and diminished renal blood flow. The urinary bladder decreases in size, and the tone of the detrusor muscle decreases. This may result in the need to urinate more often or in residual urine in the bladder after voiding. Older adults are also more subject to infections of the urinary tract, and the changes of aging may influence medication therapy for older adults ("Gerontological Issues").

Gerontological Issues

Age-Related Renal Changes. Changes typically occur in the renal system as people age and include the following:

- Decreased filtration efficiency of the kidneys, affecting the body's ability to eliminate drugs
- Decreased renal function slowing the excretion of certain drugs so they remain in the body longer

Consequently, dehydration, which the older adult is prone to having, and the changes in renal function are a serious consideration for older adults who need drug therapy. The risk of adverse drug reactions, such as toxicity and overdose, is increased. It is important to monitor kidney function (such as serum creatinine and blood urea nitrogen [BUN] levels) in an older adult receiving drug therapy.

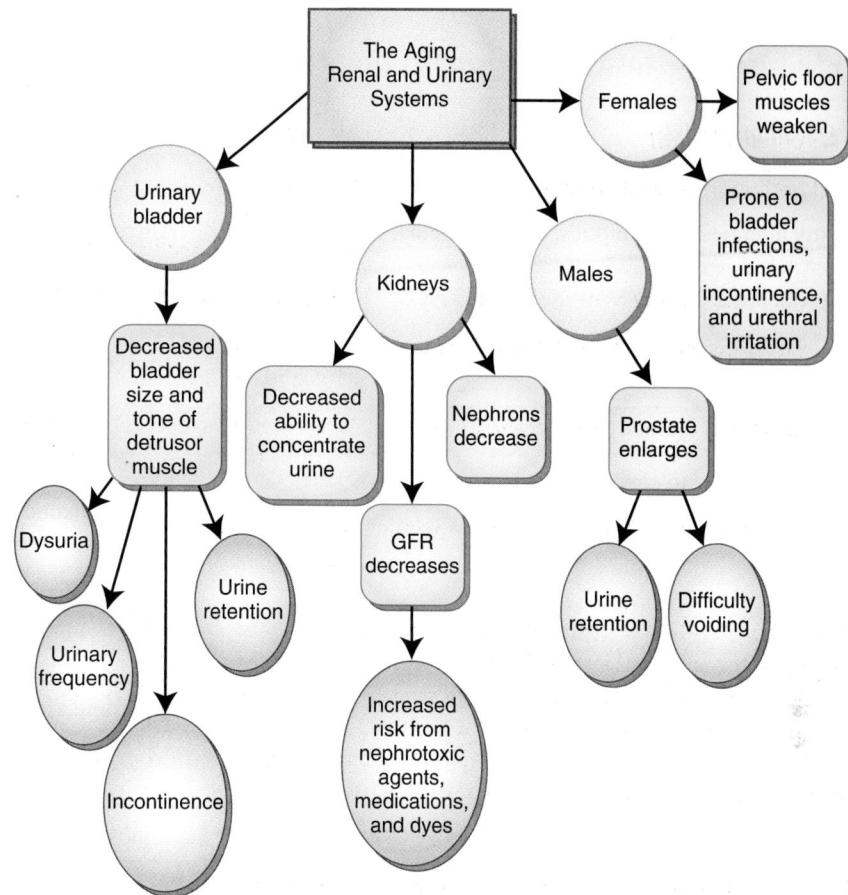

FIGURE 36.4 Aging and the urinary system. This concept map shows effects of the aging process on the urinary system.

NURSING ASSESSMENT OF THE URINARY SYSTEM

Health History

If the patient has impaired kidney function, head-to-toe data collection is needed because kidney disease can affect every system of the body. Table 36.2 describes sample questions to ask for a health history to use along with the *WHAT'S UP?* format (see Chapter 1) for symptoms.

Physical Examination

Table 36.3 lists objective data that should be collected on all body systems.

Daily Weights

Weight is the best indicator of fluid balance in the body. Patients with renal disease often have fluid imbalances. Weigh the patient at the same time each day, in the same or similar clothing, and with the same scale. Look for trends in weight gain or loss. If the patient's daily weight continues to increase, fluid is being retained and should be reported.

Intake and Output

The patient with kidney disease is often on a fluid restriction. Intake and output (I&O) should be carefully measured. Intake

includes oral, intravenous (IV), irrigation, tube feeding, and other fluids. Output includes urine, emesis, nasogastric effluent, wound drainage if it is copious, and any other drainage.

I&O totals are recorded and analyzed usually every 8 to 12 hours or more often for unstable patients. The nurse notes trends in retention or loss of fluid to report to the health care provider (HCP). Accurate documentation is vital. The HCP may order medications and IV fluids based on I&O results.

CRITICAL THINKING

Mr. Nolan is your patient. As you empty Mr. Nolan's urinary collection bag after 4 hours, you find that it has only 50 mL of concentrated urine in it. What do you do?
Suggested answers are at the end of the chapter.

DIAGNOSTIC TESTS FOR THE URINARY SYSTEM

Laboratory Tests
Urine Tests

URINALYSIS. A urinalysis (urine analysis) is a commonly performed diagnostic test for the urinary system, kidney disease, and systemic diseases that may affect the kidneys (Table 36.4).

Table 36.2

Subjective Data Collection for the Urinary System

Questions to Ask	Rationale/Significance
Allergies	
Any allergies to antibiotics, contrast media, or dyes?	Allergies to medications such as antibiotics, contrast media, and dyes can result in impaired kidney function.
Lifestyle Habits	
Do you smoke?	Tobacco use increases risk of bladder cancer.
Occupation	
Any exposure to chemicals in jobs or hobbies?	Exposure to nephrotoxic chemicals can cause cancer (e.g., bladder: arsenic, chemicals to make dyes, leather, rubber, paint, textiles; kidney: cadmium, herbicides, trichloroethylene).
Medical History	
What medical conditions have you been diagnosed with?	Diabetes and hypertension are common causes of chronic kidney disease. Streptococcal infection (strep throat) may precede renal disease. Lupus can cause glomerulonephritis in up to 50% of those with lupus.
Surgical History	
Any kidney/bladder surgery?	Indicates prior conditions to correlate with current condition.
Family History	
Does anyone in your family have hypertension, diabetes, or kidney or urinary problems?	Some causes of renal conditions and renal disorders are hereditary.
Medications/Supplements	
What prescription or over-the-counter medications or herbs do you take?	Nonsteroidal anti-inflammatory drugs (NSAIDs), vasopressors, and angiotensin-converting enzyme (ACE) inhibitors can impair renal perfusion and kidney function. Nephrotoxic drugs can damage the kidneys. Herbs with aristolochic acid may be renal toxic.
Renal/Urinary Issues	
Do you have pain, urgency, frequency, or burning with urination?	Pain, urgency, frequency, or burning with urination can indicate an infection. Urgency with diminished amounts of urine suggests urinary retention.
Is there blood in your urine? Are there any changes in color, odor, clarity, or amount of urine?	**Hematuria** may indicate an infection or cancer. Cloudy urine or foul odor indicates possible infection. Decreased amount may indicate renal disease; increased amount (**polyuria**) may indicate diabetes mellitus or inability to concentrate urine.

• WORD • BUILDING •

hematuria: hemat—blood + uria—urine

Table 36.2
Subjective Data Collection for the Urinary System—cont'd

Questions to Ask	Rationale/Significance
Do you have difficulty starting urine stream, **nocturia**, incontinence, or a urinary catheter?	Difficulty starting urination may indicate prostate obstruction. Nocturia can occur with loss of kidney's concentrating ability, nephrotic syndrome, diabetes, and heart failure.
Do you have pain in the costovertebral angle (area formed by rib cage and vertebral column)?	Renal calculus (stone) may produce a dull ache in kidney area or colicky pain radiating to genital area or leg on affected side.
Do you have swelling in the ankles or around eyes?	Edema occurs with fluid retention; periorbital edema is noted around the eyes in the morning.
Nutrition/Fluid Balance	
Describe your appetite, weight loss/gain, fluid intake, and usual diet.	Anorexia occurs with renal disease. Fluid retention can result in weight gain. Large intake of protein or dairy products may lead to kidney stone formation.

Table 36.3
Objective Data Collection for the Urinary System

Possible Abnormal Findings	Possible Causes
Vital Signs	
Hypertension	Renal disease
Elevated respiratory rate	Fluid volume overload
Irregular heart rate/rhythm	Hyperkalemia; magnesium or calcium imbalance
Level of Consciousness	
Decreased level	Fluid or electrolyte imbalances, urinary tract infection
Neurologic	
Diminished deep tendon reflexes, hyperesthesia, paresthesia, peripheral neuropathy	Altered fluid balance; increased urea, creatinine, ammonia, or parathyroid hormone
Skin	
Pallor, yellow or gray	Anemia, chronic kidney disease
Skin crystals (uremic frost)	Azotemia
Excoriation	Pruritus, dryness
Poor turgor	Dehydration
Eyes	
Conjunctival pallor	Anemia

Continued

• WORD • BUILDING •
nocturia: nox—night + uria—urine

Table 36.3

Objective Data Collection for the Urinary System—cont'd

Possible Abnormal Findings	Possible Causes
Cardiovascular	
Weight gain	Fluid retention
Edema, jugular vein distension, pulmonary edema	Increased fluid volume, decreased serum albumin
Friction rub	Azotemia
Respiratory	
Shortness of breath, tachypnea, crackles	Fluid volume overload.
Kussmaul respirations	Metabolic acidosis seen in renal disease
Hematologic	
Anemia	Decreased erythropoietin production
Bruising, bleeding	Thrombocytopenia
Gastrointestinal	
Uremic fetor (urine breath odor)	Ammonia from urea breakdown
Constipation, diarrhea	Renal disease
Urinary	
Anuria (less than 100 mL urine/24 hours)	Acute or end-stage renal disease
Oliguria (100 to 400 mL/24 hours)	Severe dehydration, shock, transfusion reaction, end-stage renal disease
Incontinence	Urological or neurologic disease
Polyuria (more than 3 L/24 hours)	Diabetes mellitus, diabetes insipidus, diuretics, caffeine, ethanol, excessive intake, urinary tract infection
Musculoskeletal	
Fractures	Bone and mineral disease from low calcium, high phosphorus, decreased activated vitamin D

Table 36.4

Urinalysis Results

Urinalysis	Baseline information	Used to plan further testing or treatment or to monitor an existing condition
Test	**Normal Results**	**Significance of Abnormal Results**
Color of urine	Light yellow to deep amber	Dark amber: dehydration Brown or green: excessive bilirubin Orange: use of phenazopyridine (Pyridium) Red or pink: hemoglobin present Smoky: hematuria
Appearance	Clear	Cloudiness: bacteria, amorphous phosphates, urates, blood, fat, or white blood cells

Table 36.4

Urinalysis Results—cont'd

Test	Normal Results	Significance of Abnormal Results
Odor of urine	Aromatic	Infection: foul smell Diabetic ketoacidosis: fruity odor
pH	4.5 to 8.0	Low pH: metabolic acidosis, starvation, diarrhea High pH: infection, renal disease, vomiting
Specific gravity	1.005 to 1.030	Low specific gravity: excessive fluid intake, diabetes insipidus High specific gravity: dehydration, heart failure, shock Specific gravity fixed at 1.010: kidney dysfunction
Protein	Less than 20 mg/dL; 24-hour urine: 30 to 150 mg	Persistent proteinuria creates foamy urine due to damage to glomerulus; significant sign of renal disease. Intermittent protein results from strenuous exercise, dehydration, or fever. Vaginal secretions can contaminate urine giving a positive reading.
Glucose	Negative	Diabetes mellitus, excessive glucose intake, or low renal threshold for glucose reabsorption
Ketones	Negative	Diabetes mellitus, starvation from breakdown of body fats into ketones, carbohydrate-free diets, severe diarrhea, dehydration, vomiting
Bilirubin	Negative	Liver disorders causing jaundice; may appear in the urine before jaundice is visible
Nitrite	Negative	Infection
Red blood cells	Less than 5/hpf (high-power field)	Kidney stones, infection, cancer, renal disease, trauma
White blood cells	Less than 5/hpf	Infection or inflammation
Leukocyte esterase	Negative	Infection
Casts	None to rare hyaline	Renal damage or infection; tube-shaped proteins formed when abnormal urine contents settle into molds of the renal tubules

A urine specimen for routine analysis may be collected at any time of day; however, the first morning specimen is best. First-morning specimens are usually concentrated and more likely to contain abnormal constituents if they are present. The specimen should be examined within 1 hour of collection or refrigerated. Urine standing at room temperature longer than 2 hours has more bacteria present, changes in pH, and hemolysis of red blood cells (RBCs). A random urine specimen collected for cytology should not be a first-morning specimen due to changes in epithelial cells in urine held overnight. If a urinalysis is ordered for a patient with an indwelling urinary catheter, the nurse obtains the sterile urine specimen (see the procedure "Urine Specimen Collection from Urinary Drainage System" on Davis Edge).

Composite urine specimens (e.g., a 24-hour urine test) are collected usually from 2 to 24 hours; Table 36.5 lists collection steps (also see the procedure "Collecting a 24-hour Urine Specimen" on Davis Edge). These specimens examine the urine for specific components such as catecholamines, creatinine, electrolytes, glucose, 17-ketosteroids, minerals, protein, and urea nitrogen. These specimens usually need refrigeration. Preservatives may be added to the collection container.

Renal Function Tests

Several blood and urine tests reflect kidney function (see Table 36.5). If the kidneys are not filtering adequately, the serum test values, such as the creatinine and blood urea nitrogen (BUN), will be elevated. These tests are useful because they provide information about the severity of a patient's kidney disease as well as the patient's response to treatments. Renal function test values may remain within the normal range until the GFR is less than 50% of normal.

Table 36.5

Laboratory Tests for the Urinary System

Test	Definition/Normal Value	Significance of Abnormal Findings
Urine Studies		
Residual urine	Shows amount of urine left in the bladder after voiding. *Normal value:* Less than 50 mL (increases with age)	Bladder ultrasound equipment may be used to determine amount of urine remaining after voiding. Increased residual volume may occur in urethral strictures, sphincter impairment, or neurogenic bladder.
Urine culture	Identifies number of bacteria in urine and organism causing urinary tract infection. Sensitivity test determines most effective antibiotic against offending bacteria. *Normal value:* Negative if less than 10,000/mL of urine. Positive if 100,000 or more/mL of urine. An amount less than 100,000 may result from contamination during specimen collection.	Urine should be collected before antibiotic treatment starts to avoid altering results. Catheterized specimen may be ordered to avoid risk of contamination from vagina if female patient is menstruating or patient is incontinent.
Composite urine specimen: Creatinine clearance	Measures amount of creatinine cleared from blood in a specified time (often 24 hours) by comparing amount of creatinine in blood with creatinine in urine. An excellent indicator of renal function. *Normal value:* Male: 85–125 mL/min/1.73m^2 Female: 75–115 mL/min/1.73m^2	Creatinine clearance is computed in the laboratory and is expressed in volume of blood that is cleared of creatinine in 1 minute. Minimum creatinine clearance of 10 mL per minute is needed to live without dialysis. Collection key points: 1. To begin the test, patient is directed to urinate and discard the urine (bladder is empty). This time is recorded and becomes the test start time. 2. All urine voided is collected for 24 hours (or specified time frame) in a large container provided by the laboratory and kept refrigerated or on ice. Remind patient/staff to save all urine for accurate results. 3. Exactly 24 hours after test began, patient is to void again (empty bladder). This urine is added to the container and the test ends.
Urine cytology	Microscopic examination of urine to detect atypical epithelial cells shed from the surface of the urinary tract. *Normal value:* No abnormal cells or inclusions seen	Used to screen people at high risk for cancer in the urinary system. Atypical cells indicate need for further testing.
Bladder tumor antigen (a bladder cancer marker)	Measurement of a protein produced by bladder tumor cells. *Normal value:* Negative	No special preparation needed. A single voided specimen collected before noon is taken directly to the laboratory.
NMP22 (a bladder cancer marker)	Measurement of a protein deposited into urine during nuclear disruption (apoptosis) of bladder cells. *Normal value:* Less than 6 units/mL	No special preparation needed. A single voided specimen collected before noon is taken directly to the laboratory.

Table 36.5

Laboratory Tests for the Urinary System—cont'd

Test	Definition/Normal Value	Significance of Abnormal Findings
Blood Chemistry Studies—Kidney Function		
Blood urea nitrogen (BUN)	Urea is a waste product of protein metabolism that is excreted by the kidneys. *Normal value:* Adult: 8–21 mg/dL Over age 90: 10–31 mg/dL	Not as sensitive an indicator of kidney function as creatinine level because BUN is affected by increased protein intake, dehydration, and other factors in the body. Elevated level: kidney disease, shock, severe heart failure, dehydration, high-protein diet, gastrointestinal bleeding, steroid use.
Serum creatinine	Creatinine is a waste product from muscle metabolism and is released into the bloodstream at a steady rate. *Normal value:* Male: 0.61–1.21 mg/dL Female: 0.51–1.11 mg/dL	Very good indicator of kidney function. The higher the creatinine level, the more impaired the kidney function.
BUN-to-creatinine ratio	Evaluates hydration status. *Normal value:* 10:1 to 20:1	An elevated ratio occurs in hypovolemia. A normal ratio with an elevated BUN and creatinine occurs in intrinsic renal disease.
Cystatin C (Cys C)	Proteinase inhibitor produced by all nucleated cells, filtered out of blood by the glomerulus membrane. Marker for kidney damage and monitors function in kidney transplant. *Normal value:* Age 1 to 50 years: 0.56–0.9 mg/L 50 years and older: 0.58–1.08 mg/L	Cystatin C is a sensitive marker that reflects glomerular filtration rate independent of weight, height, diet, age, gender, and muscle mass. Cystatin C level increases with impaired renal function.
Uric acid	Uric acid is an end product of purine metabolism and the breakdown of body proteins. It can be used to identify the cause of renal calculi. *Normal value:* Adult male: 4–8 mg/dL Adult female: 2.5-7mg/dL Male older than 60 years: 4.2–8.2 mg/dL Female older than 60 years: 3.5–7.3 mg/dL	Elevated uric acid levels can be caused by renal disease.
Blood Chemistry Studies		
Sodium (Na+)	Extracellular electrolyte related to hydration status. *Normal value:* 135–145 mEq/L	Remains within normal range until late stages of renal disease. Increased with azotemia and dehydration. Decreased with fluid retention (dilutional effect) and nephrotic syndrome. Monitor for seizures with values below 120 or above 160 mEq/L.
Potassium (K+)	Intracellular electrolyte excreted by kidneys. *Normal value:* 3.5–5.3 mEq/L	In renal disease, K+ is one of the first electrolytes to become abnormal. Level greater than 6 mEq/L can lead to muscle weakness and cardiac arrhythmias.

Continued

Table 36.5

Laboratory Tests for the Urinary System—cont'd

Test	Definition/Normal Value	Significance of Abnormal Findings
Calcium, total (Ca2+)	Main mineral stored in bones and teeth. Regulated by vitamin D and parathyroid glands. Aids in muscle contraction, neurotransmission, and blood clotting. *Normal value:* Adult: 8.2–10.2mg/dL Adult older than 90 years: 8.2–9.6mg/dL	Decreased in renal disease, causing bone and mineral disease.
Phosphorus	Mineral found in bone, teeth, bloodstream, and cells. Many functions. *Normal value:* 2.5–4.5 mg/dL	Phosphorus balance is inversely related to calcium balance. Increased in renal disease.
Bicarbonate (HCO$_3^-$)	An alkaline ion that indicates status of acid–base system. Reabsorbed and excreted by the kidneys. *Normal value:* Arterial: 22–26 mmol/L	With renal disease, metabolic acidosis and low serum HCO$_3^-$ levels can occur.
Magnesium	Found in bone and intracellularly, and excreted by the kidney. *Normal value:* 1.6–2.2 mg/dL	Elevated in chronic renal disease; can result in lethargy, nausea, vomiting, and slurred speech.
Albumin	Plasma protein maintaining oncotic pressure in vascular system. *Normal value:* Age 20 to 40 years: 3.7–5.1 g/dL Age 41 to 60 years: 3.4–4.8 g/dL Age 61 to 90 years: 3.2–4.6 g/dL Age older than 90 years: 2.9–4.5 g/dL	Low level occurs in nephrotic syndrome and renal disease and leads to edema.

Diagnostic Procedures

Table 36.6 summarizes diagnostic procedures for the urinary system. For explanations of computed tomography (CT) scan, magnetic resonance imaging (MRI), and ultrasound testing and nursing care, see Appendix A.

Contrast-Induced Nephropathy

Contrast media used in diagnostic testing and procedures can be **nephrotoxic** and cause contrast-induced nephropathy. This results in acute kidney injury within 48 hours of contrast exposure. This condition is serious and can result in death. It is usually asymptomatic, with a decline in renal function as shown by a rise in serum creatinine. Treatment is the same as for acute kidney injury (see Chapter 37).

Risk factors for contrast-induced nephropathy are having **azotemia** (increased creatinine and BUN) and diabetes mellitus–associated renal impairment. Creatinine levels are checked before the procedure and should be monitored afterward. A risk assessment should be done before testing regarding allergies/allergic reactions, diabetes, kidney disease, other medical conditions, and use of oral metformin hydrochloride (Glucophage) and other medications (e.g., anti-inflammatories, antibiotics, antifungals, immunosuppressives). When contrast media are used, metformin hydrochloride must not be given before and for 48 hours after administration of contrast media. Severe lactic acidosis as well as acute kidney injury can occur.

Protective measures continue to be studied. IV hydration with normal saline or a sodium bicarbonate infusion may be one of the main preventative measures in use. Acetylcysteine (Mucomyst) before and after the procedure is also used.

Renal Biopsy

A renal biopsy diagnoses or provides information about kidney disease. A CT scan or ultrasound is done first to locate the kidney for biopsy. A small section of the renal cortex is obtained for laboratory analysis either **percutaneously** (local anesthetic, needle through skin) or with a small flank incision. Patients with bleeding tendencies, uncontrolled hypertension, or a solitary kidney generally do not undergo renal biopsy.

• **WORD • BUILDING** •

percutaneous: per—through + cutaneous—skin

Table 36.6

Diagnostic Procedures for the Urinary System

Procedure	Uses and Possible Abnormal Findings	Nursing Management
Noninvasive		
Renal ultrasound or ultrasonography	Congenital disorders of the kidney, abscesses, hydronephrosis, kidney stones or tumors, kidney enlargement, structural changes with chronic infection.	No special preparation or aftercare. No radiation exposure.
Bladder ultrasound	Portable ultrasound instrument computes residual urine volume, bladder wall thickness, bladder calculi, tumors, diverticula.	Determines postresidual voiding accurately to reduce catheterizations for bladder distention.
Kidney-ureter-bladder x-ray	Renal calculi, kidney size, masses in the kidney.	If done as preliminary study, bowel prep may be done.
Computed tomographic (CT) scan (with/without contrast)	Evaluation of kidneys, ureters, bladder, abdominal and pelvic organs for kidney size, tumors, cysts, abscesses, malignant masses, metastases, lymph node enlargement; nonfunctioning kidneys, renal stones, obstructions, infections.	See Appendix A.
Magnetic resonance imaging (MRI) (with/ without contrast media)	Staging of cancers of the kidney, bladder, prostate.	See Appendix A.
Invasive		
Pyelogram: X-ray examination of renal tissue, calyces, pelvises, ureters, and bladder (with/without contrast media)	Abnormal size or shape of kidneys, absent kidneys, polycystic kidney disease, tumors, hydronephrosis, renovascular hypertension (Fig. 36.5).	See Appendix A. *Precare:* Enemas may be given the evening before the test to empty the colon. *Postcare:* Monitor urine output.
Renal angiography or arteriogram with contrast media	Visualizes renal blood vessels. Hypervascular tumors, renal cysts, renal artery stenosis, renal artery aneurysms, pyelonephritis, obstructions, renal infarction, renal trauma evaluation. May be used during renal angioplasty.	See Appendix A. *Precare:* Enemas may be given the evening before the test. *Postcare:* Bedrest up to 12 hours to prevent bleeding at injection site. Check distal pulses in leg every 30–60 minutes and monitor vital signs and dressing frequently. Teach patient not to bend leg or raise head of bed more than 45 degrees.
Nephrotomogram: Series of x-rays with contrast media creating three-dimensional image of the kidney	Renal cysts, tumors, areas of nonperfusion, renal fractures or lacerations following renal trauma.	See Appendix A. *Precare:* Enemas may be given the evening before the test to empty the colon. Monitor fluid intake and output before and after test. *Postcare:* Maintain hydration.

Continued

• WORD • BUILDING •

pyelogram: pyelo—pelvis of the kidney + gram—radiograph

Table 36.6

Diagnostic Procedures for the Urinary System—cont'd

Procedure	Uses and Possible Abnormal Findings	Nursing Management
Renal scan	Assesses kidneys' ability to perfuse blood and secrete urine. Renovascular hypertension diagnosis; kidney function; renal blood flow; glomerular filtration rate; tubular function; excretion of urine; kidney size and shape; abscesses, cysts, and tumors, which may appear as cold spots because of nonfunctioning kidney tissue. Determination of vascular supply to the kidneys in patients with renal trauma, dissecting aneurysm, and other disorders affecting blood flow to the kidneys.	*Precare:* Determine whether any of patient's medications will interfere with test, such as nonsteroidal anti-inflammatory drugs (NSAIDs) or antihypertensives. Patient may be asked to drink two glasses of water before test. Level of radiation is very low. Pregnant and nursing mothers are advised to be cautious. If captopril is given, monitor for hypotension.
Renal biopsy	Microscopic examination of kidney tissue for diagnosis or treatment of renal disorder, benign and malignant masses, causes of renal disease, renal transplant rejection, lupus.	*Precare:* Before biopsy, patient NPO (nothing by mouth) 6 to 8 hours. Mild sedative given. No anticoagulants. Complete blood count (CBC), coagulation studies. *During:* Prone position, with sandbag under the abdomen, for a biopsy through flank area. Patient instructed to hold breath while needle is inserted to prevent kidney from moving. *Postcare:* Pressure dressing applied. Vital signs and urine output monitored. Signs of bleeding to report immediately: Grossly bloody urine, falling blood pressure, and increasing pulse. Encourage fluids. *Teach:* No heavy lifting for 2 weeks.
Cystoscopy and pyelogram: Minor surgical procedure with lighted fiberoptic cystoscope	Diagnostic: Inspect inside of bladder, collect urine specimen from either kidney, take x-rays or biopsy growths. Therapeutic: Remove small bladder tumors, polyps, stones from bladder/ureters; dilation of ureters; treat enlarged prostate or congenital abnormalities.	*Precare:* Surgical preparation. *Postcare:* Measure urine output to detect retention from swelling of urinary meatus. Encourage fluid intake. Expect initial voidings to be blood tinged and dysuria to be present for 24 hours.
Cystogram or voiding cystourethrogram: x-ray of bladder/lower urinary tract with contrast media or radioisotope instilled into bladder via catheter or cystoscope	Evaluates bladder filling and emptying. Incomplete bladder emptying, distention, reflux, obstruction to urine outflow identified.	*Precare:* No special prep. *Postcare:* Bright red urine, fever, or persistent discomfort should be reported to the health care provider. *Teach:* After the scan, can have slight dysuria and pink urine for 1–2 days.

• WORD • BUILDING •

cystoscopy: cysto—bladder + scopy—to examine

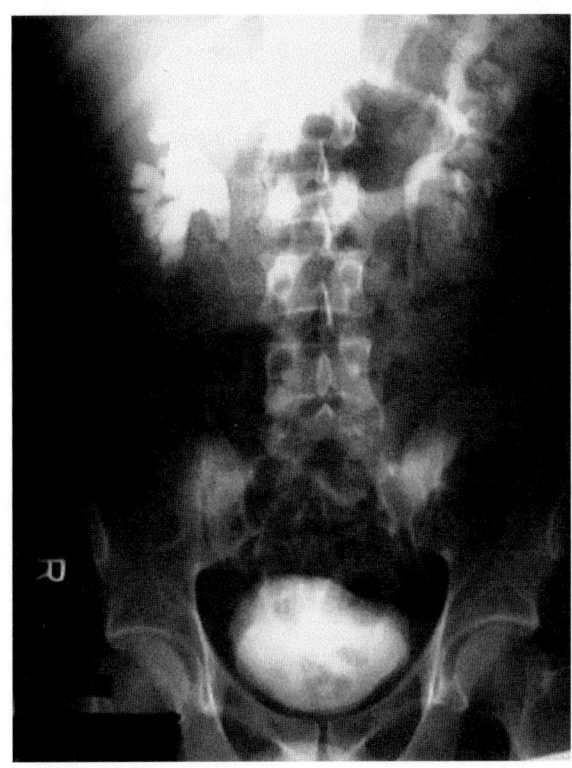

FIGURE 36.5 IV pyelogram x-ray. Contrast media injected intravenously with x-ray images taken as the contrast is excreted by the kidneys.

Nursing Process for Diagnostic Tests of the Urinary System Assessment

The patient's baseline understanding of testing procedures is determined to plan teaching sessions. Identified contraindications to testing are reported to the HCP.

Nursing Diagnoses, Planning, and Implementation

Anxiety related to unfamiliar environment, procedure, diagnostic test, health status, or severity of disease

EXPECTED OUTCOME: The patient will have reduced anxiety concerning health status or severity of disease before a procedure or test.

- Collect data of signs and symptoms for patient anxiety (e.g., verbalization, tenseness, tachycardia, elevated blood pressure, facial pallor, self-focused behaviors). *A high level of fear will interfere with teaching and learning as well as diminish cooperation during testing.*
- Acknowledge the patient's anxiety and the perceived threat of the situation *to facilitate communication and trust.*
- Encourage the patient to verbalize feelings, concerns, or specific stressors *to provide a baseline of information to develop an individualized teaching plan.*
- Reinforce explanations and correct misconceptions the patient has about diagnostic tests or disease condition *to facilitate trust and promote comfort.*

- Engage support from the patient's family throughout diagnostic testing *for the patient's coping.*
- Maintain a calm, supportive, and confident environment and manner when interacting with the patient *to reduce anxiety.*
- Instruct the patient in relaxation techniques and facilitate their use *to reduce anxiety.*
- Respond to the patient's request for assistance as soon as possible *to reduce anxiety.*
- Provide the patient with access to timely information regarding outcome of diagnostic testing *to facilitate trust and promote comfort.*

Deficient Knowledge related to diagnostic test or procedure and health status

EXPECTED OUTCOME: The patient will report understanding of the diagnostic test or procedure prior to having it.

- Collect data on the patient's understanding of the diagnostic test or procedure *to provide a baseline for teaching.*
- Include family members or significant others in teaching sessions *to encourage their support of the patient.*
- Reinforce the HCP's explanations and correct misconceptions about the diagnostic test or procedure *to help alleviate anxiety.*
- Introduce staff members who will be caring for the patient. *Familiarity with staff will decrease anxiety.*
- Orient the patient to the testing environment, equipment, and routines *to increase understanding.*
- Explain all activities that will take place before, during, and after diagnostic test or procedure *to reduce fear and promote cooperation.*
- Provide information about self-care following procedure or diagnostic test *to facilitate the patient in self-care.*

Acute Pain related to infection, edema, obstruction, or bleeding along the urinary tract or to invasive diagnostic tests

EXPECTED OUTCOME: The patient will report pain at a tolerable level within 30 minutes of report of pain.

- Identify location and level of pain, **dysuria,** burning on urination, or abdominal or flank pain *to provide baseline data to evaluate progression of pain and effectiveness of treatment plan.*
- Provide comfort measures *to relieve pain.*
- Provide analgesics and antispasmodics as prescribed *for pain relief.*
- Report severe pain to HCP. *Severe pain may indicate that complications are present or the need for a change in pain control medications.*

Impaired Urinary Elimination related to complications from diagnostic tests of the urinary system

EXPECTED OUTCOME: The patient will maintain urine output greater than 30 mL per hour in the postprocedure period.

• Maintain hydration with ordered IV infusion before and after diagnostic testing *to protect kidneys or facilitate contrast removal from the body.*
• Monitor fluid I&O closely *to ensure adequate renal function.*
• Monitor serum creatinine level and GFR *to assess for complications from diagnostic testing.*
• Observe the patient for hypersensitivity reactions to contrast media (e.g., pruritus, rashes, breathing difficulties, generalized edema, urinary retention) *to detect possible reaction symptoms and protect renal function.*

Evaluation

If interventions have been effective, the patient will have reduced anxiety, pain at a tolerable level, and increased understanding of the procedure, and will maintain urine output greater than 30 mL per hour.

THERAPEUTIC MEASURES FOR THE URINARY SYSTEM

Management of Urinary Incontinence

Urinary **incontinence** is defined as the involuntary leakage of urine. There are several types of incontinence. The incidence is rising and affects both men and women. Urinary incontinence is underreported because many people are embarrassed to talk about the problem. Most people do not seek treatment until their quality of life is affected. With incontinence, a voiding diary should be kept for several days to show when incontinence occurs and the predisposing events. The patient should be referred to a urologist specializing in incontinence or a continence clinic for treatment.

Stress Incontinence

Stress incontinence is the involuntary loss of less than 50 mL of urine associated with increasing abdominal pressure during coughing, laughing, sneezing, or other physical activities. Stress incontinence is seen in women after childbirth and menopause. In men, stress incontinence can occur after prostatectomy and radiation. Kegel exercises can increase perineal muscle tone for both stress and urge incontinence (Box 36.1).

Urge Incontinence

Urge incontinence is the involuntary loss of urine associated with an abrupt and strong desire to void. The patient typically reports being "unable to make it to the bathroom in time." It is the most common type of urinary incontinence in older adults.

Functional Incontinence

Functional incontinence is the inability to get to the toilet because of environmental barriers, physical limitations, loss of memory, or disorientation. People with functional incontinence are often dependent on others and have no other urinary problems. This is a common cause of incontinence in those who are institutionalized.

Overflow Incontinence

Overflow incontinence is the involuntary loss of urine associated with overdistention of the bladder. It occurs with acute or chronic urinary distention with dribbling of urine. The bladder is unable to empty normally despite frequent urine loss. Spinal cord injuries or an enlarged prostate can be a cause.

Total Incontinence

Total incontinence is a continuous and unpredictable loss of urine. It usually results from neurologic impairment, surgery, trauma, or a malformation of the ureter. Bladder training has been proven ineffective. The nurse's priority is to keep the patient clean and dry using absorptive products. For some male patients, an external condom catheter can be effective.

Nursing Process for the Patient With Incontinence

The medical diagnoses of stress and urge incontinence are also nursing diagnoses. See "Nursing Care Plan for the Patient With Stress or Urge Incontinence" and "Nursing Care Plan for the Patient with Functional Incontinence."

Nursing Care Plan for the Patient With Stress or Urge Urinary Incontinence

Nursing Diagnosis: *Stress Urinary Incontinence* or *Urge Urinary Incontinence* related to decreased tone of perineal muscles
Expected Outcomes: The patient will be continent of urine and will state three actions that can be taken to decrease incidence of stress or urge incontinence.
Evaluation of Outcomes: Is the patient continent? Is the patient able to state three actions that can be taken to decrease the incidence of stress or urge incontinence?

Stress Incontinence or Urge Urinary Incontinence

Intervention	Rationale	Evaluation
Collect data about the history of incontinence with a patient voiding journal.	*A journal helps identify the severity and timing of incontinence.*	Does patient complete the voiding journal?
Instruct patient on how to perform Kegel exercises (see Box 36.1).	*Kegel exercises increase perineal muscle tone to help prevent incontinence.*	Does patient correctly explain how to perform Kegel exercises?
Encourage patient to drink at least 2,000 mL of fluid per day, preferably 3,000 mL per day unless medical reason for fluid restriction.	*Concentrated urine is irritating to the urinary tract and can increase the incidence of urge incontinence and dribbling*	Is urine dilute?
Encourage patient to avoid alcohol and caffeine.	*Alcohol serves as a diuretic. Caffeine is irritating to the urinary tract.*	Does patient explain the need to avoid alcohol and fluids containing caffeine?
Discuss use of small adhesive peripads to wear in underclothing.	*Peripads provide protection in case of incontinence.*	Does patient have and use peripads if desired?
Refer patient to a continence clinic or to a health care provider specializing in incontinence.	*Specialists in the area of incontinence can use medical or surgical interventions to decrease incontinence.*	Does patient understand what resources are available to further assist with treatment of incontinence?
Refer patient to supportive and educational groups such as National Association for Continence (www.nafc.org).	*Support groups can help patients deal with the embarrassment of incontinence and learn preventive methods.*	Does patient know support groups to help with incontinence?

Urge Urinary Incontinence

Intervention	Rationale	Evaluation
Teach patient to void at frequent intervals (every 2 hours) and then gradually increase the length of time between voidings.	*By emptying the bladder at frequent intervals, the incidence of urge incontinence can be decreased.*	Does patient follow a frequent voiding schedule?
Teach urge inhibition techniques (distraction), such as counting back from 100 by sevens and relaxation breathing.	*Distraction techniques can help patients reach the bathroom in time to prevent incontinence.*	Do distraction techniques help patient prevent incontinence?

Nursing Care Plan for the Patient With Functional Incontinence

Nursing Diagnosis: *Functional Urinary Incontinence* related to interference with rapid voiding
Expected Outcomes: The patient will be continent of urine and will state three measures to increase continence.
Evaluation of Outcomes: Is the patient continent of urine? Is the patient able to state three measures to increase continence?

Intervention	Rationale	Evaluation
Ask about the history of incontinence. Keep a voiding log of when patient is incontinent.	*A voiding log helps determine the cause of incontinence and show when incontinence is most likely to occur.*	Does the patient keep a voiding log?
Identify potential acute causes of incontinence, including new onset of urinary tract infection, constipation or impaction, medication effect, or poor fluid intake.	*There are many treatable causes of incontinence.*	Does patient have any treatable causes of incontinence?
Determine whether clothing is inhibiting timely voiding. If needed, Velcro fasteners or sweatshirts and sweatpants can be helpful.	*Clothing can be difficult to remove for older adults, resulting in incontinence before the clothing can be removed. Clothing can be modified so that it comes off quickly.*	Does patient have easy-to-remove clothing?
Determine whether there are any obstacles to reaching appropriate urine receptacle, such as poor lighting, busy bathroom, lack of assistive devices.	*Obstacles can make it impossible for patient to reach the voiding receptacle in time to prevent incontinence.*	Does patient have ready access to a voiding receptacle?
Provide appropriate urinary receptacles, such as a three-in-one commode, female or male urinal, or no-spill urinal.	*Assistive devices can be helpful for patient to increase continence.*	Does patient need and have access to an appropriate assistive device?
Initiate a voiding schedule for every 2 hours, or base schedule on voiding log.	*Frequent scheduled voiding using prompting techniques can increase continence.*	Does patient receive help to do bladder training with prompted voiding?
Always assist patient to the toilet when patient first awakens and before sleep.	*These are the primary times when toileting is needed.*	Are patient's toileting needs met?
Use prompted voiding techniques, including checking patient regularly, providing positive reinforcement if dry, prompting patient to toilet, praising patient after toileting, and returning patient to toilet in a specified time.	*Maintaining a regular toileting schedule will help patient remain dry.*	Does patient remain dry?
Teach patient to set up schedule of voiding using environmental cues such as meals, bedtime, and television shows.	*Environmental cues help patient remember when it is time to void.*	Can patient indicate cues throughout the day that prompt voiding?

Management of Urine Retention

Urinary retention is the inability to empty the bladder completely during attempts to void. It can be acute, with a sudden onset of retention and no urine output, or chronic, with a slower onset of retention of urine and some urine being expelled. Acute retention often results from surgery. It is caused by anesthesia, medications, or local trauma to the urinary structures. Acute retention can be a medical emergency causing extreme pain, an enlarged bladder, and the possibility of acute kidney injury or bladder rupture. Chronic urine retention may be related to an enlarged prostate gland, diabetes, pregnancy, a medication effect, strictures, or other causes of obstruction of the urinary tract.

Gentle palpation and percussion of the bladder may be done by the nurse if urine retention is suspected. If the patient has a feeling of fullness but is unable to urinate, the nurse gently palpates the suprapubic area to identify a full bladder or performs a bedside bladder ultrasound. Normally, the bladder is not palpable. If the fluid-filled bladder is percussed, it sounds dull over the bladder and may extend up to and beyond the umbilicus.

A bladder scan assesses the volume of urine in the bladder (Fig. 36.6). Sound waves estimate the amount of urine in the bladder. It is painless and noninvasive, and it requires no patient preparation. The nurse performs this scan at the bedside. It helps guide the need for urinary catheterization, thereby reducing unnecessary catheterizations and associated risks. The bladder scan may be used instead of catheterization (the gold standard for determining urine retention) after the patient urinates to determine the amount of urine remaining in the bladder. Normally, the bladder contains less than 50 mL after urination. A residual volume of 150 to 200 mL of urine indicates a need for treatment for urine retention. Bladder scanning may also be used as a tool for incontinent patients to plan their care.

Urinary Catheters
Indwelling Catheters

Indwelling urinary catheters can be used for justifiable reasons, such as burns, shock, heart failure, or urinary tract

obstruction. Urinary incontinence is not a justification for insertion of an indwelling urinary catheter. The Joint Commission (2016) recommends using indwelling urinary catheters short term and only when necessary because of the risk of urinary tract infections (UTIs). Indwelling catheters result in UTI the longer they are in place. The incidence of infection is decreased when intermittent straight urinary catheterization is used instead of an indwelling urinary catheter.

With an indwelling urinary catheter, bacteria enter the bladder mainly in one of two ways: (1) through the outlet at the end of the collection bag contaminating the urine, which is then inadvertently drained back into the bladder, or (2) around the catheter up the urethra and into the bladder (Box 36.2). Routine perineal care during the daily bath is enough to minimize infection from an indwelling urinary catheter (see also "Home Health Hints").

Home Health Hints

- When inserting a urinary catheter, use a flashlight if lighting in the home is dim. Have an extra catheter kit and a sterile specimen container available. Secure pets in another room when performing sterile procedures such as catheter changes.
- Teach the caregiver to notify the nurse if the catheter is plugged as well as how to take the catheter out if it becomes plugged and the nurse is not readily available. Leave a syringe in the home and teach the caregiver not to cut the valve stem.
- Teach the patient and caregiver to keep a sports bottle full of water next to their chair. Patients can use the TV commercials as a reminder to take a sip.
- Teach the patient and caregiver signs and symptoms of dehydration.

After an uncircumcised male is catheterized, the foreskin must be properly repositioned over the glans penis. It cannot be left retracted to prevent injury. When left retracted, subsequent swelling may make it impossible to pull the foreskin over the glans penis later. This can then cause ischemia of the glans penis, which is a medical emergency. The HCP must be notified immediately. An emergency circumcision may be needed if the foreskin cannot be properly positioned. Always ensure that the foreskin is positioned properly after catheterization or perineal care.

BE SAFE!

Prevent Infection: Use proven guidelines to prevent infections of the urinary tract that are caused by catheters. (The Joint Commission's 2018 National Patient Safety Goals. © The Joint Commission, 2018. Reprinted with permission.)

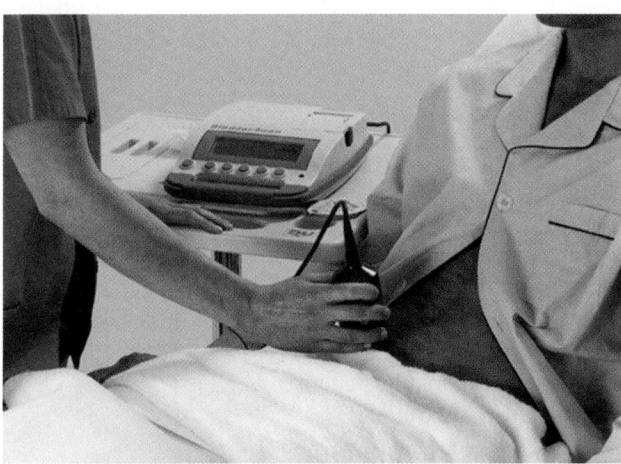

FIGURE 36.6 A bladder scan can be used to determine the volume of urine in a patient's bladder.

Box 36.2

Guidelines for Care of the Patient With an Indwelling Urinary Catheter

1. Maintain a closed system. Do not separate the catheter from the tubing of the bag. Instead, sterilely collect specimens and irrigate through the specimen port in the tubing.
2. Secure the catheter with tape or fastener as directed. This decreases traction on the catheter and the back-and-forth movements of the catheter that can help bacteria enter the bladder.
3. Encourage fluid consumption to naturally irrigate the catheter, if fluids are not contraindicated.
4. Use aseptic technique when emptying the collection bag by washing hands, wearing clean gloves, and using a clean container for single-patient use to collect the urine.
5. Wash the perineum with soap and water once a day and again if there is any bowel incontinence.
6. Keep the tubing coiled on the bed and positioned to allow free urine flow. Keep the catheter bag below the level of the bladder at all times.
7. Do not clamp catheters. Clamping a catheter results in obstruction and increases risk of infection. Periodic clamping has not been found to be effective in bladder retraining.
8. Replace the urine collection system as required.
9. Remove indwelling catheters as soon as possible.

Intermittent Catheterization

For the patient who is unable to void, the best intervention is intermittent catheterization. Those who are postoperative, have a neurologic disorder, or experience urine retention may benefit from intermittent catheterization. The risk of infection is reduced if the bladder is not allowed to overfill. Intermittent catheterization involves the use of a straight plastic or rubber catheter that is inserted into the urethra about every 3 hours to empty the bladder. After the bladder is empty, the catheter is removed. Patients may be taught to do intermittent self-catheterization (ISC) at home. Patients doing ISC may be taught to wash and reuse the same catheter repeatedly when they are in their own environment. In the health care agency, however, sterile technique is used.

Suprapubic Catheter

After certain surgeries of the urinary tract and in some long-term situations, a suprapubic catheter may be used. This is an indwelling catheter that is inserted through a surgical incision in the lower abdomen directly into the bladder.

Nursing care of a suprapubic catheter involves keeping the area clean and dry, changing the dressing when the site is new, and keeping the catheter taped to prevent tension. A skin barrier such as Stomahesive may help protect the skin from urine leakage. All other care is the same as for any indwelling urinary catheter.

SUGGESTED ANSWERS TO CRITICAL THINKING

Mr. Nolan

A total of 50 mL of concentrated urine for 4 hours is not normal or adequate output. Further investigation is needed to identify potential causes for the low output. If a problem is identified, inform the health care provider. Consider the following:

• What is Mr. Nolan's diagnosis? Is he now experiencing acute kidney injury? Is he severely dehydrated?
• Has anyone emptied Mr. Nolan's urinary bag without recording the output?

• Look at the trends in Mr. Nolan's intake and output record. Is his intake adequate? Has his output been decreasing? Is this a change?
• Look at trends in daily weights. Is Mr. Nolan's weight increasing due to fluid retention? Is this an expected finding?
• Listen to Mr. Nolan's lung sounds for crackles. Check for edema. Do findings indicate fluid retention?
• Palpate Mr. Nolan's bladder. Is it distended? Is the catheter blocked?

Review Questions

1. A home health nurse visits a patient who is 82 years old, uses a cane, and is continent. Which of the following interventions should be included in the plan of care, based on normal age-related changes of the urinary system, to promote patient safety?
   1. Encourage fluids after 6 p.m.
   2. Limit fluids to 1,000 mL per day.
   3. Provide a nightlight in the bathroom.
   4. Provide adult briefs to absorb dribbling.

2. The nurse is caring for a patient with acute kidney injury. Which of the following actions should the nurse take to obtain the most accurate assessment of fluid balance for the patient?
   1. Document voiding pattern.
   2. Obtain daily weight.
   3. Review creatinine levels.
   4. Observe skin turgor.

3. The nurse is caring for a patient who is to have a urine culture and sensitivity done. Which of the following should be included in patient teaching for collecting a midstream clean-catch urine specimen for culture and sensitivity?
   1. A second voided specimen is preferred.
   2. A 24-hour urine specimen is needed.
   3. As soon as the urine starts to flow, it should be collected in a sterile container.
   4. Women should keep the labia separated while voiding.

4. The nurse is caring for a patient who has had a pyelogram with intravenous contrast. Which of the following care should the nurse provide? **Select all that apply.**
   1. Maintain nothing by mouth.
   2. Encourage fluids.
   3. Check gag reflex.
   4. Measure urine output.
   5. Position patient prone.
   6. Maintain bedrest for 24 hours.

5. A patient is experiencing stress incontinence with frequent involuntary loss of urine. Which of the following directions would be most appropriate when teaching the patient how to perform Kegel exercises?
   1. "Tighten your rectum at frequent intervals throughout the day."
   2. "Keep your abdominal muscles tightened; do this every time you stand up."
   3. "Do 20 sit-ups per day."
   4. "Empty bladder then tighten the pelvic floor muscles for 8 seconds, then relax 10 seconds."

6. The nurse is caring for a patient with a urinary catheter. Which of the following is the most important nursing action for the nurse to take to prevent urinary tract infection in this patient?
   1. Encourage fluids to 4,000 mL every 24 hours.
   2. Empty the Foley bag every 4 hours around the clock.
   3. Maintain a closed catheter system.
   4. Wash the perineum every 8 hours.

7. The nurse is documenting the patient's shift output. What is the patient's total output as recorded during 0700 to 1500?
   • 0800 voided 165 mL
   • 1130 voided 450 mL
   • 1300 emesis 42 mL
   • 1500 voided 255 mL
   Answer: _____ mL

8. The nurse is reviewing the urinalysis of a patient. Which of the following are abnormal findings to report to the health care provider? **Select all that apply.**
   1. Blood 7/hpf
   2. Glucose none
   3. Protein 4 mg/dL
   4. White blood cells 11/hpf
   5. Nitrites positive
   6. pH 9.0

Answer rationales available in your online resources.

ANSWERS 1. 3; 2. 3, 4; 4. 2, 4; 5. 4; 6. 3; 7. 912;
8. 1, 4, 5, 6

Key Points

Find the chapter key points in your online resources available through Davis Edge.

Additional Resources

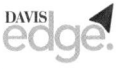 Use the scratch off code on the inside front cover of your book to access online quizzes that will help you to improve your scores on course exams and prepare for the NCLEX-PN®.

 Study Guide

CHAPTER 37

Nursing Care of Patients With Disorders of the Urinary System

Maureen McDonald

KEY TERMS

anuria (an-YOO-ree-ah)
azotemia (AH-zoh-TEE-mee-ah)
calculi (KAL-kyoo-lye)
cystitis (sis-TY-tis)
glomerulonephritis (gloh-MUR-yoo-loh-neh-FRY-tis)
hemodialysis (HEE-moh-dy-AH-lih-sis)
hydronephrosis (HY-droh-neh-FROH-sis)
nephrectomy (neh-FREK-tuh-mee)
nephrolithotomy (NEH-froh-lih-THAW-tuh-mee)
nephropathy (neh-FROP-uh-thee)
nephrosclerosis (NEH-froh-skleh-ROH-sis)
nephrostomy (neh-FRAW-stoh-mee)
nephrotoxins (NEH-froh-TOK-sins)
oliguria (AW-lih-GYOO-ree-ah)
peritoneal dialysis (PEAR-ih-toh-NEE-uhl dy-AL-ih-sis)
polyuria (PAW-lee-YOOR-ee-ah)
pyelonephritis (PY-eh-loh-neh-FRY-tis)
stent (STENT)
uremia (yoo-REE-mee-ah)
urethritis (YOO-reh-THRY-tis)
urethroplasty (yoo-REE-throw-PLAS-tee)
urosepsis (YOO-roh-SEP-sis)

CHAPTER CONCEPT

Elimination

LEARNING OUTCOMES

1. Explain the predisposing causes, symptoms, laboratory abnormalities, and treatment of urinary tract infections.
2. Explain the predisposing causes, symptoms, treatment, and teaching for kidney stones.
3. List risk factors and signs and symptoms of cancer of the bladder.
4. List risk factors and signs and symptoms of cancer of the kidneys.
5. Discuss nursing care for a patient with an ileal conduit or continent reservoir.
6. Explain the pathophysiology and nursing care for diabetic nephropathy, nephrosclerosis, hydronephrosis, and glomerulonephritis.
7. Describe the signs and symptoms for patients with acute kidney injury.
8. Describe the signs and symptoms for patients with chronic kidney disease.
9. Plan nursing care for patients with acute kidney injury.
10. Plan nursing care for patients with chronic kidney disease.
11. Discuss nursing care for a vascular access site.
12. Plan nursing care for patients on hemodialysis.
13. Plan nursing care for patients on peritoneal dialysis.

Disorders of the urinary tract involve the urethra, bladder, ureters, and kidneys. These disorders include infection, obstruction, cancer, hereditary disorders, and metabolic, traumatic, or chronic diseases. Some disorders lead to chronic kidney disease (CKD) if not treated.

URINARY TRACT INFECTIONS

A urinary tract infection (UTI) is an invasion of the urinary tract by bacteria. Normally, the urinary tract is sterile beyond the urethra. UTIs are most often caused by an ascending infection, starting at the external urinary meatus and moving up toward the bladder and kidneys. Most UTIs are caused by the bacterium *Escherichia coli,* which is commonly found in feces. Other less common pathogens include *Staphylococcus saprophyticus, Klebsiella* spp., and *Enterobacter.* Lower UTIs include urethritis, prostatitis, and cystitis. Upper UTIs include pyelonephritis and ureteritis. UTIs are the most common hospital-acquired infection (HAI). People who have one UTI commonly develop repeat infections. It is important that such patients receive education to prevent repeated infections of the urinary tract.

Risk Factors for Urinary Tract Infections
Stasis of Urine
Stasis of urine in the bladder results from voiding infrequently or obstruction. Urine stasis promotes bacterial growth, which can ascend to higher structures. The urine overdistends the bladder. The blood supply to the wall of the bladder is decreased. White blood cells (WBCs) are kept from fighting contamination that may have entered the bladder.

Contamination in Perineal and Urethral Areas
Contamination of the perineal and urethral areas can occur from fecal soiling; sexual intercourse, during which bacteria are massaged into the urinary meatus; infection in the area, such as vaginitis, epididymitis, or prostatitis; or genital piercing, which passes through the urethral meatus (Davis & Rantell, 2017).

Instrumentation Infection
Instruments or tubes inserted into the urinary meatus can cause infection. The most common cause of instrumentation infection is insertion of a urinary catheter. Bacteria ascend around or within the catheter. Bacterial colonization begins within 48 hours of indwelling catheter insertion.

Faulty Valves Causing Reflux of Urine
Faulty valves that do not maintain one-way flow cause reflux of urine from the urethra to the bladder or the bladder to the ureter. Reflux can be congenital or acquired because of previous infections.

Previous Urinary Tract Infections
Prior UTIs might provide a reservoir of bacteria that can cause reinfection.

Female Anatomic and Genetic Differences
Women are most susceptible to UTIs because of the short length of the female urethra and its proximity to the anus and vagina. Some women with recurrent UTIs have a shorter distance from the urethra to anus. Genetic factors may play a role in women who have a certain phenotype for developing UTIs.

Aging and the Urinary Tract
Older adults have an increased incidence of UTIs. This is due to diminished immune function, diabetes, and a neurogenic bladder that fails to completely empty. UTI is the most common cause of acute bacterial sepsis in patients over age 65. Older men are predisposed to infection because an enlarged prostate obstructs urine flow. In older women, the decline in estrogen contributes to the risk of UTI.

> ## NURSING CARE TIP
> When caring for a patient at risk for a catheter-associated urinary tract infection (CAUTI), limit the use of a urinary catheter, use infection control procedures at all times, and discontinue the use of the catheter as soon as possible. CAUTI is a "never event"—that is, hospitals will not be paid by Medicare for the costs of care provided if this condition occurs during hospitalization.

Signs and Symptoms
UTIs are characterized by shared signs and symptoms along with specific ones based on the UTI location (Table 37.1). A decline in mental status and fever in any patient with an indwelling catheter meets the diagnostic criteria for a UTI. In the older adult, the typical presenting symptom of UTI is generalized fatigue. New-onset confusion or delirium may also be present in the older adult, but a fever may not be.

Types of Urinary Tract Infections
Urethritis
Urethritis is inflammation of the urethra that may result from a chemical irritant, bacterial infection, trauma, or exposure to a sexually transmitted infection (STI). Posttraumatic urethritis can occur with intermittent catheterization or instrumentation of the urethra. Bubble bath and bath salts are common urethral irritants. They should be avoided by anyone with a history of UTIs. Urethritis can also be caused by spermicidal agents. Gonorrhea and chlamydia are STIs that can cause urethritis in men. Signs and symptoms are listed in Table 37.1. The male patient may have discharge from the penis. A urinalysis and urine culture diagnoses urethritis. Urethritis is treated based on the cause. If urethritis resulted from sexual transmission, the sexual partner(s) must also be treated. Phenazopyridine (Pyridium), a urinary analgesic, treats dysuria. Tell the patient that urine turns orange while taking phenazopyridine.

Cystitis
Cystitis is inflammation of the bladder wall. It is usually caused by a bacterial infection. *E. coli* is the cause of most UTIs. Cystitis can also be caused in noninfectious ways, such as catheter use, chemical irritants, medications, or radiation therapy. Chronic interstitial cystitis, whose cause is unknown, is known as painful bladder syndrome. Signs and symptoms are listed in Table 37.1. Urinalysis and sometimes cystoscopy is used for diagnosis. Urinalysis findings for cystitis include cloudy urine, WBCs, bacteria, sometimes red blood cells (RBCs), positive nitrites, and positive leukocyte esterase

---

• **WORD · BUILDING** •

urethritis: urethr—urethra (canal that discharges urine from bladder) + itis—inflammation

cystitis: cyst—closed sac containing fluid + itis—inflammation

Table 37.1

Urinary Tract Infection (Urethritis, Cystitis, Pyelonephritis) Summary

Signs and Symptoms	Shared: Voiding urgency, frequency, and burning; cloudy, foul-smelling urine; hematuria Older adult: Also fatigue, confusion, and delirium Cystitis: Also pelvic pain or pressure Pyelonephritis: Also costovertebral tenderness, high fever, chills, nausea/vomiting
Diagnostic Tests	Urinalysis: White blood cells, red blood cells, casts, bacteria, positive for nitrites Urine culture: Positive
Therapeutic Measures	Antimicrobial for causative organism Encourage fluids
Complications	Pyelonephritis Urosepsis
Priority Nursing Diagnoses	*Acute Pain* *Impaired Urinary Elimination* *Ineffective Health Maintenance*

(pyuria). A urine culture and sensitivity are then done. Bacterial cystitis is often treated with nitrofurantoin (Furadantin, Macrobid, Macrodantin), sulfamethoxazole and trimethoprim (Bactrim, Septra), or fosfomycin (Monurol). Instruct the patient to finish all prescribed medications to prevent bacterial resistance and to have a follow-up urinalysis or culture. Encourage fluids to flush the bladder.

Pyelonephritis

Pyelonephritis is infection of one or both kidneys, which can be serious. Bacteria can travel from the ureters to the bladder and then kidneys. Young women and older adults experience this infection most. Risk factors for uncomplicated pyelonephritis include history of UTIs within the past year, sexual intercourse, or spermicide use. Complicated pyelonephritis risk factors are diabetes, weak immune system, or structural or obstruction problems. In addition to the shared UTI signs and symptoms, high fever, chills, nausea/vomiting, flank (the side between the ribs and the pelvic bones) pain, and costovertebral tenderness (tenderness at the angle where rib and vertebrae join with palpation) indicate pyelonephritis. Urinalysis will show cloudy urine, bacteria, WBCs, pyuria, positive nitrites, and casts. The urine culture will have more than 100,000 colony-forming units per milliliter. In acutely ill patients, blood cultures may be obtained. Antibiotics are given orally or via intravenous (IV) route if

hospitalized (Table 37.2). After treatment, there is usually no lasting kidney damage. Frequent kidney infections can result in scarring and loss of kidney function.

Urosepsis

Urosepsis is sepsis caused by a UTI. Septic shock and death can result so prompt treatment is essential. Older adults are at greater risk for urosepsis.

Nursing Process for the Patient With a Urinary Tract Infection
Data Collection

Ask what the patient's usual pattern of voiding is and if there have been changes. Document the presence of a catheter, recent urinary instrumentation, or surgery. Note the presence of signs or symptoms (see Table 37.1) Inspect the urine for volume, color, concentration, cloudiness, blood, or foul odor. Review urinalysis and culture results.

Nursing Diagnoses, Planning, and Implementation

Acute Pain related to inflammation and infection of urinary structures

EXPECTED OUTCOME: The patient will report relief from pain and discomfort.

- Administer antimicrobial therapy as ordered *to treat infection and thus relieve pain and discomfort.*
- Administer phenazopyridine (Pyridium) as ordered *to relieve pain.*
- Apply heat to suprapubic area *to relieve discomfort.*

Impaired Urinary Elimination related to frequency

EXPECTED OUTCOME: The patient will return to previous voiding patterns.

- Ask patient normal urinary pattern and monitor pattern *to identify signs of a UTI or monitor resolution of UTI.*
- Avoid caffeine and alcohol *because they are urinary irritants.*

Ineffective Health Maintenance related to lack of knowledge on preventing or resolving UTIs

EXPECTED OUTCOME: The patient will be free from UTIs.

- Teach to drink adequate fluids, including water to produce clear-colored urine, *to prevent dehydration and flush bacteria from urinary tract.*

· WORD · BUILDING ·

pyelonephritis: pyelo—pelvis + nephr—kidney + itis—inflammation

urosepsis: uro—urine + sepsis—infection in the blood

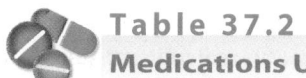

Table 37.2
Medications Used to Treat Urinary Tract Infections

Medication Class/Action

Antibiotics	
Example	**Nursing Implications**
Effective against *Escherichia coli, Klebsiella* spp., and *Serratia:* aztreonam (Azactam)	Contraindicated in patients allergic to penicillins and cephalosporins or if creatinine clearance is less than 30 mL/min. Check serum blood urea nitrogen (BUN) and serum creatinine before administration.
Effective against *E. coli* and *Enterococcus faecalis:* fosfomycin (Monurol)	Dissolve packet in 3–4 oz of cold water.
Effective against *E. coli,* enterococci, *Staphylococcus aureus, Klebsiella* spp., and *Enterobacter:* nitrofurantoin (Furadantin, Macrobid, Macrodantin)	*Teach:* Take with food or milk and full glass of water. Avoid antacids.

Fluoroquinolones	

Effective against E. coli, Klebsiella *spp., Pseudomonas,* and other organisms.

Example	**Nursing Implications**
ciprofloxacin (Cipro) levofloxacin (Levaquin)	Absorption may be decreased if given within 2 hr of aluminum antacids. Give with large amounts of water. *Teach:* Avoid sunlight or wear sunscreen of 30 HPF or more; report tendon aches promptly.

Sulfonamides	

Effective against E. coli *and* Pseudomonas; *used for uncomplicated UTIs.*

Example	**Nursing Implications**
trimethoprim-sulfamethoxazole (Bactrim, Septra)	Contraindicated in severe renal or liver disease. *Teach:* Avoid sunlight or wear sunscreen of 30 HPF or more; Take with large amounts of water.

Urinary Analgesic	

Topical analgesic; relieves pain urgency and frequency associated with UTI.

Example	**Nursing Implications**
phenazopyridine (Pyridium)	Urine color changes to red-orange. Avoid in renal insufficiency. Changes urine glucose testing.

- Suggest use of foods that may help prevent UTIs, including polyphenols (cranberry or blueberry products, coffee, black tea, and dark chocolate) *for their potential preventative action against UTIs.*
- Teach to void as soon as the urge occurs or every 3 hours while awake *to empty the bladder and lower bacterial counts, reduce stasis, and prevent infection.*
- Teach females to wipe from front to back *to prevent spreading bacteria from anal area to urinary meatus.*

- Teach to wear cotton crotch underwear and avoid constricting clothing such as tight jeans *to allow air circulation to reduce moisture.*
- Teach to avoid perfumed feminine hygiene products, bubble bath and bath salts, scented toilet paper, and tub baths, *which can irritate the urethra or introduce bacteria into the urinary meatus.*
- Teach to void after sexual intercourse *to flush bacteria from the urinary tract that entered the urinary meatus.*

- Teach signs and symptoms of UTI to report *so patient can detect UTI, recurrence, or complications.*
- Teach to finish all prescribed medications as directed *to prevent recurrent infection or resistance to antibiotics.*

Evaluation

The outcomes have been met if the patient verbalizes relief of pain and burning, returns to previous voiding patterns, and describes ways to prevent UTI.

CRITICAL THINKING

Mrs. Milan is a 25-year-old woman who recently had a weekend getaway with her husband. On Monday, she notices symptoms of dysuria, frequency, and urgency. She visits her health care provider and is diagnosed with a UTI. She is placed on an oral antibiotic.

1. What do you think predisposed Mrs. Milan to developing a UTI?
2. What should Mrs. Milan be taught to prevent further occurrences of a UTI?
3. What urinalysis findings would you expect for Mrs. Milan?
4. What should you include in her teaching plan based on her therapeutic regimen?

   Suggested answers are at the end of the chapter.

UROLOGICAL OBSTRUCTIONS

Urinary tract obstruction interferes with the flow of urine along the urinary tract. The obstruction can be partial or complete or unilateral or bilateral. It can develop rapidly or slowly. It is always a significant problem. Urine will back up from the point of the blockage, eventually distending the kidney (**hydronephrosis**) and increasing pressure on the structures of the kidney. This pressure can damage the kidney, impair its function, and ultimately lead to CKD.

Urethral Strictures

A urethral stricture is a narrowing of the lumen of the urethra from scar tissue. The patient with a urethral stricture has a diminished urinary stream, dysuria and frequency, and frequent UTIs. Strictures occur from injury, STIs, tissue trauma from use of catheters or surgical instruments, cancer, or enlarged prostate (see Chapter 43). It occurs most commonly in men. The problem becomes more apparent when attempts to insert a urinary catheter are unsuccessful because of the narrowed lumen. Treatment of a urethral stricture includes catheterization to drain the obstructed urine; mechanical dilation by the urologist, who inserts dilators over a wire to stretch open the urethra; endoscopic urethrotomy, which removes the stricture: surgical repair (**urethroplasty**); and rarely implantation of a **stent** (a tiny tube).

Renal Calculi (Urolithiasis)

Renal calculi (urolithiasis) are stones (**calculi;** one stone is a *calculus*) in the urinary tract (Table 37.3). Stones usually begin in the kidney. When stones occur in the kidney, it is nephrolithiasis (Fig. 37.1). When found in the ureter, it is ureterolithiasis.

Pathophysiology

Crystals start to form when (1) the urine is too concentrated with minerals and salts, resulting in high levels of calcium, oxalate (from plants), or phosphorus; (2) high uric acid levels; and (3) substances such as citrate that inhibit stone formation are low (see Table 37.3). The crystals bind together with other substances and form a calculus that enlarges unless it is flushed from the urinary system. There are four main types of stones: calcium (with oxalate or phosphate), uric acid, struvite (rare, large, fast-growing stone found in alkaline urine caused by bacteria in chronic UTIs), and cystine (rare stone that is hereditary; cystine is an amino acid found in foods). The majority of stones are made of calcium oxalate. Renal calculi can form in the renal pelvis and calyces, or in the ureter or bladder. They can range from the size of a grain of salt to staghorn (fill renal pelvis and calyces and area caused by urease-producing bacteria in chronic UTIs).

Etiology

Causes of stone formation may include a family history of stones; drinking too few fluids; living in a warm climate (causing sweating and resulting in more concentrated urine); consuming a diet high in sodium, sugar, or protein; obesity; and a UTI. Contributing causes for calcium-type stones include dietary factors ("Nutrition Notes: Renal Calculi"), calcium supplements between meals, and some medications (Table 37.4). The incidence of stones is on the rise, although the cause is unclear. Stones are more common in men than women. The risk for stone development peaks between ages 30 and 50. After having one stone, the risk of having other stones is increased.

Signs and Symptoms

Table 37.5 summarizes renal calculi and signs and symptoms. Stones within the kidney often produce no pain unless the stone moves or flow of urine is blocked. Typically, the pain that occurs with a stone is intense. With an infection, chills and fever may be present.

Complications

Obstructed urine flow leads to hydroureter and hydronephrosis over time. If the obstruction is not relieved, shock and

---

- **WORD** · **BUILDING** ·

hydronephrosis: hydro—pertaining to water + nephrosis— degenerative change in kidney

urethroplasty: urethro—urethra + plasty—surgical repair

Nutrition Notes

Renal Calculi. Concentrated urine enhances the formation of crystals, so adequate fluid should be consumed. Drinking six to eight 8-oz glasses of fluids daily, including plenty of water and citrus beverages, which help block renal calculi formation, can help prevent renal calculi. Three quarts of fluids are recommended daily for those with a kidney stone history to prevent a new kidney stone (read more at www.kidney.org/atoz/content/diet). The DASH diet (www.dashdiet.org) and maintaining a normal weight also reduce risk for renal calculi. For those who have had renal calculi, the type of stone determines the type of dietary changes to make to prevent new renal calculi.

Calcium oxalate stones. The most common renal calculi are composed of calcium oxalate. Reducing dietary oxalate, sodium, and animal protein, and getting adequate calcium to bind with oxalate and prevent oxalate levels from rising help prevent these types of stones. If a low-oxalate diet is prescribed, a long list of foods may be restricted, including beets, chocolate, spinach, rhubarb, nuts, peanuts, tea, wheat bran, and strawberries.

Calcium phosphate stones. Reducing dietary sodium and animal protein, avoiding colas, and getting adequate calcium helps prevent these types of stones.

Uric acid stones. Renal calculi can be a complication of gout, which is a disorder of purine metabolism. Purines are end products of the digestion of certain proteins. High-purine foods to limit include organ meats, anchovies, herring, sardines, meat extracts, consommé, and gravies. Other foods to limit are dairy products and eggs.

sepsis can occur. CKD can result if damage is caused by the stone and increased pressure from obstructed urine flow.

Prevention

For fluid and dietary guidelines, see "Nutrition Notes: Renal Calculi" and "Cultural Considerations." Encourage the patient to walk, which promotes the excretion of stones and reduces bone calcium resorption (release). Urocit-K (potassium citrate), which restores chemicals in the urine that prevent crystals from forming to decrease calcium oxalate and uric acid stones, might be prescribed.

Cultural Considerations

Calculi Development

- Caucasians have the highest incidence of renal calculi, followed by Mexican Americans. Prevalence of stones is increased in the southern United States and lowest in the western United States.
- Filipinos who immigrate to the United States are at high risk for developing renal stones due to hyperuricemia and gout. A shift from a traditional Filipino diet to an American diet likely increases the occurrence of hyperuricemia and gout development. The nurse may need to assist Filipino patients new to the United States to identify food choices that will help prevent these conditions.

Diagnostic Tests

Types of imaging for renal stones include helical (spiral) noncontrast computed tomography (CT), renal ultrasound,

Table 37.3

Overview of Renal Calculi

Type of Stone	Features	Possible Causes	Therapeutic Interventions
Calcium oxalate, calcium phosphate, or mixture	Accounts for two-thirds of stones Small, rough, and hard Shaped like needles Colors vary from gray to white	Excessive calcium Excessive urea Hyperparathyroidism, Cushing disease, immobility, and osteolysis from tumors of the breast and lung	Encourage fluids. Restrict protein and sodium in the diet. Administer hydrochlorothiazide. Treat hyperparathyroidism. Cellulose sodium phosphate (Calcibind) may prevent calcium stones by binding calcium from food in the gastrointestinal system.
Uric acid stones	Dye enhancement needed for x-ray visualization Small Color varies from yellow to red Hard	Gout High uric acid levels Decreased fluid intake	Encourage fluids. Administer sodium citrate to alkalinize urine. Administer allopurinol to reduce urinary uric acid levels.

Continued

Table 37.3
Overview of Renal Calculi—cont'd

Type of Stone	Features	Possible Causes	Therapeutic Interventions
			Teach to use low-purine diet and to avoid shellfish, anchovies, asparagus, organ meats, and mushrooms.
Struvite: magnesium ammonium phosphate	Calculi crumble easily Yellow color	Infection by urea splitting microbes, usually *Proteus*. May cause abscess formation in the kidney.	Encourage fluids. Decrease urine pH. Administer antibiotics.
Cystine stones	Small, smooth calculi Smooth, waxy stones	Cystine-containing crystals appear in the urine.	Encourage fluids. Use low-protein diet; urine is alkalinized. Give penicillamine to decrease amount of cystine in urine.

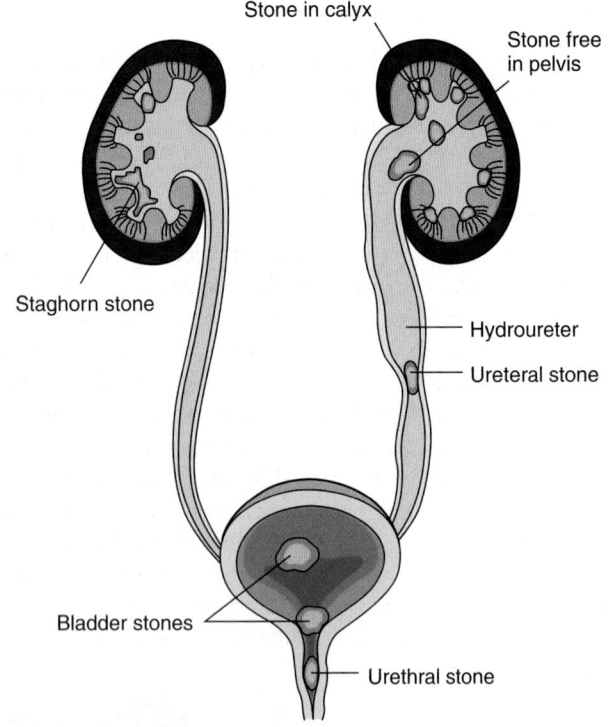

FIGURE 37.1 Location of calculi in the urinary tract.

abdominal x-ray, or MRI. Renal ultrasound is the preferred test for pregnant women.

Blood tests can show elevations of calcium or uric acid and renal function status. Urinalysis may indicate gross or microscopic hematuria and could indicate abrasion of the urinary tract. The presence of crystals or urinary pH may indicate calculus type. Two consecutive 24-hour urine collections

Table 37.4
Medications Affecting Stone Formation

Acetazolamide (Diamox)	Decreases urinary citrates and increases urinary uric acid.
Adrenocorticosteroids	Increases urinary calcium.
Allopurinol (Zyloprim)	Used to prevent uric acid calculi. May cause the rarer xanthine calculi.
Antacids such as magnesium trisilicate (Gaviscon)	May cause rare silicon-based calculi. Phosphate-binding nonabsorbable antacids can increase urinary calcium.
Aspirin	Increases urinary uric acid levels in presence of hyperuricemia.
Chemotherapeutic agents and external radiation	May cause cellular breakdown and cause acute hyperuricemia.
Hydrochlorothiazide (used to prevent calcium calculi)	Increases urinary uric acid levels.
Furosemide (Lasix)	May cause hyperuricemia.
Vitamin C in large doses	Increases oxalate excretion in urine.
Vitamin D	Increases calcium and oxalate excretion in urine.

Table 37.5
Renal Calculi Summary

Signs and Symptoms	*Nephrolithiasis:* Costovertebral angle pain Hematuria *Ureterolithiasis:* Severe, colicky (wavelike) pain from obstructed urine flow Flank, side, or lower abdomen pain radiating to genitalia Intense urge to void Frequency, dysuria, reduced output Hematuria due to irritation from stone Nausea/vomiting with severe pain *Bladder stones:* Hematuria Oliguria with obstruction of bladder outlet
Diagnostic Tests	Helical computed tomography (CT) Renal ultrasound Abdominal x-ray *Blood tests:* Calcium, uric acid, blood urea nitrogen (BUN), creatinine *Urinalysis:* Hematuria, crystals, urine pH Two 24-hour urine collections
Therapeutic Measures	*Small stones:* Hydration, analgesics, alpha-blocker (Tamsulosin) *Large stones, symptomatic:* IV fluids Pain control Thiazide diuretic Allopurinol (Zylorprim) Lithotripsy Surgery: Percutaneous nephrolithotomy, ureteroscopy, cystoscopy, cystolitholapaxy
Complications	UTI Hydroureter Hydronephrosis Shock Sepsis Chronic kidney disease
Priority Nursing Diagnoses	*Acute Pain* *Risk for Infection* *Deficient Knowledge*

can be done to identify excess minerals or reduced substances to prevent stones. The 24-hour urine collection measures total urine volume, calcium, oxalate, citrate, uric acid, sodium, potassium, phosphorus, pH, and creatinine as well as cystine and magnesium.

Therapeutic Measures

Renal calculi are treated medically if possible. Most small stones (up to 6 mm) can be flushed out of the body during urination. Drinking 2 to 3 quarts of fluids; taking analgesics for pain, such as acetaminophen (Tylenol) or ibuprofen (Motrin), or prescribed narcotics for severe pain, and using a prescribed alpha-blocker medication (such as tamsulosin [Flomax]) to relax ureter muscles help pass smaller stones.

Patients who develop severe renal colic are usually admitted to the hospital. IV fluids are given to hydrate the patient and help flush the stone out of the body. Pain medication is given. All urine is strained to detect passage of stones. The solubility of stone-forming substances can be changed by altering the pH of the urine. Calcium stones may be treated with thiazide diuretics and allopurinol (Aloprim, Zyloprim). Medical intervention is needed when the patient is unable to pass the stone, infection is present, urinary function is impaired, or severe pain continues.

LITHOTRIPSY. **Lithotripsy** is the use of sound shock waves or laser energy to break the stone into small fragments. Examples of types of lithotripsy include extracorporeal shock-wave lithotripsy (ESWL; most common), laser lithotripsy, and percutaneous ultrasonic lithotripsy.

For ESWL, the patient is sedated or anesthetized. Ultrasonic shock waves applied outside the body are focused on the stone to break it up into sandlike particles (Fig. 37.2). The particles are then flushed out with urination over time, with varying degrees of discomfort or pain. Occasionally, a stent is placed in the ureter to facilitate the passage of the stone fragments. ESWL is most effective with stones 2 centimeters or less that are in the kidney. After the outpatient procedure, the patient is usually discharged home. Blood-tinged urine (pink) for about 1 to 3 days and back soreness for several days are common. Bruising may occur on the back or abdomen. Discharge instructions include increase fluid intake to help flush out the stone particles, strain the urine to catch stone fragments for analysis, and notify the urologist if there are any problems.

SURGERY FOR RENAL CALCULI. Some patients may need surgery with local or general anesthesia for stone removal.

For kidney stones that are large and cannot be removed in other ways, a percutaneous **nephrolithotomy** is performed. A small incision is made in the back through which a nephroscope

---

• WORD • BUILDING •

lithotripsy: litho-stones + tripso-breaking stones
nephrolithotomy: nephro—kidney + lith—stone + otomy—incision

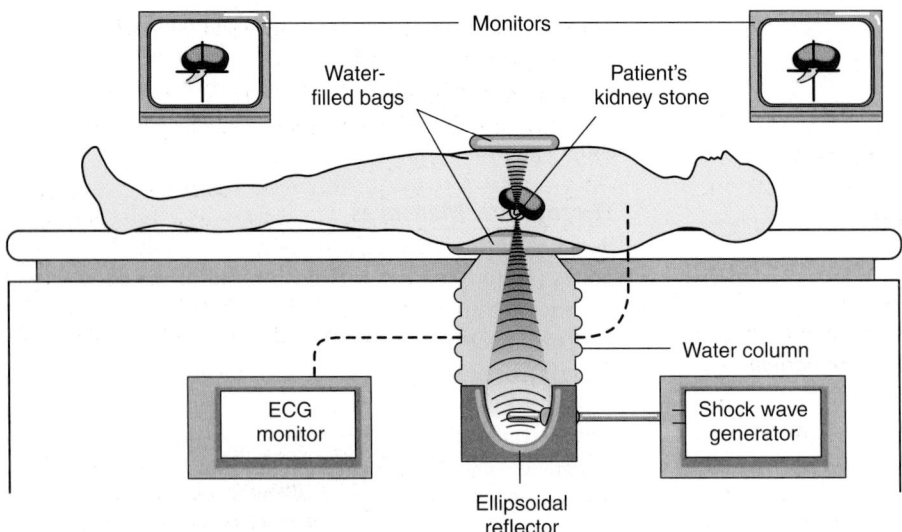

Monitors

Water-filled bags

Patient's kidney stone

Water column

ECG monitor

Shock wave generator

Ellipsoidal reflector

FIGURE 37.2 Extracorporeal shock-wave lithotripsy.

is inserted into the area of the kidney where the stone is located. The stone is broken up and removed. A temporary **nephrostomy** tube or stent can be placed to help ensure unobstructed urine flow.

Ureteroscopy is used for stones in the lower area of the kidney or the ureter. The ureteroscope is inserted into the bladder and then the ureter to allow viewing of the stone. The stone can then be removed with a wire basket or broken up with a laser or electrohydraulic energy to be flushed out in the urine. A stent may be placed for up to 2 weeks. Postoperative care is similar to cystoscopy care.

For stones in the bladder, cystoscopy for small stones (wire basket removal) and cystolitholapaxy for larger stones are used. In cystolitholapaxy, an instrument is inserted through the urethra to the bladder to crush the stone. The stone is then washed out with an irrigating solution. See postoperative care for cystoscopy in Chapter 36.

Nursing Process for the Patient With Renal Calculi

DATA COLLECTION. The health history may identify a family or patient history of previous stone formation. The patient is asked about a recent history of UTI, diet or activity changes, or other risk factors for renal calculi. If the cause is identified, specific teaching can be done to help prevent recurrent calculi.

Patients with stones often experience extreme pain, which should be monitored for pain management. Flank pain may radiate to the genitals. All urine must be strained to detect stones. If a stone is found, it is sent to the laboratory for analysis. Precise measurement of intake and output (I&O) is important. Obstruction may occur at the bladder neck or urethra. With obstruction, **anuria** (less than 50 mL of urine output daily) or **oliguria** (less than 400 mL of urine output daily) might occur. Obstruction is an emergency and must be reported and treated immediately to preserve kidney function. Urine is observed for hematuria. Temperature is monitored for fever, which would indicate an infection.

NURSING DIAGNOSIS, PLANNING, AND IMPLEMENTATION.

Acute Pain related to the presence of, obstruction by, or movement of a stone within the urinary system

EXPECTED OUTCOME: The patient will verbalize the relief of pain or ability to tolerate pain.

- Monitor severity, location, and duration of pain using a pain rating scale. *Pain typically occurs in the flank or costovertebral angle and may radiate to the abdominal, pelvic, and genital areas.*
- Administer pain medication as ordered *to promote comfort.*
- Apply heat to painful area *to reduce pain and promote comfort.*
- Ambulate if possible *to facilitate the passage of the stone through the urinary system.*
- Strain urine through strainer *to identify stones that may have been passed to provide pain relief.*

Risk for Infection related to the introduction of bacteria from obstructed urinary flow and instrumentation

EXPECTED OUTCOME: The patient will remain infection free.

- Monitor vital signs and temperature and observe for chills *as abnormalities may indicate infection.*
- Monitor urine amount, color, clarity, and odor *to ensure patency of urinary system or drainage tubes. Cloudy, bloody, foul-smelling urine may indicate an infection.*
- Encourage fluid intake *to flush bacteria and stones.*

- **WORD · BUILDING** -

nephrostomy: nephr—pertaining to the kidney + ostomy—surgically formed artificial opening to the outside

anuria: an—without + uria—urine

oliguria: olig—small + uria—urine

Deficient Knowledge related to lack of knowledge about prevention of stone recurrence, diet, and symptoms of renal calculi

EXPECTED OUTCOME: The patient will verbalize an understanding of the factors related to the recurrence of renal calculi, infection, and treatment options.

- Note if condition is a recurrence of renal stones. *Recurrence may indicate knowledge deficit.*
- Note family history of renal stones and explain relevance to patient. *Stones have a higher incidence in patients with a positive family history.*
- Determine the relationship between activity and stones. *Sedentary lifestyle or limited mobility may increase risk of stone formation.*
- Ask about patient's understanding of therapy to treat renal stones *to establish baseline knowledge.*
- Consult dietitian after stone analysis and reinforce dietary teaching *to prevent formation of specific stones.*
- Teach need for fluid intake of 2 to 3 quarts per day. *Dilute urine helps prevent stone formation.*
- Teach patient about medications used to prevent recurrence of renal stones:
  - Diuretics (thiazide type) increase tubular reabsorption of calcium, making it less available for calculi formation in the urinary tract.
  - Allopurinol (Zyloprim) reduces uric acid production.
  - Antibiotics prevent chronic UTIs, which may precede renal calculus formation.
- Teach the patient about management of stones. *Most stones pass spontaneously. There may be pain, nausea, and vomiting. Medical management consists of fluids, pain management, and antibiotics. Mechanical interventions with percutaneous catheters and nephroscopic procedures, lithotripsy, or surgery can be used to eliminate stones.*
- Teach the patient to strain all urine. *Stone fragments may continue to pass for weeks after stone crushing or lithotripsy.*
- Teach the patient to report signs of infection or cloudy, foul-smelling urine and unrelieved pain or gastrointestinal (GI) distress *for treatment.*

EVALUATION. Outcomes have been achieved if the patient remains comfortable, free from infection, and verbalizes how to prevent renal calculi.

Hydronephrosis

Hydronephrosis is distention of the renal pelvis and calices. This condition results from untreated obstruction of urine flow in the urinary tract. Hydronephrosis is usually treatable once the condition is detected. Obstruction of urine flow can result from a stricture in a ureter or the urethra, renal calculi, tumors, or an enlarged prostate. Because of the unrelieved obstruction, urine backs up and distends the ureter and then the kidney (Fig. 37.3). The capacity of the renal pelvis is normally 5 to 8 mL. As urine builds up, the kidney enlarges and pressure within the kidney increases. One or both kidneys can be affected, depending on the location of the obstruction. Unrelieved pressure within the kidneys causes the kidneys to become sacs filled with urine instead of functioning kidneys. In a matter of hours, the blood vessels and renal tubules can be damaged extensively if the pressure is not relieved.

If the onset of obstruction is gradual, the patient initially may be asymptomatic. Patients commonly develop UTIs with obstruction of urine flow. They may have symptoms of frequency, urgency, and dysuria. If the obstruction continues, flank and back pain may occur.

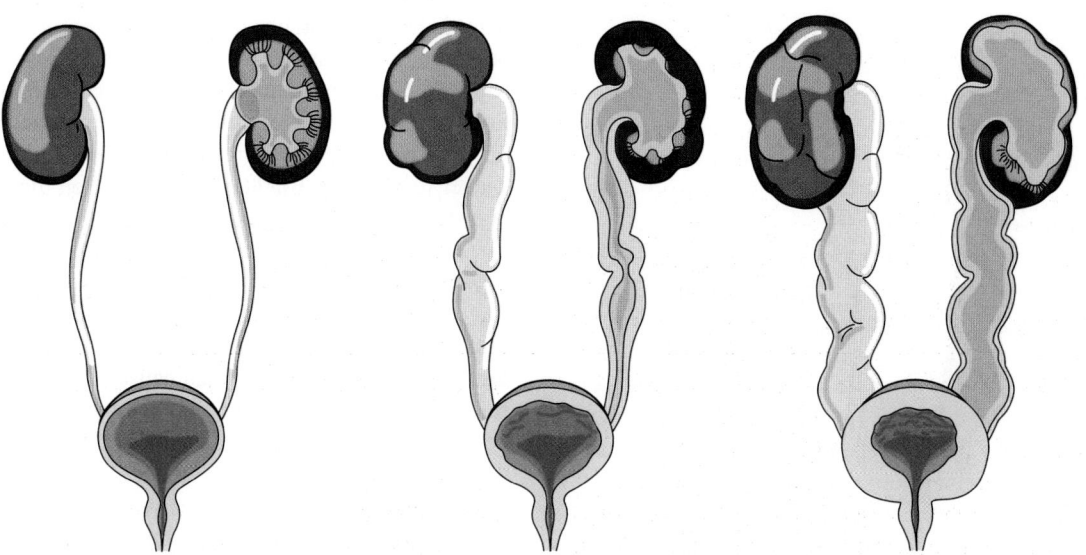

FIGURE 37.3 Hydronephrosis. Progressive thickening of bladder wall and dilation of ureters and kidneys result from obstruction of urine flow.

Immediate treatment of hydronephrosis is to relieve the urinary retention. This may be done by inserting a urinary catheter. The cause of the obstruction must be treated medically or surgically. Sometimes stents are placed inside the ureters during cystoscopy to hold the ureters open to allow passage of urine (Fig. 37.4). To relive kidney pressure, a nephrostomy tube can be inserted directly into the kidney pelvis for draining urine (see Fig. 37.4). This tube exits through an incision in the flank area. It allows urine to drain into a collecting bag to relieve kidney pressure and prevent kidney damage. Monitor the nephrostomy tube to ensure it drains adequately. It should not be kinked or clamped, which results in continuation of the hydronephrosis and possible kidney damage.

I&O is carefully measured. If both a nephrostomy tube and urinary catheter are present, output from each should be

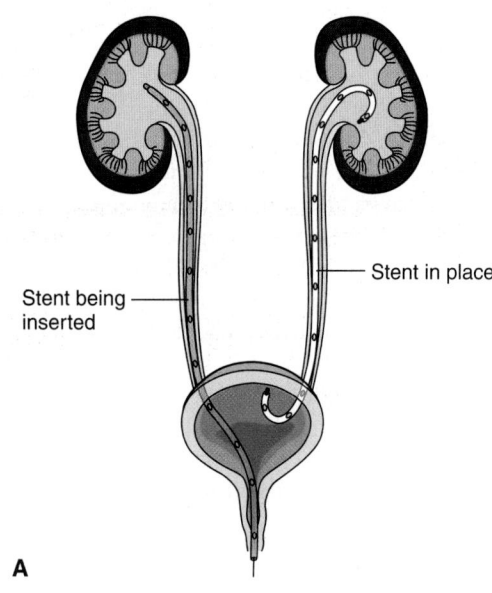

Stent being inserted

Stent in place

A

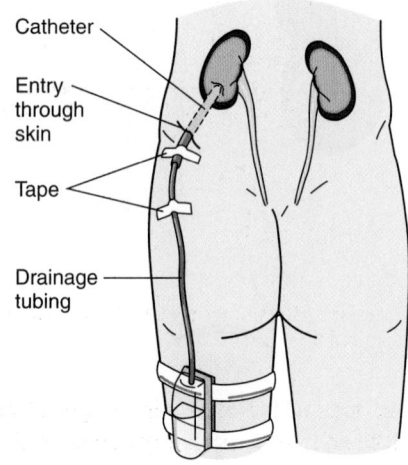

Catheter

Entry through skin

Tape

Drainage tubing

B   **Posterior view**

FIGURE 37.4 (A) Ureteral stents. (B) Nephrostomy tube inserted into renal pelvis; catheter exits through an incision on flank.

measured and documented separately. Urine retention can worsen the condition and must be recognized and reported promptly.

 TUMORS OF THE RENAL SYSTEM

Cancer of the Bladder

Cancer of the bladder is the most common kind of cancer of the urinary tract. The American Cancer Society (2018a) estimates more than 81,000 new bladder cancer cases in the United States in 2018. It occurs most commonly in men and in older adults, with the average age being 73. It is more common in Caucasians than in African Americans or Hispanics.

Pathophysiology

Cancer of the bladder often starts as a benign growth on the bladder wall that undergoes cancerous changes. Most bladder cancers begin in the inner lining of the bladder called the urothelium. They are called *transition cell cancers*. They come in a variety of forms and can behave in different ways. Some occur as small, wartlike growths on the inside of the bladder. Others form large tumors that grow into the muscle wall of the bladder and require surgical removal. If the cancer affects only the inner lining of the bladder, it is known as a superficial cancer. If it has spread to the muscle wall, it is called an invasive cancer. Common sites for metastasis include the liver, bones, and lungs.

Etiology

There is a strong correlation between cigarette smoking and bladder cancer. Those who smoke get bladder cancer twice as often as people who do not smoke. Specific chemicals that cause bladder cancer have been found in cigarette smoke. The lung absorbs chemicals from tobacco. These chemicals are then passed via the bloodstream to the kidneys and collected in the urine. From there, they accumulate in the urine and damage the cells that line the bladder. Exposure to industrial pollution, such as aniline dyes, benzidine and naphthylamine, leather finishers, metal machinery, and petroleum-processing products, also increases the incidence. It can take about 25 years after the exposure to these chemicals for bladder cancer to develop. Bladder cancer is often diagnosed at a late stage in women.

Signs and Symptoms

Cancer of the bladder usually causes painless hematuria. The urine may appear dark or reddish in color. Initially the bleeding is intermittent, which often causes the patient to delay seeking treatment. As the cancer progresses, the patient develops frank hematuria, bladder irritability, urine retention from clots obstructing the urethra, and fistula formation (an opening between the bladder and an adjoining structure such as the vagina or bowel). Other common signs and symptoms of bladder cancer include pelvic pain, pain in the lower back, painful urination, changes in bladder habits, and inability to void.

Diagnostic Tests

Routine urinalysis can detect evidence of bladder cancer. A urine test for the enzyme telomerase has been found to be 90% accurate in detecting bladder cancer in early and late stages. Urine for cytology can be obtained to determine whether cancer cells are present in the urine. Urine culture should also be done. Symptoms of bladder infection may be similar to those of bladder cancer. Diagnosis of bladder cancer may also be made with cystoscopy and transurethral biopsy. An IV pyelogram or CT scan also may be done.

Therapeutic Measures

Treatment depends on the type and staging (severity) of the bladder cancer. For early stage cancers that affect the inside lining of the bladder, intravesical therapy with chemotherapy or immunotherapy may be used. Chemotherapeutic agents are instilled into the bladder through a urinary catheter, allowed to dwell, and then removed along with the catheter. Bacillus Calmette-Guérin (BCG) therapy is used in the bladder to trigger the immune system to attack the BCG germ as well as cancer cells. Photodynamic therapy, in which drugs are given that make tumors sensitive to light, may be used. When light is applied to the tumor area, cancer cells are killed.

Surgical treatment options for bladder cancer include several procedures. A cystoscopy and pyelogram with fulguration (destruction of tissue with electrical current) may be done to burn off cancerous tissue. An alternate method is use of a laser to destroy tumor tissue. Robotic and laparoscopic surgical techniques may be used. Partial cystectomy can be done for cancer limited to one area. Complete removal of the bladder and creation of a urinary diversion may be needed. A urinary diversion means that urine leaves the body in a different manner.

INCONTINENT URINARY DIVERSION. A urostomy or ileal conduit is one type of urinary diversion. It is an involved surgery in which a 6- to 8-inch section of the ileum or colon is removed and used as a conduit for urine. The remaining portions of the bowel are stitched back together. The surgeon is careful to keep the blood and neurologic supply intact to the section of bowel that has been removed. The isolated section of bowel is closed off on one end, the ureters are stitched into it, and the other end is brought out as a stoma on the abdomen (urostomy) that almost continuously drains urine (Fig. 37.5). The urine from an ileal conduit contains mucus because it travels through the ileum, which normally secretes mucus. The patient must wear an ostomy appliance bag to collect urine at all times as urine continually flows into the bag from the stoma. This is why it is referred to as an incontinent urinary diversion. Box 37.1 explains how to apply an appliance to an ileal conduit stoma.

CONTINENT URINARY DIVERSION. Continent urinary diversion surgeries are being done for patient convenience. One version is the Kock pouch (continent internal ileal reservoir), which is created from a segment of ileum that has been made into a reservoir for urine (see Fig. 37.5B). The ureters are

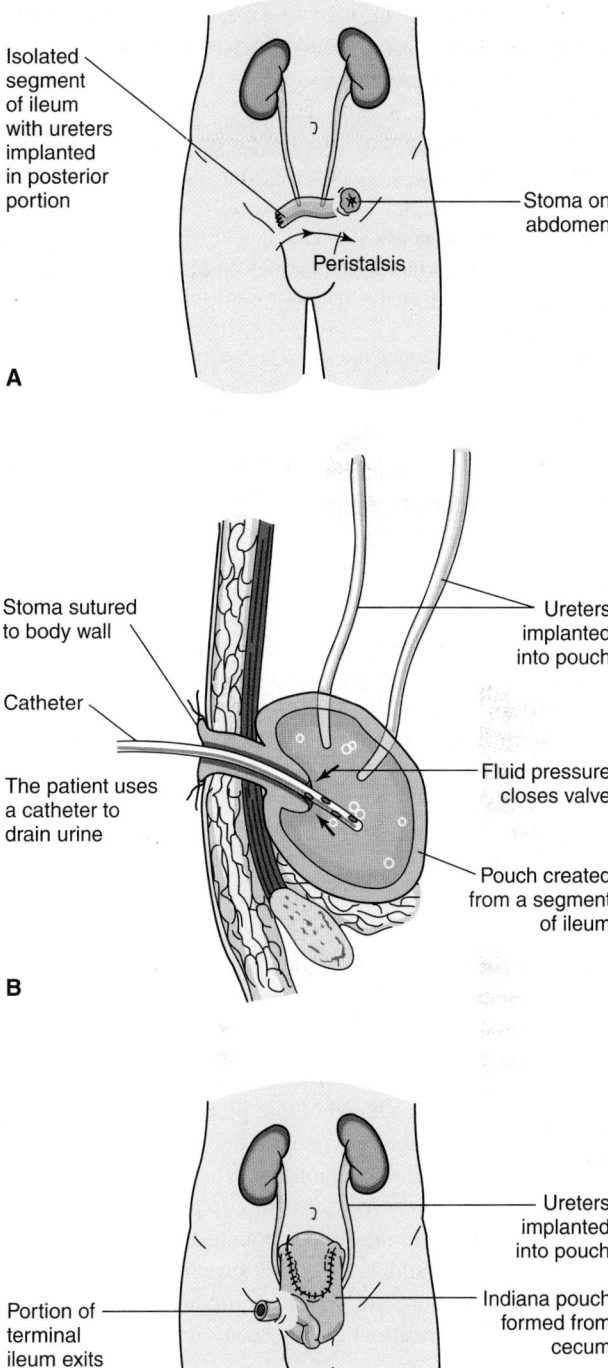

FIGURE 37.5 Urinary diversion surgery. (A) Ileal conduit. (B) Kock pouch. (C) Indiana pouch.

implanted into the side of the reservoir. A special nipple valve is constructed and is the passageway through which the patient inserts a catheter at 4- to 6-hour intervals to drain urine. Another version of this surgery is the Indiana pouch (see Fig. 37.5C). A reservoir is created using a portion of the ascending colon and terminal ileum, making a larger pouch

Box 37.1

Application of a Disposable Pouch to an Ileal Conduit

1. Gather all supplies, including a washcloth, towels, and water; a pouch to apply with a Stomahesive flange; and wicks such as gauze to absorb continually flowing urine. Wear clean gloves.
2. Empty the old pouch.
3. Gently remove the soiled pouch by pushing down on skin while lifting up on the flange. Discard soiled pouch and flange.
4. Place a towel around the stoma to catch urine.
5. Mold or cut an opening in the flange that is only 1/16 to 1/8 inch larger than the stoma. Once stomal shrinkage is complete, a presized pouch can be used that fits the stoma.
6. Remove paper backing from the Stomahesive and set the flange to one side.
7. Clean the skin around the stoma with water. Pat dry. Immediately wrap the stoma in wicks to absorb urine. Otherwise urine will leak onto the skin, and the flange will not adhere.
8. Center the flange over the stoma, remove the wick, and immediately apply the flange. Then snap the pouch onto the flange. *Note:* The flange and pouch may be snapped together before application to the stoma.
9. Use the heat of your hand to compress the flange against the skin to ensure a good seal.
10. Ensure that the bottom of the pouch is closed off or connected to a urinary catheter bag at night or if patient is in bed most of the time.

than the Kock pouch. Additional versions of this type of surgery use other parts of the bowel and include the Mainz pouch or Florida pouch.

ORTHOTOPIC BLADDER SUBSTITUTION. This surgery involves formation of an orthotopic bladder using a section of the intestine to make a neobladder (*neo* = "new") and implanting both the ureters and the urethra into the neobladder. Various types of orthotopic bladder substitution surgery include the Studer pouch, hemi-Kock pouch, and ileal W-neobladder. After this surgery, the patient can void through the urethra, although incontinence may be a problem and intermittent catheterization may be needed.

Nursing Care

Nursing care of the postoperative urological patient is similar to care following any major surgical procedure (see Chapter 12). It is important to ensure adequate urinary output and to report any obstruction of urine drainage early to prevent complications. A consultation with a nurse who specializes in wound, ostomy, and continence (WOC) care or an ostomy support group may be helpful both before and after surgery. The patient is taught how to monitor the stoma and care for the urinary diversion and surrounding skin after surgery. This may involve frequent draining of the continent pouch with a catheter or by wearing an ostomy appliance. Be sensitive to the patient's anxiety about caring for the urinary

diversion. Body image disturbance may occur because of the change in body function. Assist the patient with coping interventions. Teach the patient signs and symptoms of infection to report to the health care provider (HCP).

Cancer of the Kidney

Cancer of the kidney is among the 10 most common cancers in both men and women. The American Cancer Society (2018b) estimates more than 63,000 new cases of kidney cancer will occur in 2018. Most patients with kidney cancer are over age 55 and rarely under age 45. Men have twice the incidence of women. Risk factors include smoking, obesity, hypertension, long-term kidney dialysis, genetics (although rarely), and exposure to radiation, asbestos, and industrial pollution.

Signs and Symptoms

The three classic symptoms of kidney cancer are hematuria, dull pain in the flank area, and a mass in the area. Often, symptoms of kidney cancer do not occur until the tumor invades surrounding tissue. Less specific symptoms include fever, weight loss, night sweats, hypertension, anemia, polycythemia, swelling in the legs, fatigue, anorexia, and constipation. Often the cancer has metastasized before it is diagnosed. This is because the kidney has such a large volume of circulating blood, which increases the risk of tumor spread. In addition, the disease has few early symptoms. Symptoms of metastasis may be the first evidence of kidney cancer and include weight loss, cough, bone fractures, liver abnormalities, and increasing weakness.

Diagnostic Tests

Diagnostic tests include an IV pyelogram, cystoscopy and pyelogram, ultrasound examination of the kidneys, CT scans of the abdomen, and magnetic resonance imaging (MRI). A definitive diagnosis is made with a renal biopsy.

Therapeutic Measures

Surgery is the commonly used treatment for cancer of the kidney. A radical **nephrectomy** removes the entire kidney along with the adrenal gland and other surrounding structures, including fascia, fat, and lymph nodes, in the area. Radiation therapy, immunotherapy, or chemotherapy may be used after the surgery. In nephron-sparing surgery, only the tumor is removed, and the healthy part of the kidney is saved.

Nursing Care

After nephrectomy, provide postoperative nursing care as for any major surgery (see Chapter 12). Monitor urine output. Report changes in urine amount or color, bleeding, or signs of infection. The patient should be assessed for shortness of breath or diminished breath sounds on the affected side.

• WORD • BUILDING •
nephrectomy: nephr—kidney + ectomy—excision

Surgically induced or spontaneous pneumothorax may occasionally occur after a nephrectomy. Reinforce discharge teaching for wound care, pain management, medications. and follow-up care.

RENAL SYSTEM TRAUMA

Causes of trauma to the kidney, ureters, and bladder include motor vehicle accidents, sports injuries, falls, and gunshot and stab wounds.

Data collection includes a history of the injury and inspection of the abdomen and flank for asymmetry and bruising or swelling. Flank pain and hematuria may be present. Diagnostic tests include urinalysis, IV pyelogram, ultrasound, CT, and MRI. Treatment depends on the extent of the injury and ranges from bedrest to surgical intervention. Nursing care includes monitoring vital signs, measuring intake and output, providing IV fluids, and pain management.

Bladder trauma may occur with pelvic fractures and multiple trauma from a blow to the lower abdomen when the bladder is full. The weakest part of the bladder wall, which is the dome located at the top of the bladder, may rupture. Urine leaks out of the peritoneal cavity and around the bowel. The patient can have symptoms of hematuria, abdominal pain, inability to void, shock, and pelvic hematoma noted on rectal examination. IV pyelogram and x-ray of the abdomen may be done. A urinary or suprapubic catheter is placed until the bladder heals.

POLYCYSTIC KIDNEY DISEASE

Polycystic kidney disease is a hereditary disorder that can result in CKD. The disease affects men and women equally. Polycystic kidney disease is characterized by formation of multiple cysts in the kidney that can eventually replace normal kidney structures. The cysts are grapelike and contain serous fluid, blood, or urine. The patient typically first shows signs of the disease in adulthood. The initial symptoms include a dull heaviness in the flank or lumbar region and hematuria. Other symptoms include hypertension and UTIs. People with inherited polycystic kidney disease may also experience aneurysms in the brain and diverticulosis in the colon. As the disease progresses, the patient develops symptoms of CKD (discussed later). The renal cysts are usually diagnosed with ultrasound imaging. Ultrasound uses no dyes or radiation, so it is safe for all patients, including pregnant women.

There is no treatment to stop the progression of polycystic kidney disease. Complications such as UTIs are treated as needed. Headaches that are severe due to hypertension or seem to feel different might be caused by aneurysms in the brain. A patient with severe or recurring headache should see an HCP. As the disease progresses, treatment for hypertension and eventual CKD may be needed. Because polycystic kidney disease is hereditary, patients should be counseled about the risks of children inheriting it.

CHRONIC RENAL DISEASES

Diabetic Nephropathy

Diabetic **nephropathy** is the most common cause of CKD. It is a long-term complication of diabetes mellitus in which the effects of diabetes result in damage to the small blood vessels in the kidneys. Microalbuminuria may be detected within 5 years of the onset of type 1 diabetes and 10 to 15 years after the onset of type 2 diabetes. Renal damage appears about 15 to 20 years after onset of type 1 diabetes, but it may also be a complication of type 2 diabetes. Risk factors for development of diabetic nephropathy include hypertension, genetic predisposition, smoking, and chronic hyperglycemia. Careful control of blood glucose levels reduces the risk of nephropathy in patients with diabetes.

Pathophysiology

Multiple factors contribute to diabetic nephropathy. It begins with increased osmotic pressure from hyperglycemia, increased diuresis and compensatory cell growth and expansion, and increased glomerular filtration rate (GFR). Widespread atherosclerotic changes occur in the blood vessels of patients with diabetes, decreasing the blood supply to the kidney. Abnormal thickening of glomerular capillaries damages the glomerulus, allowing protein to leak into urine. Patients with diabetes also commonly develop pyelonephritis and renal scarring. Another complication of diabetes, neurogenic bladder, causes incomplete bladder emptying. This results in urine retention, which can cause infection or obstruction of urine, further damaging the kidneys.

Initially, patients lose only small amounts of protein in their urine (microalbuminuria). This disease can be detected only with frequent examinations of the urine by the HCP. As the disease progresses, high-output CKD (nonoliguria) can develop. Large amounts of diluted urine are excreted without the usual amounts of waste products dissolved in the urine. The patient can lose large amounts of protein in the urine and develop nephrotic syndrome. This causes massive edema because of low levels of albumin in the blood.

Symptoms

The progression of nephropathy is marked by microalbuminuria advancing to proteinuria. Hypertension accelerates renal damage. As diabetic nephropathy progresses, urine output decreases, waste products accumulate, and eventually the patient develops CKD. For symptoms, see the discussion of CKD in a later section.

Complications

Patients with diabetic nephropathy often have a guarded prognosis because they are vulnerable to all the complications

• WORD • BUILDING •
nephropathy: nephro—pertaining to the kidney + pathy—disease

of long-term diabetes in addition to kidney disease. The risk of cardiovascular disease is significant as protein spilling in the urine progresses.

Diagnostic Tests

Diabetic nephropathy is diagnosed by carefully watching the patient with diabetes for onset of protein spillage or microalbuminuria in the urine, which is an early sign of the disease. Serum creatinine levels and 24-hour creatinine clearance tests are then done to confirm the presence and extent of diabetic nephropathy.

Therapeutic Measures

In the early stages of diabetic nephropathy, strict control of blood glucose levels and blood pressure can help slow the progress of the disease and reduce symptoms. Angiotensin-converting enzyme (ACE) inhibitors or angiotensin II receptor blockers (ARBs) may be given to slow the decline of the GFR and microalbuminuria. As the disease progresses, the patient may need dialysis. Kidney or kidney-pancreas transplant, when available, is the treatment of choice for the patient with diabetic nephropathy.

A healthy lifestyle should be encouraged to help manage this disease (Onyenwenyi & Ricardo, 2015). Smoking should be avoided. Regular physical activity, maintaining normal weight, and individualized dietary planning are helpful.

Nephrotic Syndrome

Nephrotic syndrome is the excretion of 3.5 grams or more of protein in urine per day. In nephrotic syndrome, large amounts of protein are lost in the urine from increased glomerular membrane permeability. As a result, serum albumin and total serum protein are decreased. Normally, albumin and other serum proteins maintain fluid within the vascular space. When levels of these proteins are low, fluid leaks from the blood vessels into tissues, resulting in edema. With very low levels of protein, ascites and massive widespread edema (anasarca) occur. In response to the low protein levels, the liver produces lipoproteins. As a result, serum cholesterol, low-density lipoproteins, and triglyceride levels are elevated. Urine may appear foamy from lipoproteinemia. Loss of immunoglobulins may lead to increased susceptibility to infection. Elevated blood pressure occurs.

Treatment is focused on the cause and symptoms of nephrotic syndrome. To control edema, diuretics may be used and sodium intake restricted. Protein intake is based on the severity of urinary protein loss. Lipid-lowering drugs may be tried. Anticoagulants are given for thrombosis prevention. In some cases, corticosteroids may be used to reduce inflammation.

Complications of nephrotic syndrome include impaired immune function, nutritional imbalances, and, most important, increased blood coagulation. The latter is due to urinary loss of clotting inhibitors such as antithrombin III and plasminogen along with protein.

Nursing care focuses on edema and preventing infection. For edema, daily weights, careful I&O measurements, and abdominal girth measurements are documented. Edematous tissue must be protected from injury. Preventing malnutrition due to protein loss is challenging but important to maintain normal body functions.

Nephrosclerosis

Hypertension damages the kidneys by causing sclerotic changes in the small arteries and arterioles, such as arteriosclerosis with thickening and hardening of the renal blood vessels (**nephrosclerosis**). Arteriosclerotic changes in the kidney blood vessels result in a decreased blood supply to the kidney (ischemia of the kidney), which can eventually destroy the kidney. The remaining nephrons try to compensate with vasodilation to increase blood flow to the glomeruli. This results in increased glomerular pressure and filtration, which thickens the blood vessels. High pressure in the kidneys causes the vessels to weaken and hemorrhage. Large areas of the kidney become damaged. Symptoms of nephrosclerosis include proteinuria, hyaline casts in the urine, and, as it progresses, symptoms of CKD.

The treatment for nephrosclerosis is to control the hypertension with medications. The patient is placed on a low-sodium diet. Dialysis may be required.

Prognosis is often poor. By the time the patient develops nephrosclerosis, there is widespread arteriosclerosis throughout the body. Arteriosclerosis makes the patient prone to myocardial infarctions or cerebrovascular accidents.

The priority nursing diagnosis that is relevant when the patient develops nephrosclerosis is *Ineffective Health Maintenance*. The goal is to help the patient manage the hypertension. The patient should also be taught the symptoms of CKD to report.

CRITICAL THINKING

Mr. Stevens is a 35-year-old African American man admitted to the intensive care unit with uncontrolled hypertension. His blood pressure is controlled by intravenous medication. His laboratory tests show protein and hyaline casts in the urine. He is diagnosed with nephrosclerosis.

1. What data should the nurse collect as part of the morning evaluation of the patient's condition?
2. What other renal function tests are appropriate for the nurse to check?
3. What teaching does Mr. Stevens need when his condition is more stable?

Suggested answers are at the end of the chapter.

• WORD • BUILDING •

nephrosclerosis: nephro—pertaining to the kidney + sclerosis—hardening

GLOMERULONEPHRITIS

Pathophysiology

Glomerulonephritis is an inflammatory disease of the glomerulus. It can be caused by a variety of factors, including immunological abnormalities, toxins, vascular disorders, and systemic diseases. Inflammation occurs as a result of the deposition of antigen-antibody complexes in the basement membrane of the glomerulus or from antibodies that specifically attack the basement membrane. The resulting immune reaction in the glomerulus causes inflammation, which in turn causes the glomerulus to be more porous, allowing proteins, WBCs, and RBCs to leak into the urine.

Etiology

Acute Poststreptococcal Glomerulonephritis

Glomerulonephritis is most commonly associated with a group A beta-hemolytic streptococcal infection following a streptococcal infection of the throat or skin. This is the most common cause in children and young adults. Antibodies form complexes with the streptococcal antigen and are deposited in the basement membrane of the glomerulus, inducing damage from inflammation. Damaged glomeruli become unable to filter blood correctly, and protein leaks into the urine. Edema, oliguria, and hypertension result. Glomerulonephritis typically develops about 6 to 10 days after the preceding infection. The disease has an abrupt onset. Other kinds of bacteria and viruses can also be the causative infectious agent.

Goodpasture Syndrome

Occasionally, glomerulonephritis is caused by an autoimmune response. In this case, the person, for unknown reasons, forms antibodies against his or her own glomerular basement membrane. Glomerulonephritis caused by an autoimmune response usually progresses rapidly and often leads to CKD.

Chronic Glomerulonephritis

Chronic glomerulonephritis occurs over years as a result of glomerular inflammatory disease. There may be no history of renal disease before the diagnosis. Often, proteinuria and hematuria may have been noted before the diagnosis. Systemic lupus erythematosus and type 1 diabetes mellitus may precede chronic glomerular injury. It is often discovered during an examination for another concern. Ultrasound, CT scan, or renal biopsy is used to diagnose the cause.

Symptoms

Symptoms of glomerulonephritis include oliguria, hypertension, electrolyte imbalances, and edema (Table 37.6). Edema may begin around the eyes (periorbital edema) and face and progress to the abdomen (ascites), lungs (pleural effusion), and extremities. Flank pain may be present.

Complications

Adults who develop glomerulonephritis may recover renal function or progress to chronic glomerulonephritis. Some

Table 37.6
Glomerulonephritis Summary

Signs and Symptoms	Fluid volume overload Hypertension Electrolyte imbalances Edema Periorbital edema Flank pain
Diagnostic Tests	Urinalysis shows red cells, white blood cells, protein, and casts Urine dark or cola-colored Foamy urine Serum creatinine elevated Serum blood urea nitrogen (BUN) elevated Renal biopsy
Therapeutic Measures	Symptomatic treatment Nonsteroidal anti-inflammatory drugs (NSAIDs) Steroids Antibiotics prophylactically to prevent further kidney damage
Complications	Chronic kidney disease
Priority Nursing Diagnoses	*Excess Fluid Volume*

patients develop rapidly progressive glomerulonephritis. This can quickly lead to acute renal injury. Chronic glomerulonephritis is a slow process characterized by hypertension, gradual loss of renal function, and eventual CKD.

Diagnostic Tests

Glomerulonephritis is diagnosed with urinalysis, which shows protein, casts, or RBCs. The urine is dark or cola-colored from old RBCs and may be foamy because of proteinuria. Serum blood urea nitrogen (BUN) and serum creatinine levels may be elevated. Kidney ultrasound, x-ray, or biopsy may be done to determine abnormal kidney shape, size, blood flow, inflammation, or scarring of the glomeruli.

Therapeutic Measures

Most cases of acute glomerulonephritis resolve spontaneously in about a week. However, some cases progress to CKD. Sodium and fluid restrictions may be ordered, along with diuretics to treat fluid retention. Medications may be given to control hypertension. If associated with a streptococcal

• WORD • BUILDING •
glomerulonephritis: glomerulo—glomerulus + nephr—kidney + itis—inflammation

infection, antibiotics are given. If fluid overload is severe, dialysis may be required.

Nursing Care

Nursing care for a patient with glomerulonephritis focuses on symptom relief. Vital signs are monitored because the patient may be critically ill. During the acute phase, rest is encouraged. Edema is controlled with fluid and sodium intake restrictions. Protein intake may be limited if the kidneys are not filtering protein waste products (as shown by increased serum BUN and serum creatinine levels). Additional care is discussed in the section on CKD. Teaching the patient how to prevent glomerulonephritis is important. Antibiotics for diagnosed streptococcal throat infections should be taken for prevention.

ACUTE KIDNEY INJURY OR CHRONIC KIDNEY DISEASE

Kidney disease is diagnosed when the kidneys are no longer functioning adequately to maintain normal body processes and homeostasis. This results in dysfunction in almost all body systems as a result of imbalances in fluid, electrolytes, and calcium levels as well as impaired RBC formation and decreased elimination of waste products. Kidney disease can be acute (acute kidney injury) with sudden onset of symptoms, or it can be chronic (CKD), occurring gradually over time. For more information on kidneys, visit the American Kidney Fund (www.kidneyfund.org), the National Kidney Foundation (www.kidney.org), and the American Association of Kidney Patients (www.aakp.org).

Acute Kidney Injury

Acute kidney injury (AKI) is the sudden (hours to days) loss of the kidneys' ability to clear waste products and regulate fluid and electrolyte balance. Rapid accumulation of toxic wastes from protein metabolism in the blood (**azotemia**) occurs. In azotemia, the serum creatinine level and serum urea level (measured by BUN) are elevated. AKI may or may not be associated with reduced urine output. AKI affects up to 5% to 7.5 % of hospitalized patients and 20% of patients in the intensive care unit (Park, 2017). Many patients with AKI recover completely.

Pathophysiology

There are three major mechanisms of injury in AKI. These mechanisms are hypoperfusion, direct tissue injury, and hypersensitivity reactions causing renal inflammation. In AKI, rapid damage to the kidney causes waste products to accumulate in the bloodstream. The patient may become oliguric depending on the cause of the AKI. Potassium imbalances may lead to arrhythmias. AKI can affect other organs, leading to dysfunction (Shiao et al., 2015).

AKI may progress through four stages (if urine output decreases), with an intrarenal cause taking a longer recovery time because there is actual renal damage.

INITIATING PHASE. In this onset phase, an event occurs that causes AKI. It begins at the time of renal injury and lasts until the occurrence of symptoms. This phase lasts for hours to days.

OLIGURIC PHASE. In the oliguric phase, less than 400 mL of urine is produced in 24 hours. Fifty percent of those with AKI experience this phase, which occurs from 24 hours to 7 days after the initial phase. This phase can last from up to 2 weeks to several months. Renal function recovery decreases the longer this phase lasts.

In the oliguric phase, fluid is retained, electrolytes become imbalanced, and waste products are not excreted as urine output decreases. Signs of fluid overload arise. Serum potassium rises while sodium is lost in the urine, creating a normal or low serum sodium level. The longer this phase lasts, the more effects that are seen. These may include metabolic acidosis from reduced hydrogen ion excretion and sodium bicarbonate levels, increased phosphate and decreased calcium levels, abnormal blood cells (RBCs, WBCs, platelets), neurologic effects ranging from confusion to seizures to coma, and, finally, effects on all body systems as is seen in CKD (discussed later).

DIURETIC PHASE. As the kidneys begin to excrete waste products again, 1 to 3 L/day of urine is produced. Osmotic

• WORD • BUILDING •
azotemia: azo—nitrogenous waste products + temia—blood

diuresis occurs from the elevated waste products (urea), which the body is attempting to eliminate. The kidneys are not yet able to concentrate urine, so dehydration and hypotension are a concern. It is important to monitor for hypovolemia, hyponatremia, hypokalemia, and hypotension in this phase. Serum BUN and serum creatinine levels are high until the end of this phase. This phase may last 1 to 3 weeks.

RECOVERY PHASE. In this final phase, recovery begins as the GFR rises. Serum waste product levels (BUN, creatinine) decrease greatly within the first 2 weeks of this phase. This phase can last up to a year. Those who recover usually do so without complications. Older adults are more at risk for reduced recovery of renal function. In those who do not recover renal function, CKD occurs.

Etiology

AKI is often classified as prerenal, intrarenal, or postrenal. These categories relate to the causes leading to the injury. Each category is associated with the location of the cause in the kidney. Understanding the cause can point to the direction of treatment plans helpful to the patient.

PRERENAL INJURY. Prerenal (before the kidney) injury, the most common cause of AKI, is associated with a decrease or interruption of blood supply to the kidneys. Causes may include decreased blood pressure from dehydration, surgery, blood loss, shock, or trauma to or blockage in the arteries that carry blood to the kidneys. When the nephrons receive an inadequate blood supply, they are unable to produce urine, and waste products are not adequately removed. Use of nonsteroidal anti-inflammatory drugs (NSAIDs) and cyclooxygenase-2 (COX) inhibitors can also lead to prerenal injury. These drugs impair the autoregulatory responses of the kidney by blocking prostaglandin, which is needed for renal perfusion.

Prerenal injury can be diagnosed by evaluating possible causes. If dehydration is the cause, then an IV fluid challenge may be given. With increased IV fluid, more blood flows to the kidneys for filtering, which increases urine output and waste product filtering. An arteriogram of the renal arteries is helpful to determine whether the blood supply to the kidneys is decreased or blocked; angioplasty may be used to open the blockage. Serum creatinine increases and creatinine clearance decreases. Urinalysis may be helpful in determining the cause as well.

Kidney injury biomarkers such as interleukin-18, neutrophil gelatinase–associated lipocalin (NGAL), and kidney injury molecule-1 (KIM-1) can provide information on the type and severity of kidney injury.

INTRARENAL INJURY. Intrarenal (inside the kidney) injury occurs when there is damage to the nephrons inside the kidney. The most common causes are ischemia, reduced blood flow, and toxins. Other causes are infectious processes leading to glomerulonephritis, trauma to the kidney, exposure to **nephrotoxins,** allergic reactions to contrast agents, and

severe muscle injury, which releases substances that are harmful to the kidneys.

A number of substances can be toxic to the kidneys (nephrotoxic) when they enter the body (Table 37.7). Kidney damage is most likely to occur when these substances enter the body in high concentrations or when pre-existing kidney damage is present for some other reason. Many commonly administered medications can be nephrotoxic. Aminoglycosides are nephrotoxic antibiotics; when they are administered, blood levels of the drugs are carefully monitored to avoid toxic levels.

CONTRAST-INDUCED NEPHROPATHY. Contrast agents used during tests such as IV pyelograms and CT scans can cause kidney damage, especially when the patient is dehydrated, the GFR is below 60 mL/min, or there is pre-existing renal damage. The incidence increases with age greater than 60 years, decreased renal function, poor renal perfusion, or exposure to nephrotoxic drugs. Contrast media may cause renal vasoconstriction, hypoxia, and alteration of renal blood flow. Loss of regulation of renal blood flow causes decreased oxygen transport, which causes increasing renal medullary hypoxia, necrosis, and renal cell tubular collapse (Gallegos et al., 2016; Lambert et al., 2017). Before administration of contrast media, patients should be assessed for risk factors (e.g., diabetes mellitus, hypertension, dyslipidemia, advanced age over 70, renal surgery). Anemia, proteinuria, hyperuricemia, and the use of diuretics and other nephrotoxic drugs increase the likelihood of contrast-induced nephropathy. Prevention strategies should focus on screening patients for dehydration and risk factors. IV hydration with normal saline is inexpensive and usually without risks. Studies are being done on the use of sodium bicarbonate infusion as well as the use of N-acetylcysteine to prevent contrast-induced nephropathy (Gallegos et al., 2016; Lambert et al., 2017).

POSTRENAL INJURY. Postrenal (after the kidney) injury is associated with an obstruction that blocks the flow of urine out of the body. Only 5% of AKIs are classified as postrenal. The blood supply to the kidneys and nephron function initially may be normal, but urine is unable to drain out of the kidney. This results in the backup of urine and impaired nephron function. Common causes of obstruction are kidney stones, tumors of the ureters or bladder, and an enlarged prostate that blocks the flow of urine (discussed earlier). Surgical intervention may be needed to correct the problem.

Therapeutic Measures

AKI is treated by correcting the cause if possible. Prevention of permanent damage is the goal of treatment. Signs and symptoms are managed as they develop, and supportive care is given. Treatment may include restoring fluid and electrolyte

• WORD • BUILDING •
nephrotoxin: nephro—kidney + toxin—poison

Table 37.7
Common Nephrotoxins

Antibiotics	Aminoglycosides
	Amphotericin B
	Cephalosporins
	Sulfonamides
	Tetracyclines
Analgesics	Acetaminophen
	Nonsteroidal anti-inflammatory drugs (NSAIDs)
	Salicylates
Other Drugs	Angiotensin-converting enzyme (ACE) inhibitors
	Amphetamines
	Cisplatin
	Dextran
	Heroin
	Interleukin-2
	Mannitol
Heavy Metals	Arsenic
	Copper
	Gold
	Lead
	Lithium
	Mercury
Contrast Media	Contrast agents used for diagnostic testing, such as intravenous pyelograms and cardiac catheterizations
Organic Solvents	Gasoline
	Glycols
	Kerosene
	Tetrachloroethylene
	Turpentine

balance, discontinuing nephrotoxic drugs, bypassing urinary tract obstructions with catheters to relieve urine retention, or using short-term continuous renal replacement therapy to filter blood and restore potassium and other electrolytes to normal. The care of the patient with AKI is similar to care of the patient with CKD.

CONTINUOUS RENAL REPLACEMENT THERAPY. Continuous renal replacement therapy (CRRT) is used to remove fluid and solutes in a controlled, continuous manner in unstable patients with AKI. Unstable patients may not be able to tolerate the rapid fluid shifts that occur in **hemodialysis,** so CRRT provides an alternative therapy that results in less dramatic fluid shifting. CRRT can be used with hemodialysis, which is needed if severe symptoms of **uremia**

(hyperkalemia) are present. CRRT is not as complex as hemodialysis. It can be done for more than a month, if needed, via temporary vascular access.

During CRRT, a permeable hemofilter is attached to the vascular access. Blood flows through the hemofilter, and excess fluids and solutes move into a collection bag. The remaining blood returns to the patient via the venous access. If desired, replacement fluid and electrolytes can be given through the vascular access. Monitoring I&O, fluid and electrolytes, daily weights, hourly vital signs, and vascular access is important.

Chronic Kidney Disease

Kidney disease is the ninth leading cause of death in the United States (Kochanek, Murphy, Xu, & Tejada-Vera, 2016). CKD affects about 26 million people, and the incidence is on the rise. CKD is a progressive, irreversible deterioration in renal function in which the body is unable to maintain metabolic, fluid, and electrolyte balance. It occurs with a gradual decrease in the function of the kidneys over time. The result is accumulation of nitrogenous waste products in the blood and uremia. CKD affects each body system (Table 37.8).

Healthy People 2020 has 14 objectives related to CKD, including its goal of reducing new cases of CKD and its associated burdens (Office of Disease Prevention and Health Promotion, 2018).

Pathophysiology

When a large proportion of the body's nephrons are damaged or destroyed, AKI or CKD occurs. As the nephrons die off, the undamaged ones increase their work capacity. The patient may experience significant kidney damage without showing symptoms. CKD is a progressive disease process. In the early, or silent, stage (decreased renal reserve), the patient is usually without symptoms, even though up to 50% of nephron function may have been lost (Table 37.9).

The renal insufficiency stage occurs when the patient has lost 75% of nephron function and some signs of mild kidney disease are present. Anemia and the inability to concentrate urine may occur. Serum BUN and serum creatinine levels are slightly elevated. These patients are at risk for further damage caused by infection, dehydration, drugs, heart failure, and use of diagnostic x-ray dyes. The goal of care is to prevent further damage, if possible, through control of blood glucose levels and blood pressure.

End-stage renal disease occurs when 90% of the nephrons are lost. Patients at this stage experience chronic and persistent abnormal kidney function. Serum BUN and serum creatinine levels are always elevated. These patients may

• WORD • BUILDING •
hemodialysis: hemo—blood + dialysis—passage of a solute through a membrane
uremia: ur—urea + emia—in the blood

Table 37.8
Chronic Kidney Disease Summary

Signs and Symptoms	See Figure 37.6.
Diagnostic Tests	Urinalysis Glomerular filtration rate (GFR) Serum creatinine elevated Serum blood urea nitrogen elevated Urine sodium level less than 10 mEq/L Acidosis Anemia Electrolyte abnormalities Serum magnesium elevated Serum potassium elevated
Therapeutic Measures	Diet Dialysis Transplant
Complications	Accelerated atherosclerosis Anemia Anorexia Dry itchy skin, ecchymosis Subcutaneous bruises Headache Heart failure Hypertension Impotence Osteomalacia Osteoporosis Platelet Dysfunction Pulmonary edema Uremic encephalopathy (lethargy, coma, seizures) Uremic pericarditis
Priority Nursing Diagnoses	*Excess Fluid Volume* *Risk for Electrolyte Imbalance* *Anxiety* *Imbalanced Nutrition: Less Than Body Requirements* *Risk for Infection* *Sexual Dysfunction*

Table 37.9
Stages of Chronic Kidney Disease

Stage	*Kidney Function Description*	*Glomerular Filtration Rate (GFR) mL/min*
1	Slight decrease	90 or greater
2	Mild decrease	60–89
3	Moderate decrease	30–59
4	Severe decrease	15–29
5	Dialysis/Transplant	Less than 15

Etiology

The causes of CKD are numerous. The most common include diabetes mellitus resulting in diabetic nephropathy, chronic high blood pressure causing nephrosclerosis, glomerulonephritis, and autoimmune diseases.

Symptoms of Kidney Disease

Patients with either AKI or CKD have multiple symptoms ("Evidence-Based Practice"). Figure 37.6 illustrates symptoms; some of the more common ones are explained next.

Evidence-Based Practice

Clinical Question

Does chronic kidney disease (CKD) affect cognition in patients?

Evidence

This systematic review included 44 studies that measured cognitive function in persons with CKD. Results show that the cognitive changes that occur with the decline of glomerular function and progression of CKD are unique and not like those associated with other disease processes such as dementia or brain injury. Those with CKD scored lower than those without CKD, especially in the areas of orientation (attending to one's environment) and attention (focus on information or tasks) as well as language (understand, produce, use appropriately) (Berger et al., 2016).

Implications for Nursing Practice

Health care providers should be aware that cognitive changes associated with CKD are not only unique but may impair a person's ability to make decisions about their care and treatment.

Reference

Berger, I., Wu, S., Masson, P., Kelly, P. J., Duthie, F. A., Whiteley, W., ... Webster, A. C. (2016). Cognition in chronic kidney disease: A systematic review and meta-analysis. *BMC Medicine, 14*(1), 206. doi:10.1186/s12916-016-0745-9

make urine but not filter out the waste products, or urine production may cease. Dialysis or a kidney transplant is required to survive.

Uremia (urea in the blood) is present in CKD. Patients eventually develop problems in all body systems (Table 37.10). If left untreated, the patient with uremia dies within a short time.

Table 37.10

Effects of Chronic Kidney Disease on Body Systems

Body System	Disease Process
Cardiovascular	Hypertension due to fluid overload and accelerated arteriosclerosis Congestive heart failure/pulmonary edema due to fluid overload, increased pulmonary permeability, left ventricular failure Angina due to coronary artery disease, anemia Arrhythmias due to electrolyte imbalance, coronary artery disease Edema due to fluid overload and a decrease in osmotic pressure Pericarditis due to presence of waste products in the pericardial sac
Gastrointestinal	Stomatitis due to fluid restriction, presence of waste products in the mouth, secondary infections Anorexia, nausea, vomiting due to uremia Gastritis/gastrointestinal bleeding due to urea decomposition in gastrointestinal tract releasing ammonia that irritates and ulcerates the stomach or bowel; patient is also under stress, increasing ulcer formation, and may have platelet dysfunction Constipation due to electrolyte imbalances, decrease in fluid intake, decrease in activity, phosphate binders Diarrhea, hypermotility due to electrolyte imbalance
Hematopoietic	Anemia due to impaired synthesis of erythropoietin, a substance needed by the bone marrow to stimulate formation of red blood cells (RBCs); also due to decreased life span of RBCs from uremia and interference in folic acid action Bleeding tendency due to abnormal platelet function from effects of uremia Prone to infection due to a decrease in immune system function from uremia; renal patients can rapidly become septic and die from septic shock
Integumentary	Dry, itchy, inflamed skin due to calcium-phosphate deposits in the skin Pale yellow skin color due to urobilins, which give urine its yellow color Skin will have an odor of urine because skin is an organ of excretion and the body attempts to remove toxins Decreased function of oil and sweat glands
Neurologic	Confusion due to uremic encephalopathy from an increase in urea and metabolic acids Peripheral neuropathy due to effects of waste products on neurologic system Cerebrovascular accidents due to accelerated atherosclerosis
Pulmonary	Pleurisy/pleural effusion due to waste products in the pleural space, causing inflammation with pleurisy pain and collection of fluid resulting in effusion
Reproductive	Loss of libido, impotence, amenorrhea, infertility due to a decrease in hormone production
Skeletal	Bone and mineral disease due to hyperphosphatemia and hypocalcemia

Disturbance in Water Balance

Disturbances in the removal and regulation of water balance in the body occur with signs of fluid accumulation. An early symptom is edema (swelling), which is seen in the extremities, abdomen, and sacral area when supine. Patients may report shortness of breath. Crackles and wheezes (signs of fluid accumulation) may be present on auscultation of the lungs. The patient may be hypertensive. These patients may produce a large amount of dilute urine (**polyuria**), small amounts of urine (oliguria), or no urine (anuria).

Disturbance in Electrolyte Balance

As kidney function decreases, the kidneys lose their ability to absorb and excrete electrolytes. Important electrolytes are sodium, potassium, and magnesium. When the kidneys are unable to maintain normal amounts of electrolytes in the blood, these substances accumulate at high levels and may be life threatening.

• WORD • BUILDING •

polyuria: poly—much + uria—urine

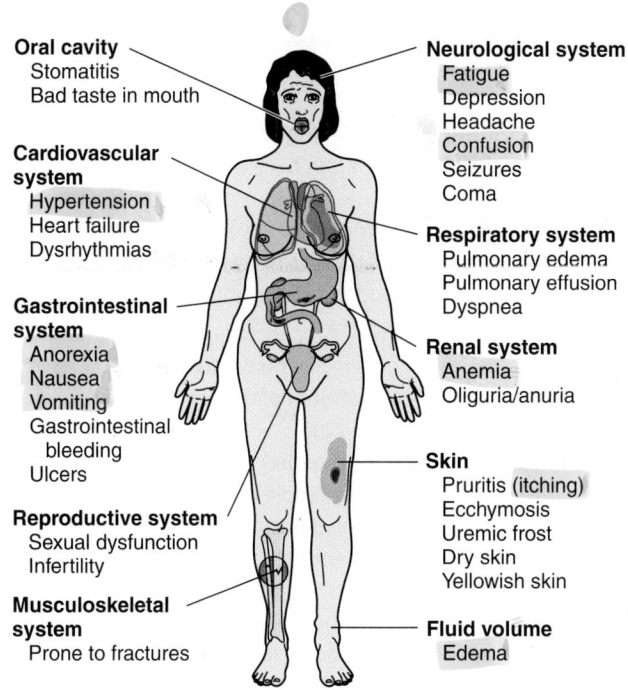

Oral cavity
Stomatitis
Bad taste in mouth

Cardiovascular system
Hypertension
Heart failure
Dysrhythmias

Gastrointestinal system
Anorexia
Nausea
Vomiting
Gastrointestinal
  bleeding
Ulcers

Reproductive system
Sexual dysfunction
Infertility

Musculoskeletal system
Prone to fractures

Neurological system
Fatigue
Depression
Headache
Confusion
Seizures
Coma

Respiratory system
Pulmonary edema
Pulmonary effusion
Dyspnea

Renal system
Anemia
Oliguria/anuria

Skin
Pruritis (itching)
Ecchymosis
Uremic frost
Dry skin
Yellowish skin

Fluid volume
Edema

FIGURE 37.6 Symptoms of chronic kidney disease.

When the kidneys are unable to regulate sodium levels adequately, the patient may show signs of hypernatremia (excessive sodium in the blood), which causes water retention, edema, and hypertension. Hyponatremia (too little sodium) may occur when too much sodium is lost. This can occur when the patient has experienced prolonged episodes of vomiting or diarrhea or is urinating large amounts of diluted urine. Patients with hyponatremia may show signs of confusion. The sodium may be normal or low due to being diluted from excess fluid.

Hyperkalemia (potassium level exceeding 5 mEq/L) can be life threatening if the level goes above 7 mEq/L. The patient may have arrhythmias or cardiac arrest if the potassium level is too high. Patients with hyperkalemia report muscle weakness, abdominal cramping, and diarrhea. The nurse may identify that the patient is confused or disinterested in care. These patients should be placed on a cardiac monitor and observed for cardiac arrhythmias while in treatment to reduce the potassium level is implemented.

A high potassium level in the patient with CKD may be caused by a diet high in potassium-rich foods, injuries, or blood transfusions. Monitoring daily laboratory values, restricting potassium intake, and reporting abnormalities are important. IV insulin with glucose or calcium gluconate may be used as a temporary measure to drive excess potassium into the cells. Sodium polystyrene sulfonate (Kayexalate) may be given either orally or as a retention enema; it causes potassium to be eliminated through the stool. Patiromer (Veltassa) is an oral powdered medication that is mixed with water; it binds potassium in the GI tract so that it cannot be absorbed. Patiromer must be taken 6 hours apart from other medications as it can interfere with their absorption. The

definitive treatment for hyperkalemia is hemodialysis, which removes potassium from the body. Dietary education is extremely important. The patient is instructed to avoid foods that are high in potassium (Box 37.2).

Calcium levels decrease because the kidneys are unable to produce the hormone that activates vitamin D, the vitamin needed for calcium absorption. Hypocalcemia exists when the calcium level falls below 8.5 mg/dL. Also associated with a low calcium level is hyperphosphatemia, a phosphorus level above 5 mg/dL. These imbalances cause the bones to release calcium, increasing the risk of fractures. These patients should ambulate regularly to prevent further calcium loss from the bone. Many patients who are on dialysis develop hypercalcemia due to hyperparathyroidism (excess release of parathyroid hormone). Cinacalcet (Sensipar) reduces excess levels of parathyroid hormone, which then reduces calcium levels.

Phosphates are also found in many foods. Medication to bind phosphates, known as phosphate binders, is taken by patients with high phosphate levels. Patients must take these medications with meals so they can bind with the phosphates and be eliminated in the stool. High phosphorus levels may cause severe itching, and patients may have open sores from scratching, placing them at risk for infections. Patients also may have muscle cramps and aches.

Disturbance of Removal of Waste Products

With azotemia (rapid accumulation of toxic wastes in the blood), the patient may show signs of weakness and fatigue, confusion, seizures, twitching movements of extremities (asterixis), nausea, vomiting, and lack of appetite. They may report a metallic or bad taste in the mouth, and there may be a smell of urine on the patient's breath. The patient may have yellowish pale skin and report itching due to urea crystals on the skin. Dialysis to remove excessive waste products in the blood is the only treatment for the underlying causes of these symptoms.

Disturbance in Maintaining Acid–Base Balance

Hydrogen ion excretion is affected, causing a disturbance in the acid–base balance that results in metabolic acidosis.

Box 37.2

Foods High in Potassium

- Beans: lima, lentils, kidney, navy, northern, pinto, refried, soy
- Chocolate
- Dairy products: cheese, ice cream, milk, yogurt
- Dried fruit: apricots, dates, figs, prunes, raisins
- Fruit: avocado, banana, kiwi, mango, melons (cantaloupe, honeydew), nectarine, oranges, orange juice, papaya, pumpkin, tomato paste
- Juice: carrot, prune, tomato, vegetable
- Nuts
- Vegetables: beet greens, potatoes (chips, sweet, white, yams), spinach, squash
- Salt substitutes
- Seeds

Patients may report headache, fatigue, weakness, nausea, vomiting, and lack of appetite. As metabolic acidosis progresses, the patient shows signs of lethargy, stupor, and coma. Respirations become fast and deep as the lungs attempt to blow off carbon dioxide to correct the acidosis (Kussmaul respirations). See Chapter 6 for a more detailed discussion of acid–base balance.

Disturbance in Hematologic Function

Anemia is seen mainly in CKD, which causes disturbances in blood cells over time. Damaged kidneys do not produce adequate erythropoietin, the hormone that stimulates RBC production. Nutritional deficiencies and blood loss during dialysis also contribute to anemia. Injections of epoetin (Epogen, Procrit), a synthetic form of erythropoietin, help restore RBC production and prevent anemia. Impaired WBC and immune functions contribute to an increased risk for infection. The patient should be protected from potential sources of infection. Impaired platelet function creates a risk for bleeding. The patient should be protected from injury, and signs of bleeding, such as blood in stool or emesis, must be reported.

Therapeutic Measures for Kidney Disease

Kidney insufficiency and early kidney disease are treated based on symptoms with a restricted diet and fluid intake, medications, and careful monitoring for onset of serious problems that warrant initiation of dialysis. In later stages, dialysis is necessary to replace lost kidney function. A kidney transplant, when available, may return the patient to a nearly normal state of health.

Diet

Dietary recommendations are individualized by the dietitian and HCP based on the patient's needs. Calories are high to maintain weight and energy needs. Protein is usually restricted to limit nitrogen intake but is increased for a patient on dialysis because protein is lost during the dialysis process. Sodium is restricted to minimize sodium and fluid retention. Potassium is restricted, especially later in the disease when the kidneys are unable to eliminate it. Calcium may be increased or supplemented because of poor absorption related to faulty vitamin D activation. Phosphorus is restricted because of high blood levels related to hypocalcemia. Saturated fat and cholesterol are restricted for patients with hyperlipidemia. Fluids are restricted to prevent overload. Most patients are given iron, folic acid, vitamins, and minerals to supplement the restricted diet ("Nutrition Notes: Understanding Dietary Changes in Renal Disease").

Because restrictions are complex, the diet may be a source of frustration for patients. The nurse should assist the patient to identify foods that are palatable yet within the diet plan. The dietitian should be consulted for instruction and assistance.

Nutrition Notes

Understanding Dietary Changes in Renal Disease

Patients with renal disease can have complex dietary requirements and need the guidance of a dietitian who specializes in renal treatment. Dietary restrictions will vary based on the patient's renal disease type and treatment. General guidelines include the following:

- Fluid restriction may vary daily according to the amount of urine output. Patients receiving hemodialysis may have 1,000 mL daily plus the amount of the previous day's urine output, if they still void.
- Adequate caloric intake is needed to maintain ideal body weight and protein stores. Simple carbohydrates and monounsaturated and polyunsaturated fats are given freely because their end products, carbon dioxide and water, are less likely to tax the kidney than protein.
- Low-protein diet is prescribed when the patient has renal function impairment to reduce damage to the nephrons. Protein is increased for dialysis to compensate for losses into the dialysate solution. Proteins of high biological value (eggs and meat) can be prescribed because they are more easily converted to body protein than those of low biological value. Vegetarian diets may be used to provide adequate protein as well as lower lipids. Plant proteins are chosen carefully to manage potassium and phosphorus serum levels.
- Potassium is restricted for patients with oliguria. Salt substitutes are often potassium compounds that patients need to be educated to avoid.
- Sodium is restricted, based on elevated blood pressure, degree of edema, and laboratory findings.

Renal diets are individualized. Teaching patients to associate adherence to their diet with relief of symptoms is important to encourage patients to manage their health.

Source: Lutz, C. A., Mazur, E., & Litch, N. (2015). *Nutrition and diet therapy* (6th ed.). Philadelphia, PA: F.A. Davis.

Medications

Early in the disease, diuretics are given to increase output, and ACE inhibitors, ARBs, calcium channel blockers, or beta blockers may be used to control hypertension. Phosphate binders are given with meals to reduce phosphate levels. Calcium and vitamin D supplements are used to raise calcium levels. Both the active and storage forms of vitamin D should be considered to decrease fractures, cancer, and infection rates and to improve cardiac function. Agents to lower potassium levels are used if needed. All drug therapy is closely monitored because diseased kidneys are unable to effectively remove medications from the body. As renal function decreases, the patient who requires insulin may need smaller doses of some long-acting insulins.

Dialysis

Dialysis is started when the patient develops symptoms of severe fluid overload, high potassium levels, acidosis, pericarditis, vomiting, lethargy, fatigue, or symptoms of uremia that are life threatening. Both peritoneal dialysis and hemodialysis involve the movement and diffusion of particles from an area of high concentration to an area of low concentration through a semipermeable membrane. Substances move from blood through the semipermeable membrane into the dialysate. Fluid and electrolyte imbalances can be corrected with dialysis. Dialysis can also be used to treat drug overdoses.

HEMODIALYSIS. Hemodialysis involves the use of an artificial kidney to remove waste products and excess water from the patient's blood. During the dialysis procedure, the patient's blood and the dialyzing solution flow in opposite directions through the dialyzer across an enclosed semipermeable membrane. The dialysate contains electrolytes and water in a balanced mix that resembles blood plasma. On the other side is the patient's blood with metabolic waste products, excess water, and electrolytes. The waste products from the patient's blood move into the dialysate by diffusion through the membrane because of the difference in their concentrations. The dialysate solution carries the waste products away, and the cleansed blood is returned to the patient's body through another tube (Fig. 37.7). A hemodialysis treatment takes 3 to 4 hours and is usually done three or four times a week at a hemodialysis center (Fig. 37.8). In-center self-care hemodialysis is offered in some centers. Patients often do better when they are involved in their treatments. The level of participation can range from doing some tasks to conducting the entire dialysis session after being trained. Hemodialysis can also be done at home with training.

Hemodialysis provides a rapid and efficient way to remove waste products from the blood. It is also excellent for correcting excessive fluid-overloaded states such as those that occur in heart failure.

Hemodialysis is not without side effects. After a treatment, the patient often feels weak and fatigued, sometimes even too tired to eat. Sudden drops in blood pressure may cause the patient to become weak, dizzy, and nauseated. Cardiac

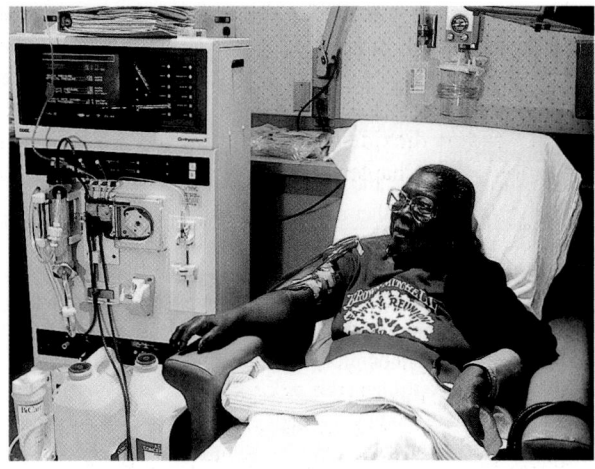

FIGURE 37.8 Patient undergoing hemodialysis at dialysis center.

arrhythmias and angina may occur. Fluid and electrolyte levels drop rapidly and can cause the patient to feel lethargic and have muscle cramps. Patients are given large amounts of heparin, an anticoagulant, to keep the blood from clotting while it is in the artificial kidney; this may cause bleeding from the puncture sites, GI tract, nose, or other sites if injury occurs. Box 37.3 reviews nursing care for patients having hemodialysis.

Vascular Access. Hemodialysis requires a permanent way to access the bloodstream for blood removal and return to the body during dialysis. Typical permanent vascular access options are an arteriovenous (AV) fistula (considered to be the gold standard) or a vascular access graft. Fistulas or grafts are placed in the arm when possible.

NURSING CARE TIP

It is important to save the veins of patients with chronic kidney disease for possible future fistula creation. The nondominant patient arm should not be used for intravenous lines, blood draws, or blood pressure to avoid damage to the veins because it will likely be the arm used for the fistula. Early consultation with a nephrologist can identify which veins to protect.

Early referral to a nephrologist can allow for the establishment of vascular access so that it is matured (developed) before the need for dialysis. If this does not occur, then a temporary access is used until a fistula or graft is placed and usable. A central venous catheter with two or three ports (the third port can be used for medications by trained staff) is placed in a central vein for temporary access. Central catheters should not be used long term because of the risk of infection.

An AV fistula is made by sewing a vein and artery together under the skin (Fig. 37.9). AV fistulas may take several weeks

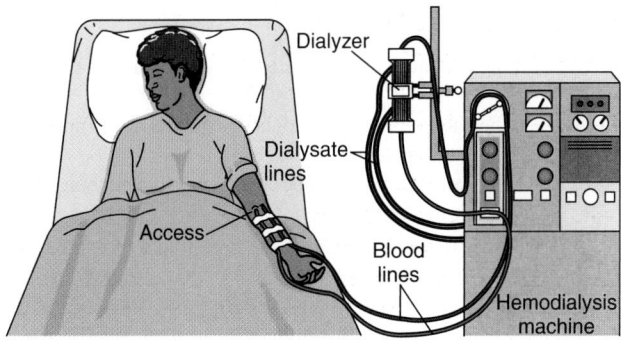

FIGURE 37.7 Hemodialysis.

Box 37.3

Nursing Care for Hemodialysis

1. Consult with the health care provider about medications to hold before hemodialysis. Some medications, such as antihypertensives, can be harmful when they become effective during dialysis and can reduce blood pressure to dangerously low levels. Other medications are water soluble and will be dialyzed out of the body, losing their effect.
2. Ensure that the patient is weighed both before dialysis in the morning and after dialysis to document weight loss as a result of fluid removal.
3. If the patient has laboratory tests ordered and blood needs to be drawn, coordinate this process with the dialysis nurse, who can obtain the blood samples and save the patient unnecessary needlesticks. To prevent painful needlesticks or other invasive procedures, a device that creates vibration to disrupt pain transmission can be held on the skin above the site of the procedure for 30 seconds. It is easy and fast to do, and patients are very appreciative. Some patients have their own devices and can teach you about it! An example of a pain-blocking vibration device can be seen at https://buzzyhelps.com/.
4. Try to get morning care done early and breakfast given before dialysis, if the patient tolerates eating before dialysis. For some patients, eating can cause hypotension by diverting blood flow to the gastrointestinal system for digestion during dialysis. After dialysis, patients are often exhausted and need rest.
5. When the patient returns from dialysis, weigh the patient, assess the access site for bleeding, and make sure that vital signs are stable. Administer medications that were held if not contraindicated and vital signs are stable.
6. Protect the patient's dialysis access as outlined in Box 37.4.

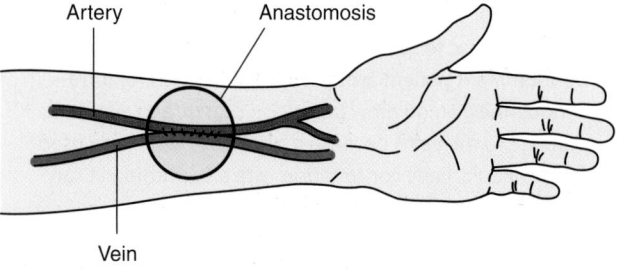

A

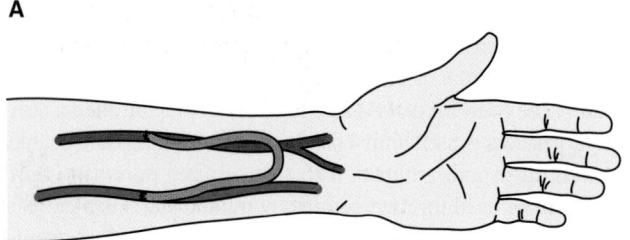

B

FIGURE 37.9 Hemodialysis access sites. (A) Arteriovenous fistula. (B) Arteriovenous graft.

to mature. The surgeon determines when the fistula is mature for use.

An AV graft uses a tube of synthetic material to attach to an artery and a vein. Needles are inserted into the graft to access the patient's blood. Traditional graft material is not self-sealing and requires time for tissue growth to serve as a plug for the hole that the needle makes before it can be used. This may take 1 to 2 weeks. The Vectra vascular access graft is self-sealing and does not require tissue growth so it can be used almost immediately after surgical implantation. This self-sealing property also decreases post-dialysis bleeding time and reduces the time required for the dialysis session.

Vascular Access Care. AV fistulas and grafts are regularly checked for patency by palpating for a thrill (a tremor) and auscultating for a bruit (swishing sound) at the site of the graft or fistula. Any decrease or cessation of bruit or thrill indicates occlusion. If a thrill or bruit is diminished or not present, the HCP is notified immediately. Special care of the access site must be taken because this is the patient's only way to eliminate waste products (Box 37.4). It is important for the site to be carefully monitored per institution policy to detect any clotting or problems. Early detection of clotting allows the surgeon an opportunity to save the access by performing a declotting procedure rather than a total revision.

Box 37.4

Care of Blood Access Fistula or Graft

Fistulas or grafts that are created for dialysis access should not be used for any purpose other than dialysis.

1. Watch for signs of bleeding or infection at the access site.
2. Listen for a bruit at the access site by placing the diaphragm of a stethoscope gently on the site. A bruit is a swishing sound made as the blood passes through the access site.
3. Gently palpate the site for a thrill, which is a buzzing or pulsing feeling that indicates good blood flow through the access site.
4. Do not take blood pressure, use a tourniquet, draw blood, give an injection, or start any intravenous lines in an arm with an access site.
5. Many hospitals have indicators (such as a red arm bracelet) to signify that an arm should be protected. A sign above the bed may also be used.
6. Teach the patient to keep the access site clean and not to bump or cut it.
7. Teach the patient to follow weight restrictions for lifting with the access arm.
8. Teach the patient to avoid wearing constrictive clothing or jewelry over the access site.
9. Teach the patient to avoid prolonged bending or sleeping on the arm with an access site.
10. Notify the health care provider if signs of bleeding, reduced circulation, or infection occur in an access site extremity (e.g., coldness, numbness, weakness, redness, fever, drainage, or swelling).

Postoperative Care. Initially, neurovascular checks are performed hourly for vascular surgery. Neurovascular checks include extremity movement and sensation, presence of numbness or tingling, pulses, temperature, color, and capillary refill (normally less than 3 seconds). Peripheral pulses are palpated to feel the thrill and auscultated to hear the bruit. If a pulse is absent or weak or the extremity is cool or dusky, the HCP is notified immediately. Dressings or incisions are checked, and any drainage, hematoma, or infection is documented and reported as needed. Vascular surgery pain is usually mild. Severe pain may indicate an occlusion of the graft. AV grafts can cause distal ischemia or "steal syndrome" because too much of the arterial blood is being "stolen" from the distal extremity. This is usually seen postoperatively and may require surgical correction to restore blood flow to the extremity.

Blood pressure readings and IVs should not be done in the extremity in which the access is placed. The extremity with the vascular access should be elevated postoperatively. Range-of-motion exercises should be encouraged. Patients are taught care of the access (see Box 37.4).

PERITONEAL DIALYSIS. **Peritoneal dialysis** provides continuous dialysis treatment and is done by the patient or family in the home. The peritoneal membrane is used as a semipermeable membrane across which excess wastes and fluids move from blood in peritoneal vessels into a dialysate solution that has been instilled into the peritoneal cavity. A peritoneal catheter is placed into the patient's peritoneal space between the two layers of the peritoneum below the waistline. This catheter is used to perform an exchange. The exchange process has three steps: (1) filling, (2) dwell time, and (3) draining.

The fill step involves instilling sterile dialyzing solution (dialysate) into the patient's peritoneal cavity through the catheter. The amount of solution is individualized by body weight. The solution is left to dwell in the abdomen for several hours, allowing time for the waste products from the blood to pass through the peritoneal membrane into the dialysate solution (Fig. 37.10).

The solution is then drained out of the body and discarded. This process is repeated three or four times a day and is continuous for the patient. Several treatment plans use this exchange process. The treatment plan that best suits the patient's needs is determined by the patient and the dialysis team.

Continuous ambulatory peritoneal dialysis is the most commonly used treatment plan. Usually, three exchanges are done during the day and one before bedtime. Other treatment plans allow for the use of a computerized machine called a cycler to regulate the exchanges during sleeping hours. Sometimes, medications are added to the dialyzing solutions, such as heparin to prevent clotting of the catheter, insulin for the patient with diabetes, or antibiotics if there is infection.

Patient and family education is extremely important for peritoneal dialysis to be successful. The patient must be taught and able to demonstrate that he or she is able to do a successful exchange. Sterile technique while performing the exchanges is imperative, and the exchanges should be done in a clean environment. A major complication is peritonitis (infection of the peritoneum), which can be life threatening. The major cause of peritonitis is poor technique when connecting the bag of dialyzing solution to the peritoneal catheter. The first sign of peritonitis is usually abdominal pain. (See Chapter 34 for additional signs and symptoms of peritonitis.) If any symptoms of peritonitis occur, the patient must contact the HCP immediately so antibiotic treatment can begin. The patient should be taught to care for the exit site (the site where the catheter comes out of the abdomen) and the need to inspect both the site and the dialysate solution for any signs of infection.

Dietary education is also important. A dietitian can assist the patient in making appropriate choices for adequate calories, protein, and potassium intake. The peritoneal dialysis patient typically has fewer dietary and fluid restrictions than the patient on hemodialysis because peritoneal dialysis is continuous and maintains serum waste levels. Proteins are lost through the peritoneal membrane into the dialysate fluid, so increased dietary protein is needed. This loss increases with peritonitis, which further increases permeability.

LEARNING TIP

Differences among hemodialysis, peritoneal dialysis, and continuous renal replacement therapy (CRRT) include the following:

- **Patient access:** Hemodialysis requires vascular access. Peritoneal dialysis requires insertion of a catheter into the peritoneal cavity. CRRT requires temporary vascular access such as a central line.
- **Equipment:** Hemodialysis requires a specialized complex dialyzer. Peritoneal dialysis and CRRT do not require the specialized dialyzer, although machines are available for these therapies.
- **Training:** Hemodialysis requires a skilled hemodialysis nurse. CRRT can be done by a nonhemodialysis nurse in a critical care setting. Peritoneal dialysis can be done by the patient.
- **Timing:** Hemodialysis is intermittent. Peritoneal dialysis and CRRT are continuous.
- **Solute removal:** Hemodialysis and peritoneal dialysis use the principles of osmosis and diffusion, which require a dialysate solution. CRRT uses convection, so no dialysate is needed.
- **Cardiovascular effects:** Hemodialysis may cause hypotension, which is a risk in the unstable patient. Peritoneal dialysis and CRRT have few cardiovascular effects. CRRT can be used for the unstable patient.

• WORD • BUILDING •

peritoneal dialysis: peritoneal—peritoneum + dialysis— passage of a solution through a membrane

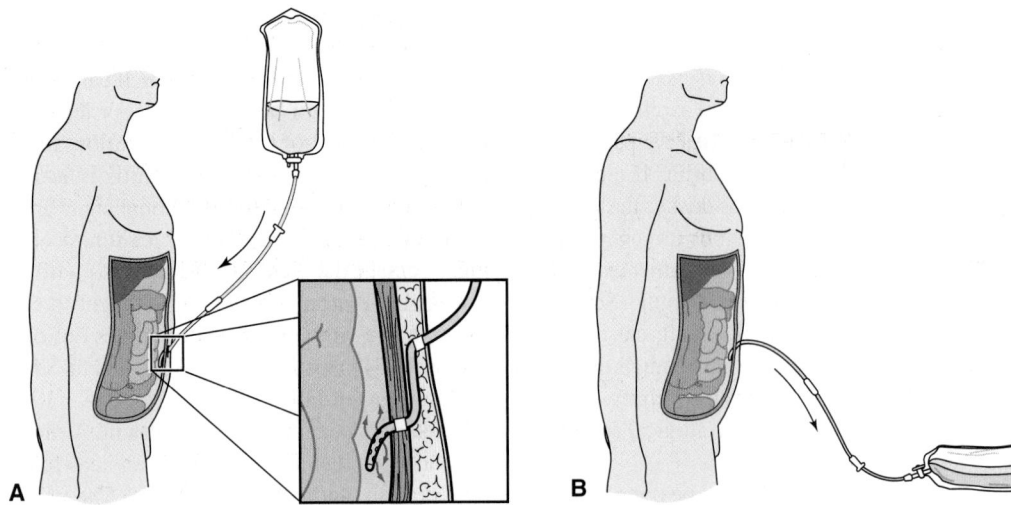

FIGURE 37.10 (A) Peritoneal dialysis works inside the body. Dialysis solution flows through a tube into the abdominal cavity, where it collects waste products from the blood. (B) Periodically, the used dialysis solution is drained from the abdominal cavity, carrying away waste products and excess water from the blood.

CRITICAL THINKING

Ms. Jackson is a single, 56-year-old woman with a 20-year history of type 1 diabetes, hypertension, hyperlipidemia, chronic anemia, and a total knee replacement. She has been diagnosed with chronic kidney disease (CKD). She is admitted to a medical unit for treatment of shortness of breath and CKD. Treatment will include hemodialysis. Ms. Jackson has increasing shortness of breath, pitting edema, and urine output of about 375 mL/day. She is having premature ventricular contractions as seen on the cardiac monitor. Her admitting serum laboratory values are sodium (Na) 131, potassium (K) 6, chloride (Cl) 97, calcium (Ca) 10, iron (Fe) 64, white blood cell 4,000, red blood cell 3.12, hemoglobin (Hgb) 10.1, hematocrit (Hct) 32, creatinine 7, and blood urea nitrogen (BUN) 30. Her blood glucose levels yesterday were as follows: 07:00, 154 mg/dL; noon, 122 mg/dL; 17:00, 188 mg/dL. She has sliding-scale insulin ordered, and an echocardiogram and chest x-ray will be done. Ms. Jackson is having a two-tailed subclavian catheter placed for vascular access. Ms. Jackson is withdrawn and quiet.

1. What would be the first thing the nurse would address after getting the report?
2. What do Ms. Jackson's physical symptoms indicate and the laboratory values reflect?
3. What should the nurse say to Ms. Jackson in relation to her withdrawn behavior?
4. What should the nurse identify related to Ms. Jackson's understanding of self-care?
5. What teaching is needed for the diagnostic tests?
6. What nursing care is required for the vascular access?
7. What type of insulin is used for sliding-scale insulin coverage? Why?
8. With what members of the health care team would the nurse anticipate collaborating?

   Suggested answers are at the end of the chapter.

Kidney Transplantation

Kidney transplantation is extremely successful. It frees the patient with CKD from dialysis and dietary restrictions. During kidney transplantation, a donor kidney is placed in the abdomen of the recipient (Fig. 37.11). The patient's native kidneys remain in place unless there is a reason to remove them. The transplanted kidney functions as a normal kidney does. The donated kidney can come from a living family member, a non-related donor, or a cadaver donor ("Cultural Considerations: Organ Donation" and "Patient Perspective"). Tissue and blood types must be matched to help prevent the body's immune

---

Cultural Considerations

Organ Donation

• Some Vietnamese Americans believe that the body must be kept intact even after death. Therefore, they may object to removal of body parts or organ donation.

• Jewish law views organ transplantation from a different viewpoint for the recipient, the living donor, the cadaver donor, and the dying donor. See "Cultural Considerations" in Chapter 36.

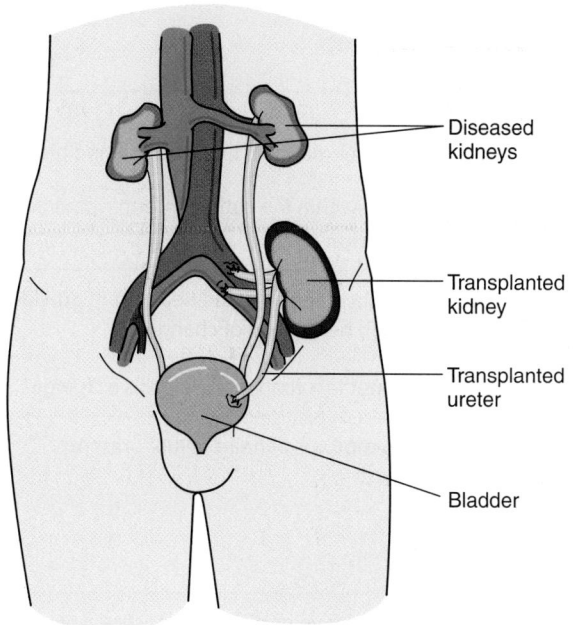

FIGURE 37.11 A transplanted kidney is placed in the abdomen.

system from rejecting the donated kidney. Patients receive immunosuppressant medications to help prevent rejection, which usually must be taken for the rest of the life of the transplanted kidney. Sometimes even with these drugs, the body rejects the kidney, and the patient must go on dialysis.

Patient Perspective

James. The cause of my chronic kidney disease (CKD) remains a mystery. I was healthy and active until my first symptom of ankle edema occurred. Over the next 3 years, my kidney function declined. When my glomerular filtration rate (GFR) was 12 mL/min, I was started on dialysis 3 days a week for 4 hours. Some people tolerated it well and could even go to work afterward, but it was a nightmare for me. I never tolerated it and dreaded going. An hour after the dialysis session, I would ache all over, be extremely fatigued and unable to move well. As soon as I arrived home from the dialysis center, I would go to sleep for several hours.

So, understand that your patients may want to be tucked in and allowed to sleep after dialysis. My entire day of dialysis was lost to other activities, and this happened 3 days a week! Family activities always had to be planned around my dialysis schedule. My family was supportive but it certainly affected them as well. Families need support just as much as the patient. I appreciated that dialysis was keeping me alive but I prayed for a kidney transplant. I was on the kidney transplant waiting list for two and half years. I had just begun home dialysis training when I got the call that a kidney was available. I was overjoyed but sad for the donor, who was on life support. My transplant surgery went smoothly. My own kidneys were left in place. The new kidney began making urine right away. In the recovery room, my urinary catheter bag was nearly full! It was liquid gold to me! The morning after surgery, I felt wonderful. I had so much energy and was walking up and down the halls, outpacing the nurses. They told me to slow down, but I felt so good for the first time in years that nothing could slow me down. The registered nurse transplant coordinator, pharmacist, and dietitian all taught me about follow-up care, my two antirejection medications that I must take for the life of the transplanted kidney, and healthy eating. I no longer had a daily 1,000-mL fluid limit (which is not much!) or dietary restrictions, which was fantastic! My recovery progressed with no complications. I had frequent follow-up lab work and clinic visits in the beginning. Three years later, all is well. I take my medications faithfully, and I have yearly clinic visits and monthly lab work. I am grateful to the donor and the donor's family for the gift I received.

Nursing Process for the Patient With Kidney Disease
Data Collection

Kidney disease progressively affects all body systems. If AKI is short term, fewer effects may be seen as some effects will not have time to develop. Nursing care for AKI is similar to CKD nursing care for effects that have occurred. In CKD, more effects are seen because the disease has time to progress. Data should be collected for signs and symptoms in all body systems. Family history of kidney disease and patient history of health problems such as hypertension, diabetes, systemic erythematous lupus, or urinary disorders are noted in the history. Also noted are medications the patient takes because they may be nephrotoxic and require adjustments. Recent changes in weight are documented.

Signs and symptoms vary depending on the severity of CKD and its cause. Common signs are hypertension, abnormal serum laboratory values (creatinine, BUN, anemia), or changes in urine output. See the signs and symptoms section for other effects.

Nursing Diagnosis, Planning, Intervention, and Evaluation

See "Nursing Care Plan for the Patient With Chronic Kidney Disease."

Nursing Care Plan for the Patient With Chronic Kidney Disease

Nursing Diagnosis: *Excess Fluid Volume* related to kidney's inability to excrete fluid
Expected Outcomes: Fluid volume will be stable as evidenced by stable weight, absence of edema, clear lung sounds, and blood pressure within the patient's normal parameters.
Evaluation of Outcomes: Is weight stable? Is edema absent? Are lungs clear? Is blood pressure within the patient's normal parameters?

Intervention	Rationale	Evaluation
Monitor weight daily at same time; report gain of more than 2 pounds.	*Those retaining fluid will have weight gain.*	Is weight stable? Should health care provider (HCP) be notified of change?
Monitor intake and output.	*This reveals degree of fluid retention.*	Is output less than intake? Is this a change?
Monitor and report shortness of breath, tachycardia, crackles in lungs, frothy sputum, heart irregularities, hypotension, and cold, clammy skin.	*These are symptoms of heart failure that may accompany fluid overload.*	Are symptoms of heart failure present?
Watch for new onset of jugular vein distention with patient's head raised to 30- to 45-degree angle.	*Fluid overload causes right-sided heart failure, resulting in distended jugular veins.*	Are jugular veins distended? Is this a new finding?
Monitor vital signs, including orthostatic blood pressure.	*Blood pressure changes reflect fluid volume.*	Is blood pressure increased?
Monitor for edema.	*Edema is a symptom of fluid overload.*	Is edema present? Is this a change?
Monitor serum protein and albumin levels.	*Low serum protein and albumin levels contribute to edema.*	Are levels within normal limits?
Maintain sodium and fluid restrictions (often 600 mL plus the previous day's urine output) as ordered. Develop a plan with specific allotted amounts of fluid at each meal and for medications. Teach patient the importance of each.	*For those on dialysis, fluid intake is adjusted so that weight gains are no more than 1 to 3 kg between dialysis sessions.*	Does patient understand and maintain sodium and fluid restriction?

Nursing Diagnosis: *Impaired Skin Integrity* related to dryness, excess fluid, and crystal deposits
Expected Outcome: The patient will maintain intact skin.
Evaluation of Outcome: Does the patient report no itching or dryness? Is the patient's skin intact?

Intervention	Rationale	Evaluation
Observe skin for open areas and signs of infection.	*Detects early signs of problems.*	Is skin intact?
Bathe with tepid water, oils, or oatmeal.	*Bathe regularly to reduce crystals with nondrying items to reduce itching and dryness and promote comfort.*	Does patient report no itching or skin dryness?
Apply lotion to skin after bathing.	*Lotion is used for itching to reduce dry skin.*	Is skin dry?

Nursing Care Plan for the Patient With Chronic Kidney Disease—cont'd

Nursing Diagnosis: *Activity Intolerance* related to anemia secondary to impaired synthesis of erythropoietin by the kidneys
Expected Outcome: The patient will be able to perform activities important to him or her.
Evaluation of Outcome: Does the patient state satisfaction with level of activity tolerance?

Intervention	Rationale	Evaluation
Identify pale mucous membranes, dyspnea, and chest pain.	*These are signs and symptoms of anemia.*	Does patient exhibit symptoms of anemia?
Monitor hemoglobin (Hgb) and hematocrit (Hct).	*Low Hgb and Hct indicate anemia.*	Are Hgb and Hct within normal limits?
Observe for signs of bleeding.	*Bleeding will worsen with anemia.*	Are signs of bleeding present?
Administer erythropoietin as ordered. Assist with blood transfusion as needed.	*Erythropoietin stimulates production of red blood cells by bone marrow.*	Are Hgb and Hct rising with use of erythropoietin?
Schedule rest periods between patient activities.	*Rest periods decrease demand for oxygen.*	Is patient able to tolerate activities with rest periods?

Nursing Diagnosis: *Risk for Injury* related to bleeding tendency from platelet dysfunction, use of heparin during dialysis, or gastrointestinal (GI) bleeding
Expected Outcomes: The patient will not experience bleeding. If bleeding occurs, it will be recognized and stopped quickly.
Evaluation of Outcomes: Are signs and symptoms of bleeding absent or recognized and reported quickly?

Intervention	Rationale	Evaluation
Observe for and report blood in stool or emesis, easy bruising, or bleeding from mucous membranes or puncture sites, and report immediately if present.	*Bleeding must be recognized quickly to prevent complications.*	Does patient have signs of bleeding?
Monitor Hgb, Hct, clotting studies, and platelets, and report results.	*Declining Hgb and Hct indicate blood loss. Declining platelet count or rising clotting times indicate increased risk of bleeding.*	Are lab results stable?
Monitor vital signs.	*Falling blood pressure and rising pulse may indicate volume deficit from bleeding.*	Are vital signs stable?
Avoid giving injections if possible.	*Injections can cause bleeding into tissue.*	Can medications be given by another route?
If bleeding, apply gentle pressure to site if possible.	*Pressure promotes hemostasis.*	Does pressure stop bleeding?
Teach patient to prevent injury to self and symptoms of bleeding to report.	*Injury can cause bleeding. Understanding symptoms of bleeding promotes early reporting.*	Does patient verbalize understanding of need to prevent injury and report bleeding?

(nursing care plan continues on page 770)

Nursing Care Plan for the Patient With Chronic Kidney Disease—cont'd

Nursing Diagnosis: *Risk for Infection* related to impaired immune system function
Expected Outcomes: The patient will not develop infection as evidenced by white blood cells (WBCs) and temperature within normal limits as well as no signs and symptoms of infection.
Evaluation of Outcomes: Are WBCs and temperature within normal limits?

Intervention	Rationale	Evaluation
Monitor for signs and symptoms of infection, and report promptly to HCP.	*Early recognition of infection and prompt treatment help prevent complications.*	Does patient have signs or symptoms of infection?
Protect patient from sources of infection, including roommates, visitors, or caregivers.	*Exposure to pathogens increases risk for infection.*	Does anyone in contact with the patient have an infection?
Maintain skin integrity.	*Intact skin protects against infection.*	Is skin intact?
Consult with HCP about the need for influenza and pneumonia vaccines.	*Patients with impaired immune function are at risk for influenza and pneumonia.*	Has patient been vaccinated?
Teach patient and caregivers to practice good handwashing technique.	*Handwashing helps control spread of infection.*	Is good handwashing being practiced?
Teach patient and family signs and symptoms of infection to report to HCP.	*Early reporting of symptoms allows for prompt treatment.*	Do patient and family verbalize understanding of symptoms to report?

Nursing Diagnosis: *Imbalanced Nutrition: Less Than Body Requirements* related to restricted diet, anorexia, nausea, vomiting, and stomatitis secondary to effect of excessive urea on the GI system
Expected Outcomes: The patient will maintain ideal weight, and serum protein and albumin levels will be within normal limits.
Evaluation of Outcomes: Are weight and lab values at desired levels?

Intervention	Rationale	Evaluation
Monitor weekly weight and serum protein and albumin levels.	*Weight and laboratory results provide information about nutrition status.*	Are weight and laboratory values stable?
Consult dietitian for renal diet restriction planning and teaching.	*Renal diets have restrictions such as low-protein to decrease formation of waste products (urea, creatinine).*	Does patient understand renal diet restrictions?
Initiate a calorie count; consult dietitian for assistance.	*A calorie count can provide information about the adequacy of the patient's diet.*	Is patient receiving adequate calories?
Provide frequent oral care.	*Oral care reduces urine taste in mouth and enhances appetite.*	Does oral care enhance appetite?
Offer medications ordered for nausea before meals.	*Nausea reduces appetite and must be controlled.*	Are antiemetics effective?
Offer frequent small feedings and dietary supplements.	*Smaller feedings are better tolerated and reduce risk of nausea.*	Does patient tolerate small feedings?

SUGGESTED ANSWERS TO CRITICAL THINKING

Mrs. Milan

1. Sexual intercourse can be a predisposing factor to urinary tract infection, especially if the patient does not urinate after intercourse.
2. Mrs. Milan should be cautioned to always urinate after intercourse (see UTI nursing process section).
3. The urinalysis will show white blood cells (WBCs), bacteria, red blood cells (RBCs), and positive nitrites.
4. Teaching should include the need to take all of the medication until it is gone, even if she feels better. The reason for this is to ensure that the infection is completely resolved so it does not return because of some remaining bacteria. She should return for a urine culture after the therapy is complete.

Mr. Stevens

1. Weight, intake and output (I&O), blood pressure, and laboratory tests should be assessed as part of the morning evaluation.
2. Serum blood urea nitrogen (BUN), serum creatinine, and serum potassium levels should also be checked.
3. Mr. Stevens should be taught that he needs to take antihypertensive medications, keep his follow-up visits to his health care provider, follow a low-sodium diet, and restrict fluids if ordered.

Ms. Jackson

1. Collect data related to Ms. Jackson's breathing and respiratory status first. Then address the cardiovascular system to see how she is tolerating the arrhythmia. Obtain Ms. Jackson's weight and I&O to monitor fluid balance.
2. Shortness of breath and pitting edema are related to fluid overload; urine output 375 mL/day is due to chronic kidney disease (CKD); premature ventricular contractions are due to elevated potassium. Sodium is low due to dilutional effect of excess fluid. Potassium is retained due to CKD. WBCs are low due to CKD. RBCs, hemoglobin (Hgb), and hematocrit (Hct) are low due to anemia. Creatinine and urea are not being excreted adequately due to CKD. Blood glucose is elevated due to diabetes.
3. Therapeutic communication suggestions: "Ms. Jackson, would you like to talk about your diagnosis?" "How do you feel about your diagnosis?" "Do you have questions or concerns?" "What are your usual coping methods?" Provide explanations for procedures and interventions.
4. Determine Ms. Jackson's understanding of what CKD is, how it is treated, how to follow the renal diet and fluid restrictions, and the action and importance of medications. Identify barriers to self-care and her support systems.
5. Teaching includes that the chest x-ray and echocardiogram require no preparation and are not painful.
6. A two-tailed subclavian vascular access is dedicated for hemodialysis. It is not used for any other purpose. Monitoring includes observing the site for signs of infection (e.g., redness, warmth, swelling, tenderness, drainage, fever).
7. Regular insulin is the only type of insulin used for a sliding scale because it is a rapid-acting insulin that affects current blood glucose levels. Sliding-scale insulin is ordered at intervals to monitor and treat the current blood glucose level.
8. The registered nurse, licensed practical nurse/licensed vocational nurse, surgeon, nephrologist, dietitian, pharmacist, and social worker.

Review Questions

1. The nurse is planning a patient teaching session on preventing urinary tract infections. Which of the following information should the nurse include in the teaching plan? **Select all that apply.**
   1. Void frequently.
   2. Drink large amounts of citrus juices.
   3. Avoid bubble baths.
   4. Wash the perineum every 8 hours.
   5. Void after sexual intercourse.
   6. Drink cranberry juice.

2. The nurse is planning care for a patient with a diagnosis of a kidney stone. Which of the following interventions would the nurse implement? **Select all that apply.**
   1. Restrict fluids.
   2. Strain all urine.
   3. Increase calcium intake.
   4. Maintain bedrest.
   5. Teach to increase fluid intake.
   6. Give analgesics as ordered.

3. The nurse is obtaining a history on a patient with a diagnosis of bladder cancer. Which of the following would the nurse expect to find in the patient's history?
1. Tobacco use
2. Vegetarian diet
3. Caffeine use
4. Alcohol use

4. While changing the pouch at the stoma site of an ileal conduit, the nurse notes the stoma is constantly spilling urine. Which of the following actions should the nurse take?
1. Notify the physician of the constant spillage.
2. Continue changing the pouch.
3. Remove the overflow of urine with a straight catheter.
4. Irrigate the stoma with a sterile solution of normal saline.

5. The nurse is contributing to the plan of care for a patient with glomerulonephritis. Which of the following interventions would the nurse recommend be included in the patient's plan of care?
1. Increase fluid intake.
2. Decrease sodium intake.
3. Increase potassium intake.
4. Decrease carbohydrate intake.

6. The nurse is caring for a postoperative patient who is receiving 0.9% normal saline intravenously at 125 mL/hour, morphine intravenously for pain control, and gentamicin (Garamycin) intravenously every 8 hours for 24 hours. The patient is allergic to iodine. Morning labs are white blood cell 8,500, hemoglobin 12.4 g/dL, and serum creatinine 2.2 mg/dL. Which of these findings is a priority for the licensed vocational nurse to report to the registered nurse?
1. White blood cell 8,500
2. Intravenous rate 125 mL/hour
3. Allergy to iodine
4. Serum creatinine 2.2 mg/dL

7. A patient with chronic kidney disease who is on hemodialysis asks for a snack in the afternoon. The patient's potassium level is 6.0 mEq/L. Which of the following foods can the nurse offer? **Select all that apply.**
1. Banana
2. Gelatin dessert
3. Clear carbonated beverage
4. Cranberry juice
5. Nectarine
6. French fries

8. The nurse is checking patency of a new right arm arteriovenous fistula. What action does the nurse use to do this? **Select all that apply.**
1. Auscultate bruit over the right arm fistula.
2. Auscultate the right brachial pulse.
3. Auscultate the right radial pulse.
4. Measure blood pressure in the right arm.
5. Palpate the right radial pulse.
6. Palpate for thrill over the right arm fistula.

9. A patient has completed a dialysis session. The nurse notes bleeding from the patient's vascular access in the left arm. Which of the following is the nurse's first action?
1. Call the physician.
2. Notify the dialysis nurse.
3. Apply pressure to access site.
4. Take patient's blood pressure.

10. A patient is to receive 1,600 mg of sevelamer (Renagel) orally with meals. Renagel 400-mg tablets are available. How many tablets should the nurse give?
Answer: _____tablets

Answer rationales available in your online resources.

ANSWERS 1. 1, 3, 5, 6; 2. 2, 5, 6; 3. 1; 4. 2; 5. 1; 6. 4; 7. 2, 3, 4; 8. 1, 6; 9. 3; 10. 4

Key Points

Find the chapter key points in your online resources available through Davis Edge.

Additional Resources

 Use the scratch off code on the inside front cover of your book to access online quizzes that will help you to improve your scores on course exams and prepare for the NCLEX-PN®.

 Study Guide

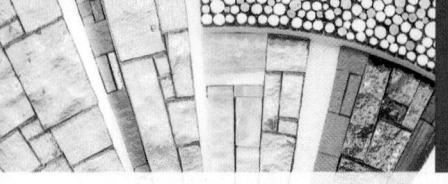
CHAPTER 38

Endocrine System Function and Assessment

Alene Homan, Paula D. Hopper, Janice L. Bradford

KEY TERMS

affect (AF-feckt)
exophthalmos (EKS-off-THAL-mus)

CHAPTER CONCEPTS

Fluid and Electrolyte Balance
Metabolism

LEARNING OUTCOMES

1. Identify the glands of the endocrine system.
2. Explain the function of each of the hormones in the endocrine system.
3. Describe the effects of aging on endocrine system function.
4. List data to collect when caring for a patient with a disorder of the endocrine system.
5. Plan nursing care for patients undergoing testing for an endocrine disorder.

NORMAL ENDOCRINE SYSTEM ANATOMY AND PHYSIOLOGY

The endocrine system consists of the endocrine (ductless) glands, which secrete hormones. Unlike other organ systems, the glands of the endocrine system are anatomically separate (Fig. 38.1). Their hormones are involved in fluid balance; metabolism, energy balance, growth, and development; contraction of smooth and cardiac muscle; glandular secretion; reproduction; and the establishment of circadian rhythms. Each hormone is secreted in response to a specific stimulus, is circulated by the blood, and affects target cells that have receptors for that hormone. Some hormones are secreted in response to hormones from other endocrine glands. Most hormone levels are regulated by negative feedback systems.

Hypothalamus and Pituitary Gland

The hypothalamus connects the nervous system to the endocrine system by way of the pituitary gland (hypophysis). The hypothalamus is above the midbrain, and the pituitary gland is suspended from the hypothalamus by a short stalk (Fig. 38.2). There are two primary lobes or portions of the pituitary gland: anterior and posterior.

Anterior Pituitary Gland

The anterior pituitary gland secretes its hormones in response to releasing hormones from the hypothalamus (Fig. 38.3).

Secretion of growth hormone (GH) is regulated by growth hormone–releasing hormone (GHRH) and by growth hormone–inhibiting hormone (GHIH, or somatostatin), both produced by the hypothalamus. GHRH is produced during hypoglycemia or when there is a high blood level of amino acids. GHIH is secreted during hyperglycemia, when carbohydrates are available for energy production and the mobilization of fat is not needed. See Figure 38.3 for the effects of GH on the body.

Thyroid-stimulating hormone (TSH) stimulates growth and secretions of the thyroid gland. TSH secretion is stimulated by thyrotropin-releasing hormone (TRH).

Adrenocorticotropic hormone (ACTH) stimulates secretion of cortisol and related hormones from the adrenal cortex. Corticotropin-releasing hormone (CRH) from the hypothalamus stimulates the release of ACTH. CRH is produced during any type of stress such as injury, disease, exercise, or hypoglycemia.

See Figure 38.3 for other hormones of the anterior pituitary gland.

Posterior Pituitary Gland

The posterior pituitary gland stores and releases antidiuretic hormone (ADH; sometimes called vasopressin) and oxytocin (Fig. 38.4). Axon tracts from the hypothalamus transmit the hormones to the posterior pituitary and signal their release.

ADH increases water reabsorption by the kidney tubules, which decreases urine output. The water is reabsorbed back into the blood, thereby maintaining normal blood volume and pressure. In cases of great fluid loss, such as severe hemorrhage, the large amount of ADH secreted is especially

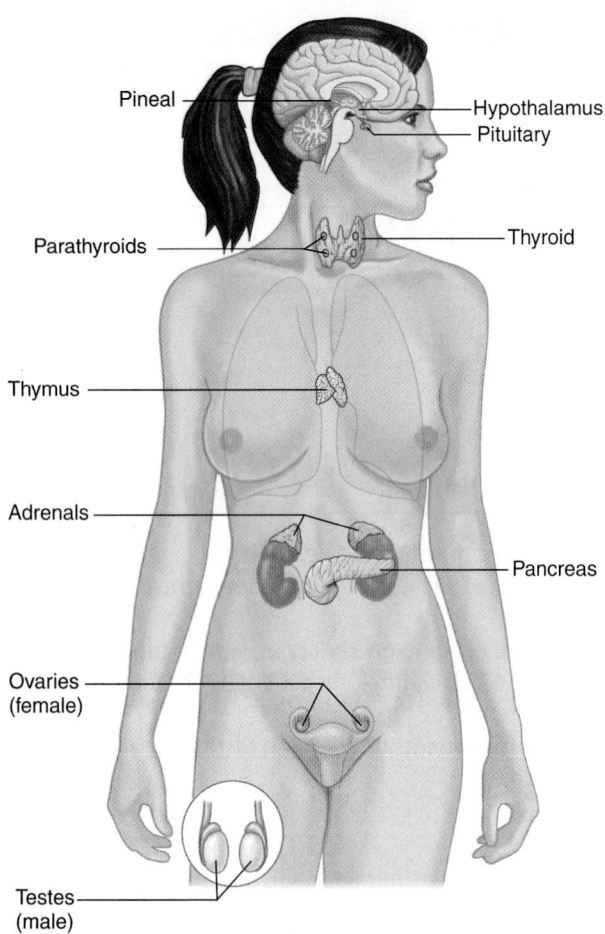

Pineal
Hypothalamus
Pituitary
Parathyroids
Thyroid
Thymus
Adrenals
Pancreas
Ovaries (female)
Testes (male)

FIGURE 38.1 Endocrine organs.

production and raise the metabolic rate. Negative feedback decreases the secretion of TRH from the hypothalamus until the metabolic rate decreases again.

The third thyroid hormone, calcitonin, targets bone tissue and is especially important during childhood when bone growth is accelerated. Resorption of calcium and phosphorous into the blood is inhibited by calcitonin so these minerals are retained in the bones. This one function of calcitonin has two important results: the maintenance of normal blood levels of calcium and phosphate, and the maintenance of a strong, stable bone matrix. The stimulus for secretion of calcitonin is hypercalcemia.

> **LEARNING TIP**
>
> Confused between resorption and reabsorption? *Resorption* breaks down bone tissue and releases calcium ions into circulation when parathyroid hormone is secreted. *Reabsorption* is the process of absorbing a substance into the blood again, such as when antidiuretic hormone causes water to be reabsorbed from the kidney tubules back into the blood supply.

> **LEARNING TIP**
>
> An easy way to remember the function of calcitonin is to remember calciTONin TONes down serum calcium.

important because it causes arteriole vasoconstriction, which increases blood pressure to homeostatic levels.

Oxytocin causes contractions of the myometrium to bring about delivery of a newborn and placenta. Release of oxytocin operates on a positive feedback loop. During breastfeeding, the subsequent release of oxytocin causes contraction of the smooth muscle cells around the mammary ducts. This release of milk is called milk ejection (or letdown).

Thyroid Gland

The thyroid gland consists of two lobes connected by a piece of tissue called the isthmus (Fig. 38.5). Three hormones are produced by the thyroid gland: triiodothyronine (T_3), thyroxine (T_4), and calcitonin.

T_3 and T_4 increase cellular respiration of glucose and fatty acids, which increases the metabolic rate—that is, energy and heat production. They are essential for normal physical growth, mental development, and reproductive maturation. Sufficient iodine intake is required for T_3 and T_4 production.

The direct stimulus for secretion of T_3 and T_4 is TSH from the anterior pituitary. A decrease in metabolic rate causes the hypothalamus to secrete TRH. TRH stimulates the anterior pituitary to secrete TSH, which stimulates the thyroid to increase secretion of T_3 and T_4. This then increases energy

Parathyroid Glands

There are usually four parathyroid glands, two on the back of each lobe of the thyroid gland (Fig. 38.6). They produce parathyroid hormone (PTH), an antagonist to calcitonin. Besides bone, the target organs of PTH are the small intestine and kidneys. The overall effect of PTH is to raise the blood calcium level and lower the blood phosphate level.

Homeostasis of blood calcium level is regulated by calcitonin and PTH (see the animation on Davis Edge). Calcium ion delivery through the blood is essential for normal excitability of neurons and muscle cells and for the process of blood clotting.

Adrenal Glands

The adrenal glands are located superior to each kidney. The inner adrenal medulla is surrounded by an outer adrenal cortex (Fig. 38.7).

Adrenal Medulla

The catecholamines (epinephrine and norepinephrine), released by the adrenal medulla, are sympathomimetic, meaning they mimic the sympathetic nervous system. During stress, the hypothalamus stimulates their release to prolong the body's stress (fight or flight) response.

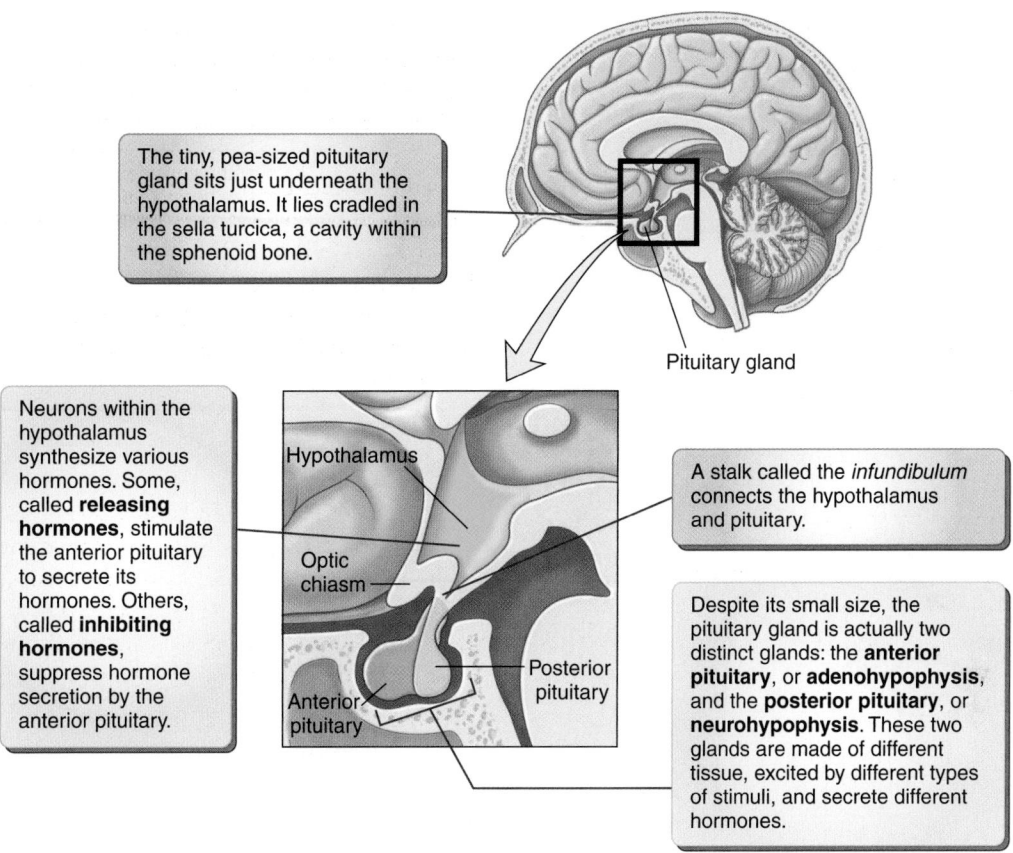

The tiny, pea-sized pituitary gland sits just underneath the hypothalamus. It lies cradled in the sella turcica, a cavity within the sphenoid bone.

Pituitary gland

Neurons within the hypothalamus synthesize various hormones. Some, called **releasing hormones**, stimulate the anterior pituitary to secrete its hormones. Others, called **inhibiting hormones**, suppress hormone secretion by the anterior pituitary.

Hypothalamus

Optic chiasm

Anterior pituitary

Posterior pituitary

A stalk called the *infundibulum* connects the hypothalamus and pituitary.

Despite its small size, the pituitary gland is actually two distinct glands: the **anterior pituitary**, or **adenohypophysis**, and the **posterior pituitary**, or **neurohypophysis**. These two glands are made of different tissue, excited by different types of stimuli, and secrete different hormones.

FIGURE 38.2 Pituitary gland and hypothalamus.

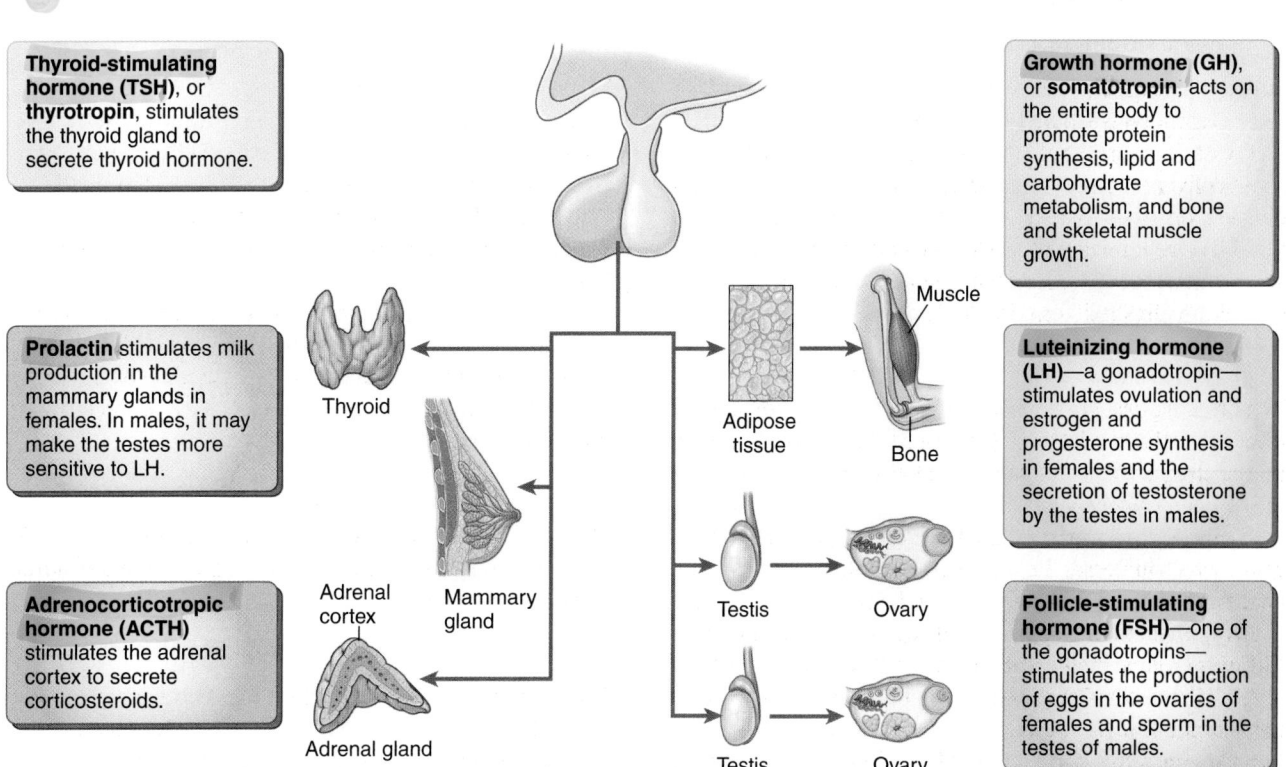

Thyroid-stimulating hormone (TSH), or **thyrotropin**, stimulates the thyroid gland to secrete thyroid hormone.

Prolactin stimulates milk production in the mammary glands in females. In males, it may make the testes more sensitive to LH.

Adrenocorticotropic hormone (ACTH) stimulates the adrenal cortex to secrete corticosteroids.

Growth hormone (GH), or **somatotropin**, acts on the entire body to promote protein synthesis, lipid and carbohydrate metabolism, and bone and skeletal muscle growth.

Luteinizing hormone (LH)—a gonadotropin—stimulates ovulation and estrogen and progesterone synthesis in females and the secretion of testosterone by the testes in males.

Follicle-stimulating hormone (FSH)—one of the gonadotropins—stimulates the production of eggs in the ovaries of females and sperm in the testes of males.

Thyroid

Mammary gland

Adrenal cortex

Adrenal gland

Adipose tissue

Muscle

Bone

Testis

Ovary

Testis

Ovary

FIGURE 38.3 Hormones of anterior pituitary.

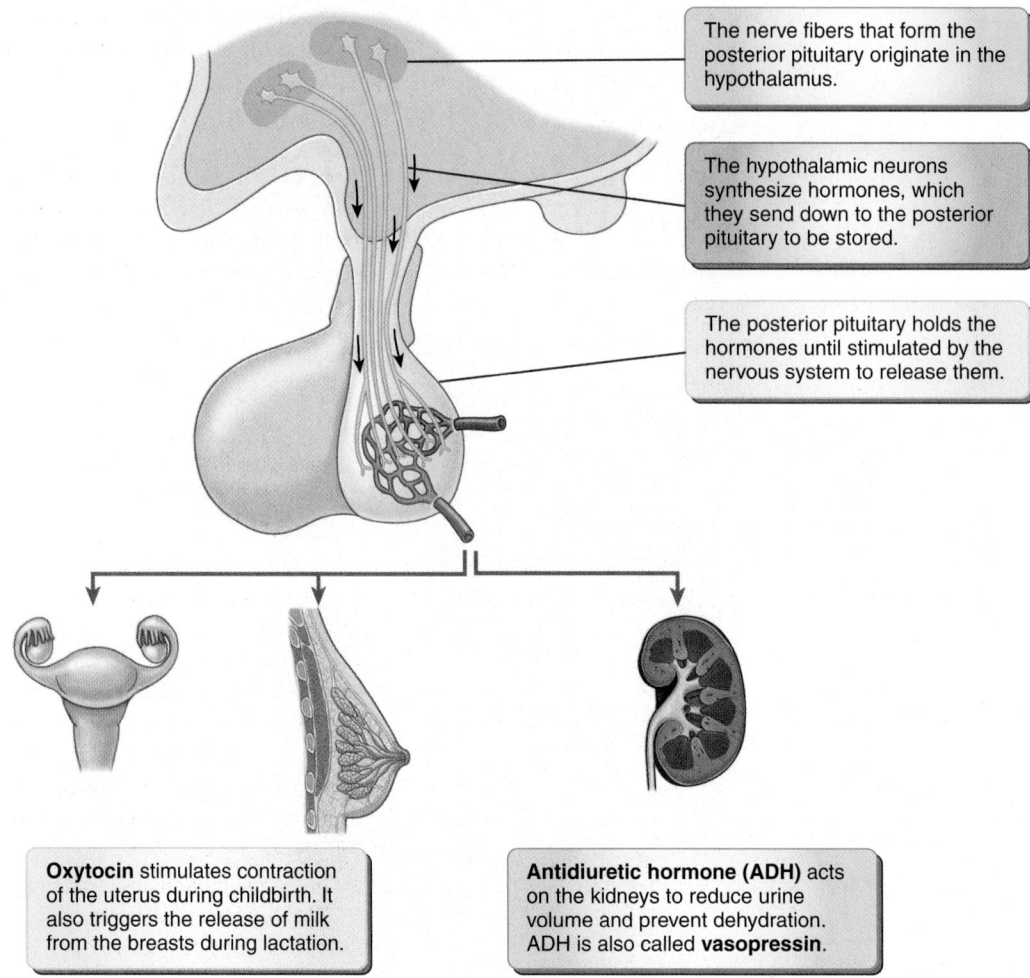

The nerve fibers that form the posterior pituitary originate in the hypothalamus.

The hypothalamic neurons synthesize hormones, which they send down to the posterior pituitary to be stored.

The posterior pituitary holds the hormones until stimulated by the nervous system to release them.

Oxytocin stimulates contraction of the uterus during childbirth. It also triggers the release of milk from the breasts during lactation.

Antidiuretic hormone (ADH) acts on the kidneys to reduce urine volume and prevent dehydration. ADH is also called **vasopressin**.

FIGURE 38.4 Posterior pituitary and hormones.

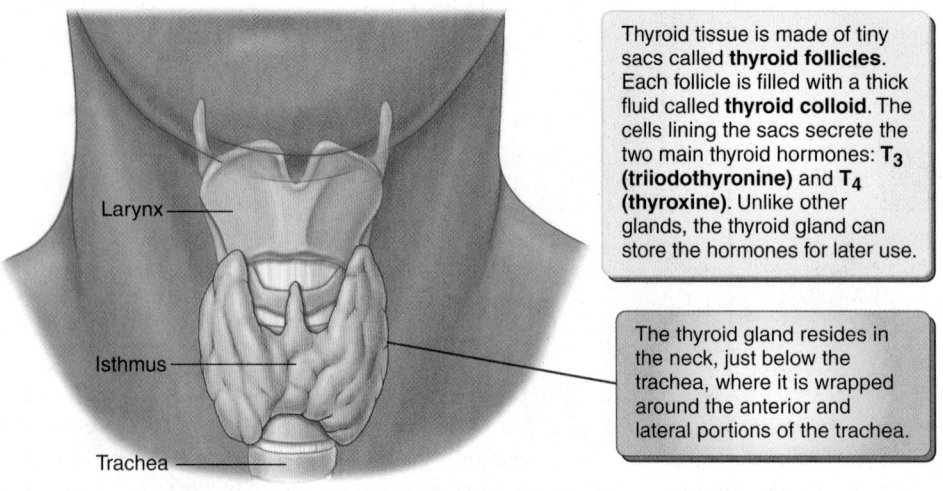

Larynx

Isthmus

Trachea

Thyroid tissue is made of tiny sacs called **thyroid follicles**. Each follicle is filled with a thick fluid called **thyroid colloid**. The cells lining the sacs secrete the two main thyroid hormones: T_3 **(triiodothyronine)** and T_4 **(thyroxine)**. Unlike other glands, the thyroid gland can store the hormones for later use.

The thyroid gland resides in the neck, just below the trachea, where it is wrapped around the anterior and lateral portions of the trachea.

FIGURE 38.5 Thyroid.

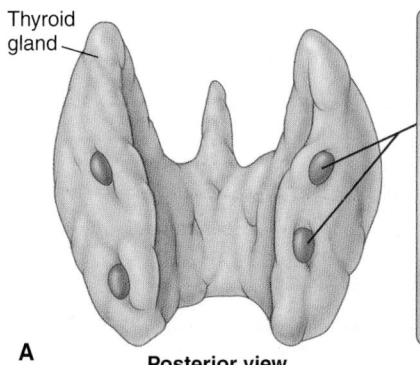

Thyroid gland

The parathyroid glands are embedded in the posterior corners of the lobes of the thyroid. Most people have four parathyroid glands, but the number of glands, as well as their locations, can vary.

A   **Posterior view**

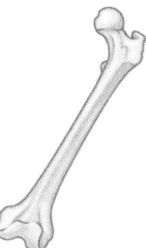

PTH inhibits new bone formation while stimulating the breakdown of old bone, causing calcium (and phosphate) to move out of bone and into the blood.

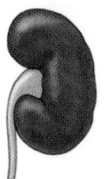

PTH encourages the kidneys to reabsorb calcium—blocking its excretion into the urine—while promoting the secretion of phosphate. PTH also prompts the kidneys to activate vitamin D, necessary for intestinal absorption of calcium.

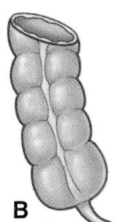

After its activation by the kidneys, vitamin D allows the intestines to absorb calcium from food; the calcium is transported through intestinal cells and into the blood.

B

FIGURE 38.6 (A) Parathyroid. (B) Effectors/targets of parathyroid hormone.

Adrenal Cortex

The adrenal cortex secretes three types of steroid hormones: mineralocorticoids, glucocorticoids, and gonadocorticoids ("sex steroids").

Aldosterone is the most abundant of the mineralocorticoids, and its target organs are the kidneys. Aldosterone increases the reabsorption of sodium ions and the excretion of potassium ions by the kidney tubules. As sodium ions are reabsorbed, hydrogen ions may be excreted in exchange. This is one mechanism to prevent the accumulation of hydrogen ions, which would lead to acidosis. Also, as sodium ions are reabsorbed, water follows; this is important for maintaining normal blood volume and blood pressure.

Cortisol is the most abundant of the glucocorticoids and has many target tissues. It stimulates gluconeogenesis in the liver and increases lipolysis and protein catabolism for energy production. By providing energy sources to body tissues, cortisol ensures that glucose will be available for the brain (glucose-sparing effect).

Cortisol release is increased during response to stress. The hypothalamus causes secretion of ACTH by the anterior pituitary, which increases cortisol secretion by the adrenal cortex. The resultant increase in energy availability is necessary for stress-induced changes. Cortisol also has an anti-inflammatory effect. However, excess cortisol decreases the immune response and can delay healing of damaged tissue.

The gonadocorticoids are small amounts of male androgens. In females, they are converted to estrogens. They are the only source of estrogen after menopause. In both genders, they contribute to libido (sexual desire).

Pancreas

The pancreas is both an exocrine and endocrine gland. As an endocrine gland, the pancreas secretes insulin and glucagon for blood glucose homeostasis. It also secretes somatostatin, which inhibits both insulin and glucagon (Fig. 38.8).

Hypoglycemia stimulates alpha cells to release glucagon. Glucagon raises blood glucose, making it available to cells.

Hyperglycemia stimulates beta cells to release insulin. Insulin increases the movement of glucose from the blood into cells. This lowers blood glucose and makes glucose available to cells for energy.

Hyperglycemia occurs after meals, especially those high in carbohydrates. Insulin and glucagon function as antagonists; normal secretion of both hormones ensures a blood glucose level that varies within normal limits (Fig. 38.9). Table 38.1 reviews endocrine hormone function.

Aging and the Endocrine System

Most of the endocrine glands decrease secretion with age, but normal aging usually does not lead to serious hormone deficiencies or illness (Fig. 38.10). Unless specific pathological conditions develop, the endocrine system continues to function adequately in old age.

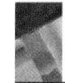 **NURSING ASSESSMENT OF THE ENDOCRINE SYSTEM**

Health History

When performing a health history, a number of questions can be asked to determine whether an endocrine problem exists. Often, however, you might be aware of a history of an endocrine disorder, such as diabetes or hypothyroidism. When a disorder exists or is suspected, you can do more focused data collection. Assessment of individual disorders is provided in Chapters 39 and 40. Table 38.2 offers general questions that can help you identify new problem areas. If the data reveal abnormalities, they should be reported to the registered nurse or health care provider (HCP).

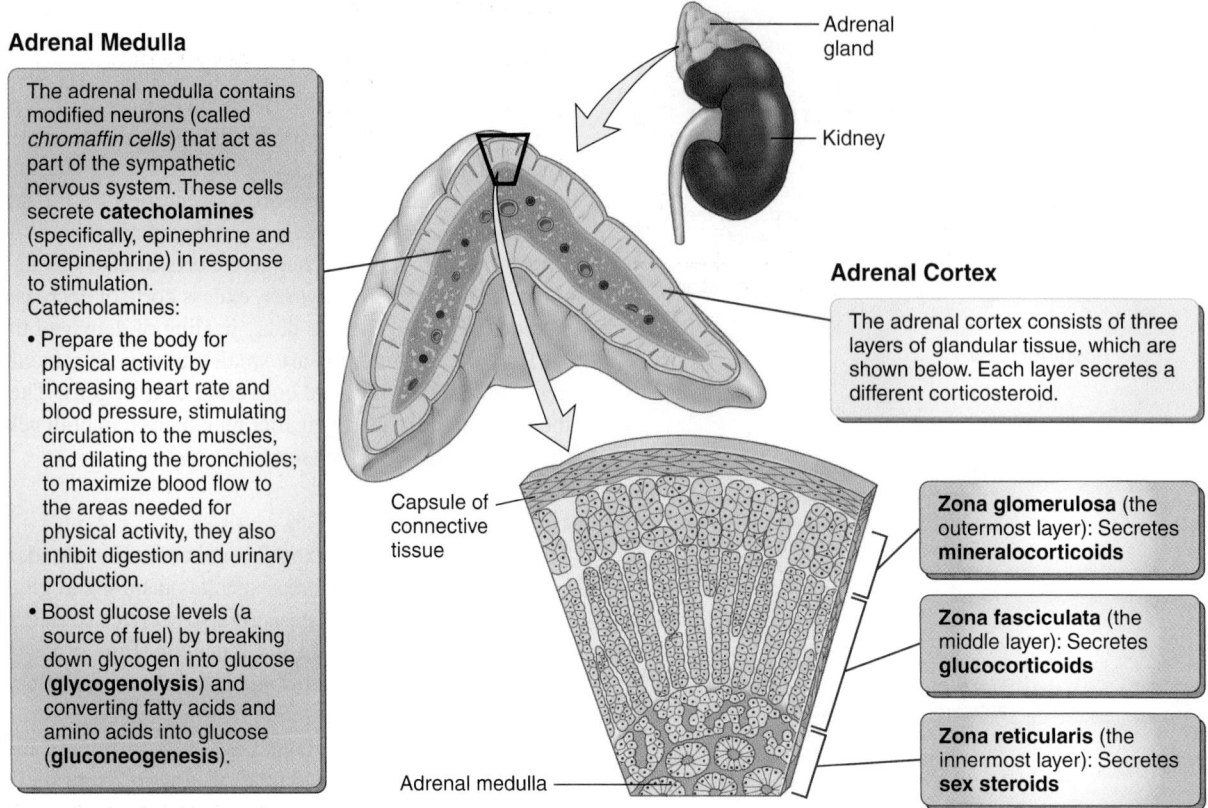

Adrenal Medulla

The adrenal medulla contains modified neurons (called *chromaffin cells*) that act as part of the sympathetic nervous system. These cells secrete **catecholamines** (specifically, epinephrine and norepinephrine) in response to stimulation.
Catecholamines:

• Prepare the body for physical activity by increasing heart rate and blood pressure, stimulating circulation to the muscles, and dilating the bronchioles; to maximize blood flow to the areas needed for physical activity, they also inhibit digestion and urinary production.

• Boost glucose levels (a source of fuel) by breaking down glycogen into glucose (**glycogenolysis**) and converting fatty acids and amino acids into glucose (**gluconeogenesis**).

Adrenal gland

Kidney

Adrenal Cortex

The adrenal cortex consists of three layers of glandular tissue, which are shown below. Each layer secretes a different corticosteroid.

Capsule of connective tissue

Zona glomerulosa (the outermost layer): Secretes **mineralocorticoids**

Zona fasciculata (the middle layer): Secretes **glucocorticoids**

Zona reticularis (the innermost layer): Secretes **sex steroids**

Adrenal medulla

FIGURE 38.7 Adrenal gland.

Physical Examination

The physical examination starts with height, weight, and vital signs. Compare findings with the patient's baseline assessment if available. Table 38.3 includes common endocrine-related causes of physical examination abnormalities.

Inspection

Observe the patient for mood and **affect** (emotional tone) throughout the physical assessment. Inspect the neck for thyroid enlargement. Look for eyes that bulge (**exophthalmos**). Note posture, body fat, and presence of tremor. Observe skin and hair texture and moisture. Note the presence of a moon-like face or "buffalo hump" on the upper back. Observe the lower extremities for skin and color changes that might indicate circulatory impairment. See Table 38.3 for the rationales for these observations.

Palpation

The thyroid gland is the only palpable endocrine gland. The licensed practical nurse/licensed vocational nurse may assist an HCP to palpate the thyroid gland. The practitioner stands behind or in front of the seated patient and palpates the gland while the patient swallows a sip of water. You can assist with positioning the patient, providing water, and instructing the patient to take a sip of water and hold it in his or her mouth until told to swallow. The thyroid gland should never be palpated in a patient with uncontrolled hyperthyroidism because this can stimulate secretion of additional thyroid hormone.

Palpate all peripheral pulses. The posterior tibial and dorsalis pedis pulses may be diminished in patients with circulatory impairment. Palpate skin turgor by gently pinching a small piece of skin. The sternum is a good place to check. If a "tent" of skin remains in place, the patient may be dehydrated as a result of water loss, as in ADH deficiency.

Auscultation and Percussion

Auscultation and percussion are not usually part of an endocrine assessment.

 DIAGNOSTIC TESTS FOR THE ENDOCRINE SYSTEM

Hormone Tests

Serum Hormone Levels

Many hormones can be measured from a simple blood specimen. This is useful in diagnosing hypofunctioning or hyperfunctioning gland states. See Table 38.4 for some commonly measured hormones.

• WORD • BUILDING •

exophthalmos: exo—outward + ophthalmos—relating to the eye

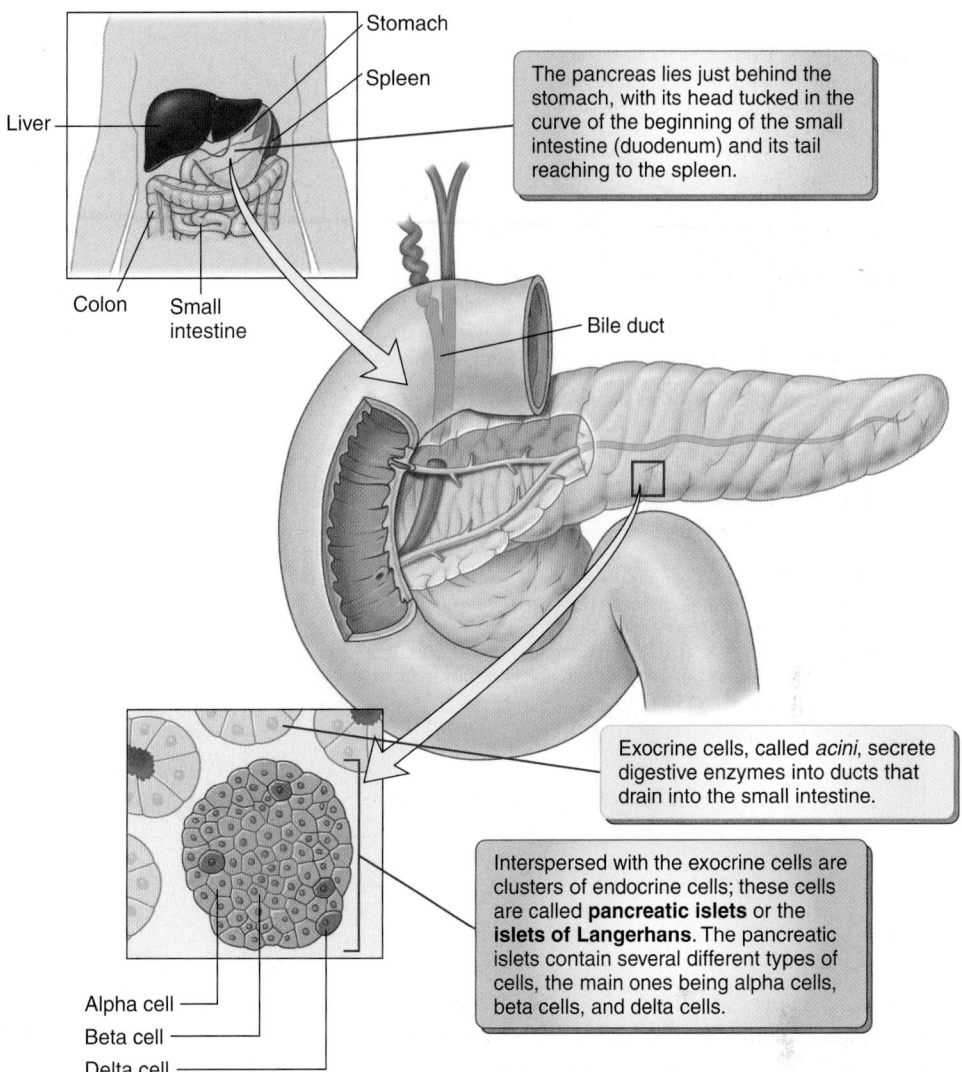

Stomach

Spleen

Liver

The pancreas lies just behind the stomach, with its head tucked in the curve of the beginning of the small intestine (duodenum) and its tail reaching to the spleen.

Colon

Small intestine

Bile duct

Exocrine cells, called *acini*, secrete digestive enzymes into ducts that drain into the small intestine.

Interspersed with the exocrine cells are clusters of endocrine cells; these cells are called **pancreatic islets** or the **islets of Langerhans**. The pancreatic islets contain several different types of cells, the main ones being alpha cells, beta cells, and delta cells.

Alpha cell

Beta cell

Delta cell

FIGURE 38.8 Pancreas.

Stimulation Tests

Stimulation tests may also help determine endocrine gland function. For this type of test, a substance is injected to stimulate a gland. The hormone secreted by that gland is then measured in the blood to determine how well it responded to the stimulation. For example, in a TRH stimulation test, TRH is injected. If the pituitary gland responds appropriately, TSH is secreted. If the thyroid gland responds appropriately to TSH, T_3 and T_4 levels rise. Failure of TRH to stimulate TSH and thyroid hormone indicates a pituitary or thyroid condition. Further studies might be done to determine the cause.

Suppression Tests

Suppression tests are the opposite of stimulating tests. For this type of test, a substance is injected that is expected to suppress a hormone's release. For example, if dexamethasone (a steroid hormone) is injected, cortisol release from the adrenal cortex is expected to be suppressed via a negative feedback mechanism. If the cortisol level is not suppressed, adrenal cortex dysfunction is suspected.

CRITICAL THINKING

Ms. Hackworth is tired all the time. The nurse practitioner orders a thyroid-stimulating hormone level drawn. The result is higher than normal.

1. You make the call to have Ms. Hackworth come in to the clinic for further evaluation. She asks, "If my thyroid level is high, then why am I so tired?" How should you respond?
2. After further testing, the nurse practitioner places Ms. Hackworth on levothyroxine (Synthroid) 50 mcg daily. Her pharmacist supplies Synthroid 0.05 mg. Is her dose correct?

Suggested answers are at the end of the chapter.

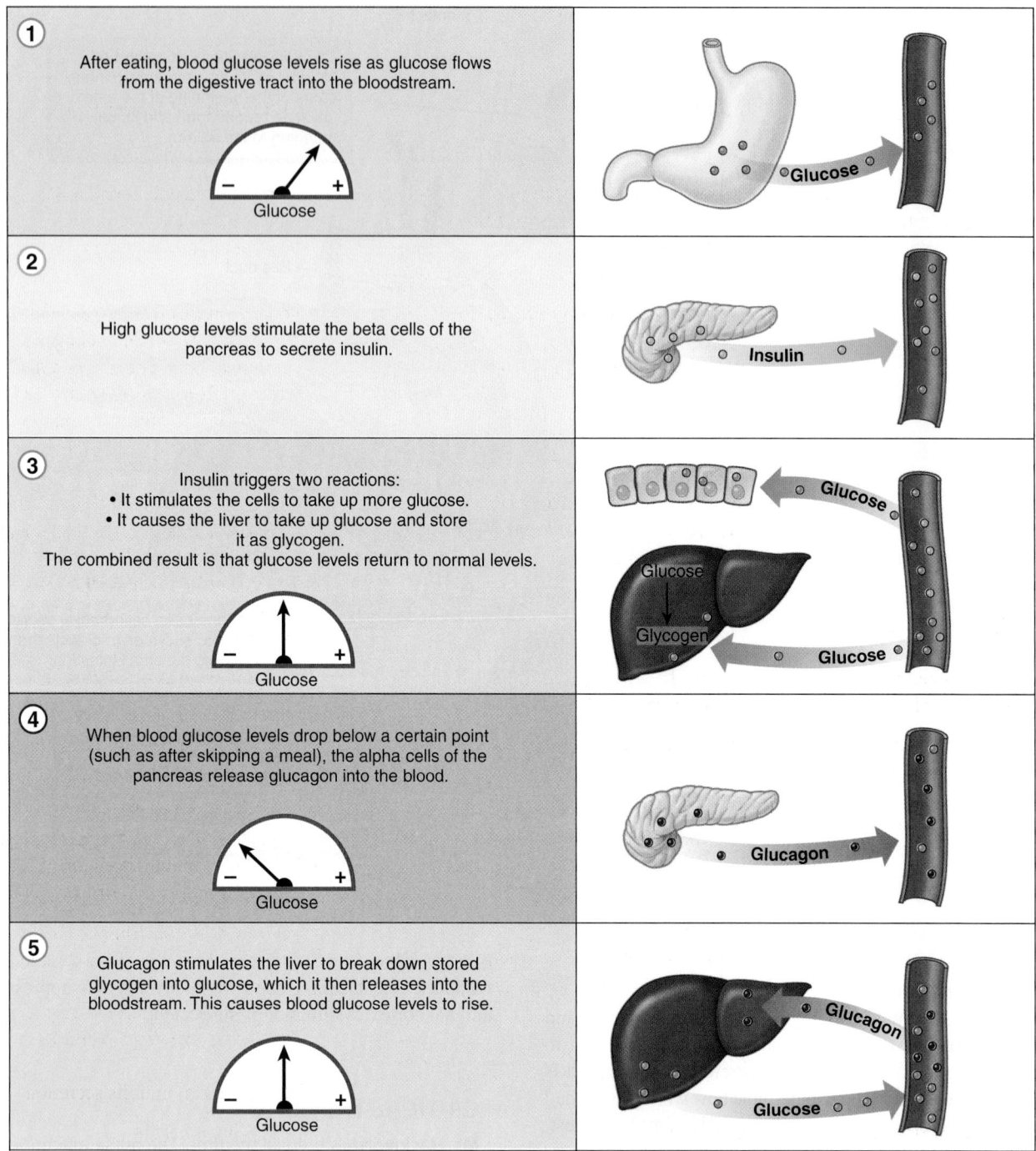

FIGURE 38.9 Regulation of blood glucose.

Urine Tests

Sometimes it is helpful to measure the amount of hormone or hormone by-product excreted in the urine during a 24-hour period. One example is the urine test for cortisol. It can help diagnose Cushing syndrome and Addison disease. See Davis Edge for the procedure for collecting a 24-hour urine specimen.

Other Laboratory Tests

Some laboratory tests may indirectly reflect the function of an endocrine gland. For example, a serum calcium level helps indicate PTH or calcitonin secretion, and a blood glucose level reflects insulin secretion.

Nuclear Scanning
Thyroid Scan

A thyroid scan may be done to determine the presence of tumors or nodules. For this test, a radioactive material is given orally or by injection. The material is taken up by the thyroid gland. After a specified time, the thyroid gland is scanned with a scintillation camera. The scan will show hot spots

Table 38.1

Review of Endocrine Function

Hormone	Function(s)	Regulation of Secretion
Hormones of the Posterior Pituitary Gland		
Antidiuretic hormone (ADH, or vasopressin)	Increases water reabsorption by the kidney tubules (water returns to the blood) Decreases sweating Causes vasoconstriction (in large amounts)	Decreased water content in the body stimulates secretion Alcohol inhibits secretion
Oxytocin	Promotes contraction of myometrium of uterus (during labor) Promotes release of milk from mammary glands	Nerve impulses from hypothalamus, the result of stretching of cervix or stimulation of nipple Secretion from placenta at the end of gestation—stimulus unknown
Hormones of the Anterior Pituitary Gland		
Growth hormone (GH)	Increases rate of mitosis Increases amino acid transport into cells Increases rate of protein synthesis Increases use of fats for energy	Growth hormone–releasing hormone (GHRH; hypothalamus) stimulates secretion Growth hormone–inhibiting hormone (GHIH, or somatostatin; hypothalamus) inhibits secretion
Thyroid-stimulating hormone (TSH)	Increases secretion of triiodothyronine (T_3) and thyroxine (T_4) by thyroid gland	Thyrotropin-releasing hormone (TRH; hypothalamus)
Adrenocorticotropic hormone (ACTH)	Increases secretion of cortisol by the adrenal cortex	Corticotropin-releasing hormone (CRH; hypothalamus)
Prolactin	Stimulates milk production by the mammary glands	Prolactin-releasing hormone (PRH; hypothalamus) stimulates secretion Prolactin-inhibiting hormone (PIH; hypothalamus) inhibits secretion
Follicle-stimulating hormone (FSH)	*In women:* Initiates growth of ova in ovarian follicles Increases secretion of estrogen by follicle cells *In men:* Initiates sperm production in the testes	Gonadotropin-releasing hormone (GnRH; hypothalamus) stimulates secretion Inhibin (ovaries) inhibits secretion GnRH (hypothalamus) stimulates secretion Inhibin (testes) inhibits secretion
Luteinizing hormone (LH)	*In women:* Causes ovulation Causes the ruptured ovarian follicle to become the corpus luteum Increases secretion of progesterone by the corpus luteum *In men:* Increases secretion of testosterone by the interstitial cells of the testes	GnRH (hypothalamus) GnRH (hypothalamus)

Continued

Table 38.1

Review of Endocrine Function—cont'd

Hormone	Function(s)	Regulation of Secretion
Hormones of the Thyroid Gland		
Thyroxine and triiodothyronine (T_4 and T_3) Calcitonin	Increase energy production from all food types Increase rate of protein synthesis Decrease the reabsorption of calcium and phosphate from bones to blood	TSH (anterior pituitary) Hypercalcemia
Hormones of the Parathyroid Glands		
Parathyroid hormone (PTH)	Increases the reabsorption of calcium and phosphate from bone to blood Increases absorption of calcium and phosphate by the small intestine Increases the reabsorption of calcium and the excretion of phosphate by the kidneys; activates vitamin D	Hypocalcemia stimulates secretion Hypercalcemia inhibits secretion
Hormones of the Adrenal Medulla		
Epinephrine, norepinephrine	Increases heart rate and force of contraction Dilates bronchioles Decreases peristalsis Increases conversion of glycogen in glucose in the liver Causes vasodilation in skeletal muscles Causes vasoconstriction in skin and viscera Increases use of fats for energy Increases the rate of cell respiration	Sympathetic impulses from the hypothalamus in stress situations
Hormones of the Intestine (Incretins)		
Glucagon-like peptide (GLP-1) Gastric inhibitory polypeptide (GIP)	Regulate blood sugar by increasing insulin secretion and decreasing glucagon secretion from the pancreas	Food ingestion
Hormones of the Pancreas		
Glucagon (alpha cells)	Increases conversion of glycogen to glucose in the liver Increases the use of excess amino acids and fats for energy	Hypoglycemia
Insulin (beta cells)	Increases glucose transport into cells and the use of glucose for energy production Increases the conversion of excess glucose to glycogen in the liver and muscles Increases amino acid and fatty acid transport into cells, and their use in synthesis reactions	Hyperglycemia
Somatostatin (delta cells)	Decreases secretion of insulin and glucagon Slows absorption of nutrients	Rising levels of insulin and glucagon

Table 38.1

Review of Endocrine Function—cont'd

Hormone	Function(s)	Regulation of Secretion
Hormones of the Adrenal Cortex		
Aldosterone	Increases reabsorption of Na$^+$ (sodium) ions by the kidneys to the blood Increases excretion of K$^+$ (potassium) ions by the kidneys in urine	Low blood Na+ level Low blood volume or blood pressure High blood K+ level
Cortisol	Increases use of fats and excess amino acids for energy Decreases use of glucose for energy (except for the brain) Increases conversion of glucose to glycogen in the liver Anti-inflammatory effect: stabilizes lysosomes and blocks the effects of histamine	ACTH (anterior pituitary) during physiological stress

Source: Adapted from Scanlon, V. C., & Sanders, T. (2019). *Essentials of anatomy and physiology* (8th ed.). Philadelphia, PA: F.A. Davis.

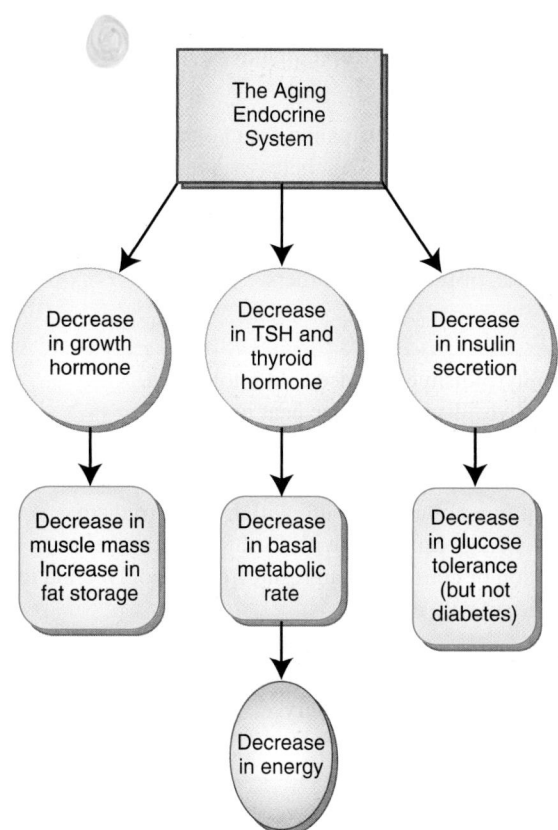

FIGURE 38.10 Effects of aging on the endocrine system.

(nodules), which are not malignant, or cold spots (areas that do not take up the radioactivity), which indicate malignancy. Cold spots can then be biopsied to confirm a diagnosis. Because such a small amount of radioactive material is used, the risk to the patient is minimal. The patient should be aware that the test takes approximately 30 minutes to complete. See Appendix A for nursing care pre- and postprocedure.

Radioactive Iodine Uptake

A radioactive iodine uptake test is similar to a thyroid scan and is done to evaluate thyroid function. Several scans are taken over a 24-hour period after administration of radioactive iodine. The amount of iodine taken up by the thyroid indicates the activity of the gland. This is especially helpful in diagnosing hyperthyroidism.

PET Scan

Positron emission tomography (PET) scanning is another type of scan that can be done to differentiate between benign and malignant endocrine tumors. PET scans are helpful because they can show metabolic changes in organs or tissues.

Radiographic Tests

A computed tomography (CT) scan or magnetic resonance imaging (MRI) may be done to locate a tumor or identify hypertrophy of a gland.

Ultrasound

Ultrasound may be done of the thyroid or parathyroid glands to determine whether they are enlarged or to find masses.

Biopsy

Biopsy is done to obtain tissue to examine for possible cancerous cells. The thyroid gland can be biopsied either by needle aspiration under local anesthesia or using a surgical incision.

Table 38.2

Subjective Data Collection for the Endocrine System

Questions to Ask During the Health History	Rationale
Neuromuscular	
Have you noticed muscle spasms or twitching?	These symptoms may be associated with syndrome of inappropriate antidiuretic hormone (SIADH) secretion or calcium depletion resulting from hypoparathyroidism.
Do you have numbness, tingling, or pain in your feet, legs, or hands?	These can be associated with neuropathy resulting from diabetes mellitus. Numbness and tingling can also indicate hypocalcemia related to hypoparathyroidism.
Nutrition/Fluid Balance	
Have you gained or lost weight without trying?	Actual weight gain may be associated with hypothyroidism. Weight gain due to water retention may result from Cushing syndrome or SIADH. Weight loss may result from uncontrolled diabetes or hyperthyroidism. Weight loss due to dehydration may be related to Addison disease.
Have you noticed excessive thirst or urination?	Excessive thirst and urination are classic symptoms of diabetes mellitus and diabetes insipidus.
Have you noticed a change in your energy level?	Lack of energy may be associated with uncontrolled diabetes, hypothyroidism, hyperthyroidism, Addison disease, or pituitary disorders.
Metabolic	
Do you generally tolerate changes in environmental temperature?	Hypothyroidism can cause cold intolerance. Hyperthyroidism can cause heat intolerance.
Mood/Memory	
Have you noticed a change in your mood or memory?	Mental function may be dull with hypothyroidism. Mood swings can occur with Cushing syndrome. Agitation or confusion can result from hypoglycemia in a person with diabetes.
Family History	
Does anyone in your family have a thyroid problem, diabetes, or another endocrine disorder?	Some disorders are hereditary.

Table 38.3

Endocrine-Related Causes of Abnormal Physical Examination Findings

Abnormal Examination Finding	*Possible Causes*
Mood	
Depressed mood or affect	Hypothyroidism
Nervousness	Hyperthyroidism, pheochromocytoma
Agitation	Low blood glucose level
Nutrition/Fluid Balance	
Weight gain	Decreased metabolic rate in hypothyroidism, fluid excess
Weight loss	Increased metabolic rate in hyperthyroidism; uncontrolled diabetes, dehydration
Poor skin turgor	Dehydration due to water loss in Addison disease, diabetes mellitus, diabetes insipidus
Integumentary	
Hyperpigmentation of skin	Addison disease
Dry, scaly skin	Hypothyroidism
Dusky lower extremities with weak peripheral pulses	Circulatory changes in diabetes mellitus
Vital Signs	
Change in pulse rate or temperature	Elevated due to increased metabolic rate in hyperthyroidism Decreased due to slowed metabolic rate in hypothyroidism
Elevated blood pressure	Increased catecholamine release in pheochromocytoma or fluid retention in Cushing syndrome
Decreased blood pressure	Sodium and water loss in Addison disease
Neuromuscular	
Tremor	Hyperthyroidism, hypoglycemia, or pheochromocytoma
Head and Neck	
Exophthalmos (bulging eyes)	Fat deposits and edema behind the eyes in Graves disease
Fat pads on neck and shoulders ("buffalo hump"), round "moon" face	Accumulation of fat in Cushing syndrome
Enlarged thyroid gland	Excessive stimulation by thyroid-stimulating hormone in hypothyroidism or hyperthyroidism

Table 38.4

Common Endocrine-Related Laboratory Tests

Test	Normal Values*	Significance of Abnormal Findings
Thyroid Tests		
Thyroid-stimulating hormone	0.4–4.2 microinternational units/mL	↑ in primary hypothyroidism ↓ in primary hyperthyroidism
Triiodothyronine (T_3), total	70–204 ng/dL	↓ in hypothyroidism ↑ in hyperthyroidism
Triiodothyronine (T_3), free	260–480 pg/dL	
Thyroxine (T_4), total	*Male:* 4.6–10.5 mcg/dL *Female:* 5.5–11 mcg/dL	↓ in hypothyroidism ↑ in hyperthyroidism
Thyroxine (T_4), free	0.8–1.5 ng/dL	
Parathyroid Tests		
Parathyroid hormone	8–24 pg/mL	↑ in primary hyperparathyroidism ↓ in primary hypoparathyroidism, parathyroid trauma during thyroid surgery
Calcium, blood	8.2–10.2 mg/100 mL *Over age 90:* 8.2–9.6 mg/dL	↑ in some cancers, hyperparathyroidism ↓ in hypothyroidism
Phosphorus	2.5–4.5 mg/dL	↑ in hypoparathyroidism ↓ in hyperparathyroidism
Pituitary Tests		
Growth hormone	*Male:* 0–5 ng/mL *Female:* 0–10 ng/mL	↑ in acromegaly ↓ in small stature
Antidiuretic hormone (vasopressin)	0–4.7 pg/mL	↑ in syndrome of inappropriate antidiuretic hormone (SIADH) secretion ↓ in diabetes insipidus
Urine specific gravity	1.001–1.029	↓ in diabetes insipidus
Adrenocorticotropic hormone (ACTH)	9–52 pg/mL in a.m. *Women on oral contraceptives:* 5–29 pg/mL	↑ in Addison disease ↓ in Cushing syndrome, long-term corticosteroid therapy
Adrenal Tests		
Aldosterone	*Supine:* 3–16 ng/dL *Upright:* 7–30 ng/dL	↑ in heart failure, chronic obstructive pulmonary disease (COPD), hypovolemia ↓ in Addison disease, hypoaldosteronism
Cortisol, blood	5–25 mcg/dL at 0800 3–16 mcg/dL at 1600	↑ in Cushing syndrome, stress ↓ in Addison disease, steroid withdrawal
Cortisol, urine	3.5–45 mcg/24 hr	↑ in Cushing syndrome, stress ↓ in Addison disease, steroid withdrawal

Table 38.4

Common Endocrine-Related Laboratory Tests—cont'd

Test	Normal Values*	Significance of Abnormal Findings
Pancreas Tests		
Fasting blood glucose (FBG)	70–100 mg/dL	↑ in stress, Cushing syndrome 100–125 mg/dL = prediabetes 126 mg/dL or greater = diabetes mellitus ↓ in hypoglycemia, Addison disease
Ketones, blood and urine	Negative	Positive in acidosis, fasting or starvation, diabetic ketoacidosis
Oral glucose tolerance test	Blood glucose level less than 140 mg/dL at 2 hr	140–199 mg/dL at 2 hr = prediabetes 200 mg/dL or greater at 2 hr = diabetes mellitus
Glycosylated hemoglobin	< 5.7%	5.7%–6.4% = prediabetes 6.5% or greater = diabetes mellitus

*All normal values are for a fasting test.

SUGGESTED ANSWERS TO CRITICAL THINKING

Ms. Hackworth

1. "It's not your thyroid hormone that is high. It's your thyroid-stimulating hormone. That means your pituitary gland has to work extra hard to try to stimulate your thyroid gland."

2.
$$\frac{50 \text{ mcg}}{} \frac{1 \text{ mg}}{1,000 \text{ mcg}} = 0.05 \text{ mg}$$

Review Questions

1. Which hormones are secreted by the posterior pituitary gland? **Select all that apply.**
   1. Antidiuretic hormone
   2. Thyroid-stimulating hormone
   3. Growth hormone
   4. Luteinizing hormone
   5. Oxytocin
   6. Calcitonin

2. A patient is started on levothyroxine (Synthroid) to replace thyroxine (T_4) for a new diagnosis of hypothyroidism. What effect can the patient expect as the medication begins to work?
   1. Increased urination
   2. Improved blood sugar
   3. Lower blood pressure
   4. Increased energy

3. Which nursing action is appropriate when assisting the health care provider with palpation of the thyroid gland during a routine physical examination?
   1. Ask the patient to take a deep breath.
   2. Give the patient a sip of water.
   3. Have the patient look up toward the ceiling.
   4. Help the patient to lie back on a pillow.

4. The nurse is doing an admission assessment on a new resident to a long-term care facility. The patient's face and shoulders seem to have a lot of fat, but the patient's arms and legs are thin. Which of the patient's routine medications might be involved?
   1. Prednisone (Deltasone, a glucocorticoid)
   2. Calcitonin
   3. Insulin
   4. Thyroid hormone (levothyroxine/Synthroid)

5. When explaining a thyroid scan to a patient, which of the following statements is correct?
   1. "You will take a special pill, and then an ultrasound will be taken of your neck."
   2. "You will receive an injection of radioactive material, and then a special camera will take pictures of your thyroid gland."
   3. "You will be placed into a special machine, and x-rays will be taken of your neck. It may be noisy."
   4. "You will be given a special drink, and then magnetic energy is used to visualize the thyroid area."

Answer rationales available in your online resources

ANSWERS 1. 1; 5; 2. 4; 3. 2; 4. 1; 5. 2

Key Points

Find the chapter key points in your online resources available through Davis Edge.

Additional Resources

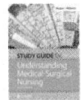 Study Guide

CHAPTER 39

Nursing Care of Patients With Endocrine Disorders

Alene Homan and Paula D. Hopper

KEY TERMS

amenorrhea (ay-MEN-uh-REE-ah)
ectopic (ek-TOP-ik)
euthyroid (yoo-THIGH-royd)
goitrogenic (GOY-troh-JEN-ik)
goitrogens (GOY-troh-jenz)
hyperplasia (HY-per-PLAY-zee-ah)
hypophysectomy (HY-pah-fi-SEK-tuh-mee)
myxedema (MIK-suh-DEE-mah)
nocturia (nok-TYOO-ree-ah)
osmolality (ahs-moh-LAL-ih-tee)
pheochromocytoma (FEE-oh-KROH-moh-sigh-TOH-mah)
polydipsia (PAH-lee-DIP-see-ah)
polyuria (PAH-lee-YOO-ree-ah)
tetany (TET-uh-nee)

CHAPTER CONCEPTS

Fluid and Electrolyte Balance
Growth and Development
Metabolism
Nutrition

LEARNING OUTCOMES

1. Identify disorders caused by variations in the hormones of the pituitary, thyroid, parathyroid, and adrenal glands.
2. Explain the pathophysiology of each of the endocrine disorders presented.
3. Describe the etiologies, signs, and symptoms of each of the endocrine disorders.
4. Describe current therapeutic measures used for each of the selected endocrine disorders.
5. List data to collect when caring for patients with each of the endocrine disorders discussed.
6. Plan nursing care for patients with each of the disorders.
7. Explain how you will know if nursing interventions have been effective.

The endocrine system is subject to a variety of disorders. Although the causes vary, the pathophysiology usually involves either too little or too much hormone activity. Insufficient hormone activity may be the result of hypofunction of an endocrine gland or insensitivity of the target tissue to its hormone. Excessive hormone activity may be the result of a hyperactive gland, **ectopic** hormone production, or self-administration of too much replacement hormone (Table 39.1). If you remember the function of each hormone in the body, understanding the problems involved with an altered amount of each hormone becomes easier.

Most endocrine disorders are either primary or secondary. A primary disorder is a problem within the gland that is out of balance. Secondary disorders are caused by problems outside the gland, such as an imbalance in a tropic hormone, certain drugs, trauma, surgery, or a problem in the feedback mechanism. For example, if the thyroid gland is diseased and causing hypothyroidism, it would be considered a primary problem. Sometimes hypothyroidism is caused by a lack of thyroid-stimulating hormone from the pituitary gland, even though the thyroid gland is healthy. This would be considered a secondary problem.

> **LEARNING TIP**
> Most symptoms of hormone hyperactivity are the opposite of the symptoms of that same hormone's hypoactivity.

Table 39.1
Causes of Endocrine Problems

Insufficient hormone activity	Gland hypofunction
	Lack of tropic or stimulating hormone
	Target tissue insensitivity to hormone
Excess hormone activity	Gland hyperfunction
	Excess tropic or stimulating hormone
	Ectopic hormone production
	Self-administration of too much replacement hormone

 PITUITARY DISORDERS

Pituitary disorders often involve several hormone imbalances at once. They are caused by general hypopituitarism or hyperpituitarism. Problems involving all of the pituitary hormones at once, however, are rare. For simplicity, imbalances are considered separately here.

Disorders Related to Antidiuretic Hormone Imbalance

Antidiuretic hormone (ADH; also called arginine vasopressin [AVP]) is synthesized in the hypothalamus and stored and secreted by the posterior pituitary gland. Recall that ADH is responsible for reabsorption of water by the distal tubules and collecting ducts in the kidneys. A decrease in ADH activity results in diabetes insipidus (DI). An increase in ADH activity is called syndrome of inappropriate antidiuretic hormone (SIADH). Table 39.2 compares DI and SIADH. Note how symptoms of too little ADH (water loss) are the opposite of symptoms of too much ADH (water retention).

Diabetes Insipidus
PATHOPHYSIOLOGY. It is important to understand that DI is unrelated to diabetes mellitus. Diabetes mellitus is caused by insulin-resistant tissue or insufficient insulin production. DI is caused by a deficiency of ADH. If ADH is lacking, adequate reabsorption of water is prevented, leading to diuresis. Patients can urinate from 3 to 15 L per day. This leads to dehydration and increased serum **osmolality** (concentrated blood). The increased osmolality and decreased blood pressure normally trigger ADH secretion, which causes water retention and dilutes the blood; in patients with DI, this does not happen. Increased osmolality also leads to extreme thirst, which usually causes the patient to drink enough fluids to maintain fluid balance. In an unconscious patient or a patient with a defective thirst mechanism, however, dehydration can quickly occur if the problem is not recognized and corrected.

ETIOLOGY. DI has a variety of causes. Tumors, trauma, or other problems in the hypothalamus or pituitary gland can lead to decreased production or release of ADH. Surgery in the area of the pituitary and certain drugs, such as glucocorticoids or alcohol, can also cause DI.

SIGNS AND SYMPTOMS. The patient with DI urinates frequently (**polyuria**), and night time urination (**nocturia**) is present. This results in high serum osmolality and low urine osmolality. Urine specific gravity is decreased, making the urine dilute and light in color.

The patient experiences extreme thirst (**polydipsia**), and consumes large volumes of water. Often patients crave ice-cold water. If urine output exceeds fluid intake, dehydration occurs, with characteristic symptoms of hypotension, poor skin turgor, and weakness. Hypovolemic shock occurs if fluid balance is not restored. Dehydration and electrolyte imbalances result in a decrease in level of consciousness and death if the problem is not corrected.

DIAGNOSTIC TESTS. Diagnosis is based initially on a history of risk factors and reported symptoms. Urine specific gravity will be less than 1.005 (normal: 1.005 to 1.03) and can be monitored by laboratory tests or by using reagent strips at the bedside. Plasma and urine osmolality are measured and compared with each other. Serum sodium level appears to be high. The actual amount of sodium in the blood may be normal, but it appears elevated in relation to the decreased amount of water. Computed tomography (CT) scanning or magnetic resonance imaging (MRI) is used to determine whether a pituitary tumor is present.

A water-deprivation test may be done. For this test, the patient is deprived of water for up to 6 hours. Body weight and urine osmolality are tested hourly. If the urine continues to be diluted, even though the patient is not drinking and is losing weight as a result of volume depletion, DI is suspected.

ADH levels can be measured in plasma or urine after administration of hypertonic saline or fluid restriction. The normal response would be elevated ADH; if it is not elevated, DI is suspected. The urine glucose level may also be checked to rule out diabetes mellitus.

THERAPEUTIC MEASURES. Hypotonic intravenous (IV) fluids such as 0.45% saline solution may be ordered to replace intravascular volume without adding extra sodium. IV fluids are especially important if the patient is unable to take oral fluids.

Medical treatment of DI involves replacement of ADH. In acute cases, vasopressin, a synthetic form of ADH, is given via the IV or subcutaneous route, along with IV fluid replacement. In patients who require long-term therapy, synthetic ADH (desmopressin, or DDAVP) can be administered orally, subcutaneously, or intranasally. Thiazide diuretics may decrease urine flow in the absence of ADH (even though they

· **WORD · BUILDING** ·
polyuria: poly—much + uria—urine
nocturia: noct—night + uria—urine
polydipsia: poly—much + dipsia—thirst

Table 39.2

Antidiuretic Hormone Disorders Summary

	Insufficient Antidiuretic Hormone	*Excess Antidiuretic Hormone*
Disorder	Diabetes insipidus	Syndrome of inappropriate antidiuretic hormone
Signs and Symptoms	Polyuria, polydipsia, dehydration, dilute urine	Fluid retention, weight gain, concentrated urine
Diagnostic Tests	Urine specific gravity, urine and plasma osmolality, water deprivation test	Serum and urine sodium and osmolality, water load test
Therapeutic Measures	Synthetic antidiuretic hormone replacement	Treat cause
Priority Nursing Diagnoses	*Deficient Fluid Volume*	*Excess Fluid Volume*

usually are used to increase urine output). If a pituitary tumor is involved, treatment usually involves removal of the pituitary gland (**hypophysectomy**).

NURSING PROCESS FOR THE PATIENT WITH DIABETES INSIPIDUS.

Data Collection. When collecting data for a patient with DI, pay special attention to fluid balance. Daily weights are the most reliable method for monitoring the amount of fluid that is being lost. Taking accurate intake and output (I&O) measurements is also helpful. Skin turgor will be poor, and mucous membranes will be dry and sticky if the patient is becoming dehydrated. Monitor skin integrity because dehydration increases risk of breakdown. Monitor vital signs for signs of shock. Use a reagent strip (dipstick) or urinometer to measure urine specific gravities. Monitor serum electrolytes and osmolality as ordered, and watch for changes in level of consciousness. Assess the patient's understanding of his or her disease and treatment. Once treatment is initiated, continue to monitor fluid balance, being especially alert to signs of fluid overload.

> **LEARNING TIP**
>
> Remember from Chapter 6 that "a pint's (about) a pound the world around." If your patient has gained 4 pounds, that is 4 pints or a half gallon of extra water!

Nursing Diagnoses, Planning, and Implementation.

Deficient Fluid Volume related to failure of regulatory mechanisms

EXPECTED OUTCOME: The patient's fluid balance will be maintained as evidenced by urine specific gravity between 1.005 and 1.03, skin turgor within normal limits, and stable daily weight.

- Monitor daily weight, I&O, vital signs, and urine specific gravity. *Decreased weight, output greater than intake,*

low blood pressure, elevated pulse rate, and high urine specific gravity can all indicate fluid deficit.
- Monitor patient for restlessness or weakness. *These can indicate significant fluid deficit with electrolyte imbalance.*
- Provide free access to oral fluids. If the patient's thirst mechanism is not intact, give the patient fluids every hour. *Oral fluids are essential to replace the excess lost in diuresis.*
- Report a significant drop in blood pressure and an increase in pulse rate to the registered nurse (RN) or health care provider (HCP) *as these may be signs of hypovolemic shock.*
- Encourage the patient to participate in maintaining I&O records, monitoring weight, and checking urine specific gravity, if able. *This involves the patient and helps prepare him or her for self-monitoring at home.*
- Teach the patient to monitor daily weights at home; losses or gains of greater than 2 pounds in a day should be reported to the HCP. *Weight loss or gain can indicate fluid imbalance and the need for a change in medication regimen.*
- Advise the patient to wear identification, such as a medical alert bracelet, that identifies the disorder. *Faster treatment can be initiated if emergency personnel are aware of a DI diagnosis.*

Evaluation. If treatment has been effective, signs of dehydration will be absent, and weight and vital signs will be stable.

Syndrome of Inappropriate Antidiuretic Hormone

PATHOPHYSIOLOGY. SIADH results from too much ADH in the body. This causes excess water to be reabsorbed by the kidney tubules and collecting ducts and back into the blood, leading to decreased urine output and fluid overload. As fluid builds up in the bloodstream, osmolality decreases, and the blood becomes diluted. Normally, decreased serum osmolality inhibits release of ADH. In SIADH, however, ADH continues to be released, adding to the fluid overload.

ETIOLOGY. Causes of SIADH can be categorized into four groups: nervous system disorders such as head trauma and meningitis, cancers such as lung and brain cancer (some tumors actually secrete an ADH-like substance), pulmonary diseases such as cystic fibrosis and chronic obstructive pulmonary disease (COPD), and medications such as antipsychotics and histamines. Whatever the cause of SIADH is, the result is increased secretion of ADH, which results in fluid overload.

SIGNS AND SYMPTOMS. Symptoms of SIADH include symptoms of fluid overload, such as weight gain (usually without edema) and dilutional hyponatremia (Box 39.1). The actual amount of sodium in the blood may be normal, but it appears to be low because of the diluting effect of the extra fluid. Serum osmolality is less than 275 mOsm/kg. The urine is concentrated because water is not being excreted. Electrolyte imbalance can cause muscle cramps and weakness. Because the osmolality of the blood is low, fluid can leak out of the vessels and cause brain swelling. If untreated, this results in lethargy, confusion, seizures, coma, and death.

DIAGNOSTIC TESTS. Serum sodium and osmolality are low, and urine sodium and osmolality are high. Serum ADH is high. Additional testing may be done to diagnose the cause.

THERAPEUTIC MEASURES. Treatment is aimed at the underlying cause. If a tumor is secreting ADH, surgical removal may be indicated. Symptoms can be alleviated by restricting fluids to 800 to 1000 mL per 24 hours. Hypertonic saline fluids may be administered via IV, and an oral sodium tablet may be prescribed to maintain the serum sodium level. A loop diuretic such as furosemide (Lasix) increases water excretion. A vasopressin receptor antagonist such as conivaptan (Vaprisol) may be used to block the action of ADH in the kidney.

NURSING PROCESS FOR THE PATIENT WITH SIADH.
Data Collection. Excess fluid volume with hyponatremia is the primary concern for the patient with SIADH. To monitor fluid balance, assess vital signs, daily weight, I&O, urine specific gravity, and skin turgor. Edema and pulmonary crackles are not typically present. Determine the patient's ability to maintain a fluid restriction. Assess level of consciousness and neuromuscular function. Monitor laboratory tests, including serum sodium level, as ordered by the HCP. Assess the patient's understanding of the disease process and treatment.

Box 39.1

Manifestations of Dilutional Hyponatremia

• Bounding pulse
• Elevated or normal blood pressure
• Muscle weakness
• Headache
• Personality changes
• Nausea
• Diarrhea
• Convulsions
• Coma

Nursing Diagnoses, Planning, and Implementation.

Excess Fluid Volume related to compromised regulatory mechanism

EXPECTED OUTCOME: The patient's fluid balance will be maintained as evidenced by weight, I&O, and serum sodium within normal limits.

• Monitor daily weight, I&O, vital signs, and laboratory values. *Increased weight, intake greater than output, elevated blood pressure, bounding pulse, crackles, and low serum sodium may all indicate fluid overload.*
• Maintain fluid restriction as ordered *to reduce serum dilution and normalize serum sodium.*
• Offer hard candy *to reduce sensation of thirst.*
• Provide ice chips (count as half the volume of fluid; that is, 100 mL of ice chips equals approximately 50 mL of water). *Ice chips take longer to consume than water and may be more satisfying to some patients.*
• Provide calibrated cups *to help the patient maintain the restriction independently if able.*
• Allow the patient to participate in planning the types and times of fluid intake. *Fluid restrictions are not pleasant for patients; patients who feel in control may be more likely to comply with restriction.*
• Report a change in level of consciousness immediately, and monitor the patient for seizures. *These are signs of serious fluid imbalance.*
• Instruct the patient to report any weight gain greater than 2 pounds in 1 day, a change in urine output, or acute thirst. *These are signs of fluid overload or risk for overload.*
• Encourage use of a medical alert bracelet or other identification *so emergency personnel will be aware of SIADH if needed.*

Evaluation. Weight should stabilize at the pre-illness level once treatment is begun. Serum sodium level should be within normal limits.

CRITICAL THINKING

Mrs. Jackson is a 78-year-old woman who has just returned to your unit after hip surgery. During the next 2 days, you notice that her weight increases from 118 to 124 pounds and that she seems lethargic, but the nurse's report didn't indicate any concerns. You check her ankles and sacrum for edema but find none. In the afternoon, her son rushes out of the room and tells you she is becoming confused, adding that this is not like her at all.

1. What assessment should you do?
2. What do you suspect?
3. What should be your next steps?
4. Based on her weight gain, about how much water is Mrs. Jackson retaining?

Suggested answers are at the end of the chapter.

Disorders Related to Growth Hormone Imbalance

Growth hormone (GH), also called *somatotropin*, is responsible for normal growth of bones, cartilage, and soft tissue. GH is synthesized and secreted by the anterior pituitary gland. An excess or deficiency of GH may be related to a more generalized problem with the pituitary gland or hypothalamus. A deficit of GH results in short stature if not corrected in childhood, and a variety of problems in adulthood. Excess GH results in gigantism (Fig. 39.1) or acromegaly.

Growth Hormone Deficiency

PATHOPHYSIOLOGY. When GH is deficient in childhood, a condition called short stature occurs. In the past, this was referred to as dwarfism (see Fig. 39.1). A deficiency of GH in adults does not affect growth, but in recent years GH has been found to have important functions even during adulthood.

ETIOLOGY. GH deficiency may be due to tumors, surgery, heredity, or trauma to the pituitary gland or hypothalamus. It may also be deficient in some cases of neglect or severe emotional stress. Malnutrition is the most common cause worldwide. Sometimes the cause is not known ("Cultural Considerations: Ellis–van Creveld Syndrome").

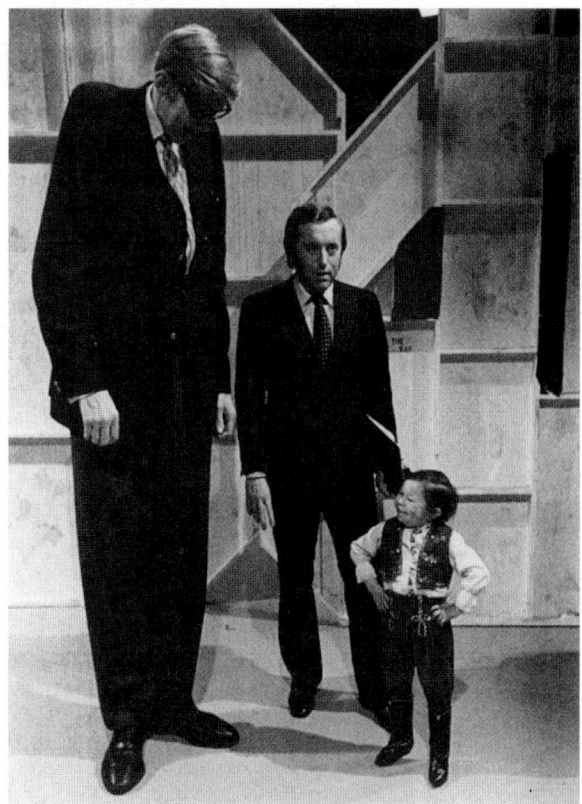

FIGURE 39.1 Gigantism and dwarfism.

Cultural Considerations

Ellis–van Creveld Syndrome. Ellis–van Creveld syndrome is prevalent among the Amish communities of Lancaster County, Pennsylvania. This inherited type of dwarfism is characterized by short stature and an extra digit on each hand, with some affected people having a congenital heart defect and nervous system involvement resulting in a degree of mental disability.

SIGNS AND SYMPTOMS. Children may grow to only 3 to 4 feet in height but have normal body proportions. Sexual maturation may be slowed, related to involvement of additional pituitary hormones. Short stature in children is sometimes accompanied by mental retardation.

In adults, symptoms of GH deficiency include fatigue, weakness, excess body fat, decreased muscle and bone mass, sexual dysfunction, high cholesterol, and increased risk for cardiovascular and cerebrovascular disease. Headaches, mental slowness, and psychological disturbances may also occur. All of these signs and symptoms can lead to decreased quality of life.

DIAGNOSTIC TESTS. GH levels in the blood can be measured by a routine laboratory test, but the results may be unreliable because GH is not evenly secreted over the course of a day. A more reliable test is a GH stimulation test that measures GH in response to induced hypoglycemia. An MRI scan can help determine the presence of a tumor; radiographic studies may be used to determine bone age. Genetic testing may also be done.

THERAPEUTIC MEASURES. Treatment of GH deficiency is administration of GH. In the past, GH was derived from human pituitary glands, so treatment was expensive and risky. Now GH, or somatropin (Humatrope), can be made in a laboratory using recombinant DNA technology, so it is more readily available to those who need it. It is administered by subcutaneous injection. Surgery may be indicated if a tumor is the cause.

NURSING PROCESS FOR THE PATIENT WITH GROWTH HORMONE DEFICIENCY.

Data Collection. Assessment of the adult with GH deficiency includes mental status, ability to cope with the effects of the disorder, and understanding of the treatment plan. Assess all patients for signs of cardiovascular disease and other complications of the disorder.

Nursing Diagnoses, Planning, and Implementation. If GH deficiency has been present since childhood, most related problems will not be new to the patient. The priority for the nurse then is to approach the patient with respect while assessing current problems that may need attention. Nursing diagnoses in the adult with GH deficiency will depend on assessed needs. These may include diagnoses such as *Ineffective Health Management, Fatigue, Deficient Knowledge, Imbalanced Nutrition: Less Than Body Requirements, Risk for Injury,* or *Risk for Spiritual Distress.*

An excellent resource for people with short stature is the Little People of America organization (www.lpaonline.org).

Ineffective Health Management related to deficient knowledge

EXPECTED OUTCOME: The patient will have necessary knowledge to be able to manage self-care as evidenced by statements and demonstration of self-care activities.

• Assess the patient's understanding of his or her disease process and treatment. *Teaching should build on baseline knowledge.*

• Explain and demonstrate self-care measures as needed to the patient, including administration of GH injections. *The patient must understand the treatment to participate in it.*

• Help the patient explore the meaning of the disorder. *Talking about the disorder may help the nurse and patient identify needs that can be addressed.*

Evaluation. Nursing care has been effective if the patient is able to demonstrate self-administration of GH and describe plans for related self-care activities.

CRITICAL THINKING

Three siblings were adopted to a loving home after having been in several foster homes. After a year in their new home, each child suddenly grew 6 to 8 inches. What do you think happened?

Suggested answers are at the end of the chapter.

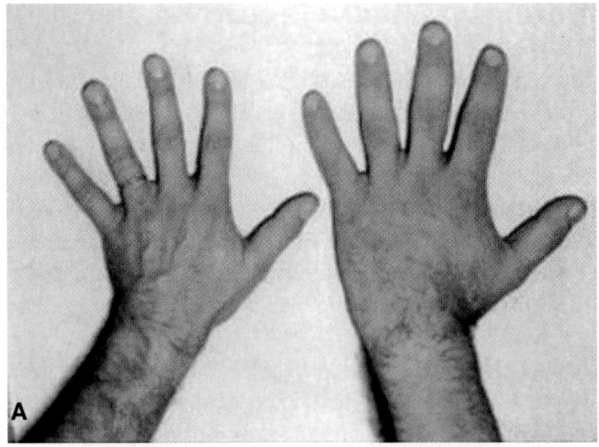
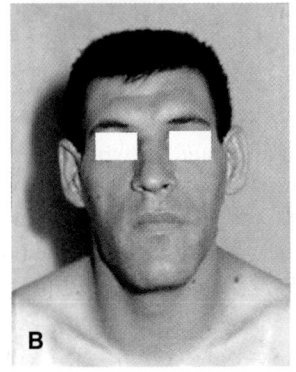
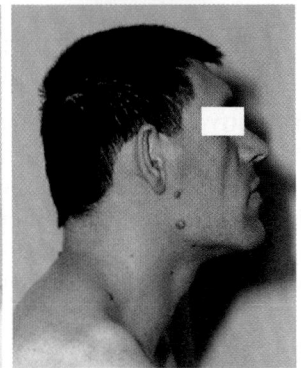

FIGURE 39.2 Patient with acromegaly. (A) Hands and (B) face.

Acromegaly

Acromegaly is a rare excess of GH that affects adults, usually in their 30s or 40s. If GH excess occurs in children, the result is gigantism.

PATHOPHYSIOLOGY. Acromegaly occurs because of overproduction of GH in an adult. Bones increase in size, leading to enlargement of facial features, hands, and feet. Long bones grow in width but not length because the epiphyseal disks are closed. Subcutaneous connective tissue increases, causing a fleshy appearance. Internal organs and glands enlarge. Impaired tolerance of carbohydrates leads to elevated blood glucose.

ETIOLOGY. Excess secretion of GH can be caused by pituitary **hyperplasia,** a benign pituitary tumor, or excess of GH-releasing hormone (GH-RH) due to hypothalamic dysfunction.

SIGNS AND SYMPTOMS. Symptoms develop very slowly, and the disorder may be present for years before it is recognized. Often the first symptom noticed is a change in ring or shoe size. The nose, jaw, brow, hands, and feet enlarge (Fig. 39.2). The teeth may be displaced, causing difficulty chewing, or dentures may no longer fit. The tongue becomes thick, causing difficulty in speaking and swallowing

(dysphagia). The patient may develop sleep apnea. Visual disturbances can occur because of tumor pressure on the optic nerve. Headaches result from tumor pressure on the brain. Diabetes mellitus may develop because GH increases blood glucose and causes an increased workload for the pancreas (see Chapter 40). With treatment, soft tissues reduce in size, but bone growth is permanent.

DIAGNOSTIC TESTS. GH levels are measured. A CT scan or an MRI is done to locate a pituitary tumor.

THERAPEUTIC MEASURES. Treatment may include medications to block GH or hypophysectomy. Radiation may be indicated if a tumor is the cause.

Pituitary Tumors

Most tumors of the pituitary gland are benign adenomas. However, even benign tumors in the brain can cause many symptoms, including visual disturbances, symptoms of increased pressure in the brain, and symptoms related to hormone imbalances, as described earlier. Treatment for pituitary tumors is usually hypophysectomy. Radiation may also be used, either alone or as an adjunct to surgery.

• WORD • BUILDING •

hyperplasia: hyper—excessive + plasia—formation or deviation

Nursing Care of the Patient Undergoing Hypophysectomy

Removal of the pituitary gland is called hypophysectomy. The procedure is most often done using minimally invasive endoscopic surgery, via the nose or a small incision just under the upper lip. This allows access through the sphenoid sinus to the pituitary gland, without disturbing brain tissue. Figure 39.3 shows the transsphenoidal approach to the gland through the upper lip. Some large tumors may need removal via transfrontal craniotomy (entry through the frontal bone of the skull).

PREOPERATIVE CARE. Make sure the patient understands the HCP's explanation of surgery. Perform and document a baseline neurologic assessment. Prepare the patient for what to expect following surgery. Explain that it will be important after surgery to avoid any actions that increase pressure on the surgical site, such as coughing, sneezing, nose blowing, straining to move bowels, or bending from the waist. Because coughing can raise intracranial pressure and is therefore contraindicated, instruct the patient in deep-breathing exercises or use of an incentive spirometer. Patients can usually expect to stay in the hospital about one day.

POSTOPERATIVE CARE. Perform routine neurologic assessments to monitor the patient for changes from the baseline assessment. Check urine for specific gravity because DI can occur following pituitary surgery. If a patient has had transsphenoidal surgery, nasal packing and a "mustache dressing" will be present. These are left in place and not removed unless ordered by the HCP. Monitor the dressing for signs of cerebrospinal fluid (CSF) leakage. CSF contains glucose, so glucose testing strips can be used to determine whether drainage is actually CSF or just nasal discharge. Remind the patient to avoid any actions that increase pressure on the surgical site. The patient is placed on hormone replacement therapy after hypophysectomy. Pituitary hormones are difficult to replace, so target hormones are generally given. These may include thyroid hormones, glucocorticoids, intranasal desmopressin, and sex hormones.

PATIENT EDUCATION. Instruct the patient before discharge according to agency guidelines. These usually include instructions to prevent increased pressure on the surgical site as well as instructions on how to administer the hormones and side effects to report. Examples include the following:

- Expect a small amount of bloody or mucous drainage from your nose.
- If you must blow your nose, do so very gently. Blowing can injure the surgical site and cause bleeding or spinal fluid leakage.
- Take stool softeners as needed to prevent straining for bowel movements.
- Take cough suppressants as directed to prevent coughing.
- If an upper lip incision was used, wait until the incision line is healed to brush teeth with a toothbrush. Floss and mouth rinses can be used instead.
- Take all medications as prescribed. You will be on lifelong hormone therapy to replace the hormones made by your pituitary gland.
- Call immediately if you develop a fever, if you have more than a small amount of blood drainage from the incision site, if you have clear drainage, if you feel very thirsty or urinate more than usual (a sign of diabetes insipidus), or if any other symptoms that concern you.

DISORDERS OF THE THYROID GLAND

Triiodothyronine (T_3) and thyroxine (T_4) are thyroid hormones secreted by the thyroid gland. These hormones may be collectively referred to as the thyroid hormone (TH). Deficient secretion of TH results in hypothyroidism; excess TH results in hyperthyroidism. For more information on disorders of the thyroid gland, visit the American Thyroid Association (www.thyroid.org).

Hypothyroidism

Hypothyroidism occurs primarily in women over 50 years old. If hypothyroidism occurs in an infant, severe problems with growth and development occur. All babies born in the United States are tested for hypothyroidism at birth.

Pathophysiology

Primary hypothyroidism occurs when the thyroid gland fails to produce enough TH even though enough thyroid-stimulating hormone (TSH) is being secreted by the pituitary gland. The pituitary gland responds to the low level of TH by producing more TSH. Secondary hypothyroidism is caused by low levels of TSH, which fail to stimulate release of TH. Tertiary hypothyroidism results from inadequate release of thyrotropin-releasing hormone (TRH), secreted by the hypothalamus. Most cases of hypothyroidism are primary (Table 39.3).

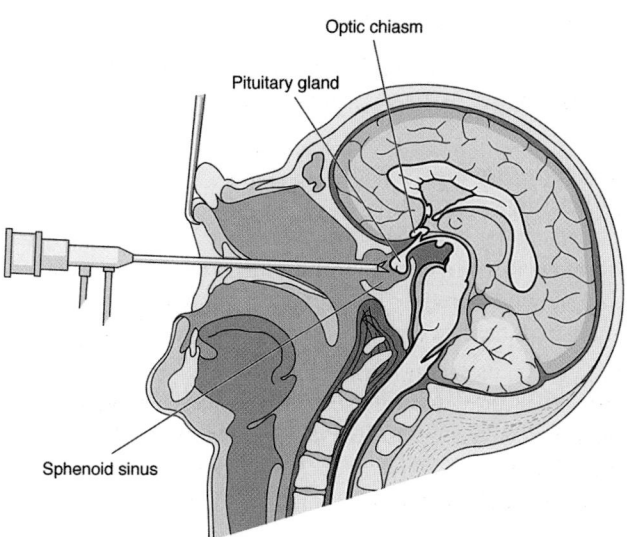

FIGURE 39.3 Transsphenoidal approach to pituitary gland for hypophysectomy.

Table 39.3

Thyroid Hormone Abnormalities

	Hyperthyroidism	Hypothyroidism
Primary	↑ thyroid hormone (TH) ↓ thyroid-stimulating hormone (TSH)	↓TH ↑TSH
Secondary (pituitary cause)	↑TH ↑TSH	↓TH ↓TSH

Because thyroid hormones are responsible for metabolism, low levels of these hormones result in a slowed metabolic rate, which causes many of the characteristic symptoms of hypothyroidism.

Etiology

Primary hypothyroidism may be a result of a congenital defect, inflammation of the thyroid gland, or iodine deficiency. Hashimoto thyroiditis, also called chronic lymphocytic thyroiditis, is an autoimmune disorder that eventually destroys thyroid tissue, leading to hypothyroidism. Secondary or tertiary hypothyroidism can be caused by a pituitary or hypothalamic lesion. Treatment of hyperthyroidism, whether with medication or thyroidectomy, can lead to secondary hypothyroidism. Peripheral resistance to TH may also occur.

Signs and Symptoms

Manifestations are related to the reduced metabolic rate and include fatigue, weight gain, bradycardia, constipation, mental dullness, feeling cold, shortness of breath, decreased sweating, and dry skin and hair (see "Patient Perspective" and Table 39.4). Heart failure may occur because of decreased pumping strength of the heart. Altered fat metabolism causes hyperlipidemia, which can lead to cardiovascular disease. In advanced disease, **myxedema** develops, which is a nonpitting edema of the face, hands, and feet.

Patient Perspective

Mary. When I turned 40-something, I began to notice a few changes in my body. I seemed to be easily fatigued, but I attributed that to moving our family across country and all the adjustments that needed to be made. I also noticed weight gain, most notably around my waist. Again, I thought, "Well, I *am* 40-something," but it seemed no matter how much I exercised and watched what I ate, I couldn't lose weight. Worse, I was gaining! One day a friend of mine pointed out that I always seemed tired. Each time she called

to do something, my reply was always the same, "I'd love to, but not today. I'm just so tired."

Things started to get worse. I began losing hair by the handfuls each time I shampooed. I began to notice dry skin (I thought it was just our hard water) and constipation (I thought I had irritable bowel syndrome). Finally, I went to the doctor for a physical, including laboratory tests, which included thyroid-stimulating hormone and free thyroxine (T_4). The diagnosis came back: I had hypothyroidism and was started on levothyroxine (Synthroid). I noticed the effect on my energy almost immediately. Now I am able to exercise effectively. I have lost nearly all the weight I gained, and my husband no longer complains about having to clean out the drain in our shower every time I wash my hair. I am thankful for the diagnosis and treatment because I feel like myself again.

Complications

If the metabolic rate drops so low that it becomes life threatening, the result is myxedema coma. This usually occurs in patients with long-standing, untreated hypothyroidism and can be triggered by stress such as infection, trauma, or exposure to cold. The patient becomes hypothermic, with a temperature less than 95°F (35°C), and has a decreased respiratory rate, depressed mental function, and lethargy. Blood glucose drops. Cardiac output drops, which in turn can reduce perfusion of kidneys. Death can occur as a result of heart or respiratory failure. If you note changes in mental status or vital signs, contact the RN or HCP immediately. Treatment of myxedema coma involves intubation and mechanical ventilation. The patient is slowly rewarmed with blankets. IV fluids and IV levothyroxine (Synthroid) are given, and the underlying cause is treated.

Diagnostic Tests

The levels of T_3 and T_4 are low, and the level of TSH may be high or low, depending on the cause. If the pituitary gland is functioning normally, TSH is elevated in an attempt to stimulate an increase in TH. Serum cholesterol and triglycerides are elevated. Antibodies are usually present in autoimmune disease.

Therapeutic Measures

Primary hypothyroidism is easily treated with oral thyroid replacement hormone. Most patients now take synthetic thyroid hormone (levothyroxine [Synthroid]). Doses are started low and slowly increased to prevent symptoms of hyperthyroidism or cardiac complications.

Nursing Process for the Patient With Hypothyroidism

See "Nursing Care Plan for the Patient With Hypothyroidism." For nursing care of the patient with constipation, refer to Chapter 34.

• WORD • BUILDING •
myxedema: myx—mucus + edema—swelling

Nursing Care Plan for the Patient With Hypothyroidism

Nursing Diagnosis: *Activity Intolerance* related to fatigue
Expected Outcomes: The patient will be able to tolerate activity as evidenced by (1) reports of lessening fatigue after treatment initiated and (2) the ability to carry out usual activities of daily living.
Evaluation of Outcomes: (1) Does patient report lessening fatigue? (2) Is patient able to carry out activities of daily living?

Intervention	Rationale	Evaluation
Assess level of fatigue.	*Assessment guides nursing care.*	What is patient's fatigue level?
Assist patient with self-care activities.	*Patients with fatigue may have difficulty carrying out activities independently.*	Are patient's self-care needs being met? Is assistance needed?
Allow for rest between activities.	*Rest periods will enable patient to conserve energy for activities.*	Does patient state rest is adequate?
Slowly increase patient's activities as medication begins to be effective.	*As thyroid replacement therapy becomes effective, patient's fatigue will lessen.*	Does patient tolerate increases in activity?

Geriatric

When getting older patients up, watch for orthostatic hypotension.	*Orthostatic hypotension is common in older adults and may cause falls.*	Does patient's blood pressure drop when changing positions?

Nursing Diagnosis: *Risk for Impaired Skin Integrity* related to dry skin, inactivity
Expected Outcome The patient's skin will remain intact as evidenced by soft moist skin without lesions
Evaluation of Outcome: Is skin soft, moist, and intact?

Intervention	Rationale	Evaluation
Assess skin daily for breakdown and risk for breakdown.	*Skin lesions are more effectively treated when identified early.*	Is breakdown present? Is patient at risk?
Use soap-free products for bathing and nondrying lotion after.	*Regular soap is drying to skin, and lotion helps trap moisture in the skin.*	Does use of soap-free products and lotion help?
Avoid daily tub baths and showers. Bathe at the sink most days.	*Full body contact with water can be drying for the skin.*	Does patient understand importance of limiting tub baths and showers?
Encourage/assist with position changes at least every 2 hours.	*Changing position enhances circulation to the skin, promoting healing and preventing breakdown.*	Does patient change position at least every 2 hours? Are pressure areas prevented?

Nursing Diagnosis: *Imbalanced Nutrition: More Than Body Requirements* related to decreased metabolic rate
Expected Outcomes: (1) Nutrition will be balanced as evidenced by return to patient's pre-illness weight. (2) The patient will verbalize understanding of dietary recommendations.
Evaluation of Outcomes: (1) Is the patient approaching pre-illness weight? (2) Is the patient able to explain dietary recommendations and a plan for implementation?

Intervention	Rationale	Evaluation
Weigh weekly and record.	*Weekly weights record progress without the frustration of daily fluctuations.*	Is patient approaching ideal weight?
Consult dietitian for therapeutic diet until hypothyroidism is controlled.	*The dietitian can provide food choices for gradual weight loss if necessary.*	Does patient verbalize understanding of and ability to follow diet?

Geriatric

Allow patient to help determine acceptable diet modifications.	*Older patients may have long-standing dietary habits that are hard to change.*	Is patient satisfied with weight loss plan?

Table 39.4

Symptoms of Thyroid Disorders

Hypothyroidism	*Hyperthyroidism*
Cardiovascular	
Bradycardia, decreased cardiac output, cool skin, cold intolerance	Tachycardia, palpitations, increased cardiac output, warm skin, heat intolerance
Neurologic	
Lethargy, slowed movements, memory loss, confusion	Fatigue, restlessness, hyperactive reflexes, tremor, insomnia, emotional instability
Pulmonary	
Dyspnea, hypoventilation	Dyspnea
Integumentary	
Cool, dry skin; brittle, dry hair	Diaphoresis; warm, moist skin; fine, soft hair
Gastrointestinal	
Decreased appetite, weight gain, constipation, increased serum lipid levels	Increased appetite, weight loss, frequent stools, decreased serum lipid levels
Skeletal	
Increased bone density but poor bone quality and increased fracture risk	Reduced bone density, increased fracture risk
Reproductive	
Decreased libido, erectile dysfunction	Decreased libido, erectile dysfunction, amenorrhea

CRITICAL THINKING

Mrs. Maino is a 59-year-old woman who is tired all the time and has gained 16 pounds during the past year. Laboratory results show low triiodothyronine (T$_3$) and thyroxine (T$_4$) and elevated thyroid-stimulating hormone (TSH) levels. Her health care provider prescribes levothyroxine by mouth (PO).

1. Why is Mrs. Maino's TSH elevated?
2. What will happen to Mrs. Maino's caloric requirements as she begins treatment? Why?
3. The nurse asks you to teach Mrs. Maino to check her pulse. Why is this important?
4. Which team members are important to involve in Mrs. Maino's care?

   Suggested answers are at the end of the chapter.

Patient Education

Instruct the patient in the importance of consistent use of thyroid replacement medication and regular blood tests to monitor TSH. The patient needs to be aware that too much TH will cause symptoms of hyperthyroidism. Such symptoms should be reported to the HCP immediately. In addition, if the patient is experiencing mental status changes, discuss the need to avoid driving or operating machinery until symptoms are resolved.

Hyperthyroidism

Hyperthyroidism is most often diagnosed in women. Graves disease, which is one cause of hyperthyroidism, is more common in young women. Multinodular goiter, another cause, is more common in older women.

Pathophysiology

Hyperthyroidism results in excessive amounts of circulating TH (thyrotoxicosis). Primary hyperthyroidism occurs when a problem within the thyroid gland causes excess hormone release. Secondary hyperthyroidism occurs because of excess TSH release from the pituitary gland, causing overstimulation of the thyroid gland. Tertiary hyperthyroidism is caused by excess TRH from the hypothalamus. A high level of TH increases the metabolic rate. It also increases the number of beta-adrenergic receptor sites in the body, which enhances the activity of epinephrine and norepinephrine. The resulting fight-or-flight response is the cause of many of the symptoms of hyperthyroidism.

Etiology

A variety of disorders can cause hyperthyroidism. Graves disease is the most common cause. It is an autoimmune disorder in which thyroid-stimulating antibodies cause the thyroid gland to make too much TH.

Other causes include thyroid nodules that secrete excess TH (multinodular goiter and toxic adenoma), inflammation of the thyroid (thyroiditis), or a thyroid tumor. A pituitary tumor can secrete excess TSH, which overstimulates the thyroid gland. Patients taking TH for hypothyroidism may take too much. Each of these problems can cause excess circulating TH and symptoms of hyperthyroidism.

Heredity can also play a role in autoimmune hyperthyroidism. Women who smoke nearly double their risk of Graves disease.

Signs and Symptoms

Many signs and symptoms are related to the hypermetabolic state, such as heat intolerance, increased appetite with weight loss, and increased frequency of bowel movements. Nervousness, tremor, tachycardia, and palpitations are caused by the increase in sympathetic nervous system activity and may be more common in younger patients. Heart failure can occur because of tachycardia and the resulting inefficient pumping of the heart. See additional signs and symptoms in Table 39.4.

If treatment is not begun, the patient can become manic or psychotic. Additional signs that occur only with Graves disease include thickening of the skin on the anterior legs and exophthalmos (bulging of the eyes; Fig. 39.4) caused by swelling of the tissues behind the eyes. Other eye changes include photophobia and blurred or double vision.

Older adult patients may not have the typical signs and symptoms of hyperthyroidism, so be especially alert for this. These patients may present with heart failure, atrial fibrillation, fatigue, apathy, and depression.

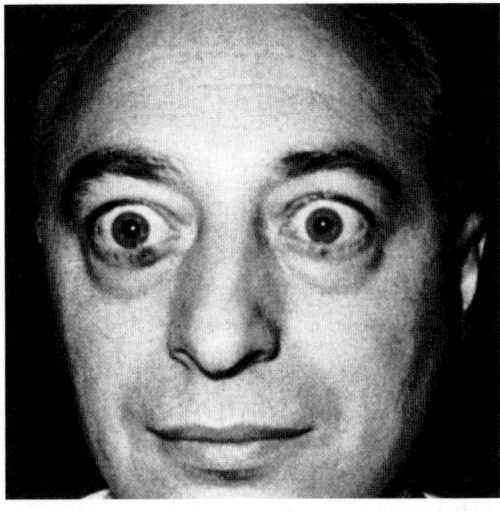

FIGURE 39.4 Exophthalmos caused by Graves disease.

Complications

THYROTOXIC CRISIS. Thyrotoxic crisis (sometimes called thyroid storm) is a severe hyperthyroid state that can occur in hyperthyroid people who are untreated or who develop another illness or stressor. It also may occur after thyroid surgery in patients who have been inadequately prepared with antithyroid medication. Thyrotoxic crisis can result in death in as little as 2 hours if untreated. Symptoms include tachycardia, high fever, extreme hypertension (with eventual heart failure and hypotension), dehydration, restlessness, delirium, or coma.

If thyrotoxic crisis occurs, treatment is first directed toward relieving the life-threatening symptoms. Acetaminophen is given for the fever. Aspirin is avoided because it binds with the same serum protein as T_4, freeing additional T_4 into the circulation. IV fluids and a cooling blanket may be ordered to cool the patient. A beta-adrenergic blocker such as propranolol is given for tachycardia and symptom control. Oxygen is administered, and the head of the bed is elevated because the high metabolic rate requires more oxygen. Once symptoms are controlled and the patient is safe, the underlying thyroid problem is treated.

HYPOTHYROIDISM. Another complication of hyperthyroidism can be hypothyroidism. This can occur as a result of long-term disease or as a result of treatment. Patients with a history of hyperthyroidism should be monitored for recurrent hyperthyroidism or the onset of hypothyroidism.

Diagnostic Tests

Serum levels of T_3 and T_4 are elevated. TSH is low in primary hyperthyroidism or high if the cause is pituitary. A radioactive iodine uptake test or a thyroid scan can be done to determine hyperactivity of the gland or to locate a nodule or tumor. The thyroid gland may be enlarged; palpation of the thyroid in a patient suspected to have hyperthyroidism should only be performed by a HCP. Thyroid-stimulating immunoglobulin is present in Graves disease.

Therapeutic Measures

Methimazole (Tapazole) inhibits the synthesis of TH, but it may take several months to be effective and must be continued for 12 to 18 months. Beta blockers relieve sympathetic nervous system symptoms. Calcium and vitamin D are given to protect bones.

Radioactive iodine (^{131}I, or RAI) may be used to destroy a portion of the thyroid gland. The patient takes one oral dose of RAI. Dietary iodine normally goes to the thyroid gland, where it is used to make TH. When RAI is given, the radioactivity destroys some of the cells that make TH.

Sometimes medications or RAI alone can control hyperthyroidism. If this does not occur, surgery is planned. Prior to surgery, antithyroid medications are prescribed to calm the thyroid. They help slow the heart rate and reduce other symptoms, making surgery safer. Oral iodine reduces the vascularity of the thyroid gland, decreasing the risk of bleeding during surgery. Adequate preparation of the patient is important because a **euthyroid** state helps prevent a postoperative thyrotoxic crisis.

Thyroidectomy can be done with a traditional, open approach or with newer minimally invasive techniques that use a combination of a tiny incision and an endoscope. Patients can usually go home the same day and have a faster recovery time with minimally invasive surgery. The surgeon may choose to leave some of the thyroid gland intact, to continue to secrete some hormone. Following surgery, the patient will likely be hypothyroid and will require thyroid replacement hormone (levothyroxine [Synthroid]). Nursing care of the patient undergoing a thyroidectomy is discussed later in this chapter.

If vision is impaired from exophthalmos, surgical orbital decompression can be done. Current endoscopic techniques have made this a safer option than in the past.

Nursing Process for the Patient With Hyperthyroidism

DATA COLLECTION. Monitor the patient with hyperthyroidism closely until normal thyroid activity is restored. Assess vital signs and lung sounds, and report changes to the RN or HCP. Assess level of anxiety and ability to cope with symptoms. Monitor weight, bowel function, and ability to sleep. Assess eyes for risk for injury caused by exophthalmos, and note degree of muscle weakness. Never palpate the thyroid gland of a patient with hyperthyroidism because palpation can stimulate release of thyroid hormone and precipitate a thyrotoxic crisis.

NURSING DIAGNOSES, PLANNING, AND IMPLEMENTATION.

Hyperthermia related to hypermetabolic state

EXPECTED OUTCOME: The patient's body temperature will be within normal limits.

- Monitor temperature. *Temperature may be elevated due to hypermetabolic state.*
- Administer acetaminophen as ordered (avoid aspirin) to reduce temperature. *Aspirin can cause an increase in circulating thyroid hormone.*
- Apply cooling blanket as ordered. *External cooling may be needed if acetaminophen is not effective.*
- If a cooling blanket is needed, set it to 1 to 2 degrees below the current temperature, and wrap the extremities with towels to prevent shivering, *which can further increase temperature.*
- Offer fluids *to replace fluids lost through diaphoresis.*

Diarrhea related to increase in peristalsis

EXPECTED OUTCOME: The patient will maintain fluid and electrolyte balance.

- Provide small, frequent meals of low-fiber foods such as bananas, rice, and applesauce. *Low-fiber foods decrease peristalsis and stooling.*

- Monitor electrolytes, especially sodium and potassium. *Diarrhea can cause electrolyte loss.*
- Monitor for dehydration. *Diarrhea causes fluid loss.*
- Keep skin clean and dry. Apply barrier cream *to protect skin from injury from stool.*

Imbalanced Nutrition: Less Than Body Requirements related to increased metabolism

EXPECTED OUTCOME: The patient will have balanced nutrition as evidenced by stable weight in proportion to height.

- Determine healthy weight for height *so that the expected outcome is realistic for the patient.*
- Monitor weight weekly *to make sure interventions are working.*
- Consult dietitian for high-calorie diet and supplements *to meet caloric requirements.*

Disturbed Sleep Pattern related to sympathetic stimulation

EXPECTED OUTCOME: The patient will have improved sleep as evidenced by stating feeling rested upon awakening.

- Provide a quiet, restful environment *to help the patient to fall asleep.*
- Ask the patient if music or earplugs are desired *to mask environmental noise.*
- Administer propranolol or sedative as ordered *to reduce sympathetic stimulation and calm patient.*

Anxiety related to sympathetic stimulation

EXPECTED OUTCOME: The patient will experience reduced anxiety as evidenced by the patient's statement that anxiety is controlled.

- Provide the patient with accurate information about the disorder and treatment, and explain that proper treatment will correct symptoms. *Fear of the unknown can produce anxiety.*
- Administer propranolol or antianxiety agent as ordered *to reduce sympathetic stimulation and calm patient.*
- Offer massage, music, or other relaxation techniques preferred by the patient. *These may promote relaxation.*

Risk for Injury related to hypermetabolic state and bone and eye involvement

EXPECTED OUTCOME: The patient will remain safe and without injury.

- Report changes in vital signs to RN or HCP. *Prompt treatment can reduce complications.*

• WORD • BUILDING •
euthyroid: eu—normal, healthy + thyroid

- Encourage all patients with Graves disease to stop smoking if they are smokers. *Smoking is a risk factor for exophthalmos.*
- Administer lubricating saline eye drops as ordered *to protect eyes from drying.*
- Advise use of dark, tight-fitting glasses *to protect eyes from light and injury.*
- Gently tape eyes shut with nonallergic tape for sleeping. *Exophthalmos may prevent the patient from fully closing the eyes.*
- Elevate the head of the bed *to reduce edema behind the eyes.*
- Provide a low-sodium diet. *This may decrease edema behind the eyes.*
- Teach the patient to notify the HCP immediately if eye pain or vision changes occur. *These can be signs of pressure from edema on optic nerve, which can cause permanent damage if not corrected.*
- Protect from injury and falls. *Reduced bone density increases risk for fractures.*

PATIENT EDUCATION. Teach the patient about the disease and symptoms of hyperthyroidism or hypothyroidism to report. Also teach the patient how to take medications and the importance of routine follow-up laboratory testing.

EVALUATION. If the plan of care is effective, the patient will remain free from complications and injury. Vital signs will be within normal limits. Diarrhea will be controlled, and complications of diarrhea such as skin breakdown and dehydration will be avoided. The patient's weight should remain stable. The patient should report that he or she is rested on awakening and that anxiety is controlled.

Nursing Care of the Patient Receiving Radioactive Iodine

If RAI is used, it is usually given orally in one dose. If the dose is high, such as for the patient with thyroid cancer, the patient is hospitalized. Patients receiving lower doses may be treated as outpatients. Limit time spent with the patient and maintain a safe distance when providing direct care (see Chapter 11). Pregnant caregivers should avoid caring for patients receiving RAI. Urine, vomitus, and other body secretions are contaminated and should be disposed of according to hospital policy. Flush the toilet twice after disposal of contaminated material. The radiation safety officer and hospital policy should be consulted for specific precautions.

At home, the patient is instructed to avoid close contact with family members and to use careful hand hygiene after urinating. Oral contact with others should be avoided, and eating utensils should be washed thoroughly with soap and water. Pregnancy should be avoided for a year. Hospital teaching protocols should be used for specific patient teaching. The amount of time patients must avoid contact with others depends on the dose of radiation received. If the treatment is being administered for hyperthyroidism, inform the patient that symptoms should subside in about 6 to 8 weeks.

Side effects can include sore throat, dry mouth or eyes, and nausea. Sore throat is easily treated with acetaminophen, and nausea usually lasts only a day or two. Dry eyes can be relieved with moisturizing eye drops. Encourage the patient to drink plenty of fluids and void frequently to help remove RAI from the body and reduce radiation exposure to the bladder. In addition, the patient should be aware of symptoms of hypothyroidism to report because hypothyroidism can occur up to 15 years after the treatment.

Goiter
Pathophysiology and Etiology
Enlargement of the thyroid gland is called a goiter. The thyroid gland may enlarge in response to increased TSH levels or sometimes in response to the autoimmune process that occurs in Graves disease. TSH is elevated in response to low TH, iodine deficiency, pregnancy, or viral, genetic, or other conditions. When a goiter is caused by iodine deficiency or other environmental factors, it is called an endemic goiter.

Some medications are **goitrogens.** These substances interfere with the body's use of iodine. Some **goitrogenic** medications include propylthiouracil, sulfonamides, lithium, and salicylates (aspirin).

A goiter can be associated with a hyperthyroid, hypothyroid, or euthyroid state. A goiter that occurs with hyperthyroidism is sometimes called a toxic goiter. Once the cause of the goiter is removed, the gland usually returns to normal size.

Signs and Symptoms
The thyroid gland is enlarged, and swelling may be apparent at the base of the neck (Fig. 39.5). Alternatively, the gland may enlarge posteriorly, which can interfere with swallowing or breathing. The patient may have a full sensation in the neck. Symptoms of hypothyroidism or hyperthyroidism may be present.

Diagnostic Tests
Serum TSH, T_3, and T_4 levels are measured to determine thyroid function. An ultrasound or a thyroid scan may be done to determine the cause or evaluate the size of the gland.

Therapeutic Measures
Treatment is aimed at the cause. Consult the HCP if goitrogenic medications are being used. If iodine deficiency is a problem, it is added to the diet with supplements or iodized salt. Hypothyroidism or hyperthyroidism is treated if indicated. Levothyroxine (Synthroid) may be given to reduce TSH levels via negative feedback. RAI therapy or thyroidectomy may be needed to treat hyperthyroid symptoms

• WORD • BUILDING •

goitrogenic: goitro—goiter + genic—producing

Nutrition Notes

Iodine Deficiency. Iodine is an essential element, needed by the thyroid to produce hormones. Iodine is found in soil and seawater at various levels throughout the world. Foods differ in their iodine content depending on the concentration of iodine in the soil and water. If an individual consumes an inadequate amount of iodine, the thyroid has to work harder to produce hormones and may enlarge, which is termed a goiter. The United States fortifies salt with iodine. Globally, approximately 40% of people are at risk for iodine deficiency (American Thyroid Association, 2018). Consuming a wide variety of foods normally prevents a deficiency in iodine. Because of iodine supplementation in chicken and dairy cattle feed, eggs and dairy products are good sources of iodine in the diet, as are saltwater fish, seaweed, shellfish, and iodized salt (American Thyroid Association, 2018; Lee, 2017).

Iodine Excess. The American Thyroid Association (2018) recommends against the ingestion of supplements that contain iodine and kelp. Excessive iodine may cause thyroid dysfunction.

References

American Thyroid Association. (2018). Iodine deficiency. Retrieved from www.thyroid.org/iodine-deficiency

Lee, S. L. (2017). Iodine deficiency. *Medscape.* Retrieved from http://emedicine.medscape.com/article/122714-overview

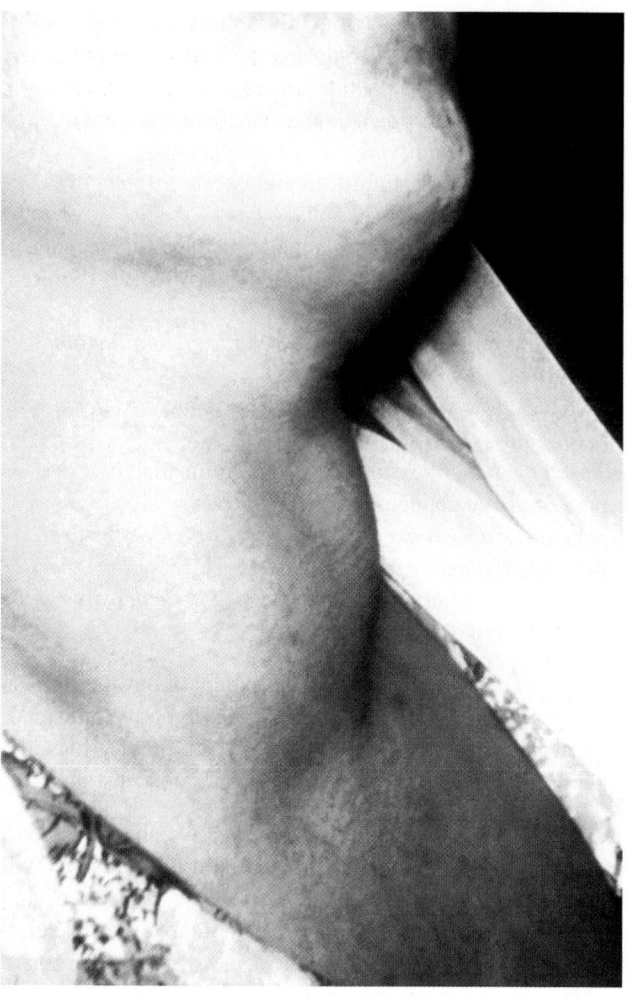

FIGURE 39.5 Goiter caused by iodine deficiency.

or if the enlarged gland is interfering with breathing or swallowing.

Nursing Care for the Patient With a Goiter

Be careful to assess the effect of the goiter on breathing and swallowing. Stridor, a whistling sound, may be heard if the airway is obstructed. Stridor is an ominous sign and should be reported to the HCP immediately. If the patient experiences difficulty swallowing, notify the HCP and collaborate with the dietitian to provide soft foods that are easy to swallow. A swallowing study might be ordered. This will assist a speech pathologist or other expert in making specific recommendations for safe swallowing.

Cancer of the Thyroid Gland

Thyroid cancer is the most common cancer of the endocrine system. Women are affected more often than men. Most tumors of the thyroid gland are not malignant. See Chapter 11 for cancer pathophysiology.

Etiology

Thyroid hyperplasia or exposure to radiation ("Cultural Considerations: Chernobyl Nuclear Disaster") can lead to thyroid cancer. The tendency to develop some forms of thyroid cancer may be inherited.

Cultural Considerations

Chernobyl Nuclear Disaster. Because of the Chernobyl nuclear disaster in Russia in 1986, Russian immigrants to the United States and other countries are at exceptionally high risk for developing pituitary, thyroid, and parathyroid disorders and cancers. The proximity of Estonia, Latvia, Lithuania, Poland, and other Eastern European countries to Russia places immigrants and long-term visitors from these countries at risk as well. Be alert for endocrine disorders among these populations and assist patients to arrange genetic counseling for those who desire it.

Signs and Symptoms

A hard, painless nodule may be palpable on the thyroid gland. Difficulty breathing or swallowing, persistent cough, or changes in the voice may occur if the tumor is near the esophagus and trachea. Most patients with cancer of the thyroid have normal TH levels.

Diagnostic Tests

A thyroid scan shows a "cold" nodule. This is because malignant tumors of the thyroid do not take up RAI administered for the scan. A "hot" nodule indicates a benign tumor. A fine-needle aspiration biopsy confirms the diagnosis.

Therapeutic Measures

A partial or total thyroidectomy may be done. Chemotherapy, RAI therapy, or external beam radiation may also be used, alone or following surgery.

Nursing Care

Nursing care is determined by the symptoms the patient is experiencing. See Chapter 11 for care of the patient with cancer.

Evidence-Based Practice

Clinical Question
Does weight affect thyroid function?

Evidence
A systematic review of 21 studies including more than 12,000 thyroid cancer cases revealed that the risk for thyroid cancer is increased in overweight individuals by 25% and in obese individuals by 55% compared with individuals of normal weight (Schmid, Ricci, Behrens, & Leitzmann, 2015).

Implications for Nursing Practice
Although being overweight is known to have serious health consequences, it is now known to put persons at risk for thyroid cancer as well. It is important to encourage persons to eat healthy diets and manage weight to prevent serious negative health outcomes, including thyroid cancer.

Reference
Schmid, D., Ricci, C., Behrens, G., & Leitzmann, M. F. (2015). Adiposity and risk of thyroid cancer: A systematic review and meta-analysis. *Obesity Reviews, 16*(12), 1042–1054.

Nursing Process for the Patient Undergoing Thyroidectomy

A thyroidectomy may be performed for cancer of the thyroid gland, for hyperthyroidism, or if the patient is suffering from dyspnea or dysphagia from a goiter. See Chapter 12 for general care of a patient having surgery.

A total thyroidectomy is usually performed if cancer is present. After a total thyroidectomy, lifelong replacement hormone must be taken. A subtotal (partial) thyroidectomy might be done for hyperthyroidism, leaving a portion of the thyroid gland to continue to secrete TH.

Preoperative Care

The patient should be in a euthyroid state before undergoing a thyroidectomy in order to avoid complications during and after surgery. This is accomplished with the use of antithyroid medication such as methimazole (Tapazole). A saturated solution of potassium iodide may also be administered to decrease the size and vascularity of the gland, reducing the risk of bleeding during surgery.

Perform a baseline assessment of vital signs and voice quality, so you can compare findings postoperatively. Explain what the patient can expect before, during, and after surgery. Preoperative teaching should include how to perform gentle range-of-motion exercises of the neck, how to support the neck during position changes, and how to use an incentive spirometer after surgery.

Postoperative Care

DATA COLLECTION. Monitor vital signs, oxygen saturation, drain (if present), and dressing every 15 minutes initially, progressing to every 4 hours, as directed, if the patient is stable. Decreased blood pressure with increased pulse can indicate shock related to blood loss. Tachycardia and fever, along with mental status changes, can indicate thyrotoxic crisis. Check the back of the neck for pooling of blood. Because of the location of the surgery, observe for signs of respiratory distress, including an increase in respiratory rate, dyspnea, or stridor. Ask the patient to speak to detect hoarseness of the voice, which can indicate trauma to the recurrent laryngeal nerve. Monitor the patient's serum calcium levels and watch for evidence of tetany (discussed later in this chapter). Report abnormal findings to the RN or HCP immediately.

NURSING DIAGNOSES, PLANNING, AND IMPLEMENTATION.

Ineffective Airway Clearance related to edema at surgical site

EXPECTED OUTCOME: The patient will maintain a clear airway as evidenced by unlabored respirations without stridor.

- Notify HCP about respiratory distress immediately; keep a tracheostomy set at the bedside. *Although not common, a tracheostomy may be needed in an emergency if edema obstructs the airway.*
- Maintain the patient in a semi-Fowler position *to help reduce edema at the surgical site and maximize respiratory effort.*
- Monitor neck dressing. *If the dressing seems to get tighter, it may be a sign that the patient's neck is swelling, which could impair the airway.*
- Use a room humidifier or humidified oxygen *to keep airways and secretions moist.*
- Remind the patient to do coughing and deep-breathing exercises every hour. *This keeps the airway clear of secretions.*
- Have suction equipment available *in case the patient is unable to cough up secretions effectively.*
- Encourage the patient to use the incentive spirometer *to assist with deep breathing.*
- Assess the patient's swallowing and gag reflexes before offering clear liquids *to guard against aspiration.*

Risk for Injury (tetany, thyrotoxic crisis) related to surgical procedure

EXPECTED OUTCOME: Complications will be recognized and treated quickly.

- Monitor the patient for muscle spasms or numbness or tingling around the mouth, and report immediately if they occur. *These are symptoms of tetany, which must be treated immediately. Tetany is most likely to occur 24 to 72 hours postoperatively.*
- Monitor vital signs often, and report changes immediately. *Elevated vital signs may be signs of thyrotoxic crisis, which is most likely to occur up to 18 hours postoperatively.*

Acute Pain related to surgical procedure

EXPECTED OUTCOME: The patient's pain will be controlled as evidenced by the patient stating that his or her pain rating is acceptable.

- Administer acetaminophen or opioids as ordered. Avoid aspirin products. *Aspirin binds to the same protein as thyroid hormone and can precipitate a thyrotoxic crisis.*
- Use pillows or sandbags to support the patient's head. *Unexpected movement may be painful.*

Ineffective Health Management related to knowledge deficit

EXPECTED OUTCOME: The patient will be able to effectively manage self-care needs as evidenced by (1) the patient verbalizes understanding of follow-up care, (2) body weight stabilizes at appropriate weight for height, and (3) TH levels are within normal limits.

- Teach the patient to do gentle range-of-motion exercises, avoiding hyperextension of the neck, which can cause strain on the incision line. *Avoidance of neck movement due to pain can result in contracture.*
- Consult dietitian to assist the patient with potential dietary changes needed following surgery. *With correction of metabolic alterations, dietary needs may be significantly altered.*
- Teach the patient the importance of follow-up care *to avoid complications:*
  - How to administer replacement hormone if ordered
  - How to change the dressing and to report bleeding or signs of infection at the site
  - Importance of immediately reporting unusual irritability, fever, palpitations, or signs of tetany
  - Importance of follow-up laboratory work for thyroid function and medication adjustment

EVALUATION. If the plan has been effective, complications caused by surgery will not occur or will be recognized and reported early. Pain will be prevented or controlled, and the patient will demonstrate understanding of postoperative self-care.

Complications of Thyroid Surgery

THYROTOXIC CRISIS. Thyrotoxic crisis can result from manipulation of the thyroid gland during surgery, with the subsequent release of large amounts of TH. This is a rare complication since the use of antithyroid drugs before surgery has become routine. For more information on thyrotoxic crisis, see the section on hyperthyroidism earlier in this chapter.

TETANY. Tetany is caused by low calcium levels and is characterized by tingling in the fingers and perioral area (around the mouth), muscle spasms, twitching, and cardiac arrhythmias. Muscle spasms in the larynx can lead to respiratory obstruction. Watch carefully for symptoms of tetany and report them immediately if they occur because, if the problem is not recognized quickly, death can result.

Tetany can occur if the parathyroid glands are accidentally removed during thyroid surgery. Because of the proximity of the parathyroid glands to the thyroid, it is sometimes difficult for the surgeon to avoid them. In the absence of the parathyroid hormone (PTH), serum calcium levels drop and tetany results. IV calcium gluconate is given to treat acute tetany.

DISORDERS OF THE PARATHYROID GLANDS

Recall that the parathyroid glands secrete PTH in response to low serum calcium levels. PTH raises serum calcium levels by promoting calcium movement from bones to blood, increasing absorption of dietary calcium, and increasing resorption of calcium by the kidneys. Decreased PTH activity is called hypoparathyroidism. Increased PTH activity is called hyperparathyroidism.

Hypoparathyroidism
Pathophysiology

A decrease in PTH causes a decrease in bone resorption of calcium, a decrease in calcium absorption by the gastrointestinal tract, and decreased resorption in the kidneys. This means that calcium stays in the bones instead of being moved into the blood, and more calcium is excreted from the body. The result is a decreased serum calcium level, called hypocalcemia. As calcium levels fall, phosphate levels rise.

Etiology

The most common causes of hypoparathyroidism are heredity and the accidental removal of the parathyroid glands during thyroidectomy or other neck surgeries. Hypoparathyroidism also occurs following purposeful removal of the parathyroid glands for hyperparathyroidism or cancer. Another cause is hypomagnesemia, which impairs secretion of PTH. Hypomagnesemia can occur with chronic alcoholism or certain nutritional problems.

Signs and Symptoms

Calcium plays an important role in nerve cell stability. Hypocalcemia causes neuromuscular irritability. In acute cases, tetany can occur, with numbness and tingling of the fingers, tongue, and lips; muscle spasms; and twitching (Table 39.5). Positive Chvostek and Trousseau signs are early indications of tetany. See Figures 6.4 and 6.5 in Chapter 6 for illustrations of these tests.

Chronic hypocalcemia can lead to lethargy; calcifications in the brain, leading to psychosis; cataracts; and convulsions. Bone changes may be evident on x-ray examination. Electrocardiogram (ECG) changes and heart failure can develop because of the importance of calcium to cardiac function. Death can result from laryngospasm if treatment is not effective.

Diagnostic Tests

Laboratory studies show decreased serum calcium and PTH levels and increased serum phosphorus. An ECG is done to evaluate cardiac function. Radiographs show bone changes.

Therapeutic Measures

Acute cases of hypoparathyroidism are treated with IV calcium gluconate. Long-term treatment includes a high-calcium diet (Box 39.2), with oral calcium and vitamin D supplements. Magnesium is given if hypomagnesemia is present.

Nursing Process for the Patient With Hypoparathyroidism

DATA COLLECTION. The patient at risk for hypoparathyroidism should be closely monitored for symptoms of tetany. If you suspect tetany, check for Chvostek and Trousseau signs. Monitor respirations closely for stridor, a sign of laryngospasm.

NURSING DIAGNOSES, PLANNING, AND IMPLEMENTATION.

Risk for Injury related to hypocalcemia and tetany

EXPECTED OUTCOME: The patient will remain free from injury. Signs of tetany will be recognized and treated quickly.

• Monitor the patient for signs of tetany, and report immediately to RN or HCP *so that treatment can begin quickly.*

• Make sure a tracheostomy set, endotracheal tube, and IV calcium are available *for emergency use if laryngospasm occurs.*

• Consult a dietitian for high-calcium diet teaching. *The patient may need a lifelong high-calcium diet.*

• Teach the patient about the importance of long-term diet, medication therapy, and follow-up laboratory testing. *The patient needs to understand self-care for follow-up at home.*

EVALUATION. Injury is prevented through early recognition and reporting of signs and symptoms of tetany. The patient should be able to describe correct treatment and self-care measures for home.

Hyperparathyroidism
Pathophysiology

Overactivity of one or more of the parathyroid glands causes an increase in PTH, with a subsequent increase in the serum calcium level (hypercalcemia). This is achieved through movement of calcium out of the bones and into the blood, absorption in the small intestine, and reabsorption by the kidneys. PTH also promotes phosphorus excretion by the kidneys.

Etiology

Hyperparathyroidism is usually the result of hyperplasia or a benign tumor of the parathyroid glands. It may also be hereditary. Parathyroid cancer is rare. Secondary hyperparathyroidism occurs when the parathyroid glands secrete excessive PTH in response to low serum calcium levels. Serum calcium may be reduced in kidney disease because of the kidneys' failure to activate vitamin D. Vitamin D is necessary for absorption of calcium in the small intestine.

Signs and Symptoms

Signs and symptoms of hyperparathyroidism are caused primarily by the increase in the serum calcium level, although

Table 39.5
Parathyroid Disorders Summary

	Insufficient Parathyroid Hormone	*Excess Parathyroid Hormone*
Disorder	Hypoparathyroidism	Hyperparathyroidism
Signs and Symptoms	Hypocalcemia, neuromuscular irritability, tetany, positive Chvostek and Trousseau signs	Hypercalcemia, fatigue, pathological fractures
Diagnostic Tests	Serum parathyroid hormone, calcium, and phosphate	Serum parathyroid hormone, calcium, and phosphate
Therapeutic Measures	Calcium and vitamin D replacement; high-calcium, low-phosphorus diet	Calcitonin, parathyroidectomy
Priority Nursing Diagnoses	*Risk for Injury* related to tetany	*Risk for Injury* related to bone demineralization

Box 39.2

Dietary Sources of Calcium
- Milk
- Cheeses
- Yogurt
- Sardines
- Oysters
- Salmon
- Cauliflower
- Green leafy vegetables
    See Chapter 6, Table 6.3, for a more detailed list.

many patients are asymptomatic. Symptoms include fatigue, depression, confusion, increased urination, anorexia, nausea, vomiting, kidney stones, and cardiac arrhythmias. The increased serum calcium level also causes gastrin secretion, resulting in abdominal pain and peptic ulcers. Because calcium is being removed from bones, bone and joint pain and pathological fractures can occur. Severe hypercalcemia can result in coma and cardiac arrest.

Diagnostic Tests
Laboratory studies include serum calcium, phosphorus, and PTH levels. Radiographs or bone density testing may show decreased bone density. A 24-hour urine test might be used to test how much calcium is being excreted in the urine. Nuclear scanning or ultrasound may be used to help locate the parathyroid glands if surgical removal is planned.

Therapeutic Measures
Mild hyperparathyroidism with asymptomatic hypercalcemia may be treated conservatively, with extra fluids to dilute calcium, monitoring for bone changes and decline in renal function, and weight-bearing exercise to keep calcium in the bones. Oral calcium and vitamin D supplements may be prescribed. Estrogen therapy might be used in women, although side effects must be considered. Cinacalcet (Sensipar) is a newer drug that acts like calcium in the blood, fooling the parathyroid glands into reducing PTH secretion.

In acute hypercalcemia, IV normal saline is given to hydrate the patient. Furosemide (Lasix) is given to increase renal excretion of calcium. Alendronate (Fosamax) or calcitonin may be given to prevent calcium release from bones. These drugs are covered in the osteoporosis section in Chapter 46.

Surgery will likely be done to remove the diseased parathyroid glands (parathyroidectomy). If possible, some parathyroid tissue is left intact to continue to secrete PTH. Minimally invasive radio-guided parathyroidectomy can be done under local anesthesia through a small incision.

Preoperative and postoperative care is similar to that of the patient undergoing thyroid surgery, with special attention paid to calcium and PTH levels. The patient will likely be on calcium and vitamin D supplements following surgery.

Nursing Process for the Patient With Hyperparathyroidism

DATA COLLECTION. Assess the patient for symptoms related to hypercalcemia, including muscle weakness, lethargy, bone pain, anorexia, nausea, vomiting, behavioral changes, and renal insufficiency. Monitor serum calcium levels as ordered.

NURSING DIAGNOSES, PLANNING, AND IMPLEMENTATION. Nursing diagnoses depend on assessment findings. *Risk for Injury* usually takes priority.

Risk for Injury (fracture, complications of hypercalcemia) related to calcium imbalance

EXPECTED OUTCOME: The patient will remain free from injury.

- Monitor the patient for signs or symptoms of calcium imbalance and report promptly. *Prompt treatment can prevent serious complications.*
- Encourage oral fluids *to prevent dehydration and kidney stones and help excrete calcium.*
- Encourage strengthening and weight-bearing exercises *to help keep calcium in the bones.*
- Provide a safe environment for ambulation; assist the patient with ambulation if needed. *A fall could result in fracture if bones are demineralized.*
- Encourage smoking cessation. *Smoking causes bone loss.*
- Teach the patient symptoms to report and use of long-term medications *so that the patient can manage self-care at home.*

EVALUATION. If the plan is effective, symptoms of hypercalcemia will be recognized and reported quickly, and complications and injury will be prevented.

DISORDERS OF THE ADRENAL GLANDS

Adrenal disorders can involve the adrenal medulla or the adrenal cortex. A rare tumor of the adrenal medulla, called a **pheochromocytoma,** causes hypersecretion of epinephrine and norepinephrine. Hyposecretion of epinephrine is rare and generally causes no symptoms. Hypersecretion of cortisol from the adrenal cortex results in Cushing syndrome. Hypofunction of the adrenal cortex results in Addison disease.

Pheochromocytoma
Pathophysiology
A pheochromocytoma is a rare tumor of the adrenal medulla that secretes excess catecholamines (epinephrine and norepinephrine). Most pheochromocytomas are benign.

• WORD • BUILDING •
pheochromocytoma: pheo—dark + chromo—color + cyt—cell + oma—tumor

Etiology

The cause of most cases of pheochromocytoma is unknown. About one-third of cases are hereditary.

Signs and Symptoms

Because norepinephrine is the fight-or-flight hormone, patients with a pheochromocytoma have exaggerated fight-or-flight symptoms. Manifestations include hypertension, tachycardia (with heart rate greater than 100 beats per minute), palpitations, tremor, diaphoresis, feeling of apprehension, and severe pounding headache. The most prominent characteristic is intermittent unstable hypertension. Diastolic pressure may be greater than 115 mm Hg. If hypertension and tachycardia are not controlled, the patient is at risk for stroke, heart attack and heart failure, vision changes, seizures, psychosis, and organ damage.

Diagnostic Tests

Patients with a suspected pheochromocytoma will have a 24-hour urine test for metanephrines and vanillylmandelic acid (VMA). These are end products of catecholamine metabolism. A blood test for metanephrines may also be done. If results are elevated, a CT scan or an MRI is done to locate the tumor.

Therapeutic Measures

Treatment for pheochromocytoma is surgical removal of one or both adrenal glands. Calcium channel blockers, alpha blockers, and beta blockers are used to control symptoms. Teach the patient to avoid caffeine and other stimulants prior to surgery.

After surgery, the patient is at risk for hypotension, hypertension, and hypoglycemia. Monitor vital signs and blood glucose, and report variations from normal. If both adrenal glands have been entirely removed, the patient will require lifelong replacement hormones. (See section on adrenalectomy later in this chapter.)

Adrenocortical Insufficiency/Addison Disease

Adrenocortical insufficiency (AI) is the insufficient production of the hormones of the adrenal cortex. Primary AI is called Addison disease.

Pathophysiology

AI is associated with reduced levels of cortisol, aldosterone, or both hormones. A deficiency in androgens may also exist. In primary disease, adrenocorticotropic hormone (ACTH) levels from the pituitary gland can be elevated in an attempt to stimulate the adrenal cortex to synthesize more hormone. In secondary disease, deficient ACTH fails to stimulate adrenal steroid synthesis. In most cases, the adrenal glands are atrophied, small, and misshapen and are unable to produce adequate amounts of hormone.

Etiology

Addison disease is thought to be an autoimmune disease; that is, the gland destroys itself in response to conditions such as tuberculosis, fungal infection, infection related to AIDS, or metastatic cancer. It can also be associated with autoimmune diseases. Bilateral adrenalectomy also results in AI.

Secondary AI may be caused by dysfunction of the pituitary gland or hypothalamus. In addition, prolonged use of corticosteroid drugs can depress ACTH and corticotropin-releasing hormone production, which in turn reduces steroid hormone production. A patient receiving long-term corticosteroid therapy is particularly at risk for AI if the drugs are abruptly discontinued. Because the pituitary gland has been suppressed for a prolonged period, it may take up to a year before ACTH is produced normally again.

> **NURSING CARE TIP**
> Always taper long-term corticosteroid therapy slowly to avoid adrenal crisis.

Signs and Symptoms

The most significant sign of Addison disease is hypotension. This is related to the lack of aldosterone. Remember that aldosterone causes sodium and water retention in the kidney and potassium loss. If aldosterone is deficient, sodium and water are lost and hypotension and tachycardia result. Low cortisol levels cause hypoglycemia, weakness, fatigue, weight loss, confusion, and psychosis. In primary AI, increased ACTH may produce hyperpigmentation of the skin, causing the patient to have a tanned or bronze appearance. Anorexia, nausea, and vomiting may also occur, possibly as the result of electrolyte imbalances. Women may have decreased body hair because of low androgen levels. Patients may report craving salt.

Complications

If a patient is exposed to stress, such as infection, trauma, or psychological pressure, the body may be unable to respond normally with secretion of cortisol (our natural stress hormone), and an adrenal crisis can occur. Loss of large amounts of sodium and water and the resulting fluid volume deficit cause profound hypotension, dehydration, and tachycardia. Potassium retention can cause cardiac arrhythmias. Hypoglycemia may be severe. Coma and death result if treatment is not initiated. Treatment of adrenal crisis involves rapidly restoring fluid volume and cortisol levels. IV fluids (containing glucose) and large doses of IV glucocorticoids are administered. Electrolytes are replaced as needed. The cause of the crisis should be identified and treated.

Diagnostic Tests

Serum and urine cortisol and blood glucose levels are all low. Blood urea nitrogen (BUN) and hematocrit levels may appear to be elevated because of dehydration. Antibodies may be present in the blood in autoimmune disease. An ACTH stimulation test helps determine whether the adrenal glands are functioning. Serum sodium and potassium levels are monitored. A CT scan or an MRI may be done to evaluate the size of the adrenal glands or to locate a pituitary tumor in secondary disease.

Therapeutic Measures

Long-term treatment consists of replacement of glucocorticoids (hydrocortisone) and mineralocorticoids (fludrocortisone [Florinef]). Some patients also receive androgen therapy. Patients will need hormone replacement therapy for the rest of their lives. Hormones are given in divided doses, with two-thirds of the daily dose given in the morning and one-third in the evening to mimic the body's own diurnal rhythm. Remember that steroid hormones are our natural stress hormones and so are naturally elevated during times of stress. Therefore, during times of stress or illness, doses need to be increased to two to three times normal. The patient may also be placed on a high-sodium diet. If the patient is ill and can't tolerate oral medication, hormones must be injected.

Nursing Process for the Patient With Addison Disease

DATA COLLECTION. The patient with Addison disease should be assessed for understanding of and adherence to the treatment regimen. Monitor vital signs and daily weights or I&O to track fluid status. Monitor serum glucose levels and symptoms of hyperkalemia and hyponatremia. Report changes in mental status. If the patient is in crisis, monitor vital signs closely and report any signs of fluid volume deficit such as orthostatic hypotension or poor skin turgor to the HCP immediately.

NURSING DIAGNOSES, PLANNING, AND IMPLEMENTATION.

Risk for Deficient Fluid Volume related to deficient adrenal cortical hormones

EXPECTED OUTCOME: The patient's fluid volume will be stable as evidenced by stable weights and vital signs, and skin turgor within normal limits.

- Monitor vital signs, and report change promptly. *Hypotension and tachycardia indicate hypovolemia.*
- Monitor fluid status, and report changes promptly *to prevent complications of fluid deficit.*
- Administer steroid replacements as ordered *to maintain fluid and electrolyte balance.*

Ineffective Health Management related to deficient knowledge about self-care of Addison disease

EXPECTED OUTCOME: The patient will verbalize understanding of self-monitoring and self-medication at home.

- Assess the patient's understanding of his or her disease process and treatment. *Teaching should build on baseline knowledge.*
- Teach the patient the importance of hormone replacement as ordered. *The patient who does not secrete endogenous adrenocortical hormones must rely on replacements for survival.*

- Help the patient identify the causes and symptoms of stress, and explain the need to increase medication dosage during times of stress or illness according to the HCP's instructions. *Because these hormones are normally increased during times of stress, it is important that the patient understand how to increase the dose during stress to prevent adrenal crisis.*
- Advise the patient that he or she may need to increase salt intake in hot weather *because of fluid and salt losses.*
- Recommend medical alert identification. *A patient in adrenal crisis may not be able to provide a medical history to emergency personnel, and identification can prevent delay of treatment.*
- If ordered by the HCP, teach the patient and family members how to use an emergency intramuscular (IM) hydrocortisone injection kit. *IM medication may be needed during stress or times when the patient is unable to take oral medications.*

EVALUATION. If nursing care is effective, the patient's fluid status will be stable, and the patient and family will be able to carry out proper self-care of Addison disease.

Cushing Syndrome

Cushing syndrome is caused by exposure to excess cortisol. This can occur because of an adrenal or pituitary gland problem, or from treatment with exogenous corticosteroids. See Table 39.6 for a comparison of adrenal insufficiency and Cushing syndrome.

Pathophysiology

Recall that cortisol, aldosterone, and androgens are the three steroid hormones secreted by the adrenal cortex. Cortisol is essential for survival and is normally secreted in a diurnal rhythm, with levels increasing in the early morning. Secretion is increased during times of stress. In Cushing syndrome, cortisol is hypersecreted without regard to stress or time of day. When levels of cortisol are very high, effects related to excess aldosterone and androgens are also seen.

> **LEARNING TIP**
>
> An easy way to remember the hormones of the adrenal cortex is to think *salt, sugar,* and *sex.* Aldosterone promotes salt retention, cortisol affects sugar (carbohydrate) metabolism, and androgens are sex hormones.

Etiology

Cushing syndrome can be caused by hypersecretion of ACTH by the pituitary gland. This is most often the result of a benign pituitary adenoma. Sometimes ACTH is produced by a tumor in the lungs or other organs. The high levels of ACTH cause adrenal hyperplasia, which in turn increases production and release of cortisol. A problem within the adrenal gland, such as an adrenal adenoma or carcinoma, can also produce excess cortisol.

Table 39.6

Adrenal Cortex Hormone Summary

	Hypofunction	*Hyperfunction*
Disorder	Adrenocortical insufficiency, Addison disease	Cushing syndrome
Signs and Symptoms	Sodium and water loss, hypotension, hypoglycemia, fatigue	Weight gain, sodium and water retention, hyperglycemia, buffalo hump, moon face
Diagnostic Tests	Serum and urine cortisol	Serum and urine cortisol
Therapeutic Measures	Glucocorticoid and mineralocorticoid replacement	Alter steroid therapy dose or schedule, surgery if tumor
Priority Nursing Diagnoses	*Risk for Deficient Fluid Volume*	*Risk for Excess Fluid Volume* *Risk for Unstable Blood Glucose Level* *Risk for Infection*

The most common cause of Cushing syndrome is prolonged use of glucocorticoid medication (e.g., prednisone) for chronic inflammatory disorders such as rheumatoid arthritis, COPD, and Crohn disease. The use of smaller doses of glucocorticoids (in inhalers for asthma) or topical creams does not usually cause a problem.

Signs and Symptoms

Most signs and symptoms of Cushing syndrome are related to excess cortisol levels. Weight gain, central obesity with thin arms and legs, fat pads on the upper back (buffalo hump), and a round, moon-shaped face result from deposits of adipose tissue at these sites (Fig. 39.6).

Cortisol also causes insulin resistance and stimulates gluconeogenesis, which results in glucose intolerance. Some patients develop secondary diabetes mellitus (see Chapter 40). Muscle wasting and thin skin with purple striae occur as a result of cortisol's catabolic effect on tissues. Catabolic effects on bone lead to osteoporosis, pathological fractures, and back pain from compression fractures of the vertebrae. Because cortisol has anti-inflammatory and immunosuppressive actions, the patient is at risk for infection. Hyperpigmentation of the skin may occur. About half of patients develop mental status changes, from irritability to psychosis (sometimes referred to as steroid psychosis). Sodium and water retention are related to the mineralocorticoid effect. As sodium is retained, potassium is lost in the urine, causing hypokalemia. (See Chapter 6 to review these electrolyte imbalances.) Androgen effects include acne, growth of facial hair, and **amenorrhea** (absence of menses) in women.

Diagnostic Tests

Suspicion of Cushing syndrome may initially be based on a cushingoid appearance and history of taking steroid medication. Plasma and urine cortisol and plasma ACTH are measured. A 24-hour urine test for cortisol may be collected.

Levels of cortisol in the saliva may also be measured. A dexamethasone suppression test may be done. Serum potassium is measured. Additional tests to locate the cause of excess endogenous cortisol may be done.

Therapeutic Measures

If a pituitary or ACTH-secreting tumor is present, surgical removal or radiation therapy to the pituitary gland may be employed. If the adrenal glands are the primary cause of the problem, radiation or removal of the adrenal gland or glands may be performed. Drugs such as ketoconazole can be used to block production of adrenal steroids.

If the cause of Cushing syndrome is administration of steroid medication, a lower dose, an every-other-day schedule, or once-a-day dosing in the morning may reduce side effects. Usually steroids are prescribed as a last resort for chronic disorders that are unresponsive to other treatment. The patient and HCP must weigh the risks and benefits of continuing the medication. The HCP may order a high-potassium, low-sodium, high-protein diet. Potassium supplements may be ordered. If the patient has high blood sugar, appropriate therapy for diabetes is instituted (see Chapter 40).

Nursing Process for the Patient With Cushing Syndrome

DATA COLLECTION. Assess the patient's medication history. Monitor vital signs and complications related to fluid and sodium excess. Auscultate the lungs for crackles, and assess extremities for edema. Assess skin integrity, and monitor capillary glucose as ordered by the HCP. Watch for signs of infection.

• **WORD** • **BUILDING** •
amenorrhea: a—not + men—month + orrhea—flow

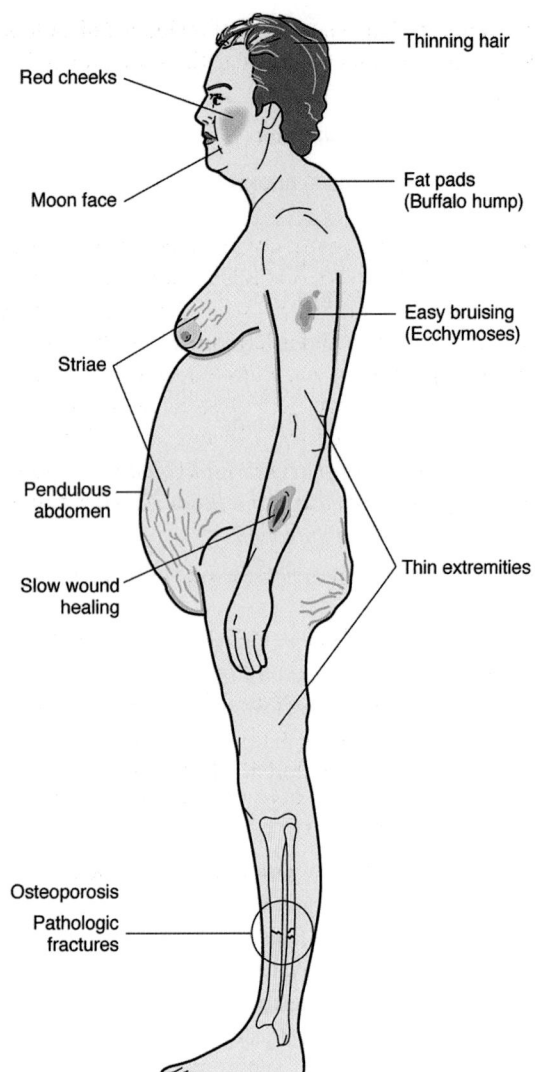

Thinning hair

Red cheeks

Moon face

Fat pads
(Buffalo hump)

Easy bruising
(Ecchymoses)

Striae

Pendulous
abdomen

Thin extremities

Slow wound
healing

Osteoporosis
Pathologic
fractures

FIGURE 39.6 Physical manifestations seen in Cushing syndrome.

NURSING DIAGNOSES, PLANNING, AND IMPLEMENTATION.

Excess Fluid Volume related to sodium and water retention

EXPECTED OUTCOME: The patient's fluid volume will be stable as evidenced by stable daily weights.

• Monitor daily weights, and report changes promptly *to prevent complications related to fluid excess.*
• Teach the patient ordered dietary modifications. *A low-sodium, high-potassium diet may help keep electrolytes in balance.*

Risk for Impaired Skin Integrity (thin, fragile skin) related to protein breakdown

EXPECTED OUTCOME: The patient's skin will remain intact.

• Observe skin, and monitor for breakdown with every position change. *Early recognition and treatment of a problem can prevent further breakdown.*

• Assist the patient in changing positions at least every 2 hours *to prevent pressure injuries.*
• Use a lift sheet to move the patient in bed *to prevent friction and shear.*
• Avoid harsh soaps and hot water. *These can dry skin and increase risk for injury.*
• Use moisturizing cream *to keep skin from drying.*
• Secure IVs and dressings without tape whenever possible. *Removal of tape can tear fragile skin.*
• Consider a specialty pressure-reducing mattress if the patient is very thin or unable to move *to reduce the risk of pressure injury.*
• Consult a dietitian if nutritional status is poor. *Poor nutrition further increases risk for skin breakdown and poor healing.*

Risk for Infection related to immune suppression

EXPECTED OUTCOME: The patient will be free from infection as evidenced by a white blood cell count and temperature within normal limits.

• Monitor the patient for signs of infection and report promptly *so appropriate treatment can be ordered.*
• Use good hand hygiene before and after patient care. *Hand washing is important in reducing exposure to pathogens.*
• Instruct the patient in good hand washing and in the importance of avoiding others who are ill. *A patient with an impaired immune system is more likely to contract illness from others.*
• Consult a dietitian if nutritional status is poor. *Poor nutrition further impairs immune function.*
• Encourage flu and pneumonia vaccinations *to help prevent illness in event of exposure.*

Risk for Unstable Blood Glucose Level related to impaired glucose tolerance

EXPECTED OUTCOME: The patient's blood glucose level will remain within normal limits.

• If glucose intolerance occurs, be prepared to administer insulin *because oral hypoglycemics are not usually effective.*
• Refer the patient and family to diabetes education classes *because diabetes is a complex disease that requires knowledge of self-care.*

See Chapter 40 for care of the patient with diabetes.

Disturbed Body Image related to cushingoid appearance

EXPECTED OUTCOME: The patient will express feelings of acceptance of self.

• Approach the patient with an attitude of acceptance and caring *to help develop a trusting nurse–patient relationship.*
• Provide an opportunity for the patient to verbalize feelings. *Expressing feelings may help reduce anxiety.*

EVALUATION. If care has been effective, complications of fluid overload will be recognized and treated early. The patient will have intact skin and be free from signs of infection. The patient will demonstrate skill in self-care of diabetes if indicated and will verbalize acceptance of self despite changes in appearance.

Nursing Care of the Patient Undergoing Adrenalectomy

Preoperative Care

Monitor the patient for electrolyte imbalance and hyperglycemia. Abnormalities must be corrected before surgery. To prevent adrenal crisis, glucocorticoids are administered because removal of the adrenals causes a sudden drop in adrenal hormones. Prepare the patient for adrenalectomy or hypophysectomy, depending on which surgery will be performed.

Postoperative Care

See "Nursing Care of the Patient Undergoing Hypophysectomy" earlier in this chapter. Following adrenalectomy, the patient receives routine postoperative care. In addition, the patient is closely monitored for changes in fluid and electrolyte balance and adrenal crisis. Patients who undergo bilateral adrenalectomy must take replacement glucocorticoid and mineralocorticoid hormones for the rest of their life. If only one adrenal gland is removed, the remaining gland should eventually produce enough hormone to enable the patient to discontinue replacement hormone.

See Table 39.7 for a summary of endocrine disorders and Table 39.8 for a summary of medications used for endocrine disorders.

CRITICAL THINKING

Mrs. Tercini is a 62-year-old woman admitted to your unit in addisonian crisis. She is lethargic, with a blood pressure of 86/48 mm Hg, pulse of 112 beats per minute, and respirations of 18 breaths per minute. While interviewing her daughter, you learn that Mrs. Tercini has a history of Cushing syndrome treated with bilateral adrenalectomy 25 years ago. She has been taking 150 mcg fludrocortisone (Florinef) and 200 mg hydrocortisone daily ever since. Three days ago, she developed the flu.

1. Why is an adrenalectomy done to treat Cushing syndrome?
2. What is the most effective schedule for Mrs. Tercini's medication?
3. What might have precipitated this addisonian crisis?
4. Why is Mrs. Tercini's blood pressure low?
5. How could this crisis have been prevented?
6. Fludrocortisone is available as 0.1-mg tablets. How many should you administer?

Suggested answers are at the end of the chapter.

Table 39.7

Summary of Endocrine Disorders

Hormone	Hypofunction	Hyperfunction
Antidiuretic hormone	Diabetes insipidus	Syndrome of inappropriate antidiuretic hormone
Growth hormone	Short stature	Acromegaly, gigantism
Thyroid hormone	Hypothyroidism	Hyperthyroidism
Epinephrine	Rare	Pheochromocytoma (hypertension)
Parathyroid hormone	Hypoparathyroidism	Hyperparathyroidism
Cortisol	Addison disease	Cushing syndrome

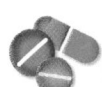

Table 39.8

Medications Used for Endocrine Disorders

Medication Class/Action

Medications for Antidiuretic Hormone (ADH) Disorders

Examples	**Nursing Implications**
vasopressin (Pitressin – subcutaneous [SC] or intramuscular [IM]): replaces ADH	Check daily weights and urine specific gravity. Do not give demeclocycline with dairy products or antacids.

Continued

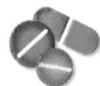

Table 39.8
Medications Used for Endocrine Disorders—cont'd

Medication Class/Action

desmopressin (DDAVP – inhaled, oral, intravenous [IV],
  SC): replaces ADH
conivaptan (Vaprisol – IV), tolvaptan (Samsca – oral):
  blocks action of ADH in the kidney
demeclocycline (Declomycin – oral): reduces ADH release

Medications for Growth Hormone (GH) Disorders

Examples	**Nursing Implications**
bromocriptine (Parlodel): reduces GH release	Monitor blood pressure, serum GH.
octreotide (Sandostatin): suppresses GH	Teach patient self-administration.
pegvisomant (Somavert): blocks the effect of GH on receptor sites	Monitor growth.
somatropin (Humatrope): replaces GH	

Medications for Thyroid Disorders

Examples	**Nursing Implications**
levothyroxine (Synthroid): replaces thyroxine (T_4)	Monitor vital signs and thyroid laboratory results.
propylthiouracil: inhibits synthesis of thyroid hormones	Monitor white blood cell count and differential, thyroid function, liver function.
methimazole (Tapazole): inhibits synthesis of thyroid hormones	

Medications for Adrenal Disorders

Examples	**Nursing Implications**
hydrocortisone: replaces cortisol in adrenal insufficiency	Teach patient to take with food and not to discontinue abruptly.
fludrocortisone (Florinef): replaces aldosterone in adrenal insufficiency	Monitor daily weights, vital signs, and serum potassium.

SUGGESTED ANSWERS TO CRITICAL THINKING

Mrs. Jackson

1. Assess mental status and level of consciousness. Assess edema, lung sounds, and vital signs. Check intake and output during the past 2 days. Check recent laboratory work to see whether her serum sodium is low. Recall that anesthetics are possible causes of syndrome of inappropriate antidiuretic hormone (SIADH). Opioids, which Mrs. Jackson is likely taking after surgery, can also cause confusion.
2. Her weight gain is most likely caused by fluid retention, which can be a result of heart failure or SIADH, among other things.
3. Notify the registered nurse (RN) of your findings and suspicions. Be prepared to place Mrs. Jackson on a fluid restriction. Reassure her son that the health care provider (HCP) is being notified of the changes he noted.
4. Remember that "a pint's (about) a pound." A pint is 2 cups or 480 mL:

$$\frac{6 \text{ pounds}}{1 \text{ pound}} \quad \frac{480 \text{ mL}}{} = 2{,}880 \text{ mL or almost } 3 \text{ L}$$

Three Siblings

The children's growth hormone secretion was probably suppressed because of psychosocial stress. Once they felt secure in a loving environment, growth hormone levels returned to normal.

Mrs. Maino

1. Mrs. Maino's thyroid-stimulating hormone (TSH) levels are elevated because her pituitary gland is working overtime to try to stimulate the underactive thyroid gland.
2. Mrs. Maino's metabolism has been slow, so she has been burning fewer calories. When she starts on thyroid replacement hormone, her metabolic rate will return to normal, and she will need more calories. Intake of calories should be balanced with the possible need for weight loss.
3. If Mrs. Maino receives too much thyroid hormone, she will have symptoms of hyperthyroidism, including an increased pulse rate. She should know how to check her pulse and to call her HCP if it is elevated.

SUGGESTED ANSWERS TO CRITICAL THINKING—cont'd

4. The nurse, HCP, and dietitian are essential. A physical therapist may be helpful if mobilization and exercise recommendations are needed. A social worker or discharge planner can help with discharge needs.

Mrs. Tercini

1. Cushing syndrome is caused by too much cortisol. The adrenal cortex is responsible for secreting cortisol.

2. Mrs. Tercini should take two-thirds of her daily dose of hydrocortisone and fludrocortisone in the morning and one-third in the evening, or as ordered. This most closely mimics the body's natural corticosteroid secretion.

3. The flu probably triggered this crisis. Illness is a stressor, and normally the body secretes steroids during stress.

Because Mrs. Tercini's body is unable to produce steroids, she experiences symptoms of hypoadrenalism during stressful times.

4. Mrs. Tercini's blood pressure is low because she has insufficient circulating mineralocorticoids. Without aldosterone, sodium and water are lost and blood pressure drops.

5. Mrs. Tercini should have taken extra medication when she became ill. Her HCP should provide guidelines for dosing during stress and illness.

6.

$$\frac{150 \text{ mcg}}{1{,}000 \text{ mcg}} \left| \frac{1 \text{ mg}}{0.1 \text{ mg}} \right| \frac{1 \text{ tab}}{} = 1.5 \text{ tablets}$$

Review Questions

1. Which assessment finding in a patient who has just returned from having a thyroidectomy should be immediately reported to the health care provider?
   1. Neck discomfort
   2. Sore throat
   3. Tingling fingertips
   4. Sleepiness

2. A patient with syndrome of inappropriate antidiuretic hormone asks the nurse why he has gained 10 pounds. Which response is best?
   1. "The syndrome causes an increase in appetite. As soon as you are effectively treated, the weight should drop back to normal for you."
   2. "You are retaining a lot of sodium and potassium and that causes you to gain water weight."
   3. "You have too much of a hormone in your system that causes you to retain water. The extra 10 pounds is likely water weight."
   4. "Your kidneys are not working correctly, so they can't get rid of extra water from your system."

3. Which assessment finding should the nurse expect to see in the patient with uncontrolled diabetes insipidus? **Select all that apply.**
   1. Edema
   2. Polyuria
   3. Heat intolerance
   4. Diarrhea
   5. Polydipsia
   6. Dehydration

4. Which of the following instructions should the nurse provide to the patient who is being discharged after a thyroidectomy?
   1. "You must take your thyroid replacement every day just as the health care provider prescribed."
   2. "You must weigh yourself daily and report any gain or loss of more than 1 pound."
   3. "You will need to return to the health care provider's office for a weekly blood pressure check."
   4. "You will need to restrict your sodium and potassium intake."

5. Which of the following nursing assessments is most important in the patient with hyperthyroidism and risk for thyrotoxic crisis?
   1. Intake and output
   2. Breath sounds
   3. Bowel sounds
   4. Vital signs

6. Which action by the nurse is most important following hypophysectomy?
   1. Performing a routine neurologic assessment
   2. Encouraging the patient to cough and deep breathe
   3. Monitoring for tracheal edema
   4. Assisting with use of an incentive spirometer

7. Which of the following statements by the patient with hypothyroidism indicates to the nurse that the plan of care has been effective?
   1. "I feel so much better now that my energy is returning."
   2. "I'm really glad the diarrhea has stopped."
   3. "I'm so glad I won't have to take medication for very long."
   4. "My fingers aren't tingling anymore."

Answer rationales available in your online resources.

Key Points

Find the chapter key points in your online resources available through Davis Edge.

Additional Resources

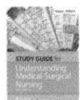

Use the scratch off code on the inside front cover of your book to access online quizzes that will help you to improve your scores on course exams and prepare for the NCLEX-PN®.

Study Guide

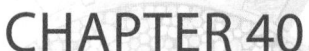

CHAPTER 40

Nursing Care of Patients With Disorders of the Endocrine Pancreas

Paula D. Hopper

KEY TERMS

diabetes mellitus (DYE-ah-BEE-tis mel-EYE-tus)
endogenous (en-DAW-jen-us)
gastroparesis (GAS-troh-puh-REE-sus)
glycosuria (GLY-kos-YOO-ree-ah)
hyperglycemia (HY-per-gly-SEE-mee-ah)
hypoglycemia (HY-poh-gly-SEE-mee-ah)
ketoacidosis (KEE-toh-as-ih-DOH-sis)
Kussmaul respirations (KOOS-mahl RES-per-AY-shuns)
nephropathy (neh-FROP-uh-thee)
neuropathy (new-RAW-puh-thee)
nocturia (nok-TYOO-ree-ah)
polydipsia (PAH-lee-DIP-see-ah)
polyphagia (PAH-lee-FAY-jee-ah)
polyuria (PAH-lee-YOO-ree-ah)
postprandial (POHST-PRAN-dee-uhl)
preprandial (PREE-PRAN-dee-uhl)
retinopathy (RET-ih-NAW-puh-thee)

CHAPTER CONCEPTS

Collaboration
Health Promotion
Metabolism
Nutrition
Patient-Centered Care

LEARNING OUTCOMES

1. Explain the pathophysiologies of type 1 and type 2 diabetes mellitus.
2. Identify risk factors for type 1 and type 2 diabetes mellitus.
3. Describe the signs and symptoms of diabetes mellitus.
4. Describe causes, signs and symptoms, and treatment of high and low blood glucose levels.
5. Discuss how diabetes mellitus increases risk of complications such as heart disease, blindness, and kidney failure.
6. Identify diagnostic tests used to diagnose and monitor diabetes mellitus and its complications.
7. Identify therapeutic measures to help patients with diabetes mellitus control blood glucose levels.
8. Differentiate the action of insulin and oral hypoglycemic agents in lowering blood glucose levels.
9. Plan nursing care and education for the patient with diabetes mellitus.
10. List measures to increase the safety of the patient with diabetes mellitus who is undergoing surgery.
11. Explain reactive hypoglycemia and its treatment.

 DIABETES MELLITUS

Diabetes mellitus is a group of metabolic diseases in which defects in insulin secretion or action result in elevated blood (or plasma) glucose (**hyperglycemia**). Be careful not to confuse diabetes mellitus with diabetes insipidus, which is a disorder of antidiuretic hormone (see Chapter 39.) In this chapter, *diabetes* or *DM* refers to diabetes mellitus. According to the most recent Centers for Disease Control and Prevention (CDC) data,

more than 30 million people in the United States have DM. Another 84 million have prediabetes, up from 70 million in 2011. Direct and indirect costs of diabetes in the United States total $245 billion per year (CDC, 2017).

• WORD • BUILDING •
diabetes mellitus: diabetes—passing through + mellitus—sweet
hyperglycemia: hyper—excessive + glyc—glucose + emia—in the blood

Diabetes is a serious disease that can cause complications such as blindness, kidney failure, heart attack, stroke, and cognitive decline. It is a leading cause of lower limb amputations in the United States. With good education and self-care, patients with diabetes can prevent or delay these complications and lead full, productive lives. Nurses play a major role in helping patients learn to care for themselves effectively.

Pathophysiology and Etiology

Body tissues, and the cells that compose them, use glucose for energy. Glucose is a simple sugar provided by the foods we eat. When carbohydrates are eaten, they are digested into sugars, including glucose, which is then absorbed into the bloodstream. Carbohydrates provide most of the energy used by the body. Glucose is able to enter the cells only with the help of insulin, a hormone produced by the beta cells in the islets of Langerhans of the pancreas (Fig. 40.1). When insulin comes in contact with the cell membrane, it combines with a receptor that allows activation of special glucose transporters in the membrane. By helping glucose enter the body's cells, insulin (1) allows glucose to be used for energy; (2) lowers the glucose level in the blood; and (3) helps the body store excess glucose in the liver in the form of glycogen.

Another hormone, glucagon, is produced by the alpha cells in the islets of Langerhans. Glucagon raises the blood glucose (BG) when needed by releasing stored glucose from the liver and muscles. Insulin and glucagon work together to keep the BG at a constant level.

Diabetes results from deficient production of insulin by the beta cells in the pancreas or from inability of the body's cells to use insulin. When glucose is unable to enter body cells, it stays in the bloodstream; hyperglycemia results, and the cells are denied their energy source. Abnormal glucagon secretion also plays a role in type 2 diabetes (see Fig. 40.1).

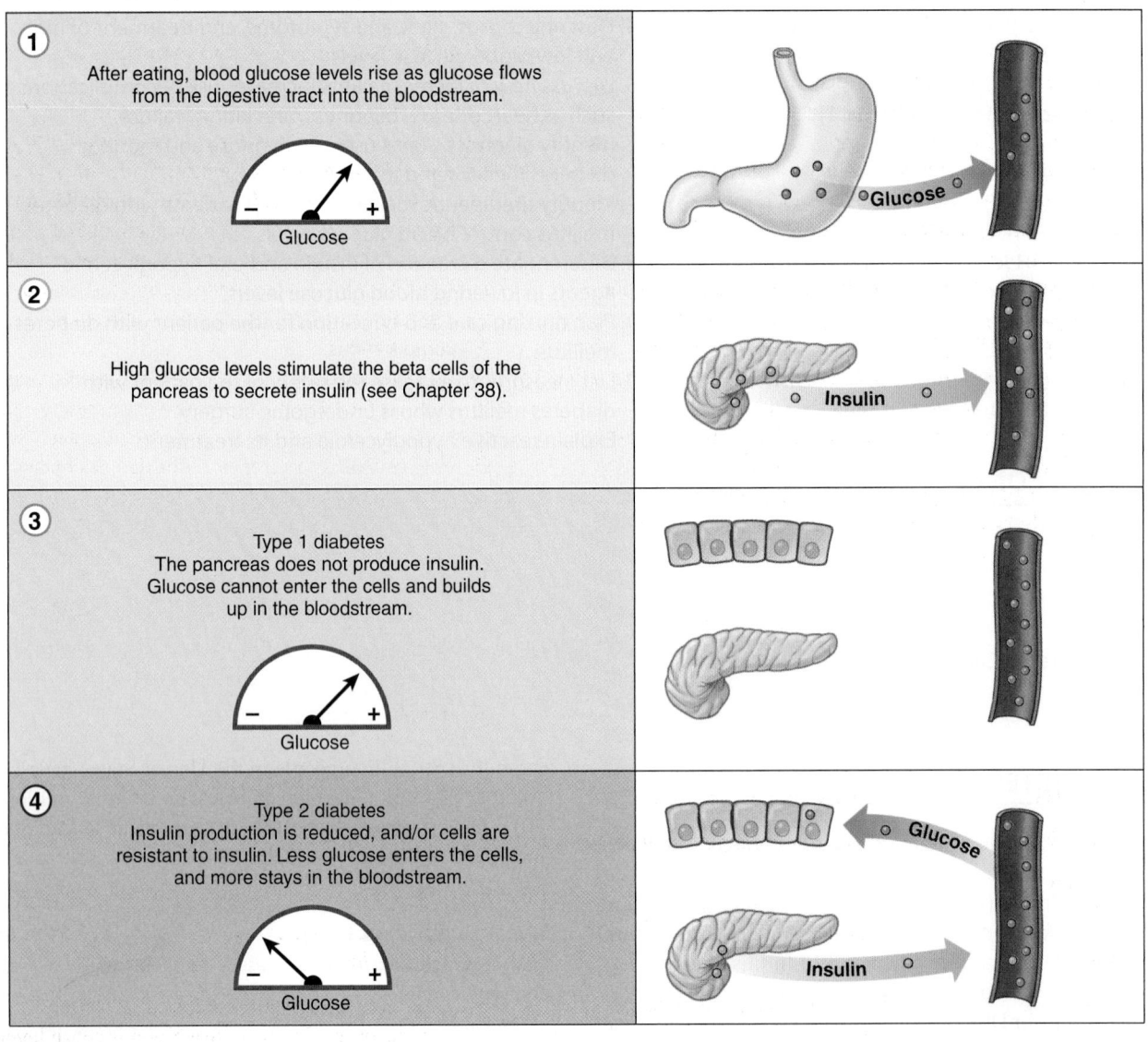

(1) After eating, blood glucose levels rise as glucose flows from the digestive tract into the bloodstream.

Glucose

(2) High glucose levels stimulate the beta cells of the pancreas to secrete insulin (see Chapter 38).

Insulin

(3) Type 1 diabetes
The pancreas does not produce insulin. Glucose cannot enter the cells and builds up in the bloodstream.

Glucose

(4) Type 2 diabetes
Insulin production is reduced, and/or cells are resistant to insulin. Less glucose enters the cells, and more stays in the bloodstream.

Glucose

Insulin

Glucose

FIGURE 40.1 Regulation of blood glucose.

Types of Diabetes

Type 1 Diabetes

Type 1 diabetes (formerly called juvenile diabetes or insulin-dependent diabetes mellitus [IDDM]) is caused by destruction of the beta cells in the islets of Langerhans of the pancreas. When the beta cells are destroyed, they are unable to produce insulin. Insulin must then be injected for the body to use food for energy. Only about 5% of people with diabetes have type 1 diabetes.

It is believed that the pancreas may attack itself following certain viral infections or administration of certain drugs. This is called an autoimmune response. Almost 90% of patients newly diagnosed with type 1 diabetes have islet cell antibodies in their blood. These antibodies might be present for years before actual symptoms of diabetes develop. About 10% of people with type 1 diabetes cases also have a genetic predisposition to its development. The patient diagnosed with type 1 diabetes is most often young and thin and is prone to develop ketoacidosis (discussed later) when BG is elevated. Table 40.1 provides a comparison of type 1 and type 2 diabetes.

Type 2 Diabetes

Ninety-five percent of people with diabetes have type 2 diabetes (formerly called adult-onset diabetes or non–insulin-dependent diabetes mellitus [NIDDM]). In type 2 diabetes, tissues are resistant to insulin. Insulin is still made by the pancreas but in inadequate amounts. Sometimes, the amount of insulin is normal or even high, but because the tissues are resistant to it, hyperglycemia results. As the disease advances, the pancreas eventually wears out, leading to little or no insulin secretion. When this occurs, the patient with type 2 diabetes will require insulin injections. Simply using insulin, however, does not mean the patient has type 1 diabetes. He or she has type 2 diabetes and needs insulin to control the BG level.

Heredity is responsible for about 90% of cases of type 2 diabetes. Obesity is a major contributing factor. Often the patient with a new diagnosis of type 2 diabetes is obese, relates a family history of diabetes, and has had a recent life stressor, such as the death of a family member, illness, or loss of a job ("Patient Perspective: Jim").

Patient Perspective

Jim. I am a 70-year-old white man of European descent. I was diagnosed with type 2 diabetes 5 years ago, and it was a complete and unexpected shock. At the time, I considered myself to be moderately overweight, moderately active, and in reasonably good general health. My physician assistant took the time to explain how he came to the diagnosis (my hemoglobin A_{1c} [HbA_{1c}] was 11.7, and my fasting blood glucose [BG] was 221) and what we could do together to address it. Having him take the time to have this discussion with me reassured me that I would not be facing this new reality alone.

He gave me a booklet detailing the carb content of common foods and instructed me to limit my total carb intake to about 6 to 8 units a day. He prescribed 1,000 mg of metformin daily, with 2.5 mg of lisinopril for kidney protection and 20 mg of atorvastatin as a precaution against future heart disease.

I followed his dietary recommendations religiously. I lost 40 pounds and 6 inches off my waist over the following 6 months! At the end of 18 months, I had reduced my HbA_{1c} to 5.4 and my average fasting BG to about 85. Now, 5 years later, my weight has leveled off at about 140 lb, my HbA_{1c} is 5.0, and I am no longer taking any diabetes medication! The physician assistant keeps me on the lisinopril and atorvastatin as a precaution against future diabetes-related complications.

I would never say that this kind of control has been easy. I struggle to keep a disciplined approach to my eating and to intentionally find ways to stay active. But whenever I feel deprived or start to get lazy, I think of the consequences of uncontrolled diabetes. I don't want to face them, ever.

Table 40.1

Comparison of Type 1 and Type 2 Diabetes

	Type 1	Type 2
Onset	Rapid	Slow
Age at onset	Usually younger than 40	Usually older than 40
Risk factors	Virus, autoimmune response, heredity	Heredity, obesity
Usual body type	Lean	Overweight or obese
High blood glucose complication	Ketoacidosis	Hyperosmolar hyperglycemic state; may develop ketoacidosis
Treatment	Diet, exercise; must have insulin to survive	Diet, exercise; may need oral hypoglycemic agents or insulin to control blood glucose level

TYPE 2 DIABETES IN YOUTH. More and more children and adolescents are developing type 2 diabetes, which in the past only occurred in adults. This is related to increasing obesity and decreasing activity levels in children today. Earlier onset of diabetes increases the risk of early complications and death.

Gestational Diabetes

Gestational diabetes mellitus (GDM) occurs in nearly 1 in 10 pregnancies, especially in women with risk factors for type 2 diabetes. The extra metabolic demands of pregnancy trigger the onset of diabetes. BG usually returns to normal after delivery, but the mother has a higher risk of developing type 2 diabetes. If the mother with GDM is overweight, she should be counseled that weight loss and exercise will decrease her risk of developing diabetes. Mothers with GDM require specialized care and should be referred to an expert in this area.

Prediabetes

Prediabetes refers to BG levels that are above normal but do not meet the criteria for diagnosing diabetes. Prediabetes occurs before the onset of type 2 diabetes. It is diagnosed by evaluating fasting BG level, oral glucose tolerance test (see "Diagnostic Tests" section), or hemoglobin A_{1c} (HgA$_{1c}$). It is important to identify patients with prediabetes, because with lifestyle changes progression to type 2 diabetes can be prevented.

OTHER TYPES OF DIABETES. Secondary diabetes can develop as a result of another chronic illness that damages the islet cells, such as pancreatitis or cystic fibrosis. Prolonged use of some drugs, such as steroid hormones, phenytoin (Dilantin), thiazide diuretics, and thyroid hormone, can also impair insulin action and raise BG. Less common causes include pancreatic trauma and other endocrine disorders.

Metabolic Syndrome

Prediabetes has been linked to a condition called metabolic syndrome. According to the American Heart Association (2015), metabolic syndrome affects about 34% of adults. It is diagnosed when at least three of the following criteria are met:

1. Central or abdominal obesity (measured by waist circumference): men—greater than 40 inches; women—greater than 35 inches
2. Fasting blood triglycerides greater than or equal to 150 mg/dL

3. Blood high-density lipoprotein (HDL) cholesterol: men—less than 40 mg/dL; women—less than 50 mg/dL
4. Blood pressure greater than or equal to 130/85 mm Hg
5. Fasting glucose greater than or equal to 100 mg/dL

Other risk factors include physical inactivity, aging, hormonal imbalance, and genetic predisposition. A major factor is the growing obesity epidemic in the United States.

Any patient who fits this profile should be monitored closely for the onset of type 2 diabetes and heart disease. Patients should be counseled on the importance of a heart-healthy diet, weight loss, physical activity, and control of blood pressure and cholesterol levels.

Signs and Symptoms

Classic symptoms of diabetes include **polydipsia** (excessive thirst), **polyuria** (excessive urination), and **polyphagia** (excessive hunger). The excess glucose in the blood causes an increase in serum concentration, or osmolality. The renal tubules are unable to reabsorb all the extra glucose that is filtered by the glomeruli, and **glycosuria** results. Large amounts of body water are required to excrete this glucose, causing polyuria, **nocturia** (nighttime urination), and dehydration. Increased osmolality and dehydration cause polydipsia. Because glucose is unable to enter the cells, the cells starve, causing polyphagia. High BG can also cause fatigue, blurred vision, abdominal pain, and headaches. Ketones (acidic by-products of fat breakdown) can build up in the blood and urine of patients with type 1 diabetes or late in the course of type 2 diabetes (**ketoacidosis**).

Diagnostic Tests
Fasting Blood Glucose Level

Diagnosis of diabetes is based on BG levels measured by a laboratory. A normal BG level is less than 100 mg/dL. When the fasting BG (drawn after at least 8 hours without eating) is 126 mg/dL or higher, diabetes is diagnosed. A second test may be required if the first test is not clearly diagnostic. If the fasting BG is between 100 and 125 mg/dL, the patient has impaired fasting glucose (IFG) and prediabetes (Fig. 40.2).

• WORD • BUILDING •

polydipsia: poly—many or much + dipsia—thirst
polyuria: poly—many or much + uria—urine
polyphagia: poly—many or much + phagia—to eat
glycosuria: glyc—glucose + uria—urine
nocturia: noc—by night + uria—urine
ketoacidosis: keto—ketones + acid—acidic + osis—condition

Random Blood Glucose

Sometimes, it is not feasible to check a fasting BG. A random BG (RPG) is checked without regard to the last meal. Diabetes is diagnosed if the RPG is 200 mg/dL or greater, with symptoms of diabetes.

Oral Glucose Tolerance Test

Another test to diagnose diabetes is the oral glucose tolerance test (OGTT). An OGTT measures BG at intervals after the patient drinks a concentrated carbohydrate drink. Diabetes is diagnosed when the BG level is 200 mg/dL or higher after 2 hours. A result between 140 and 199 mg/dL at 2 hours leads to a diagnosis of impaired glucose tolerance (IGT) and prediabetes (see Fig. 40.2).

Glycohemoglobin

The glycohemoglobin test, referred to in this chapter as the glycosylated hemoglobin or HbA_{1c}, is used to diagnose diabetes and also to monitor diabetes control. Glucose in the blood attaches to hemoglobin in the red blood cells, which live about 3 months. When the glucose that is attached to the hemoglobin is measured, it reflects the average BG level for the previous 2 to 3 months. This is a helpful measurement when BG levels fluctuate and a single measurement would be misleading. It also assists in monitoring the effectiveness of a patient's treatment plan. A normal HbA_{1c} is less than 5.7%. An HbA_{1c} of 6.5% or higher is diagnostic for diabetes. An HbA_{1c} between 5.7% and 6.5% indicates prediabetes. Once diagnosed, most patients with diabetes are advised to keep their HbA_{1c} below 7% (see Fig. 40.2).

Newer methods allow this test to be done in a health care provider's (HCP's) office while the patient waits. See Table 40.2 for average fasting BG levels based on HbA_{1c} results.

Glycohemoglobin testing might be inaccurate in some people, such as those with anemia. These patients may instead be tested for fructosamine, which is a similar test that indicates glucose levels over a period of 1 to 2 weeks instead of 3 months.

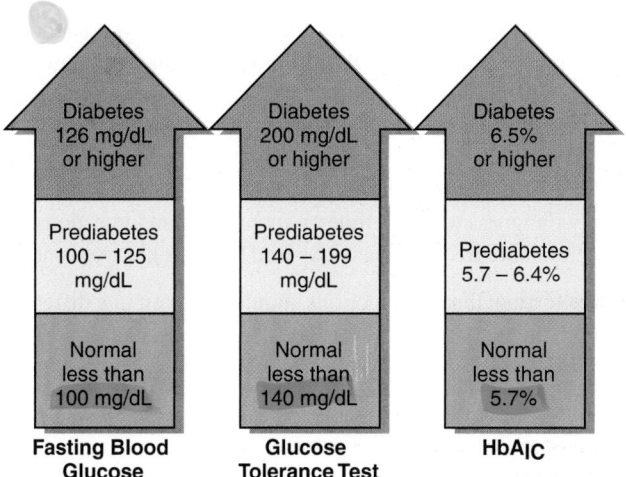

FIGURE 40.2 Tests used to determine whether a patient has normal blood glucose levels, high-risk prediabetes, or diabetes include fasting blood glucose, oral glucose tolerance, and hemoglobin A_{1c}.

Table 40.2

Correlation Between HbA_{1c} and Mean Fasting Blood Glucose

HbA_{1c} (%)	Fasting Blood Glucose (mg/dL)
6	126
7	154
8	183
9	212
10	240
11	269
12	298

Estimated Average Glucose

Some HCPs use a calculation to convert HbA_{1c} results to estimated average glucose (eAG) numbers, which may be more meaningful to patients. The formula is as follows:

$$28.7 \times HbA_{1c} - 46.7 = eAG$$

Here is an example for a patient whose HbA_{1c} is 8.6:

$$28.7 \times 8.6 - 46.7 = 200.12$$

This can be rounded to 200 mg/dL.

Additional Tests

Because diabetes affects so many body systems, additional tests recommended for baseline data include a lipid profile, serum creatinine, and urine microalbumin levels to monitor kidney function, urinalysis, and electrocardiogram.

CRITICAL THINKING

Mr. McMillan is a 50-year-old patient brought into the emergency department with extreme fatigue and dehydration. After the health care provider (HCP) sees him, you ask Mr. McMillan some additional questions. Based on his answers, you request that the HCP add a random glucose level to the laboratory tests ordered. The result is 1,400 mg/dL.

1. What questions would you ask Mr. McMillan if you suspected diabetes?
2. Why was Mr. McMillan fatigued?
3. Why was he dehydrated?

Suggested answers are at the end of the chapter.

Prevention

It is possible to prevent type 2 diabetes. Research studies have shown that patients who have prediabetes can prevent or delay the onset of diabetes with loss of 7% of body weight and moderate physical activity for at least 150 minutes per week (American Diabetes Association [ADA], 2018). Use of the diabetes medication metformin can also help prevent diabetes in patients with prediabetes. Patients at risk should have their BG level checked regularly. Research studies are ongoing to try to find ways to prevent type 1 diabetes once antibodies have been detected.

Therapeutic Measures

The only cure for diabetes is a pancreas or islet cell transplant. However, diabetes can be controlled. Treatment begins with diet and exercise. Insulin is added for patients with type 1 diabetes, and, for those with type 2 diabetes, insulin or oral hypoglycemic medication is added as needed. Weight loss is essential for patients who have type 2 diabetes and are overweight or obese. BG monitoring and education are also important for good diabetes control.

To monitor the effectiveness of treatment, patients should have regular health care follow-up visits. The ADA (2018) suggests the following goals and recommendations:

• HbA$_{1c}$ (every 3 to 6 months): Less than 7%
• Preprandial capillary glucose: 80 to 130 mg/dL
• Peak postprandial capillary glucose: Less than 180 mg/Dl
• Blood pressure: Less than 140/90 mm Hg

Target levels for blood glucose are different in hospitalized patients.

Goals of Treatment

The ADA (2018) recommends that most patients maintain a **preprandial** (premeal) BG level of 80 to 130 mg/dL, a peak **postprandial** (postmeal) BG level of less than 180 mg/dL, and HbA$_{1c}$ level of less than 7% to prevent or delay complications of diabetes. Because of the risk for cardiovascular disease, the ADA also recommends maintaining blood pressure of less than 140/80 mm Hg. All goals should be adjusted to individual circumstances. For example, the patient who is unable to feel symptoms of **hypoglycemia** (low BG) might have a higher preprandial glucose goal to prevent undetected hypoglycemic episodes.

Nutrition Therapy

Because the patient with diabetes has a limited amount of insulin, either **endogenous** (from within the body) or injected, it is important to eat foods that will not exceed the insulin's ability to carry it into the cells. Because carbohydrates contribute most to the BG level, the amount of carbohydrates consumed is especially important. If a patient eats a small amount of carbohydrate one day and a large amount the next, the BG will fluctuate, leading to complications. It is possible to create a more flexible nutrition plan if the patient is able to test BG frequently at home and adjust treatment accordingly.

The ADA recommends a complete assessment by a specially trained dietitian and an individualized nutrition therapy plan and teaching (see "Nutrition Notes"). The education of the patient with diabetes is a process that may take months and cannot be accomplished in a single visit or with a paper handout or referral to a web site.

Exercise

Exercise lowers BG by reducing insulin resistance and improving insulin action in the muscles and liver. The effects can last up to 48 hours. Exercise also improves blood lipid levels and circulation, which is important because diabetes increases risk of cardiovascular disease. Patients are instructed to engage in moderate aerobic exercise at least 150 minutes per week, spread over at least 3 days in a week. In addition, it is important to avoid a sedentary lifestyle and to interrupt prolonged sitting with light activity at least every 30 minutes. Resistance exercise also improves glycemic control, strength, and ability to perform daily activities (ADA, 2018).

Patients with complications of diabetes must be careful in their exercise choices (see "Long-Term Complications" later in this chapter). The HCP or an exercise physiologist should be consulted for an individualized exercise plan.

Persons with diabetes who take insulin or medications that increase insulin secretion should check their BG before exercise and always carry a quick source of glucose when exercising in case the BG drops too low. They should also be cautious about exercising at the time of day when their BG is at its lowest point (i.e., when insulin or medication action is peaking) and to have a carbohydrate snack before exercising if BG is less than 100 mg/dL.

Caution patients to avoid exercise if they have ketones in their blood or urine. This indicates that insufficient insulin is available and glycogen may be released during exercise, further increasing the serum glucose.

Medication

INSULIN. The person with type 1 diabetes has no endogenous insulin and, therefore, must inject insulin daily. At this time, insulin cannot be taken by mouth because it is a protein and is, therefore, digested. Inhaled insulin is available but is not widely used; the hope is that researchers will find a way to create oral insulin in the near future. Insulin is typically given subcutaneously; fast-acting insulin may be ordered via the intramuscular or intravenous (IV) route in urgent situations. Several types of insulin are available with various schedules by which they may be given. The type and schedule are determined by the HCP in collaboration with the patient based on the patient's lifestyle and willingness to spend time on monitoring and injections. In general, more frequent injections lead to better glucose control.

Site Rotation. Insulin injections should be given in a different subcutaneous site with each dose to avoid tissue injury. A

• WORD • BUILDING •
preprandial: pre—before + prandial—meal
postprandial: post—after + prandial—meal
hypoglycemia: hypo—deficient + glyc—glucose + emia—in the blood
endogenous: endo—within + genous—to produce

Nutrition Notes

Diabetic Meal Plans. Nutrition is integral to the management of diabetes and can be a challenging aspect of treatment for patients. No single approach is suitable for everyone but should be individualized based on the patient's health status and lifestyle, cultural preferences ("Cultural Considerations"), ability to learn, and willingness to change (Lutz, Mazur, & Litch, 2015).

Overall goals and strategies differ by type of diabetes. In general:

- Patients with type 1 diabetes need to prevent wide swings in blood glucose (BG) levels through careful timing of meals and snacks in relation to insulin therapy and activity.
- Patients with type 2 diabetes use diet modifications with medication as needed to maintain near-normal glucose, blood pressure, and lipid levels and to lose weight as needed.

People with diabetes usually benefit from eating on a regular basis (every 4 to 5 hours while awake). Evidence has shown that the use of sucrose (table sugar) as part of the meal plan does not impair BG control in individuals with diabetes.

A certified diabetes educator (CDE) can create a meal plan based on the patient's abilities, past dietary habits, and commitment. Several meal-planning approaches are described next.

Create Your Plate. The American Diabetes Association (ADA, 2016) has devised a simple method of meal planning that divides a plate into one half and two quarters. Half the plate is filled with nonstarchy vegetables. One quarter is filled with starchy foods, such as whole grains and starchy vegetables. The last quarter is used for meats and meat substitutes. Finally, a serving of fruit and an 8-ounce glass of nonfat or low-fat milk completes the meal (Fig. 40.3).

Examples of foods suitable for each section of the plate are provided at www.diabetes.org/food-and-fitness/food/planning-meals/create-your-plate/?loc=ff-diabetesmealplans.

Carbohydrate Counting. Because the carbohydrate is the energy nutrient that has the greatest influence on BG levels, the amount and timing of carbohydrate intake directly affect diabetes control. Only carbohydrates are counted with this system, but patients are counseled to eat about the same amount of protein each day and to choose low-fat foods. Reading labels is mandatory (e.g., some fat-free products are higher in carbohydrates than the items they replace). A patient is taught to read food labels (each 15 grams of carbohydrate equals 1 carbohydrate exchange). The patient is then prescribed a number of carbohydrate exchanges for each meal and snack.

Carbohydrate counting classifies all carbohydrates together, whether from starch, fruit, or milk (Table 40.3). This method offers more flexibility both in food choices within a day's meal plan and in insulin dosage than other systems and may achieve better control of BG.

Despite those advantages, carbohydrate counting may entail the following:

- Weighing and measuring food
- Keeping food records
- Monitoring BG before and after eating
- Controlling body weight

This system does not permit carbohydrate intake as desired. Patients should maintain their carbohydrate intake at the same level each day to keep BG as close to normal as possible (ADA, 2017).

Glycemic Index/Glycemic Load. All carbohydrates are not metabolized identically. Foods containing equal amounts of carbohydrate affect BG levels differently. The glycemic index (GI) is a classification of foods according to the speed and degree of change they produce in BG levels. The standard is commonly set with glucose given a value of 100; other foods are then compared with glucose. Whether the food is in a raw or cooked state affects the GI of the food. For example, raw carrots have a GI of 16, and cooked carrots have a GI of 60. A GI less than 55 is low, 56 to 69 is moderate, and 70 to 100 is high. The GIs of foods are based on the same portion of food and not necessarily on a normal portion size. When determining how portion size affects the GI of a food, a glycemic load (GL) is calculated by multiplying GI times the carbohydrate per serving divided by 100. An 80-g serving of raw carrots has 8 g of carbohydrate, and an 80-g serving of boiled cooked carrots has 6 g of carbohydrates; therefore, the GL of raw carrots is 1 and 3.6 for cooked carrots. A GL of less than 10 is considered low, 11 to 19 is medium, and 20 or greater is high. Both forms of carrots would be appropriate for individuals following a low GI/GL diet. Motivated patients can incorporate low GI/GL foods into the successful management of their disease (ADA, 2014).

References

American Diabetes Association. (2014). Glycemic index and diabetes. Retrieved from www.diabetes.org/food-and-fitness/food/what-can-i-eat/understanding-carbohydrates/glycemic-index-and-diabetes.html

American Diabetes Association. (2016). Create your plate. Retrieved from www.diabetes.org/food-and-fitness/food/planning-meals/create-your-plate/?loc=ff-diabetesmealplans

American Diabetes Association. (2017). Carbohydrate counting. Retrieved from www.diabetes.org/food-and-fitness/food/what-can-i-eat/understanding-carbohydrates/carbohydrate-counting.html

Lutz, C., Mazur, E., & Litch, N. (2015). *Nutrition and diet therapy* (6th ed.). Philadelphia, PA: F.A. Davis Company.

Cultural Considerations

African Americans, Hispanics and Latinos, American Indians, Pacific Islanders, and some Asian Americans are more at risk for type 2 diabetes than whites (Centers for Disease Control and Prevention, 2017). The "standard" diabetic diet may need significant adjustment to consider foods from various cultures; the typical food exchange list may prove unhelpful because it may not include foods common in a patient's culture. In such cases, the patient may be considered to be nonadherent to therapy when, in reality, the health care provider has not considered cultural food preferences. Helping the patient choose a meal plan that considers his or her culture is important. Some helpful web sites include www.diabetes.org and www.eatright.org.

sample rotation chart is shown in Figure 40.4. Because each area absorbs insulin at a slightly different rate, it is advisable to use one area for a week, then move on to the next area. Within that area, each injection should be spaced at least 2 inches from the previous injection. Some experts recommend using primarily the abdomen to provide more uniform absorption. Aspirating for blood before injection and rubbing the site after injection are not recommended with insulin injections.

Insulin Pumps. Patients who desire tighter control of BG levels and a more flexible lifestyle may choose to use an insulin pump (Fig. 40.5). A pump delivers insulin via a tiny catheter continuously in small (basal) amounts. The catheter is placed in subcutaneous tissue and remains in place for 2 to 3 days. The patient can then add a bolus of insulin with the push of a button before meals or snacks. This provides insulin levels that are more normal, like those of a person without diabetes.

Table 40.3
Example of Carbohydrate Counting

Prescribed Carbohydrate Choices (1,200 to 1,500 kilocalories/day)	Carbohydrate Selected*
Breakfast	
3	¾ cup dry cereal
	8 oz skim milk
	½ cup unsweetened orange juice
Lunch	
3	8-oz regular cola
	1 cup melon
	1 slice whole-wheat bread
Dinner	
3	½ cup cooked potato
	½ cup corn
	½ cup regular ice cream
Snack	
1	8 oz skim milk

*Additional proteins and fats are added in moderate amounts but need not be counted. Each item selected is approximately 15 grams carbohydrate or 1 carb exchange.

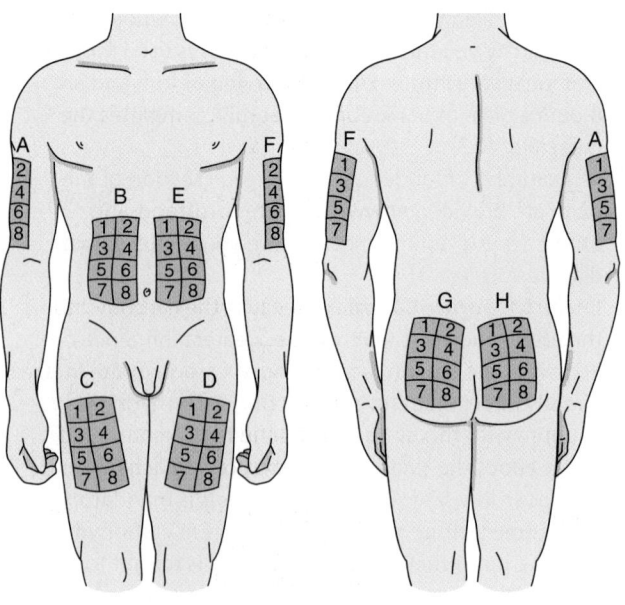

Rotation sites for injection of insulin.

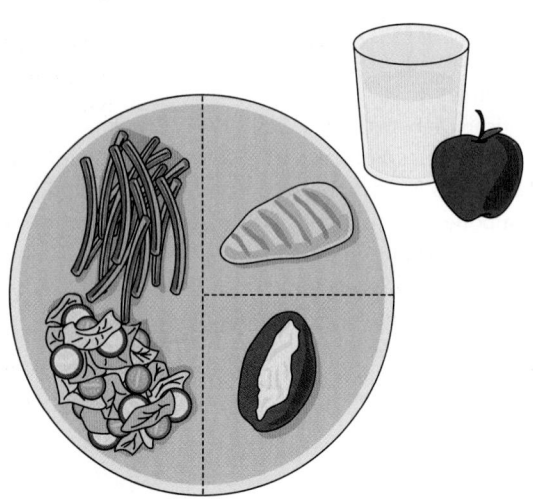

FIGURE 40.3 An example of the diabetes plate method.

FIGURE 40.4 Sample insulin rotation chart.

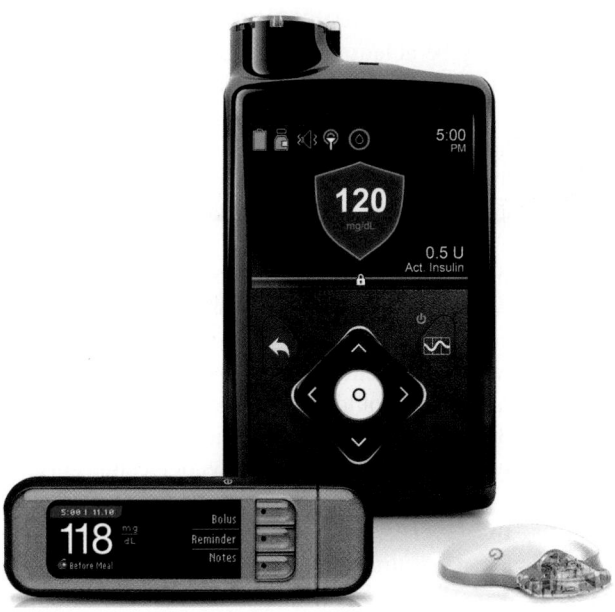

FIGURE 40.5 MINIMED™ insulin pump with optional glucose monitor.

A pump typically is worn on the abdomen or buttocks. Some models receive input from continuous glucose monitors.

Insulin Sources. Insulin is synthetically produced in a laboratory. It is either identical to human insulin or different by one or two amino acids (called insulin analogs). In the past, insulin was derived from cows and pigs; this type of insulin is no longer available in the United States but may be available from other countries. Be careful to check the source when preparing insulin for injection, especially if you work in home health care situations in which patients could purchase their insulin online from another country. Insulins from different sources may act slightly differently. Some people may be allergic to beef or pork preparations or may refuse them based on cultural beliefs.

Onset, Peak, and Duration. Once insulin is injected, a period elapses before it begins to lower BG. This time is called the *onset of action.* The *peak action* occurs when the insulin is working at its hardest and the BG is at its lowest point. It is during this peak time that the patient is most at risk for an episode of low BG. *Duration of action* is the length of time the insulin works before it is used up. Onset, peak, and duration are determined by whether the insulin is short, intermediate, or long acting (Table 40.4). It is important for the individual with

Table 40.4
Onset, Peak, and Duration of Insulins

Insulin Type	Example	Onset	Peak	Duration	When to Give
Very short-acting	Insulin lispro (Humalog)	5–15 min	30–90 min	5 hr or less	Not more than 15 minutes before meal
	Insulin aspart (NovoLog)	10–20 min	1–3 hr	3–5 hr	
	Insulin glulisine (Apidra)	15 min	60 min	2–4 hr	
	Inhaled insulin (Afrezza)	15 min	30 min	2–3 hr	
Short-acting	Insulin regular (Humulin R, Novolin R)	30 min	2–5 hr	5–8 hr	Not more than 30 minutes before meal
Intermediate-acting	Insulin neutral protamine Hagedorn (NPH) (Humulin N, Novolin N)	1–2 hr	6–12 hr	18–26 hr	Not more than 30 minutes before meal
Basal	Insulin glargine (Lantus AE) Insulin detemir (Levemir)	1–2 hr	No peak	Up to 24 hr	The same time each day

Note: A variety of premixed formulas is also available.

diabetes and the nurse to be aware of the onset, peak, and duration of any insulin given. This informs decisions about certain situations, such as when to give insulin in relation to meals, when to exercise, and when to be alert to low BG symptoms.

Insulin Regimens. Patients work with their HCPs to determine the best regimen to meet their needs and fit their lifestyles. Some patients are only willing to take one or two injections a day. More patients are now choosing to take more frequent injections to achieve better, "tighter" control of BG. These patients are often taught to adjust their insulin dose based on BG level and the amount of carbohydrates eaten. Although patients who choose tight control have to be more cautious about risk for hypoglycemia, it can significantly reduce the risk of long-term complications.

A common regimen called *basal-bolus therapy* mimics normal insulin secretion. This consists of an injection of a basal insulin (such as insulin glargine [Lantus]) once a day, often at bedtime, to provide a constant small amount of insulin in the bloodstream. Then an injection of very short-acting insulin (such as insulin lispro [Humalog]) is given before meals to mimic the extra insulin that is secreted normally with meals.

Sliding-Scale Insulin. Some patients receive varying doses of short-acting insulin before meals based on their BG reading. An example of a sliding scale might read as follows: "BG <140, 0 units; BG 141–170, 2 units; BG 171–200, 4 units; >200 call HCP." This is useful when the patient is ill and glucose levels are unstable or when adjustments need to be made. However, routine use of sliding-scale insulin is not recommended because, although it corrects an already-high BG, it is preferable to prevent hyperglycemia before it happens with routine insulin doses.

Mixing Insulins. When two insulins need to be given at the same time, they can often be mixed together to prevent having to give more than one injection (see Davis Edge for the procedure). Preset mixtures of intermediate- and short-acting insulins are also available.

CRITICAL THINKING

Mrs. Evans is a 78-year-old woman with type 2 diabetes who resides in the long-term care facility at which you work. She is on 42 units of insulin glargine (Lantus) every evening and 10 units of insulin lispro (Humalog) before each meal.

1. What time should you administer her Lantus insulin? If she eats her meals at 0800, 1200, and 1700, when should her Humalog insulin be administered? (*Hint:* See Table 40.4.)
2. At what time of day should she be alert for symptoms of low blood glucose?
3. What could happen if Mrs. Evans feels ill and misses her lunch?
4. Mrs. Evans receives an apple with her meal but cannot eat it because her dentures do not fit well. She is on a carbohydrate-counting meal plan. What should you do?

Suggested answers are at the end of the chapter.

ORAL HYPOGLYCEMIC MEDICATION. The patient with type 2 diabetes may be able to control BG levels with nutrition therapy and exercise alone. If needed, oral hypoglycemic medication or insulin will also be prescribed. Oral hypoglycemic agents are not insulin pills but work to produce more insulin (e.g., by stimulating the pancreas) or make the tissues more sensitive to insulin. Because many oral hypoglycemic agents depend on at least a partially functioning pancreas, they are not useful for patients with type 1 diabetes. Table 40.5 lists commonly used oral hypoglycemic agents and their mechanisms of action.

Most oral hypoglycemic agents should be administered before meals. Care should be taken to prevent passage of more than 30 minutes between medication administration and the meal because this may result in a hypoglycemic episode. Check individual drugs for specific timing.

If the BG level is not controlled with an oral hypoglycemic agent, insulin may be needed for the person with type 2 diabetes. However, the goal of insulin use is different than for the person with type 1 diabetes: While insulin may be needed to control BG, insulin is not needed to sustain life as is the case for the person with type 1 diabetes.

INJECTABLE HYPOGLYCEMIC MEDICATION. A newer group of medications is the incretin mimetics. These are injectable drugs that were first isolated in the saliva of the Gila monster, a poisonous lizard native to the United States and Mexico. See Table 40.5 for examples.

Another injectable drug, pramlintide (Symlin), is used with insulin. It is a synthetic analog of amylin, a naturally occurring hormone that reduces glucose levels following meals. It may also promote weight loss in individuals who are overweight. Patients using Symlin have an increased risk of hypoglycemia.

NATURAL REMEDIES. Many herbs and other natural remedies have been promoted for diabetes treatment. Some patients have tried cinnamon for blood sugar control, but there is no scientific evidence that it is effective. If your patient wishes to try a natural remedy, it is essential to encourage a conversation with his or her HCP first.

Self-Monitoring of Blood Glucose

The ability to test BG levels at home has been a major advance in diabetes care. BG can be better controlled because of the availability of monitoring at any time, in any place. A variety of BG monitors are on the market at reasonable prices (Fig. 40.6). Most of the cost involved in monitoring is in the test strips that must be used. Health insurance programs may cover this cost.

Self-monitoring schedules are based on specific patient needs and abilities. A patient taking multiple daily injections of insulin will usually test before meals and snacks, occasionally postprandially, at bedtime, before exercise, when experiencing low BG, and before critical activities such as driving (ADA, 2018). Less frequent schedules may be prescribed for patients who are unable or unwilling to test so often or for patients who take oral hypoglycemic agents.

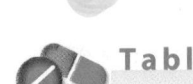
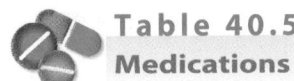

Table 40.5

Medications for Type 2 Diabetes Mellitus

Medication Class/Action

Alpha-Glucosidase Inhibitors (AGIs) – Oral

Lower postprandial glucose by reducing rate of carbohydrate digestion and absorption.

Examples	Nursing Implications
acarbose (Precose) miglitol (Glyset)	Give at start of each meal. No weight gain or hypoglycemia risk. Multiple dosing is less convenient. If used in combination with another drug and hypoglycemia occurs, treat with milk or glucose tablets, not table sugar.

DPP-4 Inhibitor – Oral

Inhibits DPP-4, an enzyme that breaks incretins. Incretins are hormones secreted by the gastrointestinal system in response to food; they reduce glucagon secretion and increase insulin synthesis and release.

Examples	Nursing Implications
sitagliptin (Januvia) saxagliptin (Onglyza) linagliptin (Tradjenta)	Administer once a day. Only works when blood glucose is high so does not cause hypoglycemia when used alone. Watch for allergic reactions.

Biguanide – Oral

Decreases glucose production by liver; increases glucose uptake by muscle.

Examples	Nursing Implications
metformin (Glucophage, Glucophage XR, Fortamet, Riomet, Glumetza)	Give with meals. May enhance weight loss. Withhold if patient is having tests involving contrast dye. Contraindicated in renal and hepatic disease and heart failure. Monitor serum creatinine level. Notify health care provider of early symptoms of lactic acidosis (e.g., hyperventilation, myalgia, malaise).

Sulfonylureas – Oral

Stimulate insulin secretion by pancreas and increase insulin receptor sensitivity.

Examples	Nursing Implications
glipizide (Glucotrol) glimepiride (Amaryl) glyburide (Micronase, Diabeta, Glynase Prestab)	Monitor patient for hypoglycemia. Teach patient to avoid alcohol.

Incretin Mimetics – Injected

Mimic natural incretins in the body to (1) stimulate insulin release and (2) reduce glucagon release in response to nutrients in the intestine.

Examples	Nursing Implications
exenatide (Byetta, Bydureon) liraglutide (Victoza) dulaglutide (Trulicity)	Administered as a subcutaneous injection. Check individual agent information or web sites for instructions on use of pens and auto-injectors. May promote weight loss. Slows gastric emptying, so may alter absorption of oral medications.

Continued

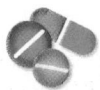

Table 40.5

Medications for Type 2 Diabetes Mellitus—cont'd

Medication Class/Action

Sodium-Glucose Cotransporter-2 (SGLT2) Inhibitors – Oral

Reduce reabsorption of glucose by kidneys, increasing glucose excretion in urine.

Examples	Nursing Implications
canagliflozin (Invokana)	Monitor for hypotension, hyperkalemia, urinary tract infection, and vaginal yeast infection.
empagliflozin (Jardiance)	Monitor renal function.
dapagliflozin (Farxiga)	

Combination Agents – Oral

Examples	Nursing Implications
metformin and glyburide (Glucovance)	See individual agents.
metformin and rosiglitazone (Avandamet)	
glipizide and metformin (Metaglip)	

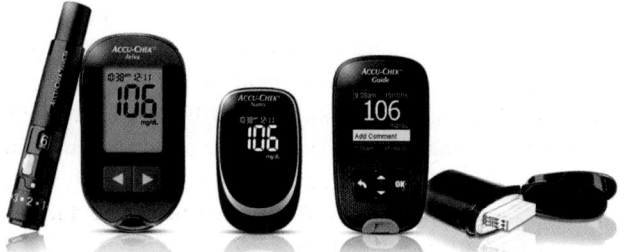

FIGURE 40.6 Glucose meters.

New devices are available that continuously monitor glucose via a small catheter inserted into the abdomen. The device records the glucose level at frequent intervals on a monitor that is worn like a pager on a belt. It can be set to alarm if the BG level drops too low.

The diabetes provider should be consulted for desirable BG ranges because these may differ for each patient. The ADA recommends a preprandial goal of 80 to 130 mg/dL for most patients. Patients who are prone to hypoglycemia or small children or older adults may have higher goal ranges,

such as 100 to 150 mg/dL. Lower BG levels for these populations could increase the risk of hypoglycemia.

An important aspect of BG monitoring is the interpretation of results. Monitoring is useless if the results are not used to improve BG control. The patient should be instructed to keep a diary of BG levels (Fig. 40.7). Some patients have computer software that graphs results. The patient may be taught by a diabetes educator to interpret the trends in the results, or the diary may be taken on a regular basis to the HCP for interpretation and adjustment of the treatment plan.

Urine Glucose and Ketone Monitoring

Urine also may be tested for glucose and for ketones. Urine glucose testing was done routinely before the development of self-monitoring of BG. A variety of dipsticks and tape products are available for urine testing. Glucose in the urine makes the patient aware that the BG is elevated, but the actual level is unknown. Most people have glucose in their urine when their BG is more than about 180 mg/dL, although this can be highly variable. It is difficult to base treatment on urine glucose levels, so routine urine testing for glucose is no longer recommended.

Day			Break-fast	Lunch	Supper	Bedtime	Urine Ketones	Notes
Sunday		Time	7:00	11:30	6:00	11:00		
		Glucose	186	108	116	142		
		Insulin	10 units Humalog	10 units Humalog	10 units Humalog	32 units Lantus		
Monday		Time	7:30	12:00	6:00	10:30	6:00–neg	Ate cake at
		Glucose	171	97	302	180		Betty's party
		Insulin	10 units Humalog	10 units Humalog	10 units Humalog	32 units Lantus		at 3 pm–oops!
Tuesday		Time						
		Glucose						
		Insulin						

FIGURE 40.7 Sample diary of blood glucose results and insulin use.

Urine should be tested for ketones (ketonuria) during acute illness or stress, when BG levels are elevated in ketosis-prone patients, or when symptoms of ketoacidosis are present (see later in this chapter). If ketones are present, the patient knows an insulin deficiency is present and should notify the HCP. Patients with type 1 diabetes are most at risk for developing ketoacidosis; however, it is wise for the patient with type 2 diabetes to test for ketones if risk factors are present. Table 40.6 provides a review of diabetes symptoms, diagnosis, and treatment.

Weight Loss

Weight loss can help the patient with type 2 diabetes control BG, blood pressure, and blood lipid levels. Weight loss can even help prevent the need for medication in some patients. In obese patients who have difficulty losing weight with usual measures, bariatric (weight loss) surgery may be considered. There are several bariatric surgeries that may be effective; see Chapter 33 for more information.

Transplant

If the patient is evaluated to be an appropriate candidate, a pancreas transplant may be considered. This is especially beneficial in the patient with kidney disease, who can receive both a kidney and pancreas transplant at the same time. Another promising treatment is the implantation of pancreatic islet cells.

Table 40.6
Diabetes Summary

Signs and Symptoms	• Polyuria • Polydipsia • Polyphagia • Fatigue • Blurred vision • Headache
Diagnostic Tests	Fasting blood glucose (BG) HbA$_{1c}$ (glycosylated hemoglobin) Oral glucose tolerance test (OGTT) Additional testing for complications
Therapeutic Measures	Nutrition therapy Exercise Insulin Oral hypoglycemic medication Self-monitoring of BG levels Education
Complications	Hypoglycemia, hyperglycemia Diabetic ketoacidosis, hyperosmolar hyperglycemia Long-term complications
Priority Nursing Diagnosis	*Risk for Unstable Blood Glucose Level*

Acute Complications of Diabetes

A person with diabetes is at risk for a variety of complications. Acute complications related to high and low BG levels are treatable and can be prevented with appropriate care.

Hyperglycemia

When calories eaten exceed insulin available or glucose used, high BG (hyperglycemia) occurs. A common cause of hyperglycemia is eating more than the meal plan prescribes. Another major cause is stress. Stress causes the release of counterregulatory hormones, including epinephrine, cortisol, growth hormone, and glucagon. These hormones all increase the BG level. In a person without diabetes, this is an adaptive function. However, the patient with diabetes is unable to compensate for the increased BG with increased insulin secretion, and hyperglycemia results.

Patients must be able to recognize signs and symptoms of high BG levels and know what to do if they occur (Table 40.7). For many patients, these are similar to the symptoms they experienced when they were first diagnosed with diabetes. Chronic high BG levels can lead to long-term complications (discussed later in this chapter).

MORNING HYPERGLYCEMIA. Sometimes, patients experience elevated morning BG levels even though they have not eaten all night. *Dawn phenomenon* is caused by normal hormone fluctuation during the night as well as release of stored glucose, leading to morning hyperglycemia. The *Somogyi effect* occurs when BG drops too low during the night due to a missed snack or too much insulin. The body responds by releasing counterregulatory hormones (epinephrine, glucagon, corticosteroids, growth hormone), which then cause rebound hyperglycemia in the morning.

The patient might be asked to monitor BG between 0200 and 0400 in addition to bedtime and morning testing to assess whether the Somogyi effect or the dawn phenomenon is occurring. The patient and HCP will work together to adjust meal and insulin timing and stabilize BG.

Hypoglycemia

Low BG, or hypoglycemia, occurs when there is not enough glucose available in relation to circulating insulin. This is sometimes referred to as an *insulin reaction*. Hypoglycemia is usually defined as a BG level below 70 mg/dL, although patients may feel symptoms at higher or lower levels. Occasionally, symptoms occur as a result of a rapid drop in BG, even though the actual glucose level is normal or high. Common causes of hypoglycemia are skipping a meal, exercising more than usual, or accidentally administering too much insulin. An occasional hypoglycemic episode, treated promptly, should not lead to chronic complications. Repeated or extremely low BG levels can cause neurologic damage because there is not enough glucose for brain function. It is, therefore, important to teach patients and families how to recognize, prevent, and treat low BG (see Table 40.7).

Initial symptoms of hypoglycemia are caused by activation of the sympathetic nervous system. These may include

Table 40.7

Comparison of High and Low Blood Glucose Levels

	Hyperglycemia	*Hypoglycemia*
Causes	Overeating Stress Illness Too little insulin or medication	Undereating, skipping a meal Too much insulin or medication Exercise
Symptoms	Polyuria Polydipsia Polyphagia Blurred vision Headache Lethargy Abdominal pain Ketonuria Coma	Hunger Sweating Tremor Blurred vision Headache Irritability Confusion Seizures Coma
Treatment	Confirm hyperglycemia with glucose meter; if patient is at risk, check urine for ketones and increase fluid intake. Assess cause of hyperglycemia, and teach prevention. Return to prescribed treatment plan if applicable. Call health care provider (HCP) for medication adjustment if indicated or if blood glucose exceeds 180 mg/dL for 2 days. Call HCP if patient is ill or vomiting.	Confirm hypoglycemia with glucose meter (if able). Administer 15 g fast-acting carbohydrate. Recheck glucose in 15 minutes. If still low, readminister carbohydrate. Continue cycle of checking glucose and administering fast sugar until hypoglycemia subsides. If symptoms worsen, call HCP or emergency help. Administer glucagon subcutaneously or dextrose 50% via intravenous route if ordered. Assess cause of hypoglycemia, and teach prevention.

hunger, sweating, pallor, tremor, palpitations, and headache. As hypoglycemia progresses, the brain is deprived of glucose (called *neuroglycopenia*). Neurologic symptoms, such as irritability, confusion, seizures, and coma, may occur.

BE SAFE!

BE VIGILANT! You can prevent hypoglycemia in your patients by being aware of who is at risk and when they are most at risk, and monitoring for early symptoms. If you recognize early symptoms, such as shaking or hunger, and respond quickly, you can prevent a much more serious complication for your patient.

CRITICAL THINKING

Jeff is a 16-year-old who is having trouble with repeated episodes of hypoglycemia. He says he has not had this trouble before, and it is interfering with his new job. What questions might you ask as you do your assessment to help him figure out how to prevent future episodes?

Suggested answers are at the end of the chapter.

To treat hypoglycemia, administer a "fast sugar" (15 to 20 grams of carbohydrate that will enter the bloodstream quickly). Examples of fast sugars include the following:

- 4 oz orange juice
- 4 oz regular (not diet) soda
- 8 oz low-fat milk
- Miniature box of raisins
- Commercial glucose tablets or gel
- 6–8 Life Savers® (or other hard candies)

If the patient is not alert or is unable to safely swallow, subcutaneous glucagon can be given. If the patient is hospitalized, IV 50% dextrose can be administered by the registered nurse (RN). Recheck the BG in 15 minutes. If it does not return to at least 70 mg/dL, repeat the procedure every 15 minutes until 70 mg/dL is reached, even if the patient is feeling better. Do not overtreat hypoglycemia with too much sugar because this can cause hyperglycemia and rebound hypoglycemia.

If you find someone with symptoms of altered BG but are unable to identify whether it is high or low, do a BG test. However, if the patient has neurologic symptoms, treat for low BG immediately. The BG may then be checked and further treatment provided as indicated.

NURSING CARE TIP

Avoid the temptation to add sugar to orange juice to treat hypoglycemia. This practice can raise the blood glucose (BG) too much. Also avoid giving a form of sugar that has fat in it (such as chocolate). This will slow down its digestion and delay recovery of the BG level.

Once the hypoglycemic episode is resolved, the patient should eat a complex carbohydrate to prevent recurrence, unless the next meal is within a half hour. If symptoms worsen instead of improving, call 911 or contact the RN or HCP. Always be aware of agency protocol for treating hypoglycemic episodes.

Some older adult patients with poor autonomic nervous system function or patients taking beta-adrenergic blocking medication such as propranolol or atenolol (which block the sympathetic response) may not feel the symptoms of hypoglycemia. These patients should check glucose levels more often and keep the levels in a safe range to prevent hypoglycemic episodes.

All people with diabetes should be instructed to keep a fast sugar in their purse or pocket at all times ("Patient Perspective: Dave"). Fast sugars may also be stored in bedside tables, cars, and desks at work.

Patient Perspective

Dave. Right after eating lunch, I headed for the woods on a cloudy mid-March afternoon. I began sawing firewood, splitting it, and loading up the trailer. I did not take insulin with lunch like I normally would because the extra activity increases the risk of hypoglycemia. I've had type 1 diabetes for nearly 60 years, so I have a lot of experience with hypoglycemia. After a short time of working, I began to sense that feeling. For me, it is an interruption of clear thinking. I immediately stopped work, went to my stash of hard candies and shoved 10 pieces into my mouth, and began to head home. My house is only a very short distance from the woods. I started up the tractor and headed home. As I pulled down the trail to the main road, the tractor quit. I spent maybe 2 minutes attempting to start it, so, with a sense of apprehension, I decided to walk the short distance to the house. Six hours later, I awakened in the emergency room. I had decided after walking only 40 yards to lie down in my neighbor's yard and take a nap. I obviously do not remember any of this. The neighbor had arrived home and saw a body in her yard and called for help. My body temperature was so low the ER staff was not sure whether I was going to make it. I am still feeling blessed and thankful to God that I survived this and have learned valuable lessons. I do not ever cut wood alone anymore. I have since begun using a continuous glucose monitor and an insulin pump that has a threshold suspend feature that stops the flow of insulin in the event of hypoglycaemia.

Diabetic Ketoacidosis

PATHOPHYSIOLOGY. Diabetic ketoacidosis (DKA) occurs when BG levels are very high and insulin is deficient. This most commonly occurs in people with type 1 diabetes, but it may occur in type 2 diabetes when insulin deficiency exists, usually late in the disease process. DKA symptoms are often the reason a person with undiagnosed type 1 diabetes first seeks help. It may also be the result of stress or illness in a person with previously diagnosed diabetes. When there is insufficient insulin to allow glucose into cells, the cells starve. The body then breaks down fat to be used for energy. The fat breakdown releases an acid substance called *ketones*. As ketones build up in the blood, ketoacidosis occurs.

The body attempts to compensate for acidosis by deepening respirations to blow off excess carbon dioxide. Because carbon dioxide combines with water in the body to form carbonic acid, blowing off carbon dioxide is like blowing off acid. (See the section on metabolic acidosis in Chapter 6.) This deep, sighing respiratory pattern is called **Kussmaul respirations.** The expired air has a fruity odor caused by the ketones and may be mistaken for alcohol. Some nurses have likened the odor to Juicy Fruit® chewing gum.

With such high BG and the accompanying polyuria, the body becomes dehydrated very quickly. Tachycardia, hypotension, and shock can result. Acidosis also causes potassium to leave the cells and accumulate in the blood (hyperkalemia). Potassium is then lost in large amounts in the urine, which can lead to hypokalemia. The combination of dehydration, potassium imbalance, and acidosis causes the patient to develop flu-like symptoms, including abdominal pain and vomiting. The patient loses consciousness and death occurs if DKA is not treated. The mortality rate for DKA is about 2%.

THERAPEUTIC MEASURES. Treatment includes IV fluids, IV or subcutaneous insulin, and BG monitoring, often initially in an intensive care unit setting. Glucose is added to the IV when the BG drops to about 180 mg/dL to avoid hypoglycemia. Potassium should also be monitored closely because it is essential to have normal levels for cardiac function. Arterial blood gases help monitor acidosis. The cause of the DKA should be identified and treated.

Prevention of ketoacidosis involves careful monitoring of BG levels at home. Teach at-risk patients to use a urine dipstick (Ketostix) to check for ketones if BG is elevated or if they are ill or under stress. If ketones are present, the HCP should be notified. Instruct patients never to stop their insulin without an HCP's supervision.

Hyperosmolar Hyperglycemic State

PATHOPHYSIOLOGY. Hyperosmolar hyperglycemic state (HHS; also called hyperosmolar hyperglycemic nonketotic syndrome [HHNKS]) occurs mainly in type 2 diabetes, when BG levels are high and the patient has reduced fluid intake as a result of stress or illness. Because the person with type 2 diabetes has some insulin production, cells do not starve, and DKA usually does not occur. HHS occurs more often in older adults.

As BG level rises (hyperglycemia), polyuria causes profound dehydration, producing the hyperosmolar (concentrated) state. BG may rise as high as 1,500 mg/dL, and electrolyte imbalances occur. Because ketoacidosis is not present, the patient may not feel as physically ill as the patient with DKA and may delay seeking treatment. Symptoms of HHS develop slowly and include extreme thirst, lethargy, and mental confusion. Shock, coma, and death occur if it is left untreated. The mortality rate for HHS is higher than for DKA.

THERAPEUTIC MEASURES. Treatment includes IV fluids and insulin as well as glucose monitoring. Electrolytes are closely monitored. The cause of HHS should be identified and treated. HHS can be prevented with careful monitoring of glucose levels at home. Instruct patients to drink plenty of fluids if BG levels are beginning to rise, especially in times of stress and illness. They should also know when to call their HCP with high BG results.

NURSING CARE TIP

Government insurers (Medicare and Medicaid) consider diabetic ketoacidosis, hyperosmolar hyperglycemic state, and hypoglycemic coma to be preventable problems. They will no longer pay hospitals for the extra expense of caring for patients who develop these conditions after they are hospitalized. You can help control costs by being vigilant for early signs and symptoms of these complications and reporting them promptly.

Source: www.cms.gov/HospitalAcqCond

Long-Term Complications

Over time, chronic hyperglycemia causes a variety of serious complications in persons with diabetes. These involve the circulatory system, eyes, kidneys, skin, and nerves. Most of the complications involve either the large blood vessels in the body (macrovascular complications) or the tiny blood vessels, such as those in the eyes or kidneys (microvascular complications). The Diabetes Control and Complications Trial (DCCT), a large classic research study completed in 1993, showed that individuals with type 1 diabetes who maintain tight control of BG experience fewer long-term microvascular complications than individuals who take traditional care of their diabetes (Diabetes Control and Complications Trial Research Group, 1993). Similarly, the United Kingdom Prospective Diabetes Study (UKPDS), completed in 1998, showed that individuals with type 2 diabetes who maintain an HbA_{1c} below 7% can significantly reduce complications. In fact, for every percentage of decrease in HbA_{1c}, there were 25% fewer deaths from diabetes-related complications (United Kingdom Prospective Diabetes Study Group, 1998). Unfortunately, tight control can be accompanied by an increased risk of hypoglycemia, and even tight control does not guarantee the prevention of all long-term complications.

Macrovascular Complications

CIRCULATORY SYSTEM. People with diabetes develop atherosclerosis and arteriosclerosis faster than the general population. They are more likely to have hypertension and elevated low-density lipoprotein (LDL) cholesterol and triglyceride levels. High BG can also affect platelet function, leading to increased clotting. These problems lead to a higher incidence of stroke, heart attack, and poor circulation in the feet and legs. The risk of cardiovascular disease and stroke is two to four times more common in persons with diabetes than in the general population.

Control of BG, blood pressure, and cholesterol levels is vital to help prevent these deadly complications. Patients should also avoid smoking, maintain normal weight, and exercise regularly. All patients should be evaluated by their HCP for treatment with aspirin or other antiplatelet medication, angiotensin-converting enzyme (ACE) inhibitor, or angiotensin-receptor blocker (ARB) therapy for blood pressure control and statin therapy for control of blood lipids.

Microvascular Complications

EYES. Small blood vessels can become diseased, eventually leading to some degree of retinopathy in most patients with diabetes. **Retinopathy** involves damage to the tiny blood vessels that supply the eye. Small hemorrhages occur, which can cause blindness if not corrected. Diabetes is a leading cause of blindness in adults in the United States (CDC, 2017). Good control of BG and blood pressure can reduce the risk of retinopathy. Newer laser surgery techniques may help improve vision after hemorrhages occur. Diabetes is also associated with a high incidence of cataracts. Patients with diabetes should have a yearly dilated eye examination.

KIDNEYS. Nephropathy is caused by damage to the tiny blood vessels in the kidneys. Native Americans, Hispanics, and African Americans have the highest risk. A primary risk factor for diabetic nephropathy is poor control of BG. If nephropathy occurs, the kidneys are unable to remove waste products and excess fluid from the blood. Diabetes is the leading cause of end-stage renal (kidney) disease (ESRD) in the United States. When the kidneys have lost most of their function, patients may have their blood cleansed artificially by either hemodialysis or peritoneal dialysis (see Chapter 37). The only cure for ESRD is a kidney transplant.

Patients should be taught the importance of BG control to prevent or delay kidney disease. ACE inhibitor and ARB medications have been shown to slow the development of kidney problems in patients with diabetes. Patients who have both diabetes and hypertension should be placed on an ACE inhibitor or ARB. Routine urine tests are done to check for albumin in the urine. A trained renal dietitian should work with the patient and HCP to determine the best diet for protecting the kidneys.

• WORD • BUILDING •
retinopathy: retino—nervous tissue of the eye + pathy—illness
nephropathy: nephro—of the kidney + pathy—illness

Nerve Complications

Another complication of diabetes is **neuropathy,** which is damage to nerves as a result of chronic hyperglycemia. Neuropathy can cause numbness and pain in the extremities, erectile dysfunction (impotence) in men, sexual dysfunction in women, **gastroparesis** (delayed stomach emptying), and other problems. Unfortunately, neuropathic pain is difficult to treat with traditional analgesics. Anticonvulsant agents gabapentin (Neurontin) and pregabalin (Lyrica) help reduce painful nerve impulses. Certain antidepressant agents may also help control nerve pain. Improved control of BG levels may also help.

Infection

Persons with diabetes are prone to infection for several reasons. If injuries occur, healing may be slow because of impaired circulation. There may not be enough blood supply to heal the wound or fight an infection. For the same reason, it may be difficult for IV antibiotics to reach an infected site, and topical antibiotics may be preferable. In the presence of hyperglycemia, white blood cells become sluggish and ineffective, further reducing the body's ability to fight infection.

The incidence of periodontal (gum) disease, caused by bacteria in plaque, is also increased in individuals with diabetes. Patients must be taught to maintain good oral hygiene and make regular visits to the dentist. The ADA recommends all patients with diabetes follow guidelines for routine vaccinations against flu, pneumonia, and hepatitis.

Foot Complications

The combination of macrovascular disease, neuropathy, and risk for infection makes patients with diabetes prone to foot problems. Consider the patient who has no feeling in his or her feet because of neuropathy. If the patient has a foot injury, it may be not noticed right away. Vascular disease will prevent good blood supply from preventing infection and promoting healing. If infection sets in, it is slow to resolve and may progress to necrosis and gangrene. Pressure points on the feet also increase risk for pressure injuries (Fig. 40.8). One woman had a pen in her shoe all day and did not realize it! Neuropathy can also lead to deformities of the feet, further increasing the risk of injuries.

For these reasons, diabetes is the leading cause of nontraumatic amputation of the lower extremities in the United States. Teaching patients how to care for their feet and prevent complications is an important role for the licensed practical nurse/licensed vocational nurse (LPN/LVN) (Box 40.1). If any sores are noted, the patient should not delay in seeking

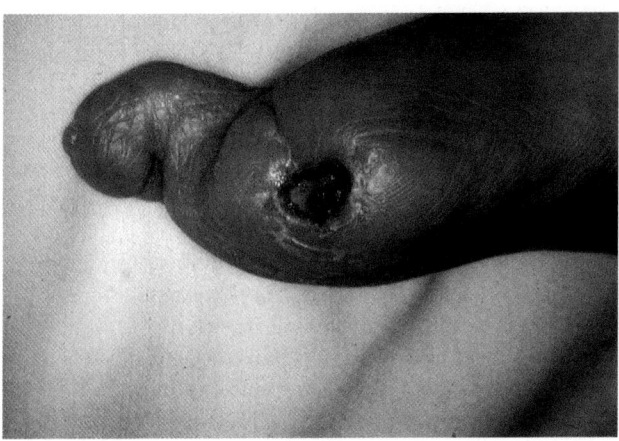

FIGURE 40.8 Diabetic foot ulcer at site of amputated toe.

Box 40.1

Foot Care Tips

- Wash and dry feet every day. Use warm (not hot) water to avoid burns.
- Apply lotion that does not contain alcohol, avoiding areas between toes.
- Inspect feet for sores or red areas daily (have a family member help if necessary).
- Report any abnormalities immediately.
- Wear leather shoes and white or light-colored cotton socks.
- Never go barefoot.
- Avoid garters and tight socks.
- Avoid crossing legs.
- Cut toenails to natural shape of nail (not into corners).
- See a podiatrist for calluses or problem toenails (avoid "bathroom surgery").
- Have feet checked at least once a year (preferably three to four times a year) for loss of sensation.

treatment. During routine visits to the HCP, teach the patient to be sure to remove shoes and socks so the feet can be thoroughly examined. The HCP or diabetes specialist can test sensation in the feet with tiny filaments. Loss of protective sensation is an early risk factor for amputation, so any reduction in sensation is a warning sign that extra care must be taken. Patients should be referred to a podiatrist (foot doctor) or specialized wound treatment center if problems occur. (See Davis Edge for "Ethical Considerations.")

NURSING CARE TIP

When you do routine patient assessments, **always** look carefully at your patients' feet. Remove shoes and socks, examine all skin surfaces, and look between toes. Report any redness, lesions, or other suspicious areas. **You** could make the difference between a small, treatable wound and an amputation!

NURSING CARE TIP

Encourage patients to wear white or light-colored socks. One woman did not know she had a wound on her foot till she saw blood coming through her white cotton socks.

• **WORD • BUILDING •**

neuropathy: neuro—nervous system + pathy—illness
gastroparesis: gastro—stomach + paresis—partial paralysis

CRITICAL THINKING

Mr. Jones is a 54-year-old banker with type 2 diabetes admitted to your unit with a tiny red area on his right heel. His admitting blood glucose is 360 mg/dL. The lesion is so small you wonder what the fuss is about. While doing his assessment, you find that he wore a new pair of shoes to work all day about a month ago and has been avoiding seeing his health care provider about the resulting red area. He is placed on intravenous (IV) antibiotics, and, within 3 days, the red area has broken open and has yellow drainage. He is sent home with topical antibiotics and crutches, to be followed by a visiting nurse. The wound takes 6 months to fully heal.

1. List three risk factors for foot problems.
2. Why did the sore take so long to heal?
3. Why do you think crutches are necessary?
4. Why might topical antibiotics work better than IV antibiotics?
5. The nurse documents the following description of Mr. Jones's wound: "Small red open area on heel, with yellow drainage on dressing." What is wrong with this charting? How can you improve it?
6. What team members should be involved with Mr. Jones's care?

Suggested answers are at the end of the chapter.

Special Considerations for the Patient Undergoing Surgery

Surgery is a stressor. The counterregulatory hormones released during stress cause the BG to rise, even if the patient has been fasting. High BG levels interfere with immune function and healing and can increase the patient's risk for infection.

Critically ill patients also do not tolerate low BG. Therefore, glucose levels in critically ill hospitalized patients should be maintained between 140 and 180 mg/dL, preferably with the use of IV insulin (ADA, 2018).

Check with the HCP for actual insulin orders. Often, patients are placed on IV infusions of glucose and insulin during and immediately after surgery, in place of longer-acting insulins. Monitor BG levels every 2 to 4 hours or as ordered, and monitor carefully for signs and symptoms of hypoglycemia or hyperglycemia. If a patient uses a pump at home, check with a diabetes resource nurse to determine whether the patient can continue to use it during hospitalization.

Patients who were not previously on insulin may be placed on insulin during surgery and postoperatively. They can generally return to their presurgical treatment plan after the stress of surgery is past.

Nursing Process for the Patient With Diabetes Mellitus
Data Collection

A complete nursing history and physical examination should be carried out because diabetes affects every body system. Some areas on which to focus are listed in Table 40.8. It is especially important to assess each patient's knowledge of diabetes and its care so that appropriate teaching can be done.

Nursing Diagnoses, Planning, and Implementation

Because diabetes affects so many different areas, nearly any nursing diagnosis may be appropriate. See "Nursing Care Plan for the Patient With Diabetes Mellitus" for an example of the diagnosis *Risk for Unstable Blood Glucose Level*. The actual presence of the defining characteristics should be confirmed with the patient before choosing any nursing diagnosis.

Table 40.8
Data Collection for the Patient With Diabetes Mellitus

Subjective Data	• Age and symptoms at onset • Understanding of diabetes (type 1 or type 2) and self-care • Current treatment plan (medication, nutrition therapy, exercise) and adherence to plan • Frequency of blood glucose (BG) self-monitoring and pattern of BG levels (check diary if patient has kept one) • History of diabetes-related complications • Involvement of family or other support systems
Objective Data	• Vital signs • Height, weight, body mass index • Skin: integrity, turgor, condition of injection sites • Feet: pulses, color, temperature, skin integrity, pressure points, sensation • Laboratory results: BG, HbA$_{1c}$, creatinine, lipid profile, albuminuria, urine and serum ketones

Nursing Care Plan for the Patient With Diabetes Mellitus

Nursing Diagnosis: *Risk for Unstable Blood Glucose Level*
Expected Outcomes: The patient will maintain at all times an HbA$_{1c}$ less than 7%, a preprandial glucose of 80 to 130 mg/dL, and a postprandial glucose less than 180 mg/dL. The critically ill hospitalized patient treated with insulin will maintain blood glucose (BG) measurements between 140 and 180 mg/dL. The noncritically ill hospitalized patient treated with insulin will maintain a preprandial glucose level of less than 140 mg/dL and a random glucose level of less than 180 mg/dL. Verify individual goals with the health care provider (HCP).
Evaluation of Outcomes: Are BG levels within predetermined parameters? Does the patient show understanding of diabetes self-care?

Intervention	Rationale	Evaluation
Assess knowledge of diabetes self-care.	*Teaching should be initiated only if a knowledge deficit exists.*	Does patient exhibit knowledge of diabetes self-care?
Assist patient to collaborate with HCP to determine appropriate BG levels and action to be taken if BG level is too high or too low.	*Appropriate BG levels may be different for each patient. The patient should know what BG levels require notification of the HCP.*	Does patient state appropriate BG levels and action to take if glucose is high or low?
Teach patient to assess glucose levels before meals and at bedtime or as ordered by HCP. Ensure that patient knows how to obtain glucose monitor and instruction for home use.	*Good BG control depends on knowledge of glucose levels and trends.*	Does patient demonstrate correct use of glucose monitor or state how monitor and instruction will be obtained?
In a hospitalized patient who is taking nothing by mouth (NPO) or on continuous feeding, check glucose level every 4 to 6 hours around the clock. Check patient on insulin drip every 1 to 2 hours.	*Regular BG monitoring is needed for scale insulin administration and maintaining glucose levels within safe parameters.*	Is BG monitoring carried out on an appropriate schedule?
Teach patient how to administer insulin or oral hypoglycemic agent after evaluating BG. Ensure that meals are timed appropriately with medications. Replace any uneaten carbohydrate foods to prevent hypoglycemia.	*If most medications are taken without appropriate food to supply calories, hypoglycemia can occur. Check individual medication for specific instructions.*	Does patient state appropriate meal and medication schedule?
Teach technique for administering insulin if indicated.	*Patient and family will be administering insulin independently at home.*	Does patient demonstrate correct injection technique?
Observe for symptoms of hypoglycemia and hyperglycemia, and treat as needed. Teach causes, prevention, recognition, and treatment of hypoglycemia and hyperglycemia.	*If patient has a good understanding of hypoglycemia and hyperglycemia, most episodes can be prevented. If hypoglycemia or hyperglycemia does occur, prompt treatment is essential to prevent complications.*	Does patient state causes, prevention, symptoms, and treatment of hypo- and hyperglycemia? Does patient carry fast sugar at all times?
Administer 15 to 20 g of glucose or carbohydrate if BG level falls below 70 mg/dL or according to institution hypoglycemia guidelines. Contact registered nurse or HCP if BG is above 180 mg/dL.	*A "fast sugar" provides prompt treatment of hypoglycemia to prevent complications. Glucose levels over 180 mg/dL are associated with poor outcomes.*	Does "fast sugar" resolve hypoglycemic episode within 15 minutes? If not, repeat. Are glucose levels within safe range?

(nursing care plan continues on page 834)

Nursing Care Plan for the Patient With Diabetes Mellitus—cont'd

Intervention	Rationale	Evaluation
Consult with dietitian for nutrition therapy instruction.	*The dietitian is trained to provide in-depth meal plan instruction.*	Is patient able to state plan for obtaining appropriate meals?
Teach patient on insulin to eat additional complex (not fast-acting) carbohydrate before exercise if glucose is less than 100 mg/dL.	*Exercise can further lower BG.*	Does patient state appropriate plan for eating additional carbohydrate?
Consult with social worker or case manager as needed.	*Some patients may not have the resources or support to carry out effective self-care.*	Does patient state availability of adequate resources for self-care at home?
Provide patient with information for obtaining comprehensive diabetes education.	*Instruction provided in the hospital usually is not comprehensive. Outpatient diabetes classes can provide additional self-care and health promotion information.*	Does patient state plan for obtaining further diabetes education after discharge?
Assist patient to obtain medical alert card or tag that identifies diabetes.	*If the patient is ever unresponsive for any reason, the HCP would need to be aware of diabetes condition.*	Does patient state plan to carry or wear identification at all times?
Geriatric		
Assess ability to see and manipulate syringe, glucose monitor, and other equipment. Obtain assistive devices as needed.	*The older adult patient may have poor eyesight or other sensory deficits.*	Is patient able to manipulate equipment to safely care for self?

Once diagnoses have been identified, planning should be done with both the patient and family. Diabetes affects not only the person with the disease, but the entire family. The desired outcomes for the plan of care are for the patient to be knowledgeable about and able to care for his or her disease and to prevent complications. Consult the dietitian, social worker, certified diabetes educator, home health nurse, outpatient education programs, and other resources as needed ("Home Health Hints").

Evaluation

The best indicator of the success of a care plan for diabetes is controlled BG and HbA_{1c} within target levels. The patient should be without symptoms of hypoglycemia or hyperglycemia and be able to state what to do if they do occur. Long-term complications should be minimized. Another important indicator is the patient's statement of satisfaction and comfort with the plan and his or her ability to carry it out on a daily basis.

Diabetes Self-Management Education

The individual with diabetes must receive diabetes self-management education if at all possible. No amount of care

from an HCP or nurse can replace the self-care required of the person with diabetes. The involvement of family or significant others is also important for the successful treatment and well-being of the person with diabetes.

If the patient is hospitalized at diagnosis, initial instruction is done in the hospital. However, hospital stays are so short, you cannot waste any time. Begin assessing baseline knowledge and teaching as soon as the patient is feeling physically well enough to learn. Depending on your state nurse practice act, this may be the responsibility of the primary or registered nurse, although aspects of the instruction may be delegated to the LPN/LVN. Some hospitals have a certified diabetes educator who provides classroom or bedside instruction. The dietitian should be contacted to provide nutrition instruction.

Most hospitals have policies or management plans describing the instruction to be provided by the nurse. Generally, this encompasses *survival skills*, which include the basic information the patient needs initially to survive at home. Survival skills include medication administration, glucose monitoring, meal plan basics, and what to do if high or low BG levels occur. A variety of helpful aids, such as pamphlets and videos, is available. Diabetes equipment suppliers provide

Home Health Hints

• Call the patient the day before performing a venipuncture for a fasting blood glucose (BG) and remind him or her not to eat after midnight.

• Record a blood sugar at every visit. If patient has not yet taken the blood sugar, have him or her take it while you are there. This will allow you to see whether the patient can use the glucometer independently, that the glucometer is working, and that the patient has adequate strips and lancets. If supplies are needed, assist the patient in ordering.

• Some home glucose monitoring devices have a memory that the nurse can access during the visit. It gives the date, time, and BG result. This is a good indication of adherence with self-monitoring performed by patient or caregiver.

• Even if patients have had diabetes for many years, observe them preparing and injecting their insulin. This provides an opportunity to praise good technique or correct bad habits.

• Patients with newly diagnosed diabetes may be anxious and overwhelmed. Have the patient repeat instructions to you and perform return demonstrations.

• Store prefilled syringes in the refrigerator flat or with needles pointing up. This prevents crystals from settling and clogging the needles. Allow syringes to come to room temperature before injecting.

• If the patient has a visual or dexterity problem, suggest a syringe magnifier (check with the pharmacy) or a prefilled insulin pen. A referral to occupational therapy may also be appropriate.

• Patients with vision problems can become isolated and depressed. Assist your patient with obtaining vision aids that can help improve social outlets.

• Teach the patient not to skip meals. Assist the patient to identify easy but nutritious meals, such as frozen dinners that are low in sodium. Another option is Meals on Wheels, which can deliver meals that are tailored to special diets. If part of the treatment is weight loss, encourage the patient to keep a food diary for 3 days to track areas in need of change.

• Teach patients to discard used syringes and needles in a hard plastic container (e.g., a Clorox bottle with a screw top) if red needle boxes are not available.

• Teach patients to use a mirror to look at the bottom of the feet or have a family member examine the patient's feet regularly.

• Teach patients to wear comfortable shoes and avoid sandals, high heels, and flip flops. If necessary, the health care provider can request a podiatry consult. A podiatrist can arrange for the patient to be measured and fitted with special shoes that reduce pressure on problem areas. Special shoes may be covered by Medicare.

• Teach patients to keep a pair of nonskid slippers at the bedside. If the patient needs to get up in the night to use the restroom, putting on secure slippers can help prevent the possibility of stepping on something and causing a foot injury.

• Teach the caregiver that hot water heaters should be set below 120°F (48.8°C) to avoid a possible burn, because many patients with diabetes have decreased skin sensation.

kits that are full of samples and information. These are a significant help when you are teaching a patient. Also advise the patient to purchase a medical alert bracelet or necklace.

It is difficult to know how to operate and teach glucose monitoring with the variety of glucose monitors available. Many drugstores and medical supply stores not only sell the monitors but also provide training for the patient and family. You can obtain this information by calling local medical suppliers or by contacting the certified diabetes educator or discharge planner at your institution.

After discharge, the patient should be referred to outpatient diabetes classes for further instruction. If classes are unavailable or if the patient is unable to leave home, a referral to a visiting nurse should be made. It is usually advisable to have a nurse present for the patient's first insulin injection at home. The American Association of Diabetes Educators recommends that diabetes self-management education include information about the following:

• Diabetes pathophysiology and treatment options
• Healthy eating
• Physical activity
• Medications usage
• Monitoring and using patient-generated health data (such as BG)
• Preventing, detecting, and treating acute and chronic complications
• Healthy coping with psychosocial issues and concerns
• Problem-solving (Beck et al., 2017)

The American Diabetes Association has helpful resources for both you and your patients at www.diabetes.org.

Because many people with diabetes are older, it is important to be aware of the special needs of the older population ("Gerontological Issues").

 REACTIVE HYPOGLYCEMIA

Reactive hypoglycemia, also called postprandial hypoglycemia, occurs when BG drops below a normal level following meals, usually below 50 mg/dL. Hypoglycemia is most often a complication of diabetes treatment, but at times it may occur without the presence of diabetes. It may be a warning sign of impending diabetes.

Pathophysiology and Etiology

Low BG can occur as an overreaction of the pancreas to eating. The pancreas senses the BG level rising and produces more

Evidence-Based Practice

Clinical Question
What are the most helpful strategies for glucose control in patients with diabetes?

Evidence
A systematic review of 775 studies found that self-efficacy, dietary adherence, and stress management were strong predictors of metabolic control as measured by HbA_{1c} levels (Brown et al., 2016).

Implications for Nursing Practice
This study stresses keeping the number of clinical goals and behavioral changes to a minimum to achieve success. Patients who feel they have the ability to manage health behavior change will have a higher rate of success in reaching goals. In addition, it is important for patients to understand that dietary control and stress management are key in the management of diabetes and HbA_{1c} levels.

Reference
Brown, S. A., Garcia, A. A., Brown, A., Becker, B. J., Conn, V. S., … Cuevas, H. E. (2016). Biobehavioral determinants of glycemic control in type 2 diabetes: A systematic review and meta-analysis. *Patient Education and Counseling, 99*(10), 1558–1567.

Gerontological Issues

Diabetes and Older Adults. Diabetes care can be a challenge for many older adults:

- Blood glucose goals can be relaxed in some older adults, as long as acute hyperglycemic complications are avoided.
- Older adults with diabetes should be assessed for cognitive impairment and depression; both conditions can make self-management difficult.

- Syringe magnifiers and talking glucose meters are available for those with impaired vision.
- Family members can be taught to draw up a week's supply of insulin for the patient to store in the refrigerator. Family members should also be able to recognize signs and symptoms of hypo- and hyperglycemia.
- Home meal programs can help ensure an adequate diet.
- Older adults should have an emergency call system in the home and regular contact with family members or other support people.

insulin than is necessary for the use of that glucose. As a result, the BG drops to below normal. It may be due to abnormally low levels of glucagon or, alternatively, to high levels of insulin. True reactive hypoglycemia is a rare condition and many "hypoglycemic" episodes are instead related to activation of the sympathetic nervous system for other reasons, without true hypoglycemia.

Signs and Symptoms
Low BG causes release of epinephrine, which in turn causes the BG to rise. Epinephrine release causes a fight-or-flight reaction, which may produce shaking, sweating, and palpitations. Headache, chills, and confusion may also occur. Symptoms are the same as those described earlier related to hypoglycemia in diabetes.

Diagnosis
Patients can test for hypoglycemia with a home glucose monitor when they have symptoms. These results may then be taken to the HCP for interpretation.

Therapeutic Measures
Treatment includes frequent small meals and avoidance of fasting. Simple sugars are avoided because they can aggravate symptoms. High-fiber foods, complex carbohydrates, and proteins are recommended.

SUGGESTED ANSWERS TO CRITICAL THINKING

Mr. McMillan
1. "Have you been eating or drinking more than usual? Have you been urinating more than usual? Do you get up at night to urinate? How is your appetite? Does anyone in your family have diabetes?"
2. Fatigue occurs because the glucose is unable to enter the cells without insulin, so they are starving.
3. Mr. McMillan is dehydrated because he is losing excessive amounts of urine as his kidneys lose excess glucose.

Mrs. Evans
1. Insulin glargine (Lantus) should be given the same time each day. The order says each evening; any time in the evening is okay as long as it is consistent. Insulin lispro (Humalog) is very fast acting so it should be given no more than 15 minutes before eating, ideally when her food is ready to eat so no delay can occur.
2. She should be alert for low blood glucose (BG) 30 to 90 minutes after she receives her Humalog dose, the peak action time for Humalog. Eating her meal after her insulin dose should prevent hypoglycemia.
3. If Mrs. Evans receives insulin and misses her meal, she will likely develop hypoglycemia. If you know she is not feeling well, it would be best to hold her insulin for that meal until you speak with the health care provider.

SUGGESTED ANSWERS TO CRITICAL THINKING—cont'd

4. She can eat another fruit that has the same amount of carbohydrate. Applesauce, canned sugar-free peaches or pears, or other soft fruits would be appropriate.

Jeff

What kind of new job is it? What schedule is he working? Is it more physically strenuous than his previous job? Does it interfere with his usual meal schedule? What other changes has he experienced in his life that may have affected his BG?

Mr. Jones

1. Poor circulation, neuropathy, and slow wound healing place Mr. Jones at risk for problems.
2. Circulation to the foot may be poor, and white blood cells are sluggish if the BG is high.

3. Any pressure on the foot while walking may further impair circulation. He should not bear weight on the affected foot.
4. If circulation to the area is poor, intravenous antibiotics may not reach the sore.
5. "Small red open area on right posterior heel, 1 cm × 1.5 cm, 2 mm deep, 2-cm area of yellow drainage on dressing." In addition, many agencies are now taking instant photos of wounds to include in the chart. If no camera is available, a drawing of the size and shape is helpful.
6. Mr. Jones might benefit from involvement with a wound care nurse, dietitian, certified diabetes educator, and home health nurse. Assess for the need for a referral to a comprehensive diabetes education center.

Review Questions

1. The nurse knows a patient with type 1 diabetes needs more education when the patient makes which of the following statements?
   1. "I must take insulin pills for the rest of my life."
   2. "I will count my carbohydrates at each meal and snack."
   3. "I will monitor my feet carefully every day."
   4. "I will try to keep my blood glucose between 70 and 130 mg/dL before meals."

2. Diabetes is diagnosed when the fasting blood glucose is greater than ____ mg/dL. Fill in the blank.

3. An obese adult patient is admitted to the hospital for shoulder repair. The nurse notes that the patient gets up four times during the night to urinate. Which action by the nurse is most important at this time?
   1. Offer a bedside commode to the patient.
   2. Request an order for a fasting blood glucose test.
   3. Contact the dietitian for weight loss counseling.
   4. Provide thorough perineal care after voiding.

4. A nursing home resident with a long history of diabetes requests a heating pad for cold, numb feet. What is the best response by the nurse?
   1. "Let's soak your feet in hot water instead; that might be safer."
   2. "Let's elevate your feet to promote circulation and provide more warmth."
   3. "I will bring you a heating pad; it will help your circulation in your feet."
   4. "A heating pad can cause burns, but I can bring you some extra socks."

5. Which statements by the patient with a new diagnosis of diabetes show understanding of instruction related to leading a healthy life and preventing complications? **Select all that apply.**
   1. "I should have a yearly eye examination."
   2. "I must check my feet daily."
   3. "I should aim to keep my premeal blood glucose readings under 130 mg/dL."
   4. "I will avoid all sweets and simple carbohydrates."

6. Which breakfast menu is most appropriate for a patient with diabetes?
   1. Two eggs, two strips bacon, orange juice, coffee
   2. Oatmeal with artificial sweetener, whole-grain toast, tea
   3. One half grapefruit, cranberry juice, bagel with sugar-free jelly
   4. One slice whole-grain toast with peanut butter, skim milk, orange juice

7. For which of the following blood glucose results would the nurse administer a "fast sugar"?
   1. 48
   2. 80
   3. 126
   4. 223

8. A patient who is preparing for surgery asks the nurse why the health care provider discontinued oral hypo-glycemic agent orders and initiated sliding-scale insulin. Which response by the nurse is best?
    1. "It helps us maintain better control of your blood glucose during surgery. You will most likely be back on your pills before you go home."
    2. "The stress of surgery often exacerbates diabetes. We will teach you how to give insulin before you go home."
    3. "Oral hypoglycemics are ineffective during times of stress. Insulin is the only way to keep your blood glucose under control."
    4. "The oral agents must not be controlling your blood glucose any longer. I will check and see which insulin you will be going home on."

9. Which meal plan is best for the patient with reactive hypoglycemia?
    1. High-carbohydrate meals
    2. Small, frequent meals
    3. Avoidance of fats and proteins
    4. Three medium to large meals daily

Answer rationales available in your online resources.

ANSWERS 1. 1; 2. 126; 3. 2; 4. 4; 5. 1; 2, 3; 6. 4; 7. 1; 8. 1; 9. 2

Key Points

Find the chapter key points in your online resources available through Davis Edge.

Additional Resources

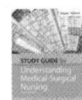 **Study Guide**

CHAPTER 41

Genitourinary and Reproductive System Function and Assessment

Laura L. McCully, Jaime Crabb, Janice L. Bradford

KEY TERMS

adnexa (ad-NEK-sah)
bimanual (by-MAN-yoo-uhl)
circumcised (SIR-kum-sized)
colposcopy (kul-PAHS-koh-pee)
conization (KOH-ni-ZAY-shun)
culdoscopy (kul-DOS-kuh-pee)
curet (kyoo-RET)
cystic (SIS-tik)
ejaculation (ee-JAK-yoo-LAY-shun)
epispadias (EP-ih-SPAY-dee-ahz)
erection (ee-REK-shun)
gravida (GRA-vid-ah)
gynecomastia (JY-neh-koh-MAS-tee-ah)
hydrocele (HY-droh-seel)
hypospadias (HY-poh-SPAY-dee-ahz)
hysterosalpingogram (HISS-tur-oh-SAL-pinj-oh-gram)
hysteroscopy (HISS-tur-AW-skoh-pee)
insufflation (in-suf-LAY-shun)
libido (lih-BEE-doh)
mammography (mah-MAW-grah-fee)
menarche (meh-NAR-kee)
menopause (MEN-oh-pawz)
orgasm (OR-gazm)
para (PAR-ah)
salpingoscopy (SAL-ping-JOS-koh-pee)
transillumination (TRANS-ih-loo-mih-NAY-shun)
varicocele (VAR-ih-koh-seel)

CHAPTER CONCEPTS

Health Promotion
Sexuality

LEARNING OUTCOMES

1. Explain the normal structures and functions of the reproductive system.
2. Identify the effects of aging on the reproductive system.
3. List data you should collect when caring for a patient with a disorder of the reproductive system.
4. Identify commonly performed tests used to diagnose disorders of the reproductive system.
5. Plan nursing care for patients undergoing each of the diagnostic tests.

NORMAL GENITOURINARY AND REPRODUCTIVE SYSTEM ANATOMY AND PHYSIOLOGY

The male and female reproductive systems produce gametes (sperm and egg cells [ova]) and facilitate the union of gametes in fertilization following sexual intercourse. The uterus provides for the developing embryo/fetus until birth.

Female Reproductive System

The female reproductive system consists of paired ovaries and fallopian tubes, a single uterus and vagina, and external genitalia (Fig. 41.1). The mammary glands may be considered accessory organs to the system.

Ovaries

The ovaries are a pair of oval structures, about 5 cm long and 2.5 cm wide, located on either side of the uterus in the pelvic cavity. The ovarian ligaments and the broad ligament help keep the ovaries and uterus in position.

The ovaries produce egg cells by oogenesis (meiosis), which begins and then pauses in the fetus, resumes at puberty, and ends at menopause. This process is cyclical. Typically, one mature ovum with its 23 chromosomes is produced and released approximately every 28 days, under hormonal control. Ovarian follicles produce estrogen and later, as the corpus luteum, secrete progesterone as well.

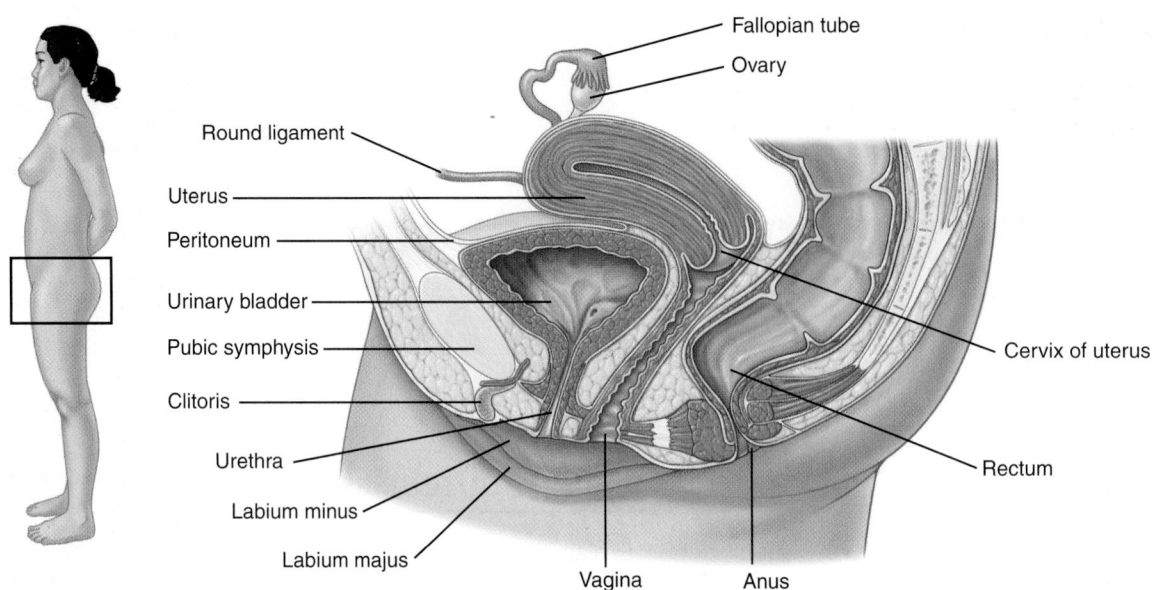

FIGURE 41.1 Female reproductive system in a midsagittal section

Fallopian Tubes

Each fallopian (uterine) tube is about 10 cm in length and extends from near the ovary to the uterus (Fig. 41.2). Its fimbriae draw an ovum into the tube, and ciliated epithelium transport the ovum (or zygote if fertilized) toward the uterus.

Uterus

The uterus is a muscular organ about 8 cm long and 5 cm wide. Ligaments help keep the uterus in position, tilted anteriorly over the top of the bladder. During pregnancy, the uterus increases greatly in size and contains the placenta, which nourishes the fetus until birth. Rising oxytocin levels increases uterine contractions to bring about birth.

The uterus is divided into three layers: the external perimetrium, the myometrium, and the internal endometrium. The endometrium is a highly vascular mucous membrane, part of which is lost and regenerated with each menstrual cycle. During pregnancy, the endometrium helps form the maternal side of the placenta.

Vagina

The vagina extends from the uterine cervix to the vaginal orifice in the perineum. It lies between the urethra and the rectum.

After puberty, the vaginal mucosa is relatively resistant to infection. The normal bacterial flora of the vagina creates an acidic pH, which retards microbial growth. While present, the hymen provides mechanical protection.

External Genitalia

Also called the vulva, the female external genitalia include the clitoris, mons pubis, and labia majora and minora (Fig. 41.3).

Mammary Glands

Enclosed within the breasts and surrounded by adipose tissue, the mammary glands produce milk after pregnancy (Fig. 41.4). During pregnancy, high levels of estrogen and progesterone prepare the glands for milk production. Prolactin causes the production of milk after pregnancy. Breastfeeding stimulates the release of oxytocin, which in turn stimulates the release of milk and contraction of the uterine muscle.

The Ovarian and Menstrual Cycles

The female reproductive cycles depend on follicle-stimulating hormone (FSH), luteinizing hormone (LH), estrogen, and progesterone (Table 41.1). These hormones bring about changes in the ovaries and uterus.

The menstrual cycle begins with the loss of the endometrium during menstruation, which lasts an average of 5 days. After the endometrium begins to proliferate again due to estrogen, FSH increases and several ovarian follicles begin to develop, although typically only one will dominate. The secretion of LH also increases, peaking to cause ovulation.

After ovulation, the ruptured follicle becomes the corpus luteum, which begins to secrete progesterone in addition to estrogen. Progesterone stimulates further development of the endometrium. If the ovum is not fertilized, the secretion of progesterone decreases. Without progesterone, the endometrium cannot be maintained and begins to slough off in menstruation. FSH secretion begins to increase as estrogen and progesterone decrease, and the cycle begins again. An average cycle is 28 days, but it is normal to have a cycle that is shorter or longer.

Male Reproductive System

The male reproductive system consists of bilateral testes and a series of tubules, ducts, and glands. The glands contribute secretions to the sperm, producing semen.

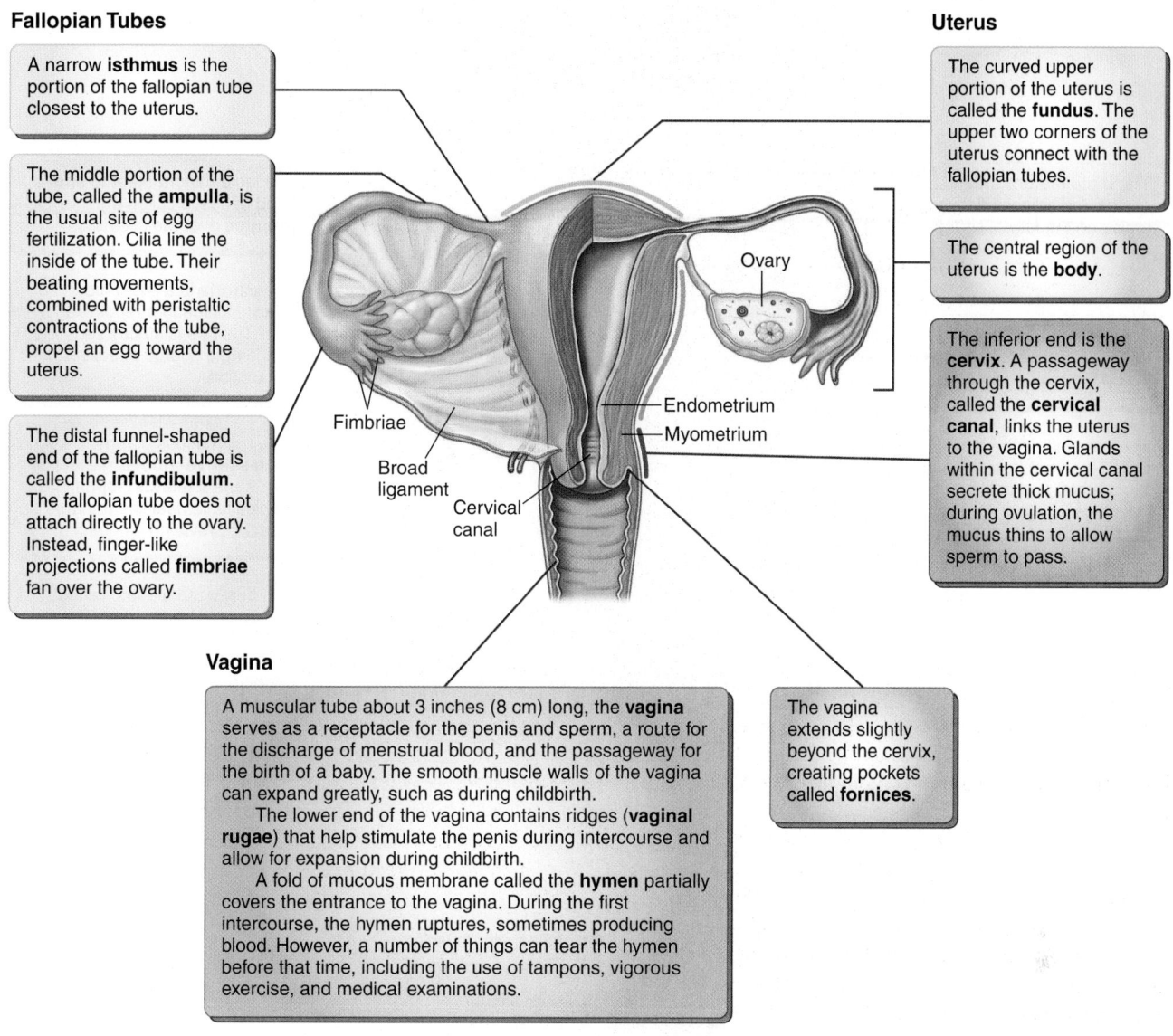

Fallopian Tubes

A narrow **isthmus** is the portion of the fallopian tube closest to the uterus.

The middle portion of the tube, called the **ampulla**, is the usual site of egg fertilization. Cilia line the inside of the tube. Their beating movements, combined with peristaltic contractions of the tube, propel an egg toward the uterus.

The distal funnel-shaped end of the fallopian tube is called the **infundibulum**. The fallopian tube does not attach directly to the ovary. Instead, finger-like projections called **fimbriae** fan over the ovary.

Uterus

The curved upper portion of the uterus is called the **fundus**. The upper two corners of the uterus connect with the fallopian tubes.

The central region of the uterus is the **body**.

The inferior end is the **cervix**. A passageway through the cervix, called the **cervical canal**, links the uterus to the vagina. Glands within the cervical canal secrete thick mucus; during ovulation, the mucus thins to allow sperm to pass.

Ovary

Fimbriae

Broad ligament

Cervical canal

Endometrium

Myometrium

Vagina

A muscular tube about 3 inches (8 cm) long, the **vagina** serves as a receptacle for the penis and sperm, a route for the discharge of menstrual blood, and the passageway for the birth of a baby. The smooth muscle walls of the vagina can expand greatly, such as during childbirth.

The lower end of the vagina contains ridges (**vaginal rugae**) that help stimulate the penis during intercourse and allow for expansion during childbirth.

A fold of mucous membrane called the **hymen** partially covers the entrance to the vagina. During the first intercourse, the hymen ruptures, sometimes producing blood. However, a number of things can tear the hymen before that time, including the use of tampons, vigorous exercise, and medical examinations.

The vagina extends slightly beyond the cervix, creating pockets called **fornices**.

FIGURE 41.2 Female internal genitalia.

Testes

The testes are located in the scrotum between the upper thighs, where the temperature is slightly lower than body temperature. This is necessary for the production of viable sperm. Each testis is about 5 cm long and 3 cm wide and contains the seminiferous tubules in which spermatogenesis (meiosis) takes place. In contrast to oogenesis, once started at puberty, spermatogenesis is a constant rather than cyclical process and usually continues throughout life. FSH initiates spermatogenesis. LH stimulates the secretion of testosterone, which contributes to the maturation of sperm. The secretion of inhibin is stimulated by testosterone; inhibin decreases the secretion of FSH, which helps keep the rate of spermatogenesis fairly constant. The functions of these hormones are summarized in Table 41.2.

Epididymis, Ductus Deferens, and Ejaculatory Ducts

A series of ducts lead sperm into and through the pelvic cavity where secretions are added; semen then exits the body via the urethra. The comma-shaped epididymis is a tube about 6 meters long that is coiled on the posterior side of a testis. Smooth muscle within its wall propels sperm from the testes into the ductus deferens. Also called the vas deferens, the ductus deferens extends from the epididymis in the scrotum to the ejaculatory duct within the pelvic cavity. Each of the two ejaculatory ducts receives sperm from the ductus deferens and the secretion of the seminal vesicle bilaterally. Both ejaculatory ducts propel semen through the urethra.

Seminal Vesicles, Prostate Gland, and Bulbourethral Glands

The male reproductive system includes bilateral seminal vesicles and bulbourethral glands, and a singular prostate (Fig. 41.5).

The mostly alkaline secretions of the male reproductive glands ensure that many sperm remain viable in the acidic environment of the vagina. The normal bacterial flora of the

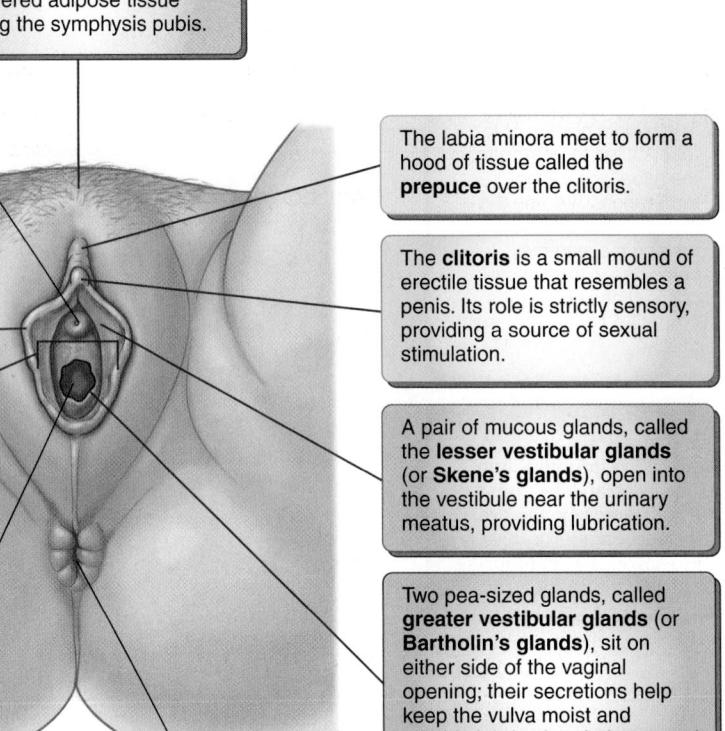

The **mons pubis** is a mound of hair-covered adipose tissue overlying the symphysis pubis.

Urethral opening

The **labia majora** are thick folds of skin and adipose tissue; hair grows on the lateral surfaces of the labia majora while the inner surfaces are hairless.

The **labia minora** are two thinner, hairless folds of skin just inside the labia majora.

The area inside the labia is called the **vestibule**; it contains the urethral and vaginal openings.

The labia minora meet to form a hood of tissue called the **prepuce** over the clitoris.

The **clitoris** is a small mound of erectile tissue that resembles a penis. Its role is strictly sensory, providing a source of sexual stimulation.

A pair of mucous glands, called the **lesser vestibular glands** (or **Skene's glands**), open into the vestibule near the urinary meatus, providing lubrication.

Two pea-sized glands, called **greater vestibular glands** (or **Bartholin's glands**), sit on either side of the vaginal opening; their secretions help keep the vulva moist and provide lubrication during sexual intercourse.

Vaginal opening

Anus

FIGURE 41.3 Female external genitalia.

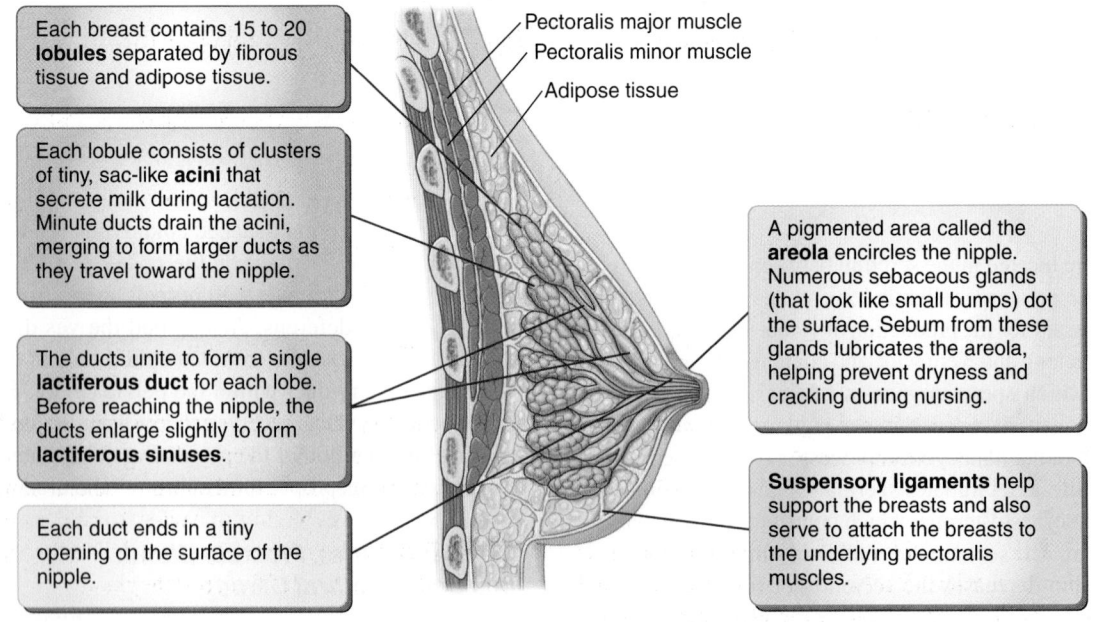

Each breast contains 15 to 20 **lobules** separated by fibrous tissue and adipose tissue.

Each lobule consists of clusters of tiny, sac-like **acini** that secrete milk during lactation. Minute ducts drain the acini, merging to form larger ducts as they travel toward the nipple.

The ducts unite to form a single **lactiferous duct** for each lobe. Before reaching the nipple, the ducts enlarge slightly to form **lactiferous sinuses**.

Each duct ends in a tiny opening on the surface of the nipple.

Pectoralis major muscle
Pectoralis minor muscle
Adipose tissue

A pigmented area called the **areola** encircles the nipple. Numerous sebaceous glands (that look like small bumps) dot the surface. Sebum from these glands lubricates the areola, helping prevent dryness and cracking during nursing.

Suspensory ligaments help support the breasts and also serve to attach the breasts to the underlying pectoralis muscles.

FIGURE 41.4 Breasts/mammary glands.

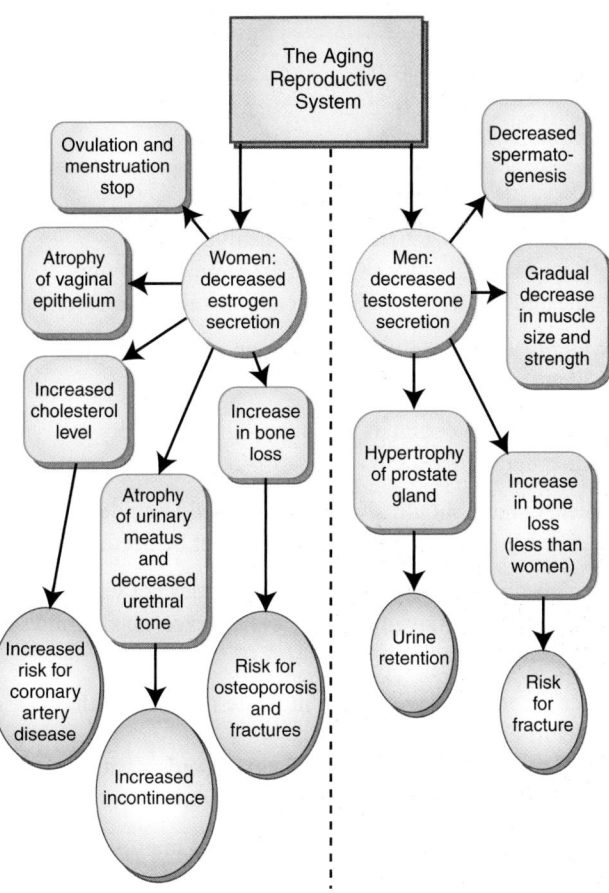

FIGURE 41.7 Aging and the reproductive system.

moods and mental functioning. Reproduction involves physical processes as well as relationships, role identification, and self-esteem issues.

Normal Function Baselines

Knowing about expected functioning of the reproductive system is your best preparation for data collection. Regular, relatively pain-free shedding of the endometrial lining of the uterus (menstruation) is expected from puberty through midlife. Intercourse is normally expected to be free of pain and infection, to occur when desired by both partners, to be satisfying, and generally to result in pregnancy within a few months unless precautions are taken. A pregnancy is expected to last approximately 40 weeks and to produce a healthy child. Physical and psychological sexual characteristics and function, including **libido** (sexual desire), are expected to be adequately maintained by hormones. Sexual functioning, desire, and fertility are expected to change throughout the process of aging. Individuals may vary somewhat from these expected descriptions. Chapter 42 further defines specific female reproductive system disorders.

Much of what happens in female reproductive system disorders occurs inside the body and may not show external signs. Skill in asking appropriate questions, documenting patient statements, and describing observations is essential. Descriptions of symptoms should be thorough. Follow the

WHAT'S UP? format described in Chapter 1. Because many signs and symptoms of reproductive system disorders occur in a cyclic fashion, you or the health care provider (HCP) may ask the patient to keep an accurate written record of occurrences, noting times and dates to identify patterns.

Health History

Subjective data related to the female reproductive system include general personal information as well as menstrual, obstetrical, gynecological, sexual, family, and psychosocial histories. See Table 41.3 for specific data to collect.

> ### NURSING CARE TIP
> It is helpful to have women maintain a monthly calendar of their menstrual cycles and bring it to any appointment during which discussion of the cycle may take place.

An obstetrical history includes number of pregnancies, pregnancy outcomes, and complications. These are generally documented using abbreviations of Latin words: G (for the Latin word *gravida*) = number of pregnancies; P (for the Latin word *para*) = births, whether alive or stillborn (regardless of number of fetuses) after 20 weeks' gestation; A (from the Latin word *abortus*) = abortions, whether spontaneous or therapeutic; a spontaneous abortion is sometimes called a miscarriage. Roman numerals follow the letters to specify the number of each. For example, three pregnancies resulting in twins, one single birth, and one spontaneous abortion are recorded as GIII, PII, AI. This may also be written as G3P2A1. Some hospitals use additional notations such as number of premature or full-term births, number of living children, and number of therapeutic abortions. Be sure to follow your institution's documentation policy.

> ### LEARNING TIP
> Remember the word *gravida* by thinking of gravity and knowing that a woman typically is heavier when pregnant.

Many nurses feel awkward asking reproductive history questions, and patients may also feel some uneasiness with this line of questioning. A matter-of-fact attitude, an assurance of confidentiality, and an adequate explanation about why the information is needed tend to encourage patient comfort and cooperation.

Breast Examination
Palpation
Palpation is the most important technique for breast examination because it can be used to identify alterations from normal consistency, to confirm the presence of lumps, and to locate areas of tenderness. Even mammograms are not sensitive enough to detect a small percentage of masses that can be felt by the patient or HCP.

Table 41.3

Subjective Data Collection for the Female Reproductive System

Questions to Ask During the Health History	Rationale/Significance
Personal History	
Have you ever been diagnosed or treated for any health problems?	Data may reveal general state of health, knowledge/practice of health promotion behaviors, meaning of health, and expectations related to care.
Have you had any recent weight changes?	Weight changes may reflect physical or psychological pathology.
Are you experiencing pain? (Use *WHAT'S UP?* questions if patient reports pain.)	Subjective indication of pain may signal a variety of disorders.
Do you have any allergies? (If so, what is the agent/type of reaction?)	Allergy status should always be assessed to guide possible intervention should treatment be needed.
Are you using any medications (prescription, over-the-counter, herbal remedies)?	A medication list may lead to health issues not yet revealed and may guide possible interventions should treatment be needed.
Do you smoke, consume caffeine, drink alcohol, or use recreational drugs? How much/how often?	Recreational behaviors can indicate risk of health disorders. Smoking increases risk of coagulation disorders with use of contraceptives containing estrogen in women over age 35.
Do you exercise? What type of exercise do you do? How often?	Exercise is recognized as an activity that improves health status, in general, and for many disorders.
How many hours of sleep do you get in a 24-hour period of time? Do you feel you get enough rest?	May indicate state of health or lead to discussion of social issues that lead to stress and, ultimately, physical disorders.
Do you feel under stress? How do you deal with stress?	Can indicate social issues that may lead to physical disorders.
Have you been hit, kicked, slapped, or made to do anything sexually against your will since your last visit?	Abuse screening should be considered during all primary care visits; may indicate need for intervention or guide care.
Menstrual History	
At what age did you begin menstruating (**menarche**)? How often do you menstruate, and how long do your periods last? How heavy is your flow?	May reveal abnormalities of cycle and lead to a diagnosis of benign/malignant tumors, endometriosis, pregnancy, anemia, and endocrine disorders.
At what age did you enter menopause [if applicable]? If menopausal, has bone density screening been done? What is your calcium/vitamin D intake?	May determine need for bone density screening and teaching related to calcium and vitamin D intake.
Obstetric/Gynecological History	
How many pregnancies and deliveries have you had? Were they full-term or pre-term? Were your deliveries vaginal or by cesarean section? How much did your largest baby weigh? Did you have any complications following your deliveries?	May indicate health of reproductive system, knowledge/meaning of health maintenance practice, and risk for disease.

• WORD • BUILDING •

menarche: men—month + arche—beginning

Table 41.3

Subjective Data Collection for the Female Reproductive System—cont'd

Questions to Ask During the Health History	*Rationale/Significance*
Have you had previous treatment/surgery on your reproductive organs?	May indicate past health issues related to the reproductive organs and need for current evaluation related to issues.
Have you had any itching of your perineum, or have you noted any unusual vaginal discharge (describe)?	Subjective report of itching or discharge may indicate disorder of inflammation or lead to diagnosis of a sexually transmitted infection (STI).
When was your last Pap/pelvic exam? What were the results?	May reflect meaning of health and guide current care.
Do you do breast self-examination? How often? Have you noticed any breast changes? When was your last mammogram [if applicable]?	If changes have been noted by the patient, they should be evaluated by the primary care provider for possible pathology.
Did you breastfeed? How long?	Breastfeeding may offer some protection against breast cancer. If patient is currently breastfeeding, may help guide care and diagnosis.

Sexual History	
Are you sexually active? How many partners do you have? Of what gender? What is your lifetime number of partners? Is your sexual activity satisfying?	May indicate risk of STIs and/or unintended pregnancy as well as state of sexual satisfaction/intimacy.
At what age did you become sexually active? What contraceptive method(s) do you use (if sexually active with a male)? How do you use them? How long have you used this method?	Early onset of sexual activity increases risk of STIs and cervical cancer. May reflect meaning of health, high-risk health behaviors, and risk for unintended pregnancy or STI. Asking length of use of a particular method allows assessment of need for replacement, as in an intrauterine device, or need for a bone density exam.
Have you ever been diagnosed with an STI? If so, when, what type, and how was it treated? Are you aware if the treatment was successful?	May indicate high-risk sexual behavior patterns or potential for active disease and, therefore, indicate need for diagnostic testing and treatment.

Family History	
Do you have a family history of cardiovascular problems, cancer, osteoporosis, diabetes, or thyroid abnormalities?	May indicate underlying cause of or risk for sexual/physical abnormalities of the reproductive system.

Psychosocial History	
Are you married or in a significant relationship? Is the relationship satisfying?	Relevant to determine financial, social, and emotional support.

Breast Self-Examination

Self-palpation during breast self-examination (BSE), if done regularly and thoroughly, may be even more sensitive than HCP or nurse palpation. This is because the patient becomes so familiar with her own breasts that she is more likely to notice subtle changes that an HCP might overlook. Because recent studies of BSE have failed to show a reduction in cancer deaths, some HCPs are now simply urging women to be familiar with their breasts and report changes, rather than teaching them to do monthly examinations. Other providers, however, continue to teach and recommend monthly BSE because they have seen it make a significant difference for many women. Table 41.4 lists additional objective data to collect.

Table 41.4

Objective Data Collection for the Female Reproductive System

Physical Examination Findings	*Possible Abnormal Findings/Causes*
Clinical Breast Examination (CBE) Observe and palpate for presence of swelling, lumps, skin changes, and nipple exudate.	Changes may indicate breast cancer or fibrocystic breast disease.
External Genitalia Observe for color, symmetry, hair distribution, lesions, swelling, and exudate.	Changes may indicate vulvar cancer, developmental abnormalities, infection, or injury.
Vagina Observe for shape, bulges, color changes, lesions, and exudate.	Changes may indicate infection, structural abnormalities, or injury.
Internal Genitalia (performed by trained personnel) Palpate for tenderness, size, shape, and mobility. Observe for color, lesions, exudate, and bleeding.	Changes may indicate infection, structural abnormalities, cervical cancer, polyps, endometriosis, fibroid/malignant tumors, pregnancy, or injury.
Perineum Observe for lesions and shape.	Abnormalities may indicate infection, structural abnormalities, or injury.
Anus Observe for shape, color changes, and lesions.	Abnormalities can indicate hemorrhoids or injury.
Inguinal Nodes Palpate for swelling and tenderness.	May indicate infectious process or regional malignancy.

Note: A female physical examination is typically done by a health care provider or other trained provider.

Patient Education

If BSE is to be done monthly, a good time to perform it is 1 week after menses, when swelling of normal breast tissue is at a minimum. For women who no longer have a regular menstrual period, any regular monthly schedule is fine. Although most women's breasts are not exactly the same size, marked differences between the breasts or a change in the size of one breast should be checked with an HCP. Puckering or dimpling of skin, asymmetrical movement, and different pointing position of the nipples should also be reported. Whether the breasts are examined in parallel lines, a spiral formation, or a wedge pattern is not important. It is important, however, for the examination to be methodical and cover all areas of the breast, including the tail of Spence, which extends into the axilla (Fig. 41.8).

NURSING CARE TIP

Some women do breast self-examination the day their electric bill (or other bill) arrives each month because it is a dependable monthly reminder.

CRITICAL THINKING

Jilli, age 24, states, "Why should I do breast exams at my age? I probably won't get breast cancer until I'm older, if I get it at all."

1. What should your response to Jilli include?
2. Why would this be a good time to provide education about health maintenance?

   Suggested answers are at the end of the chapter.

Diagnostic Tests of the Breasts
Ultrasound and Mammography

Ultrasound can determine the density of the tissues and map the breast structures. This is mainly useful for distinguishing fluid-filled (**cystic**) lumps from solid tumors. It can also be

• WORD • BUILDING •
cystic: baglike

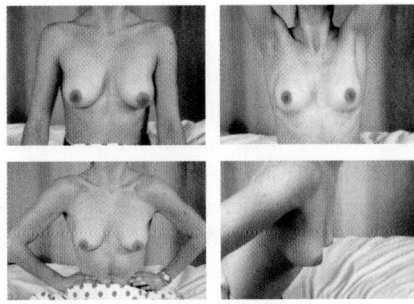
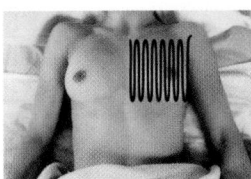
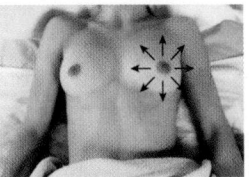
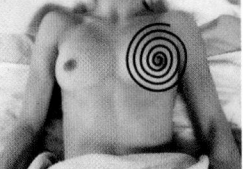

Inspection

BREAST SELF-EXAMINATION
Palpation

FIGURE 41.8 Breast self-examination.

used to guide a needle for fine-needle aspiration of cystic fluid or core needle biopsies.

Mammography is a radiographic (x-ray) examination of the breasts. A special machine is used that spreads and flattens the breast tissue to a thin layer to more effectively show benign and malignant growths that might be hidden by breast structures on typical chest examination (Fig. 41.9). New digital technology is now available that may be more effective in detecting cancers in younger women and women who have dense breasts. The procedure is the same for a digital mammogram, but the image is computerized, allowing the radiologist to look more closely at problem areas.

The American Cancer Society (2017) recommends the following for average risk women:

• Women aged 40 to 44 have the option to start screening mammogram yearly.

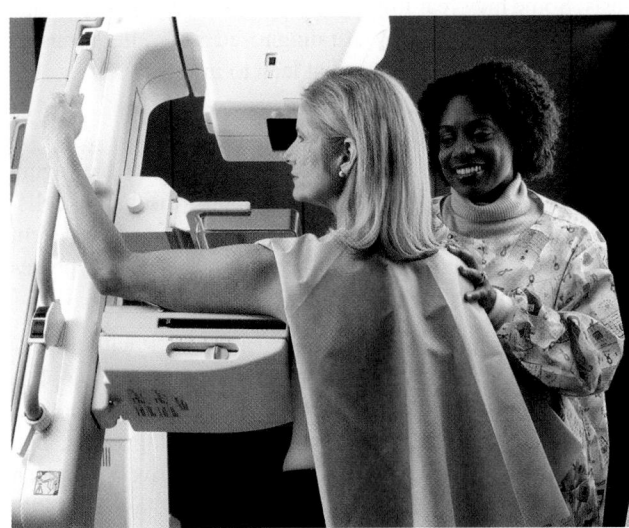

FIGURE 41.9 Mammogram machine.

• Women aged 45 to 54 should get mammograms yearly.
• Women aged 55 and older can switch to every other year or continue yearly.
• All women should be familiar with how their breasts normally look and feel and should report any changes to an HCP right away. A regular clinical breast examination (CBE) and BSE is not recommended.
• All women should understand what to expect when getting a mammogram for breast cancer screening.

Magnetic resonance imaging (MRI) and a mammogram every year are recommended for women with a high risk for breast cancer, such as those with *BRCA1* or *BRCA2* genetic mutations or a strong family history. See Chapter 11 for more information.

PATIENT EDUCATION. Advise patients preparing for mammography to bathe and not to apply deodorant, powder, or any other substance to the upper body because these can cause false shadows on the test.

Thermography, Computed Tomography Scan, and MRI
Several other methods for diagnosis of breast disorders are available but are not commonly used. Thermography is a method of mapping the breast using photographic paper that records temperature variations throughout the tissue in different colors. A computed tomography (CT) scan or MRI can offer precise location of tumors without the displacement caused by flattening the breast for a mammogram.

Biopsy
If suspicious lesions are found, they will be further assessed with a biopsy. This may be done by surgically removing a

• WORD • BUILDING •
mammography: mammo—breast + graphy—recording

portion of tissue or by aspirating fluid or cells through a needle that is placed into the lesion.

Assessment of the patient's psychological condition during breast diagnosis procedures is essential. Most women know someone who has had breast cancer. Although breast cancer screening procedures can seem routine to health care workers, they can be the cause of much anxiety for patients and their families. An understanding and calm nurse who can explain the procedures can help the assessment phase to be less traumatic.

> ### BE SAFE!
> **BE VIGILANT!** Use at least two patient identifiers when providing care, treatment, and services. Label containers used for blood and other specimens in the presence of the patient. (The Joint Commission's 2018 National Patient Safety Goals, © The Joint Commission, 2018. Reprinted with permission.)

Laboratory Tests

A blood test can be done to identify mutations in *BRCA1* and *BRCA2*, genes that are associated with breast and ovarian cancer. By reviewing a woman's family history, risk factors can be determined and testing can be offered. Women who test positive for either gene can discuss preventive treatments with their HCPs and also make their sisters and daughters aware of potential risk.

Bone Health Assessment

Bone health assessment is important for women of all ages. Teaching women early about the importance of good calcium and vitamin D intake will be of benefit later in life. Women of childbearing age produce estrogen, which helps prevent bone loss and works with calcium and other minerals to build bone. As women age and approach menopause, estrogen production slowly decreases, which in turn decreases the processes of building and remodeling bone. Menopausal women produce very little estrogen and, therefore, have little bone protection. In fact, the body tends to break down more bone than it rebuilds. At this point in a woman's life, dietary calcium and vitamin D requirements increase unless the woman is on hormone replacement therapy.

There is current debate about calcium and vitamin D supplementation for menopausal women. The U.S. Preventive Services Task Force (2017) issued a statement, based on research, against supplementation with vitamin D of 400 IU or less and calcium of 1,000 mg or less because of the increased kidney stone risk and no evidence of preventing fractures. More research is needed in this area, but for now, women should aim to get recommended calcium and vitamin D amounts through diet. If a woman is diagnosed with osteoporosis, she should speak to her HCP about a treatment plan. Table 41.5 provides recommendations for calcium and vitamin D intake from the National Institutes of Health's Office of Dietary Supplements. See Chapter 6 for the calcium content of selected foods.

Diagnostic Tests of the Bones

In addition to recommending increasing the dietary intake of calcium and vitamin D, menopausal women older than age 50 who are not on hormone replacement therapy should be assessed for bone loss. The National Osteoporosis Foundation (visit www.nof.org) recommends bone density testing for all women over age 65 and for postmenopausal women under age 65 if they are at high risk (see Chapter 46).

The best test for bone density is a dual energy x-ray absorptiometry (DEXA) scan, which measures bone density at the hip or spine. This is a specialized x-ray that takes only 5 to 10 minutes to complete. A quantitative computed tomography (QCT) scan can also be done to determine bone density. Pharmacies or other outpatient facilities may offer tests of peripheral locations such as the heel. These are less sensitive but may still provide useful information that can be followed up with more extensive testing if indicated.

Additional Diagnostic Tests of the Female Reproductive System
Hormone Tests

Hormone tests are commonly used to assess endocrine system function as it relates to reproduction. Tests may be used to measure potential fertility, find reasons for abnormal menses, assess hormone-producing tumors, and determine whether treatments to adjust hormone levels have been effective. Some hormone tests are time specific, so the samples can be rendered useless if not gathered within a certain time range.

NURSING CARE. Consult institution policy for specific instructions for each test. Explain the procedure to the patient and provide support. Women who are undergoing hormone tests may feel embarrassed, worried about their femininity and potential fertility, and depressed because of repeated tests. Some may fear loss of their spouse's love (and perhaps the relationship) if they are diagnosed with alterations in hormone levels or function that lead to infertility.

Pelvic Examination

The pelvic examination allows visual inspection of the vagina and cervix as well as sampling of mucus, discharge, cells, and exudates. Palpation of portions of the reproductive system and some treatments may also be done as part of the procedure (Fig. 41.10).

NURSING CARE. Be prepared to assist the HCP with the examination. Explain the procedure as you set out the supplies according to policy or HCP preference. Have the patient empty her bladder and then remove her clothing and change into a gown (socks can remain on, and often give a woman a tiny bit of comfort!). When the HCP is ready, assist the patient into the lithotomy position, with her feet in stirrups. If the HCP is using a metal speculum, warm it under warm

Table 41.5

Adult Calcium and Vitamin D Recommendations

Age (years)	Male	Female	Pregnant	Lactating
Recommended Dietary Allowances for Calcium				
14–18 years	1,300 mg	1,300 mg	1,300 mg	1,300 mg
19–50 years	1,000 mg	1,000 mg	1,000 mg	1,000 mg
51–70 years	1,000 mg	1,200 mg	—	—
71 years or older	1,200 mg	1,200 mg	—	—
Recommended Dietary Allowances for Vitamin D				
14–18 years	600 IU (15 mcg)	600 IU (15 mcg)	600 IU (15 mcg)	600 IU (15 mcg)
19–50 years	600 IU (15 mcg)	600 IU (15 mcg)	600 IU (15 mcg)	600 IU (15 mcg)
51–70 years	600 IU (15 mcg)	600 IU (15 mcg)	—	—
71 years or older	800 IU (20 mcg)	800 IU (20 mcg)	—	—

Source: Office of Dietary Supplements, National Institutes of Health. (2018). Vitamin D fact sheet for professionals. Retrieved from https://ods.od.nih.gov/factsheets/VitaminD-HealthProfessional; and Office of Dietary Supplements, National Institutes of Health. (2017). Calcium fact sheet for professionals. Retrieved from https://ods.od.nih.gov/factsheets/Calcium-HealthProfessional

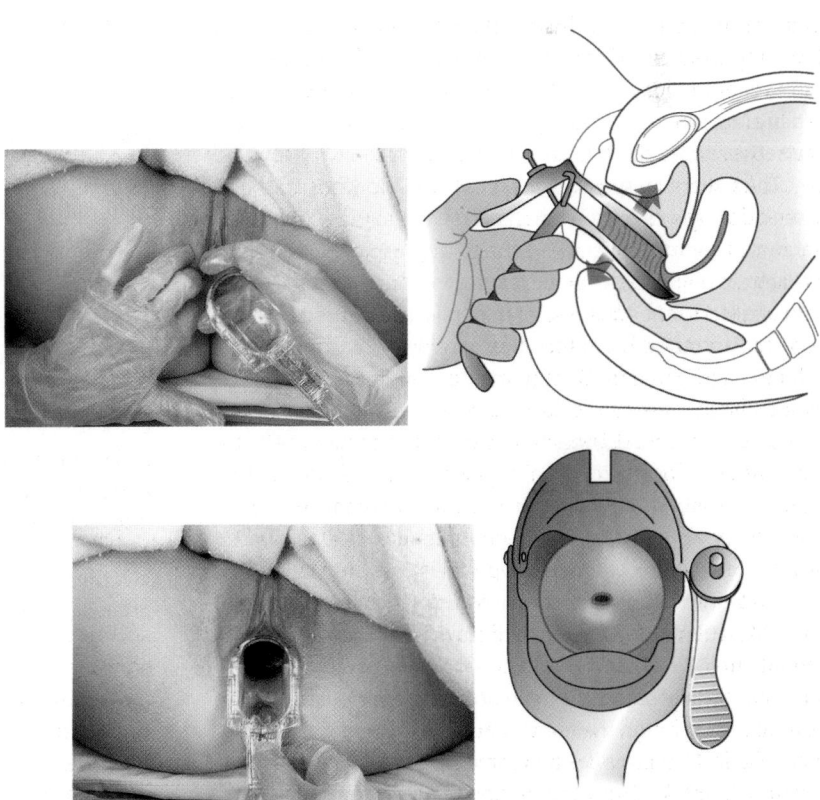

FIGURE 41.10 Pelvic exam with Pap smear.

water to make it a little more comfortable for the patient. Have the patient take a deep breath and blow out as the speculum is being inserted, to help her relax. Being in lithotomy position may make some women feel embarrassed and exposed. Be sure to provide privacy. Ideally, the examination table faces away from the door.

Bimanual Palpation

Because much of the reproductive system is not visible even with a speculum, **bimanual** palpation is often done during a pelvic examination. One hand is placed on the abdomen and the other gloved hand is inserted deeply into the vagina. The uterus and **adnexa** are moved about between the two hands to feel the size, shape, and consistency of the uterus and adnexa and to check for any abnormal growths.

NURSING CARE. Explain the procedure, and support the patient. Some women may be fearful, embarrassed, or tense and may find the procedure uncomfortable ("Patient Perspective"). Active relaxation strategies may decrease discomfort.

Patient Perspective

Jacqueline. I am a sexual assault nurse examiner. When patients come in to see me, they are in crisis. They are unsure how or what to feel and whom to trust. They are very apprehensive. As patients give me the history of their assaults, they begin to trust me. They see someone who is interested in them and who believes them. By the time I actually start the head-to-toe physical examination, they know they are safe. Often, when I am performing the physical examination, I start small talk and take an interest in their lives that has nothing to do with the assault. When they are discharged from my care, they are more animated, talkative, and sometimes smiling.

The patient I remember the most is a child whose father was molesting her when her mother went to work. She was about 6 years old. When she came to the hospital, she wasn't talking to anybody, let alone a nurse in a scary hospital at midnight. I spent 4 hours with this child. We colored, played, and talked about her brothers. By the end of the night, she allowed me to examine her, and she trusted me enough to let the physician come in and look at her. Unfortunately, in her young life, she had a reason to be scared. Her life became much worse before it got better. Her father tried to kill her mother and himself as a result of this.

So many of us have grown up with pop culture television, and we think of forensic examiners as professionals working with dead people. In fact, forensic nursing is caring for patients as it applies to the law. As a sexual assault nurse examiner, I care for people who have experienced interpersonal violence. I care for this special population of patients through the nursing process. I care not only for their physical trauma but also for their spiritual needs; finally, I collect evidence for the prosecution of a crime.

I advocate for their safety needs, and I help provide for their physical needs. I provide a bridge to the legal and mental health systems.

I began forensic nursing years ago when the concept was still new. We were navigating uncharted waters and were unsure what the result would bring. What we quickly learned is that when you deliver good nursing care to patients, the result can be a positive change in their lives. That is the reward of the job: making a positive difference in patients' lives and giving them some tools to help in their recovery process. Having the patient and family look at you and say "thank you for helping me" is what we all went into nursing for.

Becoming a sexual assault nurse examiner has made me become a more empathetic person, a more compassionate nurse, and a better citizen of my community.

Cytology

Cytology is the study of cells taken as tissue samples. Cells required for microscopic examination can be removed from the reproductive system in several ways. During a Papanicolaou (Pap) smear, one or more small samples of cells are gently scraped away from the surface of the cervical canal. They are then smeared or rolled onto microscope slides and sprayed with a fixative to preserve them for viewing, or they placed into a fixative solution for later preparation and viewing in a laboratory. Cells may also be collected by **conization,** which involves removing a small cone-shaped sample from the cervical canal, or by punch biopsy, which removes a small core of cells. Endometrial biopsy specimens are samples of cells taken from the lining of the uterus by scraping with a small spoon-shaped tool called a **curet** that is inserted through the cervix. Small biopsy specimens may also be taken by cutting or removing a suspicious lesion. Cells can be observed for changes indicative of hormonal secretion, cellular maturation, or abnormalities such as are seen with viral growths and cancerous or precancerous conditions. Results are reported simply as "normal," "unclear," or "abnormal."

NURSING CARE. Consult the procedure manual or HCP concerning specific types of instruments to set up for biopsies and Pap smears. Cells die and degrade rapidly once removed from the patient, so they must be packaged securely for transport to laboratory facilities. Always label specimens carefully.

Prepare the patient by explaining the procedure and providing support. The woman may be fearful of cancer or other abnormality. Removal of the sample may cause pain, bleeding, swelling, or, later, inflammation, so the patient is monitored after the procedure and alerted to report these complications

• WORD • BUILDING •
bimanual: bi—two + manual—hands
adnexa: ad—together + nexa—to tie (usually refers to ovaries and tubes)
conization: coniz—cone-forming + ation—process

if they occur. After the procedure, document the woman's status on the chart, and record that the sample was sent to the laboratory. Advise the woman that, if results are unclear or abnormal, additional testing will be done. Assure her that abnormal results have many causes and typically do not mean a cancer diagnosis.

CRITICAL THINKING

Reproductive Assessment. How might the age of the patient change your approach, plans, and teaching for patients who have disorders of the reproductive system? Consider each of the following scenarios:

1. A 2-year-old child is brought into the clinic by her mother because she has a foul-smelling discharge coming from her perineal area and a slight yellowish discharge from her vagina.
2. A 21-year-old woman comes to the health care provider's office where you work to obtain a renewal of her annual birth control pill prescription. Your employer enforces regular checks for cervical changes by renewing the prescription only after a Pap smear is done. As you start setting out the Pap smear materials, your patient expresses some reluctance to have it done today because she is so sore already.
3. Your 56-year-old patient comes in to "get things checked out" because she has pain every time that she and her husband have intercourse.

Suggested answers are at the end of the chapter.

Swabs and Smears

Swabs and smears are done to determine which microorganisms are causing infection and, consequently, which antibiotics should be used.

NURSING CARE. If infection is suspected, add sample collection materials, including swabs, slides, and sterile saline in site-specific receptacles, and a gonorrhea/*Chlamydia* collection kit, to the pelvic examination equipment. *Chlamydia* samples are especially difficult to transport to laboratories, and special kits are available for this pathogen. Some microorganisms, such as yeasts and *Trichomonas,* can be identified well from smears on slides. Wet mounts are smears of discharge spread onto a slide. These must be taken to the microscope immediately after they are obtained. Sodium chloride and potassium hydroxide are dropped onto individual wet-mount slides before they dry to aid in identification of some microorganisms. Support the patient, who may be anxious about possible sexually transmitted infections (STIs) and effects on relationships.

Sonography

Ultrasound assessment (also called *sonography*) may be done to determine size, shape, development, and density of structures associated with the female reproductive system as well as fetal measurements and some types of prenatal diagnoses. This procedure is especially useful for differentiating cysts from solid tumors and for locating ectopic pregnancies and intrauterine devices. Ultrasound may also be used to guide needles for obtaining samples of fluid or cells. Either external or vaginal transducers may be used to send and receive the signals. Vaginal transducers are placed in a plastic sheath before insertion into the vagina. A full bladder may be required for some ultrasound tests.

NURSING CARE. Explain the procedure and support the patient. The pressure of the transducer on the skin or in the vagina may be painful if the adjacent structures are inflamed or swollen or if the bladder is very full.

Radiographic Procedures

Several radiographic procedures may be used for diagnosis of reproductive system problems. CT scan and MRI are used to locate tumors of the reproductive system. Structures of the female reproductive system may also be outlined by taking x-ray pictures of cavities that have been filled with a radiopaque substance. During a **hysterosalpingogram,** dye is injected into the uterus until it comes out the ends of the fallopian tubes. This test is useful for identifying congenital abnormalities in the shape or structure of the uterus and blockages of the fallopian tubes.

NURSING CARE. Prepare the patient for a radiographic test according to agency policy, which may include a laxative, suppository, or enema. Ensure that the patient understands the procedure and that appropriate consents are signed as required. Ask about allergies to dye or iodine. Notify the supervisor immediately if the patient reports an allergy. After the procedure, assess for nausea, light-headedness, and signs of allergic reaction and promote comfort, because some cramping can occur. Discharge teaching should include signs of infection and advice that the x-ray dye can stain clothing. Provide a perineal pad following the procedure and advise the patient to wear a perineal pad until vaginal drainage stops.

> ### NURSING CARE TIP
> No one is really allergic to iodine—iodine is an essential element in our bodies. But some people may be allergic to dyes that contain iodine. It is still important to ask about iodine allergy, because that is how some women identify an allergy to dye.

Endoscopic Examinations

Several types of endoscopic examinations are done to visually inspect internal areas to diagnose (and sometimes treat)

• WORD • BUILDING •
hysterosalpingogram: hystero—womb + salpingo—tube + gram—record

reproductive system disorders. The names of the tests vary according to the area inspected, but all generally make use of a fiber-optic light and lens system, which is inserted through a tube called a *cannula* into a small incision. A laparoscopy is done to view the abdominal cavity and is useful for identifying problems such as endometriosis (Fig. 41.11). A **salpingoscopy** is performed to see the inside of the fallopian tubes. A **hysteroscopy** is done to see the inside of the uterus. A binocular microscope is used with an endoscope that is introduced into the vagina to closely study lesions of the cervix during a **colposcopy.** During **culdoscopy,** an endoscope is introduced into the vagina and through a small incision in the vagina into the cul-de-sac of Douglas, a cavity behind the uterus, to observe for abnormalities in this region (Fig. 41.12).

NURSING CARE. Preoperatively, the patient is prepared for an endoscopic examination according to agency protocol. This generally involves asking the patient whether she has fasted as instructed, assessing vital signs, recording the time of last voiding, helping the patient into a gown, and ensuring that the consent form has been signed. General anesthesia may be given for some endoscopic procedures. Explain what to expect, and provide support for the woman. She may be anxious about possible disorders.

Postoperatively, provide comfort measures. The woman may experience pain in the neck, shoulders, and upper back if carbon dioxide (CO_2) gas was pumped into the body compartment being examined. This is called **insufflation** and is done to increase the distance between structures, so that it is easier for the HCP to visualize structures. If small incisions were made through the abdominal wall for insertion of the endoscope and for insufflation, a Band-Aid® or small dressing is applied.

PATIENT EDUCATION. Advise the patient to observe the incision sites for redness, bleeding, or drainage, notifying the HCP promptly if these should occur. The patient will need to visit the HCP as directed for suture removal. If the endoscopic procedure was done transvaginally, provide a perineal pad following the procedure and advise the patient to wear a pad until the drainage stops. Also, instruct the patient to report any bright bleeding after the operative day and to report any fever or foul-smelling discharge. Table 41.6 provides a summary of diagnostic tests.

MALE REPRODUCTIVE SYSTEM DATA COLLECTION

As with the female reproductive system, the male reproductive system is a complex interaction of both physical and psychosocial factors. Unlike women, however, men may find it much more difficult in our society to talk about or admit to having problems related to reproductive health. From toilet training through adulthood, men are expected to exhibit behaviors associated with maleness. Unfortunately, by the time some boys reach manhood, their male identity is often defined by the successful functioning of their sex organs.

One of the important first steps in obtaining a male reproductive assessment is to provide a comfortable, nonjudgmental, confidential atmosphere for discussion. This means you must first be knowledgeable and comfortable with sexual issues. Although it may be challenging to ask questions about **erection** or ejaculation history, such questions may allow men to talk about difficulties they are experiencing. Be open and straightforward with all questions and answers. It may be necessary at times to use more commonly expressed sexual words instead of medical terminology. You will discover that many men do not know the function of their prostate gland or the difference between ejaculation and **orgasm.** Use the assessment as an

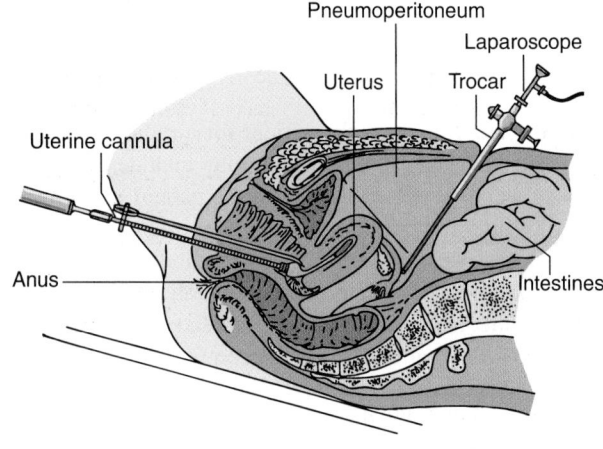

FIGURE 41.11 Laparoscopy.

Labels: Pneumoperitoneum, Laparoscope, Uterus, Trocar, Uterine cannula, Anus, Intestines

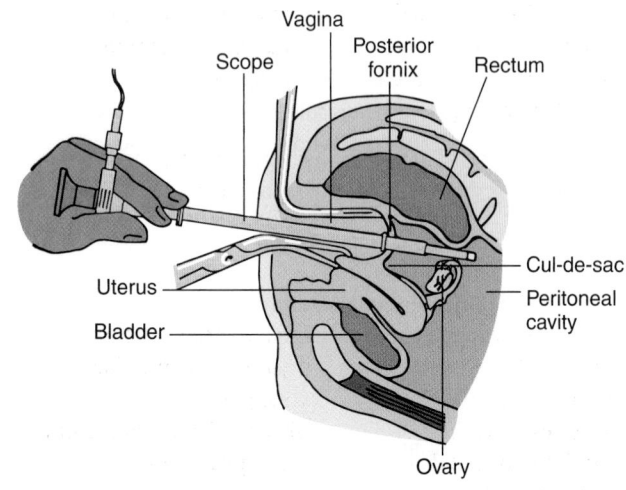

FIGURE 41.12 Culdoscopy.

Labels: Vagina, Posterior fornix, Scope, Rectum, Uterus, Cul-de-sac, Peritoneal cavity, Bladder, Ovary

• WORD • BUILDING •

salpingoscopy: salpingo—tube + scopy—looking
hysteroscopy: hystero—womb + scopy—looking
colposcopy: colpo—vagina + scopy—looking
culdoscopy: culdo—cul de sac + scopy—looking
insufflation: in—in + suffl—to blow + ation—process

Table 41.6

Diagnostic Procedures for the Female Reproductive System

Procedure	Definition/Normal Finding	Significance of Abnormal Findings	Nursing Management
Noninvasive			
Breast self-examination (BSE) or clinical breast examination (CBE)	Assessment of breast tissue by patient (BSE) or health care provider (HCP) (CBE) through inspection and palpation	Abnormal findings during physical examination may indicate pathology and indicate need for further assessment.	Educate about appropriate technique and observe a return demonstration of BSE.
Ultrasound/sonography	High-frequency sound waves bounce off tissue to map tissue structure and determine tissue density. Also may be used to guide biopsy procedure.	May help to determine abnormal lesions, abnormalities of tissue structure, or presence of abnormal fluid volume.	Follow institutional guidelines for patient preparation and support, which may be determined by testing goals.
Mammography	Radiographic examination of tissue. X-ray may be used with dye contrast injected into body before procedure.	May help to determine abnormal lesions or abnormalities of normal tissue structure.	Educate patient not to apply lotions, powders, or deodorant before test.
Thermography, computed tomography (CT) scan, magnetic resonance imaging (MRI)	Precise pictures of tissue using temperature (thermography), x-ray (CT scan), or radiofrequency (MRI)	May help to determine abnormal lesions or abnormalities of normal tissue structure.	Ask patients about presence of metal or wire inside their body before MRI because the procedure may then be contraindicated.
Hormonal tests	Assessment of endocrine function related to reproduction	Abnormal hormone levels may identify fertility potential, reasons for abnormal menses, hormone-producing tumors, or need for hormone replacement.	Explain procedure to patient and provide support.
Invasive			
Pelvic examination or bimanual examination	Inspection and palpation of external/internal reproductive organs by HCP	Abnormal physical examination may detect pathology or may indicate need for further testing.	Explain procedure to patient and provide support.
Biopsy, cytology, swabs, or smears	Obtainment of body cells/tissue through aspiration or excision or by swabbing/scrapping of tissue/exudate	May diagnose pathology or infection.	Explain procedure to patient and provide support.
Endoscopy or laparoscopy	Use of fiber-optic light and lens system to inspect internal structures	May help to determine abnormal lesions or abnormalities of normal tissue structure. Tissue biopsies may be taken during procedure.	Explain procedure to patient and provide support. Observe for postprocedure complications.

opportunity to teach men the facts about their own sexual functioning.

Health History

Some basic questions to ask a male patient during a reproductive assessment are found in Table 41.7. As mentioned earlier, a professional, matter-of-fact attitude, along with an explanation as to why the questions are necessary, can put both you and the patient at ease while collecting data.

Physical Examination

The physical examination is generally performed by an HCP trained in physical assessments. The examination begins with the patient's general appearance. He is observed for male patterns of hair growth on the head, face, chest, arms, and legs. Normal male pubic hair pattern is in a triangular shape, with hair growth up toward the umbilicus. The patient's height and muscle mass are noted. Men are commonly taller than 5 feet, 6 inches; weigh more than 135 pounds; and have shoulders

Table 41.7

Subjective Data Collection for the Male Reproductive System and Sexual Health

Questions to Ask During the Health History	*Rationale/Significance*
Medication	
Are you using any medications (prescription, over-the-counter, and herbal remedies)? How much/how often? (For medications that affect sexual desire, erection, or ejaculation, see Chapter 43.)	Loss of sexual desire, erection, ejaculation, orgasm, or fertility can occur as a result of some medication use.
Family History	
Do you have a family history of genetically transmitted diseases (e.g., heart problems, hypertension, diabetes, cancer)? Did your mother use diethylstilbestrol (DES) during pregnancy?	These conditions put men at high risk for circulation problems that interfere with erections or congenital anomalies of reproductive organs.
Personal Habits and Health Promotion Behaviors	
Do you smoke, consume caffeine, drink alcohol, use recreational drugs, or use steroids? How much/how often? Do you use hot tubs, engage in long-distance drives, or ride a bike? How much/how often? Do you use contraceptives? What type of contraceptives do you use? How do you use them? Do you do testicular self-examinations (TSEs)? Have you noticed any changes in your testicles or other reproductive organs?	These habits may lead to decreased blood flow to penis, loss of erection; decreased testosterone (male hormone) interferes with erection and fertility; excessive heat decreases sperm production. Data will reveal knowledge/practice of health promotion behaviors, meaning of health, and history of changes or abnormalities.
Personal Health History	
Did you have mumps during adolescence, or have you recently had an infection or fever?	Some infectious processes may lead to decreased sperm production.
Mental Health	
Are you experiencing stress? How do you deal with stress? Are you having problems with a sexual partner? Have you ever or are you experiencing performance anxiety or depression?	Decreased sexual desire and ability to have an erection may result from mental and/or emotional stress.
Circulatory/Respiratory	
Have you ever been diagnosed with or treated for heart problems/surgery, high blood pressure, sickle cell disease, lung disease, or sleep apnea?	Decreased circulation can lead to inability to have a usable erection; decreased respiratory function can result in activity intolerance or loss of erection.

Table 41.7

Subjective Data Collection for the Male Reproductive System and Sexual Health—cont'd

Questions to Ask During the Health History	Rationale/Significance
Gastrointestinal	
Have you ever been diagnosed with or treated for liver infection/disease or bowel problems?	Liver infections/disease can lead to decreased testosterone and increased estrogen production, and loss of erection; gastrointestinal/bowel problems can lead to pain or loss of desire; surgery may result in loss of blood flow or innervation.
Musculoskeletal	
Do you have painful joints, pelvic/lower back pain, or nerve damage?	Pain; loss of desire; limited movement/positions; and loss of erection, ejaculation, and orgasm may result from musculoskeletal problems.
Neurologic	
Have you ever experienced a stroke or suffered from multiple sclerosis, Parkinson disease, or other neurologic disorders?	Limited movement/positions, loss of sensations, and loss of control can result from neurologic problems.
Metabolic/Endocrine	
Have you ever suffered from diabetes, obesity, or thyroid problems?	Diabetes mellitus can result in circulation problems, retrograde ejaculation, and nerve damage; obesity can result in decreased male hormones and excess female hormones.
Genitourinary	
Have you ever been diagnosed with a congenital deformity of the penis/testicles, suffered from prostate problems, or experienced erection/ejaculation problems?	Difficulty with erection, penetration problems, retrograde ejaculation, or infertility may be associated with genitourinary abnormalities, stress, or medication use.
Have you ever been diagnosed with a sexually transmitted infection? When, what type, and how was it treated? Are you aware if treatment was successful?	Lesions, pain, discharge, swelling, or other abnormalities of the external reproductive organs may indicate infection, structural abnormalities such as varicocele, or other disease processes such as cancer.
Do you have any lesions, pain, discharge, or swelling of the reproductive organs? Have you noticed any abnormalities/changes in size, shape, or color of your external reproductive organs (Describe)?	
Do you practice monthly TSEs?	Adolescent and adult men should be encouraged to perform monthly TSEs as a cancer prevention measure.
For patients older than age 50: When was the last time you had a prostate examination?	A digital rectal examination (DRE) should be a regular part of a man's routine physical after age 50. Prostate cancer is treatable when detected early.
Sexual Practices	
Are you sexually active? How many partners do you have? Of what gender? Is the amount/type of sexual activity satisfying?	Some sexual practices can lead to a decrease in quality and quantity of sperm that reach the female egg.

that are broader than their hips. The presence of excess breast tissue may indicate **gynecomastia,** from an excess of female hormones. Abnormal findings in either hair patterns or muscle mass often indicate a hormone imbalance.

The penis, scrotum, and testes (testicles) are examined by observation and palpation. On observation, the penis is normally flaccid (soft) and hanging straight down. The size can vary greatly and should not be a concern unless it is unusually small (microphallus) or edematous. The left testis typically hangs slightly lower in the scrotum than the right.

The penis is examined for warts, sores (evidence of STIs), swelling, curves, or lumps along the shaft. The examiner also makes sure the urethral opening is at the tip of the penis and not on the underside of the shaft (**hypospadias**) or on the dorsum of the shaft (**epispadias**). If the man is not **circumcised** (surgical removal of the foreskin), the foreskin should be pulled back carefully and the glans inspected for signs of inflammation or foul-smelling discharge. The HCP should be sure to replace the foreskin in the forward position after the examination is completed.

The scrotum and testes are carefully examined and palpated. Both testes should be present and a normal size (approximately 2 to 4 cm). The testes are egg shaped and should feel smooth and rubbery when lightly palpated between the thumb and fingers. The epididymis can be felt along the top edge and posterior section of each testis. The testes and scrotum are palpated for any lumps, cysts, or tumors. If a fluid-filled mass (**hydrocele**) is found, further evaluation should be done.

A simple noninvasive test called **transillumination** is used to determine whether a mass is fluid filled or solid. With the room lights out, a flashlight is held behind the scrotum. If the mass is fluid, a red glow appears; if it is solid, it appears opaque. Each spermatic cord (made up of veins, arteries, lymphatics, nerves, and the vas deferens) is palpated and should feel firm and threadlike. If a condition called a **varicocele** is present, the area feels like a bag of worms. A varicocele, which is swelling of the veins of the spermatic cord, is one of the most common problems associated with male infertility.

BE SAFE!

Wrap the flashlight with clear plastic wrap to decrease the risk of contamination. Change the wrap between patients.

The male patient is also examined for inguinal hernias by pressing up through the scrotum into each of the inguinal rings while asking him to cough or bear down. Each side is examined separately while he is in the standing position. A hernia feels like a pulsation against the examiner's fingertips.

A digital rectal examination (DRE) may be done by an experienced practitioner. During DRE, the prostate gland is palpated by inserting a gloved, lubricated finger into the rectum while the man is in the Sims position or standing and bending at a right angle over the exam table. The entire posterior lobe of the gland can be felt this way. The gland should feel slightly firm and without any lumps. If the prostate gland feels very hard or soft, feels enlarged, or contains any lumps, a rectal ultrasound with needle biopsy may be ordered. A swollen, painful prostate generally indicates that an infection is present.

Many men are under the impression that, if they have had prostate surgery, the gland has been completely removed. When simple surgery is performed, prostate tissue is left in the body and will begin to regrow over time. This prostatic tissue can become cancerous and needs to be monitored with a yearly DRE.

Remind all men age 50 and older to talk to their HCPs about prostate cancer screening. There are many pros and cons to screening, and each man should make a decision that is best for him. Table 41.8 provides a summary of objective data to collect for the male reproductive system.

Testicular Self-Examination

All men after puberty should do a monthly testicular self-examination (TSE) to detect any tumors or other changes in the scrotum (Figure 41.13). See Box 41.1 for instructions that can be used to teach a man how to examine his testicles.

CRITICAL THINKING

Tony is a 20-year-old who reports a "bump" on his right testicle. He comes into the health clinic and asks whether he can take any medication for his "disease."

1. What would be the best action?
2. What should your health assessment include?

Suggested answers are at the end of the chapter.

Breast Self-Examination

Although breast cancer in men is rare, it can occur. Men, like women, should be familiar with their breasts and report changes.

Diagnostic Tests of the Male Reproductive System
Ultrasound

An ultrasound may be done to diagnose or evaluate a variety of male reproductive or genitourinary problems. A transrectal ultrasound may be done to help diagnose prostate cancer.

• WORD • BUILDING •

gynecomastia: gyneco—female + mastia—breast
hypospadias: hypo—under + spadias—span, to draw
epispadias: epi—upon + spadias—span, to draw
circumcised: circum—around + cised—cut
hydrocele: hydro—water + cele—hernia
transillumination: trans—across + illumin—light + ation—process
varicocele: varico—twisted vein + cele—swelling

Table 41.8

Objective Data Collection for the Male Reproductive System

Physical Examination Findings	Possible Abnormal Findings/Causes
Clinical Breast Examination (CBE) Observe and palpate for presence of swelling, lumps, skin changes, and nipple exudates.	Changes may indicate breast cancer, although it is rare in males.
Glans of Penis Observe for lesions, exudate, and tenderness. Observe for placement of the urethra. If foreskin is present, attempt to reduce to observe for lesions, exudate, and inflammation. (Be sure to replace when finished to prevent paraphimosis.)	Lesions, exudate, and tenderness can indicate presence of infective or disease process and injury. Epispadias/hypospadias may be noted when observing for placement of the urethra.
Shaft of Penis Observe for lesions, tenderness, and shape.	Lesions, exudate, and tenderness can indicate presence of infectious or disease process or injury. Irregularity of shape may indicate structural abnormalities/disease.
Scrotum Visualize and palpate for swelling, pain, and lesions.	Inguinal herniation may be noted. Swelling may occur with heart or renal failure, local inflammation, or injury.
Testes Palpate for descent, pain, lesions, size, and shape, consistency. Palpate for lesions/swelling of epididymitis.	Absence of palpated testes may indicate nondescent. Testicular lesion can indicate testicular cancer. Swelling and pain can indicate infectious process.
Spermatic Cord Palpate for swelling, size, consistency, and pain.	Presence of swelling or pain can indicate infection or varicocele.
Inguinal Ring (exam performed by trained personnel) Palpate for bulge and pain.	Bulge or pain may indicate inguinal hernia.
Inguinal Lymph Nodes Palpate for swelling and pain.	Swelling or pain may indicate infectious process or regional malignancy.
Digital Rectal Exam (DRE; exam performed by trained personnel) Observe external rectum for lesions and exudate. Palpate for pain, swelling, and penile exudate.	Pain, swelling, or exudate may indicate benign changes, infectious process, cancer, or injury.

Note: A male physical examination is typically done by a health care provider or other trained provider.

For this procedure, a rectal probe transducer is inserted into the rectum; sound waves are used to evaluate the prostate gland.

Pelvic or scrotal ultrasound helps evaluate and locate masses. Ultrasound may also be done to guide a needle during a fine-needle biopsy.

NURSING CARE. Explain the procedure to the patient. An enema may be ordered before the procedure. No special after-care is needed.

Cystourethrography

A cystourethrogram may be done to evaluate the degree of obstruction by an enlarged prostate gland. For this procedure, a Foley catheter is inserted, and a dye is injected into the bladder. Radiographs are taken with the dye in the bladder and while voiding after the catheter has been removed.

NURSING CARE. Explain the procedure to the patient and assess for allergy to dye. Instruct the patient to void before the procedure. A sedative or analgesic may be ordered to help the

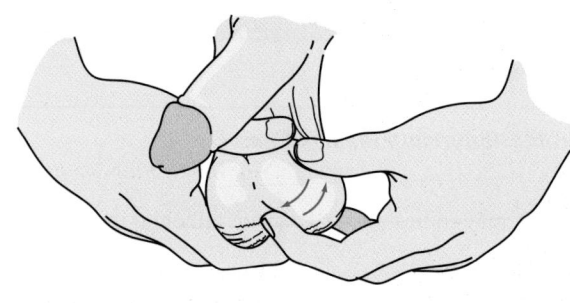

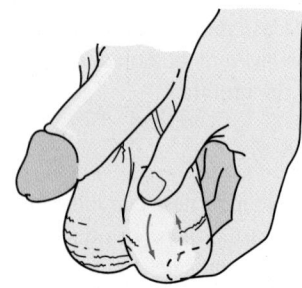

FIGURE 41.13 Testicular self-examination.

Box 41.1

Guidelines for Monthly Testicular Self-Examination

A testicular self-examination is easiest during or right after a warm shower or bath, when the scrotum is relaxed and the testicles are hanging low. Choose the same day each month to do the examination.

1. Raise the penis up out of the way and look for any difference in size or shape of each side of the scrotum (sac). The left side usually hangs a little lower than the right.
2. Using both hands, hold the scrotum in the palms. Begin, one at a time, to gently roll each testicle between the thumb and first three fingers, feeling for any lumps or hard spots.
3. Identify the parts. The testicles should feel round, smooth, and egg shaped. The epididymis along the top and back side should feel soft and a little bit tender. The spermatic cord is a tube that runs from the epididymis and usually feels firm, smooth, and movable.
4. See your health care provider immediately if you feel any lumps or unusual changes.

patient relax during the procedure. If an analgesic is used, the patient will need to have someone available to drive him home.

After the procedure, intake and output are measured for 24 hours. Alteration from the patient's normal pattern, such as blood in the urine or absence of urination, is reported to the HCP. Fluids are encouraged to promote excretion of the dye. A warm, moist cloth held over the urethra can assist with mild pain.

Laboratory Tests

PROSTATE-SPECIFIC ANTIGEN. Prostate-specific antigen (PSA) is a glycoprotein produced by prostate cells. The normal value of PSA is less than 4 ng/mL. An elevated level indicates prostatic hypertrophy or cancer.

PROSTATIC ACID PHOSPHATASE. Prostatic acid phosphatase (PAP) is an enzyme that normally affects metabolism of prostate cancer cells. The normal value of PAP is less than 3 ng/mL. An elevated level indicates possible prostate cancer.

OTHER TESTS. If prostate cancer is suspected or diagnosed, additional tests may be done. Acid phosphatase may be elevated in metastatic prostate cancer. Alkaline phosphatase and serum calcium levels may be elevated if metastasis to the bone has occurred. Table 41.9 provides a summary of diagnostic procedures.

Tests for Infertility

Various hormone levels may be measured, including FSH, LH, testosterone, and adrenocorticotropic hormone (ACTH), to help determine causes of infertility in male patients.

Semen analysis may be done to provide information about causes of infertility or to evaluate whether a vasectomy has been effective. Semen may be analyzed for sperm count, motility, and shape. Other tests determine whether the semen contains adequate nutrients to support sperm, whether antibodies to the sperm are present, and the ability of the sperm to penetrate an ovum.

NURSING CARE. The patient is instructed to refrain from ejaculation for 3 days before collecting the semen sample to avoid altering findings. Generally, specimens are collected on three separate occasions over a period of 4 to 6 days. Masturbation and ejaculation directly into a sterile container are recommended to avoid loss of semen. Condoms and lubricants should be avoided. The sample should be taken to the laboratory within 1 hour of collection. Additional tests of the male reproductive system are discussed in Chapter 43.

Table 41.9

Diagnostic Procedures for the Male Reproductive System

Procedure	Definition/Normal Finding	Significance of Abnormal Findings	Nursing Management
Noninvasive			
Testicular self-examination (TSE)	Palpation of testes by patient.	Abnormalities may indicate pathology and require further evaluation.	Instruct patient on appropriate technique and witness a return demonstration.
Ultrasound	High-frequency sound waves bounce off tissue to map tissue structure and determine tissue density. Also may be used to guide biopsy procedure.	May help to determine abnormal lesions, abnormalities of tissue structure, or presence of abnormal fluid volume.	Follow institutional guidelines for patient preparation and support.
Hormonal tests and antigen level testing	Blood test to measure hormone or antigen levels.	Abnormal hormone levels may reflect fertility potential. Abnormal antigen levels may indicate pathology.	Consult institutional policies for specific instructions for each test. Explain procedure to patient and provide support.
Invasive			
Digital rectal examination (DRE)	Palpation of internal reproductive organs, especially prostate gland, through rectum.	Abnormal physical exam may indicate pathology and indicates need for further testing.	Educate patient about procedure and provide support.
Cystourethrography	Insertion of a Foley catheter and dye into the bladder to evaluate for obstruction (usually an enlarged prostate) by radiography.	Obstruction may cause difficulty with urination.	Educate patient about the procedure and postprocedure care. Instruct patient to void before procedure. Measure intake and output for 24 hours following procedure. Observe for allergic reaction.

SUGGESTED ANSWERS TO CRITICAL THINKING

Jilli

1. The answer should include basic breast health statistics and risks as well as proper assessment practice and techniques, as discussed in this chapter. She should be informed that, although monthly breast self-examination is not absolutely necessary, knowing her breasts and reporting changes are essential. Technique should be demonstrated and a return demonstration done during the visit.

2. Questions about breast health and self-assessment practices provide an opportunity for the nurse to educate a patient about health facts and technique. Patient questions can also be a cue to patient readiness and willingness to learn.

Reproductive Assessment

1. Calm fears. Explain simply. Allow the parent to stay with the child during the examination if appropriate. Consider whether it is possible that the child has been abused. If so, evidence needs to be collected and a report filed with the

SUGGESTED ANSWERS TO CRITICAL THINKING—cont'd

appropriate child protection authorities. Check with your supervisor if you believe this is a possibility. Teach the child that this is a normal part of the body that is to be protected and taken care of.

2. Assess knowledge and maturity. Prepare the patient for a Pap smear and for swabs and smears. Teach while getting supplies ready. Explain that vaginal soreness usually needs to be treated and that the health care provider (HCP) must know more about the problem to do so effectively. Explain that inflammation can interfere with Pap smear results, so testing may have to be repeated after treatment. Explain culture and sensitivity testing. Teach about risk reduction and inform that oral contraceptives do not offer a barrier against sexually transmitted infections (STIs).

3. Try to put the woman at ease through general conversation. Set out supplies for a Pap smear (if needed) and for swabs and smears. Teach while getting supplies ready. Discuss aging and the effects of decreased estrogen in general and specifically on vaginal tissues. Inform her that there are several ways to deal with problems resulting from decreased estrogen, such as oral hormonal replacements, water-soluble vaginal lubricants, vaginal creams, estrogen patches, and selective estrogen receptor modulators.

Tony

1. Palpable scrotal changes can result from a variety of reproductive and/or genitourinary abnormalities. Before Tony's question can be answered, a complete history needs to be obtained and a clinical exam of the genitalia performed.

2. The history should explore if:
   • testicular self-examinations are regularly performed and if changes have been noted;
   • Tony is sexually active and has, recently or in the past, been knowingly exposed to an STI; and
   • there has been pain associated with the "bump" or exudate noted from the penis.

The assessment, done by an HCP should include:
• visual inspection of the size, shape, symmetry, and color of the scrotum and its contents;
• palpation to assess for abnormalities and pain;
• cultures to rule out STIs; and
• An inguinal exam to rule out herniation.

   Ultimately, based on the patient's report, a testicular tumor should be ruled out.

Review Questions

1. When obtaining the history of a 17-year-old male during a sports physical, what important screening practice should be discussed?
   1. Yearly digital rectal examination
   2. Monthly testicular self-examination
   3. Yearly prostate-specific antigen
   4. Bimonthly bimanual examination

2. Which of the following problems can occur with reduced estrogen secretion in aging women? **Select all that apply.**
   1. Increased cholesterol level
   2. Breast swelling
   3. Bone loss
   4. Urinary incontinence
   5. Muscle spasms

3. A 66-year-old woman is seen in an outpatient clinic for routine care. What teaching should the nurse provide related to bone health?
   1. "You should be taking in at least 1,200 mg of calcium and 600 international units of vitamin D in your diet."
   2. "The benefit of eating red meat outweighs the risk as you age. You should eat 6 ounces three times a week."
   3. "Your bones are protected by the calcium you ate in your younger years; increasing intake now will not help your bones."
   4. "It is important to take a calcium and vitamin D supplement, because it is difficult to get enough in your diet."

4. How would the nurse document the reproductive history of a pregnant woman who is in her fourth pregnancy, has two living children ages 3 and 5, and had one miscarriage?
   1. P4G2M1
   2. G4P3P5M1
   3. P4G35A1
   4. G4P2A1

5. What is the role of the licensed practical nurse/licensed vocational nurse in physical assessment of the male and female genitals?
   1. Perform a complete history and physical assessment of the genital area.
   2. Collect specimens under the supervision of the registered nurse.
   3. Prepare the patient for what to expect during the practitioner's examination.
   4. The licensed practical nurse/licensed vocational nurse does not have a role in assessment of the reproductive system.

Answer rationales available in your online resources.

ANSWERS 1. 2; 2. 1, 3, 4; 3. 1; 4. 4; 5. 3

Key Points

Find the chapter key points in your online resources available through Davis Edge.

Additional Resources

Use the scratch off code on the inside front cover of your book to access online quizzes that will help you to improve your scores on course exams and prepare for the NCLEX-PN®.

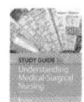 Study Guide

CHAPTER 42

Nursing Care of Women With Reproductive System Disorders

Laura L. McCully

KEY TERMS

agenesis (ay-JEN-uh-sis)
amenorrhea (AY-men-oh-REE-ah)
anteflexion (AN-tee-FLEK-shun)
anteversion (AN-tee-VER-zhun)
augmentation (AWG-men-TAY-shun)
colporrhaphy (kohl-POOR-ah-fee)
contraceptive (KON-truh-SEP-tiv)
cryotherapy (KRY-oh-THER-uh-pee)
culdocentesis (KUL-doh-sen-TEE-sis)
culdotomy (kul-DOT-uh-mee)
cystocele (SIS-toh-seel)
dermoid (DER-moyd)
dilation and curettage (DIL-AY-shun and kyoor-e-TAHZH)
dysmenorrhea (DIS-men-oh-REE-ah)
dyspareunia (DIS-puh-ROO-nee-ah)
dysplasia (dis-PLAY-zee-ah)
fibrocystic (FY-broh-SIS-tik)
hypertrophy (hy-PER-truh-fee)
hypoplasia (HY-poh-PLAY-zee-ah)
hysterectomy (HISS-tuh-REK-tuh-mee)
hysterotomy (HISS-tuh-RAH-tuh-mee)
imperforate (im-PER-foh-rate)
in vitro fertilization (in-VEE-troh FER-ti-li-ZAY-shun)
laparotomy (LAP-uh-RAH-tuh-mee)
leiomyoma (LYE-oh-my-OH-mah)
lumpectomy (lump-EK-tuh-mee)
mammoplasty (MAM-oh-PLAS-tee)
marsupialization (mar-SOO-pee-al-ih-ZAY-shun)
mastalgia (mass-TAL-jee-ah)
mastectomy (mass-TEK-tuh-mee)
mastitis (mass-TY-tis)
mastopexy (MAS-toh-PEKS-ee)
myomectomy (MY-oh-MEK-tuh-mee)
oophorectomy (oo-fur-EK-tuh-mee)
perimenopause (PER-ee-MEN-oh-PAWS)
phytoestrogens (FY-toh-ES-troh-jenz)
postcoital (post-KOH-ih-tal)
rectocele (REK-toh-seel)

LEARNING OUTCOMES

1. Explain the pathophysiology of each of the disorders of the female reproductive system.
2. Describe the etiologies, signs, and symptoms of each disorder.
3. Identify tests used to diagnose female disorders.
4. Describe current therapeutic management for each disorder.
5. List data to collect when caring for patients with disorders of the female reproductive system.
6. Plan nursing care for female patients with reproductive disorders.
7. Explain how you will know whether nursing interventions have been effective.
8. Compare different forms of contraceptives and their effectiveness.

retroflexion (RE-troh-FLEK-shun)
retrograde (RE-troh-grade)
retroversion (RE-troh-VER-zhun)
salpingectomy (sal-pin-JEK-tuh-mee)
teratoma (ter-uh-TOH-muh)
vaginitis (VAJ-in-EYE-tis)
vaginosis (VAJ-in-OH-sis)

CHAPTER CONCEPTS

Health Promotion
Family Dynamics
Self
Sexuality

Reproductive system disorders can be frightening, irritating, frustrating, embarrassing, and, in some cases, fatal. They involve not just body parts but also roles, relationships, and sense of identity and purpose in life. Nurses can play an important role in helping women with these disorders. Women's health is an area in which much research is being done. The Nurses' Health Study, conducted at Harvard Medical School, is a large ongoing study on many topics related to women's health. You can learn about it at www.nurseshealthstudy.org.

BREAST DISORDERS

Benign Breast Disorders
Cyclic Breast Discomfort
PATHOPHYSIOLOGY, ETIOLOGIES, AND SIGNS AND SYMPTOMS. The most common breast symptoms result from cyclic variations in hormone levels. Swelling, tenderness, and sometimes pain (**mastalgia**) can be related to hormone-mediated changes within the breast tissues that prepare them for their potential role of breastfeeding.

TREATMENT. If persistent or severe, these symptoms can be treated with oral contraceptives that modify hormone levels or nonsteroidal anti-inflammatory drugs (NSAIDs) to control pain. Explaining that cyclic discomfort is temporary and not from a disease process helps to reduce fears.

Fibrocystic Breast Disease
PATHOPHYSIOLOGY, ETIOLOGIES, AND SIGNS AND SYMPTOMS. Fibrocystic breast disease is common in women between the ages of 30 and 50. Overresponsiveness of cells in the breasts to hormonal stimulation (especially estrogen) can cause long-term changes resulting in replacement of normal tissue with fibrous tissue, overdevelopment of cells, and blockage of ducts so that cysts form around trapped fluid. This makes the breasts feel hard, lumpy, and sometimes painful. These changes often occur during the reproductive years and can be responses to hormonal variations during the menstrual cycle. Fibrocystic changes usually subside with menopause.

DIAGNOSIS AND TREATMENT. Fibrocystic breast changes can be identified on palpation. A mammogram or ultrasound may be done to aid in diagnosis. A biopsy may be done to rule out cancer. Treatment for fibrocystic breast changes is based on patient symptoms. Often, no treatment is necessary. Analgesics, primarily NSAIDs, help reduce discomfort. Herbal remedies, such as evening primrose oil, or supplemental vitamin therapy may offer symptomatic relief, but these therapies remain controversial. Limitation of dietary fat and caffeine and addition of oral contraceptive use may help control hormonal changes.

Although fibrocystic changes are not cancerous, more frequent mammography or ultrasound may be advised because fibrocystic changes can make it more difficult to feel early cancerous lumps during breast examination. Some types of breast cysts are associated with a higher cancer risk. Needle aspiration may be used to treat cystic lesions.

Mastitis
PATHOPHYSIOLOGY, ETIOLOGIES, AND SIGNS AND SYMPTOMS. Mastitis is breast infection with inflammation. It occurs as a result of injury and introduction of bacteria into the breast. This condition most commonly occurs while breastfeeding. The breast becomes swollen, hot, red, and painful; an abscess can form.

TREATMENT. Mastitis can be treated either with antibiotics or by incision and drainage of the abscessed area. NSAIDs, warm packs, and breast supports are often used to control pain and swelling.

NURSING CARE AND PATIENT EDUCATION. Teach the patient to wash her hands carefully to prevent the spread of infection. If the patient is breastfeeding, it is often continued to promote drainage of the breast, mother–infant bonding, and infant nutrition. The infant is often already colonized with the bacteria so further exposure is not thought to be harmful.

> ### NURSING CARE TIP
> To help prevent mastitis in a breastfeeding mother, recommend frequent changes in feeding positions to empty all portions of the breast as well as good hand hygiene techniques when handling the breasts. Also recommend breastfeeding frequently and not restricting the length of feeds.

Malignant Breast Disorders
Pathophysiology and Etiology
Breast cancer is an abnormal growth of breast cells. It can arise from the milk-producing glands, the ductal system, or the fatty and connective tissues of the breast. It is the most commonly diagnosed cancer in women (Centers for Disease Control and Prevention, 2017).

Research has identified factors that increase the risk of breast cancer. These include increasing age; personal or family history of breast, ovarian, or prostate cancer; a high-fat diet; high alcohol intake; treatment with estrogens (especially when used without progestins); early menarche; late menopause; and first pregnancy after age 30.

Signs and Symptoms
A lump or thickening of breast tissue or a change in the shape or contour of a breast can indicate breast cancer. A tumor can also cause dimpling of the overlying skin or retraction of the nipple. Clear or bloody nipple discharge can occur. Swelling, tenderness, or discoloration of the breast can indicate inflammatory breast cancer, a rare but deadly form. Breast symptoms have many causes, but all should be investigated by a health care provider (HCP).

Prevention
Breast cancer risk can be reduced by exercising, moderating fat and alcohol consumption, and using nonhormonal methods for birth control and menopausal symptoms. Breastfeeding may also reduce risk, even in women who have late first

• WORD • BUILDING •
mastalgia: mast—breast + algia—pain
fibrocystic: fibro—fibrous + cystic—sac-like
mastitis: mast—breast + itis—inflammation

pregnancies. However, many factors cannot be controlled, so the importance of early detection cannot be overemphasized. Certain genes (*BRCA1* and *BRCA2)* are linked with susceptibility to breast cancer. Genetic testing offers the possibility of very early identification of women at the highest risk of developing breast cancer (as well as ovarian cancer for those with *BRCA1*). These women can then be monitored closely for breast changes and receive early treatment if cancer develops. Some women choose to have bilateral prophylactic (or risk-reducing) mastectomy.

Before genetic testing, patients should be counseled by a professional who is qualified to explain and interpret the results. It is also important to review risks and benefits of testing. Some insurance plans don't cover the cost of such testing. More information regarding *BRCA* testing can be found at www.cancer.gov/about-cancer/causes-prevention/genetics/brca-fact-sheet.

Diagnostic Tests

Breast self-examination (BSE) and clinical breast examination (CBE) may play an important role in cancer identification. Cancerous growths tend to be harder, less mobile, less painful, and more irregularly shaped. They also have less clearly defined borders than benign growths. The prognosis is good for women who have breast cancer removed in the early stages but gets worse when treatment begins during later stages of the disease process. Teaching and encouraging regular use of BSE and appropriate use of mammography can save lives. See Chapter 41 for more about BSE and for explanations about diagnostic tests used to assist in determining whether tumors of the breast are malignant.

Staging

The spread (metastasis) of cancerous cells from the primary site to other areas of the body by way of the blood or lymph is denoted by staging classifications 0 to IV (see Chapter 11). Lower numbers indicate less cancer spread.

Therapeutic Measures

The five main treatment options for breast cancer are surgery, radiation therapy, chemotherapy, hormone therapy, and targeted therapies. These options may be used separately or in combination depending on the condition of the patient and the stage of the disease. Patients may also choose complementary and holistic therapies. Immunotherapy is a new and promising field of breast cancer treatment that uses the body's immune system to fight cancer. A number of immunotherapies are currently being studied, including the use of vaccines.

SURGERY. A **lumpectomy** removes just the tumor and a margin around it. A **mastectomy** may be partial (removing only part of the breast), simple (removing the breast tissue of one or both breasts), or radical (removing breast tissue, underlying muscle, and surrounding lymph nodes). The amount of tissue removed varies depending on the size, nature, and invasiveness of the cancer. Surgical practice has shifted from radical mastectomies to more breast-conserving surgeries with the addition of radiation therapy, resulting in survival rates similar

to those for radical mastectomy. Surgeries to remove cancerous breast tissue can be disfiguring and have profound effects on a patient's body image and self-esteem.

RADIATION THERAPY. Radiation can be administered externally or internally to attack the rapidly dividing cells of a tumor. Although radiation affects all rapidly dividing cells in its path, including healthy cells, radiation to an area of the breast just surrounding the tumor bed reduces the incidence of side effects. It is usually used after surgery to reduce the risk of cancer recurrence or spread.

CHEMOTHERAPY. Chemotherapy kills all rapidly dividing cells, not just breast cancer cells, which leads to many side effects. It may be used alone or in combination with other therapies. Newer chemotherapy options use higher doses over a shorter treatment period to reduce side effects (see Chapter 11).

HORMONE THERAPY. Hormone therapy may be used to deprive cancer cells of hormones that stimulate their growth. Because breast cancer cells are often estrogen sensitive, this may be accomplished by decreasing circulating estrogen levels with drugs or by blocking the use of estrogen by cancer cells. Interference with estrogen levels, however, may produce menopausal symptoms and increase the risk of osteoporosis and heart disease. Table 42.1 lists estrogen antagonists.

TARGETED THERAPIES. Targeted therapies attack specific molecular agents or pathways involved in the development of cancer. Some targeted therapies are given to intensify positive body responses (e.g., stimulate the immune system) or to decrease negative body responses. Because they target cancer cells, they are less toxic to normal cells. Examples include biological response modifiers such as interferons, tumor necrosis factor, interleukins, and various experimental immunotherapy formulations. Three drugs that target the protein HER2, which is found on the surface of breast cancer cells, are trastuzumab (Herceptin), pertuzumab (Perjeta), and lapatinib (Tykerb).

Alternative therapies are also available for many cancers. See Chapter 5 for information about helping patients evaluate alternative and complementary therapies. The American Cancer Society and cancer treatment centers also have staff who can answer questions about experimental and alternative therapies and discuss research findings. For more information about breast cancer, visit the American Cancer Society at www.cancer.org. Other helpful sites are www.breastcancer.org and ww5.komen.org.

Nursing Care

See "Nursing Care Plan for the Patient Undergoing a Mastectomy." In addition to the diagnoses covered, the patient will need care for postoperative pain. See Chapters 10 and 12, respectively, for additional interventions for pain and postoperative patients. Table 42.2 provides a breast cancer summary.

• WORD • BUILDING •

lumpectomy: lump + ec—away + tomy—cutting
mastectomy: mast—breast + ec—away + tomy—cutting

Nursing Care Plan for the Patient Undergoing a Mastectomy

Nursing Diagnosis: *Anxiety* related to uncertainty about diagnosis, prognosis, and treatments
Expected Outcomes: The patient will verbalize and demonstrate a decrease in anxiety.
Evaluation of Outcomes: Does the patient report a decrease in anxiety following education and explanation of the procedure? Do the patient's vital signs and verbal and nonverbal behaviors suggest a decrease in anxiety?

Intervention	Rationale	Evaluation
Assess vital signs and observe verbal and nonverbal behavior.	*An increase in blood pressure, pulse, and respirations as well as observation of mild to severe agitation may indicate anxiety.*	Are patient's vital signs within normal range for the patient? Is verbal and nonverbal behavior consistent with anxiety?
Assess patient's current knowledge of the procedure and level of anxiety related to the procedure.	*Assessment of current knowledge provides a baseline for teaching.*	What does patient know? What teaching is needed?
Teach patient what to expect about the surgical experience based on patient's understanding, concerns, and willingness to learn.	*Knowledge dispels unreasonable fears and helps patient to prepare to cope with stressors.*	Does patient evidence adequate understanding of the procedure and what to expect afterward?
Support and clarify the health care provider's (HCP's) explanations, answer questions, and refer to knowledgeable sources.	*The patient may not remember or understand what the HCP said.*	Does patient have accurate information? Are appropriate referrals made?

Nursing Diagnosis: *Ineffective Breathing Pattern* related to pain with chest movement following surgery
Expected Outcome: The patient will have an effective breathing pattern with clear lung sounds and oxygen saturation (Spo_2) of 95% or above.
Evaluation of Outcome: Are respirations regular, easy, and unlabored? Are respiratory rate and Spo_2 within a normal range for the patient? Are lung sounds clear?

Intervention	Rationale	Evaluation
Assess patient's vital signs, Spo_2, pain level, and lung sounds.	*Pain contributes to shallow breathing, which can affect vital signs, Spo_2, and lung sounds*	Are patient's vital signs and Spo_2 within normal range for the patient? Does patient report pain at an acceptable level? Are lung sounds clear?
Medicate to relieve pain as ordered. Remember that opioids can depress respirations and continue to monitor breathing.	*Pain may inhibit deep breathing efforts.*	Does patient evidence pain or guarding during chest movement? Does analgesic help?
Encourage deep breathing and coughing each hour.	*This helps to loosen secretions and to prevent atelectasis, pneumonia, and inadequate oxygenation of tissues.*	Does chest sound clear? Are skin color and Spo_2 adequate?
Encourage use of an incentive spirometer each hour when awake.	*To encourage deep breathing.*	Does patient use spirometer correctly?

Nursing Diagnosis: *Risk for Ineffective Peripheral Tissue Perfusion* related to damage to blood and lymph vessels and tension at surgical incision site
Expected Outcome: The patient's incision will heal by primary intention without excessive bleeding or swelling.
Evaluation of Outcome: Are edges of the incision well approximated, with scant bleeding/serous drainage and mild edema/erythema?

Intervention	Rationale	Evaluation
Monitor vital signs and Spo_2 according to agency policy and as necessary.	*Vital signs and Spo_2 affect tissue perfusion and oxygenation.*	Are vital signs and Spo_2 stable and within normal range? Are extremities pink and warm?

(nursing care plan continues on page 868)

Nursing Care Plan for the Patient Undergoing a Mastectomy—cont'd

Intervention	Rationale	Evaluation
Avoid use of the affected arm for blood pressures, venipunctures, and injections.	*Restrictive and invasive procedures might further compromise tissue integrity of the affected arm.*	Is arm protected?
Assess incision for bleeding, amount and color of drainage, and swelling. Empty drain device as needed.	*Excessive bleeding or swelling can compromise tissue perfusion.*	Does incisional area look swollen, smooth, or shiny? Are drainage amount and color appropriate?
Measure circumference of arms daily and compare. Report changes.	*Swelling causes an increase in circumference and impairs circulation.*	Is affected arm larger than unaffected arm?
Elevate affected arm if swelling occurs.	*Gravity aids fluid return to the heart.*	Does elevation reduce swelling?
Place items where patient can easily reach them.	*Excessive movement of the affected arm may exert tension on incision and increase bleeding.*	Can patient reach items without abducting the arm more than 90 degrees?
Encourage postmastectomy exercises of affected arm according to agency policy.	*Appropriate exercise promotes circulation, preserves muscle and joint function, and increases self-care ability.*	Is patient moving arm appropriately and gradually increasing range of motion and self-care ability?
Teach postoperative self-care and signs and symptoms of ineffective healing to report.	*Early assessment and intervention help prevent the development of serious complications.*	Does patient demonstrate and verbalize understanding of appropriate postoperative self-care?

Nursing Diagnosis: *Ineffective Coping* related to cancer threat and body image disturbance
Expected Outcomes: The patient will verbalize ability to cope and will seek help and support appropriately.
Evaluation of Outcomes: Does the patient take an interest in care of condition? Does the patient ask appropriate questions related to care and verbalize appropriate concerns?

Intervention	Rationale	Evaluation
Observe patient's interest in self-care, ability to problem solve, and level of family or other support.	*Poor self-care, problem-solving skills, and lack of support may indicate a risk for ineffective coping.*	Does patient solve problems appropriately? Are family members or other support persons present? Is patient taking an active interest in her personal appearance?
Use therapeutic communication and listening skills to allow patient to share concerns.	*Loss of a breast disturbs many aspects of body image, and cancer threatens one's sense of security and stability in life.*	Is patient able to share concerns?
Help patient remember previous successes in coping and strategies used.	*Memory of prior success can encourage hope for future success.*	Does patient possess appropriate coping strategies?
Provide accurate information according to agency policy.	*Fear of the unknown can increase anxiety and reduce coping.*	Does patient relate understanding of follow-up treatment?
Refer to appropriate agencies for further support as needed (e.g., American Cancer Society, Reach to Recovery, local support groups).	*Social support can assist individuals to meet their needs while developing effective coping skills and strategies.*	Does patient have resources to call on as needed?

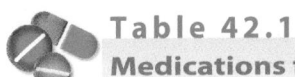

Table 42.1

Medications for Disorders Related to Hormonal Alterations (Breast Disorders, Menstrual Disorders, Menopause)

Medication Class/Action

Contraceptives

Interfere with the release of gonadotropin-releasing hormone (GnRH), luteinizing hormone (LH), and follicle-stimulating hormone (FSH); also maintain stable hormonal levels, relax uterus, and limit endometrial proliferation.

Examples

Progesterone and estrogen:
Oral:
norethindrone acetate and ethinyl estradiol (Loestrin)
drospirenone and ethinyl estradiol (Yasmin, Yaz)
levonorgestrel and ethinyl estradiol (Aviane)
ethinyl estradiol/norgestimate (Ortho Tri-Cyclen)
Patch:
norelgestromin and ethinyl estradiol (Ortho Evra)
Vaginal ring:
etonogestrel and ethinyl estradiol (NuvaRing)
Progesterone only:
norethindrone (Micronor)
medroxyprogesterone Acetate (Depo-Provera)
levonorgestrel-releasing intrauterine system (Mirena,
    Skyla, Kyleena)
etonogestrel implant (Nexplanon)

Nursing Implications

Teach:
About use and side effects (see ACHES side effects in
    Learning Tip).
Smoking increases risk of blood clots; advise to stop
    smoking while on these medications.

Hormone Replacement Therapy (HRT)

Interferes with GnRH, LH, and FSH release; also maintains stable hormonal levels, relaxes uterus, limits endometrial proliferation, promotes vasomotor stability, and prevents bone loss.

Examples

Progesterone and estrogen:
conjugated estrogens and medroxyprogesterone (Prempro)
estradiol and norethindrone acetate (Activella)
Estrogen only:
conjugated estrogens (Premarin, Cenestin)
estradiol (Estrace, Climara)
Vaginal preparations:
conjugated estrogens (Premarin cream)
estradiol (Estrace cream, Vagifem, Estring)
Progesterone only:
norethindrone (Micronor)
medroxyprogesterone acetate (Provera)
Estrogen and testosterone:
esterified estrogens and methyltestosterone (Estratest)

Nursing Implications

Teach:
About use and side effects (see ACHES side effects in
    Learning Tip).
Smoking increases risk of blood clots; advise to stop
    smoking while on these medications.

Nonsteroidal Anti-inflammatory Drugs (NSAIDs)

Inhibit prostaglandin synthesis, therefore interrupt pain receptors and produce anti-inflammatory effect.

Examples

ibuprofen (Motrin, Nuprin, Advil)
naproxen (Aleve)
ketoprofen (Orudis)
ketorolac (Toradol)

Nursing Implications

Avoid with aspirin allergy.
Administer with milk or food.
Ketorolac is reserved for acute pain due to bleeding
    risk.

Continued

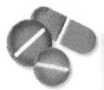

Table 42.1

Medications for Disorders Related to Hormonal Alterations (Breast Disorders, Menstrual Disorders, Menopause)—cont'd

Medication Class/Action	
	Teach: About side effects, use during pregnancy, and use when on anticoagulant therapy.

Estrogen Antagonists

Inhibit growth of estrogen-dependent tumors.

Examples	**Nursing Implications**
tamoxifen (Nolvadex)	Promote use of nonhormonal contraceptives during use.
anastrozole (Arimidex)	*Teach:*
toremifene (Fareston)	Report vaginal bleeding, leg cramps, shortness of breath, and weakness.
exemestane (Aromasin)	Smoking increases risk of blood clots; advise to stop smoking during use.
letrozole (Femara)	
fulvestrant (Faslodex)	

Table 42.2

Breast Cancer Summary

Signs and Symptoms	Swelling, tenderness, pain, redness
	Palpable lumps
	Leakage of fluid/blood from nipple
	Changes in contour of skin of breast/nipple
Diagnostic Tests and Findings	Breast self-examination (BSE) and clinical breast examination (CBE)
	Mammography
	Excisional/fine-needle biopsy
Therapeutic Measures	Lumpectomy, mastectomy, breast reconstruction
	Radiation
	Chemotherapy
	Hormone therapy
	Targeted therapy
Complications	Metastasis
	Significant treatment side effects
	Profound negative effect on patient's self-image.
Priority Nursing Diagnoses	*Anxiety*
	Ineffective Breathing Pattern
	Risk for Ineffective Peripheral Tissue Perfusion
	Ineffective Coping

CRITICAL THINKING

Julie, age 32, reports pain and grapelike "lumps" in her breasts, and her nurse practitioner diagnoses fibrocystic changes.

1. What questions would you ask to further assess Julie's symptoms?
2. What can you teach Julie to help her control her symptoms?
3. What can Julie do to remain vigilant for more concerning changes in her breasts?

   Suggested answers are at the end of the chapter.

Breast Modification Surgeries

Mammoplasty is surgical modification of the breast. This may be done to restore a normal shape after removal of cancerous tissues. Many women, however, undergo mammoplasty electively to change the size or appearance of their breasts. Body image is an important component of quality of life.

Breast Reduction and Mastopexy

Generally, in breast reduction operations, the nipple is separated from the surrounding tissue except for a small section with the blood vessels and nerves that supply it (Fig. 42.1). A large wedge of tissue is removed from the bottom of the breast, the edges are sewn together, and the nipple is

· WORD · BUILDING ·

mammoplasty: mamm(o)—breast + plasty—to mold

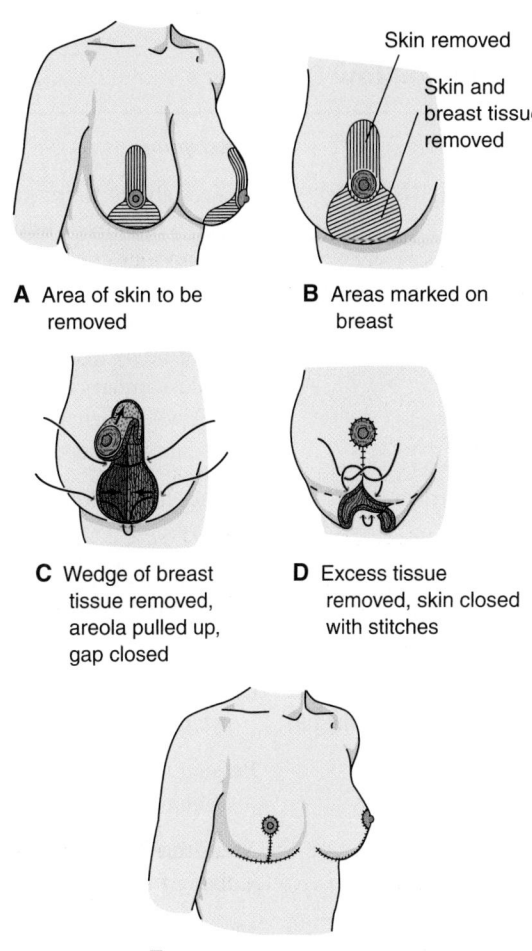

A Area of skin to be removed

B Areas marked on breast

C Wedge of breast tissue removed, areola pulled up, gap closed

D Excess tissue removed, skin closed with stitches

E Post-operative appearance

FIGURE 42.1 Breast reduction.

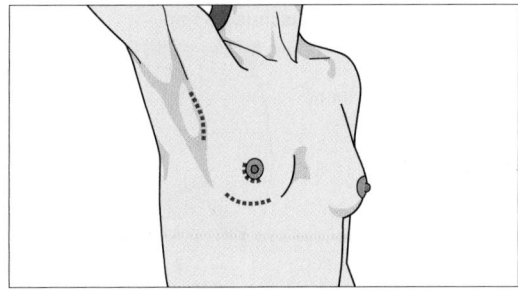

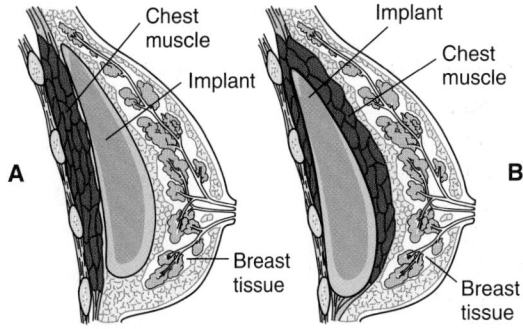

FIGURE 42.2 (A) Implant over muscle. (B) Implant under muscle.

reimplanted in a higher position. This not only decreases the overall size of the breast, which may help with back, neck, and head pain, but also corrects excessive sagging—a common problem for women with large breasts.

A **mastopexy** involves the removal of some skin and fat with subsequent resuturing so that the breast tissues are held higher on the chest to correct sagging breasts. This procedure usually does not remove as much tissue as a breast reduction.

Augmentation and Reconstruction Mammoplasty

Augmentation is a surgery to increase the size of the breasts. An implant—either a bag containing saline solution or silicone gel or a transplanted portion of the patient's own body tissues from another area—is inserted through an incision and positioned either under or over the pectoral muscles (Fig. 42.2).

For reconstructive mammoplasty, use of the patient's own tissues is generally safer than use of artificial implants because no foreign material is introduced into the body. For situations in which significant amounts of tissue are needed for reconstruction, a portion of tissue may be moved

from one area of the body to another as a pedicle graft. *Pedicle* literally means "little foot" because the graft remains attached to a stalk (containing the blood vessels and nerves) somewhat resembling a little leg with a foot (the graft) attached.

Figure 42.3 shows two options for mastectomy graft repair. Tissue from the buttock area or the abdomen may also be grafted onto a mastectomy site without a pedicle.

Complications

Any surgery can be complicated by infection or impaired healing. The use of silicone implants has been less than satisfactory for many women. Some women have experienced hardening of breast tissues, and others have developed serious autoimmune problems after receiving silicone gel implants. Although actual etiologies of all the problems are uncertain, many surgeries have been undertaken recently to remove silicone implants; saline implants are now more common.

Nursing Care and Patient Education

Carefully assess the healing process when changing dressings and explain to the patient how to assess healing, because not all tissues successfully attach at the new site. Failure of attachment can require surgical revision. Signs of poor attachment include unnatural color of the incision, graft, or surrounding tissues; swelling; drainage; gaping incision lines; and sloughing of the graft or edges of the site.

• WORD • BUILDING •

mastopexy: masto—breast + pexy—fixation

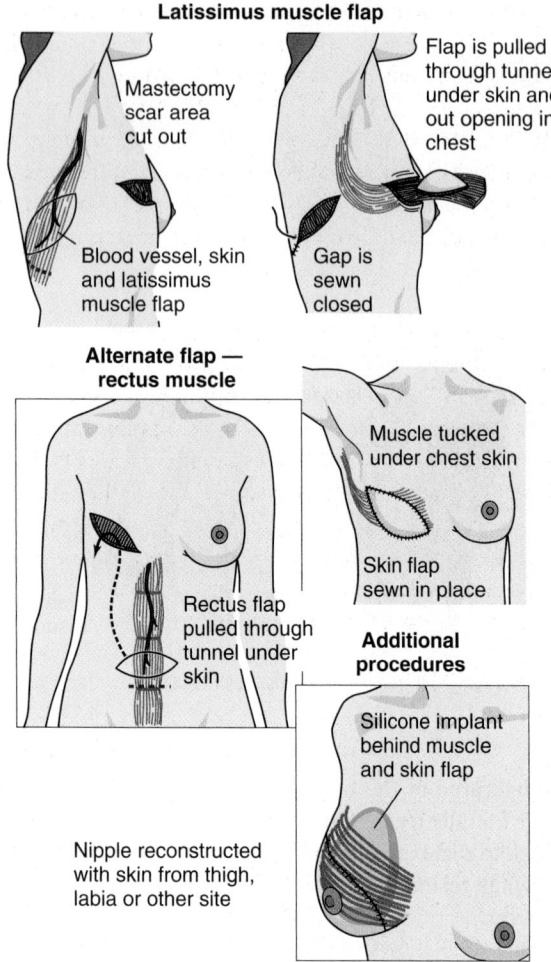

FIGURE 42.3 Mastectomy reconstruction.

Table 42.3
Menstrual Flow Disorders

Disorder	Description
Amenorrhea	Menses absent for more than 6 months or three of previous cycles Called primary amenorrhea when menarche has not occurred by age 17 Called secondary amenorrhea when menses are absent after menarche
Hypermenorrhea	Menses lasting longer than 7 days
Hypomenorrhea	Less than the expected amount of menstrual bleeding
Menometrorrhagia (also called metromenorrhagia)	Overly long, heavy, and irregular menses
Menorrhagia	Passing more than 80 mL of blood per menses
Oligomenorrhea	Menstrual cycles of more than 35 days
Polymenorrhea	Menses more frequently than 21-day intervals

 MENSTRUAL DISORDERS

Flow and Cycle Disorders
Pathophysiology, Etiologies, and Signs and Symptoms

There are many types of menstrual abnormalities (Table 42.3). Causes can include stress, pregnancy, hormonal imbalances, metabolic imbalances (such as obesity, anorexia nervosa, and excessive exercise), tumors (both benign and malignant), infections, organ diseases (such as liver, kidney, or thyroid disease), blood or bone marrow abnormalities, and the presence of foreign bodies in the uterus (such as intrauterine devices [IUDs]). Menstrual abnormalities can be distressing. They can result in anemia, persistent fatigue, and sexual dysfunction. Establishment of a comfortable and open professional relationship between a woman and her nurse or HCP is essential for communication about such concerns.

Diagnostic Tests

Appropriate testing to determine the cause of menstrual abnormalities involves a thorough history and physical examination. Papanicolaou (Pap) smear, cervical and vaginal cultures, laparoscopy, ultrasound, endometrial biopsy, pregnancy testing, urine testing, and blood testing may be done to screen for any of the disorders that can influence the menstrual cycle and flow.

Therapeutic Measures

Medical treatment of menstrual disorders often involves manipulation of hormone levels or use of NSAIDs. Surgical treatment can involve **dilation and curettage** (D&C), laser ablation of endometrial tissue, and **hysterectomy** (removal of the uterus). During D&C, the cervix is first dilated (opened wider); a curet (a sharp, spoonlike instrument) is then inserted through the cervix and used to scoop out the inner lining of the uterus. Laser ablation involves targeted burning of endometrial tissue so that scar tissue forms that does not bleed. Hysterectomy is a last-resort treatment and is described later in this chapter.

• WORD • BUILDING •
dilation and curettage: dilat(e)—to widen + ation—the process of + curet—scoop + tage—doing
hysterectomy: hyster—womb + ec—away + tomy—cutting

Nursing Care

The only accurate way to estimate menstrual flow is to weigh used sanitary pads (sealed in a biohazard bag) and then subtract the weight of the original pads. A 1-g increase in pad weight equals approximately 1 mL of blood loss. Simply counting numbers of pads used is much less accurate, because women may change pads at different intervals. You may have to rely on a woman's report of blood loss. Be sure to include "patient estimate" when you document.

D&C is typically done as an outpatient procedure. Women can expect some cramping and spotting or light bleeding for a few days afterward.

Dysmenorrhea

Pathophysiology, Etiologies, and Signs and Symptoms

Painful menstruation, or **dysmenorrhea,** is a common problem in women. Primary dysmenorrhea (menstrual cramps) is not pathological and is thought to be caused mainly by the action of endogenous prostaglandins that stimulate uterine contractions, producing cramping pain. Secondary dysmenorrhea is caused by a reproductive tract disorder such as endometriosis, pelvic infection, retroversion of the uterus, or fibroid tumors.

Diagnostic Tests

Hormonal tests of estrogen and progesterone levels may be evaluated for primary dysmenorrhea. Additional tests such as laparoscopic examination, biopsies, or cultures may be required for investigation of secondary dysmenorrhea.

Therapeutic Measures

Primary dysmenorrhea can be treated with drugs that inhibit prostaglandin synthesis, such as aspirin and NSAIDs. Correction of secondary causes of dysmenorrhea may include such measures as hormonal adjustment, usually with oral contraceptives or hormone replacement therapy, D&C, or other surgical or medical intervention based on the cause.

Nursing Care and Patient Education

A warm heating pad to the abdomen or a hot bath help reduce discomfort. If dysmenorrhea is related to uterine retroversion, assuming a knee-to-chest position may relieve the discomfort. Sudden development of dysmenorrhea in a woman with no previous menstrual discomfort should always be investigated.

Premenstrual Syndrome and Premenstrual Dysphoric Disorder

Pathophysiology, Etiologies, and Signs and Symptoms

Premenstrual syndrome (PMS) is a recurrent problem for many women. Although the exact cause is not understood, ovarian hormones, aldosterone, and neurotransmitters such as monoamine oxidase and serotonin are believed to play a role. Symptoms include water retention; headaches; discomfort in joints, muscles, and breasts; changes in affect, concentration, and coordination; and sensory changes. Few women find PMS serious enough to interfere with work or relationships.

Premenstrual dysphoric disorder (PMDD) is a condition like PMS but much more severe. Women experience symptoms of depression, irritability, and tension before menstruation. They may have mood swings, feelings of hopelessness, and suicidal ideation. Like PMS, the exact cause is unknown.

Therapeutic Measures

A variety of drugs have been given to combat PMS and PMDD with varying degrees of success. Some commonly used medications include NSAIDS, hormonal contraceptives, antidepressants, and diuretics as well as supplements of calcium, magnesium, vitamin E, and vitamin B_6. Patients should be warned, however, that dosages of vitamins should not be increased without professional advice because vitamins are medications as well as nutrients. High doses of some vitamins can lead to physiological damage. Regular exercise and eating a healthy diet help to reduce symptoms as well.

Nursing Care and Patient Education

Being understanding and nonjudgmental is especially important. Some women who suffer from severe PMS or PMDD may have been treated as if they are psychologically impaired because of outdated ideas about PMS or PMDD. You can help by providing educational materials on lifestyle measures, such as restriction of alcohol, caffeine, nicotine, salt, and simple sugars; participation in regular exercise; and development of stress management skills that may help to reduce symptoms. If the patient is experiencing severe depression, discuss the possibility of suicidal thoughts that can occur with increasing depression symptoms during the second half of the menstrual cycle. Counsel the patient to call 911 or seek medical care immediately if suicidal thoughts occur.

Endometriosis

Pathophysiology, Etiologies, and Signs and Symptoms

Endometriosis is a condition in which functioning endometrial tissue is located outside the uterus (Fig. 42.4). One cause is **retrograde** menstruation, which is a backward leakage of blood and tissue into the fallopian tubes and into the pelvic cavity. Wayward endometriotic cells then grow into tissues such as the intestinal walls, ovaries, and other abdominal structures. On a cyclic basis, mediated by ovarian hormones, these cells build up and slough just as they would in the uterus. However, the sloughing and bleeding occur in the enclosed abdominal cavity or into the tissues that they have invaded. The buildup of the blood and cells can result in pain, swelling, damage to abdominal organs and structures, scar tissue development, and infertility.

• WORD • BUILDING •

dysmenorrhea: dys—painful + men(o)—month + rrhea—flow
retrograde: retro—backward + grade—step

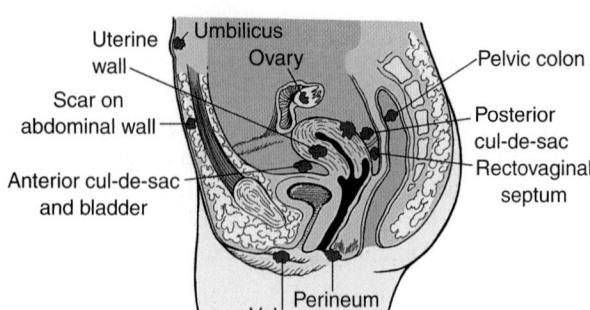

FIGURE 42.4 Possible sites of endometriosis.

Therapeutic Measures

Surgical intervention may be required, especially if scar tissue develops into tight bands that strangulate sections of bowel or ureters. Reduction of estrogen and prevention of ovulation either with medications or by surgical removal of the ovaries can be effective but result in infertility and menopausal symptoms. Analgesics may be required for pain.

Nursing Care and Patient Education

The severity and persistence of the pain of endometriosis can lead to reliance on pain medication, so it is important to teach patients alternative and complementary pain relief strategies such as relaxation exercises and application of heat to the abdomen or back.

Menopause

Pathophysiology and Signs and Symptoms

Menopause is the permanent cessation of menstrual cycles resulting from decreased hormone production. This is a natural part of aging, but related uncomfortable symptoms and conditions can occur. The climacteric (**perimenopause**) is the period of gradual decline in hormone production before the permanent end of menses. It may last from months to years. Perimenopausal physical symptoms vary widely. They can include erratic menses, atrophy of urogenital tissues with a marked decrease in the amount of natural lubrication, a pH shift toward alkalinity (encouraging yeast overgrowth), and vasomotor instability (resulting in hot flashes and night sweats; "Evidence-Based Practice").

Estrogen protects women against several disease processes. The risk of heart disease and osteoporosis increases with declining estrogen production. Mental changes can occur because of the complex interplay of reproductive hormones and neurotransmitters. It is important to acknowledge symptoms such as irritability, anxiety, insomnia, memory problems, and mild depression as a normal, temporary result of hormonal changes so that perimenopausal women do not doubt their sanity.

Therapeutic Measures

Hormone replacement therapy (HRT), also known as menopausal hormone therapy (MHT), is a controversial

Evidence-Based Practice

Clinical Question

How does menopause affect women?

Evidence

A total of 24 qualitative studies were included in a systematic review, resulting in 108 extracted findings. The findings were aggregated into 17 categories and, finally, six findings were synthesized: (1) Menopause is a natural event in a woman's life that is closely associated with psychosocial events of midlife and the aging process; (2) the physical and emotional changes of menopause strongly affect women; (3) women perceive menopause as a time characterized by gains and losses; (4) resilience is improved at the time of menopause, and coping strategies are adopted to enhance physical and emotional well-being; (5) health issues, family and marital relations, sociocultural background, and meaning attributed to one's sex life determine whether the sexual experiences during menopause are pleasant or not; and (6) women should be prepared and have their needs supported according to their perspectives (Hoga, Rodolpho, Gonçalves, & Quirino, 2015).

Implications for Nursing Practice

There is no doubt that menopause has a profound effect on the health and well-being of women, both physiologically and psychologically. Therefore, understanding the experience of menopause from a woman's perspective may help nurses. Suggestions include the following: (1) Support women during this difficult transitional period in their lives; (2) listen more closely to women's concerns regarding the changes that occur during menopause; (3) provide tailored health care according to individual needs, preferences, and expectations; and (4) help women with effective coping strategies regarding the effects of menopause.

Reference

Hoga, L., Rodolpho, J., Gonçalves, B., & Quirino, B. (2015). Women's experience of menopause: A systematic review. *JBI Database of Systematic Reviews and Implementation Reports, 13*(8), 250–337.

treatment for perimenopausal symptoms. Although HRT can reduce symptoms and protect bones, there may also be a higher risk for breast cancer, heart disease, stroke, and blood clots. A Revised Global Consensus Statement from the International Menopause Society now states that the benefits of HRT for menopause outweigh the risks in some cases, such as in controlling vasomotor symptoms and osteoporosis-related fractures in women under 60 or within 10 years after menopause (de Villiers et al., 2016). Estrogen

• WORD • BUILDING •

perimenopause: peri—around + men(o)—month + pause—stopping

alone is only indicated for women who have had a hysterectomy. All other women should receive progesterone along with estrogen. HRT can be administered orally, vaginally, or transdermally. Type and route of MHT should be individualized and based on patient preference and safety issues. See Table 42.1 for examples.

Dietary changes that include **phytoestrogens** (present in foods and herbs such as soy, tofu, flax seeds, black cohosh, and dong quai) may provide some of the benefits of estrogen replacement without HRT. However, even phytoestrogens have some risk. Women should discuss food and herb supplements with their HCP before using them.

Prevention of osteoporosis begins in early adulthood, long before perimenopause. Fair-skinned, thin women are at greatest risk for bone loss. Throughout life, adequate intake of calcium and vitamin D (preferably from foods) and regular weight-bearing exercise help to maximize bone mass. At menopause, some women may receive treatment with bone-building medications such as alendronate (Fosamax) to slow bone loss.

Complications

It is important to note that resumption of vaginal bleeding after menstruation has finally ceased can be a sign of an endometrial cell disorder caused by either benign changes, such as polyps, or malignant changes of internal reproductive organs. Any bleeding that occurs following previous cessation should always be investigated.

Nursing Care and Patient Education

Teach perimenopausal women that they can plan ahead for hot flashes by dressing in layers of clothing that may be removed. Vaginal symptoms can be treated with a water-soluble moisture restorer or lubricant or with an estrogen cream (following prescription directions). Eating a healthy diet that is light in caffeine, sugar, and alcohol can help women better control their bodies and minds. Looking forward to new challenges rather than backward to the past may help to counteract hormone-related depressive tendencies. It is important to remind perimenopausal women that they may still be fertile even after several months of **amenorrhea.** To prevent conception, they need to continue to practice birth control until they receive confirmation from their HCP that menopause is complete. Table 42.4 provides a summary of menstrual disorders.

CRITICAL THINKING

Lola, age 53, has been experiencing menopausal hot flashes during the afternoons as she works in her office.

1. What self-care measures can you suggest to help with her symptoms?
2. If she considers hormone replacement therapy, what information should you share with her?
3. With whom should you collaborate as you help Lola decide what to do?

Suggested answers are at the end of the chapter.

Table 42.4
Menstrual Disorders Summary

Signs and Symptoms	Increase or decrease in menstrual flow
	Increased pain with menses or generalized abdominal pain
	Fluid retention
	Headaches
	Breast pain, lesions, swelling
	Mood changes
Diagnostic Tests	Hormone levels
	Pregnancy test
	Pap smear
	Cervical/vaginal cultures
	Urine testing
	Ultrasound
	Laparoscopy
	Biopsy
Therapeutic Measures	Medication to stabilize hormone levels
	Nonsteroidal anti-inflammatory drugs (NSAIDs)
	Dilation and curettage (D&C), laser ablation, hysterectomy
	Treatment of underlying causes
	Vitamin/mineral supplements
	Diuretics, serotonin reuptake inhibitors (SSRIs), dietary changes
Priority Nursing Diagnoses	*Deficient Fluid Volume* related to increased bleeding
	Acute Pain related to uterine cramping
	Deficient Knowledge related to self-care measures

IRRITATIONS AND INFLAMMATIONS OF THE VAGINA AND VULVA

Various causative agents can irritate the vulva and the vagina. Signs and symptoms are often similar, but there are some differences in the discharge produced in response to the disorders. Table 42.5 lists common vaginal irritations and inflammations that are not generally sexually transmitted. See Chapter 44 for information on sexually transmitted infections (STIs).

Pathophysiology, Etiologies, and Signs and Symptoms

The normal vaginal environment is a balanced ecosystem with a pH of less than 4.2 as a result of lactic acid and hydrogen

• **WORD • BUILDING** •
phytoestrogens: phyto—plant + estrogens—hormones
amenorrhea: a—without + men(o)—month + rrhea—flow

Table 42.5

Common Vaginal Irritations and Inflammations

Disorder and Etiology	Signs and Symptoms	Discharge/ Examination	Diagnostic Tests	Usual Treatment
Candidiasis: *Candida albicans, C. glabrata,* or *C. tropicalis* overgrowth	Burning, itching, redness of vulva; burning on urination	White, cottage cheese appearance	Wet-mount slides (yeasts look like tiny, budding tree branches); may be cultured	Antifungal agents (drugs mostly ending in -*azole*)
Bacterial vaginosis: *Gardnerella vaginalis, Mycoplasma,* or anaerobe overgrowth	None or vulvar or vaginal irritation	White or gray, homogeneous, foul-smelling discharge; pH higher than 4.5	Wet-mount slides show "clue cells" or release fishy odor when potassium hydroxide is applied	Metronidazole, tinidazole, or clindamycin
Trichomoniasis: *Trichomonas vaginalis* (may be transmitted by inanimate objects or sexually)	Itching, irritation, foul odor, redness, dysuria	Discharge may be frothy; pH higher than 4.5; "strawberry cervix" resulting from petechiae	Wet-mount slides treated with normal saline show motile cells with flagella (like tiny whips); may also be cultured	Metronidazole or tinidazole
Cytolytic vaginosis: *Lactobacilli* overgrowth, stress, some medications	Burning, irritation, pain with intercourse	Nonodorous, thick, white, pasty, or dry and flaking	Lower than normal pH as tested with pH indicator tape (or litmus strip); may be cultured	Depends on cause; alkaline douches may be prescribed
Contact vulvovaginitis: contact with allergens or irritating chemicals such as contraceptive creams or bubble baths	Itching, burning, redness	Generally no change from normal discharge, though may be increased	History and physical information, recent contact with chemicals	Avoidance of the offending substance; warm sitz baths or application of hydrocortisone cream
Atrophic vaginitis: estrogen levels too low to support estrogen-sensitive vaginal tissues	Vulvovaginal irritation, dryness, dyspareunia, increased tendency for resident microbe overgrowth	May have little or increased discharge; discharge may be watery, yellow, or green; may be blood tinged	Maturation index may be determined during Pap test to identify atrophic cellular changes, but diagnosis is usually by history and physical information	Hormone replacement therapy (oral, patch, or vulvovaginal cream) or water-soluble lubricant replacing vaginal lubricants

peroxide production by vaginal cells. This acidic pH protects against the growth of many pathogenic microorganisms. A variety of microorganisms normally coexist unless the ecological balance is destroyed. Candidiasis, bacterial vaginosis, and cytolytic vaginitis are all instances of overgrowth of normally present, nonpathogenic microorganisms. Trichomoniasis also is included here because it can be transmitted nonsexually (on fomites, such as toilet seats) as well as sexually, and it grows well when the vaginal environment is disturbed.

Several conditions can predispose patients to an overgrowth of normal microbes. These include poor nutrition (especially diets high in simple sugars), inconsistent control of blood glucose levels in patients with diabetes, stress, pregnancy, marked hormonal fluctuations, pH changes, prolonged overheating of the genital area with little aeration (as happens with sitting still for long periods in restrictive clothing), and changes in the balance of vaginal flora types because of antibiotic treatment or douching. Patients who have a compromised immune system can experience overgrowth of resident microbes; conversely, vaginal infections can make women more susceptible to STIs, such as gonorrhea and HIV. Frequent and persistent yeast infections can be one sign of HIV infection. **Vaginosis** (overgrowth) and **vaginitis** (inflammation) can sometimes produce irritation and inflammation in the male sexual partner as well, leading to urethritis, excoriation, and penile inflammation or lesions. A variety of anti-infective medications are used for these disorders (Table 42.6). If the male partner is not also treated, he may reactivate the problem for the woman. Therefore, several types of medication come in "partner packs" for both partners to use.

Nursing Care and Education of the Patient Undergoing Diagnostic Testing

The patient may feel embarrassed to talk about what is bothering her. A safe way to begin with most patients is to say, "Hello. What can I write on your chart as the reason for your visit today?" If embarrassment is evident, a comment that you need to know a bit about what materials to put out for examination purposes often defuses an uncomfortable situation. As you set up materials for a pelvic examination, you can explain that some information is needed to determine how to treat the problem (see Chapter 41). Often this is a good time to ask about vaginal discharge or other signs and symptoms using the *WHAT'S UP?* format (Chapter 1). Allow the patient privacy while she changes into a gown. Return to the room if requested as a chaperone, assistant, and support for the woman.

> ### NURSING CARE TIP
> If any wet-mount slides are made, these must be taken to the laboratory immediately while still wet. Use standard precautions to transport samples. Although samples may be taken for culture, the health care provider may prescribe medication before the results are returned because such irritations are so uncomfortable.

Nursing Care and Education of the Patient Undergoing Treatment

Vaginal inflammations and infections may require oral medication or local application of medication in cream, suppository, or medicated douche form. You may apply this for patients who cannot do so themselves, or you may teach patients to self-administer. Anatomically, the vagina slopes back toward the sacrum for about the length of an adult finger (although it can stretch longer). Application is easiest when the patient is lying down ready to sleep because vaginal medications tend to run out when the patient stands or sits. Medicated douches may be administered to a hospitalized patient sitting on a bedpan in bed in the semi-Fowler position. Patients may self-administer while sitting on a toilet. Most vaginal medications come with an applicator that either injects

a dose of creamy medication or pushes a firmer, shaped dose of medication off the end of the tube when the plunger is depressed. Consult the instructions supplied with the medication. Instruct patients to use all the medication as prescribed and to wear an absorbent pad to prevent possible staining of clothing.

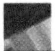

TOXIC SHOCK SYNDROME

Pathophysiology, Etiologies, and Signs and Symptoms

Toxic shock syndrome (TSS) is primarily associated with superabsorbent tampon use during menstruation but can also occur with use of nasal packings or in other individuals with no specific risk factors. It is a severe systemic infection with strains of *Staphylococcus aureus* that produce an epidermal toxin. The effect of the toxin on the liver, kidneys, and circulatory system makes TSS a life-threatening condition. A streptococcal infection can cause a similar syndrome.

Individuals with TSS may experience a sudden high fever with sore throat, headache, dizziness, confusion, redness of the palms and soles of the feet, rash, blisters, and petechiae followed by peeling of the skin. Muscle pain and weakness as well as gastrointestinal upset have been reported. Signs and symptoms of TSS should be reported to an HCP immediately.

Prevention

Tampon makers have removed the highly absorbent fibers that were most often associated with the syndrome from their product lines, and TSS is now rare. Women can also reduce their risk of developing TSS by substituting sanitary pads for tampons at least part of the time, such as at night; changing tampons every 4 hours; washing hands carefully before inserting anything into the vagina; not leaving female barrier contraceptives in place for longer than needed; and not using tampons or female barrier contraceptives in the first 12 weeks after giving birth.

Nursing Care and Patient Education

All menstruating women should be taught measures to prevent TSS. They should also be taught to recognize symptoms of TSS because early identification and treatment can save lives.

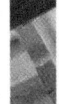

DISORDERS RELATED TO THE DEVELOPMENT OF THE GENITAL ORGANS

Pathophysiology, Etiologies, and Signs and Symptoms

Several types of congenital malformations of the reproductive organs can affect the health of female patients. Genetic or environmental factors during pregnancy can cause these.

• WORD • BUILDING •

vaginosis: vagin—vagina + osis—condition
vaginitis: vagin—vagina + itis—inflammation

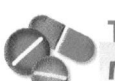

Table 42.6
Medications for Irritations and Inflammations of the Vagina and Vulva

Medication Class/Action

Antibiotics

Inhibit bacterial protein synthesis.

Examples	Nursing Implications
clindamycin (Cleocin)	*Teach:*
	Correct use.
	Use as directed, even if symptoms cease.
	Report change in symptoms.

Antifungals

Believed to bind to sterol in fungal cell membrane, thereby altering cell permeability.

Examples	Nursing Implications
fluconazole (Diflucan)	*Teach:*
miconazole (Monistat)	Correct use.
terconazole (Terazol)	Use as directed, even if symptoms cease.
clotrimazole (Gyne-Lotrimin)	Report change in symptoms.

Antiprotozoal

Enters cells of microorganisms that contain nitroreductase; interferes with DNA synthesis and causes cell death.

Examples	Nursing Implications
metronidazole (Flagyl)	*Teach:*
	Avoid alcohol use while on medication and for 48 hours after completion.
	Concurrent use of alcohol and metronidazole will induce severe nausea and vomiting.
	Use as directed, even if symptoms cease.
	Take with meals.
	Treat partner.

They may require medical or surgical treatment at some point in life. **Agenesis** of structures means that they never developed. **Hypoplasia** of reproductive tract portions means that they are underdeveloped. **Imperforate** means that expected openings do not exist. Blind pouches exist where cavities should meet but do not. The uterus can form in several configurations, including a double uterus.

Many malformations are discovered during childhood or early adolescence, but some are identified when patients seek medical help because of dysmenorrhea, **dyspareunia** (pain with intercourse), infertility, repeated spontaneous abortions (miscarriages), or preterm labor during pregnancy.

Diagnostic Tests
Procedures such as ultrasonography, hysterosalpingography, computed tomography (CT) scan, magnetic resonance imaging (MRI), and endoscopy may be used to determine the type and extent of developmental defects.

Therapeutic Measures
Some defects can be repaired surgically, while others cannot. Depending on the type and location of the defect, surgeries may be done by endoscopy or by surgical incision.

Nursing Care and Patient Education
Patients who have these problems may struggle with self-esteem issues, such as feeling that they are somehow incomplete or have been cheated of something they desire. Show that you are willing to listen if and when the patient wishes to talk, while allowing her as much privacy as she desires.

• WORD • BUILDING •
agenesis: a—without + genesis—production
hypoplasia: hypo—little + plasia—shape (or form)
imperforate: im—not + perforate—pierced
dyspareunia: dys—painful or abnormal + pareunia—mating

DISPLACEMENT DISORDERS

Pathophysiology and Etiologies

The pelvic organs are suspended in the pelvis by ligaments and supported by muscles and fascia. The pubococcygeus muscle runs from the pubis to the coccyx and supplies support from below. Pregnancies (especially those producing large babies) and rapid or traumatic deliveries may result in stretching and injury of the supporting structures. This can cause displacement of the uterus, vagina, bladder, or bowel from a normal position.

Some children have defective muscular support of the pelvic organs, and prolapse is more prevalent in some families. Such observations seem to suggest that congenital defects and genetic inheritance may influence displacement disorders, even without pregnancy. Scarring from STIs may also be a factor. Aging generally increases the problem because the effects of gravity over time contribute to stretching, and lower estrogen levels weaken estrogen-dependent supportive tissues. Chronic constipation, obesity, and lack of exercise also worsen these problems.

Diagnostic Tests

Ultrasonography, hysterosalpingography, CT scan, MRI, and endoscopy may be used to determine the type and extent of displacement disorders.

Therapeutic Measures

A *pessary* is a supportive (usually ring-shaped) device that is placed in the vagina to help support the pelvic organs. A pessary is usually removed daily at bedtime for cleaning, but some types are designed to remain in the vagina for months at a time. When pessary use is begun, it is important that the woman return to the HCP for a recheck after an initial period of use to determine whether it is causing pressure damage to tissues. Because the pessary is a foreign object in the vagina, increased vaginal discharge can be expected. Discharge should not be pink, bloody, or purulent.

Nursing Care and Patient Education

Teach patients to eat a healthy diet to avoid obesity and constipation. Also teach how to do Kegel exercises to keep the pubococcygeus muscle strong and able to support the organs in the pelvic cavity. One way to do Kegel exercises follows:

1. To find the pubococcygeus muscle, tighten while urinating so that the flow of urine stops.
2. Squeeze the muscle that stopped urinary flow tightly, holding for 10 seconds and totally relaxing the muscle afterward. Repeat 15 times per day.
3. Practice controlling the muscle by contracting and relaxing it to move the pelvic floor upward and downward very slowly. Thinking of an elevator helps some women. Repeat this 15 times per day.

> **NURSING CARE TIP**
> Teach women to do Kegel exercises during the day, for example, while waiting in lines, to use otherwise wasted time to promote their health. Another suggestion is to plan specific times of day or activities that would include Kegel exercises, such as while in a car or working at a computer. Kegel exercises can be done anywhere and are not apparent to anyone watching.

Cystocele
Pathophysiology, Etiologies, and Signs and Symptoms

Cystocele occurs when the bladder sags into the vaginal space because of inadequate support (Fig. 42.5A). A feeling of pelvic pressure and stress incontinence are common with this condition.

Therapeutic Measures

Kegel exercises or the use of a pessary may help. If these measures are ineffective, anterior **colporrhaphy,** which is a surgical repair of the anterior portion of the vagina, may be needed. Another possible surgical treatment involves resuspending the bladder.

Rectocele
Pathophysiology, Etiologies, and Signs and Symptoms

Rectocele occurs when a portion of the rectum sags into the vagina because of inadequate support (see Fig. 42.5B). A feeling of pelvic pressure as well as fecal incontinence, constipation, and hemorrhoids can result.

Therapeutic Measures

Kegel exercises can help strengthen the supporting muscles. The patient should maintain bowel regularity with a high-fiber diet to avoid further discomfort and sagging from bowel overdistention. Posterior colporrhaphy may be necessary to correct this problem.

Uterine Position Disorders
Pathophysiology, Etiologies, and Signs and Symptoms

The most common variations in position of the uterus are **anteversion, anteflexion, retroversion,** and **retroflexion**

• WORD • BUILDING •

cystocele: cysto—bag (bladder) + cele—hernia
colporrhaphy: colpo—vagina + rrhaphy—suture
rectocele: recto—rectum + cele—hernia
anteversion: ante—front + version—turning
anteflexion: ante—front + flexion—bending
retroversion: retro—back + version—turning
retroflexion: retro—back + flexion—bending

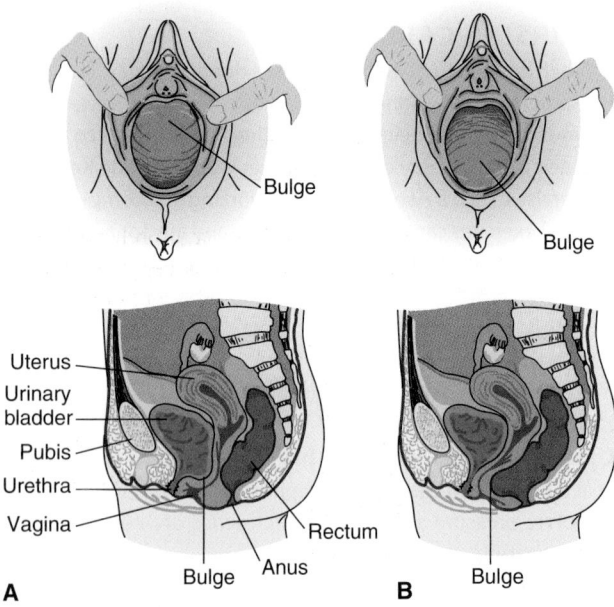

FIGURE 42.5 (A) Cystocele. (B) Rectocele.

(Fig. 42.6). In anteversion, the uterus lies too far forward, and in retroversion, it lies too far back. In anteflexion, the upper portion of the uterus bends forward, and in retroflexion, it bends backward.

Symptoms that can result from these uterine displacements include painful menstruation and intercourse, infertility, and repeated spontaneous abortion.

Therapeutic Measures

A pessary may correct some positional problems. If infertility or recurrent spontaneous abortion is involved or the condition is very painful, surgery to correct the condition may be necessary.

Uterine Prolapse
Pathophysiology, Etiologies, and Signs and Symptoms

Uterine prolapse occurs when the uterus sags into the vagina (Fig. 42.7). The amount of sagging can vary and increase over time as a result of the effects of gravity, poor pelvic support, and excessive lifting or straining. In first-degree prolapse, less than half the uterus sags into the vagina. In second-degree prolapse, the entire uterus sags into the vagina. In third-degree prolapse, the uterus sags outside the body.

Uterine prolapse can be very uncomfortable, resulting in back pain, pelvic pain, pain with intercourse (or inability to have intercourse), urinary incontinence, constipation, and development of hemorrhoids. Pressure on the uterus can compromise circulation, resulting in tissue necrosis. Vaginal vault prolapse can also occur in women who have had a hysterectomy, so that the vagina turns inside out and sags downward, causing similar signs and symptoms. This condition typically requires surgical resuspension.

Therapeutic Measures

Some minor uterine displacements may be treated with use of a pessary. Kegel exercises may be more effective in prevention of uterine prolapse than in treatment because, once

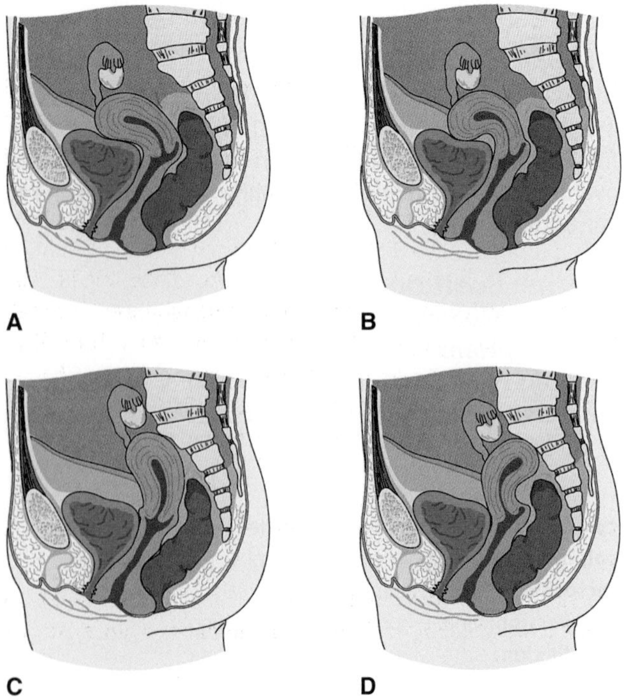

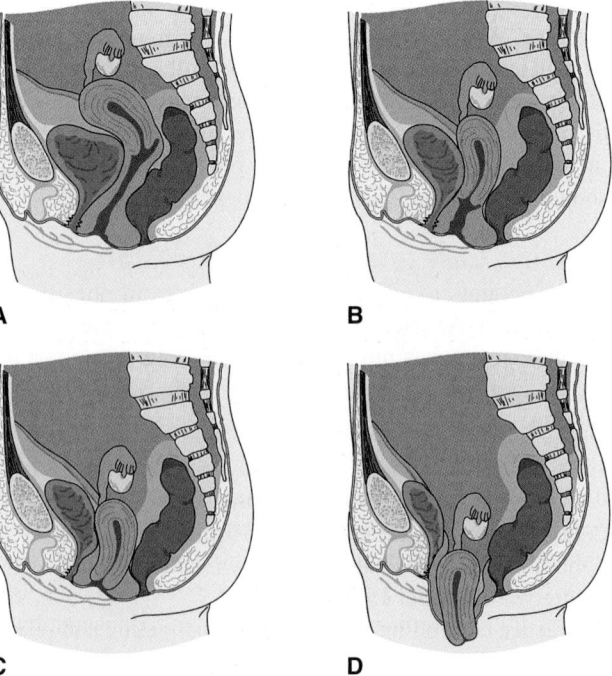

FIGURE 42.6 Uterine positions. (A) Anteversion. (B) Anteflexion. (C) Retroversion. (D) Retroflexion.

FIGURE 42.7 Uterine prolapse. (A) Normal uterus. (B) First-degree prolapse: descent within the vagina. (C) Second-degree prolapse. (D) Third-degree prolapse: vagina is completely everted.

the tissues become stretched sufficiently for the uterus to sag into the vagina, the continued weight of the uterus prevents adequate contraction of the muscles. Surgery may be done to correct the prolapse. Although the uterus can be resuspended by shortening the muscles and fascia, hysterectomy is the more common treatment unless further childbearing is desired.

See Table 42.7 for a summary of displacement disorders.

 FERTILITY DISORDERS

Infertility is a complicated problem with many causes. Some couples with infertility may have multiple reproductive problems. Both male and female partners should be examined. (See Chapter 43 for greater detail on male reproductive system disorders.) Table 42.8 provides a summary of fertility disorders and diagnostic tests.

Nursing Care and Education of the Patient Undergoing Fertility Testing

An understanding attitude is very important because infertility can be a cause of low self-esteem as well as relationship problems. Patients who have been undergoing diagnostic testing or treatment for infertility can become very discouraged with the process and the expense, especially if it has been ineffective. Having to plan one's sexual activity around an HCP's directions can compromise feelings of spontaneity, enjoyment, and privacy.

On the first infertility investigation visit, the nurse may teach or give a handout to the patient about keeping a precise record of her oral temperatures with a basal thermometer each morning on awakening, before any other activity. The first day of her menses is day 1 on the temperature chart. Changing levels of hormones result in slight temperature changes, which can be used to identify when ovulation seems to be occurring and when particular hormone levels should be tested. Because many factors can influence temperature and cycles, explain that it may take a few months of recording to clearly identify her pattern.

You may assist with office procedures such as endometrial biopsy, which can be done during a pelvic examination 2 or 3 days before menses is expected. A pregnancy test should be done before this procedure to avoid interfering with a pregnancy. The woman may receive pain medication and paracervical block anesthesia for the procedure. Assess pulse and blood pressure. A vasovagal reaction treatment kit containing epinephrine (or atropine, according to the HCP's choice), a tourniquet, and a syringe should be available for injection if a vasovagal reflex occurs during the procedure. Vasovagal reflex is a reflex stimulation of the vagal nerve that can happen when the cervix, larynx, or trachea is manipulated. It results in slowing of the heart rate and decreased cardiac output, so that the blood pressure drops markedly.

Therapeutic Measures

Treatment of infertility is designed to ensure that an adequate amount of sperm and an ovum can be in proximity in

Table 42.7

Displacement Disorders of the Genital Organs Summary

Signs and Symptoms	Pain with menses or sexual intercourse Infertility Spontaneous abortion or preterm labor Prolapse of uterus, bladder, or rectum into vagina or outside of body
Diagnostic Tests	Physical examination Ultrasound Hysterosalpingography Computed tomography (CT) scan or magnetic resonance imaging (MRI) Endoscopy
Therapeutic Measures	Kegel exercises Surgery Hormone supplements
Priority Nursing Diagnoses	*Acute* or *Chronic Pain* related to structural abnormality or surgery *Urge Urinary Incontinence* or *Constipation* related to structural abnormalities *Sexual Dysfunction* related to disturbance in self-concept *Grieving* related to absence or loss of reproductive status

the most conducive environment for fertilization. Removal of barriers such as scar tissue may require surgery. Depending on the results of blood tests and the **postcoital** test (described in Table 42.8), adjustments of environmental factors may involve such actions as sperm washing to avoid destructive antigen–antibody responses, changing the pH of the seminal fluid to encourage sperm motility, treating the female partner to prevent substances in her genital tract fluids from disabling the sperm, or adjusting her hormone levels. The number of sperm or ova available can be increased through use of fertility drugs or hormone preparations. Infertility treatments are quite complicated and expensive and change periodically as a result of ongoing research. For more information, visit www.cdc.gov/reproductivehealth/Infertility/index.htm.

Various methods can be used to bring the gametes together. If the problem involves inability to get the sperm close enough to the ovum (as may happen with ejaculatory problems), the HCP may use intrauterine insemination (IUI) to place a semen sample from the male partner closer to the

• WORD • BUILDING •

postcoital: post—after + coital—pertaining to intercourse

Table 42.8

Female Fertility Disorders

Pathophysiology/Etiology	*Diagnostic Tests*
Ovulation	
Possible anatomic and physiological abnormalities of ovaries Hormonal imbalances related to hypothalamus, thyroid, or adrenal glands Polycystic ovary syndrome (PCOS)	Basal body temperature charting Midluteal serum progesterone blood levels Luteinizing hormone (LH) levels Blood or urine testing Ultrasound monitoring of a follicle for evidence of release of ovum Endometrial biopsy Observation of male hair distribution Other hormone testing as indicated
Tubal	
Possible obstruction of the fallopian tubes resulting from anatomic variations, scarring, or adhesions; prior surgeries; or inflammatory processes involving other abdominal tissues	Hysterosalpingography (see Chapter 41) Laparoscopy
Uterine	
Possible abnormalities in shape or blockages within the uterus (rare cause of infertility but a potential cause of pregnancy loss before maturity) Menstrual disorders involving the endometrium	Hysteroscopy (see Chapter 41) Removal of tissue samples using curet or endoscope
Other Sources	
Possible reproductive environmental factors such as destructive antigen–antibody responses Inappropriate pH of seminal fluid for maximal sperm motility Substances in genital tract fluids that disable sperm	Postcoital test: Couple is advised to have intercourse when LH and estrogen levels are high; then a specimen of cervical mucus is taken from the woman 2 to 12 hours later for analysis of reproductive environment

ovum via a small catheter. **In vitro fertilization** (IVF) involves bringing ova and sperm together outside the bodies of the participants. Ova may be harvested using a long needle or an endoscope after hormonal preparation of the woman. Sperm can be obtained through masturbation; intercourse with a nonlubricated, nonspermicidal condom; or electrical stimulation of ejaculation for patients with spinal cord injuries. Once fertilized, the ova are implanted in the woman's uterus.

For those cases in which sperm is unable to successfully penetrate the ovum, procedures involving gamete micromanipulation may be done. Under a microscope, an ovum from the female partner is partially opened by removing a portion of the outer covering to facilitate sperm penetration, or sperm may be injected into the ovum. This fertilized ovum is then reinserted into the woman's body.

When measures to improve the chances of conception using the partners' own gametes are unsuccessful, gametes from donors may be used. Artificial insemination by injecting another man's sperm into the woman's genital tract is the simplest of the donor procedures. Ova also may be harvested from a donor woman and used for IVF using the male partner's sperm if possible. Both of these procedures allow for genetic inheritance from one member of the couple. If genetic inheritance is not possible or desirable (as with familial disease carriers), both donor sperm and ova may be used for IVF

• WORD • BUILDING •

in vitro fertilization: in—inside + vitro—glass + fertiliz—fruitful + ation—process

to be transferred into the female patient. Surrogacy is a situation in which an embryo from one couple is placed into a "host" mother for growth of a baby for the couple.

Nursing Care and Education of the Patient Undergoing Treatment

Patients who are undergoing infertility treatment may experience many upsetting and distressing feelings. If the infertility was caused by something the patient perceives as avoidable, such as an STI, guilty feelings may add to the psychological discomfort. Any or all of the previously described tests may be completed and even repeated many times without success in identifying an underlying etiology for infertility, resulting in repeated disappointments. The beginning of menses may signal a time of mourning for these couples. Depression may result after failed IVF attempts. Strained relationships may develop between marriage partners, especially if there is disagreement about the value of testing or the importance of having biological children.

In IVF, usually more than the desired number of embryos is implanted because it is expected that not all will survive and because this is more cost effective with less physical risk for the mother. However, this requires heart-wrenching decisions of whether to "reduce" (abort) extra pregnancies or to risk having more than the desired number of children at once as a result of the fertility treatments.

Many varieties of assistive reproductive technology are available, and the number is increasing with research. Most of the procedures are known by their acronyms. For example, GIFT stands for gamete intrafallopian transfer, during which gametes are placed together in the fallopian tube with the hope that fertilization will occur. ZIFT stands for "zygote intrafallopian transfer," during which fertilization of gametes occurs outside of the body; the conceptus is then placed into a woman's fallopian tube to make the journey to the uterus. Acronyms can be useful shortcuts but can be confusing to patients. Most nurses probably do not need to know all acronyms or infertility treatments unless they work in a gynecologist's office or infertility clinic.

 REPRODUCTIVE LIFE PLANNING

Reproductive life planning is a more comprehensive term than *contraception* and implies reasoned decisions related to pregnancy timing and whether or not to have children. Nurses can contribute to the overall health and quality of life for women and families by helping them to find the information they need to make wise choices.

Many types of birth control are available, and several additional types are in developmental and testing stages. General categories of agents are discussed in this section. Understanding of how the different types of contraceptives work can assist the nurse in answering patients' questions or helping patients find additional information.

Methods are introduced in the order of usual effectiveness, from most to least effective (with the exception that experimental methods are discussed at the end regardless of their efficacy). Consult your clinic or HCP for an approved, current comparison list of methods for distribution.

For some patients, the distinction of whether a birth control method actually prevents conception or only interferes with implantation or maintenance of a pregnancy is an important factor in their decision. If a patient believes life begins at conception, any action other than prevention of conception would be considered equivalent to abortion.

Oral Contraceptives

Oral **contraceptive** medications are among the most widely used forms of birth control in North America. Most contain an estrogen and a progestin in combination, although some (mini-pills) contain only a progestin. Some work to prevent conception by inhibiting ovulation or changing the environment of the reproductive tract so that activity of the sperm is inhibited. Others do not prevent conception but make implantation less likely and hasten the breakdown of the corpus luteum so that pregnancy-sustaining hormones are not produced. Many of the adverse effects that occurred in the past have been overcome by adjustment of dosage levels.

Oral contraceptives can also be used in some instances to regulate irregular menses, decrease menorrhagia or dysmenorrhea, or decrease the symptoms associated with endometriosis or cyclic breast changes. Oral contraceptives do not prevent STIs; advise women about the risks of contracting STIs and using condoms for the prevention of STIs while taking an oral contraceptive.

Advantages, Disadvantages, Side Effects, and Risks

Oral contraceptives are very effective. Improvement of dysmenorrhea, endometriosis, increased regularity of menses, and decrease in menstrual flow may occur; however, some women experience menstrual changes such as amenorrhea, irregular or prolonged menses, and intermenstrual spotting.

Oral contraceptives require a great deal of commitment because irregular use decreases their effectiveness. To encourage regular use, oral contraceptives are generally dispensed in containers labeled with the days of the week. In addition, some companies include unmedicated pills in the package to be taken during the time of hormone cessation for menses so that the woman only has to remember to take a daily pill, instead of timing the taking of the pills with her cycle. Some oral contraceptives are now available to be taken continuously. Women should speak to their HCPs to determine which method is best for them.

• WORD • BUILDING •

contraceptive: contra—against + ceptive—taking in (conceiving)

Some women experience side effects such as acne, fluid retention, headaches, breast swelling and discomfort, midcycle bleeding, and sometimes depression. Use of an oral contraceptive also has some risks. Higher rates of blood clot formation, stroke, high blood pressure, heart attack, and worsening of diabetes are rare occurrences with some hormonal contraceptives. These are generally related to pre-existing risk factors. Women who smoke or have diabetes, high blood pressure, heart disease, or a history of thrombophlebitis should receive information about the risks of oral contraceptives and alternative methods of contraception.

Oral contraceptives decrease the risk of endometrial and ovarian cancer. However, there is debate about risk of breast cancer and cervical **dysplasia** (cell changes that may become cancerous) sometimes occurs among oral contraceptive users. Women should be advised to have regular Pap smears while taking oral contraceptives.

Many medications can alter the effectiveness of oral contraceptives. Women should be warned to always alert HCPs and pharmacists that they are using oral contraceptives when a new medication is started or a regular medication is discontinued. Use of hormonal contraceptives increases the risk of vitamin B deficiencies, so a healthy diet with good sources of B vitamins is advisable.

LEARNING TIP

Side effects of oral contraceptives can be serious. Teach your patient to watch for "ACHES" and to contact her health care provider immediately if they occur. ACHES stands for:

Abdominal pain
Chest pain
Headache
Eye pain
Severe leg pain

Contraceptive Implant and Injectable Medications

Contraceptive implants are small permeable tubes surgically implanted through a small incision under the skin; they slowly release hormones for long-term contraception. Implants have been used with varying success; an example is etonogestrel implant (Nexplanon).

Medroxyprogesterone acetate (Depo-Provera) is a contraceptive agent available in a slow-release depot form that can be injected intramuscularly. Medication is continuously released for 3 months.

Advantages, Disadvantages, Side Effects, and Risks

The main advantage of progesterone-only medications and implants is that the woman does not have to remember to take daily medication. Disadvantages are that the medications may not be immediately effective, so another method may be necessary for 1 to 2 weeks after the initial injection. Another disadvantage is that fertility may not return for several months to 1 year after discontinuation.

Alterations in menstrual flow, especially amenorrhea, are the most commonly noted side effects with both depot medications and implants. Weight gain of 5 to 10 pounds is also common, which can lead to discontinuation of use. Other side effects and risks are similar to those encountered with oral contraceptives that contain progesterone only.

Estrogen-Progestin Contraceptive Ring

A newer method is an estrogen-progestin contraceptive ring (NuvaRing). It works in much the same manner as other hormonal contraceptives by slowly releasing hormones. The user inserts the ring into the vagina. The ring is left in place for 3 weeks; it is then removed for 1 week in order for menses to occur, after which a new ring is placed.

Advantages, Disadvantages, Side Effects, and Risks

Not having to remember daily medication can be an advantage of the contraceptive ring. However, failing to remove it at the right time may disrupt the regularity of the menstrual cycles. With consistent use, it is very effective in preventing pregnancy. Because it does not provide a barrier over the cervix, there is less risk of infection than with a diaphragm or cervical cap. A common side effect is an increase in normal vaginal discharge. Other side effects and risks are similar to other low-dose hormonal contraceptives.

Transdermal Contraceptive Patch

Transdermal patches contain estrogen and progestin. The patch is placed on the abdomen, upper arm, or buttock after a menstrual period and left in place for 1 week. A new patch is placed on the body each week for 3 weeks. After 3 weeks, the patch is removed and not replaced for 1 week in order for menses to occur.

Advantages, Disadvantages, Side Effects, and Risks

The contraceptive patch has been found to be similar to oral contraceptives in effectiveness, side effects, and risks, but with the advantage of not having to remember to take a pill each day. The patch remains in place during bathing, swimming, and other activities.

CRITICAL THINKING

Jessica, who appears to be about 13 years old, announces loudly at the clinic reception desk that she is "ready to be a responsible adult" and would like some birth control.

1. What information should be gathered from her?
2. What do you think she needs to know before making a decision?
3. How can you base your teaching on her desire to be a responsible adult?

    Suggested answers are at the end of the chapter.

• WORD • BUILDING •

dysplasia: dys—painful or abnormal + plasia—shape or form

Barrier Methods

Barrier methods of birth control are less effective in preventing pregnancy than most of the previously mentioned methods when used alone. Barriers are intended to prevent sperm from reaching the ovum. Used in combination, barrier methods with spermicidal preparations have effectiveness close to that of oral contraceptives. Barrier methods and spermicidal preparations may be purchased without a prescription.

Condoms

Condoms are barriers that are used once and then discarded into an appropriate waste receptacle. Condoms used with contraceptive jelly or spermicide are most effective at decreasing risk of pregnancy. They should be stored in a cool, dry place before use and should not be stored where heat or pressure can weaken them. Storage in a wallet or glove compartment is not advisable. Petroleum-based substances, such as Vaseline, can also weaken condoms, so use of water-soluble lubricants (preferably spermicides) should be advised.

ADVANTAGES, DISADVANTAGES, SIDE EFFECTS, AND RISKS OF MALE CONDOMS. Male condoms have long been used for contraception because they are a relatively inexpensive, totally reversible method that men can control at the time of intercourse. They also provide some barrier protection against transmission of STIs. An electron microscopic study of a sample of nonlubricated latex condoms, however, found that most of those viewed had surface abnormalities, including cracking and melted areas. Patients should be informed that barrier methods can reduce risk but do not absolutely prevent transmission of STIs, especially in areas of contact not covered by the barrier.

The main disadvantages of condom use are interruption of foreplay for application, decreased sensation, and the possibility of slippage or breakage during intercourse. These disadvantages may be overcome by incorporating application of the condom by the female partner as a part of foreplay; using thinner, lubricated, or textured condoms to increase sensation; using the correct size condom with a reservoir or application that leaves about a half-inch at the tip of the condom loose enough to serve as a reservoir for semen (Fig. 42.8); and removal from the vagina before relaxation of the erection.

ADVANTAGES, DISADVANTAGES, SIDE EFFECTS, AND RISKS OF FEMALE CONDOMS. Female condoms are a more recent innovation that allows female initiation of contraception as well as some barrier protection against STIs. Coverage of the labia by the condom may provide more of a barrier than male condoms (Fig. 42.9). Disadvantages are similar to those of male condoms; they are also more expensive than male condoms.

Diaphragms and Cervical Caps

Diaphragms and cervical caps work in the same manner as condoms, by blocking the entry of sperm through the cervix (Fig. 42.10). The barrier effect is enhanced by simultaneous use of a spermicide. Application of a spermicide to the edge of the device and placement of a small amount in the cup before use increases effectiveness.

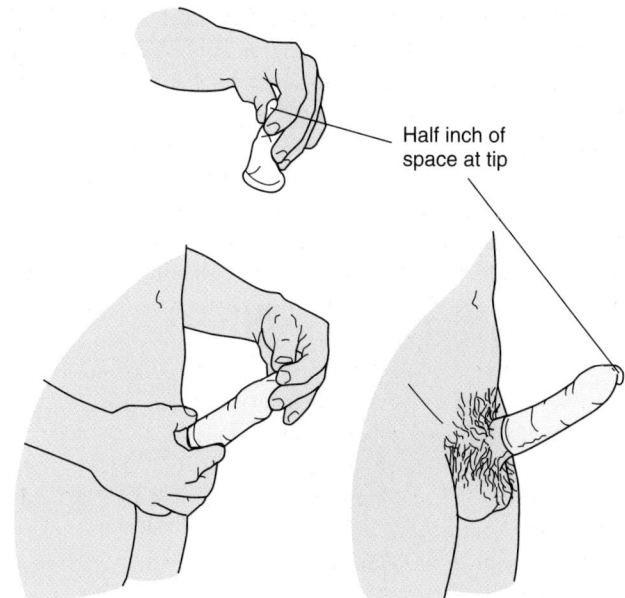

Half inch of space at tip

FIGURE 42.8 Correct application of a male condom.

ADVANTAGES, DISADVANTAGES, SIDE EFFECTS, AND RISKS. Diaphragms and cervical caps are relatively inexpensive, are female initiated, and work without systemic medication. Diaphragms and cervical caps require initial fitting and a prescription to buy them, may need to be refitted after childbirth and the loss or gain of weight, and can last for years. They should be replaced periodically based on manufacturer recommendations or whenever there is any evidence of hardening, cracking, or thin spots. They need to be washed with soap and water, dried, and stored in a case away from heat and sunlight between uses.

Women and their partners can experience irritation or allergic reaction to the spermicide or the contraceptive device material, which would require changing birth control methods. These types of methods require that the device be inserted before intercourse and left in place for several hours afterward. (See package inserts for specific recommendations.) An increase in incidence of urinary tract infection has been reported with use of the diaphragm, and risk of TSS increases with prolonged uninterrupted use of cervical barriers. Adequate fluid intake, voiding shortly after intercourse, and removal of the device as directed following intercourse all help to prevent these potential problems. If urinary tract infections are recurrent using the diaphragm, changing to a cervical cap may decrease the occurrence because there is less pressure against the bladder through the anterior vagina.

Spermicides

Spermicidal agents may be used alone, although use in combination with a barrier method is much more effective. They come in a variety of forms, such as creams, gels, foams, and suppositories, that kill or disable sperm so that fertilization does not occur.

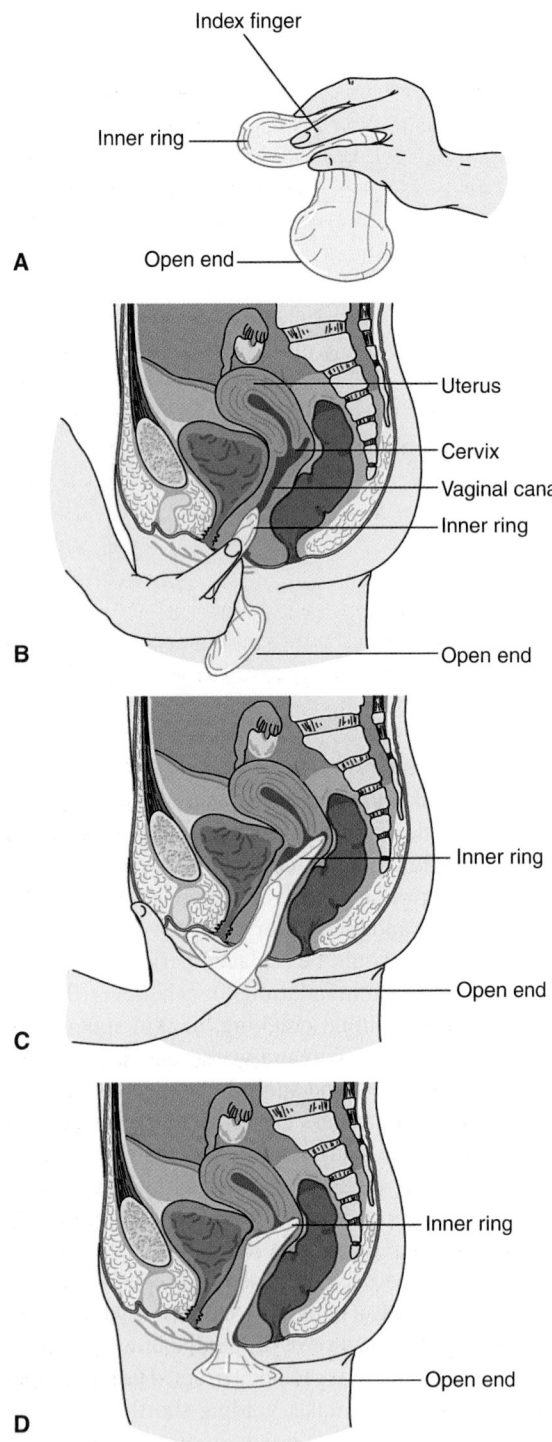

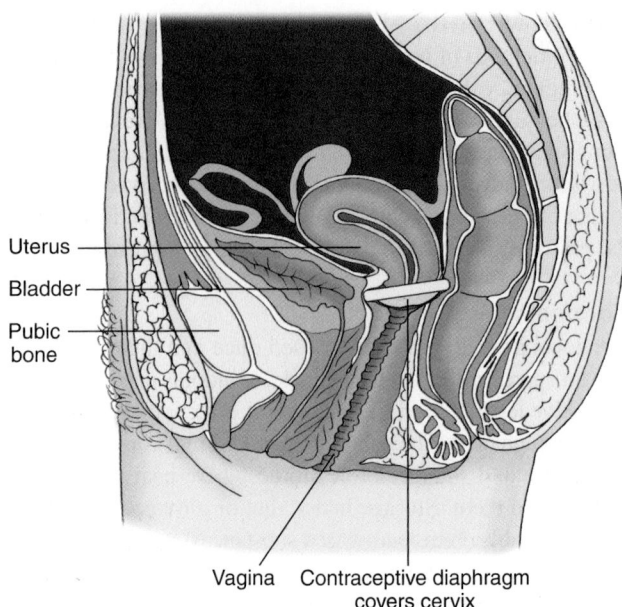

FIGURE 42.10 Contraceptive diaphragm.

FIGURE 42.9 Female condom application. (A) Inner ring is squeezed for insertion. (B) Sheath is inserted similar to a tampon. (C) Inner ring is pushed up as far as it can go with index finger. (D) Condom in place.

Advantages, Disadvantages, Side Effects, and Risks

Spermicidal preparations are relatively inexpensive and can be male- or female-initiated. They do not produce systemic effects, and no hormones are involved. Spermicides require application before each act of intercourse, and some patients consider them to be somewhat messy. Many contain the same ingredient: nonoxynol 9. If genital irritation or a rash occurs with a spermicide, the patient should read labels carefully to avoid future contact with the same ingredient.

Intrauterine Devices

The presence of a foreign object in the uterus is thought to alter the environment so that implantation is less likely to occur. IUDs are generally made from a form of plastic. They may contain copper wire (such as ParaGard) or a supply of a progestin (e.g., Mirena) that is slowly released into the system to further alter the uterine environment to hinder fertilization or implantation.

Advantages, Disadvantages, Side Effects, and Risks

The main advantage of an IUD is continuous contraception without the necessity of remembering to take medication and without the side effects associated with medications. Para-Gard is effective for 10 years, and Mirena is effective for 5 years. Mirena may help lighten and potentially eliminate menstrual bleeding in women who have a history of anemia or heavy menstrual flow.

Disadvantages are changes in menstrual bleeding, cramping, and increased risk of pelvic inflammatory disease (PID). Rarely, an IUD has caused a uterine perforation. IUDs should be avoided in women with uterine abnormalities, those with PID, and those who currently have STIs. Expulsion or displacement of the IUD can occur, so women should be taught to feel for the presence of the external string before intercourse.

Insertion Procedure

Insertion of an IUD typically is done in an HCP's office, usually during the first 7 days of the menstrual cycle because the cervix is slightly dilated at this time. The IUD is inserted into the cervix through a tube that comes packaged with the IUD, which temporarily holds the IUD flat or folded for insertion. When the IUD is pushed out the end of the tube, it springs into a shape that helps to keep it inside the uterus. One potential danger of IUD insertion is vasovagal reflex stimulation (previously described in association with endometrial biopsy). Periodically assess pulse or blood pressure during the procedure and notify the HCP of slowing of the heart rate or a decrease in blood pressure.

Natural Family Planning

Periodic abstinence (natural family planning) is less effective than the previously described methods. It is a method by which couples control their fertility by restricting intercourse to "safe periods" during which risk of conception is low. Many signs can be assessed to determine "safe" days, including temperature changes, cervical consistency and mucus changes, calendar timing, and awareness of symptoms of fertility.

Slight body temperature changes can indicate ovulation. During the first half of the menstrual cycle, the temperature remains low, with a marked drop just before ovulation occurs. With ovulation, the temperature rises and stays higher for the last half of the cycle. Women who use this assessment method should use a basal body temperature thermometer when they awaken, before doing anything else, and record it on a chart.

Cervical consistency and mucus changes can also help pinpoint ovulation. As hormone levels change, the consistency of cervical mucus changes. As ovulation approaches, there is an increase in the amount of mucus. The mucus also becomes more clear, thin, slippery, and stretchable than at other times of the month. Around the time of ovulation, the cervix becomes softer to touch and more open than at other times of the cycle.

Following the calendar can work fairly well if a woman's menstrual periods are regular, but becoming aware of her pattern may take time. Symptoms such as breast tenderness and midcycle discomfort (*mittelschmerz*) can also help identify ovulation. Users of this method should be advised to abstain from intercourse for approximately 3 days before ovulation and 3 to 4 days after because the sperm and ovum can survive for a long period in the female genital tract.

Advantages and Disadvantages

The advantage of this method is that it requires no expense or medication. For those who adhere to Catholicism, it is the only birth control method currently approved by the Catholic Church. The disadvantages are that it requires the cooperation of both partners and may interfere with spontaneity of sexual expression. It is generally not very effective as a means of birth control. It may be difficult to accurately identify ovulation times because infectious and inflammatory processes can affect temperature readings, infections and feminine hygiene products can affect cervical mucus, and irregularity of flow and symptoms may make prediction difficult.

Less Effective Methods
Coitus Interruptus

Coitus interruptus involves removal of the penis from the vagina before ejaculation occurs. Although this method requires no expense or preparation, it is not very effective. Excellent control of ejaculation is required, and even the small amount of sperm that may be present in pre-ejaculatory fluid can result in pregnancy.

Postcoital Douching

The intended purpose of postcoital douching is to wash sperm out of the reproductive tract or to kill or immobilize sperm that the douche solution contacts. This is relatively inexpensive and female-initiated, but it is not very effective. Sperm move very rapidly once deposited, and douching may actually push the sperm upward.

Lactational Amenorrhea Method (Breastfeeding)

Breastfeeding is sometimes used as a method of birth control because the high blood levels of prolactin that occur with breastfeeding may suppress ovulation. This may be effective in the first 6 months after delivery. It requires "full or nearly full" breastfeeding and that the woman has not experienced her first postpartum menses (any bleeding 56 days postpartum). This method costs nothing but is not very effective. Prolactin levels can vary widely, and ovulation may resume at any time without any noticeable signs, resulting in pregnancy before even experiencing a menstrual period after the birth.

Sterilization

Permanent sterilization can be accomplished by interrupting the fallopian tubes, by interrupting the vas deferens (by vasectomy, as discussed in Chapter 43), or by removing the uterus (hysterectomy). Tubal interruption may be done by tying a suture or placing a ring or clip around each fallopian tube, by coagulating a section of the tubes, or by surgically removing a portion of the tube and suturing the ends. These procedures are usually done by laparoscope in an outpatient setting, as an additional procedure performed during a cesarean delivery, or within a few days after a vaginal delivery. A nonsurgical procedure (Essure) uses an endoscope to implant a tiny insert into each fallopian tube to block patency.

Advantages, Disadvantages, Side Effects, and Risks

Although sterilization is not absolutely certain to be permanent, the failure rate is low and has been decreasing recently with newer surgical methods.

Patient Education

Patients should be advised by their surgeon about the complications of the surgery and reversal before they sign a consent form for sterilization. If any uncertainty about the surgery is evident, the HCP should be notified promptly.

PREGNANCY TERMINATION

Termination of pregnancy (abortion) is a difficult topic. Discussions about it are often highly charged with emotion. Both prolife and prochoice advocates argue on the basis of human rights—the former based on rights of the fetus and the latter on rights of the mother—because of the humanity of each party.

Reasons for Therapeutic Abortion
Ectopic Pregnancy
An ectopic pregnancy is the implantation of a fertilized ovum in an area other than the uterus. This can occur because of an abnormally shaped uterus or fallopian tubes that are obstructed as a result of abnormal development, scarring from STIs or other inflammatory processes, or for unknown reasons. It is a life-threatening situation for the mother; currently, a therapeutic abortion is the only treatment.

Prenatal Abnormalities
Development of a variety of prenatal testing methods has introduced the possibility of knowing many things about a baby before birth. Prenatal testing may be done using ultrasound, samples of fluid taken from the amniotic sac or the placental villi, or blood samples from the mother. From these tests, some genetic diseases and congenital deformities can be identified. After anomalies are diagnosed, some patients choose to abort the baby. This is a very difficult decision to consider, even in instances in which the baby has a fatal defect that will not allow it to live outside the uterus. It is important to provide information about alternatives to abortion and possible treatments for the child when a patient has a serious prenatal diagnosis. No one should feel pressured to make the decision quickly to abort, but legal requirements and increasing risk for the mother may limit the time to decide. Abortion because of fetal abnormality may result in much grieving and guilt for the patient and her family.

Methods of Abortion
Several methods are available. The method is determined primarily by the length of the gestation and the goal of inflicting as little trauma to the mother's reproductive system as possible while still inducing pregnancy loss. Time periods for the different abortion methods and the allowable reasons for legal abortion vary according to the laws of the state, province, or country.

Chemical Agents
For emergency contraception, treatment consists of postcoital administration of sufficient estrogen and progestin, or levonorgestrel (Plan B, also sometimes called the "morning-after pill"), to prevent ovulation and possibly to prevent fertilization if ovulation has already occurred. The drug also prevents a fertilized ovum from implanting in the uterine lining. If a fertilized ovum has already implanted when the patient takes the drug, the pregnancy will not be terminated. For this reason,

there is some disagreement about whether Plan B is a form of contraception or a form of abortion.

Plan B is available at pharmacies without a prescription. Typically, it is used after unexpected, unprotected sexual intercourse (as with sexual assault) or with unexpected risk of conception (as with condom failure). For the medication to be effective, the initial dose typically is given within 72 hours after intercourse and preferably within the first 24 hours. Because no advance planning is required before intercourse, Plan B can be misused as a casual form of birth control. Patients who use it in this way need education about more appropriate birth control methods. Side effects of Plan B can include nausea, vomiting, headaches, and breast tenderness.

Another type of postcoital medication prevents the binding of progestins at their receptors, which causes a chemically induced abortion up to the 10th week of pregnancy. This is known as a medical abortion. Medication can be given orally and/or vaginally. You may recall the controversial RU-486, or mifepristone (Mifeprex). Mifepristone causes the blockage of progesterone from the uterine lining, causing the lining to break down. The patient is also then given a dose of misoprostol, which causes the uterus to empty. It must be used within 70 days after the first day of the woman's last period. Pregnancy must be confirmed along with how far pregnant a woman is before medical abortion. Nausea and cramping can accompany expulsion of the uterine contents.

Abortion Methods for Early Pregnancy
Early in a pregnancy (during approximately the first 13 weeks), there are three primary means of pregnancy termination: menstrual extraction, vacuum aspiration, and D&C. Menstrual extraction is removal of the endometrial lining by manual suction and can be done during the first 7 weeks following the last menstrual period. This can be done without anesthesia and without cervical dilation by inserting a small cannula into the cervix and aspirating with a large syringe. Vacuum aspiration is a similar process that is used from confirmation of pregnancy through the first 13 weeks. It requires cervical dilation and usually is done with local anesthesia. The patient returns home 1 to 4 hours after the procedure. D&C also may be used during the first 13 weeks. In this procedure, the cervix is dilated, and the uterine contents are scooped away with a curet. This is done as an outpatient procedure under general, regional, or local anesthesia.

Abortion Methods for Later Pregnancy
During the second trimester, the fetus is much larger, so more dilation is required. A dilation and evacuation (D&E) may be performed in much the same manner as a D&C. Dried laminaria (a type of seaweed) or some other absorbent substance is placed inside the cervical canal. This absorbs fluid and swells, thus gradually dilating the cervix. Prostaglandin may be administered either by suppository into the vagina or by injection into the amniotic sac; this usually induces uterine

contractions and results in delivery a few hours later. Unfortunately, a live fetus too premature to survive may be born by this method and continue to breathe for a time until death.

An induction with either a saline or urea injection may be used for pregnancies beyond 16 weeks. A portion of amniotic fluid is removed and replaced with concentrated saline or urea solution, which kills the fetus and stimulates contractions. Sometimes saline and prostaglandins are used in combination to terminate a pregnancy.

Hysterotomy involves removal of the uterine contents through an abdominal incision in the same manner as a cesarean delivery. This procedure is rarely done for pregnancy termination.

Risks and Complications

Abortion involves risks. Some are the same risks inherent in childbirth, such as possible hemorrhage or introduction of infection. However, there are additional risks related to the interruption of natural processes and the aggressiveness with which the products of conception are removed during abortion. During an uncomplicated childbirth, the uterine lining is not scraped or forcefully emptied by suction. Natural hormonal preparation for term childbirth contributes to uterine contraction after the birth, which decreases blood loss, but no such preparation occurs for abortion. Artificial dilation of the cervix may cause injury, as may introduction of the instruments used for abortion. Injured tissues can become sites for growth of microorganisms. Finally, the possibility of infertility as a result of complications related to abortion, although relatively uncommon, is a risk.

Some possible physical complications following abortion are injuries to the uterus or cervix, excessive bleeding, infection, retention of some products of conception, and possible failure of abortion. Rarely, second-trimester abortions can be complicated by amniotic fluid embolism, in which amniotic fluid is absorbed into the uterine circulation because of disruption of placental attachments with instruments. Amniotic fluid in the mother's circulatory system can result in circulatory collapse and disseminated intravascular coagulation (DIC). DIC is a serious derangement of the body's blood clotting controls and, although rare, can be fatal.

Nursing Care and Patient Education

Care after abortion is very important. Patients rarely stay overnight, and complications can occur after they are discharged. Patients should be carefully assessed after the procedure for signs of bleeding. Instruct the patient that bleeding should not exceed that of a heavy period, that passage of clots larger than a quarter may be a sign of complications, and that discharge should not become foul smelling. Patients should be given a phone number to call 24 hours per day, 7 days per week in case fever, chills, excessive bleeding, or foul-smelling discharge occur. The patient should be advised to abstain from sexual intercourse for the time specified by the HCP (usually about 3 weeks).

A grief response may occur after a pregnancy termination, even if the baby was unwanted and the patient does not have strong beliefs against abortion. There is debate about frequency of postabortion syndrome or whether such a condition exists. However, loss and trauma have occurred in any case and can result in higher rates of anxiety, depression, alcohol abuse, and suicidal behavior (Coleman, 2011). Availability of psychological counseling for women after abortion is very important. Women should be given a number to call if they experience psychological discomfort. The need for birth control should be assessed.

Ethical Issues

Ethically, an individual nurse should not be required to assist in any treatment that demands he or she act in a way that contradicts personal moral beliefs. This would violate the nurse's rights. However, there is also an ethical duty to provide care to patients for whom the nurse is responsible. Therefore, it is wise for nurses who have moral objections to abortion to carefully choose their work setting. For example, choosing to work in day surgery in a hospital that performs abortions and refusing to care for abortion patients is not a legitimate option (see "Ethical Considerations" on Davis Edge). One way nurses can positively influence the abortion situation is by teaching about family planning, which may lower the number of requests for abortions. Another way might be to become involved with agencies that help pregnant women find viable alternatives to abortion.

 ## TUMORS OF THE REPRODUCTIVE SYSTEM

Benign Growths
Fibroid Tumors

PATHOPHYSIOLOGY, ETIOLOGIES, AND SIGNS AND SYMPTOMS. A fibroid tumor, or **leiomyoma** (plural: leiomyomas or leiomyomata), is a benign tumor made up of endometrial cells that have implanted on or within the walls of the uterus. These tumors can grow very large and may cause pain or menstrual disorders, exert pressure on the bladder or bowel, cause necrosis because of pressure on the blood supply to tissues, and interfere with fertility. Although the exact cause is unknown, heredity and hormones play a role.

THERAPEUTIC MEASURES. Because fibroid tumors are estrogen sensitive, medical treatment may involve hormone suppression. Uterine artery embolization (also called fibroid embolization) involves introduction of tiny spongelike particles into the artery that supplies the fibroid. This cuts off the blood supply to the tumor and causes it to shrink. Surgical options include myomectomy or hysterectomy.

• WORD • BUILDING •
hysterotomy: hystero—womb + tomy—cutting
leiomyoma: leio—smooth + myom(a)—fibroid

Myomectomy is removal of only the fibroid tumor. It may be chosen to preserve fertility. Myomectomy may be done surgically through an abdominal or vaginal incision or with a laser introduced through a laparoscope. Hysterectomy may be necessary for very large fibroids or those that cause severe bleeding or discomfort.

Polyps

PATHOPHYSIOLOGY, ETIOLOGY, AND SIGNS AND SYMPTOMS. Polyps are benign growths that grow inside the uterus or on the cervix. They may bleed after intercourse or between menstrual cycles. They are generally teardrop shaped and are attached by a stalk. The cause is unknown, but estrogen plays a role in their development.

THERAPEUTIC MEASURES. Polyps are generally removed vaginally or transcervically by separating the stalk from the uterus and then stopping the bleeding by use of chemical, electrical, or laser cautery. Removal of polyps in the vagina can be done without anesthetic in an HCP's office. Removal of polyps transcervically requires cervical dilation and is more likely to be done in a hospital with anesthesia.

Reproductive System Cysts

PATHOPHYSIOLOGY, ETIOLOGIES, AND SIGNS AND SYMPTOMS. Several types of cysts can affect women's health. Cysts of the ovaries can develop associated with incomplete ovulation, **hypertrophy** of the corpus luteum after ovulation, or inflammation of the ovary. Most ovarian cysts will eventually shrink spontaneously and merely cause discomfort for a time. "Chocolate" cysts are formed when endometrial cells bleed into an enclosed space, as occurs with endometriosis. They are filled with old blood that has become the color of chocolate. Cystadenomas are benign growths that can sometimes undergo cellular transformation and become cancerous. Any pelvic mass in a postmenopausal woman should be investigated for malignancy.

THERAPEUTIC MEASURES. Most cysts are not surgically removed, but excessive size, interference with fertility, and high cancer potential may make needle drainage, biopsy, laparoscopic surgery, or **laparotomy** necessary. If cysts are painful, application of heat to the abdomen or back can help promote comfort.

Polycystic Ovary Syndrome

PATHOPHYSIOLOGY AND ETIOLOGY. Polycystic ovary syndrome (PCOS) is a complex abnormality of endocrine balance of unknown etiology. Multiple cysts on the ovaries are a sign that was discovered early and for which the disease was named, but they are not present in all cases. There seem to be strong genetic links with such family history as too much or too little hair (especially for women), severe acne, diabetes, irregular menses, and infertility. Many of the symptoms of PCOS are a result of insulin resistance with excessive levels of insulin in the blood, which in turn stimulates secretion of androgens.

SIGNS AND SYMPTOMS. Women with PCOS often have infertility, obesity, and menstrual disturbances. They also may have masculinization because of the excess androgen secretion. They have an increased risk of diabetes mellitus, elevated blood pressure, coronary artery disease, and endometrial cancer.

DIAGNOSTIC TESTS. Diagnostic tests can include blood tests to rule out other causes of endocrine abnormality, tests to determine whether ovulation is occurring (such as midluteal progesterone levels and basal body temperature graphing), endometrial biopsies to determine the level of proliferation and to check for endometrial cancer, and blood tests to determine lipid levels and glucose tolerance.

THERAPEUTIC MEASURES. Medical treatments can involve blood pressure medications, lipid control medications, and oral hypoglycemic agents such as metformin (Glucophage). Diet and exercise may be recommended for weight reduction, control of lipid levels, and cardiac health. Oral contraceptives may be used to normalize hormone levels and protect the endometrium for those not desiring to conceive. Ovulation-inducing medication may be used for women who desire to conceive; treatment with metformin may also prompt ovulation.

If masculinization is a problem, antiandrogen medication such as spironolactone (Aldactone) may be prescribed. In severe cases, gonadotropin-releasing hormone (GnRH) agonists may be used to produce medical suppression of the ovaries, with results similar to removal of the ovaries. This is followed 6 months later with an estrogen-progestin combination to protect the bones from osteoporosis.

If medications and lifestyle changes are ineffective, laparoscopic surgery or laser treatments may be used to trigger ovulation or destroy some of the cysts.

Bartholin Cysts

PATHOPHYSIOLOGY, ETIOLOGY, AND SIGNS AND SYMPTOMS. Bartholin cysts are actually infected Bartholin glands at either side of the vaginal opening that occur due to obstruction of the glands. Excessive swelling of Bartholin glands results in pain with sitting and with intercourse.

THERAPEUTIC MEASURES. Incision and drainage can alleviate the discomfort. If Bartholin cyst formation occurs often, **marsupialization** (the surgical formation of a pouch around an opening made into a gland to facilitate drainage) may be needed. Sitz baths may be ordered to cleanse the area and to promote comfort and healing.

• WORD • BUILDING •

myomectomy: myom(a)—fibroid + ec—away + tomy—cutting

hypertrophy: hyper—too much + trophy—nourishment (growth)

laparotomy: laparo(o)—abdominal wall + tomy—cutting

marsupialization: marsupial—pouch + ization—process of making

Dermoid Cysts

PATHOPHYSIOLOGY, ETIOLOGY, AND SIGNS AND SYMPTOMS. Rarely and for unknown reasons, a **dermoid** cyst (also called a cystic **teratoma**) may develop from a germinal cell of an ovary. This cell divides and differentiates into various tissue types such as skin, teeth, bones, hair, and even extremities in a disordered arrangement. This type of cyst may grow quite large and may occur on both ovaries at the same time.

THERAPEUTIC MEASURES. Dermoid cysts are removed by laparoscopy or laparotomy. If the cyst contains glandular tissue that is secreting hormones, adjustment of hormone levels to normal may take some time. Although most teratomas are benign, some are malignant, especially in postmenopausal women, so a biopsy is generally done on the tissue.

NURSING CARE AND PATIENT EDUCATION. Growth of a dermoid cyst can be a frightening experience for a woman. Reassurance that this is a disordered group of cells identical to the other cells in her body, rather than a deformed baby, is important.

Malignant Disorders

It is difficult to distinguish benign growths from malignant growths without biopsy results. Also, some benign growths can become cancerous. Malignancies can occur in all parts of the reproductive system and at all ages. Although reproductive system cancers are more common in older age-groups, ovarian tumors can occur even in young children. Both male and female children of women who were given diethylstilbestrol (DES) in the past to prevent premature delivery in high-risk pregnancies have experienced a high incidence of developmental defects and cancers of the reproductive organs.

This section presents a general overview of the most common cancers. If investigated and treated early enough, cure is often possible.

Vulvar Cancer

PATHOPHYSIOLOGY, ETIOLOGIES, AND SIGNS AND SYMPTOMS. Although vulvar cancer is not common, alertness to changes in visible parts of the reproductive system such as the vulva can result in early diagnosis, require less drastic treatment, and end with more positive results. Persistent itching of the vulva or appearance of white or red patches, rough areas, skin ulcers, or wartlike growths should not be ignored; these can be signs of precancerous or cancerous changes. Risk factors for development of vulvar cancer are having an STI of any type, precancerous or cancerous changes of the anus or genitalia, immune system depression, and smoking.

DIAGNOSTIC TESTS. Regular Pap smears and physical examinations can identify lesions. Biopsy of suspicious lesions is necessary to diagnose vulvar cancer.

THERAPEUTIC MEASURES. If discovered early, vulvar cancer may be treated with removal or destruction of cancerous cells. If diagnosed late, it may require surgical removal of the entire vulva and associated lymph nodes (a radical vulvectomy) with subsequent skin grafting from other areas of the body for repair.

> **LEARNING TIP**
>
> "Three C" changes that may indicate cancer are changes in color, contour, and consistency of a tissue.

Cervical Cancer

PATHOPHYSIOLOGY, ETIOLOGIES, AND SIGNS AND SYMPTOMS. Changes in cervical cells seen with a Pap smear are called cervical dysplasia. Abnormal cells are most often caused by human papillomavirus (HPV). If abnormal cells are found on a biopsy of the cervix, then it is called cervical intraepithelial neoplasia. Without treatment, severe dysplasia can turn into invasive cancer. The severity of the dysplasia determines the treatment plan.

Some risk factors for development of cervical cancer include having multiple sex partners, having three or more pregnancies, smoking, being overweight, long-term use of oral contraceptives, and being infected with chlamydia, HPV, or herpes simplex virus type II (HSV-II). Although some women experience slight spotting or serosanguineous discharge with cervical cancer, many are asymptomatic until the cancer is widespread.

DIAGNOSTIC TESTS. Pap smears are the best method of screening for cervical cancer currently available, but some work is being done on self-tests that women can collect. A Pap smear determines the degree of cellular change, or dysplasia. Colposcopy is done to obtain more information following an abnormal Pap smear (see Chapter 41). Stages of cervical cancer range from stage I (confined to the cervix) to stage IV (spread to other areas of the body). Guidelines introduced in 2012 (the most recent) recommend Pap smears starting at age 21 and then every 3 years through age 65, unless abnormalities develop (U.S. Preventive Services Task Force, 2012). After a period of normal Pap smears, some HCPs advocate longer intervals for low-risk women.

THERAPEUTIC MEASURES. Treatments for preinvasive neoplasia include **cryotherapy** (freezing), laser therapy (burning), and surgical removal of the involved area with a loop excision instrument or by conization (Fig. 42.11). All of these procedures are done through the vagina, so there are no external incisions. After any of these treatments, the patient is advised not to douche, use tampons, or have intercourse for approximately 2 weeks to allow healing to take place. She should be advised to report immediately if fever, bloody vaginal discharge, or foul-smelling vaginal discharge occurs.

• **WORD • BUILDING** •
dermoid: derm—skin + oid—form
teratoma: terat—monster + oma—growth
cryotherapy: cryo—cold + therapy—treatment

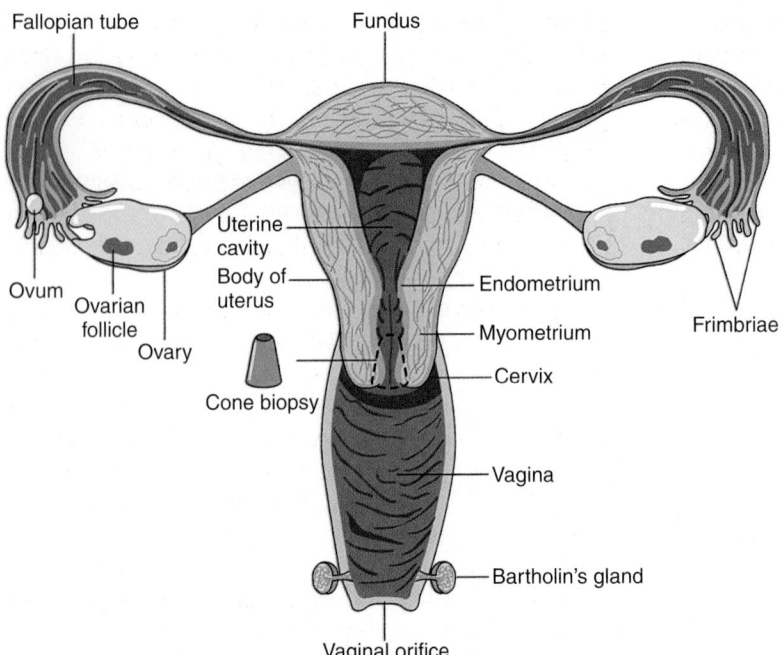

FIGURE 42.11 Conization.

For invasive cancers, hysterectomy, radiation implant, or chemotherapy may be done.

PREVENTION. An HPV vaccination (Gardasil) is available to help protect against many types of HPV. It is recommended for both males and females aged 9 to 26, regardless of sexually activity status or exposure to HPV.

Endometrial Cancer

PATHOPHYSIOLOGY, ETIOLOGIES, AND SIGNS AND SYMPTOMS. Endometrial cancer is the most common type of uterine cancer. Most develop in response to relative estrogen excess. Abrupt changes in bleeding patterns, especially bleeding in a menopausal woman, can indicate endometrial cancer development. Estrogen excess can develop for many reasons. Estrogen levels fluctuate widely in the perimenopausal period. Obesity results in increased estrogen production that is not balanced by progestins. Estrogen replacement therapy for menopausal symptoms without the addition of progestins also has been associated with an increase in endometrial cancer. However, addition of a progestin may decrease the risk of endometrial cancer to less than that of untreated women. Alcohol consumption may increase the risk of endometrial cancer by interfering with estrogen metabolism, but this is still a matter of debate. Some endometrial cancer is unexplained by any currently known risk factors.

DIAGNOSTIC TESTS. Diagnosis is generally done by endometrial biopsy, but MRI may be used to evaluate invasiveness and involvement of lymph nodes.

THERAPEUTIC MEASURES. Depending on the stage of endometrial cancer and metastasis, treatment with hysterectomy, radiation, or chemotherapy may be used.

Ovarian Cancer

PATHOPHYSIOLOGY, ETIOLOGIES, AND SIGNS AND SYMPTOMS. Ovarian cancer is an especially insidious killer because cellular changes in the ovaries often are asymptomatic until the cancer is advanced. Little is known about what prompts these cells to undergo malignant changes. Risk factors are not definitely identified, but some proposed factors include low fertility and number of children, late menopause, a family history of reproductive or colon cancers, and a diet rich in animal fats. Use of hormonal contraception may help prevent ovarian cancer because it results in less ovulation during a woman's lifetime.

DIAGNOSTIC TESTS. Identification of abnormal growths on the ovaries may begin with bimanual examination, so it is important for women, especially in the older age-groups, to continue to have regular pelvic examinations even if they are not sexually active and even if they have had a hysterectomy. Various blood tests measuring tumor marker substances, ultrasonography, CT scan, and MRI may also be used to assist in diagnosis.

THERAPEUTIC MEASURES. Treatment may involve surgical removal of the ovaries by laparoscopy or laparotomy. Sometimes the ovaries are removed to prevent the disease in women who have a high familial risk. Radiation and combination chemotherapy may also be used.

Nursing Care and Education of Patients With Malignant Disorders

Radiation therapy for cancers of the reproductive system may involve the placement of radioactive implants into the patient's body for 24 to 72 hours. Prevent inappropriate radiation of the patient's other body parts by such actions as maintaining patency of a urinary catheter to avoid unnecessary exposure of the bladder. Follow institutional guidelines for radiation precautions. A foul-smelling vaginal discharge is expected after radiation by implant because of tissue destruction caused by the radiation; document the amount and character of the discharge. Chemotherapy treatments often cause severe nausea as well as anorexia and sores of the mouth, vagina, and anus. See Chapter 11 for care of patients receiving radiation or chemotherapy.

See Table 42.9 for a summary of tumors of the reproductive system.

 GYNECOLOGICAL SURGERY

Endoscopic Surgeries

Many of the surgeries performed on the reproductive system can be done using an endoscope. The endoscopes used contain

Table 42.9
Tumors of the Reproductive System Summary

Signs and Symptoms	Menstrual pain/dysfunction
	Infertility
	Constipation
	Vaginal bleeding
	Abdominal/perineal pain/swelling
	Androgen characteristics
	Obesity
	Diabetes
	Coronary artery disease
Diagnostic Tests	Physical examination
	Laparoscopy
	Ultrasound
	Computed tomography (CT) scan or magnetic resonance imaging (MRI)
	Biopsy
	Hormone levels
Therapeutic Measures	Surgery
	Chemical, electrical, or laser cautery
	Oral contraceptives and medications
	Incision, drainage, marsupialization
	Chemotherapy
	Radiation therapy
Priority Nursing Diagnoses	*Acute* or *Chronic Pain* related to lesion/surgery
	Urge Urinary Incontinence or *Constipation* related to lesion or surgery
	Disturbed Body Image related to body structure abnormality
	Sexual Dysfunction related to disturbance in self-concept

not only magnifying lenses and a light source but may also include tiny tools for performing surgery, removing small areas of diseased tissue and samples, suction, and cauterizing bleeding vessels. Because endoscopic surgeries require tiny incisions (usually less than 1 inch long), there is less tissue disruption and little bleeding compared with traditional surgical techniques. Smaller incisions also present less risk of infection than traditional methods, and recuperation is usually faster with fewer complications.

The danger to the patient is generally low for endoscopic surgeries; however, not all surgical situations can be satisfactorily handled in this way. The size of the cannula restricts the size of tissues that can be removed, unless they can be divided into smaller sections and then pulled out through the cannula. If affected areas are widespread, the endoscope may not be able to reach all sites. Traditional surgery still may have to be done when endoscopic surgery has been ineffective; this can be frustrating to patients. However, information gained through the previous endoscopic surgery may decrease the time required for a traditional surgery.

Laparoscopies are the most common type of endoscopic surgical procedure used for women's reproductive system surgeries. This method can be used for access to the abdominal cavity and the anterior portions of the reproductive organs. Tubal ligations, tubal repairs, removal of ectopic pregnancy implantations, removal of small tumors, removal of endometriotic tissue, and aspiration of fluid-filled cysts can all be done by this method.

The newest method of surgery uses computers and robots and is minimally invasive (see Chapter 12). This method allows the surgeon to make several of 1- to 2-cm incisions to gain access and three-dimensional visualization into the pelvic cavity. Gynecologically, this method can be used for hysterectomy and myomectomy. The benefits of this method versus other surgical methods are a shorter hospital stay and less pain and scarring for the patient. There is also less risk of infection, less blood loss, fewer transfusions, faster recoveries, and quicker return to normal activities.

Culdoscopies may be done to access the area at the back of the uterus. A **culdotomy,** which is an incision into the upper posterior portion of the vagina, is necessary to insert the cannula. A **culdocentesis,** which is the removal of fluid from the cul-de-sac of Douglas, may be done during a culdoscopy. Aftercare is much the same as it is for a laparoscopy. The patient should be informed that a small amount of vaginal spotting may be expected from the incision but that heavy, purulent, or foul-smelling discharge should be reported because it could indicate infection.

Colposcopies typically are used to screen, diagnose, or treat problems of the cervix. The binocular microscope attached to the scope cannula, which is introduced into the vagina, allows the HCP to examine dysplastic cells while they are still in

• WORD • BUILDING •
culdotomy: culdo—cul-de-sac + tomy—cutting
culdocentesis: culdo—cul-de-sac + centesis—puncturing

their normal place and to treat cervical dysplasia as previously described.

Hysteroscopy may be used to treat problems within the uterus. Removal of polyps and other growths, modification of congenital malformations such as septa (walls of tissue where there should be none), and laser ablation of endometrial tissue may all be done during hysteroscopy. The endoscope may be inserted further into the fallopian tubes to perform a salpingoscopy, allowing surgical or laser opening of blocked tubes.

Nursing Care and Patient Education

Postoperative care involves careful assessment for signs of possible excessive internal bleeding, including assessment of vital signs, skin color and temperature, and pain. Discharge teaching includes instruction about signs of complications to report, medications, and when and where to go for suture removal.

Hysterectomy

Removal of the uterus (hysterectomy) may be done for a variety of reasons, including abnormally heavy or painful menstruation, large fibroid or other benign tumors, severe uterine prolapse, and cancer of the uterus. It should not be done merely as a sterilization procedure because the risks involved in hysterectomy are much greater than the risks associated with tubal ligation. The surgery can be done through an abdominal incision (total abdominal hysterectomy [TAH]), vaginally, laparoscopically, or robotically. The vagina is left intact, and the proximal end (which had been attached to the uterus) is sutured, forming a blind pouch. Although less vaginal lubrication is present after hysterectomy, nerve routes are maintained, and satisfactory sexual intercourse is expected to continue.

There are three types of hysterectomy: *Total hysterectomy* is the removal of the uterus and cervix. *Supracervical hysterectomy* (also known as partial or subtotal) removes just the upper part of the uterus, while the cervix is left in place. A *radical hysterectomy,* which is the removal of the whole uterus, the tissue on the both sides of the cervix, and the upper part of the vagina, is done when cancer is present.

Sometimes, the choice is made to remove the fallopian tubes (**salpingectomy**) and ovaries (**oophorectomy**), which is known as a bilateral salpingo-oophorectomy (BSO). If the ovaries are removed, the woman undergoes immediate menopause. She may suffer from symptoms associated with menopause, including the increased risks of cardiovascular disease and osteoporosis. If removal of the ovaries is done because of the presence of estrogen-dependent cancer, then estrogen replacement is not usually feasible. Extra care, comfort, and explanation from nurses is needed.

See "Nursing Care Plan for the Patient Undergoing Hysterectomy." In addition to the nursing diagnoses covered, also assess for *Anxiety* related to surgery, *Disturbed Body Image*, and *Ineffective Coping*. See Chapters 10 and 12, respectively, for additional interventions for pain and postoperative patients.

• WORD • BUILDING •

salpingectomy: salpingo—tubal + ec—from + tomy—cutting
oophorectomy: oophor—ovary + ec—from + tomy—cutting

Nursing Care Plan for the Patient Undergoing Hysterectomy

Nursing Diagnosis: *Risk for Impaired Tissue Perfusion* related to surgical incision and removal of the uterus (and possibly the ovaries)
Expected Outcome: The patient's incision(s) will heal by primary intention without excessive bleeding.
Evaluation of Outcome: Is dressing dry and intact, and/or does perineal pad show less than 3-cm stain every hour? Are edges of the incision well approximated, with scant bleeding/serous drainage, and mild edema/erythema (if applicable)?

Intervention	Rationale	Evaluation
Monitor vital signs and oxygen saturation according to hospital policy and as necessary.	*Vital signs and oxygen saturation reflect tissue perfusion status.*	Are vital signs stable and within normal range?
Assess for bleeding or other discharge on perineal pad and on abdominal dressing (if applicable).	*Excessive bleeding may compromise tissue perfusion and slow healing. Vaginal discharge gives clues to healing of incision at the proximal end of the vagina.*	Is pad or dressing dry? Is discharge foul smelling?
Assess wound healing (if applicable) twice a day and as needed, and report any evidence of infection or inadequate healing promptly.	*Early treatment of inadequate wound healing decreases postoperative complications.*	Is incision area swollen, reddened, or draining purulent material?
Teach patient to report changes in incision site or excessive bleeding.	*Patients are discharged quickly and should know what to monitor at home.*	Does patient verbalize understanding of instruction?

Nursing Care Plan for the Patient Undergoing Hysterectomy—cont'd

Nursing Diagnosis: *Urinary Retention* related to manipulation of the bladder and ureters during surgery, anticholinergic drugs, fluid intake changes, and fear of pain
Expected Outcome: The patient will void 30 mL/hr or more without difficulty.
Evaluation of Outcome: Is the patient able to void and effectively empty bladder when voiding? Is the patient voiding at least 30 mL/hr?

Intervention	Rationale	Evaluation
Assess urinary output after surgery. Report to registered nurse or health care provider (HCP) if less than 30 mL/hr or unable to void.	*Inadequate urinary output can be an evidence of dehydration, low glomerular perfusion, kidney dysfunction, damage to ureter, or urinary retention.*	Is output greater than 30 mL/hour? Is patient able to void without discomfort?
Assess bladder fullness using Doppler monitoring or scratch test (listening with a stethoscope, lightly scratch abdomen as you move downward from xiphoid until you hear change in sound indicating top of the bladder).	*Urine retention can cause infection and damage to kidneys, ureters, and bladder. The scratch test and Doppler monitoring cause less discomfort and pressure than palpation of the abdominal incision area.*	Does patient feel she is emptying fully when voiding? Does Doppler or scratch test indicate residual urine after voiding?
Medicate for pain on a fixed schedule for operative day and first postoperative day (unless patient declines).	*Maintenance of a consistent blood level of medication in the immediate postoperative period provides relief of pain and promotes voiding without fear of discomfort.*	Does patient state that she is comfortable?

Nursing Diagnosis: *Risk for Constipation* related to manipulation of the bowel during surgery, use of opioid analgesics and anticholinergic drugs, diet changes, less exercise than usual, and fear of pain when passing stool
Expected Outcome: The patient will pass soft, formed stool without excessive gas discomfort by third postoperative day.
Evaluation of Outcome: Are bowel sounds active in all four quadrants? Is the patient passing gas without difficulty? Is the patient able to have a soft, formed bowel movement within 3 days of surgery?

Intervention	Rationale	Evaluation
Assess for active bowel sounds in all four abdominal quadrants before giving anything orally.	*Manipulation of the bowel during surgery and anesthetics or other medications can interfere with bowel function.*	Are bowel sounds within normal limits?
Encourage high fluid intake, and graduate diet toward a high-fiber, regular diet as soon as patient is able to tolerate it (or HCP orders prescribe).	*Adequate fluid and fiber in the diet softens the stool for easy passage*	Is patient able to tolerate fluids and high-fiber foods?
Encourage adequate exercise.	*Reasonable exercise promotes peristalsis and relieves gas discomfort.*	Has patient dangled legs at bedside the day of surgery and then walked increasing amounts each following day?
Assess quantity and quality of pain. Control pain with analgesics, especially before administering a suppository or enema.	*The presence of pain may inhibit defecation.*	Is pain controlled? Does patient express concern about pain with bowel movement?
Administer stool softeners, laxatives, suppositories, or enemas as ordered (check bowel protocol or standing orders).	*Soft stool is easier to pass.*	Has patient passed soft, formed stool by the third day after surgery?

SUGGESTED ANSWERS TO CRITICAL THINKING

Julie

1. Questions to further assess Julie's symptoms should include the following: How long have you been noticing the lumps? Do you do breast self-examination (BSE)? Has there been a change in the characteristics of the lumps? Are the lumps mobile or fixed? Have you noticed any breast skin or nipple changes? Have you noticed any leakage of fluid or blood from your breasts? Are you breastfeeding or have you recently delivered an infant? Have you had a fever? Are the pain and lumps related to your menstrual cycle? Is there anything that makes the symptoms better or worse?

2. You can teach Julie to continue to do BSE because she is the best person to detect changes. Teach her that limiting fat and caffeine in her diet may help reduce symptoms. Reinforce any information or treatments provided by the nurse practitioner.

3. If Julie is doing BSE every month, then she knows her breasts better than anyone. She should be vigilant for changes that do not feel like her usual tissue.

Lola

1. Interventions that can help control Lola's discomfort related to hot flashes include possible hormone replacement therapy (HRT), including phytoestrogens in her diet with her health care provider's (HCP's) direction, limiting caffeinated foods or beverages, dressing in layers so that some may be removed as needed, and lowering the thermostat as needed.

2. Information that should be shared with Lola concerning HRT includes the risks as well as benefits according to most recent studies. Risks include increased risk of stroke, cardiovascular disease, breast cancer, and thromboembolism. Benefits include symptomatic relief and decreased risk of complications from osteoporosis.

3. Collaborate with the HCP, because even herbal remedies can interact with medications and should be recommended by an HCP.

Jessica

1. Some important information from Jessica would include her true age (laws vary concerning birth control for minors), her intentions, her family situation, whether she is already sexually active, and what information she wants.

2. She needs to know that being sexually active involves more risks than just pregnancy. Discussion of sexually transmitted infections (STIs) is vital. Early sexual activity may also be associated with abuse and psychological suffering. The choices of birth control should be explained, including the risks, effectiveness, disadvantages, and advantages of each method. Follow clinic protocol to determine your role in teaching the patient.

3. Potential scenarios can be presented for her "responsible" consideration, such as the following: What would she do if contraceptive failure resulted in a pregnancy? How would she feel if she contracted an incurable or permanently damaging STI that she might pass on to someone else? How would she react to a breakup with her partner after she has engaged in sexual intercourse? Ask about her goals and plans in life. Counseling that evidences concern for the individual at this stage may do a lot to postpone sexual activity until the patient is more mature. It is important for her to realize that choosing to delay sexual activity at this time may be the most responsible and health-promoting life decision she can make.

Review Questions

1. A patient who is breastfeeding her baby says, "My doctor said I have mastalgia. What does that mean?" Which response by the nurse is best?
   1. "That means you may have an infection in your breasts."
   2. "Mastalgia is the normal discomfort that is associated with breastfeeding."
   3. "The word *mastalgia* means breast pain; it can occur with monthly cycles of hormone levels."
   4. "Mastalgia is the medical term for fibrocystic breast disease. It is important to have it treated promptly."

2. Which response by the nurse is most appropriate when a 60-year-old woman who has been menopausal for several years relates that she has begun having vaginal bleeding again?
   1. "Don't be concerned. It is perfectly normal."
   2. "Try taking some ibuprofen. That may reduce the bleeding."
   3. "You should see your health care provider to have that checked as soon as possible."
   4. "Give it time. Bleeding after menopause usually goes away within a month."

3. During an endometrial biopsy, for which of the following signs and symptoms of vasovagal response should the nurse observe?
   1. Pain in the chest and abdomen
   2. Cramping and diaphoresis
   3. High blood pressure and tachycardia
   4. Bradycardia and falling blood pressure

4. Which of the following medications can be used to treat vasovagal response during gynecological procedures? **Select all that apply.**
   1. Atropine
   2. Morphine
   3. Epinephrine
   4. Metoprolol
   5. Naproxen

5. The nurse is discharging a patient with endometriosis from an office visit. The patient says her medication helps but does not relieve all her discomfort. What other measures can the nurse recommend?
   1. "Check with the health food store. There are several herbal remedies that can be very effective."
   2. "Try using the relaxation exercises you learned in your childbirth classes. A warm compress to your abdomen might also help."
   3. "You can double up on your pain medication on occasion, but you shouldn't do it on a regular basis."
   4. "If the medications aren't effective, then it is time to talk to the physician about a hysterectomy."

6. The nurse enters the room of a patient who is 1-day postoperative left-sided mastectomy and notes a phlebotomist taking blood from her left antecubital space. What should the nurse do first?
   1. Nothing; the nurse is not the phlebotomist's supervisor.
   2. Nothing; blood pressures should be avoided in the affected arm, but blood draws are safe.
   3. Stop the phlebotomist and ask that the blood be drawn from the right arm.
   4. Notify the health care provider.

7. Following a total hysterectomy with bilateral salpingo-oophorectomy, what should the nurse teach the patient to expect?
   1. Heavy bleeding for a week
   2. Symptoms of menopause
   3. Painful intercourse for approximately 6 months
   4. Monthly cramping but no menstrual flow

8. A patient who has just returned from a transabdominal hysterectomy is at risk for impaired urinary elimination. At least how many milliliters should be in her catheter bag 8 hours postoperatively? Fill in the blank.
   Answer: _____ mL

9. Which of the following is the least effective form of contraception?
   1. Douching
   2. Condom with spermicide
   3. Diaphragm with spermicide
   4. Oral contraceptive medication

Answer rationales available in your online resources.

ANSWERS 1. 3; 2. 3; 3. 4; 4. 1, 3; 5. 2; 6. 3; 7. 2; 8. 240; 9. 1

Key Points

Find the chapter key points in your online resources available through Davis Edge.

Additional Resources

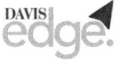

Use the scratch off code on the inside front cover of your book to access online quizzes that will help you to improve your scores on course exams and prepare for the NCLEX-PN®.

Study Guide

CHAPTER 43

Nursing Care of Male Patients With Genitourinary Disorders

Jaime Crabb, Michelle Johnson

KEY TERMS

cryptorchidism (kript-OR-ki-dizm)
epididymitis (EP-i-DID-i-MY-tis)
erectile dysfunction (ee-REK-tile dis-FUNK-shun)
hydrocele (HY-droh-seel)
orchiectomy (or-ki-EK-toh-mee)
orchitis (or-KY-tis)
paraphimosis (PAR-uh-fih-MOH-sis)
phimosis (fih-MOH-sis)
priapism (PRY-uh-pizm)
prostatectomy (PRAHS-tah-TEK-tuh-mee)
prostatitis (PRAHS-tuh-TY-tis)
retrograde (REH-troh-GRADE)
suprapubic (SOO-pruh-PEW-bik)
urodynamic (YOO-roh-dy-NAM-ik)
urosepsis (YOO-roh-SEP-sis)
vasectomy (va-SEK-tuh-mee)

CHAPTER CONCEPTS

Elimination
Health Promotion
Sexuality

LEARNING OUTCOMES

1. Explain the pathophysiology associated with each male genitourinary and reproductive disorder discussed in this chapter.
2. Describe the etiologies, signs and symptoms, and treatments of prostate disorders.
3. Plan nursing care for men with genitourinary and reproductive disorders.
4. Describe disorders of the testicles and penis and how they affect sexual function.
5. List selected physical and emotional causes of erectile dysfunction.
6. Discuss the nurse's role in helping men cope with loss of sexual function.
7. Identify disorders of the male reproductive system that interfere with fertility.
8. List treatment options available for male infertility.

Problems affecting the male genitourinary system are sensitive in nature for both the patient and the nurse because of the sexual nature of the male anatomy. To provide holistic care, the nurse must acknowledge patients' sexuality and become skilled in assessing and caring for problems related to sexual and genitourinary health. The nurse has a great opportunity to provide important sexual health care teaching. Discussions about sexual health can be positive learning experiences for both the patient and the nurse if approached in an appropriate manner.

PROSTATE DISORDERS

The prostate gland sits at the base of the bladder and wraps around the upper part of the male urethra like a doughnut. The primary purpose of the prostate is to provide alkaline secretions to semen and to aid in ejaculation. The prostate is prone to increasing in size as the male ages. The prostate does not contain any hormones; however, many men fear that prostate problems and treatment will cause problems with their erections or sexual activities.

Prostatitis

Pathophysiology

Prostatitis, or inflammation of the prostate gland, can occur any time after puberty. The problem can be chronic or a single, acute episode. The inflammation causes the prostate gland to swell, resulting in pain, especially when standing. It can eventually lead to difficulty in passing urine as a result of an inward squeezing on the urethra and restricted urine flow.

Etiology

According to the National Institutes of Health, there are four basic types of prostatitis: (1) acute bacterial prostatitis, (2) chronic bacterial prostatitis, (3) chronic prostatitis/chronic pelvic pain syndrome, and (4) asymptomatic inflammatory prostatitis (National Institute of Diabetes and Digestive and Kidney Diseases, 2014). Bacterial prostatitis is most common in older men. It results in edema and inflammation of all or part of the prostate gland.

Any bacteria that can cause a urinary tract infection (UTI) can also cause infectious prostatitis. Common bacteria are organisms such as *Escherichia coli* and *Staphylococcus aureus.* Sexually transmitted infections (STIs) can also cause prostatitis. The prostate gland may become infected in the following ways:

- Bacteria ascending the urethra
- Infected urine refluxing from the bladder into the prostatic ducts
- Bacteria in the blood or lymph supply to the gland
- Surgical instrumentation or other forms of urethral trauma

Prevention

Ways to prevent prostatitis are regular and complete emptying of the bladder to prevent UTIs, avoiding excess alcohol (alcohol is a bladder irritant), and avoiding high-risk sexual practices, such as multiple partners.

Signs and Symptoms

The most common symptoms are those that occur with any UTI: urgency, frequency, hesitancy, dribbling, and dysuria. Because of the location and function of the prostate gland, the patient may report low-back, perineal, and postejaculation pain. Other symptoms may include nocturia, fever, and chills.

Complications

One complication of acute bacterial prostatitis is urinary retention. If the prostate is extremely swollen, the bladder cannot be completely emptied. Another complication may be a temporary problem with erections. Ascending infections, prostatic abscess, epididymitis, and prostatic calculi (stones) are some of the more serious and rare complications of prostatitis.

Diagnostic Tests

Initial diagnosis is based on symptoms. The first test performed is a digital rectal examination of the prostate. The health care provider (HCP) examines the prostate gland by inserting a lubricated, gloved finger into the rectum. Findings may include a warm, irregular, swollen, or painful prostate gland. A urine culture tests for bacteria. The examiner may massage the prostate gland to express prostate secretions, which can be tested for bacteria and white blood cells. Cystoscopy, a visualization of the urethra and bladder, may be done to rule out other urological conditions.

Therapeutic Measures

Acute bacterial prostatitis is treated with antibiotics. Additional treatments may include anti-inflammatory agents, stool softeners, warm sitz baths, prostatic massage, and dietary changes such as decreasing spicy foods and alcohol. Alpha-adrenergic blockers such as alfuzosin (Uroxatral) can help relax the bladder neck and reduce pain associated with urination (Table 43.1). In some cases, prostate surgery is needed to remove the obstruction.

BE SAFE!

BE VIGILANT! Patients with prostate disorders should avoid alpha-adrenergic agonist and anticholinergic medications, which can cause urine retention.

Nursing Process for the Patient With Prostatitis

DATA COLLECTION. Begin the assessment by asking the patient to describe signs and symptoms that indicate evidence of a UTI, such as sudden fever, chills, and reports of urgency, frequency, hesitancy, dysuria, and nocturia. The patient may also have pain in the lower back, in the perineum, or after ejaculating. Ask the patient whether he has ever had a UTI or prostate infection in the past. Be sure to assess urinary retention resulting from obstruction. Obtain a urine culture and assist with collection of the expressed prostate secretion specimen as needed.

NURSING DIAGNOSES, PLANNING, AND IMPLEMENTATION.

Urinary Retention related to obstruction as evidenced by residual urine in bladder after voiding

EXPECTED OUTCOME: The patient will be able to void effectively as evidenced by residual urine of less than 25% of bladder capacity.

- Evaluate the patient's medications for urinary retention as a side effect. *Many medications, especially those with anticholinergic effects, can cause urinary retention.*
- If suspicion of urine retention is present, determine residual urine volume by catheterizing the patient (according to HCP order) or obtaining a bladder ultrasound immediately after voiding. *Incomplete emptying of the bladder may lead to increased discomfort or ascending infection.*

- WORD · BUILDING -

prostatitis: prostat—prostate gland + itis—inflammation

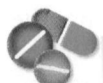

Table 43.1

Medication Used to Treat Disorders of the Male Reproductive Organs

Medication Class/Action

Testosterone Suppressing/Blocking Agents

Examples	**Nursing Implications**
Initially stimulates and then inhibits follicle-stimulating hormone (FSH) and luteinizing hormone (LH) to suppress testosterone: leuprolide (Lupron) Analog to luteinizing-releasing hormone; works on pituitary to decrease FSH to decrease sex hormones: goserelin (Zoladex) Inhibits androgen uptake and/or binding in tissues: flutamide (Eulexin)	Store drug at room temperature and protect from light. Monitor for side effects. Inject into upper abdominal wall. Do not aspirate syringe. Monitor hepatic function tests. *Teach:* Signs and symptoms may increase initially. Medication may increase testosterone initially and thus also increase signs and symptoms. Urine color changes to amber/yellow-green. Avoid excess exposure to sun. Promptly report side effects.

Alpha-Adrenergic Antagonists and Alpha-Reductase Inhibitors

Alpha-Adrenergic Antagonists
Relax smooth muscle and produce vasodilatation.

Examples	**Nursing Implications**
tamsulosin (Flomax) terazosin (Hytrin) alfuzosin (Uroxatral) doxazosin (Cardura)	Monitor blood pressure/pulse. *Teach:* Dizziness may occur with onset of use. Report side effects. Do not to crush or chew tablets. Do not drive or use heavy machinery.

Alpha-Reductase Inhibitors
Inhibit enzyme responsible for formation of potent androgen from testosterone.

Examples	**Nursing Implications**
finasteride (Proscar) dutasteride (Avodart)	Obtain baseline prostate-specific antigen (PSA) and perform digital rectal examination before use. Caution with liver dysfunction. *Teach:* Side effects. Do not to chew or crush tablets.

Vasodilators, Smooth Muscle Relaxers, and Hormone Replacement

Examples	**Nursing Implications**
Relax smooth muscle and produce vasodilation: sildenafil (Viagra) tadalafil (Cialis) vardenafil (Levitra)	Some are taken daily and also help with symptoms of benign prostatic hyperplasia. Assess cardiovascular status before use; may be contraindicated. *Teach:* Avoid use when taking nitroglycerin preparations. Take about 1 hour before sexual activity (may be taken .5 to 4 hours before). If erection lasts more than 4 hours, seek emergency care.

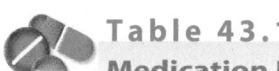

Table 43.1
Medication Used to Treat Disorders of the Male Reproductive Organs—cont'd

Medication Class/Action	
Relax smooth muscle and produce vasodilation: alprostadil (Caverject injection or MUSE suppository) prostaglandin E1 *Herbal vasodilator:* yohimbine	Monitor vital signs. Assess for other medical conditions before use. Monitor blood pressure as well as renal and hepatic function. *Teach:* Erection should occur in 2 to 5 minutes and not last more than 4 hours. Report side effects immediately.
Testosterone replacement; produce androgen effects: testosterone transdermal (Testoderm, Androderm) testosterone cypionate (DEPO-testosterone injection)	Rule out cancer before use. Monitor hepatic function and red blood cell count. *Teach:* Report side effects, prolonged erection, or difficulty urinating. Women should avoid contact with medication.

• Have the patient complete a bladder log including patterns of elimination and related symptoms as well as volume/type of fluid consumed for 3 to 7 days. *This will provide an objective verification of intake and output volumes and aid in determination of urinary retention.*

• Educate the patient about avoidance of risk factors for urine retention (e.g., alpha-adrenergic agonists, anticholinergic agents, overfilling of the bladder). *These are modifiable variables that may limit retention of urine.*

• Report urine retention to the registered nurse (RN) or HCP. *Catheterization may be needed to empty the bladder and prevent complications.*

Deficient Knowledge about cause, treatment, and prevention of prostatitis

EXPECTED OUTCOME: The patient will verbalize understanding of the disorder and demonstrate appropriate self-care.

• Determine the patient's current knowledge and understanding about cause and treatment of prostatitis. *This will allow for additional and/or correct information to be provided about the disorder for appropriate understanding.*

• Provide the patient with additional and/or correct information about the cause and treatment of prostatitis. *This will allow the patient to have a full understanding of the etiology and care related to the disorder and increase likelihood of patient adherence to treatment.*

• Teach avoidance of risk factors such as urinary catheterization, poor hygiene, risky sexual practices, and excessive intake of bladder irritants such as alcohol, caffeine, or citrus juices. *Avoiding risk factors is important to resolving or preventing prostatitis.*

• Encourage the patient to wash his hands and sitz bath equipment before and after each treatment *to prevent infection.*

• Encourage the patient to empty his bladder every 2 to 3 hours even if he does not feel the urge to urinate. *An overstretched bladder increases risk of infection.*

• Encourage fluids up to 2,500 to 3,000 mL/day unless contraindicated by heart failure or other chronic illness. *Fluids help flush the bladder and prevent infection.*

• Include the patient's partner in care. *Some treatment options may also include treatment of the partner (e.g., for STIs such as gonorrhea, chlamydiosis, or trichomoniasis; see Chapter 44).*

• Explain use of antibiotics as directed, and advise the patient to take the complete course of medication even if he is feeling better. *The entire course of antibiotics is essential to treat bacterial infection and prevent development of antibiotic-resistant bacteria.*

Acute Pain related to swelling and irritation of the prostate gland as evidenced by pain rating

EXPECTED OUTECOME: The patient's pain will be controlled as evidenced by the patient's statement that comfort is at an acceptable level.

• Use a culturally appropriate pain scale to help the patient identify his comfort level. *This will aid in understanding the comfort level as defined by the patient and aid in guiding appropriate interventions.*

• Encourage appropriate use of anti-inflammatory medication as ordered. *This will decrease inflammation and promote comfort.*

- Encourage use of comfort measures such as warm sitz baths, sitting on a pillow, or prostatic massage, as needed. *These measures help to decrease swelling and promote patient comfort.*
- Teach the patient to avoid irritants, such as spicy and acidic foods, alcohol, or caffeine. *These irritants can exacerbate symptoms.*
- Consult the HCP about the need for stool softeners. *Firm stool will further irritate the prostate during defecation and increase discomfort.*

EVALUATION. A clean urine culture with the absence of all symptoms of prostatitis is the desired outcome. If interventions have been effective, the patient will have an acceptable comfort level and understand the cause and treatment plan. Prevention of chronic prostatitis can generally be achieved with patient education.

Benign Prostatic Hyperplasia

Enlargement of the prostate gland is a normal process in older men. Benign prostatic hyperplasia (BPH) is a common nonmalignant growth of the prostate that gradually causes urinary obstruction. According to current data, BPH does not increase a man's risk of developing cancer of the prostate.

Pathophysiology

A slow increase in the number of cells in the prostate gland is generally the result of aging and the male hormone dihydrotestosterone. As the size of the prostate gland increases, it begins to compress or squeeze the urethra. This narrowing of the urethra makes it difficult to empty the bladder. Eventually the narrowing causes an obstruction, which leads to urine retention or distention of the kidney with urine (hydronephrosis).

The location of the enlargement, rather than the size, determines symptoms. A small growth in the prostate gland closest to the urethra can cause more problems with urination than a growth the size of an orange in the outer portion of the gland.

Etiology

There is no known cause of BPH other than normal aging. Some men think they may have caused the problem by certain sexual practices; however, there is no scientific proof of that at this time. Obesity may play a role in increasing risk. Exercise can reduce risk.

Signs and Symptoms

Symptoms of BPH are identified in two ways: problems related to obstruction or problems related to irritation. Symptoms related to obstruction include a decrease in the size or force of the urinary stream, difficulty in starting a stream, dribbling after urination is complete, urinary retention, and a feeling that the bladder is not empty. The patient may also experience overflow incontinence or an interrupted stream, where the urine stops midstream and then starts again.

Symptoms related to irritation include nocturia, dysuria, and urgency. HCPs may use a standardized symptom score index tool with patients to assess symptoms and determine treatment options.

Complications

When BPH is untreated and obstruction is prolonged, serious complications can occur. Urine that sits in the bladder for too long can back up into the kidneys, causing hydronephrosis, renal insufficiency, or **urosepsis** (UTI with septicemia). It can also damage the bladder walls, leading to bladder dysfunction, recurrent UTIs, or calculi (stones). Acute urine retention with total inability to urinate can occur. This is a medical emergency that requires catheterization.

NURSING CARE TIP

It can be difficult to catheterize a man with an enlarged prostate gland. If you try once and are unable to advance the catheter, contact the registered nurse or health care provider.

Diagnostic Tests

The first test is usually digital rectal examination of the prostate to assess for enlargement and whether the gland is hard, lumpy, or "boggy" (soft). Additional tests include urinalysis, blood urea nitrogen (BUN), serum creatinine, and prostate-specific antigen (PSA). Secondary tests include **urodynamic** flow studies, which may show a decreased urine flow rate. Transrectal ultrasound of the prostate and cystoscopy can reflect structural abnormalities.

Therapeutic Measures

If the patient has no symptoms or mild symptoms, the current medical approach is "watchful waiting." The HCP watches for any increase in symptoms that suggest the urethra is becoming obstructed. Treatment of symptoms may include use of a catheter (indwelling or intermittent), encouraging oral fluids, and antibiotics for UTI.

Conservative medical treatment includes the use of medication to either relax the smooth muscles of the prostate and bladder neck or block the male hormone to prevent or shrink tissue growth. Alpha-adrenergic antagonists, such as tamsulosin (Flomax) and alfuzosin (Uroxatral), are medications that relax the smooth muscles. These medications are also used to treat high blood pressure; therefore, patients need to work closely with their HCPs to avoid overdose or the negative side effects of postural hypotension (see Table 43.1).

The most commonly used medications to block the action of the male hormone in the prostate gland are finasteride

- WORD • BUILDING •
urosepsis: uro—urine + sepsis—systemic infection
urodynamic: uro—urine + dynamic—force

(Proscar) and dutasteride (Avodart). These medications must be taken on a long-term, continuous basis to achieve results. Conservative measures are used initially unless the patient is experiencing recurring infections, repeated gross hematuria, bladder or kidney damage, evidence of cancer, or unsatisfactory lifestyle changes.

Nonsurgical invasive treatments are available; however, some are experimental and may have limited accessibility. Nonsurgical treatments include transurethral microwave therapy (heat is applied directly to the gland to inhibit growth), transurethral needle ablation (radiofrequency waves are used to destroy excess prostate tissue), and high-intensity focused ultrasound (radio or sound waves are used to destroy parts of the prostate). Urethral stents can be used to open the passageway for urine obstructions.

Complementary and Alternative Therapies
Many herbal supplements such as allium, saw palmetto, and echinacea have been used for management of BPH. However, research has been unable to show any benefit with these or other herbs (Keehn & Lowe, 2015). Accupuncture is currently being researched as a treatment for BPH.

Surgical Treatment
Because so many other treatments are available now, surgery is not needed as often. When symptoms are severe enough to require surgery, several types are available.

TRANSURETHRAL RESECTION OF THE PROSTATE. Transurethral resection of the prostate (TURP) is used most often to relieve obstruction caused by an enlarged prostate (Fig. 43.1). Several other transurethral options also exist. Transurethral incision of the prostate (TUIP) uses surgical incisions into the gland to relieve obstruction. Transurethral

ultrasound-guided laser-induced prostatectomy (TULIP) uses a laser to relieve obstruction.

For TURP, the patient is anesthetized. The surgery is performed using an instrument called a resectoscope. The resectoscope is inserted into the urethra, and the prostate gland is "chipped" away a piece at a time. Special surgical instruments are used to "vaporize" or "microwave" the pieces and cut down on the amount of bleeding during surgery. During routine TURP, the "chips" are flushed out using an irrigating solution. They are then sent to the laboratory to be analyzed for possible evidence of cancer. The prostate gland is not completely removed but peeled away like the rind of an orange. The prostatic tissue that remains eventually grows back. It can cause obstruction again at a later time. Patients need to be reminded to continue having yearly prostate examinations.

Bleeding occurs during a TURP. A Foley catheter will be inserted and left in place with 30 to 60 mL of sterile water inflating the balloon. This overfilled balloon is secured tightly to the leg or abdomen to tamponade (compress) the prostate area and stop the bleeding. Irrigation solution generally flows continuously (Fig. 43.2); manual irrigation may be done for the first 24 hours to help remove clots and chips, and to maintain catheter patency. The Foley catheter is removed after the danger of hemorrhage has passed.

You may need to save "serial urines" to monitor for bleeding. To do this, each time the patient urinates or the catheter

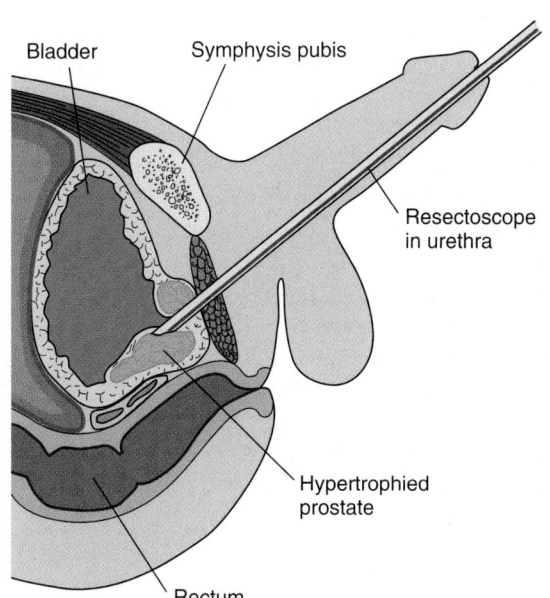

FIGURE 43.1 Transurethral resection of the prostate.

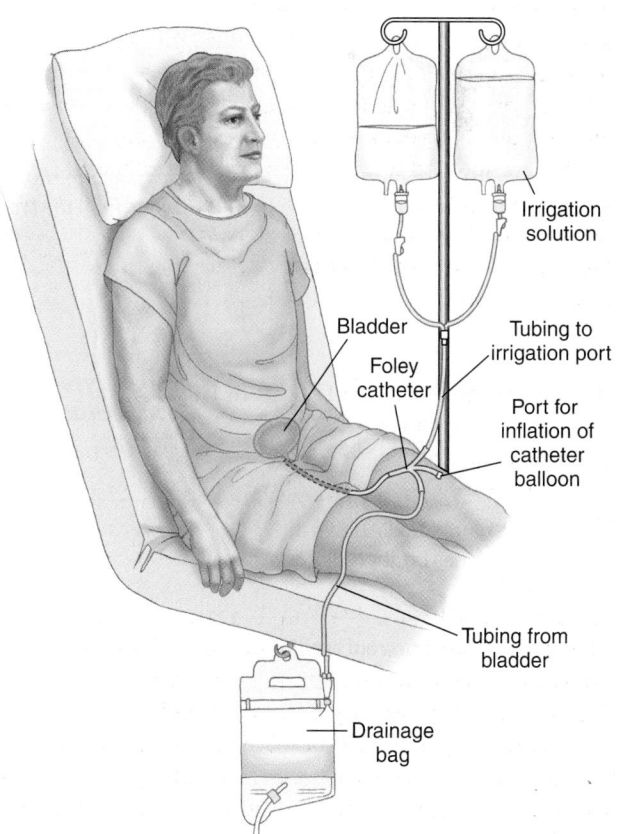

FIGURE 43.2 Bladder irrigation.

bag is emptied, save a sample of urine in a transparent cup. Place it in a safe place, such as on a shelf in the bathroom. With each subsequent urination, place the new cup to the right of the previous cup. When five or six cups are lined up, you can start over at the left side, replacing the oldest cup with the newest one. This allows the nurse or HCP to examine the urine for progressively less blood with each void.

Complications associated with prostate surgery depend on the type and extent of the procedure performed. The main medical complications include clot formation, bladder spasms, and infection. Less common complications are urinary incontinence, hemorrhage, and erectile dysfunction (see "Nursing Care Plan for the Postsurgical Patient Having Transurethral Resection of the Prostate for Benign Prostatic Hyperplasia").

Nursing Care Plan for the Postsurgical Patient Having Transurethral Resection of the Prostate for Benign Prostatic Hyperplasia

Nursing Diagnosis: *Risk for Bleeding* related to surgical intervention
Expected Outcome: The patient's bleeding will be minimal as evidenced by urine becoming progressively more clear.
Evaluation of Outcome: Is urine clearing? Is bleeding reported promptly?

Intervention	Rationale	Evaluation
Closely monitor urinary output in terms of amount, color, and presence of clots at least every hour for the first 24 to 48 hours postoperatively. Monitor serial urines.	*Careful monitoring and reporting of changes can help prevent major complications.*	Is urine becoming progressively less bloody and more clear with each void?
Explain to the patient that some bloody urine is normal after a transurethral resection of the prostate (TURP), as long as it does not suddenly get much worse. Also explain that a little blood mixed with irrigating fluid in a Foley bag may look worse than it actually is.	*Seeing the catheter bag filled with bloody drainage may be upsetting to the patient or his family.*	Is the patient aware of what to expect in a Foley bag?
Encourage the patient to drink up to 2,500 mL/day (unless contraindicated by other medical conditions) of water, noncitrus juices, and other noncaffeinated, nonalcoholic beverages.	*Increasing urine flow can help flush blood from the bladder.*	Is the patient drinking adequate amounts?
Teach the patient to avoid constipation (e.g., suggest stool softener, fluids, prune juice) and heavy lifting.	*These can increase pressure in the abdomen and increase risk of bleeding.*	Does the patient verbalize understanding of instructions?
Advise the patient to lie down if urine becomes bright red or has large clots.	*Activity can increase bleeding.*	Does the patient reduce activity if bleeding increases?
Teach the patient to avoid aspirin and nonsteroidal anti-inflammatory drugs (NSAIDs) until risk of bleeding is over.	*Aspirin and NSAIDs inhibit platelet function and increase risk of bleeding.*	Does the patient verbalize understanding?

Nursing Care Plan for the Postsurgical Patient Having Transurethral Resection of the Prostate for Benign Prostatic Hyperplasia—cont'd

Nursing Diagnosis: *Acute Pain* related to bladder spasms, obstruction, or surgical process as evidenced by patient pain rating
Expected Outcome: The patient's pain will be controlled as evidenced by patient statement of lower pain rating.
Evaluation of Outcome: Does the patient state that pain is decreased to an acceptable level?

Intervention	Rationale	Evaluation
Monitor pain on an appropriate scale every 2 to 4 hours for first 48 hours and within 30 minutes after any intervention.	*A pain scale is the most accurate measure of pain.*	Does the patient verbalize pain as increasing or decreasing on the scale?
Monitor for signs of pain related to bladder spasms, obstruction, or surgical process. Look for facial grimaces, irrigation solution that does not flow into bladder, urinating around catheter, or multiple clots.	*Relief of the mechanical cause of pain promotes comfort, rest, and healing.*	Is the patient free from signs of pain related to bladder spasms, obstruction, or surgical process?
Administer prescribed medication (analgesics or antispasmodics such as belladonna and opium [B&O] suppository) and monitor response.	*B&O suppositories relieve bladder spasms.*	Does the patient state relief when medications are given?
Irrigate catheter as ordered.	*Irrigation promotes removal of clots to reduce spasms and pain.*	Does irrigating solution flow in and out easily?
Educate the patient regarding nonpharmacological methods to control pain, such as relaxation and deep breathing techniques. Nonpharmacological measures should be used with, not in place of, medication.	*Relaxation calms spasms and relieves pain.*	Are clots being removed? Is the patient able to relax?

Nursing Diagnosis: *Urge Urinary Incontinence* related to poor sphincter control as evidenced by inability to control urination
Expected Outcome: The patient will be able to prevent incontinence.
Evaluation of Outcome: Is the patient experiencing incontinence?

Intervention	Rationale	Evaluation
Teach Kegel (pelvic floor) exercises (see Chapter 42), to be practiced every time the patient urinates and throughout the day.	*Kegel exercises strengthen muscle tone to hold urine after the catheter is removed.*	Is the patient able to start and stop urine stream?
Discuss use of a condom catheter or penile pads.	*These can keep the patient dry until incontinence can be controlled.*	Does the patient indicate an informed choice of incontinence products?
Instruct the patient to continue drinking 2,000 to 4,000 mL of noncaffeinated, nonalcoholic beverages each day.	*Adequate nonirritating fluid intake is important for healing and preventing urinary tract infection (UTI).*	Does the patient drink adequate fluids even though he dribbles?
Encourage the patient to discuss long-term (longer than 6 months) incontinence problems with the health care provider (HCP).	*The patient may need to learn self-catheterization or try medication.*	Does the patient verbalize understanding of what to do if incontinence continues?

(nursing care plan continues on page 906)

Nursing Care Plan for the Postsurgical Patient Having Transurethral Resection of the Prostate for Benign Prostatic Hyperplasia—cont'd

Intervention	Rationale	Evaluation
Refer the patient to national incontinence support group if indicated.	*Support groups can provide information and emotional support.*	Does the patient show interest in a support group?

Nursing Diagnosis: *Deficient Knowledge* related to lack of experience with postoperative restrictions and care
Expected Outcomes: The patient will avoid activities that increase intra-abdominal pressure resulting in excessive bleeding. The patient will verbalize understanding of how to prevent postoperative infection.
Evaluation of Outcomes: Does the patient verbalize understanding of how to prevent bleeding? Is infection prevented?

Intervention	Rationale	Evaluation
Teach the patient to avoid lifting heavy objects (more than 10 pounds), stair climbing, driving, strenuous exercise, constipation, straining during bowel movements, and sexual activities until approved by the HCP (about 6 weeks).	*Heavy lifting or straining can disrupt the healing process and result in tissue damage or excess bleeding.*	Does the patient verbalize understanding of reasons for limitation of heavy lifting and straining?
Instruct the patient on proper catheter care if the patient will be discharged with a catheter. Include the following information: Keep catheter tubing secured to abdomen or thigh, and keep bag below bladder; wash catheter/meatus junction with soap and water once daily; use clean technique with good hand hygiene to change from leg bag to night drainage bag; report signs and symptoms of UTI to HCP immediately; and encourage oral fluids.	*UTIs are extremely dangerous and can cause death following genitourinary surgery in an older patient.*	Can the patient give a return demonstration of proper catheter care? Is the patient free from signs and symptoms of infection?
Teach the patient to report bleeding that is not stopped with resting, fever, swelling, or difficulty urinating to HCP promptly.	*These are signs of complications that may require prompt medical intervention.*	Does the patient verbalize understanding of signs and symptoms to report?

Nursing Diagnosis: *Anxiety* related to concerns over loss of sexual functioning following prostate surgery as evidenced by patient statement
Expected Outcomes: The patient will verbalize normal sexual changes that happen after prostate surgery. The patient will identify available support systems if needed.
Evaluation of Outcomes: Is the patient able to verbalize understanding of expected body function after prostate surgery? Does the patient access support systems?

Intervention	Rationale	Evaluation
Explain to the patient that he will probably have retrograde ejaculation into the bladder after surgery. It is not harmful, and semen will come out when he urinates.	*Removal of the prostate gland often results in retrograde ejaculation.*	Does the patient understand what will happen when he ejaculates?
Instruct the patient to talk with the urologist if erection problems occur.	*Urologists who specialize in treatment of erectile dysfunction can provide information and treatment.*	Is the patient aware of local support services?

Retrograde ejaculation is a common result of prostate surgery. When any of the prostate gland is removed, there is a decrease in the amount of semen produced. Also, a part of the ejaculatory ducts may be removed. This results in less semen being pushed outside the body. Instead, it "falls back" into the bladder. This causes no harm. The semen is simply passed during the next urination.

It is important to understand that erection, ejaculation, and orgasm are all separate actions. Erection means the penis becomes hard, ejaculation is the release of semen, and orgasm is felt as pulsations along the urethra. Unless additional problems are present, the patient continues to have erections and orgasmic sensations but decreased or no ejaculation.

RADICAL PROSTATECTOMY. When the prostate gland is very large, causes obstruction, or is cancerous, a radical **prostatectomy** may be performed to remove the entire prostate gland.

Open Prostatectomy. Several approaches may be taken during traditional radical surgery (Fig. 43.3). In the **suprapubic** approach, an incision is made through the lower abdomen into the bladder. The gland is removed, and the urethra is reattached to the bladder. The retropubic approach is similar, except there is no incision into the bladder. A perineal prostatectomy involves making an incision between the scrotum and anus to remove the gland. This procedure is rarely done because of the increased risk of contamination of the incision (close to the rectum). There is also risk of urinary incontinence, erectile dysfunction, or injury to the rectum.

An open prostatectomy means a longer hospital stay compared with other BPH surgeries. The presence of a suprapubic catheter (a catheter that is placed in the lower abdomen to drain the bladder) and care for an abdominal incision increase the length of stay and risk for complications. Follow-up home health care for wound and catheter care is important for these patients.

Minimally Invasive Prostatectomy. Newer techniques use laparoscopy and tiny robot arms to perform radical prostatectomy through five small "porthole" incisions in the abdomen. The surgeon makes all the decisions about the surgery while guiding the robotic arms from a computer. The robotic arms allow for precision and an ability to maneuver in small areas. The robotic surgery is much less invasive. Patients experience better results with less postoperative bleeding, incontinence, and nerve damage as well as shorter hospital stays.

Nursing Process for the Patient With BPH Who Undergoes a TURP Procedure

DATA COLLECTION. Begin by asking the patient whether he has ever had treatment or surgery for prostate trouble. Assess amount and type of fluid intake per day. Ask whether the patient has noticed any of the symptoms of BPH. Monitor output. If the patient is not catheterized, ensure that urine retention is being managed appropriately.

NURSING DIAGNOSES, PLANNING, AND INTERVENTIONS. For nursing care of the patient following TURP, see "Nursing Care Plan for the Postsurgical Patient Having Transurethral Resection of the Prostate for Benign Prostatic Hyperplasia." Each patient experience is different. Care plans must be individualized. Keep in mind that the majority of these patients are older and have secondary medical problems such as cardiovascular disease.

EVALUATION. A patient should be discharged home with minimal bladder discomfort, light pink to clear urine, no evidence of UTI, and knowledge related to self-care at home. Home health care nursing may be required if the patient lives alone or does not have the capacity to provide for meals, toileting, or transportation for the follow-up visit. Table 43.2 provides a summary of BPH.

CRITICAL THINKING

Mr. Atkinson is a 68-year-old African American farmer with an enlarged prostate gland. He lives on a 75-acre farm with his wife and one son. He is scheduled for a transurethral resection of the prostate in 6 weeks.

1. Mr. Atkinson is currently taking terazosin (Hytrin). His health care provider wants him to increase his dose from 2 to 5 mg daily until surgery. He has a bottle at home of 2-mg tablets. How should you instruct him to take his medication? What side effect should he be advised to watch for?
2. What special postoperative instructions should he be given because of his occupation?
3. What should you tell him if he asks about how the surgery will affect his "nature" (sexual activities)?
4. What other health team members can you collaborate with and anticipate Mr. Atkinson might need while in the hospital or when he goes home?

Suggested answers are at the end of the chapter.

Cancer of the Prostate

Cancer of the prostate is the most common cancer in American men. Most prostate cancers grow very slowly and often do not cause a major threat to health or life. Many treatment options are available, and the prognosis is often very good.

Pathophysiology

Prostate cancer depends on testosterone to grow. The cancer cells are usually slow growing. They begin in the posterior (back) or lateral (side) part of the gland. The cancer spreads by one of three routes. If it spreads by local invasion, it will

---

• WORD • BUILDING •

retrograde: retro—backward + grade—step
prostatectomy: prostat—prostate gland + ectomy—excision
suprapubic: supra—above + pubic—pubic bone

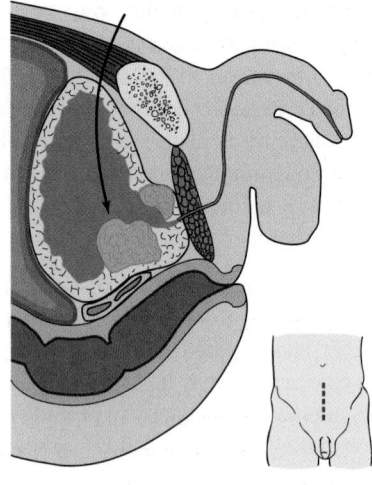

Suprapubic prostatectomy
A

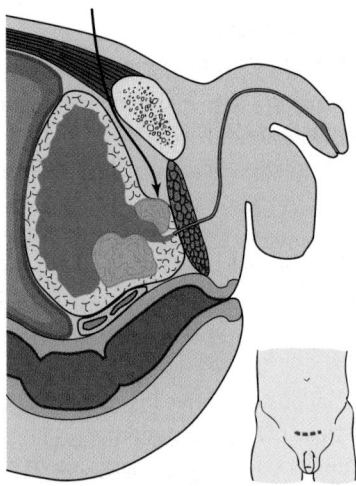

Retropubic prostatectomy
B

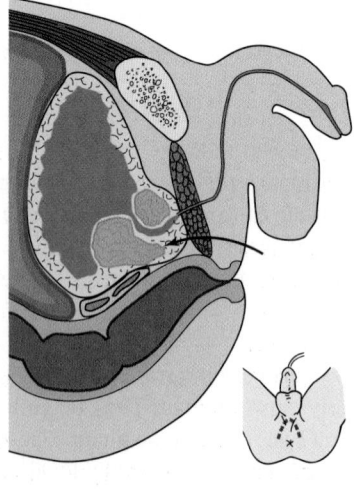

Perineal prostatectomy
C

FIGURE 43.3 (A) Suprapubic prostatectomy. (B) Retropubic prostatectomy. (C) Perineal prostatectomy.

Table 43.2

Benign Prostatic Hyperplasia Summary

Signs and Symptoms	*Related to obstruction:* Decrease in size/force of stream, difficulty in starting stream, dribbling, interrupted stream, urinary retention, overflow incontinence *Related to irritation:* Nocturia, dysuria, urgency
Diagnostic Tests	*Primary:* Digital rectal examination, urinalysis, blood urea nitrogen (BUN), serum creatinine, prostate-specific antigen (PSA) *Secondary:* Urodynamic flow studies, transrectal ultrasound, cystoscopy
Therapeutic Measures	*Conservative:* Alpha-adrenergic blockers, testosterone blockers *Nonsurgical:* Transurethral microwave therapy, prostatic balloon, prostatic stents *Transurethral:* Transurethral incision of the prostate (TUIP), transurethral ultrasound-guided laser-induced prostatectomy (TULIP), transurethral resection of the prostate (TURP) *Radical prostatectomy:* Suprapubic, retropubic, perineal, laparoscopic, or robotic resection
Complications	Ascending or localized infection Injury to surrounding tissues during surgery Impaired sexual function related to tissue injury
Priority Postoperative Nursing Diagnoses	*Risk for Bleeding* *Acute Pain* *Urge Urinary Incontinence* *Deficient Knowledge* *Anxiety*

move into the bladder, seminal vesicles, or peritoneum. The cancer may also spread through the lymph system to the pelvic nodes and may travel as far as the supraclavicular nodes. The third route is through the vascular system to bone, lung, and liver. Prostate cancer is staged or graded based on the growth or spread.

Etiology

Age is the primary risk factor. Prostate cancer is found most often in men older than age 65 and is rare in men younger than age 40. Other risk factors are higher levels of testosterone, a high-fat diet, and immediate family history. About one in seven men is diagnosed with prostate cancer during his lifetime. Some types of occupational exposures (e.g., to polyaromatic hydrocarbons and fire smoke) have been found to contribute to increased risk of prostate cancer.

Signs and Symptoms

Symptoms are rare in the early stage of prostate cancer. Later stages include symptoms of urinary obstruction, hematuria, and urinary retention. Advanced (metastatic) stage symptoms can include pain in the back, hip, abdomen, or bone; anemia; weakness; weight loss; and overall fatigue.

Complications

Early complications of prostate cancer are related to bladder problems, such as difficulty urinating, and bladder or kidney infection. Erectile dysfunction can occur as a result of the cancer or its treatment.

If the cancer metastasizes, the patient may develop problems such as pain, bone fractures, weight loss, and depression; eventually death can occur if treatment is not successful.

Diagnostic Tests

A routine digital rectal examination of the prostate is the first test; often the examiner finds a hard lump or hardened prostate lobe. If a palpable abnormality is found, the HCP may order a transrectal ultrasound and biopsy for confirmation. Bone scans and other tests may be ordered to determine if the cancer has spread outside the prostate gland.

Measuring the PSA via a blood sample can indicate prostate cancer but may also indicate other conditions. In the past, the PSA test was used to screen men for prostate cancer. However, more recently, the U.S. Preventive Services Task Force withdrew this recommendation because routine screening was not found to save lives. Screening led to slow-growing, noninvasive prostate cancers being discovered and treated. If prostate cancer is not aggressive, the treatment may be worse than the disease. A new blood test, the IsoPSA, is more specific for prostate cancer and may reduce the occurrence of unnecessary biopsies.

Therapeutic Measures

Prostate cancer in the early stages may be treated with testosterone-suppressing medications, such as leuprolide (Lupron) or goserelin (Zoladex), or with drugs that block testosterone's action on the prostate gland, such as bicalutamide (Casodex). Surgery, such as TURP or radical prostatectomy, or a combination of medication and radiation therapy may be done. In later stages, the treatment is usually a radical prostatectomy, radiation therapy, or implantation of radioactive "seeds" into the prostate (brachytherapy). A new immune stimulant, sipuleucel-T (Provenge), slows the growth and aggressiveness of some prostate cancers.

Metastatic prostate cancer treatment involves relief of symptoms through blocking testosterone by bilateral **orchiectomy,** administration of antiandrogen (flutamide [Eulexin]),

or use of agents such as leuprolide and goserelin. Sometimes chemotherapy is used to help relieve symptoms resulting from spread of the cancer.

Unfortunately, any therapy that reduces androgen activity in a man can cause side effects, such as hot flashes, breast tenderness and growth, impaired sexual function, osteoporosis, and loss of muscle mass. These, in turn, can cause significant concerns with body image.

RADICAL PROSTATECTOMY. A radical prostatectomy (described earlier in this chapter) is done for patients with cancer of the prostate or when the gland is too large to resect using a less invasive method.

The patient returns from surgery with a large indwelling catheter in the urethra and potentially a suprapubic catheter. A wound drain may be placed to remove fluids and promote wound healing from the inside outward. Keep dressings, drains, and incisions clean and dry according to institution policy using sterile technique.

Radical prostatectomy has more complications associated with it than any other treatment option. The major complications are hemorrhage, infection, loss of urinary control, and erectile dysfunction.

Patient Education

All men older than age 40 should be educated regarding prostate screening, including the risks and benefits of screening.

PENILE DISORDERS

Problems of the penis, aside from those caused by STIs, are fairly rare but may cause great concern and worry for the patient. Many men have difficulty seeking help for such a personal problem. It is important to be sensitive when assessing or providing care for these patients.

Peyronie Disease

Peyronie disease gives the penis a curved or crooked look when it is erect. Fibrous bands or plaques form mainly on the dorsal (top) part of the layer of tissue that surrounds one of the corpora cavernosa of the penis. The plaque may be caused by injury or inflammation of the penile tissue. Also, it may come and go spontaneously. If the plaque is thick enough, it can cause curvature, painful erection, difficulty in vaginal penetration, and erectile dysfunction. When conservative treatments such as oral vitamin E, colchicine, or potassium aminobenzoate do not work, surgery may be needed to remove the plaque. Another option is injections into the scar tissue to break it down. Patients need to be reassured that the problem is not life-threatening and can be treated.

• WORD • BUILDING •

orchiectomy: orchi—testicles + ectomy—excision

Priapism

Priapism is a painful erection that lasts longer than 4 hours. If not relieved, it can become a medical emergency. The small veins in the corpora cavernosa spasm, so blood cannot drain back out of the penis as it should. When the blood cannot drain, penile tissue does not get oxygen. Permanent tissue damage can result. There may be a complete loss of erection ability after the priapism episode. Prolonged priapism can also prevent the patient from passing urine, which can lead to painful bladder and kidney problems. Some causes of priapism are sickle cell anemia, leukemia, widespread cancer, spinal cord injury or tumors, and use of medications to manage erectile dysfunction (such as sildenafil [Viagra]) or recreational drugs (such as crack cocaine). Treatment in the emergency department may include ice packs, sedatives, analgesics, injection of medications directly into the penis to relax the vein spasms, needle aspiration, and irrigation of the corpora. Surgery to implant a shunt that reroutes blood flow can also be done.

Phimosis and Paraphimosis

Phimosis is a condition in which the foreskin of an uncircumcised male becomes so tight that it is difficult or impossible to pull back away from the head of the penis. It may make it impossible to clean the area underneath. Smegma, a cottage cheese–like secretion made by the glands of the foreskin, becomes trapped under the foreskin. This is prime place for the growth of bacterial and yeast infections. Antibiotics and warm soaks may be ordered if infection is present. Topical steroid ointment and stretching exercises for the foreskin may be prescribed. A circumcision may be recommended if the problem continues. Phimosis is generally prevented by teaching uncircumcised males to pull the foreskin back carefully, wash with mild soap and water daily, and replace the foreskin to its normal position.

Paraphimosis occurs when the uncircumcised foreskin is pulled back, during intercourse or bathing, and not replaced in a forward position. This can lead to compression of vessels of the penis and potentially gangrene. Prevention requires good hygiene and returning the foreskin back over the glans of the penis when it has been retracted.

Cancer of the Penis

Cancer of the penis has been found in men who were not circumcised as infants or adolescents or who have acquired the human papillomavirus (HPV). The tumor is typically a squamous cell carcinoma. It may look like a small, round raised wart, induration, or red area. This form of cancer can be spread to a sexual partner. Several research studies have found a link between cancer of the penis and cancer of the uterine cervix. Cancer of the penis may be treated with minor surgery, such as a circumcision or laser removal of the growth. If the cancer has spread, sections of the penis may be surgically removed. Penile reconstruction can be done if necessary after surgery. Radiation or chemotherapy may also be done. Teach male patients the importance of early reporting of any lesions, HPV vaccination, and good hygiene if not circumcised.

 TESTICULAR DISORDERS

Cryptorchidism

Cryptorchidism (undescended testicles) is a congenital condition in which an infant boy is born with one or both of his testicles not in the scrotum. The testicles normally drop down (descend) into the scrotum in the last 1 to 2 months before a boy is born. Often, undescended testicles descend into the scrotum on their own in the first few months of life. If they do not descend during that time, surgery should be done to correct the problem, typically before age 1. Testicles that are not brought down into the scrotum may lead to infertility. Also, the risk of testicular cancer is higher if the condition is not corrected before the child reaches his teen years.

Hydrocele

A **hydrocele** is a painless collection of fluid in the scrotal sac. The cause is not known. It can happen at any point during a man's lifetime. No treatment is necessary unless the hydrocele is so large that it causes discomfort or embarrassment, or is a threat to the blood supply to the testicles. In cases that require treatment, the patient may have surgery to remove the hydrocele, or a needle aspiration of the fluid may be performed.

Varicocele

A varicocele is a condition sometimes called varicose veins of the scrotum. The main blood supply to the testicles travels along the spermatic cord. The veins become dilated, and when the man is standing, the area in the scrotum begins to feel like a "bag of worms." The patient may report a pulling sensation, a dull ache, or scrotal pain. The sensations are most often felt when standing up. Most varicoceles occur on the left side because of the way the scrotal vein enters at a sharp angle from the left renal vein.

A varicocele is often not discovered until a couple is unable to conceive. It is believed that the varicose veins may increase the temperature of the testicles and cause damage to the sperm. The most successful treatment is surgical repair of the varicose veins.

Epididymitis

The epididymis is a small tube along the back of the testicles where sperm is matured for its last 10 to 12 days before it is ready to be ejaculated. **Epididymitis** is inflammation or

---

- **WORD · BUILDING ·**

priapism: priap—phallus + ism—condition of
phimosis: phimo—muzzling + osis—condition
paraphimosis: para—abnormal + phimo—muzzling + osis—condition
cryptorchidism: crypt—hidden + orchid—testicle + ism—condition
hydrocele: hydro—water + cele—swelling
epididymitis: epididymis + itis—inflammation

infection of the epididymis that can be caused by bacteria, viruses, parasites, chemicals, or trauma. Risk factors include sexual or nonsexual contact, STIs, a complication of some urological procedures, or reflux (backflow) of urine. The problem can also be associated with prostate infections. It is usually painful, with the scrotal skin being tender, red, and warm to the touch.

Epididymitis is treated with antibiotics; the partner is also treated if it was sexually transmitted. Depending on the severity of the pain, the patient may be placed on bedrest with the scrotum elevated, possibly on ice packs, and given analgesics. The pain and tenderness usually go away in about a week, although the swelling may last for several weeks. Complications include chronic epididymitis, abscess formation, and sterility.

Orchitis

Orchitis is a rare inflammation or infection of the testicles. The problem may be caused by trauma or infection from epididymitis, UTIs, STIs, or systemic diseases such as influenza, infectious mononucleosis, tuberculosis, gout, pneumonia, or mumps (after puberty). The patient has swollen, extremely tender testicles, red scrotal skin, and a fever. Interventions are basically the same as for epididymitis. Sterility is a complication of orchitis caused by mumps. This complication can be prevented by giving boys the mumps vaccine at an early age.

Cancer of the Testicles
Pathophysiology and Etiology

Cancer of the testicles is the most common cancer in men between ages 15 and 35 in the United States. The etiology of testicular cancer is unknown. Some of the known risk factors are cryptorchidism, family history, white race, and high socioeconomic status. Some older studies showed a link between testicular cancer and a mother's use of diethylstilbestrol (DES; an estrogen preparation once used to prevent spontaneous abortion) while pregnant. However, current research has not shown this risk to be significant. The tumors are mostly a germ cell type of cancer formed during normal embryo development.

Prevention

The best prevention is early detection with a monthly testicular self-examination (TSE). The American Cancer Society does not necessarily recommend monthly TSE for all men. This is because not enough studies have been done to show that it reduces death. However, men should be aware of what is normal for them so that they can recognize changes if they occur. The TSE procedure is simple and easy to learn. It makes sense to teach it to all men until more data are available. See Chapter 41 for instructions on TSE.

Signs and Symptoms

Early warning signs of cancer can include a small, usually painless lump on the testicle. The patient may also notice that the scrotum is swollen and feels heavy. Some tumors produce hormones that cause breast enlargement and tenderness.

Complications

Emotional complications can range from fear of cancer and death to feelings of loss of masculine body image and sexual function. Physical complications may involve dealing with pain and the effects of metastasis to areas such as the lungs, abdomen, or lymph nodes. Other less common areas of cancer spread are the liver, brain, and bone.

Diagnostic Tests

When a lump is found, several laboratory and radiographic tests are done. An ultrasound of the testicles is done first, to differentiate a possible tumor from a hydrocele or other noncancerous condition. Blood is drawn to look for tumor markers. An example of a tumor marker for testicular cancer is human chorionic gonadotropin (hCG). A surgical biopsy or removal of the testicle is done to determine the stage of the tumor. If cancer is confirmed, a chest x-ray examination is done to look for spread to the lungs. A scan of the lymph nodes, liver, brain, and bones also may be ordered. Testicular tumors are staged according to the TNM [Tumor, Node, Metastasis] Classification of Malignant Tumors system introduced in Chapter 11.

Therapeutic Measures

Intervention depends on the stage of the cancer. All treatment begins with complete removal of the cancerous testicles, spermatic cord, and local lymph nodes. Based on the stage of the cancer, radiation or chemotherapy may be done in addition to surgery. If the cancer is found in the beginning stages, the chances for complete recovery are very good. All patients should have regular follow-up testing.

Nursing Care

Nursing care is directed first at prevention, by teaching young men to practice TSE and to see their HCP if they notice any changes. If a diagnosis of cancer has been made, provide emotional support for the patient. If the patient wants to have children, he should be encouraged to make deposits in a sperm bank before any surgery or treatment is started. The patient and his partner may have many questions about sexual activities as they go through treatment. Encourage them to talk with their HCP or a sex therapist about ways to express love and tenderness toward one another. Helping patients deal with pain and the side effects of chemotherapy or radiation therapy are also important nursing interventions. See Chapter 11 for care of the patient with cancer.

• WORD • BUILDING •
orchitis: orch—testicle + itis—inflammation

CRITICAL THINKING

Mr. Cunningham is a 23-year-old college student engaged to be married next spring. While taking a shower one day, he discovers a lump on his left testicle.

1. What should he do?
2. What are the treatment options if Mr. Cunningham has testicular cancer?
3. How can you help Mr. Cunningham cope with the diagnosis?

Suggested answers are at the end of the chapter.

 SEXUAL FUNCTIONING

Vasectomy

A **vasectomy** uses tiny clamps or cauterization to seal off the vas deferens to prevent sperm from reaching the outside of the body (Fig. 43.4). This 15- to 30-minute surgery is done through a small puncture in the upper part of the scrotum. It is performed as an outpatient sterilization method for men. The patient should carefully discuss the surgery with his physician so that there is a clear understanding of the results following the procedure.

After the procedure, the testicles continue to produce sperm and the male hormone testosterone. The prostate gland, along with the seminal vesicles, still ejaculates semen. However, the semen does not contain sperm. There should be no major change in the way the ejaculate looks or feels after the procedure. The patient should be encouraged to continue using another birth control method for about 3 months after surgery to be sure there are no sperm left in the tract above the surgical site. A semen sample should be evaluated for the absence of sperm before the procedure is considered successful. Sperm continue to be produced in the testicles but are absorbed by the body.

Vasectomy Reversal

Sometimes a man may decide he wants to have more children and asks to have a vasectomy reversed. The surgical procedure to reverse a vasectomy is called a vasovasostomy. Using microscopic instruments, the surgeon reconnects the vas deferens. If this is not possible, the surgeon may reconnect the vas deferens to the epididymis. During the surgery, the physician typically tries to determine whether the testicles are still producing good sperm. Vasectomy reversal is more successful if it is done soon after the vasectomy. Success rates drop as the period between vasectomy and reversal grows longer.

Erectile Dysfunction

A problem getting or keeping an erection can happen at any age. It has been a concern of men and their partners for centuries. It is a unique problem because it affects not only the man but his partner as well. Most men experience a temporary erection problem at some time during their lives. It can be caused by stress, illness, fatigue, or an excessive use of alcohol or drugs. When the problem becomes persistent, it is time to seek medical help.

Before the 1980s, 90% of men who went to their HCPs for help were told the problem was emotional, not physical. Because of improved testing methods, however, researchers now believe that 80% to 90% of erection problems have a physical cause.

Pathophysiology

The term *impotence* means "powerlessness." This term is being replaced with the more accurate term **erectile dysfunction,** or ED, which describes a physical condition. Erectile dysfunction means that a man cannot obtain or keep a usable erection that is firm enough and long-lasting enough for satisfactory sexual intercourse. For a man to have a usable erection, several conditions must be met:

1. *Circulatory system.* The blood supply coming into the penis from the arteries must be sufficient to fill the corpus cavernosa (spongy erectile tissue inside the penis), causing the penis to become rigid. The veins in the penis must then be able to constrict to trap the blood in the corporal bodies to keep the penis erect. The most common cause of erectile dysfunction is failure in the circulatory system.
2. *Nervous system.* Both the sympathetic and parasympathetic nerves are involved in the erection, ejaculation, orgasm, and resting phases of the penile response cycle. There are many nerve receptors and transmitters in the spinal cord and the penis that must be intact for a usable erection. Spinal cord injury is the most common neurologic cause of erectile dysfunction.
3. *Hormonal system.* There are three basic male hormones involved with an erection. The most important hormone, testosterone, affects a man's sex drive and desire. Luteinizing hormone (LH) stimulates testosterone production. Prolactin in large amounts may block testosterone.
4. *Limbic system.* This is the center in the brain that affects how we feel emotionally. It works with our five senses to stimulate the desire for sex.

All of these systems can be influenced by physical, emotional, and chemical factors. A good assessment is important to determine the cause of erectile dysfunction.

Etiology

Erectile dysfunction has many psychological and physical causes. It can also be caused by many medications and chemicals that interfere with desire, blood supply, or nerve transmission (Table 43.3). The most common types of medications that cause problems are those prescribed for high blood pressure and cardiovascular disease. Obstructive sleep apnea has been found to be related to erectile dysfunction, but it is unclear which condition might come first.

• WORD • BUILDING •
vasectomy: vas—vas deferens + ectomy—excision

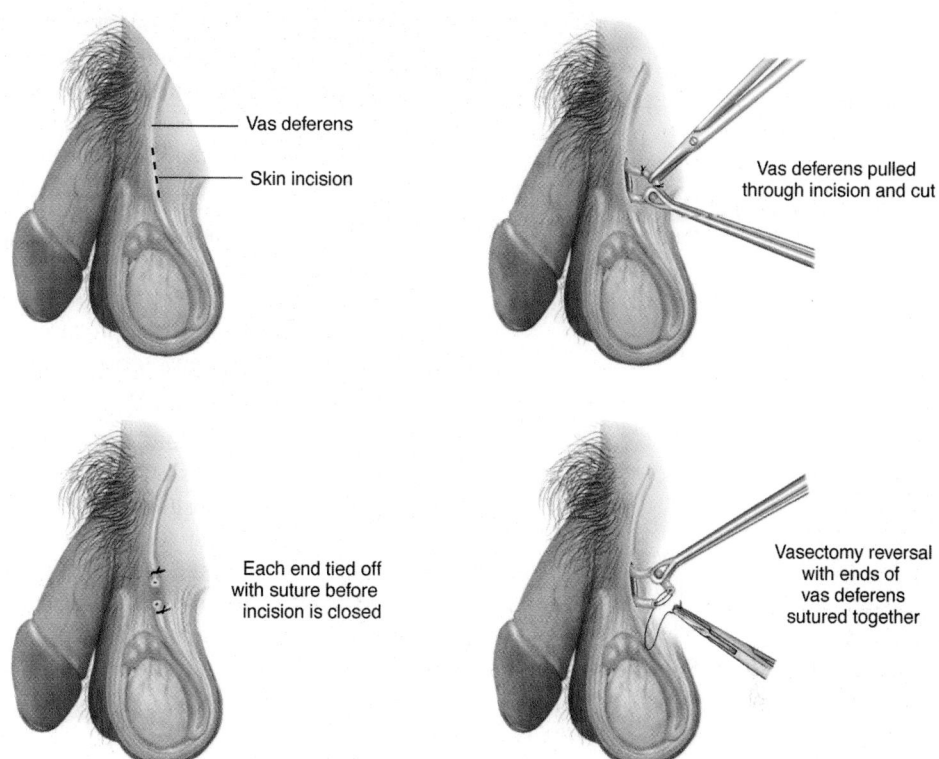

Vas deferens

Skin incision

Vas deferens pulled through incision and cut

Each end tied off with suture before incision is closed

Vasectomy reversal with ends of vas deferens sutured together

FIGURE 43.4 Vasectomy and reversal.

Diagnostic Tests

In the first step of the assessment process, the HCP obtains a history, including medical-surgical history; use of medications, including any substance abuse; lifestyle patterns; and sexual history. During physical examination, the HCP looks for evidence of genital disorders, hormonal imbalance (such as hair patterns or enlarged breasts), surgical interventions, decreased circulation, and lack of nerve sensation. Blood tests evaluate glucose levels; testosterone; evidence of liver, heart, or kidney disorders; signs of infection; or blood disorders. Some HCPs may use intracorporeal injection of vasoactive medications that can create an erection to test the blood flow in the penis. A psychosocial evaluation may be recommended to rule out relational or emotional problems that may contribute to erectile dysfunction or affect the treatment outcome.

A second level of testing may involve the use of vascular flow studies to locate areas where either the blood vessels are narrowed or the veins allow the blood to drain out of the penis too rapidly. Other testing can monitor erections during sleep. A healthy man typically has erections every 60 to 70 minutes while he sleeps. Absence of erections during sleep indicates a physical cause for erectile dysfunction. Because of the expense of vascular flow studies and sleep studies, they are used on a limited basis.

Therapeutic Measures

One of the most important treatment options begins with a couple being able to share intimate communication. No matter what is causing the problem, if the patient and his partner are not touching, talking, and sharing feelings with one another, treatment options are going to have limited success.

When the problem has clearly been identified as psychological, counseling or therapy is the treatment of choice. If long-term therapy has been tried with only limited success, the addition of oral medication or even intracorporeal injection therapy may be added to provide a boost in confidence and self-esteem. Medical treatment for physical erection problems begins with conservative, nonsurgical treatment. It then progresses to surgical options if needed. See Table 43.1 for additional information on medications.

MEDICATION CHANGES. Sometimes all that is needed to correct the problem is a change in medication. It is important for the patient to talk with his HCP before stopping any medication. Some men have stopped taking their blood pressure medication and risked a stroke or heart attack because it interfered with their sexual activity.

ORAL MEDICATIONS. Oral medications (sildenafil [Viagra], tadalafil [Cialis], and vardenafil [Levitra]) are now the first line of therapy used to treat erectile dysfunction. These medications cause the arterioles and cavernous tissue to relax. This allows more blood to flow into the penis in response to sexual stimulation. The pill is usually taken 30 to 60 minutes before anticipated sexual intercourse. Men using nitrate medication (antianginal agents) should avoid using the pills because of risk for severe low blood pressure.

Table 43.3

Causes of Erectile Dysfunction

Psychological	Stress
	Anxiety
	Depression
	Fatigue
Urological	Peyronie disease
	Kidney failure
	Treatment for prostate disease
Endocrine	Low testosterone levels
	Diabetes mellitus
Respiratory	Obstructive sleep apnea
Cardiovascular	Heart disease
	Atherosclerosis
	Metabolic syndrome
	Stroke
Neurologic	Spinal cord injury
	Parkinson disease
	Multiple sclerosis
Lifestyle	Tobacco use
	Alcohol use
	Drug use (e.g., marijuana, cocaine, others)
	Excessive caffeine use
Medications*	Angiotensin-converting enzyme (ACE) inhibitors
	Antianxiety agents
	Antidepressants
	Antihistamines
	Antineoplastic agents
	Beta blockers
	Diuretics
	Estrogen
	Histamine (H_2) antagonists
	Muscle relaxants
	Nonsteroidal anti-inflammatory drugs (NSAIDs)
	Opioids
	Drugs for Parkinson disease

*Note: Not all drugs in a category cause erectile dysfunction.

HORMONE TREATMENT. If the patient's testosterone level is low, replacement hormone may be needed. The HCP should first examine the patient carefully for any evidence of prostate cancer; testosterone replacement can cause the cancer to grow and spread. Testosterone replacement can be given by intramuscular injection, topical gel, or transdermal patch. Testosterone levels must be monitored closely for both positive and negative effects.

HERBAL REMEDIES. Several herbal remedies may be effective, including yohimbine, dehydroepiandrosterone (DHEA; a steroid hormone), ginseng, ginkgo, and others. Herbal remedies have side effects, just like prescription medications. They should not be taken without an HCP's recommendation.

INJECTED MEDICATION. After careful evaluation, a patient or his partner may be taught how to inject a medication into the penis using a 26- or 27-gauge needle on a tuberculin syringe or a prefilled autoinjector. The injections are nearly painless and produce a natural erection in 10 to 15 minutes. The most serious side effect is priapism, which requires immediate reversal in a physician's office or emergency room.

TRANSURETHRAL SUPPOSITORY. To facilitate medication dispersion and absorption, a patient may choose to use a suppository. The patient is instructed to urinate before use of the suppository. A tiny pellet (microsuppository) is inserted into the urethra using a specialized single-dose applicator. The medication usually begins to work in 5 to 10 minutes. The effects last for about 30 to 60 minutes.

OTHER NONSURGICAL TREATMENTS.

Sexual Devices and Techniques. A variety of mechanical sexual aids may be considered by patients who do not want or cannot afford expensive medical treatment. Men should be encouraged to talk with an HCP or qualified sex therapist before trying these alternatives.

Suction devices are one nonsurgical treatment option. An external cylinder vacuum device fits over the penis and draws the blood up into the corporeal bodies, causing an erection. A penile ring is then slipped onto the base of the penis. Once the cylinder is removed, sexual intercourse can begin. Special care must be taken to remove the penile ring within 15 to 20 minutes to prevent tissue damage.

SURGICAL TREATMENTS.

Penile Implants (Prostheses). Penile implants are a pair of solid or fluid-filled chambers that are surgically placed into the corporeal bodies in the penis to produce an erection. There are two basic types of implants: noninflatable and inflatable (Fig. 43.5).

Vascular Surgery. If a younger man has an erection problem caused by poor blood flow into the penis or from blood leaking out of the penis, rapidly causing the loss of the erection, corrective surgery may be performed. A bypass graft may be done to increase blood flow into the penis or to go around a blockage (as occurs, for example, with Peyronie disease).

Nursing Process for the Patient With Erectile Dysfunction

DATA COLLECTION. Your role as a nurse may vary based on your work setting. It is always appropriate to ask a man if he has any concerns related to sexual health. It may open the door for him to talk further. It is important to provide privacy and confidentiality. Ask questions about possible psychosocial causes, including use of medications, street drugs, alcohol, or nicotine. If a problem is identified, alert the HCP, who will continue a more thorough assessment.

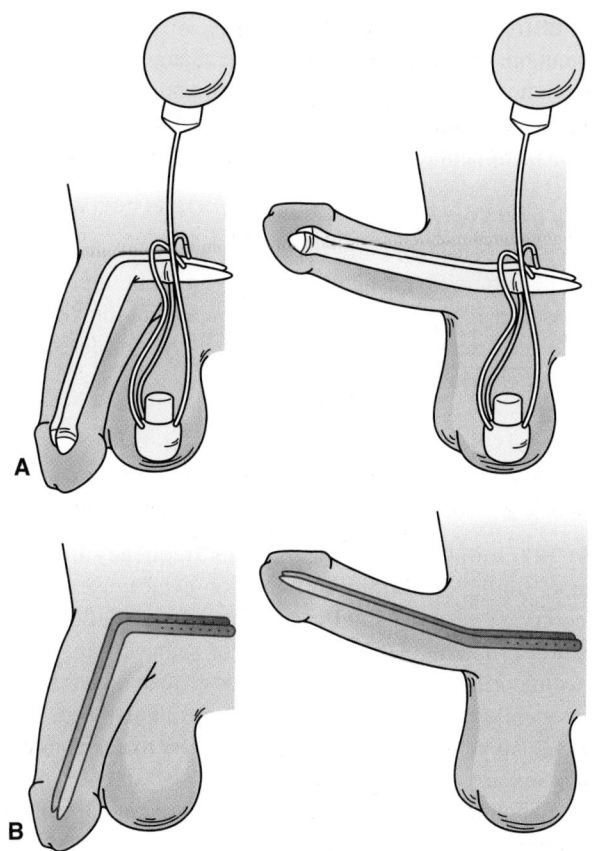

FIGURE 43.5 Penile implants. (A) Inflatable penile implant. Inflatable cylinders are implanted in the penis, the small hydraulic pump in the scrotum, and the fluid-filled reservoir in the lower abdomen. Sterile radiopaque saline from the reservoir fills the cylinders to provide an erection. (B) Malleable penile implant. Malleable rods are implanted into the penis. The penis is always firm, but the rods can be bent close to the body when erection is not desired.

NURSING DIAGNOSES, PLANNING, AND IMPLEMENTATION.

Sexual Dysfunction related to physical or psychosocial alterations

EXPECTED OUTCOME: The patient will verbalize understanding of the cause and treatment options for erectile dysfunction.

• Determine the patient and partner's current knowledge and understanding about cause and treatment of the disorder. *This will allow for additional and/or correct information to be provided about sexual dysfunction for appropriate understanding.*
• Provide the patient and partner with additional and/or correct information about cause and treatment of disorder. *This will allow the patient to have a full understanding of the etiology and care related to the disorder, and will increase likelihood of patient adherence to and success of treatment.*
• Refer the patient and partner (as appropriate) for medical treatment, psychological treatment, or counseling. *An individualized treatment plan (determined by the*

etiology) is needed to move toward restoration of sexual functioning.

EVALUATION. The best indicator of a positive outcome is restoration of erectile function with a verbal account of understanding the disorder and satisfaction with the treatment process. Sometimes the physical problem is easier to correct than the emotional scars that the problem has created. It is important to evaluate both the physiological and emotional outcomes of treatment.

PATIENT EDUCATION. The nurse plays an important role in public education related to erectile dysfunction. Men need to know that they are not alone with their problem. More than 30 million men in the United States experience ongoing problems with erections. Usually, the cause is physical. Help is available through HCPs who specialize in treating erectile dysfunction. See Table 43.4 for a summary of male sexual dysfunction.

CRITICAL THINKING

Mr. Kittle presents to the clinic saying that he is not able to sustain an erection long enough for sexual intercourse that is satisfactory for himself and his partner.

1. You have never had a patient tell you his sexual problems, and you feel a little uncomfortable. How should you respond?
2. What will your assessment include?
3. What is an appropriate role for the licensed practical nurse/licensed vocational nurse in helping Mr. Kittle?

Suggested answers are at the end of the chapter.

Table 43.4

Male Sexual Dysfunction Summary

Signs and Symptoms	Report of problems with obtaining and keeping an erection Reported dissatisfaction with sexual performance
Diagnostic Tests	*Primary:* History, physical *Secondary:* Vascular flow evaluation, sleep studies
Therapeutic Measures	Counseling Medication to increase blood flow to the penis Surgical implants or repair of structural disorders
Priority Nursing Diagnosis	*Sexual Dysfunction*

Infertility

A growing number of couples in the United States are having difficulty conceiving children. Several factors can interfere with a man's ability to father a child.

Physiology

Many conditions must be present in the man for conception to occur. Endocrine function, autonomic nervous system function, and male reproductive structures must all be functioning properly. Normal healthy sperm in a concentration of at least 20 million per milliliter of semen are needed.

Etiology

The factors related to infertility are divided into three general categories: pretesticular, testicular, and post-testicular.

PRETESTICULAR (ENDOCRINE) FACTORS. The first factor involves the proper functioning of the hypothalamus, the pituitary gland, and the testicles. These endocrine functions are complex and are a rare cause of infertility. Examples of endocrine causes might be pituitary or adrenal tumors, thyroid problems, or uncontrolled diabetes.

TESTICULAR FACTORS. The two most common causes of male infertility are varicoceles (40% to 50%) and idiopathic causes (40%). It is believed that a varicocele lowers the sperm count by raising the blood flow and temperature in the testicles. Sperm cannot live if the temperature is too high or too low.

Congenital anomalies such as Klinefelter syndrome (a chromosomal defect) or cryptorchidism result in absent or damaged testicles. Certain disease or inflammatory processes may cause damage to the storage area (e.g., epididymitis) or to the testicles themselves (e.g., mumps orchitis). Any high fever or viral infection can interfere with the production of sperm for up to 3 months.

Medications, radiation, substance abuse, environmental hazards, and lifestyle practices have all been identified as possible factors that can interfere with spermatogenesis (sperm production). Excessive use of hot tubs and saunas, wearing tight jeans, and long-haul truck driving have all been identified as raising the temperature level in the scrotum to the extent that sperm production is decreased.

POST-TESTICULAR FACTORS. The most common factor in post-testicular infertility is the result of surgery or injury along the pathway from the testicles to the outside of the man's body. Examples of surgical causes are vasectomy, bladder neck reconstruction, pelvic lymph node removal, or any surgery that causes retrograde ejaculation. Congenital anomalies and various types of infections may also cause infertility problems.

Prevention

Prevention involves possible lifestyle changes to avoid excessive heat to the scrotum, substance abuse, exposure to toxins, and environmental hazards. Problems related to medication or infections should be discussed with the HCP.

Signs and Symptoms

A couple is considered infertile if they have been unsuccessful at becoming pregnant after at least 1 year of unprotected intercourse. If pregnancy has occurred during the year but there was no delivery, the problem usually is considered a female rather than a male factor.

Diagnosis

Diagnosis begins with a detailed history and physical examination that looks for known male causes of infertility.

HISTORY. Initial assessment includes frequency of intercourse, timing (according to ovulation cycle), use of contraceptives, problems with premature ejaculation, and erection problems. Use of hot tubs or saunas; tight jeans; use of nicotine, caffeine, alcohol, or marijuana; and the desire for children on the part of the man are all assessed. High stress, long periods of sitting, and exposure to environmental toxins are determined. The patient also may be questioned about STIs, endocrine problems, congenital urinary problems, serious illnesses or groin injuries, cancer, and treatment with chemotherapy or radiation.

PHYSICAL EXAMINATION. The HCP will observe for normal hair pattern and growth, muscle development, size of testicles, and any evidence of a varicocele or hydrocele.

DIAGNOSTIC TESTS. Analysis is done on several semen specimens to see if they contain the right amount and type of healthy sperm needed for a pregnancy. Infection should be ruled out. Several other tests may be done, including hormone tests, genetic testing, and ultrasound, depending on the level of desire and the financial resources of the couple. Many insurance companies do not pay for testing or treatment for infertility.

Therapeutic Measures

Treatment may be as simple as making a change in sexual or lifestyle practices. Surgery to correct a varicocele or obstruction may be done. If the couple is able to handle the emotional and financial strain, they may try a variety of in vitro fertilization (IVF) procedures. IVF is very costly, and success rates vary. Another option that may be presented to the couple is adoption.

You can play an important role in the emotional support a couple needs during infertility studies. It is important that the couple feel comfortable in communicating their feelings and frustrations with one another and their HCP. It also may help them to attend a support group designed for couples experiencing infertility.

SUGGESTED ANSWERS TO CRITICAL THINKING

Mr. Atkinson

1. $\dfrac{5\,mg \mid 1\,tablet}{\mid 2\,mg} = 2.5$ tablets

   Mr. Atkinson should be alert for signs of hypotension, such as dizziness or lightheadedness on arising. He should not drive until effects and side effects of the medication are known.
2. Mr. Atkinson should be instructed not to lift anything heavier than 10 pounds for the first 6 weeks. He will not be able to plow or drive for the first 6 weeks. It is important that his son understand his father's limitations and how important it is for him or someone else to help out with the farm chores.
3. Mr. Atkinson will notice a change in his ejaculation (either very little ejaculate or none at all). If he could have an erection before surgery, the chances are very good that he will continue to be able to have intercourse; however, he will not ejaculate.
4. A home health care nurse can assist Mr. Atkinson with care at home, such as catheter care and removal, possible dribbling postsurgery, and reinforcement of activity level. A dietitian can help with dietary instructions related to foods high in dietary fiber and fluids to avoid such as caffeine, citrus juices, and alcohol beverages.

Mr. Cunningham

1. Mr. Cunningham should be encouraged to see his health care provider (HCP) immediately for an evaluation to rule out testicular cancer.
2. Depending on the stage of the cancer, he will have the cancerous testicle, cord, and lymph nodes removed.

He may need chemotherapy or radiation treatments as well.
3. Mr. Cunningham should be encouraged to make deposits at a certified sperm bank before any treatments. It is also important to include his future wife and his family in the decision-making process. They should be encouraged to share their feelings and concerns with one another. Cancer support groups may also be helpful to Mr. Cunningham.

Mr. Kittle

1. It is okay to "pretend" here! Act like you are perfectly comfortable and that you hear this sort of thing every day. (Of course, you would never pretend to know something you don't—it is always okay to say you don't know.) Have a matter-of-fact communication style. If you get nervous and forget what questions you should ask, start with something general such as, "Can you tell me more about your symptoms?"
2. Begin a psychosocial assessment to identify presence of stress, fear, depression, fatigue, or problems with interpersonal relationships; also ask about medication, alcohol, and nicotine use. Assure him you will alert the HCP to follow up with further assessment.
3. After alerting the HCP, encourage Mr. Kittle to share openly so that an accurate diagnosis can be made. Reassure Mr. Kittle that many men have the same problem and that he is not alone. Let him know there are many treatments available and that his HCP will work with him to find what is best for him.

Review Questions

1. The nurse is caring for a patient with benign prostatic hyperplasia who expresses concern that he has cancer. Which of the following would be the best response by the nurse?
   1. "Don't worry. Prostatic hyperplasia is not the same thing as cancer."
   2. "Since it is called benign, you don't have to worry about it. No treatment should be necessary. You will just need to have it watched."
   3. "Hyperplasia means your prostate is growing too many cells. They are not cancerous, but they could interfere with your ability to urinate, so it is important to have it treated."
   4. "You are correct. It is a form of cancer, but it is very slow growing and very treatable. Your doctor will recommend treatments for you."

2. The nurse is discharging a man after treatment for priapism. Which of the following statements by the patient shows understanding of discharge instructions?
   1. "I should use hot packs three times a day for the next 3 days."
   2. "I should be seen immediately if I have another erection lasting more than 2 hours."
   3. "The Viagra I took may have caused this problem."
   4. "I should avoid having sex for 1 month."

3. The nurse is caring for a patient who is 1-day post–transurethral resection of the prostate. He says he is having pain in his bladder. The nurse notices urine leakage around his catheter. Which of the following would be the best response from the nurse?
   1. "Bladder spasms are common after your surgery. Take some deep breaths while I get a belladonna and opium suppository."
   2. "You should not be experiencing spasms. I will notify the registered nurse right away."
   3. "Spasms can be very painful. Would you like an injection of morphine?"
   4. "Your catheter is leaking. We will need to replace it right away."

4. A nurse working in a nursing home notes that it is difficult but not impossible to retract the foreskin for washing on an older gentleman. Which action is correct?
   1. Avoid retracting the foreskin for cleaning to prevent paraphimosis.
   2. Gently retract the foreskin for cleaning, and then replace it and notify the health care provider.
   3. Retract the foreskin for cleaning, and leave it retracted to prevent infection.
   4. Retract the foreskin and leave it retracted until the health care provider can evaluate it.

5. Which statement by a patient shows the need for more education about erectile dysfunction?
   1. "I may have blood flow problems that are causing the dysfunction."
   2. "I can try some herbal remedies such as ginseng before consulting my physician."
   3. "Some men inject drugs into their penis to cause an erection."
   4. "My sleep apnea could be a factor in erectile dysfunction."

6. The nurse is caring for a patient admitted for complications of diabetes. The nurse asks if he is satisfied with his level of sexual functioning, and he becomes tearful. Which of the following is the best initial response by the nurse?
   1. "You seem upset with my question. Are you having a problem you would like to talk about?"
   2. "Impotence is common with diabetes. Don't let it worry you."
   3. "What kind of sexual dysfunction are you experiencing?"
   4. "I am sorry you are having problems with your sexual functioning. Would you like a referral to a sex therapist?"

7. What are common complications of varicocele? **Select all that apply.**
   1. Infertility
   2. Infection
   3. Erectile dysfunction
   4. Pain
   5. Priapism
   6. Cancer

8. Which of the following should the nurse anticipate teaching about when caring for a man with infertility?
   1. Penile implants
   2. Prostatectomy
   3. Transurethral resection of the prostate
   4. Decrease in nicotine and alcohol use

Answer rationales available in your online resources.

ANSWERS 1. 3; 2. 3; 3. 1; 4. 2; 5. 2; 6. 1; 7. 1, 4; 8. 4

Key Points

Find the chapter key points in your online resources available through Davis Edge.

Additional Resources

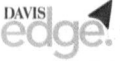 Use the scratch off code on the inside front cover of your book to access online quizzes that will help you to improve your scores on course exams and prepare for the NCLEX-PN®.

 Study Guide

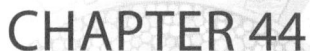

CHAPTER 44

Nursing Care of Patients With Sexually Transmitted Infections

Laura L. McCully, Debra Perry-Philo

KEY TERMS

cervicitis (SIR-vih-SY-tis)
chancre (SHANK-er)
condylomata acuminata (KON-dih-LOH-mah-tah ah-KYOOM-in-AH-tah)
condylomatous (KON-dih-LOH-mah-tus)
conjunctivitis (kon-JUNK-tih-VY-tis)
cytotoxic (SY-toh-TOK-sik)
electrocautery (ee-LEK-troh-CAW-tur-ee)
endometritis (EN-doh-meh-TRY-tis)
gummas (GUH-mahs)
hepatosplenomegaly (heh-PAT-oh-SPLEH-noh-MEG-ah-lee)
herpetic (her-PET-ik)
lymphadenopathy (lim-FAD-deh-NAW-puh-thee)
mucopurulent cervicitis (MYOO-koh-PYOO-ruh-lent SIR-vih-SY-tis)
ophthalmia neonatorum (awf-THAL-mee-ah NEE-oh-nuh-TOR-uhm)
proctitis (prok-TY-tis)
puerperal (pyoo-UR-pur-uhl)
sacral radiculopathy (SAY-krul ra-DIK-yoo-LAW-puh-thee)
salpingitis (SAL-pin-JY-tis)
serological (SEAR-uh-LAW-jih-kuhl)
urethritis (YOO-reh-THRY-tis)
verrucous (veh-ROO-kus)
vesicular (veh-SIK-yoo-lur)
vulvovaginitis (VUL-voh-VAJ-ih-NY-tis)

CHAPTER CONCEPTS

Health Promotion
Infection
Sexuality

LEARNING OUTCOMES

1. Identify the pathogens involved with each of the common sexually transmitted infections (STIs).
2. Describe the signs and symptoms of each of the common STIs.
3. Plan teaching to promote STI prevention.
4. Describe treatment options for common STIs.
5. Plan nursing care for patients with STIs.
6. Explain how you will know whether your nursing interventions have been effective.

Sexually transmitted infections (STIs) are infections that can be transmitted through intimate contact with the genitals, mouth, or rectum of another individual. Some STIs can also be spread by other routes such as blood or body fluids. A nurse's best protection against catching diseases from blood and body fluids of infected patients is the strict practice of standard precautions and maintaining his or her own healthy, intact skin.

Healthy People 2020 (Office of Disease Prevention and Health Promotion, 2017) recognizes the burden of STIs on individuals and society, and has developed a goal to "promote healthy sexual behaviors, strengthen community capacity, and increase access to quality services to prevent [STIs] and their complications." Physically, STIs can cause tremendous suffering because of pain, scarring of genitourinary structures, damage to other body organs, infertility, birth defects, nervous system damage, development of cancer, and even death of infected patients and sometimes their children. Psychologically and socially, these infections also have profound effects on individuals, families, and relationships. Guilt about passing on an incurable infection to a loved one or feelings of betrayal because of being infected because of someone else's choices are some of the emotional consequences of STIs.

Changing social norms have been associated with increasing incidence of almost all types of STIs, including some previously rare infections related to anal intercourse. Coexistence of more than one STI in an individual is also occurring more often. Many infections and syndromes are associated with STIs. The more common ones are discussed in this chapter; HIV and AIDS are discussed separately in Chapter 20.

One of the most important ways you can help those who experience STIs is by being kind, nonjudgmental, and sensitive to the patient's communication. Maintaining an open posture and eye contact (if appropriate for the patient's culture) relays a sense of openness and willingness to talk, and preserves the possibility of continuing health promotion with these individuals in the future. For more information on STIs, visit www.cdc.gov/std/healthcomm/fact_sheets.htm.

> ### BE SAFE!
> Observe standard precautions and careful hand hygiene to avoid contact with infectious organisms. Go to www.cdc.gov and type in "hand hygiene" for complete guidelines.

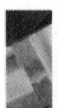

DISORDERS AND SYNDROMES RELATED TO SEXUALLY TRANSMITTED INFECTIONS

Vulvovaginitis
Vulvovaginitis is an inflammation of the vulva and vagina. It can be asymptomatic or involve redness, itching, burning, excoriation, pain, swelling of the vagina and labia, and discharge. A variety of sexually and nonsexually transmitted infectious agents can cause vulvovaginitis. The odor, consistency, and color of the discharge vary with the different microbes involved. Nonsexually transmitted vaginitis, vulvovaginitis, and vaginosis are described in Chapter 42. Bartholin glands can develop abscesses as a result of infection with nonsexually transmitted microbes or STIs such as gonorrhea and chlamydia.

Urethritis
Both STIs and nonsexually transmitted microorganisms can cause **urethritis** in men and women. In men, inflammation of the urethra, prostate, and epididymis can result in difficult, painful, and frequent urination and a urethral discharge. The discharge may be clear, cloudy, or yellow. Female partners of men with urethritis may also suffer from urethritis. They may also develop mucopurulent cervicitis. Some causative agents for urethritis include *Neisseria gonorrhoeae, Chlamydia trachomatis, Ureaplasma urealyticum, Trichomonas vaginalis, Candida albicans,* and herpes simplex virus.

Mucopurulent Cervicitis
Mucopurulent cervicitis (MPC) is an inflammation of the cervix. It may produce a mucopurulent yellow exudate on the cervix or may have no noticeable symptoms. MPC during pregnancy can result in **conjunctivitis** and pneumonia in newborn infants. It can also cause **puerperal** infection in the mother. MPC can be caused by the same organisms that cause urethritis. MPC may spread to become pelvic inflammatory disease.

Proctitis and Enteritis
Proctitis is inflammation of the rectum and anus. It may be due to either nonsexually transmitted microbes or STIs. It is especially prevalent among those who practice anal intercourse. Enteritis is inflammation of the lining of the intestine. Enteritis may occur as a result of contamination during anal intercourse. *Giardia lamblia* is the most common infecting organism. Care of patients who have gastrointestinal disorders is discussed in Unit 8.

Genital Ulcers
Genital ulcers are formed when papules or macules erode and leave painful, raw, pitted, or excoriated areas on or around the genitals. Not all genital ulcers are caused by STIs. STIs that can produce genital ulcers include syphilis, herpes, and HIV. Although the ulcerations can look similar in these STIs, a distinctive difference is that a syphilitic ulcer is painless. Genital ulcers from one type of disease may increase the risk of infection with other STIs during sexual activity. This is because the open areas present easy access for the infecting organism.

Cellular Changes
Cellular changes can also be caused by STIs, including **condylomatous** (wartlike) growths and dysplasia or neoplasia. These may result in precancerous or cancerous conditions. Herpes viruses, HIV, and human papillomavirus have all been linked to the development of cancer.

Pelvic Inflammatory Disease
Pathophysiology and Etiology
Pelvic inflammatory disease (PID) is an infection of the upper genital tract that can cause chronic pelvic pain due to inflammation. The primary sources of infection include *C. trachomatis* and *N. gonorrhoeae*. It may also result from any organism that is associated with an STI. These organisms can invade the endocervical canal, resulting in inflammation of the cervix (**cervicitis**), and move upward, resulting in infection of the endometrium (**endometritis**), fallopian tubes (**salpingitis**), and pelvic cavity. The chronic inflammation results in extensive scarring and adhesions. This can cause

• WORD • BUILDING •
vulvovaginitis: vulvo—vulva + vagin—vagina + itis—inflammation
urethritis: ureth—urethra + itis—inflammation
mucopurulent cervicitis: muco—involving mucus + purulent—involving pus + cervic—cervix + itis—inflammation
conjunctivitis: conjunctiv(a)—lining of the eyelids and sclera of the eye + itis—inflammation
puerperal: puer – child + parere – to give birth
proctitis: proc—anus + itis—inflammation
condylomatous: condyl—rounded projection + oma(t)—growth + ous—like
cervicitis: cervic—cervix + itis—inflammation
endometritis: endo—inside + metr—womb + itis—inflammation
salpingitis: salping—tube + itis—inflammation

infertility and increase the risk of ectopic pregnancy. Increased risk for PID occurs with a history of multiple sexual partners, STIs, substance abuse, frequent vaginal douching, and insertion of an intrauterine device (IUD). The risk of PID at the time of IUD insertion is as much as 2% when no cervical infection is present and as much as 5% when cervical infection is present. Testing for STIs can be done at the time of IUD insertion; if results come back positive, the patient can be treated without removal of the IUD (American College of Obstetricians and Gynecologists, 2012).

Signs and Symptoms

Women may present with lower abdominal pain and tenderness, purulent vaginal discharge or vaginal bleeding, pain with sexual intercourse, fever, nausea and vomiting, and pain with urination. They may also present with no symptoms at all. Findings during physical examination include adnexal tenderness upon palpation, and pain in the uterus and cervix when moved during a bimanual examination.

Diagnostic Tests

Laboratory tests reveal a positive culture of the causative organism(s) and leukocytosis. Urinary tract infection may need to be ruled out.

Therapeutic Measures

With serious infection, hospitalization and intravenous (IV) antibiotics may be needed. IV therapy can be changed to oral therapy after 48 hours if status improves. Outpatient therapy with oral antibiotics is used with minor infections. Laparoscopic surgery may be done to release adhesions and reduce complications. Testing and treatment for other STIs should be considered for both the patient and partner. Education on the cause of the infection and prevention of future episodes is essential.

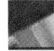 ## SEXUALLY TRANSMITTED INFECTIONS

Chlamydia
Etiology and Signs and Symptoms
Chlamydia is a commonly diagnosed STI in the United States. (Table 44.1 provides a summary of this and other common STIs.) It can be transmitted sexually and by blood and body fluid contact. There are several strains of the bacteria *C. trachomatis*. Chlamydia is often asymptomatic (a "silent" STI) in women, but it can cause urethritis, MPC, and conjunctivitis. Fitz-Hugh-Curtis syndrome, a surface inflammation of the liver, can also be caused by *C. trachomatis*. This inflammation can cause nausea, vomiting, and sharp pain at the base of the ribs that sometimes refers to the right shoulder and arm. Chlamydia is a frequent cause of PID and infertility. It also increases the risk of ectopic pregnancy. The infection can be passed from mother to baby during birth, resulting in neonatal pneumonia and conjunctivitis. It also increases the risk of HIV infection.

Lymphogranuloma venereum (LGV) is also caused by some strains of *C. trachomatis*. LGV is more commonly seen in tropical climates or among people who emigrated from tropical areas. This disease also causes urethritis and proctitis. It inflames lymph nodes that drain the pelvic area, resulting in draining sores and fistula development. Scarring from LGV can complicate vaginal deliveries.

Diagnostic Tests
Several tests for chlamydia are available. Samples are gathered in a special collection tube to send to a laboratory for culture. Nucleic acid amplification testing (NAAT) identifies the presence of chlamydial DNA or RNA in urine, cervical, or urethral specimens. If the health care provider (HCP) is performing a Papanicolaou (Pap) test, the chlamydia NAAT screening can be done with the ThinPrep specimen. The Centers for Disease Control and Prevention (CDC) recommends that all sexually active females under the age of 25, older women with risk factors such as new or multiple sex partners, or women with sex partners who have had an STI be tested annually (CDC, 2015).

Therapeutic Measures
Antibiotics are given to treat chlamydia in adults and their sexual partners (Table 44.2). Erythromycin or azithromycin is used during pregnancy because other antibiotics may pose a risk to the fetus. Use of an erythromycin ophthalmic ointment is recommended to treat the neonate shortly after birth to prevent conjunctivitis, though efficacy for prevention of chlamydial ophthalmia is unclear. Institutional policies and state regulations determine whether administration of the medications requires specific consent of the parents.

Gonorrhea
Etiology and Signs and Symptoms
According to the CDC (2015), 820,000 new cases of gonorrhea infections occur each year. It is caused by the bacterium *N. gonorrhoeae*. Transmission can occur vaginally, rectally, orally, via contact with other mucous membranes, or through contact with blood and body fluids. It can produce a variety of signs and symptoms. Men may be asymptomatic or may have urethritis with a yellow urethral discharge. Women may have either no noticeable symptoms or have a sore throat, MPC, urethritis, or abnormal menstrual symptoms such as bleeding between periods. Many cases of PID are caused by gonorrhea. Intercourse with an infected partner during menstruation may be especially risky for development of PID. This is because removal of the cervical mucous barrier can promote the growth of the gonococcus in the higher reproductive tract. Gonorrhea can also cause Fitz-Hugh-Curtis syndrome. Fever, nausea, vomiting, and lower abdominal pain may be present. Gonorrhea may also infect the throat and the rectum. In addition, it may cause widespread gonococcal infection, resulting in inflammation of the joints, skin, meninges, and lining of the heart.

Table 44.1

Common Sexually Transmitted Infections Summary

	Chlamydia	Gonorrhea	Syphilis	Trichomoniasis	Herpes Simplex	Condylomata (HPV)
Signs and Symptoms	Conjunctivitis; in men, urethritis, epididymitis, prostatitis; in women, MPC, urethritis	In men, urethritis, penile discharge, epididymitis, prostatitis; in women, MPC, urethritis, abnormal menses	*Primary syphilis:* chancre; *secondary syphilis:* flu-like symptoms, rashes, condylomatous growths	Genital redness, swelling, itching, burning, foul discharge; in men, urethritis, prostatitis; in women, "strawberry cervix"	Vesicles/ ulcerations in mouth, genitals, flu-like symptoms, lymphadenopathy, urethritis, cystitis, MPC	Fleshy tumors, primarily on genitalia
Diagnostic Tests	NAAT culture, urine	NAAT culture, urine	VDRL test, ELISA, RPR test, FTA-ABS	Microscopic examination	Culture, Western blot, ELISA	Visualization of lesions, biopsy
Therapeutic Measures	Antibiotics (see Table 44.2)	Antibiotics (see Table 44.2)	Penicillin	Metronidazole (Flagyl) or tinidazole (Tindamax)	Antiviral medication (see Table 44.2)	Wart removal, topical therapies, interferon therapy
Complications	Fitz-Hugh-Curtis syndrome, increased susceptibility to HIV infection, PID, infertility, transmission to baby at birth, co-infection with gonorrhea	PID, disseminated gonococcal infection, Fitz-Hugh-Curtis syndrome, transmission to baby at birth, co-infection with chlamydia	Tertiary syphilis; gumma damage to heart, circulatory system, nervous system; transmission to fetus during pregnancy	Preterm delivery, infertility, increased risk of HIV transmission	Lifelong infection, disseminated infection, nervous system invasion, increased risk of cervical cancer, transmission to baby at birth	Long-term complications are rare

Note: ELISA = enzyme-linked immunosorbent assay; FTA-ABS = fluorescent treponemal antibody absorption; HPV = human papillomavirus; MPC = mucopurulent cervicitis; NAAT = nucleic acid amplification testing; PID = pelvic inflammatory disease; RPR = rapid plasma reagin; VDRL = Venereal Disease Research Laboratory.

Newborns born to mothers who have gonorrhea can develop **ophthalmia neonatorum.** This involves inflammation of the conjunctivae and deeper parts of the eye, and can result in blindness. All newborns are treated with erythromycin ophthalmic ointment to prevent this complication. The newborn may also experience a gonorrheal infection at other sites following birth. Abscesses may develop where fetal scalp monitors were attached during labor, and infection of the nose, lungs, and rectum may occur.

Diagnostic Tests

Diagnosis is made by microscopic examination of smears and cultures of the discharge or identification of bacterial DNA (NAAT) from urine, the vagina, or the endocervix. Testing

• WORD • BUILDING •
ophthalmia neonatorum: ophthalmia—eye disease + neonatorum—of the newborn

Table 44.2

Medications Used to Treat Sexually Transmitted Infections

Medication Class/Action

Chlamydia Antibiotics

Macrolides
Inhibit bacterial protein synthesis.

Examples
erythromycin
azithromycin

Nursing Implications
Administer on empty stomach.
Do not administer with antacids.
Use caution with hepatic disorders.

Tetracyclines
Examples
Inhibits protein synthesis by binding to ribosomes:
doxycycline
Binds to bacterial cell wall, causing cell death:
amoxicillin

Nursing Implications
Do not administer during pregnancy due to bone/teeth
    effects.
Do not give with antacids or dairy products.
Administer on empty stomach.
Teach:
Avoid unnecessary exposure to sunlight.

Fluoroquinolones
Inhibit cell wall synthesis.

Examples
ofloxacin
levofloxacin

Nursing Implications
Safety under age 18 is not established.
Do not administer with antacids.
Use caution with other medications and with renal,
    hepatic, or central nervous system (CNS) disorders.

Gonorrhea Antibiotics

Cephalosporins
Inhibit cell wall synthesis.

Examples
ceftriaxone
cefixime

Nursing Implications
Use caution with penicillin allergies or renal or hepatic
    dysfunction.
Teach:
Avoid excess sun exposure.

Syphilis Antibiotics

Penicillin
Inhibits cell wall synthesis.

Examples
penicillin G

Nursing Implications
Administer deep intramuscularly or slow intravenously.
Apply ice packs to injection site as needed.
Administer orally on empty stomach.
Avoid tetracycline in children and pregnant women.
Teach:
Report fever/rash.

Tetracyclines
Examples
tetracycline
doxycycline

Nursing Implications
See above under *Penicillin.*

Continued

Table 44.2

Medications Used to Treat Sexually Transmitted Infections—cont'd

Medication Class/Action

Trichomoniasis Amebicides/Antiprotozoals

Bind to DNA to inhibit synthesis and cause cell death.

Examples
metronidazole (Flagyl)
tinidazole (Tindamax)

Nursing Implications
Administer with food.
Treat partner as well as patient.
Teach:
Avoid alcohol; abstain for a minimum of 48 hours
  following treatment to prevent severe flu-like
  reaction.

Herpes Antivirals

Inhibit DNA synthesis.

Examples
acyclovir
valacyclovir
famciclovir

Nursing Implications
Use systemic preparations cautiously with CNS, hepatic,
  or renal disorders.
Infuse IV slowly.
Maintain hydration.
Caution patient that viral transmission can still occur
  during treatment.
Some patients take daily as suppressive therapy.

Genital Warts – Acidic Agents

Acids burn and erode affected area.

Examples
trichloroacetic acid (TCA)
bichloracetic acid (BCA)

Nursing Implications
Teach:
Return for repeated applications as needed.
Avoid medication contact with eyes or tissue surrounding
  lesion.

Genital Warts – Antimitotic Agent

Exact mechanism of action unknown. Causes necrosis of wart tissue.

Examples
podofilox solution

Nursing Implications
Can be applied by patient at home with cotton-tipped
  applicator.
Teach:
Apply to warts only and allow to dry completely, or as
  ordered by health care provider.

Genital Warts – Antiviral/Immune Response Modifier

Stimulates patient's immune system to destroy warts

Examples
imiquimod

Nursing Implications
Can be applied by patient at home.
May take up to 16 weeks to completely clear warts.
Teach:
Apply thin film to clean dry skin at bedtime, as ordered
  by provider.

can also be obtained with ThinPrep, if a Pap specimen is collected.

Therapeutic Measures

Development of antibiotic resistance by *N. gonorrhoeae* and co-infection with other microorganisms, such as *C. trachomatis,* has made treatment more complicated. Cephalosporin antibiotics are recommended for the treatment of gonorrhea (see Table 44.2). It is also recommended that the patient be treated for chlamydia because co-infection is common. It is important that the patient's partner is treated as well. Ophthalmia neonatorum can be prevented by use of erythromycin eye ointment. It is recommended that all infants be treated shortly after birth regardless of the diagnostic status of the mother. The treatment is simple and may prevent a devastating outcome for the newborn. Institutional policies and state regulations determine whether administration of the ointment requires consent of the parents.

CRITICAL THINKING

Mrs. Miller delivered an infant boy 1 hour ago. The nurse is currently applying erythromycin ointment to the infant's eyes bilaterally. Mrs. Miller asks whether the medication is necessary.

1. How will you respond?
2. Should all infants receive prophylactic eye treatment at birth?

Suggested answers are at the end of the chapter.

Syphilis
Pathophysiology, Etiology, and Signs and Symptoms

Syphilis is an ancient infection that has not disappeared, although it is overshadowed by more commonly occurring infections such as chlamydia. It occurs in stages. The primary stage of syphilis begins with the entry of the *Treponema pallidum* spirochete through the skin or mucous membranes. Between 3 and 90 days later, a papule develops at the site of entry and then sloughs off, leaving a painless, red, ulcerated area called a **chancre** (Fig. 44.1). Chancres can also develop in other areas of the body at this time. Chancre formation typically is the only symptom of this stage of syphilis. The chancre eventually heals, but the spirochete remains active in the infected individual and can be passed on to others.

Secondary syphilis begins 2 to 8 weeks later. It affects the body more generally, causing such problems as flu-like symptoms, joint pain, hair loss, skin rashes (primarily on the soles of the hands and feet), mouth sores, **lymphadenopathy,** and condylomatous growths in moist areas of the body.

Serious damage can occur if syphilis is untreated in the early stages. About 15% of infected individuals will progress

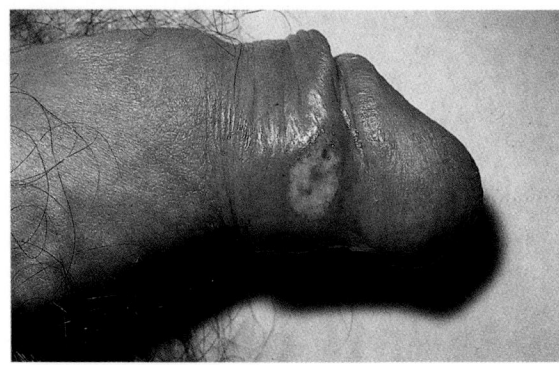

FIGURE 44.1 Syphilis chancre.

to the tertiary (or late) stage, up to 10 to 20 years later. At this stage, it can involve any organ system of the body. The spirochete can form **gummas,** which are tumors of a rubbery consistency that can break down and ulcerate, leaving holes in body tissues. The gummas can damage the heart, circulatory system, and nervous system (called neurosyphilis). Ulceration of gummas can destroy areas of vital tissue and lead to mental and physical disability or early death.

Syphilis can be passed on to the unborn children of women who carry the spirochete, resulting in **hepatosplenomegaly,** increase in bilirubin, destruction of red blood cells, birth defects (especially of the face), lymphadenopathy, and a baby who can transmit the spirochete through nasal drainage. If left untreated, syphilis during pregnancy can cause lesions in various organs of the unborn baby and result in higher rates of spontaneous abortion, stillbirth, and premature birth.

Diagnostic Tests

Several tests for syphilis exist, and a combination may be used for accurate diagnosis. Cultures may be done but are difficult to grow. **Serological** (blood) tests include the Venereal Disease Research Laboratory (VDRL) test, the rapid plasma reagin (RPR) test, and the automated reagin test (ART). These tests indirectly check for syphilis by detecting the presence of antibodies to *Treponema.* Diagnosis of neurosyphilis is even more difficult because some testing of cerebrospinal fluid may result in false-negative results. Enzyme-linked immunosorbent assay (ELISA), fluorescent treponemal antibody absorption (FTA-ABS), and polymerase chain reaction (PCR) tests for treponemal DNA are some newer methods that reduce the risk of false results. Latent syphilis infections can be detected by serologic testing even when patients have no symptoms.

• WORD • BUILDING •
lymphadenopathy: lymph—lymph nodes + adeno—node + pathy—disorder
gummas: from the word meaning "rubber"—rubbery tumors
hepatosplenomegaly: hepato—liver + spleno—spleen + megaly—enlargement
serological: sero—blood + logical—science

Therapeutic Measures

Penicillin G is the treatment of choice for patients diagnosed with syphilis (see Table 44.2). For those who are allergic to penicillin, doxycycline and tetracycline are treatment options. When HIV and syphilis are diagnosed in the same individual, symptoms of neurosyphilis are more likely to occur.

Trichomoniasis
Pathophysiology and Etiology

Trichomoniasis is an STI caused by a protozoan parasite. It can also be transmitted through nonsexual contact with infected articles because it can survive for a long time outside the body. Carriers of *T. vaginalis* can be asymptomatic for several years until changes in vaginal or urethral conditions encourage an outbreak of the infection. A decrease in resident bacteria, injuries to the vaginal tissues, or development of lesions from other STIs can activate the organism.

Signs and Symptoms

Symptoms include redness, swelling, itching, and burning of the genital area; pain with intercourse and voiding; and a frothy, foul-smelling discharge that can be clear, white, yellowish, or greenish. Men with trichomonal infection can develop prostatitis and infertility. Men who are also infected with HIV are more likely to transmit HIV to others. Women with *T. vaginalis* are more susceptible to HIV infection if exposed. Women who are pregnant risk preterm delivery and babies with low birth weights.

Diagnostic Tests

A Pap smear, NAAT, or antigen testing can be done on secretions or on urine in men. Visualization of the cervix during female pelvic examination shows a characteristic "strawberry cervix." When wet-mount slides of discharge are viewed under a microscope, the organisms can be identified by their motility and whiplike flagella. Because trichomoniasis can produce abnormal Pap smear readings, more frequent Pap smears must be done to provide adequate surveillance of cellular changes.

Therapeutic Measures

Metronidazole (Flagyl) or tinidazole (Tindamax) are used to treat trichomoniasis (see Table 44.2). Because some people carry the organism without symptoms, sexual partners should also be treated regardless of symptoms.

Herpes
Pathophysiology, Etiology, and Signs and Symptoms

Herpes infection is caused by the herpes simplex virus types 1 and 2 (HSV-1 and HSV-2). Herpes viruses have an affinity for the skin and nervous system. They can lie dormant in nervous system tissues and then reactivate when the body undergoes stress, fever, or immune system compromise. Both HSV-1 and HSV-2 can cause fever blisters of the mouth (Fig. 44.2) as well as genital lesions. However, HSV-1 is more

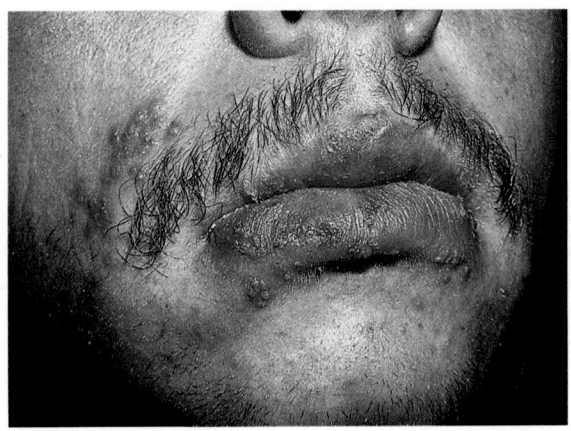

FIGURE 44.2 Herpes simplex.

CRITICAL THINKING

Kerri presents to the health clinic with a report of generalized redness, swelling, itching, and burning of her external genitalia. Following history and physical and microscopic examinations, trichomoniasis is diagnosed. Kerri is upset, stating she has been in a monogamous relationship for 2 years.

1. What should your response to Kerri include?
2. Kerri is placed on metronidazole (Flagyl), but you are not comfortable with the dose prescribed, so you look it up. How do you approach the health care provider with what appears to be an error?
3. What patient education is important for Kerri?

   Suggested answers are at the end of the chapter.

frequently associated with oral lesions and HSV-2 with genital lesions.

Genital HSV-2 outbreaks are more severe than genital HSV-1 outbreaks. After infection, vesicles develop, spontaneously rupture, and produce painful ulceration of the underlying skin tissues. Asymptomatic latent periods are generally interspersed between the **vesicular** outbreaks. Although not as common, the virus may still be transmitted even during latent periods.

An initial outbreak following infection with HSV occurs 2 days to 2 weeks after exposure and can produce a flu-like condition. Urethritis, cystitis, or MPC with vaginal discharge can also occur. Infection of the spinal nerve roots by HSV can result in **sacral radiculopathy** (damage of the sacral spinal nerves), causing retention of urine and feces. Although

• WORD • BUILDING •
vesicular: vesicul—blister + ar—type
sacral radiculopathy: sacral—sacrum + radiculo—root + pathy—disorder or disease

rare, disseminated herpes infection can result in inflammation of the spinal cord, meninges, nerve pathways, and lymph nodes as well as urethral strictures and increased risk for development of cervical cancer in women.

It is estimated that one in five pregnant women carry herpes, although most of their babies do not develop **herpetic** disease. If infected, the baby's skin, eyes, mucous membranes, and nervous system can be involved, and death from disseminated herpes infection is possible. The greatest risk of herpes transmission from mother to child during pregnancy occurs if the mother has an active genital lesion at the time of delivery.

Diagnostic Tests

Clinical diagnosis of herpes can be difficult because the lesions that are associated with HSV are absent in many infected persons. Testing for HSV requires special viral collection kits for swabbed or scraped specimens from lesions. Cell cultures and PCR are the preferred HSV tests. Follow the directions on the viral collection kit as well as institutional policies. Blood tests are used to test specifically for HSV-1 or HSV-2 antibodies.

Therapeutic Measures

There is currently no known cure for herpes infection, although antiviral medications may be given to decrease the severity of symptoms (see Table 44.2). The same discussion and treatment options should be had with patients who only test positive with blood testing. Pregnant women with a history of HSV are treated prophylactically with antiviral medication starting at 36 weeks' gestation (CDC, 2015). If an active genital lesion is present when a woman is close to the time of delivery, a cesarean delivery is likely to be performed. However, an active lesion at any time during pregnancy poses a risk for transmission. See "Nursing Care Plan for the Patient With a Sexually Transmitted Infection" later in the chapter.

Human Papillomavirus

Human papillomavirus (HPV) can be either high risk or low risk. High-risk HPV can cause cervical, vaginal, and vulvar cancers in women, penile cancers in men, and anal and oropharyngeal cancers in both men and women. Low-risk HPV does not cause cancer but can cause genital warts (condyloma). More than 100 types of HPV have been identified, and several have been closely linked to the development of cancers.

The Gardasil vaccine was introduced in 2006 for the prevention of four types of HPV. The current Gardasil formulation protects against the low-risk types 6 and 11, which cause 90% of genital warts, and high-risk types 16, 18, 31, 33, 45, 52, and 58, which are known to cause 70% of cervical cancers. Women and men can receive the vaccine between the ages of 9 and 26, with age 11 or 12 being the recommend age for routine vaccination. If the vaccine is initiated between 9 and 14, only two doses are needed. The second dose is administered 6 to 12 months after the first dose. If initiated on or after a child turns 15, then the three-dose schedule is recommended. The first dose is given, followed by the second dose 2 months after initiation, and the third dose 6 months after initiation. The vaccine does not prevent many of the other types of both high- and low-risk HPV (Meites, Kempe, & Markowitz, 2016).

Genital Warts (Low-Risk HPV)

SIGNS AND SYMPTOMS. **Condylomata acuminata** (genital warts) is a common sexually transmitted viral infection, with incidence increasing rapidly. Infection with HPV produces condylomata. These are soft, raised, **verrucous** fleshy tumors, which may also have finger-like projections and resemble cauliflower (Fig. 44.3). Lesions most commonly develop on the external genitalia and perineum as well as on the internal vaginal wall and cervix in women. However, lesions can also develop on other areas of the body after contact with the virus. Some people remain asymptomatic but can still transmit the infection.

The latent period from the time of exposure to development of the warts can be as long as 3 years. HPV can be passed from a pregnant woman to her fetus, resulting in HPV infection of the baby's respiratory tract. Genital warts tend to grow more rapidly in pregnant women and bleed more easily with injury than in nonpregnant women. Vaginal delivery is an option unless the pelvic outlet is blocked with warts or the warts would cause excessive bleeding.

DIAGNOSTIC TESTS. Diagnosis of condyloma is usually by visual inspection. Biopsy can be used to confirm diagnosis but is only done if lesions are atypical. HPV testing is not recommended for condyloma since the results are not reliable (CDC, 2015).

THERAPEUTIC MEASURES. There is currently no known cure for HPV. Genital warts can be treated by freezing, burning, or chemically destroying them or by manipulating the patient's immune system to attack the virus. Cryotherapy (freezing) of the warts can be done by touching each wart with a cryoprobe or a liquid nitrogen–soaked swab. Warts may also be burned or electrocoagulated with an **electrocautery** or a laser. Heat causes the proteins to coagulate, resulting in death of the wart tissue. Several topical agents are also available (see Table 44.2).

Some treatment options are not appropriate for use during pregnancy because of their **cytotoxic** effects, which might damage the fetus. However, cryosurgery and laser destruction of wart tissue can be done during pregnancy. All treatments

---

• **WORD • BUILDING •**

herpetic: herpet—herpes + ic—pertaining to

condylomata acuminata: condyl—rounded projection + oma—growth + ta—pluralizes the word (singular form is condyloma) + acuminata—genital growths

verrucous: verruc—wart + ous—like

electrocautery: electro—electrical + cautery—branding iron

cytotoxic: cyto—cell + toxic—poison

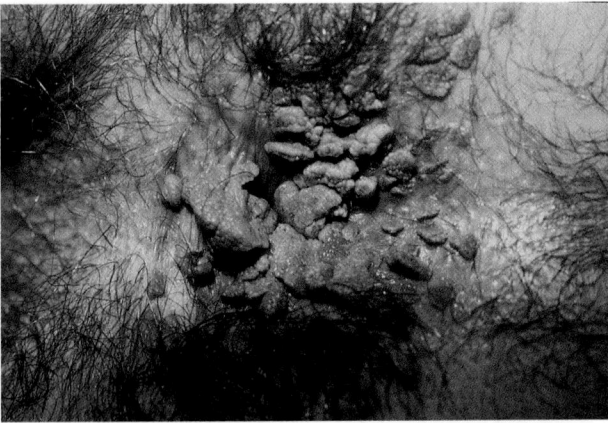

FIGURE 44.3 Condylomata, commonly known as genital warts.

may require multiple applications and generally result in a great deal of discomfort as the warts degenerate, ulcerate, and slough over a long period. Wart removal does not cure the infection, and new wart growth can occur after treatment.

HOME CARE. Patients who have genital warts burned off need to recuperate at home. Multiple areas may be treated. If the burns are near the urethra or rectum, the patient may need a Foley catheter inserted to avoid contamination and irritation of the lesions after treatment. The patient is instructed to increase dietary roughage and fluids to prevent constipation. Consult the HCP for care of the burns. Teach the patient to premedicate for pain control as needed and to use sterile technique for dressing changes.

High-Risk HPV

High-risk HPV is known to cause cervical, anal, penile, and oropharyngeal cancers.

DIAGNOSIS. The only cancer screening done routinely is cervical cancer screening on women from ages 21 to 65. Testing can be performed using conventional Pap or liquid-based Pap cytologic tests. Annual screening is no longer recommended. From ages 21 to 29, screening is recommended every 3 years. From ages 30 to 65, screening may continue every 3 years or Pap tests with high-risk HPV co-testing every 5 years.

TREATMENT. If the results of the Pap test are abnormal, follow-up care should be provided by the HCP. Depending on the severity of the findings, repeating the Pap, a colposcopy, a diagnostic excision of the lesion, or hysterectomy may be done.

Hepatitis B

Hepatitis B is an infection of the liver caused by the hepatitis B virus. It deserves mention here because it can be transmitted through sexual contact with blood and body fluids. During pregnancy, hepatitis B virus may be transmitted to the unborn baby. This can result in acute hepatitis and the possibility of becoming a chronic carrier of hepatitis B. See Chapter 35 for a full discussion on hepatitis.

Genital Parasites
Etiology and Signs and Symptoms

Genital parasites are not a true STI, but they may be transmitted during close body contact. The two most commonly seen parasites are pubic lice (*Phthirus pubis,* commonly called "crabs" because of the shape of the lice) and scabies (*Sarcoptes scabiei*). These parasites cause itching, redness, and, for scabies, tracks under the skin where the females burrow to lay their eggs.

Diagnostic Tests

History, physical examination, and direct visualization or magnified view of the parasites aid in diagnosis.

Therapeutic Measures

Parasites are treated with topical insecticides such as permethrin (Elimite or Acticin for scabies) or malathion (Ovide for pubic lice). Advise the patient to refer to package inserts for application instructions and precautions to avoid reinfection.

 ## REPORTING OF SEXUALLY TRANSMITTED INFECTIONS

The nurse may be required to facilitate the reporting and public health follow-up of STIs by filling in patient information on an STI reporting form and placing the form in the patient's chart for completion by the HCP. The requirements for reporting STIs may vary for different states, provinces, and countries. In some areas, laboratories are also required to submit a report form for positive reportable STI results. The report form has spaces for listing of sexual contacts that should be notified of possible STI exposure. Depending on state law, contacts may be notified by the HCP, patient, or a public health authority.

 ## NURSING PROCESS FOR SEXUALLY TRANSMITTED INFECTIONS

Data Collection

STIs are usually assessed, diagnosed, and treated in HCP offices and in clinics. It is important to evaluate the patient's reason for seeking health care with every outpatient visit. Sometimes patients visit clinics or HCP offices for stated reasons other than STIs, yet their real concern is an STI.

If a patient presents with signs and symptoms that could lead to an STI diagnosis, inquire about irritation, pain, lesions, or discharge in the genital region. Explain to the patient that you need to know what examination supplies to prepare for an appropriate assessment, as this may allow him or her to share concerns and true reasons for the visit. Establishing rapport and conveying acceptance may also facilitate communication. You may be asked to be present during the examination to assist the HCP and to serve as a chaperone or patient support person.

STIs may also be discovered in hospitalized patients. Nurses are often the ones who bathe and provide perineal care to patients. It is important to be aware of signs and symptoms in older adults as well as younger people ("Gerontological Issues"). Unusual discharge, redness, blisters, swollen areas, ulcers, and evidence of parasites in the genital area may be observed during patient care. STI awareness can also sensitize you to the possible significance of patient reports of persistent pelvic pain, dysuria, discharges, and rectal soreness. Such problems should be accurately documented and reported, so that further investigation and treatment can take place.

Nursing Diagnoses, Planning, and Implementation

See "Nursing Care Plan for the Patient With a Sexually Transmitted Infection."

Gerontological Issues

Older Adults and Sexual Activity. Older adults retain interest in and are capable of engaging in sex. Do not assume that because an older adult is single or widowed that he or she is not sexually active. Older adults who have enjoyed active and fulfilling sex lives with a previous spouse or partner may seek that in new relationships. Older adults who engage in high-risk sexual behaviors (e.g., multiple partners, genital-anal sex, no use of barriers during sexual intercourse) are also at risk for STIs.

NURSING CARE TIP

Neighbors, friends, or family members may seek information from you because they know nurses are educated about health issues. Such questions may be stated in indirect terms, such as "I have a friend who is having a problem." You can provide accurate information and stress the importance of diagnosis and treatment to prevent the serious consequences of untreated sexually transmitted infections without asking probing or embarrassing questions.

CRITICAL THINKING

Stephanie is sitting in the exam room of the clinic where you work. She comments, "I am new to this area, and I've heard that there are three guys in this town who have syphilis and are spreading it around. Is that true?"

1. What are some concerns this question might reflect?
2. You find out that Stephanie knows very little about syphilis. List in outline form a teaching plan that includes the information that is important for Stephanie to know about syphilis.

Suggested answers are at the end of the chapter.

Nursing Care Plan for the Patient With a Sexually Transmitted Infection

Nursing Diagnosis: *Acute Pain* related to inflammation and skin lesions as evidenced by patient pain rating
Expected Outcome: The patient will experience relief as evidenced by a decrease in pain rating to a level that is acceptable to patient.
Evaluation of Outcome: Does the patient state relief of pain level is acceptable?

Intervention	Rationale	Evaluation
Assess pain using the *WHAT'S UP?* format.	*Assessment of the characteristic of the pain assists the nurse in providing appropriate relief measures.*	Can patient describe the pain characteristics?
Recommend pain relief measures appropriate to the type and location of the pain (both alternative measures, such as heat, ice, and change of position, and medication may be offered).	*Not all types of pain respond well to the same treatment.*	Does patient express satisfactory relief of pain? Does patient move and rest without evidence of pain?
Document results of pain relief measures.	*Documentation alerts other caregivers about what works and does not work, thus providing more consistent, effective pain relief.*	Have you gained sufficient information from patient to document results?
Instruct patient about self-care for pain and sexually transmitted infection (STI) follow-up at home	*Patient must understand self-care in order to comply with treatment.*	Does patient verbalize understanding of self-care measures?

(nursing care plan continues on page 930)

Nursing Care Plan for the Patient With a Sexually Transmitted Infection—cont'd

Nursing Diagnosis: *Risk for Infection* (transmission to others) related to lack of knowledge about transmission, symptoms, and treatment
Expected Outcome: The patient will verbalize understanding of measures to prevent transmission to others.
Evaluation of Outcome: Does the patient verbalize understanding of transmission prevention? Does the patient practice preventive behaviors?

Intervention	Rationale	Evaluation
Assess patient's understanding of transmission, symptoms, complications, and treatment of STIs.	*New instruction should be based on patient's previous knowledge.*	Is patient's current understanding accurate? What teaching is needed?
Assess whether patient is engaging in high-risk behaviors.	*If patient is continuing to engage in high-risk behaviors, risk for infection of others is high.*	Is patient protecting self and others appropriately?
Use standard precautions and strict aseptic technique for all procedures involving blood and body fluids.	*The health care team, in addition to other patient contacts, must be protected.*	Are standard precautions observed?
Instruct patient in appropriate strategies to reduce risk of infecting others, including abstinence, monogamy (if no active infection), use of barrier methods and spermicides, and adherence to treatment regimen.	*These measures may help prevent transmission of infection to others.*	Does patient verbalize understanding of methods to prevent transmission and intent to practice them?
Teach patient signs and symptoms of STIs to report immediately.	*Prompt treatment of patient and his or her partners further reduces risk of transmission of infection.*	Does patient verbalize understanding of signs and symptoms to report?
Explain importance of a follow-up evaluation.	*Follow-up is essential to affirm that treatment was successful.*	Does patient make a follow-up appointment?

Nursing Diagnosis: *Readiness for Enhanced Health Management* related to lack of knowledge about STIs as evidenced by the patient requesting information
Expected Outcome: The patient will verbalize realistic and accurate information about disease prevention.
Evaluation of Outcome: Does the patient relate accurate knowledge and plans for prevention?

Intervention	Rationale	Evaluation
Assess patient's health beliefs and correct misconceptions.	*Many myths about sexual activity are sincerely believed by some patients.*	Does patient have an accurate understanding of STI prevention?
Explain importance of patient knowing the sexual and lifestyle history of any potential partner before sexual activity occurs.	*Having a sexual relationship with someone is the epidemiological equivalent of engaging in sexual activity with each of that person's previous partners.*	Can patient relate a plan to approach this subject with a potential partner?
Provide pamphlets or other materials. (Make sure patient is able to read.)	*Written materials can reinforce teaching.*	Is patient observed viewing materials offered?
Explain that abstinence or lifelong monogamy of both sexual partners in a relationship is the only sure prevention against STIs.	*These practices eliminate risk of exposure.*	Does patient relate understanding of monogamy?

Nursing Care Plan for the Patient With a Sexually Transmitted Infection—cont'd

Intervention	Rationale	Evaluation
Educate patient that consumption of alcohol or other psychoactive drugs can reduce inhibitions and may result in unintended sexual encounters, which can transmit STIs.	*Avoiding or limiting alcohol and other drug consumption when with potential partners may help prevent STI infection from occurring.*	Does patient relate a plan to limit the effect of substances on sexual encounters?

Nursing Diagnosis: *Ineffective Sexuality Pattern* related to infection and risk for transmission of infectious organism
Expected Outcome: The patient will describe acceptable, alternative sexual practices and safer sex practices.
Evaluation of Outcome: Does the patient relate safer sex practices?

Intervention	Rationale	Evaluation
Provide privacy. Be verbally and nonverbally nonjudgmental when allowing patient and his or her partner to express concerns about sexual practice.	*Treatment success rates are generally higher when a rapport is established with the health care provider and when the partner is included in the decision-making process.*	Do patient and partner express concerns?
When teaching the patient, use *safer sex* terminology.	*Safer sex practices may decrease the risk of (but not absolutely prevent) transmission of STIs (Table 44.3). Safe sex and STI prevention are misnomers, since no practices provide absolute protection.*	Does patient exhibit understanding of the concept of safer sex?
Discuss alternative means of sexual expression, as appropriate.	*This may allow for intimacy when the desired sexual expression is not recommended, such as during treatment.*	Can patient identify some acceptable (to patient) alternative means of sexual expression?
Support realistic expectations about treatment and outcomes.	*Unrealistic expectations may lead to additional undesired issues related to sexuality pattern.*	Does patient have realistic expectations?

Table 44.3

Barrier Methods for Safer Sex

Barrier	*Related Information*
Male condoms	Latex condoms are less likely than other types to break during intercourse.
	Lubrication decreases the chance of breakage during use. Only water-soluble lubricants should be used because substances such as petroleum jelly (Vaseline) may weaken the condom.
	Condoms should never be inflated to test them; doing so can weaken them.
	Condoms should be applied only when the penis is erect.
	Condoms should have a reservoir tip or should be applied while holding about a half inch of tip flat between the fingertips to allow room for ejaculate; otherwise, the condom might break.
	The penis should be withdrawn after ejaculation and before the erection begins to subside while holding the condom securely around the penis to avoid spillage.
	Condoms should never be reused and should be discarded properly after use so that others will not come in contact with contents.

Continued

Table 44.3

Barrier Methods for Safer Sex—cont'd

Barrier	Related Information
Female condoms	Female condoms should be applied before any penetration occurs; even pre-ejaculation fluid can contain microorganisms. Lubrication decreases the chance of breakage during use, but only water-soluble lubricants should be used because substances such as petroleum jelly (Vaseline) may weaken the condom. Female condoms should never be reused and should be discarded properly after use so that others will not come in contact with contents.
Cervical caps or diaphragms	These may provide some protection for the cervix only. They are not effective barriers against sexually transmitted infections (STIs).
Rubber gloves, rubber dental dams, split (opened) male condoms	These may provide some barrier protection for manual and oral sex. Although some groups suggest that male condoms may be split down one side and opened or that rubber dental dam material may be taped over areas that have lesions to avoid direct contact with blood and body fluid, this very high-risk behavior is not recommended.
Double condoms	Anal intercourse is a very high-risk activity for transmission of many types of STIs as well as many intestinal organisms; it is not recommended. Wearing double condoms and using water-soluble lubricants, preferably containing nonoxynol-9, to decrease risk somewhat is advised if engaging in this type of sexual activity.

SUGGESTED ANSWERS TO CRITICAL THINKING

Mrs. Miller

1. You can educate Mrs. Miller about the possibility of neonatal infections from *Neisseria gonorrhoeae* and *Chlamydia trachomatis,* especially of the eyes. Institutional and governmental policies related to treatment should be explained. Care should be taken to explain to Mrs. Miller that treatment is widely used, so as not to make her feel she has a condition she has not been told about.
2. Because the benefits of prophylactic eye treatment of the neonate for *C. trachomatis* and *N. gonorrhoeae* exposure are generally seen as greater than the risks, it is recommended by governmental agencies and supported by most institutional policies to treat all newborns, regardless of known exposure, shortly after birth.

Kerri

1. Explain to Kerri that trichomoniasis is often a sexually transmitted infection but that the organism that causes the infection can be transmitted through infected articles during nonsexual contact and can survive a long time outside the body. Also explain that a person can be asymptomatic for many years following exposure to the organism before an outbreak occurs. Her partner could also have an undiagnosed infection.
2. You don't want to assume the health care provider is wrong. An approach might sound something like,

"I noticed in the drug guide that the usual dose is 2 grams, but I see you have written it for 4 grams."
3. Teach Kerri that treatment should be provided to her partner regardless of symptoms. Also, reinfection may occur if both partners are not treated. Teach her how the infection is spread and how to avoid it in the future. She and her partner should use condoms or remain abstinent until treatment is effectively completed. Be sure to tell her that she should abstain from alcohol while on metronidazole and for at least 48 hours following its completion. Patients who drink alcohol while taking it are very likely to vomit.

Stephanie

1. Concerns might include (a) the wish to speak with a health care worker, (b) uncertainty about whether patient information will be kept confidential (give assurance that if you knew about anyone with syphilis, it would be your professional responsibility to keep it confidential), (c) fear that she might have become infected through heterosexual contact, (d) a desire to protect herself by avoiding those who have syphilis, and (e) a desire for information about syphilis and its transmission routes.
2. The teaching plan might include information about the spirochete that causes syphilis, signs and symptoms, diagnostic tests, means of transmission, strategies for risk reduction, treatment, research, and rights and responsibilities of those who have the disease.

Review Questions

1. What signs and symptoms of sexually transmitted infections should nurses assess for in all patients? **Select all that apply.**
   1. Itching
   2. Discharge
   3. Dysuria
   4. Genital ulcers
   5. Genital warts
   6. Rectal pain

2. A young woman is seen at a walk-in clinic and is diagnosed with a sexually transmitted infection. She says, "How could I have one? I only have sex with my boyfriend. I don't sleep around!" Which of the following responses by the nurse is best?
   1. "You are right. That should have kept you safe. There just are no guarantees."
   2. "If your boyfriend is not infected, then it is apparent that you have had sex with someone else."
   3. "You or your boyfriend could be infected from past sexual encounters. He should also be tested at this time."
   4. "Even lifelong monogamy cannot prevent many sexually transmitted infections."

3. A home health care nurse is preparing to change a dressing on a patient who had genital warts removed the previous day. Which intervention should be completed first?
   1. Clean the wounds.
   2. Remove the old dressing.
   3. Assess for drainage.
   4. Administer an analgesic.

4. An older man is admitted to the hospital with mental status changes. As the nurse begins the shift assessment, the patient begins to cry and says his doctor thinks his problems stem from an untreated syphilis infection when he was in the military as a young man. Which response by the nurse is best?
   1. "Why didn't you have it treated when it occurred?"
   2. "What's done is done. It's unfortunate that treatment is too late now."
   3. "That must be upsetting for you. Do you want to talk about it?"
   4. "Don't cry. I am sure there is treatment that can help now."

5. A nurse has completed instruction related to sexually transmitted infection risk reduction with a 17-year-old woman. Which statement by the patient indicates that teaching has been effective?
   1. "I should avoid drinking alcohol when I will be in situations with potential sex partners."
   2. "If I make sure my partners wear condoms, I will be protected."
   3. "Use of a barrier method of birth control will prevent infection."
   4. "As long as I know my partner well, I am safe."

Answer rationales available in your online resources.

ANSWERS 1. 1, 2, 3, 4, 5, 6; 2. 3; 3. 4; 3. 4; 5. 1

Key Points

Find the chapter key points in your online resources available through Davis Edge.

Additional Resources

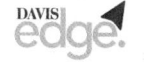 Use the scratch off code on the inside front cover of your book to access online quizzes that will help you to improve your scores on course exams and prepare for the NCLEX-PN®.

 Study Guide

CHAPTER 45

Musculoskeletal Function and Assessment

Cindy Leffel, Janice L. Bradford

KEY TERMS

arthrocentesis (AR-throw-sen-TEE-sis)
arthrogram (AR-throw-gram)
arthroscopy (ar-THROW-scop-ee)
articular (ar-TIK-yoo-lar)
bone (BOWN)
bursae (BUR-sah)
cartilage (car-TIL-ij)
crepitation (crep-ih-TAY-shun)
diaphysis (dye-uh-piff-uh-sis)
epiphyses (e-piff-uh-sees)
gout (GOWT)
hemarthrosis (heem-ar-THROW-sis)
joint (JOYNT)
ligament (LIG-uh-ment)
muscle (MUH-suhl)
osteoblast (ahs-TEE-oh-blast)
osteoclast (ahs-TEE-oh-clast)
periosteum (PEAR-ih-ahs-TEE-um)
resorption (ree-SORP-shun)
synarthrosis (sin-AR-throw-sis)
synovitis (sin-oh-VY-tis)
tendons (TEN-duns)
vertebrae (VER-teh-bray)

CHAPTER CONCEPT

Mobility

LEARNING OUTCOMES

1. Explain the anatomy and function of the musculoskeletal system.
2. Describe the effects of aging on the musculoskeletal system.
3. List subjective data that are collected when caring for a patient with a disorder of the musculoskeletal system.
4. List the objective data that are collected when caring for a patient with a disorder of the musculoskeletal system.
5. List areas included in a neurovascular assessment for the musculoskeletal system.
6. Identify diagnostic tests for musculoskeletal problems.
7. Describe the nursing care provided for patients undergoing diagnostic tests of the musculoskeletal system.

MUSCULOSKELETAL SYSTEM ANATOMY AND PHYSIOLOGY

The skeletal and muscular systems can be considered as one system because together they move the body. The skeleton is the framework of the body to which the voluntary **muscles** are attached. The framework includes the **joints,** or articulations, between **bones.** Contraction of a muscle stabilizes or changes the angle of a joint. Movement would not be possible without the proper functioning of the nervous, cardiovascular, and respiratory systems. Voluntary muscles require nerve impulses to contract, a continuous supply of blood provided by the circulatory system, and oxygen provided by the respiratory system.

MUSCULOSKELETAL SYSTEM TISSUES AND THEIR FUNCTIONS

The tissues that make up the skeletal system are primarily bone tissue, **articular** (joint) **cartilage** (cushions joint and reduces friction), and fibrous connective tissue that forms the **ligaments** (that connect bone to bone) and other structures within joints. The tissues of the muscular system include skeletal muscle tissue and fibrous connective tissue. The fibrous connective tissue forms **tendons** (which connect muscle to bone) and *fasciae* (the strong membranes enclosing individual muscles).

Besides its role in movement, the skeleton has other functions. It protects organs and tissues from mechanical injury. The brain is protected by the skull, and the heart and lungs are protected by the thoracic cage. Flat and irregular bones as well as the ends of long bones contain red bone marrow, the hematopoietic (blood-forming) tissue. These bones also store excess calcium, which may undergo **resorption** (bone broken down with minerals including calcium released into blood) for blood calcium homeostasis. Calcium in the blood is needed for blood clotting and for the proper functioning of nerves and muscles.

Although the primary function of the muscular system is to move or stabilize the skeleton, the voluntary muscles collectively contribute significantly to heat production, which maintains normal body temperature. Another important function of the muscular system is to aid in the return of blood from the legs through muscular compression on the leg veins.

Bone Tissue and Bone Growth

Bone tissue is composed of bone cells, called osteocytes, within a strong, nonliving matrix made of calcium salts and the protein collagen. In compact bone, the osteocytes and matrix are in precise, densely structured arrangements called osteons. In spongy bone, the arrangement of cells and matrix is more irregular and sparse. This gives the bone a spongy appearance. Compact bone forms the diaphyses (shafts) of the long bones, covers the spongy bone of the epiphyses of long bones, and covers the spongy bone that forms the bulk of short, flat, and irregular bones. The **periosteum** (connective tissue) covers all outer bone surfaces except at the joints, where cartilage covers the end of the bone. The periosteum provides protection, is involved in bone growth and repair (producing osteoblasts), and participates in the blood supply of bone.

Osteoblasts produce bone matrix during growth and replace matrix during normal remodeling or in repair of fractures. Other cells called **osteoclasts** resorb bone matrix when more calcium is needed in the blood or during repair when excess bone must be removed as bone changes shape.

The growth of bone from fetal life until final adult height depends on many factors. Proper nutrition (particularly vitamins and minerals) provides the raw material to produce bone matrix, comprising calcium, phosphorus, and protein. Vitamin D is essential for the efficient absorption of calcium and phosphorus in the small intestine. Vitamins A and C are required for the production process of bone matrix. Hormones directly needed for growth include growth hormone (GH) from the anterior pituitary gland, thyroxine from the thyroid gland, and insulin from the pancreas. GH increases mitosis and protein synthesis. Thyroxine stimulates osteoblasts and increases energy production. Insulin is essential for the efficient use of glucose to provide energy. If a child is lacking any of these hormones, growth is slower, and the child may not reach his or her genetic potential for height.

Bone is not a fixed tissue, even when growth in height has ceased. Calcium and phosphate are constantly being removed and replaced (remodeled) to maintain normal blood levels of these minerals. Parathyroid hormone, secreted by the parathyroid glands, increases the removal of calcium and phosphate from bones. The hormone calcitonin from the thyroid gland promotes the retention of calcium in bones.

Structure of the Skeleton

The 206 bones of the adult human skeleton are in two divisions: the axial and appendicular skeleton (Fig. 45.1; axial in white, appendicular in turquoise). The axial bones are flat or irregular bones and contain red bone marrow (hematopoietic tissue). Within the appendicular skeleton, the limbs consist of long bones (except the carpals, tarsals, and patella). All long bones have the same general structure: a central **diaphysis,** or shaft, with two ends called **epiphyses.**

Skull

The skull consists of eight cranial bones and 14 facial bones. It also contains the three auditory bones found in each middle ear cavity. All of the joints between the cranial bones and those between most of the facial bones are immovable joints called sutures (**synarthrosis**).

Vertebral Column

The vertebral column (or spinal column) is made of 33 individual bones called **vertebrae** (Fig. 45.2). *Atlas,* the first of seven cervical vertebra, articulates with the occipital bone of the skull and forms a pivot joint with the *axis,* the second cervical vertebra. The 12 thoracic vertebrae articulate with the posterior ends of the ribs. The five lumbar vertebrae are the largest and strongest. The *sacrum,* consisting of five fused sacral vertebrae, articulates with the *os coxae* at the sacroiliac joints. The coccyx, composed of four fused coccygeal vertebrae, serves as an attachment point for some muscles of the perineum.

The vertebrae as a unit form a flexible backbone that supports the trunk and head and that contains and protects the spinal cord. Spinal nerves and vessels exit via intervertebral foramina. Intervertebral discs cushion and permit movement of the column.

Thoracic Cage

The thoracic cage consists of 12 pairs of ribs and the sternum. The thoracic cage protects the heart and lungs as well as upper abdominal organs, such as the liver and spleen, from mechanical injury. During breathing, the flexible thoracic cage is pulled upward and outward by the external intercostal muscles to expand the chest cavity and bring about inhalation.

• **WORD · BUILDING** •

periosteum: peri—surrounding + osteo—bone
osteoblast: osteo—bone + blastanō—germinate
osteoclast: osteo—bone + klastēs—breaker
epiphyses: epi—upon + phyein—to grow
synarthrosis: sun—together + arthrosis—jointing

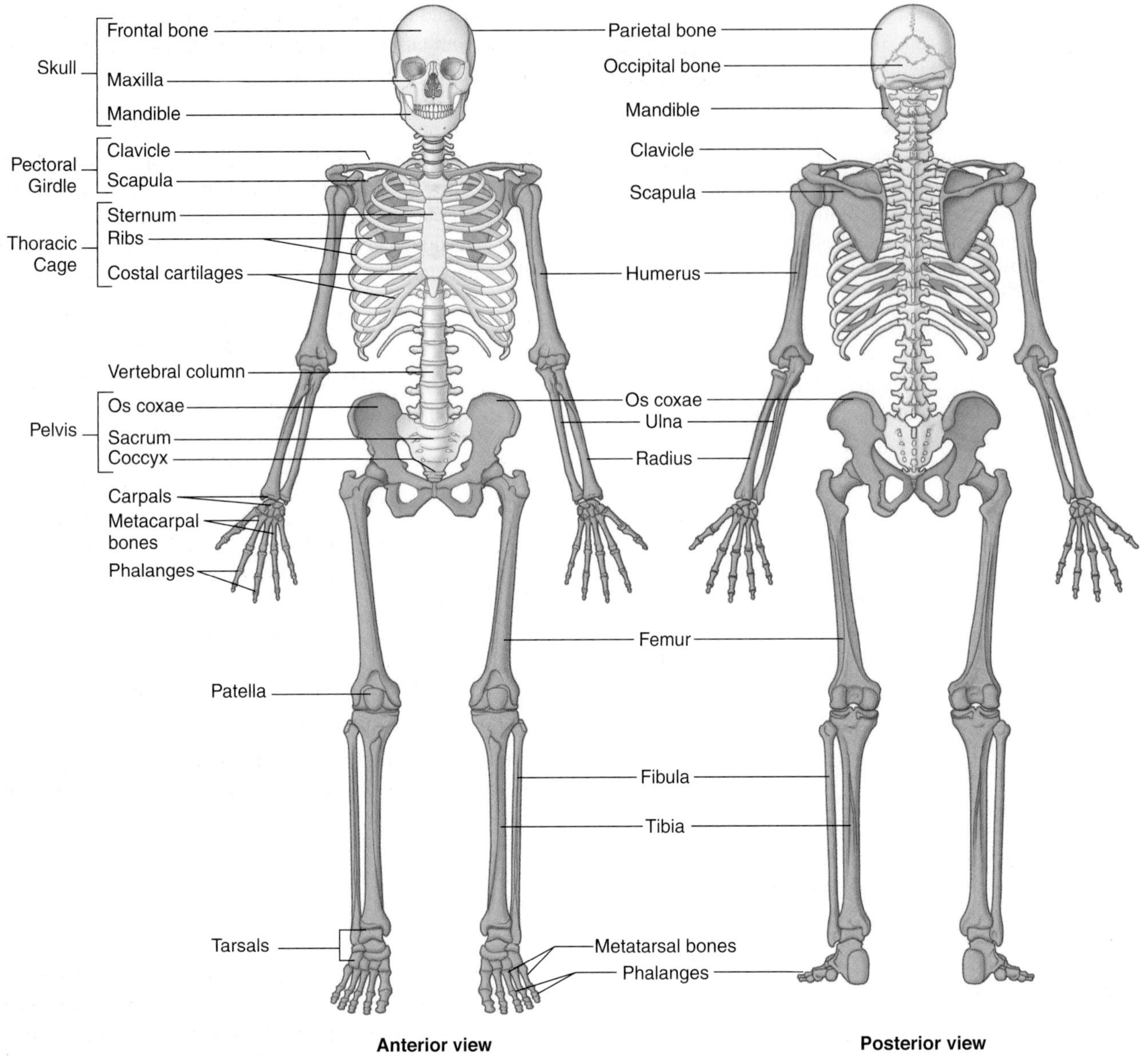

Skull
- Frontal bone
- Maxilla
- Mandible

Pectoral Girdle
- Clavicle
- Scapula

Thoracic Cage
- Sternum
- Ribs
- Costal cartilages

Vertebral column

Pelvis
- Os coxae
- Sacrum
- Coccyx

Carpals
Metacarpal bones
Phalanges

Patella

Tarsals

Parietal bone
Occipital bone
Mandible
Clavicle
Scapula
Humerus
Os coxae
Ulna
Radius
Femur
Fibula
Tibia
Metatarsal bones
Phalanges

Anterior view

Posterior view

FIGURE 45.1 Adult skeleton—anterior and posterior views.

Synovial Joints

The primary joints of the appendicular skeleton are summarized in Table 45.1. All freely movable joints (diarthroses) are synovial joints (Fig. 45.3). Many synovial joints also have **bursae** (small sacs of synovial fluid between the joint and structures that cross over the joint). Bursae lessen wear in areas of friction.

Muscle Structure and Arrangements

One muscle can consist of thousands of skeletal muscle cells (fibers), which are specialized for contraction. When a muscle contracts, it shortens and exerts force on a bone. Each muscle fiber receives its own motor nerve ending. The number of fibers that contract depends on the workload. Muscles are anchored to bones by tendons, which are made of fibrous connective tissue. A muscle usually has at least two tendons, each attached to a different bone. The more stationary muscle attachment is called its origin; the more movable attachment is the insertion.

The muscle itself crosses the joint formed by the two bones to which it is attached. When the muscle contracts, it pulls on the insertion, moving the bone in a particular direction. The muscle causing this particular action is termed the agonist.

There are approximately 700 skeletal muscles in the body (Fig. 45.4). The general type of arrangement is the agonist with opposing antagonists and the cooperative synergists. Without synergism, maintaining balance or having fine motor control for writing or talking would be difficult, if not impossible.

 ROLE OF THE NERVOUS SYSTEM

Skeletal muscles are voluntary: conscious control initiates nerve impulses to cause contraction. Nerve impulses originate in the motor areas of the frontal lobes of the cerebral cortex. The coordination of voluntary movement is a function of the cerebellum. Neurons in the central nervous system

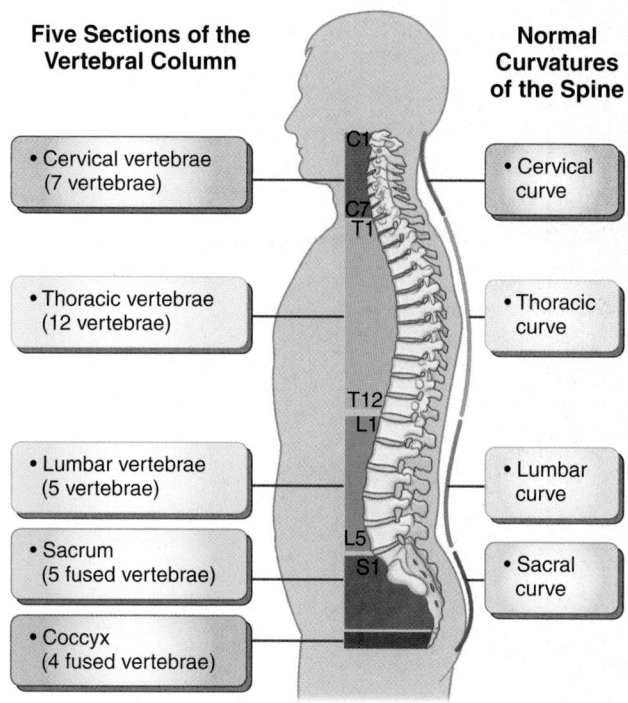

Five Sections of the Vertebral Column

- Cervical vertebrae (7 vertebrae)
- Thoracic vertebrae (12 vertebrae)
- Lumbar vertebrae (5 vertebrae)
- Sacrum (5 fused vertebrae)
- Coccyx (4 fused vertebrae)

Normal Curvatures of the Spine

- Cervical curve
- Thoracic curve
- Lumbar curve
- Sacral curve

FIGURE 45.2 Vertebral column.

Table 45.1
Joints of the Appendicular Skeleton

Type of Joint and Description	Examples
Symphysis—disk of fibrous cartilage between bones	Between vertebrae Between pubic bones
Ball and socket—movement in all planes	Scapula and humerus (shoulder) Pelvic bone and femur (hip)
Hinge—movement in one plane	Humerus and ulna (elbow) Femur and tibia (knee) Between phalanges (fingers and toes)
Combined hinge and planar	Temporal bone and mandible (lower jaw)
Pivot—rotation	Atlas and axis (neck) Radius and ulna (distal to elbow)
Gliding—side-to-side movement	Between carpals (wrist)
Saddle—movement in several planes	Carpometacarpal of thumb

Source: Modified from Scanlon, V. C., & Sanders, T. (2019). *Essentials of anatomy and physiology* (8th ed.). Philadelphia, PA: F.A. Davis.

(CNS) act involuntarily to regulate muscle tone, the state of slight contraction usually present in muscles. Healthy muscle tone is important for posture and coordination.

Neuromuscular Junction

Each of the fibers in a muscle has its own motor neuron ending. The neuromuscular junction is the termination of the motor neuron at the muscle fiber (synapse). The neuron releases the neurotransmitter acetylcholine (ACh), which signals the muscle to contract. Figure 45.5 illustrates the following steps:

1. When an impulse reaches the end of a motor neuron, it causes small vesicles in the axon terminal to release a neurotransmitter (chemical messenger) called acetylcholine (ACh) into the synaptic cleft (narrow space between the motor neuron and muscle fiber).
2. The ACh diffuses across the synaptic cleft, where it stimulates receptors in the sarcolemma (muscle fiber membrane).
3. This sends an electrical impulse over the sarcolemma and inward along the T tubules. The impulse in the T tubules causes the sacs in the sarcoplasmic reticulum to release calcium.
4. The calcium binds with the troponin on the actin filament to expose attachment points. In response, the myosin heads of the think filaments grab onto the thin filaments and muscle contraction occurs.

If a muscle has little work to do, few of its many muscle fibers contract; but if the muscle has more work to do, more of its muscle fibers contract.

AGING AND THE MUSCULOSKELETAL SYSTEM

The amount of calcium in bones depends on several factors. Good nutrition is certainly one factor, but age is another, especially for women. One function of estrogen (or testosterone in men) is the maintenance of a strong bone matrix. For women, after menopause, bone matrix loses more calcium than is replaced. The loss can be offset by weight-bearing physical exercise, which stimulates bone matrix deposition, increasing bone density.

Weight-bearing joints are also subject to damage after many years. Often the articular cartilage wears down and becomes rough, leading to pain and stiffness.

Muscle strength declines with age as protein synthesis decreases. Such loss of strength need not be exaggerated because aging muscles also benefit from regular exercise. Furthermore, maintenance of muscle strength reduces falls and accidents. Figure 45.6 presents a concept map that shows the effects the aging process has on the musculoskeletal system.

MUSCULOSKELETAL SYSTEM DATA COLLECTION

Practicing in a health care reform environment requires the delivery of patient-centered care and an interdisciplinary

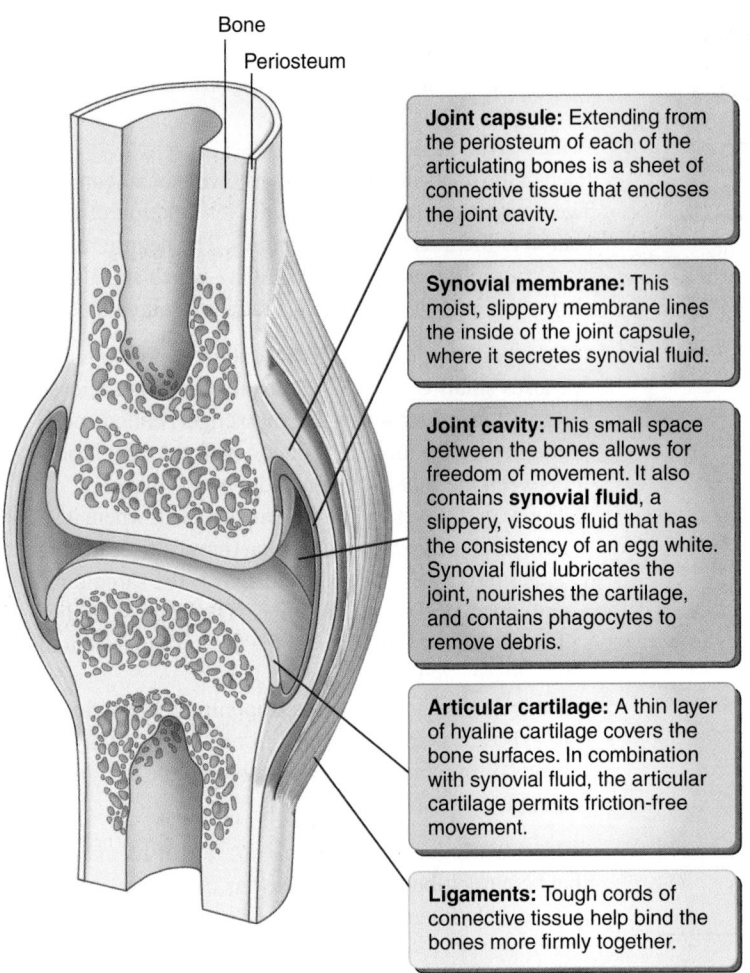

Bone

Periosteum

Joint capsule: Extending from the periosteum of each of the articulating bones is a sheet of connective tissue that encloses the joint cavity.

Synovial membrane: This moist, slippery membrane lines the inside of the joint capsule, where it secretes synovial fluid.

Joint cavity: This small space between the bones allows for freedom of movement. It also contains **synovial fluid,** a slippery, viscous fluid that has the consistency of an egg white. Synovial fluid lubricates the joint, nourishes the cartilage, and contains phagocytes to remove debris.

Articular cartilage: A thin layer of hyaline cartilage covers the bone surfaces. In combination with synovial fluid, the articular cartilage permits friction-free movement.

Ligaments: Tough cords of connective tissue help bind the bones more firmly together.

FIGURE 45.3 Synovial joints.

team approach. By working together, the interdisciplinary team can meet the patient and family needs as well as provide quality outcomes in a cost-efficient way.

Health History

Subjective data collection on the patient begins with a history that includes the condition's impact on the patient's life (Table 45.2). The **WHAT'S UP?** model can be used to assess the patient's pain (see Chapter 1).

Deformities resulting from arthritis or other musculoskeletal disorders can affect a patient's body image and self-concept and may result in social withdrawal (see Chapter 46). Chronic pain may keep the patient from working or socializing. Data collection should include questions related to the psychological effects of the musculoskeletal disorder. Patients may experience psychological stress from withdrawal from friends and family, pain, and loss of income. Determine the patient's ability to cope by asking what coping strategies have been used in the past for other life stressors and about support systems for the patient. As needed, consult the appropriate member(s) of the health care team (social work, clergy, support groups) to ensure that the patient's psychosocial needs are being met.

Physical Examination

Three areas of musculoskeletal data collection are important: inspection, range of motion (ROM), and muscle tone and palpation (Table 45.3). If the patient can walk, inspect posture and gait, noting poor posture or alterations in movement, such as limping. Note the use of mobility aids, such as a cane or walker. Document other gross deformities, such as unequal limbs, malalignment, or contractures. Spinal deformities are especially significant because they can compromise breathing and balance. Inspect the joints and muscles of the arms, hands, legs, and feet for deformity, redness, and swelling. Listen for **crepitation** (grating sound as joint or bone moves). Also note the patient's general nutritional status (e.g., normal, obese, emaciated).

Observe ROM and muscle tone as the patient performs activities of daily living. To check ROM in the hands, ask the patient to touch each finger, one by one, to the thumb (known as opposition) and then make a fist. Note the size, shape, strength, and tone of muscles. Evaluate bilateral muscle strength by asking the patient to grip your hands. This enables you to feel the strength and equality. The push of an extremity against your hand provides a general indication of muscle strength. More specific evaluation is performed by a physical therapist or an occupational therapist.

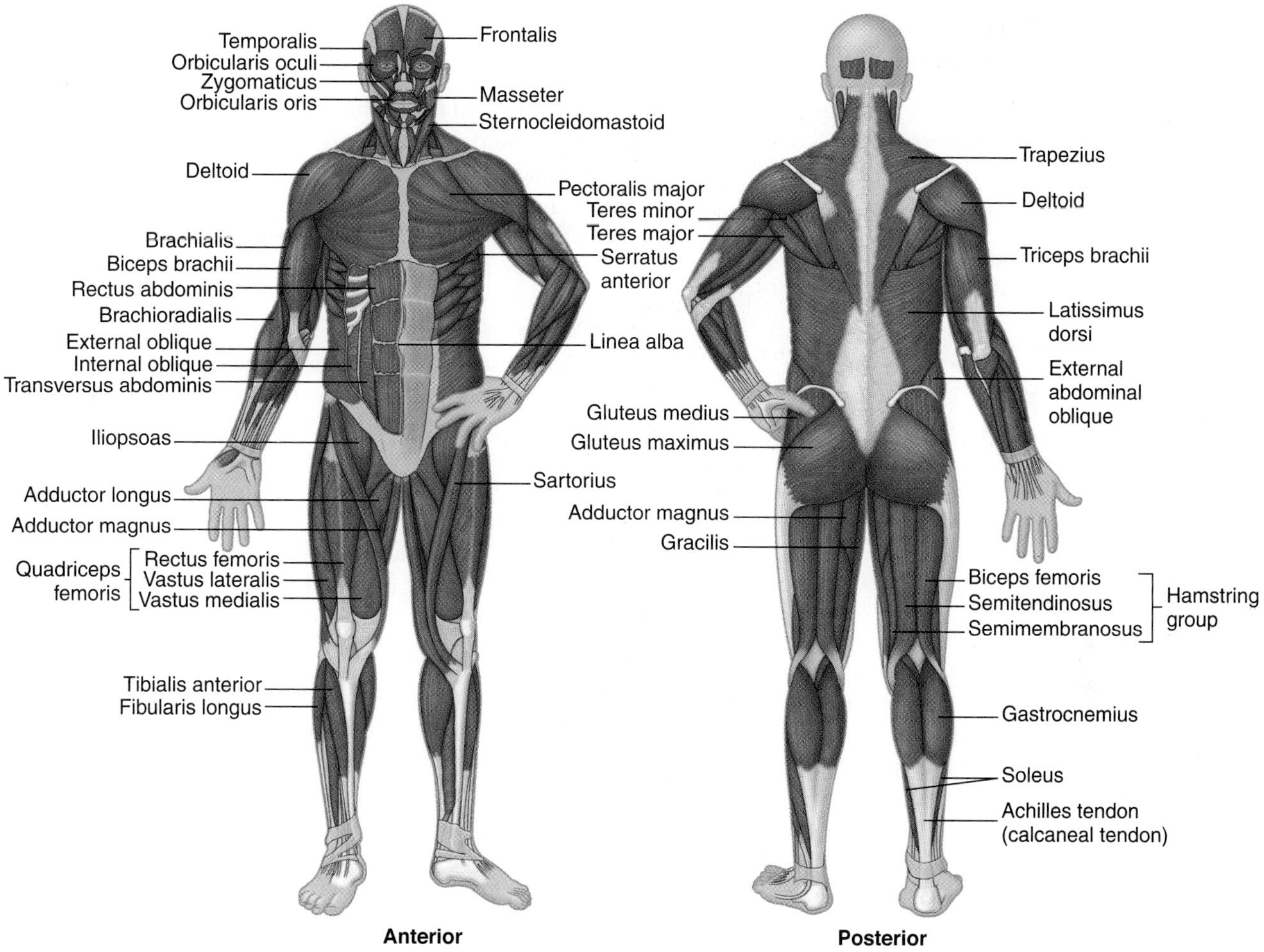

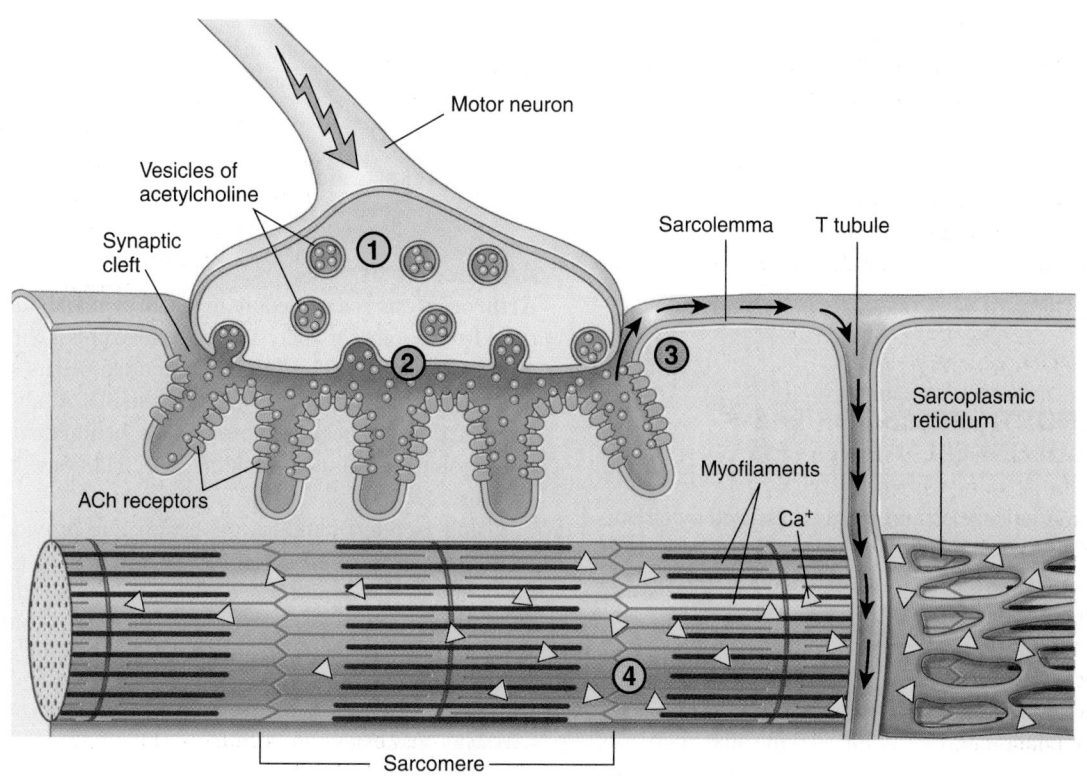

FIGURE 45.4 Superficial muscles.

Anterior

Posterior

Temporalis
Orbicularis oculi
Zygomaticus
Orbicularis oris
Frontalis
Masseter
Sternocleidomastoid
Deltoid
Pectoralis major
Teres minor
Teres major
Serratus anterior
Brachialis
Biceps brachii
Rectus abdominis
Brachioradialis
External oblique
Internal oblique
Transversus abdominis
Linea alba
Iliopsoas
Adductor longus
Adductor magnus
Sartorius
Quadriceps femoris { Rectus femoris, Vastus lateralis, Vastus medialis
Tibialis anterior
Fibularis longus

Trapezius
Deltoid
Triceps brachii
Latissimus dorsi
External abdominal oblique
Gluteus medius
Gluteus maximus
Adductor magnus
Gracilis
Biceps femoris
Semitendinosus
Semimembranosus } Hamstring group
Gastrocnemius
Soleus
Achilles tendon (calcaneal tendon)

FIGURE 45.5 How muscle fibers contract.

Motor neuron
Vesicles of acetylcholine
Synaptic cleft
Sarcolemma T tubule
ACh receptors
Sarcoplasmic reticulum
Myofilaments
Ca⁺
Sarcomere

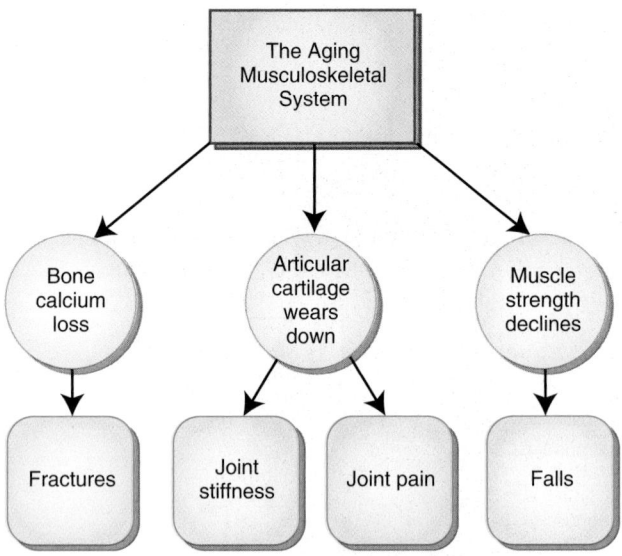

FIGURE 45.6 Aging and the musculoskeletal system.

Next, gently palpate for warmth and tenderness in the areas of swelling and in areas where the patient reported pain (being careful to minimize the pain this may cause). For example, reddened joints should be palpated for **synovitis** (swollen synovial tissue within the joint) or the presence of bony nodes. In some cases, joints and muscles may seem healthy but are tender when palpated. Frequent neurovascular assessments may be needed if there is a risk of circulation impairment, such as might happen if the patient has a fracture or has had musculoskeletal surgery (Table 45.4).

CRITICAL THINKING

Mrs. O'Donnell, age 80, is brought to the emergency department with a fractured left hip. She is positioned for comfort while you collect data.

1. What health history and subjective data should you collect for Mrs. O'Donnell?
2. What should be checked in Mrs. O'Donnell's physical examination?

   Suggested answers are at the end of the chapter.

DIAGNOSTIC TESTS FOR THE MUSCULOSKELETAL SYSTEM

Diagnosis of musculoskeletal problems is assisted by laboratory tests and diagnostic imaging and procedures (Table 45.5; see Appendix A). Specific tests for connective tissue diseases are described in Chapter 46.

Laboratory Tests
Alkaline Phosphatase
Alkaline phosphatase (ALP) is an enzyme that increases when bone is damaged. In metabolic bone diseases and bone cancer, ALP increases to reflect osteoblast (bone-forming cell) activity.

Calcium and Phosphorus
Bone disorders commonly cause changes in calcium and phosphorus (or phosphate) levels. In a healthy person, calcium and phosphorus have an inverse relationship. This means that when serum calcium increases, serum phosphorus decreases, and vice versa.

Muscle Enzymes
When muscle tissue is damaged, many serum enzymes are released into the bloodstream, including skeletal muscle creatine kinase (CK-MM [CK3]), aldolase (ALD), aspartate aminotransferase (AST), and lactate dehydrogenase (LDH).

Myoglobin
Myoglobin is a protein found in striated (skeletal or cardiac) muscle. It is what causes the red color of muscle. When skeletal muscle is damaged, myoglobin levels rise in the blood.

RHABDOMYOLYSIS. Rhabdomyolysis is a very serious and potentially fatal condition associated with muscle destruction due to an injury (such as crush syndrome), high fever, convulsions, or prolonged muscle compression. Creatine kinase (CK) levels can be five times greater than normal. If the patient has muscle destruction, look for elevated CK, myoglobin, and serum potassium levels to monitor for rhabdomyolysis. Observe for dark urine, muscle weakness, and myalgia (muscle pain). The goal of treatment is to restore normal fluid and electrolyte balance.

Uric Acid
Uric acid is normally found in blood. When uric acid levels rise in the serum, a condition called **gout** can occur (Chapter 46).

Other Tests
Additional explanations for some of the following diagnostic tests can be found in Appendix A.

Arthrocentesis
Arthrocentesis is a procedure in which synovial fluid is aspirated from a joint for analysis or to relieve pressure (improves pain and mobility). The fluid buildup often occurs secondary to an inflammatory process such as bursitis. Analysis of the synovial fluid can help diagnose crystals, **hemarthrosis** (blood in the joint cavity), noninflammatory conditions, and septic arthritis.

Using aseptic technique, the health care provider (HCP) administers a local anesthetic. A needle is used to aspirate the contents of the joint space. For analysis, the fluid is sent to the lab. If required, the HCP can instill medications such as corticosteroids, anti-inflammatories, or antibiotics. The site

• WORD • BUILDING •
synovitis: synovia—joint + itis—inflammation

Table 45.2

Subjective Data Collection for the Musculoskeletal System

Questions to Ask During the Health History	*Rationale/Significance*
Demographic	
What is your age, gender, socioeconomic status?	Increased age, being female, and lower socioeconomic status can increase risk of musculoskeletal injury/problems.
What is your occupation?	Enables discharge planning if occupation may be affected by condition.
Where do you live geographically?	Regions where sunlight is limited increases the risk of vitamin D deficiency, leading to increased risk for skeletal injuries.
Prior Health History	
Do you have allergies?	Prevents exposure to medication or compounds used in diagnostic tests, treatments, and therapies.
What prior medical conditions, surgeries, or problems with anesthesia (e.g., malignant hyperthermia) have you had?	Identifies any pre-existing conditions that may influence the musculoskeletal system.
What activities do you participate in, and how often?	Provides baseline information regarding the level of activity of the patient before the problem.
What risk factors for musculoskeletal problems are present (e.g., smoking, sedentary lifestyle, weight gains/losses)?	Smoking and a sedentary lifestyle are risk factors for musculoskeletal problems.
What is your nutritional intake?	Nutritional intake of calcium and vitamin D influences some musculoskeletal disorders.
What is your family's medical history?	Some musculoskeletal conditions or anesthesia problems have genetic and familial tendencies.
Injury or Present Concern	
What is the history of the injury or current concern?	Provides information that helps in the diagnosis of the problem as well as possible complications of the injury.
What is your pain level (use pain assessment scale)? What medications, treatments, and procedures are used to alleviate pain?	Pain or related stiffness and tenderness may be acute or chronic and may limit the patient in everyday life.
Psychosocial	
Are deformities, changes in body image, or self-concept present?	The patient may need assistance with strategies to cope with the stress of a possible chronic musculoskeletal condition.
What coping skills do you use? Who do you consider your support system?	Some musculoskeletal conditions require lifestyle alterations that can cause increased stress and difficulties in coping.

Table 45.3

Objective Data Collection for the Musculoskeletal System

Data to Collect	*Rationale/Significance*
Inspect, palpate, and observe range of motion (ROM) of area of concern or injury. Check asymmetry, limb length, deformity, swelling, and ecchymosis.	The nature and severity of an injury is identified. Altered gait, tone, size, shape, posture, contractures, deformities, ROM, pain, and effects on activities of daily living can be determined.
Check color, warmth, circulation, and movement of affected areas.	Nerve function, sensation, movement, weakness, and the potential development of compartment syndrome can be determined.
Palpate all pulses below involved area.	Alterations may indicate altered vascular integrity (and, therefore, tissue integrity) of affected area or demonstrate developing compartment syndrome.

Table 45.4

Neurovascular Data Collection

Monitor	*Report*
Movement	Alterations in movement
Sensation	Alterations in feeling; tingling or paresthesias
Capillary refill	Nailbed that does not blanch in 3–5 seconds
Color	Pallor, cyanosis, redness, or discoloration
Pulses	Diminished or absent distal pulses
Temperature	Unusual coolness or warmth
Pain	Pain that is worse on passive motion; pain that no longer responds to analgesics

is covered with a sterile dressing to prevent infection. Monitor the injection site for increased bruising, bleeding, redness, and warmth.

Arthroscopy

An arthroscope allows the surgeon to directly visualize a joint. The knee and shoulder are the joints most often evaluated. Because **arthroscopy** is an invasive procedure performed under local or light general anesthesia, the patient is treated as a surgical candidate in a same-day surgery setting.

The surgeon makes several small incisions and distends the joint with injected saline. The scope is inserted, and the joint is visualized from different angles. The joint is moved through ROM so tears, defects, or other soft tissue damage can be assessed and/or repaired through the scope using special instrumentation. Depending on the extent of the procedure, a bulky or small dressing wrapped with an elastic bandage may be applied.

The perianesthesia care nurse monitors the neurovascular status of the surgical limb frequently (see Table 45.4). A mild analgesic usually relieves pain. The patient resumes activities, as ordered, usually within 24 to 48 hours. If a surgical repair was performed, the patient may have activity restrictions and need a stronger analgesic.

Although complications are not common, teach the patient the following signs to report to the surgeon:

- Thrombophlebitis (extremity warmth, redness, swelling, tenderness, pain)
- Infection (fever or warmth, pain, redness, swelling at surgical site)
- Increased joint pain

If a repair was done during the surgery, the patient is seen by the surgeon in 1 week to check for complications and progress. Physical or occupational therapy may be ordered (see "Home Health Hints").

Bone or Muscle Biopsy

Bone or muscle tissue can be extracted for microscopic examination to confirm cancer, damage (muscle biopsy), infection (bone biopsy), or inflammation. A sterile pressure dressing is applied because bone is highly vascular. The nurse inspects the biopsy site for bleeding, swelling, and hematoma formation. Increased pain that is unresponsive to analgesic

• WORD • BUILDING •
arthroscopy: arthro—joint + scopy—to examine

T a b l e   4 5 . 5

Diagnostic Laboratory Tests for the Musculoskeletal System

Test (Serum)	Normal Value	Significance of Abnormal Findings
Alkaline phosphatase (ALP), total	*Male:* 35–142 units/L *Female:* 25–125 units/L	↑ Paget disease, metastatic bone cancer, new bone formation
Calcium, total	8.2–10.2 mg/dL	↑ bone cancer, extended immobilization, hypophosphatemia, Paget disease ↓ hyperphosphatemia, nutritional deficiency, osteomalacia
Creatine kinase (CK)	*Male:* 50–204 units/L *Female:* 36–160 units/L	↑ cellular destruction of cells that store CK, intramuscular injections
CK3 (MM) isoenzyme	96%–100%	↑ conditions that cause cellular damage
Phosphorus	2.5–4.5 mg/dL	↑ hypocalcemia, bone cancer ↓ hypercalcemia, gout, vitamin D deficiency
Myoglobin	*Male:* 28–72 ng/mL *Female:* 25–58 ng/mL	↑ skeletal muscle destruction
Uric acid	*Male:* 4–8 mg/dL *Female:* 2.5–7 mg/dL Over 60 years: *Male:* 4.2–8.2 mg/dL *Female:* 3.5–7.3 mg/dL	↑ gout

medication may indicate bleeding into the soft tissue. Vital signs and neurovascular assessments are monitored (see Table 45.4).

Bone Density Scan

A bone density test measures bone strength. There are several types of scans. One example that uses a special x-ray process is the dual-energy x-ray absorptiometry (DEXA). This test measures the spine, hip, and total body bone density. Other tests measure other body areas such as the heel, fingers, or wrist. DEXA is used to diagnose osteoporosis (see Chapter 46).

Computed Tomography

Computed tomography (CT) scan is helpful for diagnosing problems of the joints or vertebral column (Fig. 45.7).

Magnetic Resonance Imaging

Magnetic resonance imaging (MRI) diagnoses musculoskeletal problems, especially those involving soft tissue ("Patient Perspective"). An MRI is more accurate than a CT scan for diagnosing many problems of the vertebral column (Fig. 45.8). If the patient has had previous spinal surgery, a contrast medium is used. See patient teaching guidelines for screening and preparation information for MRI on Davis Edge.

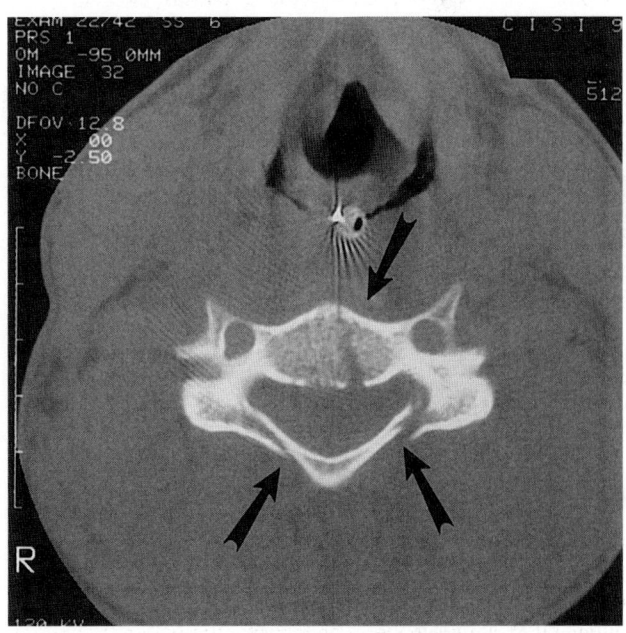

FIGURE 45.7 Computed tomography (CT) scan of fifth cervical vertebra showing a burst fracture of the vertebral body (*top arrow*) and both laminae (*bottom arrows*).

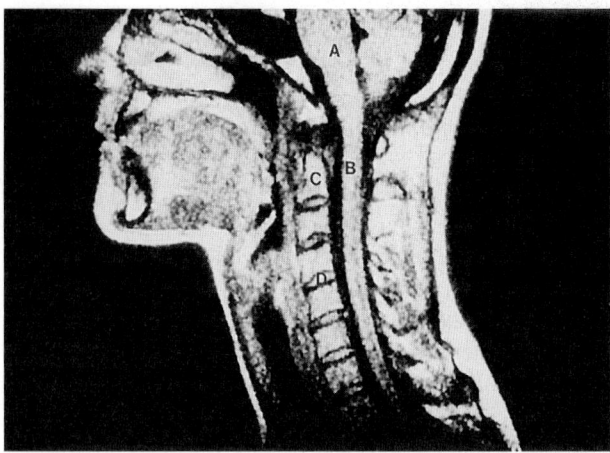

FIGURE 45.8 Magnetic resonance image (MRI) of a normal cervical spine. (A) Cerebellum. (B) Spinal cord. (C) Marrow of C2 vertebral body. (D) C4–5 intervertebral disk.

Patient Perspective

Emily. After a traumatic injury, I had magnetic resonance imaging (MRI) and was instructed on the procedure. I knew I had to lie still and not move. I knew if I opened my eyes, I would be scared, so I kept them closed. I did take a peek and saw part of the machine just inches from my face. I closed my eyes and repeated in my head, "Inhale, exhale, relax. Inhale, exhale, relax," a mantra I had learned in yoga class. I could feel myself going in and out of consciousness, but when I was conscious, I repeated my mantra, the only thing that helped me hang on to reality. I didn't feel any pain. Before I knew it, the test was over, and I felt relieved. My personal coping techniques really helped me through the MRI so that I could complete the test. Providing information to your patients on what to expect during the test as well as coping methods to use can help them successfully complete an MRI.

BE SAFE!

Ensure patient has no contraindications for magnetic resonance imaging (MRI) related to metal in the body, such as implants, shrapnel, or a pacemaker, to prevent injury to the patient.

Myelography

Myelography is usually reserved for patients unable to have a CT scan or MRI or for complicated spinal surgery revisions. Inform patients that they may be positioned head down for a short period to allow injected contrast medium to flow up to the level of the neck.

Nerve Conduction Studies

Electromyography (EMG) measures a muscle's electrical impulses. This helps diagnosis muscle diseases or nerve damage, which may follow a traumatic injury. Instruct the patient not to apply lotions before the test and to remove all jewelry. Occasionally, slight discomfort and bruising occur at the site where the study occurred. Warm compresses or mild analgesics can be offered for pain relief.

Nuclear Medicine Scans

A bone scan allows visualization of the entire skeleton. The patient is injected with a radioisotope. The radioisotope is attracted to bone and travels to bone tissue. Images are taken at various intervals to see how the radioisotope has collected in the bone. Gallium and thallium are radioisotope examples. Gallium concentrates in areas of tumors, inflammation, and infections. Thallium identifies bone cancer, especially osteosarcoma.

Patients are instructed to remove all jewelry before the test. For an accurate test, the patient must be able to lie still for up to 90 minutes during scanning. Patients who are older adults, restless, agitated, or in pain may, therefore, find this test uncomfortable. Sedatives or analgesics may have to be administered before or during the procedure.

The HCP looks for "hot spots" on the test results. Hot spots are created by increased circulation in abnormal bone areas that concentrates the radioactive substance there. Hot spots indicate bone disease.

Radiographs (X-Rays)

X-ray examination is used to determine bone alignment, density, erosion, swelling, and soft tissue damage (e.g., ligaments and tendons) because of alterations in bone position and spacing.

Arthrogram (or arthrography) is an x-ray examination of a synovial joint, most often the knee and shoulder, after joint trauma. Air or a contrast medium is injected into a synovial joint, which is then x-rayed. Inform the patient that the test is uncomfortable during injection. Joint swelling is common after the procedure. Apply ice, elevate the limb, and inform the patient to rest the joint for 12 to 24 hours after procedure as ordered.

Ultrasonography

Sound waves are used to detect osteomyelitis (bone infection), soft tissue disorders, traumatic joint injuries, and surgical hardware placement.

• WORD • BUILDING •
arthrogram: arthro a—joint + gram a—diagram

CRITICAL THINKING

Mrs. Gardenio, 84 years old, fell when using a step stool in her home. She was taken to the hospital, where it was determined that she had a femoral neck fracture of her left hip.

1. What data should you obtain from Mrs. Gardenio?
2. What possible condition may be the cause of her fracture?
3. What tests may be performed to identify the condition creating her problem?
4. Mrs. Gardenio is to receive morphine 4 mg by intramuscular injection now. You have available morphine 5 mg/mL. How many milliliters will you give?
5. What should be included in a teaching plan for home safety for Mrs. Gardenio?

Suggested answers are at the end of the chapter.

Home Health Hints

- According to the Social Security Act, to be considered homebound, a Medicare patient must meet the following criteria:

    1. Because of illness or injury, the patient needs the aid of supportive devices such as crutches, canes, wheelchairs, and walkers; the use of special transportation; or the assistance of another person to leave his or her place of residence. Or, the patient must have a condition such that leaving his or her home is medically contraindicated.

    2. Additionally, there must exist a normal inability to leave home, and leaving home must require a considerable and taxing effort.

- If it is determined that the patient is not homebound, then services such as physical and occupational therapy can be performed in an outpatient setting.
- Observe patients performing their activities of daily living to determine their functional abilities. Observe the patient's dress and hygiene. Do not rely on the patient's self-report of functional abilities. Older patients may try to hide their deficits out of fear that they will not be allowed to stay in their own homes.
- If the home health nurse identifies that the patient is at risk for falls or if the patient has had recent falls, request a physical therapy referral.
- Teach caregivers to use sand or cat box litter on icy steps to increase traction, preventing slips and falls.

SUGGESTED ANSWERS TO CRITICAL THINKING

Mrs. O'Donnell

1. Determine whether Mrs. O'Donnell has any allergies to medications, how and when the injury occurred, whether she has had any previous surgeries, what medications she takes, her medical history, and any past problems with anesthesia (including her family).
2. Inspect and compare her left leg with her right leg, including limb length, deformity, pain, loss of range of motion, edema, and ecchymosis. Perform neurovascular checks, including movement, sensation (numbness/tingling), presence of pulses, skin temperature, color, and capillary refill.

Mrs. Gardenio

1. Identify Mrs. Gardenio's age, allergies, her nutritional intake, what she was doing at the time of the injury, whether anything like this has happened before, whether anything similar has happened to any of her relatives, her pain level, when she ate last, her medications, her medical history, and whether she uses tobacco products.
2. Mrs. Gardenio may have osteoporosis that has resulted in a pathological fracture from decreased bone density. This is common in postmenopausal women.
3. X-ray examinations, bone scans, bone density tests, and laboratory tests, including serum alkaline phosphatase, calcium, phosphorus, thyroid, and vitamin D levels, are tests that might be performed.
4. Unit analysis method:

$$\frac{4 \text{ mg}}{} \left| \frac{1 \text{ mL}}{5 \text{ mg}} = \frac{4 \text{ mL}}{5} = 0.8 \text{ mL} \right.$$

5. Discuss home safety and ways to avoid the use of a step stool to keep the patient free from injury.

Review Questions

1. The nurse is assigned to care for a patient who has been diagnosed with a musculoskeletal disease that causes decreased bone density. Which data collection questions are most appropriate by the nurse? **Select all that apply.**
   1. "Do you have any broken bones?"
   2. "Has your doctor informed you not to exercise so you will not break a bone?"
   3. "What forms of physical activity are you able to participate in?"
   4. "Does your spouse have bone problems?"
   5. "Do you exercise regularly?"
   6. "What is typically included in your daily diet?"

2. The nurse is caring for a patient with a fractured left leg. Which of the following findings during a neurovascular assessment of the lower extremities would the nurse recognize as a priority to report to the health care provider?
   1. Strong bilateral left leg post tibial pulse
   2. Right foot capillary refill less than 2 seconds
   3. Bilateral dorsal flexion
   4. Pallor of the left leg

3. A patient is scheduled for magnetic resonance imaging of the pelvis. Which of the following actions would the nurse take if during data collection it was revealed that the patient had had a previous surgery for heart problems?
   1. Ask if there is any metal in the patient's body.
   2. Obtain an order for a chest x-ray
   3. Cancel the magnetic resonance imaging.
   4. Inform the physician.

4. The nurse is caring for a patient who has undergone a right knee arthroscopy. Two hours after the procedure, the patient's right pedal pulse is diminished compared with the previous assessment. What action should the nurse take?
   1. Take vital signs.
   2. Notify the surgeon.
   3. Perform neurovascular assessment in 30 minutes.
   4. Change the dressing and rewrap the elastic wrap.

5. The nurse is caring for a patient who is undergoing an arthroscopy of the knee with ligament repair. Which of the following would be included in nursing preoperative care for the patient the morning of surgery? **Select all that apply.**
   1. Provide toast and clear juice 6 hours before surgery.
   2. Provide clear liquids up to 2 hours before surgery.
   3. Explain the surgical procedure.
   4. Explain the anesthetic agents.
   5. Reinforce how to perform coughing and deep-breathing exercises.
   6. Teach the patient to perform straight-leg raises.

Answer rationales available in your online.

ANSWERS 1. 3, 5, 6; 2. 4; 3. 1; 4. 2; 5. 1, 2, 5

Key Points

Find the chapter key points in your online resources available through Davis Edge.

Additional Resources

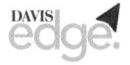 Use the scratch off code on the inside front cover of your book to access online quizzes that will help you to improve your scores on course exams and prepare for the NCLEX-PN®.

 Study Guide

CHAPTER 46

Nursing Care of Patients With Musculoskeletal and Connective Tissue Disorders

Cindy Leffel

KEY TERMS

arthritis (ar-THRY-tis)
arthroplasty (AR-throw-PLAS-tee)
avascular necrosis (ah-VAS-cue-lar neh-KROW-sis)
fasciotomy (fash-ee-OTT-oh-mee)
hemipelvectomy (heh-mee-pel-VEC-tuh-mee)
hyperuricemia (HY-purr-yoor-eh-SEE-mee-ah)
osteomyelitis (AWS-tee-oh-my-eh-LY-tis)
osteosarcoma (AWS-tee-oh-sar-KOH-mah)
replantation (ree-plan-TAY-shun)
rhabdomyolysis (rab-DOE-my-oh-LY-sis)
synovitis (sin-oh-VY-tis)

CHAPTER CONCEPTS

Mobility
Self

LEARNING OUTCOMES

1. Explain the pathophysiology, signs and symptoms, and complications of fractures.
2. Plan nursing care for a patient in a splint, cast, traction, or external fixation.
3. Describe the causes and prevention of osteomyelitis.
4. Plan nursing care for osteomyelitis.
5. Describe risk factors, pathophysiology, treatment, and nursing care for osteoporosis.
6. Describe the pathophysiology, treatment, and nursing care for gout.
7. Compare the care for osteoarthritis and rheumatoid arthritis.
8. Plan nursing care for the patient with a fractured hip.
9. Plan nursing care for a patient having a total joint replacement.
10. Explain patient teaching for a patient with a lower extremity amputation and prosthesis.

 BONE AND SOFT TISSUE DISORDERS

Strains

A strain is a soft tissue injury that occurs when a muscle or tendon is excessively stretched. Causes of strains include falls, excessive exercise, and lifting heavy items. A mild strain causes minimal inflammation. Swelling and tenderness are present. A moderate strain involves partial tearing of the muscle or tendon fibers. Pain and inability to move the affected body part result. The most severe strain occurs when a muscle or tendon is ruptured, with separation of muscle from muscle, tendon from muscle, or tendon from bone. Severe pain and disability result from this injury.

RICE is an acronym for *R*est, *I*ce, *C*ompression, and *E*levation, which is the therapy for strain injuries. Immediately after a strain, the injured area should be *R*ested to protect it. *I*ce should be applied to decrease swelling and pain. Applying an elastic bandage for *C*ompression and *E*levating the affected area (if appropriate) provide support to the strained

area and reduce swelling. After swelling stops, heat application (15 to 30 minutes four times a day) brings increased blood flow to the injured area for healing. Activity is limited until the soft tissue heals. Nonsteroidal anti-inflammatory drugs (NSAIDs) and muscle relaxants may be prescribed. For severe strains, surgical repair may be needed.

Sprains

A sprain is excessive stretching of ligaments from twisting movements during a sports activity, exercise, or fall. A mild sprain involves the tearing of a few ligament fibers, which causes tenderness. RICE and NSAIDs are used for several days until swelling and pain diminish. In a moderate sprain, more fibers are torn, but the stability of the joint is not affected. Moderate sprains may need immobilization with a brace or cast. A moderate sprain is uncomfortable, especially with activity. A severe sprain causes instability of the joint and usually requires surgical intervention for tissue repair or grafting. Pain and inflammation restrict mobility.

Dislocations

A dislocation is a common injury in which the ends of the bones (joints) are moved out of their normal position. This is usually caused by trauma or a disease such as rheumatoid arthritis. Severe pain, loss of range of motion of the joint, and joint deformity occur. Keep the joint immobile and apply ice. Immediate medical treatment is required to preserve function. Do not move the joint because blood vessels, muscles, and nerves could be damaged.

BE SAFE!

For patients with disease processes that could result in a dislocation or fracture, careful moving is essential. Use lifting devices such as draw sheets and mechanical devices when moving a patient rather than pulling on the patient's extremities to avoid patient injury. Follow institutional policy for moving patients to avoid patient injury and liability for a patient's injury.

Bursitis

Bursae (fluid-filled sacs) cushion tendons during movement to prevent friction between the bone and tendon. Several joints have bursae (e.g., shoulder, elbow, hip, knee, ankle, heel). Inflammation of a bursa is called bursitis. It occurs from **arthritis,** gout, repetitive movement, or sleeping on one's side that compresses the shoulder bursa. Prevention is key because bursitis may become harder to cure over time. Teach patients to stretch and strengthen muscles, move frequently, avoid repetitive movements for long periods, use cushioned seats, and avoid leaning on the elbows.

Symptoms of bursitis include achy pain, stiffness, or burning pain over the joint area that worsens with activity. Usually pain decreases in about a week. The condition can become chronic if it lasts more than 6 months. Treatment includes resting the joint and application of ice 20 minutes several times per day until joint warmth is gone and then switching to heat. Other treatment options include elevating the joint, ultrasound, massage, NSAIDs, or physical therapy.

Rotator Cuff Injury

Short tendons that are connected to muscles around the shoulder form the rotator cuff. The cuff covers the top, front, and back of the shoulder. Muscle contraction causes these tendons to tighten and move or rotate the shoulder. Various cuff injuries can occur. With chronic impingement syndrome, the top tendon of the cuff (supraspinatus tendon) and bursae become impinged in the narrow space under the acromion bone. This causes inflammation when the arm is repeatedly moved forward, and pain results. Over time, the tendon can tear from the bone.

Symptoms of rotator cuff injury include shoulder aching, increased pain with lifting the arm, pain that is greater at night, weakness, and sometimes limited range of motion. Magnetic resonance imaging (MRI) diagnoses the injury. For minor injury, resting the shoulder, ice, NSAIDs, and physical therapy are recommended. For a severe injury, arthroscopic and/or small-incision surgery relieves the impingement or repairs the tear. A sling or special brace is worn after surgery. Physical therapy is ordered for rehabilitation.

Carpal Tunnel Syndrome

Carpal tunnel syndrome results in the compression of the median nerve within the carpal tunnel when there is swelling in the tunnel. The swelling can result from edema, trauma, rheumatoid arthritis, or repetitive hand movements (repetitive motion injury) used in some occupations such as typing or factory work. Preventative measures include alternating nonrepetitive tasks with repetitive movements and using ergonomically appropriate devices to minimize the pressure placed in the area of the wrist. Slow-onset finger, hand, and arm pain and numbness may occur. Painful tingling and paresthesia may also be present. Eventually, fine motor deficits and then muscle weakness may develop. Diagnosis is based on signs and symptoms, patient history, and a positive Phalen test (numbness with wrist flexion). Electromyography detects nerve abnormalities.

Treatment initially aims to relieve the inflammation and rest the wrist using a splint. NSAIDs or cortisone injection into the tunnel reduce inflammation and pain. Endoscopic or open incision surgery may be needed to release the median nerve from compression. After surgery, elevate the patient's hand. Explain the use of a splint as ordered. Teach the patient that lifting is restricted for several weeks as well as signs and symptoms of neurovascular compromise to report. These include numbness and tingling, coolness, lack of pulse, pale skin or nailbeds, or limited movement. Physical therapy helps recover extremity function.

Fractures

A fracture is a break in a bone that can be minor and treated on an ambulatory basis or complex with surgical intervention and rehabilitation.

Pathophysiology

Bone is a dynamic, changing tissue. When it is broken, the body immediately begins to repair the injury (Fig. 46.1). For an adult, within 48 to 72 hours after the injury, a hematoma (blood clot) forms at the fracture site because bone has a rich blood supply. Various cells that begin the healing process are attracted to the damaged bone. In about a week, a nonbony union called a callus develops and is seen on x-ray examination. As healing continues, osteoclasts (bone-destroying cells) resorb necrotic bone, and osteoblasts (bone-building cells) make new bone as a replacement. This process is referred to as bone remodeling. Young, healthy adult bone completely heals in about 6 weeks; however, it can take up to a year

• WORD • BUILDING •
arthritis: arthr(on)—joint + itis—inflammation

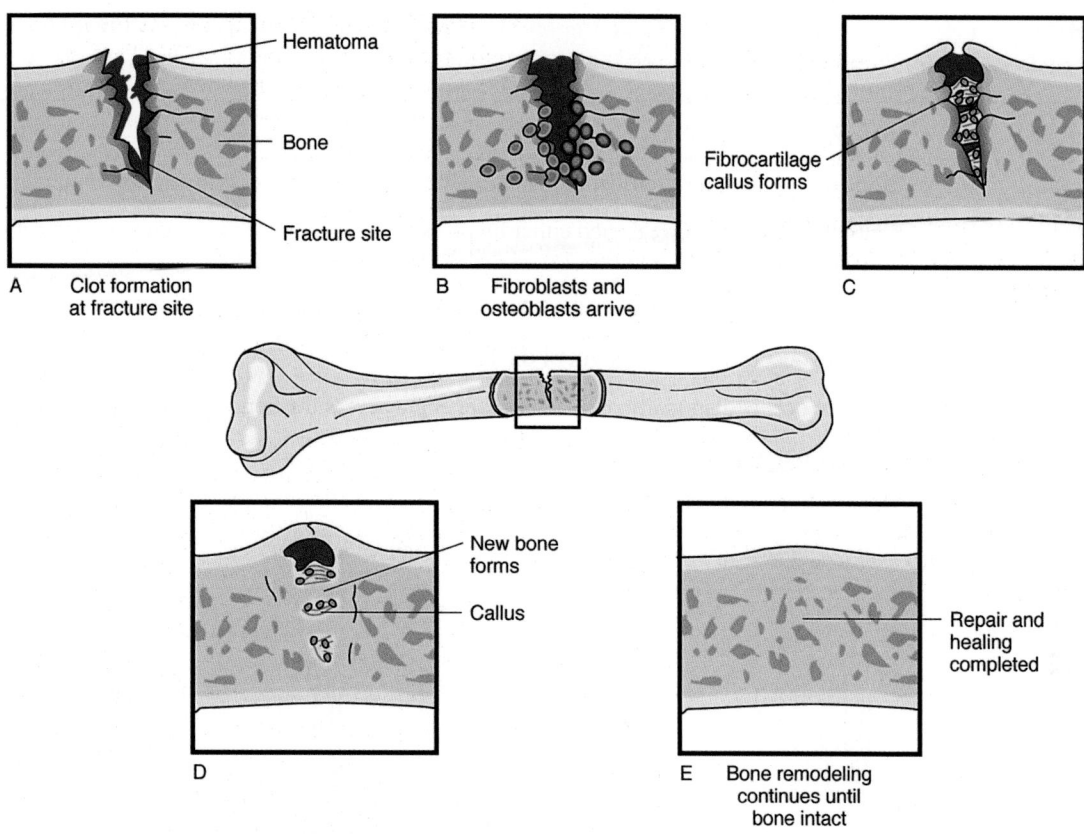

FIGURE 46.1 Fracture healing phases.

before the whole process of remodeling is complete. An older person's bones take longer to heal. Adequate nutrition that includes vitamins, minerals, and protein is essential to heal fractures (see Chapter 45).

Etiology and Types

Fractures are caused by a fall, an accident, or a crushing injury. Bone disease, such as osteoporosis; metastatic bone cancer; malnutrition; and regular intake of carbonated beverages containing phosphoric acid (which may interfere with calcium absorption) can lead to fractures. Side effects from some medications can cause a decrease in bone density,

resulting in fracture. When fractures result from disease, they are referred to as pathological fractures.

There are many types of fractures (Table 46.1) Fractures can be described by the way the bone breaks (spiral or oblique; Fig. 46.2). In a complete fracture, the bone is broken into two separate pieces. Complete fractures have the potential to be life threatening because sharp bone fragments can sever blood vessels and nerves. In an incomplete fracture, the bone does not divide into two pieces. With a displaced fracture, the bone sections are out of alignment. In a closed fracture, the bone does not disrupt the skin. In an open fracture, the bone breaks the skin. Open fractures create a risk for infection.

Table 46.1
Types of Fractures

Fracture Type	Description
Avulsion	A piece of bone is torn away from the main bone while still attached to a ligament or tendon.
Comminuted	Bone is splintered or shattered into numerous fragments. Often occurs in crushing injuries.
Impacted	Bone is forcibly pushed together, resulting in bone being pushed into bone.
Greenstick	Bone is bent and fractures on the outer arc of the bend. Often seen in children.
Interarticular	Fracture involves bones within a joint.

Continued

Table 46.1

Types of Fractures—cont'd

Fracture Type	Description
Displaced	Bone pieces are out of normal alignment. One or more pieces may be out of alignment.
Pathological (also called neoplastic)	Caused when bone is weakened either by pressure from a tumor or an actual tumor within the bone.
Spiral	Fracture curves around the shaft of the bone.
Longitudinal	Fracture occurs along the length of the bone.
Oblique	Fracture occurs diagonally or at an oblique angle across the bone.
Stress	Results in the bone being fractured across one cortex. This is an incomplete fracture.
Transverse	Bone is fractured horizontally.
Depressed	Bone is pushed inward. Often seen with skull and facial fractures.

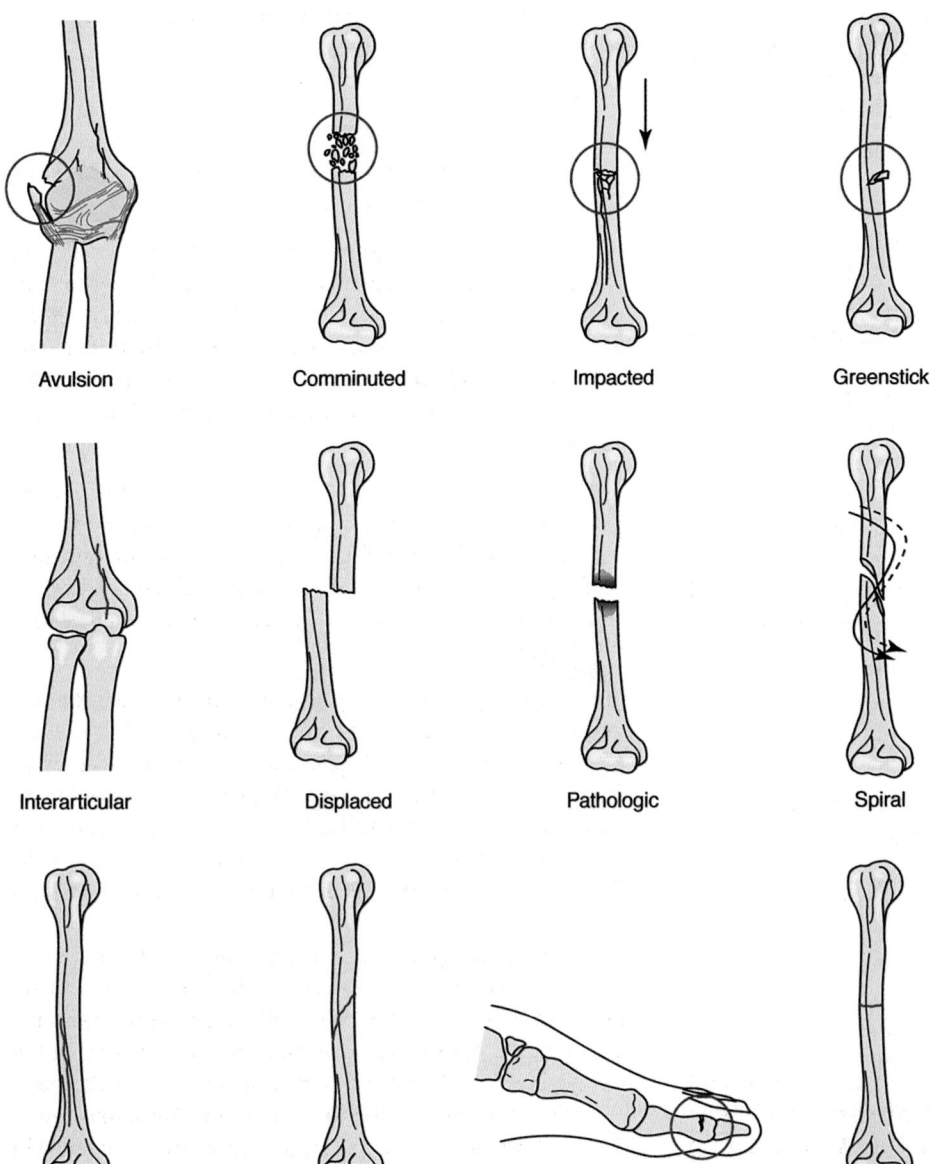

Avulsion   Comminuted   Impacted   Greenstick

Interarticular   Displaced   Pathologic   Spiral

Longitudinal   Oblique   Stress   Transverse   **FIGURE 46.2** Types of fractures.

Signs and Symptoms

This section focuses on fractures of upper and lower extremities. If the patient sustains a hairline (microscopic) fracture, the signs and symptoms are not readily observable. The patient may report tenderness over the site of the injury or more severe pain when moving the affected part of the body. The patient with a hip fracture usually experiences pain either in the groin area (the hip is a deep joint) or at the back of the knee (referred pain). If the fracture is complete, the limb is often shortened because of contraction of the muscles pulling on the bone sections.

In addition to pain, patients with more complex fractures experience limb rotation or deformity and shortening of the limb (if a limb bone is broken). Range of motion is decreased. With movement, a continuous grating sound (crepitation) caused by bone fragments rubbing on each other may be heard. Do not move the extremity as damage could occur to nerves and blood vessels.

Inspect the skin for intactness. A patient with a closed fracture may have ecchymosis (bruising) over the fractured bone from bleeding into the soft underlying tissue. Swelling may also be present and can impair blood flow, causing marked neurovascular compromise. In an open fracture, one or more bone ends pierce the skin, causing a wound.

Diagnostic Tests

An x-ray examination can visualize bone fractures and show bone malalignment or disruption. A computed tomography (CT) scan detects fractures of complex areas such as the hip and pelvis. MRI shows the extent of associated soft tissue damage. A serum calcium level may be ordered to determine baseline values for bone repairs. With moderate to severe bleeding, hemoglobin and hematocrit levels are checked.

Emergency Treatment

Box 46.1 describes urgent care for the patient with an extremity fracture. A patient with a fracture often has other injuries. Observe the patient for respiratory distress, bleeding, and head or spine injury. Emergency care for these problems is provided prior to fracture care.

LEARNING TIP

For emergency care of a suspected fracture, do not try to reposition the limb. Remember: Splint it as it lies. Also ensure that the limb is secured above and below the fracture to minimize movement and bone grating (crepitation).

Fracture Management

The goals of fracture management are reduction (alignment) of bone ends; immobilization of the fractured bone; preservation or restoration of surrounding soft tissue structures, such as vessels, tendons, ligaments, and muscles; prevention of

---

Box 46.1

Urgent Management of Fractures

1. Immediately immobilize the affected limb. If movement is required for splinting, support the limb above and below the fracture.
2. Unless there is bleeding, apply splints and padding above and below the fracture site, directly over the clothing. For bleeding, the site may need to be seen before pressure can be applied to the origin of the bleeding. Keep the patient covered to preserve body heat.
3. If the fracture is in the leg, the other leg can be used as a splint by bandaging both legs together. An arm can be bandaged to the chest or put into a sling to minimize further tissue damage.
4. Assess color, warmth, circulation, and movement of the limb distal to the fracture.
5. For an open fracture, the protruding bone should be covered with a clean (sterile preferred) dressing.
6. Do not attempt to straighten or realign a fractured extremity. Move the affected limb as little as necessary.
7. If not in a hospital, transport for emergency medical care as soon as possible.

---

deformity or further injury; preservation or restoration of function; promotion of early healing; and pain relief.

CLOSED REDUCTION. Closed reduction is the most common treatment for simple fractures. Analgesia and/or procedural sedation is given before the procedure. While manually pulling on the bone (limb), the health care provider (HCP) manipulates the bone ends into alignment. An x-ray confirms that the bone ends are aligned before the area is immobilized by a splint or cast.

SPLINTS. An elastic wrap and splint may be used to immobilize the bone during the healing phase. Splints are used when there is a wound to care for or a need to allow for swelling. Perform neurovascular checks hourly to monitor adequate blood flow to the area until the concern for swelling is over (see Chapter 45).

CASTS. Casts provide stronger support for fractured bones. Plaster or fiberglass casts are typically used. As casts dry, heat is produced. Plaster cast drying can take 24 to 72 hours. The plaster cast is dry when it feels hard and firm, is odorless, and is shiny white. Synthetic material casts such as fiberglass harden quickly and dry in less than 2 hours. Box 46.2 and Figure 46.3 present care for a patient with a cast.

A serious complication of a cast being too tight is compartment syndrome (discussed later). If the cast becomes too tight, the HCP orders it to be cut (bivalved) with a cast saw. This relieves pressure and prevents pressure necrosis of the underlying skin. If a wound is present or an odor is detected, a window opening into the cast is created. This allows treatment of the skin. The cast window should always be taped in place when wound care is not being provided to prevent the

Box 46.2

Nursing Interventions for a Patient With a Cast

1. Monitor:
   a. Neurovascular checks every 1 to 2 hours for 24 hours and then four times a day and as needed.
   b. Cast for tightness (ask patient) and ask patient to move all digits distal to the cast.
   c. Patient comments about cast and take action to prevent complications.
2. With newly applied casts (wet):
   a. Do not grasp a wet cast to hold or move it. Use only the palms of the hands, as finger pressure on a wet cast can cause pressure points on the inside cast surface.
   b. Position cast on absorbent surface; do not place it on a surface that can cause an indentation. Placing on a pillow while drying traps heat and increases thermal injury risk.
   c. Inform the patient that the cast creates heat when drying. Thermal injuries can occur. Ensure a cast air dries (may require 24 to 72 hours for complete drying). Do not cover a cast but keep it open to the air. Do not use drying aids such as hot blow dryers, which add more heat.
   d. If the patient is lying, assist the patient to turn every 1 to 2 hours to prevent flattening of a plaster cast surface during drying.
3. Reduce swelling (essential for the first 48 hours):
   a. Elevate extremity above the patient's heart level. Elevate casted arm while walking.
   b. Ice cast (first 48 hours). Use bags of frozen vegetables or leakproof plastic bags of ice wrapped with a towel.
   c. For casted arm, pump fingers 10 times per hour while awake.
4. Maintain tissue integrity within the cast:
   a. Check visible skin for signs of impaired integrity.
   b. Ensure cast edges are smooth; cover with stockinet or gauze to prevent rubbing of skin.
   c. Teach patient to keep cast dry; during bathing, cover with plastic and rubber band or tape ends.
   d. Monitor for signs and symptoms of infection, such as foul odor, warmth, redness, and pain.
   e. Do not use skin products on affected limb.
   f. Monitor visible blood on the surface of the cast. Outline area with a pen to observe for increasing size. Shadowing of blood not quite reaching the surface of the cast is fairly common but also should be circled and monitored.
   g. Never place an object inside the cast, and instruct patient not to do so. Explain the risk of tissue damage and infection.
   h. For itching, teach patient to try a blow dryer to blow cool air into the cast or tapping on the cast. Benadryl may be helpful.

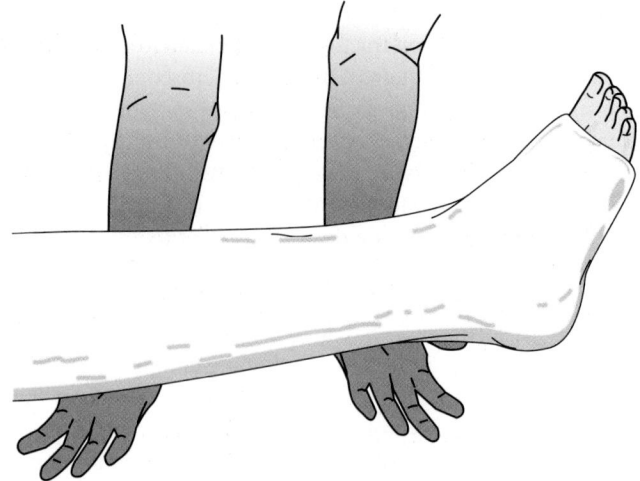

FIGURE 46.3 A wet plaster cast is moved with the palms of the hand to prevent making indentations in the plaster that could become pressure points.

skin from "popping up" through the window and developing pressure points and ischemia.

TRACTION. Traction is the application of a pulling force with prescribed weights to part of the body to position and hold bone fragments in correct alignment. Advances in orthopedic surgery have greatly decreased traction use. Buck traction is *skin traction,* with 5- to 10-pound (2.2- to 4.5-kg) weights; it is used for patients with hip fractures to relieve muscle spasms. *Skeletal traction* uses pins, wires, or tongs inserted into the bone for bone alignment as the fracture heals. Extremity skeletal traction is maintained with 20- to 40-pound (9- to 18-kg) weights that must hang freely at all times.

OPEN REDUCTION WITH INTERNAL FIXATION. The fractured bone ends are reduced (aligned) by direct visualization through a surgical incision (open reduction). The bone ends are held in place by internal fixation devices such as metal plates and screws or by a prosthesis with a femoral component similar to that used for total joint replacement (Fig. 46.4). For hip surgery, the internal fixation device is not removed after the fracture heals. For ankle or long-bone surgery, the hardware may be removed after healing due to loosening or pain.

One of the most common indications for this surgical procedure is a fractured hip. Hip fractures involve the proximal femur. They affect older adults more than any other age-group. Healthy People 2020's objective is to reduce hip fractures in adults over age 65 by 10% (Office of Disease Prevention and Health Promotion, 2017). Open reduction with internal fixation of the hip allows early ambulation while the bone is healing. See "Nursing Care Plan for the Patient After Open Reduction With Internal Fixation of the Hip."

EXTERNAL FIXATION. External fixation is used when bone damage is severe, as in crushed or splintered fractures, or if the bone has numerous breaks. After the fracture is reduced, the surgeon inserts pins into the bone. The pins are held in place by an external metal frame to prevent bone movement (Fig. 46.5). External fixation allows visualization of soft tissue damage that also requires treatment. See "Nursing Care Plan for the Patient With External Fixation of the Lower Extremity."

Nursing Care Plan for the Patient After Open Reduction With Internal Fixation of the Hip

Nursing Diagnosis: *Acute Pain* related to surgical incision
Expected Outcome: The patient will state that pain relief is satisfactory.
Evaluation of Outcome: Does the patient state that pain is absent or at a tolerable level (pain rated 0 to 2 on pain assessment scale)?

Intervention	Rationale	Evaluation
Monitor patient's rating of pain level every 2 to 4 hours or as needed and with each interaction.	*Frequent pain checks provide baseline and ongoing data and allow for timely interventions.*	Does the patient indicate pain is tolerable or relieved?
Administer analgesics as ordered and required; anticipate need for pain relief.	*Analgesics relieve pain, especially when administered before pain becomes severe.*	Does the patient indicate pain is tolerable or relieved?
Administer analgesics before activity (e.g., session with physical therapist).	*Increased activity can cause pain.*	Is the patient restless or agitated during activity?
Use pain relief measures, such as distraction, guided imagery, other relaxation techniques.	*Analgesic therapy is enhanced with complementary pain relief measures.*	Does the patient report that pain relief occurs with music or relaxation?
Use fracture bedpan as applicable.	*Fracture bedpans are more comfortable and easier to position.*	Is the patient able to use fracture pan comfortably?

Nursing Diagnosis: *Impaired Physical Mobility* related to surgical pain
Expected Outcome: The patient will maintain desired level of activity.
Evaluation of Outcome: Does the patient maintain activity level desired?

Intervention	Rationale	Evaluation
Observe level of physical mobility with each interaction and as needed.	*Early and frequent data collection provides baseline data and allows for timely interventions.*	Is the patient able to transfer and ambulate? With or without assistance?
Monitor the patient for and take measures to prevent complications of immobility: turn patient every 2 hours and check skin; keep heels off bed; teach patient to deep breathe and cough every 2 hours; and teach use of incentive spirometer.	*Immobility complications can occur without preventive measures.*	Does the patient experience complications of immobility?
Apply thigh-high elastic stockings or sequential compression device to unaffected limb as ordered. Remind patient to practice leg exercises. Administer anticoagulants as ordered. Ambulate patient as early as possible.	*These activities help prevent blood clots.*	Is the patient free from blood clots?

Nursing Care Plan for the Patient With External Fixation of the Lower Extremity

Nursing Diagnosis: *Risk for Infection* related to open skin at pin site
Expected Outcome: The patient does not develop an infection.
Evaluation of Outcome: Does the patient remain free from infection?

Intervention	Rationale	Evaluation
Inspect pin sites and dressings for signs and symptoms of infection (e.g., warmth, redness, heat, edema, drainage, pain).	*Early and frequent inspection allows for timely intervention to prevent infection.*	Are pin sites infected?
Provide pin site care per agency policy to remove crusting using strict aseptic technique.	*The pin is a pathway for microorganisms to directly enter bone tissue and cause osteomyelitis. Aseptic technique reduces risk of infection.*	Are pin sites clean with no crusting?

Nursing Diagnosis: *Impaired Physical Mobility* related to the limb injury
Expected Outcome: The patient will maintain desired level of mobility and activity.
Evaluation of Outcome: Has the patient maintained desired level of mobility and activity?

Intervention	Rationale	Evaluation
Monitor the patient's mobility with external fixation (EF) device in place.	*Data concerning the patient's abilities allow intervention planning.*	Does the patient transfer and ambulate with or without assistance?
Collaborate with other disciplines in teaching and promoting ambulation.	*Physiotherapy can provide initial teaching or reinforce education needed to promote ambulation (e.g., with crutch walking).*	Has the patient used information learned from other disciplines to aid ambulation?
Teach the patient how to move limb with EF device.	*Providing the patient with instruction on moving the extremity promotes independence and minimizes pain.*	Does the patient move the extremity with EF device?
Reinforce transfer and ambulation techniques for safety.	*Depending on severity of fracture and size of EF device, there may be special needs to transfer and ambulate.*	Does the patient transfer and ambulate as instructed?

Nursing Diagnosis: *Disturbed Body Image* related to EF device appearance.
Expected Outcome: The patient will demonstrate acceptance of body image while EF device is in place.
Evaluation of Outcome: Does the patient adjust to new image resulting from EF device?

Intervention	Rationale	Evaluation
Reinforce preoperatively EF device's purpose and what it will look like.	*Educating the patient increases the likelihood of acceptance and minimizes anxiety.*	Was the patient able to verbalize why EF device is to be used and what device will look like?
Observe the patient's reaction to EF device.	*Identifying the patient's reaction will guide further nursing responses.*	How does the patient react to EF device?
Reinforce that EF device will decrease discomfort and allow for earlier ambulation.	*Promoting increased comfort that allows early ambulation enhances acceptance.*	Does the patient understand the benefit of EF device as allowing for increased comfort and early ambulation?
Assist with coping.	*Allowing discussion of concerns promotes a sense of well-being and acceptance of EF device.*	Did the patient feel comfortable expressing concerns related to body image?

CRITICAL THINKING

Mrs. Martinez, a rehabilitation center resident, was found at 1000 lying on her left side, moaning and holding her left leg. She cried out with any movement and said she fell and broke her leg. Vital signs are blood pressure 150/84 mm Hg, pulse 100 beats per minute, and respirations 20 breaths per minute. Her left leg is noticeably shorter than her right leg. The supervisor notified paramedics and the health care provider. The licensed practical nurse (LPN) remained with Mrs. Martinez and instructed her not to move until help arrived. The LPN got blankets and a pillow for her head. At 1025, the paramedics took Mrs. Martinez to the hospital, where she was diagnosed as having an incomplete femoral neck (hip) fracture. Five pounds of Buck traction until surgery the next morning was ordered.

   Later, Mrs. Martinez is restless and picking at her bedcovers when the registered nurse arrives to collect data at the beginning of the shift.

1. How should the LPN document the incident of Mrs. Martinez's fall at the care center?
2. What is the purpose of Buck traction for Mrs. Martinez?

   Suggested answers are at the end of the chapter.

CRITICAL THINKING

Mr. Schnell, age 18, was in a motor vehicle accident that resulted in a fractured pelvis and an open right femoral fracture.

1. Identify four priority nursing diagnoses related to Mr. Schnell's care.
2. What are nursing interventions and rationales for these diagnoses?
3. How can the constipating effects of opioids be balanced with the benefits of pain relief to manage bowel elimination (see Chapter 10)?

   Suggested answers are at the end of the chapter.

NURSING CARE TIP

When moving a limb that has an external fixation device, grasp the device and lift, raise, or move the limb as needed. By grasping the device, there is less movement of the healing bone and therefore less trauma to the healing site and less pain with movement. Care must be taken not to loosen any fasteners holding the pins in place.

NON-UNION MODALITIES. Most bones heal properly with treatment. However, malunion (malalignment of healed bone) or non-union (delayed or no healing) can occur. Bone healing is affected by age, nutritional status, and diseases that alter the healing process, such as diabetes mellitus.

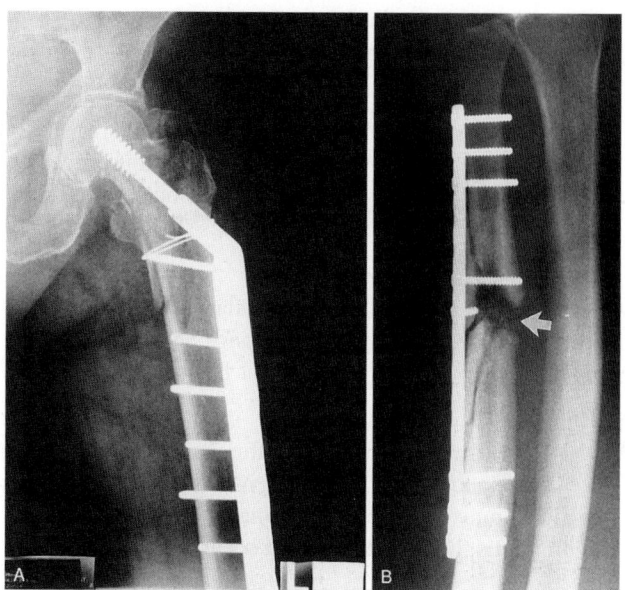

FIGURE 46.4 Internal fixation. (A) Intertrochanteric fracture of the hip with fracture fixation via a side plate and screw combination device. (B) Side plate and screw fixation of radial fracture.

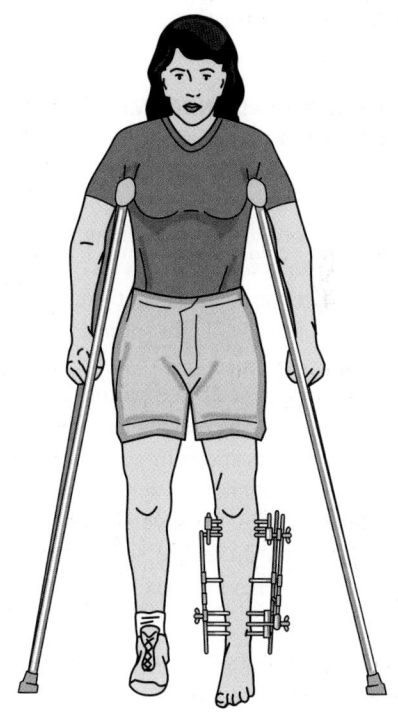

FIGURE 46.5 External fixation for complex fractures and wound care.

Identification of the reason for non-union allows the appropriate treatment selection. Treatment methods for non-union can include electrical bone stimulation, bone grafting, or external fixation.

Complications of Fractures

Monitor the patient for possible complications. Although rare, acute compartment syndrome and fat embolism syndrome (more common with fractures of long bones) can be life-threatening complications of fractures.

NEUROVASCULAR STATUS. Neurovascular checks are done to detect abnormalities. Decreased or absent pulses, cool skin temperature, and dusky color show circulation problems. Numbness and tingling, decreased sensation, and mobility show neurologic changes. These findings should be reported to the HCP right away.

HEMORRHAGE. Bone is highly vascular. Damage to or surgery on bone (particularly the large long bones of the extremities) can cause bleeding. Check for bleeding and monitor vital signs.

INFECTION. Trauma can lead to infection, especially when the skin, the body's first line of defense, is not intact. Wound infections, pin-site infections, drainage tube infections, and **osteomyelitis** (bone infection) can occur.

THROMBOEMBOLITIC COMPLICATIONS. Deep vein thrombosis (DVT) or pulmonary embolus (see Chapter 31) can develop in patients having orthopedic surgery. Leg exercises, early ambulation, and prophylactic anticoagulant therapy (such as with dalteparin [Fragmin], enoxaparin [Lovenox], fondaparinux [Arixtra], or rivaroxaban [Xarelto]) help prevent them.

ACUTE COMPARTMENT SYNDROME. Compartments are sheaths of fibrous tissue that support and partition nerves, muscles, and blood vessels, primarily in the extremities (Fig. 46.6). Each extremity has several compartments. Acute compartment syndrome is a limb-threatening condition in which pressure in limb compartments increases. This causes reduced circulation to the compartment's muscles and nerves. Trauma is a common cause. Tight splints, casts or dressings are another cause.

The early symptom of acute compartment syndrome is the patient's report of severe, increasing pain that is not relieved with opioids and occurs more in active movements than passive movements. Decreased sensation follows before ischemia becomes severe. To save the limb, don't wait to report early symptoms! In severe acute compartment syndrome, the patient may have the six *P*s if treatment does not prevent late symptoms:

1. Pain (severe, unrelenting, and increased with passive stretching)
2. Paresthesia (painful tingling or burning)
3. Pallor (but there may be warmth or redness over the area)
4. Paralysis (late symptom)
5. Pulselessness (late and ominous sign)
6. Poikilothermia (temperature matches environment; i.e., the extremity is cool to touch).

Immediate relief of pressure is the goal. This may be done by removing the source of pressure, such as by bivalving a cast or by performing a **fasciotomy,** which is an incision into the fascia enclosing the compartment. Fasciotomy allows compartment tissue the ability to expand, which

relieves the pressure. These surgical incisions are left open until the pressure decreases. They are then closed. If this condition continues without pressure relief, tissue necrosis, infection, Volkmann contracture (permanent flexion of hand at wrist), **rhabdomyolysis** (muscle breakdown releases myoglobin, which is harmful to the kidneys), or acute kidney injury may result.

CRITICAL THINKING

Mr. Kardos has a fracture of his right tibia. He has a cast on his right leg. An hour ago, he received 10 mg of morphine intravenously. He is reporting continued and increasing pain.

1. What data should the nurse collect now?
2. What might be happening with Mr. Kardos?
3. What patient-centered care interventions may be needed?

Suggested answers are at the end of the chapter.

FAT EMBOLISM SYNDROME. Fat embolism syndrome is a serious complication of fractures. Small fat droplets are released from yellow bone marrow into the bloodstream (Table 46.2). The droplets then travel to the lung fields, causing respiratory insufficiency. This can lead to respiratory failure. This process occurs with long bone fractures (especially the femoral shaft) and perhaps when the patient has multiple fractures. The older adult patient with a fractured hip is also at a high risk for fat embolism syndrome. This condition can occur up to 72 hours after the initial injury.

The three primary manifestations of fat embolism syndrome are respiratory failure, cerebral involvement, and skin petechiae. Pulmonary dysfunction is the earliest sign and includes tachypnea, dyspnea, and cyanosis. Cerebral changes are often seen and include confusion or drowsiness. A petechial (red, measles-like) rash on the chest, neck, axilla, and conjunctiva appears in some patients. Other signs include tachycardia, fever, and retinal changes. If a fat embolism is suspected, notify the HCP immediately. Treatment interventions may include:

1. Promote oxygenation by administering oxygen at 2 L/min via nasal cannula, and apply a pulse oximeter.
2. Place the patient in high-Fowler position or raise the head of the bed as tolerated.

• WORD • BUILDING •

osteomyelitis: osteo—bone + myel—bone marrow + itis—inflammation
fasciotomy: fascia—fibrous tissue + otomy—opening into
rhabdomyolysis: rhabdo—striped + myo—muscle + lysis—break down

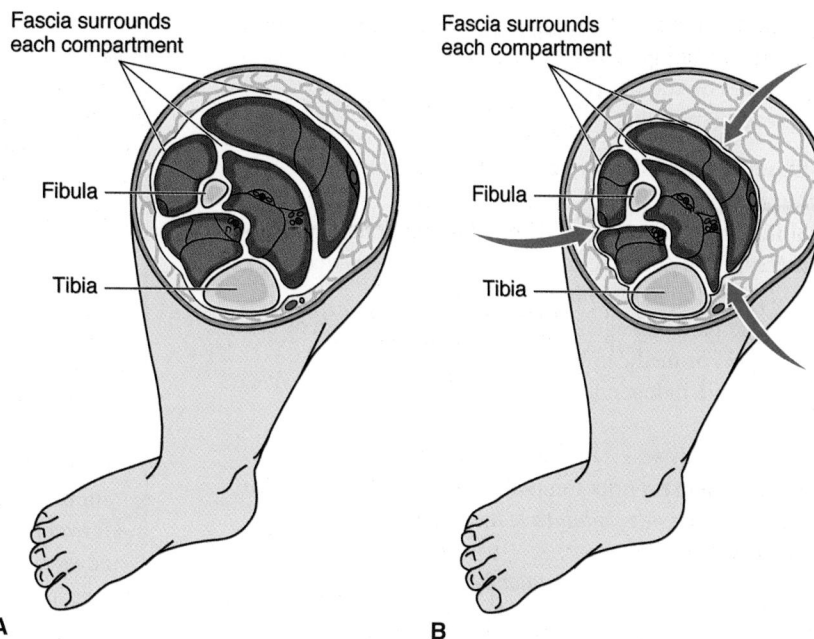

FIGURE 46.6 (A) Lower leg compartments. Each compartment contains muscles, an artery, a vein, and a nerve. (B) Compartment syndrome. Increased pressure in a compartment compresses structures within the compartment.

Table 46.2

Fat Embolism Syndrome vs. Pulmonary Embolism

	Fat Embolism Syndrome	*Pulmonary Embolism*
Origin	Multiple small fat droplets	Large clot or fat globule
Cause	Long bone fractures; surgical fracture repair; multiple fractures Hip fracture	Complication of deep vein thrombosis
Signs and Symptoms	Gradual onset with tachycardia, dyspnea, and cyanosis	Sudden onset, shortness of breath, and chest pain

3. Maintain bedrest, and minimize movement of the extremity.
4. Obtain arterial blood gas.
5. Initiate venous access for medications.
6. Administer corticosteroids.
7. Prepare patient for a chest x-ray and an MRI of the brain.
8. Provide emotional support and calm environment.

Nursing Process for the Patient With a Fracture

Caring for the patient with a fracture requires collaborative care with other health team members.

DATA COLLECTION. Frequent checking of neurovascular status (e.g., circulation, sensation, mobility) distal to a fracture is vital to detect problems (see Chapter 45). Pain is monitored using appropriate pain rating scales.

NURSING DIAGNOSES, PLANNING, AND IMPLEMENTATION. Determination of the appropriate nursing diagnosis depends on the location and type of fracture. See "Nursing Care Plan

for the Patient After Open Reduction With Internal Fixation of the Hip."

Acute Pain related to fractured bone

EXPECTED OUTCOME: The patient will report pain relief on a scale of 0 to 10 or be rated as pain-free using a pain rating scale for those who cannot report pain.

- Identify pain level using appropriate pain rating scale *to establish baseline for further interventions.* (See "Nursing Care Tip.")
- Provide regularly scheduled analgesic administration for those who cannot report pain *to ensure pain is relieved.*
- Administer analgesics and NSAIDs as ordered *to relieve pain and swelling.*
- Ensure proper positioning and alignment *to promote pain relief and future functioning.*
- Teach complimentary methods for pain relief *to maximize relief of pain.*

Impaired Physical Mobility related to bone fracture

EXPECTED OUTCOME: The patient will demonstrate increased mobility.

- Observe the patient's mobility level *to provide baseline data.*
- Utilize other disciplines, such as occupational and physiotherapy, and equipment, such as crutches, *to encourage and promote patient mobility.*
- Provide pain management prior to mobility such as heat, massage, or medication *to improve mobility.*
- Encourage independence *to prevent contributing to immobility.*
- Provide chair seat 3 inches above height of knee and raised toilet seat or commode with arms *to improve the ability of the older adult to stand up.*

Risk for Peripheral Neurovascular Dysfunction related to increased tissue volume or restrictive envelope

EXPECTED OUTCOME: The patient will maintain peripheral pulses, warm skin, sensation, and ability to move extremity.

- Monitor for swelling of affected limb (especially if the patient has a cast, splint, or tight dressing) *to detect complications.*
- Monitor for increasing pain even after analgesic administration *to detect complications.*
- Monitor for compartment syndrome *to allow prompt reporting of abnormalities to HCP.*
- Place limb at heart level if developing compartment syndrome detected *to prevent decrease in arterial blood flow.*
- Apply ice to fracture site as ordered *to decrease swelling and pain.*
- Administer NSAIDs as ordered *to reduce pain and swelling.*
- Act on the patient's reports of pain, limb symptoms, or cast status *to prevent complications.*

EVALUATION. The outcome is met if the patient reports or demonstrates that pain is within tolerable levels on a pain rating scale, peripheral pulses, warm skin, sensation, and the ability to move extremity are maintained, and the patient demonstrates increased physical mobility.

PATIENT EDUCATION. For the patient with a cast, teach cast care (see Box 46.2), wound care, and care of the extremity after cast removal (Box 46.3). Teach patient signs and symptoms of infection to report. Explain the importance of adequate intake of protein, calories, vitamins, and minerals in healing.

Osteomyelitis

Osteomyelitis is an infection of bone that can be either acute (lasts less than 4 weeks) or chronic (lasts more than 4 weeks).

NURSING CARE TIP

- A patient who is confused or comatose may not be able to report pain. This can be problematic because the most reliable indicator of pain is the patient's report. Nonverbal indicators (e.g., grimacing, restlessness, elevated blood pressure, and heart rate) are not reliable for pain identification and should not be used to assume the absence of pain.
- Use pain assessment tools designed for those who are cognitively impaired to ensure that their pain is adequately relieved. The Pain Assessment in Advanced Dementia (PAINAD) scale, for example, was developed for this purpose. Share pain research findings with institution administrators to establish policies that support proactive pain management for all patients.
- Prevent pain by anticipating it and treating it in advance. This can be done by recognizing causes of pain and understanding that the effects of mild but repetitive pain (as in turning several times a day) can adversely affect the patient (e.g., by leading to exhaustion).
- Causes of pain include conditions or diseases (such as fractures, trauma, or cancer), procedures (such as surgery, turning, or wound care), and biomedical devices (such as orthopedic fixation devices, wound drains, urinary catheters, nasogastric tubes, and chest tubes).
- With few patients being medicated before painful procedures (some of which, like turning, may be done several times a day), patients who are confused or comatose are at greater risk for lack of pain relief. To keep patients comfortable, administer analgesics as ordered before painful procedures and on a regular basis when pain is assumed to be present. For anticipated pain, use the acronym APP (assume pain present).

Pathophysiology

Bone infection results from invasion of bacteria into the bone and surrounding soft tissues. Inflammation occurs, followed by ischemia (decreased blood flow; Fig. 46.7). Bone tissue then becomes necrotic (dies), which retards healing and causes more infection, often as a bone abscess.

Box 46.3

Extremity Care After Cast Removal

- Cleanse skin by soaking rather than rubbing skin to remove dry scales.
- The extremity may be weak, with decreased range of motion. Move it gently and administer analgesics as needed.
- Support extremity when not in use with pillows or orthotic device until strength and movement return.
- Ensure active and passive range of motion are performed as recommended by physical therapist.
- Lower extremity swelling can be prevented with elastic support stockings.

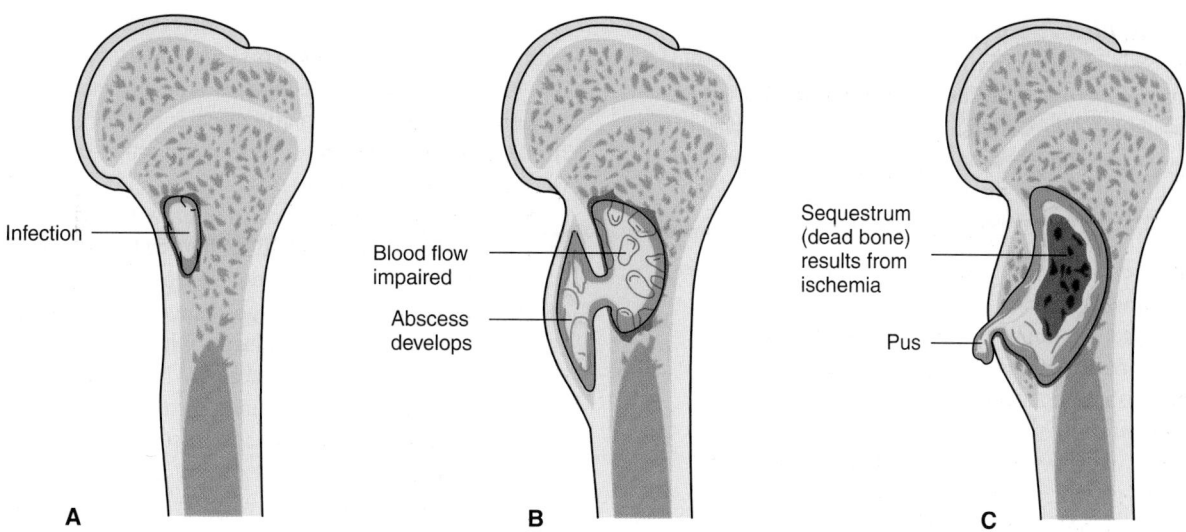

FIGURE 46.7 Sequence of osteomyelitis development. (A) Infection begins. (B) Blood flow is blocked in the area of infection. An abscess with pus forms. (C) Bone dies within the infection site, and pus formation continues.

Etiology

Injury to the body, such as an open fracture, allows pathogens direct access to bone tissue. Infection in another part of the body can travel to a bone. For instance, a patient with a total hip replacement may acquire osteomyelitis from a urinary tract infection. The most common pathogen causing osteomyelitis is *Staphylococcus aureus.*

Signs and Symptoms

The patient with acute osteomyelitis has site pain, redness, warmth, and swelling as well as fever. Ulceration, drainage, and localized pain are signs and symptoms of chronic osteomyelitis.

Diagnostic Tests

The patient with osteomyelitis may have an elevated white blood cell count, an elevated erythrocyte sedimentation rate (ESR), positive bone biopsy for infection, and a positive blood culture. MRIs, x-rays, and CT scans show infected areas.

Therapeutic Measures

Infection in bone tissue is difficult to resolve. Treatment is individualized. Curative therapy can include surgical debridement, reconstruction, and antibiotics. Palliative therapy is provided with chronic suppressive antibiotic therapy. Amputation is used for patients who have massive infections that have not responded to one or more of the conventional treatments.

Nursing Care

Patients on long-term IV antibiotics can receive them at home. The home health nurse teaches side effects, toxicity, interactions, and precautions for antibiotic therapy. If a soft tissue wound is present, sterile technique is used for dressing changes. The home health nurse teaches the patient and family how to perform dressing changes, the importance of hand hygiene before dressing changes, and how to avoid the spread of pathogens.

Osteoporosis

Osteoporosis (porous bone) is a metabolic disorder in which there is low bone mass and deterioration of bone structure, resulting in fragile bones that are prone to fracture. The spine, wrist, and hip are most commonly involved, although all bones can be affected.

Prevalence

More than 54 million Americans have osteoporosis or low bone density (National Osteoporosis Foundation, 2017). Women are at greatest risk because their bones are smaller than men's bones. As the U.S. population ages, the incidence and cost of osteoporosis will rise. Healthy People 2020's objective is to reduce the proportion of adults over age 50 with osteoporosis from 5.9 to 5.3% (Office of Disease Prevention and Health Promotion, 2017). This is important because hip or vertebral fractures are associated with reduced quality of life, increased disability, and increased risk of death, especially within the year after the fracture.

Pathophysiology

Bone is living tissue that is constantly resorbing (breaking down) old bone tissue (osteoclast cells) and building new bone tissue (osteoblast cells). Normally, the bone remodeling process is balanced. In osteoporosis, there is an imbalance. Bone density (mass) peaks between ages 30 and 35. After these peak years, the rate of bone breakdown exceeds the rate of bone buildup. For postmenopausal women, decreased estrogen appears to slow the absorption of calcium, leading to increased bone loss.

Types and Risk Factors

Osteoporosis is categorized as either primary or secondary. Primary osteoporosis is the most common and is not associated with another disease. Some risk factors for primary osteoporosis can be modified but others cannot. Those that are nonmodifiable include the following:

- Female gender
- Aging
- Caucasian or Asian
- Small-boned, petite body build
- Postmenopausal status
- Low testosterone and estrogen in men
- Family history of osteoporosis or fractures
- History of fractures

Risk factors related to lifestyle that are modifiable include the following:

- Anorexia nervosa
- Cigarette smoking
- Excessive alcohol use
- Nutrition (e.g., low calcium or vitamin D intake; excessive caffeine, protein, or sodium intake)
- Sedentary lifestyle

Secondary osteoporosis results from an associated medical condition or procedure, such as hyperparathyroidism; renal dialysis; medication therapy with steroids, certain antiseizure medications, sleeping medications, aluminium-containing antacids, hormones for endometriosis, or cancer medications; and prolonged immobility, such as that seen with patients who have a spinal cord injury.

Prevention

To protect against osteoporosis, practicing healthy lifestyle and nutritional habits that build bone are especially important through age 30, before bone mass begins to decrease. These habits should include consuming recommended amounts of calcium (1,000 mg/day for ages 19 to 50 and 1,200 mg/day for ages 50+) and vitamin D (600 IU [15 mcg]/day for ages 1 to 70 and 800 IU [20 mcg] for ages 71 and over) (National Institutes of Health, 2017). Additional healthy habits include performing weight-bearing exercises, avoiding alcohol, and not smoking.

Signs and Symptoms

Most people do not realize they have osteoporosis until they fracture a bone, have vertebral compression fractures, lose height (up to 6 inches), or develop a forward curvature of the spine (kyphosis). Pain may not be present. The patient may be embarrassed by the change in body image and may curtail social activities. Some patients have difficulty finding clothes that fit comfortably.

General effects of the disease go beyond the obvious bone deformities. Quality of life can be affected. Acute or chronic pain may occur. Physiological effects can include decreased respiratory capacity due to spinal deformities. It can be difficult to expand the lungs because of curvature of the spine or painful vertebral fractures. This can increase fatigue and the risk of pneumonia. Osteoporosis can be associated with chronic obstructive pulmonary disease, or COPD, because of limited activity related to dyspnea and corticosteroid therapy (which breaks down bone).

Functional abilities (activities of daily living [ADLs] and instrumental activities of daily living [IADLs]) may be limited. This increases the patient's dependence. Emotional effects may relate to body image changes, depression, or fear of breaking a bone such as during intimacy. Socialization may be reduced because of activity limitations or fear of injury. Because these effects are interrelated, data should be collected on the whole person, not just the disease for treatment that will improve quality of life.

Diagnostic Tests

Dual-energy x-ray absorptiometry (DEXA) is the standard screening tool to measure bone density ("Gerontological Issues: Osteoporosis"). This noninvasive scan is a low-dose x-ray and takes about 5 minutes to perform while the patient lies on a table. A DEXA scan identifies low bone density at the hip and spine. It shows response to treatment.

Serum calcium and vitamin D values can be decreased, and serum phosphorus may be increased. With severe bone loss, alkaline phosphatase levels may be elevated, confirming bone damage.

Gerontological Issues

Osteoporosis. Bone mineral density testing can be helpful in determining the risk of fractures for residents in long-term care. Providing treatment for osteoporosis can reduce the risk of hip fractures.

Therapeutic Measures

There is no cure for osteoporosis, but it can be treated. The cornerstone of treatment for osteoporosis is medication and controlling risk factors to prevent bone loss.

MEDICATION. Supplements and medication are used for prevention or treatment. These include calcium supplements, vitamin D, antiresorptive medications, and bone-forming medications.

Calcium is important to prevent bone loss. If serum calcium falls below normal levels, the parathyroid glands stimulate bone to release calcium into the bloodstream. The result is demineralized bone. Therefore, calcium supplements to maintain normal levels are important. The patient is taught to drink plenty of fluids to prevent calcium-based urinary stones. Vitamin D supplementation, to aid calcium absorption, also may be needed. This is especially important for patients who have reduced exposure to sunlight (residents of long-term care facilities or northern geographical areas, for example) or who cannot metabolize vitamin D.

Antiresorptive Medications. Bisphosphonates bind to bone and suppress osteoclast activity. This prevents or reduces the bone breakdown process in osteoporosis. Bisphosphonates include alendronate (Fosamax, Fosamax Plus D), ibandronate (Boniva), risedronate (Actonel, Actonel with calcium), and zoledronic acid (Reclast).

Side effects of bisphosphonates include bone, muscle, or joint pain; gastrointestinal upset; gastric ulcers; and, rarely, osteonecrosis (bone death) of the jaw. Teach the patient exactly how to take the medication to reduce side effects. The tablet or solution form is taken after arising in the morning on an empty stomach with 6 to 8 ounces of water only. The patient should wait 30 minutes before taking other medications. To prevent esophageal reactions, the patient should remain upright for at least 30 minutes after taking the medication. Older adults should be monitored for increased risk of gastrointestinal reactions.

The synthetic thyroid hormone calcitonin (Fortical, Miacalcin) treats osteoporosis by decreasing bone loss. It is used for women who have been menopausal for 5 years. The monoclonal antibody denosumab (Prolia) inhibits the protein that signals bone removal. Raloxifene (Evista) is a selective estrogen receptor modulator (SERM) that increases bone mass by 2 to 3% each year. SERM medications are designed to mimic estrogen in some parts of the body while blocking its effects elsewhere.

Estrogen therapy may be used to prevent the bone loss that occurs with menopause as estrogen levels fall. However, other treatments should be considered first due to risk factors associated with estrogen therapy.

Anabolic (Bone-Forming) Medications. Teriparatide (Forteo) is used for men and women who are at great risk for fracture. Teriparatide increases bone mass by increasing the action and number of osteoblasts that form bone. It should not be taken for more than 2 years.

DIET. Increasing calcium and vitamin D intake are the main dietary considerations. Teach patients which foods are high in calcium, such as dairy products (yogurt and skim milk may have low levels) and dark green, leafy vegetables.

EXERCISE. Weight-bearing exercise, especially walking, stimulates bone building. The patient should wear well-supporting, nonskid shoes and avoid uneven surfaces that could cause falls. Exercise such as weight training is also beneficial ("Gerontological Issues: Falls").

Gerontological Issues

Falls. Falls become more common as people age. Exercise that focuses on strength, balance, agility, and coordination is one way of reducing falls in older adults.

Fall Prevention

Osteoporotic bone may cause a pathological hip fracture, in which the hip breaks and causes the fall. On the other hand, a fall can cause a hip or other fracture. Therefore, fall prevention programs in health care facilities are important.

In collaboration with other health care team members, the patient's home environment is checked for safety. The patient and caregivers are taught to create a hazard-free environment. This includes avoiding scatter rugs and slippery floors, and keeping walking paths free of clutter to prevent falls. A walker or cane provides support.

Nursing Care

Nursing care for osteoporosis focuses on education for prevention, providing pain relief and support for symptoms, and medication teaching. For more information, visit the National Osteoporosis Foundation at www.nof.org.

Paget Disease

Paget disease is a rare metabolic bone disease. Increased breakdown and formation of bone results in abnormally formed, weak bones. This causes severe bone pain, deformities and fractures, and osteoarthritis. There is no cure for Paget disease. Older adults and men are mainly affected. X-rays show bones with punched-out areas. Increased serum alkaline phosphatase levels occur due to osteoblast activity. NSAIDs are given for pain control, and bisphosphonates reduce bone resorption. Calcitonin (Fortical, Miacalcin) decreases bone loss. Exercise helps maintains bone health and joint mobility. Nursing care promotes pain relief, teaching, and promotion of quality of life.

Bone Cancer

Bone tumors may be benign or malignant. Malignant tumors are either primary (begin in the bone) or metastatic (migrate to bone from another site). Metastatic lesions often affect older adults.

Primary Malignant Tumors

Osteosarcoma, or osteogenic sarcoma, is the most common primary malignant bone tumor. It is the most fatal bone tumor. It typically metastasizes to the lung within 2 years of diagnosis. It usually affects young people between ages 10 and 25. Males are twice as likely to develop it. Long bones of the legs and arms are most often the sites of origin.

Ewing sarcoma is the most malignant bone tumor. In addition to local pain and swelling, low-grade fever, leukocytosis, and anemia are common. The pelvis and legs are most often affected in children and young men.

METASTATIC BONE DISEASE. Primary malignant tumors that occur in the prostate, breast, lung, and thyroid gland are called bone-seeking cancers because they migrate to bone more than any other primary cancer. With metastasis, multiple sites in the bone are typically seen. Pathological fractures

• WORD • BUILDING •
osteosarcoma: osteo—bone + sarc—flesh + oma—tumor

and severe pain are major concerns in managing metastatic disease (see Chapter 11).

Signs and Symptoms

Primary tumors cause pain and swelling at the site. A tender, palpable mass is often present. Metastatic disease is not as visible, but the patient reports diffuse severe pain, eventually leading to marked disability.

Diagnostic Tests

Diagnosis of bone cancer is made with x-ray, CT scan, bone scan, bone biopsy, or MRI (see Chapter 45). Patients with metastatic disease have elevated alkaline phosphatase levels and possibly an elevated ESR, indicating secondary tissue inflammation.

Therapeutic Measures

Treatment of primary bone tumors is usually surgery with chemotherapy or radiation. Chemotherapy and surgical excision of the affected bone with bone grafting or amputation of the affected limb are common treatments for osteosarcoma. For patients with Ewing sarcoma or early osteosarcoma, external radiation may be the treatment of choice to reduce tumor size and pain. For metastatic bone disease, surgery is not appropriate. External radiation is given, primarily for palliation to shrink the tumor and reduce pain.

Nursing Care

Nursing care for the patient with bone cancer is similar to care for other types of cancer (see Chapter 11). Care of the postoperative patient is similar to that for any patient undergoing musculoskeletal surgery. Monitoring the neurovascular status of the operative limb is a vital nursing intervention (see Chapters 12 and 45).

CONNECTIVE TISSUE DISORDERS

Connective tissue disorders comprise a group of more than 100 diseases in which the major signs and symptoms result from joint involvement. Some of these diseases affect only one part of the body; others affect many body organs and systems. Gout, osteoarthritis, and rheumatoid arthritis are discussed.

Gout

Gout is an easily treated systemic connective tissue disorder occurring from the buildup of uric acid. Men, especially those middle aged and older, are most affected.

Pathophysiology

Uric acid is a waste product resulting from the breakdown of proteins (purines) in the body. Urate crystals are formed because of excessive uric acid buildup (**hyperuricemia**). They are deposited in joints and other connective tissues, causing severe inflammation (Fig. 46.8). The inflammation may resolve in several days, with or without treatment. Urate

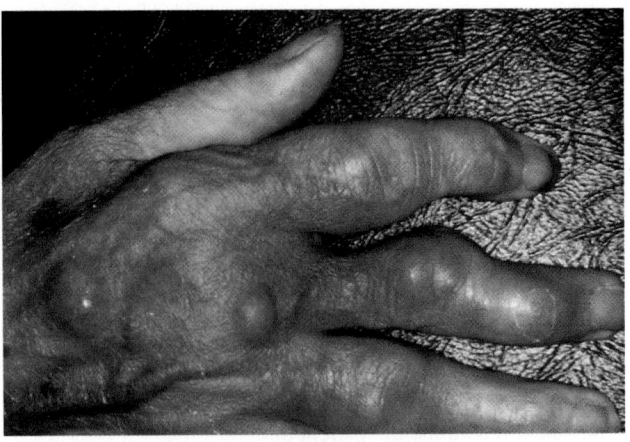

FIGURE 46.8 Gout: subcutaneous nontender lesions near joints.

deposits (tophi) occasionally appear under the skin (outer ear, commonly) or in the kidneys or urinary system, causing stone (calculi) formation (see Chapter 37).

Etiology and Types

Primary gout, the most common type of gout, is caused by an inherited problem with purine metabolism. Uric acid production is greater than the kidneys' ability to excrete it. Therefore, the amount of uric acid in the blood increases. Acute attacks of gout may be triggered by stress, alcohol consumption, illness, trauma, dieting, or certain medications such as aspirin and diuretics.

Uric acid is also increased in secondary gout. However, the increase is related to a health issue. Examples include renal insufficiency or medications, such as diuretic therapy and certain chemotherapeutic agents.

Signs and Symptoms

ACUTE GOUT. When an "attack" of gout occurs, the patient has severe pain and inflammation due to the uric acid crystals in one or more small joints, usually the great toe. The joint is swollen, red, hot, and usually too painful to be touched.

CHRONIC GOUT. Patients with chronic gout may not have obvious signs and symptoms. Renal stones can develop from elevated uric acid.

Diagnostic Tests

Diagnosis of gout is based on an elevated serum uric acid level. Joint fluid aspiration analysis can also identify uric acid crystals in the synovial fluid.

Therapeutic Measures

Medication therapy is the first-line treatment for primary gout. Treatment for secondary gout involves management of the underlying cause. For an acute gout episode NSAIDs,

• WORD • BUILDING •

hyperuricemia: hyper—excessive + uric—uric acid + emia—in blood

colchicine (Colcrys), or steroids are prescribed until the joint inflammatory response subsides. For chronic gout patients for whom other medications are not effective, pegloticase (Krystexxa) by IV infusion can be given every 2 weeks.

Uricosuric medications are used to prevent increased serum uric acid levels. Febuxostat (Uloric) and allopurinol (Zyloprim) decrease uric acid production. Probenecid (Benemid) increases renal excretion of uric acid. Serum uric acid level is monitored during medication use.

Prevention and Nursing Care

Interventions to teach the patient to help prevent gout include the following:

- Drink plenty of fluids, especially water.
- Consider eating cherries or drinking cherry juice.
- Avoid high-purine (protein) foods, such as organ meats, shellfish, and oily fish (e.g., sardines).
- Avoid alcohol.
- Avoid all forms of aspirin and medications containing aspirin.
- Avoid diuretics.
- Avoid excessive physical or emotional stress.

Osteoarthritis

Osteoarthritis (OA) is the most common type of arthritis, affecting more than 30 million people in the United States (Centers for Disease Control and Prevention, 2017). It is more common with age. OA is also known as degenerative joint disease.

Pathophysiology

OA is a disease of the joint that affects all the joint's structures (Table 46.3). The cartilage and bone ends slowly break down. The joint space narrows, bone spurs develop, and the joint lining becomes inflamed. Ligaments and tendons may also be affected. The body's repair process is not able to overcome this loss of cartilage and bone. Weight-bearing joints (e.g., hips and knees), hands, and the vertebral column are most often affected (Fig. 46.9).

Etiology

Risk factors for OA include heredity, being overweight, and physical activities that create mechanical stress on synovial joints, such as long periods of standing or repetitive motions. OA may also develop as a result of trauma, sepsis, congenital anomalies, certain metabolic diseases, or rheumatoid arthritis.

Table 46.3

Osteoarthritis and Rheumatoid Arthritis Summary

	Osteoarthritis	Rheumatoid Arthritis
Pathophysiology	Articular cartilage and bone ends deteriorate. Joint is inflamed.	Inflammatory cells cause synovitis. Synovium becomes thick and fluid accumulates, causing swelling and pain. Joint becomes deformed.
Etiology	*Primary (idiopathic):* • Cause unknown. • Risk factors include age, obesity, activities causing joint stress. *Secondary:* • Causes include trauma, sepsis, congenital abnormalities, metabolic disorders, rheumatoid arthritis.	Periodontal disease may be a cause. Is an autoimmune disease. Can occur at any age (including juvenile rheumatoid arthritis). Familial history possible.
Signs and Symptoms	Joint pain and stiffness occur. Pain increases with activity and decreases with rest. Nodes on joints of fingers appear (Heberden nodes, Bouchard nodes).	Symptoms vary according to disease process. *Early symptoms:* • Bilateral and symmetrical joint inflammation • Redness, warmth, swelling, stiffness, pain • Stiffness after resting (morning stiffness) • Activity decreases pain and stiffness • Low-grade fever, weakness, fatigue, anorexia (mild weight loss) • Organ system involvement *Late symptoms:* • Joint deformity • Secondary osteoporosis

Continued

Table 46.3

Osteoarthritis and Rheumatoid Arthritis Summary—cont'd

	Osteoarthritis	Rheumatoid Arthritis
Therapeutic Measures	Medication • Nonsteroidal anti-inflammatory drugs (NSAIDs) • Acetaminophen • Muscle relaxants. Balanced rest and exercise Splinting of joint to promote rest Heat and cold Diet for weight loss Complementary therapies Surgery for total joint replacement	Medication • Antibiotics • NSAIDs • Biological response modifier • Prednisone • Disease-modifying antirheumatic drug (DMARD) • T-cell modulators Heat and cold Balanced rest and activity Surgery for total joint replacement
Priority Nursing Diagnoses	*Chronic Pain* *Impaired Physical Mobility* *Disturbed Body Image*	*Chronic Pain* *Self-Care Deficits* *Ineffective Health Maintenance*

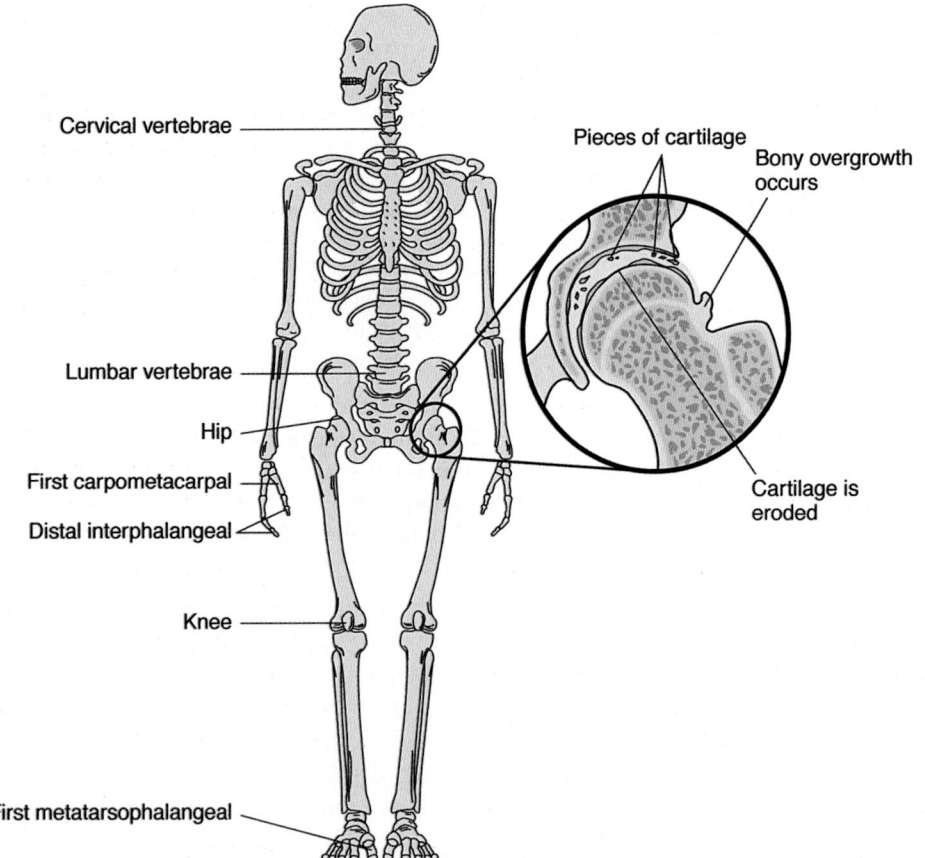

Cervical vertebrae

Lumbar vertebrae

Hip

First carpometacarpal

Distal interphalangeal

Knee

First metatarsophalangeal

Pieces of cartilage

Bony overgrowth occurs

Cartilage is eroded

FIGURE 46.9 Common joints affected by osteoarthritis and the changes that result in the joint.

Signs and Symptoms

Pain and stiffness, especially upon arising, commonly occur. Joint pain and swelling increase after activity. Stiffness is reduced with movement. The patient usually seeks medical attention when symptoms are severe or range of motion is limited while performing everyday activities. Painful bony nodes on the finger joint, called Heberden and Bouchard nodes, may occur. Women tend to have them more often than men. If the vertebral column is involved, the patient reports radiating pain and muscle spasms in the extremity innervated by the area affected.

Diagnostic Tests

X-ray examinations can outline the joint structure and detect bone changes. MRI is helpful in showing joint structure abnormalities. Analysis of synovial fluid aids in the diagnosis of OA.

Evidence-Based Practice

Clinical Question

Can exercise effectively relieve chronic low back pain?

Evidence

In this systematic review, 39 quantitative studies examined the effectiveness of exercise for relieving chronic lower back pain (Searle, Spink, Ho, & Chuter, 2015). The results showed exercises that targeted strength/resistance and coordination/stabilization were most effective. Cardiorespiratory exercise was not effective.

Implications for Nursing Practice

Chronic low back pain is a commonly reported health issue. In the majority of cases, the mechanism is poorly understood, which leads to challenges in treating it. Nurses can encourage patient participation in exercise programs to improve strength/resistance and coordination/stabilization.

Reference

Searle, A., Spink, M., Ho, A., & Chuter, V. (2015). Exercise interventions for the treatment of chronic low back pain: A systematic review and meta-analysis of randomized controlled trials. *Clinical Rehabilitation, 29*(12) 1155–1167.

CRITICAL THINKING

Mr. Finn, a 59-year-old hardware store manager, is 5'11" and weighs 250 pounds. He visits his health care provider because of knee pain. He has noticed that it is becoming increasingly difficult to bend to pick up heavy boxes. The health care provider suspects osteoarthritis.

1. What data collection questions should you include in Mr. Finn's history?
2. What risk factors does the patient have?
3. What other signs and symptoms might Mr. Finn have?
4. What are patient-centered care interventions for Mr. Finn?
5. What health care team members can provide collaborative care along with you?

Suggested answers are at the end of the chapter.

Therapeutic Measures

There is no cure for OA. Symptom control is the focus of treatment. An interdisciplinary approach is needed to prevent decreased mobility and preserve joint function.

EXERCISE. Joint pain from OA tends to decrease with rest; therefore, pain is less severe in the morning. Activities should be scheduled at this time. A severely inflamed joint may be splinted by the occupational therapist or physical therapist to promote rest to a selected joint. However, rest must be balanced with exercise to prevent muscle atrophy from disuse. Exercise has been identified as a means to maintain general health and weight, range of motion, and muscle strength, while decreasing anxiety and depression. To minimize muscle atrophy and to stabilize and protect arthritic joints, patients should be encouraged to perform exercises to strengthen their quadriceps if they have OA of the knee. Yoga and tai chi are helpful for gently stretching the joints to reduce stiffness.

Joints should always be placed in their functional position—that is, a position that does not lead to contractures. For example, only a small pillow should be placed under the head when sleeping to prevent excessive neck flexion.

WEIGHT CONTROL. Obese or overweight patients benefit from losing weight to decrease stress on weight-bearing joints and thereby reduce pain. If the patient is on medications that can alter fluid volumes (corticosteroids), a diet low in sodium may be appropriate.

MEDICATION. Medication therapy is commonly used to reduce pain in patients with OA. Often, it is combined with other pain-reducing therapies. The most commonly used medications are NSAIDs (Table 46.4). NSAIDs have analgesic and anti-inflammatory effects. Common side effects include gastrointestinal distress and bleeding, which can be severe, and sodium and fluid retention. NSAIDs also may increase the risk of cardiovascular events, such as myocardial infarction or stroke. Older patients taking NSAIDs on a routine basis should be carefully monitored for heart failure and hypertension from fluid retention. Other analgesics such as acetaminophen or corticosteroids may be used. Over-the-counter topical creams such as capsaicin (Arthricare) can be applied to the joints.

Synvisc-One (one injection) or SYNVISC (three injections) is injected directly into osteoarthritic knees to replace the cushioning synovial fluid (visit www.synviscone.com). Pain can be relieved and flexibility restored for up to 6 months.

HEAT AND COLD. The patient with OA usually prefers heat therapy unless the joint is acutely inflamed. Hot packs, warm compresses, warm showers, moist heating pads, and paraffin dips provide sources of heat. Cold therapy minimizes inflammation while altering cutaneous pain receptors, thereby decreasing pain. Cold packs should be applied for no longer than 20 minutes at a time.

COMPLEMENTARY AND ALTERNATIVE THERAPIES. Complementary and alternative therapies can reduce pain. Acupressure, acupuncture, hydrotherapy, imagery, music therapy, massage, and other holistic modalities that foster the mind-body-spirit connection work well for many people.

SURGERY. If the patient's pain cannot be managed successfully, a total joint replacement may be indicated. Total joint replacement is the most common type of arthroplasty (see later section on musculoskeletal surgery).

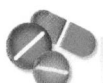

Table 46.4
Common Medications Used to Treat Connective Tissue Diseases: Osteoarthritis, Rheumatoid Arthritis, and Others

Medication Class/Action

Biological Response Modifiers

Interleukin-1 inhibitors that reduce inflammation and cartilage degradation.

Examples	**Nursing Implications**
anakinra (Kineret)	Monitor neutrophils.

Corticosteroids

Reduce inflammation and swelling.

Examples	**Nursing Implications**
prednisone (Deltasone, Orasone)	Take daily weight.
	Monitor intake and output.
	Monitor for infection.
	Give with food/milk.
	Recommend patient obtain medic alert ID.
	Not used for osteoarthritis.

Disease-Modifying Antirheumatic Drugs (DMARDs)

For use in rheumatoid arthritis and ankylosing spondylitis, reduce symptoms, prevent joint damage, and preserve joint function by suppressing immune or inflammatory systems. Slow-acting and may take months for effect; other medications used to control symptoms until effective. Effect ends when medication stopped.

Pyrimidine Synthesis Inhibitors

Examples	**Nursing Implications**
leflunomide (Arava)	Screen for tuberculosis before starting.
	Monitor blood pressure, complete blood count, liver function.
	Teach patient to report rash promptly.

Gold Preparations

Examples	**Nursing Implications**
auranofin (Ridaura)	Give test dose and monitor for allergic reaction for about
aurothioglucose (Solganal)	1 hour.
	Lab testing for gold toxicity recommended.

Immunosuppressives

Examples	**Nursing Implications**
azathioprine (Imuran)	Protect from infection.
cyclophosphamide (Cytoxan)	Monitor for infections.
cyclosporine (Sandimmune, Neoral)	
leflunomide (Arava; *for rheumatoid arthritis only*)	
methotrexate (Mexate)	
d-penicillamine (Cuprimine, Depen)	

Tumor Necrosis Factor Inhibitors

Examples	**Nursing Implications**
adalimumab (Humira)	Screen for tuberculosis.
etanercept (Enbrel)	

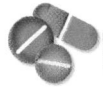

Table 46.4

Common Medications Used to Treat Connective Tissue Diseases: Osteoarthritis, Rheumatoid Arthritis, and Others—cont'd

Medication Class/Action

Antimalarials

Examples	Nursing Implications
chloroquine (Aralen)	Report vision problems.
hydroxychloroquine (Plaquenil)	Promote safety due to dizziness.

Nonsteroidal Anti-Inflammatory Drugs (NSAIDs)

Block activity of enzyme cyclooxygenase (COX-1, COX-2), which makes prostaglandins that produce inflammation, fever, and pain; support platelets; and protect stomach lining (COX-1 only).

Examples	Nursing Implications
acetylsalicylic acid (aspirin)	Those with asthma at higher risk for allergic reaction.
diclofenac sodium (Voltaren)	Teach patient there is a risk of gastrointestinal bleeding.
diflunisal (Dolobid)	
etodolac (Lodine; *for osteoarthritis only*)	
fenoprofen (Nalfon)	
flurbiprofen (Ansaid)	
ibuprofen (Motrin)	
indomethacin (Indocin)	
ketoprofen (Orudis)	
naproxen (Aleve, Naprosyn)	
oxaprozin (Daypro)	
piroxicam (Feldene)	
nabumetone (Relafen)	
sulindac (Clinoril)	
tolmetin (Tolectin)	

T-Cell Modulators

Reduce activation of T cells in the inflammatory process.

Examples	Nursing Implications
abatacept (Orencia)	Screen for tuberculosis.
	Use silicone-free syringe only.
	Infuse over 30 minutes.
	Monitor for serious infections.

Nursing Process for the Patient With Osteoarthritis

DATA COLLECTION. The patient's report of pain is documented. Affected joints are observed for signs of inflammation or deformity. Also examined are joint function, ADL performance, and mobility.

NURSING DIAGNOSES, PLANNING, IMPLEMENTATION, AND EVALUATION.

Acute Pain related to movement

EXPECTED OUTCOME: The patient will report pain is tolerable or relieved on a scale of 0 to 10 or be rated as pain-free using a pain rating scale for those who cannot report pain.

• Use appropriate pain rating scale for patient *to determine level of pain and need for pain relief.*

• Administer analgesics as ordered *to help alleviate painful sensations.*
• Collaborate with an interdisciplinary team, such as a pain clinic, *to explore alternative pain relief measures.*
• Consider complimentary methods for pain relief such as guided imagery, distraction, acupuncture, and biofeedback *to use all possible methods of pain control.*

Activity Intolerance related to pain

EXPECTED OUTCOME: The patient will participate in ADLs as tolerated.

• Provide pain relief measures before activity *to enable an increase in activity level.*

- Monitor pain during activity *to provide baseline data.*
- Encourage independence as able *to promote activity.*
- Assist with ADLs as needed *to prevent patient exhaustion.*
- Group nursing interventions together *to conserve patient energy.*
- Collaborate with an interdisciplinary team, such as an occupational therapist and home health physiotherapist, *to develop patient plan of care.*

Chronic Sorrow related to altered body image, altered role, pain, and ongoing losses

EXPECTED OUTCOME: The patient will verbalize improvement in feelings of sorrow.

- Observe patient's affect and mood connected to pain and loss *to provide baseline data.*
- Allow time to discuss feelings and anticipate trigger events *to ensure the patient is aware of what may increase feelings of sorrow.*
- Encourage use of interdisciplinary team, such as a social worker, psychologist, clergy, or spiritual adviser, *to provide alternate methods of dealing with sorrow.*
- Encourage use of support groups *to enable the patient to discuss concerns with others experiencing the same problems.*

Disturbed Body Image related to changes in joint function and structure

EXPECTED OUTCOME: The patient will demonstrate acceptance of changes in body image.

- Encourage the patient to discuss feelings and concerns *to allow the nurse to understand what the patient is experiencing.*
- Provide information and clarify misconceptions *to ensure that the patient is aware of expected problems and concerns.*
- Encourage socialization *to improve the patient's perceptions of how he or she appears to others.*

Impaired Physical Mobility related to altered joint function and pain

EXPECTED OUTCOME: The patient will demonstrate improved physical mobility.

- Observe mobility capabilities *to provide baseline data.*
- Administer analgesics and NSAIDS as ordered *to improve joint function and decrease pain.*
- Encourage active range-of-motion exercises *to prevent or minimize further alteration in joint function.*
- Ensure proper positioning and alignment *to promote joint function and decrease pain.*
- Collaborate with an interdisciplinary team, such as a physiotherapist and occupational therapist, *to incorporate their resources and knowledge into the plan of care.*

Self-Care Deficit (Bathing, Dressing, Feeding, Toileting) related to degenerative joint disease

EXPECTED OUTCOME: The patient will be able to provide his or her own self-care.

- Observe the patient's self-care abilities *to gather baseline data for planning care.*
- Encourage independence *to decrease feelings of despair about being unable to care for self.*
- Assist when necessary *to minimize frustration when the patient cannot perform self-care.*
- Teach the patient about assistive devices to help with ADL living *to promote self-care.*
- Collaborate with an interdisciplinary team, such as a home health nurse, occupational therapist, or physiotherapist, *to acquire assistive devices and use alternate resources.*

EVALUATION. The pain outcome is met if pain is rated at a tolerable level on an appropriate pain scale. Other outcomes are met if the patient is able to participate in ADLs, verbalizes improvement in feelings of sorrow, demonstrates acceptance of changes in body image, demonstrates improved physical mobility, and is able to provide own self-care.

PATIENT EDUCATION. A vital function of each member of the health care team is health teaching. The patient with OA is seldom admitted to the hospital for treatment of OA unless surgery is scheduled. However, many patients with OA are admitted for other reasons. Their arthritis needs must also be considered in the plan of care. Most patients residing in long-term care facilities also have OA, which can affect their participation in ADLs and recreational activities.

Patients should be taught ways to protect their joints and conserve energy. For educational materials and self-help courses, visit the Arthritis Foundation at www.arthritis.org.

Rheumatoid Arthritis

Rheumatoid arthritis (RA) is a chronic, progressive, systemic inflammatory disease that destroys synovial joints and other connective tissues, including major organs.

Pathophysiology

Inflammatory cells and chemicals cause **synovitis,** an inflammation of the synovium (the lining of the joint capsule). As the inflammation progresses, the synovium becomes thick. Fluid accumulation causes joint swelling and pain. A destructive pannus (new synovial tissue growth infiltrated with inflammatory cells) erodes the joint cartilage and eventually destroys the bone within the joint (Fig. 46.10). Ultimately the pannus is converted to bony tissue, resulting in loss of mobility. Joint deformity and bone loss are common in late RA (see Table 46.3).

Any connective tissue may be affected in RA, including blood vessels, nerves, kidneys, pericardium, lungs, and subcutaneous tissue. Dysfunction or failure of the organ or system can occur. Death can result if the disease does not respond to treatment.

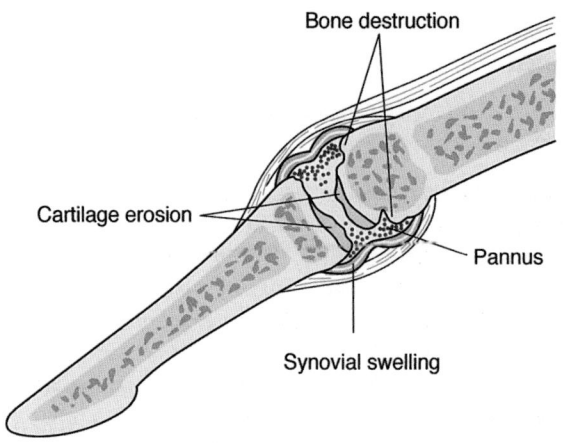

FIGURE 46.10 Rheumatoid arthritis.

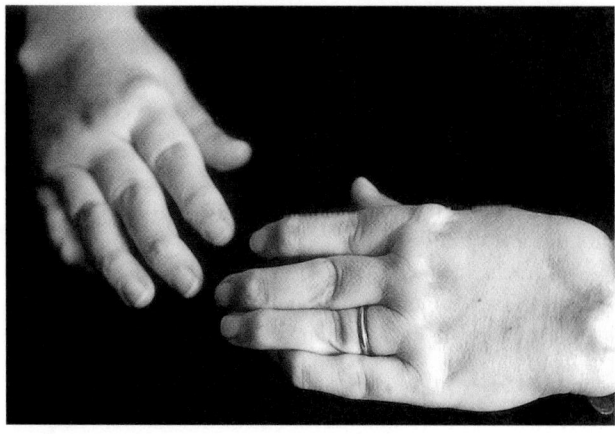

FIGURE 46.11 Joint abnormalities in hands of patient with rheumatoid arthritis.

Many patients experience spontaneous remissions and exacerbations (flare-ups) of RA. Symptoms may disappear without treatment for months or years. Then the disease flares up just as unpredictably, often due to physical or emotional stress.

Etiology

RA affects people with a family history of the disease two to three times more often than the rest of the population. Oral pathogens might be a cause of RA. Studies have shown that the symptoms of RA improve with antibiotic treatment (Erickson, 2016). In RA, an autoimmune response occurs that affects the synovial membrane of the joints. Antibodies (called rheumatoid factor; RF) are often found in patients with RA. It is suggested that these antibodies join with other antibodies and form antibody complexes. These complexes lodge in synovium and other connective tissues, causing local and systemic inflammation. They may be responsible for the destructive changes of RA in body tissues.

Signs and Symptoms

Signs and symptoms vary because the disease presents differently in each patient. In general, the signs and symptoms can be divided into early and late manifestations.

The typical pattern of joint inflammation is bilateral and symmetrical. The disease usually begins in the upper extremities and progresses to other joints over many years (Fig. 46.11). Affected joints are slightly reddened, warm, swollen, stiff, and painful. The patient with RA often has morning stiffness lasting for up to an hour. Those with severe disease may report having stiffness all day. Generally, activity decreases pain and stiffness.

Because of the systemic nature of RA, the patient may have a low-grade fever, malaise, depression, lymphadenopathy, weakness, fatigue, anorexia, and weight loss. As the disease worsens, major organs or body systems are affected. Joint deformities occur as a late symptom. Secondary osteoporosis (bone loss) can lead to fractures.

Diagnostic Tests

No specific diagnostic test confirms RA. An increase in white blood cells and platelets is typical. Immunological tests findings for patients with RA usually include the following:

- Presence of RF in serum
- Decreased red blood cell count
- Decreased C4 complement
- Increased ESR
- Positive antinuclear antibody test
- Positive C-reactive protein test

RF can indicate the aggressiveness of the disease. However, it is not specific to RA. The ESR test screens for inflammation. It measures the amount of time it takes for red blood cells to settle to the bottom of a test tube. In the presence of inflammation, red blood cells settle faster in the tube. Therefore, the ESR increases with the presence of inflammation. It also evaluates the effectiveness of treatment. If the disease responds to treatment, the ESR decreases.

> **LEARNING TIP**
> Avoid shaking hands with people who have rheumatoid arthritis. A simple "Nice to meet you" can be more appropriate and will avoid the pain caused by even a weak handshake.

X-ray examination and MRI detect joint damage and bone loss, especially in the vertebral column. A bone or joint scan assesses the extent of joint involvement throughout the body. With arthrocentesis, the synovial fluid is found to be cloudy, milky, or dark yellow with inflammatory cells present.

Therapeutic Measures

Antibiotics may improve the symptoms of RA. Chronic joint pain can interfere with mobility or the ability to perform

ADLs. Medication therapy can relieve or reduce pain as well as slow the progression of the disease. Disease-modifying antirheumatic drugs (DMARDs) can prevent joint destruction, deformity, and disability with early single or combination medication use. NSAIDs and corticosteroids are also used (see Table 46.4). Many of these medications have potentially serious side effects, such as severe infection, and must be monitored carefully.

Complementary therapies that may help decrease inflammation or pain include capsaicin cream, fish oil, and antioxidants such as vitamin C, vitamin E, and beta carotene (see Chapter 5).

HEAT AND COLD. Heat applications or hot showers help decrease joint stiffness and make exercise easier for the patient. For acutely inflamed, or "hot," joints, cold applications are preferred. A program that balances rest and exercise is most beneficial for the patient.

SURGERY. If nonsurgical approaches are not effective in relieving arthritic pain, the patient may have a total joint replacement (discussed later).

Nursing Process for the Patient With Rheumatoid Arthritis

DATA COLLECTION. A complete history and physical examination is needed for the patient with RA because the disease can involve every system of the body. In addition to identifying physical signs and symptoms, explore the patient's psychosocial, functional, and vocational needs.

After having the disease for approximately 15 years, fewer than half of RA patients are totally independent in their ADLs. These limitations may place a burden on family members, who must be included in the care of the patient with RA. Many patients with the disease are young or middle-aged. RA can impair their ability to work, depending on the type of job they have. Occupational therapy assesses the patient's work skills to determine the need for changes in the workplace or a need to train for a new type of work.

NURSING DIAGNOSES, PLANNING, AND IMPLEMENTATION.

Acute Pain related to chronic disease process

EXPECTED OUTCOME: The patient will report pain is tolerable or relieved on a scale of 0 to 10 or be rated as pain-free using a pain rating scale for those who cannot report pain.

• Use appropriate pain rating scale for patient *to determine level of pain and need for pain relief.*
• Administer analgesics as ordered *to relieve pain.*
• Teach complimentary pain relief methods *to maximize means to relieve pain.*
• Encourage maintenance of normal weight *to prevent excess stress on joints.*

Disturbed Body Image related to changes resulting from disease process

EXPECTED OUTCOME: The patient will accept alterations in body.

• Encourage the patient to discuss feelings and concerns *to provide the nurse with an understanding of what the patient is experiencing.*
• Provide information and clarify misconceptions *to ensure that the patient is aware of the expected problems and concerns.*
• Encourage socialization *to improve on the patient's perceptions of how he or she "looks" to others.*
• Encourage sharing with support groups *so that the patient discusses his or her concerns with others experiencing the same problems.*

Fatigue related to chronic pain and limited mobility

EXPECTED OUTCOME: The patient will have decreased episodes of fatigue.

• Monitor levels of fatigue throughout the day *to determine the patient's reaction to various activities.*
• Provide assistance as required *to conserve the patient's energy.*
• Ensure regular rest periods throughout the day *to not overexert the patient.*
• Teach the patient the need to delegate *to avoid overexertion.*
• Teach energy conservation techniques *to reduce workload.*

Self-Care Deficit (Bathing, Dressing, Feeding, Toileting) related to chronic degenerative disease process

EXPECTED OUTCOME: The patient will be able to provide own self-care.

• Observe the patient's ability to care for self *to determine level of ability and adjust the patient's plan of care.*
• Encourage independence *to decrease feelings of despair about self-care deficits.*
• Assist when necessary *to minimize frustration when the patient is unable to perform self-care function.*
• Teach patient about assistive devices *to help with ADLs and promote self-care.*
• Collaborate with an interdisciplinary team, such as a home health nurse and occupational or physical therapists, *for adaptive resources.*

Impaired Physical Mobility related to chronic inflammation of joints

EXPECTED OUTCOME: The patient will have improved physical mobility.

• Administer analgesics and NSAIDs *to reduce pain and increase mobility.*

- Administer heat and cold therapy *to aid in joint function and movement.*
- Encourage continued mobilization *to minimize complications of immobility.*
- Collaborate with other disciplines *to assist with maintaining mobility.*

EVALUATION. The outcomes are met if the patient has pain relief within acceptable levels on a pain assessment scale. The patient must also demonstrate acceptance of changes in body image and have decreased episodes of fatigue. In addition, the patient must be able to provide own self-care and demonstrate improved physical mobility.

PATIENT EDUCATION. The patient with RA needs extensive patient education regarding the disease process, medication management, and the comprehensive plan of care. In collaboration with health team members, help the patient plan a daily schedule that balances rest and exercise. A vocational counselor may be necessary for job training if the patient needs to pursue a different occupation. Patients who are unable to work may be able to qualify for disability benefits through the federal Social Security program. Inform the patient about community resources such as support groups (visit www.arthritis.org).

CRITICAL THINKING

Mrs. Harris is a 48-year-old nurse who has had upper extremity joint pain and swelling for about 4 years. She was recently diagnosed with rheumatoid arthritis but has no systemic involvement. She has extreme fatigue at this time. She is concerned that she will have to give up providing direct patient care on a busy medical unit in the local hospital.

1. What questions might you ask her about her illness?
2. What should you discuss with Mrs. Harris about pain management?

Suggested answers are at the end of the chapter.

 MUSCULOSKELETAL SURGERY

Some health problems cannot be managed conservatively and require surgery. The most common orthopedic surgeries are discussed here.

Total Joint Replacement

Total joint replacement (TJR) is most often performed for patients who have some type of connective tissue disease in which their joints become severely deteriorated. TJR may also be needed after long-term steroid therapy. Long-term use of steroids, trauma, and complications of joint replacement can cause **avascular necrosis,** a condition in which bone tissue dies (usually the femoral head) as a result of impaired blood supply. Advanced avascular necrosis is very

painful and usually does not respond to conservative pain relief measures. The primary goal of TJR is to relieve severe chronic pain and improve ability to carry out ADLs when no other treatment is successful.

Total hip replacement and total knee replacement are the most common replacement surgeries. Any synovial joint can be replaced. Another term used for joint replacement is **arthroplasty.** The replacement devices, sometimes referred to as prostheses, are made of metal, ceramic, plastic, or a combination of these materials. Some prostheses are held in place by cement. Others are secured by the patient's bone as it grafts and connects to the prosthesis. Bone substitutes, also called biologics, are used when the amount of available bone is insufficient to provide a good base of support for the replacement devices.

Total Hip Replacement

Total hip replacement (THR) uses two components: an acetabular cup that is inserted into the pelvic acetabulum and a femoral component that is inserted into the femur to replace the femoral head and neck (Fig. 46.12). A THR can last 15 years to a lifetime.

PREOPERATIVE CARE. THR is an elective procedure. It is scheduled to allow time for preoperative teaching and screening. A case manager (e.g., registered nurse or social worker) may assess the patient's needs and support systems available postoperatively. Preoperatively, the nurse checks the neurovascular status of the operative extremity, level of pain, and mobility. The patient is taught about the surgery and what to expect postoperatively. Some patients are scheduled to meet with a physical therapist to learn postoperative exercises and how to ambulate with a walker or crutches.

Since some patients receive postoperative blood transfusions due to blood loss in surgery, the HCP may order an autologous blood donation by the patient. The patient donates blood before surgery per guidelines (e.g., time frames specified, hemoglobin levels normal). This blood is then available for reinfusion postoperatively if needed. The predeposited blood donation is cost-effective. It can reassure patients who are concerned about receiving blood from other donors.

A prophylactic antibiotic given just prior to the surgery reduces the chance of an infection. The patient's length of stay is about 2 to 5 days. Some hospitals have joint camp programs where a group of patients undergoing joint replacements are admitted on the same day, undergo surgery, and then support each other during recovery in activities such as physical therapy.

POSTOPERATIVE CARE. Care for the patient having a THR is interdisciplinary. The patient usually gets out of bed and into a chair the night of surgery or early the next day. Ensure that the patient does not adduct or hyperflex the surgical hip during transfer to the chair. The chair should have a straight

• WORD • BUILDING •
arthroplasty: arthro—joint + plasty—creation of

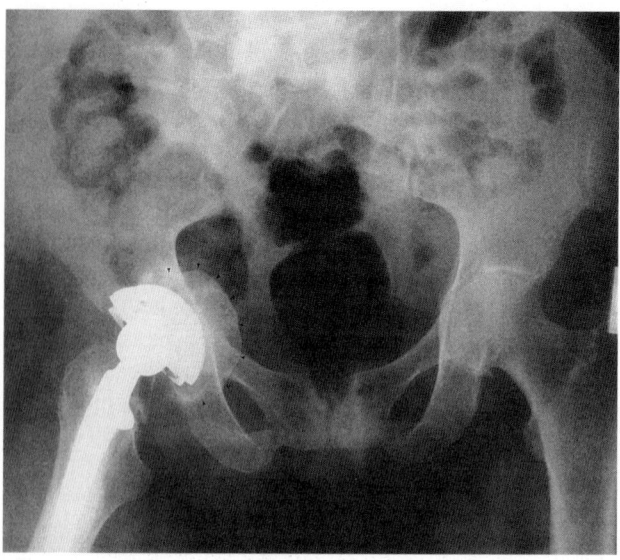

FIGURE 46.12 Total hip arthroplasty of arthritic right hip.

back and be high enough to prevent excessive flexion. The toilet seat should also be raised for the same purpose. The HCP orders the amount of weight bearing permitted. Initially, pain is managed by epidural analgesia, patient-controlled analgesia, or IV analgesics. After the first postoperative day, the patient usually progresses to an oral analgesic. Early ambulation helps prevent postoperative complications, such as atelectasis and DVT. The physical therapist works with the patient for ambulation or assistive devices.

In addition to providing the general postoperative care that all patients undergoing general or epidural anesthesia require, plan and implement interventions to help prevent the following common complications of THR (see Chapter 12).

Hip Dislocation. The most common postoperative complication for the patient having a THR is subluxation (partial dislocation) or total dislocation. Dislocation occurs when the femoral component becomes dislodged from the acetabular cup. Often, if a dislocation occurs, there is an audible "pop" followed by immediate pain in the affected hip. In addition to pain, the patient experiences shortening and possibly internal rotation of the surgical leg. If any of these signs and symptoms occur, notify the surgeon immediately and keep the patient in bed. Additional analgesics may be ordered until the patient can be taken to the operating room. Under anesthesia, the surgeon manually manipulates the hip back into alignment.

Preventing dislocation is a major nursing responsibility. Correct positioning of the surgical leg is critical. The primary goals are to prevent hip adduction (across the body's midline) and hyperflexion (bending forward more than 90 degrees). To accomplish these goals, place the patient after surgery in a supine position with the head slightly elevated. A trapezoid-shaped abduction pillow (called a triangular pillow), splint, wedge, or regular bed pillows may be ordered to be placed between the legs to prevent adduction. The patient can be turned to the side of the body specified by the HCP, with

hip adduction avoided. The patient is turned with the abductor pillow or three regular pillows (one proximal and two distal) in place between the legs. When turning, it is important that the hip and legs turn together to minimize the chance of dislocation. Supporting the leg and abductor pillow during turning is required to decrease the chance of dislocation.

To prevent hyperflexion, surgeons initially may allow the patient to sit at no more than a 60-degree angle in a reclining chair. The patient's positioning is progressed to 90 degrees, the maximum allowed to prevent hyperflexion (Fig. 46.13). While the patient is on bedrest, the use of a fracture bedpan is recommended to reduce discomfort and dislocation.

Because of restrictions in hip flexion, patients are instructed not to bend forward to tie shoes or put on pants. The occupational therapist provides adaptive or assistive devices, such as dressing sticks and long-handled shoe horns, to assist the patient in being independent in ADLs.

Skin Breakdown. Because most patients having THR are older, skin breakdown prevention is a major part of postoperative care. Turning the patient at least every 2 hours (more often if high risk) and keeping the heels off the bed help prevent pressure injuries. Heels, elbows, and the sacrum are vulnerable and can break down within 24 hours. A reddened area that does not blanch is a stage 1 pressure injury and must be treated aggressively to prevent progression to other stages. Prophylactic application of cushioning dressings and the use of heel protectors help to decrease the chance of skin breakdown of the heels.

Patients who are incontinent must be kept clean and dry. Assisting the patient to use the toilet every 2 hours and using a protective barrier cream also help prevent skin problems related to incontinence. Adequate diet and hydration are also important to prevent skin breakdown. Box 46.4 describes additional nursing interventions that meet the needs of postoperative patients recovering from THR.

Infection. Orthopedic surgery patients are at an increased risk for infection because of the nature of the surgery and their age. In addition to a preoperative prophylactic IV antibiotic, the surgeon can irrigate the incision with antibiotics

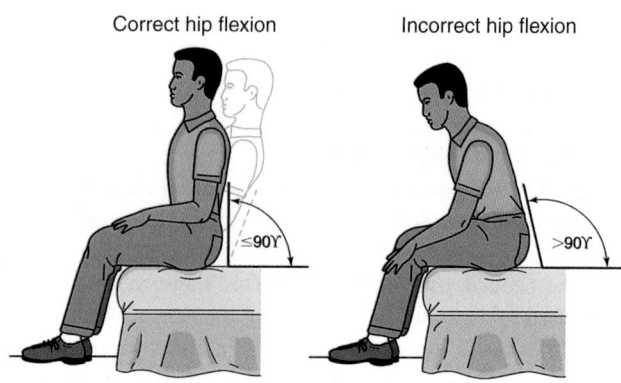

Correct hip flexion   Incorrect hip flexion

≤90Y   >90Y

FIGURE 46.13 Hip flexion after total hip replacement should be 90 degrees or less to prevent dislocation.

Box 46.4

Nursing Interventions Following Total Hip Replacement

- Ensure the hip is not allowed to become adducted. Can use abductor pillow or pillows.
- Turning the patient requires abduction to be maintained. Turn the patient as a whole, not allowing hip or legs to fall forward or backward. Use pillows to support raised limb.
- Monitor for skin integrity of the opposite heel, which often is used to help mobilize in bed and so is prone to friction and pressure sores. Apply protective devices for heels.
- Make sure limb remains in abduction when moving the patient out of bed.
- Prevent postoperative pneumonia by encouraging deep breathing and coughing and use of incentive spirometer.
- Pain control is of utmost importance. Administer regularly scheduled analgesics, and make sure breakthrough analgesia is provided as needed. Decreased pain allows for earlier mobilization and fewer complications of immobility.
- Monitor level of consciousness and orientation. Many older patients have alterations in mental status after surgery because of anesthetics, analgesics, blood loss, and environmental changes.

intraoperatively, place antibiotic beads in the incision, or continue IV antibiotics postoperatively.

Many institutional policies permit only the surgeon or their designate to remove the initial dressing. Regardless of who removes the dressing, meticulous aseptic care of the surgical wound is important to minimize the chance of infection. When performing dressing changes, observe the incision for signs and symptoms of infection (e.g., redness, swelling, warmth, odor, pain, or yellow, green, or brown-tinged drainage). Monitor the patient's temperature. An older patient with an infection might not experience a fever but may exhibit confusion due to the infection.

Infection may not occur during the patient's hospital stay but can occur 1 or more years later. If this late infection does not respond to antibiotics, the prosthesis may be removed and replaced.

CRITICAL THINKING

Mrs. Adam is 78 years old and had a left total hip replacement 3 days ago. When changing her dressing, the nurse notices a purulent discharge. Cefaclor (Ceclor) 500 mg by mouth every 8 hours is ordered. It is available as a 375-mg/5-mL suspension. How many milliliters should Mrs. Adam be given?

Suggested answers are at the end of the chapter.

Bleeding. In THR, up to two-thirds of any blood loss can occur postoperatively. The patient might have a surgical drain (e.g., Hemovac or Jackson-Pratt) that is emptied every 8 to

12 hours as ordered for the first day or two, although the use of drains has decreased to prevent infection. Monitor dressings for drainage and report large or unexpected amounts. Reinforce it as needed. On the second or third postoperative day, the patient's hemoglobin and hematocrit levels may decrease to the point that blood transfusion is needed. The patient might receive autologous blood or salvaged operative or postoperative blood. By using an orthopedic patient autotransfusion (such as OrthoPAT) during surgery, about 50% of blood that is lost can be recovered and saved for reinfusion into the same patient. Postoperatively, blood can be replaced by collecting shed blood via suction into a reservoir and then filtering and reinfusing it within 6 hours of collection. Monitoring for blood loss and signs of shock is an important nursing action.

Neurovascular Compromise. For any musculoskeletal surgery or injury, frequent neurovascular checks for circulation (e.g., color, warmth, pulses), sensation, and movement are performed distal to the surgical procedure or injury (and compared with the unaffected side) when vital signs are checked. The procedure and significance of these assessments are described in Chapter 45.

Venous Thromboembolitic Complications. Patients having hip surgery are at the greatest risk for DVT or pulmonary embolus. Older adult patients, obese patients, and those with a history of thromboembolitic problems are also at a high risk for potentially fatal problems. Thigh-high elastic stockings and intermittent pneumatic compression devices may be used while the patient is hospitalized (see Chapter 12). Anticoagulant medication is given to help prevent clot formation.

NURSING CARE TIP

When giving anticoagulant medications such as enoxaparin (Lovenox) or dalteparin (Fragmin), follow manufacturer's instructions for administration. The air bubble should not be removed from the prefilled syringe before administration to ensure the entire dose is given.

Because DVT occurs mostly in the lower extremities, leg exercises are started in the immediate postoperative period and continued until the patient is fully ambulatory. The physical therapist teaches the patient how to perform foot and ankle exercises per facility guidelines. Once the foot and ankle exercise routine has been determined, the nurse then reinforces the teaching and monitors the patient for compliance.

If the patient is medically stable, he or she is discharged home for rehabilitation or to a subacute care unit, rehabilitation unit, or nursing home for short-term rehabilitation, lasting a week or less. The rehabilitation program that began in the hospital continues after discharge until the patient is independent in ambulation and self-care.

Before hospital discharge, the interdisciplinary team provides patient education for home care, including hip precautions that need to be used until the surgeon reevaluates the patient at the 6- to 8-week follow-up visit (Box 46.5).

Total Knee Replacement

The knee is the second most commonly replaced joint. It requires three components for total replacement: a femoral component, a tibial component, and a patellar button (Fig. 46.14). For patients who do not yet need a total replacement, partial knee resurfacing is available.

Care for the patient with a total knee replacement (TKR) is similar to that required for a patient with a THR, except that dislocation and, therefore, preventive positioning are not a concern. Postoperatively, a bulky dressing and possibly a surgical drain are in place. Once again, it is important to monitor for bleeding along with the usual postoperative interventions. Medical complications described for THR, such as DVT, may be seen in the patient undergoing knee replacement (see Box 46.4).

Amputation

An amputation is the removal of a body part. It can be as limited as removing part of a finger or as devastating as removing nearly half the body. Amputations may be *surgical* as a result of disease or *traumatic* as a result of an accident.

Surgical Amputation

The main reason for surgical amputations is ischemia from peripheral vascular disease occurring in the older adult. The rate of lower extremity amputation is much higher in the diabetic patient than in the nondiabetic patient (see Chapter 40). Surgical amputations may also be done for bone tumors, thermal injuries (e.g., frostbite, electric shock), crushing injuries, congenital problems, or infections.

Traumatic Amputation

Traumatic amputations occur from accidents, often in young and middle-aged adults. Industrial machinery, motor vehicles,

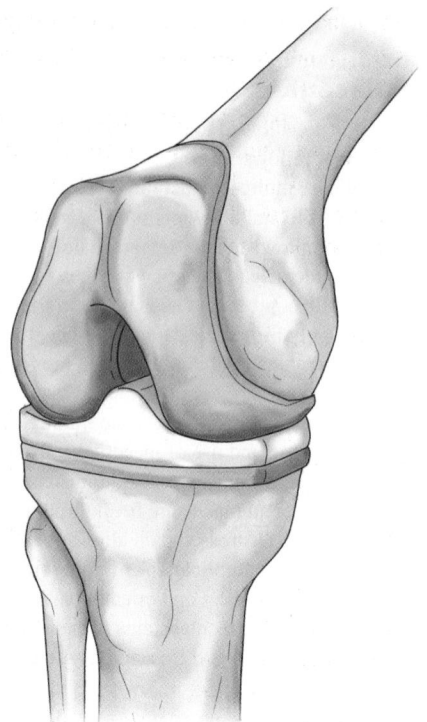

Total knee
replacement

FIGURE 46.14 Total knee replacement.

lawn mowers, chain saws, and snow blowers are common causes of accidental amputation.

Because in these patients the amputated part is usually healthy, attempts at **replantation** can occur. One of the most common replantations is one or more fingers. Prehospital care of the severed body part includes rinsing if dirty and wrapping in a clean, moist cloth that is placed in a sealed plastic bag. The bag should then be placed into ice cold water until the body part is transported to the hospital. The surgical procedure is performed by specialists who operate using a microscope. Nerves, vessels, and muscle must be reattached.

Levels of Amputation

The most common surgical amputation site is the lower extremity. The loss of the great toe affects balance and gait. Midfoot amputations are preferred over below-the-knee amputations for patients with peripheral vascular disease. The more proximal the amputation, the more disability is present.

If the lower leg is amputated, a below-the-knee amputation is preferred over an above-the-knee amputation to preserve joint function. The higher the level of amputation, the more energy required for ambulation. Hip disarticulation

---

Box 46.5

Patient Education After Total Hip Replacement

Teach patients to follow these safety measures to prevent hip dislocation:

• Keep legs abducted (away from center of body) with pillows.
• Sleep with pillows between legs per health care provider's instructions.
• Do not bend at the waist (hip) more than 90 degrees per health care provider's instructions.
• Get up from a sitting position by pushing straight up off of the chair or bed without leaning forward.
• Use a walker, if desired, to assist walking.
• Physiotherapy and occupational therapy can provide equipment that aids in putting on socks and shoes.
• Sexual activity can be started when tolerated, provided hip safety measures are followed.

• WORD • BUILDING •

replantation: re—again + plant—to plant + ation—process

(removal through the hip joint) and **hemipelvectomy** (removal through part of the pelvis) are reserved for young patients who have cancer or severe trauma.

Upper extremity amputations are usually more significant than lower extremity amputations and more often result from trauma. The arms and hands are necessary for performing ADLs. Early replacement with a prosthesis is crucial for the patient with an upper extremity amputation.

Preoperative Care
Patients who are scheduled for elective amputations have the advantage of time for preoperative teaching, prosthesis fitting, and adjustment to the loss of part of their bodies. Preoperative teaching is started in the surgeon's office. Postoperative and rehabilitative care is reviewed with the patient and family or significant other. Those patients experiencing a traumatic amputation have no opportunity to prepare for the significant changes that will result from the accident. Preoperative care will not only involve physical needs being met; significant psychological and emotional concerns also have to be addressed. This continues postoperatively.

Preoperatively, the patient should be referred to a certified prosthetist-orthotist to begin plans for replacing the removed body part with a prosthesis.

Disturbed Body Image is a common nursing diagnosis for the patient having an amputation. If possible, it is helpful for the preoperative patient to meet with a rehabilitated amputee. Note the patient's reaction to having an amputation with the expectation that the patient will experience many of the stages of loss and grieving. Support systems and coping mechanisms are identified that can help the patient through the surgery and postoperative period. Ensure that appropriate support is provided by other disciplines such as social work and clergy.

Postoperative Care
In addition to the general postoperative care described here, plan and implement interventions to help prevent postoperative complications, including hemorrhage and infection (see Chapter 12).

PREVENTION OF HEMORRHAGE AND INFECTION. When a patient loses part of the body, because of either trauma or surgery, blood vessels are severed or damaged. The patient returns from surgery with a large pressure dressing that is secured with an elastic wrap. Monitor the closest proximal pulse between the heart and the amputated body part for strength. Compare findings with the nonsurgical extremity. Check the bulky dressing for bloody drainage. If blood is on the dressing when the patient is admitted to the postanesthesia care unit or the surgical unit, circle, date, and time the area of drainage, and closely monitor for enlargement. If bleeding continues, notify the surgeon immediately. A tourniquet should be readily available in case severe hemorrhage occurs.

After the dressing is removed, observe for adequate perfusion to the skin flap at the end of the residual limb, referred to as the stump. The skin should be pink in a patient who has light skin and not discolored (lighter or darker than other skin pigmentation) in a patient who has dark skin. The residual limb temperature should be warm but not hot to touch.

Infection of the wound can be problematic, especially if the infection enters the bone (osteomyelitis). Inspect the wound for intense redness or drainage. Localized infections usually do not cause an increase in body temperature. If temperature is elevated, it could indicate a serious wound infection, a systemic infection, or some other type of infection. Traumatic amputations are at risk for developing infection due to the nature of the injury and the likelihood of exposure to environmental pathogens from the source of the amputation.

PAIN CONTROL. Phantom pain arises from the spinal cord and brain. The patient reports severe pain usually distal to the removed body part. The pain may be described as intense burning, cramping, shooting, stabbing, or throbbing. Phantom pain can be triggered by touching the residual limb, fatigue, emotional stress, or weather changes. It may improve over time.

Never doubt that a patient is experiencing phantom pain. Phantom sensation is different from phantom pain in that the patient feels as if the limb is still present rather than being painful. Treat phantom pain with prescribed medication and complementary and alternative therapies. Medications used include anticonvulsants, such as gabapentin (Gralise, Neurontin) or pregabalin (Lyrica); beta-blocking agents, such as propranolol (Inderal); and antidepressants, such as amitriptyline (Elavil). To complement traditional therapy, alternative therapies may be useful, including biofeedback, nerve stimulation, myoelectric prosthesis, massage, mirror box (watching unaffected limb while moving), imagery, acupuncture, and spinal cord or brain stimulation (during which a small electric current is used). Future therapy may involve virtual reality goggles (during which it appears as if no amputation occurred).

MOBILITY AND AMBULATION. To reduce surgical swelling, cold application may be ordered. Alternately, the residual limb may be elevated on a pillow for 24 hours or less. Continued use of a pillow for elevation can lead to flexion contractures, especially for patients with a below-the-knee or above-the-knee amputation. If the hip becomes contracted, the patient will not be able to walk so using a prosthesis will not be possible. Check the limb periodically to ensure that it lies completely flat on the bed. The patient should avoid positions of flexion, such as sitting for long periods. If the patient is able, lying prone (on the stomach) for 30 minutes four times daily helps prevent hip contracture (abnormal shortening of muscle or scar tissue).

Postoperative care after amputation is interdisciplinary. It often requires an extensive rehabilitation program. The

• WORD • BUILDING •
hemipelvectomy: hemi—half + pelv—pelvis + ectomy—
    removal of

physical therapist teaches the patient muscle-strengthening exercises that help with ambulation and transfers and prevent flexion contractures. A trapeze bar on an overhead bed frame aids in strengthening the arms and helps the patient move around in bed.

PROSTHESIS CARE. The residual limb must be prepared for wearing the prosthesis. A temporary prosthesis may be worn until the swelling subsides. A shrinker sock is commonly used to decrease swelling and prepare the residual limb for the prosthesis. It is also worn with the prosthesis. There are several brands of shrinker socks. It is important to perform neurovascular checks and check the residual limb for infection and alterations in tissue integrity each time the shrinker sock is removed.

The prosthesis requires special care. The patient should be taught to do the following:

- Clean the prosthesis socket with mild soap and water and then dry it.
- Clean inserts and liners regularly.
- Use garters to keep socks in place.
- Grease prosthesis parts as instructed by prosthetist.
- Replace shoes when they wear out with shoes of the same height and type.

LIFESTYLE ADAPTATION. The patient may feel that life will be markedly changed as a result of amputation. If the case manager thinks it is needed, a job analysis may be conducted by a vocational analyst or specialized case manager. With technological advances in prostheses, most patients who worked before surgery are able to return to their jobs after surgery. Many patients with amputations are able to bowl, ski, hike, and continue with all of the recreational hobbies that they were able to do before surgery.

A supportive family or significant other is vital to help the patient adjust to body image change. Consider the need for a sexual counselor or psychologist if indicated. For any patient with an amputation, help the patient set realistic expectations.

For the patient who is not a candidate for a prosthesis, home adaptations for a wheelchair may be needed. The patient must have access to toileting facilities and areas necessary for self-care ("Home Health Hints"). Structural changes in the living environment may be needed before the patient can be discharged from rehabilitation.

Home Health Hints

- The home health nurse frequently removes staples and sutures. Always have several of each type of removal device on hand. Remember that staples, scissors, or other items that are "sharp" need to be disposed of in a biohazard container or sturdy plastic container such as a detergent bottle.
- If equipment or modifications to the home are needed following hospitalization for an orthopedic adaptation, it is best if they can be obtained or arranged before discharge.
- Physical and/or occupational therapy are often ordered for the orthopedic patient discharged from the hospital to help with strengthening, ambulation, activities of daily living, and obtaining and use of assistive devices (e.g., raised toilet seats, handheld reachers, walkers, canes, wheelchairs, and hand rails).
- Teach the patient to wear padded cycling gloves if the walker is making his or her hands sore.
- Teach the patient to wear flat, sturdy, rubber-soled shoes to prevent slipping, tripping, or turning an ankle.
- Teach the patient to remove all throw rugs, unnecessary furniture, and other possible fall hazards in the home.
- Teach the patient that the risk of deep vein thrombosis (DVT) after hip or knee surgery is highest by the postoperative day five and that the risk persists for up to 12 weeks. Teach the patient to be alert for such signs as warmth, redness, edema, and increased pain of the affected leg.
- Teach the patient how to put on their open-toed compression stockings more easily. Using a plastic bag, instruct the patient to tie a knot on the closed end. Slip the bag over the foot, and then put the stocking on over the bag. Once the stocking is on over the heel, the patient or caregiver can grab the knot in the plastic bag and pull the bag out through the toe opening. Another example is the Doff N' Donner, a rubberized device filled with water that slides up the leg and unrolls the stocking in place (www.doffanddonner.com).
- Teach a family member or patient how to give their injections to prevent DVT formation. If the patient cannot do this and no one is available to teach him or her, the home health nurse can make visits to administer the injection.

SUGGESTED ANSWERS TO CRITICAL THINKING

Mrs. Martinez

1. When documenting, answer the questions what, why, where, who, and how to make the charting complete.
   What = Patient found on the floor on her left side, moaning and holding her left leg, crying out with any movement.
   Why = fall
   When = Date/Time: 7/2, 1000

   Where = day room
   Who = Mrs. Martinez (patient)
   How = unknown, was not witnessed.
   Date/Time: 7/2; 1000. Found on floor in day room lying on left side, moaning and holding left leg, crying out with any movement. Stated, "I fell. I think my leg is broken." Supervisor immediately notified paramedics and health care provider notified. BP [blood pressure]

SUGGESTED ANSWERS TO CRITICAL THINKING—cont'd

150/84, P [pulse] 100, R [respirations] 20. Left leg shorter than right. Remained with patient and instructed not to move until paramedics arrived. Blankets applied and pillow under head. Taken to Memorial Hospital by ambulance at 1025. I. Smith, LPN

2. To help reduce muscle spasms and therefore pain.

Mr. Schnell

1. Possible priority nursing diagnoses include:
   - *Acute Pain* related to injury and immobility
   - *Risk for Constipation* related to opioids and immobility
   - *Risk for Impaired Skin Integrity* related to extended recovery time
   - *Social Isolation* related to hospitalization
   - *Decreased Diversional Activity* related to extended need for bedrest
2. Nursing interventions may include the following:
   - Monitor pain level; administer analgesics as ordered; check pain relief; check position for comfort; provide backrubs.
   - Ensure Mr. Schnell's diet includes fiber and adequate hydration (1.5 to 2 L/day); give stool softener as ordered; monitor daily bowel movements.
   - Ensure Mr. Schnell does the exercises recommended by occupational and physical therapists; reposition him every 2 to 3 hours; have trapeze bar set up for him to use; use skin assessment tool to determine risk for skin breakdown; check for pressure points and signs and symptoms of skin breakdown.
   - Encourage Mr. Schnell's family and friends to alternate visits; have an occupational therapist assess his social needs.
   - Encourage him to listen to music; encourage visitors; ensure access to hobbies, videos, books, magazines, and comics.
3. Because opioids are an essential part of pain management and can cause constipation when used long term, planning is necessary to prevent it. Monitor daily bowel movements. Give medications to prevent opioid constipation as ordered, such as lubiprostone (Amitiza), or opioid antagonists, such as methylnaltrexone. Be proactive in ensuring normal elimination. Report lack of bowel movements promptly for intervention. Reduce opioid dosage and move to nonopioids promptly as pain relief allows.

Mr. Kardos

1. Data collection: neurovascular check including the six Ps; pain level; vital signs.
2. He might be experiencing compartment syndrome.
3. Interventions may include the need for a bivalved cast or a fasciotomy.

Mr. Finn

1.
   - "What is your typical day on the job like?"
   - "Do certain activities increase joint pain?"
   - "When is your pain worse: after activity or after rest?"
   - "How long have you experienced joint pain?"
   - "What relieves the joint pain?"
2. Risk factors include that he is overweight, is in late middle age, and has a physically demanding job.
3. Other signs and symptoms may include bony nodules on his fingers (such as Heberden nodes) and secondary inflammation causing joint swelling.
4. Patient-centered care interventions include pain management, weight loss, restoring and maintaining functional ability (i.e., bending ability for work).
5. Health care provider, occupational therapist, pharmacist, physical therapist, registered nurse.

Mrs. Harris

1. Ask what is the nature of her pain, whether it is worse after activity or rest, and whether she experiences joint stiffness and, if so, when. Follow the *WHAT'S UP?* method of pain assessment.
2. Teach Mrs. Harris to balance rest with exercise; use ice for very hot, swollen joints; and use heat to decrease stiffness.

Mrs. Adam

Unit analysis method:

$$\frac{500 \text{ mg} \mid 5 \text{ mL}}{375 \text{ mg}} = 6.7 \text{ mL}$$

Review Questions

1. The nurse is caring for a patient being transferred into bed who has just had a plaster long-leg cast applied. The patient reports pain of 6 on a scale of 0 to 10. Place the nursing interventions in order of priority.
   1. Expose cast to air dry.
   2. Administer ordered analgesic.
   3. Check circulation, sensory, and mobility status.
   4. Palm cast as positioned upon pillow.
   5. Obtain vital signs.

2. The nurse is caring for a patient with an external fixation device. Which of the following actions should the nurse implement? **Select all that apply.**
   1. Avoid touching the pins.
   2. Follow agency protocol for pin care.
   3. Cleanse pins with hydrogen peroxide four times daily.
   4. Loosen screws holding the pins during cleaning.
   5. Monitor pin sites at least daily.
   6. Use strict aseptic technique for pin care.

3. The nurse is caring for a patient with an open fracture. Which of the following actions are essential for the nurse to perform to help prevent osteomyelitis? **Select all that apply.**
   1. Perform hand hygiene before dressing change.
   2. Wear a protective gown.
   3. Use aseptic technique.
   4. Wear goggles.
   5. Wear sterile gloves to apply new dressing.
   6. Wear mask.

4. The nurse is caring for a patient who is 72 years old, postmenopausal, has osteoporosis, lost 2 inches of height, is thin, and has never exercised regularly. Which of these interventions should be included in the plan of care to prevent further bone loss?
   1. Avoid weight-bearing activities.
   2. Avoid smoking.
   3. Encourage muscle strengthening exercise.
   4. Encourage weight gain.
   5. Encourage calcium 1,000 milligrams daily
   6. Encourage vitamin D 800 IU daily

5. The nurse is caring for a male patient with gout. Which of the following lab values would be a priority for the nurse to report to the physician?
   1. White blood cell count 6.2 cells/mL
   2. Potassium 5 mEq/L
   3. Uric acid 10.2 mg/dL
   4. Ammonia 34 (mol/L

6. A patient with osteoarthritis who had a right total knee replacement tells the nurse that the other knee is becoming painful. Which of the following is the most appropriate instruction to help the patient preserve function of the left knee?
   1. Reduce dietary purines.
   2. Maintain ideal body weight.
   3. Maintain normal uric acid levels.
   4. Begin a jogging program.

7. A patient is scheduled for a right total hip replacement. The nurse should teach which of the following postoperative leg positions?
   1. Maintain legs in adduction.
   2. Maintain legs in abduction.
   3. Maintain internal leg rotation.
   4. Maintain more than 90-degree hip flexion.

8. The nurse is caring for a patient immediately after a below-the-knee amputation. Which data collection should the nurse consider a priority?
   1. Sacral edema
   2. Emotions
   3. Stump dressings
   4. Blood sugar level

9. The nurse is collecting data on a patient with a left tibia fracture. Which of the following findings is a priority finding?
   1. Increased red blood cell count
   2. Decreased body temperature
   3. Decreased lymphocyte count
   4. Absent left pedal pulse

10. A patient who has a 36-hour-old fractured femur had morphine 5 mg intramuscularly 1 hour ago and is now reporting severe unrelieved pain. Which nursing action is most appropriate?
    1. Administer an analgesic.
    2. Apply Buck traction.
    3. Raise head of bed.
    4. Notify the health care provider.

Answer rationales available in your online resources.

ANSWERS 1. 4; 1, 3, 5; 2; 2, 5, 6; 3; 1, 3, 5; 4; 2, 3, 6; 5, 3; 6, 2; 7, 2; 8, 3; 9, 4; 10, 4

Key Points

Find the chapter key points in your online resources available through Davis Edge.

Additional Resources

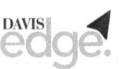 Use the scratch off code on the inside front cover of your book to access online quizzes that will help you to improve your scores on course exams and prepare for the NCLEX-PN®.

 Study Guide

CHAPTER 47

Neurologic System Function, Assessment, and Therapeutic Measures

Linda K. Cook, Deborah L. Weaver, Janice L. Bradford

KEY TERMS

anisocoria (an-ih-suh-KOR-ee-ah)
aphasia (ah-FAY-zee-ah)
contractures (kon-TRAK-churs)
decerebrate (dee-SER-eh-brayt)
decorticate (dee-KOR-tih-kayt)
dysarthria (dis-AR-three-ah)
dysphagia (dis-FAYJ-ee-ah)
electroencephalogram (ee-LEK-troh-en-SEF-uh-
   loh-gram)
myelogram (MY-eh-loh-gram)
nystagmus (nih-STAG-mus)
paresis (puh-REE-sis)
paresthesia (PAR-es-THEE-zee-ah)
subarachnoid (SUB-uh-RAK-noyd)

CHAPTER CONCEPTS

Cognition
Neurologic Regulation

LEARNING OUTCOMES

1. Describe the normal structures and functions of the nervous system.
2. Identify the effects of aging on the nervous system.
3. List data to collect when caring for a patient with a disorder of the nervous system.
4. Identify tests used to diagnose disorders of the nervous system.
5. Plan nursing care for patients undergoing diagnostic tests for disorders of the nervous system.
6. Describe common therapeutic measures used for patients with disorders of the nervous system.

NORMAL NEUROLOGIC SYSTEM ANATOMY AND PHYSIOLOGY

The nervous system has two divisions: the central nervous system (CNS), which consists of the brain and spinal cord, and the peripheral nervous system (PNS), which includes the nerves of the autonomic nervous system (ANS). Electrical impulses are transmitted through the nervous system to permit sensory, motor, and integrative activity. Actions are either automatic by reflex or a result of gathering, organizing, and processing data.

Nerve Tissue

Nerve tissue consists of neurons and support cells called neuroglia. Neurons are diverse, including unipolar, bipolar, and multipolar anatomy. Most common is the multipolar neuron with multiple dendrites and a singular axon (Fig. 47.1).

Myelination of axons increases their conduction speed. The level of myelination correlates to the necessity of speed. For example, neurons involved in protective reflexes are heavily myelinated, whereas processing neurons of the CNS lack myelin.

Neuroglial cells include oligodendrocytes, which produce myelin; microglia, which perform phagocytosis; astrocytes, which contribute to the blood-brain barrier; and ependyma, which are involved in production of cerebrospinal fluid (CSF).

Types of Neurons

Functional classification of neurons considers their position and direction of signal: a neuron is a sensory neuron (afferent), a motor neuron (efferent), or an interneuron (between the afferent and efferent neurons; Fig. 47.2). Receptors are specialized to detect external or internal changes and then generate electrical impulses. Sensory neurons from receptors

The **cell body** (also called the **soma**) is the control center of the neuron and contains the nucleus.

Dendrites, which look like the bare branches of a tree, receive signals from other neurons and conduct the information to the cell body. Some neurons have only one dendrite; others have thousands.

The **axon**, which carries nerve signals away from the body, is longer than the dendrites and contains few branches. Neurons have only one axon; however, the length of the fiber can range from a few millimeters to as much as a meter.

The axons of many (but not all) neurons are encased in a **myelin sheath**. Consisting mostly of lipid, myelin acts to insulate the axon. In the peripheral nervous system, Schwann cells form the myelin sheath. In the CNS, oligodendrocytes assume this role.

Gaps in the myelin sheath, called **neurofibral nodes** (previously called **nodes of Ranvier**), occur at evenly spaced intervals.

The end of the axon branches extensively, with each axon terminal ending in a **synaptic knob**. Within the synaptic knobs are vesicles containing a neurotransmitter.

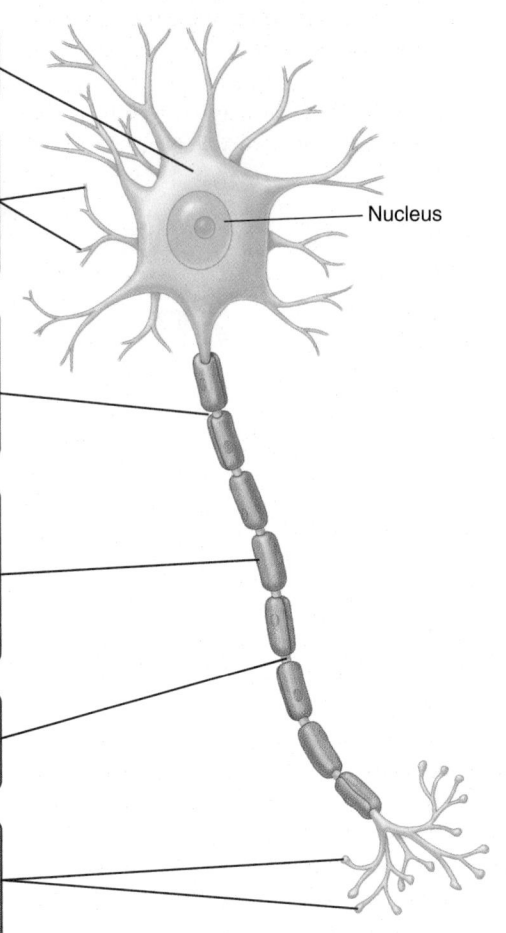

Nucleus

FIGURE 47.1 Multipolar neuron structure.

Interneurons

Interneurons, which are found only in the CNS, connect the incoming sensory pathways with the outgoing motor pathways. Besides receiving, processing, and storing information, the connections made by these neurons make each of us unique in how we think, feel, and act.

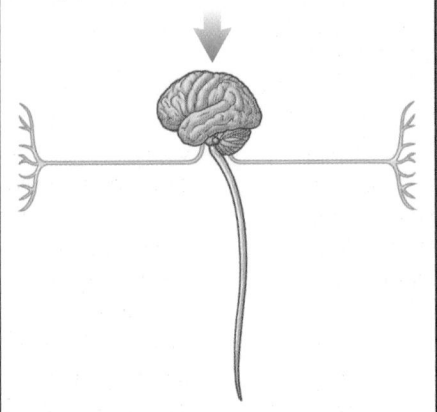

Sensory neurons

Sensory (afferent) neurons detect stimuli—such as touch, pressure, heat, cold, or chemicals—and then transmit information about the stimuli to the CNS.

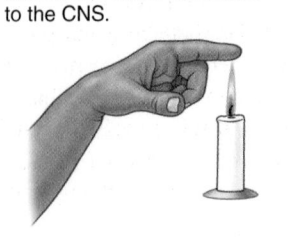

Motor neurons

Motor (efferent) neurons relay messages from the brain (which the brain emits in response to stimuli) to the muscle or gland cells.

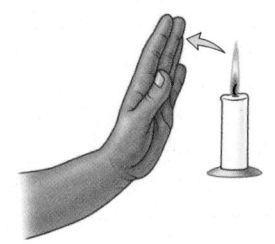

FIGURE 47.2 Neurons: sensory, interneurons, motor.

in the skin, skeletal muscles, and joints are called somatic. Sensory neurons from receptors in internal organs are called visceral sensory neurons. Motor neurons that innervate skeletal muscle are called somatic. Motor neurons that innervate smooth muscle, cardiac muscle, and glands are called visceral.

LEARNING TIP

To remember the difference between *afferent* and *efferent*, try these clues:

- **A**fferent: A is for affect or sense.
- **E**fferent: E is for effect (action).
- Or, think of the alphabet—**A** before **E**: You have to feel or sense (afferent) a stimulus before you can take action (efferent).

Nerve Impulses

A nerve impulse, which is also called an *action potential*, is an electrical change brought about by the movement of ions across the neuron cell membrane. When a neuron is at rest, it is polarized with a positive charge outside the membrane and a relatively negative charge inside the membrane. A threshold stimulus will cause a reversal in charge (action potential). A wave of depolarization travels the length of the neuron as a positive feedback loop. Repolarization occurs immediately after, restoring the positive charge outside and the negative charge inside. After a *refractory period* (the brief time after being stimulated when a nerve cannot react to another stimulus), the neuron is polarized again and ready to respond to another stimulus. A myelinated neuron is capable of transmitting hundreds of impulses per second and at speeds of more than 100 meters per second.

Synapses

Neurons typically work in a circuit. When the axon of a neuron must transmit an impulse to the dendrite or cell body of another neuron, the impulse must cross a small gap called a *synapse*. An electrical impulse is incapable of crossing this microscopic space, so when an impulse reaches the synapse, impulse transmission becomes chemical.

At chemical synapses, impulse transmission is one way because the neurotransmitter is released only by the presynaptic neuron; the impulse cannot go backward. This is important for the normal activity of functional neurons. The relative complexity of synapses also makes them a potential target for the actions of medications. For example, some antidepressants block the reuptake (reabsorption) of serotonin, a neurotransmitter, back into the proximal nerve endings, increasing the mood-elevating serotonin levels in the synapse.

Nerves and Nerve Tracts

A nerve (whether cranial, spinal, or peripheral) is a group of axons with blood vessels, wrapped in connective tissue. Most nerves are mixed; that is, they contain both sensory and motor neurons. Some, however, are not mixed. For example, the optic nerve for vision is sensory only, and autonomic nerves are purely motor.

A nerve tract is a group of thickly myelinated neurons within the CNS; such tracts within white matter appear white due to the myelin sheaths. A nerve tract within the spinal cord carries either sensory or motor impulses; those within the brain may have sensory, motor, or integrative functions.

Spinal Cord

The spinal cord transmits impulses to and from the brain. It is the integrating center for spinal cord reflexes. The spinal cord is within the vertebral canal formed by the vertebrae of the skeleton. It extends from the foramen magnum of the occipital bone to the intervertebral disk between the first and second lumbar vertebrae. The spinal nerves emerge from the intervertebral foramina.

In cross section, the spinal cord is oval shaped; internally, it has an H-shaped mass of gray matter surrounded by white matter (Fig. 47.3). Each spinal nerve attaches to the cord by two roots: dorsal and ventral. Meninges (three concentric, external layers of connective tissue) and circulating CSF offer further protection to the spinal cord.

Spinal Nerves

There are 31 pairs of spinal nerves, named according to their respective vertebrae: eight cervical pairs, 12 thoracic, five lumbar, five sacral, and one coccygeal (Fig. 47.4). These nerves are often referred to by letter and number: the second cervical nerve is C2, the tenth thoracic is T10, and so on.

Spinal Cord Reflexes

A reflex is a fast, involuntary, automatic, and predictable response to a stimulus. A spinal cord reflex uses a neural circuit, independent of the brain, called a spinal reflex arc. Sensory input triggers motor output.

The somatic spinal cord reflexes include stretch reflexes and flexor reflexes (Fig. 47.5). In a stretch reflex, a muscle that is stretched automatically contracts (e.g., the familiar patellar reflex), but all skeletal muscles have such a reflex. Because gravity exerts a constant force on the body, the purpose of these reflexes is to keep the body upright without requiring conscious processing. They also prevent potential injury from overstretching a muscle. Flexor reflexes may also be called withdrawal reflexes: the stimulus is painful trauma to tissue, and the response is to pull away from it. Again, this occurs without the need for conscious thought; the brain is not directly involved.

The clinical testing of spinal cord reflexes provides a way to assess the functioning of their reflex arcs. For example, if the patellar reflex is absent, the problem might be in the quadriceps femoris muscle, the femoral nerve, or the spinal cord itself. If the reflex is present, it indicates that all parts of the reflex arc are functioning normally.

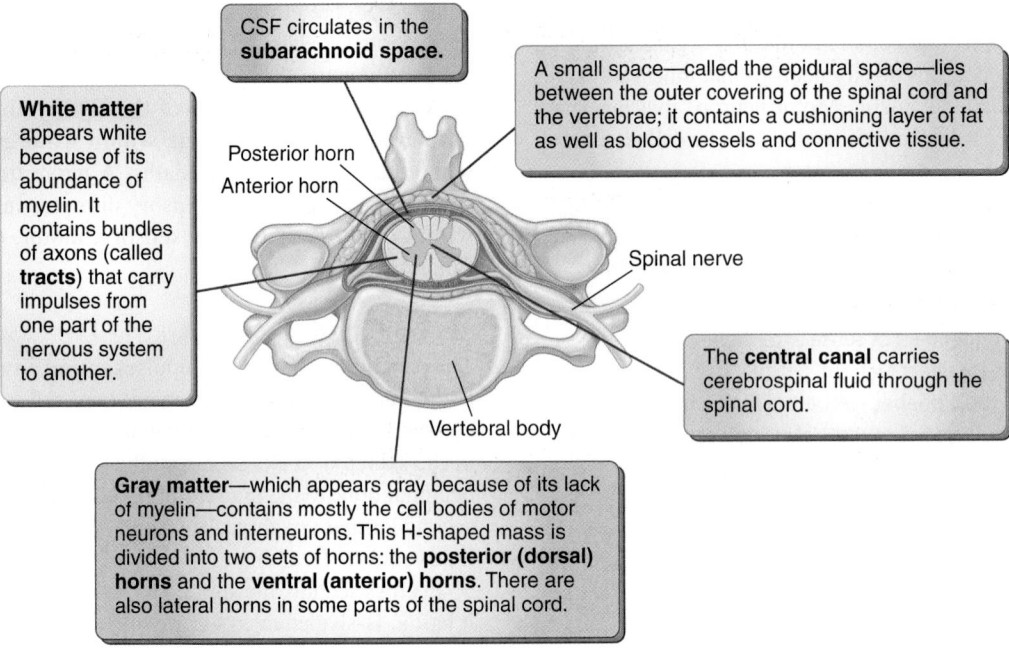

CSF circulates in the **subarachnoid space.**

A small space—called the epidural space—lies between the outer covering of the spinal cord and the vertebrae; it contains a cushioning layer of fat as well as blood vessels and connective tissue.

White matter appears white because of its abundance of myelin. It contains bundles of axons (called **tracts**) that carry impulses from one part of the nervous system to another.

Posterior horn

Anterior horn

Spinal nerve

The **central canal** carries cerebrospinal fluid through the spinal cord.

Vertebral body

Gray matter—which appears gray because of its lack of myelin—contains mostly the cell bodies of motor neurons and interneurons. This H-shaped mass is divided into two sets of horns: the **posterior (dorsal) horns** and the **ventral (anterior) horns**. There are also lateral horns in some parts of the spinal cord.

FIGURE 47.3 Spinal cord—internal anatomy, cross section, superior view.

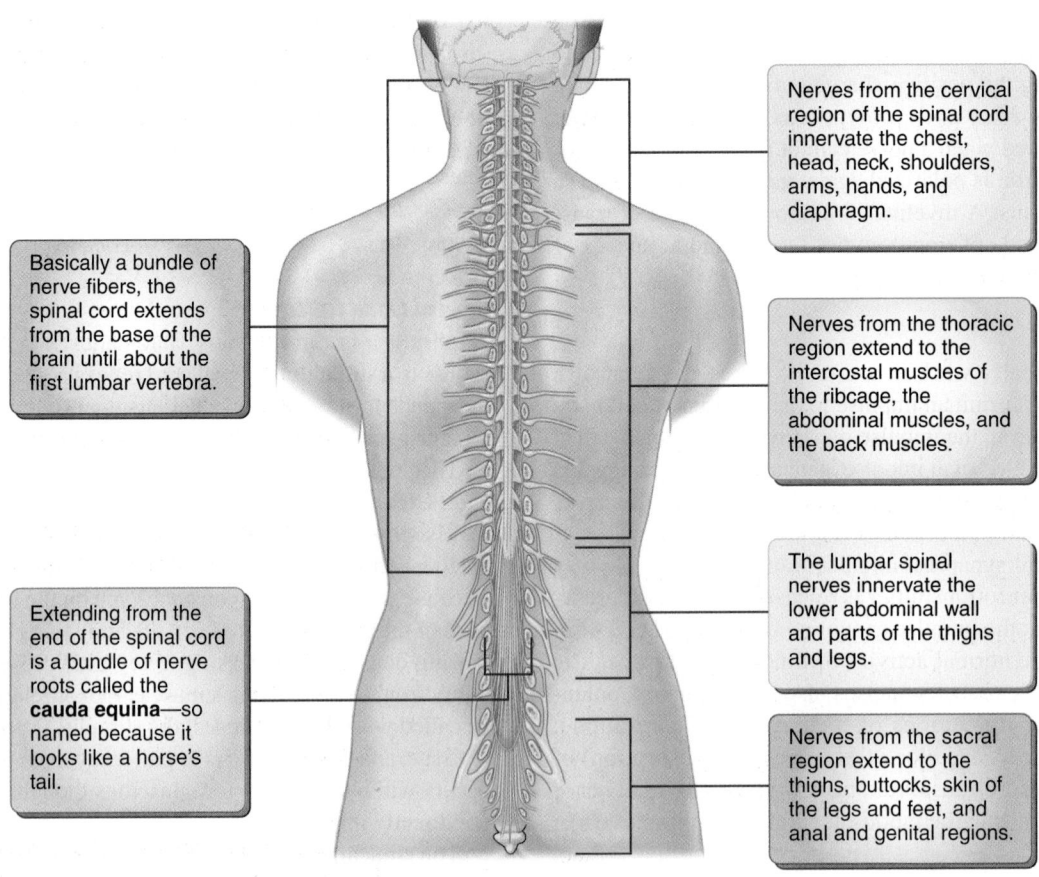

Nerves from the cervical region of the spinal cord innervate the chest, head, neck, shoulders, arms, hands, and diaphragm.

Basically a bundle of nerve fibers, the spinal cord extends from the base of the brain until about the first lumbar vertebra.

Nerves from the thoracic region extend to the intercostal muscles of the ribcage, the abdominal muscles, and the back muscles.

The lumbar spinal nerves innervate the lower abdominal wall and parts of the thighs and legs.

Extending from the end of the spinal cord is a bundle of nerve roots called the **cauda equina**—so named because it looks like a horse's tail.

Nerves from the sacral region extend to the thighs, buttocks, skin of the legs and feet, and anal and genital regions.

FIGURE 47.4 Spinal cord—full length, posterior view.

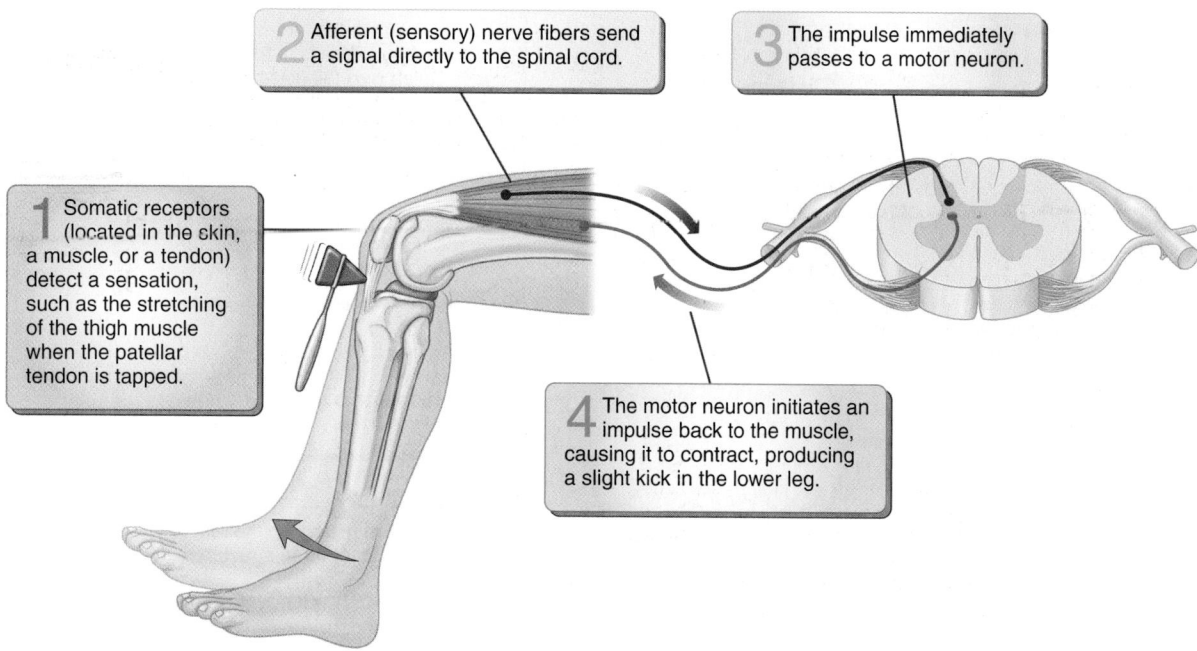

FIGURE 47.5 Somatic spinal reflex.

Brain

The brain consists of many parts that function as an integrated whole. The four principle areas are the cerebrum, dien-cephalon (thalamus and hypothalamus), brainstem (midbrain, pons, and medulla oblongata), and cerebellum (Fig. 47.6).

Meninges

The meninges are the three layers of connective tissue that cover the CNS. Where they enclose the brain, they are referred to as cranial meninges.

Ventricles and Cerebrospinal Fluid

The ventricles are four cavities within the brain: two lateral ventricles are located within the cerebral hemispheres, the third ventricle lays midline within the thalamus, and the fourth ventricle is midline between the brainstem and cere-bellum. CSF is formed from capillaries of the choroid plexus within and circulates through the four ventricles. Circulation of CSF moves inferiorly within the CNS, into the **subarach-noid** space, and ultimately superiorly to drain into the dural venous sinuses. CSF permits the exchange of nutrients and wastes between the blood and CNS neurons. It also acts as a cushion or shock absorber for the CNS. The pressure and constituents of CSF may be determined by means of a lumbar puncture (spinal tap) and may be helpful in the diagnosis of diseases such as meningitis.

Brainstem: Midbrain, Pons, and Medulla Oblongata

Primarily a reflex center, the midbrain regulates visual re-flexes (coordinated movement of the eyes), auditory reflexes (turning the ear toward a sound), and righting reflexes that keep the head upright and contribute to balance. Within the pons are two respiratory centers that work with those in the medulla oblongata to produce a normal breathing rhythm. The medulla oblongata lies just superior to the spinal cord. It regulates the most vital life functions.

Cerebellum

The cerebellum is posterior to the brainstem. The functions of the cerebellum include the involuntary aspects of voluntary movement: coordination, appropriate direction and endpoint of movements, and maintenance of posture and balance. For maintenance of balance, the cerebellum uses input from vision, proprioceptors, and equilibrium receptors in the inner ear to detect movement and changes in position.

Diencephalon: Thalamus and Hypothalamus

Deep beneath the cerebral hemispheres, the diencephalon consists primarily of the thalamus and hypothalamus. Above the brainstem, the thalamus acts as a gateway for nearly every sensation traveling to the cerebral cortex. The thalamus filters sensory input, permitting the cerebrum to concentrate on more important sensations with less distraction. The hypothalamus suspends the pituitary gland from a stalk called the infundibu-lum; they are anatomically and physiologically connected.

Cerebrum

The two cerebral hemispheres form the largest part of the human brain. The right and left hemispheres are connected

- **WORD** · **BUILDING** ·

subarachnoid: sub—below + arachnoid—middle layer of the meninges

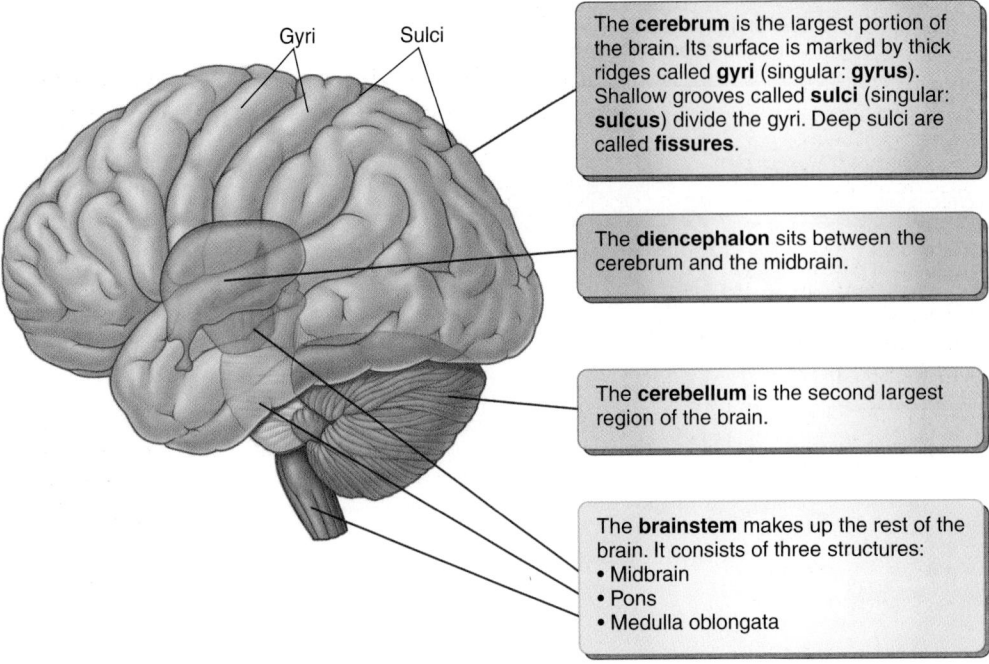

Gyri   Sulci

The **cerebrum** is the largest portion of the brain. Its surface is marked by thick ridges called **gyri** (singular: **gyrus**). Shallow grooves called **sulci** (singular: **sulcus**) divide the gyri. Deep sulci are called **fissures**.

The **diencephalon** sits between the cerebrum and the midbrain.

The **cerebellum** is the second largest region of the brain.

The **brainstem** makes up the rest of the brain. It consists of three structures:
• Midbrain
• Pons
• Medulla oblongata

FIGURE 47.6 General structures of the brain—external, left lateral view.

primarily by the corpus callosum, a band of about 300 million nerve fibers. The cerebral cortex is folded extensively into convolutions (or gyri) that create more surface area for neurons. The deep grooves between the folds are called fissures; shallow grooves are called sulci. The cerebral cortex is divided into lobes, whose functions have been extensively mapped (Fig. 47.7).

Collectively, the cerebral cortex has areas that enable learning, memory, and thought. It also helps form our individual personalities with complex behaviors that require integration of several cerebral and lower brain areas.

Deep within the white matter of the cerebral hemispheres are masses of gray matter called the basal nuclei (*ganglia*). Their functions are concerned with certain subconscious aspects of voluntary movement: regulation of muscle tone, inhibiting tremor, and use of accessory movements such as arm swinging when walking.

Cranial Nerves

The 12 pairs of cranial nerves emerge from the brainstem with the exception of pair one, which originates from the temporal lobe, and pair two, which originates from the occipital lobe. Some are purely sensory nerves, whereas others are mixed nerves. The impulses for sight, smell, hearing, taste, equilibrium, and somatic senses of supplied areas are all carried by cranial nerves to their respective sensory areas in the brain. Other cranial nerves carry motor impulses to muscles of the face, neck, shoulders, and tongue or to glands. Cranial nerves III, VII, IX, and X contain axons of both the somatic and autonomic nervous systems. The functions of all the cranial nerves are summarized in Table 47.1.

LEARNING TIP

The cranial nerves are easier to remember when a mnemonic device is used:

On	Olfactory
Old	Optic
Olympus'	Oculomotor
Towering	Trochlear
Top	Trigeminal
A	Abducens
Finn	Facial
Very	Vestibulocochlear
Graciously	Glossopharyngeal
Viewed	Vagal
A	Accessory
Hop	Hypoglossal

Autonomic Nervous System

The ANS motor output provides dual innervation to effectors—that is, smooth muscle, cardiac muscle, and glands that produce the response (effect). These two divisions (sympathetic and parasympathetic) function in opposition to one other. Their activity is integrated by the hypothalamus. Table 47.2 summarizes both ANS divisions.

Sympathetic Division

The cell bodies of the sympathetic preganglionic neurons are thoracolumbar (in the thoracic and lumbar segments of the spinal cord; Fig. 47.8). The sympathetic division is dominant in stressful situations such as fear, anger, anxiety, excitement,

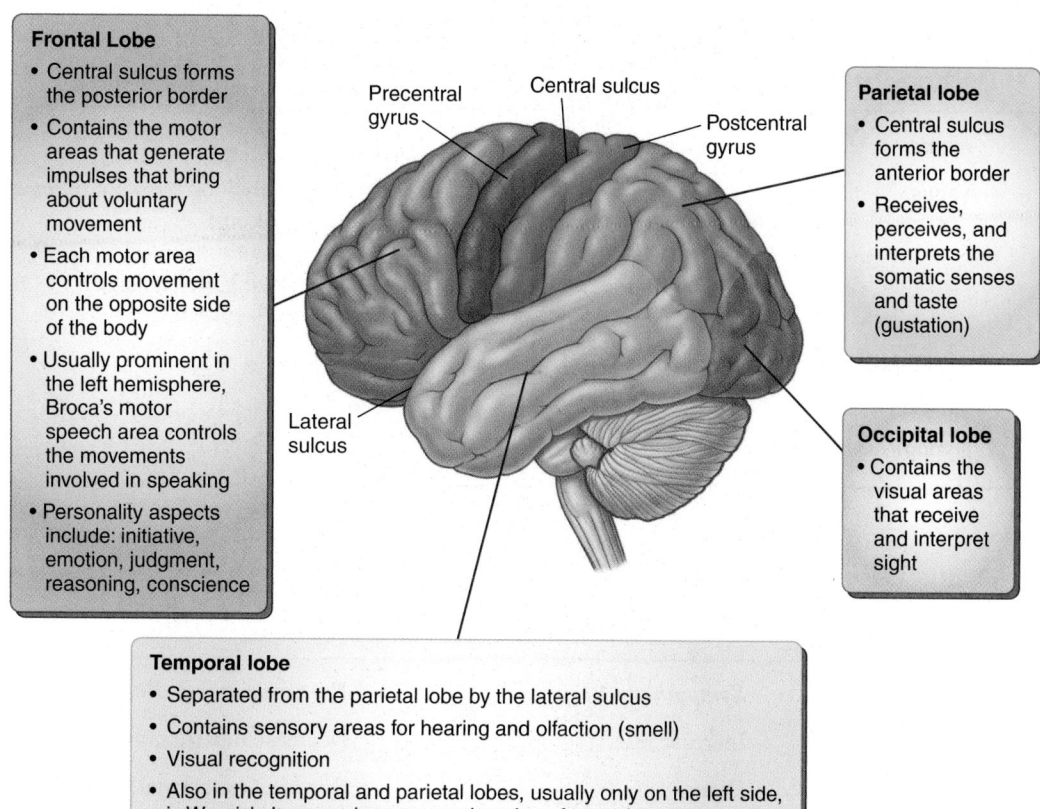

Frontal Lobe
- Central sulcus forms the posterior border
- Contains the motor areas that generate impulses that bring about voluntary movement
- Each motor area controls movement on the opposite side of the body
- Usually prominent in the left hemisphere, Broca's motor speech area controls the movements involved in speaking
- Personality aspects include: initiative, emotion, judgment, reasoning, conscience

Parietal lobe
- Central sulcus forms the anterior border
- Receives, perceives, and interprets the somatic senses and taste (gustation)

Occipital lobe
- Contains the visual areas that receive and interpret sight

Temporal lobe
- Separated from the parietal lobe by the lateral sulcus
- Contains sensory areas for hearing and olfaction (smell)
- Visual recognition
- Also in the temporal and parietal lobes, usually only on the left side, is Wernicke's area where comprehension of speech occurs.

Precentral gyrus   Central sulcus   Postcentral gyrus   Lateral sulcus

FIGURE 47.7 Cerebrum—lobes, left lateral view.

Table 47.1

Cranial Nerves

Number	Name	Function
I	Olfactory	Sense of smell
II	Optic	Sense of sight
III	Oculomotor	Movement of eyeball Constriction of pupil for bright light or near vision
IV	Trochlear	Movement of eyeball
V	Trigeminal	Sensation in face, scalp, and teeth Contraction of chewing muscles
VI	Abducens	Movement of eyeball
VII	Facial	Sense of taste Contraction of facial muscles Secretion of saliva
VIII	Vestibulocochlear	Sense of hearing Sense of equilibrium
IX	Glossopharyngeal	Sense of taste Secretion of saliva Sensory input for cardiac, respiratory, and blood pressure reflexes Contraction of pharynx, swallowing

Continued

Table 47.1

Cranial Nerves—cont'd

Number	Name	Function
X	Vagus	Sensory input in cardiac, respiratory, and blood pressure reflexes Sensory and motor input to larynx (speaking) Decreased heart rate Contraction of alimentary tube (swallowing, peristalsis) Increased digestive secretions
XI	Accessory	Contraction of neck and shoulder muscles Motor input to larynx (speaking)
XII	Hypoglossal	Movement of the tongue

Table 47.2

Functions of the Autonomic Nervous System

Organ	Sympathetic Response	Parasympathetic Response
Heart (cardiac muscle)	Increase rate	Decrease rate (to normal)
Bronchioles (smooth muscle)	Dilate	Constrict (to normal)
Iris (smooth muscle)	Dilate pupil	Constrict pupil (to normal)
Salivary glands	Decrease secretion	Increase secretion (to normal)
Stomach and intestines (smooth muscle)	Decrease peristalsis	Increase peristalsis for normal digestion
Stomach and intestines (glands)	Decrease secretion	Increase secretion for normal digestion
Internal anal sphincter	Contract to prevent defecation	Relax to permit defection
Urinary bladder (smooth muscle)	Relax to prevent urination	Contract for normal urination
Internal urethral sphincter	Contract to prevent urination	Relax to permit urination
Liver	Change glycogen to glucose	None
Sweat glands	Increase secretion	None
Blood vessels in skin and viscera (smooth muscle)	Constrict	None
Blood vessels in skeletal muscle (smooth muscle)	Dilate	None
Adrenal glands	Increase secretion of epinephrine and norepinephrine	None

Source: From Scanlon, V. C., & Sanders, T. (2015). *Essentials of anatomy and physiology* (7th ed.). Philadelphia, PA: F.A. Davis.

and exercise. The responses prepare the body for physical activity, whether or not it is actually needed. Heart rate increases, vasodilation in skeletal muscles increases oxygen and glucose supply, bronchioles dilate to take in more oxygen, and the liver converts glycogen to glucose to provide energy. The neurotransmitters of the sympathetic division are acetylcholine and norepinephrine. Acetylcholine is released by sympathetic preganglionic neurons; its inactivator is acetylcholinesterase. Norepinephrine is released by most sympathetic postganglionic neurons at the synapses with the effector cells; its inactivator is catechol O-methyltransferase (COMT) or monoamine oxidase (MAO).

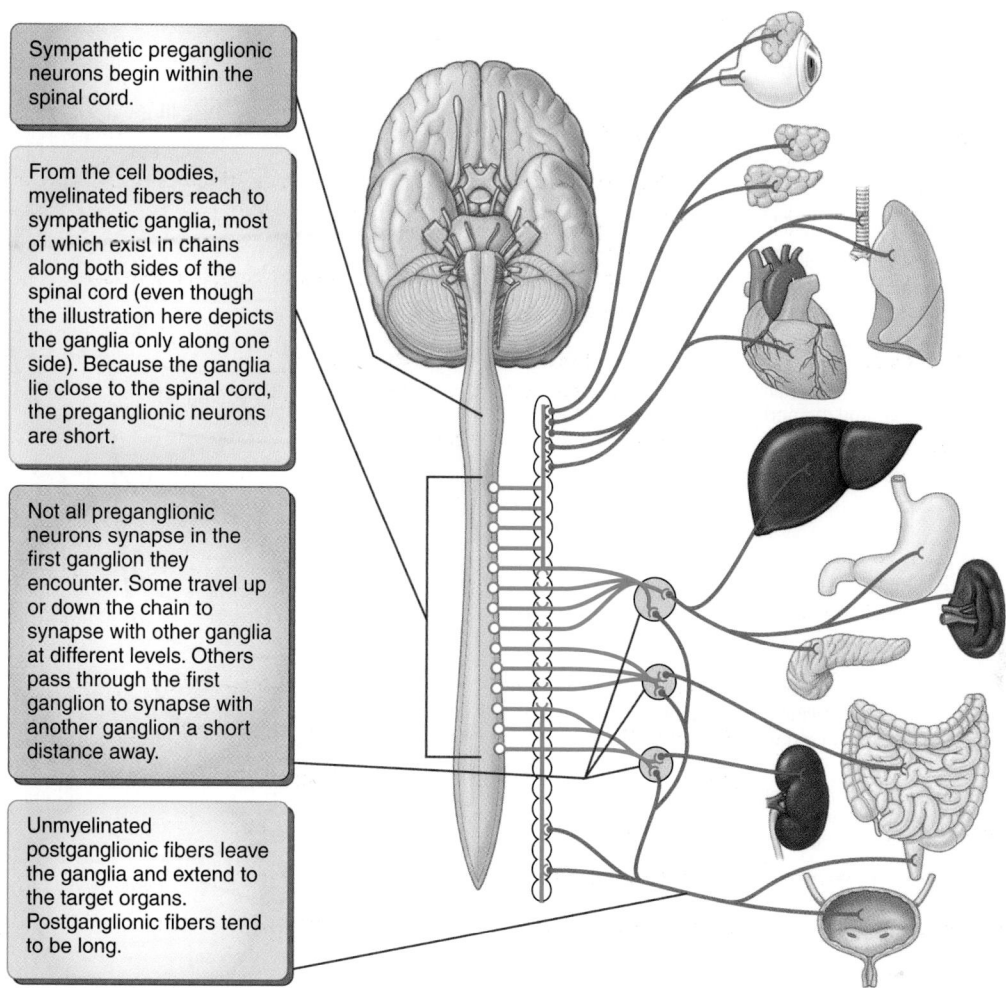

Sympathetic preganglionic neurons begin within the spinal cord.

From the cell bodies, myelinated fibers reach to sympathetic ganglia, most of which exist in chains along both sides of the spinal cord (even though the illustration here depicts the ganglia only along one side). Because the ganglia lie close to the spinal cord, the preganglionic neurons are short.

Not all preganglionic neurons synapse in the first ganglion they encounter. Some travel up or down the chain to synapse with other ganglia at different levels. Others pass through the first ganglion to synapse with another ganglion a short distance away.

Unmyelinated postganglionic fibers leave the ganglia and extend to the target organs. Postganglionic fibers tend to be long.

FIGURE 47.8 Sympathetic nervous system.

Parasympathetic Division

Cell bodies of the parasympathetic preganglionic neurons are craniosacral—that is, in the brainstem and sacral segments of the spinal cord (Fig. 47.9). The parasympathetic division dominates during relaxed, nonstressful situations to promote normal functioning of several organ systems. Digestion proceeds normally, with increased secretions and peristalsis; defecation and urination may occur; and the heart beats at a normal resting rate (see Table 47.2). Acetylcholine is the neurotransmitter at all parasympathetic synapses,

both preganglionic and postganglionic; it is inactivated by acetylcholinesterase.

Aging and the Nervous System

With age, the brain loses neurons. However, it loses only a small percentage of the total, so this is not the usual cause of mental impairment in older adults. Far more common causes of mental changes include depression, malnutrition, infection, hypotension, and side effects of medications. Some forgetfulness is to be expected, as is a decreased ability for problem-solving. Figure 47.10 presents a concept map that shows the effects that the aging process has on the neurologic system.

NURSING ASSESSMENT OF THE NEUROLOGIC SYSTEM

The focus of a nursing neurologic assessment is to establish the present function of the patient's neurologic system and to detect changes from previous assessments. A complete neurologic assessment, intended to determine the existence

CRITICAL THINKING

Mrs. Stevens receives albuterol treatments for her chronic obstructive pulmonary disease (COPD). The medication opens her airways effectively, but after her treatments, she often reports that her heart is racing. What part of the parasympathetic nervous system do you think this medication affects?

Suggested answers are at the end of the chapter.

Parasympathetic fibers leave the brainstem by joining one of the following cranial nerves:

- **Oculomotor nerve (III):** Parasympathetic fibers carried in this nerve innervate the ciliary muscle, which thickens the lens of the eye, and the pupillary constrictor, which constricts the pupil.
- **Facial nerve (VII):** These parasympathetic fibers regulate the tear glands, salivary glands, and nasal glands.
- **Glossopharyngeal nerve (IX):** The parasympathetic fibers carried in this nerve trigger salivation.
- **Vagus nerve (X):** This nerve carries about 90% of all parasympathetic preganglionic fibers. It travels from the brain to organs in the thoracic cavity (including the heart, lung, and esophagus) and the abdominal cavity (such as the stomach, liver, kidneys, pancreas, and intestines).

Parasympathetic fibers leave the sacral region by way of pelvic nerves and travel to portions of the colon and bladder.

Unlike the ganglia of the sympathetic division, the ganglia of the parasympathetic division reside in or near the target organ. As a result, the preganglionic fibers of the parasympathetic division are long while the postganglionic fibers are short.

Because the ganglia are more widely dispersed, the parasympathetic division produces a more localized response than that of the sympathetic division.

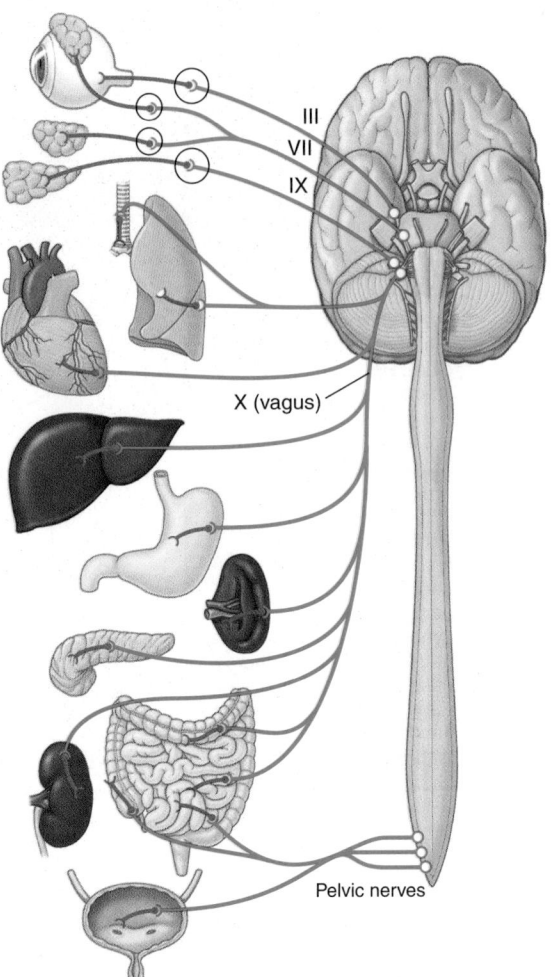

FIGURE 47.9 Parasympathetic nervous system.

LEARNING TIP

Sympathetic—*S* is for STRESS RESPONSE. The sympathetic response is referred to as the fight-or-flight response. When thinking of the sympathetic nervous system, imagine getting away from a lion. You need dilated pupils to see the path better, copious production of sweat to lose heat through evaporation, increased rate and force of heart contraction to ensure that enough blood gets to the extremities so you can run faster, dilated bronchioles to get more oxygen to your muscles, decreased digestion because that would be wasted energy, decreased urine output so you won't have to stop for the restroom, and increased mental alertness so you are always aware of where the lion is.

Parasympathetic—*P* is for PEACEFUL. The parasympathetic nervous system brings the body back to balance and rest. It is sometimes referred to as the rest-and-digest response. Think, "There is no longer a lion. Now my body can go back to normal and start digesting and urinating again!"

of neurologic disease, is performed by a health care provider (HCP). A baseline neurologic assessment should be performed on every patient admission (Box 47.1). In addition to providing valuable information about the current functioning of the patient's neurologic system, the assessment provides baseline data for later comparison. This is especially important if the patient has chronic neurologic deficits on admission.

Consider a patient admitted for surgery who has had a previous stroke resulting in **paresis** (weakness or partial paralysis) of the right arm. A complete neurologic assessment would document that the right arm is weaker than the left. If during the postoperative course you assess that both arms are equal in strength, you would want to notify the HCP so the patient could be further assessed for possible causes of weakening of the left arm.

The results of the baseline assessment are invaluable in planning and implementing safe care. For example, a patient who has a history of seizures needs a safe environment and careful monitoring, and all staff members who interact with such patients should be aware of how to respond to a seizure.

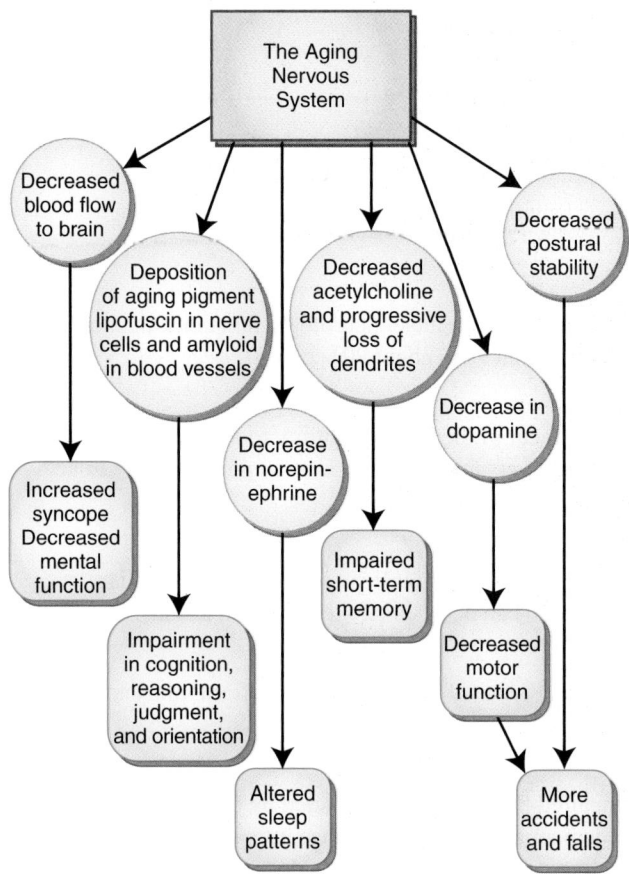

FIGURE 47.10 Aging and the neurologic system.

Patients with **dysphagia** (difficulty swallowing) may need to have restrictions placed on the types of food or fluids they can have. This information must be consistently communicated to all staff involved in the patient's care.

The frequency of neurologic assessments depends on the patient's admitting diagnosis, presence of any chronic neurologic disorders, and current functioning of the patient's neurologic system. Orders for neurologic assessments vary from every 15 minutes for an acutely ill or injured patient, to every 8 hours for a patient who is close to being discharged, to every 24 hours for a resident living in long-term care. It is always appropriate to assess a patient more often than ordered, based on observed changes in the patient's condition, and to

Box 47.1

Basic Neurologic Assessment

• Determine history of neurologic problems.
• Assess level of consciousness (patient's response to verbal or tactile stimulation) and orientation.
• Obtain vital signs (specifically blood pressure, pulse, and respirations).
• Check pupillary response to light.
• Assess strength and equality of hand grip and movement of extremities.
• Determine ability to sense touch or pain in extremities.

communicate the findings of those assessments to the HCP. Rapid detection and intervention may mean the difference between chronic dysfunction and recovery or even between life and death for the patient.

Health History

To understand the patient's neurologic status, ask about past and current diagnoses and symptoms, use of prescription and over-the-counter medications, use of recreational drugs, past surgeries, treatments, and risk factors such as family history, diet, exercise, sedentary lifestyle, caffeine intake, and recent stressors. Assessment of symptoms, as with other body systems, includes asking the *WHAT'S UP?* questions.

Obtain a history of the patient's general health and then focus on any neurologic symptoms. Symptoms of neurologic disorders vary in type, location, and intensity. It is important to remember that some neurologic disorders can affect the patient's ability to think, remember, speak, or interpret stimuli. It may be necessary to question significant others about duration and severity of symptoms. Table 47.3 presents sample questions to ask if the patient has a change in mental status.

In addition to questioning the patient, the nurse observes the patient during the health history. Is he or she shifting positions and exhibiting signs of discomfort? Is the patient able to move about freely? Is the patient able to carry on a coherent conversation?

Physical Examination

The physical examination begins when you first meet the patient and evaluate the patient's mental and physical status. The neurologic system is assessed using inspection, palpation, and percussion (with a reflex hammer). When conducting the mental status and cognitive portions of the examination, be aware that fatigue, illness, or medications can alter findings. When interpreting neurologic findings, be sure to consider the patient's age, educational background, and cultural background.

Level of Consciousness

Level of consciousness (LOC) exists along a continuum from full wakefulness, alertness, and cooperation to unresponsiveness to any form of external stimuli. A fully conscious patient responds to questions spontaneously. As consciousness becomes impaired, a patient may show irritability, a shortened attention span, or an inability to cooperate. LOC should be the first thing assessed during a neurologic examination because the information obtained can be used to modify the remainder of the examination if necessary. Keep in mind that a decrease in LOC can be caused by problems such as hypoxia, hypoglycemia, medications, or intoxication, and not just dysfunction of the neurologic system.

• **WORD • BUILDING •**
dysphagia: dys—difficult + phagia—eating

Table 47.3

Data Collection Related to Mental Status

Questions to Ask During the Health History	*Rationale/Significance*
Mental Status What is your name? What is the month? Year? Where are you now?	Disorientation is often an initial sign of a neurologic disorder.
Intellectual Function Subtract 7 from 100, then 7 from that answer, and so on (serial 7s).	Most people with intact neurologic function can complete serial 7s in about 90 seconds.
Thought Content What would you do if you smelled smoke? Where would you put milk?	Assessment of the patient's ability to interpret information and act appropriately is an important safety issue and activity of daily living.
Perception Show the patient a pencil and pen and ask what each is.	Agnosia (inability to interpret or recognize familiar objects) can occur in stroke and brain lesions.
Language Ability Read the following sentence: ____.	Different types of aphasia can result from injury to different parts of the brain.
Memory Repeat these four or five words: ____. Repeat them again in 5 minutes.	Impaired memory can be affected by both delirium and dementia. Delirium can cause impaired immediate and short-term memory, whereas dementia not only affects immediate and short-term memory but also the ability to learn new information. It also may be related to stroke.
Pain On a scale of 0 to 10, with 0 as no pain and 10 as the worst you have ever had, what is your pain level?	Pain perception may be altered or impaired by spinal injury, medications, alcohol, stress, and level of consciousness. Some spinal injuries may be critical, but the patient will not report pain.

GLASGOW COMA SCALE. Many health care institutions use the Glasgow Coma Scale (GCS), which is an international scale used to assess LOC and document findings (Table 47.4). The GCS is used to evaluate patients who have a potential for rapid deterioration in consciousness. When assessing LOC, consider the patient's physical ability to respond, taking into consideration trauma, medical condition, and medications. For example, a patient who cannot open his or her eyes because of facial trauma may still have an intact neurologic system.

Motor response is scored in the GCS based on following commands, responding to pain, or displaying abnormal postures. Abnormal postures include decorticate and decerebrate. In **decorticate,** or flexion, posturing, the patient's arms are flexed at the elbow, the hands are raised toward the chest, and the legs are extended (Fig. 47.11A). This posture indicates significant impairment of cerebral functioning. In **decerebrate,** or extension, posturing, both the arms and legs are extended, and the arms are internally rotated (Fig. 47.11B). This abnormal posturing indicates damage in the area of the brainstem.

The total possible score on the GCS ranges from 3 to 15. A score of less than 7 indicates a comatose patient and a score of 15 indicates the patient is fully alert and oriented. When used to score the effects of a head injury, a score of 13 or 14 indicates mild head injury, 9 to 12 indicates moderate injury, and any score of 8 or below indicates severe head injury. For all categories of the GCS, the type of painful stimuli required to elicit a response should be documented. Deterioration in the patient's condition (i.e., a lowering of the GCS score) should be reported to the HCP promptly ("Evidence-Based Practice").

• WORD • BUILDING •

decorticate: de—down + corticate—cerebral cortex
decerebrate: de—down + cerebrate—cerebrum

Table 47.4
Glasgow Coma Scale

Assessment	Findings	Score
Eye opening	Spontaneous	4
	To verbal stimulus	3
	To painful stimulus	2
	No response	1
Verbal response	Normal conversation	5
	Confused conversation	4
	Inappropriate words	3
	Incomprehensible sounds	2
	No response	1
Motor response	Obeys commands	6
	Localizes pain	5
	Withdraws from pain*	4
	Abnormal flexion	3
	Abnormal extension	2
	No response	1

Note: This scale is for adults only. Criteria specific to children should be used for pediatric cases.

*To elicit pain, place pressure on a nailbed or on the trapezius muscle. Be sure to apply the stimulus long enough to elicit a response.

FOUR SCORE SCALE. The Full Outline of UnResponsiveness (FOUR) Score Coma Scale is a newer tool that has been introduced into many critical care and emergency department areas. It has been shown to be as effective as if not better than the GCS. A major benefit of using the FOUR score scale is that no evaluation of verbal response is necessary, which is a problem when using the GCS with intubated patients. The FOUR score scale uses four categories: eye response, motor movement, reflexes, and breathing pattern. A maximum of four points can be earned in each of the four areas. The terms *decorticate* and *decerebrate* are not used when assessing the motor response to prevent confusion. In addition, the brainstem is evaluated using both pupillary reflexes and corneal reflexes along with the cough reflex. Once each of the components is

Evidence-Based Practice

Clinical Question

Is the Glasgow Coma Scale (GCS) a reliable tool for assessing level of consciousness?

Evidence

A systematic review of research related to the GCS was conducted to determine whether it is a reliable scale across clinical settings—that is, does it consistently produce the same results when used by different practitioners? After reviewing 41 studies, authors found that factors that can influence reliability include education and training for using the scale, the level of consciousness of the patient, and the type of stimuli used. Conflicting results were found in patients who are intubated and sedated (Reith, Synnot, ven den Brande, Gruen, & Maas, 2017).

Implications for Nursing Practice

Make sure you have been formally trained to use the scale before using it and documenting results. If you are caring for an intubated patient, consider using the FOUR score scale (covered next).

Reference

Reith, F. C., Synnot, A., ven den Brande, R., Gruen, R. L., & Maas, A. I. R. (2017). Factors influencing the reliability of the Glasgow Coma Scale: A systematic review. *Neurosurgery, 80*(6), 829–830.

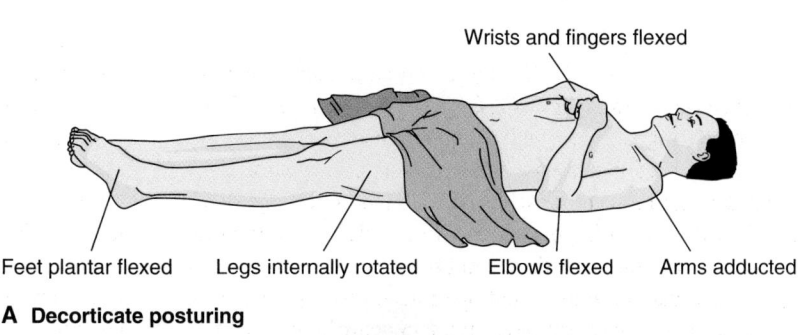

A Decorticate posturing

Wrists and fingers flexed — Feet plantar flexed — Legs internally rotated — Elbows flexed — Arms adducted

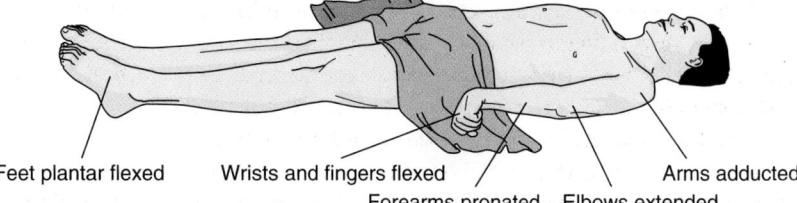

B Decerebrate posturing

Feet plantar flexed — Wrists and fingers flexed — Forearms pronated — Elbows extended — Arms adducted

FIGURE 47.11 Abnormal posturing. (A) Decorticate posturing. (B) Decerebrate posturing.

assessed and assigned a numerical value, the components are totaled. In general, the lower the FOUR score scale is, the worse the patient is neurologically and the poorer the prognosis. Conversely, the higher the score, the better the prognosis will be (Fig. 47.12).

Mental Status

Mental status can be affected not only by the aging process but by a variety of neurologic disorders and injuries. A traumatic brain injury (TBI) can result in memory impairment, delayed amnesia, affective (mood) disorders, and dementia. To assess for cognitive impairment, the Mini-Mental State Examination (MMSE) or Confusion Assessment Method (CAM) can be used. The MMSE is an assessment tool that tests orientation, registration, attention and calculation, recall, and language. Your clinical site should have an example of the MMSE.

CAM uses the following criteria to help diagnose delirium (Hartjes, Meece, & Horgas, 2016):

• Acute onset and fluctuating course
• Inattention
• Disorganized thinking
• Altered LOC

Find more about CAM at https://consultgeri.org/try-this/general-assessment/issue-13.pdf.

A change in mental status should be taken seriously, especially when the patient takes multiple medicines or has had a recent change in medicines. A primary cause of delirium and acute states of confusion is adverse effects from medications. Other causes of acute delirium include vision or hearing impairment, infection, pain, electrolyte or kidney or liver disorders, sleep deprivation, or being in an unfamiliar environment.

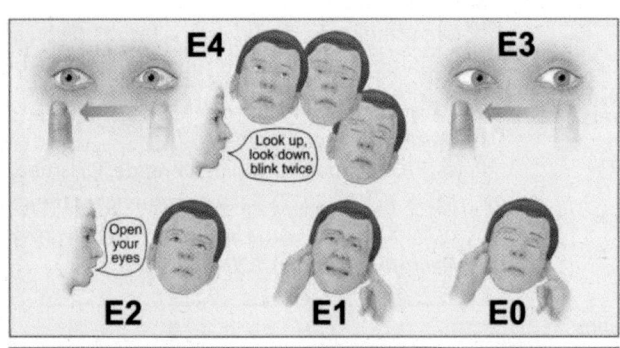

Eye response
4 = eyelids open or opened, tracking, or blinking to command
3 = eyelids open but not tracking
2 = eyelids closed but open to loud voice
1 = eyelids closed but open to pain
0 = eyelids remain closed with pain

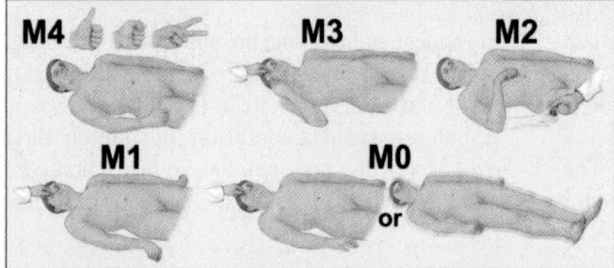

Motor response
4 = thumbs-up, fist, or peace sign
3 = localizing to pain
2 = flexion response to pain
1 = extension response to pain
0 = no response to pain or generalized myoclonus status

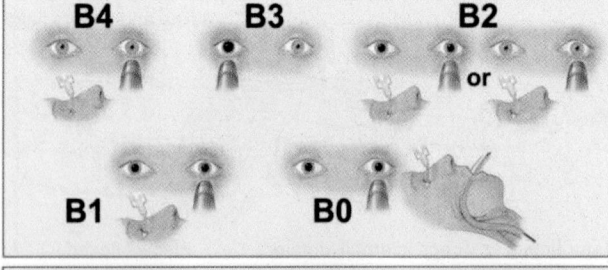

Brainstem reflexes
4 = pupil and corneal reflexes present
3 = one pupil wide and fixed
2 = pupil or corneal reflexes absent
1 = pupil and corneal reflexes absent
0 = absent pupil, corneal, and cough reflexes

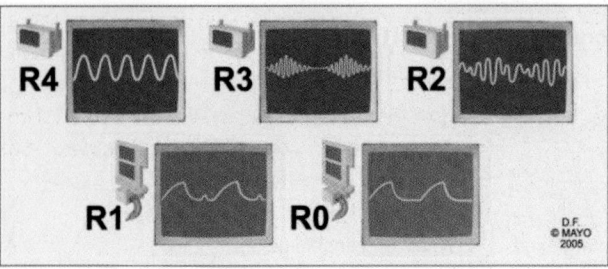

Respiration
4 = not intubated, regular breathing pattern
3 = not intubated, Cheyne-Stokes breathing pattern
2 = not intubated, irregular breathing
1 = breathes above ventilator rate
0 = breathes at ventilator rate or apnea

FIGURE 47.12 FOUR Score Coma Scale.

Pupil gauge (mm)

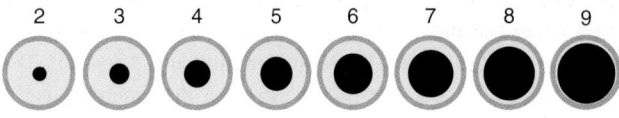

FIGURE 47.13 Assessment of pupil size.

When you assess cognitive function, you are evaluating the patient's thinking capacity. You want to determine the length of attention span, ability to concentrate, judgment, memory, orientation, perception, problem-solving ability, and motor function.

You can learn a great deal about a patient's mental capacities and emotional state by simply interacting with the patient. Behavior, mood, hygiene, grooming, and choice of dress reveal pertinent information about mental status. Mental status examinations can be performed to determine patients' cognitive functioning, thought processes, and perceptions by observing the patient's verbal and nonverbal responses to questions and specific requests. See Table 47.3 for some ways to assess these areas.

Orientation refers to the patient's ability to comprehend himself or herself in relation to person, location (place), and time. A patient who is fully oriented is often referred to as "oriented times three." Typical questions include, "What is your name? Where are you? What day is it?" (Keep in mind that we all forget the date from time to time!) You can also ask whether the person knows what season it is (spring, fall, etc.). A resident of a long-term care facility who says he or she is "at home" may consider the facility to be home and is not necessarily disoriented. Be sure that questions are appropriate to the patient's age, culture, living conditions, lifestyle, and medical condition. If the patient is unable to speak because of a stroke (expressive **aphasia**) or being intubated, do not rule out the possibility that the patient is oriented. Give expressively aphasic patients yes-or-no questions such as "Are you in a grocery store? Are you in a bowling alley? Are you in a hospital?" Patients may be able to answer with a shake of the head, eye blinks, or hand squeezes as instructed.

Examination of the Eyes

Examination of the pupils is an important part of the neurologic assessment and cranial nerve evaluation. The size of the pupils at rest is documented in millimeters (Fig. 47.13). If the patient's pupils are unusually large or small, determine whether the patient has received any medications that can affect pupil size. If the patient's pupils are unequal in size (**anisocoria**), without a correlating diagnosis or symptoms, ask the patient or significant others whether the patient normally has unequal pupils. Anisocoria may be congenital; it can also be caused by cataract surgery. Development of unequal pupils in a patient who previously had equal pupils is an emergency and should be reported to the HCP immediately. Any deviation from the normal round shape of the pupils is documented.

The next step is to assess pupillary response to light. In a darkened room, a light source (such as a flashlight) is directed at the pupil from the lateral aspect of the eye. This allows the examiner to see the direct and consensual responses to the light. A consensual response means that when one pupil is exposed to direct light, the other pupil also constricts. Absence of a consensual response may indicate a pathological condition in the area of the optic chiasm. Typically, the speed of the reaction to light is described as brisk, sluggish, or absent. Differences in the speed or size of constriction between the two pupils should be reported to the HCP.

Accommodation is the process of visual focusing from far to near. To evaluate for accommodation, have the patient focus on an object at a distant point and then refocus on the object at a near point. Pupils should constrict with the adjustment to the near object, and the eyes should converge. Upon completion of the assessment of the pupils, document your findings. PERRLA is a commonly used acronym to note that *p*upils are *e*qual, *r*ound, and *r*eactive to *l*ight and *a*ccommodation. (If assessment for accommodation is not performed, then do not include the A in the acronym.)

Next, evaluate for range of motion and for smoothness and coordination of movements. Eyes that move in the same direction in a coordinated manner are said to have a *conjugate* gaze. Conversely, a *dysconjugate* gaze is movement of the eyes in different directions. Some patients may be unable to move one or both eyes in a specific direction; this is called *ophthalmoplegia*. It is often documented as "limited extraocular movements." Always document what the limitation is (e.g., "Patient is unable to look laterally with left eye"). This allows colleagues to compare findings and recognize changes.

Nystagmus is involuntary movement of the eyes. Nystagmus varies in the speed of the movement and direction. Horizontal nystagmus is the most common. Common causes of nystagmus are phenytoin (Dilantin) toxicity and injury to the brainstem.

Examination of Muscle Function

Examine muscle groups systematically in the upper extremities and then lower extremities, comparing right to left. Compare muscle groups for symmetry of size and strength. Keep in mind the patient's age and general physical condition when evaluating muscle strength. (You would not expect the same

• **WORD • BUILDING •**

aphasia: a—absence + phasia—speech
anisocoria: aniso—unequal + coria—pupil

amount of strength from a 75-year-old woman as from a 20-year-old man.) If the patient has chronic neurologic deficits, ask whether the results of the assessment are different from his or her usual level of function.

Many HCPs use a 5-point scale to document muscle strength. A score of 5 describes a patient who is able to move the extremity against gravity and against the resistance of the examiner, displaying normal muscle strength. If the examiner is able to provide more resistance than the patient can overcome with active movement, the score is 4. If the patient can move the extremity only against gravity but not resistance, the score is 3. If gravity must be eliminated by having the examiner support the extremity to allow the patient to move the extremity, the score is 2. A score of 1 is given if there is no active movement of the extremity but a minimum muscular contraction can be palpated. If the examiner is unable to detect any muscular function, a score of 0 is given.

To test the deltoid muscles, ask the patient to raise his or her arms at the shoulder. Have the patient resist as you push down on the upper arms. The biceps are tested by having the patient flex the arm at the elbow and bring the palm toward the face, and then resist as you attempt to straighten the arm by pulling on the forearm. With the arm similarly flexed, ask the patient to straighten the arm while you resist the movement.

Hand grasps are tested by having the patient squeeze your fingers. Remember to cross your index and middle fingers to prevent the patient from hurting your fingers. If the patient does not release the grasp when told to, it is a reflex grasp, not a response to command. A reflex palmar grasp may indicate a pathological condition of the frontal lobe.

Assess for arm drift by asking the patient to hold both arms straight in front with the palms upward while keeping the eyes closed. A downward drift of the arm or rotation so that the palm is down indicates impairment of the opposite side of the brain. If a pathological condition is present, arm drift may be apparent before differences in muscle strength can be detected.

Assessment of leg muscle strength begins with the iliopsoas muscle. Place your hand on the patient's thigh and ask the patient to raise the leg, flexing at the hip. Hip adductors are tested by having the patient bring his or her legs together against your hands. The hip abductors and gluteus medius and minimus are tested by having the patient move the legs apart against resistance. Hip extension by the gluteus maximus is tested by placing the hand under the thigh and having the patient push down with the leg. The quadriceps femoris extends the knee and is tested by having the patient attempt to straighten the leg at the knee. The hamstrings are responsible for knee flexion and are evaluated by having the patient attempt to keep the heel of the foot against the bed or chair rung. Dorsiflexion is tested by having the patient pull the toes toward the head against resistance. Plantar flexion is tested by having the patient push against the examiner's hand with the ball of the foot.

The Babinski reflex is tested by firmly stroking the sole of the foot. Normal response is flexion of the great toe. If the great toe extends and the other toes fan out, neurologic dysfunction should be suspected if the patient is more than 6 months old. Deep tendon reflexes are not usually part of a routine nursing assessment. The patient's gait should be assessed to detect any neurologic dysfunction and to assess ability to ambulate safely. Patients who stagger, weave, or bump into objects may need assistance with walking.

> **BE SAFE!**
> If your patient has an unsteady gait during your assessment, place him or her on "Fall Precautions" based on facility policy. This will trigger procedures to keep the patient safe.

The Romberg test is performed by having the patient stand with feet together and eyes closed. A negative Romberg test means that the patient experiences minimal swaying for up to 20 seconds. A patient who sways or leans to one side is said to have a positive Romberg test, which may be seen in cerebellar dysfunction.

> **BE SAFE!**
> A positive Romberg test in an older adult is expected as a result of normal aging changes in the cerebellum. Be sure to protect the patient with a positive result from falls. A gait belt may be helpful when assisting the patient with ambulation.

Examination of Cranial Nerves
The cranial nerves are usually not examined in depth during a routine bedside neurologic assessment. Testing requires a patient who is able to cooperate with the examiner. Table 47.5 provides testing techniques for a basic assessment of cranial nerve function.

Summary of Examination Findings
In all cases, the findings of the neurologic examination should be correlated with the remainder of the physical examination findings. A decreased LOC coupled with a decreased oxygen saturation on pulse oximetry points to hypoxia as a cause. Correlation of vital signs with neurologic signs is particularly important. Bradycardia, increasing systolic blood pressure with widening pulse pressure, and irregular respirations, commonly referred to as the Cushing triad, are late indications of increasing intracranial pressure. These findings, in conjunction with a unilateral dilated pupil, may indicate impending herniation of the brain (discussed further in Chapter 48).

Table 47.5

Data Collection Related to Cranial Nerve Function

Nerve	Test
Olfactory nerve	Ask patient to identify common scents, such as cinnamon and coffee.
Optic nerve	Ask patient to read something or tell how many fingers you are holding up.
Oculomotor nerve	Check pupils for reaction to light and accommodation.
Oculomotor, trochlear, and abducens nerves	Ask patient to follow your finger while moving it in front of his or her eyes in the positions of a clock: 1, 3, 5, 7, 9, and 11 o'clock.
Trigeminal nerve	Ask patient to identify touch on different parts of the face with eyes closed.
Facial nerve	Ask patient to frown, smile, and wrinkle forehead; check for symmetry.
Vestibulocochlear nerve	Have patient identify a whisper close to each ear. Observe gait for balance.
Glossopharyngeal and vagus nerves	Watch for uvula and palate to rise when patient says "ahh." Touch back of throat with cotton-tipped applicator to elicit gag reflex.
Spinal accessory nerve	Ask patient to turn head and shrug the shoulders against resistance.
Hypoglossal nerve	Ask patient to stick out tongue and move it from side to side.

CRITICAL THINKING

Tim Thompson is a 78-year-old man admitted with heart problems. As you enter his room with his afternoon medications, you find Tim confused. He thinks he is at home and that the year is 1968, and he does not understand who you are or why you are there. He recognizes his wife, who is at his bedside, and he knows his own name.

1. How would you describe and document his mental status?
2. What additional data do you need to decide how to proceed?
3. What may have contributed to his confusion?
4. What members of the health care team can you collaborate with in caring for Tim?

Suggested answers are at the end of the chapter.

DIAGNOSTIC TESTS FOR THE NEUROLOGIC SYSTEM

Laboratory Tests

Specific diagnostic blood tests do not exist for neurologic disorders. However, depending on the history and physical examination, the HCP may include laboratory tests to look for underlying causes of symptoms. Possible tests include thyroid hormone levels, vitamin B_{12}, complete blood count (CBC), electrolytes, creatine kinase (CK) and isoenzymes, venereal disease research lab (VDRL) test (for syphilis), liver function, and renal function. Measurement of erythrocyte sedimentation rate (ESR) and white blood cell (WBC) count may indicate an infection, such as meningitis. Hormone levels, such as prolactin or cortisol, may indicate dysfunction of the pituitary gland related to a brain tumor. Anticholinesterase testing and antibody titers are useful in diagnosing myasthenia gravis. New blood tests and genetic testing procedures are being developed to predict Alzheimer disease risk.

Lumbar Puncture

CSF may be obtained via lumbar puncture and evaluated for glucose and protein levels, presence of bacteria and WBCs, levels of immunoglobulin, antibodies, and culture and sensitivity. See Appendix A for nursing care of a patient undergoing lumbar puncture.

> ### NURSING CARE TIP
> The idea of a needle being introduced into the spinal canal is frightening to many people. Give simple, clear directions to the patient; help the patient maintain his or her position; and provide emotional support throughout the procedure.

X-Ray Examination

Spinal x-ray (radiograph) examinations are done to determine the status of individual vertebrae and their relationship to one another. If the patient experiences pain with certain movements, he or she may be asked to flex and extend the area of the spine being examined while the radiographs are taken. This allows detection of abnormal movement of the vertebrae. Skull radiographs may be taken to detect skull fractures or foreign bodies. No special nursing care is required.

Computed Tomography

A computed tomography (CT) scan is used for diagnosing neurologic disorders of the brain or spine. A CT scan can detect hemorrhage, altered ventricle size, cerebral atrophy, tumors, skull fractures, and abscesses. A CT scan is used when magnetic resonance imaging (MRI) is contraindicated because of metal aneurysm clips or other metal implants.

The scan may be performed with or without radiopaque contrast material to enhance the clarity of the images. Contrast material is most commonly used if a tumor is suspected or following surgery in the area to be scanned. CT scans are commonly used in emergency evaluations because they can be done quickly, an important consideration if the patient is mechanically ventilated or has unstable vital signs.

Nursing Care

During a CT scan, the patient must lie still on a movable table. Noncontrast scans take about 10 minutes; contrast scans take 20 to 30 minutes. Patients who are receiving dye should be warned that they may feel a sensation of warmth following the injection; warmth in the groin area might make them feel as though they have been incontinent of urine. Nausea, diaphoresis, itching, or difficulty breathing can indicate allergy to the dye and should be reported immediately to the HCP. Sedation may be required for patients who are agitated or disoriented. Patients who are in pain may need pain medication before the examination. See Appendix A for nursing care of a patient undergoing a CT scan.

Magnetic Resonance Imaging

MRI is used for diagnosis of degenerative diseases such as multiple sclerosis, arteriovenous malformations, small tumors, hemorrhages, and cerebral and spinal cord edema. An MRI of the mediastinal cavity will determine whether the thymus gland is enlarged and facilitate diagnosis of myasthenia gravis. It is a longer procedure and may be difficult for unstable, disoriented, or mechanically ventilated patients. As with CT scan, MRI can be done with or without contrast material. Some facilities have the capability to perform magnetic resonance angiograms (MRAs). This test allows visualization of blood vessels and assessment of blood flow without being as invasive as a traditional angiogram. See Appendix A for nursing care of a patient undergoing MRI.

Angiogram

An angiogram in an x-ray following injection of dye that provides information about the structure of specific vessels as well as overall circulation to an area. See Appendix A for nursing care of a patient undergoing an angiogram.

Myelogram

A **myelogram** is an x-ray examination of the spinal canal and its contents after injection of contrast material. Compression of nerve roots, herniation of intravertebral disks, and blockage of CSF circulation can all be detected by myelogram. See Appendix A for nursing care of a patient undergoing a myelogram.

Electroencephalogram

Electrodes are placed on the scalp to record brain activity during an **electroencephalogram** (EEG). Analysis of the tracing can identify areas of abnormality, such as a seizure focus or areas of slowed activity. See Appendix A for nursing care of a patient undergoing an EEG.

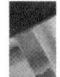

THERAPEUTIC MEASURES FOR THE NEUROLOGIC SYSTEM

Moving and Positioning

Patients who have pain may need help changing positions and ambulating. Use of heat, cold, or analgesics may allow the patient to be more independent in mobility.

If the patient has sensory loss, make sure that no part of the body is inadvertently compressed (e.g., a hand caught under a hip or the scrotum compressed between the legs). Pressure injuries are a primary concern with the patient who is unable to move independently. Collaborate with the physical therapist to determine positioning techniques that maximize the potential for recovery.

Patients with paresis, paralysis, or **paresthesia** (abnormal sensation such as burning or tingling) may be partially or completely dependent in moving and body positioning. Take care to maintain the body in functional positions when routine position changes are made. This means keeping the trunk, extremities, hands, and feet in usable positions. For example, hands can be splinted to keep the thumb and fingers opposed, or high-top tennis shoes can be used to keep the feet in an appropriate position for standing or walking.

Contractures and foot drop are complications that are often associated with neurologic disorders. Contractures are permanent muscle contractions with fibrosis of connective

---

• WORD • BUILDING •

myelogram: myelo—referring to the spinal cord + gram—picture

electroencephalogram: electro—electrical activity + encephalo—referring to the brain + gram—picture

paresthesia: para—beside + asthesia—sensations

tissue that occur from lack of use of a muscle or muscle group. They cause permanent deformities and prevent normal functioning of the affected part. Foot drop occurs when the feet are not supported in a functional position and become contracted in a position of plantar flexion (Fig. 47.14). Use high-top tennis shoes and splints to help prevent foot drop. Splints are commonly used to prevent contractures of the upper and lower extremities and to keep the affected parts in a functional position. If splints are used, the patient must be evaluated for and protected from discomfort and skin breakdown at the splint site.

Mobilization should begin as soon as a patient is medically stable. Initially, this may involve the use of a lift device if the patient is unable to bear weight. Transfer of the patient to a bedside chair or use of ambulation aids may require a multidisciplinary approach. Be careful to recognize any physical or cognitive deficits that might affect safety and adjust the environment to protect the patient. This includes communicating safety concerns to unlicensed personnel who interact with the patient.

Activities of Daily Living

The effects of neurologic disorders on activities of daily living (ADLs) can range from an inconvenience to complete dependence. Patients may have trouble bending over to put on their shoes and socks, lifting a full cooking pot, or caring for an infant. A quadriplegic patient may be completely unable to perform ADLs but can be taught to direct his or her own personal care. Encourage patients to use strategies they learned in occupational or physical therapy.

Assessment of a hospitalized patient should include a discussion of strategies the patient normally uses at home to accomplish ADLs. Every attempt should be made to continue to use these strategies. This is particularly true if the patient is admitted to a long-term care facility. Patients who have intact cognitive function should be included in care planning and encouraged to work collaboratively with caregivers. If strategies the patient uses during ADLs must be changed (e.g., if the patient's transfer technique is unsafe), be sure to explain the rationale for the changes to the patient and significant others. If patients have impaired cognitive function,

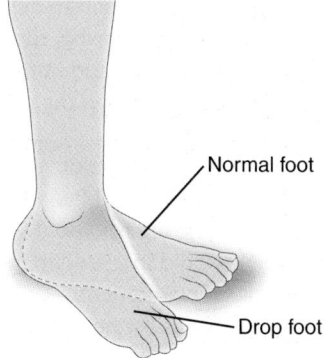

FIGURE 47.14 Contractures, foot drop.

try to maintain a specific routine that is as close to their normal environment as possible. Normalizing routines may help patients adapt to a change in environment and maximize their ability to function.

Communication

Communication problems associated with neurologic disorders have a variety of etiologies. Some neurologic disorders cause difficulty speaking (**dysarthria**). Dysfunction of the lips, tongue, or jaw makes speech difficult or impossible to understand. When dysarthric individuals know what they want to say but cannot be understood, they can become very frustrated. This frustration is compounded if the patients are treated as if they have cognitive deficits merely because they have difficulty communicating.

Patients who have had a stroke can experience different types of aphasia. *Expressive aphasia* is difficulty or inability to verbally communicate with others. The patient may be able to speak in sentences but inappropriately substitutes words, such as "The sky is dish." Word-finding difficulty is another type of expressive aphasia. These patients may tell you, "I want a …" and then be unable to complete the sentence. In severe cases of aphasia, the patient may make sounds that resemble words or may only utter sounds. For individuals with no intelligible speech or with word-finding difficulty, a picture board with commonly used items may facilitate communication. (See an example of a picture board in Chapter 49.) Keep in mind that patients with expressive aphasia may answer yes to all questions rather than just those for which yes is correct. The same is true of answering no. This is one reason why a nurse should never ask a patient, "Are you Mrs. Gonzalez?" An aphasic patient may say yes even if that is not her name. Instead, ask the patient to state her name. Always check the identification band.

For patients who substitute words, simply correct the substitution and continue the conversation. Patients with expressive aphasia are often very aware of and frustrated by their difficulty communicating. Give them time to try to express themselves. If you cannot understand them, offer possibilities based on the situation. If the patient is sitting in the chair, ask whether he or she wants to go back to bed or wants to use the bathroom. If the patient is restless, ask whether he or she is in pain.

Some patients use the same word in response to all questions, and, for a few patients, that word is a profanity. This is very difficult for significant others to deal with, particularly if a patient did not normally use profanity in the past. Make it clear to the family that you understand that this behavior is part of the patient's illness.

Receptive aphasia affects the patient's ability to understand spoken language. Again, the severity of the aphasia

• **WORD** • **BUILDING** •

dysarthria: dys—dysfunctional + arthria—movement of the joints used in speech

varies. Some patients may understand simple directions such as "sit down" or "squeeze my fingers." In other cases, the nurse may need to pantomime the action the nurse wants the patient to perform, such as showing the patient pills and then mimicking taking the pills and drinking water.

BE SAFE!

If the patient has receptive aphasia, assume that he or she cannot understand or follow safety instructions, such as "Do not stand up until I get back." Even going around the corner to get water can give a patient enough time to try to stand up and subsequently fall.

Nutrition

Alterations in the ability to maintain an adequate nutritional intake can have many causes. LOC may be depressed enough that the patient does not recognize that she or he is hungry or thirsty. Decreased LOC or cranial nerve dysfunction may impair the patient's ability to swallow safely. Severe weakness may limit the patient's ability to take in enough food to meet the body's requirements. These conditions are often compounded by the increased metabolic rate that accompanies neurologic injury or illness.

If there is any question of the patient's ability to swallow, a swallowing evaluation should be performed by a speech therapist. Some institutions also use a radiological examination to evaluate the ability to swallow. A small amount of barium is added to food or fluid, and fluoroscopy is used while the patient swallows. This allows visualization of the path of the food or fluid. Patients with swallowing difficulty (dysphagia) may have better success with foods or thick liquids rather than thin fluids. Liquids may be thickened with special thickening agents to allow easier swallowing. All patients should be positioned as upright as possible while eating or drinking. Patients who have difficulty swallowing should be monitored during eating and not left alone.

If weakness or fatigue is the cause of decreased nutritional intake, several modifications are possible. Serving small portions of food more frequently can increase intake. Using high-protein, high-calorie foods and supplements increases the nutritional content of small amounts of foods.

For patients who cannot swallow or who cannot swallow enough food, enteral (tube) feedings may be needed. If enteral feedings are anticipated to be for a short duration, a nasogastric tube may be used. Disadvantages of nasogastric tubes include impairment of the integrity of nasal skin and risk of aspiration. The risk of aspiration in neurologically impaired patients who have cognitive impairments is increased because these patients may pull out the nasogastric tube due to their lack of understanding the purpose of the tube. If long-term enteral feedings are anticipated, a gastrostomy tube may be placed directly through the abdominal wall into the stomach. This feeding method has the advantage of reducing the risks of aspiration and eliminating nasal skin breakdown.

Family

When working with patients who have a neurologic deficit, whether acute or chronic and whether in the hospital, in a long-term care facility, or at home, the family should be included in their care and rehabilitation. Depending on the patient's diagnosis and prognosis, the family will need support from staff. It is rewarding to see the patient who has had an accident recover with rehabilitation, but it is also rewarding to promote quality of life for the patient with Alzheimer disease and his or her family. Communication with the family regarding patient improvements and information about the illness is important. Include the family in the patient's care, such as bathing, feeding, and grooming. Suggest that the family participate in physical, occupational, and speech therapy sessions. Education is of vital importance, especially if the patient is going to be discharged home. Direct the patient and family to support groups and case managers for information regarding financial assistance and community resources during rehabilitation.

SUGGESTED ANSWERS TO CRITICAL THINKING

Mrs. Stevens

Albuterol is an adrenergic agonist (sometimes called a sympathomimetic), which is given to stimulate the sympathetic nervous system, resulting in open airways in patients with respiratory disease. However, it can also stimulate the cardiac system and cause a rapid heart rate and increased blood pressure. Be sure to monitor vital signs in patients receiving medications that affect the autonomic nervous system.

Tim Thompson

1. He is alert but confused, oriented to person only.
2. The nurse should ask his wife whether this has ever happened before, check his medical history for any disorders that may contribute to neurologic dysfunction,

do a quick neurologic examination to determine whether any additional deficits exist, check vital signs and pulse oximetry if available, and notify the health care provider (HCP) immediately if the symptoms are a new finding.

3. Some possible explanations to explore include hypoxemia, stroke, worsening heart problems causing inadequate flow of blood to the brain, hypoglycemia, or acute confusion (delirium) related to a sudden transition from home to an unfamiliar environment.
4. Consider based on further assessment (as noted in #2 and #3) if there may be a need to contact the HCP for evaluation. Involve a respiratory therapist, electrocardiogram technician, or others based on assessed needs.

Review Questions

1. What assessments are included in the FOUR score coma scale? **Select all that apply.**
   1. Eye response
   2. Motor response
   3. Brainstem reflexes
   4. Respiration
   5. Verbal response

2. Which instruction would the nurse provide for the patient when testing the trigeminal nerve?
   1. "Stick out your tongue."
   2. "Turn your head side to side."
   3. "I am going to shine a light into your eyes and observe your pupils."
   4. "Close your eyes and tell me where you feel the cotton touching your face."

3. When performing a neurologic assessment, which of the following is a symptom of increasing intracranial pressure that the nurse should immediately to the primary care provider?
   1. Constricted pupils
   2. Decreasing level of consciousness
   3. Narrowing pulse pressure
   4. Bradypnea

4. The nurse identifies which of the following as normal effects of aging on the central nervous system? **Select all that apply.**
   1. Increased postural stability
   2. Reduced blood flow to the brain
   3. Impaired short-term memory
   4. Sleep disturbances
   5. Loss of deep tendon reflexes
   6. Decrease in acetylcholine

5. The nurse knows the patient understands teaching about an angiogram when the patient makes which of the following statements?
   1. "A small needle will be inserted into my spinal column to withdraw fluid for examination."
   2. "I will be in a large machine that uses magnetic energy to create images; it has a noisy knocking sound."
   3. "Electrodes will be placed on my head to monitor electrical activity in my brain."
   4. "A catheter will be placed in an artery in my groin, and dye will be injected that will make my vessels show up on x-ray."

6. A patient has returned from having a computed tomography scan with contrast. Which of the following should be a priority in the hours after the scan?
   1. Ambulation
   2. Drinking fluids
   3. Turning side to side
   4. Coughing and deep breathing

7. Which of the following nursing interventions should be included in the plan of care for a patient at risk for foot drop?
   1. Position the patient in the left lateral position.
   2. Provide daily foot massage.
   3. Apply high-top tennis shoes.
   4. Maintain the patient in an upright position as much as possible.

Answer rationales available in your online resources.

ANSWERS 1. 1, 2, 3, 4; 2. 4; 3. 2; 4. 2, 3, 4, 6; 5. 4; 6. 2; 7. 3

Key Points

Find the chapter key points in your online resources available through Davis Edge.

Additional Resources

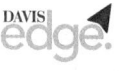 Use the scratch off code on the inside front cover of your book to access online quizzes that will help you to improve your scores on course exams and prepare for the NCLEX-PN®.

 Study Guide

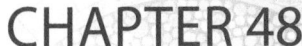

CHAPTER 48

Nursing Care of Patients With Central Nervous System Disorders

Deborah L. Weaver, Linda K. Cook

KEY TERMS

akinesia (AH-kin-EE-zee-ah)
ataxia (ah-TAK-see-ah)
bradykinesia (BRAY-dee-kin-EE-zee-ah)
contralateral (KON-truh-LAT-er-uhl)
craniectomy (KRAY-nee-EK-tuh-mee)
cranioplasty (KRAY-nee-oh-plas-tee)
craniotomy (KRAY-nee-AH-toh-mee)
delirium (de-LEER-ee-um)
dementia (dee-MEN-cha)
dysreflexia (DIS-re-FLEK-see-ah)
encephalitis (en-SEF-uh-LYE-tis)
encephalopathy (en-SEF-uh-LAHP-ah-thee)
hemiparesis (hem-ee-puh-REE-sis)
hydrocephalus (HY-droh-SEF-uh-luhs)
ipsilateral (IP-sih-LAT-er-uhl)
laminectomy (LAM-ih-NEK-toh-mee)
meningitis (MEN-in-JY-tis)
neurodegenerative (new-roh-de-JEN-er-uh-tiv)
nuchal rigidity (NEW-kuhl re-JID-ih-tee)
paraparesis (PAR-ah-puh-REE-sis)
paraplegia (PAR-ah-PLEE-jee-ah)
photophobia (FOH-tuh-FOH-bee-ah)
postictal (pohs-TIK-tuhl)
prodromal (proh-DROH-muhl)
quadriparesis (KWA-drih-puh-REE-sis)
quadriplegia (KWA-drih-PLEE-jee-ah)
sciatica (sye-AT-ik-ah)
turbid (TER-bid)

CHAPTER CONCEPTS

Cellular Regulation
Cognition
Infection
Mobility
Neurologic Regulation
Sexuality
Trauma

LEARNING OUTCOMES

1. Explain causes, risk factors, and pathophysiology of central nervous system infections, including meningitis and encephalitis.
2. Plan nursing interventions for a patient with a central nervous system infection.
3. Differentiate between the various types of headaches.
4. Identify teaching to be provided for a patient experiencing headaches.
5. List the causes and types of seizures.
6. Describe appropriate interventions for an individual experiencing a seizure.
7. Recognize symptoms in a patient who is developing increased intracranial pressure.
8. Identify nursing interventions that can help prevent increased intracranial pressure.
9. Explain the causes, risk factors, and pathophysiology of injuries to the brain and spinal cord.
10. Plan nursing care for a patient with an injury to the brain or spinal cord.
11. Explain causes, risk factors, and pathophysiology associated with neurodegenerative disorders such as Parkinson, Huntington, and Alzheimer diseases.
12. Plan nursing care for a patient with a neurodegenerative disorder.
13. Plan nursing interventions for the patient with dementia.

Disorders of the central nervous system (CNS) include problems originating in the brain and spinal cord. Because the CNS is the control center for the entire body, disorders in this system can cause symptoms in any part of the body, including pain, confusion, paralysis, and coma. This chapter presents nursing care of patients with these disorders. Care of patients with cerebrovascular disorders is covered in Chapter 49.

CENTRAL NERVOUS SYSTEM INFECTIONS

Infectious agents can enter the CNS via a variety of routes (Table 48.1). Anything that depresses the patient's immune system, such as steroid

Table 48.1

Routes of Entry for Central Nervous System Infections

Route of Entry	Examples
Bloodstream	Insect bite Otitis media
Direct extension	Fracture of frontal or facial bones
Cerebrospinal fluid	Dural tear Poor sterile technique during procedure
Nose or mouth	Meningococcus meningitis
In utero	Contamination of amniotic fluid Rubella Vaginal infection

Table 48.2

Cranial Nerves Affected by Meningitis

Cranial Nerve Affected	Manifestation
III, IV, VI	Ocular palsies Unequal and sluggishly reactive pupils
VII	Facial weakness
VIII	Deafness and vertigo

administration, chemotherapy, radiation therapy, or malnutrition, can make the patient more vulnerable to infection.

Meningitis

Pathophysiology and Etiology

Meningitis is an inflammation of the meninges that surround the brain and spinal cord. It can be caused by either bacterial or viral infection. Any microorganism that enters the body can result in meningitis. Bacterial meningitis is a serious infection that is spread by direct contact with discharge from the respiratory tract of an infected person. Viral meningitis, also called aseptic meningitis, is more common and rarely serious. It usually presents with flu-like symptoms, and patients recover in 1 to 2 weeks.

The most common bacteria that cause meningitis are *Neisseria meningitidis, Streptococcus pneumoniae,* Group B *Streptococcus,* and *Haemophilus influenzae* type b (Hib). With current immunization standards in the United States, Hib has decreased in recent years. Bacterial infection generally begins in another area, such as the upper respiratory tract, enters the blood, and invades the CNS, causing the meninges to become inflamed and intracranial pressure (ICP) to increase. Vessel occlusion and necrosis of areas in the brain can occur. Cranial nerve function can be transiently or permanently affected by meningitis (Table 48.2).

Prevention

Vaccines are available against some pathogens. Hib vaccinations are begun during infancy. A vaccine against *S. pneumoniae* is recommended for people over age 65 and those who have a chronic medical condition. Currently, the Centers for Disease Control and Prevention (CDC, 2017) recommends two doses of meningococcal vaccine (MCV4) for adolescents,

one at age 11 or 12 and a booster at age 16. Other groups at increased risk who should be vaccinated are college freshmen living in dormitories, U.S. military recruits, anyone with compromised immunity, laboratory personnel, and those traveling to areas of the world where meningococcal disease is common.

Prophylactic treatment is recommended for those who have had significant exposure to anyone currently infected with meningitis. To destroy the organism from the nasopharynx, antimicrobials such as rifampin (Rifadin), quinolones, or sulfonamides are used.

Signs and Symptoms

The most common symptom of meningitis is a severe headache, caused by tension on blood vessels and irritation of the pain-sensitive dura mater. A high fever and stiff neck are present, and the patient may experience photophobia (light sensitivity). The patient with meningococcal meningitis usually presents with petechiae on the skin and mucous membranes.

Nuchal rigidity (pain and stiffness when the neck is moved) is caused by spasm of the extensor muscles of the neck. Positive Kernig and Brudzinski signs are often seen in patients suffering from meningitis. Both signs are caused by inflammation of the meninges and spinal nerve roots. To elicit the Kernig sign, the examiner flexes the patient's hip to 90 degrees and tries to extend the patient's knee. The sign is positive if the patient experiences pain and spasm of the hamstring. The Brudzinski sign is positive when flexion of the patient's neck causes the hips and knees to flex (Fig. 48.1). Nausea and vomiting associated with meningitis are caused by irritation of brain tissue and by increased ICP.

Encephalopathy refers to the mental status changes seen in patients with meningitis. These are manifested as short attention span, poor memory, disorientation, difficulty following commands, and a tendency to misinterpret environmental stimuli. Late signs of meningitis include lethargy and seizures.

• WORD • BUILDING •

meningitis: mening—membranous covering of the brain + itis—inflammation

photophobia: photo—light + phobia—fear or intolerance

encephalopathy: encephalo—brain + pathy—illness

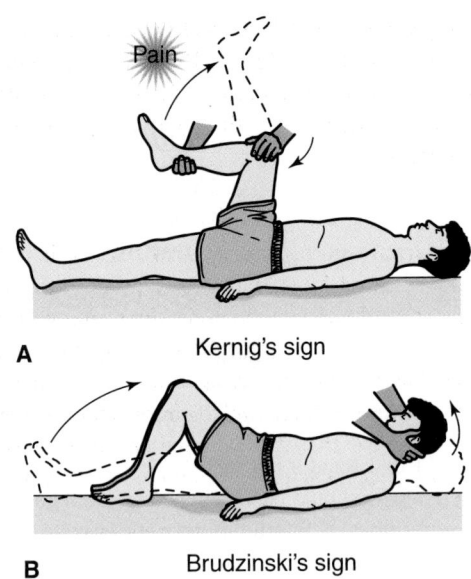

FIGURE 48.1 (A) Kernig sign. (B) Brudzinski sign.

Complications

Resolution of meningitis depends on how quickly and effectively the disease is treated. Viral meningitis usually has no lasting effects; however, bacterial meningitis can be fatal. Cranial nerve damage can leave a patient blind or deaf. Seizures can continue to occur even after the acute phase of the illness has passed. Cognitive deficits ranging from memory impairment to profound learning disabilities can occur.

Diagnostic Tests

A lumbar puncture is the most informative diagnostic test for a patient with suspected meningitis (see Chapter 47). Viral meningitis is characterized by clear cerebrospinal fluid (CSF) with normal glucose level and normal or slightly increased protein level. No bacteria are seen, but the white blood cell (WBC) count is usually increased. In contrast, the CSF of an individual with bacterial meningitis is **turbid**, or cloudy, because of the elevated number of WBCs. Bacteria are identified by Gram stain and culture, and a sensitivity test is done to identify the most effective antibiotic. The bacteria use the glucose normally found in CSF, thereby lowering the glucose level. The amount of protein in the CSF is elevated. Magnetic resonance imaging (MRI) or computed tomography (CT) scan can be done to evaluate for complications.

Therapeutic Measures

Antibiotics such as vancomycin and cephalosporins are administered for bacterial meningitis. It is important to note the sensitivity report when it is complete to confirm that the antibiotic in use is the best choice. Symptom management is the same for viral or bacterial meningitis. Antipyretics such as acetaminophen are used to control fever; a cooling blanket also can be used. Care should be taken to avoid cooling the patient too much because shivering increases the metabolic demand

for oxygen and glucose. Analgesics are given to lessen head and neck pain. Corticosteroids and anti-inflammatory agents are given to decrease cerebral swelling. Nausea and vomiting are controlled with antiemetic medications. The patient with meningococcal meningitis should be placed in droplet isolation for at least the first 24 hours of medication administration to prevent transmission to others.

Patients can become agitated. A quiet, dark environment lessens the stimulation of a patient who has a headache or photophobia and who is agitated, disoriented, or at risk for seizures. An important aspect of nursing care focuses on keeping patients from harming themselves. It is very upsetting to families to see a loved one acting agitated or disoriented. Therefore, it is important to teach the family about symptoms and treatment goals for the patient (Table 48.3).

Table 48.3
Meningitis Summary

Signs and Symptoms	Nuchal rigidity
	Positive Kernig and Brudzinski signs
	Fever
	Photophobia
	Petechial rash on skin and mucous membranes
	Encephalopathy
Diagnostic Tests	Lumbar puncture with cerebrospinal fluid, analysis, culture and sensitivity (C&S)
	Complete blood count (CBC)
	C&S nose and throat
Therapeutic Measures	Antimicrobials (if bacterial)
	Seizure precautions
	Antipyretics
	Pain management
	Reduction of environmental stimuli
	Education
Complications	Seizures
	Increased intracranial pressure
	Hearing loss
	Vision impairment
	Cognitive defects
Priority Nursing Diagnoses	*Hyperthermia*
	Risk for Acute Confusion
	Self-Care Deficit (Dressing/Feeding/Toileting)
	Acute or *Chronic Pain*
	Risk for Injury
	Impaired Physical Mobility

Encephalitis
Pathophysiology
Encephalitis is an inflammation of brain tissue. Nerve cell damage, edema, and necrosis cause neurologic findings in the specific areas of the brain affected. Hemorrhage in the brain can occur in some types of encephalitis. Increased ICP can lead to herniation of the brain (see later section on increased ICP).

Etiology
Viruses are the most common cause of encephalitis. They can be specifically related to a particular time of year or geographic location. Some viruses, such as West Nile virus, are carried by ticks or mosquitoes. Others are systemic viral infections, such as infectious mononucleosis or mumps, which spread to the brain.

Herpes simplex virus (HSV) is the most common non–insect-borne virus to cause encephalitis. The majority of individuals harbor HSV type 1 in a dormant state. This is the virus responsible for sores on the oral mucous membranes, commonly called cold sores. Communicable diseases, fever, and emotional stress are possible reasons for the virus becoming active, but the exact mechanism is not known.

Signs and Symptoms
As with many viruses, symptoms of headache, general malaise, nausea, vomiting, and fever develop over a period of several days. Additional symptoms include nuchal rigidity, confusion, decreased level of consciousness (LOC), seizures, photophobia, **ataxia** (lack of muscle coordination), abnormal sleep patterns, and tremors. The patient may also have **hemiparesis** (weakness on one side of the body).

The patient with herpes encephalitis develops edema and necrosis (sometimes associated with hemorrhage), most commonly in the temporal lobes. This significant cerebral edema causes increased ICP and can lead to herniation of the brain. If the patient becomes comatose before treatment is begun, the mortality rate can be as high as 70% to 80%. Risk of death is highest in the first 72 hours.

Complications
Patients who have had encephalitis are often left with cognitive disabilities and personality changes. Ongoing seizures, motor deficits, and blindness can occur. Changes in cognition and personality are particularly stressful for family members. The patient's behavioral control is a major factor in determining discharge plans. You can assist family members to realistically assess the patient's functional level as well as their ability to care for the patient. In-home care, outpatient therapy, and adult day care are options to explore. For some severely impaired individuals, long-term care in a facility may be the only feasible and safe discharge option.

Diagnostic Tests
CT scan, MRI, lumbar puncture to obtain CSF, and electroencephalogram (EEG) are used to diagnose encephalitis. CSF analysis typically reveals increased WBC count and protein level and normal glucose levels. Breakdown of blood after cerebral hemorrhage results in yellow-colored CSF. Viral serology can be useful to identify the type of virus and guide treatment options.

Therapeutic Measures
No specific treatment is currently available for insect-borne encephalitis. Careful neurologic assessment and treatment of symptoms can help prevent complications and improve survival. Anticonvulsants, antipyretics, and analgesics are administered to reduce seizures, fever, and headache. Corticosteroids are used to decrease cerebral swelling from inflammation. Sedatives may be given for irritability. Antiviral medications such as acyclovir (Zovirax) may also be used, especially for HSV.

Nursing Process for the Patient With a Central Nervous System Infection
See "Nursing Process for the Patient With a Communicable or Inflammatory Neurologic Disorder" later in this chapter.

 INCREASED INTRACRANIAL PRESSURE

Pathophysiology and Etiology
The skull is a rigid compartment containing three components: brain, blood, and CSF. ICP is the pressure exerted inside the cranial cavity by these components. Normal ICP is 0 to 15 mm Hg. ICP fluctuates with normal physiological changes, such as arterial pulsations, changes in position, and increases in intrathoracic pressure (e.g., coughing or sneezing).

If an increase in one component is not accompanied by a decrease in one or both of the other components, the result is increased ICP (Fig. 48.2). Any patient with a pathological intracranial condition is at risk for increased ICP. Common causes of increased ICP include brain trauma, intracranial hemorrhage, and brain tumors. Prompt detection of changes in neurologic status indicating increased ICP allows intervention aimed at preventing permanent brain damage.

The consequences of increased ICP depend on the degree of elevation and the speed with which the ICP increases. Patients with slow-growing tumors can have significantly increased ICP before they develop symptoms. Conversely, patients with a subarachnoid hemorrhage can sustain a sudden sharp increase in ICP.

The normal functioning body has several methods of compensating for increased ICP. CSF can be shunted into the spinal subarachnoid space. Hyperventilation can trigger constriction of cerebral blood vessels, decreasing the amount of blood within the cranial vault. These compensatory mechanisms are temporary and not particularly effective if the increase in ICP is sudden or severe.

• WORD • BUILDING •
encephalitis: encephalo—brain + itis—inflammation
hemiparesis: hemi—one side + paresis—partial paralysis

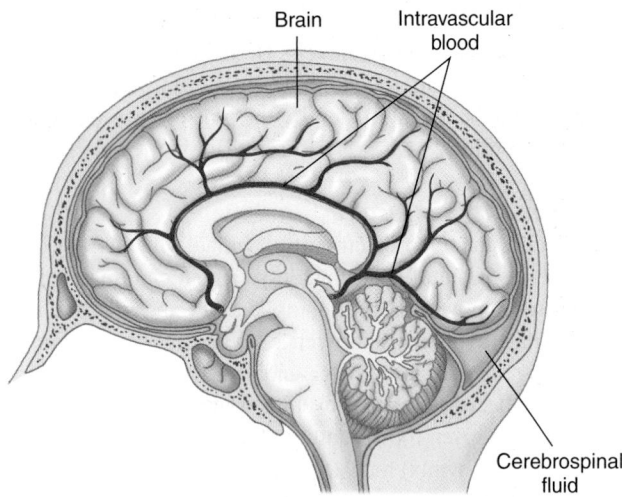

FIGURE 48.2 Any increase in brain tissue, blood, or cerebrospinal fluid can increase intracranial pressure.

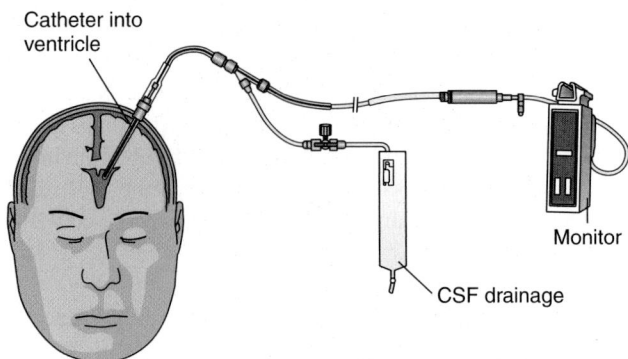

FIGURE 48.3 Ventricular drain. A catheter into the ventricle allows intracranial pressure monitoring and cerebrospinal fluid (CSF) drainage.

Signs and Symptoms

Initial symptoms of increased ICP include restlessness, irritability, and decreased LOC because cerebral cortex function is impaired. If not intubated, the patient can hyperventilate, causing vasoconstriction as the body attempts to compensate. As the pressure increases, the oculomotor nerve can be compressed on the side of the impairment. Compression of the outermost fibers of the oculomotor nerve results in diminished reactivity and dilation of the pupil. As the fibers become increasingly compressed, the pupil stops reacting to light. If the compression continues and the brain tissue exerts pressure on the opposite side of the brain from the injury, both pupils become fixed and dilated.

Vital sign changes are a late indication of increasing ICP. The Cushing triad is a classic late sign of increased ICP. It is characterized by bradycardia, irregular respirations, and arterial hypertension (increasing systolic blood pressure while diastolic blood pressure remains the same), resulting in widening pulse pressure. By the time these symptoms appear, the ICP is significantly increased, and interventions may not be successful.

Monitoring

ICP monitoring allows for early detection of changes in the pressure on the brain, before changes in symptoms are seen. The most common method of monitoring ICP in adults is by placing a catheter in a ventricle of the brain, in the cerebral parenchyma, or in the subdural or subarachnoid space. This can be done at the bedside or in an operating room. Each of these methods requires anesthetizing the scalp and drilling a hole, called a *burr hole,* into the skull.

Placement of a catheter into one of the lateral ventricles is referred to as external ventricular drainage (Fig. 48.3). This method allows for pressure monitoring as well as drainage of CSF to reduce ICP. Disadvantages to this method include difficulty in locating the ventricle for insertion of the catheter and clotting of the catheter by blood in the CSF.

To allow communication with the subarachnoid space, a subarachnoid bolt can be tightly screwed into the burr hole after the dura has been punctured (Fig. 48.4). The advantage of a subarachnoid bolt is ease of placement. Disadvantages include occlusion of the sensor portion of the bolt with brain tissue and inability to drain CSF. An intraparenchymal monitor is placed directly into brain tissue. Some physicians believe that this most accurately reflects the actual situation within the skull. These monitors cannot be used to drain CSF and can become occluded by brain tissue.

Patients with ICP monitors are cared for in an intensive care unit (ICU) and require aggressive nursing care to prevent complications. These patients are often mechanically ventilated and may be pharmacologically paralyzed and sedated. In addition to meeting the patient's physiological needs and preventing complications, education and emotional support for family members are important.

Nursing Process for the Patient With a Communicable or Inflammatory Neurologic Disorder
Data Collection

Collaborate with the registered nurse (RN) to obtain a complete history from the patient, if feasible, and from family members. Pay particular attention to exposure to risk factors. The physical examination must include all body systems because neurologic impairment affects the entire person. Following the initial examination, serial neurologic assessments continue to be important to detect and report changes promptly. You can assist with monitoring pupil response, LOC, and vital signs for signs of increased ICP (Box 48.1). Monitor headache on a pain scale or the Pain Assessment in Advanced Dementia (PAINAD) scale if necessary. The Glasgow Coma Scale or the FOUR Score Coma Scale, presented in Chapter 47, are valuable tools to use to monitor LOC.

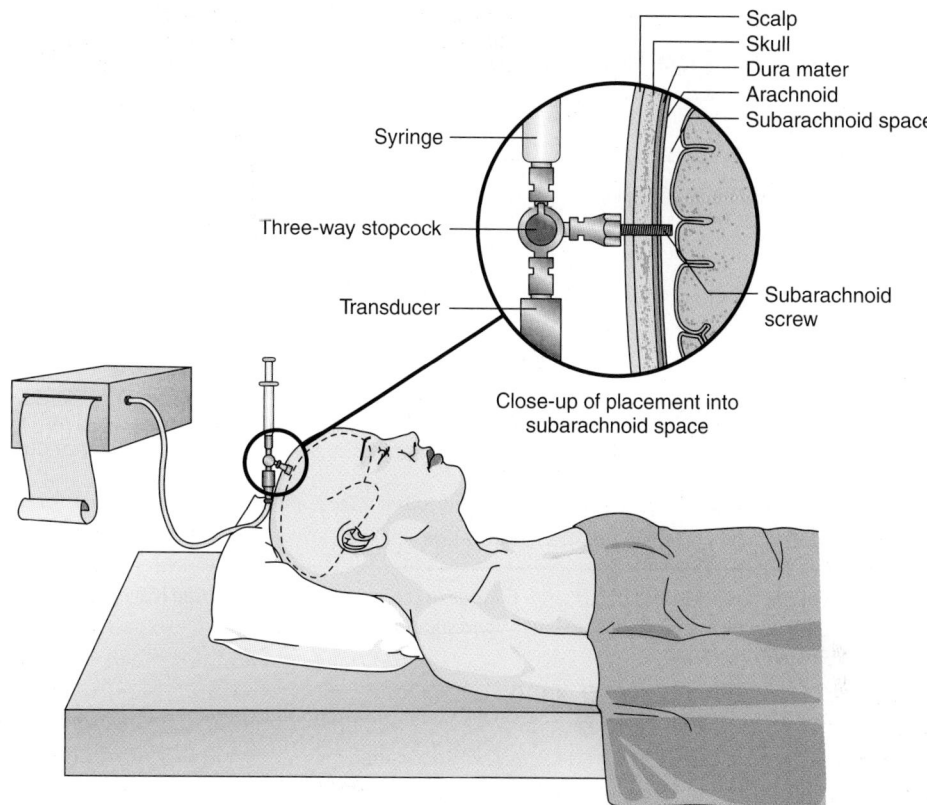

Scalp
Skull
Dura mater
Arachnoid
Subarachnoid space

Syringe

Three-way stopcock

Transducer

Subarachnoid screw

Close-up of placement into subarachnoid space

FIGURE 48.4 Subarachnoid bolt monitor.

Signs and Symptoms of Increased Intracranial Pressure

- Vomiting
- Headache
- Dilated pupil on affected side
- Hemiparesis or hemiplegia
- Decorticate then decerebrate posturing
- Decreasing level of consciousness
- Increasing systolic blood pressure
- Increasing then decreasing pulse rate
- Rising temperature

Nursing Diagnoses, Planning, and Implementation

The licensed practical nurse/licensed vocational nurse (LPN/LVN) collaborates with the RN in implementing care. For additional interventions for patients with communicable or inflammatory disorders, see "Nursing Care Plan for the Patient With a Brain Infection or Injury."

Patient Education

The nature and focus of teaching depend on the patient's LOC and cognitive status. When appropriate, both the patient and family members should be included in the education process. If the patient is not able to participate, family members become the focus of teaching.

Nursing Care Plan for the Patient With a Brain Infection or Injury

Nursing Diagnosis: *Hyperthermia* related to infectious process or damage to hypothalamus
Expected Outcome: The patient will not exhibit evidence of hyperthermia.
Evaluation of Outcome: Is temperature controlled?

Intervention	Rationale	Evaluation
Assess temperature every 4 hours and as needed (prn).	*An elevated temperature can increase risk for seizures.*	Is temperature controlled?
Administer acetaminophen or aspirin as ordered.	*Antipyretic agents reduce fever.*	Are antipyretics effective?

(nursing care plan continues on page 1006)

Nursing Care Plan for the Patient With a Brain Infection or Injury—cont'd

Intervention	Rationale	Evaluation
Provide a cooling mattress or tepid sponge baths as necessary.	*A cooling mattress may be necessary to reduce fever. Cooling blankets are uncomfortable for the patient. Comfort can be increased and shivering reduced by cooling the patient gradually and wrapping extremities in bath blankets during cooling mattress therapy.*	Is cooling mattress or tepid bath effective? Is patient comfort maintained?

Nursing Diagnosis: *Risk for Acute Confusion* related to cerebral edema and increased intracranial pressure (ICP)
Expected Outcomes: The patient will be oriented to person, place, and time; if this is not possible, the patient's safety will be maintained.
Evaluation of Outcomes: Is the patient oriented to self, place, and time and able to ask for help appropriately to prevent injury?

Intervention	Rationale	Evaluation
Assess level of consciousness (LOC) using Glasgow Coma Scale or the FOUR Score Coma Scale.	*Change in LOC can indicate increased ICP and should be reported.*	Is patient alert and responsive? Is LOC stable?
Monitor orientation and reorient as needed.	*Giving correct information to patient will assist in orientation.*	Can patient identify who he/she is, location, and month, year, or season?
Observe patient's reaction to simple commands such as "raise your hand."	*This helps distinguish between reflexes and purposeful movement.*	Is patient able to follow simple commands?
Monitor patient's capabilities as activities increase.	*Patient can experience dizziness, imbalance, and confusion; patient will need assistance with mobilization until stable.*	Can patient safely sit up and ambulate to a chair?
If patient is not able to be reoriented, assess for safety and implement appropriate safety measures.	*Depending on patient's prognosis, orientation may not be a realistic goal.*	Is patient's safety maintained?

Nursing Diagnosis: *Self-Care Deficit (Dressing/Feeding/Toileting)* related to mental status changes and inability to perform activities of daily living (ADLs) independently
Expected Outcome: The patient will maintain as much independence with ADLs as possible.
Evaluation of Outcome: Is the patient able to participate in self-care at an appropriate level?

Intervention	Rationale	Evaluation
Assess what the patient was able to do before admission/injury.	*Patient's potential for participation will depend on what he or she was able to do before injury.*	What was patient able to do? How does that compare with what he or she can do now?
Provide all supplies and equipment needed to carry out ADLs.	*Assembling equipment for patient reserves energy for performing self-care.*	Is patient able to perform the majority of bath and hygiene tasks with appropriate setup?
Encourage patient to perform activities at own pace.	*Patient may need more time to perform activities*	Does patient gradually increase performance of self-care in a timely fashion?
Teach and encourage family to participate with care.	*Including the family in the patient's care promotes support and family interaction.*	Is the family involved? Is patient accepting of their assistance?
Refer to occupational therapy if indicated.	*An occupational therapist is trained to assist patients to manage ADLs within health limitations.*	Is occupational therapist able to assist patient with strategies to maintain independence?

Nursing Care Plan for the Patient With a Brain Infection or Injury—cont'd

Nursing Diagnosis: *Acute* or *Chronic Pain* related to cerebral edema and headache as evidenced by the patient's pain rating or evidence of painful behaviors
Expected Outcomes: The patient's pain is controlled as evidenced by statement that pain level is acceptable, or decrease in painful behaviors.
Evaluation of Outcomes: Does the patient state that the pain level is acceptable? Are pain behaviors reduced?

Intervention	Rationale	Evaluation
Assess pain using a scale of 0 to 10 or PAINAD scale (see Chapter 10).	*The patient's self-report is the best measure of the patient's pain.*	Is patient able to rate pain? Is there evidence that pain is present?
Monitor vital signs.	*Pulse and blood pressure can be elevated in acute pain.*	Are vital signs elevated?
Administer appropriate pain medication as ordered.	*Nonnarcotic medications are preferred because they do not alter LOC. If these are not effective, codeine preparations, which have a minimal effect on LOC, may be prescribed.*	Does patient state pain has decreased? Is sedation minimized?
Implement measures to reduce ICP. Table 48.4 provides measures and rationales.	*Increased ICP can increase pain.*	Do measures to reduce ICP help prevent pain?
Provide alternative comfort measures such as dim lights, a quiet environment, and positioning for comfort.	*Decreasing stimuli in the room by dimming lights and decreasing noise can have a calming effect.*	Is patient resting quietly, with no evidence of pain?

Nursing Diagnosis: *Risk for Injury* secondary to *Disturbed Sensory Perception* related to brain infection or injury and cranial nerve involvement as evidenced by alterations in response to stimuli
Expected Outcome: The patient will be kept safe from injury related to reduced sensation.
Evaluation of Outcome: Is the patient safe? Is skin intact?

Intervention	Rationale	Evaluation
Monitor patient's ability to perceive stimuli.	Changes in patient's perceptions must be incorporated into the plan of care.	What can the patient feel?
Turn patient and assess skin at least every 2 hours while in bed; provide moisturizer as needed. Protect bony prominences.	If patient cannot feel pressure or dryness, the nurse must evaluate and act to prevent skin breakdown.	Is skin intact, pink, warm, dry, and without redness?
Assist patient out of bed and into a different environment.	This can help prevent sensory deprivation and social isolation.	How does patient respond to being in a chair or wheelchair and taken to sunroom or common area?
Teach patient to monitor own position and skin, and to direct position changes.	This provides a way for the patient to maintain some control over his or her body and to take part in preventing complications.	Is patient able to direct care activities effectively?

(nursing care plan continues on page 1008)

Nursing Care Plan for the Patient With a Brain Infection or Injury—cont'd

Nursing Diagnosis: *Impaired Physical Mobility* related to motor deficits as evidenced by weakness and inability to change position
Expected Outcomes: The patient will maintain maximum mobility and be free from complications of immobility.
Evaluation of Outcomes: Is the patient kept mobile without contractures? Is skin intact?

Intervention	Rationale	Evaluation
Assess degree of mobility limitation.	*A good assessment can help determine how much the patient can actively participate in a plan for mobilization.*	How much can patient do independently? Is physical/occupational therapy evaluation indicated?
Turn patient every 1 to 2 hours; if postoperative, avoid positioning on the operative site unless specifically permitted by the surgeon.	*Turning helps prevent skin and respiratory complications.*	Is a turning schedule maintained? Is skin free from redness and breakdown?
Position patient in correct body alignment. High-top tennis shoes, trochanter rolls, and slings can be used to keep the body in alignment.	*This keeps patient in functional position in case function is regained in the future.*	Are all joints maintained in correct alignment?
Perform range-of-motion (ROM) exercises; consult physical therapy as ordered.	*ROM exercises help prevent contractures*	If patient is unable to perform active ROM exercises, are passive ROM exercises provided on a regular schedule?
Consult occupational therapist to assist patient in learning to perform ADLs.	*Patient may be able to participate in self-care with assistive devices.*	Do assistive devices help patient mobilize and maintain independence?

Nursing Diagnosis: *Risk for Injury* related to seizures
Expected Outcome: The patient will remain free of injury if a seizure occurs.
Evaluation of Outcome: Is safety maintained? Is skin intact, without bruising or discoloration?

Intervention	Rationale	Evaluation
Observe patient's behavior and time the length of the seizure. When patient is alert following seizure, determine whether an aura occurred and what it was.	*Observing the seizure can provide clues for teaching the patient to recognize the warning signs of a future seizure and how to maintain safety.*	What did patient experience? What can be taught to help keep patient safe in the future?
If patient loses consciousness during the seizure, lay patient on his or her side or turn head to the side.	*This helps prevent oral secretions from being aspirated.*	Did patient maintain a patent airway without respiratory distress?
Remove objects from patient's surroundings to prevent injury during a seizure. If patient must have side rails, pad them with blankets or foam (see also Table 48.6, later in chapter).	*During a tonic-clonic seizure, the patient can be harmed by hitting furniture or other objects.*	Is patient protected from objects that could cause injury during a seizure?

Table 48.4

Measures to Prevent Increased Intracranial Pressure

Preventive Measures	Rationale
Keep head of bed elevated 30 degrees unless contraindicated.	Head elevation reduces intracranial pressure (ICP) in some patients.
Avoid flexing the neck; keep head and neck in midline position.	Neck flexion can obstruct venous outflow.
Administer antiemetics and antitussives as necessary to prevent vomiting and cough.	Coughing and vomiting can increase ICP.
Administer stool softeners.	Straining for bowel movement can increase ICP.
Minimize suctioning. If absolutely necessary, oxygenate first and limit suction passes to one or two.	Suctioning can increase ICP.
Avoid hip flexion.	Hip flexion can increase intra-abdominal and thoracic pressure, which can increase ICP.
Prevent unnecessary noise and startling the patient.	Noxious stimuli can increase ICP in some patients.
Space care activities to provide rest between each disturbance.	Clustering care activities can increase ICP.

CRITICAL THINKING

Mr. Chung is an 18-year-old college student. He comes to the emergency department with a headache, stiff neck, and fever. On physical assessment, you notice a petechial rash on his legs and torso. The health care provider diagnoses meningococcal meningitis.

1. What tests are likely to be performed?
2. What patient education should be planned for Mr. Chung?
3. What infection control practices should be instituted?
4. What comfort measures might you offer to Mr. Chung?
5. What concerns do you have about how Mr. Chung contracted his illness?

Suggested answers are at the end of the chapter.

HEADACHES

Headache is a common symptom of neurologic disorders. However, most headaches are transient events and do not indicate a serious pathological condition. If headaches are recurrent, persistent, or increasing in severity, the patient should undergo a neurologic evaluation. This section addresses the most common types of headache.

Types of Headaches

Headaches are divided into three major types: (1) primary, (2) secondary, and (3) cranial neuralgias, central and primary facial pain, and other headaches. Primary headaches are discussed in this section. Secondary headaches are caused by trauma, infection, or other disorders. Cranial neuralgias and facial pain are discussed in Chapter 50. For more information, visit the International Headache Society at www.ichd-3.org.

Migraine Headaches

Migraine headaches are a neurologic disorder involving brain chemicals and neurologic pathways. Current thought is that a trigger stimulates a release of chemicals that cause an inflammatory response and overstimulation of the trigeminal nerve, resulting in pain. A migraine may or may not involve an aura, such as vision changes or tingling, that precedes an attack. The tendency to develop migraine headaches is often hereditary. Children who have one or both parents who experience migraines are more likely to experience them as well. Migraines frequently begin in childhood or adolescence and are more common in women. Common migraine triggers include hormones (menses related), changes in barometric pressure, specific foods, noise, bright light, alcohol, and stress.

There are two major types of migraine: migraine with aura and migraine without aura. There are four phases generally associated with migraine headaches: prodromal, aura, headache, and resolution. The pre-headache (**prodromal**) phase can include symptoms such as irritability, sleepiness, or food cravings. The aura stage might include visual disturbances, difficulty speaking, and/or numbness or tingling. The

• WORD • BUILDING •

prodromal: pro—before + dromos—running

headache that follows is often accompanied by nausea and sometimes vomiting; it can last for hours to days. Commonly used descriptors of migraine pain include *throbbing, boring, viselike,* and *pounding.* The pain is usually on one side of the head. Noise and light tend to worsen the headache, leading patients to find a dark, quiet environment. The final stage, resolution, might be accompanied by sluggishness or confusion.

Treatment of migraine may be prophylactic or directed at an acute episode. Prophylactic treatment is usually reserved for those patients experiencing one or more migraine headaches per week. Patients who experience 15 or more days a month with a migraine headache may be treated with botulinum toxin (Botox). Small doses of Botox are injected into specific areas of the head and neck around pain fibers that stimulate the release of the inflammatory chemicals. It may take two or three treatments of Botox for the patient to experience relief. The treatments are repeated every 3 months.

Dietary restrictions can be helpful if precipitating foods or beverages can be identified.

Several types of medications are available to treat acute migraine headaches. Nonsteroidal anti-inflammatory drugs (NSAIDs) such as naproxen (Naprosyn, Aleve) may be tried first. Ergot (Cafergot), a vasoconstrictor, is effective only if taken before the vessel walls become edematous, usually within 30 to 60 minutes of headache onset. Triptans, such as sumatriptan (Imitrex) and zolmitriptan (Zomig), work at the serotonin receptor sites and have a vasoconstricting action. Treximet combines naproxen and sumatriptan. Opioids are habit forming and are used only as a last resort. The potentially additive effects of multidrug regimens require careful monitoring.

A new class of medication is under development for the treatment of migraine headaches. Calcitonin gene-related peptide (CGRP) spikes during migraine attacks. The new medications are aimed at neutralizing CGRP or at blocking its receptor sites.

Tension or Muscle Contraction Headaches

Persistent contraction of the scalp and facial, cervical, and upper thoracic muscles can cause tension headaches. A cycle of muscle tension, muscle tenderness, and further muscle tension is established. This cycle may or may not be associated with vasodilation of cerebral arteries. Tension headaches can be associated with premenstrual syndrome or psychosocial stressors such as anxiety, emotional distress, or depression. Symptoms typically develop gradually. Radiation of pain to the crown of the head and base of the skull, with variations in location and intensity, is common. *Pressure, aching, steady,* and *tight* are some of the words patients use to describe the pain of tension headaches.

Care must be taken to thoroughly rule out physical causes before attributing the headache to psychosocial origins. Symptom management may include the use of relaxation techniques, massage of the affected muscles, rest, localized heat application, nonopioid analgesics, and appropriate counseling.

Cluster Headaches

Vascular disturbance, stress, anxiety, and emotional distress are all proposed causes of cluster headaches. As indicated by the name, these headaches tend to occur in clusters during a time span of several days to weeks. Months or even years can pass between episodes. Alcohol consumption may worsen the episodes.

The patient may state that the headache begins suddenly, typically at the same time of night. *Throbbing* and *excruciating* are often the adjectives used by the patient. The headache tends to be unilateral, affecting the nose, eye, and forehead. A bloodshot, teary appearance of the affected eye is common.

Because of the brief nature of cluster headaches, treatment is difficult. A quiet, dark environment and cold compresses can lessen the intensity of the pain. NSAIDs or tricyclic antidepressants may be prescribed.

Diagnosis of Headaches

Most headaches are diagnosed based on the patient's history and symptoms. MRI, CT scan, skull x-ray, arteriogram, EEG, cranial nerve testing, and lumbar puncture to test CSF may be done to rule out other causes for the headaches.

Nursing Process for the Patient With a Headache

Data Collection

The *WHAT'S UP?* mnemonic is particularly useful in helping the patient provide useful information regarding the headache:

- **W**—Where is the pain? Does it remain in one place or radiate to other areas of the head? Does the headache consistently start in one place?
- **H**—How does the headache feel? Is it throbbing, steady, dull, or bandlike, or does it have other qualities?
- **A**—Aggravating or alleviating factors should be assessed. Some aggravating factors include red wine, caffeine, chocolate, and foods containing nitrates or monosodium glutamate (MSG). Other factors include particular stages of the menstrual cycle, emotional stress, and tension. Alleviating factors might include lying down in a dark room, cold compresses, or medications.
- **T**—Timing can help with diagnosis. When does it typically occur? How long does it last?
- **S**—Ask the patient to rate the severity on a scale of 0 to 10. Is the severity consistent or does it vary from headache to headache?
- **U**—Ask about other useful data. For example, are there associated symptoms, such as nausea, vomiting, or bloodshot eyes?
- **P**—Determine the patient's perception of the headache. Does it interfere with the patient's life? If so, how? Has the patient had a previous evaluation of headaches?

Nursing Diagnoses, Planning, and Implementation

Acute Pain related to physiological mechanisms of headache as evidenced by the patient's pain rating

EXPECTED OUTCOME: The headache will be prevented or controlled as evidenced by the patient statement of no pain or acceptable pain rating.

- Assist the patient to identify and reduce or eliminate aggravating factors. Have the patient keep a headache diary for a time, recording the time of day the headache occurs, foods eaten or other aggravating factors, description of the pain, identification of associated symptoms such as nausea or visual disturbances, and other factors related to headache symptoms. *Identification of triggers can help the patient lessen the frequency and intensity of attacks.*
- Encourage the patient to use alleviating techniques such as warm or cold compresses, biofeedback, or stress reduction. *This helps the patient participate in the treatment of the headache and provides a sense of control over his or her illness.*
- Teach the patient to use relaxation exercises. *Relaxation may be helpful for tension headaches.*
- Provide a dark room and rest *to reduce stimulation during a migraine headache.*
- Teach the patient about medications, appropriate dosage, expected action, side effects, and consequences of misuse. *The patient will need to understand medication administration for appropriate use at home.*

Evaluation

If interventions have been effective, the patient will understand self-care to prevent and treat headaches and report a reduction in headache pain and occurrences.

SEIZURE DISORDERS

A seizure can be a symptom of epilepsy or other neurologic disorders such as a brain tumor or meningitis. Epilepsy is a chronic neurologic disorder characterized by recurrent seizure activity.

Pathophysiology

The normal stability of the neuron cell membrane is impaired in individuals with seizures. This instability allows for abnormal electrical discharges to occur, causing the characteristic symptoms seen during a seizure.

Seizures can be classified as partial or generalized. Partial seizures begin on one side of the cerebral cortex. In some cases, the electrical discharge spreads to the other hemisphere and the seizure becomes generalized. Generalized seizures are characterized by involvement of both cerebral hemispheres.

Etiology

Epilepsy can be acquired or idiopathic (unknown cause). Causes of acquired epilepsy include traumatic brain injury and anoxic events. No cause has been identified for idiopathic epilepsy. The most common time for idiopathic epilepsy to begin is before age 20. New-onset seizures after this age are most commonly caused by an underlying neurologic disorder. As the population ages, more older adults are having first-time seizure as a result of bleeding or bruising in the brain related to a fall. Multiple medications in the elder population and untreated hypertension can increase the risk of falls as well as brain injury after a fall.

Signs and Symptoms

Symptoms of seizure activity correlate with the area of the brain where the seizure begins. Some patients experience an aura or sensation that warns that a seizure is about to occur. An aura can be a visual distortion, a noxious odor, or an unusual sound. Patients who experience an aura may have enough time to sit or lie down before the seizure starts, thereby minimizing the risk of injury.

Partial Seizures

Repetitive, purposeless behaviors, called *automatisms,* are the classic symptom of partial seizures. The patient appears to be in a dreamlike state while picking at his or her clothing, chewing, or smacking his or her lips. Patients may be labeled as mentally ill, particularly if automatisms include unacceptable social behaviors such as spitting or fondling themselves. Patients are not aware of their behavior or that it is inappropriate. If the patient does not lose consciousness, the seizure is labeled as simple partial and usually lasts less than 1 minute. Older terms for simple partial seizures include *Jacksonian* and *focal motor.* If consciousness is lost, it is called a complex partial seizure or psychomotor seizure; it can last from 2 to 15 minutes.

Partial seizures arising from the parietal lobe can cause paresthesias on the side of the body opposite the seizure focus. Visual disturbances are seen if the seizure originates in the occipital lobe. Involvement of the motor cortex results in involuntary movements of the opposite side of the body. Typically, movements begin in the arm and hand and can spread to the leg and face.

The **postictal** period is the recovery period after a seizure. Following a partial seizure, the postictal phase may be no more than a few minutes of disorientation.

Generalized Seizures

Generalized seizures affect the entire brain. Two types of generalized seizures are absence seizures and tonic-clonic seizures. Absence seizures, sometimes referred to as petit mal seizures, occur most often in children. They are manifested by a period of staring that lasts several seconds.

Tonic-clonic seizures are what most people envision when they think of seizures; they are sometimes called grand mal

• WORD • BUILDING •
postictal: post—after + ictal—seizure

seizures or convulsions. Tonic-clonic seizures follow a typical progression. Aura and loss of consciousness may or may not occur. The tonic phase, lasting 30 to 60 seconds, is characterized by rigidity, causing the patient to fall if not lying down. The pupils are fixed and dilated, the hands and jaws are clenched, and the patient may temporarily stop breathing. The clonic phase is signaled by contraction and relaxation of all muscles in a jerky, rhythmic fashion. The extremities can move forcefully, causing injury if the patient strikes furniture or walls. The patient is often incontinent. Biting the lips or tongue can cause bleeding.

The postictal period is usually longer after a tonic-clonic seizure. Patients may sleep deeply for 30 minutes to several hours. Following this deep sleep, patients may report headache, confusion, and fatigue. Patients may realize that they had a seizure but not remember the event itself.

Diagnostic Tests

An EEG is the most useful test for evaluating seizures. An EEG can determine where in the brain the seizures start, the frequency and duration of seizures, and the presence of subclinical (asymptomatic) seizures. Sleep deprivation and flashing light stimulation may be used to evaluate the seizure threshold. See Appendix A for more information on EEGs.

Therapeutic Measures

If an underlying cause for the seizure is identified, treatment focuses on correcting the cause. If no cause is found or if the seizures continue despite treatment of concurrent disorders, treatment focuses on stopping or preventing seizure activity.

Numerous anticonvulsant medications are available (Table 48.5). Typically, the patient is started on one medication, and the dosage is increased until therapeutic levels are attained or side effects become troublesome. If seizures are not controlled on a single medication, another medication is added. Many anticonvulsants require periodic blood tests to monitor serum levels as well as kidney and liver function. Most of these medications can cause drowsiness, so teach the patient to avoid driving or operating machinery until the effects of the drug are known. Driving is also contraindicated until seizures are under control.

If a patient must discontinue an anticonvulsant, it should be tapered slowly according to manufacturer directions. Stopping an anticonvulsant abruptly can result in status epilepticus, discussed later. If seizures continue despite anticonvulsant therapy, surgical intervention may be considered.

Surgical Management

The success of surgical intervention for epilepsy depends on identification of an epileptic focus within nonvital brain tissue. The surgeon attempts to resect the area affected to prevent spread of seizure activity. In some cases, seizures can be cured, but in others, the goal is to reduce the frequency or severity of the seizures. If no focus is identified or if it is in a vital area such as the motor cortex or speech center, surgery is not feasible.

The preoperative assessment for epilepsy surgery is an extensive multistage process. Thorough assessment and teaching are essential. To adequately identify seizure foci, the patient is weaned off anticonvulsant therapy. Increasing the frequency of seizures with weaning is anxiety provoking for patients and family members.

Emergency Care

Emergency care is required when a seizure occurs. The prime objective is to prevent injury during a seizure. Side rails, if used, should be padded to prevent injury if the patient strikes his or her extremities against them. If the patient falls to the floor, move furniture out of the way. Maintain a patent airway, and, if possible, turn the patient on his or her side to prevent aspiration if vomiting occurs. Do not force an airway or anything else into the patient's mouth once the seizure has begun. Do not restrain the individual because this can also increase the risk of injury ("Patient Perspective: Mrs. Rowley"). Observe and document the patient's behavior during the seizure (e.g., which part of the body was first involved, progression of the seizure, length of time the seizure lasted). After the seizure, assess the patient for breathing, suction the oral pharynx if necessary, and, in rare cases, initiate rescue breathing or cardiopulmonary resuscitation (CPR) as indicated.

Patient Perspective

Mrs. Rowley. I have had seizures for 35 years and, as a result of falling during seizures, have experienced cuts, bruises, and a broken bone. I usually have an aura that lets me know a seizure is about to occur. This is helpful if I can get myself to a safe place to prevent falling or being injured. When a patient is having a seizure, you can best help by using padding such as pillows or blankets for protection, talking calmly, and using gentle touch to prevent injury. You should not sit on or hold down someone during a seizure. I have had the frightening experience of waking up with a nurse sitting on me and holding down my arms. After you have protected the patient, let the person come out of the seizure naturally. When the seizure is over, I usually want to sleep because seizures are exhausting.

Status Epilepticus

Status epilepticus is characterized by at least 30 minutes of repetitive seizure activity without a return to consciousness. This is a medical emergency and requires prompt intervention to prevent irreversible neurologic damage. Abruptly stopping anticonvulsant therapy is the usual cause of status epilepticus.

Seizure activity precipitates a significant increase in the brain's need for glucose and oxygen. This metabolic demand is even greater during status epilepticus. Irreversible neuronal

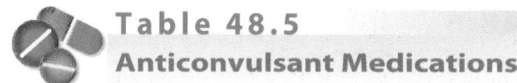

Table 48.5
Anticonvulsant Medications

Medication Class/Action

Anticonvulsants—Preventive Agents

Suppress abnormal discharge of neurons and suppress spread of seizure activity from focus to other parts of brain.

Examples	*Nursing Implications*
carbamazepine (Tegretol)	Monitor complete blood count (CBC). Therapeutic level is 6–12 mcg/mL. Do not crush sustained-release (SR) forms.
lacosamide (Vimpat)	Injectable form available. May increase risk of suicidal ideation.
ezogabine (Potiga)	May cause retinal abnormalities. Vision exam necessary at baseline and every 6 months. Monitor for urinary retention. Blood levels not necessary.
gabapentin (Neurontin)	Blood levels not necessary.
levetiracetam (Keppra)	May need reduced dose for older adults. Assess white blood cell, red blood cell, and liver function tests.
lamotrigine (Lamictal)	Discontinue therapy and notify health care provider if rash appears. Monitor blood levels.
topiramate (Topamax)	Blood levels not necessary.
phenytoin (Dilantin)	Regular dental care essential. Therapeutic level is 10–20 mcg/mL. Binds to tube feedings; hold tube feeding 1 hr before and 2 hr after dose.
phenobarbital (Luminal)	Monitor vital signs. Therapeutic level is 15–40 mcg/mL.
valproic acid (Depakote)	Therapeutic level is 50–100 mcg/mL. Do not crush SR form.

Benzodiazepines—Emergency Agents

Potentiate gamma-amino butyric acid (GABA), an inhibitory neurotransmitter in the central nervous system.

Examples	*Nursing Implications*
lorazepam (Ativan) diazepam (Valium, Diastat)	Given to stop a seizure that has not resolved within 5 minutes. Given via intramuscular or intravenous push route by emergency personnel. Diastat may be given rectally at home.

damage can occur if cerebral metabolic needs cannot be fulfilled. Adequate oxygenation must be maintained, if necessary, by intubating and mechanically ventilating the patient. These patients are also at significant risk for aspiration. Therefore, it is important that the nurse assist in airway maintenance and suction as needed to prevent hypoxia and aspiration pneumonia.

Intravenous (IV) diazepam (Valium) or lorazepam (Ativan) is administered to stop active seizures. Diazepam can also be given rectally. Because both of these drugs can cause respiratory depression, careful airway management is required. After obtaining serum drug levels, anticonvulsant therapy is adjusted to achieve therapeutic levels.

If seizures remain resistant to treatment, a barbiturate coma may be induced with IV pentobarbital. The last line of treatment for status epilepticus is general anesthesia or pharmacological paralysis. Both of these therapies require intubation, mechanical ventilation, and management in an ICU setting. Continuous EEG monitoring is used to verify that the seizures have actually stopped. A patient treated with neuromuscular blockade drugs can still be seizing but have no visible manifestations.

For more information on seizures, visit the Epilepsy Foundation at www.efa.org.

Psychosocial Effects

Finances can be a major concern to patients with seizure disorders. Some patients with epilepsy experience hiring discrimination or may not qualify for some jobs in which safety is a concern. Remind patients that falsifying information on job applications may be grounds for dismissal. Health insurance coverage issues can create financial hardships for patients on long-term medications. Most patients whose seizures are controlled can work and lead productive lives. A social worker can help explore options for financial assistance if needed.

Patients with poorly controlled seizures should not operate motor vehicles. In today's society, a driver's license is a sign of adulthood and independence, and patients who cannot drive can experience lowered self-esteem. Job opportunities may be limited for patients who depend on public transportation. Encourage the patient to obtain a state identification card. This can be used in place of a driver's license for identification.

Patients may limit interpersonal relationships out of fear of having a seizure. The involuntary movements, sounds, and possible incontinence that occur with seizures are embarrassing to patients and can be frightening to laypeople. Role-playing may help the patient determine when and how to confide in others.

Nursing Process for the Patient With Seizures

Data Collection

Perform a general neurologic examination of the patient with a history of seizures. Determine the type of seizure manifestations and type of aura, if any. Assess the patient's knowledge of the disease and its treatment. It is important to assess whether the patient has the resources to purchase prescribed anticonvulsant medications and whether the medication regimen is adhered to. Drug levels can help determine degree of adherence to therapy.

Nursing Diagnoses, Planning, and Implementation

Risk for Injury related to seizure activity

EXPECTED OUTCOME: The patient will remain free from injury.

- Instruct the patient with generalized seizures to recognize an aura and to get to safety if it occurs. This may mean lying down away from furniture or other objects. *This helps prevent injury during involuntary movements.*
- Institute seizure precautions for the patient admitted to a health care institution. Table 48.6 lists precautions and interventions *to prevent injury.*
- Encourage all patients to wear medical alert jewelry or other identification *to alert others to the presence of seizure disorder.*

Table 48.6

Interventions for Seizures

Seizure Precautions

- Pad side rails of hospital bed with commercial pads or bath blankets folded over and pinned in place.
- Keep call light within reach.
- Assist patient when ambulating.
- Keep suction and oral airway at bedside.

Nursing Care During a Seizure

- Stay with patient.
- Do not restrain patient.
- Protect from injury (move nearby objects).
- Loosen tight clothing.
- Turn to side when able to prevent occlusion of airway or aspiration.
- Suction if needed.
- Monitor vital signs when able.
- Be prepared to assist with breathing if necessary.

- Assist patients to identify conditions that trigger seizures. Hypoglycemia, hypoxia, and hyponatremia are all potential triggers of hypersensitive neurons. Teach the patient the importance of a consistent schedule of eating and sleeping. *The patient may be able to prevent seizures by avoidance of triggers.*

Ineffective Health Management related to complex regimen and possible lack of resources

EXPECTED OUTCOME: The patient will follow medication regimen as evidenced by therapeutic drug levels and controlled seizure activity.

- Assess the patient's ability to obtain and pay for medication. *Stopping a medication suddenly can result in status epilepticus.*
- Refer the patient to a case manager or social worker, if needed, *to assist with obtaining resources for medications.*
- Teach the patient about medication action, dose, side effects, schedule, and importance of not stopping treatment suddenly. *Patients with seizures can have several medications to take several times each day. Patients who understand their regimens are more likely to comply.*
- Teach the patient about the importance of regular blood tests if required. *Therapeutic blood levels help prevent seizures (too low) and toxicity (too high).*

Evaluation

Successful care of a patient with epilepsy results in a decrease in seizures to the lowest possible frequency. Patient verbalization of understanding needed lifestyle changes is another indication of success. Patients should be able to state measures to prevent injury if a seizure should occur and should verbalize understanding of all medications and their administration schedules. Therapeutic drug levels can be measured to evaluate adherence to the medication regimen.

TRAUMATIC BRAIN INJURY

Traumatic brain injury (TBI) is a major cause of death and disability in adults. Young men make up a large proportion of brain injury victims.

Pathophysiology

TBI is a complex phenomenon with results ranging from no detectable effect to a persistent vegetative state. Trauma can result in hemorrhage, contusion or laceration of the brain, and damage at the cellular level. In addition to the primary insult, the brain injury can be compounded by cerebral edema, hyperemia, or hydrocephalus.

Etiology

Motor vehicle collisions account for the largest percentage of TBIs. Falls, sports-related injuries, and violence are also common causes of TBI.

The brain is susceptible to various types of injury that can be classified in several ways. The term *closed head injury* or *nonpenetrating injury* is used when there has been rapid back and forth movement of the brain that causes bruising and tearing of brain tissues and vessels, but the skull is intact. An *open head injury* or *penetrating injury* refers to a break in the skull. *Acceleration injury* is the term used to describe a moving object hitting a stationary head. An example of this type of injury is a patient who is hit in the head with a baseball bat. A *deceleration injury* occurs when the head is in motion and strikes a stationary surface. This type of injury is seen in patients who trip and fall, hitting their head on furniture or the floor.

A combination *acceleration-deceleration injury* occurs when the stationary head is hit by a mobile object and the head then strikes a stationary surface. A soccer player who sustains a blow to the head and then hits the ground with his or her head can sustain an acceleration-deceleration injury.

Rotational injuries have the potential to cause shearing damage to the brain as well as lacerations and contusions. Rotational injuries can be caused by a direct blow to the head or can occur during a motor vehicle collision in which the vehicle is struck from the side. Twisting of the brainstem can damage the reticular activating system, causing loss of consciousness. Movement of the brain within the skull can result in bruising or tearing of brain tissue where it comes in contact with the inside of the skull.

Types of Brain Injury and Signs and Symptoms
Concussion

Cerebral concussion is considered a mild brain injury. If there is loss of consciousness, it is for 5 minutes or less. Concussion is characterized by headache, dizziness, or nausea and vomiting. The patient may describe amnesia of events before or after the trauma. On clinical examination, there is no skull or dura injury and no abnormality detected on CT scan or MRI.

Contusion

Cerebral contusion is characterized by bruising of brain tissue, possibly accompanied by hemorrhage. There can be multiple areas of contusion, depending on the causative mechanism. Severe contusions can result in diffuse axonal injury. The symptoms of a cerebral contusion depend on the area of the brain involved.

Brainstem contusions affect LOC. Decreased LOC can be transient or permanent. Respirations, pupil reaction, eye movement, and motor response to stimuli can also be affected. The autonomic nervous system can be affected by edema or by hypothalamic injury, causing rapid heart rate and respiratory rate, fever, and diaphoresis.

Hematoma

SUBDURAL HEMATOMA. Subdural hematomas are classified as acute or chronic based on the time interval between injury and onset of symptoms. Acute subdural hematoma is characterized by appearance of symptoms within 24 hours following injury. The bleeding is typically venous in nature and accumulates between the dura and arachnoid membranes (Fig. 48.5). About 24% of patients who sustain a severe brain injury develop an acute subdural hematoma. Damage to the brain tissue can cause an altered LOC. Therefore, it can be difficult to recognize a subdural hematoma on the basis of clinical examination alone. As the subdural hematoma increases in size, the patient may exhibit one-sided paralysis of extraocular movement, extremity weakness, or dilation of the pupil. LOC can deteriorate further as ICP increases.

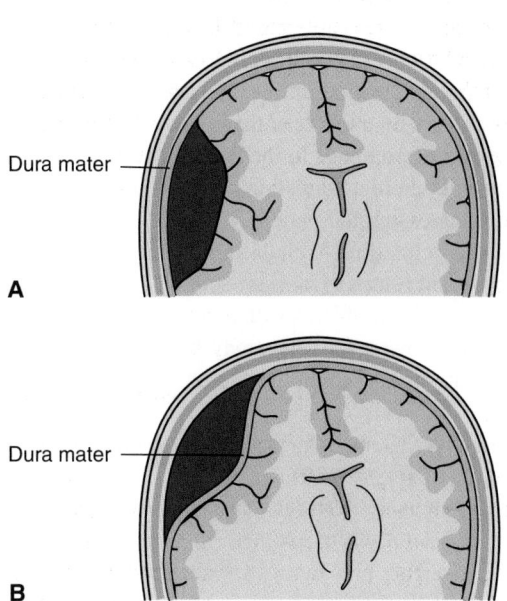

FIGURE 48.5 (A) A subdural hematoma is usually venous and forms between the dura and the arachnoid membranes. (B) An epidural hematoma is usually from an arterial bleed and forms between the dura mater and the skull.

Older adults and people with alcoholism are particularly prone to chronic subdural hematomas. Atrophy of the brain, common in these populations, stretches the veins between the brain and dura. A seemingly minor fall or blow to the head can cause these stretched veins to rupture and bleed. Often, there are no other injuries associated with the trauma. Because a chronic subdural hematoma can develop weeks to months after the injury, the patient may not remember an injury occurring.

The patient with a chronic subdural hematoma may be forgetful, lethargic, or irritable or may report a headache. If the hematoma persists or increases in size, the patient can develop hemiparesis and pupillary changes. The patient or family members may not associate the symptoms with a previous injury and, therefore, may delay seeking medical care.

EPIDURAL HEMATOMA. About 10% of patients with severe brain injuries develop epidural hematomas. Blood collects between the dura mater and skull. The blood is usually arterial in nature and is often associated with skull fracture (see Fig. 48.5). Arterial bleeding can cause the hematoma to become large very quickly. Patients with epidural hematoma typically exhibit a progressive course of symptoms. The patient loses consciousness directly after the injury; he or she then regains consciousness and is coherent for a brief period. The patient then develops a dilated pupil and paralyzed extraocular muscles on the side of the hematoma and becomes less responsive. If there is no intervention, the patient becomes unresponsive. Seizures or hemiparesis can occur. Once the patient has symptoms, deterioration can be rapid. Airway management and control of ICP must be instituted immediately, or the patient will die.

Diagnostic Tests

A CT scan is usually the first imaging test performed on a patient with a TBI (Table 48.7). It is faster and more accessible than MRI. This is particularly important for unstable patients or those with multiple injuries. It is easier to identify skull fractures on a CT scan than on MRI. MRI can be used later to identify damage to the brain tissue.

Neuropsychological testing by a trained specialist can be useful in assessing the patient's cognitive function. This information helps direct rehabilitation placement, discharge planning, and return to work or school. Neuropsychological testing identifies problems with memory, judgment, learning, and comprehension. Patients may be able to learn compensation strategies based on the results.

Therapeutic Measures
Surgical Management
Surgical treatment of hematomas is discussed under intracranial surgery later in this chapter.

Medical Management
Medical management of TBI involves control of ICP and support of body functions. Patients with brain injuries can be partially or completely dependent on assistance with respiration, nutrition, elimination, movement, and skin integrity.

Table 48.7
Traumatic Brain Injury Summary

Signs and Symptoms	Loss or decrease in level of consciousness (LOC), depending on severity and type of injury Loss of memory before or after the injury Increased intracranial pressure Headache, dizziness Nausea and vomiting Unequal pupils Tachycardia, tachypnea Diaphoresis Hemiparesis
Diagnostic Tests	Computed tomography (CT) scan, magnetic resonance imaging (MRI) Skull x-rays Routine laboratory tests (hemoglobin, electrolytes, coagulation studies, type and crossmatch) Neuropsychological testing
Therapeutic Measures	Control intracranial pressure Surgical management of hematoma Maintain respiratory function Maintain diet/nutrition Maintain skin integrity Prevent complications Education
Complications	Increased intracranial pressure Diabetes insipidus Acute hydrocephalus Post-traumatic syndrome Cognitive and personality changes
Priority Nursing Diagnoses	*Risk for Ineffective Cerebral Tissue Perfusion* *Ineffective Airway Clearance* *Ineffective Breathing Pattern*

A variety of techniques are used to control ICP in the patient with moderate or severe brain injury. The first step is to insert an ICP monitor to allow measurement of the ICP. Refer to the section on increased ICP earlier in this chapter for further information.

If ICP remains elevated despite drainage of CSF, the next step is use of an osmotic diuretic. The most commonly used drug is IV mannitol (Osmitrol). Mannitol uses osmosis to pull fluid from the brain into the intravascular space and eliminate it via the renal system. Serum osmolarity and electrolytes must be carefully monitored when mannitol is being administered. Some patients experience a rebound increase in ICP after the mannitol wears off.

Mechanical hyperventilation may be used if the patient is still experiencing increased ICP. Hyperventilation is effective in lowering ICP because it causes cerebral vasoconstriction. Vasoconstriction allows less blood into the cranium, thereby lowering ICP. Research has demonstrated, however, that aggressive hyperventilation, particularly within the first 24 hours after injury, can induce ischemia in the already compromised brain. Therefore, hyperventilation is now reserved for increased ICP that does not respond to other treatments.

High-dose barbiturate therapy may be used to induce a therapeutic coma, which reduces the metabolic needs of the brain during the acute phase following injury. These patients are completely dependent for all of their needs and care. They must be mechanically ventilated and cared for in an ICU setting. Vasopressors may be required to maintain blood pressure, and the patient's temperature should be kept as normal as possible.

Complications

Brain Herniation

If interventions to control ICP are unsuccessful, the patient can experience uncontrolled edema or herniation of brain tissue (Fig. 48.6). Herniation is displacement of brain tissue out of its normal anatomical location. This displacement prevents function of the herniated tissue and places pressure on other vital structures, most commonly the brainstem. Herniation usually results in brain death.

Patients who experience brain death may be suitable organ donor candidates. For some family members, the opportunity to donate their loved one's organs provides some sense of purpose in the death.

Diabetes Insipidus

Edema or direct injury that affects the posterior portion of the pituitary gland or hypothalamus can result in inadequate release of antidiuretic hormone, causing diabetes insipidus. This results in polyuria and, if the patient is awake, polydipsia. Fluid replacement and IV vasopressin are used to maintain fluid and electrolyte balance. See Chapter 39 for more information on diabetes insipidus.

Acute Hydrocephalus

Cerebral edema can interfere with CSF circulation, causing **hydrocephalus.** Initial treatment is use of an external ventricular drain, followed by a ventriculoperitoneal shunt if necessary. A shunt drains excess CSF into the peritoneum, where it is reabsorbed into circulation and excreted.

Labile Vital Signs

Direct trauma to or pressure on the brainstem can cause fluctuations in blood pressure, cardiac rhythm, or respiratory pattern. Treatment is aimed at control of ICP.

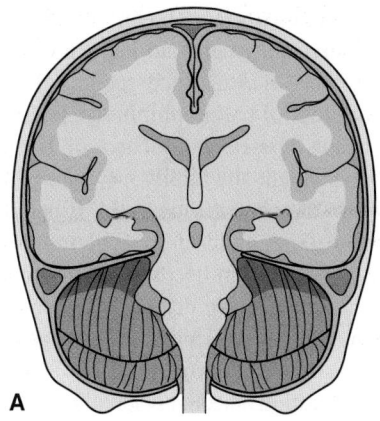

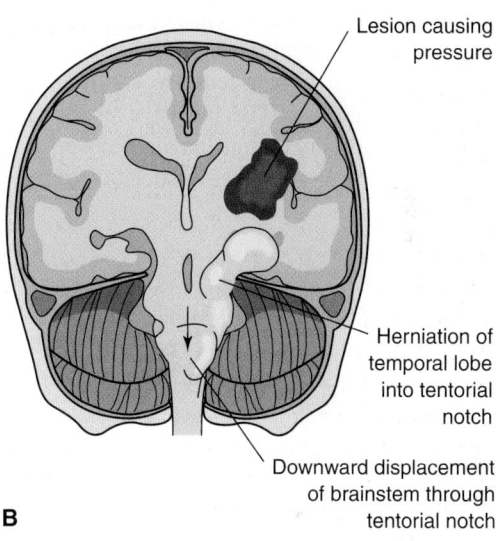

FIGURE 48.6 Herniation of the brain. (A) Normal brain. (B) Herniation of brain tissue into tentorial notch.

Post-Traumatic Stress Disorder

Patients who sustain a concussion can experience ongoing, somewhat vague symptoms. They may report headache, fatigue, difficulty concentrating, depression, or memory impairment. Symptoms can be severe enough to interfere with work, school, and interpersonal relationships. Neuropsychological testing can provide objective evidence of cognitive dysfunction and establish the need for cognitive rehabilitation for post-traumatic stress disorder, or PTSD (see Chapter 57 for more about PTSD). Symptoms can take 3 to 12 months to resolve.

Cognitive and Personality Changes

Alterations in personality and cognition may be the most difficult long-term complication for patients and family members to adjust to. The patient can have significant short-term memory impairment. This limits his or her ability to learn

• WORD • BUILDING •

hydrocephalus: hydro—water + cephalus—head

new information and can interfere with ability to function at work or school. Impaired judgment can make the patient a safety risk to self or others. It also affects social functioning.

Emotional lability, loss of social inhibitions, and personality changes may occur. These consequences of TBI have a profound effect on the patient and family members. Spouses may state, "This is not the person I married." If behavior is violent, bizarre, or profane, children may be unwilling to bring their friends home and can become socially isolated. Young children in particular have difficulty understanding why a parent is behaving so differently. Disintegration of relationships is not uncommon following TBI.

Neuropsychological testing objectively identifies problems. These deficits can then be addressed with cognitive rehabilitation. Individual and family counseling can be helpful. Support groups for patients and family members may also help.

Motor and speech impairment are additional possible long-term complications of TBI. Intensive rehabilitation provides the best opportunity for maximizing recovery. For more information, visit the Brain Injury Association of America at www.biausa.org.

Nursing Process for the Patient With Traumatic Brain Injury

Acute care is presented here. Also see "Nursing Care Plan for the Patient With a Brain Infection or Injury" earlier in this chapter.

Data Collection

After stabilization in the emergency department, care of the patient with a severe TBI takes place in the ICU setting, where ICP can be carefully monitored. Frequent data collection is essential, including a Glasgow Coma Scale score or the FOUR Score (see Chapter 47), pupil responses, muscle strength, and vital signs. Review Box 48-1 for additional signs of increased ICP for which to monitor. Once the patient is stabilized, neurologic damage is assessed. Identification of deficits guides nursing care. Assessment of discharge needs should begin as soon as possible. The patient may require extensive rehabilitation, and early referral can speed transfer to an appropriate setting.

Nursing Diagnoses, Planning, and Implementation

Risk for Ineffective Cerebral Tissue Perfusion related to increased ICP

EXPECTED OUTCOME: Changes in cerebral tissue perfusion will be prevented or recognized and reported promptly.

• Monitor vital signs for widening pulse pressure or irregular respirations. *These are signs of increased ICP and should be reported promptly.*
• Monitor Glasgow Coma Scale or FOUR Score Coma Scale and report worsening status promptly. *Decreasing LOC can indicate increased ICP and may necessitate emergency intervention.*

• Implement measures *to prevent increased ICP.* See Table 48.4 for preventive measures and rationale.

Ineffective Airway Clearance related to reduced cough reflex and decreased LOC as evidenced by adventitious lung sounds and dropping SpO₂.

EXPECTED OUTCOME: The patient will maintain a clear airway as evidenced by clear breath sounds and SpO₂ of 90% or above.

• Monitor airway and breath sounds. *If the patient has excess secretions and is unable to cough effectively, oropharyngeal suctioning may be necessary.*
• Limit suction passes to one or two at a time for a maximum of 5 to 10 seconds each time. *Suctioning can increase ICP.*
• Keep head of bed elevated 20 to 30 degrees *to reduce risk of aspirating oral secretions and reduce ICP.*
• Turn the patient frequently *to help mobilize secretions and prevent other complications of immobility.*

Ineffective Breathing Pattern related to pressure on respiratory center

EXPECTED OUTCOME: The patient will maintain oxygen saturation (SpO₂) of 90% or above.

• Monitor respiratory rate and depth, arterial blood gases (ABGs), and SpO₂ and report changes. *If respiratory status is deteriorating, mechanical ventilation may be necessary.*
• Elevate head of bed 20 to 30 degrees *to allow chest expansion and ease work of breathing.*
• Administer oxygen as ordered and needed *to prevent hypoxia. Hypoxia promotes brain death.*

Evaluation

The plan of care has been successful if the patient shows no unexpected worsening of neurologic function and injuries and complications are prevented. The patient's airway should be clear and SpO₂ level should be 90% or above. The patient is kept comfortable, and self-care needs are met.

Rehabilitation

Once the patient is stabilized, evaluation for discharge to a rehabilitation facility is completed. The patient must be able to physically tolerate the rehabilitation program, in which the patient will be taught to function as independently as possible. The family must be prepared for changes in the patient's ability to function and possible changes in personality. It can take months to years before the patient reaches his or her maximum potential. In some cases of severe brain damage or continued comatose state, rehabilitation is not feasible and the patient is discharged to home or a long-term facility for custodial care.

CRITICAL THINKING

Mr. Evans is a 24-year-old white male who was involved in a motor vehicle collision. His blood alcohol level was 0.24. Mr. Evans has no pre-existing medical problems. Emergency medical services personnel report that Mr. Evans was unconscious on their arrival at the scene and then became alert and combative. A computed tomography (CT) scan shows a left-sided epidural hematoma. Mr. Evans is admitted to your unit for observation.

1. What symptoms would you expect to see if Mr. Evans's hematoma increases in size?
2. What emergency preparations should you have ready?
3. What psychosocial data should you collect?
4. What other members of the health care team should be consulted?

Suggested answers are at the end of the chapter.

 BRAIN TUMORS

Brain tumors are neoplastic growths of the brain or meninges. Brain tumors can be characterized by vague symptoms such as headache or visual changes or by focal neurologic deficits such as hemiparesis or seizures.

Pathophysiology and Etiology

Brain tumors cause symptoms by either compressing or infiltrating brain tissue. Tumors can arise from CNS cells or can metastasize from other locations in the body. Primary brain tumors rarely metastasize; however, if they do, it is to the spine.

There is no established cause for primary brain tumors. It is unclear what causes the cells to begin reproducing in an uncontrolled fashion. Risk factors include age (45 and older), exposure to radiation or industrial chemicals, and family history. Whites are more likely to be diagnosed with a brain tumor than other racial or ethnic groups.

Brain tumors can be classified in several ways. The traditional distinction of benign and malignant is less helpful when classifying brain tumors than when classifying other cancers. A benign tumor in the brainstem can be fatal, whereas a malignant tumor in the frontal lobe may not be. Location of the tumor can be just as important a factor in outcome as the cell type.

Primary tumors are those arising from cells of the CNS. Intra-axial tumors are those that arise from the glial cells within the cerebrum, cerebellum, or brainstem. These tumors infiltrate and invade brain tissue. Extra-axial tumors arise from the skull, meninges, pituitary gland, or cranial nerves; they place pressure on the brain.

Most brain tumors are secondary; that is, they have metastasized from a primary malignancy somewhere else in the body (Fig. 48.7). These tumors commonly spread via the arterial system. If untreated, they cause increased ICP. This can be the cause of the patient's death rather than the primary malignancy.

Signs and Symptoms

The symptoms of a brain tumor are directly related to the location of the tumor in the brain and to the rate of growth. Slow-growing types of tumors such as meningiomas (a tumor arising from the meninges; Fig. 48.8) can get to be quite large before causing symptoms. Conversely, glioblastoma multiforme or metastatic tumors can abruptly cause seizures or hemiparesis. Other types of tumors include oligodendroglioma, astrocytoma, and acoustic neuroma. The suffix *-oma* refers to tumor. The prefix denotes the type of cell from which the tumor arises.

The most common early symptom of a brain tumor is fatigue. Other symptoms can include seizures, motor and sensory deficits, nausea and vomiting, headaches, personality changes, confusion, and speech and vision disturbances. If the pituitary gland is involved, additional symptoms related to changes in hormone secretion occur, such as abnormal growth or fluid volume imbalances.

Diagnostic Tests

MRI gives the clearest images of a brain tumor. If the tumor appears to be highly vascular or in proximity to major blood vessels, an angiogram may be performed. It is now possible to do a magnetic resonance angiogram (MRA), which involves IV administration of contrast material. MRA is much less invasive than a traditional angiogram. If the tumor is in the region of the pituitary gland, serum hormone levels are evaluated. Biopsy may be done during surgical removal of the tumor or using needle aspiration. Additional tests may be carried out to find a primary cancer site.

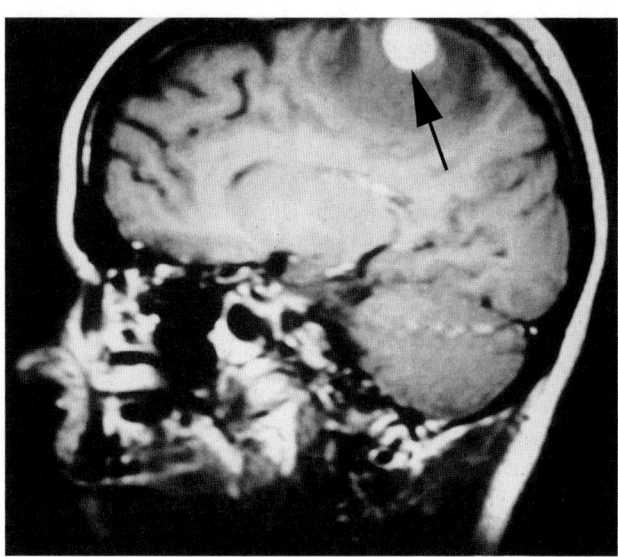

FIGURE 48.7 Metastatic brain tumor. This patient's primary cancer was in the lung.

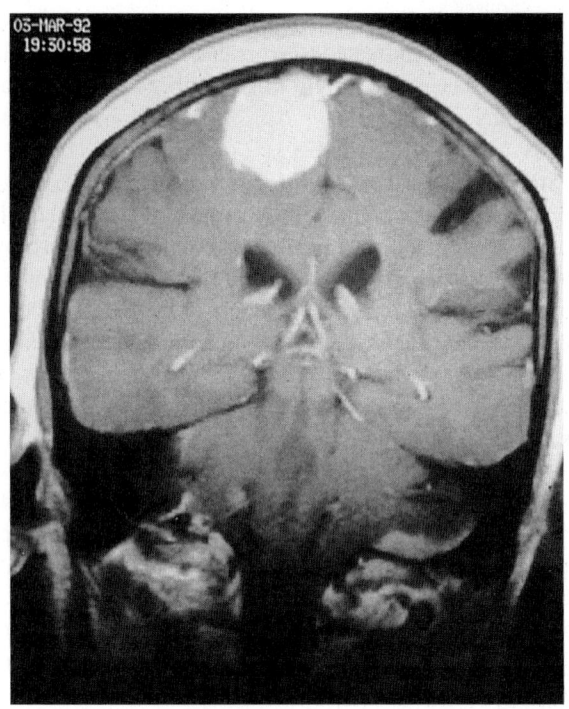

FIGURE 48.8 Meningioma.

Therapeutic Measures

Surgery

Surgical treatment involves removal of the tumor or as much of the tumor as possible. Care of the patient undergoing intracranial surgery is discussed later in this chapter.

Medical Treatment

Medical treatment is aimed at controlling symptoms. Patients who have a seizure are placed on anticonvulsants. If significant cerebral edema is noted on MRI or if the patient is suffering from headaches or other symptoms, a steroid such as dexamethasone (Decadron) may be prescribed to lessen edema and reduce symptoms. Typically, patients do not require narcotics for pain relief.

Radiation Therapy

External beam radiation therapy is standard treatment for many patients with a brain tumor. The therapy is typically given 5 days a week for 6 weeks. Some clinicians use a hyperfractionated schedule, in which the patient has therapy twice a day for less time. Brachytherapy is a means of delivering radiation therapy directly to the tumor. Small catheters are implanted in the tumor, and then tiny radioactive particles are inserted into the catheters. The treatment typically takes 3 to 5 days. During this time, the patient is confined to a private room. Interaction with visitors and staff is kept to a minimum to reduce exposure to radioactivity. This therapy is not appropriate for confused individuals because they may not be able to cooperate with restrictions.

Stereotactic radiosurgery is a technique that uses small amounts of radiation directed at the tumor from different angles. A metal frame is affixed to the patient's skull, and the tumor is visualized within the framework on a CT scan or MRI. A computer plan is generated to direct the radiation. Because multiple small sources are used, the normal brain tissue receives very little radiation, while the majority of the radiation accumulates in the tumor.

Chemotherapy

The blood–brain barrier is a protective mechanism that prevents many injurious substances from reaching brain tissue. Unfortunately, it is also effective in preventing most chemotherapy agents from reaching the brain. To penetrate the blood–brain barrier, large doses of chemotherapy may be required. These doses may not be well tolerated by other body systems. New treatments are currently being investigated. Chemotherapy substances may be placed in the cavity left by surgical resection. Other treatments disrupt the blood–brain barrier with mannitol (an osmotic diuretic) and then deliver intra-arterial chemotherapy under general anesthesia. Targeted drug therapy uses a drug such as bevacizumab (Avastin), which stops formation of new blood vessels that support the tumor. Gene therapy is also being used in an effort to kill malignant cells.

Complementary and Alternative Therapies

The rate of success for treatment of brain tumors is not as high as treatment of other neoplasms. Patients may be drawn to nontraditional therapies both as potential cures and for treatment of symptoms. Encourage patients to look at each option in a rational manner. Some questions they should ask themselves include the following:

- Will this interfere with any of my other treatments or medications?
- What is the cost?
- What are the side effects?
- Is there any objective information (research) available?
- What does my physician think of this?

Additional information on evaluation of complementary and alternative therapies is found in Chapter 5.

Acute and Long-Term Complications

It is difficult to distinguish between symptoms of a brain tumor and complications of treatment. Seizures, headaches, memory impairment, cognitive changes, and ataxia can be symptoms of the tumor or the result of surgery or radiation therapy. Patients can experience hemiparesis or aphasia following surgery. If the tumor continues to grow despite treatment, the patient will experience further decline in function. Gradually, the patient becomes more lethargic and unresponsive. Once the patient becomes comatose, death can occur within a matter of days, particularly if artificial nutrition and hydration are not administered.

Nursing Process for the Patient With a Brain Tumor

Nursing care of the patient with a brain tumor is similar to that for the patient with a brain injury because both experience neurologic deficits. See "Nursing Care Plan for the Patient With a Brain Infection or Injury" earlier in this chapter.

 INTRACRANIAL SURGERY

The primary purpose of intracranial surgery is to remove a mass lesion. These types of lesions include hematomas, tumors, arteriovenous malformations, and, occasionally, contused brain tissue. Other indications for surgery include elevation of a depressed skull fracture, removal of a foreign body, debridement of a wound, or resection of a seizure focus. The term **craniotomy** refers to any surgical opening in the skull. A burr hole is an opening into the cranium made with a drill. **Craniectomy** is the term used to describe removal of part of the cranial bone. **Cranioplasty** refers to repair of bone or use of a prosthesis to replace bone following surgery.

The goal of intracranial tumor surgery is gross total resection (removal) of the tumor. This involves removal of all visible tumor, called *debulking*. Even with the use of an operative microscope, viable tumor cells can be left behind that can give rise to recurrence. If the entire tumor cannot be removed, the surgeon debulks as much as possible, giving radiation therapy or chemotherapy less of a burden to combat. In some cases, it is not feasible to attempt more than a biopsy of the tumor. Location of the tumor or the patient's age or medical condition may not allow the patient to tolerate a full craniotomy. A biopsy may be done under local or general anesthesia, depending on the patient's condition. The goal of a biopsy is to obtain tissue that allows pathological diagnosis of the tumor, which then guides further treatment.

Intracranial surgery is usually performed under general anesthesia. Occasionally, a procedure requires that the patient be awake and cooperative.

Preoperative Care

Preoperative care of the patient undergoing intracranial surgery is similar to that of patients having other surgeries (see Chapter 12). The patient undergoes a laboratory workup and anesthesia evaluation. If the patient has cognitive impairments, it is important that a family member be available to provide information and sign consents. A thorough baseline neurologic assessment should be documented.

Patient education is important preoperatively. The extent of education depends on the patient's ability to absorb new information, which is influenced by the disease process, cognitive functioning, anxiety, and education level. Family members are involved as needed. Information about the disease process and surgery is provided by the surgeon. The nurse can play an important role in reinforcing and clarifying the information presented.

Anxiety is also a significant concern before surgery. The patient is anticipating serious surgery as well as an unknown outcome. Allow time for the patient and family members to express their fears and ask questions. Honest and accurate information should be provided.

Family members should be prepared for how the patient will look after surgery. A preoperative visit to the ICU may help prevent some anxiety postoperatively. Family members should be accompanied on this visit by a knowledgeable nurse who can explain what they are seeing.

Surgery can last 2 hours for a biopsy to 12 hours or longer for more involved procedures. Patients and family members should be prepared for the idea that some or all of the patient's hair will be shaved off. Some people prefer to have all their hair shaved rather than just part. The patient should be prepared to see his or her face swollen after surgery, particularly around the eyes; the periorbital region may be bruised. Many patients wish to wear a scarf or scrub cap after the dressing is removed.

Nursing Process for the Postoperative Care of the Patient Having Intracranial Surgery

Acute care of the postoperative patient is presented here. Also see "Nursing Care Plan for the Patient With a Brain Infection or Injury" earlier in this chapter.

Data Collection

After intracranial surgery, the patient will be cared for in the ICU. Plan to assist the RN with frequent neurologic assessments in addition to routine postoperative monitoring. Patients should have their neurologic status assessed every hour for the first 24 hours or as ordered by the health care provider (HCP). Many patients undergo a CT scan within the first 24 hours following surgery to assess cerebral edema. Once the patient is awake and alert, plan to assess the patient's response to changes in body image and knowledge base related to care that will be required following discharge.

Nursing Diagnoses, Planning, and Implementation

The primary goal after intracranial surgery is prevention of complications. Once the patient is stabilized, goals can change to longer-term outcomes such as acceptance of changes in body image and understanding of self-care following discharge. If the patient has severe deficits following surgery, rehabilitation or long-term care may become necessary. A consultation with a social worker can help with planning for this transition. Priority nursing diagnoses are discussed next.

> **Risk for Ineffective Cerebral Tissue Perfusion related to edema of the operative site**
>
> **EXPECTED OUTCOME:** The patient will have adequate cerebral tissue perfusion as evidenced by stable or improving neurologic assessments.

• Monitor neurologic status as ordered. Report changes promptly. *Deteriorating status can signify increased ICP.*

• WORD • BUILDING •
craniotomy: crani—skull + otomy—incision
craniectomy: crani—skull + ectomy—excision, removal
cranioplasty: crani—skull + plasty—to form

- Implement measures *to prevent increased ICP*. See Table 48.4 for preventive measures and rationales.
- Position the patient with the head of the bed at 30 degrees or higher, unless ordered otherwise, *to promote venous drainage and minimize increases in ICP*. The exception to this is patients who have had a chronic subdural hematoma removed; these patients must remain flat. Patients can turn from side to side or lie on their back but should not lie on the operative side.
- Implement seizure precautions *because the patient is at risk for seizures due to cerebral edema.*
- Use caution to protect the many monitoring systems being used. The patient may have an intracranial monitor in place following surgery *to monitor ICP*. Some patients may also have central venous pressure catheters or pulmonary artery catheters *to monitor fluid status*. Urinary catheters are used during the immediate postoperative period *to accurately monitor fluid balance.*
- Monitor dressings for drainage. *Drainage that is blood-tinged in the center with a yellowish ring around it can be CSF leakage. A suspected CSF leak should be reported to the RN or HCP immediately.*

Risk for Infection related to surgical procedure

EXPECTED OUTCOME: The patient will remain free from infection as evidenced by temperature and WBC count within normal limits and incision sites clean and dry.

- Monitor patient for rise in temperature, purulence at incision site, and increase in WBC count. *These are signs of infection and should be reported immediately.*
- Use strict aseptic technique for care of the incision, dressing, and monitoring equipment sites *to reduce risk of infection.*
- Use appropriate hand hygiene *to reduce risk of transmitting infection.*

Disturbed Body Image related to changes in appearance or function as evidenced by patient statement of disturbance or unwillingness to observe changes

EXPECTED OUTCOME: The patient will display an open attitude toward change in appearance, as evidenced by willingness to look in mirror and/or be seen by others.

- Offer a turban, scarf, or hat if the patient desires *to help conceal a shaved head.*
- Portray an accepting attitude toward the patient. *Patients are likely aware of nurses' nonverbal behavior.*
- Allow the patient to express his or her feelings if desired. *Talking may help the patient work through feelings, but it should not be forced.*

Deficient Knowledge related to change in treatment regimen after surgery as evidenced by patient statement

EXPECTED OUTCOME: The patient and family members will verbalize correct information for follow-up care at home.

They will state they have the resources to manage care effectively.

- Teach the patient and family members home management, including medication regimen, wound care, and ordered activity restrictions, including driving. Have the patient and family members verbalize the signs of infection or other possible complications to report. *The patient and family members will assume responsibility for care after discharge, unless the patient is being transferred to another facility.*
- Teach the patient and family members seizure precautions and the importance of taking anticonvulsants as ordered. *The patient may be on anticonvulsants to prevent seizures after surgery. If seizure free for 1 year, the HCP may discontinue anticonvulsants.*
- Consult a social worker or case manager for resources if needed. *The patient may need discharge planning if transfer to another facility is planned. If discharge home is expected, the patient and family members will benefit from a home health care nurse follow-up. Assistance with obtaining medications can also be provided if necessary.*

Evaluation

Interventions have been effective if the patient's neurologic status is stable and infection and other complications have been prevented. The patient may begin to show evidence of acceptance of changes in body image, although this may not happen until after discharge from the hospital. The patient or family members should be able to demonstrate appropriate follow-up care.

SPINAL DISORDERS

Herniated Disks

Herniated intravertebral disks are a common health problem. They are characterized by pain and paresthesias that follow a radicular (nerve path) pattern. It is not uncommon for patients to have more than one herniated disk or to have herniated disks in different areas of the spine.

Pathophysiology

When the disk between two vertebrae herniates, it moves out of its normal anatomical position. In most cases, the annulus fibrosus, the tough outer ring of the disk, tears. This allows escape of the nucleus pulposus, the soft inner portion of the disk. Displacement of the disk compresses one or more nerve roots, causing the characteristic symptoms (Fig. 48.9).

Etiology

In some cases, a specific event can be correlated with a herniated disk. The patient may describe a fall, lifting a heavy object, or a motor vehicle collision. In other instances, the patient cannot identify a triggering incident.

Signs and Symptoms

Cervical disk herniation causes pain and muscle spasm in the neck. The patient may have decreased range of motion

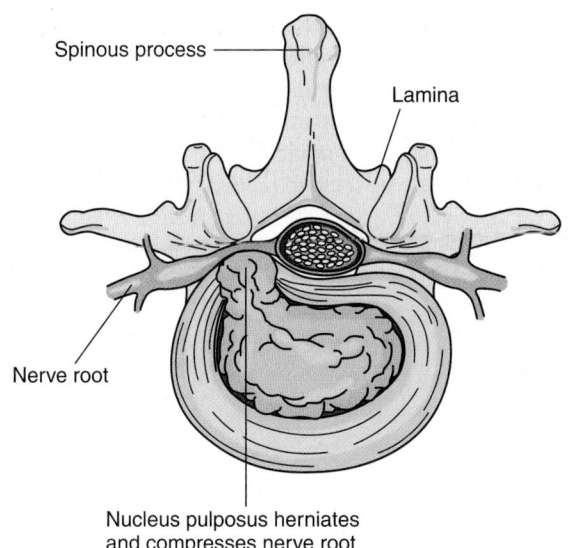

Spinous process

Lamina

Nerve root

Nucleus pulposus herniates
and compresses nerve root

FIGURE 48.9 A herniated disk places pressure on a spinal nerve root.

(ROM) secondary to pain. Hand and arm pain is unilateral (one sided) and follows the distribution of the spinal nerve root. Patients often report numbness or tingling in the extremity. Asymmetrical weakness and atrophy of specific muscle groups may be detected. The severity of the pain or paresthesia does not correlate directly with the severity of the nerve compression. However, weakness and atrophy are indicators of significant nerve compression.

Thoracic herniated disks are not common. This portion of the spine is the least mobile; therefore, less stress is exerted on the disks. Patients with herniated thoracic disks may report pain in the back. It is uncommon to detect muscular weakness.

A herniated lumbar disk is typically characterized by low back pain, pain radiating down one leg, paresthesias, and weakness. Often the sciatic nerve is affected, thus the term **sciatica**. The patient may limp on the affected leg or may have difficulty walking on his or her heels or toes. Muscle spasm is often present. Pain and muscle spasm can limit the patient's ROM. Depending on the disk affected, the knee or ankle deep tendon reflex may be decreased or absent. A severely herniated L5–S1 disk can affect bowel or bladder continence. This is an emergency situation and should be reported immediately.

The *WHAT'S UP?* mnemonic can be used to assess symptoms of herniated disks at any level:

- **W**—Where is the pain? Does it radiate into an extremity? In what distribution?
- **H**—How does it feel? Sharp, stabbing, burning?
- **A**—Do certain positions or activities alleviate or aggravate the pain? Holding the affected arm above the head can alleviate cervical pain. Sitting places pressure on disks and aggravates lumbar pain; lying down may relieve it.
- **T**—Is there a correlation between time and pain? Some patients have more pain at the end of the day. Is the pain constant or intermittent?

- **S**—Ask the patient to rate the severity of the pain on a scale of 0 to 10. Which is the most painful, the spine or extremity?
- **U**—Ask the patient to identify other useful data, such as symptoms of numbness, tingling, or weakness.
- **P**—What is the patient's perception of the pain? Is it interfering with work or other aspects of the patient's life?

Diagnostic Tests

MRI will detect herniation of a disk and compression or abnormality of the spinal cord. If the patient has previously had surgery in the area of the suspected herniation, the MRI is done with and without contrast to differentiate between scar tissue and a herniated disk.

If the patient cannot tolerate MRI or if MRI does not provide enough information, a myelogram can be done. Refer to Appendix A for a description of both tests.

Therapeutic Measures

Most HCPs and patients prefer to try conservative medical therapy before performing surgery for a herniated disk.

MEDICAL TREATMENT.

Rest. The typical recommendation is 1 or 2 days of bedrest, followed by a careful, gradual increase in activity.

Physical Therapy. Physical therapy can be very useful for some patients. A gradually progressive course of exercise strengthens the muscles. This is particularly important in the lumbar area, where the muscles help stabilize the spine. Techniques such as ultrasound, electrical stimulation, heat, ice, and deep massage can decrease pain and muscle spasm and allow for increased ROM. Instructions in proper body mechanics and strategies for avoiding re-injury are important components of physical therapy.

Traction. Cervical traction is a noninvasive technique sometimes used by physical therapists for patients with herniated cervical disks. The patient's head is placed in a halter-like device. A series of ropes and pulleys connects the halter to a weight. This gently pulls the head away from the shoulders. The rationale is that this traction slightly separates the vertebral bodies and can allow the disk to return to its proper position. If it is effective in relieving the patient's pain, cervical traction can be done at home on an as-needed basis. Traction is discontinued immediately if it increases the patient's pain. Lumbar traction is not particularly effective because the lumbar paraspinal muscles are large and strong. The amount of traction needed to overcome the muscular resistance can cause injury.

Medication. Muscle relaxants are often prescribed as a short-term therapy for patients who are experiencing muscle spasms. These medications decrease pain by decreasing the spasm, helping the patient increase ROM and activity. Muscle spasm is actually a protective mechanism. Muscles tighten and become painful, causing the patient to limit movement. This lessens the chance that the disk will be further injured. However, chronic spasm can cause tearing and scarring of the muscles. Patients should be warned that drowsiness is a common side effect of many muscle relaxants. They should be cautioned against driving or operating machinery until they determine how well they tolerate the medication. Diazepam (Valium) is an effective muscle relaxant; however, it has a strong potential for addiction, so it is usually used only if muscle spasm cannot be adequately treated with other medications.

Inflammation of the nerve root is caused by compression and irritation from the herniated disk. NSAIDs can be effective in reducing this inflammation, but there is no way to predict response to a given drug. It may be necessary for the patient to try several NSAIDs before an effective one is found. Because several of these drugs are now available without prescription, the patient should be cautioned not to use a nonprescription NSAID at the same time as a prescription NSAID. Patients should be instructed to report any stomach upset to the HCP because NSAIDs can cause gastric bleeding. Occasionally, oral steroids are used on a short-term basis for patients with severe inflammation that does not respond to other treatments. A rapidly tapering dose of steroid over 1 week is often prescribed. Steroids can also cause gastric upset as well as elevated serum glucose levels. Instruct patients with diabetes to monitor glucose levels closely and to consult their HCP if the levels are outside their normal parameters.

Epidural injections may be tried for patients who have no relief with more conservative measures. A mixture of medications, typically a steroid, a long-acting anesthetic, and a long-acting pain reliever, is injected into the epidural space. The anesthetic provides immediate relief, while the steroid reduces swelling for a longer lasting effect. If relief is obtained, the injection can be repeated every 3 to 4 months.

The use of opioid pain medication is a subject of concern in the treatment of patients with herniated disks. Opioids generally are appropriate for short-term treatment of acute pain. However, if treatment is not effective, the pain can become chronic. In that circumstance, the HCP and patient must discuss the potential complications of long-term opioid use, such as constipation, tolerance, and dependence. A referral to a pain clinic for alternative strategies may be appropriate.

Some alternatives to long-term use of opioids include topical lidocaine patches or NSAID patches as well as the use of agents for neuropathic pain such as gabapentin (Neurontin) or pregabalin (Lyrica).

Complementary and Alternative Therapy. A transcutaneous electrical nerve stimulator (commonly called a TENS unit) is a noninvasive pain-relief technique. Small electrodes are placed on the skin around the area of the pain. The device then transmits a low-voltage electrical current through the skin. The patient feels a tingling or buzzing sensation, which can help block the pain impulses. A physical therapist or pain specialist teaches the patient where to place the electrodes and how to operate the unit. The patient decides when to use it and at what settings. This allows the patient to actively participate in his or her care and have some control over the pain level.

SURGICAL MANAGEMENT. Surgeries are less common today than in the past, because conservative measures have been found to be successful for most patients. If surgery is indicated, several options are available. A **laminectomy** removes one of the laminae, the flat pieces of bone on each side of a vertebra. This may be done to relieve pressure or to gain access for removal of a herniated disk. A *diskectomy* removes the entire disk. A spinal fusion uses a bone graft to fuse two vertebrae together if the area is unstable. Surgery can be done through a microscope for less scarring and faster recovery. Most patients are discharged within 24 hours of surgery.

A diskectomy is generally done for a herniated cervical disk. This can be accomplished via an anterior or posterior approach. Most surgeons replace the disk with bone or another material. This prevents collapse of the disk space and creates a spinal fusion. If bone is used, it may be harvested from the patient's iliac crest or donated from a cadaver. Mobility of the spine is lost in the area of a fusion. Spinal fusions may also be done to correct instability of the spine from other causes, such as scoliosis or degenerative disorders.

A posterior approach is used for a herniated lumbar disk. Typically, the vertical incision is 1 to 2 inches long. It is necessary to pull some of the muscle away from the bone, which accounts for some of the postoperative pain that patients experience. A laminectomy is done, and the herniated portion of the disk is resected. The remainder of the disk continues to provide a cushion between the intravertebral bodies. The surgeon removes any free fragments and any disk material that appears unstable.

Percutaneous diskectomy involves insertion of a large needle into the disk under local anesthesia to aspirate herniated disk material. This technique is not used for severely herniated disks. Laser disk surgery may be used to disintegrate the herniated tissue. Laparoscopic techniques may also be used.

An artificial disk may be used in select patients. It is made of two plastic disks designed to slide so that mobility is not impaired as with spinal fusion. The artificial disk is attached to the vertebra above and below after the damaged disk is removed. This alternative to spinal fusion has been effective for those with single-disk problems.

Complications After Surgery. Hemorrhage. As with any surgery, intraoperative hemorrhage is possible, although it is not common in disk surgery. If a postoperative hemorrhage occurs in a patient who has had an anterior cervical diskectomy, the airway can become occluded. Monitor the patient for bleeding from the incision and respiratory distress.

Nerve Root Damage. If the nerve root is severed during surgery, the patient experiences loss of motor and sensory functions in that nerve's distribution area. This can result in decreased use of the extremity. If the nerve root is damaged

• WORD • BUILDING •

laminectomy: lamin—posterior portion of the vertebra + ectomy—excision, removal

or excessive scarring occurs, the patient can experience pain, weakness, or paresthesias. In some cases, physical therapy and NSAIDs may be effective in improving function and reducing pain.

Reherniation. Lumbar disks can reherniate. This can occur anywhere from 1 week to several years after the initial surgery. If the reherniation occurs within a few weeks to months after the first surgery, the patient usually undergoes a microdiskectomy. Reherniation of a cervical disk does not occur because the entire disk is removed.

Herniation of Adjacent Disk. Fusion of the cervical spine results in loss of movement at that motion segment. This can place increased stress on the disks above and below the fusion. This can increase the risk of another herniated disk, especially if the patient already has degeneration of other disks. The patient should be instructed to maintain an exercise program and to frequently move the spine through ROM exercises.

Spinal Stenosis

Spinal stenosis is a condition in which the spinal canal compresses the spinal cord (Fig. 48.10). Arthritis is a major cause of spinal stenosis. The facet joints of the spine become inflamed and enlarged, narrowing the diameter of the spinal canal and compressing the spinal cord. Patients may report pain and weakness. Compression of the cervical portion of the spinal cord can result in hyperreflexia and weakness of the arms and hands.

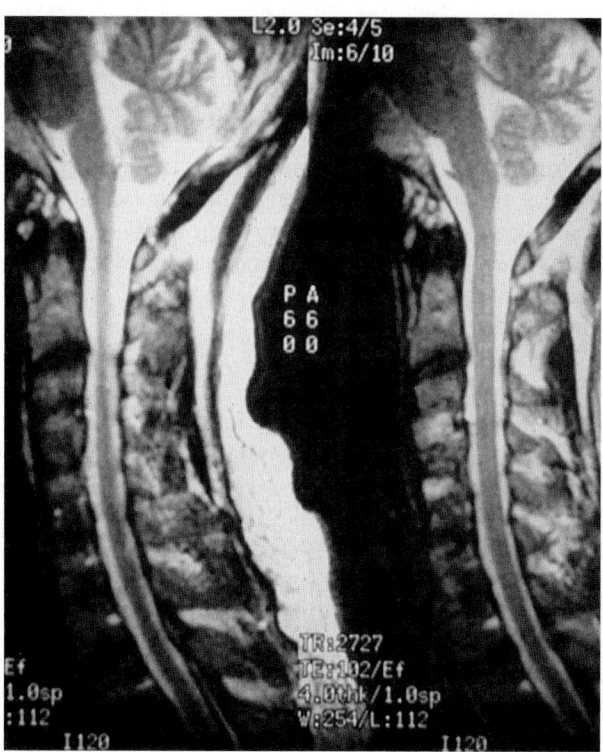

FIGURE 48.10 Stenosis of the cervical spine (left). Compare with normal spinal column (right).

A laminectomy may be done to relieve pressure on the spinal cord. The size of the incision depends on the number of vertebrae involved. These patients are often older and may have concurrent illnesses. They may require inpatient rehabilitation before returning home.

Nursing Process for the Patient Having Spinal Surgery

Preoperative Care

In addition to routine teaching, instruct the patient in how to logroll following surgery. This procedure involves keeping the body in alignment and rolling as a unit, without twisting the spine, to prevent injury to the operative site.

Postoperative Care

DATA COLLECTION. In addition to routine postoperative data collection, monitor extremities for changes in circulation, movement, and sensation. Monitor color, warmth, and presence of pulses in the extremities. Assess movement by asking the patient to move the extremities. Assess sensation by gently touching the patient's extremity and asking if feeling is present. Report any changes immediately to the HCP because this can indicate nerve or circulatory damage.

Monitor pain frequently. The pain that necessitated surgery should be relieved, but the patient can still have muscular and incisional pain. Reassure the patient that it will gradually subside. Monitor the surgical dressing and drain (if present) for CSF drainage or bleeding. Any sign of CSF drainage or significant bleeding should be reported to the HCP immediately. If bone was taken from a separate donor site, this site must also be monitored. Intake and output are measured to ensure that the patient is able to void. Notify the HCP if the patient has difficulty voiding.

NURSING DIAGNOSES, PLANNING, AND IMPLEMENTATION. Goals of nursing are to keep the patient safe and free from injury or complications and free from pain. Gradual return to normal physical activity is expected. Possible postoperative diagnoses are discussed next.

> *Acute Pain related to surgical procedure as evidenced by the patient's pain rating*
>
> **EXPECTED OUTCOME:** The patient will verbalize an acceptable pain level.

• Monitor pain following surgery using an appropriate pain scale. *The patient's self-report is the most reliable method for assessing pain.*

• Administer muscle relaxants, analgesics, and NSAIDs as ordered. If a local anesthetic was injected into the surgical site during surgery, the patient may not have pain immediately postoperatively. *Medications to relieve pain help the patient to mobilize following surgery, which helps prevent complications.*

• Position the patient in bed in correct body alignment. If ordered, keep the patient flat for 6 to 8 hours. *Correct alignment avoids twisting and injury to the operative site.*

- Place a pillow between the legs when lying on the side *to promote alignment and comfort.*

Impaired Urinary Elimination related to effects of surgery

EXPECTED OUTCOME: The patient will be able to empty bladder without assistance.

- Monitor urine output for retention. *Patients may have difficulty voiding following lumbar surgery because of anesthesia, immobility, or occasionally because of nerve damage related to surgery.*
- If activity orders allow, assist the patient to get up to urinate (or to stand for men). *This may help the patient urinate.*
- If unable to void, try running warm water over the perineum or having the patient take a warm bath or shower. *This may stimulate voiding.*
- If difficulty urinating continues, contact the HCP for an order for intermittent catheterization until the problem resolves. *Urine retention that is not resolved can lead to bladder rupture. Intermittent catheterization is a safe way to empty the bladder.*

Impaired Physical Mobility related to neuromuscular impairment

EXPECTED OUTCOME: The patient will be able to ambulate and prevent complications of immobility after surgery.

- Assess mobility of affected extremities following surgery. *A reduction in expected mobility following surgery indicates nerve damage in surgery and should be reported immediately.*
- Assist the patient to logroll to get out of bed and ambulate on the first postoperative day, as ordered. If spinal fusion has been done, the fused area of the spine will be immobile. *Early mobilization after surgery helps prevent complications.*
- Apply a soft cervical collar to the patient with a cervical laminectomy as ordered *for neck support.*

EVALUATION. The patient is expected to be free of complications and pain, be able to urinate, be able to move all extremities, and return gradually to pre-illness activity level.

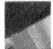 **SPINAL CORD INJURIES**

Injuries to the spinal cord affect people of all ages but take their greatest toll on young people. Spinal cord injuries are characterized by a decrease or loss of sensory and motor functions below the level of the injury.

Pathophysiology

The spinal cord is made up of nerve fibers that allow communication between the brain and the rest of the body. Damage to the spinal cord results in interference with this communication process. Damage may be caused by bruising, tearing, cutting, edema, or bleeding into the cord. The damage can be caused by external forces or by fragments of fractured bone.

Etiology and Types

The causes of spinal cord injury are similar to those of TBI. It is not uncommon for a patient to have both a spinal cord injury and TBI. Motor vehicle collisions are the most common causes of spinal cord injury in the United States. Females are more often injured by falls, and males are more often injured during acts of violence or contact sports. Assaults can cause cord injury if a knife or bullet penetrates the spinal cord. Diving into shallow water is a common cause of cervical cord injury.

Spinal cord injuries can be classified by location or by degree of damage to the cord. A complete spinal cord injury means that there is no motor or sensory function below the level of the injury. With an incomplete lesion, some function remains. This does not necessarily mean that the remaining function will be useful to the patient. Some patients find that having areas where sensation is intact may be more painful than useful.

The cervical and lumbar portions of the spine are injured more often than the thoracic or sacral segments. This is because the cervical and lumbar areas are the most mobile portions of the spine.

Signs and Symptoms
Cervical Injuries

Signs and symptoms depend on the level at which the cord is damaged (Fig. 48.11). Cervical cord injuries can affect all four extremities, causing paralysis and paresthesias, impaired respiration, and loss of bowel and bladder control. Paralysis of all four extremities is called **quadriplegia;** weakness of all extremities is called **quadriparesis.** If the injury is at C3 or above, the injury is usually fatal because muscles used for breathing are paralyzed. An injury at the fourth or fifth cervical vertebra affects breathing and may necessitate some type of ventilatory support. Such patients typically need long-term assistance with ADLs.

Thoracic and Lumbar Injuries

Thoracic and lumbar injuries affect the legs, bowel, and bladder. Paralysis of the legs is called **paraplegia;** weakness of the legs is called **paraparesis.** Sacral injuries affect bowel and bladder continence and may affect foot function. Individuals with thoracic, lumbar, and sacral injuries can usually learn to perform ADLs independently.

> • WORD • BUILDING •
>
> **quadriplegia:** quad—four + plegia—paralysis
> **quadriparesis:** quad—four + paresis—partial paralysis
> **paraplegia:** para—beside + plegia—paralysis
> **paraparesis:** para—beside + paresis—partial paralysis

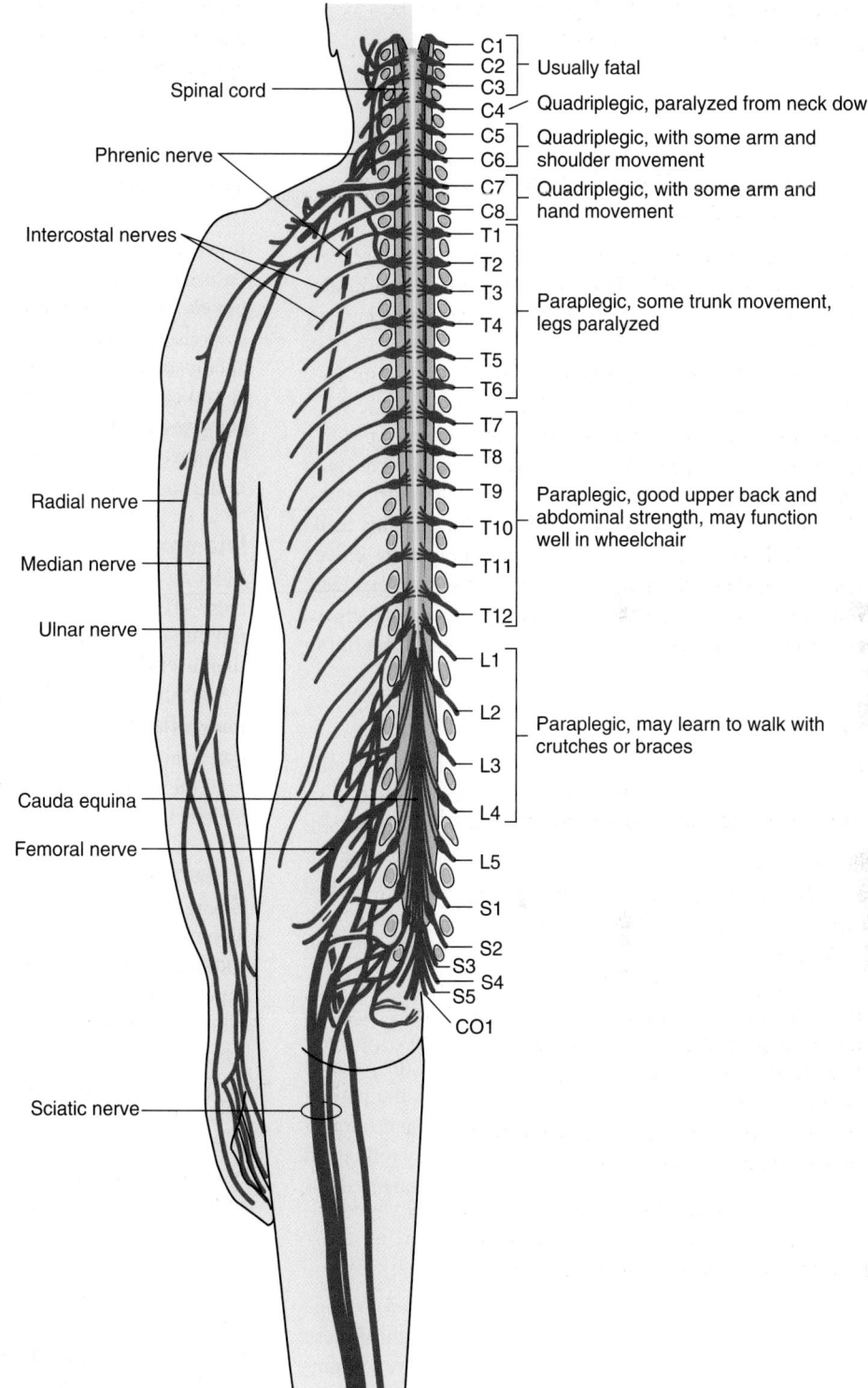

FIGURE 48.11 Spinal cord injury—quadriplegia versus paraplegia.

Spinal Shock

Spinal cord injury has a profound effect on the autonomic nervous system. Immediately after injury, the cord below the injury stops functioning completely. This causes a disruption of sympathetic nervous system function, resulting in vasodilation, hypotension, and bradycardia, called *neurogenic shock* or *spinal shock*. Dilation of the blood vessels allows more blood flow just beneath the skin. This blood cools and is circulated throughout the body, causing hypothermia. The patient is unable to maintain control of body temperature. In addition, all reflexes below the level of the injury are lost, and retention of urine and feces occurs. Spinal shock can last from a week to many weeks in some patients.

Complications

Infection

Impaired respiratory effort, decreased cough, mechanical ventilation, and immobility all predispose a patient with a spinal cord injury to pneumonia. Urinary catheterization, whether indwelling or intermittent, places patients at risk for urinary tract infection.

Deep Vein Thrombosis

Lack of movement in the legs inhibits normal blood circulation. Compression stockings, sequential compression devices, and anticoagulant medications may be used to reduce the risk of deep vein thrombosis.

Orthostatic Hypotension

Most patients with spinal cord injuries no longer have muscular function in their legs to promote venous return to the heart. They also have impaired vasoconstriction. This leads to pooling of the blood in the legs when the patient moves from a supine to a sitting position. If the movement is sudden, the patient can become dizzy or light-headed. Gradual elevation of the head, use of elastic stockings, and a reclining wheelchair help lessen this response.

Skin Breakdown

Patients or their caregivers must be diligent about relieving pressure on the skin by position changes and cushioning of bony prominences. It is important to realize that the patient may not be able to feel pain and, therefore, may not ask for position changes. Development of pressure injuries can lead to infection and loss of skin, muscle, or bone. Treatment of pressure injuries is time consuming and expensive and can interfere with work or school.

Renal Complications

Urinary tract infections are an ongoing concern for patients with spinal cord injuries. Caregivers as well as the patient need to be taught to observe the color, clarity, and odor of urine and to report changes promptly. Both urinary reflux and untreated urinary tract infections can cause permanent damage to the kidneys.

Depression and Substance Abuse

Patients with spinal cord injury have a higher than average incidence of depression and substance abuse. Both of these factors can interfere with the patient's ability to care for himself or herself. Individual or family counseling may be helpful. Some rehabilitation centers have support groups for patients with spinal cord injuries.

Autonomic Dysreflexia

This life-threatening complication occurs in patients with injuries above the T6 level. The spinal cord injury impairs the normal equilibrium between the sympathetic and parasympathetic divisions of the autonomic nervous system.

If a noxious stimulus below the spinal cord injury causes activation of the sympathetic system, it will continue unchecked because the parasympathetic responses cannot descend past the spinal cord injury.

The most common cause of autonomic **dysreflexia** is bladder distention. Other causes include bowel impaction, urinary tract infection, ingrown toenails, pressure injuries, pain, and labor in a pregnant woman. Stimulation of the sympathetic nervous system results in cool, pale skin, gooseflesh, and vasoconstriction below the level of the injury. Blood pressure can rise as high as 300 mm Hg systolic. The parasympathetic response results in vasodilation, causing flushing and diaphoresis above the lesion, and bradycardia as low as 30 beats per minute. The patient reports a pounding headache and nasal congestion secondary to the dilated blood vessels.

Care of the patient with autonomic dysreflexia is discussed in the care plan later in this section.

Diagnostic Tests

Plain radiographs are done to identify fractures or displacement of vertebrae. A CT scan is also useful for identifying fractures. MRI can demonstrate lesions within the cord.

Therapeutic Measures

Patients with spinal cord injuries typically are brought to the emergency department. They should be kept immobilized until they are assessed by an HCP. If injury to the spinal cord is detected, the patient needs to remain immobilized.

Emergency Management

Emergency management involves careful monitoring of vital signs and airway as well as keeping the patient immobilized. Intubation and mechanical ventilation may be necessary, especially with cervical spine injuries. IV normal saline may be used for fluid replacement and to provide an access site for medication administration. The physician does not rely on fluid administration alone to correct hypotension. It is possible to administer enough fluid to cause pulmonary edema and not correct the hypotension. Vasoactive drugs may be required. The use of various medications to reduce the extent of injury, including IV steroids, is routine. Often treatment is started by emergency medical services (EMS) personnel before arrival at the emergency department.

Respiratory Management

Patients with injuries above C4–C5 have some degree of respiratory impairment. The patient may require a tracheostomy and continuous mechanical ventilation or require a ventilator only at night or when fatigued. Some patients are able to breathe by using a phrenic nerve stimulator. This device, similar to a pacemaker, artificially stimulates the phrenic nerve, causing the diaphragm to contract. These patients use

• WORD • BUILDING •

dysreflexia: dys—abnormal + reflexia—reflex activity

a mechanical ventilator at night to lessen the stress on the phrenic nerve and remove the risk of the system failing while the patient is asleep.

Patients can be breathing independently when they first arrive in the emergency department and then experience respiratory compromise as the spinal cord becomes edematous. Edema can compress the spinal cord above the lesion, leading to symptoms at a higher level. This deterioration is usually temporary. Fatigue of the accessory muscles can also cause respiratory compromise. The intercostal muscles are not normally of major importance in respiration. However, if the diaphragm is paralyzed, the intercostal muscles become very important. As these muscles fatigue, the patient's breathing becomes shallow and rapid. Elective intubation and mechanical ventilation protect the patient from expending huge amounts of energy trying to breathe. Feeling their breathing becoming more labored is terrifying, and patients need to be reassured that it is probably a temporary setback. As the edema recedes and the accessory muscles become stronger, the patient may be weaned from the ventilator.

Gastrointestinal Management

Absence of bowel sounds is a common finding on examination. Oral or enteral feedings are not started until bowel function resumes. The metabolic needs of the patients are influenced by the work of breathing and the extent of other injuries. If oral or enteral feedings are not possible, parenteral nutrition is begun.

Genitourinary Management

An indwelling urinary catheter is placed to prevent bladder distention and protect skin integrity until spinal shock resolves. Once it is determined what degree of hand function the patient will have, a bladder management program is devised.

Immobilization

The cervical spine can be immobilized with skeletal traction such as Crutchfield or Gardner-Wells tongs (Fig. 48.12). Some patients have a halo brace, a device that attaches to the skull with four small pins. The skull ring attaches to a rigid plastic vest by four poles (Fig. 48.13). This device keeps the head and neck immobile while fusion and healing take place. The advantage over traction is that the patient is not confined to bed.

Surgical Management

The goal of surgery following spinal cord injury is to stabilize the bony elements of the spine and relieve pressure on the spinal cord. Surgery may or may not improve functional outcome. Stabilization of the spine allows for earlier mobilization of the patient. This decreases the risk of complications from immobility and speeds the transition to a rehabilitation setting. Patients who have been in cervical traction before surgery may be placed in a halo brace postoperatively.

Unstable thoracic and lumbar fractures may also be treated with surgical implantation of rods to stabilize the spine. It is more difficult to stabilize these areas in the postoperative recovery period. Patients may wear a supportive corset, a rigid brace, or occasionally a body cast to supplement the support provided by the internal fixation devices. For more information, visit the Spinal Cord Injury Model System Information Network at www.spinalcord.uab.edu.

Research is being conducted now with stem cells to help with nerve regeneration. Stem cells can be harvested and then processed in a laboratory before reinjection into the body. The goal is improvement in mobility and/or sensation.

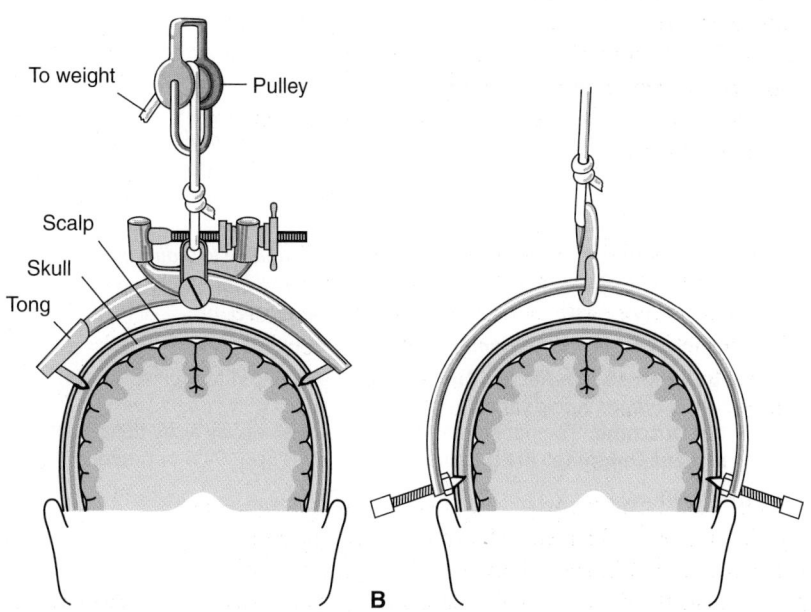

FIGURE 48.12 Skeletal traction for cervical injuries. (A) Crutchfield tongs. (B) Gardner-Wells tongs.

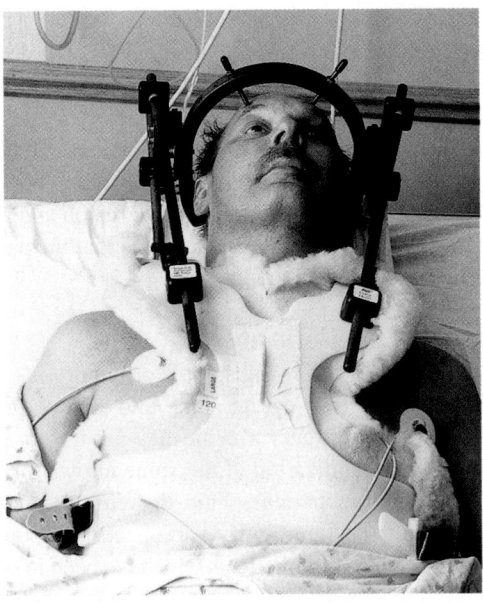

FIGURE 48.13 Halo brace.

Nursing Process for the Patient With a Spinal Cord Injury

Patients with spinal cord injury need ongoing evaluation of all body systems. Frequent neurologic and respiratory assessments are essential. Early assessment of the patient's support systems can help with discharge and rehabilitation planning. Initial goals for the patient include maintenance of safety and prevention of complications. Long-term goals include rehabilitation and maximizing remaining function.

See "Nursing Care Plan for the Patient With a Spinal Cord Injury," "Gerontological Issues," and Table 48.8.

Gerontological Issues

Aging With Spinal Cord Injury. Individuals aging with a spinal cord injury have an increased risk for developing complications in the following areas:

- Blood pressure control
- Abnormalities in carbohydrate and lipid metabolism related to immobilization
- Cardiovascular disease
- Respiratory complications
- Osteoporosis
- Bladder infections
- Skin injuries
- Chronic pain

Nursing Care Plan for the Patient With a Spinal Cord Injury

Nursing Diagnosis: *Impaired Gas Exchange* related to respiratory muscle weakness as evidenced by oxygen saturation (Spo_2) less than 90% and abnormal arterial blood gases (ABGs)
Expected Outcome: The patient will maintain oxygenation as evidenced by Spo_2 of 90% or greater, partial pressure of oxygen (Pao_2) of 75 mm Hg or greater, and partial pressure of carbon dioxide ($Paco_2$) of 45 mm Hg or less.
Evaluation of Outcome: Are ABGs and Spo_2 within acceptable limits?

Intervention	Rationale	Evaluation
Monitor respiratory rate, effort, ABGs, and Spo_2.	*These are indicators of respiratory function. Patient may have difficulty maintaining normal respiration if diaphragm or accessory muscles are weak related to injury.*	Are ABGs and Spo_2 within normal limits? Does patient appear distressed?
Notify health care provider (HCP) immediately if Spo_2 or Pao_2 drops, or if $Paco_2$ rises.	*If patient is unable to maintain normal blood gases, mechanical ventilation may be needed.*	Are changes recognized and reported promptly?

Nursing Diagnosis: *Ineffective Airway Clearance* related to ineffective cough and decreased muscle control as evidenced by adventitious breath sounds and Spo_2 less than 90%
Expected Outcome: The patient will maintain a clear airway as evidenced by clear breath sounds and Spo_2 of 90% or greater.
Evaluation of Outcome: Are breath sounds clear? Is Spo_2 90% or greater?

Intervention	Rationale	Evaluation
Monitor cough and lung sounds.	*Patient may not have adequate muscle strength to cough effectively.*	Is patient able to cough up secretions? Is there evidence that secretions are retained?

Nursing Care Plan for the Patient With a Spinal Cord Injury—cont'd

Intervention	Rationale	Evaluation
Suction patient as needed (prn) if unable to cough effectively.	*To keep the airway clear.*	Is suctioning effective in clearing airway?
Once patient is stable, try assisting him or her to cough to clear secretions. Gently push upward and inward on patient's chest while he or she coughs as strongly as possible.	*This can help patient clear secretions without invasive suctioning. This is similar to the Heimlich maneuver but not as forceful.*	Does the assisted cough technique help patient to clear the airway?
Provide humidified air and oral or enteral fluids.	*Humidification helps keep secretions thin and mobile.*	Are secretions thin and easily expectorated?

Nursing Diagnosis: *Risk for Autonomic Dysreflexia* related to stimuli below the level of injury
Expected Outcomes: The patient will not demonstrate signs of autonomic dysreflexia as evidenced by stable vital signs. If dysreflexia occurs, it is recognized and corrected promptly.
Evaluation of Outcomes: Is the patient free of signs, or are signs recognized and promptly treated?

Intervention	Rationale	Evaluation
Monitor for signs of autonomic dysreflexia (e.g., sudden high blood pressure, bradycardia, headache, pale skin below the injury, gooseflesh). Remember that patients with spinal cord injury are typically hypotensive, so a finding of even mild hypertension can represent a dramatic increase from their baseline blood pressure.	*Autonomic dysreflexia must be recognized quickly to remove cause and prevent complications such as seizures, intracerebral hemorrhage, or death.*	Are signs of autonomic dysreflexia present?
If you suspect autonomic dysreflexia, immediately take patient's blood pressure and continue to monitor it every 5 minutes.	*Blood pressure must be continually monitored until it is under control, to prevent complications.*	Is blood pressure higher than normal for patient? Are emergency interventions warranted?
Place patient in high-Fowler position. Remove elastic stockings or any other garment that could prevent blood from pooling in the periphery.	*High-Fowler position uses the effect of orthostasis to control blood pressure. Allowing blood to pool in the periphery can help reduce blood pressure.*	Does position change reduce blood pressure?
Evaluate the indwelling catheter for patency. If it is not patent or a catheter is not in place and the bladder is full, obtain an order to insert a catheter immediately. Monitor blood pressure during catheterization.	*A full bladder can be the cause of the stimuli causing the autonomic dysreflexia.*	Is catheter patent? Is bladder full? Does emptying bladder resolve autonomic dysreflexia?
Perform a rectal examination to determine whether an impaction is present. Apply anesthetic ointment to the rectum before disimpaction. Have another nurse monitor blood pressure, and stop disimpaction if the blood pressure increases.	*Fecal impaction can be the stimulus causing the autonomic dysreflexia. Anesthetic is used because further rectal stimulation can exacerbate symptoms.*	Is impaction present? Does removal resolve autonomic dysreflexia?

(nursing care plan continues on page 1032)

Nursing Care Plan for the Patient With a Spinal Cord Injury—cont'd

Intervention	Rationale	Evaluation
If bowel or bladder distention is not present, examine the patient for other causative mechanisms. If a cause cannot be identified or removal of the cause does not relieve hypertension, notify the HCP immediately.	*If the cause cannot be found and removed, an antihypertensive agent may be ordered.*	Are other causes identifiable? Is an antihypertensive agent ordered?
If hypertension is treated with medication, continue to carefully monitor blood pressure.	*Blood pressure can decrease rapidly once the cause of the autonomic dysreflexia is corrected.*	Is blood pressure stabilized?
Once the acute episode is past, work with patient and family members to devise a plan to prevent reoccurrence. Teach patient how to direct caregivers in treating autonomic dysreflexia.	*Episodes of autonomic dysreflexia can recur, and most can be prevented.*	Do patient and caregivers verbalize understanding of how to prevent and treat future episodes of autonomic dysreflexia?

Nursing Diagnosis: *Reflex Urinary Incontinence* related to spinal cord damage and no sensation to void as evidenced by inability to control flow of urine
Expected Outcomes: The patient's skin will be dry and free of urine; urine elimination will be controlled.
Evaluation of Outcomes: Is the patient clean and dry at all times?

Intervention	Rationale	Evaluation
Assess patient's ability to control urination.	*If patient has some control, a bladder training program may be effective.*	Is patient able to sense need to urinate? Is any degree of control present?
Implement a bladder training program, using set times for voiding.	*Following a voiding schedule can help reduce incontinence.*	Is patient able to avoid incontinence with regular voiding?
Use bladder ultrasound to scan bladder for residual urine.	*Incomplete voiding can increase risk for urinary tract infection.*	Is patient effectively emptying bladder?
Teach the patient or caregiver self-catheterization as ordered, if bladder training is not effective.	*Intermittent self-catheterization is associated with fewer complications than an indwelling catheter.*	Is patient able to perform self-catheterization correctly?
Monitor appearance of urine, temperature, and white blood cell count.	*Cloudy urine with an increase in temperature and white blood cell count indicates urinary tract infection.*	Is urine clear, and temperature and white blood cell count within normal limits?
Consult with HCP regarding indwelling Foley catheter if patient is not a candidate for intermittent self-catheterization.	*An indwelling catheter can increase risk for infection but may be necessary as a last resort for some patients.*	Is Foley catheter necessary? Are signs of infection avoided?

Nursing Diagnosis: *Constipation* related to immobility and nerve damage as evidenced by passage of hard, dry, or infrequent stools
Expected Outcome: The patient will return to preinjury bowel pattern.
Evaluation of Outcome: Does the patient pass soft stool at regular intervals?

Intervention	Rationale	Evaluation
Assess previous and current bowel pattern and continence.	*Decreased or absent sphincter tone, inability to detect the need to defecate, and immobility put patient at risk for incontinence and constipation.*	What was previous pattern? How can it be maintained for the patient?

Nursing Care Plan for the Patient With a Spinal Cord Injury—cont'd

Intervention	Rationale	Evaluation
Monitor bowel sounds and abdominal distention.	*These are indicators of bowel function.*	Are bowel sounds present? Is abdomen soft?
Institute a bowel management program as soon as oral feedings are resumed. Include a suppository on a scheduled daily or every-other-day basis as ordered.	*A management program including stool softeners and routine suppository use can help to restore regular defecation.*	Does management program keep bowel movements soft and regular and maintain continence?
If possible, have patient sit on a toilet or bedside commode to move bowels.	*Sitting allows gravity to help evacuate the bowel.*	Does sitting help patient move bowels?
Provide a high-fiber diet with adequate fluid intake.	*Fiber and fluids help keep stool soft.*	Is patient receiving adequate fiber and fluids?

Nursing Diagnosis: *Impaired Physical Mobility* related to hemorrhage, ischemia, and edema of cord as evidenced by paresis or paralysis
Expected Outcomes: The patient will maintain maximum mobility and be free from complications of immobility.
Evaluation of Outcomes: Is the patient kept mobile without contractures? Is skin intact? Can the patient complete activities of daily living (ADLs) with assistance?

Intervention	Rationale	Evaluation
Determine patient's ability to move independently.	*Assessment should guide interventions.*	What can patient do independently?
Assess patient's ability to feel pressure and pain.	*If patient is unable to feel pain or pressure, it will be even more important to monitor skin and prevent prolonged pressure.*	Can patient feel pressure and pain?
Reposition every 2 hours, using supportive devices.	*Unrelieved pressure on the skin, especially bony prominences, will result in ischemia and necrosis.*	Is skin intact without redness?
Change positions slowly; have patient sit at side of bed before standing (if able) or getting up to a chair.	*Patients with cervical spine injuries or patients remaining immobile for long periods are prone to orthostatic hypotension.*	Does patient become dizzy when getting up?
Perform active or passive range-of-motion (ROM) exercises at least once every 8 hours. If patient has arm mobility, teach patient to participate in doing as many ROM exercises as possible.	*ROM exercises maintain mobility and prevent contractures.*	Is patient able to perform ROM exercises with minimal difficulty?
Teach patient importance of repositioning self at least every 2 hours.	*Patients with some mobility can learn to reposition themselves; this helps prevent total dependence on caregivers.*	Does patient demonstrate correct repositioning every 2 hours?
Teach patient to direct own care, if unable to reposition independently.	*This allows patient some control over his or her situation.*	Does patient direct own care and prevent complications of immobility?

(nursing care plan continues on page 1034)

Nursing Care Plan for the Patient With a Spinal Cord Injury—cont'd

Nursing Diagnosis: *Self-Care Deficit (Dressing/Feeding/Toileting/Bathing)* related to paralysis
Expected Outcome: The patient's self-care needs will be met by self or caregivers.
Evaluation of Outcome: Are the patient's needs met? Does the patient verbalize satisfaction with care?

Intervention	Rationale	Evaluation
Determine patient's level of function and ability to perform ADLs.	*Patient should be encouraged to be as independent as possible.*	What is patient able to do? Is it incorporated into plan of care?
Explain rationale for nursing activities, and encourage patient and family members to participate in hands-on care as much as possible.	*This will help prepare the patient and family members to assume responsibility for care at home.*	Do patient and family members verbalize understanding of care? Are they able to demonstrate procedures correctly?
If patient will not be able to perform self-care, assist him or her to learn to direct care.	*This allows patient some control over his or her care.*	Does patient participate by directing care?
Consult with physical and occupational therapists.	*Physical and occupational therapists can help patient learn to adapt to physical limitations; they can provide a wheelchair or other mobility aids.*	Is patient adapting to limitations with help?
Discuss discharge to a rehabilitation facility with patient, HCP, and discharge planner.	*A rehabilitation facility can teach the patient to function independently. Some patients may require long-term care.*	Is patient a candidate for rehabilitation?
Assist patients and caregivers to determine contingency plans. These include what to do in the event of a power failure, fire, or illness of the caregiver.	*Planning ahead for what to do in an emergency can mean the difference between life and death for an immobile patient.*	Do patient and caregivers have a plan to keep the patient safe?
Encourage patient to establish a relationship with an HCP who is familiar with spinal cord injury.	*Patients with spinal cord injuries experience the same basic health care needs as individuals without injuries, in addition to unique needs related to the injury.*	Does patient have an HCP who understands his or her unique needs?

Nursing Diagnosis: *Risk for Impaired Skin Integrity* related to immobility and possible paresthesias
Expected Outcome: The patient's skin will remain intact without redness or breakdown.
Evaluation of Outcome: Is the patient's skin intact?

Intervention	Rationale	Evaluation
Monitor skin frequently. When permitted by the HCP, turn patient frequently and assess bony prominences for redness.	*The patient who does not have sensation is at increased risk of developing pressure injuries.*	Is patient turned and repositioned at least every 2 hours? Is skin intact?
Start preventive measures in the emergency department by being sure to remove anything between patient and the backboard.	*Patients have developed pressure injuries from lying on keys or other objects in their pockets.*	Are skin surfaces protected from pressure?
Use a pressure-reducing mattress.	*Specialty mattresses or beds can reduce pressure but do not reduce the need to turn the patient.*	Is patient on an appropriate mattress?

Nursing Care Plan for the Patient With a Spinal Cord Injury—cont'd

Intervention	Rationale	Evaluation
If on a self-turning bed, make sure patient is not sliding as the bed turns. Avoid pulling and friction on skin when repositioning patient in bed.	*Sliding can cause friction and shearing damage to the skin.*	Is friction damage to skin avoided?
Ensure that patient's extremities do not get caught in side rails or wheelchair spokes.	*Patient may not be aware this is happening, and a pressure injury can result.*	Are all patient's body parts accounted for and safe?
If patient is in skeletal traction or a halo brace, assess pin sites frequently. Keep the sites clean and dry, and report any sign of infection.	*Skin sites are at risk for infection and breakdown.*	Are pin sites clean and dry?
Monitor temperature of bath water (no more than 102°F).	*Patient may not be able to feel burning if water is too hot.*	Are burns prevented?

Nursing Diagnosis: *Ineffective Role Performance* related to effects of injury
Expected Outcome: The patient will identify new ways to carry out essential roles.
Evaluation of Outcome: Is the patient able to identify ways to carry out roles?

Intervention	Rationale	Evaluation
Allow patient to verbalize concerns about his or her roles if desired.	*This can help to clarify potential role problems for the patient and begin the process of developing a plan.*	Is patient able to identify roles he or she has filled in the past that will be difficult to carry out due to injury?
Help patient and family members to identify resources.	*Interpersonal relationships can be significantly stressed by spinal cord injury. Friends, family members, and members of the patient's religious affiliation can provide emotional and physical help.*	Does patient have adequate support systems in place to provide help?
Consult a social worker to help the patient gain access to appropriate physical and financial assistance.	*Loss of income can be temporary or permanent and can add to the burden of spinal cord injury. Not all insurance policies cover the extensive inpatient rehabilitation needed by patients with spinal cord injuries. Adaptive equipment is expensive and may not be covered by insurance.*	Is patient able to access appropriate financial assistance if needed?
Provide information about area support groups.	*Individuals who have been through similar experiences can provide support and information for the patient and family.*	Is patient willing to contact support groups?

(nursing care plan continues on page 1036)

Nursing Care Plan for the Patient With a Spinal Cord Injury—cont'd

Nursing Diagnosis: *Risk for Sexual Dysfunction* related to autonomic nervous system dysfunction
Expected Outcome: The patient will state he or she has an acceptable means for sexual expression.
Evaluation of Outcome: Does the patient state satisfaction with sexual function?

Intervention	Rationale	Evaluation
If a male patient has an erection during a bath or catheterization, discontinue the procedure and continue at a later time if possible. Maintain a matter-of-fact attitude.	*Male patients with quadriplegia may develop an erection during any penile stimulation.*	Is patient's dignity maintained during personal care?
Allow patient to voice concerns about sexual function if desired.	*Male patients with paraplegia can have difficulty achieving and maintaining an erection.*	Is patient able to voice concerns? Is a consult with a urologist or other specialist needed?
Encourage patient and his or her partner to explore alternative methods of sexual expression.	*Closeness and touching may be a satisfying alternative.*	Is patient able to discuss alternative methods with his or her partner?
If a male patient wishes to have children, encourage a consult with a fertility specialist or urologist.	*Men with spinal cord injuries may not ejaculate in the normal manner. A specialist can provide some help for conception if desired.*	Is patient given information about conception if desired?

Nursing Diagnosis: *Anxiety* related to change in health status as evidenced by behavioral changes such as insomnia, poor eye contact, and irritability
Expected Outcomes: The patient will participate in rehabilitation activities. The patient will be able to verbalize fears, concerns, and expectations.
Evaluation of Outcomes: Is the patient able to participate in rehabilitation? Does the patient verbalize that anxiety is controlled?

Intervention	Rationale	Evaluation
Allow patient to voice feelings of fear and anxiety.	*Communication is vital to assess patient's coping abilities.*	Is patient able to verbalize anxiety?
Provide information about what is happening to the patient physiologically and about procedures.	*Understanding of what is happening can help the patient cope with changes.*	Does patient verbalize understanding of what is happening? Does information help keep patient less fearful?
Consult a social worker, pastoral care, and/or support groups.	*A social worker or pastor can help provide emotional and spiritual support. Discussing rehabilitation with patients and family members who have had similar experiences can provide insight and encouragement.*	Does patient state talking with support persons helps reduce anxiety?
Encourage patient to participate in physical and occupational therapy.	*Seeing progress toward becoming independent can help reduce anxiety and fear about the future.*	Does patient participate in therapies? Is anxiety lessening?

Table 48.8
Spinal Cord Injury Summary

Signs and Symptoms	Paralysis and paresthesias (depending on level of the lesion) Loss of reflex activity below the level of the lesion Spinal shock initially Risk for autonomic dysreflexia (injuries above sixth thoracic vertebra)
Diagnostic Tests	Radiograph Computed tomography (CT) scan Magnetic resonance imaging (MRI)
Therapeutic Measures	Immobilization Maintenance of airway and respiratory status Bowel and bladder training Nutrition/diet Activity/rehabilitation Prevention of dysreflexia Prevention of skin breakdown Sexual counseling Education
Complications	Infection Deep vein thrombosis Paralysis Orthostatic hypotension Pressure injuries Depression
Priority Nursing Diagnoses	*Impaired Gas Exchange* *Ineffective Airway Clearance* *Risk for Autonomic Dysreflexia* *Reflex Urinary Incontinence* *Constipation* *Impaired Physical Mobility* *Self-Care Deficit (Dressing/Feeding/Toileting/Bathing)* *Risk for Impaired Skin Integrity* *Ineffective Role Performance* *Risk for Sexual Dysfunction* *Anxiety*

NEURODEGENERATIVE AND NEUROCOGNITIVE DISORDERS

Neurodegenerative is a term that can apply to any nervous system disorder that causes degeneration, or wasting, of the neurons in the nervous system. The disorders discussed in this section are some of the most common neurodegenerative disorders. *Neurocognitive* is the term used to describe acquired neurologic disorders that cause cognitive decline. Management of chronic conditions does not focus on the short-term stay in the hospital as a result of an exacerbation of the disease process but rather on the long-term goal of helping the patient and family to cope with the disease process and to maintain the patient's independence for as long as possible. Nursing care involves providing information on management of the illness, prevention and treatment of complications, and referrals to support groups or case managers. As patients decline, there will come a time when family members can no longer care for their loved one in their homes and must consider care in a long-term care facility.

Dementia

Dementia is not a disease but rather a symptom of a number of neurocognitive disorders. According to the National Institute of Neurological Disorders and Stroke (2017), patients with dementia have "significantly impaired intellectual functioning that interferes with normal activities and relationships. They also lose their ability to solve problems and maintain emotional control, and they may experience personality changes and behavioral problems, such as agitation, delusions, and hallucinations. While memory loss is a common symptom of dementia, memory loss by itself does not mean that a person has dementia." Some patients can have mild mental status changes that do not interfere significantly with day-to-day functioning. This is sometimes referred to as mild cognitive impairment (MCI). However, patients with MCI are more likely to go on to develop Alzheimer disease than those without MCI.

Etiology and Pathophysiology

There are many causes of dementia, including Parkinson, Huntington, and Alzheimer diseases, which are discussed later in this chapter. Multiple "mini-strokes" (multi-infarct dementia or vascular dementia) are another common cause. Chronic alcoholism, neurologic infections, head injuries, and many medications (Box 48.2) also can cause changes in mental status, leading to dementia. Although aging is associated with more frequent dementia diagnoses, dementia is not a normal part of aging. In general, thinking is affected by changes in the brain that result from reduced blood flow or from structural changes related to disease states.

Much research has been done to determine factors related to dementia and its prevention. Some studies indicate that patients who have more education, have higher socioeconomic status, and engage in stimulating intellectual and leisure activities are less likely to develop dementia. Some experts believe these individuals develop a sort of cognitive reserve that keeps them functioning at a high level, even when changes in their brains

• WORD • BUILDING •

neurodegenerative: neuro—nervous system + degenerative—deteriorating

dementia: de—down or from + mentia—the mind

on autopsy indicate dementia. People with less education, fewer leisure activities, and less intellectual stimulation are more likely to develop symptoms of Alzheimer disease.

Signs and Symptoms

Have you ever forgotten something important? Most people have occasional memory lapses, but they do not typically have dementia. In patients with dementia, recent memories are usually affected first. Patients may have difficulty recalling whether they ate breakfast or may accuse a family member of not calling when in reality they called just a few hours earlier. This same patient, however, may easily recall an event or a phone number from childhood.

As patients become more forgetful, they may ask the same questions repeatedly. They can get lost driving or walking in a familiar neighborhood. They can become disoriented to time and not be aware of the year. Patients might say that Eisenhower is president, for example, because they remember that as true when they were younger. As the disease progresses, they may not recognize where they are, and, eventually, they can lose recognition of even their own family members.

Later in the course of the dementia, remote memory can be lost. Patients can forget how to perform simple tasks, such as doing the dishes or making a phone call. They may wander and become lost. Safety is a significant issue with a wandering patient; patients have been found wandering in their nightclothes in the middle of a road, unaware of what they are doing. Patients can develop aphasia and become unable to communicate their needs or follow simple instructions. This can become frustrating to both the family and nursing caregivers. Behavioral problems may necessitate admission to a long-term care facility. In very late stages, the patient becomes totally dependent on caregivers.

Diagnostic Tests

Diagnosis of dementia is twofold. First, dementia must be identified; then the focus moves to finding the cause of the mental status change. Early diagnosis is essential, because some causes of MCI may be reversible, and early treatment may

delay progression. Neuropsychological testing can determine the degree of memory, personality, and behavior change. The patient should also be tested for depression, which can cause mental status changes but is often easily treated. A review of medications by a knowledgeable nurse, HCP, or pharmacist may reveal a medication that is contributing to the mental changes. MRI, CT scan, positron emission tomography (PET) scan, and blood tests help diagnose underlying causes.

Therapeutic Measures

Medical interventions depend on the cause of the dementia. Table 48.9 lists medications that can be used to delay progression of Alzheimer-related dementia. If medical treatment cannot alter the course of the disease, the focus will shift to delaying progression of symptoms and maintaining patient safety. Excellent nursing care becomes essential for both the patient and family at this point. An important aspect of care in early dementia is determination of the patient's wishes while the patient is still able to make decisions. Some difficult decisions relate to the patient's continued ability to drive and live alone. Other decisions related to resuscitation, guardianship, and powers of attorney for health care and finances are essential to discuss.

Nursing Process for the Patient With Dementia

See "Nursing Care Plan for the Patient With Dementia."

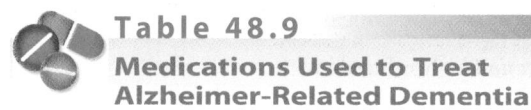

Table 48.9

Medications Used to Treat Alzheimer-Related Dementia

Medication Class/Action

Cholinesterase Inhibitors	
Inhibit cholinesterase, to improve function of acetylcholine in the central nervous system. May improve cognitive function but will not alter course of disease.	
Examples	**Nursing Implications**
donepezil (Aricept) tacrine (Cognex) rivastigmine (Exelon) galantamine (Reminyl)	Must be taken regularly; patient may need reminders to take, or family member may need to assist. Monitor for weight loss and report to health care provider.

N-Methyl-D-Aspartate (NMDA) Antagonist	
Reduces binding of glutamate, an excitatory neurotransmitter.	
Examples	**Nursing Implications**
memantine (Namenda, Namenda XR, Axura)	Teach patient and family that improvements may take months.

Nursing Care for the Patient With Dementia

Nursing Diagnosis: *Risk for Injury* related to impaired memory, thought processes, and judgment
Expected Outcome: The patient will remain free from injury.
Evaluation of Outcome: Is the patient safe and free from injury? Is environment safe?

Intervention	Rationale	Evaluation
Monitor patient's ability to maintain safety.	*As dementia worsens, the patient's needs will change.*	Is patient able to make decisions and negotiate the environment safely?
Keep environment simple and familiar; label doors and objects. Keep patient in familiar environment as long as possible.	*Change can result in confusion; even a minor change in furniture arrangement can result in falls.*	Is patient able to remain in the home with minimum confusion and without injury?
Remove harmful objects (e.g., scissors, matches); store medicines in a locked cabinet; remove knobs from stoves.	*Impaired judgment can make safety a major concern for patients who live at home.*	Is the environment safe for the patient?
Make sure patient has eyeglasses and hearing aids if necessary.	*Impaired sensory perception can increase confusion and risk for falls.*	Is patient able to see and hear effectively?
Use nightlights; remove throw rugs; use safety gates on stairs.	*These can reduce the risk for falls.*	Is environment set up to reduce risk for falling?
Have identification bracelet on patient and identification tags sewn into clothes; put locks on doors to prevent patient from leaving.	*Patients can wander, making them prone to injury.*	Is wandering confined to a monitored area? Is environment set up to allow movement within a safe area?
Provide daily walks or exercise.	*Exercise can decrease wandering.*	Does exercise reduce wandering?

Nursing Diagnosis: *Imbalanced Nutrition: Less Than Body Requirements* related to impaired thought processes and lack of interest in eating or refusal to eat
Expected Outcomes: The patient will maintain adequate food intake and weight within normal limits for height.
Evaluation of Outcomes: Does the patient maintain appropriate weight?

Intervention	Rationale	Evaluation
Monitor intake and weight.	*Loss of weight may indicate poor nutrition.*	Is weight stable and within normal limits?
Develop meal plan to include patient preferences, snacks, and supplements, as necessary.	*Using patient's favorite foods will encourage eating.*	Is patient consuming an adequate amount?
Offer larger meal when patient has the greatest appetite or serve small meals five to six times a day.	*A lot of food at one time can feel overwhelming to the patient.*	Is patient eating meals that are served?
Offer one food at a time if patient is not successful with a whole plate full.	*Too many choices on a plate can feel overwhelming to the patient.*	Does patient eat more if only one food at a time is offered?
Offer finger foods.	*Utensils can be difficult for patient to use and can discourage eating.*	Does patient eat more when finger foods are offered? (See "Nutrition Notes.")

(nursing care plan continues on page 1040)

Nursing Care for the Patient With Dementia—cont'd

Nursing Diagnosis: *Chronic Confusion* related to dementia
Expected Outcome: The patient will function at optimal cognitive level.
Evaluation of Outcome: Is the patient maintaining optimum cognitive function?

Intervention	Rationale	Evaluation
Monitor changes in thought processes.	*As cognitive function declines, care plan will need to be revised.*	Is patient able to correctly identify objects, remember tasks, speak clearly, and identify person, place, and time?
Provide a box of safe, familiar items, such as empty thread spools or pretty handkerchiefs for women.	*Patients often rummage through drawers, closets, or boxes. Patients may not recognize the difference between their own possessions and those of others. Keeping them occupied with a box of safe items may decrease their need to look for things.*	Does a box of items keep patient occupied and content?
Place calendars, clocks, personal items, and seasonal decorations in patient's environment.	*These provide orientation to the present.*	Can patient identify the season or year?
If patient hallucinates or has delusions, do not attempt to correct. Focus instead on the feelings related to the hallucinations, such as "Do you feel frightened?"	*Having feelings validated can help develop trust while not validating the hallucination.*	Does patient respond to refocusing on feelings?
Reduce stressors such as fatigue, overstimulation, or pain.	*Stress may increase dysfunctional behaviors.*	Are stressors eliminated as much as possible? Is patient's behavior calm?
Maintain patient's usual routines as much as possible.	*Familiar routines of activities, sleeping, and eating are more comfortable for patients. Change can be stressful.*	Are routines organized around patient rather than the staff?
Communicate clearly. Make eye contact, speak slowly and directly to the patient, and use nonverbal gestures. Use a tone of voice conveying respect and sincerity.	*Unclear communication can increase confusion and stress. Tone of voice plays a role in the ability of the patient to cooperate.*	Do all staff members communicate clearly and respectfully with the patient?
Involve family in care planning and implementation.	*The family knows the patient's preferences and routines best.*	Does family presence help patient stay calm and function at optimum level?
Provide video or audiotapes of patient's family members.	*Familiar sounds and pictures can reduce agitation when family is not present.*	Do video or audiotapes help calm the patient?

Nursing Diagnosis: *Risk for Caregiver Role Strain* related to demands of caring for patient with declining mental status while balancing other demands
Expected Outcomes: The caregiver will have the support needed to safely manage care of the patient. The caregiver will be able to identify when the patient is too difficult to care for and requires more structured care.
Evaluation of Outcomes: Is the caregiver managing demands of caring for the patient? Is the patient safe? Is additional support or a change in environment for the patient indicated?

Intervention	Rationale	Evaluation
Allow caregiver to verbalize concerns related to burden of caring for patient.	*An assessment of caregiver concerns and challenges can help the nurse plan appropriate support.*	Does caregiver share concerns? What are caregiver's current support systems?

Nursing Care for the Patient With Dementia—cont'd

Intervention	Rationale	Evaluation
Observe for signs of depression or stress in the caregiver.	*A stressed or depressed caregiver may have difficulty providing safe care for the patient.*	Are signs of stress present? Does patient care appear to be suffering?
Encourage caregiver to identify family and friends that can provide support. If involved in a local church or religious organization, encourage caregiver to make his or her needs known.	*There are often resources in the family or community that can be accessed without cost and can help if they know the need exists.*	Can caregiver identify potential resources to contact?
Refer for assistance with caregiving and/or day care utilizing Alzheimer support groups and resources.	*Formal support systems in the community may be available to help relieve some of the caregiver's burden.*	Is caregiver able to obtain support and take some time for himself or herself?
Encourage caregiver to use support systems identified to allow him or her time to care for self; encourage him or her to take care of own health needs, and enjoy some respite time doing something enjoyable on a regular basis.	*If the caregiver becomes ill due to the stress of caregiving, he or she will no longer be able to assist the patient.*	Does caregiver maintain own physical and emotional health?
Allow the caregiver to grieve over the losses he or she is experiencing— losses in the patient as well as loss of control over his or her own life.	*As the disease progresses, the patient gradually loses awareness of the neurologic deterioration. Occasional lucid moments can be very difficult for patient and caregiver as they realize what has been lost.*	Is the caregiver able to identify feelings of grief, anger, or sorrow?
Discuss progression of the disease process and the possibility of transferring patient to a long-term care facility.	*The caregiver may feel guilt over not being able to care for the patient and may need permission to consider placement at long-term care facility.*	Is caregiver able to identify when home care is too demanding, and choose an alternative arrangement?

Delirium

Whereas dementia is chronic and progressive, **delirium** is a mental disturbance that is temporary. It can have either a rapid or gradual onset. Delirium is considered to be a medical emergency and should be diagnosed and treated promptly. Delirium is characterized by disorganized thinking and difficulty staying focused. It is seen most commonly in older adults when experiencing stress or illness. Patients who are severely ill or who have a history of hypertension, alcoholism, or pre-existing dementia are most at risk. In many cases, response to medications is the cause (see Box 48-2). The disturbance can also be the result of anything that is a stressor to the person's body, such as pain, oxygen deficiency, urinary catheters, fluid and electrolyte imbalances, a change in environment, or nutritional deficiency. Often, the most effective nursing intervention is to have a family member present to assist with orientation and reassurance. It is beneficial to have continuity in nursing personnel when possible.

Nutrition Notes

Nutrition Issues in Dementia. The World Health Organization (WHO, 2017) estimates that 47 million people have dementia worldwide, and that figure is expected to grow to 75 million by 2030. However, there are some studies that have shown a decrease in the prevalence of dementia, which is thought to be related to increased cardiac health (American Speech-Language-Hearing Association, 2017). The immediate problem may be providing the patient with sufficient nutrients to prevent malnutrition and dehydration. Brain atrophy, changes in the sense of smell, and high levels of pro-inflammatory cytokines may negatively impact appetite and eating behaviors. Problems frequently seen in in early- to late-stage dementia patients include difficulty with grocery shopping, meal preparation, eating regularly, recognizing foods, remembering how to eat and drink independently, and wandering and pacing, which burns excessive calories. Vitamin deficiencies, such as B_6 and B_{12}, and dysphagia are also concerns (Hillard, 2013; Volkert et al., 2015).

Patients should be monitored for weight loss and dehydration as well as nutrient deficiency. However, supplements should not be given unless there is evidence of deficiencies. Meal times should be routine and in a quiet area with supervision or assistance provided by the same individual whenever possible. Changes in food textures may be necessary with diagnosed dysphagia to prevent aspiration. Oral liquid supplements may be required to improve nutritional status, as tolerated by patient, but feeding tubes are not recommended (Hillard, 2013; Volkert et al., 2015).

References

American Speech-Language-Hearing Association. (2017). Dementia: Incidence and prevalence. Retrieved from www.asha.org/PRPSpecificTopic.aspx?folderid=8589935289&section=Incidence_and_Prevalence

Hillard, L. (2013). Caring for dementia patients. *Today's Dietitian, 15*(8), 16.

Volkert, D., Chourdakis, M., Faxen-Irvin, G, Fruhwald, T., Landi, F., Suominen, M. H., … Schneider, S. M. (2015). ESPEN guidelines on nutrition in dementia. *Clinical Nutrition, 34*(6), 1052–1073.

World Health Organization. (2017). 10 facts on dementia. Retrieved from www.who.int/features/factfiles/dementia/en

Evidence Based Practice

Clinical Question

How can delirium be managed in the acute care setting?

Evidence

Delirium is associated with increased mortality in the intensive care unit (ICU) setting, prolonged hospital stays, and higher incidence of confusion following an ICU stay. Arumugam and colleagues (2017) reviewed 46 articles to develop guidelines for recognition and management of delirium. Early identification of risk factors, screening for delirium, and implementation of nondrug interventions are important nursing interventions in all settings and can help prevent the need for antipsychotic medications.

Implications for Nursing Practice

(1) Recognize risk factors such as older age, alcohol abuse, dementia, respiratory disorders, and certain medications. (2) Assess patients using a valid delirium scale. (3) Ensure that patients are using their eyeglasses and hearing aids. (4) Mobilize patients and begin physical therapy as soon as possible. (5) Reduce environmental noise and prevent sleep deprivation. (6) Avoid use of restraints whenever possible.

Reference

Arumugam, S., El-Menyar, A., Al-Hassani, A., Strandvik, G., Asim, M., Mekkodithal, A., … Al-Thani, H. (2017). Delirium in the intensive care unit. *Journal of Emergencies, Trauma, and Shock, 10*(1), 37–46. Retrieved from http://doi.org/10.4103/0974-2700.199520

NURSING CARE TIP

Patients with delirium or dementia must be kept safe, and interventions are similar for both. One important difference, however, is in how you respond to confusion. If a patient is experiencing delirium, reorient him or her to the present time and situation. If a patient with dementia is chronically confused, however, reorientation may not be effective. In this case, validate their feelings. An example would be comforting a patient who is calling for a long-lost parent rather than reminding the patient the mother has been gone for 30 years.

It is essential that delirium not be mistaken for dementia. If an older adult is hospitalized and exhibits new-onset confusion, consider that it might be delirium. Correcting electrolyte levels, controlling pain, changing medications, or administering oxygen can be helpful in reversing delirium. See "Nursing Care Plan for the Patient With Dementia" for nursing interventions.

Parkinson Disease

Parkinson disease is a chronic degenerative movement disorder that arises in the basal ganglia in the cerebrum. Parkinson disease has typically been considered a disease of older adults; however, there are many people with young-onset Parkinson disease. An example is Michael J. Fox (actor and founder of the Michael J. Fox Foundation for Parkinson's Research), who was diagnosed at age 30. The disease is characterized by tremors, changes in posture and gait, rigidity, and slowness of movements. Approximately 60,000 new cases of Parkinson disease are diagnosed each year in the United States; it ranks 14th in causes of death according to the CDC (Parkinson's Foundation, 2017).

Pathophysiology

The substantia nigra is a group of cells located within the basal ganglia, which is situated deep in the brain. These cells are responsible for the production of dopamine, an inhibitory neurotransmitter. Dopamine facilitates the transmission of impulses from one neuron to another. Parkinson disease is caused by destruction of the cells of the substantia nigra, resulting in decreased dopamine production. Loss of dopamine function results in impairment of semiautomatic movements. Parkinson disease is sometimes referred to as an extrapyramidal disorder because the extrapyramidal tracts in the spinal cord that contain motor neurons are affected.

Acetylcholine, an excitatory neurotransmitter, is secreted normally in individuals with Parkinson disease. The normal balance of acetylcholine and dopamine is interrupted in these patients, causing a relative excess of acetylcholine. This results in the tremor, muscle rigidity, and **akinesia** (loss of muscle movement) characteristic of Parkinson disease.

Etiology

The etiology of Parkinson disease is unknown. It was first described in 1817 by London surgeon James Parkinson. Although scientists now know that the symptoms are caused by death of dopamine-producing cells in the substantia nigra, they do not know what causes the cells to die. There may be a genetic component, especially in younger patients. Certain environmental toxins can also play a role. Parkinson disease-like symptoms, referred to as *parkinsonism*, can be associated with use of certain drugs, such as phenothiazines. Parkinsonism was also linked to an outbreak of encephalitis in the 1920s.

Signs and Symptoms

The onset of symptoms in patients with Parkinson disease is usually gradual and subtle. A substantial percentage of the dopamine-producing cells are nonfunctional before the patient becomes symptomatic. Symptoms may be mistakenly attributed to aging or fatigue. In retrospect, patients and their family members often identify a long period in which symptoms were present but not identified as symptoms of Parkinson disease.

The primary symptoms of Parkinson disease are muscular rigidity, **bradykinesia** (slow movement) or akinesia, changes in posture, and tremors. The brain is no longer able to direct the muscles to perform in the usual manner. This lack of communication between the brain and muscles can have a profound impact on the patient's ability to ambulate safely, perform ADLs and job functions, or enjoy leisure activities. The symptoms may also have a significant negative impact on the patient's self-esteem.

The patient may have difficulty initiating movement; this can be particularly apparent when the patient tries to start walking, rise from a sitting position, or begin dressing. Because considerable effort is required to move the rigid muscles, the patient performs voluntary movements very slowly. At times, the patient can experience freezing of gait and be unable to initiate ambulation or negotiate a turn during ambulation.

The extensor muscles are more affected by Parkinson disease than the flexor muscles. This impaired function of the extensor muscles results in the stooped posture typical of patients with Parkinson disease (Fig. 48.14). Flexion of the hips, knees, and neck shifts the center of gravity forward. The gait is characterized by short, shuffling steps that may increase in speed once the patient finally starts walking. Once in motion, the patient may have difficulty stopping. The patient maintains a broad base when making turns to try to compensate for imbalance. These changes place patients at high risk for falls. Slowness of movement and stiff muscles make it much harder for patients to catch themselves if they start to fall or to relax the muscles to minimize injury.

Tremors typically begin in the hand and then progress to the **ipsilateral** foot. In most patients, the tremor then moves

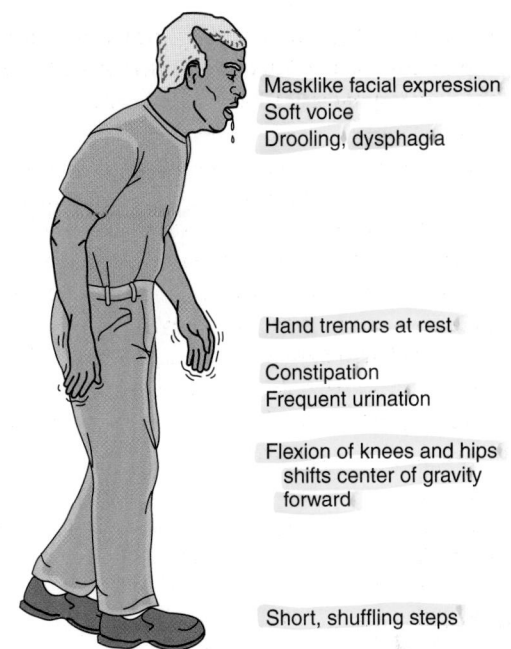

FIGURE 48.14 Manifestations of Parkinson disease.

Masklike facial expression
Soft voice
Drooling, dysphagia

Hand tremors at rest

Constipation
Frequent urination

Flexion of knees and hips shifts center of gravity forward

Short, shuffling steps

to the **contralateral** side. Many patients identify one side of the body as being more affected by the tremor than the other. Tremor of the hand has been described as a pill-rolling tremor; the thumb typically moves back and forth across the fingers and looks like the patient is rolling a pill. Tremors typically lessen or disappear during movement and are more noticeable when the extremity is at rest or when trying to hold an object still (this is called a resting tremor). The tremors disappear when the patient is asleep. The inability to hold an object still can make simple acts such as drinking a glass of water or reading a book nearly impossible. The signs and symptoms of Parkinson disease tend to increase in severity when the patient becomes fatigued. Another type of tremor, a benign familial (or essential) tremor, can sometimes be mistaken for Parkinson disease. Treatment is different for each. Table 48.10 details differentiation of these tremors.

The secondary symptoms of Parkinson disease include generalized weakness, muscle fatigue and cramping, and difficulty with fine motor activities. This fine motor dysfunction can make it difficult for the patient to button a shirt or tie shoes. Handwriting typically deteriorates as the disease progresses. A soft, monotone voice and masklike facial expression can make the patient appear to be lacking in emotional responses. It may be necessary to ask patients about their emotional status and help them develop ways to express their emotions. The normal blink response is diminished, so

• WORD • BUILDING •
akinesia: a—not + kinesia—movement
bradykinesia: brady—slow + kinesia—movement
ipsilateral: ipsi—same + lateral—side
contralateral: contra—opposite + lateral—side

Table 48.10

Symptoms of Parkinson Disease Tremor vs. Essential Tremor

Disease	Parkinson Tremor	Benign Familial (Essential) Tremor
Resting tremor	Yes	No
Intention tremor (with movement)	No	Yes
Pill-rolling tremor	Yes	No
Head/voice tremor	No	Yes
Relieved with beta-blocking medication (propranolol)	No	Yes
Relieved with anti-Parkinson medications	Yes	No

the patient and significant others must be educated about eye care to prevent corneal abrasions.

Dysfunction of the autonomic system can cause diaphoresis, constipation, orthostatic hypotension, drooling, dysphagia, seborrhea, and frequent urination. Patients who experience seborrhea and diaphoresis need frequent attention to personal hygiene. Drooling and dysphagia can make the patient reluctant to appear in public. Slowness in initiating walking, balance problems, and frequent urination place the patient at risk for urinary incontinence, which can also increase the patient's reluctance to leave home.

Late in the disease, mental function may become slowed, and the patient may develop dementia. This is compounded by the side effects of many anti-Parkinson drugs. Death is usually from complications of immobility.

Complications

The most typical acute complications of Parkinson disease are related to the patient's difficulties with mobility and balance. Patients are prone to falls, which can result in injuries ranging from bruises or fractures to head or spinal cord injuries. Constipation is common because of decreased activity, diminished ability to take in food and fluids, and side effects of anticholinergic medications. Patients are encouraged to increase fiber and fluids in their diets. If constipation is not alleviated by dietary modifications, the patient may need to use stool softeners.

Muscular rigidity and bradykinesia contribute to joint immobility, which decreases patients' ability to ambulate and care for themselves. Position changes can be painful for patients. A turning sheet and adequate personnel are necessary when turning a patient in bed to prevent stress on the joints. Tremors interfere with ADLs, consume immense amounts of energy, and can prevent the patient from working or performing leisure activities. Swallowing can become so impaired that enteral (tube) feeding is required. Depression is a common complication at any stage of Parkinson disease and may compromise communication, ability to learn, and performance of ADLs. Patients may require counseling or antidepressants.

Diagnostic Tests

No specific tests are used to diagnose Parkinson disease. The diagnosis is based on the history given by the patient and a thorough physical examination. MRI may be done to rule out alternative causes of the patient's symptoms.

Therapeutic Measures

There is no cure for Parkinson disease. Treatment is aimed at controlling symptoms and maximizing the patient's functional level. Drugs used to control symptoms are listed in Table 48.11.

Many patients with Parkinson disease experience fluctuations in motor function related to their drug therapy. This is referred to as the "on–off phenomenon." Patients may experience a decreased response to levodopa, or off period, particularly as the dose is wearing off. As the disease progresses, patients may notice that the off periods become less predictable and occur more rapidly. The patient may have a delayed or absent response to the next dose of levodopa, resulting in the patient being stuck in the off stage and being significantly disabled for that period. Fluctuations in motor function can be accompanied by other symptoms, such as pain, diaphoresis, anxiety attacks, hallucinations, or mood swings. These symptoms significantly increase the disability associated with the episodes.

Patients who are taking maximum doses of medication for Parkinson disease symptoms may benefit from a "drug holiday." During a drug holiday, patients are taken off all drugs for a time and then restarted on lower doses. Hospitalization may be necessary during this time to maintain patient safety.

Surgical Treatments

Pallidotomy may be an option for patients whose rigidity, tremor, and bradykinesia are uncontrollable by medical management. During this stereotactic procedure, a destructive lesion is created in the basal ganglia. The surgery is only performed on one side of the brain. The patient remains awake during the surgery to make sure that the lesion is being placed in the appropriate location. These patients need a great deal of education and support before and during the surgery.

Deep-brain stimulation is another surgical treatment, in which a tiny electrode is placed into brain tissue. A generator is then implanted under the skin on the chest and is connected to the electrode. The generator delivers electrical pulses to the electrode, which may help control symptoms.

Some researchers have experimented with implanting stem cells into the brain to develop into dopamine-producing cells; research into gene therapies is also ongoing. These

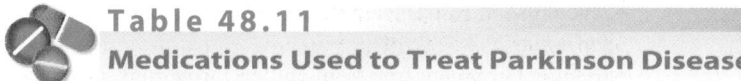

Table 48.11
Medications Used to Treat Parkinson Disease

Medication Class/Action

Dopamine Agonists

Convert into dopamine in the brain.

Examples	**Nursing Implications**
levodopa (L-dopa)	*Teach:*
levodopa/carbidopa combination (Sinemet): Carbidopa prevents peripheral breakdown of levodopa so more is available in the central nervous system (CNS).	Take food shortly after (not before or with) each dose to prevent gastric irritation.
	May discolor urine and sweat.
	Take around the clock to control symptoms.

Dopamine Agonists

Stimulate dopamine receptors in the brain.

Examples	**Nursing Implications**
pramipexole (Mirapex)	Giving with meals may reduce nausea.
ropinirole (Requip)	Caution about drowsiness and sleep attacks (falling asleep during activities that require alertness, including driving).

Monoamine Oxidase B (MAO-B) Inhibitor

Blocks metabolism of central dopamine, increasing dopamine in CNS.

Examples	**Nursing Implications**
selegiline (Eldepryl, Zelapar)	Can slow progression of Parkinson disease.
rasagiline (Azilect)	Administer daily at noon to prevent insomnia.
	Can cause dangerous interaction with meperidine (Demerol), alcohol, and CNS depressants.

Catechol-O-Methyltransferase (COMT) Inhibitor

Blocks the enzyme COMT to prevent breakdown of levodopa, prolonging levodopa action. For use with levodopa/carbidopa combination (Sinemet).

Examples	**Nursing Implications**
entacapone (Comtan)	Report elevated temperature, muscular rigidity, altered level of consciousness, and elevated creatine phosphokinase (CKP).
carbidopa/levodopa/entacapone combination (Stalevo)	

Note: With all anti–Parkinson disease agents, teach patient to check with physician before taking over-the-counter medications, especially cold preparations. Teach patient to rise slowly to prevent orthostasis.

therapies are only experimental at this time. For more information, visit the Parkinson's Foundation web site at www.parkinson.org.

Nursing Process for the Patient With Parkinson Disease

DATA COLLECTION. Ask the patient about symptoms of Parkinson disease and their effect on level of functioning. Observe ability to move, walk, and perform ADLs safely. Determine risk for injury related to immobility or falls.

Assess nutritional status and condition of skin. Identify presence of confusion and side effects of medications. Psychosocial assessment includes the patient's and caregiver's responses to the disease, coping strategies, and support systems.

NURSING DIAGNOSES, PLANNING, AND IMPLEMENTATION. The patient with Parkinson disease is at risk for many problems. Priority diagnoses are addressed next. If confusion is present, also see "Nursing Care Plan for the Patient With Dementia" earlier in this chapter.

Impaired Physical Mobility related to muscle stiffness and tremor

EXPECTED OUTCOME: The patient will maintain optimal mobility and ability to ambulate as long as possible.

- Assist the patient to plan daily activities based on anticipated response to medications. *Certain times of day may be less troublesome than others.*
- Consult with physical and occupational therapists to provide assistive devices *to help maintain mobility and provide diversional activities.*
- Provide assistance with ROM exercises *to maintain flexibility of muscles.*
- Teach patients who have difficulty initiating walking to pick up one foot as though attempting to step over something to take the first step. It may also help to take several steps in place before starting to walk. *This may help overcome freezing of gait.*

Self-Care Deficit (Dressing/Feeding/Toileting/Bathing) related to reduced mobility

EXPECTED OUTCOME: The patient's self-care needs will be met as evidenced by patient statement.

- Encourage the patient to participate in ADLs as much as possible. *This helps the patient maintain independence and self-esteem.*
- Consult an occupational therapist *to assist with devices and strategies for maintaining independence.*
- Instruct the patient or family to provide clothing without buttons and supply shoes with adherent fasteners, rather than shoelaces, *to help maintain independence.*
- Assist the patient and family to make decisions about long-term care. Consult a social worker as needed for assistance. *As the patient ages, so do the family members who are providing care. The point may be reached at which the caregiver is no longer able to meet the increasing needs of the patient. The decision to place the patient in a skilled nursing facility is extremely difficult and emotional.*

Risk for Injury related to reduced mobility and balance

EXPECTED OUTCOME: The patient will remain safe and without injury.

- If the patient is in the hospital or long-term care facility, keep the call light within reach at all times. Remind the patient to request assistance with ambulation. *The patient is at risk for injury from falls related to problems with mobility.*
- Maintain bed in the low position, with side rails raised if appropriate (side rails may be prohibited in some institutions). *Maintaining the bed in a low position reduces the risk for injury or fall when getting out of bed. Side rails can increase the risk for injury and must be used carefully.*
- Use an alarm system on the bed and chair that alerts the staff that the patient is getting up *so that staff can assist the patient to get up and ambulate.*

- Avoid use of restraints. *Restraints can increase the risk for injury.*
- Keep environment free from clutter, throw rugs, or other items *that can cause a patient to trip.*
- Provide walkers and other assistive devices *to provide support and prevent falls.*

EVALUATION. The care of the patient with Parkinson disease has been successful if the patient remains as mobile and independent as possible. Self-care needs should be met by the patient or others, and the patient should remain safe from injury.

CRITICAL THINKING

Ms. Simpson, 47 years old, has had Parkinson disease for the past 5 years, and the symptoms are becoming progressively worse. She is now admitted for a urinary tract infection.

1. What problems do you foresee when caring for Ms. Simpson?
2. What safety measures should you implement?
3. Ms. Simpson is receiving intravenous (IV) fluids of 5% dextrose in 0.45% saline, 1,000 mL over 12 hours. The registered nurse on duty is accountable for her IV, but as you are bathing her you notice that the bag is nearly full and it has been hanging for 4 hours. How many milliliters should still be in her IV bag after 4 hours?
4. What members of the health care team should you collaborate with in providing Ms. Simpson's care?

Suggested answers are at the end of the chapter.

Huntington Disease

Huntington disease is a progressive, hereditary, degenerative, incurable neurologic disorder. It was first described in 1872 by George Huntington, a general practitioner in New York. The uncontrolled movements associated with Huntington disease caused some sufferers in the 17th century to be accused of and executed for witchcraft. Many of the cases around the world can be traced back to specific individuals.

Pathophysiology and Etiology

Huntington disease (also known as Huntington chorea) is inherited in an autosomal dominant manner, which means that each offspring of an affected parent has a 50% chance of inheriting the disorder. A mutation in a specific gene has been identified; however, the cause of the mutation is not known. A protein called *rhes* may be responsible for the activation of a mutant protein that causes destruction of the cells in the corpus striatum. Destruction also occurs in the caudate nucleus and other deep nuclei of the brain and in portions of the cerebral cortex. This degeneration results in progressive loss of normal movement and intellect. The rate of disease progression varies from person to person.

Signs and Symptoms

Signs and symptoms usually begin in middle age and develop slowly, becoming progressively more apparent. Cognitive signs can be noticed before movement problems. Patients who are not aware of their hereditary risk for Huntington disease may be incorrectly diagnosed as being mentally ill.

The patient can display personality changes and inappropriate behavior. The patient may be euphoric or irritable and can rapidly alternate between moods. Paranoia is common, and behavior can become violent as dementia worsens. The patient eventually progresses to the point at which he or she is incontinent and totally dependent on others for care. These symptoms are difficult for family and friends as well as professional caregivers to cope with. The disease progression and associated symptoms are particularly devastating for offspring, who may or may not know whether they have inherited the disease.

Physical symptoms also develop slowly. Huntington disease is characterized by involuntary, irregular, jerky, dance-like (choreiform) movements. Initially, these symptoms can take the form of mild fidgeting and facial grimacing, starting in the arms, face, and neck and progressively involving the remainder of the body. Patients display hesitant speech, eye blinking, irregular trunk movements, abnormal tilt of the head, and constant motion (Fig. 48.15). The gait is wide, and the patient may appear to be dancing. Emotional upset, stress, or trying to perform a voluntary task can significantly increase the severity and rate of the abnormal movements; the movements typically diminish or disappear during sleep. Dysphagia can significantly impair the patient's nutritional status.

Depression and suicide are common in the earlier stages of the disease, when the patient still has the cognitive ability to carry out a suicidal act. As the disease progresses, the patient becomes more and more dependent. Aspiration resulting in respiratory failure is the primary cause of death. Life span following diagnosis is about 10 to 30 years.

Diagnostic Tests

Huntington disease has typically been diagnosed based on clinical examination and a family history of the disease. MRI or CT scan may be helpful. Genetic testing is available for prenatal use and to determine whether an individual has Huntington disease before he or she becomes symptomatic. This is important because Huntington disease does not become symptomatic until patients are in their 30s or 40s, when they may already have children who could be affected ("Patient Perspective: Betty").

Therapeutic Measures

Because there is no cure, treatment of Huntington disease focuses on minimizing symptoms and preventing complications. Antipsychotic, antidepressant, and antichoreic drugs may be used to treat both the involuntary movements and behavioral outbursts. Tetrabenazine (Xenazine) may help reduce involuntary movements by increasing dopamine in the brain. Physical and occupational therapy can help keep the patient mobile and independent for as long as possible.

Patient Perspective

Betty. I was born the second of six children. My mom was diagnosed with Huntington chorea (an old name for Huntington disease) after she had all of us. My brother was diagnosed with Huntington disease at the age of 60. He started out with terrible mood swings and a bad temper, but eventually he had a lot of movement problems, including pronounced facial and tongue movements.

By the time we knew the disease had affected our family, many of us had children and grandchildren of our own. My kids wanted me to be tested. It is a hereditary disease, and you have a 50/50 chance of having it if a parent has it. If I had Huntington disease, then my kids would have a 50/50 chance of having it. If I tested negative, then they and their children would not be at risk.

I was very nervous and afraid of being tested. When I went for the initial visit at the University of Michigan, they observed my movements, how I walked and talked, and my facial movements. They made me go to a psychologist to see whether I could handle the results if they did the blood test that would tell for sure. I understand the suicide rate is kind of high for people with Huntington. After talking for an hour and a half, they decided I could handle the results.

At my next visit, they just drew blood, which was sent out for testing. I had to return to the university 6 weeks later for the results. When I went back, I was a nervous wreck. A friend went with me. When the technician came in, she said the doctor would be with me soon. I immediately had bad thoughts. Then when the technician and doctor came back, they were both smiling and had tears in their eyes—I had tested negative. So my friend, the doctor, the technician, and I all hugged and cried.

It is a very hard disease to live with, whether you or another family member has it. My brother has it very bad. Out of my five siblings, four have it for sure, and we think the fifth has it because of mood swings we have observed.

I am the only one of the six who tested clear. I felt very guilty at first that they all had it and I didn't. I'm starting to get over that, but when I see one of them having a bad time with talking, or temper, or movement, the guilt starts to kick in again.

Research has been done on the benefits of transplanting stem cells into the brains of patients with Huntington disease, but this is still experimental at this time.

Nursing Care

Patients with Huntington disease are typically cared for on an outpatient basis. When a patient with Huntington disease is admitted to an inpatient facility, it is important to obtain as much information as possible about that person's response to medication, daily routine, and emotional and cognitive functioning from the caregivers. For example, knowing that

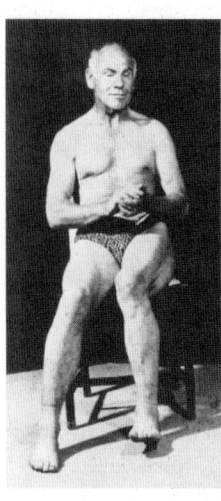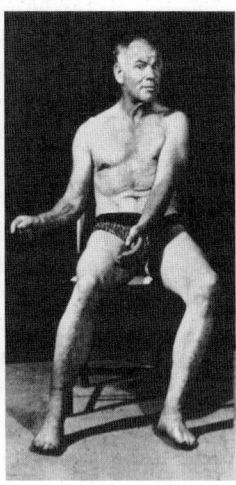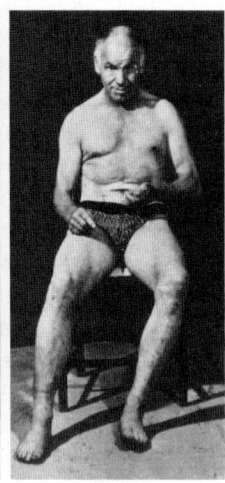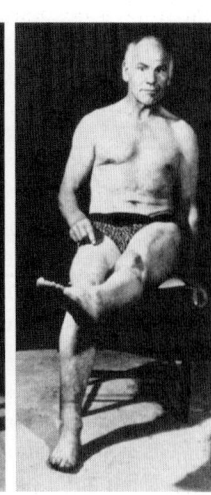

FIGURE 48.15 A 47-year-old patient with Huntington disease. Note constant fidgety movement.

a certain patient is intensely afraid of bathtubs but willingly takes showers can prevent unnecessary struggles and outbursts. Providing some objects from home can make the new environment seem less threatening. The caregivers may relate that the patient has better cognitive functioning at a particular time of day. As the dementia progresses, the patient responds less to attempts at reasoning. Giving directions in a calm but firm tone may help the patient cooperate with activities. The environment should be modified to keep the patient safe. Keep in mind that forceful, involuntary movements of the patient's extremities can happen at any time and should not be misinterpreted as an attempt to harm caregivers.

Difficulty swallowing typically begins toward the middle of the disease course. Patients exhibit trouble swallowing liquids in particular. At this stage, it may still be possible to teach the patient to hold the chin down to the chest while swallowing, which lessens the chance of aspiration. Have patients sit straight upright while eating. Thickening agents can be added to thin liquids to help prevent aspiration. Adaptive devices can prolong the patient's ability to eat independently. Soft foods that are easily manipulated in the mouth are most suitable. Patients may have difficulty taking in adequate calories to maintain a normal body weight, even if a caregiver assists with feeding them. One of the many ethical issues faced by these patients and their family members is whether artificial feeding should be used and, if so, for how long. Patients and their family members should be encouraged to discuss end-of-life decisions early in the course of the disease.

Also see "Nursing Care Plan for the Patient With Dementia" earlier in this chapter.

Alzheimer Disease

Alzheimer disease (also called dementia of the Alzheimer type [DAT]) is the most common type of dementia. Dementia is a progressive loss of mental functioning that interferes with memory, ability to think clearly and learn, and eventually ability to function (see discussion of dementia earlier in this chapter).

Alois Alzheimer, a German neurologist, first described the disease in 1907. He described pathological changes, now referred to as neurofibrillary tangles and neuritic plaques, that he discovered while performing an autopsy on a patient with dementia. Alzheimer disease is a progressively degenerative disease that is inevitably fatal. The incidence of Alzheimer disease is more common in women than men and doubles for every 5 years a person lives beyond age 65.

Etiology and Pathophysiology

Many etiologies have been theorized for Alzheimer disease, including viral or bacterial infection and autoimmune dysfunction. Markers associated with Alzheimer disease can be found on several chromosomes. Chromosome 21 in particular has been associated with Alzheimer disease and is also the location of the genetic abnormality responsible for Down syndrome. Patients older than age 40 who have Down syndrome usually develop Alzheimer disease. The exact correlation between the two disorders is still being studied. Lifestyle factors that increase risk of Alzheimer disease include hypertension, hypercholesterolemia, and poorly controlled diabetes.

Although the exact cause of Alzheimer disease is unknown, the structural changes associated with it have been well documented. An abnormality exists within the protein of the cell membrane of a neuron. As the axon terminals and dendrite branches disintegrate, they collect in neuritic plaques. Inside the normal brain is a precise arrangement of filaments and tubules that are responsible for cell integrity. Individuals with Alzheimer disease develop neurofibrillary tangles instead of the normal orderly arrangement. Instead of remaining a small area of abnormality, these neuritic plaques and neurofibrillary tangles spread via axons to other areas of the brain. In addition, patients tend to have a deficiency of acetylcholine in the cerebral cortex. Remember that acetylcholine is a neurotransmitter important for nervous system function.

Advancement of neurofibrillary tangles and neuritic plaques typically affects the hippocampus first, resulting in short-term memory dysfunction. As the tangles and plaques spread to the temporal lobe, memory impairment becomes more severe. It may be at this point that the patient accesses the health care system. Personality changes and incontinence are inevitable results of Alzheimer disease. These symptoms can be attributed to the spread of plaques and tangles to the frontal lobes of the brain.

It is believed that the younger the patient is at the time of onset, the faster the neurofibrillary tangles and neuritic plaques spread. Younger patients tend to deteriorate faster, require complete care earlier, and have a shorter life span.

One area of the brain that is left relatively untouched by Alzheimer disease is the subcortical area. This structure is responsible for our subconscious urge to survive. The needs for basic requirements such as shelter, food and water, security, and reproduction are controlled by the subcortical area, as are emotional responses to situations. The patient with Alzheimer disease may experience hunger but no longer know how to meet that basic need. Left to their own devices, these individuals would starve.

Signs and Symptoms

The signs and symptoms of Alzheimer disease are typically broken down into three stages.

STAGE 1. This early stage lasts from 2 to 4 years and is characterized by increasing forgetfulness. At this stage, the patient may attempt to cope by using lists and reminders. Interest in day-to-day activities, acquaintances, and surroundings tends to diminish. The patient is reluctant to take on tasks because of uncertainty in how to perform them. If the patient is still working, his or her performance deteriorates and can result in being terminated from the job.

STAGE 2. The second stage is the longest in duration, lasting 2 to 12 years. Progressive cognitive deterioration causes difficulty doing simple calculations or answering questions. Patients may become irritable, particularly when asked to perform a task that they know they should be able to perform but cannot. It may help the patient to break down the task into manageable steps. Depression is common. Aphasia and the resulting inability to make themselves understood can exacerbate patients' irritability. It is during the middle stage, as cognitive function significantly deteriorates, that the patient may become more physically active. The normal sleep–wake cycle is disrupted, and the patient tends to wander aimlessly, particularly at night. The patient may become lost in familiar surroundings, which compounds the anxiety that typically develops during this stage. Hallucinations and seizures can occur. Management of day-to-day activities, such as feeding a pet or paying bills, becomes overwhelming. Personal hygiene deteriorates, as does appropriate social behavior. Patients may make up stories to cover for deficits, saying that possessions they misplaced were stolen. Some patients hoard food or money.

STAGE 3. The third stage of Alzheimer disease is characterized by progression to complete dependency. The patient loses the ability to converse or control bowel or bladder function. If the patient is still mobile, constant supervision is required to protect from wandering and avoid injury. Emotional control and ability to recognize loved ones are lost. This lack of recognition is particularly devastating for family members. Eventually, the patient is unable to move independently, swallow, or express needs. Death usually occurs from complications of immobility.

The duration of the final stage of Alzheimer disease, characterized by complete dependence, depends in part on the physical stamina and general health of the individual. The healthier the patient, the longer the body will continue to function. Another factor is the decisions that have been made regarding artificial feeding and respiratory support. Few family members or HCPs advocate intubation and mechanical ventilation for patients with Alzheimer disease. The issue of enteral feedings, however, is an emotional one with few easy answers. The use of enteral feedings can prolong the patient's life, despite the absence of cognitive functioning. As with patients suffering from Huntington disease, every effort should be made to determine the patient's wishes before cognitive impairment makes that impossible.

Some experts recognize seven stages of Alzheimer disease. Individuals are evaluated using the Global Deterioration Scale for Assessment of Primary Degenerative Dementia (GDS), which presents a more detailed description of each stage. Pre-dementia (Stages 1 through 3) is characterized with no impairment to MCI. In Stages 4 and 5, patients have significant memory loss and confusion. In Stage 5, the person cannot survive without assistance with ADLs. The final stages (6 and 7) are associated with loss of verbal and basic psychomotor skills, and the brain no longer has control over the body.

Table 48.12 provides a comparison of the symptoms of Parkinson, Huntington, and Alzheimer diseases.

Diagnostic Tests

Alzheimer disease is diagnosed primarily on the basis of clinical examination, history, and elimination of other possible causes of symptoms. MRI can reveal the presence of the classic neurofibrillary tangles and neuritic plaques. PET and single-photon emission computed tomography (SPECT) scans show areas of neuronal inactivity. Genetic testing and brain imaging can help predict the risk of Alzheimer disease. New blood tests that can predict risk are also being developed.

Therapeutic Measures

There is no known cure for Alzheimer disease. Treatment has traditionally focused on minimizing the effects of the disease and maintaining independence as long as possible. Acetylcholinesterase (AChE) inhibitors such as donepezil (Aricept) or rivastigmine (Exelon) are thought to inhibit the breakdown of the neurotransmitter acetylcholine (see Table 48.9). Increased levels of acetylcholine in the brain allow better functioning of the remaining neurons. They appear to be most effective for those patients who exhibit mild to moderate symptoms of Alzheimer disease. It can take some time to notice any effects

Table 48.12

Comparisons of Parkinson, Huntington, and Alzheimer Diseases

Symptom	Parkinson	Huntington	Alzheimer
Tremors	Present	Absent	Absent
Bradykinesia/akinesia	Present	Absent	Absent
Muscle rigidity	Present	Absent	Absent
Memory dysfunction	Late	Late	Early
Cognitive dysfunction	Late	Present	Early
Inability to perform activities of daily living	Progressive	Progressive	Progressive
Involuntary movements	Absent	Present	Absent
Depression	Present	Present	Present

of the drugs. Use of AChE inhibitors diminishes the amount of medical care and social service interventions required and delays admission to skilled nursing facilities. This delay in institutionalization can result in significant positive impact on quality of life as well as financial savings for the patient and family.

Another class of medications, NMDA (N-methyl-D-aspartate) antagonists, can prevent overexcitation of NMDA receptors in the brain and allow more normal function. Memantine (Namenda, Axura) is the only drug currently available in this class. These drugs can be given at any stage of Alzheimer disease and, like AChE inhibitors, simply slow the patient's decline.

Antidepressants, antipsychotics, and antianxiety drugs can be used as a last resort to control symptoms of depression and behavioral disturbances, but they do not treat the dementia. Patients should be carefully monitored for drug interactions and side effects. For more information, visit the Alzheimer's Association web site at www.alz.org.

Nursing Process for the Patient With Alzheimer Disease

See the earlier discussion of dementia as well as "Nursing Care Plan for the Patient With Dementia" earlier in this chapter.

CRITICAL THINKING

Mrs. Johnson has just become a resident at a long-term care facility. She is diagnosed with Alzheimer disease and is in Stage 2 with some signs of Stage 3 disease. When you check on her during the evening, you find her walking around her room, talking to herself. What other signs and symptoms are typical for Stage 2 and Stage 3 Alzheimer disease? How should you address her behavior?

Suggested answers are at the end of the chapter.

Home Health Hints

- Note whether the patient's clothes are matched and properly fastened. Is the patient clean and well groomed?
- Observe the patient during bathing, grooming, or dressing to assess motor function and coordination.
- Determine energy level by noting whether the patient makes frequent requests to sit or lie down.
- Observe the patient's gait for steadiness.
- Teach the caregiver to move furniture to allow a clear path for ambulation and to remove throw rugs.
- Teach the caregiver to position frequently used items, such as a comb, glass of water, eyeglasses, books, tissues, and phone, where they are easily accessible.
- Teach the caregiver to provide shoes with Velcro closures to promote independence.
- Teach the caregiver and patient to use chairs with armrests so the patient can rise from his or her chair more easily.
- Teach the caregiver to make a clip-on bib with suspender clips attached to a piece of elastic. A clean napkin or washcloth can be attached for each meal.
- Teach the caregiver that patients with visual impairments can see contrasting colors better. Slipper color should be different from the floor, a dark-colored placemat can be used under light dishes, and the first and last steps of a stairway can be painted a contrasting color.
- Teach the caregiver to use a bath or shower seat, hand-held showerhead, and soothing music to help the patient feel safe and oriented to the task while bathing.
- Teach the caregiver to prevent the patient from getting outside alone by covering doorknobs with a piece of cloth.

SUGGESTED ANSWERS TO CRITICAL THINKING

Mr. Chung

1. Be prepared to assist with a lumbar puncture.
2. You should use short, simple sentences because he may be very anxious or disoriented. Involve his family. Further education can be provided when he is feeling better.
3. Because meningococcal meningitis is contagious, he should be placed in droplet isolation. Personal protective equipment, such as gloves, gowns, and masks, should be used. Explain the need for these practices to Mr. Chung and his visitors.
4. Comfort measures include tepid baths; a quiet, dark environment; and minimal stimulation. Administer acetaminophen and analgesics as ordered.
5. The health care service at his college should be notified of his diagnosis. Close contacts may require prophylactic treatment. If Mr. Chung lives at home rather than at college, his family members should be advised to see their health care provider and begin prophylactic treatment.

Mr. Evans

1. You might expect to see impaired speech, right-sided weakness, and a rapid decrease in consciousness if Mr. Evans's hematoma is enlarged.
2. Intubation equipment, mannitol, and intravenous access should be ready. He should be given nothing by mouth (NPO), and the results of laboratory tests should be ready in the event of emergency surgery. The location of Mr. Evans's next of kin must be known.
3. Who are Mr. Evans's support people? Was this drinking episode an isolated incident or a chronic problem that should be addressed if he is discharged safely?
4. Health care team members needed for Mr. Evans depend on the extent of his injury. They may include a social worker; physical, occupational, and speech therapists; neuropsychologist; dietitian; and others.

Ms. Simpson

1. Urinary tract infection is often accompanied by urinary urgency. Ms. Simpson may have difficulty getting to the bathroom quickly and safely.
2. Keep a bedside commode nearby if the bathroom is not close. Assist Ms. Simpson to the bathroom or commode at regular intervals to prevent urgency. Remind her to ask for help if she needs to get up. Make sure that her call light is within reach.
3.

$$\frac{1{,}000 \text{ mL}}{12 \text{ hours}} \quad \bigg| \quad 4 \text{ hours} = 333 \text{ mL}$$

After 4 hours, 1,000 mL – 333 mL = 667 mL should remain in the bag. Because it is still nearly full, the registered nurse should be notified.
4. Occupational, physical, and speech therapy may be involved in Ms. Simpson's care. Speech therapy can help with swallowing problems. Work with nursing assistants to be sure she is mobilized and protected from falls and that swallowing problems are addressed.

Mrs. Johnson

Being admitted to a new and unfamiliar facility can increase confusion. Signs of Stage 2 Alzheimer disease include memory loss, wandering at night, sleeplessness, irritability, loss of way in familiar surroundings, losing possessions and searching for them, and neglect of personal hygiene. During Stage 3 of the disease, the patient will lose weight, recognize hunger but be unable to eat, be unable to communicate verbally or in writing, lose ability to recognize family, become incontinent of urine and feces, and eventually lose ability to stand and walk. Address Mrs. Johnson by her name and ask her what she needs. Reorient her to where she is and assure her that she is safe and being cared for.

Review Questions

1. A college student is admitted to the hospital with a severe headache. Which finding in the student's history is consistent with the diagnosis of meningitis?
   1. A sore throat for 3 days
   2. A history of migraine headaches
   3. A muscle injury in the neck
   4. A recent motor vehicle accident

2. A patient with meningitis has photophobia and a severe headache. Which nursing interventions will be most helpful to relieve symptoms?
   1. Administer antibiotics as ordered, and prepare the patient for a lumbar puncture.
   2. Darken the room and administer analgesics.
   3. Administer acetaminophen as ordered and maintain isolation.
   4. Check level of consciousness with the Glasgow Coma Scale and monitor vital signs.

3. A patient makes an appointment to see a health care provider for recurrent severe headaches. Which instruction by the nurse will help gather the best additional data before the appointment?
   1. "Try relaxation and warm moist compresses for your headaches and document your response."
   2. "Call and come in the next time you have a headache so you can be examined."
   3. "Keep track of how many headaches you have before you come in."
   4. "Keep a diary of your headaches, recording symptoms, timing, and headache triggers."

4. A patient who has had a generalized tonic-clonic seizure is sound asleep 30 minutes after the seizure. Meals are about to be delivered. Which nursing action is most appropriate?
   1. Wake the patient because nourishment is essential following a seizure.
   2. Wake the patient to do a neurologic assessment before the meal.
   3. Let the patient sleep during the postictal state, and keep the meal warm.
   4. Do not attempt to wake the patient because of the risk of a repeat seizure.

5. A patient with a history of seizures reports experiencing an aura and is concerned about an impending seizure. Place the nurse's interventions in the correct order.
   1. Protect the patient from injury during the seizure.
   2. Document the events of the seizure.
   3. Help the patient lie down in a safe place.
   4. Turn the patient on his or her side to sleep.

6. Which patients should be closely monitored by the nurse for symptoms of increased intracranial pressure? **Select all that apply.**
   1. The patient who has a history of epilepsy
   2. The patient admitted with a high fever and severe headache
   3. The patient in the postanesthesia care unit following craniectomy
   4. The patient with a brain tumor who is admitted for radiation therapy
   5. The patient with a history of migraine headaches, admitted for orthopedic surgery
   6. The patient with Alzheimer disease admitted with a urinary tract infection

7. Which of the following actions should the nurse take to help prevent increased intracranial pressure in a patient following a traumatic brain injury?
   1. Cluster care so the patient can have long periods of rest.
   2. Keep the head of the bed elevated at 30 degrees.
   3. Suction frequently to keep the airway clear.
   4. Do not give anything by mouth.

8. A patient is admitted following a T4 spinal injury. When taking morning vital signs, the nurse notes that the patient appears restless and that blood pressure is elevated. Which of the following actions by the nurse is appropriate?
   1. Recheck the patient's blood pressure in 30 minutes.
   2. No action is necessary. This is an expected finding.
   3. Check for a full bladder or bowel.
   4. Encourage the patient to express any anxiety.

9. Which nursing interventions are appropriate for the patient with a neurodegenerative disorder who has difficulty swallowing?
   1. Have the patient tuck his or her chin down during swallowing.
   2. Provide clear to full liquids and avoid solid foods.
   3. Place the patient in semi-Fowler position for eating.
   4. Provide adaptive eating utensils.

10. A resident of a long-term care facility who has Alzheimer disease is sitting in a corner, crying loudly that no one is paying attention. Several staff members have tried to find out what's wrong, but the patient won't answer and just keeps rocking back and forth and crying. Which approach by the nurse might best help the patient?
    1. Say in a quiet voice, "What is wrong? We can't help you if you don't tell us what's wrong."
    2. Sit quietly by the patient and say, "I'm here. You aren't alone."
    3. Say in a firm voice, "Several staff members have asked what you need. Now it is time to stop crying."
    4. Ignore the continued crying. Continuing to respond will encourage the behavior.

Answer rationales available in your online resources.

ANSWERS 1. 1; 2. 3, 4; 3. 4; 4. 3; 5. 3, 1, 4, 2; 6. 2, 3, 4; 7. 2; 8. 3; 9. 1; 10. 2

Key Points

Find the chapter key points in your online resources available through Davis Edge.

Additional Resources

 Use the scratch off code on the inside front cover of your book to access online quizzes that will help you to improve your scores on course exams and prepare for the NCLEX-PN®.

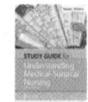 Study Guide

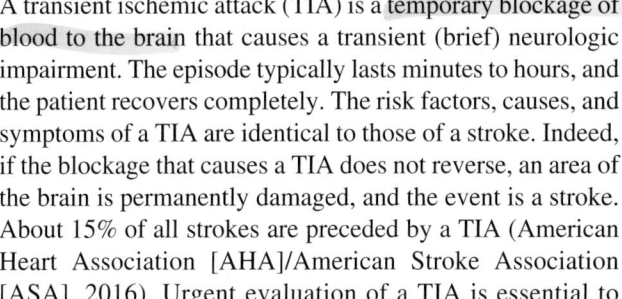

CHAPTER 49

Nursing Care of Patients With Cerebrovascular Disorders

Deborah L. Weaver, Linda K. Cook

KEY TERMS

aphasia (uh-FAY-zhuh)
ataxia (ah-TAK-see-ah)
diplopia (dip-LOH-pee-ah)
dysarthria (dis-ARTH-ree-ah)
dysphasia (dis-FAY-zhah)
embolic (em-BOL-ik)
embolism (EM-buh-lizm)
endarterectomy (end-AR-tur-EK-tuh-mee)
hemiplegia (HEM-ee-PLEE-jee-ah)
hemorrhagic (hem-uh-RAH-jik)
intracerebral (IN-trah-sur-EE-brul)
ischemic (ih-SKEE-mik)
penumbra (puh-NUM-brah)
thrombolytic (throm-buh-LIT-ik)
thrombosis (throm-BOH-sis)
thrombotic (throm-BOT-ik)

LEARNING OUTCOMES

1. Describe causes, risk factors, and pathophysiology of transient ischemic attack, ischemic stroke, and hemorrhagic stroke.
2. Identify emergency interventions for transient ischemic attack, ischemic stroke, and hemorrhagic stroke.
3. Plan therapeutic measures for transient ischemic attack, ischemic stroke, and hemorrhagic stroke.
4. Identify outcomes that can be expected for a stroke victim.
5. Plan nursing care for a patient with a cerebrovascular disorder.

CHAPTER CONCEPTS

Neurologic Regulation
Perfusion

Cerebrovascular disorders occur when the supply of blood and oxygen to brain cells is inadequate, allowing brain tissue to die and causing a stroke. The most common cerebrovascular disorders include transient ischemic attack, ischemic stroke, and hemorrhagic stroke.

TRANSIENT ISCHEMIC ATTACK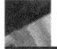

A transient ischemic attack (TIA) is a temporary blockage of blood to the brain that causes a transient (brief) neurologic impairment. The episode typically lasts minutes to hours, and the patient recovers completely. The risk factors, causes, and symptoms of a TIA are identical to those of a stroke. Indeed, if the blockage that causes a TIA does not reverse, an area of the brain is permanently damaged, and the event is a stroke. About 15% of all strokes are preceded by a TIA (American Heart Association [AHA]/American Stroke Association [ASA], 2016). Urgent evaluation of a TIA is essential to decrease the risk of stroke.

Treatment of a TIA is focused on preventing a full stroke. The cause of the TIA may be discovered with diagnostic tests, which can then guide treatment. However, there may be no clear etiology of the TIA. Treatment, therefore, is mostly centered on minimizing the patient's risk factors for a stroke.

STROKE

A stroke (also called cerebrovascular accident or CVA) is caused by the disruption of blood flow to the brain, resulting in death of brain cells. In most cases, permanent disability results. About 795,000 people of all ages are affected each year (AHA/ASA, 2016), and a stroke is more likely to happen as one ages. Because of their increased longevity, 55,000 more women have strokes each year than men (National Stroke Association, 2017). Stroke is the fifth leading cause of death and the leading cause of disability in the United States (AHA/ASA, 2016). African Americans, Hispanic Americans, and American Indian/Alaska Natives are at higher risk than Hispanics, Asian Americans, and whites (National Heart, Lung, and Blood Institute, 2017). There is also a higher incidence of stroke in people with lower levels of education,

1053

lower socioeconomic status, and those living in the south-eastern United States.

Pathophysiology

Cerebral function depends on oxygen and glucose delivery to neurons in the brain. The brain cannot store oxygen or glucose, so it relies on a constant supply of these nutrients. If the supply of oxygen and glucose is stopped, brain tissue dies. When a stroke occurs, brain cells begin dying immediately. There is an area of brain tissue surrounding the damage called the **penumbra.** It contains brain cells that are "stunned" and can be revived if the brain is reperfused quickly. However, the brain cells will die if the blood supply is not restored.

The particular vessel or vessels involved determine the area of the brain affected and symptoms that result. The duration of ischemia determines whether the symptoms are transient or permanent. TIA symptoms generally resolve within 24 hours; however, a TIA can be a warning of an impending stroke.

Etiology

Strokes are classified as either ischemic or hemorrhagic. Ischemic strokes are more common, accounting for about 87% of all strokes (AHA/ASA, 2016). Hemorrhagic strokes account for the remaining 13% of strokes.

Ischemic Stroke

Ischemic stroke occurs when the blood supply to the brain is blocked or significantly slowed. There are two major types: thrombotic or embolic (Fig. 49.1).

THROMBOTIC STROKE. Thrombotic strokes occur when an occlusion builds up in an artery until it significantly decreases

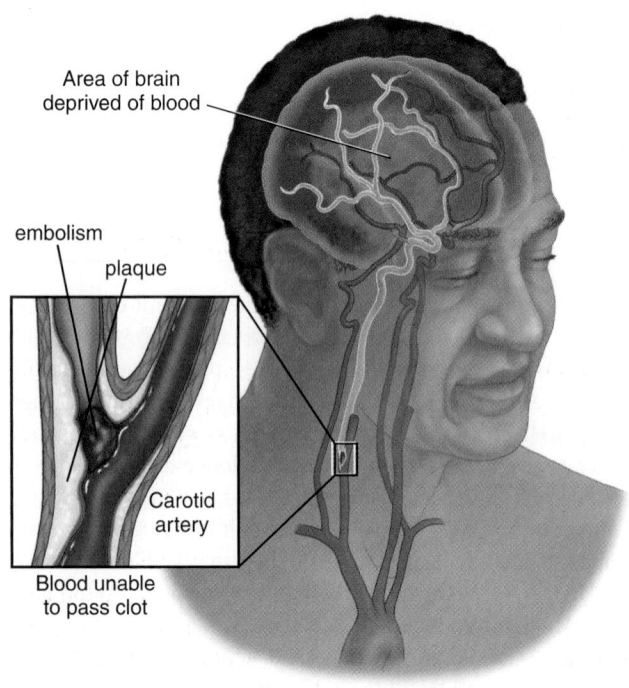

Area of brain
deprived of blood

embolism

plaque

Carotid
artery

Blood unable
to pass clot

FIGURE 49.1 Embolism and thrombosis.

or stops blood flow to the brain. Thrombotic strokes most often occur in the internal or common carotid arteries.

EMBOLIC STROKE. An **embolic** stroke is typically caused by a blood clot that is created somewhere in the body, often within the heart. It then travels through the arteries until it becomes trapped in a smaller vessel, preventing the passage of blood. Typically, the **embolism** will travel and become lodged in the middle, anterior, or posterior cerebral arteries.

RISK FACTORS. Risk factors for ischemic stroke are classified as modifiable or nonmodifiable (Box 49.1). Nonmodifiable risk factors are those that cannot be altered, such as age or gender. Modifiable risk factors are those that can be changed with treatment, such as high blood pressure. Women have additional risks due to hormone changes in pregnancy and menopause. Children with sickle cell disease, cardiac anomaly, and hyperlipidemia are also at risk for stroke. Minimizing or eliminating these modifiable risk factors can significantly lower risk of a stroke. The Stroke Risk Scorecard from the National Stroke Association (Fig. 49.2) can help you determine your risk for stroke.

> ### NURSING CARE TIP
> Print the Stroke Risk Scorecard from www.stroke.org, and keep it in your pocket for patient teaching opportunities.

Hemorrhagic Stroke

Hemorrhagic strokes are caused by the rupture of a cerebral blood vessel that allows blood to escape into brain tissue and not travel beyond the point of the rupture. It can be further classified into two major types: subarachnoid hemorrhage and intracerebral hemorrhage.

SUBARACHNOID HEMORRHAGE. A *subarachnoid* hemorrhage is a stroke that occurs on the surface of the brain. It is most often the result of a ruptured cerebral aneurysm (covered later in this chapter). Strokes caused by subarachnoid hemorrhage usually are very serious and require surgery to correct. They are often fatal.

INTRACEREBRAL HEMORRHAGE. An **intracerebral** hemorrhage is a stroke that occurs in the deeper tissues of the brain. It usually is caused by uncontrolled hypertension. Patients can experience multiple undetected intracerebral hemorrhages, with minimal deficits noted. However, damage will eventually accumulate, and the patient will develop major

---

• WORD • BUILDING •

ischemic: isch—to hold back + emia—blood + ic—relating to
thrombotic: thrombus—clot + ic—relating to
embolic: embolism—to throw (as in clot or other debris) + ic—relating to
embolism: embol—to throw + ism—condition
hemorrhagic: hemorrhage—blood loss + ic—relating to
intracerebral: intra—within + cerebral—cerebrum

Box 49.1

Modifiable Risk Factors for Stroke

Men and Women

- Cigarette smoking
- High blood pressure
- Diabetes mellitus
- Cardiovascular disease
  - High total cholesterol
  - Low high-density lipoprotein (HDL) cholesterol
  - Dyslipidemia
- Atrial fibrillation
- Asymptomatic carotid stenosis
- Sickle cell disease
- Obesity
- Excessive alcohol intake
- Poor diet (e.g., high sodium, high fat, low potassium)
- Physical inactivity

Women

- Pregnancy
- Oral contraceptives
- Hormone replacement therapy
- High triglycerides
- History of migraines
- Thick waist

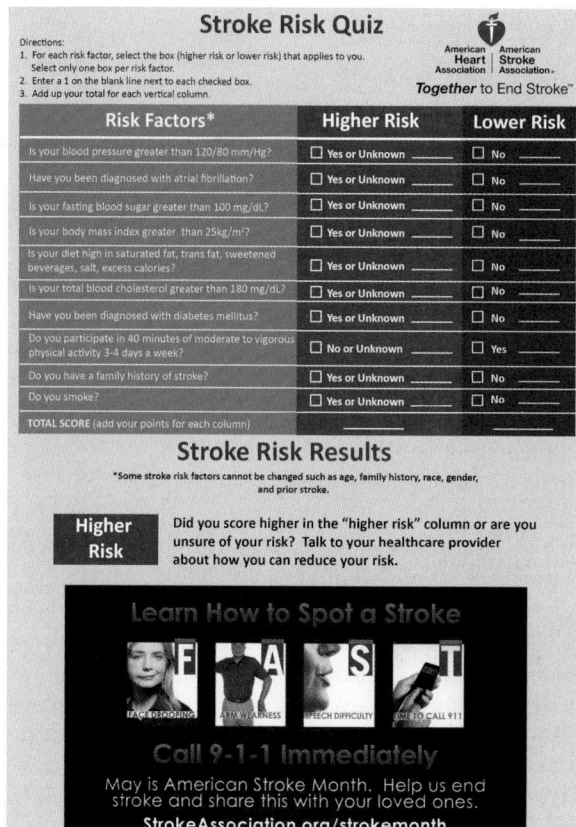

FIGURE 49.2 Stroke Risk Scorecard from the National Stroke Association – located at: https://www.stroke.org/stroke-risk-scorecard-2018. Reprinted with permission ©2018 American Heart Association, Inc.

deficits. Maintaining blood pressure below 120/80 mm Hg should be the goal for these patients. (More specific information related to special care of patients with hemorrhagic strokes will be addressed later in the chapter.)

Warning Signs of Any Type of Stroke

Patients and family members should be taught to recognize signs and symptoms and how to activate emergency medical services (EMS) if these signs occur. There is evidence that, if treatment begins within 1 hour of the onset of symptoms, permanent loss of function can be avoided or minimized.

The acronym FAST, which states for **F**ace, **A**rms, **S**peech, and **T**ime (see Fig. 49.2), can be used to teach emergency triage nurses, first responders, nonlicensed personnel, and community members to recognize a stroke and respond quickly. Time is extremely important to preserve brain cells. Quick access to the EMS is of particular importance. EMS can focus on delivering a suspected stroke patient to a stroke center for rapid assessment and care.

In addition to FAST, the following five signs or symptoms recognized by the AHA and ASA (2017b) require immediate EMS activation:

- Sudden numbness or weakness of face, arm, or leg, especially on one side of the body
- Sudden confusion or trouble speaking or understanding
- Sudden trouble seeing in one or both eyes
- Sudden trouble walking, dizziness, loss of balance, or coordination
- Sudden severe headache with no known cause

Women may have other unique symptoms, such as sudden onset of the following:

- Nausea
- Facial and limb pain
- Sudden behavioral changes
- Hallucinations
- General weakness
- Chest pain
- Shortness of breath
- Hiccups
- Palpitations (National Stroke Association, 2017)

NURSING CARE TIP

When teaching a stroke victim and family, repetition is very important. Besides the anxiety and stress they may be feeling, the patient's ability to process information can also be altered by the stroke.

Acute Signs and Symptoms

Most patients with stroke symptoms present with sudden or rapidly evolving symptoms. Symptoms are varied and depend on the area of the brain affected (Table 49.1). Common symptoms include visual disturbances, language disturbances, weakness or paralysis on one side of the body, and

Table 49.1

Clinical Manifestations of the Most Common Stroke Symptoms

Left Middle Cerebral Artery Syndrome	Right Middle Cerebral Artery Syndrome	Basilar Artery Syndrome
Weakness of the right face, arm, and leg (arm weakness greater than leg weakness).	Weakness of the left face, arm, and leg (arm weakness greater than leg weakness).	Dizziness.
Decrease in sensation on the right side of the body.	Decrease in sensation on the left side of the body.	Ataxia. Tinnitus. Nausea and vomiting.
Right homonymous hemianopsia (loss of vision in the right temporal field of vision and left nasal field of vision, requiring patients to scan an area in order to visualize objects on their right side).	Left homonymous hemianopsia (loss of vision in the left temporal field of vision and right nasal field of vision, requiring patients to scan an area in order to visualize objects on their right side).	Weakness on one side of the body that may be ipsilateral to the side of ischemia or injury or contralateral.
Dysphasia—in most patients, the language center of the brain is located in the left hemisphere. Language deficits may involve the motor speech area (Broca area) and cause patients to have difficulty expressing thoughts and to make errors in speech that they are able to detect. Injury or ischemia to the sensory speech area (Wernicke area) results in an inability to process speech input in the brain, causing patients to make errors in speech of which they are unaware.	Inattention or neglect of the left side.	Decrease in sensation on one side of the body that may be ipsilateral to the side of ischemia or injury or contralateral. Difficulty in the articulation of speech. Difficulty with swallowing and managing oral secretions.
Inattention or neglect of the right side.		

Source: Hoffman, J., & Sullivan, N. *Medical-surgical nursing: Making connections to practice* (p. 833). Philadelphia, PA: F.A. Davis.

difficulty swallowing (dysphagia). Signs and symptoms are generally the same for both ischemic and hemorrhagic stroke. Patients may have drowsiness and a severe headache, often described as "the worst headache of my life."

Language Disturbances

Difficulty with language is commonly associated with TIA and stroke. **Aphasia** refers to the absence of language; **dysphasia** refers to difficulty with speech and is not as severe as aphasia. With dysphasia, the patient may experience trouble selecting the correct words, use incomprehensible or nonsense speech, have trouble understanding others' speech, and have trouble writing or reading. Aphasia can be *expressive,* in which the patient knows what he wants to say but cannot speak or make sense, or *receptive,* which is an inability to understand spoken and/or written words. When both expressive and receptive aphasia are present, it is called *global aphasia.* Slurred or indistinct speech because of a motor problem (lack of coordination) is referred to as **dysarthria.** This speech impairment is often the cause of delay in treatment and emphasizes the importance of observation of symptoms by others.

Motor Disturbances

Motor disturbances include paralysis, weakness, and numbness. Sometimes, the first evidence of paralysis or weakness is clumsiness or a feeling of heaviness in a limb. The onset is sudden and typically involves one side of the body (the side opposite the damaged area of the brain). Deficits can appear on both sides of the body if the patient has had a brainstem or vertebrobasilar stroke.

Most commonly, paralysis or weakness affect the arm and face together. Some patients present with complete hemiparesis, with one entire side of the body flaccid. **Ataxia** may be present, which is poor balance or a stumbling, staggering gait. This can be related to damage to the cerebellum or to poor coordination due to weakness or paralysis. If the swallowing muscles are affected, the patient will have trouble swallowing (dysphagia).

• **WORD • BUILDING** •

aphasia: a—absent + phasia—speech
dysphasia: dys—difficult + phasia—speech
dysarthria: dys—difficult + arthria – joint or articulation

BE SAFFE!

BE VIGILANT! Before giving a patient with a suspected stroke anything to eat or drink, including medications, the patient should pass a swallow (dysphagia) screening test to prevent possible aspiration. Evaluate the patient's facial features; if there is any apparent weakness or asymmetry, stop and do not give the patient anything by mouth. If no weakness is evident, have the patient swallow about 30 mL of water. If the patient coughs, has difficulty swallowing, or has a wet or gurgly voice afterward, keep the patient NPO (nothing by mouth) until evaluated and cleared by a physician or speech and language pathologist.

Visual Disturbances

Visual field disturbances are also a common symptom of a stroke. The vision loss is painless and can involve loss of all or part of the vision in one eye. Patients often describe the change as a curtain dropping, as fog, or as a gray-out or blackout of vision. The involved eye is on the same side as the diseased artery. Potential visual field abnormalities are shown in Figure 49.3. When assessing the patient, stop talking and keep moving across the room. If the patient's eyes do not follow you, there is a good chance he or she has a deficit in that visual field.

Diagnostic Tests

On arrival at the emergency department (ED), a computed tomography (CT) scan will be performed immediately. The purpose of the CT scan is to identify whether symptoms are caused by a hemorrhagic stroke so that the health care provider (HCP) can determine the appropriate course of treatment. Ischemic stroke changes will not be visible on a CT until several days after the event. Interventions for hemorrhagic strokes are different than for ischemic strokes. Care for hemorrhagic strokes is discussed later in this chapter.

After the CT scan, patients may have an electrocardiogram (ECG) to determine whether atrial fibrillation is present. An echocardiogram may be done to determine the presence of other heart disease that increases the risk of thrombus formation. Other tests that may be performed in the ED include complete blood count (CBC), blood glucose level, metabolic panel, blood typing, prothrombin time (PT), international normalized ratio (INR), and serum pregnancy, if indicated. Stools and emesis may be checked for blood if indicated. The patient will be placed on a cardiac monitor and pulse oximeter. The ED nurse will complete a dysphagia screen before the patient consumes any food or fluids.

Use of the National Institutes of Health Stroke Scale (NIHSS; Fig. 49.4) is recommended to determine the patient's neurologic deficit level (found at www.ninds.nih.gov/Stroke-Scales-and-Related-Information). This 11-point scale determines

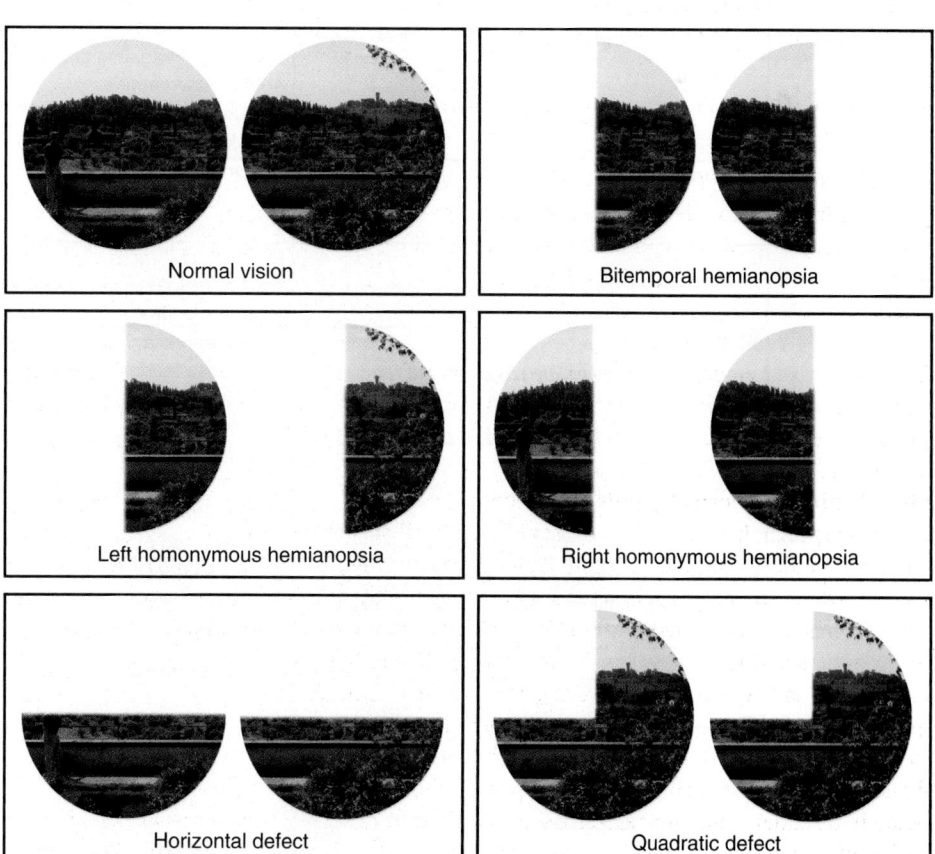

Normal vision

Bitemporal hemianopsia

Left homonymous hemianopsia

Right homonymous hemianopsia

Horizontal defect

Quadratic defect

FIGURE 49.3 Visual deficits in stroke.

Category	Scale Definition		Score
1a. Level of Consciousness (Alert, drowsy, etc.)	0 = Alert 1 = Drowsy 2 = Stuporous 3 = Coma		
1b. LOC Questions (Month, age)	0 = Answers both correctly 1 = Answers one correctly 2 = Incorrect		
1c. LOC Commands (Open/close eyes, make fist/let go)	0 = Obeys both correctly 1 = Obeys one correctly 2 = Incorrect		
2. Best Gaze (Eyes open—patient follows examiner's finger or face)	0 = Normal 1 = Partial gaze palsy 2 = Forced deviation		
3. Visual Fields (Introduce visual stimulus/threat to pt's visual field quadrants)	0 = No visual loss 1 = Partial Hemianopia 2 = Complete Hemianopia 3 = Bilateral Hemianopia (Blind)		
4. Facial Paresis (Show teeth, raise eyebrows and squeeze eyes shut)	0 = Normal 1 = Minor 2 = Partial 3 = Complete		
5a. Motor Arm—Left **5b. Motor Arm—Right** (Elevate arm to 90° if patient is sitting, 45° if supine)	0 = No drift 1 = Drift 2 = Can't resist gravity 3 = No effort against gravity 4 = No movement X = Untestable (Joint fusion or limb amp)	Left Right	
6a. Motor Leg—Left **6b. Motor Leg—Right** (Elevate leg to 30° with patient supine)	0 = No drift 1 = Drift 2 = Can't resist gravity 3 = No effort against gravity 4 = No movement X = Untestable (Joint fusion or limb amp)	Left Right	
7. Limb Ataxia (Finger-nose, heel down shin)	0 = No ataxia 1 = Present in one limb 2 = Present in two limbs		
8. Sensory (Pin prick to face, arm, trunk, and leg—compare side to side)	0 = Normal 1 = Partial loss 2 = Severe loss		
9. Best Language (Name item, describe a picture and read sentences)	0 = No aphasia 1 = Mild to moderate aphasia 2 = Severe aphasia 3 = Mute		
10. Dysarthria (Evaluate speech clarity by patient repeating listed words)	0 = Normal articulation 1 = Mild to moderate slurring of words 2 = Near to unintelligible or worse 3 = Intubated or other physical barrier		
11. Extinction and Inattention (Use information from prior testing to identify neglect or double simultaneous stimuli testing)	0 = No neglect 1 = Partial neglect 2 = Complete neglect		
		Total Score	

FIGURE 49.4 National Institutes of Health Stroke Scale.

the severity of a stroke. Nurses can be specially trained and certified to use it. Find out more about the NIHSS at www.nihstrokescale.org.

Once the patient is stabilized, additional tests can be done. Carotid Doppler testing uses ultrasound to detect stenosis of the carotid arteries. Carotid angiography can be done to further determine degree of blockage and help guide treatment.

Therapeutic Measures

Initial emergency care is supportive while test results are pending. ABCs (**A**irway, **B**reathing, and **C**irculation) are monitored. Oxygen is administered to maintain oxygen saturation at or above 94% and the patient's level of consciousness (LOC) is reduced. Vital signs and heart rhythm are monitored. A temperature greater than 99.6°F is treated because hyperthermia is associated with poorer patient outcomes. When test results verify whether the stroke is hemorrhagic or ischemic, therapeutic interventions are begun.

Some hospitals have a stroke team that evaluates all patients who arrive at the hospital within 2 hours of symptom onset. The stroke team will assess the patient within the first 15 minutes of arrival. Lab tests, ECG, and CT scans will be done, with results back within 45 minutes after assessment. The HCP will make a decision regarding thrombolytic therapy within 1 hour of arrival.

If the patient is hyperglycemic, blood glucose should be lowered to 140 to 180 mg/dL. According to the AHA/ASA 2018 guidelines, hyperglycemia during the first 24 hours following ischemic stroke is associated with worse outcomes (Powers et al., 2018). If intravenous (IV) fluids are needed, only solutions without glucose are used, such as normal saline solution.

Patients suffering from a stroke can develop increased intracranial pressure (ICP), which further adds to brain damage. Stroke patients are also at risk for repeated strokes. Careful serial neurologic assessments and vital signs are needed to promptly detect and report changes.

Thrombolytic Therapy

Some patients with ischemic stroke may be candidates for **thrombolytic** therapy. This is a "clotbuster" medication (alteplase [tissue plasminogen activator; tPA]) that can lyse (or break down) a thrombus (clot) and potentially completely reverse stroke symptoms. tPA works best when administered within 3 to 4.5 hours of symptom onset, so it is only an option if the patient arrives at the ED quickly after symptoms begin. Some patients awaken after a night's sleep to discover they have had a stroke; their symptom onset is considered the time they went to bed, so they are not candidates for thrombolytic therapy.

Thrombolytic agents can lyse a thrombus by causing conversion of plasminogen to plasmin. Plasmin is the enzyme that causes thrombi to break down. Patients treated effectively with tPA may be able to leave the hospital within 1 or 2 days with no residual effects from the stroke. Thrombolytics are associated with a significant risk of hemorrhage, so all risk

of bleeding must be ruled out before these drugs will be considered. They are used very cautiously. If a patient is experiencing an ischemic stroke involving a large blood vessel of the brain, a stent-retrieval device might be used to remove any remnants of the thrombus after the tPA is used (AHA/ASA, 2017a). The device is inserted through the groin and advanced to the affected cerebral vessel.

> ### LEARNING TIP
>
> Remember: *Time lost is brain lost*. This means the faster the patient with a stroke receives treatment, the more brain (and brain function) that can be saved. Teaching your patients to recognize the signs and symptoms of a stroke and encouraging them to call 911 if needed could mean the difference between leading a normal life and total disability. **Act FAST!**

Pharmacological Management

Blood pressure control is vital for the stroke patient. Because of the lack of perfusion to certain areas of the brain, the body's response is to increase the systolic blood pressure to force blood into the affected areas. If the patient will receive tPA, the blood pressure must be maintained below 185/110 mm Hg to reduce the risk of bleeding (Powers et al., 2018). This is often done through the use of a beta blocker (labetalol) or calcium channel blocker (nicardipine), because of their fast-acting effects and ability to be given via IV. Table 49.2 lists medications commonly used for cerebrovascular disorders.

If tPA is not being given, the HCP may allow the blood pressure to remain high for a period of time to help salvage brain tissue, depending on the source of the stroke and location of the thrombus. This "permissive hypertension" helps blood travel through collateral blood vessels in the brain to reach the affected area. Antihypertensive agents should be given if the systolic pressure exceeds 220 mm Hg or the diastolic pressure exceeds 120 mm Hg (Bowry, Navalkele, & Gonzales, 2014).

Postemergent Care

Once emergent treatment is completed, medical management focuses on controlling the cause of the TIA or stroke. The results of the diagnostic tests help the HCP determine the course of treatment. If the patient has residual physical deficits, the HCP will order physical, occupational, and speech therapy consultations to evaluate the patient's functional status and make recommendations for further treatment and rehabilitation.

The AHA/ASA guidelines recommend that patients who have a minor stroke receive dual antiplatelet therapy with aspirin and clopidogrel (Plavix) within 24 hours of symptom

• WORD • BUILDING •
thrombolytic: thromb—clot + lytic—causing breakdown

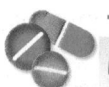

Table 49.2
Medications Used in Cerebrovascular Disorders

Medication Class/Action

Thrombolytic Agents

Dissolve existing clots.

Examples
alteplase (tissue plasminogen activator [tPA]; Activase)

Nursing Implications
Must be administered within 3 to 4.5 hours of symptom onset.
Monitor for bleeding

Antiplatelet Agents

Prevent formation of clots.

Examples
aspirin
clopidogrel (Plavix)
aspirin/dipyridamole (Aggrenox)

Nursing Implications
Monitor patient for bruising, change in level of consciousness, and prolonged bleeding time.

Anticoagulant Agents

Prolong time to form clots; prevent new clots.

Examples
warfarin (Coumadin)
heparin

Nursing Implications
Monitor patient for bruising, change in level of consciousness, and prolonged bleeding time.
For warfarin (Coumadin), monitor international normalized ratio (INR) frequently until therapeutic, and then monthly.

Cholesterol-Lowering Agents

Reduce cholesterol level.

Examples
simvastatin (Zocor)
pravastatin (Pravachol)
atorvastatin (Lipitor)
lovastatin (Mevacor)

Nursing Implications
Patient should notify health care provider if muscle pain or weakness occur.

---

onset (Powers et al., 2018). Decreasing platelet aggregation lessens the likelihood of another stroke. The patient in atrial fibrillation may also receive an anticoagulant to prevent thrombus development.

Cholesterol-lowering medication, preferably a statin, will be ordered for patients who have a low-density lipoprotein (LDL) cholesterol level greater than 100 mg/dL. This will also help minimize the development of atherosclerotic plaques. Statins also may have a neuroprotective effect and may further decrease risk of a stroke.

Deep vein **thrombosis** (DVT) is of concern when caring for patients who have had a stroke. The decrease in movement, confinement to a hospital bed, and hypercoagulable state all increase risk of DVT. Not only can DVTs cause severe pain and complications in the affected leg, but the thrombus can dislodge and travel to the lungs and cause a pulmonary embolism. Prevention involves anticoagulant medication or nondrug treatments such as sequential compression devices.

Stroke patients are at risk for respiratory complications for several reasons, such as an increase in ICP. Patients with stroke are prone to aspiration because of a decreased LOC and possibly impaired swallowing ability. Patients should be orally suctioned as needed to keep the airway clear. A patient who vomits should be turned to the side to reduce the risk of aspiration. Oral feedings should be started carefully and progressed slowly. Feedings should begin only after the patient is alert and the ability to swallow safely has been determined by an appropriate swallowing evaluation.

• WORD • BUILDING •
thrombosis: thromb—clot + osis—condition

Surgery

Patients with warning signs of stroke or patients who have been stabilized after a stroke may be candidates for surgery. In patients with significant carotid artery occlusion, a carotid **endarterectomy** may be performed. This involves a small incision in the neck and surgical removal of the occlusion from the artery.

Alternatively, a patient who is at high risk for complications with a carotid endarterectomy may have a carotid stent placed. This is placed during a carotid angiogram procedure. A catheter is advanced to the carotid artery, where a balloon is inflated to open the artery by pushing on the plaque. Then a stent (a tiny metal or polymer-based tube) is expanded inside the artery to keep it open and allow better blood flow to the brain. A risk from either procedure is an ischemic stroke.

CRITICAL THINKING

Mr. Jankowski, 56 years old, has been admitted to your orthopedic unit after knee surgery. While listening to his lungs at the start of the shift, you notice that his lung sounds are diminished. You ask whether he is a smoker and find that he has smoked for 40 years. You realize that his smoking history, postoperative status, and reduced mobility will all place Mr. Jankowski at risk for deep vein thrombosis and stroke.

1. What further data should you collect?
2. What preventive measures can you provide?
3. What resources can you provide to support smoking cessation?
4. What other interdisciplinary team members should you work with regarding your respiratory assessment?

Suggested answers are at the end of the chapter.

Prevention of Stroke

The incidence of stroke can be lessened by reducing risk factors (see Box 49-1). Keeping hypertension, cholesterol level, weight, and diabetes controlled can go a long way toward preventing strokes. Smoking cessation is essential. Emboli may be prevented with anticoagulants in people at high risk due to atrial fibrillation. Aspirin or other antiplatelet agents help prevent abnormal clotting.

It is important to educate all patients about new treatments for stroke and the potential for reversal of symptoms with the use of thrombolytic agents. Patients must be educated about risk factors for a stroke, warning signs, and the importance of immediate EMS transport if symptoms occur.

Long-Term Effects of Stroke
Impaired Motor Function and Sensation

Paresthesias and paralysis are common long-term effects of strokes that were not treated with a thrombolytic agent. The side of the body opposite the side of the cerebral infarct (contralateral side) is affected because nerve fibers cross over as they pass from the brain to the spinal cord (Fig. 49.5). Paralysis on one side of the body is called **hemiplegia** (Fig. 49.6). The affected limbs may be weak or totally paralyzed (flaccid). The arm or leg may be weaker, depending on the artery affected. These patients are particularly prone to contractures, which cause permanent immobility of a muscle or joint from fibrosis of connective tissue. Adaptation or assistance with activities of daily living (ADLs) is required.

Patients should be mobilized within 24 hours if possible to prevent complications of immobility. Physical and occupational therapy are provided to maximize functioning and to progress the patient toward a return to baseline functioning.

Motor involvement also often affects swallowing and control of urination and bowel function. Sensation changes may prevent the patient from being aware of pressure, temperature, or injuries on the affected side. Patients must be taught to be aware of these changes and protect the involved limbs.

APHASIA. If a stroke affects the temporal lobe region, especially on the dominant side, the speech center will likely be affected. Aphasia can be expressive, receptive, or global, as described earlier. Patients may be able to say words but be unable to form coherent speech, such as the patient who picks up a fork but calls it a comb. If a patient does not understand what is said, avoid the temptation to speak louder to try to help the patient understand. Remember that it is not the patient's hearing that is affected. Be patient and understanding as the patient tries to communicate. Speech therapy can help the patient relearn to communicate. See the "Nursing Process for the Patient With a Cerebrovascular Disorder" section for interventions for the aphasic patient.

Pseudobulbar Affect

Pseudobulbar affect (PBA) can manifest as emotional lability, or instability, and is a common consequence of stroke. Patients may move rapidly from profound sadness to an almost euphoric state and back again. Laughing or crying may have no relationship to the patient's situation at any given moment. Families can be upset by this behavior because they do not understand why a once happy person is now crying all the time or why the patient laughs inappropriately. You can help by explaining that these responses probably do not reflect how the patient is feeling but rather are caused by the stroke damage. Dextromethorphan/quinidine (Nuedexta) can reduce these symptoms.

Impaired Judgment

All patients who have had a stroke, in particular those with right-sided lesions, present a high safety risk. Patients may have poor understanding of their own limitations and believe

• WORD • BUILDING •

endarterectomy: endo—inside + arter—artery + ectomy—surgical removal of

hemiplegia: hemi—one side + plegia—paralysis

Left-side infarct

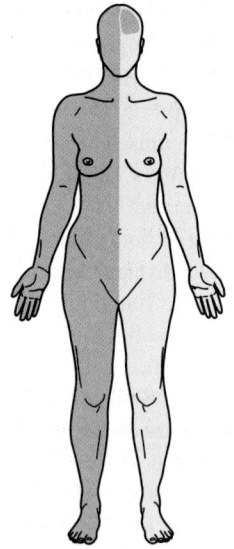

Right-side infarct

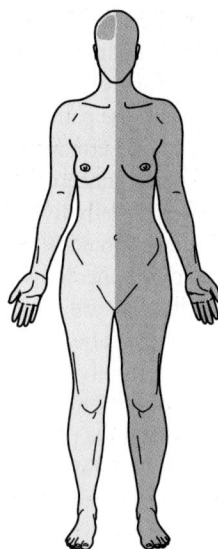

Right-sided weakness or paralysis
Aphasia (in left–brain-dominant clients)
Depression related to disability common

Left-sided weakness or paralysis
Impaired judgment/safety risk
Unilateral neglect more common
Indifferent to disability

FIGURE 49.5 The side opposite the infarct is affected by a stroke.

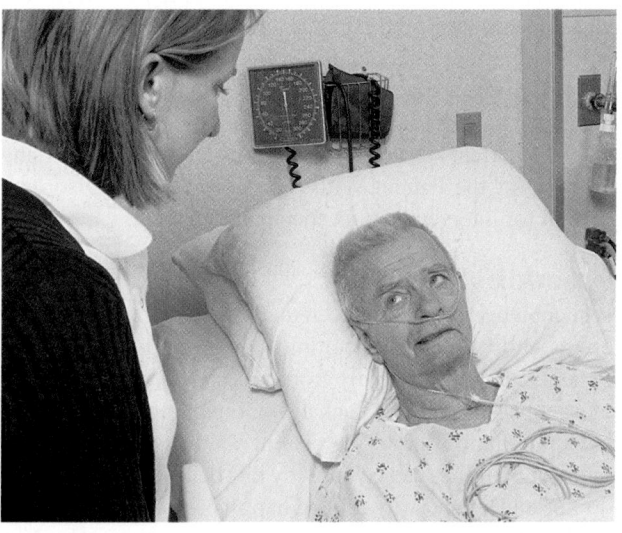
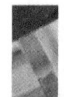

FIGURE 49.6 Hemiplegia: Note the left-sided weakness in this man's smile as result of a stroke.

that they are capable of performing tasks they did before the stroke. Those with left-sided lesions are more likely to be hesitant even to try performing ADLs. These generalizations may be the opposite if the individual is predominantly left-handed. Precautions must be taken to protect the patient from injury.

If the frontal lobes are involved, learned social behaviors may be lost. The patient may undress in public, use profanity, or make inappropriate sexual advances. These behaviors are extremely difficult for family members to cope with. Education and emotional support for significant others are essential. Allowing them to talk about their frustration and anger may

facilitate coping. Distracting the patient from inappropriate behavior may help. The patient should not be reprimanded or punished because he or she no longer has the cognitive ability to control the behaviors.

Unilateral Neglect

The phenomenon of unilateral neglect is seen predominantly in patients who have right hemisphere infarcts. It has been estimated to affect up to 30% of all patients who have had a stroke. These patients do not acknowledge the left side of their environment and may not even be aware of their own body on the affected side. Safety is a primary consideration. Essential items such as the call light and telephone should be placed on the patient's right side. Position the bed so the patient's right side is toward the door. Treatment should focus on providing stimuli to all senses on the patient's affected side and teaching the patient to focus on the left side. This involves teaching the patient to purposefully check where the left limbs are positioned and to look for safety risks. The patient can learn to turn his or her head and scan the environment. Patients may also need reminders to accomplish simple tasks, such as turning their plates during meals to recognize the food on the left side of the plate.

Other Long-Term Effects

The stroke patient may experience other complications after the acute phase of the stroke has passed. These include pneumonia, DVT, pulmonary embolism, pressure injuries, malnutrition, and depression. For the homeward-bound patient, education for the patient and family regarding prevention and recognition of these complications will assist the patient in a successful recovery. If a patient needs to receive rehabilitation in a skilled nursing facility, prevention of these issues will be a part of the care plan at the facility. For more information, visit the National Stroke Association at www.stroke.org or the American Stroke Association at www.strokeassociation.org.

CEREBRAL ANEURYSM, SUBARACHNOID HEMORRHAGE, AND INTRACRANIAL HEMORRHAGE

A cerebral aneurysm is a weakness in the wall of a cerebral artery. It may be congenital, traumatic, or the result of disease. If the aneurysm ruptures, the result is often a subarachnoid hemorrhage. It is unknown what causes the formation of congenital aneurysms or what causes them to rupture. Unruptured aneurysms are typically asymptomatic. The exception is a very large aneurysm, which can cause symptoms similar to a brain tumor. Aneurysms can affect children and young, otherwise healthy adults.

Pathophysiology and Etiology

Aneurysms can occur in any of the cerebral arteries, although most occur in the circle of Willis. The most common site is at the bifurcation of an artery. It is theorized that increased turbulence at the bifurcation can cause an outpouching of a congenitally weak arterial wall.

Subarachnoid hemorrhage is the collection of blood beneath the arachnoid mater following aneurysm rupture. Rupture of an arteriovenous malformation or head trauma may also result in subarachnoid hemorrhage (Fig. 49.7). The presence of blood outside the blood vessels is very irritating to brain tissue. It is believed that irritation from blood breakdown is the major cause of vasospasm, a common complication of subarachnoid hemorrhage.

It is unclear what causes an aneurysm to rupture. Some people develop a subarachnoid hemorrhage while performing the Valsalva maneuver, engaging in sexual activity, or physically exerting themselves. For others, the aneurysm ruptures during a quiet, inactive period. If the aneurysm rupture is associated with a particular activity, the patient may be very frightened of engaging in that activity again. This may have a negative effect on the patient's interpersonal relationships if the associated activity was sexual in nature. The patient's partner may feel guilty or responsible for the hemorrhage. Education, emotional support, and confidentiality are essential to help both the patient and significant other.

Signs and Symptoms

Some patients experience a small hemorrhage before diagnosis of subarachnoid hemorrhage. This leakage of blood may cause a mild headache, vomiting, or disorientation. The symptoms may be attributed to a flu-like syndrome. Patients may dismiss the symptoms and not seek medical care.

The most common presentation of rupture of an aneurysm is sudden onset of a severe headache. Typically, a patient will state, "I have never had a headache this bad in my life." Patients may hold their heads and moan or cry in pain. Sensitivity to light is a common finding. This may make patients reluctant to cooperate with pupil examinations.

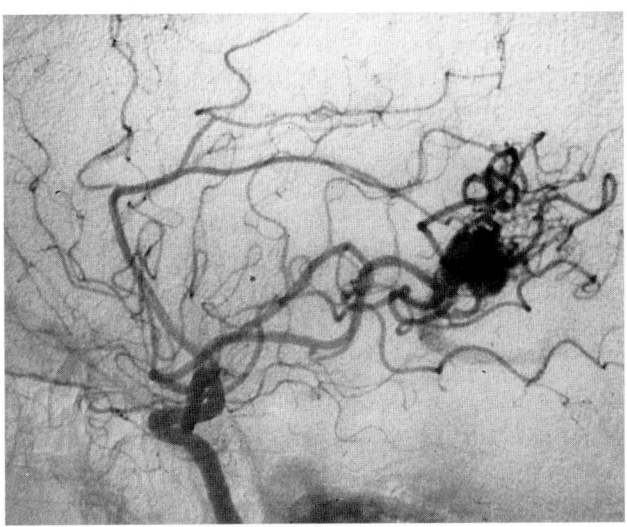

FIGURE 49.7 Arteriovenous malformation. Note tangled vessels.

LOC varies based on the severity of the hemorrhage. Patients may be alert and coherent, lose consciousness immediately, or gradually become less responsive. The decreased LOC is caused by ICP and impairment of cerebral blood flow. Patients may experience generalized seizures.

Blood in the subarachnoid space causes meningeal irritation. The patient may exhibit nuchal rigidity. The most commonly affected cranial nerves are III and VI. This is manifested as an enlarged pupil or abnormal gaze. Motor dysfunction may involve one or both limbs on the side opposite the hemorrhage.

Diagnostic Tests

Because of the severe nature of the symptoms, patients with subarachnoid hemorrhage almost always come to the ED rather than seeking care from a primary HCP. A CT scan or MRI is done to identify and locate a hemorrhage. Precise diagnosis of an aneurysm requires a cerebral angiogram. The contrast material fills the aneurysm if one exists. For a patient with a severe headache facing a life-threatening illness, this test can be very frightening. If the patient's neurologic status does not allow him or her to cooperate, sedation may be required before and during the examination.

Therapeutic Measures

Patients with subarachnoid hemorrhage are cared for in an intensive care unit (ICU) setting. They typically have an arterial line and a central venous pressure monitoring catheter. Blood pressure is carefully monitored because high pressures increase the risk of re-rupture of the aneurysm and low pressures can be associated with ischemia. Values outside parameters identified by the HCP are reported. Typically, the systolic blood pressure is kept between 120 and 160 mm Hg. Vasoactive drugs may be required to maintain blood pressure within the prescribed parameters.

There is no cure for subarachnoid hemorrhage. Treatment consists of correcting the cause of the hemorrhage if possible. Preventing or managing complications and providing supportive care are important aspects of nursing care.

Surgical Management

Definitive treatment of the aneurysm involves performing a craniotomy and exposing the aneurysm. If the aneurysm has a neck (berry aneurysm), it is identified and clamped with a metal clip (Fig. 49.8). An aneurysm without a neck may be wrapped with a sterile plastic or muslin wrap. This provides stability to the aneurysm walls, lessening the chance of rupture. In some situations, it is possible to clamp the artery on either side of the aneurysm, removing that portion of the vessel, and the aneurysm, from the circulation. After the removal, the ends are reconnected to maintain blood flow.

Nonsurgical Management

Nonsurgical intervention may be provided for aneurysms that are inoperable because of size, configuration, or the patient's medical status. A foreign material such as a metallic or

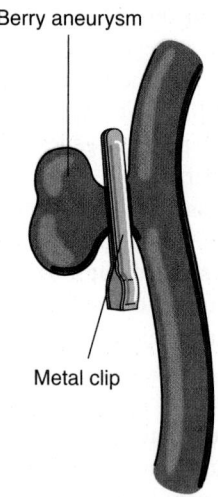

FIGURE 49.8 Surgical management of aneurysms.

polymer-based coil may be introduced into the aneurysm. A thrombus develops around the foreign body and, if the treatment is successful, occludes the aneurysm. The goal is to fill the aneurysm enough to prevent blood flowing into it, without causing rupture.

Complications
Rebleeding
Recurrent rupture of a cerebral aneurysm carries significant morbidity and mortality rates. Patients are at risk for rebleeding until the aneurysm is surgically repaired. If the aneurysm is wrapped or embolized, there is a risk of rebleeding, but risk is much lower than if the aneurysm is left untreated.

Hydrocephalus
Blood in the ventricular system interferes with the circulation and reabsorption of cerebrospinal fluid (CSF), and hydrocephalus can develop. Early in the course of subarachnoid hemorrhage, an external ventricular drain may be used to treat hydrocephalus.

About 25% of patients with subarachnoid hemorrhage require placement of a ventriculoperitoneal shunt to treat hydrocephalus (Fig. 49.9). This surgical procedure involves placement of a catheter into a ventricle in the brain. The catheter is then connected to a valve, which regulates the rate of CSF drainage. Another catheter connects to the valve and is passed down to the peritoneal cavity. The CSF drains out of the peritoneal catheter and is absorbed into the peritoneal cavity.

Vasospasm
Vasospasm is responsible for most long-term complications of subarachnoid hemorrhage. Vasospasm causes a blood vessel's diameter to narrow. Although it typically begins in the vessel, giving rise to the aneurysm, vasospasm may spread to other vessels. This explains why the ischemia or infarct caused by vasospasm can be so widespread and devastating.

The long-term complications of subarachnoid hemorrhage are similar to those of stroke.

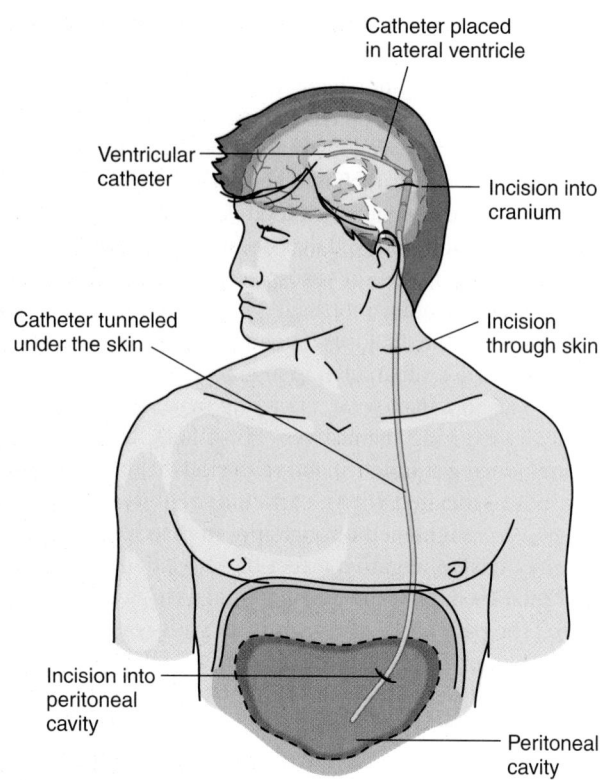

FIGURE 49.9 A ventriculoperitoneal shunt drains cerebrospinal fluid into the peritoneal cavity.

Rehabilitation
If the patient can tolerate intensive therapy, discharge from the hospital to a rehabilitation center may occur. Rehabilitation and long-term care are similar whether the patient

CRITICAL THINKING

Mrs. Washington is a 68-year-old African American woman and retired office worker. She was admitted to your unit after a right-sided intracerebral hemorrhage. Her daughter states that Mrs. Washington has taken antihypertensive medication for the past 20 years. However, she states that her mother has been forgetful lately, and that there are five more pills in the medicine bottle than expected. On admission, Mrs. Washington is oriented only to person and has hemiparesis.

1. What may have precipitated Mrs. Washington's stroke?
2. On which side do you expect Mrs. Washington's extremities to be affected?
3. List two safety concerns and strategies to promote patient safety.
4. List at least two educational needs for Mrs. Washington and her daughter.
5. What health care providers are important in the interdisciplinary team caring for Mrs. Washington? What is the role of nursing on this team?

   Suggested answers are at the end of the chapter.

has had an aneurysm, intracerebral bleed, or an ischemic stroke.

 NURSING PROCESS FOR THE PATIENT WITH A CEREBROVASCULAR DISORDER

Data Collection

Observe the patient for signs and symptoms of decreased cerebral tissue perfusion. These include decreased LOC, irritability or restlessness, dizziness, syncope, blurred or dimmed vision, **diplopia** (double vision), change in visual fields, unequal pupils or a sluggish or absent pupillary reaction to light, paresthesias, motor weakness, paralysis, or seizures. Reassess frequently and report any change or decline. Monitor vital signs and oxygen levels. Monitor laboratory tests, including CBC, lipid profile, and INR/PT if the patient takes warfarin (Coumadin). Perform a routine respiratory assessment. Monitor lung sounds for adventitious sounds or a change in breath sounds. Assess pain level. Assess swallowing ability before offering oral intake. Promptly report any changes in vital signs, laboratory values, respiratory function, or neurologic status.

Nursing Diagnoses, Planning, and Implementation

See "Nursing Care Plan for the Patient With Stroke" for nursing diagnoses during acute care. Possible postacute nursing diagnoses are listed next with outcomes and interventions.

Impaired Physical Mobility related to decreased motor function

EXPECTED OUTCOME: The patient will maintain physical mobility as evidenced by maximum physical mobility within limitations of deficits. The patient will not experience complications related to immobility.

- Consult physical and occupational therapists *to assess the patient's abilities and make specific recommendations related to mobility.*
- Discuss use of constraint therapy with physical and occupational therapists. *Constraint therapy forces the use of the affected limbs by restraining the unaffected side.*
- Maintain the patient in correct body alignment *to prevent contractures and promote comfort.*
- Support affected extremities with pillows *to prevent dislocation injuries and promote comfort.*
- Perform range-of-motion exercises as prescribed by the physical therapist *to prevent contractures and atrophy.*
- Follow physical/occupational therapy recommendations for being up in chair or ambulation. *Prolonged bedrest is associated with complications and poor outcomes.*
- If the patient is unable to get out of bed, turn and reposition at least every 2 hours *to prevent skin, respiratory, and musculoskeletal complications.*

Evidence-Based Practice

Clinical Question
What are priorities for nursing care of stoke patients?

Evidence
A review of 65 articles, including 12 systematic reviews, looked at priority nursing interventions to improve outcomes for patients following strokes (Theofanidis & Gibbon, 2016).

Implications for Nursing Practice
Strong evidence was found for nursing interventions (that can be accomplished by the licensed practical nurse/licensed vocation nurse): monitoring blood pressure and reporting blood pressure exceeding 185/110; monitoring temperature and treating with acetaminophen if it is over 99.5°F (37.5°C); requesting a swallowing evaluation within 24 hours of admission; and monitoring blood glucose and reporting elevated results. Additional interventions can be found in the referenced article.

Reference
Theofanidis, D., & Gibbon, B. (2016). Nursing interventions in stroke care delivery: An evidence-based clinical review. *Journal of Vascular Nursing, 34*(4), 144–151. doi:10.1016/j.jvn.2016.07.001

Imbalanced Nutrition: Less Than Body Requirements related to impaired swallowing and motor deficits

EXPECTED OUTCOME: The patient will maintain adequate nutrition without aspiration as evidenced by stable weight at appropriate level for height and no signs of aspiration.

- Keep patient NPO (nothing by mouth) until swallowing can be evaluated *to prevent aspiration.*
- Perform dysphagia screening. *This quick assessment can identify problems before a complete evaluation can be done.*
  - Observe for facial weakness or inability to completely close mouth.
  - Ask patient to stick out tongue and move it side to side.
  - Observe for drooling.
- If swallowing appears to be intact, have the patient swallow a sip of water from a cup before offering other foods or fluids. Observe for coughing, choking, or noisy lung sounds. *These are signs of difficulty swallowing.*
- Request speech pathologist evaluation if indicated *to diagnose specific swallowing problems and make recommendations.*

• WORD • BUILDING •
diplopia: diplo—double + opia—sight

Nursing Care Plan for the Patient With Stroke

Nursing Diagnosis: *Risk for Ineffective Cerebral Tissue Perfusion* related to interruption of blood supply
Expected Outcomes: The patient will experience improved cerebral tissue perfusion as evidenced by absence of or reduction in dizziness, syncope, and visual disturbances; improved level of consciousness; pupils equal and reactive to light; and improved motor and sensory function.
Evaluation of Outcomes: Are the patient's symptoms of ineffective perfusion improving?

Intervention	Rationale	Evaluation
Monitor neurologic status at least every 30 minutes initially and then every 4 hours or as ordered. Report changes.	*A change in status could indicate decreased perfusion.*	Is there a change in neurologic status since the previous documented assessment?
Assess vital signs every 30 minutes initially and then every 4 hours or as ordered.	*High or low blood pressure can lead to decreased tissue perfusion and recurrent stroke. Temperature above 99.6°F can worsen ischemic injury to brain tissue.*	Are vital signs within normal limits? Are changes reported?
Monitor oxygen saturation and administer oxygen as ordered for peripheral oxygen saturation (Spo$_2$) less than 92%.	*Hypoxemia can increase brain damage.*	Is Spo$_2$ 92% or greater?
Monitor blood glucose as ordered and report value greater than 140 mg/dL.	*Elevated glucose is associated with worsening of infarct and hemorrhage.*	Is glucose level greater than 140 mg/dL? Was health care provider (HCP) notified?
Keep head of bed elevated 20 to 30 degrees. Keep neck in neutral position.	*This facilitates venous return and reduces risk of cerebral edema.*	Is head of bed elevated? Is neck in neutral position?
Monitor medication for therapeutic and nontherapeutic effects. Monitor coagulation studies if appropriate.	*Anticoagulant therapy must be closely monitored to make sure it is at a therapeutic level and not increasing risk for bleeding.*	Are coagulation studies within normal or therapeutic ranges? Are signs of bleeding present?

Nursing Diagnosis: *Ineffective Airway Clearance* related to stasis of secretions associated with decreased mobility and poor cough effort and airway obstruction resulting from tongue falling back in throat
Expected Outcome: The patient will maintain an open airway as evidenced by respirations quiet and unlabored, 12 to 20 per minute, with Spo$_2$ greater than 92%.
Evaluation of Outcome: Are respirations quiet, 12 to 20 per minute, with Spo$_2$ greater than 92%?

Intervention	Rationale	Evaluation
Monitor lung sounds, cough, and respirations.	*Assessment provides the basis for intervention.*	Are lung sounds clear? Is cough effective? Are respirations quiet and easy?
Position the patient to maintain an open airway.	*Side lying may keep tongue from obstructing airway.*	Is patient positioned to keep airway clear?
Consult with registered nurse or HCP about an oral airway if airway is not clear.	*An oral airway will keep tongue from obstructing airway if needed.*	Is an airway indicated?
Encourage patient to deep breathe and cough if able.	*Coughing and deep breathing will help clear secretions from airway and prevent atelectasis.*	Is patient able to deep breathe and cough? Is cough effective?

Nursing Care Plan for the Patient With Stroke—cont'd

Intervention	Rationale	Evaluation
If cough is ineffective, suction as needed.	*Suctioning may be needed if patient is unable to swallow secretions or cough effectively.*	Is suctioning indicated? Is airway clear after suctioning?

Nursing Diagnosis: *Risk for Injury* related to seizure, repeat stroke, or hemorrhage secondary to thrombolytic therapy
Expected Outcome: The patient will remain free from injury.
Evaluation of Outcome: Is the patient free from injury? Are problems recognized and reported quickly?

Intervention	Rationale	Evaluation
Monitor neurologic status frequently and report changes promptly.	*Prompt recognition of a repeat stroke is essential.*	Are neurologic checks within normal limits? Are changes reported promptly?
Monitor for signs of hemorrhage for 24 to 36 hours following thrombolytic therapy.	*Hemorrhage is the most common side effect of thrombolytic therapy.*	Are signs of hemorrhage present? Are they reported promptly?
Administer anticonvulsant agent as ordered.	*Patient is at increased risk for seizures following a stroke.*	Is patient seizure free?
Implement seizure precautions (see Chapter 48).	*Precautions help protect patient in event of a seizure.*	Are precautions in place and patient protected? Is patient assisted with mobility?
Assist with transfers and ambulation.	*Patient is at risk for falls because of motor and sensory deficits and impaired judgment.*	Is patient able to call for help when needed?

• Implement measures to prevent aspiration. *Aspiration can lead to pneumonia, which will greatly complicate the patient's recovery.*
• Stay with the patient during meals.
• Ensure that the patient is fully alert before feeding.
• Place the patient in high-Fowler position or chair for meals.
• Avoid use of straws.
• Use a thickening agent if swallowing study recommends.
• Place food on unaffected side of mouth.
• Teach the patient to swallow twice after each bite.
• Check the patient's mouth for pocketing of food.
• Have suction equipment available.
• Notify HCP if patient is unable to take in adequate oral calories. *A feeding tube may be needed if the patient cannot take in enough calories to maintain nutrition. Advance directives should be consulted before a feeding tube is placed.*
• Assist with insertion and care of feeding tube if needed. *If the patient cannot swallow effectively, a feeding tube may be needed to maintain nutrition.*

See "Nutrition Notes" and Chapter 47 for additional interventions.

Nutrition Notes

Feeding Patients With Swallowing Disorders. Swallowing disorders (dysphagia) may occur when an individual suffers from nervous system disorders such as stroke. When dysphagia is suspected, a speech pathologist is consulted to perform comprehensive tests of an individual's ability to swallow foods and liquids. A diet prescription is recommended that includes the appropriate texture of foods (e.g., regular, soft, mechanically altered, pureed) and consistency of liquids (e.g., thin [water], nectar thick, or honey thick). Recommendations for body and head positioning while eating are also made by the speech pathologist.

Commercially prepared thickeners are designed to provide the appropriate thickness in liquids. The standardized "recipe" must be closely followed by a nurse or family member who has been properly trained and demonstrated competence. Pre-thickened liquids are available commercially in nectar and honey thick consistencies. Home recipes (e.g., using instant potato flakes or gelatin) should be avoided because it is difficult to be sure the thickness is appropriate for the patient.

Disturbed Sensory Perception related to central nervous system damage

EXPECTED OUTCOME: The patient will adapt to sensory-perceptual deficits as evidenced by avoidance of injury to affected areas.

- Assist the occupational therapist to assess for visual and/or spatial deficits and decreased sensory perception (heat and cold, position of body parts, pressure). *Identification of specific deficits is the first step in creating a plan of care.*
- Teach the patient to scan the environment *to compensate for a visual deficit.*
- Implement plans for skin integrity and mobility *to protect patient from complications related to sensory deficits.*

Risk for Impaired Skin Integrity (irritation or breakdown) related to immobility and incontinence

EXPECTED OUTCOME: The patient's skin integrity will be maintained as evidenced by absence of redness or breakdown.

- Examine the skin often for redness or breakdown, especially around bony prominences, dependent areas, and perineum. *Any signs of breakdown must be treated immediately to prevent further damage.*
- Thoroughly cleanse and dry the perineal area after each episode of incontinence. *Urine and feces can be very irritating to the skin.*
- If incontinence is unavoidable, use a barrier cream such as zinc oxide *to protect skin.*
- Turn and position the patient at least every 2 hours or more often if the patient experiences breakdown. *Pressure impairs circulation and increases risk of breakdown.*
- Use a lift sheet to move the patient in bed *to avoid damage from friction and shear.*
- Consider the use of a pressure-reducing mattress if the patient cannot be out of bed for long periods. *This helps reduce pressure but does not eliminate the need to reposition the patient every 2 hours.*
- If breakdown occurs, contact the HCP or wound care specialist *to obtain treatment recommendations.*

Incontinence (Bowel or Overflow Urinary or Functional Urinary) related to loss of voluntary control of elimination

EXPECTED OUTCOME: Episodes of incontinence are avoided, or, if unavoidable, they will be cleaned up quickly and skin complications avoided.

- Monitor for incontinence of bowel or bladder *so patient can be cleaned promptly and skin protected.*
- Determine usual pattern of urinary and bowel elimination. *Keeping the patient on his or her regular prehospitalization pattern may help prevent incontinence.*
- Provide assistance with toileting according to the patient's usual schedule. *The patient who is unable to get up unaided may wait too long for help or try to get up alone and be injured.*

- Respond quickly to requests for assistance with toileting *to avoid accidental incontinence.*

Self-Care Deficit (Bathing, Dressing, Feeding, Toileting) related to impaired motor function, spatial-perceptual alterations, and fear of injury

EXPECTED OUTCOME: Self-care will be accomplished as evidenced by the patient's ADL needs being met and the patient becoming increasingly independent.

- Determine the patient's ability to perform ADLs. *Good baseline data will guide development of a care plan.*
- Work with the patient to create a plan for meeting daily physical needs. *The patient will be more likely to participate in a plan if he or she participated in creating it.*
- Encourage the highest level of independence possible and facilitate the patient's ability to do ADLs. *Providing too much assistance can promote dependence and further loss of mobility.*
  - Place objects within reach and within visual field.
  - Place food/fluids within the patient's visual field.
  - Encourage use of assistive devices.
- Assist the patient with learning to use the nondominant side of body. *If the dominant side is affected, the patient may have to use the nondominant side.*
- Provide positive feedback *to help reduce discouragement with slow progress.*
- Provide education for family members and significant others regarding the patient's deficits and recovery plan. *The family can assist the patient with mobility if they understand what needs to be done.*

Impaired Verbal Communication (dysarthria) related to loss of motor function of the muscles of speech articulation or aphasia or dysphasia related to ischemia of the dominant hemisphere

EXPECTED OUTCOME: Communication needs will be met as evidenced by the patient communicating needs and desires effectively and by avoidance of frustration.

- Listen for difficulties in verbal communication (difficulty speaking, articulating or incorrect ordering of words, inability to find or name words and objects). *Good baseline data will guide planning of care.*
- Consult a speech pathologist for assistance in determining types of aphasia or dysphasia and need for follow-up treatment. *A speech pathologist is specially trained to diagnose and treat communication problems and can work with nursing staff to develop a plan of care.*
- Implement measures to facilitate communication. *These measures help ensure the patient has his or her immediate needs met while learning to adapt to communication impairment.*
  - Answer call light in person rather than over an intercom.
  - Assess needs frequently.
  - Listen carefully, and avoid interrupting the patient and allow ample time for communication.

- When the patient is tired, ask questions that require short answers.
- Provide appropriate aids to communication (picture board, magic slate, pencil and paper; Fig. 49.10).
- Provide education to family members and significant others regarding communication problems and interventions *so they can communicate with patient and participate in care.*
- If the patient is unable to communicate, do not assume that he or she cannot hear and understand. Make every effort to speak to the patient and to keep conversation appropriate when it is within the patient's range of hearing. *The patient may understand exactly what is being said, even if he or she is unable to respond.*
- Contact the HCP if impairment increases. *This may be a sign of stroke extension.*

Acute or Chronic Confusion related to cerebral ischemia

EXPECTED OUTCOME: The patient's thought processes will be as clear as possible within limitations of brain damage as evidenced by responses appropriate to situation; the patient's safety will be maintained, and the patient will feel calm and safe.

- Observe the patient for thought process impairment such as shortened attention span, impaired memory, confusion, slowed or quick and impulsive responses, and aggressive and/or inappropriate responses. *Disturbed thinking can be*

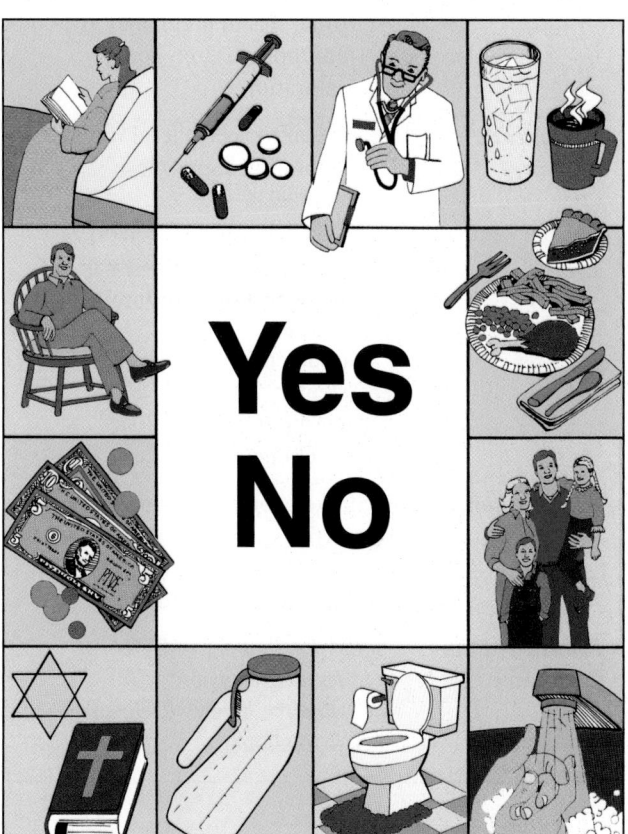

FIGURE 49.10 Picture board.

manifested in a variety of ways. See Chapter 48 for interventions for patients with disturbed thought processes.

Risk for Falls related to changes in mobility, sensation, or confusion

EXPECTED OUTCOME: The patient will remain safe and free from falls.

- Perform a fall risk assessment according to agency policy *to identify patients at risk.*
- Instruct the patient and family to call for help before the patient gets up *so staff can assist.*
- Keep call light and other essential items within the patient's reach *to prevent falls while trying to access needed items.*
- Provide frequent toileting. *Patients often fall while getting up to use the toilet.*
- Avoid restraints if at all possible. *Restraints are associated with injuries.*

Deficient Knowledge related to diagnosis and treatment

EXPECTED OUTCOME: The patient and family will have the necessary knowledge to make decisions and assist with care.

- Explain what has happened to the patient. Explain tests, procedures, and care activities. *The patient and his or her family members are likely to be very frightened about what is happening. Providing correct information about what a stroke is, tests and procedures, and rationale for care activities helps reduce anxiety.*
- Present information in small amounts and as simply as possible. *The patient may have difficulty managing large amounts of information while acutely ill or if confusion is present.*
- Orient the patient and family to the ICU or other setting and the constant monitoring provided. *This can help reduce anxiety and reassure the patient and family that the patient is receiving competent care.*
- If the patient is to be discharged to home, make sure information is provided related to medications, treatments, and follow-up care. *The patient and family need to know how to provide appropriate care at home.*
- Evaluate the need for home health care nursing, physical therapy, and occupational therapy, and request appropriate referrals. *The patient will likely need continued therapy after discharge to regain as much function as possible.*

Risk for Caregiver Role Strain related to changes in roles, responsibilities, finances, and intimacy

EXPECTED OUTCOME: The caregiver will be comfortable with his or her role as evidenced by a statement that she or he understands how to care for the patient and has the needed resources to do so. The caregiver will maintain her or his own health.

- Work with caregivers to identify how the patient's functional level will affect their lives. *Assumption of roles or responsibilities previously fulfilled by the patient may be very stressful to family members. If the caregiver can anticipate the impact, he or she can plan ahead regarding how to make sure needs are met.*

- Encourage the patient and caregiver to identify support systems and make use of community resources.
- Provide a list of resources. *If support is in place before discharge, caregivers are more likely to use it after the patient goes home.*
- Consult a social worker or case manager. *These individuals have access to many resources and can help the patient and caregiver identify appropriate sources of assistance, including a caregiver support group.*
- Provide support if transfer to a skilled nursing facility is needed. *This can be a very difficult decision for a patient and caregiver.*

Evaluation

If interventions have been effective, the patient will not experience increased deficits due to decreased perfusion of brain cells. The patient will recover as much physical ability as possible and adjust to remaining deficits to meet self-care needs. Basic needs, including safety, elimination, nutrition, and skin integrity, will be met by the patient or caregiver. The patient will be able to communicate effectively and have needs and desires understood. Caregivers will identify support systems available to help. Table 49.3 provides a summary on stroke.

Home Health Hints

- Referrals to physical, occupational, and speech therapies are often appropriate for patients during rehabilitation. Therapists can make recommendations for assistive devices that can promote the patient's independence. A home health care aid, homemaker, and respite worker may also be needed during the early stages of rehabilitation, especially if the caregiver is an elderly spouse.
- The home health care nurse can help the patient progress toward his or her goals by encouraging compliance with home exercise programs and offering frequent praise for all achievements.
- Teach the patient and caregiver to keep the home environment free of clutter to prevent falls.
- Teach the patient and caregiver that a portable phone and other frequently used items can be kept in a bag attached to the patient's walker. In the event of a fall, a portable phone can be used to call for help if the patient is unable to purchase a medical alert button.
- Teach caregivers and patients that a pureed diet can be made at home using a food processor. Baby food can also be purchased to meet swallowing guidelines.
- Teach patients to wear clothes that are easy to get on and off and shoes that fasten with Velcro.
- Teach patients and caregivers that a bedside commode cover can be kept up for easy access, with patches of Velcro attached to the seat and the frame.

Table 49.3
Stroke Summary

Signs and Symptoms	Dizziness Syncope Visual disturbances Irritability, restlessness, confusion Decreased level of consciousness Unequal pupils Paresthesias Motor weakness Paralysis Seizures Difficulty swallowing, understanding language, speaking
Diagnostic Tests	Computed tomography scan, magnetic resonance imaging MRI Electrocardiogram Carotid Doppler Echocardiogram Cerebral angiogram Laboratory: international normalized ratio/prothrombin time, metabolic panel, glucose, complete blood count, partial thromboplastin time, serum pregnancy (if appropriate), oxygen saturation
Therapeutic Measures	Oxygen for peripheral oxygen saturation (Spo_2) less than 92% Antiplatelet, anticoagulant, or thrombolytic medication Physical, occupational, or speech therapy Carotid endarterectomy or stent Knee-high antiembolism stockings
Complications	Stroke evolves, causing more deficits, aspiration pneumonia, skin breakdown, urinary tract infection, malnutrition
Priority Nursing Diagnoses	*Risk for Ineffective Cerebral Tissue Perfusion* *Ineffective Airway Clearance* *Risk for Injury*

SUGGESTED ANSWERS TO CRITICAL THINKING

Mr. Jankowski

1. Ask Mr. Jankowski about other risk factors for stroke, such as his dietary and alcohol habits. Check his chart for history of diabetes, hypertension, or heart disease. Check his weight and cholesterol levels if drawn. Educate him about risk factors for stroke and how they can be modified. Use the Stroke Risk Scorecard and teach him the FAST acronym (see Fig. 49.2). As a nurse, you will be in a position to recognize risks and help patients modify risk factors for many problems before they occur.

2. Discuss use of an anticoagulant agent or sequential compression device with the registered nurse (RN) or health care provider (HCP).

3. Provide written or audiovisual information on stroke prevention and smoking cessation. Ask the HCP about use of a nicotine patch or other medication for smoking cessation, if Mr. Jankowski is willing.

4. Involve a dietitian for dietary counseling if indicated. Consult the smoking cessation coordinator at your agency if one is on staff.

Mrs. Washington

1. Uncontrolled hypertension, in the presence of a pre-existing aneurysm, might have precipitated Mrs. Washington's stroke.

2. Her left extremities will be affected.

3. Mrs. Washington is disoriented. Her room should be as close to the nurse's station as possible. Reorient her to her surroundings and condition frequently. Keep side rails up when Mrs. Washington is alone. Mrs. Washington also has hemiparesis. Obtain a bedside commode because Mrs. Washington will probably not be able to walk to the bathroom. Place the call light and telephone on her right side. Assist Mrs. Washington with positioning to prevent injury to her affected limbs.

4. If Mrs. Washington will be going back to her home, you should teach her and her daughter about the relationship of uncontrolled hypertension to intracranial hemorrhage; options for inpatient, outpatient, and in-home therapy; and memory strategies to prevent missed medication doses (e.g., weekly pill box, keeping medications with breakfast food, or an alarm clock or watch).

5. The HCP directs the medical care, but often it is the nurse (typically an RN) who oversees the multidisciplinary team and ensures that everything is being done as ordered. Other important team members include the case manager or discharge planner; dietitian, physical, occupational, and speech therapists; as well as pastoral care if the patient desires.

Review Questions

1. Which of the following are modifiable risk factors that should be taught to patients at risk for stroke? **Select all that apply.**
   1. Heredity
   2. Age
   3. Diabetes
   4. Race
   5. High cholesterol
   6. Obesity

2. What interventions can help prevent aspiration in a post-stroke patient with dysphagia? **Select all that apply.**
   1. Ensure that the patient is fully alert before feeding.
   2. Place the patient in high-Fowler position or chair for meals.
   3. Use straws for thin liquids.
   4. Use a thickening agent.
   5. Place food on affected side of mouth.

3. How soon after symptom onset must a person who is having a stroke receive thrombolytic therapy?
   1. 30 minutes
   2. 1 hour
   3. 2 hours
   4. 4.5 hours

4. Which is the best method for the nurse to use to communicate with the patient experiencing receptive aphasia?
   1. Be patient as the patient tries to speak.
   2. Listen carefully, while making eye contact.
   3. Speak loudly toward the patient's good side.
   4. Use gestures, standing where the patient can see.

5. A nurse is caring for a patient who is recovering from an ischemic stroke. Upon entering the room to pick up the supper tray, the nurse notes that the patient has only eaten food on the left side of the tray. What should the nurse do?
   1. Turn the plate 180 degrees and observe the patient's response.
   2. Remove the tray and do not comment.
   3. Encourage the patient to eat the rest of the meal.
   4. Assist the patient by providing finger foods and feeding the patient items that require a utensil.

6. A nurse is doing an afternoon assessment on a patient transferred to a medical unit from intensive care following a subarachnoid hemorrhage. The patient was alert and oriented during the morning assessment but reported being very tired. Now the patient is difficult to arouse. What action should the nurse take?
   1. Let the patient sleep; transferring from the intensive care unit can be very strenuous.
   2. Reassess the patient in an hour. If the sleepiness continues, notify the registered nurse.
   3. Call the registered nurse immediately.
   4. Call a code.

Answer rationales available in your online resources.

ANSWERS 1. 3, 5, 6; 2. 1, 2, 4; 3. 4; 4. 5, 1; 6. 3

Key Points

Find the chapter key points in your online resources available through Davis Edge.

Additional Resources

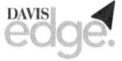 Use the scratch off code on the inside front cover of your book to access online quizzes that will help you to improve your scores on course exams and prepare for the NCLEX-PN®.

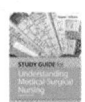 Study Guide

CHAPTER 50

Nursing Care of Patients With Peripheral Nervous System Disorders

Deborah L. Weaver, Linda K. Cook

KEY TERMS

amyotrophic (ay-MY-oh-TROH-fik)
anticholinesterase (AN-tee-KOH-lin-ESS-ter-ays)
atrophy (A-troh-fee)
demyelination (dee-MY-uh-lin-AY-shun)
fasciculation (fah-SIK-yoo-LAY-shun)
neuralgia (new-RAL-jee-ah)
neuropathies (new-ROP-uh-thees)
plasmapheresis (PLAZ-mah-fer-EE-sis)
ptosis (TOH-sis)
remyelination (ree-MY-uh-lin-AY-shun)
sclerosis (skleh-ROH-sis)

CHAPTER CONCEPTS

Mobility
Neurologic Regulation
Sensory Perception

LEARNING OUTCOMES

1. Identify disorders that are caused by disruption of the peripheral nervous system.
2. Explain the pathophysiology, major signs and symptoms, and complications of selected peripheral nervous system disorders.
3. Identify therapeutic measures used for selected peripheral nervous system disorders.
4. List common nursing diagnoses associated with peripheral nervous system disorders.
5. Plan prioritized nursing interventions for patients with peripheral nervous system disorders.
6. Evaluate the effectiveness of nursing care.

The peripheral nervous system (PNS) consists of all nervous system structures outside the central nervous system (CNS). A variety of disorders affect the PNS. Some of these disorders become chronic and cause degeneration of body systems, while others are more temporary. Two common types of PNS disorders are discussed in this chapter. The first type is neuromuscular disorders, which can include motor or sensory disorders or both. The second type is cranial nerve disorders. Both types of disorders present a challenge to the nurse caring for the patient and family.

NEUROMUSCULAR DISORDERS

Neuromuscular disorders are chronic and degenerative in nature. They involve a disruption of impulse transmission between neurons and the muscles they stimulate, resulting in muscle weakness. If the muscles of the respiratory system are affected, deadly complications can develop, including pneumonia and respiratory failure. Common neuromuscular

disorders include multiple sclerosis, myasthenia gravis, amyotrophic lateral sclerosis, and Guillain-Barré syndrome.

Multiple Sclerosis

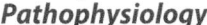

Pathophysiology

Multiple **sclerosis** (MS) is a chronic progressive degenerative disease that affects the myelin sheath of the neurons in the CNS. Myelin is responsible for the smooth transmission of nerve impulses. In MS, the myelin sheath begins to break down (Fig. 50.1) as a result of activation of the body's immune system. The affected nerves become inflamed and edematous, which interrupts impulses to the muscles. As the disease progresses, sclerosis or scar tissue damages the nerves. Nerve impulses can become completely blocked, causing permanent loss of muscle function in that area of the body.

Etiology

The cause of MS is not really understood. Damage to the myelin sheath is thought to be from an autoimmune process;

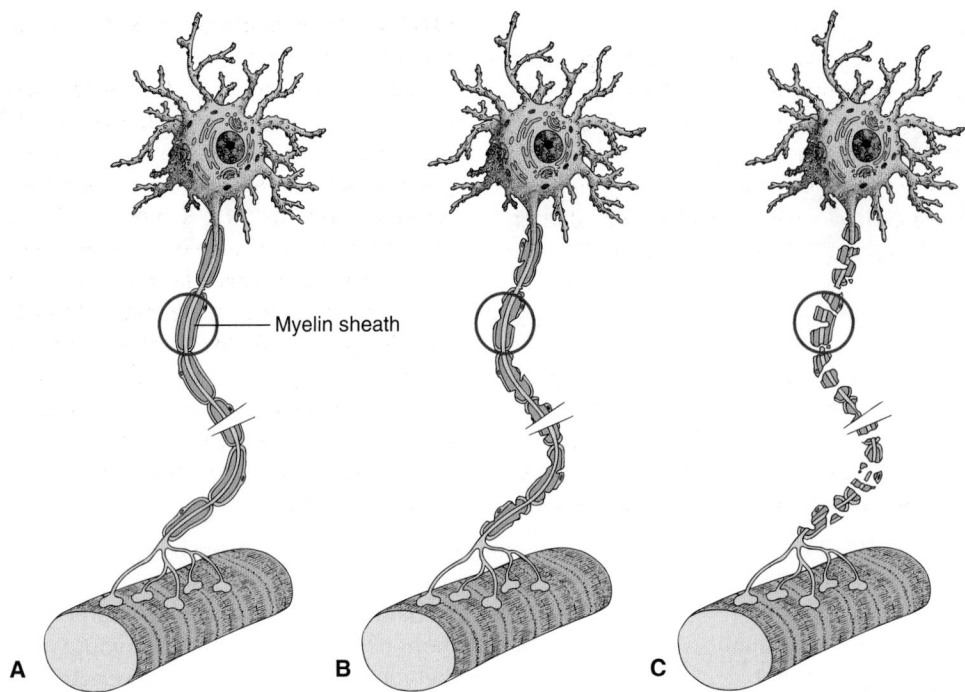

FIGURE 50.1 The myelin sheath breaks down in multiple sclerosis, interrupting transmission of nerve impulses. (A) Normal myelin sheath. (B) Myelin beginning to break down. (C) Total myelin disruption.

however, the disease can be related to viral infections, heredity, and other unknown factors. Some research indicates that there is an inherited tendency to develop MS and that the disease is triggered in the presence of environmental factors. The disease usually starts between ages 20 and 50. Women are two to three times more likely to develop MS than men and are more likely to have relapses (National Multiple Sclerosis Society, 2017). Smokers and those with vitamin D deficiency have a higher risk of MS. The course of the disease is unpredictable. There are many variations in symptoms, depending on which nerves are affected. Some individuals have mild illness, while others suffer permanent disability or rapid decline and death.

Signs and Symptoms

Symptoms of MS vary greatly among patients. Patients may present with muscle weakness, tingling sensations, numbness, or visual disturbances, usually in one eye at a time. Symptoms may begin slowly over weeks to months or start suddenly and dramatically. MS affects many body systems (Box 50.1). Many factors can trigger the onset of symptoms or aggravate the condition, including extreme heat and cold, fatigue, infection, and physical and emotional stress. Hormonal changes after pregnancy can also cause symptom onset or exacerbation.

Periods of exacerbation and remission lead patients with MS to be uncertain about when the disease will flare up and what body system will be affected. Intense fatigue is common; therefore, immobility can become a problem. Accidents and falls are common because of muscle weakness or numbness of the trunk and limbs. Some people with MS

experience symptoms such as muscle spasticity, bowel or bladder dysfunction, or paralysis. Difficulty with concentration or forgetfulness can also be problematic. Pneumonia can occur from immobility and from weakness of the diaphragm and intercostal muscles. Death, often resulting from respiratory infection, typically occurs 20 to 35 years after diagnosis.

Box 50.1

Problems Associated With Multiple Sclerosis

- Weakness/paralysis of limbs, trunk, or head
- Diplopia (double vision)
- Slurred speech
- Spasticity of muscles
- Numbness and tingling
- Patchy blindness (scotomas)
- Blurred vision
- Vertigo
- Tinnitus
- Impaired hearing
- Nystagmus
- Ataxia
- Dysarthria
- Dysphagia
- Constipation
- Spastic (uninhibited) bladder
- Flaccid (hypotonic) bladder
- Sexual dysfunction
- Anger, depression, or euphoria

Diagnostic Tests

Diagnosis is based on the patient's history and signs and symptoms. Analysis of cerebrospinal fluid (CSF) may show an increase in immunoglobulin G (IgG) antibodies. Magnetic resonance imaging (MRI) of the brain and spinal cord can detect demyelination. Evoked potential tests may be done to determine slow transmission of nerve impulses. Blood tests are being developed that may identify specific antibodies associated with MS.

Therapeutic Measures

MS has no cure, although early treatment can delay progression of the disease. Some drugs can slow disease progression by modifying the immune system, such as interferon therapy (Betaseron or Avonex) or immunoglobulins (ocrelizumab [Ocrevus]). Teriflunomide (Aubagio) and dimethyl fumarate (Tecfidera) can reduce relapses. Each of these medications has serious side effects.

Other drugs are given to control symptoms. Steroids such as adrenocorticotropic hormone (ACTH, which triggers the body to make its own steroids) and prednisone are given to decrease inflammation and edema of the neurons, which can relieve some symptoms. Anticonvulsants such as carbamazepine (Tegretol) or duloxetine (Cymbalta) help relieve neuropathic pain. The medications valium (Diazepam), baclofen (Lioresal), and tizanidine (Zanaflex) help control muscle spasms. Bladder problems are treated with parasympathetic agents such as bethanechol (Urecholine) and oxybutynin (Ditropan). Fatigue can be treated with antidepressants or an antiviral agent such as amantadine (Symmetrel). Table 50.1 reviews additional medications used to treat PNS disorders.

Table 50.1

Medications Used to Treat Peripheral Nervous System Disorders

Medication Class/Action

Cholinesterase Inhibitors

Increase acetylcholine at synapses.

Examples	**Nursing Implications**
neostigmine (Prostigmin)	Atropine is an antidote.
pyridostigmine (Mestinon)	
edrophonium (Tensilon, used in diagnosis of myasthenia gravis)	

Glucocorticoids

Reduce inflammation.

Examples	**Nursing Implications**
prednisone	Provide calcium supplement.
prednisolone	Monitor fluid balance.
prednisolone acetate or sodium phosphate	May need to treat high blood sugar levels with insulin while on medication.
methylprednisolone (Solu-Medrol)	*Teach:*
	Avoid crowds and others with infections.

Immunosuppressants

Suppress immunity and antibody formation.

Examples	**Nursing Implications**
azathioprine (Imuran)	Monitor blood counts.
cyclophosphamide (Cytoxan)	Protect from bleeding and infection.
	Administer with meals to reduce nausea.

Antispasmodics/Muscle Relaxants

Relax muscles and reduce pain.

Examples	**Nursing Implications**
dantrolene (Dantrium)	Monitor patient for respiratory depression.
baclofen (Lioresal)	*Teach:*
tizanidine (Zanaflex)	Avoid operating machinery or driving until effects are known.
benzodiazepines such as diazepam (Valium)	

Continued

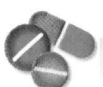

Table 50.1
Medications Used to Treat Peripheral Nervous System Disorders—cont'd

Medication Class/Action

Anticonvulsants

Treat nerve pain.

Examples	Nursing Implications
phenytoin (Dilantin)	Monitor for fall risk.
carbamazepine (Tegretol)	Monitor complete blood counts.
gabapentin (Neurontin)	*Teach:*
duloxetine (Cymbalta)	Maintain good oral hygiene with soft bristle brush, floss, and gum massage (phenytoin).

Glutamate Antagonist

Delays progression of amyotrophic lateral sclerosis (ALS).

Examples	Nursing Implications
riluzole (Rilutek)	Monitor for respiratory depression.
ocrelizumab (Ocrevus); also used for MS	Give on empty stomach.
	Monitor liver function laboratory values.
	Teach:
	Rest.
	Avoid large quantities of caffeine.
	Avoid charcoal-broiled foods.

Potassium Channel Blocker

Improves walking in patients with multiple sclerosis (MS) and some other movement disorders.

Examples	Nursing Implications
dalfampridine (Ampyra)	Monitor for urinary tract infection.
	Do not administer to patients with seizure history.

Disease Modifying Agents

Reduce relapses in relapsing-remitting MS.

Examples	Nursing Implications
alemtuzumab (Lemtrada)	Monitor complete blood count and signs of infection.
interferon beta-1a (Avonex, Betaseron)	Health care provider may recommend delaying vaccines.
glatiramer acetate (Copaxone); also used for ALS	Other implications based on individual drug action.
dimethyl fumarate (Tecfidera)	*Teach:*
fingolimod (Gilenya)	Avoid others who are ill.
teriflunomide (Aubagio)	
tysabri (Natalizumab)	

Acute exacerbations are typically treated with high doses of steroids or with ACTH. For those who suffer sudden severe attacks or do not respond to high doses of steroids, plasma exchange or **plasmapheresis** may be used to remove antibodies from the blood that are attacking the myelin (Box 50-2).

Rehabilitation after acute exacerbation includes physical, speech, and occupational therapies. Physical therapy can help with strength, coordination, and balance. An occupational therapist can help the patient and family adapt the home environment to the patient's special needs. Assistive devices such as braces, canes, wheelchairs, and splints allow the patient increased mobility and independence. Patients who develop speech difficulties benefit from speech therapy. Exercise also can be beneficial ("Evidence-Based Practice").

• WORD • BUILDING •

plasmapheresis: plasma—liquid of blood + pheresis—removal

Evidence-Based Practice

Clinical Question

Do patients with multiple sclerosis (MS) benefit from exercise?

Evidence

A review of evidence-based recommendations found that resistance exercise can improve fitness and mood as well as reduce fatigue. It can also improve mobility and exercise tolerance, which allows patients to be more socially active and improve quality of life (Canavan, 2016).

Implications for Nursing Practice

Exercise can benefit patients with MS in many ways. Be sure that patients have a physical therapy consultation for exercise recommendations.

Reference

Canavan, P. K. (2016). Evidence based therapeutic exercise recommendations for patients with multiple sclerosis: A physical therapy approach. *Journal of Gerontological and Geriatric Research, 5*(1), 271. doi:10.4172/2167-7182.1000271

Nursing Care

See "Nursing Care Plan for the Patient With a Progressive Neuromuscular Disorder."

In addition to reviewing routine care, instruct the patient to avoid factors that can exacerbate symptoms. This includes avoiding stressful situations as much as possible.

Box 50.2

Plasmapheresis

Plasmapheresis, also known as plasma exchange therapy, is a procedure that removes the plasma component from whole blood and replaces it with fresh plasma. The goal is to remove antibodies through plasma exchange, suppressing the immune response and inflammation.

Preprocedure Nursing Care

• Teach the patient about the procedure and what to expect, including what the machine looks like (similar to but smaller than a dialysis machine), the need for arterial and venous access sites, and the length of the procedure (2 to 5 hours).
• The health care provider may order medications held until after the procedure. Some patients may require premedication, especially if they have experienced complications in the past.
• Assess baseline vital signs and weight.
• Assess complete blood cell count (CBC), platelet count, and clotting studies.
• Check blood type and crossmatch for replacement blood products.

Postprocedure Nursing Care

• Observe the patient for signs of hypovolemia, such as dizziness and hypotension.
• Apply pressure dressings to the access sites.
• Monitor the patient for infection and bruits at the access site.
• Monitor electrolytes and signs of electrolyte loss. Report imbalances, and administer replacement electrolytes as ordered.
• Compare preprocedure and postprocedure laboratory data, such as CBC, platelet count, and clotting times.

Nursing Care Plan for the Patient with a Progressive Neuromuscular Disorder

Nursing Diagnosis: *Ineffective Airway Clearance* related to respiratory muscle weakness, and impaired cough and gag reflexes
Expected Outcomes: The patient will maintain a patent airway as evidenced by clear lung sounds and freedom from signs and symptoms of respiratory distress.
Evaluation of Outcomes: Is the patient's airway patent, and are lung sounds clear? Is the patient free of signs and symptoms of respiratory distress?

Intervention	Rationale	Evaluation
Monitor respiratory rate and depth, breath sounds, oxygen saturation (Spo$_2$), and arterial blood gases (as ordered). Report deterioration.	*Increasing respiratory distress indicates progressing muscle weakness that may require mechanical ventilation or end-of-life decisions.*	Is patient's respiratory rate status stable, or is intervention indicated?
Encourage patient to cough and deep breathe every 2 hours.	*Effective coughing helps keep airway clear.*	Does patient have the strength to cough effectively?
Observe patient for breathlessness while speaking.	*Inability to speak without breathlessness indicates declining respiratory function.*	Is patient able to finish sentences without needing to take a breath?

(nursing care plan continues on page 1078)

Nursing Care Plan for the Patient with a Progressive Neuromuscular Disorder—cont'd

Intervention	Rationale	Evaluation
Elevate head of bed.	*The Fowler position improves lung expansion, decreases work of breathing, improves cough efforts, and decreases risk for aspiration.*	Does elevation of head of bed help relieve dyspnea and prevent aspiration?
Evaluate cough, swallow, and gag reflexes frequently. Notify health care provider (HCP) if absent.	*Impaired reflexes place patient at risk for aspiration and possible pneumonia.*	Is patient able to cough effectively? Is gag reflex intact?
Suction secretions as needed, noting color and amount of secretions.	*Muscle weakness can result in inability to clear airway.*	Does patient require suctioning to clear airway? What color are secretions?

Nursing Diagnosis: *Impaired Physical Mobility* related to muscle weakness
Expected Outcomes: The patient will maintain optimum mobility and activity level, identify measures to help maintain mobility, and perform exercises that help promote mobility.
Evaluation of Outcomes: Is optimal activity level maintained? Can the patient identify measures that will help maintain mobility? Does the patient perform exercises that help maintain mobility?

Intervention	Rationale	Evaluation
Determine pre-illness and current level of mobility.	*Assessment guides care planning.*	What was patient able to do prior to illness or exacerbation?
Identify factors that affect ability to be mobile and active.	*Some factors that interfere with mobility can be modified.*	Are interfering factors modified effectively?
Encourage patient to perform self-care to maximum ability.	*Promotes sense of control and independence for patient.*	Does patient perform self-care activities? Is assistance required?
Consult physical therapist to provide exercise recommendations.	*Exercise can improve strength and mobility.*	Does patient follow exercise recommendations? Is mobility maintained?
Consult physical therapist or occupational therapist to provide assistive devices for walking (e.g., canes, braces, walker, wheelchair) and other activities.	*Assistive devices decrease fatigue and promote independence, comfort, and safety.*	Does patient use assistive devices safely during activities? Do they help keep patient active?
Reposition frequently if patient is immobile.	*Prevents skin breakdown and stasis of pulmonary secretions.*	Is patient free from complications of immobility?
Provide active/passive range-of-motion (ROM) exercises if needed on a regular basis.	*Prevents contractures and disuse atrophy.*	Does patient have any contractures or atrophy?
Plan activities with a balance of frequent rest periods.	*Rest decreases fatigue.*	Is fatigue controlled?

Nursing Diagnosis: *Nutrition: Less Than Body Requirements* related to weakness or lack of coordination of muscles for chewing and swallowing
Expected Outcome: The patient will maintain body weight within normal limits for height and frame.
Evaluation of Outcome: Is the patient's weight stable and within normal limits?

Intervention	Rationale	Evaluation
Evaluate cough, swallow, and gag reflexes frequently. Notify HCP if absent.	*If patient is unable to swallow, an enteral feeding tube may be indicated, depending on patient's wishes.*	Does patient eat and drink without aspirating?

Nursing Care Plan for the Patient with a Progressive Neuromuscular Disorder—cont'd

Intervention	Rationale	Evaluation
Offer soft foods that are easy to chew and swallow.	*Soft foods require less effort to chew and are less fatiguing.*	Is patient able to chew and swallow without excessive fatigue?
Request speech therapist and dietitian consultations as indicated.	*A speech therapist can evaluate swallowing and make recommendations for safe swallowing. A dietitian can recommend appropriate foods.*	Are consults indicated? Are recommendations implemented?

Nursing Diagnosis: *Impaired Verbal Communication* related to impaired respiratory and muscle function
Expected Outcome: The patient will be able to communicate needs.
Evaluation of Outcome: Does the patient indicate that needs are met with a minimum of frustration?

Intervention	Rationale	Evaluation
Assess ability to speak and communicate.	*Assessment is essential to planning appropriate communication interventions.*	Can patient speak and communicate needs?
Request referral for speech therapy if indicated.	*Speech therapist can help with speech clarity or recommend appropriate alternative communication techniques.*	Is referral completed if indicated?
Assess for nonverbal signs of pain or distress, such as restlessness, agitation, and grimacing.	*Patient may not be able to tell you if he or she is in pain or distress.*	Are signs of pain or distress present? Are they attended to?
Use a picture board or paper and pencil. Ask questions that require a yes or no answer.	*These do not require patient to speak to communicate.*	Do alternative methods help patient communicate needs?
Use a nonhurried, calm, and caring approach while providing care	*This will help decrease anxiety and provide emotional support to patient and family.*	Do patient and family appear anxious? Does calm approach help?
Explain all procedures.	*Patient can still hear and needs to know what is happening.*	Does patient indicate understanding?

Rest, exercise, and a balanced diet are important self-care steps to control symptoms. In addition, avoiding extreme temperature changes, infection, and illness are important. Any infection, especially respiratory, should be reported immediately to the health care provider (HCP). Two excellent sources of information on MS are the National Multiple Sclerosis Society at www.nationalmssociety.org and the Multiple Sclerosis Foundation at www.msfocus.org.

Myasthenia Gravis
Pathophysiology
Myasthenia gravis (MG) means "grave muscle weakness," or weakness of the voluntary or skeletal muscles of the body. MG is a chronic disease of the neuromuscular junction (Fig. 50.2). Normally, a neuron releases the chemical neurotransmitter acetylcholine (ACh) at the neuromuscular junction. Receptors on the muscle tissue take up ACh, and contraction of the muscle results. In MG, the body's immune system is activated, producing antibodies that attack and destroy ACh receptors at the neuromuscular junction. Therefore, ACh cannot stimulate muscle contraction because the number of ACh receptors has been reduced. This results in loss of voluntary muscle strength.

Etiology
MG is a chronic autoimmune process. No specific cause has been found. However, certain viruses may initiate the autoimmune process. Genetic susceptibility may also play a role. Disorders of the thymus gland are often associated with MG. All ethnic groups and both genders can develop this disease. Peak age of onset in women is ages 20 to 30. Men are affected more often after age 60. MG occurs more often in women than in men.

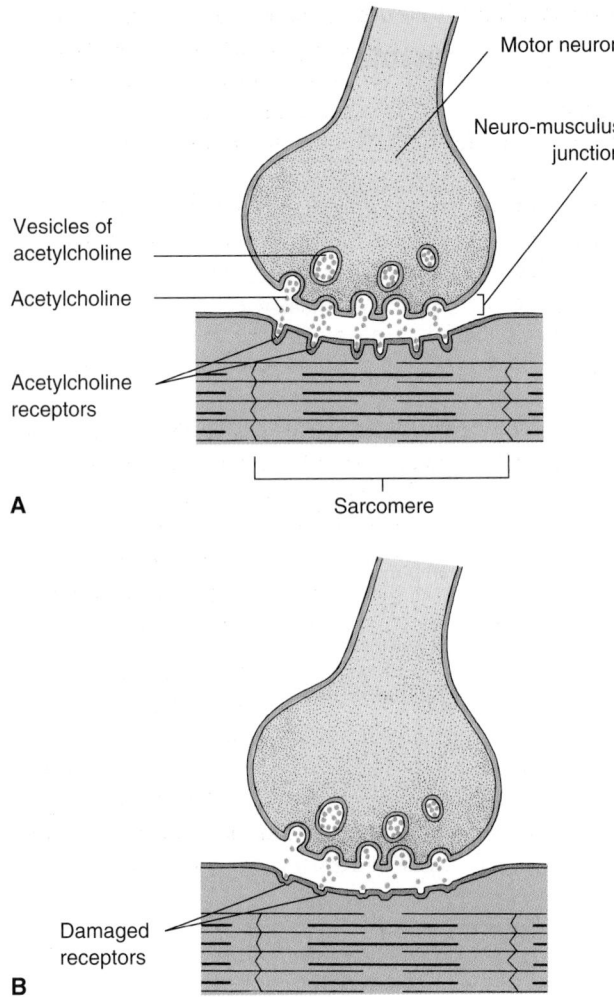

FIGURE 50.2 Myasthenia gravis. (A) Normal neuromuscular junction. (B) Note damaged acetylcholine receptor sites in myasthenia gravis.

Signs and Symptoms

MG results in progressive extreme muscle weakness. The classic sign of MG is increased muscle weakness during activity and improvement in muscle strength after rest. Muscles are strongest in the morning, when the person is rested. Activities affected by MG include eye and eyelid movements, chewing, swallowing, speaking, and breathing as well as skeletal muscle function. Patients often present with drooping of the eyelids (**ptosis**). Facial expressions become masklike. After long conversations, the patient's voice may fade. Falls occur because of weakness of the arm and leg muscles. Patients with MG experience periods of exacerbation and remission of symptoms, similar to patients with MS. Exacerbations can be caused by emotional or physical stress such as menses, illness, trauma, extremes in temperature, pregnancy, electrolyte imbalance, surgery, and drugs that block action at the neuromuscular junction.

Complications

Major complications associated with MG result from weakness of muscles that assist with swallowing and breathing.

Aspiration, respiratory infections, and respiratory failure are the leading causes of death. Sudden onset of muscle weakness in patients with MG resulting from not enough medication is called a *myasthenic crisis*. Overmedication with **anticholinesterase** drugs causes a *cholinergic crisis* (Table 50.2). Both crises require immediate medical attention.

> ### LEARNING TIP
>
> Symptoms of cholinergic crisis can be remembered with the acronym **SLUDGE**, which stands for **s**alivation, **l**acrimation, **u**rination, **d**iarrhea, **g**astrointestinal (GI) cramping, and **e**mesis. A severe crisis has been described as "liquid pouring out of every body orifice."

Diagnostic Tests

Diagnosis of MG is based on history of symptoms and physical examination of the patient. A simple test involves the patient looking upward for 2 to 3 minutes. Increased ptosis occurs if MG is present. After a brief rest, the eyelids can be opened without difficulty. Another test is done by injecting edrophonium (Tensilon), an anticholinesterase drug, intravenously (IV). If muscle strength improves dramatically (e.g., the patient can suddenly open the eyes wide), MG is diagnosed. However, improvement is only temporary. An increased number of anti-ACh receptor antibodies in the blood are present in 90% of patients with MG. Electromyography (EMG) may be done to rule out other conditions. Pulmonary function tests may be done to predict potential myasthenic crisis leading to respiratory failure.

Therapeutic Measures

No cure is currently available for MG. Treatment is aimed at controlling symptoms. Removal of the thymus gland (thymectomy) can decrease production of ACh receptor antibodies and decrease symptoms in most patients. Medications used to treat MG include the anticholinesterase drugs neostigmine (Prostigmin) and pyridostigmine (Mestinon). These drugs improve MG symptoms by destroying the acetylcholinesterase that breaks down ACh. Remember that ACh causes muscles to contract. If ACh is allowed more time to attach to remaining muscle tissue receptors, the muscle contracts and strength is increased. Steroids such as prednisone and immunosuppressants are used to suppress the body's immune response. The monoclonal antibody rituximab (Rituxan) is an IV-administered medication used in some cases of MG; it works by affecting the immune system. Plasmapheresis can be used to remove antibodies from the patient's blood. IV immunoglobulin (IVIg) helps restore normal immune function.

• WORD • BUILDING •

anticholinesterase: anti—against + cholinesterase—chemical that breaks down acetylcholine

Table 50.2

Comparison of Myasthenic Crisis and Cholinergic Crisis

	Myasthenic Crisis	Cholinergic Crisis
Cause	Too little medication	Too much medication
Signs and Symptoms	Ptosis Difficulty swallowing Difficulty speaking Dyspnea Weakness	Salivation Lacrimation Urinary incontinence Diarrhea Gastrointestinal cramping Emesis Increased bronchial secretions Sweating Miosis (constriction of pupils) Bradycardia Increasing muscle weakness Dyspnea

Nursing Process for the Patient With Myasthenia Gravis

DATA COLLECTION. Determine the patient's baseline muscle strength. Ask how much activity is tolerated before fatigue and muscle weakness occur. Identify the patient's support systems and determine whether the patient's needs are being met. Assess the knowledge base of the patient and family. Check respiratory function and swallowing ability.

NURSING DIAGNOSES, PLANNING, AND IMPLEMENTATION.

Activity Intolerance related to muscle weakness

EXPECTED OUTCOME: The patient will improve activity tolerance as evidenced by the ability to carry out necessary activities.

- Schedule anticholinesterase drugs so that peak action occurs at times when increased muscle strength is needed *so that the patient has strength for activities such as meals and physical therapy.*
- Teach the patient to schedule activities such as grocery shopping or errands at times when medication is at peak action *so that muscle strength is adequate for the activity.*
- Be aware of symptoms and treatment of myasthenic and cholinergic crises *so that quick intervention can be carried out to prevent worsening symptoms.*
- Teach the patient and family members signs and symptoms of crisis conditions *because both crises constitute medical emergencies and require immediate intervention* (see Table 50.2).

- Teach methods to conserve energy, such as sitting down to do grooming and housekeeping activities whenever possible. *This helps the patient conserve energy to manage activities of daily living (ADLs).*
- Teach the patient to rest between activities *to allow time for muscle strength to be restored.*
- Teach the importance of avoiding people with infections and exposure to cold *to minimize risk for respiratory infections, which can exacerbate symptoms and increase risk for ineffective airway clearance.*
- Instruct the patient to eat nutritious, well-balanced meals *to maintain strength and resistance to infections, which can exacerbate symptoms.*
- Teach the patient to only use medications that are prescribed by the HCP. If multiple providers are used, all medications should be checked with the HCP who is treating the MG. *Many medications can exacerbate muscle weakness or interfere with medications used to treat MG* (Box 50.3).
- Provide information about support groups *that can provide encouragement and assistance to patients and their families.*

EVALUATION. If the plan of care has been effective, the patient's activity and self-care needs will be met, either by the patient or by other support individuals.

Also see "Nursing Care Plan for the Patient With a Progressive Neuromuscular Disorder" earlier in this chapter. More information can be found at the Myasthenia Gravis Foundation of America web site at www.myasthenia.org.

CRITICAL THINKING

Jamie is referred to a neurologist because of muscle weakness.

1. What history can help differentiate between multiple sclerosis (MS) and myasthenia gravis (MG)?
2. What physical examination can be done to differentiate between MS and MG?
3. The neurologist prepares to do an edrophonium (Tensilon) test and asks you to prepare 2 mg of Tensilon for intravenous injection. It is supplied as 10 mg per milliliter. How much should you draw up?
4. In preparing for a case management meeting for a patient with a neuromuscular disease, which health care providers should be invited?

Suggested answers are at the end of the chapter.

Amyotrophic Lateral Sclerosis
Pathophysiology and Etiology

Amyotrophic lateral sclerosis (ALS; also called Lou Gehrig disease) is a progressive, degenerative condition that affects

- WORD · BUILDING ·
amyotrophic: a—without + myo—muscle + trophy—nourishment + ic—related to

Box 50.3

Medications That Can Exacerbate Symptoms of Myasthenia Gravis

- Antibiotics (some)
- Alpha interferon
- Anticholinergic agents
- Beta blockers
- Botulinum toxin
- Calcium channel blockers
- Chloroquine
- Lithium
- Magnesium
- Neuromuscular blocking agents (such as those used during surgery)
- Penicillamine
- Prednisone
- Procainamide
- Quinidine

motor neurons responsible for the control of voluntary muscles. In the brain and spinal cord, upper and lower motor neurons begin to degenerate and form scar tissue or die, blocking transmission of nerve impulses. Without stimulation, muscles **atrophy,** and muscle strength and coordination decrease. As the disease progresses, more muscle groups, including muscles controlling breathing and swallowing, become involved. The heart and gastrointestinal tract are controlled involuntarily and so are not affected by ALS. The ability to think and reason also is not affected.

ALS can occur at any age but usually does not appear until adulthood. The cause of ALS is not known, but it is believed to have a genetic component. Smoking and other toxins appear to increase risk.

Signs and Symptoms

Symptoms are vague early in the course of ALS. Primary symptoms include progressive muscle weakness and decreased coordination. This can begin in the arms, legs, or muscles of speech and swallowing. Atrophy of muscles and **fasciculation** (twitching) also occur. Muscle spasms can cause pain. Difficulty with chewing and swallowing places the patient at risk for choking and aspiration as the disease progresses. Inappropriate emotional outbursts of laughing and crying can occur. Speech becomes increasingly difficult. Bladder and bowel functions remain intact, yet problems such as constipation, urinary urgency, hesitancy, or frequency can occur.

Late in the disease, communication becomes limited to moving and blinking the eyes in response to questions. Pulmonary function becomes severely compromised to the point of requiring mechanical ventilator assistance if the patient chooses. Other complications can include extreme malnutrition, falls, pulmonary emboli, and heart failure. ALS eventually leads to death from respiratory complications such as atelectasis, respiratory failure, and pneumonia.

Diagnostic Tests

Diagnosis is made based on clinical symptoms. Additional tests such as CSF analysis, electroencephalogram (EEG), nerve biopsy, nerve conduction velocity (NCV), or EMG may be done to rule out other conditions. Blood enzymes can be increased as a result of muscle atrophy.

Therapeutic Measures

There is no cure for ALS, and treatments are palliative in nature. Goals of treatment are aimed at maintaining function as long as possible and emotionally supporting the patient and family. Glycopyrrolate (Robinul) may be administered to decrease saliva production. Quinine (Qualaquin) may be used for muscle cramps. Riluzole (Rilutek) slows the progression of the disease and can prolong life by 3 to 4 months. Edaravone (Radicava) reduces the glutamate in the body, which damages the motor nerves, slowing decline in function.

Nonpharmacological measures such as physical therapy, massage, position changes, and diversional activities can help control pain. Enteral feedings via a surgically placed gastrostomy tube help provide adequate nutrition. Prevention of infections, such as pneumonia and urinary tract infection (UTI), is vital. Meticulous skin care minimizes the incidence of pressure injuries. Physical, occupational, and speech therapies allow the patient to maximize function for as long as possible. Therapy can also decrease the occurrence of complications such as aspiration, falls, and contractures. As the disease progresses, mechanical ventilation may be needed. Patients may choose supportive hospice care instead of life-prolonging mechanical ventilation.

Patients with speech problems may benefit from the use of alternative communication. A variety of such systems are available; most involve laptop computers that patients can use to type in words or symbols to generate speech. Medicare pays at least a portion of the cost for the equipment. Support groups and counseling provide emotional support for the patient and family.

Nursing Care

See "Nursing Care Plan for the Patient With a Progressive Neuromuscular Disorder" earlier in this chapter.

PATIENT EDUCATION. Reinforce information given by the HCP to the patient and family about ALS and its prognosis. Support groups can provide emotional support as the patient and family deal with the likely reality of untimely death. Assistive devices and exercises help prevent complications. Teaching family members how to perform physical therapy and other health care activities allows the patient to spend as much time as possible at home. Teach the patient to avoid exposure to persons with infections because an infection can be deadly to a patient with a debilitating disease. Request a consultation with a palliative care specialist or other resource

• WORD • BUILDING •
atrophy: a—without + trophy—nourishment

personnel to help the patient and family develop an advance directive.

> ## NURSING CARE TIP
>
> When planning care, remember that a person with amyotrophic lateral sclerosis has an intact mind; it is the body that is deteriorating.

CRITICAL THINKING

Mr. Miller has been having difficulty swallowing. He is diagnosed with amyotrophic lateral sclerosis (ALS).

1. What are the priority nursing diagnoses for Mr. Miller?
2. How can the patient and his family be supported in coping with ALS?
3. What health care team members should be consulted for his care?

Suggested answers are at the end of the chapter.

Guillain-Barré Syndrome

Pathophysiology

Guillain-Barré syndrome (GBS) is a rare neuromuscular disease affecting only 1 in every 100,000 persons. Both men and women in the United States are affected equally. Onset is usually between 30 and 50 years of age. GBS is an inflammatory disorder characterized by abrupt onset of symmetrical paresis (weakness) that progresses to paralysis. The myelin sheath of the spinal and cranial nerves is destroyed by a diffuse inflammatory reaction. The peripheral nerves are infiltrated by lymphocytes, which leads to edema and inflammation. Segmental **demyelination** causes atrophy of the axons, resulting in slowed or blocked nerve conduction. Typically, the demyelination begins in the most distal nerves and ascends in a symmetrical fashion. **Remyelination** is a much slower process. It occurs in a descending pattern and is accompanied by a resolution of symptoms.

There are four recognized variants of GBS; however, only the most common type, ascending GBS, is addressed in this chapter. It is characterized by progressive weakness and numbness that begins in the legs and ascends up the body. The numbness tends to be mild, but the muscle weakness usually progresses to paralysis. The paralysis can ascend all the way to the cranial nerves or stop anywhere between the legs and head. Deep tendon reflexes are either depressed or absent. Respiratory function becomes compromised in approximately 50% of patients with ascending GBS.

Etiology

GBS is believed to be caused by an autoimmune response to some type of viral infection or to certain vaccines, although the exact cause is not known. Usually, the viral illness affects the respiratory or GI system and occurs within 2 weeks before onset of neurologic symptoms. The most common organism found to be associated with GBS is *Campylobacter jejuni,* a common cause of gastroenteritis.

Signs and Symptoms

GBS is divided into three stages.

STAGE 1: ONSET OF SYMPTOMS. The first stage starts with the onset of symptoms and lasts until the progression of symptoms stops. This stage can last from 24 hours to 3 weeks. It is characterized by abrupt and rapid onset of muscle weakness and paralysis, with little or no muscle atrophy. Patients with ascending GBS may gradually notice a reduced ability to take deep breaths or carry on conversations and may feel short of breath. These patients are terrified that they will not be able to breathe and may require intubation and artificial ventilation.

The autonomic nervous system is often affected by GBS. Patients can experience unstable blood pressure, cardiac arrhythmias, urine retention, or paralytic ileus. Patient reports of discomfort range from annoying numbness and cramping to severe pain. The discomfort is exacerbated by the patient's inability to move voluntarily.

STAGE 2: PLATEAU. The second stage is the plateau stage, when symptoms are most severe but progression has stopped. It can last from 2 to 14 days. Patients may become discouraged if no improvement is evident.

STAGE 3: RECOVERY. Axonal regeneration and remyelination occur during the third state, recovery. This stage lasts from 6 to 24 months, and symptoms slowly improve. Most patients with GBS recover completely within a few months to a year. A few patients experience chronic disability.

Complications

Complications that can occur include respiratory failure, infection, and depression. It is important to discuss the possible need for intubation early in the patient's illness. The decision to intubate in GBS is different from that with other PNS disorders because GBS patients are expected to recover. It is important to be vigilant in monitoring pulse oximetry, respiratory rate and depth, and dyspnea to predict the need for intervention and maintain the patient's safety.

Patients with GBS are prone to pneumonia and UTIs. Maintaining infection control practices and maximizing the patient's nutritional status help decrease the likelihood of infection. Immobility leads to such problems as skin breakdown, pulmonary embolus, deep vein thrombosis,

· WORD · BUILDING ·

demyelination: de—down or from + myelin—sheath surrounding neurons + ation—process

remyelination: re—repeat + myelin—sheath surrounding neurons + ation—process

and muscle atrophy. Patients with GBS have little time to adjust to their illness and deterioration; they often fear they will not recover function. Calm, supportive reassurance is important.

Diagnostic Tests

A lumbar puncture is performed to obtain CSF. The CSF analysis shows a normal cell count with an elevated protein level. EMG and NCV tests are done to evaluate nerve function. Pulmonary function testing helps confirm impending respiratory problems.

Therapeutic Measures

During the initial stages, patients are partially or completely dependent for all needs. They are often frightened and anxious. Oxygen and mechanical ventilation may be required. Plasmapheresis may be used to remove the patient's plasma and replace it with fresh plasma. This procedure is thought to lessen the body's immune response. Immunoglobulin therapy may help reduce the severity of the disease. Supportive interventions include anticoagulants to prevent deep vein thrombosis and analgesics for pain. Intensive rehabilitation helps the patient regain function during the recovery phase.

Nursing Care for the Patient With Guillain-Barré Syndrome

See "Nursing Care Plan for the Patient With a Progressive Neuromuscular Disorder" earlier in this chapter. Assess the patient's vital signs, arterial blood gases (ABGs), and oxygen saturation (SpO$_2$) to monitor respiratory status. Monitor gag, corneal, and swallowing reflexes to determine whether safety measures are needed to prevent aspiration or injury to the eyes. Be prepared to teach the patient and family about the disease and treatment. Table 50.3 summarizes and compares MS, MG, ALS, and GBS.

Postpolio Syndrome
Pathophysiology and Etiology

Postpolio syndrome is a condition that affects survivors of polio 20 to 40 years after they have recovered from infection caused by the poliomyelitis virus. Up to 40% of patients who previously had polio develop postpolio syndrome.

Signs and Symptoms

Postpolio syndrome involves further weakening of the muscles that were affected with the first poliovirus infection. Symptoms range from fatigue to progressive muscle weakness and atrophy. Sleeping problems, joint pain, scoliosis,

Table 50.3
Summary of Peripheral Nervous System Disorders

	Multiple Sclerosis	Myasthenia Gravis	Amyotrophic Lateral Sclerosis	Guillain-Barré Syndrome
Signs and Symptoms	Muscle weakness Muscle paralysis Visual disturbances Fatigue	Progressive severe weakness of voluntary muscles Muscles regain strength with rest Masklike face	Progressive muscle weakness Decreased coordination Muscle twitching Muscle spasms Pain Emotional outbursts Difficulty with speech	Three stages: 1. Ascending paralysis 2. Plateau 3. Descending resolution Pain, cramping, or numbness
Diagnosis	CSF analysis MRI gMS Dx (blood test)	Ptosis test Tensilon test EMG	CSF analysis EEG Nerve biopsy NCV	CSF EMG NCV
Therapeutic Measures	Interferon therapy Steroids Immunosuppressants Plasmapheresis Anticonvulsants Antiviral agents Muscle relaxants Physical therapy Speech therapy	Plasmapheresis Thymectomy Anticholinesterase agents Steroids	Antispasmodics/quinine Riluzole (Rilutek) Physical therapy Massage Muscle relaxants Diversional activities Enteral feeding Alternative communications devices	Plasmapheresis Ventilation support Physical therapy

Table 50.3

Summary of Peripheral Nervous System Disorders—cont'd

	Multiple Sclerosis	Myasthenia Gravis	Amyotrophic Lateral Sclerosis	Guillain-Barré Syndrome
Complications	Falls Muscle spasms Bowel and bladder problems; risk for UTI Forgetfulness Extreme fatigue	Aspiration Respiratory infections Respiratory failure Myasthenic crisis or cholinergic crisis	Communication problems Risk for aspiration Pain Respiratory failure	Respiratory infection Respiratory failure Depression Fatigue UTI Complications of immobility
Priority Nursing Diagnoses	Ineffective Airway Clearance Impaired Physical Mobility Imbalanced Nutrition: Less Than Body Requirements Impaired Verbal Communication			

CSF = cerebrospinal fluid; EEG = electroencephalogram; EMG = electromyography; MRI = magnetic resonance imaging; NCV = nerve conduction velocity; UTI = urinary tract infection.

and respiratory compromise can occur. Some people suffer great debilitation; others have fewer problems.

Diagnostic Tests

Diagnosis is made based on history and by ruling out other disorders.

Therapeutic Measures

No interventions have been found to be effective at this time. Physical therapy can help the patient increase exercise tolerance. An occupational therapist can help the patient with assistive devices to conserve energy.

Restless Legs Syndrome

Restless legs syndrome (RLS) is an uncomfortable sensation in the legs, causing the sufferer to constantly feel the need to move the legs. It typically occurs at rest or at night.

Pathophysiology and Etiology

RLS is believed to be related to imbalance of dopamine and serotonin in the brain. There may be a hereditary tendency to develop RLS. Some medications can aggravate RLS. Patients with chronic medical conditions such as kidney failure, iron deficiency, diabetes, Parkinson disease, and peripheral neuropathy may develop RLS. Symptoms of RLS can improve as these medications are discontinued and illnesses are treated.

Signs and Symptoms

Patients often complain of unpleasant sensations such as creeping, crawling, throbbing, pulling, or pins and needles in the legs. Symptoms occur as the person is resting and often increase in severity during sleep. Moving the legs temporarily relieves symptoms.

RLS can interfere with falling and staying asleep, resulting in daytime fatigue and exhaustion. The resulting sleep deprivation can impact work performance and ADLs.

Both men and women and all ages are affected by RLS. The incidence in women is twice as high as men. People often fail to report symptoms to their HCP as they believe their symptoms will not be taken seriously or treated.

Diagnostic Tests

There are not any specific tests to diagnosis RLS. Diagnosis is based upon the patient's report of symptoms. A blood test for iron deficiency should be done, and tests may be done to rule out other disorders. Patients should be asked about their medication history, if family members have similar symptoms, and if they experience daytime sleepiness.

Therapeutic Measures

Treatment of RLS is aimed at improving symptoms. Encourage patients to try eliminating alcohol, tobacco, and caffeine and to establish routine sleep habits and a regular exercise program. Use of heat and cold therapies, leg massages, and warm baths may also help reduce symptoms. A vibrating pad (Relaxis) was approved in 2014 by the Food and Drug Administration and has helped some RLS sufferers.

Medications such as pramipexole (Mirapex), ropinirole (Requip), and rotigotine (Neupro) may be ordered to treat moderate to severe RLS by increasing serum dopamine levels. Opioids, anticonvulsants, and benzodiazepines may also be prescribed to relieve symptoms.

Nursing Care

Nursing care is aimed at patient education about lifestyle changes and medications to control symptoms. Conduct a thorough sleep history if the patient complains of insomnia. A sleep specialist can be consulted for additional help.

CRANIAL NERVE DISORDERS

Cranial nerves are the peripheral nerves of the brain. There are 12 pairs of cranial nerves. Areas that the cranial nerves innervate include the head, neck, and special sensory structures (see Chapter 48). Cranial nerve problems are classified as peripheral **neuropathies.** Disorders can affect the sensory, motor, or both branches of a single nerve. Causes of cranial nerve disorders include tumors, infections, inflammation, trauma, and unknown causes. Two common cranial nerve problems are trigeminal neuralgia (tic douloureux) and Bell palsy.

Trigeminal Neuralgia
Pathophysiology and Etiology

Trigeminal **neuralgia** (TN), sometimes called *tic douloureux,* involves the fifth cranial (trigeminal) nerve. The fifth cranial nerve has three branches that include both sensory and motor functions. The branches innervate areas of the face, including the forehead, nose, cheek, gums, and jaw. TN affects only the sensory portion of the nerve. Irritation or chronic compression of the nerve is suspected to initiate symptoms. This condition is seen more often in women and usually begins about age 50 to 60.

Signs and Symptoms

TN causes intense recurring episodes of pain, described as sudden, jabbing, burning, or knifelike. Episodes of pain begin and end suddenly, lasting a few seconds to minutes. Attacks occur in clusters from a few times a year to up to hundreds of times daily. Pain is felt in the skin on one side of the face. A slight touch, cold breeze, talking, or chewing can trigger attacks of pain. The areas of the face where pain occurs are referred to as trigger zones. Areas affected include the lips, upper or lower gums, cheeks, forehead, or side of the nose (Fig. 50.3). Sleep provides a period of relief from the pain. Therefore, persons with TN may sleep most of the time to avoid painful attacks. They also may refrain from activities such as talking, face washing, teeth brushing, shaving, and eating to prevent pain. Frequent blinking and tearing of the eye on the affected side also occur.

Diagnostic Tests

History of symptoms and direct observation of an attack confirm diagnosis. Radiological studies, including computed tomography (CT) scan and MRI, may be used to rule out other causes of the pain.

Therapeutic Measures

Initial management includes the use of anticonvulsants such as phenytoin (Dilantin), gabapentin (Neurontin), or carbamazepine (Tegretol) to reduce transmission of painful nerve impulses. Baclofen or clonazepam (Klonopin) may also be effective in controlling symptoms. Commonly administered analgesics and opioids are typically not effective in managing the sharp, intense pain.

If medications are not effective, surgery to remove the vessel that is irritating the nerve may be done. Other methods such as radiation, injection, or heat may be used to destroy the sensory portion of the trigeminal nerve. These interventions leave the patient with varying degrees of numbness. Complementary and alternative therapies such as botulinum toxin (Botox) injection, acupuncture, electrical stimulation, and nutritional therapy have been used with varying success.

PATIENT EDUCATION POSTPROCEDURE. The patient will need to learn to protect anesthetized areas of the face after nerve procedures. If corneal sensation is lost, goggles and sunglasses should be used as needed to protect the affected eye. An eye patch may be needed at night to prevent injury during sleep. Artificial tears may also be needed to prevent corneal damage.

Bell Palsy
Pathophysiology and Etiology

In Bell palsy, the facial nerve (cranial nerve VII) becomes inflamed and edematous, causing interruption of nerve impulses. The cause is thought to be nerve trauma from a viral infection such as Epstein-Barr, herpes simplex, or herpes zoster. Loss of motor control typically occurs on one side of the face; bilateral facial palsy occurs rarely. Contracture of facial muscles can occur if recovery is slow. Men and women are affected equally. Bell palsy is more common in women in the third trimester of pregnancy, in people with immune disorders such as HIV, and in people with diabetes. It occurs in all ages (including children).

Signs and Symptoms

Onset of symptoms may be sudden or may progress over a 2- to 5-day period. Pain behind the ear may precede the

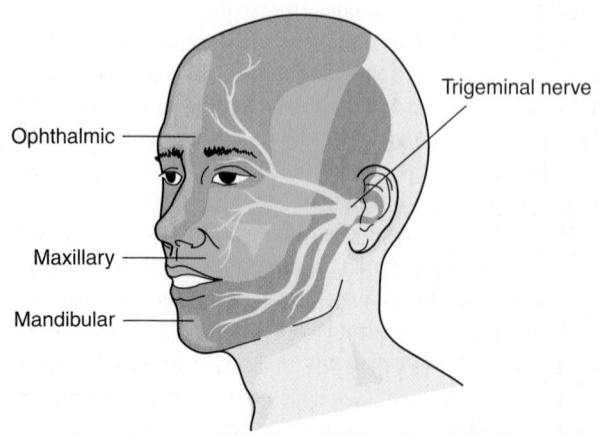

FIGURE 50.3 Areas innervated by the three main branches of the trigeminal nerve (cranial nerve V) are affected in trigeminal neuralgia.

• WORD • BUILDING •

neuropathies: neuro—nerve + pathies—disease
neuralgia: neur—nerve + algia—pain

onset of facial paralysis. Other vague initial symptoms are dry eye or tingling around the lips with progression to the more recognizable symptoms of Bell palsy. The patient may be unable to close the eyelid, wrinkle the forehead, smile, raise the eyebrow, or close the lips effectively. The mouth is pulled toward the unaffected side (Fig. 50.4). Drooling of saliva occurs, and the affected eye has constant tearing. Sense of taste is lost over the anterior two-thirds of the tongue. Speech difficulties occur. Most patients recover completely within 6 months ("Patient Perspective").

Diagnostic Tests

History of the onset of symptoms is used to diagnose Bell palsy. Observation of the patient confirms the diagnosis. EMG may be done. The possibility of a stroke must be ruled out.

Therapeutic Measures

Prevention of complications is the goal of treatment. Prednisone may be given over 7 to 10 days to decrease inflammation. Antiviral agents such as acyclovir (Zovirax) may be used to fight the virus and can shorten the course of the disease. Analgesics are given for pain control. Moist heat and gentle massage to the face and ear can ease pain. A facial sling can be used to aid in eating and support of facial muscles.

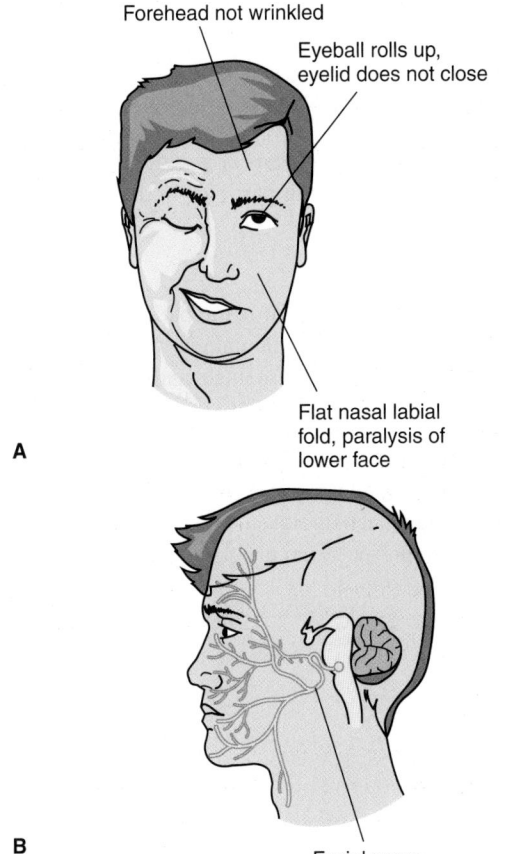

A

Forehead not wrinkled

Eyeball rolls up, eyelid does not close

Flat nasal labial fold, paralysis of lower face

B

Facial nerve

FIGURE 50.4 Bell palsy. (A) Note weakness of affected side of face. (B) Distribution of facial nerve.

Patient Perspective

Angela. I woke up that Thursday morning with the same intense pain in my forehead that I had been experiencing for the past week. When I rolled out of bed, I realized that I didn't have morning breath (or so I thought). Knowing that I had not brushed my teeth yet, I proceeded to do so and noticed that I could not taste the toothpaste. The fruit cup I ate for lunch tasted like bleach. I chomped up and down on each bite, then carefully attempted to swallow. It was like I had been injected with several shots of Novocain. My throat felt like it had closed up, and each swallow took a concentrated effort. Over the course of eating my fruit, I managed to bite my tongue three times.

I was 35 weeks pregnant and on strict bedrest due to pregnancy-induced hypertension and severe edema (which later spiraled into toxemia). We attributed the numbness in my mouth to the edema. I had already swollen up like a balloon and had experienced intense numbness in my extremities since the 12th week of pregnancy. As the afternoon progressed, I grew more and more concerned. I knew something was not quite right. By 5:30 that evening, I had lost control of the entire left side of my face. I called my obstetrician, and she said to get to the emergency room (ER) because I was either having a stroke or had developed Bell palsy. The doctor at the ER confirmed that I had Bell palsy and prescribed valacyclovir (Valtrex) and prednisone to treat it.

The symptoms of Bell palsy that I experienced were severe pain in my forehead, not being able to breathe out of the left side of my nose, and difficulty chewing, swallowing, and saying most consonants. I completely lost the ability to smile, blink, close my eye, raise my eyebrow, or use a straw or blow. My eyesight in the left eye blurred, and I could not go out at night due to the intense pain behind my eye triggered by headlights and having to use eye drops every 5 to 20 minutes.

I delivered my baby 2 weeks after being diagnosed with Bell palsy. During labor, I continuously asked for my eye drops, and the pain in my head was so fierce that it overshadowed the contractions.

After delivery, I was desperate for my face to be "fixed." I tried everything that anyone suggested—herbal supplements, chiropractic medicine, facial massage, laser treatments, facial exercise, shock treatments, a neurologist consultation, and physical therapy. The only thing that has worked for me is time (and lots of it)!

For the first 15 weeks after being diagnosed, I wanted to hide from the world. However, here it is, 7 months later, and I have come to terms with it. I am constantly aware of it, though I have regained a tremendous amount of the muscle control. I still have not shared a "real smile" with my daughter and do not blink my left eye. Covering my mouth when I smile or laugh so others do not see has become almost like a reflex now.

Nursing Process for the Patient With a Cranial Nerve Disorder

Data Collection

Assess attacks using the *WHAT'S UP?* format, being sure to include factors that trigger pain. Are sensory or motor problems associated with the pain? Assess the effect of the disorder on the patient's life, including nutritional status, general and oral hygiene, behavior, and emotional state. Carefully document all findings.

Nursing Diagnoses, Planning, and Implementation

Acute Pain related to inflammation or compression of the nerve

EXPECTED OUTCOME: The patient will state pain is controlled at an acceptable level.

- Administer medications as needed for pain. Anticonvulsant and antidepressant agents used to treat neuropathic pain must be given routinely to prevent pain. *Medications prevent or decrease pain and increase comfort.*
- Discuss and implement alternative and complementary pain relief measures *to complement medications and increase the patient's control over pain.*
- Plan hygiene activities when pain relief is at its peak *to decrease discomfort with activities.*
- Provide alternative communication methods (e.g., paper and pencil, dry erase board, communication board, visual pain scale). *The patient may not be able to speak clearly or want to speak due to pain.*
- Teach the patient to chew on the opposite side of the face *to avoid triggering pain and injury.*
- Encourage use of an electric razor rather than blades *to prevent injury to numb areas.*
- Provide measures for trigeminal neuralgia *to reduce pain triggers:*
  - Provide soft cloths for facial hygiene using lukewarm water.
  - Avoid touching the patient's face.
  - Provide a soft bristle toothbrush for oral care.
  - Teach the patient to protect face from cold or wind.
- Provide measures for Bell palsy *to reduce pain and prevent muscle atrophy:*
  - Provide warm, moist compresses as needed.
  - Massage face.
  - Assist with facial exercises as prescribed by physical therapy.
  - Provide a facial sling.

Imbalanced Nutrition: Less Than Body Requirements related to fear of triggering pain as evidenced by poor intake and weight loss

EXPECTED OUTCOME: The patient will maintain sufficient nutrition as evidenced by stable weight.

- Weigh patient twice weekly and record *to monitor weight loss or gain.*
- Provide small, frequent meals *to promote nutrition without increasing pain.*
- Provide soft, easy-to-chew foods at lukewarm temperature *to prevent triggering pain.*
- Provide a high-protein and high-calorie diet. *Protein and calories are needed for cellular repair.*
- Avoid hot or cold foods and drinks. *Temperature extremes can trigger pain. If foods are associated with pain, the patient may avoid them.*
- Encourage oral hygiene after each meal and at bedtime *to prevent gum and tooth disease as triggers for pain.*
- Insert an enteral feeding tube as ordered into the nostril on the unaffected side if nutrition is severely impaired *to provide means for nutrient intake while avoiding painful nerve areas.*

Risk for Injury to Eyes related to inability to blink (Bell palsy)

EXPECTED OUTCOME: The patient's cornea will remain intact and without injury.

- Administer eye drops or eye ointment as ordered by the HCP *to protect the eye.*
- Teach the patient to use a patch over the affected eye *to protect the eye.*
- Advise the patient to wear glasses or goggles, especially when outside or in areas with particles in the air, *to protect the eyes.*

Evaluation

Nursing care has been successful if the patient reports that pain is controlled, nutrition is maintained with no inappropriate weight loss, and the eyes are intact and without injury.

LEARNING TIP

Remember! Trigeminal neuralgia (cranial nerve V) is a sensory disorder; Bell palsy (cranial nerve VII) is a motor disorder.

SUGGESTED ANSWERS TO CRITICAL THINKING

Jamie

1. Muscle weakness caused by myasthenia gravis improves with rest, unlike multiple sclerosis.
2. Have Jamie look up for 2 to 3 minutes. If ptosis occurs, have her close her eyes for several minutes. If she can open her eyelids and look up, myasthenia gravis is likely. Of course, diagnosis will be done by a neurologist.
3.

$$\frac{2 \text{ mg}}{} \frac{1 \text{ mL}}{10 \text{ mg}} = 0.2 \text{ mL}$$

4. The team may include a nurse, occupational therapist, physical therapist, neurologist, pharmacist, dietitian, and primary HCP for other health issues.

Mr. Miller

1. Priority nursing diagnoses include *Ineffective Airway Clearance* and *Risk for Aspiration* related to muscle weakness. If a patient's respiratory system is compromised by a disease, nursing care should be focused on maintaining pulmonary function to preserve life.
2. Providing compassionate care to the patient and providing information about the disease and its prognosis to the patient and family establish an honest and supportive relationship. Support groups provide resources and emotional support.
3. The team may include a registered nurse, respiratory therapist, speech pathologist, neurologist, and dietitian. In addition, find out who at your institution helps patients make end-of-life decisions. A palliative care specialist or social worker can help the patient and family work through some difficult decisions and develop an advance directive.

Review Questions

1. A patient with trigeminal neuralgia asks the nurse why carbamazepine (Tegretol) has been ordered. Which response is best?
   1. "It will help decrease the inflammation in your nervous system."
   2. "It will depress your immune system, which can slow the progression of the disease."
   3. "Carbamazepine is used to help relieve nerve pain."
   4. "It is an anticonvulsant to prevent seizures."

2. A patient with amyotrophic lateral sclerosis expresses concern about not having enough breath to sing anymore. Which explanation by the nurse is best?
   1. "Amyotrophic lateral sclerosis can damage the nerves to your bronchi and bronchioles, causing constriction and reduced airflow."
   2. "The demyelination of your nerves caused by amyotrophic lateral sclerosis causes confusion in the impulses to your lungs."
   3. "Amyotrophic lateral sclerosis can affect your vocal cords, making it difficult to form sounds as you speak or sing."
   4. "Amyotrophic lateral sclerosis may be affecting the nerves that go to your respiratory muscles, making them weak."

3. A patient who is newly diagnosed with amyotrophic lateral sclerosis says to the nurse, "I do not want to be kept alive on machines." Which nursing action is best in response?
   1. Ask the patient whether advance directives have been prepared and provide information if indicated.
   2. Reassure the patient that decisions about machines will not have to be made for a long time.
   3. Inform the patient that individuals with amyotrophic lateral sclerosis are not candidates for artificial ventilation.
   4. Explain to the patient that a ventilator will be necessary to maintain respiratory function as the disease progresses.

4. When caring for a patient admitted with Guillain-Barré syndrome, which nursing diagnosis should take priority?
   1. *Anxiety*
   2. *Imbalanced Nutrition*
   3. *Impaired Gas Exchange*
   4. *Impaired Physical Mobility*

5. Which nursing interventions are appropriate for the patient with Bell palsy? **Select all that apply.**
   1. Administer moisturizing eye drops.
   2. Apply an eye patch.
   3. Avoid touching the patient's face.
   4. Apply warm compresses.
   5. Provide facial massage.
   6. Teach the patient to protect the face from cool breezes.

6. Which meal would be the best choice for a patient with myasthenia gravis?
   1. Baked chicken sandwich, fresh carrots, apple
   2. Meatloaf, mashed potatoes, canned green beans
   3. Steak, baked potato, green salad
   4. Tacos, fresh vegetables, sliced peaches

7. How will the home health care nurse caring for a patient with myasthenia gravis and severe muscle weakness know if interventions have been effective?
   1. The patient verbalizes satisfaction with the plan of care.
   2. The patient states understanding of the medication regimen.
   3. The patient and family state that no further home visits are needed.
   4. The patient is able to perform activities of daily living with oxygen saturation remaining at 95%.

Answer rationales available in your online resources.

ANSWERS 1. 3; 2. 4; 3. 1; 4. 3; 5. 1, 2, 4, 5; 6. 2; 7. 4

Key Points

Find the chapter key points in your online resources available through Davis Edge.

Additional Resources

Use the scratch off code on the inside front cover of your book to access online quizzes that will help you to improve your scores on course exams and prepare for the NCLEX-PN°.

Study Guide

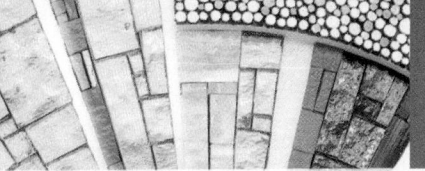

CHAPTER 51

Sensory System Function, Assessment, and Therapeutic Measures: Vision and Hearing

Lazette V. Nowicki, Janice L. Bradford

KEY TERMS

accommodation (ah-KOM-uh-DAY-shun)
arcus senilis (AR-kuss seh-NIL-iss)
cochlear implant (KOK-lee-ur IM-plant)
consensual response (kon-SEN-shoo-uhl ree-SPONS)
electroretinography (ee-LEK-troh-RET-in-AW-gruh-fee)
esotropia (ESS-oh-TROH-pee-ah)
exotropia (EKS-oh-TROH-pee-ah)
hearing aid (HEER-ing AYD)
hypotropia (HY-poh-TROH-pee-ah)
nystagmus (nye-STAG-mus)
ophthalmologist (AWF-thal-MAW-luh-jist)
ophthalmoscope (awf-THAL-muh-skohp)
optician (awp-TISH-uhn)
optometrist (awp-TOM-uh-trist)
otalgia (oh-TAL-jee-ah)
otorrhea (OH-toh-REE-ah)
ototoxic (OH-toh-TOK-sik)
ptosis (TOH-sis)
Rinne test (RIH-neh TEST)
Romberg test (RAHM-berg TEST)
Snellen chart (SNEL-en CHART)
tropia (TROH-pee-ah)
Weber test (VAY-ber TEST)

CHAPTER CONCEPT

Sensory Perception

LEARNING OUTCOMES

1. Describe the normal anatomy of the sensory system.
2. Explain the normal function of the sensory system.
3. List data to collect when caring for a patient with a disorder of the sensory system.
4. Identify diagnostic tests commonly performed to diagnose disorders of the sensory system.
5. Plan nursing care for patients undergoing diagnostic tests for sensory disorders.
6. Describe therapeutic measures for patients with disorders of the sensory system.

It is difficult to imagine what it would be like not to see or hear the world around us. Nurses assist patients in maintaining or coping with deficits in these primary senses.

 VISION

Normal Anatomy and Physiology of the Eye
External Structures
Several structures protect the eye from desiccation (extreme dryness) and debris (Figs. 51.1 and 51.2).

Structure of the Eyeball
Most of the eyeball is within the orbit, the bony socket that protects the eye from trauma. The six extrinsic muscles that move the eyeball are attached to the orbit and to the outer surface of the eyeball. There are four rectus muscles that move the eyeball side to side or up and down. Two oblique muscles rotate the eye. The cranial nerves that innervate these muscles are the oculomotor, trochlear, and abducens (third, fourth, and sixth cranial nerves, respectively). Actions of the six extrinsic eye muscles allow voluntary control of movement. They also will be innervated by the autonomic nervous system to perform convergence, an alignment of the visual axis of each eye on the same field of view.

The wall of the eyeball has three layers. They are the outer fibrous tunic (sclera and cornea), the middle vascular tunic (choroid, ciliary body that suspends the lens, and iris), and the inner nervous tunic (retina; Fig. 51.3). The lens divides the interior of the eye into two main cavities: anterior cavity and posterior cavity. Anterior to the lens is the ring-shaped curtain called the iris. The iris divides the

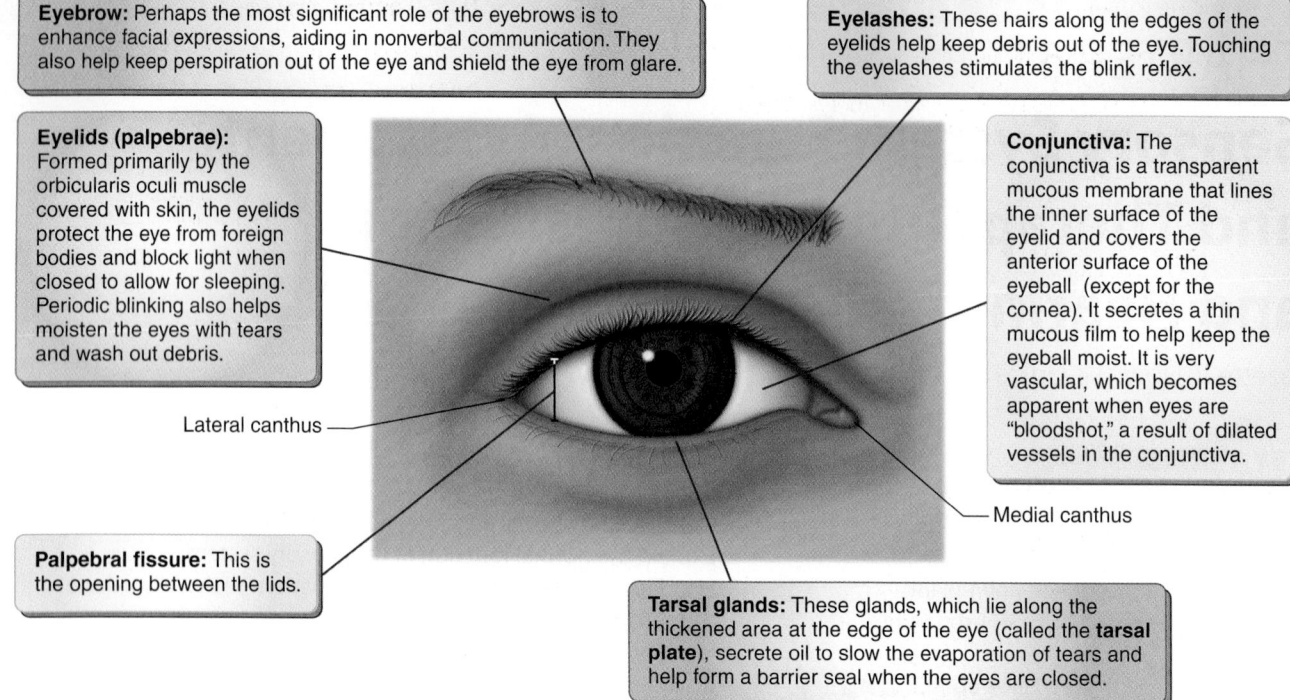

Eyebrow: Perhaps the most significant role of the eyebrows is to enhance facial expressions, aiding in nonverbal communication. They also help keep perspiration out of the eye and shield the eye from glare.

Eyelashes: These hairs along the edges of the eyelids help keep debris out of the eye. Touching the eyelashes stimulates the blink reflex.

Eyelids (palpebrae): Formed primarily by the orbicularis oculi muscle covered with skin, the eyelids protect the eye from foreign bodies and block light when closed to allow for sleeping. Periodic blinking also helps moisten the eyes with tears and wash out debris.

Conjunctiva: The conjunctiva is a transparent mucous membrane that lines the inner surface of the eyelid and covers the anterior surface of the eyeball (except for the cornea). It secretes a thin mucous film to help keep the eyeball moist. It is very vascular, which becomes apparent when eyes are "bloodshot," a result of dilated vessels in the conjunctiva.

Lateral canthus

Medial canthus

Palpebral fissure: This is the opening between the lids.

Tarsal glands: These glands, which lie along the thickened area at the edge of the eye (called the **tarsal plate**), secrete oil to slow the evaporation of tears and help form a barrier seal when the eyes are closed.

FIGURE 51.1 Accessory structures of the eye.

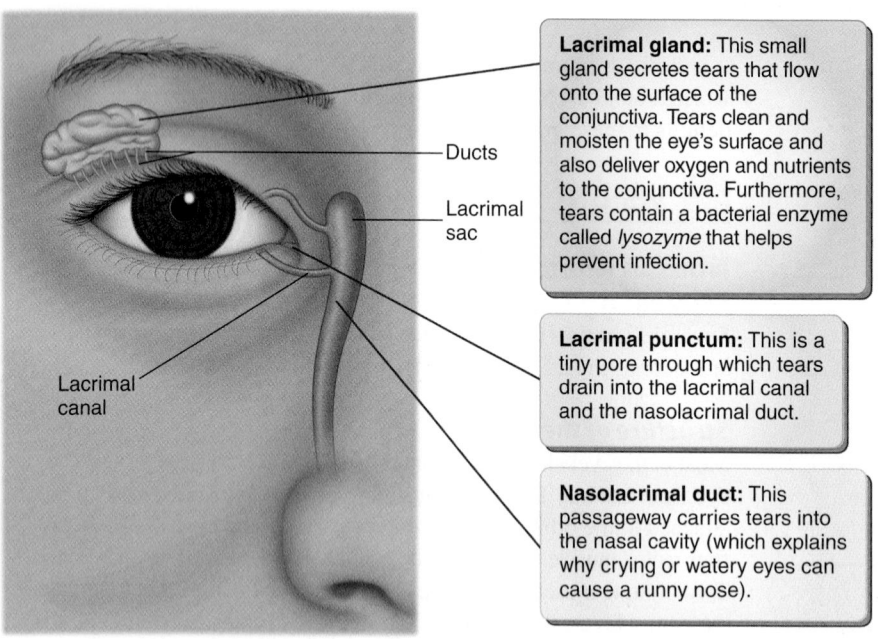

Lacrimal gland: This small gland secretes tears that flow onto the surface of the conjunctiva. Tears clean and moisten the eye's surface and also deliver oxygen and nutrients to the conjunctiva. Furthermore, tears contain a bacterial enzyme called *lysozyme* that helps prevent infection.

Ducts

Lacrimal sac

Lacrimal punctum: This is a tiny pore through which tears drain into the lacrimal canal and the nasolacrimal duct.

Lacrimal canal

Nasolacrimal duct: This passageway carries tears into the nasal cavity (which explains why crying or watery eyes can cause a runny nose).

FIGURE 51.2 Lacrimal apparatus.

anterior cavity into two chambers: anterior chamber and posterior chamber (Fig. 51.4).

The retina lines the posterior two-thirds of the eyeball and contains the photoreceptors (rods and cones). Rods detect only the presence of light, whereas cones respond to photons (the basic particle of light) of differing wavelengths. The fovea centralis is a small depression in the macula lutea of the posterior retina. It is directly behind the center of the lens and contains only cones. The fovea centralis, therefore, is the area of most acute color vision. Rods are proportionately more abundant toward the periphery of the retina. For this reason, night vision is best at the sides of the visual field.

Neurons called ganglion cells transmit the impulses generated by the rods and cones. These neurons all converge at the optic disc and pass through the wall of the eyeball as the optic nerve. The optic disc may also be called the blind spot because no rods or cones are present.

Fibrous Outer Layer

The **sclera**—formed from dense connective tissue— is the outermost layer of the eye. Most of the sclera is white and opaque; it forms what is called "the white of the eye." Blood vessels and nerves run throughout the sclera.

The **cornea** is a transparent extension of the sclera in the anterior part of the eye. It sits over the iris (the colored portion of the eye) and admits light into the eye. It contains no blood vessels.

Vascular Middle Layer

The **iris** is a ring of colored muscle; it works to adjust the diameter of the pupil (the central opening of the iris) to control the amount of light entering the eye.

The **ciliary body** is a thickened extension of the choroid that forms a collar around the lens. It also secretes a fluid called aqueous humor.

The **choroid** is a highly vascular layer of tissue that supplies oxygen and nutrients to the retina and sclera.

Neural Inner Layer

The **retina** is a thin layer of light-sensitive cells.

Exiting from the posterior portion of the eyeball is the **optic nerve** (cranial nerve II), which transmits signals to the brain.

FIGURE 51.3 Eye tissue layers—fibrous, vascular, and neural.

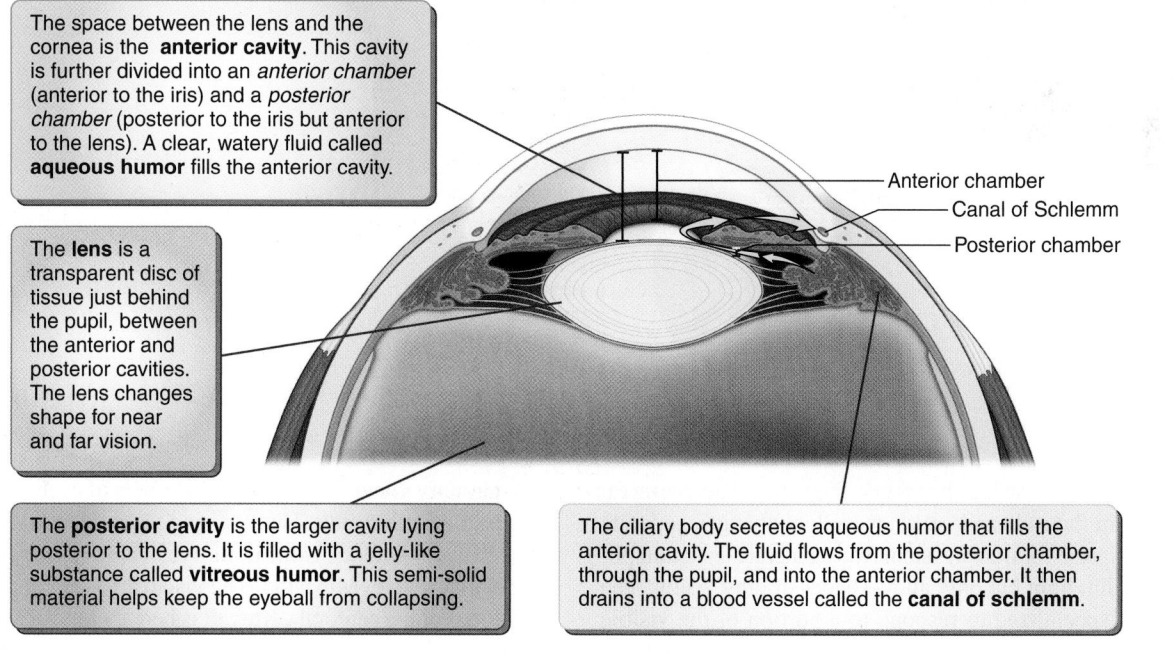

The space between the lens and the cornea is the **anterior cavity**. This cavity is further divided into an *anterior chamber* (anterior to the iris) and a *posterior chamber* (posterior to the iris but anterior to the lens). A clear, watery fluid called **aqueous humor** fills the anterior cavity.

The **lens** is a transparent disc of tissue just behind the pupil, between the anterior and posterior cavities. The lens changes shape for near and far vision.

The **posterior cavity** is the larger cavity lying posterior to the lens. It is filled with a jelly-like substance called **vitreous humor**. This semi-solid material helps keep the eyeball from collapsing.

The ciliary body secretes aqueous humor that fills the anterior cavity. The fluid flows from the posterior chamber, through the pupil, and into the anterior chamber. It then drains into a blood vessel called the **canal of schlemm**.

Anterior chamber
Canal of Schlemm
Posterior chamber

FIGURE 51.4 Chambers and fluids.

Physiology of Vision

Vision involves the focusing of light rays on the retina and the transmission of the subsequent nerve impulses to the visual areas of the cerebral cortex.

The refractive structures of the eye are, in order, the cornea, aqueous humor, lens, and vitreous humor. The lens is the only adjustable part of this focusing system. When the eye shifts focus to an object that is near, accommodation of the lens occurs (Fig. 51.5). Also, the pupil will constrict in near vision to force photons through the thickness of the lens (Fig. 51.6). Accommodation and pupil constriction increase the number of photons that strike the fovea centralis.

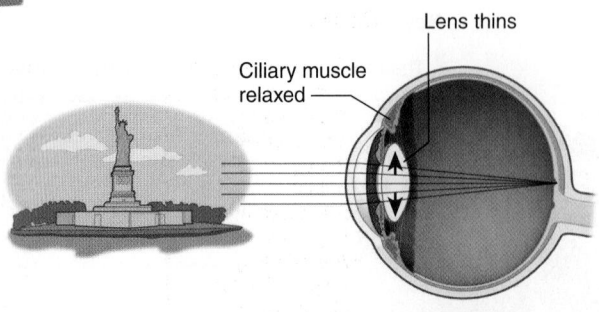

Ciliary muscle relaxed

Lens thins

The nearly parallel light rays from distant objects require little refraction. Consequently, the ciliary muscle encircling the lens relaxes and the lens flattens and thins.

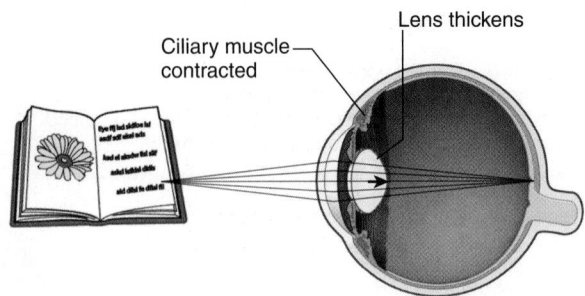

Ciliary muscle contracted

Lens thickens

The more divergent light rays from a nearby object require more refraction. To help focus the light rays, the ciliary muscle surrounding the lens contracts. This narrows the lens, causing it to bulge into a convex shape and thicken, giving it more focusing power.

FIGURE 51.5 Accommodation of the lens.

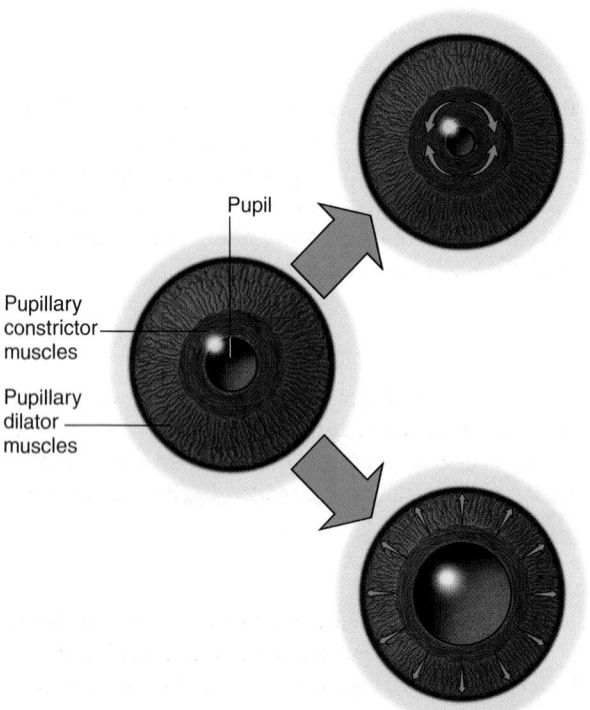

Pupil

Pupillary constrictor muscles

Pupillary dilator muscles

The **pupillary constrictor** muscle encircles the pupil. When stimulated by the parasympathetic nervous system, the muscle constricts, narrowing the pupil to admit less light.

The **pupillary dilator** looks like the spokes of a wheel. When stimulated by the sympathetic nervous system, this muscle contracts, pulling the inside edge of the iris outward. This widens the pupil and admits more light.

FIGURE 51.6 Constriction of the pupil.

When photons strike the retina, they stimulate chemical reactions in the rods and cones. Resultant changes generate a nerve impulse for transmission. Rods generate an action potential in dim light but only allow shades of gray vision. The cones are specialized to respond to a portion of the visible light spectrum; there are red-absorbing, blue-absorbing, and green-absorbing cones. Differing combinations of three cone types allow interpretation of color (Fig. 51.7).

Refraction inverts the image onto the photoreceptors in the retina. The impulses from the rods and cones are transmitted to the ganglion neurons. The ganglion neurons converge at the optic disc and become the optic nerve. The optic nerves from both eyes converge at the optic chiasma, just in front of the pituitary gland. Here, the medial fibers of each optic nerve cross to the other side. This crossing permits each visual area to receive impulses from both eyes. This is important for binocular (two eyes) vision. The visual areas are in the occipital lobes of the cerebral cortex. It is here that the upside-down retinal images are righted and the slightly different pictures from the two eyes are integrated into one image; this is binocular vision, which also provides depth perception.

Aging and the Eye

The most common changes in the aging eye are those in the lens (Fig. 51.8). With age, the lens may become partially or totally opaque. The lens also loses its elasticity with age; most

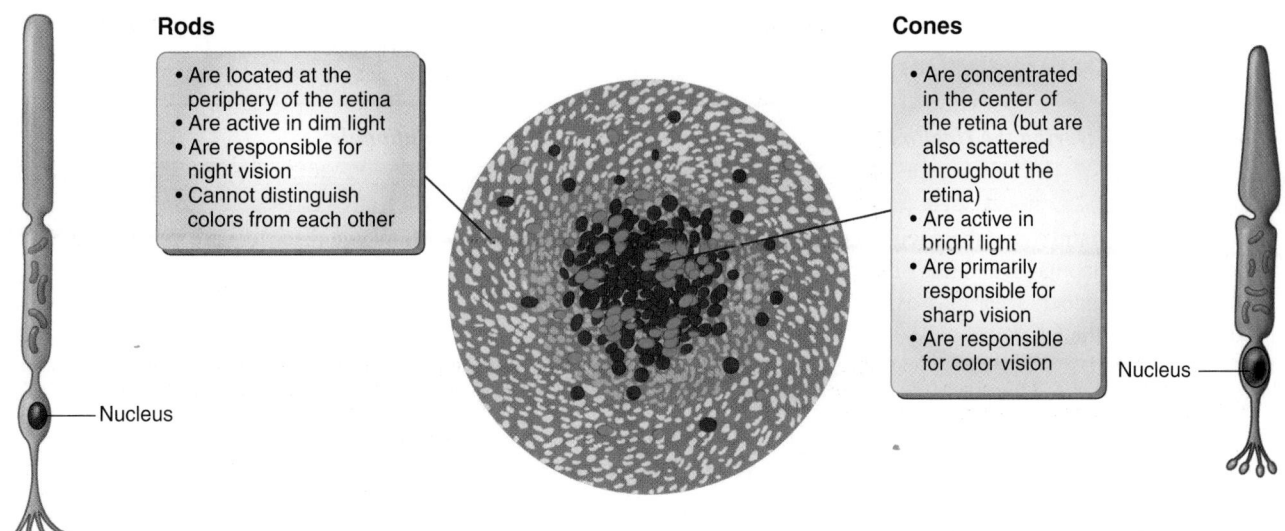

Rods

- Are located at the periphery of the retina
- Are active in dim light
- Are responsible for night vision
- Cannot distinguish colors from each other

Cones

- Are concentrated in the center of the retina (but are also scattered throughout the retina)
- Are active in bright light
- Are primarily responsible for sharp vision
- Are responsible for color vision

Nucleus

Nucleus

FIGURE 51.7 Action of photoreceptors.

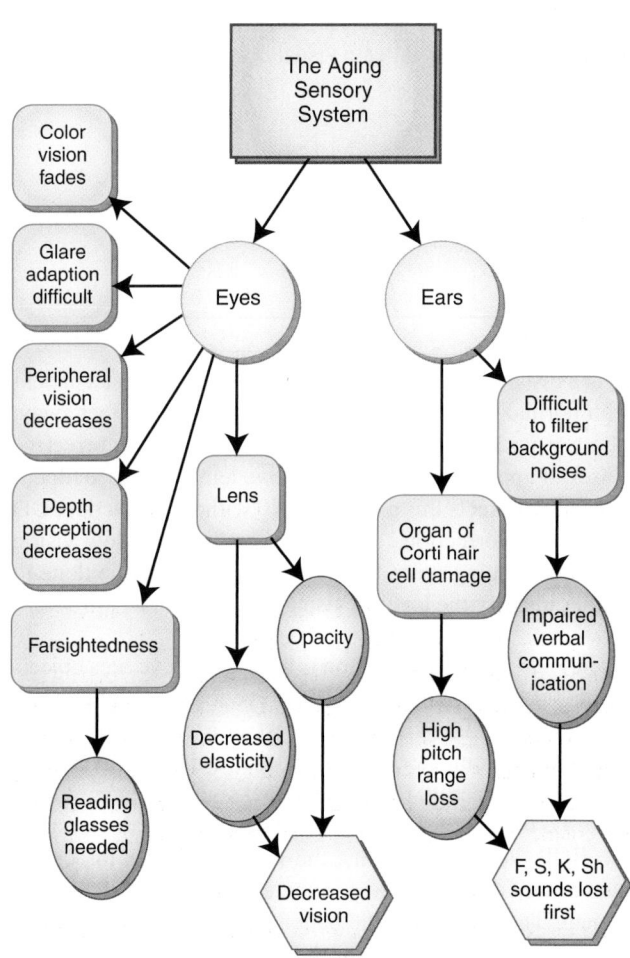

FIGURE 51.8 Aging and the sensory system.

people become farsighted as they age and by 40 years begin to need corrective lenses for near vision. Peripheral vision losses may occur. Depth perception decreases and glare is intensified, both of which can affect safety. Color vision fades with lesser discrimination of blue, green, and violet colors. Red, yellow, and orange colors are seen best.

Nursing Assessment of the Eye and Visual Status

Assessment of the eye begins with a subjective health history and objective observation, testing, and physical examination. Licensed practical nurses/licensed vocational nurses (LPN/LVNs) assist the health care provider (HCP) in conducting the physical examination.

Health History

Ask about family history that can affect vision. This includes diabetes, hypertension, glaucoma, cataracts, and blindness. Eye disorders and diseases can be genetically transmitted so this information is helpful. Patients are asked about their general health status and disorders such as diabetes and hypertension. A medication review checks for eye side effects. The patient is asked about eye symptoms or changes in visual acuity (Table 51.1).

Physical Examination

VISUAL ACUITY. Visual acuity is measured several ways (Table 51.2). It often begins with the use of a **Snellen chart** or an E chart to measure distance acuity. A handheld visual acuity chart (a Rosenbaum card) measures near acuity. The Snellen chart has lines of letters, labeled for visual acuity, that range in size (Fig. 51.9). The largest letters are at the top, with the smallest at the bottom. For the Snellen or E chart test, people stand 20 feet from the chart. They cover one eye and read aloud a line of letters. The lowest line (smallest

Table 51.1

Subjective Data Collection for the Eye

Questions to Ask During the Health History	Rationale
Family History	
Do you have any family members with a history of diabetes? Hypertension? Cataracts? Glaucoma? Blindness? Diabetes mellitus? Do any family members wear glasses or contact lenses? Is their vision corrected with the lens?	Many eye disorders are genetically transmitted.
Health History	
What health problems do you currently have? How are they treated? What health problems or trauma to your eyes have you had in the past?	Some metabolic disorders are precursors to eye disorders, such as diabetes and hypertension.
What medications do you take?	Look for ocular effects of systemic medications.
How often do you have eye examinations? When was the last time you had an eye examination? Do you wear protective eyewear (e.g., sunglasses, safety goggles) and hats in the sun?	Identify preventive practices and need for further teaching.
Visual Acuity	
Do you wear glasses or contact lenses? Have you had any changes in vision, such as difficulty seeing distances or up close, sensitivity to light, or difficulty seeing at night? Do you have double vision? Do you have clouded vision? Do you see halos around lights? Does it look like you are looking through a veil or web? Is there pain? Itching? Tearing? Burning? Do you have headaches? If so, what are the precipitating events?	Any of these signs and symptoms could indicate visual disorders/disturbances.

letters) on the chart that the patient can read accurately designates the visual acuity of that eye. The E chart is used for people with literacy issues. The patient indicates the direction of the E-shaped figure. The handheld visual acuity chart is held by the patient 14 inches from the eyes to read the letters. The LogMAR chart was created to provide better visual acuity measurement than the other visual acuity charts. It is similar to the Snellen chart and measures distance acuity.

Normal vision is defined as 20/20. This means the patient can see at 20 feet what the normal eye clearly sees at 20 feet. Moderate low vision is defined as 20/70 through 20/160. Legal blindness in the United States occurs at 20/200 in the best eye with the best possible correction. Most people defined as blind still have some sight. The LogMAR rates 20/20 vision as 0.00, low vision as 0.5 through 1.3, and higher than 1.3 as legal blindness.

The vision acuity test is done on each eye separately and then both eyes together. A documentation example of low vision acuity findings is: "oculus dexter (OD) [right eye] 20/70, oculus sinister (OS) [left eye] 20/70, oculus uterque (OU) [both eyes] 20/70." This example means that the patient must

be at a distance of 20 feet from an object to see what a patient with normal vision would be able to see from 70 feet away. The test is done with and without the patient's corrective lenses, if applicable. When corrective lenses are used, documentation reflects this as "OD 20/70 without correction, OD 20/20 with correction." Additional testing with low vision charts containing more letters and numbers can be done to further identify the level of visual impairment.

Visual Fields. Peripheral vision is how far the eye sees objects up, down, right, and left while the eye looks straight ahead. The confrontation visual field test is a basic, quick test. Perimetry is computerized testing that maps one's vision. It gives more accurate results and tracks vision changes over time. To perform the confrontation test (named this because the HCP faces the patient), the HCP compares his or her own normal ability to see peripheral objects with that of the patient. The HCP faces the patient 2 feet away. The patient covers one eye and stares at the HCP. The HCP covers his own corresponding eye (e.g., if the patient's right eye is covered, the HCP's left eye is covered). The HCP extends

Table 51.2

Objective Data Collection for the Eye

Physical Examination Findings	Possible Abnormal Findings/Causes
Visual Acuity	
Normal vision 20/20	Hyperopia, myopia, presbyopia, blurred or cloudy vision. Possible causes: refractive error, opacity, or disorder of pathway.
Visual Fields	
Full peripheral fields	Peripheral field loss.
Muscle Balance and Eye Movement	
Movement in all six cardinal fields of gaze	Nystagmus. Inability to move in all six fields can indicate cranial nerve impairment.
Corneal light reflex test (light at the same place on both pupils)	Asymmetry could mean muscle weakness.
Cover test–steady gaze	Drifting eye indicates muscle weakness.
Pupillary Reflexes	
Pupillary light reflex Accommodation	Dilated, fixed, or constricted pupils. Absence of constriction or convergence.
External Structures	
Inspection and palpation of eyebrows, orbital area, eyelids, palpebral fissure, medial canthus, irises, corneal clarity, anterior chamber	Ptosis (drooping of eyelid) usually indicates nerve dysfunction. Opaque whitening of outer rim of cornea can indicate arcus senilis. Corneal opaqueness can be from cataract or trauma.

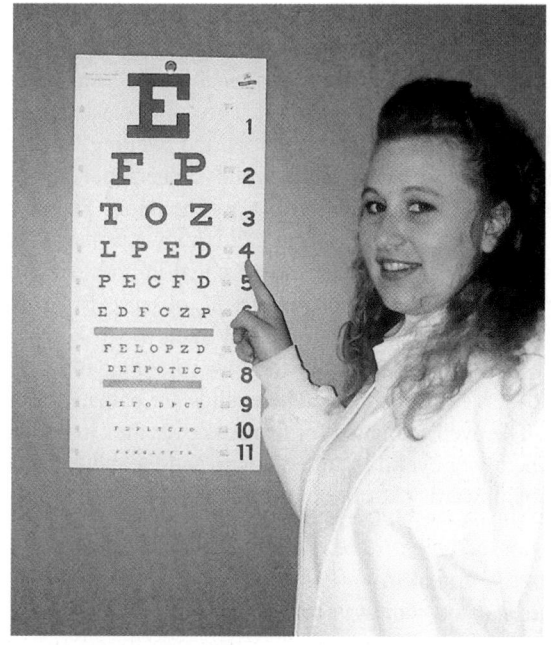

FIGURE 51.9 A Snellen chart is used to assess visual acuity.

his arm to the side and moves his fingers back into the visual field from three directions: superior, inferior, and temporal (middle). The patient indicates when the fingers are seen. The patient has full visual fields if the patient and HCP see the fingers at the same place.

MUSCLE BALANCE AND EYE MOVEMENT. To test extraocular muscle balance and cranial nerve function, the patient and HCP face each other. The patient looks straight ahead. The HCP moves his finger in the six cardinal fields of gaze, coming back to the point of origin between each field of gaze (Fig. 51.10). The patient follows the HCP's finger without moving the head. The purpose is to see if the patient's eyes can follow the HCP's finger in all fields of gaze without nystagmus. **Nystagmus** is an involuntary, cyclical, rapid movement of the eyes.

The corneal light reflex test checks muscle balance. This test is conducted by shining a penlight toward the cornea while the patient is staring at an object straight ahead. The light reflection should be at exactly the same place on both pupils. If the eyes lack symmetry, muscle weakness could be present.

The cover test is used in conjunction with an abnormal corneal light reflex test to evaluate muscle balance. The

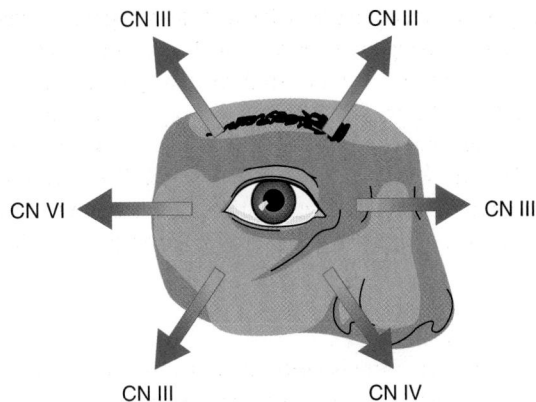

FIGURE 51.10 Six cardinal fields of gaze.

patient is asked to look straight ahead at a far object. The HCP covers one of the patient's eyes with a 3 × 5 card. The uncovered eye should have a steady gaze; if it moves, there may be muscle weakness. Next, the cover is quickly removed, and the action of this uncovered eye is observed. If this eye moves to fixate on the light instead of staring straight ahead, it indicates a drifting of the eye occurred when it was covered. This is a sign of muscle weakness. This deviation of the eye away from the visual axis is known as **tropia.** Deviation of the eye toward the nose is **esotropia.** Movement laterally is **exotropia.** Downward deviation is **hypotropia.**

PUPILLARY REFLEXES. When observed, the pupils should be round, symmetrical, and reactive to light. To test pupillary response to light, both consensual and direct examinations should be completed. A slightly darkened room works best. The patient looks straight ahead, and the size of the pupil is noted. A penlight is shone toward the pupil from the side of the eye. Movement of the pupil is observed. The pupil should quickly constrict. The size of the pupil is noted when it constricts. This is known as direct response.

To conduct a consensual pupil examination, observe the eye just tested for reaction while shining the penlight into the other eye. The observed pupil should constrict. This is known as **consensual response.** Repeat the procedure for the opposite eye.

The HCP proceeds to test for **accommodation.** This is the ability of the pupil to respond to near and far distances. The patient is told to look at an object far away. The size and shape of the pupils are observed. The HCP continues to observe the pupils as the patient focuses on a near object (the HCP's penlight or finger) held about 5 inches from the patient's face. Normally, the patient's eyes turn inward and the pupils constrict. These responses, convergence and constriction, are called accommodation ("Gerontological Issues: Age-Related Changes in Vision"). HCPs use the acronym PERRLA to indicate pupils equal, round, reactive to light, and accommodation. If accommodation is not tested along with the other tests, the acronym used is PERRL.

INSPECTION AND PALPATION OF EXTERNAL STRUCTURES. The extraocular structures are inspected. The presence of eyebrows, symmetry, hair texture, size, and extension of the brow are noted. The HCP first inspects and palpates the orbital area for edema, lesions, puffiness, and tenderness. Then the eyelids are inspected for symmetry, presence of eyelashes, eyelash position, tremors, flakiness, redness, and swelling. The patient is asked to open and close the eyelids. When open, the eyelid should cover the iris margin but not the pupil. The distance between the upper and lower eyelid, known as the palpebral fissure, is inspected; it should be equal in both eyes. If the palpebral fissure is nonsymmetrical, observe for **ptosis,** a drooping of the eyelid, commonly seen in stroke patients. Next, the medial canthus of the lower lid is gently palpated and observed for exudate. The eyelids are palpated for nodules. The eye is palpated for firmness over the closed eyelid.

The lower eyelid is pulled down, and the patient is asked to look upward. The conjunctiva and sclera are inspected for

• **WORD • BUILDING •**

esotropia: eso—inward + tropia—movement of the eye
exotropia: exo—out + tropia—movement of the eye

color, discharge, and pterygium (thickening of the conjunctiva). To inspect the upper eyelid, the upper lid is everted (turned inside out) over a cotton-tipped applicator by the HCP. The patient blinks to return the eyelid to its resting position when the inspection is complete.

The external eyes are inspected for color and symmetry of the irises, clarity of the cornea, and depth and clarity of the anterior chamber. Shining a light obliquely across the cornea shows the clearness of the cornea. The cornea should be transparent without cloudiness. In individuals older than 40 years, there may be bilateral opaque whitening of the outer rim of the cornea. This is known as **arcus senilis.** It is caused from lipid deposits and is considered normal. It does not affect vision.

INTERNAL EYE EXAMINATION. Examination of the internal eye is done by an HCP. A dark room allows the pupil to dilate. Anticholinergic mydriatic (causing dilatation) eye drops may be used but are not always necessary. An **ophthalmoscope** is a handheld instrument with a light source. It magnifies the internal structures of the eye. For the examination, the patient is asked to hold the head still while looking at a distant object. The patient is informed that the bright light could be uncomfortable. The HCP can examine the internal eye using a stationary device called a slit-lamp microscope. For this exam, the patient is seated and rests the chin on a support while a microscope and a bright light source are directed into the eye.

Intraocular Pressure. Estimation of intraocular pressure is measured by using one of several types of tonometer. The procedure may be performed using anesthetic drops. Readings above the normal range of 10 to 21 mm Hg may indicate glaucoma.

Diagnostic Eye Tests
Exudate Culture
If exudate from any portion of the eye or surrounding structure is present, an eye culture may be ordered. Results of the culture guide anti-infective treatment.

Digital Imaging
Digital imaging is a newer way of viewing most of the retina without requiring the use of dilating eye drops. The instrument takes a digital picture of the retina in 2 seconds. This assists in early detection of eye disease. A permanent photographic reference for the retina is obtained.

Optical Coherence Tomography
Optical coherence tomography takes a picture of the retina. Light beams are shone into the eye at various angles. The amount of interference is measured, creating a detailed image of the depth of the retina.

Fluorescein and Indocyanine Green Angiography
Angiography with dye is a test using special cameras to find leaking or damaged blood vessels in the retinal or deeper choroidal circulation. Fluorescein is a yellow dye that glows in visible light and is useful for showing the retinal circulation.

Indocyanine green is a green dye that shows up with invisible infrared light to highlight the choroidal circulation. The patient is asked about dye allergies (indocyanine green contains iodine). Then the pupil is dilated. The dye is injected intravenously and travels to the eye's circulation, making the blood vessels there visible. Fluorescein is used for diabetic retinopathy and retinal vascular disease. Indocyanine green is used for the wet form of macular degeneration when blood is present in the macula.

Electroretinography
Electroretinography is useful in diagnosing diseases of the rods and cones of the eye. The procedure evaluates differences in the electrical potential between the cornea and retina in response to light wavelengths and intensity. The test is conducted by placing contact lenses with electrodes directly on the eye.

Ultrasonography
Ultrasound is useful when the internal eye cannot be visualized directly because of obstructions, such as corneal opacities or bloody vitreous. The eye is anesthetized with anesthetic drops. A transducer probe is placed on the eye to perform the ultrasound.

Imaging Tests
X-ray films show bone structure and tumors. Computed tomography (CT) scan and magnetic resonance imaging (MRI) visualize ocular structures and abnormalities of the eye and surrounding tissues.

Therapeutic Measures for the Eye and Vision
Nurses have an important role in screening and educating people about care for healthy eyes and the prevention of disease and helping them cope with visual deficits. To learn more to promote vision health, visit www.lighthouseguild.org. For resources to help those persons who are blind, visit the American Foundation for the Blind at www.afb.org or the National Federation of the Blind at www.nfb.org.

Eye Examinations
The American Optometric Association (2018) guidelines suggest eye examinations for people aged 18 to 60 every 2 years. For those younger than 61 at risk for eye disease, eye examinations should be done every 1 to 2 years or as directed by the HCP. Those 61 or older should have annual or as-directed eye exams.

Eye care providers include the ophthalmologist and optometrist. An **ophthalmologist** is a physician who specializes in diagnosing and treating eye diseases. An **optometrist** (doctor of optometry) specializes in eye examinations to identify visual defects, diagnose problems, prescribe corrective lenses or other treatments, and refer for medical treatment. An **optician** is trained to grind and fit lenses prescribed by an ophthalmologist or optometrist.

Eye Hygiene

It is important to keep debris out of the eyes to prevent scratching of the eye's delicate surfaces. When a foreign object gets into the eye, such as dirt or an eyelash, teach people not to rub the eye. Tears can wash out the object by pulling the upper eyelid down over the eye briefly. When wiping the eyes, wipe from the inner canthus to the outer canthus.

Nutrition for Eye Health

Adequate nutrition is important for eye health (see "Nutrition Notes"). Inadequate vitamin intake can result in corneal damage and night blindness from a lack of vitamin A. Optic neuritis can result from a vitamin B deficiency.

Nutrition Notes

Nutrition and Eye Disease. The National Eye Institute (NEI) studied different antioxidants, vitamins, and minerals to determine which combinations may provide better eye health for those at risk of age-related macular degeneration (AMD). A lower risk of developing AMD was found in those who ate a diet rich in leafy, green vegetables. These are a good source of the antioxidants lutein and zeaxanthin. Researchers with the Age-Related Eye Disease Study (AREDS) found that a supplement containing vitamins and minerals could reduce the risk of developing advanced AMD. Ongoing studies resulted in a reformulation of the supplement, called AREDS2, which contains lutein, zeaxanthin, omega-3 fatty acids, and zinc. Vitamins haven been taken out of the original formula because of a possible increase in cancer risks in some individuals. Recent research suggests there is no benefit from supplemented omega-3 fatty acids, but that consumption of fish is associated with lower rates of AMD. NEI also studied eye health in people with diabetes and found that by maintaining intensive glycemic control, retinopathy progression was reduced by approximately one-third. Visit www.nei.nih.gov for more information.

Eye Safety and Prevention of Injury

Many people in the United States suffer eye injuries each year. Common activities such as microwave cooking, lawn care, shooting rubber bands, and BB gun use cause most injuries. Many of these injuries could be prevented with education and use of safety measures (Table 51.3).

Eye Irrigation

If it is necessary to irrigate foreign bodies or chemical substances from the eye, prepare the patient by explaining the procedure (see "Eye Irrigation" under "Procedures" on Davis Edge).

Guide Dogs for the Blind and Visually Impaired

Guide dogs are trained to lead blind and visually impaired people around obstacles. While the dogs are working, they should not

Table 51.3

Eye Safety and Injury Prevention

To Protect From:	Use These Eye Safety Measures
Foreign objects	Always wear safety goggles when working with tools or yard equipment.
Chemical splashes	Use splash shields when around body fluids or chemicals. Close eyes to avoid getting hairspray in them.
Corneal lens abrasions/ infections from contact lenses	Follow manufacturer's or eye care professional's directions for length of use and cleaning procedures. Do not wear contact lenses too long.
Ultraviolet light (UV)	Wear UV-protective sunglasses at all ages. Wear a hat to shield sun. Wear sunglasses with side shields after administration of mydriatics.
Visual deficits	Update prescription of glasses yearly. Wear glasses that fit properly, are clean, and are free of scratches.
Computer vision syndrome (digital eye strain)	Position the center of the computer screen 4 to 5 inches below eye level and the screen 20 to 28 inches from the eyes. Avoid glare on the computer screen. Blink frequently to prevent dry eyes. Rest eyes: Every 20 minutes, look 20 feet away for 20 seconds. Take a break every 2 hours for 15 minutes.
Eye injury from sports	Wear protective eyewear with polycarbonate lenses, facemasks, or helmets while participating in sports.

be approached, touched, or fed without their owner's permission. Most dogs do not like to be petted or patted on the head, so ask the owner the dog's petting preference (often the chest, back, and near the tail) if permission is given to touch the dog.

Medication Administration

Most eye medications are applied as drops, ointments, or irrigations (see Chapter 52). The nurse must know the normal dosage and strength, desired action, side effects, and contraindications of the medication for safe administration. The steps for application of eye medications ("Administration of Eye Drops" and "Administration of Eye Ointment") can be found under "Procedures" on Davis Edge. Systemic adverse reactions from eye medications can occur.

PUNCTAL OCCLUSION. After eye drop administration, the eyelids should be closed for 2 minutes without blinking, which is about the time it takes for absorption of the medication into the eye. During this same time period, the puncta (tear duct) on the eyelid of the eye in which medication was administered should have pressure applied to it, by either the nurse wearing gloves or the patient (see Fig. 51.2). The index finger is placed on the corner of the eye. Pressure is applied against the bone along the nose (not into the eye). This allows the eye drop to remain in the eye longer for greater effect. It also reduces systemic absorption and side effects of the medication. Some eye medications can have serious cardiac or respiratory effects. Teach the patient the proper instillation of eye medications.

> **NURSING CARE TIP**
>
> Older patients, when instilling their own eye drops, may not feel the drops go in. Teaching patients to refrigerate the drops, if not contraindicated, for 15 to 30 minutes before instillation helps them feel whether the drops go into the eye or miss and fall onto the face.

EYE PATCHING. After treating an injured or infected eye, the HCP may order the eye to be patched. Apply ointment or drops if ordered and ask the patient to keep the eyelid shut. Place a disposable, cotton gauze eye patch over the eye socket depression. The purpose of eye patching is to protect the eye from further damage by keeping the lids closed. Sometimes an additional metal shield is placed over the soft pads to protect the eye from external injury. The patch is taped in place and the patient instructed to rest the eyes. Suggest quiet activities, such as listening to music or an audio book, or sleeping. Watching television or reading is not recommended because the patched eye will follow the movement of the unpatched eye.

 HEARING

Normal Anatomy and Physiology of the Ear

The ear consists of three areas: the outer ear, the middle ear, and the inner ear. The inner ear contains the receptors for the senses of hearing and equilibrium.

Outer Ear

The outer ear consists of the auricle and the auditory canal (Fig. 51.11).

Middle Ear

The middle ear is an air-filled cavity in the temporal bone (see Fig. 51.11). Vibrations of the tympanic membrane caused by sound are transmitted through the three auditory bones (ossicles). The stapes then transmits vibrations to the fluid-filled inner ear at the oval window.

Inner Ear

The inner ear is a cavity in the temporal bone called the bony labyrinth, lined with membranes called the membranous labyrinth. The fluid between bone and membrane is called perilymph, and that within the membrane is called endolymph. The structures of the bony labyrinth include the semicircular canals, vestibule, and cochlea (Fig. 51.12).

The process of hearing involves the transmission of vibrations and the generation of nerve impulses. When sound waves enter the auditory canal, vibrations are transmitted by the following structures: tympanic membrane, malleus, incus, stapes, oval window of the inner ear, perilymph and endolymph within the cochlea, and hair cells of the organ of Corti. When the hair cells bend, they generate impulses that are carried by the eighth cranial nerve to the brain. The auditory areas, for both hearing and interpretation, are in the temporal lobes of the cerebral cortex.

The inner ear also has receptors for equilibrium. Dynamic equilibrium receptors are within the semicircular canals, whereas static equilibrium receptors are within the vestibule (Fig. 51.13). Within the utricle and saccule of the vestibule, the hair cells bend in response to gravity on the otoliths as the position of the head changes. The impulses generated are carried by the vestibular branch of the eighth cranial nerve to the cerebellum, medulla, and pons. The cerebellum sends this information continuously to the cerebral motor cortex. The cerebellum and brainstem use this information to maintain equilibrium at a subconscious level; the cerebrum interprets the conscious awareness of the position of the head.

When the head moves, movement of the endolymph will bend the cupula within the ampulla. The bending of the hair cells at its base generates impulses carried by the vestibular branch of the eighth cranial nerve to the cerebellum and brainstem. Then impulses are sent to the cerebral cortex. These impulses are interpreted as directional acceleration or deceleration; this information is used to maintain equilibrium during movement.

Aging and the Ear

In the ear, cumulative damage to the hair cells in the organ of Corti usually becomes apparent sometime after the age of 60 (see Fig. 51.8). Damaged hair cells cannot be replaced. Ability to hear high frequencies is usually lost first (presbycusis), whereas hearing may still be adequate for lower-pitched ranges. The high-pitched sounds *f*, *s*, *k*, and *sh* are

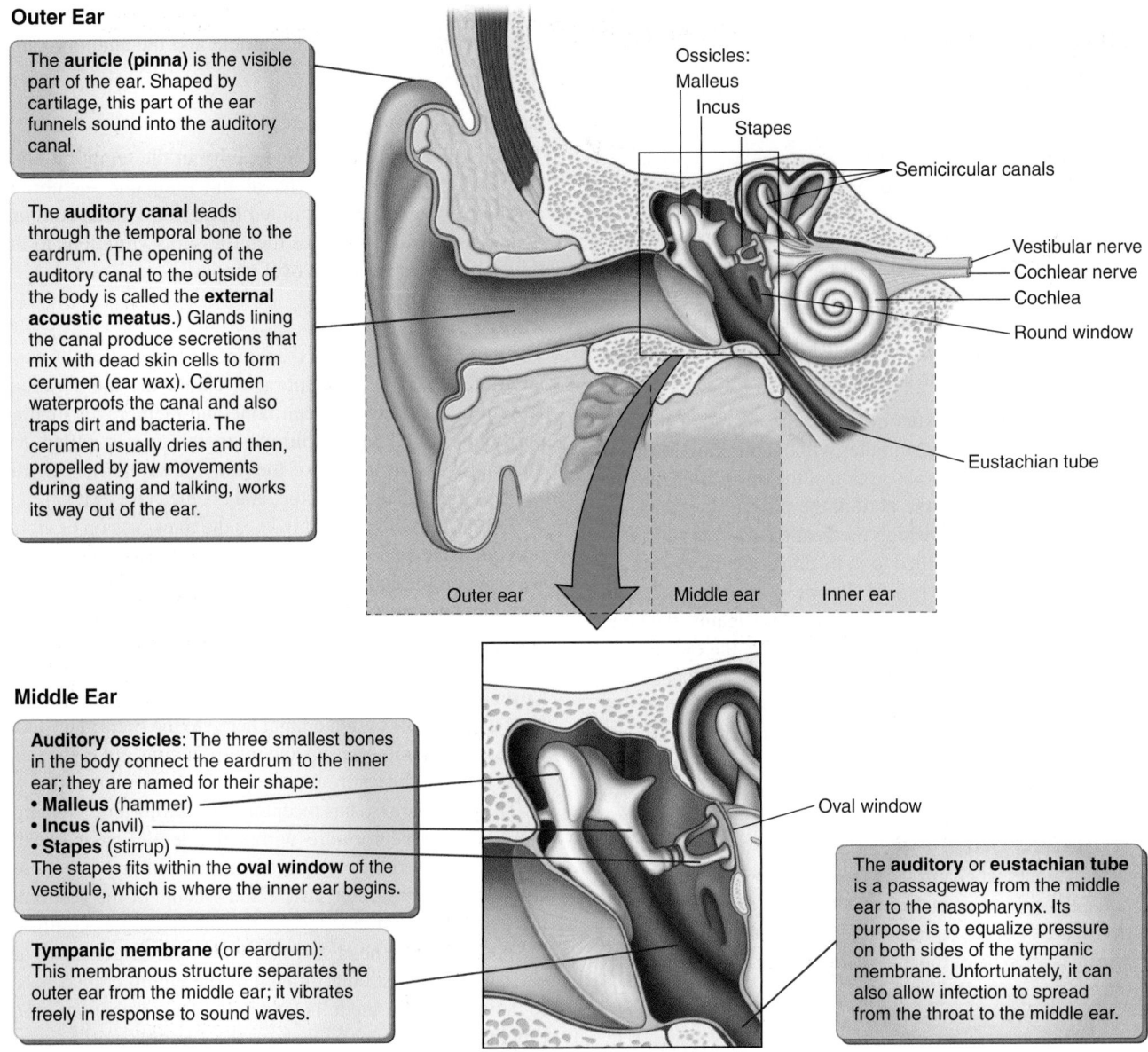

Outer Ear

The **auricle (pinna)** is the visible part of the ear. Shaped by cartilage, this part of the ear funnels sound into the auditory canal.

The **auditory canal** leads through the temporal bone to the eardrum. (The opening of the auditory canal to the outside of the body is called the **external acoustic meatus**.) Glands lining the canal produce secretions that mix with dead skin cells to form cerumen (ear wax). Cerumen waterproofs the canal and also traps dirt and bacteria. The cerumen usually dries and then, propelled by jaw movements during eating and talking, works its way out of the ear.

Ossicles:
Malleus
Incus
Stapes

Semicircular canals

Vestibular nerve
Cochlear nerve
Cochlea
Round window

Eustachian tube

Outer ear   Middle ear   Inner ear

Middle Ear

Auditory ossicles: The three smallest bones in the body connect the eardrum to the inner ear; they are named for their shape:
• **Malleus** (hammer)
• **Incus** (anvil)
• **Stapes** (stirrup)
The stapes fits within the **oval window** of the vestibule, which is where the inner ear begins.

Oval window

The **auditory** or **eustachian tube** is a passageway from the middle ear to the nasopharynx. Its purpose is to equalize pressure on both sides of the tympanic membrane. Unfortunately, it can also allow infection to spread from the throat to the middle ear.

Tympanic membrane (or eardrum): This membranous structure separates the outer ear from the middle ear; it vibrates freely in response to sound waves.

FIGURE 51.11 Outer and middle ear.

common losses. Also, it becomes more difficult to filter out background noises, so loud environments make it difficult to hear conversations ("Gerontological Issues: Age-Related Changes in Hearing").

Gerontological Issues

Age-Related Changes in Hearing. Presbycusis is an age-related change in which progressive hearing loss is caused by loss of hair cells and decreased blood supplying the ear. This results in the loss of hearing high-pitched sounds (pitch = cycles per second; loudness = decibels). Because the ability to hear pitch, rather than volume, is lost, it is not helpful to talk louder to a patient with this type of hearing

loss. In fact, talking louder can make it more difficult to discriminate sounds. The loss of high-pitched hearing causes the older adult to hear distracting background noises more clearly than conversation. It is important to know what helps a person hear best.

Deafness or decreased hearing acuity is one of the main reasons that older adults withdraw from social activities.

Older adults who have a hearing loss may need adaptive equipment in their home for safety. The use of a hearing aid may increase hearing for those who do not have nerve damage deafness. The use of flashing lights instead of buzzers or alarms increases the safety of an older adult who is not able to hear a smoke detector or fire alarm.

Inner Ear

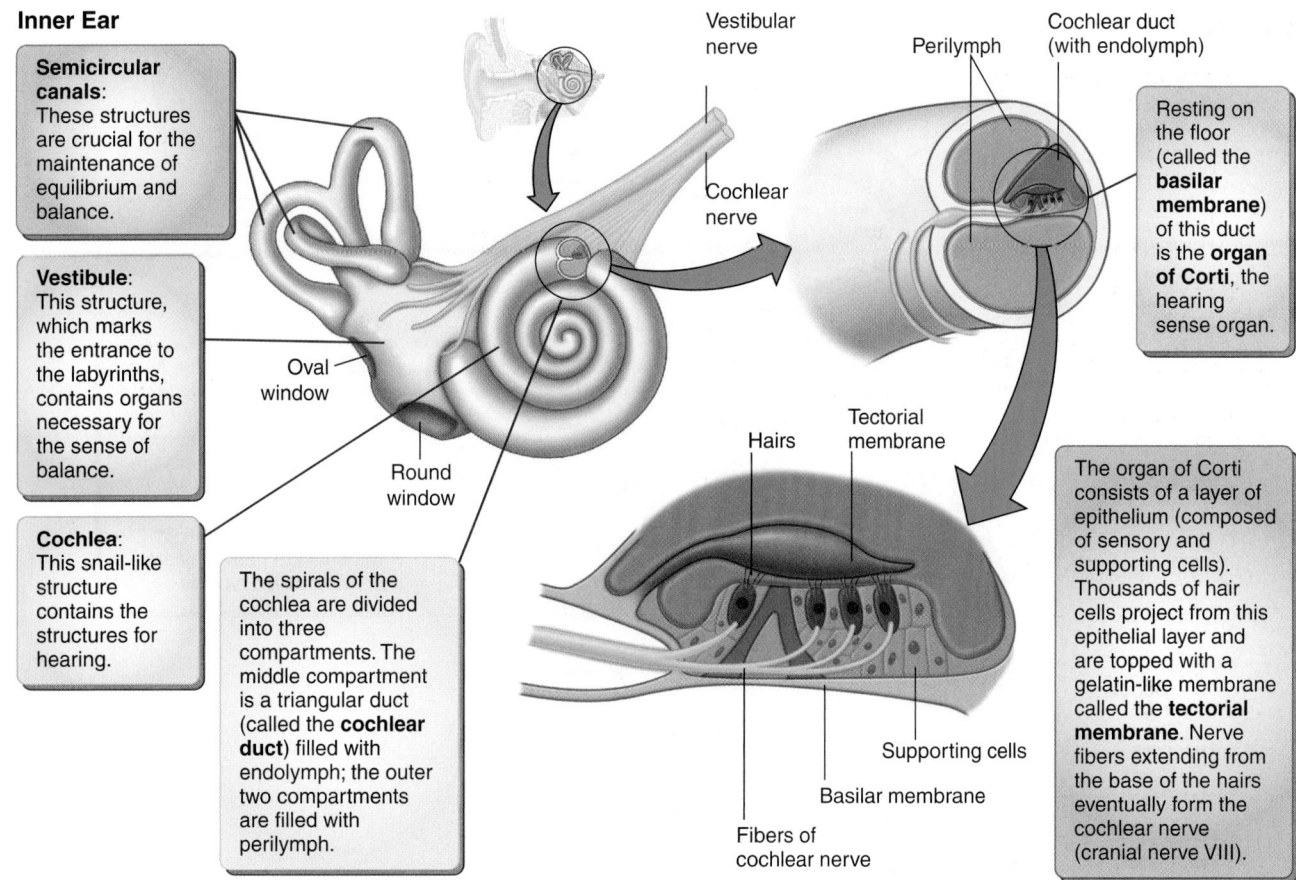

Semicircular canals: These structures are crucial for the maintenance of equilibrium and balance.

Vestibule: This structure, which marks the entrance to the labyrinths, contains organs necessary for the sense of balance.

Cochlea: This snail-like structure contains the structures for hearing.

The spirals of the cochlea are divided into three compartments. The middle compartment is a triangular duct (called the **cochlear duct**) filled with endolymph; the outer two compartments are filled with perilymph.

Oval window

Round window

Vestibular nerve

Cochlear nerve

Perilymph

Cochlear duct (with endolymph)

Resting on the floor (called the **basilar membrane**) of this duct is the **organ of Corti**, the hearing sense organ.

Hairs

Tectorial membrane

Supporting cells

Basilar membrane

Fibers of cochlear nerve

The organ of Corti consists of a layer of epithelium (composed of sensory and supporting cells). Thousands of hair cells project from this epithelial layer and are topped with a gelatin-like membrane called the **tectorial membrane**. Nerve fibers extending from the base of the hairs eventually form the cochlear nerve (cranial nerve VIII).

FIGURE 51.12 Inner ear.

Nursing Assessment of the Ear and Hearing

A quiet environment is helpful for collecting accurate hearing data. Document the patient's behavior as it may provide information related to a hearing loss.

Health History

The patient's self-appraisal of his or her hearing or related symptoms and family observations are obtained during the health history (Table 51.4). Data collection regarding symptoms includes asking **WHAT'S UP?** questions (see Chapter 1). Symptoms related to the ear that may be reported include decreased hearing or loss of hearing, **otorrhea** (discharge), **otalgia** (ear pain), itching, fullness, tinnitus (ringing, buzzing, or roaring in the ears), or vertigo (dizziness). Note exposure to medications that are potentially **ototoxic**, such as certain antibiotics or diuretics (see Chapter 52).

Physical Examination

Physical examination of the ear begins by observing the behaviors of the patient (Box 51.1). Note how the patient communicates. Observe how the patient talks. Note slurred speech. Examination of the ear includes inspection, palpation, testing of auditory acuity, balance testing, and otoscopic examination by the HCP (Table 51.5). Document all findings.

INSPECTION AND PALPATION OF THE EXTERNAL EAR. Inspection of the external ear begins with examining the auricle and the ear canal. A small bump seen on the inside of the helix (the upper external ear margin), called Darwin's tubercle, is normal. The ear canal should be inspected before obtaining an infrared ear temperature because the presence of excess cerumen can alter the accuracy of the reading. To inspect the external ear canal, tip the adult patient's head toward the opposite side of the ear. Use a penlight or otoscope to inspect the canal.

Next the auricles and mastoid process are palpated. The mastoid process (bony prominence located behind the earlobe) should be smooth and hard when palpated. It should not be tender or swollen.

AUDITORY ACUITY TESTING. Auditory function can be evaluated using three assessment tests. The whisper voice test identifies hearing function in each ear. Ask the patient to occlude one ear with a finger and rub the tragus to mask

• **WORD · BUILDING** •
otorrhea: oto—related to the ear + rrhea—to flow
otalgia: ot—related to the ear + algia—signifying pain
ototoxic: oto—related to the ear + toxic—poison

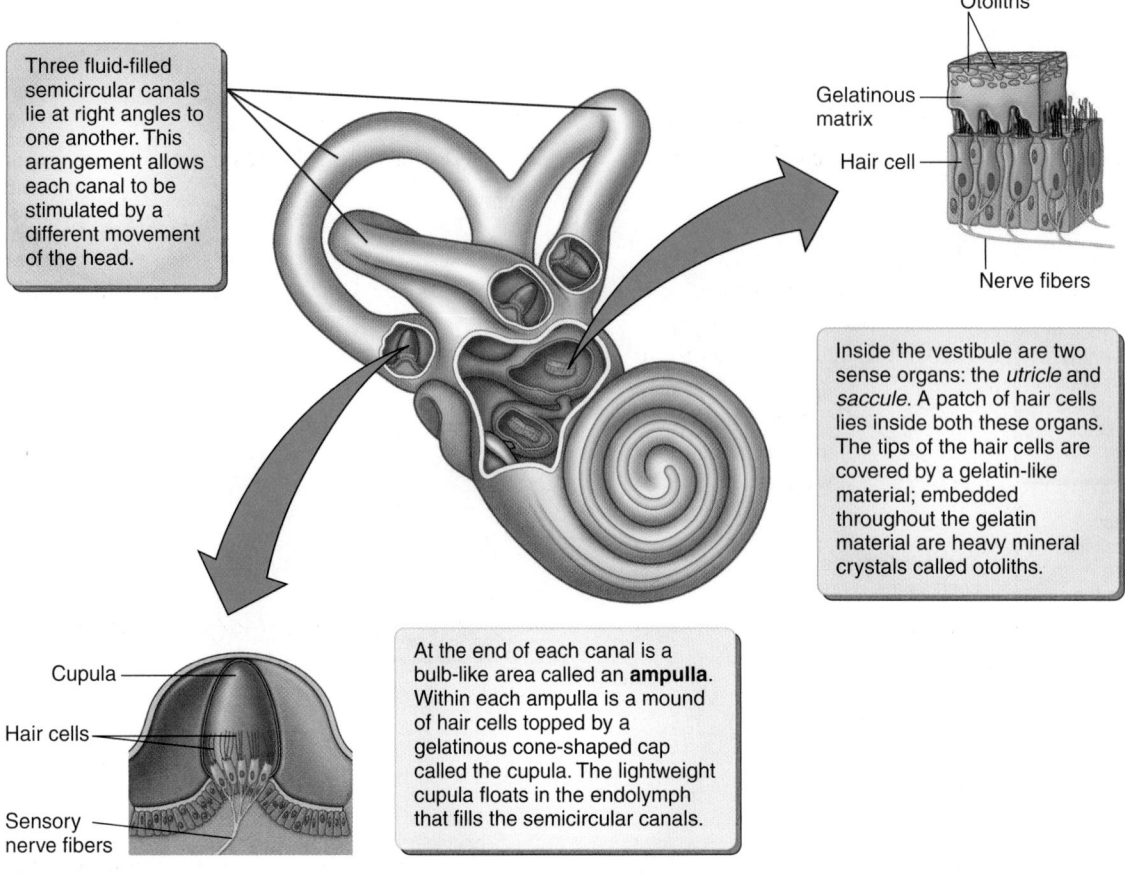

Three fluid-filled semicircular canals lie at right angles to one another. This arrangement allows each canal to be stimulated by a different movement of the head.

Otoliths

Gelatinous matrix

Hair cell

Nerve fibers

Inside the vestibule are two sense organs: the *utricle* and *saccule*. A patch of hair cells lies inside both these organs. The tips of the hair cells are covered by a gelatin-like material; embedded throughout the gelatin material are heavy mineral crystals called otoliths.

Cupula

Hair cells

Sensory nerve fibers

At the end of each canal is a bulb-like area called an **ampulla**. Within each ampulla is a mound of hair cells topped by a gelatinous cone-shaped cap called the cupula. The lightweight cupula floats in the endolymph that fills the semicircular canals.

FIGURE 51.13 Balance.

Table 51.4
Subjective Data Collection for the Ear

Questions to Ask During the Health History	Rationale
Family History	
Has any family member had any hearing problems or loss? Has any family member had Ménière disease?	Some ear diseases may be genetic.
Health History	
What childhood illnesses have you had?	Mumps, measles, or scarlet fever can affect hearing.
What current diseases do you have? Hospitalizations?	Diseases and their treatments can affect hearing.
What is your sodium intake? How much alcohol do you drink?	Sodium and alcohol intake can affect amount of endolymph in the inner ear, affecting hearing.
What medications do you take?	Many medications are ototoxic and can cause hearing loss.
What are your swimming habits?	Swimming can cause swimmer's ear.
Have you had any injuries or surgeries to the ear?	Recent trauma or surgeries can affect hearing.
Do you have any allergies? Have you had a recent or past upper respiratory or ear infection?	Allergies can cause nasal congestion, leading to middle ear congestion and/or infection.
Do you have discharge from the ear (otorrhea), ear pain (otalgia), itching, fullness, tinnitus, or vertigo? Do you have a fever, nausea, or vomiting?	These symptoms can indicate outer, middle, or inner ear infections; ototoxicity; or other ear diseases.

Table 51.4

Subjective Data Collection for the Ear—cont'd

Questions to Ask During the Health History	Rationale
Have you been exposed to pressure changes such as with flying or diving?	Barotrauma may occur due to pressure changes.

Hearing Impairment

Have you noticed any hearing loss, either gradually or suddenly?	Patient may have hearing loss in one or both ears.
Do you have difficulty understanding certain words or entire conversations?	
Do you have difficulty hearing when there is a lot of background noise?	
Do you hear better out of one ear than the other?	
Do you wear a hearing aid or other assistive device? If so, what is the device and for which ear is it used?	
Have your friends or family commented on your decreased hearing?	Others may notice hearing loss signs in patient.
How does your hearing loss affect your daily life?	Hearing loss can cause social isolation.
Do you feel frustrated or embarrassed because of your hearing loss?	
How do your friends and family react to your hearing loss?	
Are you exposed to loud noises (e.g., current/past job, transportation, machinery, or music)?	Loud noises can cause damage to the ear, leading to hearing loss over time.

Self-Care Behaviors

Have you had your hearing checked? If so, when?	Provides information about patient's ear self-care and health.
How do you clean your ears?	
How do you protect your ears from loud noises?	

Box 51.1

Behaviors Indicating Hearing Loss

Adults with hearing loss may show any or all of the following behaviors:

- Turns up volume on the television or radio.
- Frequently asks, "What did you say?"
- Leans forward or turns head to one side during conversations to hear better.
- Cups hand around ear during conversation.
- Says people are talking softly or mumbling.
- Speaks in an unusually loud or quiet voice.
- Answers questions inappropriately or not at all.
- Has difficulty hearing high-frequency consonants.
- Avoids group activities.
- Shows loss of sense of humor.
- Has strained or serious look on face during conversations.
- Appears to ignore people or does not participate.
- Is irritable or sensitive in interpersonal relations.
- Reports ringing, buzzing, or roaring noise in ears.

sound. Stand 1 to 2 feet away on the opposite side, behind the patient's field of vision to prevent lip reading. Whisper two-syllable words toward the unoccluded ear. Variability can occur in the loudness of the whisper. The patient is asked to restate the whispered words. The process is repeated on the other ear. Ask the patient if hearing was better in one ear than in the other ear. Normally, the patient should be able to hear a soft whisper equally well in both ears. Findings of one ear hearing better than the other or an inability to hear a soft whisper can indicate hearing impairment.

A second acuity test is the **Rinne test.** This test is performed with a tuning fork. It is useful for differentiating between conductive and sensorineural hearing loss. To perform the test, strike the tuning fork and place it on the patient's mastoid process (Fig. 51.14). Verify that the patient is able to hear the tuning fork. Then instruct the patient to say immediately when the sound is no longer heard. When the patient indicates that the sound is not heard, place the vibrating tuning fork 2 inches in front of the ear. Ask the patient whether he or she hears the

Table 51.5

Objective Data Collection for the Ear

Physical Examination Findings	*Possible Abnormal Findings/Causes*
Inspection and Palpation of the External Ear	
Ears should be symmetrical in size, configuration, and angle of attachment.	Asymmetrical size and placement could indicate congenital deformities.
Skin covering the ear should be intact, smooth, and without erythema or inflammation.	Breaks in the skin, discharge, inflammation, or growths can be caused by infections, a poorly fitting hearing aid, skin cancer, or trauma.
Ear canal should have minimal or no cerumen and no drainage.	Excessive cerumen or drainage may be due to infection or trauma. Color, consistency, and odor are noted, if present. Excessive cerumen can alter hearing and cause inaccurate tympanic temperature readings.
No lesions, tophi, or masses should be palpated. No foreign bodies should be seen.	Tophi (deposits of uric acid crystals in external ear margin) occur in gout. A mass could indicate cancer.
No tenderness of auricle when palpated. No odor from ear detected.	Tenderness and odor can indicate infection.
Auditory Acuity Testing	
Patient can hear whispered words at 1 to 2 feet away. Rinne and Weber tests are normal (see Table 51.6).	Abnormal results can indicate conductive, sensorineural, mixed, or neural hearing loss.
Balance Testing	
Patient can sit and walk without difficulty. Patient can perform Romberg test with minimal swaying.	Difficulty sitting and/or walking as well as increased swaying or falling with Romberg test may be due to balance difficulties. This may be due to inner ear infection or disorder.
Otoscopic Examination	
Ear canal should be smooth and empty, without redness, scaliness, swelling, drainage, excessive cerumen, or foreign objects.	Ear canal may be reddened and swollen; drainage may be present; excessive cerumen or foreign object may be present. This could be caused by infection, improper care, or excessive cerumen production.
Internal otoscope examination is completed by experienced practitioner and should reveal a slightly conical, shiny, smooth, pearly gray eardrum.	Eardrum may be dull, bulging, retracted, or reddened, possibly caused by middle ear infection or blockage.
Other	
Observe the patient's position and posture during the interview and physical exam. Does the patient watch the practitioner's mouth or lean toward the practitioner?	Behaviors may indicate hearing loss and the patient's effort to compensate.

tuning fork and then to indicate when the sound is no longer heard. Normally, air conduction (AC) is heard twice as long as bone conduction (BC). The patient reports this by hearing the tuning fork when placed in front of the ear (AC) after it is no longer heard on the mastoid process (BC). Normal results are recorded as "AC greater than BC." The test is repeated on the other ear. Abnormal findings can indicate conduction or sensorineural problems (Table 51.6).

The **Weber test** is a third test to assess hearing acuity. The Weber test is also performed using a tuning fork. Place the vibrating tuning fork on the center of the patient's forehead or head (Fig. 51.15). Verify that the patient can hear the tuning fork. If the patient says yes, ask the patient whether the sound is heard better in the left ear, better in the right ear, or the same in both ears. It is important to give the patient three choices from which to choose.

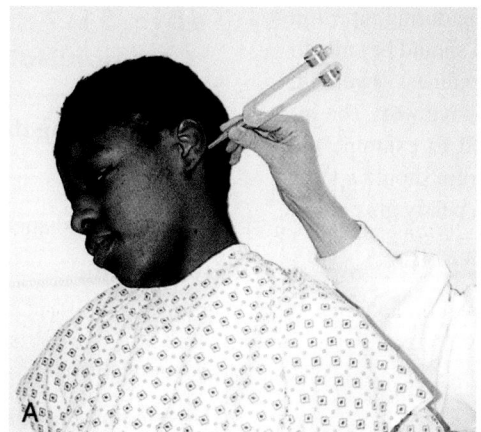
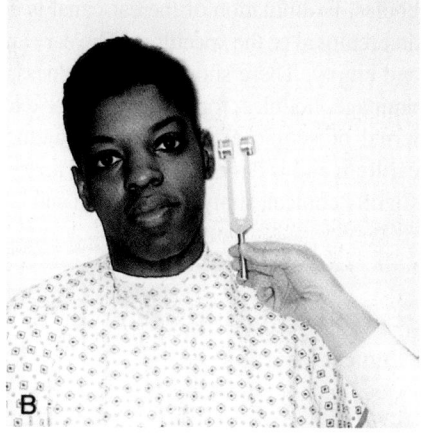

FIGURE 51.14 Rinne test. (A) Bone conduction. (B) Air conduction.

Table 51.6

Auditory Acuity Tuning Fork Tests

Test	Normal Hearing Results	Conductive	Sensorineural Hearing Loss
Rinne Test	Air conduction heard twice as long as bone conduction	Bone conduction heard longer than air conduction in affected ear	Air conduction heard longer than bone conduction in affected ear (but may be less than 2:1 ratio)
Weber Test	Tone heard in center of the head; no lateralization	Sound heard louder in affected ear	Sound heard louder in better ear

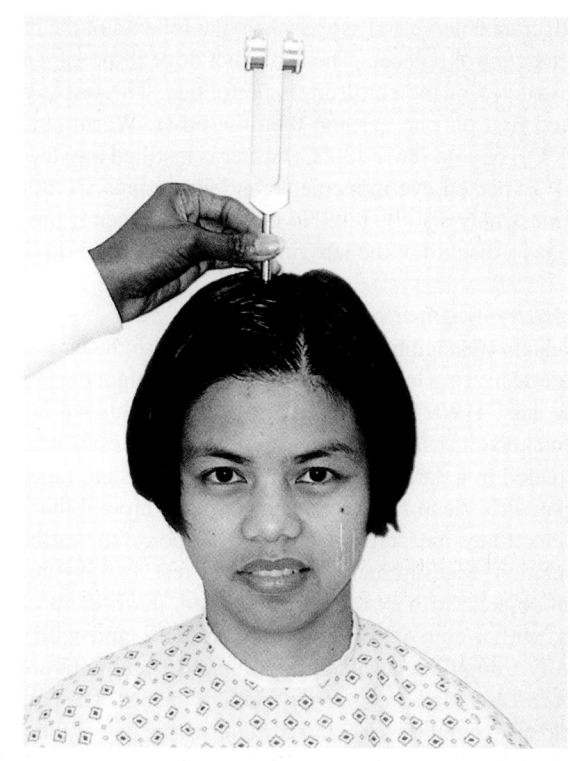

FIGURE 51.15 Weber test.

Normally, the patient hears the sound the same in both ears (see Table 51.6).

BALANCE TESTING. When the patient reports dizziness, nystagmus, or problems with equilibrium, simple tests can be performed to assess vestibular function. Plan for patient safety before testing. The first test is simply to observe the patient's gait by having the patient walk away from the HCP and then walk back. Note the patient's balance, posture, and movement of arms and legs. The patient should be able to walk in an upright position with no difficulties in balance or movement.

Romberg test (falling test) is another simple test to assess vestibular function. If a fall appears likely, be prepared to support the patient during the test to prevent injury. Instruct the patient to stand with feet together, first with eyes open and then with eyes closed. Normally, the patient has no difficulty maintaining a standing position with only minimal swaying. If the patient has difficulty maintaining balance or loses balance (a positive Romberg test), the patient may have an inner ear problem.

OTOSCOPIC EXAMINATION. An otoscope is an instrument consisting of a handle, a light source, a magnifying lens, and an optional speculum for inserting in the ear. Some otoscopes have a pneumatic device for injecting air into the canal to test the eardrum's mobility and integrity. The otoscope is used by the HCP to visualize the external ear, ear canal, and tympanic membrane. Otoscopic examination is completed to identify specific disorders or infections, remove wax, or remove foreign bodies. Examination of the ear canal is done during insertion and removal of the speculum. The ear canal should be smooth and empty. There should be no redness, scaliness, swelling, drainage, nodules, foreign objects, or excessive wax. The internal otoscopic examination is conducted to examine the eardrum and is done by the HCP. The eardrum should appear slightly conical, shiny, and smooth and be a pearly gray color.

Evidence-Based Practice

Clinical Question
Does hearing loss affect balance?

Evidence
A systematic review examining 12 cross-sectional design studies found that older adults with hearing loss were 2.39 times more likely to experience falls than those without hearing loss. It is thought that the vestibular system (balance) may be adversely affected by infections and toxins that affect the cilia in both the cochlea and vestibular systems. This is in addition to age-related changes that occur in the older adult. A positive publication bias was noted by the authors, and further studies were encouraged to strengthen the evidence for cause and effect of falls and hearing loss (Jiam, Li, & Agrawal, 2016).

Implications for Nursing Practice
Understanding and identifying risk factors for falls, including hearing loss, may help reduce the incidence of falls. Preventing falls can help keep older adults safe and reduce admissions to health care agencies.

Reference
Jiam, N. T-L., Li, C., & Agrawal, Y. (2016). Hearing loss and falls: A systematic review and meta-analysis. *Laryngoscope*, 126(2), 587–596.

Diagnostic Tests for the Ear and Hearing
Audiometric Testing
An audiologist uses audiometric testing as a screening tool to determine the type and degree of hearing loss. The audiometer produces a stimulus that consists of a musical tone, pure tone, or speech. To test AC, the patient sits in a soundproof booth, wears earphones, and signals the audiologist when and if a tone is heard. Each ear is tested separately. The patient is exposed to sounds of varying frequency or pitch (hertz) and intensity (decibels). By varying the levels of the sound, a hearing level is established (Table 51.7). Earphone testing can be used to measure AC, level of speech hearing, and understanding of speech. For BC testing, a vibrator is placed on the mastoid process, and the earphones are removed. Testing proceeds as with AC.

A patient with normal hearing should have the same AC as BC hearing levels. Differences in AC and BC hearing can provide information about the location and type of hearing loss.

Tympanometry
Tympanometry tests the movement of the tympanic membrane (ear drum) and evaluates middle ear function. The test

Table 51.7
Common Noise Levels

Human hearing threshold	**0–25 decibels (dB)**
Quiet room	30–40 dB
Conversational speech	60 dB
Heavy traffic	70 dB
Alarm clock	80 dB
Vacuum cleaner	80 dB
Unsafe noise levels begin	**90 dB**
Circular saw	100 dB
Rock music	120 dB
Jet planes	120–130 dB
Pain threshold	**130 dB**
Firearms	140 dB

is not done if the ear canal is obstructed or the ear drum is perforated. The tympanometer probe applies varying amounts of pressure to vibrate the tympanic membrane. The results are graphed on a tympanogram. The patient is informed that the tympanometry may cause transient vertigo. The patient is asked to report any nausea or dizziness felt during the test.

Caloric Test
The caloric test is used by the HCP to test the function of the eighth cranial nerve and assess vestibular reflexes of the inner ear that control balance. The test is not done if the ear canal is obstructed or the ear drum is perforated. The test is performed first on one ear and then the other. Warm (112°F [44.5°C]) or cold (86°F [30°C]) water is instilled into the ear canal. Expected eye movements and nystagmus are noted. Dizziness may also be felt. No nystagmus is seen if the patient has a disease of the labyrinth, such as Ménière disease.

Electronystagmogram
The electronystagmogram is used to diagnose the causes of unilateral hearing loss of unknown origin, vertigo, or ringing in the ears. The test is contraindicated in patients who have pacemakers. It is similar to the caloric test. The test is usually completed in a darkened room. Five electrodes are taped to the patient's clean face at certain positions around the eye. The electrodes measure nystagmus in response to vestibular stimulation. Measurements are taken at rest, looking at different objects, with eyes open and closed, in different positions, with water of different temperatures, and with air. Usually tranquilizers, alcohol, stimulants, and antivertigo agents are avoided for 1 to 5 days before the test. The patient should also avoid tobacco and caffeine on the day of the test. The patient may experience nausea, vertigo, or weakness following the test.

Computed Tomography Scan

A CT scan is useful for visualizing the temporal and mastoid bones, the middle and inner ears, and the eustachian tube.

Magnetic Resonance Imaging

MRI examines the membranous organs, nerve, and blood vessels of the temporal bone for disease.

Laboratory Tests

CULTURE. Culture of drainage from the ear canal or a surgical incision is important in diagnosis and treatment with the appropriate anti-infective agent for acute infections. Often with chronic infections, the culture is less helpful because gram-negative bacilli cover up the original pathogen. Drainage from the external ear is collected using a culture swab kit and taken to the lab immediately.

PATHOLOGY EXAMINATION. Pathology examination of tissue obtained during surgery is completed to rule out a malignancy and identify any unusual problems. A cholesteatoma (cyst of epithelial cells and cholesterol found in the middle ear) is identified by a pathology examination.

Therapeutic Measures for the Ear and Hearing

Medications

The medications most often used to treat ear disorders include anti-infectives, anti-inflammatories, antihistamines, decongestants, cerumenolytics, and diuretics. Anti-infectives can be administered systemically or as a topical solution. Ear medications are usually given as drops (see "Administration of Eardrops" under "Procedures" on Davis Edge). Anti-inflammatories, antihistamines, and decongestants are used with acute infections to reduce nasal and middle ear congestion. Cerumenolytics are used to soften cerumen and remove it from the ear canal. Diuretics are used with some inner ear disorders to reduce pressure caused by fluids.

CRITICAL THINKING

Mr. Frank is at his health care provider's office when his wife expresses concern about his changing behavior during the past 6 months. She says that Mr. Frank no longer enjoys talking to neighbors or visiting with friends and is irritable. He has also lost his sense of humor and does not always answer her questions appropriately.

1. What do you think is occurring with Mr. Frank?
2. What examination techniques or tests might you use to gather data related to Mr. Frank's signs and symptoms?
3. What would be the expected findings of these tests?
4. Which other members of the health care team might be involved in Mr. Frank's care?
5. What teaching for these symptoms and their effect on Mr. Frank's lifestyle would be helpful?
6. What safety issues should Mr. Frank be taught to address?

Suggested answers are at the end of the chapter.

Ear Health Maintenance

Safe routine cleaning and care of the ears should be taught to all patients (Fig. 51.16). All patients can also benefit from ear and hearing protection education, as found in Table 51.8.

Assistive Hearing Devices

Hearing aids are instruments that amplify sound (see Chapter 52). Certain hearing aids may be designed to amplify sounds and attenuate certain portions of the sound signal. A small battery serves as the energy source. Digital hearing aids contain computers that convert sound waves into numerical codes, before amplifying. This provides clearer and crisper sound that is programmable to each person's hearing loss. Digital hearing aids are more expensive than analog hearing aids (which convert sound waves into electrical signals for amplifying). Three types of hearing aids are commonly used today:

• The in-the-ear aid fits into the ear.
• The canal aid fits into the ear canal and is nearly unseen.
• Technology for assistive devices that involves the use of Bluetooth and smartphones and amplification apps is available.

To care for a hearing aid, ensure that it is turned off and the battery is removed when it is not in use. This reduces battery expense for the patient, who may be on a fixed income. When turning the hearing aid on, the volume should be turned up just until it squeals. Then it is turned down until the patient indicates it is at the best level for hearing. At least weekly, the patient should clean the hearing aid with a dry cloth or a damp, soapy cloth and rinse with a damp cloth. A brush may come with the hearing aid for cleaning. A cotton-tipped swab can also be used to clean the small tip that fits into the ear.

Other types of assistive hearing devices are middle ear implants and cochlear implants. The middle ear implant (visit http://www.medel.com/us) is for those with a sensorineural hearing loss. It provides sound perception by enhancing the normal middle ear hearing function. A **cochlear implant** features a microelectronic processor for converting sound into electrical signals, a transmission system to relay signals to the implanted parts,

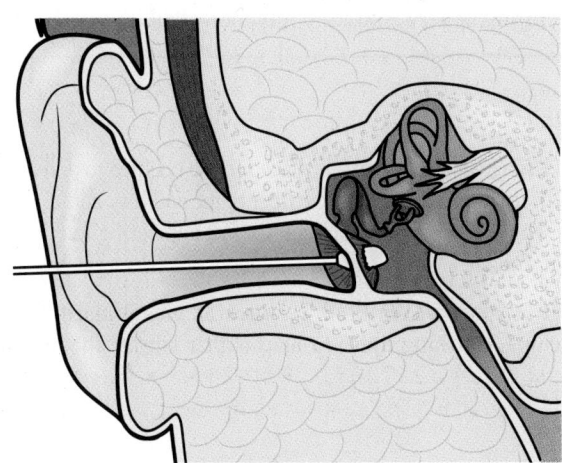

FIGURE 51.16 Ear drum perforation. Avoid putting things into the ear canal for cleaning to prevent injury.

Table 51.8

Prevention of Ear Problems

Patient Education	*Rationale*
Caring for the External Ear	
Wash external ear with soap and water only.	Keeps external ear clean.
Do not routinely remove wax from the ear canal.	Wax serves as a protective mechanism to lubricate and trap foreign material. The ear is generally self-cleaning. Wax is normally removed through talking, eating, and showering.
Preventing Ear Trauma	
Avoid inserting any objects or solutions into the ear. Avoid swimming in polluted areas.	Prevents traumatizing the ear and tympanic membrane or exposing the ear to infection.
Avoid flying when the ear or upper respiratory system is congested.	Prevents barotrauma due to pressure changes.
Preventing Damage from Noise Pollution	
Avoid exposure to excessive occupational noise levels. Avoid other causes of excessive noise such as use of firearms and high-intensity music.	Normal speech is 60 decibels (dB). Above 80 dB is uncomfortable. If there is ringing in the ear, damage may be occurring. Occupational noise is the primary cause of hearing loss.
Use protective earplugs or earmuffs if exposure to loud noise cannot be avoided.	Hearing loss can occur due to exposure to loud noises. Protects ears from hearing loss by decreasing exposure to loud noises.
Instruct adults to have hearing checked every 2 to 3 years.	Degenerative changes occur in the ear with aging.
Early Detection of Hearing Loss	
Monitor for side effects of ototoxic drugs. Instruct patient to report dizziness, decreased hearing acuity, or tinnitus.	Prevents side effects of medications from causing hearing loss.
Caution older patients who use aspirin that it is ototoxic and can cause tinnitus.	Older patients may have hearing loss and not be able to hear the tinnitus.
Instruct patient to report acute symptoms of ear pain, swelling, drainage, or plugged feeling.	Many medical problems can be prevented with prompt treatment.
Instruct patient to blow nose with both nostrils open during upper respiratory infections (colds).	Prevents infected secretions from moving up the eustachian tubes into the middle ear.

and a long, slender electrode placed in the cochlea to deliver the electrical stimuli directly to the fiber of the auditory nerve. A person who is profoundly deaf and has lost all hearing may benefit from a cochlear implant. The implant is placed surgically.

SAFETY PRODUCTS. Products such as visual-alarm smoke detectors (flashing light) or alarms that vibrate the bed as a means to alert a person with a hearing impairment of a fire are available.

Hearing Service Dogs

Hearing service dogs are trained to respond to sounds that a person who is hearing impaired cannot hear. Examples include a crying baby, smoke alarm, or oven timer.

SUGGESTED ANSWERS TO CRITICAL THINKING

Mr. Frank

1. He is exhibiting behaviors of hearing loss.
2. Ear inspection, a whisper voice test, a Rinne test, and a Weber test might be performed.
3. For inspection of ear, cerumen impaction may be found. For a whisper voice test, the whisper is not heard in the affected ear. For a Rinne test, bone conduction is heard longer than air conduction in the affected ear. For a Weber test, sound is heard louder in the affected ear.
4. An audiologist.
5. Explaining to Mr. and Mrs. Frank symptoms of hearing loss will help them understand Mr. Frank's behaviors. Explore with them the effects of these symptoms on daily life so they can develop plans for coping with the hearing loss until an intervention is implemented.
6. Mr. Frank may not hear telephones or alarms such as smoke or carbon monoxide detectors, so alternatives such as visual alarms could be considered. If he drives, he may not hear car horns or emergency vehicles, which he should be aware of so he can compensate.

Review Questions

1. In what order does a beam of light pass through the refractive structures in the eye? (Use all items, and place them in the correct order.)
   1. Aqueous humor
   2. Cornea
   3. Lens
   4. Vitreous humor

2. The nurse is asked to assist with the assessment of a patient's visual acuity. Which assessment methods would the nurse anticipate could be used? **Select all that apply.**
   1. E chart
   2. Fluorescein angiography
   3. Inspection with ophthalmoscope
   4. Confrontation test
   5. Rosenbaum card
   6. Snellen chart

3. Which patient behaviors would the nurse expect to find in the health history of a patient who has a hearing loss? **Select all that apply.**
   1. Answers questions appropriately
   2. Avoids group activities
   3. Has difficulty hearing high-frequency consonants
   4. Is irritable or sensitive in interpersonal relations
   5. Mentions that people talk too loudly
   6. Turns head to one side during conversations

4. The nurse is collecting data during a patient's clinic visit. Which question will best collect data about a patient's preventive ear health?
   1. "What symptoms are you having?"
   2. "Tell me about your ear pain."
   3. "When was your last hearing evaluation?"
   4. "What medications do you take?"

5. The nurse is assisting with a Romberg test. What is the most important nursing action during the Romberg test?
   1. Ensure a quiet environment.
   2. Ensure patient safety.
   3. Remove all cerumen from ear canal.
   4. Whisper softly into each ear.

6. The nurse teaches a patient about ear care. Which patient statement indicates to the nurse that the patient understands the ear care teaching?
   1. "I should insert a cotton swab into my ear canal for cleaning."
   2. "I should not get my external ear wet during bathing."
   3. "I should not block one nostril when blowing my nose."
   4. "I should not need to routinely remove wax from the ear canal."

7. The nurse prepares to provide an eye irrigation to a patient with a methicillin-resistant *Staphylococcus aureus* infection. Contact precautions are ordered. Which protective items will the nurse need while performing this procedure? **Select all that apply.**
   1. Gloves
   2. Gown
   3. Goggles
   4. Mask
   5. Shoe protectors
   6. Sterile gloves

8. A patient is taking aspirin. Which finding would indicate
   to the nurse that the patient is experiencing a toxic effect
   related to the medication?
   1. Halos around lights
   2. Decreased night vision
   3. Tinnitus
   4. Vertigo

Answer rationales available in your online resources.

ANSWERS 1. 2, 1. 3, 4. 2. 1, 5. 6; 3. 2, 3, 4, 6; 4. 3; 5. 2; 6.
3; 7. 1, 2, 3; 8. 3

Key Points

Find the chapter key points in your online resources
available through Davis Edge.

Additional Resources

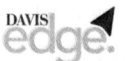 Use the scratch off code on the inside front
cover of your book to access online quizzes
that will help you to improve your scores
on course exams and prepare for the NCLEX-PN®.

 Study Guide

CHAPTER 52

Nursing Care of Patients With Sensory Disorders: Vision and Hearing

Lazette V. Nowicki

KEY TERMS

astigmatism (uh-STIG-mah-TIZM)
blepharitis (BLEF-uh-RY-tis)
blindness (BLYND-ness)
carbuncle (KAR-bun-kul)
cataract (KAT-uh-rakt)
chalazion (kah-LAY-zee-on)
conductive hearing loss (kon-DUK-tiv HEER-ing LOSS)
conjunctivitis (kon-JUNK-ti-VY-tis)
enucleation (ee-NEW-klee-AY-shun)
external otitis (eks-TER-nuhl oh-TY-tis)
furuncle (FYOOR-un-kul)
glaucoma (glaw-KOH-mah)
hordeolum (hor-DEE-oh-lum)
hyperopia (HY-per-OH-pee-ah)
macula (MAK-yoo-la)
Ménière disease (ma-NEAR di-ZEEZ)
miotics (my-AH-tiks)
myopia (my-OH-pee-ah)
myringoplasty (mir-IN-goh-PLAS-tee)
myringotomy (MIR-in-GOT-uh-mee)
otosclerosis (OH-toh-skle-ROH-sis)
photophobia (FOH-toh-FOH-bee-ah)
presbycusis (PREZ-by-KYOO-sis)
presbyopia (PREZ-by-OH-pee-ah)
retinopathy (ret-i-NAH-puh-thee)
sensorineural (SEN-suh-ree-NEW-ruhl)
stapedectomy (stuh-puh-DEK-tuh-mee)

CHAPTER CONCEPT

Sensory Perception

LEARNING OUTCOMES

1. Explain the pathophysiology of each of the disorders of the sensory system.
2. Define blindness and the refractive errors of vision.
3. Explain the etiologies, signs, and symptoms of each sensory disorder.
4. Plan nursing care for patients undergoing tests for sensory disorders.
5. Identify therapeutic measures for each sensory disorder.
6. Identify medications contraindicated for patients with acute angle-closure glaucoma.
7. List three ototoxic drugs.
8. List data to collect when caring for patients with disorders of the sensory system.
9. Plan nursing care for patients with disorders of the eye or ear.
10. Plan nursing care interventions for the patient with a hearing impairment.

VISION DISORDERS

Early detection of visual problems can lessen their impact on a person's life. Nurses play an important role in assisting patients with visual problems (Table 52.1).

Infections and Inflammation

Infections of the eye can be caused by bacteria or viruses. Bacteria include *Staphylococcus* and *Streptococcus* ("Cultural Considerations"). Viruses include herpes simplex virus, cytomegalovirus, and human adenovirus. Inflammation has several causes. Allergies to environmental substances is one. Irritation from chemicals found in perfumes, makeup, sprays, or plants is another. Mechanical irritation can occur such as with sunburn.

Conjunctivitis

Conjunctivitis is inflammation of the conjunctiva. It is caused by either a virus or bacteria. Viral conjunctivitis occurs more often than

• WORD • BUILDING •
conjunctivitis: conjunctive—joining membrane + itis—inflammation

Table 52.1

Eye Disorder Summary

Signs and Symptoms	Pain Redness, secretions, itchiness Sensation of pressure in eyes Visual disturbances
Diagnostic Tests	Visual acuity Amsler grid (identifies visual field disturbances) Ophthalmoscopic examination of internal and external eye Slit-lamp examination (identifies abnormalities on cornea and sclera) Tonometry (identifies intraocular pressure)
Therapeutic Measures	Medications to reduce intraocular pressure, treat infections, anesthetize the eye Surgery
Complications	Worsening vision or loss of vision Acute pain
Priority Nursing Diagnoses	*Anxiety* *Deficient Knowledge* *Risk for Injury*

Cultural Considerations

Trachoma, a form of conjunctivitis, is a common, chronic disease that affects millions of people worldwide. It is primarily seen among low-income persons in the Mediterranean, Africa, Brazil, and the Far East. Trachoma is caused by a viral strain of *Chlamydia trachomatis* that is highly contagious. Following the acute conjunctivitis phase, the eyelids shrink as a result of scarring. The shrinking tends to pull the eyelashes inward (entropion), which may scratch the cornea. In addition, granulations form on the inner eyelids. This painful condition may eventually lead to corneal ulceration and blindness.

bacterial conjunctivitis. It is highly contagious. The virus is usually transmitted via contaminated eye secretions on a hand that then touches or rubs an eye. This then infects the eye. The virus is hardy. It may live on dry surfaces for 2 weeks or more. Viral conjunctivitis lasts 2 to 4 weeks. Bacterial conjunctivitis (commonly called pinkeye) usually is due to staphylococcal or streptococcal bacteria. It is also highly contagious. Conjunctivitis can also be caused by the organisms *Haemophilus influenzae, Chlamydia trachomatis,* and *Neisseria gonorrhoeae.* Conjunctivitis is commonly transmitted among children and then to family members. Signs and symptoms of conjunctivitis include conjunctival redness and crusting exudate on the lids and in the corners of the eyes. Itching, pain, and excessive tearing also occur.

Viral conjunctivitis treatment includes eye washes or eye irrigations. They cleanse the conjunctiva. This relieves the inflammation and pain. Bacterial conjunctivitis is treated with antibiotic eye drops or ointments (Table 52.2). Adults generally prefer eye drops because they do not impair vision. Ointments are used when the eye is resting (at night). Hand hygiene helps prevent the spread of conjunctivitis.

Blepharitis

Blepharitis is inflammation of the eyelid edges. It is a chronic inflammatory process. The cause may include staphylococcal infection, seborrhea (dandruff), rosacea (a chronic disease of the skin usually affecting middle-aged and older adults), or abnormalities of the meibomian glands and their lipid secretions. There are two types of blepharitis: seborrheic blepharitis and ulcerative blepharitis. Seborrheic blepharitis is characterized by reddened eyelids with scales and flaking at the base of the eyelashes. Ulcerative blepharitis produces crusts at the eyelash base, reddened eyes, and inflamed corneas. Treatment requires a commitment to long-term daily cleansing. Cotton-tipped swabs dipped in diluted baby shampoo or sterile eyelid cleanser solution are used. Eyelids chronically infected with *Staphylococcus* may become thickened. Eyelashes may be lost. For infection, antibiotic ointment (e.g., bacitracin [Bactrim], erythromycin [E-Mycin]) is applied to the eyelid edges one to four times a day after the eyelids have been cleansed.

Keratoconjunctivitis Sicca (Dry Eye Disease)

Dry eye results from inadequate lubrication of the eye due to reduced quality or amount of tears. Risk increases over the age of 50. Symptoms are a scratchy feeling in the eye, excess tearing followed by dryness, burning, pain, redness, and blurred vision. Treatment includes smoking cessation, avoiding exposure to second-hand smoke, reducing screen time, taking eye breaks (closed with blinking), using warm compresses for Meibomian gland swelling, using tear duct plugs, requesting prescription medications that are nondrying, and using over-the-counter or prescribed eye drops such as cyclosporine (Restasis) or lifitegrast (Xiidra).

Hordeolum and Chalazion

Another type of eyelid infection is a **hordeolum.** An external hordeolum (also known as a sty) is a small staphylococcal abscess in the sebaceous gland at the base of the eyelash (either the glands of Zeis or glands of Moll). A sty is a small, raised, reddened area. Use of cosmetics around the eyes may contribute to hordeolum formation. A second type of abscess is a **chalazion** (internal hordeolum). It may form in the connective tissue of the eyelids, specifically in the meibomian glands. A chalazion is larger than a sty. While a sty may be tender, a chalazion often puts pressure on the cornea, causing

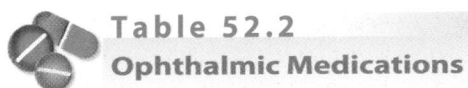

Table 52.2
Ophthalmic Medications

Medication Class/Action

Diagnostic Aids

Fluorescein Sodium
Used for staining of eye; lesions of foreign objects pick up bright yellow-orange stain.

Examples	**Nursing Implications**
fluorescein (AK-Fluor)	Irrigate stain from eye after examination with caution as stain is colorfast.

Topical Anesthetics
Provide local anesthesia to area, making examination painless. Also used to reduce pain of injury.

Examples	**Nursing Implications**
tetracaine (Pontocaine)	*Teach:* Eye must be protected as blink reflex is temporarily lost. Keep eyelid closed to keep eye moist.

Antiangiogenetics

Antivascular Endothelial Growth Factor
Inhibits growth of new blood vessels and slows progression of wet age-related macular degeneration.

Examples	**Nursing Implications**
pegaptanib (Macugen)	Monitor for 1 week after administration to detect infection early.

Eye Allergy Symptom Relief
Relieves red, itchy eyes caused by allergies.

Examples	**Nursing Implications**
nedocromil (Alocril)	Caution patient not to wear soft contact lenses while eyes are red.
azelastine (Astelin)	
naphazoline (Naphcon)	
olopatadine (Patanol)	

Anti-Infectives

Antibiotics
Treat bacterial eye infections.

Examples	**Nursing Implications**
ciprofloxacin (Ciloxan)	Follow instructions for instillation.
gatifloxacin (Zymar)	
polymyxin B and trimethoprim ophthalmic (Polytrim)	
tobramycin (Tobrex)	
sulfacetamide (Bleph-10, Isopto Cetamide, Sodium Sulamyd)	

Antivirals
Treat viral eye infections.

Examples	**Nursing Implications**
trifluridine (Viroptic)	None

Continued

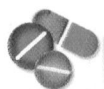

Table 52.2
Ophthalmic Medications—cont'd

Medication Class/Action

Antifungals
Treat fungal eye infections.

Examples
natamycin (Natacyn)

Nursing Implications
Follow instructions for instillation.

Anti-Inflammatories

Steroidal
Reduce inflammation of conjunctiva, cornea, or eyelids due to infection, edema, allergic reaction, cataract surgery, or burns.

Examples
dexamethasone (Decadron)
tobramycin and dexamethasone (TobraDex)

Nursing Implications
Follow instructions for instillation.

Nonsteroidal
Reduce ocular inflammation and pain after cataract surgery, usually within 2 days.

Examples
ketorolac (Acular)
bromfenac (Xibrom)

Nursing Implications
Follow instructions for instillation.

Lubricants

Moisten eyes in healthy and ill persons.

Examples
artificial tears (Lacri-Lube, Tears Plus)

Nursing Implications
Explain that ointment distorts vision.

Miotics

Lower intraocular pressure by stimulating papillary and ciliary sphincter muscles.

Examples
pilocarpine (Pilocar)
physostigmine (Isopto Eserine)

Nursing Implications
Pupil will be smaller than normal with little or no
   reaction to light.

Beta-Adrenergic Blockers

Reduce intraocular pressure by reducing aqueous humor formation and increasing its outflow.

Examples
timolol (Timoptic)
betaxolol (Betoptic)

Nursing Implications
Monitor for bradycardia, heart block, or wheezing.

Mydriatics

Dilate pupils for examination or surgical procedures.

Examples
atropine (Isopto Atropine)

Nursing Implications
Dilated pupils cannot protect eye from bright light, so
   dark glasses needed until drug effects wear off.

Cycloplegics

Paralyze muscles of accommodation for examination or surgical procedures.

Examples
cyclopentolate (Cyclogyl)

Nursing Implications
Contraindicated in patients with glaucoma as it increases
   intraocular pressure.

Evidence-Based Practice

Clinical Question
Are over-the-counter (OTC) artificial tear eye drops effective in treating dry eyes?

Evidence
A systematic review of 43 randomized control trials of 3,497 people diagnosed with "dry eyes" found that although OTC artificial tears may be a safe and effective means for treating dry eyes, eye drops containing 0.2% polyacrylic acid-based artificial tears were consistently more effective (Pucker, Ng, & Nichols, 2016).

Implications for Nursing Practice
OTC artificial tears, which can be economical, may provide relief for people suffering from dry eyes, although prescription medication may be needed for some people.

Reference
Pucker, A. D., Ng, S. M., & Nichols, J. J. (2016). Over the counter (OTC) artificial tear drops for dry eye syndrome. *Cochrane Database of Systematic Reviews, 2016*(2). CD009729. doi:10.1002/14651858.CD009729.pub2

---

greater discomfort. Hordeolums usually heal on their own within a few days. They require no treatment. Chalazions may require surgical incision and drainage if they do not drain on their own. If either type of abscess persists, administration of oral antibiotics may be prescribed. Warm compresses can aid comfort and healing.

Keratitis

PATHOPHYSIOLOGY AND ETIOLOGY. Keratitis is inflammation of the cornea. It may be acute or chronic. It can be superficial or deep. The depth of keratitis is determined by the layers of the cornea that are affected. Keratitis may be associated with bacterial conjunctivitis, a viral infection such as herpes simplex, a corneal ulcer, or diseases such as tuberculosis and syphilis. Herpes simplex keratitis is the most common corneal infection in developed countries. Bacterial and fungal infections are more common throughout the rest of the world. People who have dry eyes, have decreased corneal sensation, are immunosuppressed, or practice poor contact lens hygiene are at increased risk of keratitis.

SIGNS AND SYMPTOMS. The cornea has many pain receptors. Any inflammation of the cornea is painful. This pain increases with movement of the lid over the cornea. Other signs and symptoms of keratitis include blepharospasm (spasm of the eyelids), decreased vision, **photophobia** (eye sensitivity to light), and tearing. The conjunctiva often appears reddened. In advanced cases, the cornea may appear opaque (cloudy).

DIAGNOSTIC TESTS. Assessment of keratitis or corneal ulcer is done with a slit lamp or a handheld light. The cornea is examined by shining the light source obliquely (diagonally) across the cornea. This shows opacity in the cornea. Fluorescein stain may be used to outline the area of involvement. When the stained area is viewed with a blue light, the disruption in the corneal surface shows up clear. If the patient is having pain from blepharospasm (contraction of the orbicularis oculi muscle), a topical ophthalmic anesthetic such as proparacaine can be administered.

THERAPEUTIC MEASURES. Therapeutic measures may include topical antibiotics, topical corticosteroids, topical interferons, antiviral medications for herpes simplex, cycloplegic agents (to keep the iris and ciliary body at rest), and warm compresses. Corneal transplant may be needed for severe damage. The eye may be patched to decrease the amount of eyelid movement over the cornea during healing.

COMPLICATIONS. Corneal infections are usually serious. They often threaten eyesight. The corneal tissue may become thin. It becomes susceptible to perforation. Untreated keratitis can cause permanent scarring of the cornea. This results in permanent loss of vision.

Nursing Process for the Patient With Infection and Inflammation of the Eye

DATA COLLECTION. Table 52.3 reviews subjective data. Objective data collection includes the condition of the conjunctiva, eyelids, and eyelashes; the presence of exudate, tearing, any visible abscess on the palpebral border, or a palpable abscess in the eyelid; opacity of the cornea; and visual acuity testing comparing unaffected and affected eyes.

NURSING DIAGNOSES, PLANNING, AND IMPLEMENTATION.

Acute Pain related to inflammation or infection of the eye or surrounding tissues

EXPECTED OUTCOME: The patient's pain will be decreased or absent as evidenced by lower rating on a pain scale.

- Identify presence and level of the patient's pain. *Use of dark glasses, rubbing the eye, squinting, and avoiding light may be indicators of pain that should be assessed.*
- Administer eye medications as ordered *to relieve eye pain.*
- Apply warm or cool packs as ordered *to assist in soothing the eye.*
- Patch affected eye as ordered to help reduce pain *by decreasing the movement of the eye across the eyelid.*
- Explore additional methods of pain reduction, *such as guided imagery, relaxation techniques, music, or distraction.*

• WORD • BUILDING •

photophobia: photo—light + phobia—fear of

Table 52.3

Subjective Data Collection for Eye Inflammation, Eye Infection, or Visual Impairment

W: Where is it?	What part of the eye or visual field is affected? What characteristics can be seen? Blurry? Hazy? Dark? Halos around lights?
H: How does it feel?	Pressure? Itchy? Irritated? No pain? Painful? Headaches? How does visual impairment make the patient feel? Fearful? Anxious? Depressed? Helpless? Hopeless? Accepting?
A: Aggravating and alleviating factors	Is there photosensitivity? Is vision better at a distance or close up? Is it worse when blinking? Reading? Watching television? Only at night?
T: Timing	Was there exposure to a pathogen? Previous infection or irritation? Was onset sudden? When did the symptoms start? How long have symptoms persisted? Do they come and go? Is visual impairment progressively getting worse?
S: Severity	Does pain or visual impairment affect the patient's activities of daily living? If so, how severely? Does the patient need assistance to cook, dress, bathe, read mail, pay bills, access health care, obtain transportation, maintain household, or shop?
U: Useful data for associated symptoms	What is typical eye hygiene? Is the patient infected with lice? Immunosuppressed? Do other members of the family or peer group have infection symptoms? Is there exudate? Are the eyelids stuck together on awakening? Does the patient wear contact lenses, soft contact lenses overnight, or disposable contact lenses? Does the patient have dry eyes? Is the patient infected with tuberculosis, syphilis, or HIV? Does the patient have diabetes, hypertension, a family history of retinitis pigmentosa, a history of eye infection, or eye trauma? Has the patient recently traveled out of the country?
P: Perception of the problem by the patient	What does the patient think is wrong? How severe does the patient think visual impairment is?

Risk for Injury related to visual impairment

EXPECTED OUTCOME: The patient remains free of injury.

- Identify and plan interventions for visual impairments *to promote safety.*
- Advise the patient with one eye patched not to drive *to prevent injury because depth perception is altered.*
- Teach caution when ambulating and reaching for things *to prevent injury because inflamed eyes often do not focus well and may have exudate, tearing, or ointment present, which can interfere with vision.*

Deficient Knowledge related to eye disease, preventive measures, and treatment from lack of previous experience

EXPECTED OUTCOME: The patient will be able to explain the eye disease, preventive measures, and treatment. The patient will demonstrate correct application of eye medications.

- Identify the patient's baseline knowledge of eye disease *to plan further teaching needs.*
- Teach the patient about eye disease, preventive measures, care of the affected eye, and medication administration *for understanding and adherence to therapeutic plan.*
- Observe the patient administering eye medications after teaching *to evaluate understanding.*

- Teach the patient and his or her family how *to prevent spreading infection, including hand hygiene, if it is contagious.*
- Teach contact lens hygiene *to prevent reinfection of the eye.*
- Teach the patient not to wear contact lenses when the eye or surrounding structure is inflamed *to prevent irritation.*

EVALUATION. The plan of care has been successful if pain is reduced to an acceptable rating, vision improves or returns to pre-illness levels, injury does not occur as a result of visual impairment, and infection does not occur as a result of poor eye hygiene or wearing of contact lenses. The patient explains eye disease, preventive measures, and treatment accurately, and prescribed treatment is stated or demonstrated correctly (e.g., administering eye medications).

Refractive Errors
Pathophysiology and Etiology

Refraction is the bending of light rays as they enter the eye. *Emmetropia* is normal vision. It means that the light rays are bent to focus images precisely on the macula of the retina. *Ametropia* describes any refractive error. When an image is not clearly focused on the retina, a refractive error is present. Ametropia occurs when parallel light rays entering the eye are not refracted (bent) to focus precisely on the retina.

Refractive errors account for the largest number of impairments in vision. There are four common ametropic disorders: hyperopia, myopia, astigmatism, and presbyopia.

HYPEROPIA. **Hyperopia** (farsightedness) is caused by light rays focusing behind the retina. People who are hyperopic see far away images more clearly than images that are close. Physiologically, the globe or eyeball is too short from the front to the back, causing the light rays to focus beyond the retina. Hyperopia is corrected with convex lenses (Fig. 52.1).

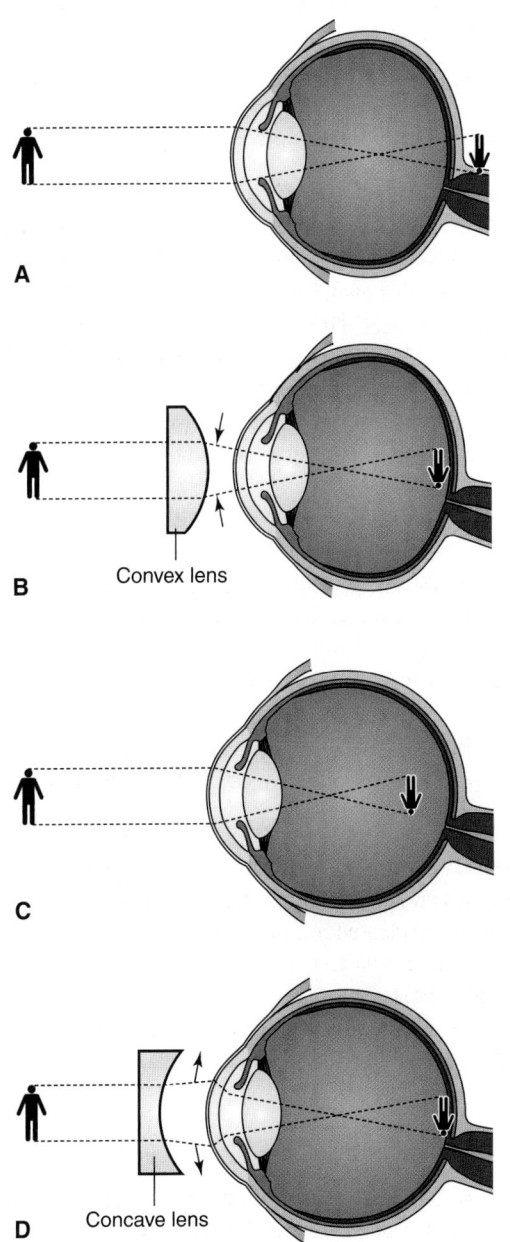

A

B Convex lens

C

D Concave lens

FIGURE 52.1 Refractive disorders. (A) Hyperopia (farsightedness). The eyeball is too short, causing the image to focus beyond the retina. (B) Corrected hyperopia. (C) Myopia (nearsightedness). A long eyeball causes the image to focus in front of the retina. (D) Corrected myopia.

MYOPIA. **Myopia** (nearsightedness) is caused by light rays focusing in front of the retina. The eyeball is elongated. The light rays do not reach the retina. Distance vision is blurred. Items close are clear. Myopia is corrected with concave lenses (see Fig. 52.1).

LEARNING TIP

To remember the type of vision a person has, use this saying: *You are what you say.* For example, if you say you are farsighted, this means that you have clear vision of far-away images but difficulty seeing images that are nearer. If you say you are nearsighted, this means that you have clear vision of images that are near but difficulty seeing images that are farther away.

ASTIGMATISM. **Astigmatism** results from unequal curvatures in the shape of the cornea. When parallel light rays enter the eye, the irregular cornea causes the light rays to be refracted to focus on two different points. This can result in either myopic or hyperopic astigmatism. The person with astigmatism has blurred vision with distortion. The corneal irregularities can be caused by injury, inflammation, corneal surgery, or an inherited autosomal dominant trait.

PRESBYOPIA. **Presbyopia** is an age-related condition in which the eye's lens gradually loses its elasticity. This makes it difficult for the lens to change shape. It is less able to focus light onto the retina to see close objects. This condition is different from the other errors of refraction as they relate to the shape of the eyeball. People often compensate for presbyopia by holding objects farther away. It occurs at about age 40. There is no way to stop the lens from becoming more rigid. Reports of eyestrain and mild frontal headache occur. Treatment includes contact lenses, eyeglasses, or surgery.

Signs and Symptoms

Difficulty reading or seeing objects is reported with errors of refraction. The eyestrain that occurs as one strains to improve visual acuity often causes a headache.

Diagnostic Tests

A refractive error can be estimated by use of a Snellen chart. A retinoscopic examination definitively identifies the refractive error. Before this examination, a cycloplegic drug is often instilled (see Table 52.2). A cycloplegic drug dilates the pupil. It temporarily paralyzes the ciliary muscle. This prevents accommodation. During the examination, the internal and external eye are examined. Trial lenses via a retinoscope are used to identify the type of lens that will correct the refractive error in each eye. With a cycloplegic agent, blurred vision might be present. Sunglasses should be worn until the agent wears off. In addition,

• WORD • BUILDING •

presbyopia: presby—old man + opia—concerning vision

the patient should be instructed that driving and reading might not be possible until the effect of the cycloplegic drug is gone.

Therapeutic Measures

Refractive errors are commonly treated with either eyeglasses or contact lenses. The corrective lenses bend the parallel light rays so that they converge on the macular portion of the retina. Laser-assisted in situ keratomileusis (LASIK) and photorefractive keratectomy (PRK) are surgical procedures also used to correct refractive error. With LASIK and PRK, laser energy is applied to reshape the cornea. The cornea is made flatter for individuals with myopia. It is made more cone shaped for those with hyperopia.

Blindness

Blindness is the complete or almost complete absence of the sense of sight. Some people consider the terms *blind* and *partially sighted* to be negative. They prefer the term *visually impaired* to describe their condition.

Pathophysiology and Etiology

Blindness in adults is caused by a variety of factors that impair nerve transmission of light images or cause damage to the optic nerve or brain. Such factors include cataracts, glaucoma, diabetes, hypertension, and trauma. Blindness may be permanent or transient. It can be complete or partial. It also may occur only in darkness (night blindness).

Signs and Symptoms

Total vision loss may be reported. In other cases, vision may be described as blurred, distorted, or absent in specific areas of the visual field. Vision may be reported as blurry or hazy with corneal visual problems, cataracts, diabetic retinopathy,

or refractive errors. Objects may appear dark or absent in the peripheral field with glaucoma or retinitis pigmentosa (rare inherited degeneration of the pigmented layer of the retina). The center of the visual field may appear dark for individuals with diabetic retinopathy or macular degeneration (Fig. 52.2). Half the visual field may be impaired in patients with hemianopia. This results from a defect in the optic pathways in the brain and occurs with stroke.

Diagnostic Tests

Diagnostic tests include a visual field examination, tonometry, and slit-lamp microscope examination. Retinal angiography follows blood flow through the retinal vessels. It detects vascular changes. Ultrasonography may be used to visualize changes in the posterior eye that cannot be directly examined because of other pathological conditions. These conditions include a cloudy cornea, a bloody vitreous, or an opaque lens.

Therapeutic Measures

Treatment for blindness centers on caring for the underlying condition. Treatment may include medications, surgical intervention, corrective eyewear, and referral to supportive services. For retinal disorders, a device similar to a bionic eye, called the Argus II, is available. This retinal prosthesis system is implanted into the eye. The patient wears special sunglasses with a video camera that transmits images to the Argus II. It sends signals to healthy retinal cells that can then send the signals to the brain.

Nursing Process for the Patient With Visual Impairment

DATA COLLECTION. Subjective data are collected (see Table 52.3). Observe the patient to gather objective data. Is there squinting? Rubbing of the eyes? Is the patient using

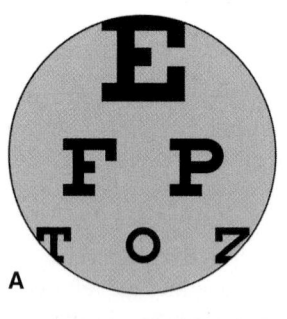 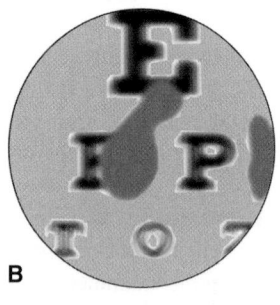 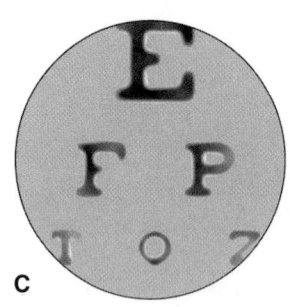

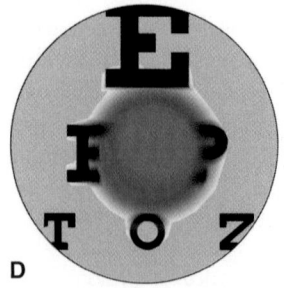 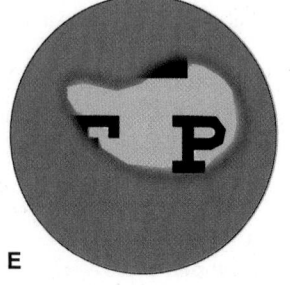

FIGURE 52.2 Visual field abnormalities. (A) Normal vision. (B) Diabetic retinopathy. (C) Cataracts. (D) Macular degeneration. (E) Advanced glaucoma.

compensatory measures (e.g., magnifying glass, sitting close to the television, using large-print reading materials, avoiding reading, using eyeglasses)? Psychosocial data are important to collect. Blind people may be withdrawn or socially isolated. They can have low self-esteem, poor coping mechanisms, or poor interpersonal skills.

NURSING DIAGNOSES, PLANNING, AND IMPLEMENTATION. Nursing care begins by understanding how to interact with a patient who is visually impaired (Box 52.1). The patient's level of independence is included in planning care. Patients with minimal visual impairment or who have attended rehabilitation may be able to function independently. Patients who have recently become visually impaired may be completely dependent. They will need to learn ways of coping to become independent.

Planning focuses on meeting several goals. They include self-care needs, keeping the patient safe from injury, and supporting the grieving process. Inform the patient of agencies, services, and devices that promote independence. Families must be included in planning. They need to understand and be supportive of the self-image and role performance changes that can occur (see "Nursing Care Plan for the Patient With Visual Impairment").

EVALUATION. The outcomes for a patient with a visual impairment are met if the patient demonstrates the ability to complete activities of daily living (ADLs) with increasing independence, remains free of injury, and demonstrates the ability to contact agencies and services for those with visual impairments.

Nursing Care Plan for the Patient With Visual Impairment

Nursing Diagnosis: *Self-Care Deficit (Bathing, Dressing, Feeding)* related to impaired vision.
Expected Outcome: The patient will demonstrate ability to perform activities of daily living (ADLs), with assistance if necessary.
Evaluation of Outcome: The patient is able to perform ADLs as independently as possible.

Intervention	Rationale	Evaluation
Identify patient's ability to perform ADLs.	*Determines patient's ability to adequately dress and feed self.*	Does patient groom, dress, and feed self independently? If does not, what level of assistance is required?
Assist with grooming and dressing (such as pre-matching coordinated clothing or laying coordinated clothing out for patient to dress) as required.	*Ensures patient's grooming and dressing needs are met.*	Is patient able to groom and dress self?
Provide assistance with preparing food and feeding as required; for severe vision loss, use the face of a clock for referencing location of foods on a plate.	*Ensures patient's feeding needs are met.*	Is patient able to eat as desired?

Nursing Diagnosis: *Risk for Injury* related to impaired vision
Expected Outcome: The patient will remain safe from injury.
Evaluation of Outcome: The patient remains injury free.

Intervention	Rationale	Evaluation
Provide for optimal care of assistive appliances such as eyeglasses, including maintenance of proper prescription, fit, and cleaning.	*Improperly fitting or dirty eyeglasses may impair vision even further. Older adults should have their eyeglass prescription checked yearly.*	Do eyeglasses fit properly? Are lenses clean? Is prescription current?
Structure environment to compensate for visual loss by adding color and contrast (e.g., chairs and carpeting in contrasting colors, bright tape or paint on stairs, medicine bottles color coded with colored dot stickers).	*Makes the environment easier to visualize and interpret, and assists in depth perception and identifying medications.*	Does the environment have clearly delineated walkways, sitting areas, and doorways? Are areas with changes in elevation clearly identified using contrasting tape or paint? Is there a way for the patient to safely self-administer medications?

(nursing care plan continues on page 1122)

Nursing Care Plan for the Patient With Visual Impairment—cont'd

Intervention	Rationale	Evaluation
Structure the environment to compensate for visual loss by use of large-print directional signs and arrows, well-lit areas, nonglare surfaces, consistent placement of objects, and traffic areas free of clutter.	*Large directional signs assist the patient in maintaining orientation. Shiny floors or areas with bright window glass can impair vision. Traffic areas free of clutter assist in preventing injury.*	Can patient identify locations such as the bathroom, dining room, and office? Can patient ambulate freely without safety hazards?
Introduce other assistive devices such as handheld magnifying glasses, tableside magnifiers, television magnifiers, large-print items, talking watches, and phones, alarm clocks, and calculators with large numbers.	*Patients may not be aware of assistive devices that could help them adapt to vision loss during activities such as watching television or reading letters and magazines. Allows patient to rely on hearing rather than vision.*	Is patient aware of assistive devices that allow participation in previously enjoyed activities such as watching television or reading? Is patient able to pay bills? Read mail? Use a phone?

Nursing Diagnosis: *Deficient Knowledge* related to new onset of impaired vision
Expected Outcome: The patient will understand resources that will allow maintenance of independence.
Evaluation of Outcome: The patient will identify resources that can be used to support independence.

Intervention	Rationale	Evaluation
Refer to an ophthalmologist, occupational therapist, or resources from such organizations as American Foundation for the Blind or Prevent Blindness.	*Specialized clinicians can provide detailed examination and treatment. Specialized resource groups assist people in coping with vision loss and maximizing abilities.*	Does patient know what resources are available? Does patient know how to access them?

Box 52.1

Interacting With a Patient Who Has a Visual Impairment

- Identify yourself when entering a room and at each contact with the patient.
- Use a normal tone of voice and do not yell, as this is not a hearing impairment.
- Speak directly to the patient, not through a companion.
- If the patient has a Seeing Eye dog, do not play with the dog, pet it, or feed it without consulting the patient—the dog is working! Make sure the patient's dog is near the bed, on a mat provided especially for the dog, preferably on the side of the bed that is less likely to be used by staff. Instruct staff and visitors about the Seeing Eye dog.
- When orienting the patient to the hospital room, explain the location of items the patient may need, such as the water pitcher, call light, bed controls, urinal, and tissues. Attempt to keep these items in the same place at all times.
- Ask the patient what his or her needs are; do not assume the patient needs help with everything.
- Explain procedures before beginning them. Speak to the patient before touching him or her.
- Explain activity occurring in the room or within the patient's auditory range.
- At mealtime, explain the location of items on the tray by comparing their position to the numbers on a clock if doing so is agreeable to the patient (e.g., milk at 2 o'clock, peas at 7 o'clock).
- When seating the patient, place the patient's hand on the arm of the chair.
- When walking with the patient, allow the patient to grasp an arm and walk a half step behind. Be aware of obstacles on either side when walking.
- Tell the patient when you leave the area so the patient does not continue conversation in an empty room, which may cause embarrassment.

Diabetic Retinopathy
Pathophysiology and Etiology

Retinopathy is a disorder in which vascular changes occur in the retinal blood vessels. It is most common in persons with diabetes. The pathological changes in diabetic retinopathy are related to excess glucose, changes in the retinal capillary walls, formation of microaneurysms, and constriction of retinal blood vessels. Three stages of diabetic retinopathy have been identified. They are background retinopathy, preproliferative retinopathy, and proliferative retinopathy.

Background retinopathy is the earliest stage. Microaneurysms form on the retinal capillary walls. These microaneurysms may leak blood into the central retina or macula. The leakage may cause edema. If it does, the patient may notice a decrease in color discrimination and visual acuity.

The second stage is preproliferative retinopathy. It is characterized by swollen and irregularly dilated veins. This results in sluggish or blocked blood flow. There are no symptoms. So, patients generally are not aware of this stage.

Proliferative retinopathy is the third stage. It is characterized by the formation of new blood vessels. They grow into the retinal and optic disc area to increase the blood supply to the retina. The newly formed blood vessels are fragile. They often leak blood into the vitreous and retina. In addition, the newer vessels may grow into the vitreous. This causes a traction effect. It pulls the vitreous away from the retina. Then it pulls the retina away from the choroid. This condition is called retinal detachment (discussed later).

Signs and Symptoms

There may be a reduction in central visual acuity or color vision due to macular edema (see Fig. 52.2). Many patients with diabetic retinopathy have no symptoms until the proliferative stage. This is when vision is lost. Visual loss at the last stage usually cannot be restored. If people with diabetes have changes in visual acuity or color discrimination, they should immediately contact their health care provider (HCP).

Complications

Early treatment for diabetic retinopathy is very successful in preventing further visual loss. However, existing visual loss cannot be reversed. Therefore, it is essential for patients with diabetes to have a comprehensive eye examination through dilated pupils at least once each year. Careful control of diabetes during the first 5 years after diagnosis is vital. It can delay onset of diabetic retinopathy.

Diagnostic Tests

Diabetic retinopathy can only be diagnosed with examination of the internal eye. First, the pupil is dilated with a cycloplegic agent. Then an ophthalmoscope is used to view the internal eye. Retinoangiography may also be used to enhance the examination. In the initial stages, vessels may appear swollen and tortuous (twisted).

Therapeutic Measures

Treatment of diabetic retinopathy is to stop the leakage of blood and fluid into the vitreous and retina. The leaking microaneurysm is sealed with a laser. Lasers can also shrink the abnormal blood vessels. If blood has already leaked into the vitreous, a vitrectomy is performed. During a vitrectomy, the vitreous humor is drained out of the eye chamber. It is replaced with saline or silicon oil (oil often removed months later). The replacement fluid is necessary to support the structures of the eyeball until healing can occur. Use of intravitreal corticosteroids is beneficial.

Nursing Process for the Patient With Diabetic Retinopathy

DATA COLLECTION. Risk factors for diabetic retinopathy are identified. The patient may not have any symptoms to report.

NURSING DIAGNOSIS, PLANNING, AND IMPLEMENTATION. The planning phase of the nursing process for diabetic retinopathy focuses on prevention of visual loss with early detection and treatment. If the patient has entered the final state and is already visually impaired, the "Nursing Care Plan for the Patient With Visual Impairment" is used.

Ineffective Health Management

EXPECTED OUTCOME: The patient will state ability to manage therapeutic regimen.

- Determine whether the patient with a visual impairment who is diabetic can monitor blood glucose and draw up and administer the correct amount of insulin. *Specialty devices are available that can be preset to draw up the correct amounts of insulin. Family members may have to assist the patient.*
- Teach the patient the importance of yearly comprehensive eye examinations *to detect visual changes for treatment.*

EVALUATION. The patient goal is met if the patient is able to manage the therapeutic regimen.

Retinal Detachment
Pathophysiology and Etiology

Retinal detachment is a separation of the retina from the choroid layer that is beneath it (see Fig. 51.3). This allows fluid to enter the space between the layers. There are three causes of retinal detachment. One cause is a hole or tear in the retina that allows fluid to flow between the two layers. Another cause is a fibrous tissue in the vitreous humor that contracts and pulls the retina away from its normal position. A third cause is fluid or exudate accumulation in the subretinal space that separates the retinal layers.

• WORD • BUILDING •

retinopathy: retino—having to do with the retina + pathy— illness, disease, or suffering

Signs and Symptoms

Patients experiencing a retinal detachment report a sudden change in vision. Initially, as the retina is pulled, patients report seeing flashing lights and then floaters. The flashing lights are caused by vitreous traction on the retina. Floaters are caused by bleeding into the vitreous fluid. When the retina detaches, patients often describe it as "looking through a veil" or "cobwebs" and finally "like a curtain being lowered over the field of vision," with darkness resulting. There is no pain. The retina does not contain sensory nerves. The patient typically has a loss of visual acuity in the affected eye. There is loss of peripheral vision.

Diagnostic Tests

Indirect ophthalmoscopy allows the examiner to visualize the retina. It may be pale, opaque, and in folds with retinal detachment. The type of detachment is diagnosed. If there are lesions in the eye, the slit-lamp examination magnifies the lesions.

Therapeutic Measures

Emergency medical treatment must be sought to help protect vision. The amount of vision restored varies. It depends on the affected area. One or more procedures are performed to treat retinal tears or detachment. They include lasers, cryopexy, pneumatic retinopexy, or scleral buckling.

LASER SURGERY. Laser surgery focuses a laser beam at the torn area of the retina. It causes a controlled burn. This forms scars around the tear and reattaches the retina to surrounding tissue.

CRYOPEXY. Cryopexy is the placement of a supercooled probe on the sclera over the affected area. The probe freezes and scars the tear or hole, a principle similar to the laser procedure.

PNEUMATIC RETINOPEXY. Pneumatic retinopexy is done in the HCP's office. It is time-consuming for the patient. It involves injecting air or gas into the eye chamber to hold the retina in place. The patient must be extremely compliant with the treatment regimen. Reclining for about 16 hours before the procedure is required to allow the retina to fall back toward the choroid. Because air rises, the patient must maintain a position that keeps the air bubble against the detached area for up to 8 hours a day for 3 weeks.

SCLERAL BUCKLING. Scleral buckling is a surgical procedure for retinal detachment. A silicon buckle under a thin band of silicon around the sclera is used. It is tightened to create an indentation that brings the choroid in contact with the retina. Cryosurgery or laser surgery is usually used to permanently adhere the retina and choroid layers together. Vitrectomy is often done as well.

Complications

With any retinal procedure, there is risk of increased intraocular pressure (IOP), retinal tears, and recurrent retinal detachment.

Nursing Process for the Patient With Retinal Detachment

DATA COLLECTION. Subjective data include patient observation of the loss of peripheral vision, changes in visual acuity, and the presence of floaters, flashing lights, cobwebs, or veil-like visual impairments. There should be no pain reported. Objective data include the patient's visual acuity, visual fields, ability to perform ADLs, and level of anxiety.

NURSING DIAGNOSES, PLANNING, IMPLEMENTATION, AND EVALUATION. See "Nursing Process for the Patient Having Eye Surgery" later in this chapter.

CRITICAL THINKING

Mr. Samuel, age 65, is working in the yard when a branch strikes his right eye. He sees flashes of light and then a short time later a dark shadow out of his right eye.

1. What should Mr. Samuel do?
2. After having a scleral buckling procedure, Mr. Samuel reports nausea. What action should the nurse take?
3. Ondansetron (Zofran) 4 mg intramuscular is ordered. Ondansetron 2 mg/mL in 2 mL/vial is available. How many milliliters should be given?

Suggested answers are at the end of the chapter.

Glaucoma

Glaucoma is a group of diseases that damage the optic nerve. In all but one type, there is increased pressure within the eye. This pressure damages the optic nerve. The optic nerve transmits visual information from the eye to the brain. The damage to it is silent, progressive, and irreversible. Loss of peripheral vision occurs. It is then followed by reduced central vision and eventually blindness (see Fig. 52.2). Normal tension glaucoma with optic nerve damage can also occur. It is a form of primary open-angle glaucoma. There is no cure for glaucoma. Treatment plans must be followed to prevent any further vision loss.

Pathophysiology

The most common form of glaucoma is primary. It consists of two types: primary open-angle glaucoma (POAG) and acute angle-closure glaucoma (AACG). Secondary glaucoma may be caused by infections, tumors, or injuries. A third form is congenital glaucoma.

POAG occurs when the drainage system of the eye, the trabecular meshwork and canal of Schlemm, degenerates and subsequently blocks the flow of aqueous humor. AACG occurs in people who have an anatomically narrowed angle at the junction where the iris meets the cornea. When nearby eye structures such as the iris protrude into the anterior chamber, the angle is occluded. This blocks the flow of aqueous fluid. AACG is considered a medical emergency. It results in partial or total blindness if not treated.

Etiology and Prevention

Incidences of POAG increase in those age 40 and older (age 40 for African Americans [Glaucoma Research Foundation, 2017] and age 50 for European Americans), in people with diabetes, and in those with a family history of glaucoma. POAG occurs four to five times more in African Americans than European Americans. The incidence of AACG is highest among Asians, women over age 45, and people who are nearsighted. Those in high-risk groups or over age 60 should have yearly eye examinations.

Signs and Symptoms

POAG develops bilaterally. The onset is usually gradual and painless. The patient may have no noticeable symptoms. After some time, there may be mild aching in the eyes, headache, halos around lights, or frequent visual changes that are not corrected with eyeglasses.

AACG is an ophthalmic emergency. It typically has a unilateral, rapid onset. The patient may report severe pain over the affected eye, blurred vision, rainbows around lights, and photophobia. Eye redness, a steamy-appearing cornea, and tearing may be seen. Increased IOP can cause nausea and vomiting.

Diagnostic Tests

Measuring IOP and identifying optic nerve damage and visual loss are done to diagnose glaucoma. Tonometry detects increased IOP (normal is 12 to 20 mm Hg). It may be present in about 50% of glaucoma cases. In AACG, IOP may exceed 50 mm Hg. The GDx Access, a laser device, detects nerve damage long before the patient has symptoms of glaucoma. A visual field examination checks for peripheral vision loss. Corneal thickness is measured, as it can affect IOP. With gonioscopy, a special lens is used to look at the angle where the iris meets the cornea. This identifies POAG or AACG.

Therapeutic Measures

The first-line treatment for POAG focuses on opening the aqueous flow. Cholinergic agents (**miotics**) such as carbachol (Isopto Carbachol) or pilocarpine (Pilocar) are given to constrict the pupil. When the pupil is constricted, the iris pulls away from the drainage canal. This allows the aqueous fluid to flow freely. A second medication may be given to slow the production of aqueous fluid. This includes adrenergic agonists such as dipivefrin (Propine) and beta blockers such as timolol (Timoptic). Slowing the production of aqueous fluid helps decrease IOP. Steroid eye drops may be ordered to reduce inflammation. The patient having an acute attack of AACG is also given these types of medications, as well as analgesics, and placed on bedrest.

Patients with glaucoma need lifelong use of eye drop medications. With no symptoms, adherence to treatment is often an issue. Other factors that cause nonadherence are the patient's age, inability to afford the medication, and lack of understanding of the seriousness of the disease. Patients should carry medical alert identification and medications for their glaucoma. This can help prevent administration of medications in emergency situations that are contraindicated for AACG.

Certain medications are contraindicated in AACG regardless of their route and can cause blindness. They include anticholinergics such as atropine, antihistamines such as diphenhydramine (Benadryl), or hydroxyzine (Vistaril). They are all mydriatics. Before a medication is given, the nurse must determine that it is not contraindicated in AACG. This can prevent blindness from occurring.

LEARNING TIP

Mydriatic medications are contraindicated in acute angle-closure glaucoma (AACG). They can cause an acute episode of increased intraocular pressure by dilating the pupil and pushing the iris back. This blocks the outflow of aqueous humor.

Miotic medications constrict the pupil. They can be given to patients with AACG.

To remember the pupillary action of mydriatic medications and miotic medications so that the appropriate medication is given and contraindicated ones are never given, think of the following:

• **D** = **d**ilate = my**d**riatic = **d**o not give.
• No D = constricts = miotic = okay to give.

Surgical Management

When medication is no longer effective, surgical intervention may be needed. Surgery can create an area where the aqueous humor can flow freely or reduce aqueous humor production. This prevents increased IOP (Fig. 52.3). Laser

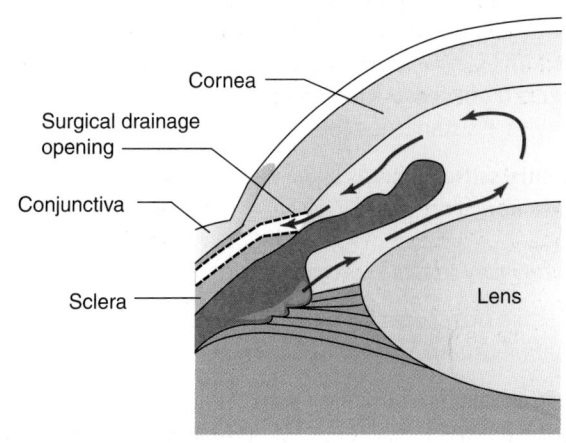

FIGURE 52.3 Flow of aqueous humor after trabeculoplasty (*arrows*).

trabeculoplasty (a narrow laser beam opens drainage angle of eye) is often used first for POAG. Traditional trabeculectomy removes part of the trabecular meshwork. Glaucoma drainage devices (shunts) carry aqueous humor away. Cyclocryotherapy (in which a cryoprobe destroys part of ciliary body to reduce production of aqueous humor) is used less often. Procedures for those with both glaucoma and cataracts can be done. The iStent Trabecular Micro-Bypass is implanted during cataract surgery. It creates a permanent opening in the trabecular meshwork for outflow of aqueous humor. For AACG, laser peripheral iridotomy or surgical iridectomy is performed. Laser iridotomy creates a small hole on the edge of the iris. This allows the aqueous fluid to flow out of the area. Prophylactic laser iridotomy may be performed on the other eye in order to prevent AACG.

Nursing Process for the Patient With Glaucoma

DATA COLLECTION. The patient should be monitored for pain, loss of central and peripheral vision, understanding of disease and adherence to treatment regimen, and ability to conduct ADLs.

NURSING DIAGNOSES, PLANNING, AND IMPLEMENTATION. The goal of nursing care for the patient with glaucoma is to prevent further visual loss and to promote comfort if the patient is experiencing pain with acute glaucoma. See "Nursing Process for the Patient With Visual Impairment" (earlier in this chapter) and "Nursing Process for the Patient Having Eye Surgery" (later in this chapter) for additional nursing diagnoses.

Acute Pain related to increased intraocular pressure

EXPECTED OUTCOME: The patient will report that pain is relieved.

• Give analgesics as needed for AACG glaucoma *to relieve pain.*

Self-Care Deficit (Bathing, Dressing, Feeding, Toileting) related to decreased vision

EXPECTED OUTCOME: The patient will be able to care for self with assistance if needed.

• Identify self-care needs and assist as needed *to ensure ADLs are met.*

Risk for Injury related to decreased vision

EXPECTED OUTCOME: The patient will not be injured as a result of visual impairment.

• Refer the patient to support services that *provide adaptive visual devices.*
• Teach the patient and his or her family to keep walking areas clutter free and not to rearrange furniture without patient knowledge *to prevent falls or injury.*

Deficient Knowledge related to medical regimen and disease process due to no prior experience

EXPECTED OUTCOME: The patient will demonstrate correct instillation of eye medications and be able to verbalize understanding of condition and treatment.

• Teach the patient the need for regular eye examinations through dilated pupils *to monitor disease and detect complications.*
• Teach how to administer medications with a return demonstration *to ensure that eye drops are administered properly.*
• Teach the patient to rest his or her hand on the forehead *if the patient has trouble keeping the hand steady when administering eye drops.*
• Consider large-print labels or audiotaped directions *if the patient is unable to see the label on the eye drop bottle.*
• Consider placing large, multicolored dot stickers on medication bottles and on corresponding instruction cards *for patients with multiple medications.*

EVALUATION. Interventions are successful if the patient maintains an acceptable level of comfort, has no further loss of vision, and is able to care for self with assistance. Also, the patient states anxieties are relieved, does not suffer injury as a result of the visual impairment, demonstrates correct instillation of eye medications, and is able to verbalize understanding of condition and treatment.

Cataracts
Pathophysiology and Etiology
A **cataract** is an opacity in the lens of the eye that may cause a loss of visual acuity (see Fig. 52.2). Vision is diminished because the light rays are unable to reach the retina through the clouded lens. Factors that contribute to cataract development may include age, ultraviolet (UV) radiation (sunlight), diabetes, smoking, steroids, nutritional deficiencies, alcohol consumption, intraocular infections, trauma, and congenital defects.

Signs and Symptoms
Cataracts are painless. Symptoms of cataract formation may include halos around lights, difficulty reading fine print or seeing in bright light, increased sensitivity to glare such as when driving at night, double or hazy vision, and decreased color vision.

Diagnostic Tests
Cataracts are diagnosed with an eye examination. Visual acuity is tested for near and far vision. The direct ophthalmoscope and slit-lamp microscope are used to examine the lens and other internal structures.

Surgical Management
When cataracts begin to interfere with daily living and quality of life, intraocular lens implant surgery is recommended. One eye is treated at a time. Outpatient laser (with a LenSx laser)

or no-stitch cataract surgery to remove the cloudy lens is performed. Implantable lenses come in various types. They are inserted after lens removal. Some lens can reduce the need for eyeglasses. There are no postoperative activity restrictions except for swimming. Complications are rare.

Nursing Process for the Patient With Cataracts

DATA COLLECTION. The patient is monitored for visual deficits to assist care planning. Knowledge needs about the disease, treatment, and postoperative care are identified.

NURSING DIAGNOSES, PLANNING, IMPLEMENTATION, AND EVALUATION. Preoperative and postoperative nursing care is the primary nursing responsibility for the patient with cataracts, as discussed next.

Nursing Process for the Patient Having Eye Surgery

DATA COLLECTION. Subjective data to be collected include type of visual impairment, which eye is affected, presence of pain, and anxiety. Objective data may include visual acuity with and without corrective lenses and peripheral field measurements. Eye tearing, redness, or swelling is noted.

NURSING DIAGNOSES, PLANNING, AND IMPLEMENTATION.

Risk for Injury related to altered visual acuity

EXPECTED OUTCOME: The patient will remain free of injury.

- Ambulate with assistance and use clearly marked stairs *to prevent injury.*

Deficient Knowledge related to preoperative and postoperative eye care

EXPECTED OUTCOME: The patient will verbalize preoperative and postoperative care directions.

- Teach the patient about disease process, preoperative and postoperative care, and how to administer eye medications as instructed *to increase patient knowledge.*
- Teach the patient to seek medical care for sudden or worsening pain, watery or bloody discharge, or sudden loss of vision *because these are signs of hemorrhage or problems.*

Anxiety related to visual alteration and surgery

EXPECTED OUTCOME: The patient will report reduced anxiety.

- Give the patient the opportunity to discuss his or her feelings about vision loss or surgery *to reduce anxiety.*

EVALUATION. The patient goals have been met if the patient is free of injury, verbalizes preoperative and postoperative directions, and reports reduced anxiety.

Macular Degeneration
Pathophysiology and Etiology

Age-related macular degeneration (AMD) is the leading cause of permanent impairment of close-up vision or reading in U.S. residents over 64 (Centers for Disease Control and Prevention, 2015). It involves deterioration and scarring within the **macula.** This is the area on the retina where light rays converge for the sharp, central vision needed for reading and seeing small objects (Fig. 52.4). The macula is also responsible for color vision. There are two types of AMD: dry (atrophic) and wet (exudative). In dry AMD, photoreceptors in the macula fail to function and are not replaced because of advancing age. This accounts for 70% to 90% of cases. In the wet form, retinal tissue degenerates, allowing vitreous fluid or blood into the subretinal space. New fragile blood vessels form (angiogenesis). This compromises the macular tissue, causing subretinal edema. Eventually, fibrous scar tissue forms, severely limiting central vision.

People at risk of developing AMD include those older than age 60, those with a family history of macular degeneration, persons with diabetes, people who smoke, those frequently exposed to UV light, and Caucasians.

NURSING CARE TIP
Most damaging exposure to ultraviolet (UV) light occurs before age 18. It is important for everyone of *all* ages to use adequate UV protective sunglasses.

Prevention

A healthful lifestyle is important. A diet that includes dark green leafy vegetables (e.g., kale, collard greens, lettuce, spinach) and orange- and yellow-colored fruits and vegetables (e.g., peppers, corn) is helpful. Measuring macula pigment optical density is an important screening tool. Taking the retinal carotenoids lutein and zeaxanthin as well as zinc supplements for a low macula pigment optical density (less than 44) can be beneficial. Doing so can raise the macula pigment optical density over time. This can prevent progression of some macular degeneration.

Signs and Symptoms

The dry type of AMD is characterized by slow, progressive loss of central and near vision (see Fig. 52.2). People usually have the condition in both eyes. Each eye may be affected in varying degrees. The wet type of AMD has the same loss of central and near vision. However, the onset is sudden. It results in more severe vision loss. The vision loss can occur in one or both eyes. This vision loss is described as blurred vision, distortion of straight lines, and a dark or empty spot in the central area of vision. Some patients may have a decreased ability to distinguish colors.

Diagnostic Tests

Visual acuity for near and far vision and an examination of the internal eye structures with an ophthalmoscope is done. The examiner uses an Amsler grid (Fig. 52.5) to detect central vision distortion. A color vision test evaluates color differentiation. Patients are given an Amsler grid to look at on a

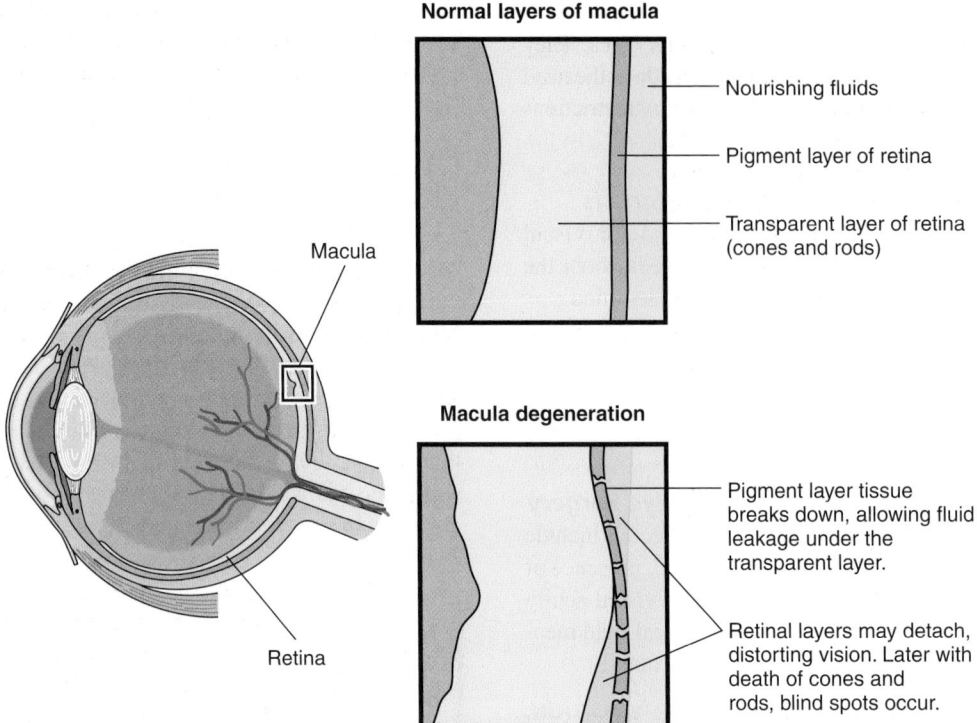

FIGURE 52.4 Macular degeneration. The macula is a small area of the retina responsible for central and color vision.

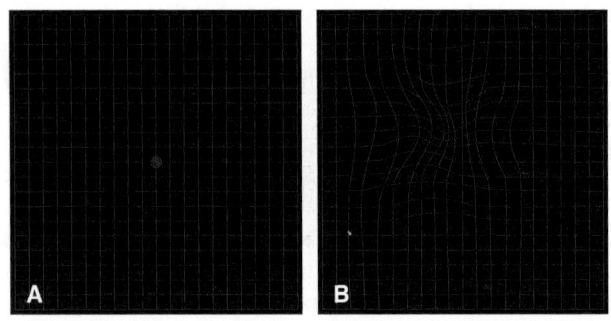

FIGURE 52.5 An Amsler grid is used for self-assessment to identify central vision blind spots or distortions. (A) Normal Amsler grid. The red on black grid was developed to increase better accuracy with the test. (B) Abnormal Amsler grid with distortion and small area of central vision loss.

regular basis. This allows them to monitor vision changes. If any of the grid lines look crooked or disappear, the patient should contact the HCP. Digital imaging, an optical coherence tomography retinal scan (similar to a computed tomography [CT] scan), or intravenous fluorescein (dye) angiography is used to evaluate blood vessel leakage or abnormalities in the eye.

Therapeutic Measures

Unfortunately, there is no treatment for the dry type of AMD. Prevention is important when possible. Most patients with dry AMD do not lose peripheral vision or become totally blind. Most are classified as legally blind (less than 20/200 vision with correction). Low-vision telescopic glasses can enhance remaining vision. There is a telescope implant for those with end-stage AMD. It is placed in only one eye after the eye's natural lens is removed. It can help restore central vision. Visit www.centrasight.com for more information.

Wet AMD is treated with intermittent injection into the eye of an antiangiogenesis medication (e.g., ranibizumab [Lucentis] or aflibercept [Eylea]). Drugs that are antiangiogenetic prevent the formation of new fragile blood vessels that can become leaky and bleed. Older treatment options are not used as much due to the availability of antiangiogenesis drugs. These include laser photocoagulation that seals the leaking blood vessels or photodynamic therapy. With either type of AMD, patients have significant visual loss and must adapt to it.

Nursing Process for the Patient With Macular Degeneration

See "Nursing Process for the Patient With Visual Impairment" earlier in this chapter.

Trauma

Emergencies and trauma of the eye must be immediately treated. Injuries to the eye include foreign bodies, chemical burns, UV exposure, direct heat sources, abrasions, lacerations from dragging something across the eye, and penetrating wounds. Penetrating wounds are the most serious eye injury. They increase the risk for infection and blindness.

Signs and Symptoms

Foreign bodies produce pain when the eyeball or eyelid moves. The eye tears excessively to irrigate the noxious substance out of the eye. Injuries that irritate or penetrate layers of the cornea result in mild to severe pain. With corneal abrasions, the pain sensation may be delayed for several hours. Other symptoms that occur with abrasions, lacerations, and foreign bodies include conjunctival redness, photosensitivity, decreased visual acuity, erythema, and pruritus. Acute pain and burning are characteristic symptoms of a burn to the eye. Penetrating wound symptoms depend on the area of the eye involved and the extent of the damage.

Diagnostic Tests

Visual acuity is tested. It is important to establish baseline acuity to evaluate effectiveness of treatment. Many patients resist acuity testing because of the discomfort. Testing includes examination by slit-lamp microscope and direct ophthalmoscope. Fluorescein staining is used to evaluate abrasions.

Therapeutic Measures

Foreign bodies are treated with a normal saline flush. This irrigates the object out of the eye or to a point where it can be removed with a swab. Topical antibiotic ointment is prescribed to prevent infection. Chemical burns must be treated immediately with a 15- to 20-minute irrigation at an eye wash station or with sterile solution at a medical facility. Topical antibiotic ointments are prescribed. Burns from heat or UV radiation are not irrigated.

Abrasions and lacerations are cleansed with normal saline. Then they are treated with anti-infective ointments or drops.

An eye specialist treats penetrating wounds. After the injury, both eyes should be covered to prevent ocular movement. If there is a protruding object, it should be stabilized but not removed until the HCP can assess the patient.

Complications

If the eye cannot be saved with medical treatment, it may be necessary to surgically remove the eye. This procedure is called **enucleation** (entire eyeball removal).

Nursing Care for the Patient With Eye Trauma

FOREIGN BODIES. The eye is inspected for foreign bodies, which may be visible on the eyeball. Assist the HCP who will evert the eyelid to examine the surface and irrigate the eye.

BURNS. Identification of the type of burn is done because treatment options vary. Immediate irrigation of the eyes is performed once it has been established that a chemical burn has taken place, unless contraindicated for the chemical. Medication and eye patching are applied as indicated.

ABRASIONS AND LACERATIONS. The eye is assessed for visible lacerations and then cleansed, medicated, and patched as indicated.

PENETRATING WOUNDS. The patient is kept calm and relaxed to minimize eye movement and increased IOP. If a protruding object is present, the object is stabilized with tape or other supports.

 HEARING DISORDERS

Hearing Loss

Hearing loss is the most common disability in the United States. It can be acquired or congenital. Hearing impairment ranges from difficulty understanding words or hearing certain sounds to total deafness (Table 52.4). It can affect communication, social activities, and work activities. It can diminish quality of life. Nurses have a responsibility to communicate with patients with hearing impairments and provide needed information regarding health care.

Conductive Hearing Loss

Conductive hearing loss is a mechanical problem. It is interference with the conduction of sound impulses to the inner ear through the external auditory canal, the eardrum, or the middle ear. The inner ear is not involved in pure conductive hearing loss. Causes of conductive hearing loss include cerumen, foreign bodies, infection, perforation of the tympanic membrane, trauma, fluid in the middle ear, cysts, tumor, and otosclerosis. Many causes of conductive hearing loss, such as infection, foreign bodies, and impacted cerumen, can be corrected. Hearing devices may improve hearing for conditions resulting in conductive hearing loss that cannot be corrected. These include scarred tympanic membrane or otosclerosis.

Sensorineural Hearing Loss

Sensory hearing loss originates in the cochlea and involves the hair cells and nerve endings. Neural hearing loss originates in the nerve or brainstem. **Sensorineural** hearing loss results from disease or trauma to the sensory or neural components of the inner ear. Some of the causes of nerve deafness are complications of infections (such as measles, mumps, and meningitis), ototoxic drugs (Table 52.5), trauma, noise, neuromas, arteriosclerosis, and the aging process.

Presbycusis is hearing loss caused by the aging process. It results from degeneration of the organ of Corti. This degenerative process often begins in the fifth decade of life. The person develops an inability to decipher high-frequency sounds (consonants *s, z, t, f,* and *g*). This interferes with the person's ability to understand what is being said, especially in noisy environments. The older adult commonly has more difficulty understanding higher-pitched female voices than lower-pitched male voices.

Other Types of Hearing Loss

Mixed hearing loss occurs when an individual has both conductive and sensorineural hearing loss. This can be caused

• WORD • BUILDING •
enucleation: e—removed from + nuclear—center

Table 52.4
Hearing Loss Summary

Signs and Symptoms	Difficulty understanding words or certain sounds Total deafness Ringing, buzzing, or roaring noise in ears Changes in social and work activities, turning up volume on the television, asking, "What did you say?" Reports that people are talking softly Speaks in a quiet or loud voice and answers questions inappropriately Avoids group activities, loss of sense of humor, appears aloof
Diagnostic Tests	Rinne and Weber tests Audiometric testing
Therapeutic Measures	Cerumenolytics Anti-infectives Anti-inflammatories Assistive devices (e.g., hearing aids, implantable middle ear hearing devices, cochlear implants)
Complications	Safety issues related to hearing impairment Withdrawal from social activities and
Priority Nursing Diagnoses	*Impaired Verbal Communication* *Impaired Social Interaction* *Ineffective Coping* *Disturbed Body Image* *Deficient Knowledge*

Table 52.5
Ototoxic Drugs

Aminoglycoside antibiotics	amikacin (Amikin) gentamicin (Garamycin) neomycin (Antibiotic Otic, Cortomycin) streptomycin tobramycin (Tobrex)
Other antibiotics	erythromycin (E-Mycin) minocycline (Minocin) vancomycin (Vancocin, Vancoled)
Diuretics	bumetanide (Bumex) furosemide (Lasix) hydrochlorothiazide (Aquazide, Hydrocot)
Other drugs	cisplatin (Platinol) methotrexate (Rheumatrex, Trexall) salicylate (Bayer, Ecotrin)

patient's hearing (see Chapter 51; visit www.nidcd.nih.gov/health/cochlear-implants for more information).

Nursing Process for the Patient With Hearing Impairment

DATA COLLECTION. Nursing care includes identifying those patients at risk for hearing impairment (Table 52.6). Patients with renal or hepatic disease, who use two or more ototoxic drugs, or who have previously used ototoxic drugs are at risk for developing hearing impairment. If the patient is using ototoxic medications, assess for tinnitus, sensorineural hearing loss, or vestibular dysfunction. These could indicate ototoxicity. The medications should be discontinued if signs of ototoxicity are present. Monitor for signs of vertigo, horizontal nystagmus (fast side to side eye movements), nausea, vomiting, and spinning or rocking sensation while sitting still. When collecting data for the patient with hearing impairment, include family members. They can often report what the patient is not able to hear.

Objective data collection should start with a normal conversation with the patient. Observe the patient for any difficulty understanding the conversation or questions. Clarity of the patient's speech is determined. Physical examination includes the whisper voice, Rinne, and Weber tests (see Chapter 51). Test results provide an estimate of conductive or sensorineural hearing loss. The patient should be assessed for the underlying cause of the problem to determine whether it is an external, middle, or inner ear problem. Examination of the external ear may reveal an external ear problem. The HCP may examine the ear canal for impacted cerumen or

by a combination of any of the disorders previously discussed. Central hearing loss occurs when the central nervous system cannot interpret normal auditory signals. This condition occurs with disorders such as cerebrovascular accidents and tumors. Functional hearing loss is a hearing loss for which no organic cause or lesion can be found. It is also called psychogenic hearing loss. It is triggered by emotional stress.

Therapeutic Measures

The goal of medical management is to improve the patient's hearing. With any permanent hearing loss, the use of a hearing aid should be considered (Fig. 52.6; see Chapter 51). Surgical intervention may be available if hearing aids do not work. Implantable middle ear hearing aids can improve sound perception for patients with moderate-to-severe sensorineural hearing loss. Cochlear implants can restore up to half of the

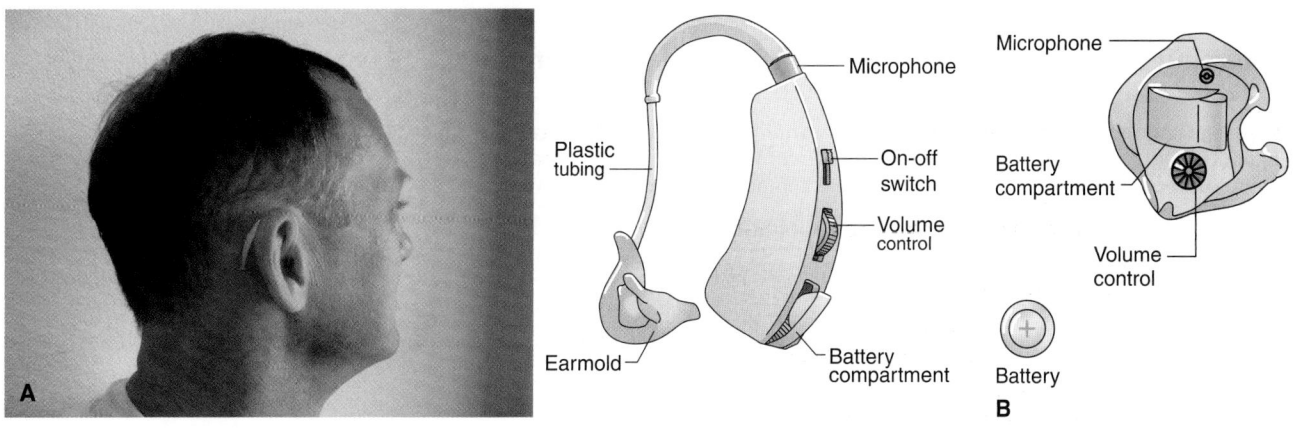

FIGURE 52.6 Hearing aids. (A) Behind-the-ear hearing aid. (B) In-the-ear hearing aid.

Table 52.6

Subjective Data Collection for Hearing Disorders

W: Where is it?	Are both ears affected? Is one side worse than the other?
H: How does it feel?	Are certain words unclear or entire conversations? Are high-frequency sounds (consonants *s, t, z, f, g,* and female voices) unclear or difficult to understand? Is any pain associated with the hearing loss? Any tinnitus or vertigo?
A: Aggravating and alleviating factors	Is hearing worse in large groups or when there is a lot of background noise? Is hearing improved in a quiet environment or when speaking only to an individual? Is it easier to understand someone when seeing the person's lips move? Does the patient own or use any assistive hearing devices? Are they effective? What type is used?
T: Timing	When did the hearing loss start? Was it gradual or sudden? Is the hearing loss associated with any illness or traumatic event? Is it associated with any recent flying? Any history of ototoxic drug use?
S: Severity	Does it cause communication impairment? How much? Does it affect activities of daily living? Does it affect or limit usual social activities? Have family or friends commented on decreased hearing? Does the patient avoid communication or social activities because of difficulty hearing? Is the patient having difficulties hearing telephone voices, radio, television, or movies?
U: Useful data for associated symptoms	Is there any fever, nausea, vomiting, or dizziness? Is there any history of occupational or environmental exposure to loud noises? What are the usual ear self-care habits? Any history of impacted cerumen? Has the patient ever had cerumen removed from ears?
P: Perception of the problem by the patient	What does the patient feel is wrong? Does the patient think that he or she has a hearing problem? How does the patient feel about hearing assistive devices? How does the patient perceive the hearing loss, and how is it influencing the patient's life?

a tympanic membrane problem. Any assistive hearing devices should be noted and inspected for proper functioning.

NURSING DIAGNOSES, PLANNING, AND IMPLEMENTATION. Planning focuses on helping the patient optimize hearing, promoting communication, and promoting adjustment to impaired hearing (Box 52.2 and Box 52.3). Nursing management for the patient with hearing impairment focuses on enhancing communication and quality of life (see "Nursing Care Plan for the Patient With Hearing Impairment"). Families should be included in discussions about therapeutic hearing devices, enhancing communication, and limiting patient social isolation.

EVALUATION. The patient's goals are met if the patient communicates effectively, engages in usual social activities, uses assistive hearing device, copes with emotional reaction to hearing impairment, and demonstrates care of a hearing aid.

Nursing Care Plan for the Patient With Hearing Impairment

Nursing Diagnosis: *Impaired Verbal Communication* related to impaired hearing
Expected Outcome: The patient will use effective communication techniques.
Evaluation of Outcome: The patient is able to communicate effectively to have needs met and reduce social isolation.

Intervention	Rationale	Evaluation
Inspect ear canals for mechanical obstruction. If cerumen is found, request order for a softening product to assist in wax removal, if not contraindicated. If canal is clear, continue assessment by using a tuning fork, loud ticking clock, or verbal cues to determine auditory ability at various distances.	*Hearing loss may result from buildup of cerumen in the auditory canal. Determination of hearing ability assists in developing interventions appropriate to patient's hearing level.*	Is ear canal free of mechanical obstruction? Is patient able to hear verbal input? If not, how severe is the impairment?
Enhance hearing by giving auditory cues in quiet surroundings.	*The presence of background noise, such as television, radio, or large numbers of people, makes hearing more difficult.*	Are auditory cues being delivered in an environment free of extraneous background noises?
Enhance understanding of auditory cues in a well-lit area but not in front of a window (which may cause glare). Get patient's attention before speaking; face patient, speak slowly, add hand gestures, and adjust voice pitch lower without shouting.	*Hearing is enhanced when additional cues assist patient in understanding the message. Use of hand gestures to point, lip-reading, facial expression, and lower pitch all assist communication.*	Are auditory cues being understood by patient? Are instructions given in a step-by-step format with written cues?
Structure environment to compensate for hearing loss by adding visual indicators to telephone ringer, doorbell, smoke detectors, and other emergency sounds.	*Assists in communication and safety.*	Is patient able to receive input in ways other than auditory?
Provide for optimal care of assistive appliances such as hearing aids by making sure that cerumen has been cleaned from the device, batteries are charged, and the appliance is placed correctly in ear.	*Appliances that are not functioning properly will not assist patient in hearing.*	Is patient's hearing aid placed correctly? Is cerumen blocking sound conduction? Do batteries work?
Introduce assistive devices such as hearing amplifiers, telephone amplifiers, telephones with extra-loud bells, written communication, and sign language.	*Patients may not be aware of assistive devices that could help them adapt to hearing loss and continue previous activities, such as talking on the telephone or listening to television.*	Is patient aware of assistive devices that will allow him or her to continue to verbally communicate with others? Is patient able to use the devices to compensate for auditory impairment?
Refer to specialized clinician such as an audiologist or occupational therapist or to specialized resources from such groups as the National Association of the Deaf or American Speech-Language-Hearing Association.	*Specialized clinicians can provide detailed examination and treatment. Specialized resource groups have networks in place to help patients cope with loss and maximize abilities.*	Does patient know whom to call for detailed examination and treatment? Does patient know that there are specialized clinicians and resource groups to help with hearing impairment? Does patient know how to access these specialists?

Box 52.2

Communicating With a Patient Who Has a Hearing Impairment

- Do not avoid conversation with a person who has hearing loss.
- Obtain the patient's attention before beginning to speak.
- If the listener uses a hearing device, ensure that it is operational and in place before beginning to communicate. Give the person time to adjust the hearing device before speaking.
- Ensure an optimal environment by reducing background noises (e.g., turn off television and radio, close the door, or move to a quieter area).
- Face and stand close to the person being spoken to and maintain eye contact.
- Do not smile, chew gum, or cover your mouth when talking.
- Avoid standing in the glare of bright sunlight or other bright lights.
- Speak clearly and at a normal rate and volume near the good ear. Do not shout or overarticulate.
- If the listener has difficulty with high-pitched sounds, lower the pitch of your voice.
- Encourage nonverbal communication, such as touch or gestures, as appropriate.
- Inform the listener of topics to be discussed and when a change of topic occurs. Stick to a topic for a while and avoid quick shifts.
- Use short sentences and check for understanding. If the listener does not understand after the message is repeated, rephrase the message.
- Allow extra time for the listener to respond and do not rush the listener.
- Use written communication if the person is unable to communicate verbally.
- Use active listening with attentive body posture, pleasant facial expressions, and a calm, unhurried manner.

Box 52.3

Care of Hearing Aids

Teach the patient the following regarding care of hearing aids:
- Apply hair or medicinal sprays before inserting hearing aid to protect the hearing aid.
- Insert hearing aid over a soft surface to prevent damage if the hearing aid is dropped during insertion.
- Turn hearing aid on and increase volume once it is inserted.
- Check battery or lower the volume if sound is not clear or is intermittent. Buzzing noise may indicate that the battery door is not completely closed.
- Minimize whistling noise by ensuring that the volume is not too high, the aid fits securely, and the aid is free from earwax.
- Remove hearing aid before showering or bathing. Do not immerse it in water.
- Clean the hearing aid's body daily with a dry, soft cloth. Clean earmold with small brush or toothpick to keep free of earwax.
- Turn the hearing aid volume down and then off when not in use to conserve battery.

External Ear

Infections

PATHOPHYSIOLOGY AND ETIOLOGY. Infection is the most common disorder of the external ear. **External otitis** is the infection that most often occurs. Exposure to moisture, contamination, or local trauma provides an ideal environment for pathological growth in the external ear. External otitis may be caused by bacterial or fungal pathogens. Staphylococci most frequently are the causative organism. *Pneumocystis* infections have been seen in patients who have HIV. A bacterial or fungal external otitis that occurs when water is left in the ear and washes away protective earwax is known as swimmer's ear. External otitis occurs more often in the summer months. However, it can be seen year-round in patients who swim indoors.

A localized infection called ear canal **furuncle** (abscess) results when a hair follicle becomes infected. A **carbuncle** forms when several hair follicles are involved in forming the abscess. Most furuncles and carbuncles erupt and drain spontaneously.

Otomycosis is an infection caused by fungal growth. It is typically seen after topical corticosteroid or antibiotic use. Otomycosis occurs more often in hot weather.

An infection of the auricle is called perichondritis. It can result in necrosis of ear cartilage.

SIGNS AND SYMPTOMS. The most common sign of infection of the external ear is pain (Table 52.7). An early indication of infection is pain with gentle pulling on the pinna (outer ear). The patient may also experience pain when moving the jaw or when the otoscope is inserted into the ear canal. Pruritus (itching) is also a common symptom and can be an early sign of infection. Signs of inflammation are present on the external ear. The ear canal may become swollen or occluded. As a result, hearing may be diminished. Redness, swelling, and drainage can be observed during otoscopic examination. If drainage is present, it usually starts out clear and becomes purulent as the disease progresses. The patient may also be febrile.

DIAGNOSTIC TESTS. A complete blood cell count, with elevated white blood cell counts, and cultures of discharge help diagnose infections. Culture and sensitivity tests isolate the specific infective organism and determine which antibiotics would be most effective to treat the infection. The Rinne and Weber tests can indicate conductive hearing impairment.

Table 52.7

Ear Disorders Summary

Signs and Symptoms	*External ear:* Pain, pruritus, swelling, redness, drainage, lacerations, contusion, hematomas, abrasion, blistering, hearing loss, foreign body *Middle ear:* Fever, earache, feeling of fullness in affected ear following upper respiratory infection, nausea, vomiting, mastoid tenderness, redness, bulging tympanic membrane, progressive hearing loss, vertigo, disorientation
Diagnostic Tests	Complete blood count (CBC) Audiometric, Rinne, Weber, and whisper voice tests Ear drainage culture Imaging studies
Therapeutic Measures	Cerumenolytics to remove earwax Anti-infectives, anti-inflammatories, analgesics *External ear:* Débridement, surgical repair, application of protective covering for trauma *Middle ear:* Myringotomy, myringoplasty, stapedectomy
Complications	*External ear:* Spread of infection to other parts of the ear, disfigurement, loss of hearing, scarring *Middle ear:* Perforation of tympanic membrane, cholesteatoma, tympanosclerosis, mastoiditis, permanent hearing loss
Priority Nursing Diagnoses	*Acute Pain* *Risk for Injury* *Deficient Knowledge*

Impacted Cerumen

PATHOPHYSIOLOGY AND ETIOLOGY. Normally, the ear is self-cleaning. However, cerumen (wax) may become impacted, blocking the ear canal. Factors that contribute to an impaction include large amounts of hair in the ear canal, exposure to dusty or dirty areas, improper ear cleaning, aging (because cerumen is drier as secretions decrease from shrinking ceruminous glands and keratin continues to collect), the use of hearing aids, and bony growths secondary to an osteophyte or osteoma.

SIGNS AND SYMPTOMS. The patient may experience hearing loss, a feeling of fullness, or a blocked ear if cerumen has become impacted (see Table 52.7). Otoscopic examination reveals cerumen blocking the ear canal.

DIAGNOSTIC TESTS. Audiometric testing reveals conductive hearing loss in the affected ear. Hearing acuity can be decreased by 45 decibels because of impacted cerumen. Whisper voice, Rinne, and Weber tests also indicate conductive hearing loss.

Masses

PATHOPHYSIOLOGY AND ETIOLOGY. Benign masses of the external ear are usually cysts resulting from sebaceous glands. Other benign masses are lipomas, warts, keloids, and infectious polyps. Infectious polyps usually arise from the middle ear and enter the external ear through a hole in the tympanic membrane. Actinic keratosis is a precancerous lesion that can be found on the auricle. It may be seen in older adults. Malignant tumors such as basal cell carcinoma on the pinna and squamous cell in the ear canal may develop and can spread.

SIGNS AND SYMPTOMS. Changes in the appearance of the skin can occur with benign or malignant masses. Usually, impaired conductive or sensorineural hearing loss occurs with masses. Pain is another symptom and is usually described as deep pain radiating inward on the affected side. Ear drainage may be present. As the condition progresses, facial paralysis may occur. Visualization of the mass may be observed during otoscopic examination.

DIAGNOSTIC TESTS. A biopsy may be obtained to determine whether the mass is benign or malignant. Imaging studies are also used to diagnose tumors. Audiometric studies reveal any hearing impairment.

Trauma

PATHOPHYSIOLOGY AND ETIOLOGY. Injuries to the external ear are commonly caused by a blow to the head, automobile accidents, burns, foreign bodies lodged in the ear canal, or cold temperatures. Cotton ball pieces and insects are the most common foreign bodies found in adult ears.

SIGNS AND SYMPTOMS. Lacerations, contusions, hematomas, abrasions, erythema, and blistering are signs seen with thermal or physical trauma. Repeated trauma to the ear can cause swelling, also known as cauliflower ear. This is more common among boxers, rugby players, martial artists, and wrestlers. Conductive hearing loss can occur if the ear canal is partially or totally blocked. Patients who have contusions or hematomas commonly report numbness, pain, and paresthesia of the auricle. Symptoms associated with foreign bodies may include decreased hearing, itching, pain, and infection. Care is taken during otoscopic examination not to push the foreign body further into the ear canal.

DIAGNOSTIC TESTS. Imaging studies may be needed to determine the extent of the trauma. Audiometric, whisper voice, Rinne, and Weber tests may demonstrate conductive hearing loss.

Complications of External Ear Disorders

If not treated, infections can spread, causing cellulitis, abscesses, middle ear infection, and septicemia. Metastasis can occur if malignant tumors are not treated. Infection, trauma, and malignant tumors may cause temporary or permanent hearing loss, disfigurement, discoloration, and scarring.

Therapeutic Measures for External Ear Disorders

For external ear infections, topical antibiotics are given. Systemic antibiotics are used for severe infections that are localized or have spread to surrounding tissues. Analgesics are used to control pain. Topical or systemic steroids may be used to treat inflammation. The ear is thoroughly cleaned before starting any topical treatment. If the external ear canal has drainage or is swollen shut, a wick may be inserted. The wick serves to aid in removing drainage or to aid in administering medication into the ear canal. Cerumen may be removed with irrigation by a trained clinician (Fig. 52.7). Irrigation is not used if the patient has a history of perforated tympanic membrane (eardrum) or other contraindications. Débridement, surgical repair, or application of a protective covering may be done when trauma occurs to the external ear. Surgical management consists of incision and drainage of abscesses. Excision of cysts or cutaneous carcinomas may also be required.

Nursing Process for the Patient With External Ear Disorders

DATA COLLECTION. Subjective data obtained in a patient history include reports of pain, fullness, previous cerumen impaction, itching, or hearing loss. Onset, duration, and severity of symptoms are also part of the data. Additional data include patient's occupation, previous ear problems, use of a hearing aid, and typical ear hygiene. Observation

for objective data includes redness, swelling, drainage, furuncles, carbuncles, lesions, abrasions, lacerations, growths, cerumen, scaliness, or crusting. The patient may report pain when the ear is palpated. Basic hearing acuity tests are conducted to evaluate hearing loss (see Chapter 51).

NURSING DIAGNOSES, PLANNING, AND IMPLEMENTATION.

Acute Pain related to inflammation or trauma

EXPECTED OUTCOME: The patient's pain will be relieved as evidenced by a lower rating on a pain scale within 30 minutes of report of pain.

- Monitor pain using a pain scale, and determine optimum analgesic schedule with the patient *to maximize pain control.*
- Implement nonpharmacological methods, such as relaxation, massage, music, guided imagery, or distraction techniques *to relieve pain.*
- Apply heat as ordered to the area *to promote comfort.*
- Offer liquid or soft foods *to relieve pain when chewing.*

Risk for Injury related to self-cleaning of external ear

EXPECTED OUTCOME: The patient will explain or demonstrate prescribed treatment.

- Explain ear care (Box 52.4) *to prevent injury.*
- Teach the patient the treatment regimen *to ensure completion of treatment.*

Deficient Knowledge related to lack of information on preventive ear care

EXPECTED OUTCOME: The patient will explain or demonstrate procedures to maintain wellness of the external ear.

- Explain the procedure before removal of cerumen *to decrease anxiety.*

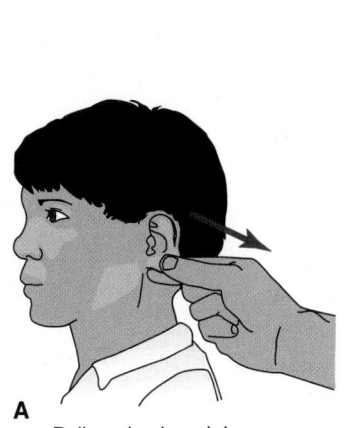
A Pull ear back and down to straighten ear canal in a child

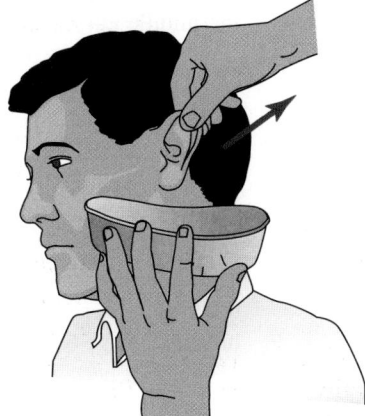
B Pull ear up and back to straighten ear canal in an adult

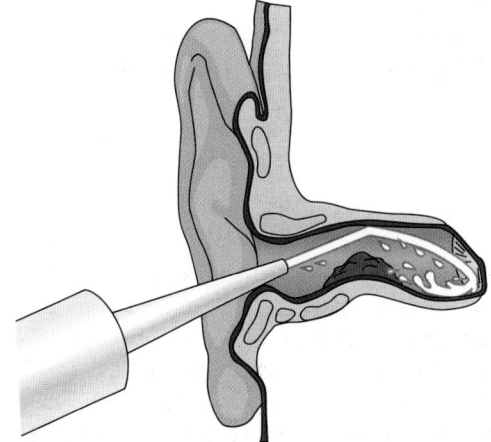
C Irrigation – Fluid is aimed off top of ear canal wall behind impacted cerumen

FIGURE 52.7 Ear irrigation. (A) Child. (B) Adult. (C) Irrigation.

Box 52.4

Ear Care

1. Cleanse the external ear with a wet washcloth. Gently cleanse the helix.
2. The ear has an effective self-cleaning system that continually moves protective earwax outward to prevent buildup. Cleaning attempts, particularly with swabs, can cause a wax impaction. Never insert anything into the ear canal, including cotton-tipped swabs, hair pins, matchsticks, safety pins, toothpicks, paper clips, or fingers. The thin skin of the ear canal is very fragile and can become abraded and then infected from being touched with these objects.
3. A person with a history of ear infections, perforated tympanic membrane, or swimmer's ear should prevent moisture from entering the ear canal and should avoid swimming in contaminated water. Moisture or water in the ear canal can be prevented by using earplugs.
4. For frequent swimming, use swim earplugs (custom or over the counter), an ear conditioner to prevent ear dryness, and an ear dryer after swimming.
5. Do not try home remedies for ear care without consulting a health care provider.
6. A person with an upper respiratory infection should gently blow the nose with both nares open to prevent microbes from being forced into the eustachian tubes.

- If a wick is inserted into the ear canal, explain to the patient that it is used *to monitor for drainage and report excessive drainage to HCP.*
- Teach the patient how to use topical antibiotics, oral antibiotics, and/or anti-inflammatory medications *to promote healing.*
- Teach the patient how to complete the prescribed treatment and maintain ear health (see Box 52.4). Include keeping the ear clean and dry, and use of earplugs or cotton with petroleum jelly *to avoid getting water in the ears during an infection.*

EVALUATION. The outcomes for the patient are met if the patient indicates pain is relieved as evidenced by a lower rating on a pain scale, hearing improves or returns to pre-illness level, the patient states or demonstrates prescribed treatment (e.g., administering ear drops or ointments), and the patient explains or demonstrates measures to maintain wellness of the external ear.

Middle Ear, Tympanic Membrane, and Mastoid Disorders

Infections

PATHOPHYSIOLOGY AND ETIOLOGY. Otitis media is the most common disease of the middle ear. Otitis media is a general term for inflammation of the middle ear, mastoid, and eustachian tube. Inflammation of the nasopharynx causes most cases of otitis media. As inflammation occurs, the nasopharyngeal mucosa becomes edematous. Discharge is produced. When fluid, pus, or air builds up in the middle ear, the eustachian tube becomes blocked. This impairs middle ear ventilation.

There are several types of otitis media in which inflammation can occur alone, with infective drainage, or with noninfective drainage. The first type is otitis media without effusion. This is an inflammation of the middle ear mucosa without drainage. The second type occurs when there is a bacterial infection of the middle ear mucosa. This is called acute otitis media, suppurative otitis media, or purulent otitis media. The infected fluid becomes trapped in the middle ear. If the infection continues longer than 3 months, chronic otitis media results. The third type is otitis media with effusion. Other names include serous otitis media, nonsuppurative otitis media, and glue ear. With this type of otitis media, noninfective fluid accumulates within the middle ear.

SIGNS AND SYMPTOMS. Acute otitis media commonly follows an upper respiratory infection. A fever, earache, and feeling of fullness in the affected ear are common symptoms (see Table 52.7). As purulent drainage forms, pain and conductive hearing loss occur. Nausea and vomiting may also be present. Purulent drainage may be evident in the external ear canal if the tympanic membrane ruptures. Mastoid tenderness indicates that the infection may have spread to the mastoid area. Otoscopic examination reveals a reddened, bulging tympanic membrane.

Symptoms of otitis media with effusion may go undetected in adults because there are no signs of infection. The patient may report fullness, bubbling, or crackling in the ear. The patient may have slight conductive hearing loss or allergies or be a mouth breather. Otoscopic examination can reveal a bulging tympanic membrane. The eardrum is not reddened.

COMPLICATIONS. A perforation may occur with an acute or chronic infection. Buildup of fluid and pressure in the middle ear can cause a spontaneous perforation of the tympanic membrane. The patient usually experiences pain before the rupture. Relief of pain occurs after the rupture. The fluid in the middle ear moves through the perforation into the ear canal. This relieves pressure and pain. A tympanic membrane perforation causes hearing loss. The location and size of the perforation determine the extent of hearing loss. Damage to ossicles can also occur with perforation.

Repeated infections in the middle ear or mastoid can cause a cholesteatoma. This is an epithelial cystlike sac that fills with debris such as degenerated skin and sebaceous material. The cholesteatoma starts in the external ear canal and spreads to the middle ear through a perforation in the tympanic membrane. Damage occurs in the middle ear structures as a result of pressure necrosis. The cholesteatoma causes conductive hearing loss. As the disease progresses, facial paralysis and vertigo may occur.

Tympanosclerosis is another complication of repeated middle ear infections. Tympanosclerosis consists of deposits of collagen and calcium on the tympanic membrane. The condition can slowly progress over time to the area around the middle ear ossicles. These deposits appear as chalky white plaques on the tympanic membrane and contribute to conductive hearing loss.

Mastoiditis can occur if acute otitis media is not treated. The infection spreads to the mastoid area, causing pain. The use of antibiotics has resulted in acute mastoiditis becoming relatively uncommon. Chronic mastoiditis is still seen with repeated middle ear infections.

DIAGNOSTIC TESTS. An elevated white blood cell count may be seen. Cultures on ear drainage identify the specific infective organism. Conductive hearing loss is usually present on audiometric studies and Rinne, Weber, and whisper voice tests. Imaging studies may be done to diagnose infection.

THERAPEUTIC MEASURES. Bacterial infections are treated with topical and systemic antibiotics. Topical antibiotics may contain steroids to help with inflammation. Oral analgesics are given to control pain.

A modified Politzer ear device can be used to help equalize pressure in the middle ear and aid fluid drainage. The device, also known as an ear popper (www.earpopper.com), emits a stream of air into the nasal cavity that gently opens the eustachian tubes. This relieves negative pressure. It allows pressure to equalize and fluid to drain.

Surgical intervention includes several techniques. Paracentesis may be performed with a needle and syringe. The tympanic membrane is punctured with the needle, and the fluid is drained from the middle ear. A **myringotomy** may also be performed. During this procedure, an incision is made in the tympanic membrane, and fluid drains out or is suctioned out of the middle ear. Another technique is laser-assisted myringotomy, which vaporizes the tympanic membrane. Various types of transtympanic tubes may be inserted to keep the incision open. With the transtympanic tube keeping the incision in the tympanic membrane open, pressure is equalized. Thus, further fluid formation and buildup is prevented. The transtympanic tubes are left in place until the infection is cured. Most tubes spontaneously extrude in 3 to 12 months. They rarely have to be removed.

Reconstructive repair of a perforated tympanic membrane is called a **myringoplasty.** One technique involves placing Gelfoam over the perforation. A graft from the temporal muscle behind the ear or tissue from the external ear is then placed over the perforation and Gelfoam. The Gelfoam is absorbed, and the graft repairs the perforation.

A mastoidectomy involves incision, drainage, and surgical removal of the mastoid process if the infection has spread to the mastoid area.

Otosclerosis

PATHOPHYSIOLOGY AND ETIOLOGY. Otosclerosis, or hardening of the ear, results from the formation of new bone along the stapes. With the new bone growth, the stapes becomes immobile. This causes conductive hearing loss. The formation of the new bone growth begins in adolescence or early adulthood and progresses slowly. Hearing loss is most apparent after the fourth decade of life. Otosclerosis is more common in women than in men. The disease usually affects both ears. Although the exact cause of otosclerosis is not known, most patients have a family history of the disease. It is therefore thought to be a hereditary disease.

SIGNS AND SYMPTOMS. The primary symptom of otosclerosis is progressive hearing loss. The patient usually experiences bilateral conductive hearing loss, particularly with soft, low tones. Usually, medical treatment is sought when the hearing loss interferes with the patient's ability to take part in conversations. The patient may also experience tinnitus. Otoscopic examination reveals a pinkish orange tympanic membrane because of vascular and bony changes in the middle ear.

DIAGNOSTIC TESTS. Audiometric testing indicates the type and extent of the hearing loss. Imaging studies indicate the location and the extent of the excessive bone growth. The whisper voice test and normal conversation show decreased hearing. The patient hears best with bone conduction in the Rinne test, whereas lateralization to the most affected ear occurs with the Weber test.

THERAPEUTIC MEASURES. There is no cure for otosclerosis. However, hearing aids may be used to improve hearing for the patient. Reconstruction of necrotic ossicles is done to restore some of the patient's hearing. Various methods are used to reposition and replace some or all of the ossicles. Unfortunately, the surgeries are not always successful over time. Ossiculoplasty is the reconstruction of the ossicles. Prostheses made of plastic, ceramic, or human bone are used to replace the necrotic ossicles. Total or partial ossicular replacement prosthesis may be used.

Stapedectomy is the treatment of choice for otosclerosis. Either part or all of the stapes is removed and replaced with a prosthesis. The prosthesis is placed between the incus and the oval window. Advances in surgical treatment include the use of lasers for improved visualization, less trauma, and greater precision during surgery. The goal is to restore vibration from the tympanic membrane to the oval window and allow sound transmission. Many patients experience improved hearing immediately; others do not have improvement until swelling subsides. Complications of ossiculoplasty and stapedectomy include extrusion of the prosthesis, infection, hearing loss, dizziness, and facial nerve damage.

NURSING CARE. Initially the patient may be on bedrest for several hours, then asked to ambulate to determine tolerance. When lying in bed, instruct the patient to lie on the side of the unaffected ear or the back during the first week. The cotton ball placed in the ear during surgery may be changed

---

• **WORD • BUILDING** •

myringoplasty: myringo—tympanic membrane + plasty—surgical repair

otosclerosis: oto—ear + sclerosis—hardening

stapedectomy: stape(s)—stirrup + ectomy—excision of

as needed if there is drainage. Occasionally, the patient may experience nausea or dizziness. Antiemetics can be used to prevent vomiting. The patient's safety should be ensured if dizziness occurs. Oral analgesics are given for pain. To prevent dislodgment or damage to the prosthesis, patients are instructed to sneeze with the mouth open, and not to blow their nose, sniff, fly in an airplane, scuba dive, exercise, lift heavy objects, or use ear plugs for several weeks as instructed. Showering and hair washing may be allowed 2 days after surgery with a cotton ball in the ear that is covered with Vaseline. If the patient develops a cold, the HCP should be contacted.

CRITICAL THINKING

Mrs. Springhorn is an 83-year-old woman who is scheduled to be discharged from the hospital after a stapedectomy. She lives alone at home and is able to care for herself.

1. How would you communicate with Mrs. Springhorn to ensure that she understands the discharge instructions?
2. What teaching methods would you use to enhance communication?
3. What ear care instructions would you give her?

   Suggested answers are at the end of the chapter.

Trauma

ETIOLOGY AND PHYSIOLOGY. Trauma, such as a blasting force, a blunt injury to the side of the head, or sudden changes in atmospheric pressure, can cause the tympanic membrane to perforate and middle ear ossicles to fracture. Blast injuries

cause injury from the direct pressure on the ear. Blunt injury to the head can cause temporal skull fractures and trauma to both the middle and inner ear. Barotrauma caused by sudden changes in atmospheric pressure in the ears can occur during scuba diving and airplane takeoffs and landings. Pressure changes can occur during normal atmospheric conditions such as nose blowing, heavy lifting, and sneezing. During these rapid changes of pressure, the eustachian tube does not ventilate because of occlusion or dysfunction. A negative pressure then develops in the middle ear. The resulting pressure can cause the tympanic membrane to rupture or cause damage to the middle and inner ear.

SIGNS AND SYMPTOMS. Pain and hearing loss are the most common symptoms associated with trauma. Other signs and symptoms of barotrauma include fullness of the ears, vertigo, nausea, disorientation, edema of the affected area, and hemorrhage in the external or middle ear. In severe cases of barotrauma when scuba diving, these symptoms can cause drowning or cerebral air embolism from an overly rapid ascent. Otoscopic examination may reveal a retracted, reddened, and edematous tympanic membrane.

DIAGNOSTIC TESTS. Audiometric studies are completed to determine the hearing loss. Imaging studies may be done to determine the extent of middle and inner ear damage. Conductive or sensorineural hearing loss may be evident, depending on the extent and location of the damage.

Nursing Process for the Patient With Middle Ear, Tympanic Membrane, and Mastoid Disorders

DATA COLLECTION. Table 52.8 reviews the subjective data that should be collected. The external ear should be inspected

Table 52.8

Subjective Data Collection for Middle Ear, Tympanic Membrane, Mastoid, or Inner Ear Disorders

W: Where is it?	Are both ears affected? Is it deep within the head?
H: How does it feel?	Is there pressure? Drainage? Fullness? Vertigo? Tinnitus? Is it painful? If so, is it sharp, dull, continuous, intermittent, throbbing, localized? No pain?
A: Aggravating and alleviating factors	Are there any allergies? Is it worse with change of position or movement? Is there relief with heat or drainage? Is there relief with analgesics or other medications?
T: Timing	When did it start? Was it a sudden onset? How long have symptoms persisted? Has there been any recent upper respiratory infection, airline travel, scuba diving, trauma, or weight lifting?
S: Severity	Does it cause hearing impairment? How much? Does it affect activities of daily living, nutritional intake, work?
U: Useful data for associated symptoms	Is there fever, headache, drainage from the ear canal, nausea, vomiting, dizziness? Is there a family history of otosclerosis? Any previous ear problems or ear surgeries?
P: Perception of the problem by the patient	What do you think is wrong? Has the problem occurred before? If so, what was the same and what was different?

and palpated to obtain objective data. Pain with palpation is indicative of external ear problems, not middle ear problems. Pain over the mastoid area can indicate a mastoid problem. The middle ear and mastoid cavity cannot be visualized directly. The tympanic membrane is the only middle ear structure that can be directly visualized with an otoscope. Objective assessment also includes vital signs, noting any elevation in temperature. Any drainage from the ear should be noted and described. Hearing acuity is screened with the whisper voice, Rinne, and Weber tests.

NURSING DIAGNOSES, PLANNING, AND IMPLEMENTATION.

Risk for Infection related to pressure necrosis or surgical procedure

EXPECTED OUTCOME: The patient will have no signs of infection (i.e., no drainage from ear, no tenderness over mastoid, negative culture, afebrile).

- Instruct the patient not to blow his or her nose by pinching off nares *to prevent spread of upper respiratory infections up the eustachian tube.*
- Teach the patient not to insert anything into the ear canal *to prevent ear damage* (see Box 52.4).
- Teach the patient how to correctly remove cerumen from ear *to prevent infection or damage.*

Acute Pain related to fluid accumulation, inflammation, or infection

EXPECTED OUTCOME: The patient will indicate pain is decreased or absent as evidenced by a lower rating on a pain scale.

- Monitor pain using a pain scale, and determine optimum analgesic schedule with the patient *to maximize pain control.*
- Use nonpharmacological measures such as heat, distraction, and relaxation techniques *for pain reduction.*
- Teach the patient how to administer ear drops or ear ointment *to help resolve infection and decrease pain.*
- Instruct the patient to take all prescribed antibiotics, even after symptoms are relieved, *to ensure that the infection is completely resolved.*

Deficient Knowledge related to no prior experience with a middle ear disorder

EXPECTED OUTCOME: The patient will state an understanding of methods for preventing problems in the middle ear, tympanic membrane, and mastoid process or impending surgery.

- Ask about the patient's knowledge regarding surgery *to determine learning needs.*
- Include the patient's family in teaching sessions *to enhance learning and assist with retention of information.*
- Teach the patient to avoid trauma to the ear, loud noise exposure, and environmental or occupational conditions *to prevent damage to the ear.*

- Teach the patient to yawn or perform jaw-thrust maneuver (opening mouth wide and moving jaw) *to equalize ear pressure, which helps maintain ear health.*
- Teach the patient methods of effective communication *to compensate for hearing loss* (see "Nursing Care Plan for the Patient With Hearing Impairment" earlier in this chapter).
- Provide preoperative and postoperative instructions *to promote patient understanding* (Box 52.5).
- Teach the patient how to avoid getting water in the ear postoperatively *to prevent moisture from reaching surgical site.*

EVALUATION. The goals for the patient are met if there is no ear drainage or pain over mastoid and if the patient has negative culture and remains afebrile. Also, the patient states that no pain is present or pain is decreased, verbalizes care of ears and methods to prevent further infection, describes signs

---

Box 52.5

Preoperative and Postoperative Nursing Interventions for the Patient Having Ear Surgery

Preoperative Care

For the patient undergoing ear surgery, the nurse collects data, determines the patient knowledge base, notes the patient's mental readiness, and obtains baseline physiological data.

- Ask about the type of surgery and anesthesia that will be used.
- Help alleviate the patient's fear by encouraging the patient to ask questions. Ensure that all questions are answered before surgery by the appropriate person.
- Explain types of pain control, packing or dressings to expect, and postoperative restrictions that may be ordered.
- Obtain and document baseline vital signs.
- Ensure that the informed operative consent is signed.
- Document the patient's current medications.
- Leave hearing devices for interactions in place until surgery.

Postoperative Care

Postoperatively, the nurse is responsible for monitoring the patient's physiological status and discharge teaching.

- Monitor vital signs.
- Explain that an occlusive dressing may decrease hearing until it is removed.
- Instruct patients with ear tubes to avoid getting water in the ear and to use a shower cap or earplugs as ordered.
- Instruct the patient to seek medical care if excessive bleeding or drainage occurs. If a cotton plug is to be left in place, instruct the patient to change it daily and as needed.
- Instruct patient to sneeze with mouth open and avoid blowing the nose.
- Explain ordered activity restrictions such as flying and heavy lifting.
- Explain use of pain medication and instruct to take antibiotics as ordered.
- Instruct the patient to call the health care provider's office for a follow-up appointment.

requiring medical attention, and verbalizes the rationale and outcome for any upcoming surgery as well as preoperative and postoperative instructions.

Inner Ear
Labyrinthitis

PATHOPHYSIOLOGY AND ETIOLOGY. Labyrinthitis is an inflammation or infection of the inner ear. It can be caused by either viral or bacterial pathogens. The bacterium or virus enters the inner ear from the middle ear, meninges, or bloodstream. Serous labyrinthitis is a type of acute labyrinthitis that sometimes follows drug intoxication or overindulgence in alcohol. It can also be caused by an allergy. Diffuse suppurative labyrinthitis occurs when acute or chronic otitis media spreads into the inner ear or after middle ear or mastoid surgery. Destruction of soft tissue structures from the infection can cause permanent hearing loss.

SIGNS AND SYMPTOMS. Vertigo, tinnitus, and sensorineural hearing loss are the most common symptoms. Vertigo, or dizziness, occurs when the vestibular structures are involved. Tinnitus, or ringing in the ear, occurs when the infection is located in the cochlea. Sensorineural hearing loss can be caused by infections in the cochlea or vestibular structures. Nystagmus on the affected side may occur. Other signs and symptoms include pain, fever, ataxia, nausea, vomiting, and beginning nerve deafness.

DIAGNOSTIC TESTS. A complete blood count (CBC) is done to diagnose infection. A hearing evaluation by an audiologist may reveal mild to complete hearing loss. Rinne and Weber tests indicate conductive or sensorineural hearing loss.

THERAPEUTIC MEASURES. Antibiotics are used to treat bacterial inner ear infections. Viral infections usually run their course in about 1 week. Mild sedation may help the patient relax. Although there is no specific medicine to relieve dizziness, antihistamines can be used if they prove helpful on an individual basis. Patients may be placed on bedrest.

NURSING CARE. Nursing management includes helping the patient manage symptoms and self-care. Educate the patient about safety issues while on bedrest and sedatives to prevent falls and injury. The patient should avoid turning the head quickly to help alleviate vertigo. The patient is assisted to cope with anxiety that may be present because of the frustration surrounding hearing loss or loss of work.

Neoplastic Disorders

PATHOPHYSIOLOGY AND ETIOLOGY. Inner ear tumors can be benign or malignant. Acoustic neuroma, a tumor of the eighth cranial nerve, is the most common benign tumor. It is slow growing, occurs at any age, and usually occurs unilaterally. As it spreads, it compresses the nerve and adjacent structures. Malignant tumors arising from the inner ear are rare. Squamous and basal carcinomas arise from the epidermal lining of the inner ear.

SIGNS AND SYMPTOMS. Early symptoms of an acoustic neuroma include progressive unilateral sensorineural hearing loss of high-pitched sounds, unilateral tinnitus, and intermittent vertigo. Headache, pain, and balance disorders may also be present. Symptoms progress as the tumor spreads to other structures. Most malignant tumors grow quickly. The symptoms vary depending on the area of the ear that is involved.

DIAGNOSTIC TEST. Neurologic, audiometric, and vestibular testing are used to diagnose neuroma. Auditory brainstem evoked response and electronystagmography are completed. Examination of the cerebrospinal fluid shows increased protein. A CT scan and magnetic resonance imaging (MRI) are used to determine the size and location of the tumor.

THERAPEUTIC MEASURES. The preferred method of treatment involves surgical removal of the tumor. The labyrinth is destroyed, with a resulting permanent hearing loss. Steroids and radiation may be used to decrease the size of the tumor or for inoperable tumors.

NURSING CARE. Nursing care focuses on preparing the patient for surgery and adjusting to the diagnosis and the resulting hearing loss (see Box 52.5).

Ménière Disease

PATHOPHYSIOLOGY AND ETIOLOGY. **Ménière disease** is a balance disorder. Its cause is unknown. With the disease, there is a dilation of the membranous labyrinth resulting from a disturbance in the fluid physiology of the endolymphatic system. The exact etiology is unknown but is thought to stem from hypersecretion, hypoabsorption, deficit membrane permeability, allergies, viral infection, hormonal imbalance, or mental stress. The disease usually develops between ages 40 and 60. The symptoms range from vague to severe and debilitating.

SIGNS AND SYMPTOMS. A triad of symptoms of vertigo, hearing loss, and tinnitus characterizes Ménière disease. Recurring episodic bouts of the incapacitating triad of symptoms and nausea and vomiting occur. The attacks may happen suddenly, or the patient may experience warning signs such as headache or fullness in the ears. During an acute episode, the patient experiences vertigo that lasts 2 to 4 hours. The vertigo is usually accompanied by nausea and vomiting, followed by dizziness and unsteadiness. The patient is uncoordinated and has gait changes when walking. Hearing loss is often described as a fluctuating fullness in the ears. Tinnitus is present. Irritability, depression, and withdrawal are common. Vital signs usually remain normal. It takes several weeks for symptoms to resolve, and hearing loss in the affected ear remains. The patient then enters a stage of remission until the next attack. The acute episodes occur two to three times yearly. Eventually the patient has complete remission with some degree of permanent hearing loss.

DIAGNOSTIC TESTS. Audiometric studies identify the type and magnitude of the hearing loss. Neurologic testing and radiographic studies are done to rule out other pathological conditions. A caloric stimulation test checks for damage to the acoustic nerve (involved in hearing and balance). The test is normal if nystagmus (fast side-to-side eye movements) occurs.

THERAPEUTIC MEASURES. Medical treatment consists of prophylactic treatment between attacks and symptomatic treatment for acute attacks. A salt-restricted diet, diuretics, antihistamines, and vasodilators are used during prophylactic treatment. The patient should avoid alcohol, caffeine, and tobacco use. Meclizine (Antivert) for vertigo, tranquilizers, and vagal blockers may be needed during acute attacks. The patient may be placed on bedrest during acute attacks. The goals of medical treatment are to preserve hearing and to reduce symptoms. Some patients who do not respond to treatment may be placed on low doses of methotrexate (Rheumatrex, Trexall).

Surgical treatment is used only when medical management has failed. When involvement is unilateral, a labyrinthectomy can be performed. This causes complete loss of hearing in that ear. Another surgical intervention establishes a shunt from the inner ear to the subarachnoid space. This procedure helps drain the fluid and prevent future hearing loss. Another surgical treatment is intratympanic gentamicin (Garamycin) injection, which is usually done in the HCP's office.

NURSING CARE. Nursing management focuses on managing the patient's symptoms and providing safety during acute attacks. Because of the unpredictability of Ménière disease, nursing care focuses on emotional support for the patient during periods of remission. Provide emotional support and resources to help the patient cope with the unpredictable nature of the disease and the physical impairments associated with the disease.

Nursing Process for the Patient With Inner Ear Disorders

DATA COLLECTION. Subjective data are collected (see Table 52.8). Objective data are collected through examination of gross hearing; the whisper voice, Rinne, and Weber tests; a physical examination; and laboratory data. The patient should be assessed for any nutritional deficiencies, including dehydration, weight loss, or weight gain. An unsteady gait or temperature is also noted.

NURSING DIAGNOSES, PLANNING, AND IMPLEMENTATION. Planning focuses on helping the patient maintain a normal lifestyle, remain free of injuries, cope with the illness or hearing loss, and maintain adequate nutrition and hydration.

Anxiety related to unpredictability of sudden and severe acute attacks

EXPECTED OUTCOME: The patient will state that anxiety is decreased.

- Encourage the patient to express concerns about hearing loss and the unpredictability of acute attacks *to identify causes of anxiety.*

- Monitor for signs of anxiety such as fidgeting, restlessness, apprehension, shakiness, and increased heart rate *to determine whether anxiety is present.*
- Explore with the patient techniques that have and have not worked in the past *to determine which techniques to use to reduce anxiety.*
- Use a calm reassuring approach *to help instill confidence.*
- Provide a quiet environment and diversional activities *to calm the patient.*
- Provide information regarding diagnosis and treatment *to promote understanding and reduce anxiety.*

Risk for Injury related to impaired equilibrium

EXPECTED OUTCOME: The patient will not be injured from falling due to alterations in equilibrium.

- Institute fall precautions *to help prevent injury.*
- Ensure that the environment is safe and free of obstacles (e.g., throw rugs, electrical cords in walkways, poor lighting) *to prevent falls.*
- Monitor for signs of headache or fullness in the ears *to detect an oncoming Ménière disease attack.*
- Instruct the patient to avoid sudden movement of the head during periods of vertigo *to prevent increasing symptoms.*
- Instruct the patient on correct dosage and administration of medications *to help ensure resolution of symptoms.*
- Instruct the patient to avoid use of alcohol, caffeine, and tobacco *to decrease disruptions of equilibrium.*
- Instruct the patient to call for assistance when ambulating *to minimize risk of falling.*
- If indicated, instruct the patient to remain on bedrest until symptoms are relieved *to prevent injury.*

Imbalanced Nutrition: Less Than Body Requirements related to nausea and vomiting

EXPECTED OUTCOME: The patient will experience adequate nutrition and hydration with relief of nausea and vomiting.

- Monitor for signs of nausea, vomiting, and inadequate hydration *to determine baseline information.*
- Instruct the patient to use deep breathing, voluntary swallowing, and eating slowly *to suppress the vomiting reflex.*
- Medicate as ordered *to relieve symptoms and prevent episodes of nausea and vomiting.*
- Institute a salt-restricted diet, if ordered, and instruct the patient on low- and high-sodium foods *to reduce fluid retention.*

EVALUATION. The goals for the patient have been met if signs of anxiety are decreased and if the patient remains free from injury and maintains weight within normal range with no signs of dehydration.

CRITICAL THINKING

Mrs. Belmont is a 48-year-old woman diagnosed with Ménière disease. She is currently in a state of remission. She states that she is fearful that the next attack will occur during her daughter's upcoming wedding.

1. What data would you collect about Mrs. Belmont's attacks?

2. What instructions would you provide to Mrs. Belmont to use during her attacks?

3. How will you handle Mrs. Belmont's fears about future attacks?

   Suggested answers are at the end of the chapter.

SUGGESTED ANSWERS TO CRITICAL THINKING

Mr. Samuel

1. Mr. Samuel should seek assistance, patch both eyes, and have someone take him to receive medical treatment immediately.
2. Ensure that an antiemetic is ordered postoperatively on the patient's return to the unit. When Mr. Samuel reports nausea, the antiemetic should be given *promptly*.
3. Did you recognize that the concentration is 2 mg/1 mL, and the volume of the vial is 2 mL? The concentration is what is required to calculate the dose:

$$\frac{4\ mg}{} \times \frac{1\ mL}{2\ mg} = 2\ mL$$

Mrs. Springhorn

1. Gain her attention, face her and stand in her visual field, avoid glare, speak clearly, inform her of topics to be discussed, assess for understanding, allow extra time for more explanation, reduce background noises, use nonverbal communication, and do not cover your mouth when talking.
2. Use active listening. Use written communication to enhance spoken words. Use demonstration and return demonstration. Allow questions. Do not hurry. Provide information in short segments. Reassess understanding at each session.

3. Place the operative ear upward or lie on back when in bed. Sneeze with the mouth open. Do not blow nose, sniff, fly in an airplane, or lift heavy objects. Exercise as instructed. Shower and wash hair as instructed. If a cold develops, call the health care provider. If dizzy, be careful when standing up.

Mrs. Belmont

1. You should ask Mrs. Belmont about specific signs she may have had before previous attacks, such as headache or fullness in the ears. You should also ask her specifically what symptoms she has during attacks. Common symptoms include the triad of vertigo, hearing loss, and tinnitus. She may also have nausea, vomiting, and unsteady gait.
2. Encourage her to ensure safety to prevent falling. Discuss treatment that Mrs. Belmont has used with previous attacks. Ask her which treatments helped. Recommend taking ordered medications such as tranquilizers and vagal blockers; maintaining adequate fluid and nutritional intake; ambulating with assistance; limiting salt in her diet; and avoiding alcohol, caffeine, and tobacco use.
3. Provide emotional support. Discuss methods to help her cope with the disease, such as counseling and relaxation techniques. Discuss with Mrs. Belmont prophylactic treatment, such as a salt-restricted diet, diuretics, antihistamines, and vasodilators.

Review Questions

1. The nurse is caring for a patient who is diagnosed with otosclerosis and asks what the disease is. Which is the most appropriate response by the nurse?
   1. "Infection of the external ear commonly caused by moisture."
   2. "It is a tumor of the eighth cranial nerve."
   3. "Hardening of the stapes due to new bone growth."
   4. "Inflammation of the inner ear caused by pathogens."

2. The nurse is caring for a patient who is diagnosed with a refractive error and asks what this means. What would be the appropriate explanation by the nurse?
   1. "You are losing your vision and will become blind."
   2. "You will need corrective lenses to see clearly."
   3. "The pressure in your eyes is higher than normal."
   4. "Your vision was measured as 20/20."

3. A patient comes to the health clinic for a suspected ear infection. Which of these data collection findings does the nurse expect with an external ear infection? **Select all that apply.**
   1. Dizziness
   2. Fullness in ears
   3. Redness
   4. Pain
   5. Pruritus
   6. Swelling

4. A patient has been prepped for an internal eye examination. Anesthetic drops and a mydriatic drug have been administered. Which instruction should the patient be taught for eye safety following the examination?
   1. "Wear sunglasses after the exam."
   2. "Rub your eye hourly to increase blood circulation."
   3. "You may reapply contact lenses when the eye exam is completed."
   4. "Flush your eye with water to remove the eye drops."

5. The nurse cares for patients after eye surgery. Which of these patients would the nurse provide specific positioning instructions to after eye surgery to prevent complications?
   1. 19-year-old after removal of congenital cataract
   2. 30-year-old woman after pneumatic retinopexy
   3. 52-year-old man after trabeculectomy
   4. 82-year-old man after corneal transplant

6. The nurse is caring for a patient with a history of acute angle-closure glaucoma. The nurse is preparing to administer the patient's medications. Which medications should the nurse question before administration? **Select all that apply.**
   1. cefazolin (Kefzol)
   2. cyclopentolate (Cyclogyl)
   3. hydroxyzine (Vistaril)
   4. ranitidine (Zantac)
   5. morphine
   6. warfarin (Coumadin)

7. The nurse is assisting with discharge instructions for a patient. Which of these medications would the nurse teach the patient can cause hearing loss? **Select all that apply.**
   1. acetaminophen (Tylenol)
   2. erythromycin (E-Mycin)
   3. furosemide (Lasix)
   4. gentamicin (Garamycin)
   5. aspirin (Bayer)
   6. tobramycin (Tobrex)

8. The nurse is caring for a patient with macular degeneration. During data collection, which symptom would the nurse anticipate the patient to report?
   1. Loss of peripheral vision
   2. Sudden darkness
   3. Dull ache in the eyes
   4. Loss of central vision

9. The nurse is contributing to the plan of care for a patient with Ménière disease. What is the primary goal for this patient that the nurse should recommend to include in the plan of care?
   1. Prevent dehydration.
   2. Decrease pain.
   3. Prevent injury.
   4. Preserve hearing.

10. The nurse is caring for a patient with presbycusis. Which technique is most important for the nurse to use to increase communication with this patient?
    1. Talk in a very loud voice.
    2. Lower voice pitch.
    3. Do not smile or chew gum when talking to the patient.
    4. Allow extra time for patient to respond.

Answer rationales available in your online resources.

ANSWERS 1. 3; 2. 3, 4, 5, 6; 4. 1; 5. 2; 6. 2, 3; 7. 2, 3, 4, 5, 6; 8. 4; 9. 3; 10. 2.

Key Points

Find the chapter key points in your online resources available through Davis Edge.

Additional Resources

 Use the scratch off code on the inside front cover of your book to access online quizzes that will help you to improve your scores on course exams and prepare for the NCLEX-PN®.

 Study Guide

CHAPTER 53

Integumentary System Function, Assessment, and Therapeutic Measures

Rita Bolek Trofino, Janice L. Bradford

KEY TERMS

alopecia (AH-low-PEE-she-ah)
ecchymosis (EK-ih-MOH-sis)
erythema (AIR-ih-THEE-mah)
petechiae (peh-TEE-kee-eye)
turgor (TUR-gur)

CHAPTER CONCEPT

Tissue Integrity

LEARNING OUTCOMES

1. Explain normal structures and functions of the integumentary system.
2. Identify the effects of aging on the integumentary system.
3. List data to collect when caring for a patient with an integumentary system disorder.
4. Identify laboratory and diagnostic tests commonly performed to diagnose integumentary disorders.
5. Describe therapeutic measures that are used for patients with integumentary disorders.

 NORMAL INTEGUMENTARY SYSTEM ANATOMY AND PHYSIOLOGY

The skin, its accessory structures, and the subcutaneous tissue form the integumentary system, the covering of the body that separates the living internal environment from the external environment. The skin itself is considered an organ. It consists of two layers: the outer epidermis and the inner dermis (Fig. 53.1).

Epidermis, Dermis, and Hypodermis

The epidermis has up to five epithelial layers. The innermost epidermal layer is called the *stratum germinativum*. This is where mitosis occurs to produce new epidermal cells. The rate of mitosis is fairly constant but increases from chronic abrasion to the skin, as in callus formation. The new cells, keratinocytes, produce the protein keratin and a water-repelling sealant. As they are pushed to the surface of the skin, they die and become the *stratum corneum,* the outermost of the epidermal layers. These cells resist abrasion and water entry and exit.

The stratum corneum consists of many layers of dead, keratinized cells. An unbroken stratum corneum is an effective barrier against pathogens and most chemicals, although even microscopic breaks are sufficient to permit their entry. As dead cells are worn off the surface of the skin (which

contributes to the removal of pathogens), they are continuously replaced by cells from beneath. Loss of large portions of the stratum corneum, as with extensive third-degree burns, greatly increases the risk for infection and dehydration.

Melanocytes are cells in the lower epidermis that produce the protein melanin. The amount of melanin is a genetic characteristic and gives color to skin and hair. When the skin is exposed to ultraviolet (UV) rays from the sun or artificial lighting, production of melanin is incorporated into the epidermal cells making the cells darker. Melanin is a pigment barrier to prevent further exposure of living cells in the stratum germinativum to UV rays. UV rays are mutagenic; that is, they are capable of damaging the DNA in cells and causing mutations that can result in malignancy.

Also in the epidermis are Langerhans cells, a type of macrophage that presents foreign antigens to immune cells. This is the first step in the destruction of pathogens that penetrate the epidermis.

Extensive collagen fibers in the dermis give the skin its strength as an organ. Elasticity results from these elastic fibers and allows stretched skin to return to its proper position.

The hypodermis (also known as the subcutaneous layer) consists of areolar and adipose tissue. This subcutaneous adipose tissue cushions, insulates, and stores energy as triglyceride. The subcutaneous tissue contains abundant leukocytes that destroy pathogens that enter through broken skin.

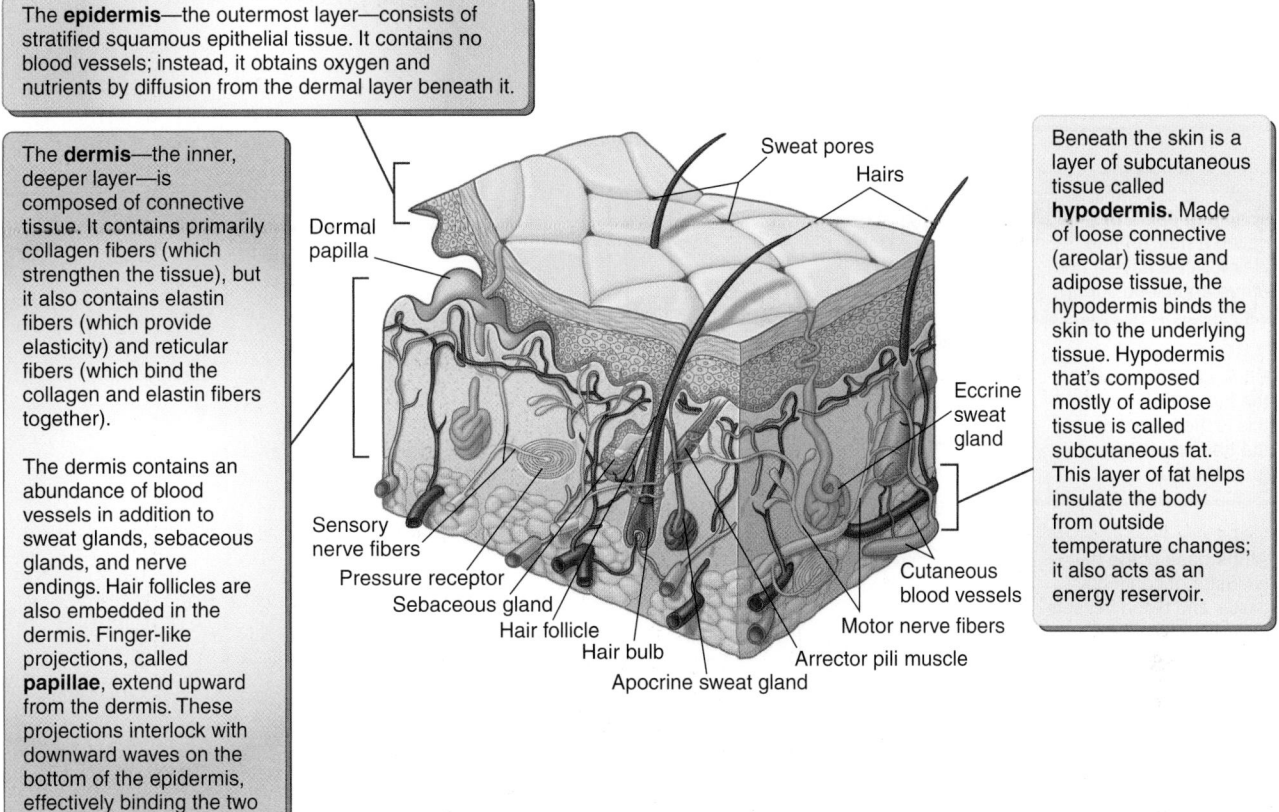

The **epidermis**—the outermost layer—consists of stratified squamous epithelial tissue. It contains no blood vessels; instead, it obtains oxygen and nutrients by diffusion from the dermal layer beneath it.

The **dermis**—the inner, deeper layer—is composed of connective tissue. It contains primarily collagen fibers (which strengthen the tissue), but it also contains elastin fibers (which provide elasticity) and reticular fibers (which bind the collagen and elastin fibers together).

The dermis contains an abundance of blood vessels in addition to sweat glands, sebaceous glands, and nerve endings. Hair follicles are also embedded in the dermis. Finger-like projections, called **papillae**, extend upward from the dermis. These projections interlock with downward waves on the bottom of the epidermis, effectively binding the two structures together.

Beneath the skin is a layer of subcutaneous tissue called **hypodermis.** Made of loose connective (areolar) tissue and adipose tissue, the hypodermis binds the skin to the underlying tissue. Hypodermis that's composed mostly of adipose tissue is called subcutaneous fat. This layer of fat helps insulate the body from outside temperature changes; it also acts as an energy reservoir.

Dermal papilla · Sweat pores · Hairs · Eccrine sweat gland · Sensory nerve fibers · Pressure receptor · Sebaceous gland · Hair follicle · Hair bulb · Apocrine sweat gland · Cutaneous blood vessels · Motor nerve fibers · Arrector pili muscle

FIGURE 53.1 Structure of the skin.

Hair

Human hair with significant function includes the eyelashes and eyebrows, which keep dust and sweat out of the eyes, and nostril hair, which filters air entering the nasal cavities. Hair on the head provides thermal insulation (Fig. 53.2).

Nails

Nail roots are found at the ends of the fingers and toes. Growth of nails is similar to growth of hair. Mitosis in the nail root is a continuous process to produce new, keratinized cells. As these cells die, they form the visible nail. Nails protect the ends of the digits from mechanical injury and are useful for picking up small objects.

Receptors

Sensory receptors for the cutaneous senses reside in the dermis. Receptors for heat, cold, and pain are free nerve endings; encapsulated nerve endings are specific for touch and pressure. The sensitivity of an area of skin is determined by the density of receptors present.

Glands

Cutaneous exocrine glands lie within the dermis and secrete to the surface of the skin through ducts. These include sudoriferous glands (both eccrine and apocrine), sebaceous (oil) glands (Fig. 53.3), ceruminous glands (cerumen), and ciliary glands (tears).

Water lost to eccrine gland secretion, at minimum, is about 500 mL per day through insensible perspiration. Excessive loss can rise to a liter per day in extreme heat or during vigorous exercise. Such dehydration and electrolyte loss must be replaced to avoid imbalances.

Blood Vessels

Blood vessels in the dermis serve the usual function of tissue nourishment, but the arterioles are also involved in maintaining body temperature. Blood carries heat produced by active organs and distributes it throughout the body. In a warm environment, dilation of blood vessels in the dermis increases blood flow and loss of heat to air. Constriction of blood vessels in a cold environment decreases blood flow to the skin and conserves body heat.

Stressful situations also cause vasoconstriction in the dermis, which allows blood to circulate to more vital organs, such as the heart, liver, brain, or muscles.

Other functions of the skin are the formation of vitamin D from cholesterol when the skin is exposed to the UV rays of the sun and the excretion of small amounts of ammonia, urea, and sodium chloride in sweat.

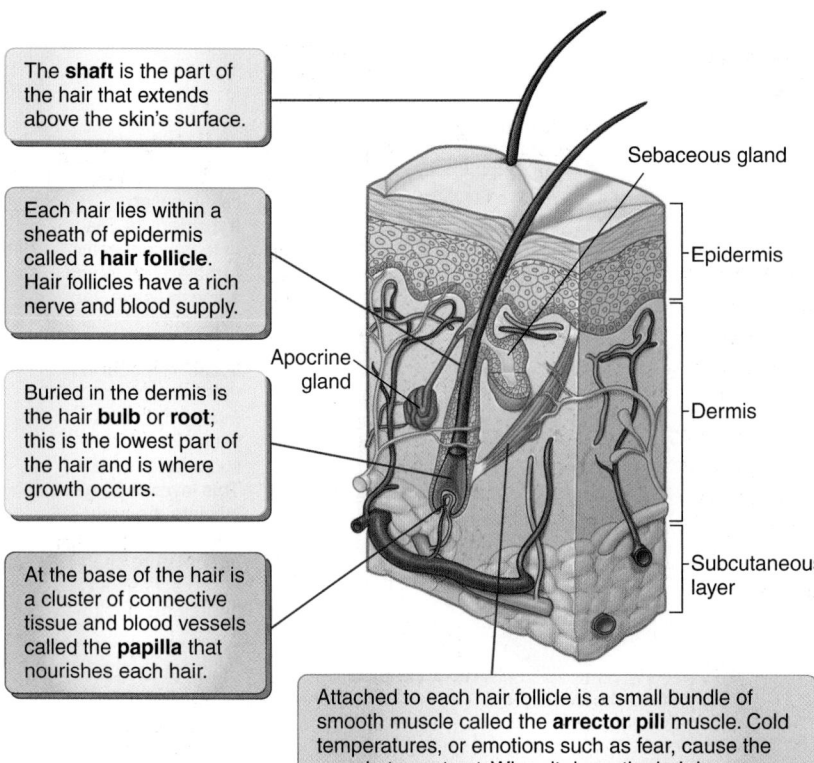

The **shaft** is the part of the hair that extends above the skin's surface.

Each hair lies within a sheath of epidermis called a **hair follicle**. Hair follicles have a rich nerve and blood supply.

Buried in the dermis is the hair **bulb** or **root**; this is the lowest part of the hair and is where growth occurs.

At the base of the hair is a cluster of connective tissue and blood vessels called the **papilla** that nourishes each hair.

Apocrine gland

Sebaceous gland

Epidermis

Dermis

Subcutaneous layer

Attached to each hair follicle is a small bundle of smooth muscle called the **arrector pili** muscle. Cold temperatures, or emotions such as fear, cause the muscle to contract. When it does, the hair becomes more upright, sometimes called "standing on end."

FIGURE 53.2 Hair.

Eccrine glands

- Contain a duct that leads from a secretory portion (consisting of a twisted coil in the dermis), through the dermis and epidermis, and onto the skin's surface
- Are widespread throughout the body, but are especially abundant on the palms, soles, forehead, and upper torso
- Produce a transparent, watery fluid called sweat, which contains potassium, ammonia, lactic acid, uric acid, and other wastes
- Sweat plays a chief role in helping the body maintain a constant core temperature and also helps the body eliminate wastes.

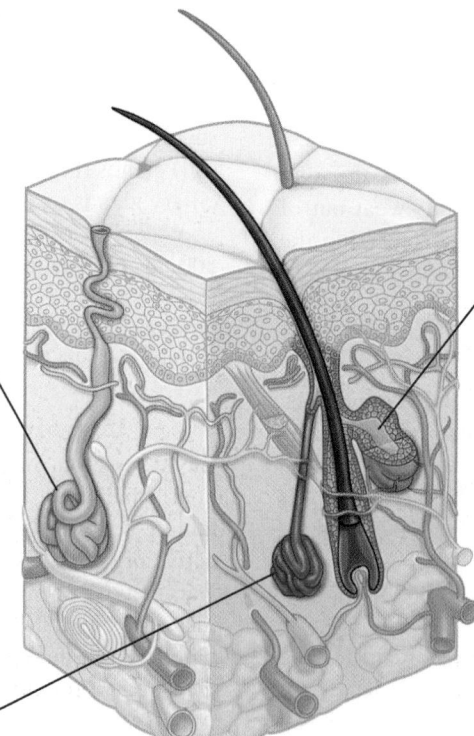

Sebaceous glands

Sebaceous glands, which open into a hair follicle, secrete an oily substance called sebum. Sebum helps keep the skin and hair from drying out and becoming brittle. Sebum has a mild antibacterial and antifungal effect. Under the influence of sex hormones, sebum production increases during adolescence. When excess sebum accumulates in the gland ducts, pimples and blackheads can form. (When the accumulated sebum is exposed to air, it darkens, forming a blackhead. A pustule results if the area becomes infected by bacteria.)

Apocrine glands

- Contain a duct that leads to a hair follicle (as opposed to opening onto the skin's surface)
- Are located mainly in the axillary and anogenital (groin) regions
- Are scent glands that respond to stress and sexual stimulation
- Begin to function at puberty
- Sweat produced by these glands does not have a strong odor unless it accumulates on the skin; when this occurs, bacteria begin to degrade substances in the sweat, resulting in body odor

FIGURE 53.3 Glands.

Aging and the Integumentary System

The effects of age on the integumentary system are often quite visible. Figure 53.4 summarizes the effects of aging.

NURSING ASSESSMENT OF THE INTEGUMENTARY SYSTEM

Health History

Many factors can influence the integumentary system. A skin problem may be the only problem a patient has, or it may be a manifestation of an underlying systemic condition or psychological stress. Most important, the skin can visibly communicate a patient's health. Therefore, a good skin assessment can help determine whether a problem is a skin disease or a sign of a more systemic disorder. Table 53.1 provides examples of general questions that can be asked of the patient to gather information.

If further assessment of a particular problem area is needed, the *WHAT'S UP?* line of questioning can be used. For example, if the patient has a rash, you can respond by pursuing the following information:

- **W**here is it? Is that the only area where you have a rash?
- **H**ow does it feel? Does it itch? Burn? Hurt?
- **A**ggravating and alleviating factors. Does scratching aggravate it? Does anything else aggravate it, such as soaps and detergents? What relieves it? How have you treated it in the past?
- **T**iming. How long have you had this problem? Does it recur?

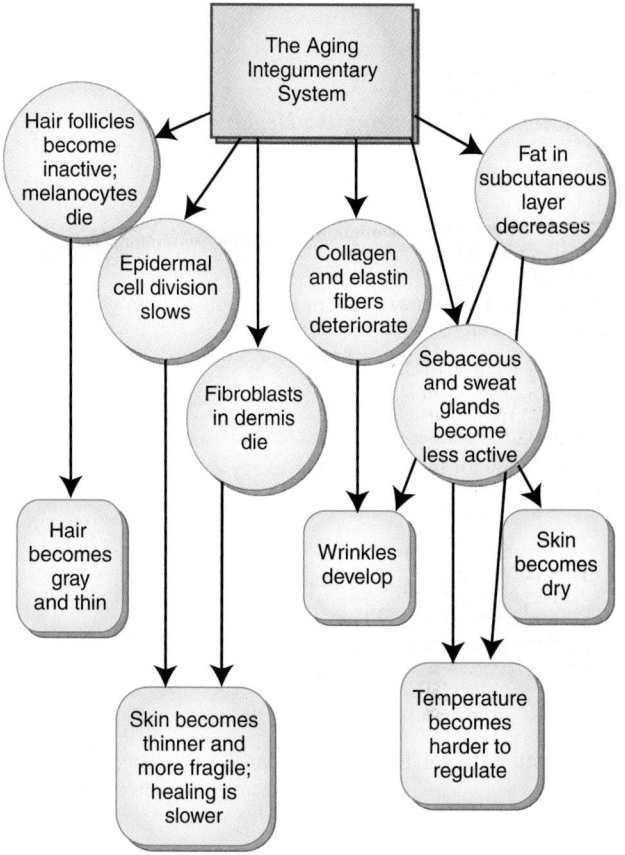

FIGURE 53.4 Aging and the integumentary system.

Table 53.1

Subjective Data Collection for the Integumentary System

Questions to Ask During the Health History	Rationale
History	
Do you (or does anyone in your family) have a history of dryness, rashes, itching, skin disease, psoriasis, eczema, dermatitis, asthma, hay fever, hives, or allergies?	These conditions may be hereditary.
Risk Factors	
Have you noticed any changes in your skin, such as a sore that does not heal, rashes, lumps, or a change in an existing mole?	Sores that do not heal, moles that change color, or lumps may indicate cancer. Slow healing can also be associated with diabetes. Brown staining of the skin in the lower legs is associated with venous stasis.
Have you had any recent trauma to your skin? Do you have a tendency to sunburn easily? Do you use sunblock? Do you go to tanning salons or use a sun lamp?	A break in skin integrity can lead to infection. Repeat sunburns and tanning are a risk factor for skin cancer.
Hair	
Do you wear a wig or hairpiece?	Adequate examination of the scalp requires permission for removal of a wig or hairpiece.

Continued

Table 53.1

Subjective Data Collection for the Integumentary System—cont'd

Questions to Ask During the Health History	*Rationale*
Have you noticed a change in hair growth or hair loss?	Hair loss can result from systemic illness or treatment or sometimes from infections or hair care products.
Nails	
Have you experienced recent trauma to or changes in your nails? Do you wear artificial nails?	Nail changes may be caused by circulatory problems. Artificial nails may mask changes.
Medications	
What medications do you take every day (prescription and over the counter)?	The patient may be taking medication for a skin disorder. Many medications cause skin reactions, from hives and photosensitivity to serious inflammatory conditions.
What medications did you take most recently? When did you take your last dose?	This might help pinpoint the cause of a new reaction.
Exposures	
What is your occupation?	Occupational exposures can lead to skin problems.
How often do you bathe or shower?	Frequent bathing can cause dry skin.
What kind of soap do you use?	Some soap may cause allergic reactions.
What recreational activities do you participate in?	Skin disorders can be caused by gym equipment that was not cleaned properly. Poison ivy may result from being in wooded areas.
Have you or any members of your immediate family or your coworkers had recent skin issues?	Some skin disorders are contagious.
Have you traveled recently?	This could help pinpoint causes of suspicious skin changes.
Is there anything in your current environment, at home or work, that may be causing any skin problems (e.g., animals, plants, chemicals, infections, new carpeting, new soaps or detergents)?	Various environmental factors cause contact dermatitis; some chemicals can cause skin disorders.
Is there anything that touches your skin that causes a rash?	This may help pinpoint causes of contact dermatitis.

- **Severity.** How bad is the discomfort on a scale of 0 to 10, with 0 being comfortable and 10 being unable to touch the area?
- **Useful other data.** Do you have other symptoms besides the rash?
- **Patient's perception.** What do you think is causing your rash?

Physical Examination

Examination of the skin involves not only the entire skin area, but also the hair, nails, scalp, and mucous membranes. The main techniques used in physical examination of the skin are inspection and palpation. Make sure the patient is undressed but adequately draped in a well-lit and warm environment.

Use a handheld magnifying glass or penlight to see small details and light the area being inspected.

Normally, the skin is intact, with no abrasions, and is smooth, dry, well hydrated, and warm. Skin **turgor** (tension) is firm and elastic. The skin surface is flexible and soft. Skin color ranges from light to ruddy pink or olive in white-skinned patients and light brown to deep brown in dark-skinned patients.

Be aware of normal developmental changes when performing an examination. The skin of the neonate is very thin and friable (easily broken). During adolescence, the skin becomes thicker, with active sebaceous, eccrine, and apocrine glands. Body hair also changes during adolescence as a result of hormonal influences. In older patients, the skin loses some of its elasticity and moisture. There is decreased activity of sebaceous and sweat glands. The older patient's skin is thinner, more fragile, and more wrinkled.

Inspection

Inspect each area of the skin for color, moisture, lesions, edema, intactness, vascular lesions, turgor, and cleanliness. This examination should be done in an orderly sequence, such as hair, scalp, buccal mucosa, nails, and then the general skin surface from head to toe.

COLOR. Skin color can be influenced by many factors, including the temperature of the patient, oxygenation, blood flow, exposure to UV rays, and positioning. Because skin color can differ genetically from very light to very dark, skin assessment can be difficult for the novice practitioner.

In general, healthy patients have an even skin tone that matches their genetic background. Light-skinned patients may have pink or yellow to olive undertones. Patients with naturally dark skin may have a reddish undertone, with pinkish buccal mucosa, tongue, nails, and lips.

Commonly noted alterations can include pallor, **erythema** (redness), jaundice, cyanosis, and brown coloring. Pallor is paleness or a decrease in color. It can be caused by vasoconstriction, decreased blood flow, or decreased hemoglobin levels from anemia. Pallor is best assessed on the face, conjunctivae, nailbeds, and lips. If a dark-skinned patient is pale, the mucous membranes have an ash-gray color, lips and nailbeds appear paler than usual, and the skin appears yellow brown to ash gray.

Erythema, or red discoloration, can be caused by vasodilation or increased blood flow to the skin from fever or inflammation. Erythema is best assessed on the face or in an area of trauma. Erythema presents in dark-skinned patients as a purplish-gray color.

Jaundice, a yellow-orange discoloration, can result from liver disease. Although skin is affected by jaundice, the best place to inspect for jaundice is in the sclera of the eye.

Cyanosis, or bluish discoloration, can indicate a cardiac, pulmonary, or perfusion problem. The best places to inspect for cyanosis are the lips, nailbeds, conjunctivae, and palms. People of Mediterranean descent normally have a bluish tone to their lips; this is not cyanosis. Cyanosis in a dark-skinned patient presents as a gray cast to the skin. The nailbeds, palms, and soles may have a bluish cast.

A brown color in an otherwise light-skinned patient may be caused by increased melanin production. It can indicate chronic exposure to sunlight or pregnancy. This is best assessed on areas exposed to the sun; changes in pregnancy can be seen on the face, areolae, and nipples. A brownish color also may result from chronic peripheral vascular disease, especially noted on the lower legs.

LESIONS. A lesion is any change or injury to tissue. Assessment of skin lesions helps determine the cause of a skin disorder. Lesions are described as primary or secondary. Primary lesions are the initial reaction to a disease process. Secondary lesions are changes that take place in the primary lesion because of trauma, scratching, infection, or various stages of a disease. Lesions are further described according to type and appearance in Figure 53.5.

When assessing and documenting skin lesions, note the color or colors of the lesion and the size (usually in centimeters), location, distribution, and configuration. Configuration refers to the pattern of the lesions, as shown in Figure 53.6. Also note any exudate, including amount, color, and odor, and any accompanying symptoms. Gently stretching the skin over the affected area makes lesions stand out more for better visualization.

MOISTURE/DRYNESS. Assessment of moisture provides clues to the patient's level of hydration. Observe the skin for dryness, moisture, scales, and flakes. Moisture may be found in skinfold areas. The skin is normally smooth and dry. Flaking and scaling of the skin can indicate dry skin or an inflammatory disorder.

EDEMA. Edema occurs because of excess fluid in the tissues. It can cause the skin to become stretched, dry, and shiny. Examine and document the location, distribution, and color of edematous areas. If edema is unilateral, compare it with the opposite side of the body. Measure edematous extremities to track changes over time. Dependent edema occurs in the part of the body that is at the lowest point, typically the feet and ankles, or in the sacrum if the patient is lying down.

VASCULAR LESIONS. Two common abnormal vascular changes result from bleeding under the skin: petechiae and ecchymosis (see Figures 28.1 and 28.2 in Chapter 28). **Petechiae** are reddish-purple spots that are smaller than 0.5 mm in diameter. In the dark-skinned patient, petechiae are usually not visible on the skin but can be visualized in the conjunctivae and oral mucosa. **Ecchymosis** is a bruise that changes color from blue black to greenish brown or yellow over time.

GENERAL INTEGRITY AND CLEANLINESS. Examine the integrity of the skin. Older adults have thin, fragile skin that is easily broken or torn. Be sure to check between toes and skinfolds and under a pendulous abdomen or breasts. Check over bony prominences for signs of pressure. Note general cleanliness and odors.

Palpation

Palpation is used with inspection. Use the dorsum (back) of the hand to palpate temperature because this part of the hand is most sensitive to changes in temperature. Use the fingertips to gently palpate over the skin to determine size, contour (flat, raised, or depressed), and consistency (soft or indurated) of lesions. If a lesion is moist or draining, wear gloves to protect against the spread of infectious organisms. Note the degree of pain or discomfort associated with light palpation of lesions.

• WORD • BUILDING •
ecchymosis: ec—out + cchymos—juice + is—condition

PRIMARY LESIONS

Macule:
Flat, nonpalpable change in skin color, with different sizes, shapes, color; usually smaller than 1 cm (e.g., rubella, scarlet fever, freckles)
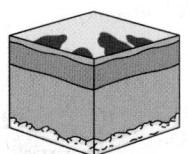

Papule:
Palpable solid raised lesion that is less than 1 cm in diameter due to superficial thickening in the epidermis (e.g., ringworm, wart, mole)
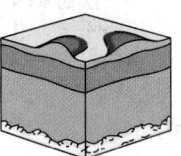

Nodule:
Solid elevated lesion that is larger and deeper than a papule (e.g., fibroma, intradermal nevi)
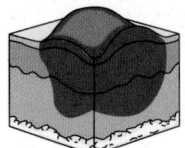

Vesicle:
A small, blisterlike raised area of the skin that contains serous fluid, up to 1 cm in diameter (e.g., poison ivy, shingles, chickenpox)
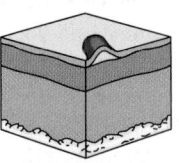

Bulla:
A fluid-filled vesicle or blister larger than 1 cm (e.g., burns, contact dermatitis)
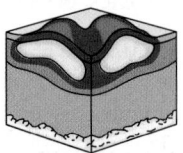

Pustule:
Small elevation of skin or vesicle or bulla that contains lymph or pus (e.g., impetigo, scabies, acne)
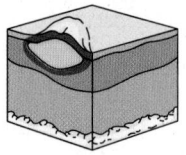

Wheal:
Round, transient elevation of the skin caused by dermal edema and surrounding capillary dilatation; white in center and red in periphery (e.g., hives, insect bites)
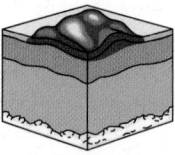

Plaque:
A patch or solid, raised lesion on the skin or mucous membrane that is greater than 1 cm in diameter (e.g., psoriasis)
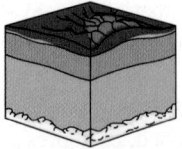

Cyst:
A closed sac or pouch which consists of semisolid, solid, or liquid material (e.g., sebaceous cyst)
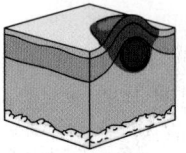

SECONDARY LESIONS

Scale:
Dry exfoliation of dead epidermis that may develop as a result of inflammatory changes (e.g., very dry skin, cradle cap, psoriasis)
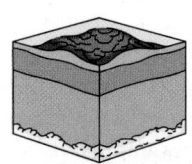

Crust:
A scab formed by dry serum, pus, or blood (e.g., infected dermatitis, impetigo)
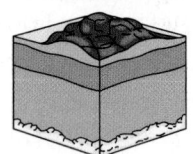

Excoriation:
Traumatized abrasions of the epidermis or linear scratch marks (e.g., scabies, dermatitis, burns)
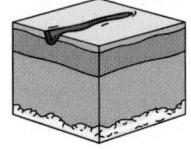

Fissure:
A slit or cracklike sore that extends into dermis, usually due to continuous inflammation and drying (e.g., athlete's foot, anal fissure)
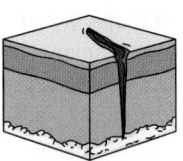

Ulcer:
An open sore or lesion that extends to the dermis (e.g., pressure sores)
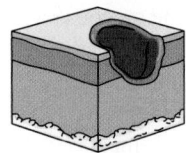

Lichenification:
Thickening and hardening of skin from continued irritation such as from intense scratching
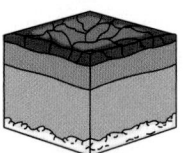

Scar:
A mark left in the skin due to fibrotic changes following healing of a wound or surgical incision
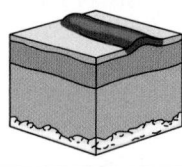

FIGURE 53.5 Description of skin lesions.

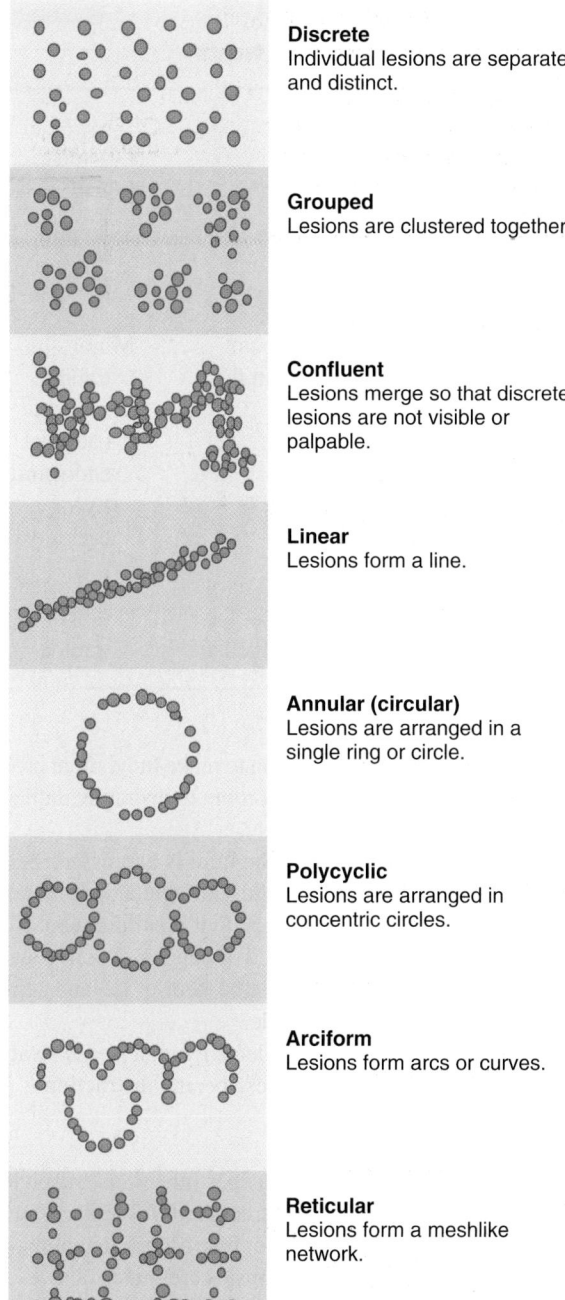

Discrete
Individual lesions are separate and distinct.

Grouped
Lesions are clustered together.

Confluent
Lesions merge so that discrete lesions are not visible or palpable.

Linear
Lesions form a line.

Annular (circular)
Lesions are arranged in a single ring or circle.

Polycyclic
Lesions are arranged in concentric circles.

Arciform
Lesions form arcs or curves.

Reticular
Lesions form a meshlike network.

FIGURE 53.6 To assess configuration, observe the relationship of the lesions to each other. Then characterize the configuration by choosing one of the patterns illustrated in the chart.

Examine for turgor and observe the texture of the skin. Skin turgor is a measure of the amount of skin elasticity. To assess for turgor, pinch the skin on the back of the forearm or over the sternum between the thumb and forefinger and then release. Normally, the skin lifts easily and then quickly returns to its normal state. Poor skin turgor is indicated by "tenting" of the skin, with more gradual return to its normal state. Poor skin turgor can indicate dehydration. Normal aging of skin produces some loss of skin elasticity; the preferred place to check skin turgor in older adults is over the sternum.

If edema is suspected, palpate those areas to assess for tenderness, mobility, and consistency. Press the edematous area (against bone, if possible) with your thumb for 5 seconds and then release. When pressure from your fingers leaves an indentation, this is called *pitting edema*. If the edema is in an extremity, measure and record the circumference in centimeters, and monitor it for increase or decrease in size.

Inspect and/or palpate the hair over the entire body for color, quantity, thickness, and texture. Note any areas of **alopecia** (hair loss). Determine any recent changes in color and growth pattern. Note cleanliness, redness, scaling, flakes, and tenderness. If lesions or lice are suspected, use disposable gloves to avoid spread of infection.

Terminal hair is the hair on the scalp, eyebrows, axillae, and pubic areas and on the face and chest of men. Vellus hair is the soft, tiny hair covering the body. Normally, body hair has a uniform distribution. Loss of hair on the extremities can indicate impaired circulation. Note male or female pubic hair distribution. Scalp hair can normally be thick, thin, coarse, smooth, shiny, curly, or straight. Describe scalp hair distribution and cleanliness.

Nails can reflect the patient's general health. Examine fingers and nails for color, shape, texture, thickness, and abnormalities. Normally, the nails appear pink, smooth, hard, and slightly convex (160-degree angle), with a firm base. Older adults' nails may have a yellowish-gray color, thickening, and ridges. Brown or black pigmentation between the nail and nail base is normal in dark-skinned patients. Abnormal findings include clubbing, which may indicate hypoxia, and spoon nails (concave nails, also called koilonychia), which can be associated with anemia. Thick nails may indicate fungal infection. Palpate for nail consistency, and observe for redness, swelling, or tenderness around the nail area. Table 53.2 describes other nail abnormalities.

Describe any abnormal skin conditions in detail. Include findings such as color of lesion, pain, swelling, redness, location, size, drainage (including amount, color, and odor), and eruption patterns. If equipment is available, an excellent way to supplement documentation is by photographing the area; serial photographs can be mounted in the chart to document healing progression. "Gerontological Issues" describes assessment and care specific to older adults.

DIAGNOSTIC TESTS FOR THE INTEGUMENTARY SYSTEM

Laboratory Tests
Cultures

Skin cultures are done to determine the presence of fungi, bacteria, and viruses. When a fungal infection is suspected, gently scrape scales from the lesion into a Petri dish or other indicated container. The specimen is then treated with a

Gerontological Issues

Care of Older Patients' Feet. Many older people are unable to bend down or bring the feet up high enough to see or care for them. Take time to assess and take special care of your older patients' feet. General guidelines for assessment include the following:

• Inspect feet for redness or pressure injuries over bony prominences.
• Inspect feet for dryness or cracking.
• Inspect between toes for cracking, wounds, or excess moisture.
• Inspect and palpate for calluses.
• Inspect toenails for thickening.
• Palpate dorsalis pedis and posterior tibial pulses for circulatory status.
• Assess patient's sensation using a wisp of cotton, monofilament, or light touch.

Actions to promote healthy feet include the following:

• Soak the patient's feet briefly in warm water and wash using a gentle soap. Test the water to be sure it is not too warm, especially for the patient with reduced sensation.
• Thoroughly dry the feet, including between the toes. Water left to evaporate can cause drying, cracking, and fungal infection.
• Use a pumice stone to help remove dry dead skin over heels or calluses. Work gently, rubbing the stone in one direction only and removing only a small amount of dead skin at any one time. Only use a pumice stone on a patient with diabetes mellitus under direction of a podiatrist.
• Use a cream or lotion that does not contain alcohol to moisturize the feet. *Do not* apply between toes. Apply it with gentle massage while moving the patient's feet through range-of-motion exercises. To prevent falls, never apply lotion before the patient steps into the tub or shower.
• Use gauze or a commercially made pad to decrease pressure and friction in areas between toes that cross or other areas where breakdown is likely.
• Encourage the patient to wear cotton or dry weave socks that allow feet to stay dry with perspiration.
• Encourage the patient to wear comfortable leather shoes or hard-soled slippers to avoid injury to the feet and prevent falls. Patients with diabetes should be encouraged to wear closed-toe shoes.
• Take extra care to assess and care for feet in patients with diabetes because of their increased risk for injury and slow healing.

NURSING CARE TIP

When scraping scales for culture, position the patient so that the skin lesion is vertical. Place the slide against the skin below the lesion. Be sure to wear gloves when collecting specimens and perform hand hygiene before and after.

Table 53.2
Abnormalities of the Nails

Physical Examination Finding	Description	Possible Causes
Beau lines	Transverse depressions in the nails	Systemic illnesses or nail injury
Splinter hemorrhages	Red or brown streaks in the nailbed	Minor trauma, subacute bacterial endocarditis, or trichinosis
Paronychia	Inflammation of the skin at the base of the nail	Local infection or trauma

10% potassium hydroxide solution to make fungi more prominent. The specimen can remain at room temperature until sent to the laboratory.

If a viral culture is ordered, the fluid is expressed (gently squeezed) from an intact vesicle, collected with a sterile cotton swab, and placed in a special viral culture tube. If the lesion has crusts, they are removed or punctured before swabbing. The viral culture tube must be kept in ice and sent to the laboratory as soon as possible.

Bacterial cultures may be collected with a sterile swab or wound culture kit. Box 53.1 gives specific instructions.

Skin Biopsy

A skin biopsy is indicated for deeper infections, suspicious lesions, or evaluation of current treatment. A biopsy is an excision of a small piece of tissue for microscopic examination. Three common types of skin biopsies are punch, shave, and incisional.

A punch biopsy uses a small, round cutting instrument, called a punch, to cut a cylinder-shaped plug of tissue for a full-thickness specimen. A shave biopsy removes just the

---

Box 53.1

Steps in Culturing a Wound

1. Use sterile saline to remove excess drainage and debris from the wound. Purulent material may have different bacteria than those actually causing the infection.
2. Using a sterile calcium alginate swab in a rotating motion, swab wound and wound edges 10 times in a diagonal pattern across the entire surface of the wound.
3. Do not swab over eschar or slough.
4. Place swab in culture tube, label, and send to lab.

area that has risen above the rest of the skin. An incisional biopsy is performed with a scalpel to make a deep incision and almost always requires sutures for closure.

For all biopsies, explain the procedure, assist in preparing a sterile field, calm and comfort the patient during the procedure, and assist in dressing the site after the procedure. The most uncomfortable part of the procedure is usually injection of a local anesthetic. Explaining the procedure and calming the patient can make the procedure less traumatic.

Other Diagnostic Tests

Wood Light Examination

A Wood light examination involves the use of UV rays to detect fluorescent materials in the skin and hair present in certain diseases such as tinea capitis (ringworm). This examination is performed with a handheld black light (Wood light) in a darkened room.

Skin Testing

Patch and scratch tests are performed when allergic contact dermatitis is suspected. These are usually done by a dermatologist on uninvolved skin, such as the upper back or arms. Any hair in the area must first be shaved.

For a scratch test, the skin is superficially scratched or pricked with an allergen for an immediate reaction. If a reaction such as a wheal occurs, the test is positive for that allergen. Resuscitation equipment should be in the immediate vicinity in the event of a severe allergic (anaphylactic) reaction.

For a patch test, allergens are applied under occlusive tape patches; a delayed hypersensitivity reaction develops in 48 to 96 hours. The skin should be free of oils to promote patch adhesion, so cleanse the skin first with alcohol. The test site must remain dry and free from moisture. The patch is removed in 2 days. Any reaction is noted, with a final reading in 2 to 5 days.

THERAPEUTIC MEASURES FOR THE INTEGUMENTARY SYSTEM

Open Wet Dressings

Wet compresses may be ordered for acute, weeping, crusted, inflamed, or ulcerated lesions. The purpose of wet dressings is to decrease inflammation, cleanse and dry a wound, and promote drainage of infected areas. They may be ordered either sterile or clean, depending on the risk for infection. The solutions commonly consist of room temperature to cool tap water or normal saline solution, aluminum acetate solution (Burow solution), or magnesium sulfate. The dressing is saturated with the solution before it is applied. Wet dressings usually are applied every 3 to 4 hours for 15 to 30 minutes.

Wet dressings should not be prescribed for more than 72 hours because the skin may become too dry or macerated. If cool compresses are used, they should be reapplied every 5 to 10 minutes because they become too warm from body heat. If warm compresses are used, monitor the skin closely to prevent burns.

> **NURSING CARE TIP**
>
> To prevent chilling, no more than one-third of the body should be treated with a wet dressing at one time. Keep the patient warm during wet dressing treatment.

Balneotherapy

Balneotherapy (therapeutic bath) is useful in applying medications to large areas of the skin as well as for débridement, or removing old crusts; for removing old medications; and to relieve itching and inflammation. The temperature of the water should be kept at a comfortable level, and hot water avoided. The bath should last for 15 to 30 minutes, all the while maintaining its warmth. Fill the tub half full. Keep the room warm to minimize chilling. Advise the patient to wear loose clothing after the bath.

Water and saline solution are utilized for weeping, oozing, and erythematous lesions. Colloidal baths (such as oatmeal or Aveeno) are used for widely distributed skin lesions, drying, and relief of itching. Medicated tar baths, such as Balnetar, are used for chronic eczema and psoriasis. Any loose skin crusts can be removed after the bath. The room should be well ventilated because tars are volatile.

To increase hydration after the bath, a lubricating agent is applied to damp skin if prescribed. Bath oils, such as Alpha Keri or Lubath, are used for lubrication and to relieve itching.

> **NURSING CARE TIP**
>
> A nonslip bath mat should be used in treatment baths because some of the treatments may make the tub slippery.

Topical Medications

Many types of topical medications are used to treat skin conditions. These include lotions, ointments and creams, powders, gels, pastes, and intralesional therapy. Systemic medications may be given for more serious conditions.

Lotions tend to cool the skin through water evaporation. They also may have a protective effect and may be antipruritic (anti-itch). Lotions are usually applied with cotton, gauze, gloves, or a soft brush.

Ointments and creams have a varied base (greasy, nongreasy, or penetrating), depending on the drug applied. These medications can protect the skin, provide lubrication, and prevent water loss. They are used for localized or chronic skin conditions. Ointments and creams can cause some reduction in blood flow to the skin. They are applied with a gloved hand or wooden tongue depressor.

Powders usually have a zinc oxide, talc, or cornstarch base. They are used to absorb moisture and reduce friction. Antifungal powders may be used in skinfolds. Powders are usually supplied with a shaker top. They should be shaken onto a gauze pad or gloved hand away from the patient's face. The powder is then applied by gently patting or rubbing onto the affected area. Avoid use of powders in patients with respiratory disease or tracheostomies.

NURSING CARE TIP
Avoid applying too much powder in skinfold areas. Dermatitis and fungal infection can occur with too much powder in these areas.

Gels, or semisolid emulsions, become liquid with topical application. They are usually greaseless and do not stain. Many topical steroids are prescribed in this manner.

Pastes are semisolid substances comprising ointments and powders. They are used for inflammatory disorders. Mineral oil can facilitate removal of pastes.

Topical corticosteroids are used to reduce or relieve pain and itching by decreasing inflammation. Steroids should be used sparingly and according to package directions. Overuse of topical corticosteroids can cause thinning of the skin. Some clinicians use steroid inhalers (usually used for patients with asthma) to apply a fine mist of medication to affected areas.

Intralesional therapy may be used for anti-inflammatory action. This procedure uses a sterile suspension of a corticosteroid injected just below the lesion with a tuberculin syringe. Local atrophy may occur if the injection is made into subcutaneous tissue. Common conditions that are treated with this therapy include psoriasis and keloids.

CRITICAL THINKING

Mr. Evans comes to the doctor's office with atrophic skin (thin, shiny, and pink, with visible vessels) at the area of psoriasis where he is applying his corticosteroid ointment. He says that he has been applying a thick layer of ointment four times a day.

1. What should you teach Mr. Evans about his treatment?
2. What should you include when you document his skin condition?

Suggested answers are at the end of the chapter.

Dressings

Dressings may be used to enhance absorption of topical medications, promote retention of moisture, prevent evaporation of medication, and reduce pain and itching. Occlusive dressings (for sealing a wound) are commonly used for skin disorders. For an occlusive dressing, an airtight plastic film is applied directly over the topical agent. Corticosteroids are also available in a special plastic surgical tape that can be cut to size. See "Nursing Care Plan for the Patient With an Occlusive Dressing."

Nursing Care Plan for the Patient With an Occlusive Dressing

Nursing Diagnosis: *Impaired Skin Integrity* related to open lesions
Expected Outcome: The patient will experience improved skin integrity as evidenced by reduction in size of lesion.
Evaluation of Outcome: Is there a decrease in wound size?

Intervention	Rationale	Evaluation
Assess areas of lesions for changes in size, color, swelling, dead skin, and drainage three times a day or as ordered.	*Areas of redness, swelling, pain, and drainage may indicate infection.*	Are lesions free of redness, swelling, pain, and drainage?
Cleanse wound as prescribed. Lightly pat dry.	*Cleansing helps provide a healthy granulation area for healing.*	Is wound clean and free of debris, crusts, and exudate?
Apply prescribed topical agent to moist skin as ordered. Apply sparingly or as directed.	*Depends on agent and reason prescribed.*	Does area exhibit signs that treatment is effective (e.g., decrease in size and numbers of lesions, free from infection, less itching)?
Cut plastic film to size and apply. Cover with an appropriate dressing to seal edges.	*Film enhances absorption of medication and helps retain moisture.*	Is the topical agent adherent to the skin?
Remove dressing for 12 of 24 hours.	*Continued use may cause skin atrophy, folliculitis, erythema, and systemic absorption of medication.*	Are there signs of healthy granulation tissue? Is skin pink? Are there fewer open areas? Is dressing removed for at least 12 hours every 24 hours?

Nursing Care Plan for the Patient With an Occlusive Dressing—cont'd

Nursing Diagnosis: *Disturbed Body Image* related to presence of lesions or wound
Expected Outcomes: The patient will verbalize acceptance of condition. The patient will be willing to participate in care of lesion or wound.
Evaluation of Outcomes: Does the patient verbalize acceptance of condition? Does the patient participate in care of lesions?

Intervention	Rationale	Evaluation
Assess patient's feelings regarding condition.	*Assessment provides a baseline for care. If patient denies condition, he or she may not comply with care.*	Does patient state willingness to follow care instructions?
Care for patient with an accepting attitude.	*Patient will be aware of nurse's response to the appearance of the skin.*	Does patient appear comfortable allowing nurse to provide care for lesion or wound?
Allow opportunities for patient to verbalize concerns about condition.	*Verbalization allows patient to begin to accept changes and problem solve.*	Does patient verbalize feelings appropriately?
Provide referrals to support groups and counselors as appropriate.	*Patient may benefit from talking to others with similar condition or to another professional for objective evaluation.*	Is patient receptive to appropriate referrals?
Assist patient in concealing lesion or wound in a safe and appropriate manner.	*Long sleeves and long pants may help conceal and protect lesions, and prevent further skin damage.*	Is patient able to conceal lesions if desired?

Nursing Diagnosis: *Self-Care Deficit (Bathing)* related to presence of lesions or wound and discomfort
Expected Outcomes: The patient will verbalize the importance of good hygiene. The patient will participate in bathing/hygiene.
Evaluation of Outcomes: Does the patient verbalize importance of good hygiene? Is the patient's skin clean and dry?

Intervention	Rationale	Evaluation
Assess patient's level of hygiene.	*Assessment provides a baseline for care.*	Is patient's level of hygiene at an acceptable level?
Instruct patient in appropriate bathing/hygiene, including: avoid strong detergents and soaps; use gentle emollient soaps or prescribed soaps; gently stroke areas of lesions; pat dry; avoid friction; maintain a little moisture on skin; maintain comfortable environmental temperature; have temperature of bath at a comfortable level to patient but not too hot.	*Patient needs to be able to properly cleanse lesions to prevent infection. Avoidance of friction and strong soaps prevents further trauma to skin. Patient will not shiver in comfortable temperatures.*	Does patient demonstrate good bathing techniques? Are lesions free of infection?

Proper application of a plastic wrap dressing includes washing the area, lightly patting it dry, applying the medication to moist skin, covering the medicated area with plastic wrap, and covering with a dressing to seal the edges. Wet dressings and ointments should only be applied to affected areas, not to healthy intact skin, because this can cause maceration of good skin. Plastic wrap dressings should be used for no more than 12 hours a day.

NURSING CARE TIP

Continued use of occlusive dressings can cause skin atrophy, folliculitis, maceration, erythema, and systemic absorption of the medication. To prevent some of these complications, the dressing is removed for at least 12 of every 24 hours.

Hydrocolloid dressings (e.g., DuoDERM, Tegaderm) can help protect areas exposed to pressure and treat pressure injuries in early stages. Gels, pastes, and granules can be used to fill in deep wounds to promote granulation and aid healing. See Chapter 54 for dressings used specifically for pressure injuries. A skin tear (superficial flap of skin exposing underlying dermis) should be covered with a nonadherent dressing such as Xeroform and wrapped with gauze. Table 53.3 summarizes various types of wound dressings.

Other items commonly used with topical treatments for skin conditions include gauze or cotton cloth held in place with the following:

- Small, stretchable tubular material (e.g., Surgitube) for fingers, toes, and extremities
- Disposable polyethylene gloves sealed at the wrist for hands
- Cotton socks or plastic bags for feet
- Disposable diapers or cotton diapers for the groin and perineal areas
- Cotton cloth held in place with dress shields for the axillae
- Cotton or light flannel pajamas for the trunk
- A shower cap for the scalp
- A facemask made from gauze and stretchable dressings with holes cut out for eyes, nose, mouth, and ears.

The patient's health care provider or a wound care specialist should specify the type of dressing and particular materials needed.

Table 53.3
Common Dressings

Dressing Type/Examples	Description	When Used
Alginates: Kaltostat SeaSorb Tegagen	Derived from brown seaweed; conform to the shape of the wound.	When packed into wound, absorb exudate and form a soft gel to maintain moist environment for wound healing.
Antimicrobial dressings: Acticoat Aquacel Ag SilvaSorb Gel Tegaderm Ag Mesh	Topical dressings derived from such agents as silver, iodine, and polyhexamethylene biguanide.	Intended for use in draining, nonhealing wounds that have bacterial contamination, such as burns, surgical wounds, diabetic ulcers, pressure injuries, and leg ulcers.
Collagen dressings: CellerateRX Gel Fibracol Plus Collagen	Collagen is the most abundant protein in the body; its fibers are found in connective tissues, skin, bone, ligaments, and cartilage.	To stimulate new tissue development.
Promogran matrix: Prisma Ag	Oxidized regenerated cellulose and collagen. Binds metalloproteases, which protect growth factors.	For diabetic foot ulcers, venous leg ulcers, and surgical wounds.
Composite dressings: Alldress Covaderm	Combine two or more distinct products into a single dressing.	May absorb and also cover a wound, for example.
Contact layers: Mepitel Conformant Wound Veil Profore	Nonadherent dressing layers often used with other products.	To allow exudate to flow through to a secondary dressing; protects wound.
Foam dressings: Allevyn Mepilex Foam Lyofoam Biatain Adhesive Dressing PolyMem	Absorbent; some have a film coating and adhesive border.	To provide a moist environment and thermal insulation.
Honey: Medihoney (various forms) TheraHoney	Medical grade honey used in a variety of dressing types.	For colonized wounds; have antimicrobial and anti-inflammatory properties.

Table 53.3

Common Dressings—cont'd

Dressing Type/Examples	Description	When Used
Hydrocolloid dressings: DuoDERM Tegaderm Absorbent Comfeel Plus	Occlusive or semiocclusive dressings made of pectin, gelatin, and carboxymethylcellulose.	Used when a moist environment is needed that allows clean wounds to granulate; provides autolytic debriding.
Hydrogels: DuoDERM Gel SAF-Gel Amerigel AquaSite CarraDres SilvaSorb	Water or glycerine-based amorphous gels, impregnated gauzes, or sheet dressings.	Used when a moist healing environment is needed to promote granulation and epithelialization and facilitate autolytic débridement.
Impregnated gauze: Mesalt Xeroform Xeroflo Adaptic Curity Non-adherent Dermagran Vaseline Petrolatum Gauze Iodoform Packing AMD Gauze	Woven or nonwoven material impregnated by the manufacturer with substances such as iodinated agents, petrolatum, zinc, bismuth tribromophenate, chlorhexidine gluconate, crystalline sodium chloride, or aqueous saline.	Used for a variety of conditions, depending on the agent added to the dressing.
Transparent films: Bioclusive Plus Tegaderm CarraFilm OpSite Mefilm Polyskin II	Adhesive semipermeable polyurethane membrane dressings that are waterproof and impermeable to bacteria and contaminants yet permit water vapor to cross the barrier.	Used when a moist healing environment is needed, promoting formulation of granulation tissue and autolysis of necrotic tissue.
Wound fillers: FlexiGel Strands Iodosorb Gel Iodoflex Pads	Sterile products that absorb exudate and conform to the shape of the wound bed.	Used when wound has exudate and would benefit from débriding.

SUGGESTED ANSWERS TO CRITICAL THINKING

Mr. Evans

1. Teach Mr. Evans to apply the ointment in a thin layer and usually only twice daily (as ordered). He may be sensitive or allergic to the medication. Most likely, he is applying too much, too often.

2. Note the size (usually in centimeters), location, color, distribution, and configuration of lesions. Describe exactly what you see, avoiding judgments about what you think it is. Document any teaching you provided related to how his medication should be applied.

Review Questions

1. When is the best time for the nurse to apply prescribed ointment to a patient with an inflamed skin rash?
   1. In the morning before the patient dresses
   2. When the patient will be resting for at least an hour
   3. After the patient bathes
   4. In the evening before bed

2. Which nursing interventions are essential to achieve maximum benefit for the patient receiving balneotherapy for widespread dermatitis? **Select all that apply.**
   1. Maintain the bath water at the hottest temperature tolerated by the patient.
   2. Keep the patient in the water for 15 to 30 minutes.
   3. Keep the tub room warm.
   4. Dry the skin vigorously following the bath.
   5. Use gentle or emollient soaps.

3. Which term should the nurse use to document a raised, fluid-filled lesion smaller than 1 centimeter?
   1. Macule
   2. Papule
   3. Vesicle
   4. Wheal

4. What equipment is most important to have readily available when a patient is undergoing skin testing for allergies?
   1. Resuscitation equipment
   2. Flashlight
   3. Measuring device
   4. Alcohol and cotton swabs

5. Which nursing intervention is essential to protecting the patient's skin integrity when applying occlusive dressings?
   1. Make sure all skin surfaces are covered.
   2. Remove the dressings for 12 of every 24 hours.
   3. Apply a thick layer of prescribed ointment before applying the dressings.
   4. Apply a gauze dressing next to the skin, underneath the plastic film.

Answer rationales available in your online resources.

ANSWERS 1. 3; 2. 2, 3, 5; 3. 3; 4. 1; 5. 2

Key Points

Find the chapter key points in your online resources available through Davis Edge.

Additional Resources

Use the scratch off code on the inside front cover of your book to access online quizzes that will help you to improve your scores on course exams and prepare for the NCLEX-PN®.

 Study Guide

CHAPTER 54

Nursing Care of Patients With Skin Disorders

Rita Bolek Trofino

KEY TERMS

cellulites (sell-yoo-LYE-tis)
comedo (KOH-meh-doh)
dermatitis (DER-mah-TYE-tis)
dermatomycosis (DER-mah-toh-my-KOH-sis)
eschar (ESS-kar)
lichenified (lye-KEN-i-fyde)
onychomycosis (ON-ih-koh-my-KOH-sis)
pediculosis (peh-DIK-yoo-LOH-si)
pruritus (proo-RY-tus)
psoriasis (suh-RY-ah-sis)
purulent (PURE-you-lent)
pyoderma (PYE-oh-DER-mah)
seborrhea (SEB-uh-REE-ah)

CHAPTER CONCEPT

Tissue Integrity

LEARNING OUTCOMES

1. Explain the pathophysiology of each of the skin disorders listed in this chapter.
2. Describe the etiologies, signs, and symptoms of each of the skin disorders.
3. Describe current therapeutic measures that are used for each of the skin disorders.
4. List data to collect when caring for patients with disorders of the integumentary system.
5. Recognize the role of the nurse in preventing pressure injuries.
6. Plan nursing care for patients with each of the skin disorders.
7. Explain how you will know whether your nursing interventions have been effective.

Skin disorders cover a wide array of diseases and conditions. They can be generalized or localized, acute, chronic, or traumatic. This chapter discusses common skin disorders encountered by nurses.

PRESSURE INJURIES

Pathophysiology and Etiology

Patients often refer to pressure injuries with old terms such as *bedsores, decubitus ulcers,* or *pressure ulcers.* Essentially, a pressure injury is a lesion caused by prolonged pressure against the skin. This can result from spending long periods in one position, causing the weight of the body to compress the capillaries against, for example, a bed or chair, especially over bony prominences. Pressure injuries are the result of tissue anoxia and begin to develop within 20 to 40 minutes of unrelieved pressure on the skin. Other causes include pressure from a tight splint or cast, traction, or other device.

Those at risk are patients who are immobile, have decreased circulation, or have impaired sensory perception or neurologic function.

Mechanical forces (e.g., pressure, friction, and shear) lead to the formation of pressure injuries. The pressure level that closes capillaries in healthy people is 25 to 32 mm Hg. When pressure applied to the skin is greater than the pressure in the capillary bed, the blood supply to the tissues is decreased, which impairs cellular metabolism. This eventually causes tissue ischemia. This reduction in blood flow causes the skin to *blanch,* or lose color. The longer the pressure lasts, the greater the risk of skin breakdown and the development of a pressure injury.

Friction is created when the skin surface rubs over a stationary surface. *Shearing* occurs when the patient slides down in bed when the head of the bed is raised or when being pulled or repositioned without being lifted off the sheets. With shearing, the skin and subcutaneous tissue remain stationary, and the fat, muscle, and bone shift in the direction of body movement. As a result, damage occurs deep within the tissues.

Any patient experiencing prolonged pressure is at risk for a pressure injury. Older adult patients have increased risk because of normal aging changes of the skin. Thin patients are at greatest risk because they have little padding when pressure is present. Obesity also is a contributing factor because adipose tissue is poorly vascularized and is therefore more likely to develop ischemic changes. Impaired peripheral circulation also makes the skin more susceptible to ischemic damage. See Chapter 24 for more information on problems caused by poor circulation.

NURSING CARE TIP

Be sure to document with photographs all pressure injuries present on admission to the hospital. Pressure injuries are classified as serious reportable events because they can be prevented. Therefore, hospitals will not be paid by Medicare for care of stage 3, stage 4, or unstageable pressure injuries acquired during hospitalization.

Prevention

USE A VALIDATED ASSESSMENT TOOL. Use an assessment tool such as the Braden Scale for Predicting Pressure Sore Risk to assess patients for physical condition, mental status, activity, mobility, and incontinence to determine the risk for pressure injuries. Advanced age, low diastolic blood pressure, elevated body temperature, and inadequate intake of protein are all risk factors associated with the development of pressure injuries. Table 54.1 shows for the Braden instrument.

BE SAFE!

BE VIGILANT! Find out which patients and residents are most likely to have pressure injuries. Take action to prevent pressure injuries in these patients and residents. From time to time, re-check patients and residents (The Joint Commission's 2018 National Patient Safety Goals © The Joint Commission, 2018. Reprinted with permission).

CLEANSE THE SKIN. Gently cleanse the skin daily with tepid water and mild soap to prevent drying. To reduce friction, pat the skin dry rather than rubbing it dry. After bathing, prevent dryness with daily lubrication of the skin with moisturizers. Thoroughly dry skin-to-skin surfaces, such as under the breasts, skinfolds (especially in the groin and abdominal folds), and between the toes, to prevent prolonged exposure to moisture.

PREVENT DAMAGE FROM INCONTINENCE. If the patient is incontinent, clean the skin promptly with tepid water and mild soap, pat dry, and apply a moisture barrier to prevent breakdown.

AVOID MASSAGING BONY PROMINENCES. Avoid massaging bony prominences or reddened skin areas. Blood vessels are damaged by massage when ischemia is present or when they lie over a bone.

MAINTAIN MOBILITY. Maintain the highest possible level of mobility, as follows:

- Teach patients to shift their weight every 15 minutes if possible when lying or sitting.
- Provide frequent active or passive range-of-motion exercises as well as turning according to a written

---

Table 54.1

Braden Scale for Predicting Pressure Sore Risk

Patient's Name:
Evaluator's Name:
Date of Assessment:

SENSORY PERCEPTION ability to respond meaningfully to pressure-related discomfort	1. Completely Limited Unresponsive (does not moan, flinch, or grasp) to painful stimuli, due to diminished level of consciousness or sedation OR Limited ability to feel pain over most of body	2. Very Limited Responds only to painful stimuli. Cannot communicate discomfort except by moaning or restlessness OR Has a sensory impairment which limits the ability to feel pain or discomfort over 1/2 of body	3. Slightly Limited Responds to verbal commands, but cannot always communicate discomfort or the need to be turned OR Has some sensory impairment which limits ability to feel pain or discomfort in 1 or 2 extremities	4. No Impairment Responds to verbal commands. Has no sensory deficit which would limit ability to feel or voice pain or discomfort.

Table 54.1

Braden Scale for Predicting Pressure Sore Risk—cont'd

MOISTURE degree to which skin is exposed to moisture	1. **Constantly Moist** Skin is kept moist almost constantly by perspiration, urine, etc. Dampness is detected every time patient is moved or turned.	2. **Very Moist** Skin is often, but not always moist. Linen must be changed at least once a shift.	3. **Occasionally Moist** Skin is occasionally moist, requiring an extra linen change approximately once a day.	4. **Rarely Moist** Skin is usually dry, linen only requires changing at routine intervals.
ACTIVITY degree of physical activity	1. **Bedfast** Confined to bed	2. **Chairfast** Ability to walk severely limited or nonexistent. Cannot bear own weight and/or must be assisted into chair or wheelchair.	3. **Walks Occasionally** Walks occasionally during day, but for very short distances, with or without assistance. Spends majority of each shift in bed or chair.	4. **Walks Frequently** Walks outside room at least twice a day and inside room at least once every two hours during waking hours
MOBILITY ability to change and control body position	1. **Completely Immobile** Does not make even slight changes in body or extremity position without assistance	2. **Very Limited** Makes occasional slight changes in body or extremity position but unable to make frequent or significant changes independently	3. **Slightly Limited** Makes frequent though slight changes in body or extremity position independently	4. **No Limitation** Makes major and frequent changes in position without assistance
NUTRITION usual food intake pattern	1. **Very Poor** Never eats a complete meal. Rarely eats more than 1/3 of any food offered. Eats 2 servings or less of protein (meat or dairy products) per day. Takes fluids poorly. Does not take a liquid dietary supplement OR Is NPO and/or maintained on clear liquids or IVs for more than 5 days	2. **Probably Inadequate** Rarely eats a complete meal and generally eats only about 1/2 of any food offered. Protein intake includes only 3 servings of meat or dairy products per day. Occasionally will take a dietary supplement. OR Receives less than optimum amount of liquid diet or tube feeding	3. **Adequate** Eats over half of most meals. Eats a total of 4 servings of protein (meat, dairy products) per day. Occasionally will refuse a meal, but will usually take a supplement when offered. OR Is on a tube feeding or TPN regimen which probably meets most of nutritional needs	4. **Excellent** Eats most of every meal. Never refuses a meal. Usually eats a total of 4 or more servings of meat and dairy products. Occasionally eats between meals. Does not require supplementation.

Continued

Table 54.1

Braden Scale for Predicting Pressure Sore Risk—cont'd

FRICTION AND SHEAR	1. Problem	2. Potential Problem	3. No Apparent Problem
	Requires moderate to maximum assistance in moving. Complete lifting without sliding against sheets is impossible. Frequently slides down in bed or chair, requiring frequent repositioning with maximum assistance. Spasticity, contractures, or agitation leads to almost constant friction.	Moves feebly or requires minimum assistance. During a move skin probably slides to some extent against sheets, chair, restraints, or other devices. Maintains relatively good position in chair or bed most of the time but occasionally slides down.	Moves in bed and in chair independently and has sufficient muscle strength to lift up completely during move. Maintains good position in bed or chair.

© Copyright Barbara Braden and Nancy Bergstrom, 1988. Reprinted with permission.
Note. IV = intravenous; NPO = nothing by mouth; TPN = total parenteral nutrition.

Total Score

INTERVENTIONS FOR SPECIFIC RISK LEVEL
AT RISK (15–18)*
FREQUENT TURNING
MAXIMAL REMOBILIZATION
PROTECT HEELS
MANAGE MOISTURE, NUTRITION, AND
FRICTION AND SHEAR
PRESSURE-REDUCTION SUPPORT SURFACE IF
BED- OR CHAIRBOUND
*If other major risk factors are present (advanced age,
fever, poor dietary intake of protein, diastolic pressure
below 60 mm Hg, hemodynamic instability) advance
to next level of risk.

MODERATE RISK (13–14)*
TURNING SCHEDULE
USE FOAM WEDGES FOR 30° LATERAL
POSITIONING
PRESSURE-REDUCTION SUPPORT SURFACE
MAXIMAL REMOBILIZATION
PROTECT HEELS
MANAGE MOISTURE, NUTRITION,
AND FRICTION AND SHEAR
*If other major risk factors present, advance to next
level of risk.

SPECIFIC CONDITION MANAGEMENT
MANAGE MOISTURE
USE COMMERCIAL MOISTURE BARRIER
USE ABSORBANT PADS OR DIAPERS
THAT WICK & HOLD MOISTURE
ADDRESS CAUSE IF POSSIBLE
OFFER BEDPAN/URINAL AND GLASS OF WATER
IN CONJUNCTION WITH TURNING
SCHEDULES

MANAGE NUTRITION
INCREASE PROTEIN INTAKE
INCREASE CALORIE INTAKE TO SPARE
PROTEINS
SUPPLEMENT WITH MULTIVITAMIN
(SHOULD HAVE VITAMINS A, C, & E)
ACT QUICKLY TO ALLEVIATE DEFICITS
CONSULT DIETITIAN

Table 54.1

Braden Scale for Predicting Pressure Sore Risk—cont'd

HIGH RISK (10–12) INCREASE FREQUENCY OF TURNING SUPPLEMENT WITH SMALL SHIFTS PRESSURE REDUCTION SUPPORT SURFACE USE FOAM WEDGES FOR 30° LATERAL POSITIONING MAXIMAL REMOBILIZATION PROTECT HEELS MANAGE MOISTURE, NUTRITION, AND FRICTION AND SHEAR	**MANAGE FRICTION AND SHEAR** ELEVATE HOB NO MORE THAN 30° USE TRAPEZE WHEN INDICATED USE LIFT SHEET TO MOVE PATIENT PROTECT ELBOWS & HEELS IF BEING EXPOSED TO FRICTION
VERY HIGH RISK (9 or below)* ALL OF THE ABOVE USE PRESSURE-RELIEVING SURFACE IF PATIENT HAS INTRACTABLE PAIN OR SEVERE PAIN EXACERBATED BY TURNING OR ADDITIONAL RISK FACTORS *Low-air-loss beds do not substitute for turning schedules.	**OTHER GENERAL CARE ISSUES** NO MASSAGE OF REDDENED BONY PROMINENCES NO DONUT TYPE DEVICES MAINTAIN GOOD HYDRATION AVOID DRYING THE SKIN

© Barbara Braden, 2001.

repositioning schedule. If patients are on bedrest, turn and reposition them at least every 2 hours but preferably more often because ischemia development begins after 20 to 40 minutes of pressure.

- When positioning patients on their side, place them at a 30-degree angle or less and not directly on the trochanter because this area is especially sensitive to pressure and can quickly break down. If patients are placed on the trochanter, they usually become restless and squirm around to get off the trochanter.
- If the patient is seated in a chair, repositioning every hour is important. A mobility program specific to the patient must be developed.

REDUCE PRESSURE, FRICTION, AND SHEAR DAMAGE. Avoid elevating the head of the bed more than 30 degrees to reduce pressure on the coccyx as well as friction and shear damage from sliding down in the bed. Use a sheet to lift and move patients. Provide a bed trapeze to help patients to move themselves.

ELEVATE HEELS AND AVOID PRESSURE ON CALVES. Elevate the patient's heels off the bed with pillows placed lengthwise under the calf or with heel elevators. Take care so pressure is not applied on the calves from the pillows.

PROTECT BONY PROMINENCES FROM PRESSURE. Be sure also to protect the patient's elbows, sacrum, scapulae, ears, and occipital area from pressure.

PREVENT ISCHEMIA. Avoid the use of donut-shaped cushions. They create a circle of pressure that cuts off the circulation to

the surrounding tissue, promoting ischemia rather than preventing it.

PROTECT SKIN CONTACT SURFACES. Pad skin contact surfaces, especially bony prominences, so they do not press against each other. (For example, place a small pillow between the knees when the patient is in a side-lying position.)

USE PRESSURE-REDUCING MATTRESSES AND CUSHIONS. Provide an appropriate pressure-relieving or pressure-reducing mattress and chair cushion for immobile patients.

PREVENT MALNUTRITION AND DEHYDRATION. Prevent malnutrition and dehydration by ensuring an adequate intake of protein, calories, and fluid. Provide 2,500 mL of fluid each day if not contraindicated by other medical problems.

"Gerontological Issues" summarizes additional preventive measures. See also "Evidence-Based Practice."

Gerontological Issues

Interventions to Prevent Skin Breakdown

- Avoid use of soap and water on dry skin areas. Use a moisture barrier cream or ointment on dry skin before bathing to protect the skin from the drying effects of water.
- Regularly wash and dry between toes.
- Toilet patient often, and institute a bowel program to prevent incontinence.
- Use perineal cleansing products to cleanse urine and feces residue from the perineum and anal area. These

products are specially designed to break down and facilitate the complete removal of urine and feces without irritating the skin.

• Use moisturizing creams that have no alcohol or perfume, which can irritate the skin.
• Avoid pressure, especially over bony areas, by assisting the older adult to change positions on a regular schedule.
• Remind the patient to change position or shift weight frequently while sitting in a chair to avoid prolonged pressure.
• Examine skin for areas of redness. If redness occurs, the positioning schedule should be more frequent.
• Keep fingernails short to avoid scratching.
• Use pillows and pads to help maintain alignment with position changes. Use specialized mattresses and chair cushions designed to decrease pressure. Keep the patient's heels off the bed with pillows under the calves for support and to prevent pressure.
• Encourage the older adult to be out of bed and active throughout the day. Remember to assess skin and reposition frequently even when out of bed because areas of pressure occur whether the patient is in or out of bed.
• Provide a high-protein, vitamin-rich diet if not contraindicated.
• Assess for dehydration and encourage fluids if not contraindicated.
• Make sure bed linens are kept dry and unwrinkled.

Evidence-Based Practice

Clinical Question
What are best practices for skin care in patients in acute and long-term care settings?

Evidence
Researchers reviewed 41 systematic reviews, intervention studies, guidelines, and best practice standards to determine the most effective, research-based methods for basic skin care (Lichterfeld-Kottner et al., 2015).

Implications for Nursing Practice
General findings include the importance of (1) assessing risk factors, (2) avoiding frequent bathing of patients with dry skin, (3) using oil-soluble moisturizers for dry skin, (4) protecting skin against exposure to urine or stool, and (5) cleaning moist areas (e.g., between toes, between skinfolds, under breasts) daily with gentle synthetic detergent (syndet) soaps that have a pH of 4 to 5. See Lichterfeld-Kottner et al. (2015) for a research-based algorithm for basic skin care.

Reference
Lichterfeld-Kottner, A., Hauss, A., Surber, C., Peters, T., Blume-Peytavi, U., & Kottner, J. (2015). Evidence-based skin care: A systematic literature review and the development of a basic skin care algorithm. *Journal of Wound, Ostomy, and Continence Nursing, 42*(5), 501–524.

Signs and Symptoms

A developing pressure injury usually begins with a reddened area, often over a bony prominence, that does not blanch with pressure. You have learned to check for capillary refill by pressing on a fingertip and watching it turn white, then red again. If redness returns within 3 seconds, then capillary refill is considered to be adequate. A pressure injury stays red and does not blanch. If pressure is not relieved and healing does not occur, it can progress to an open, ulcerated area. Stages of pressure injuries are discussed in the section on data collection.

The most common sites for pressure injuries are the sacrum, heels, elbows, lateral malleoli, greater trochanters, ischial tuberosities, base of the skull, scapulae, and ears. Most patients experience pain at the injury site. A report of pain requires continual monitoring, documentation, and treatment.

A wound may contain a mixture of black, yellow, and red colors. Necrotic wounds are the worst because they contain dead tissue. Beefy red wounds are desired because they are healing wounds. It is important to consider treating the worst color present first, or healing will be delayed. For example, if a wound is both yellow and black, the dead tissue must be removed first before the infection can be effectively treated. This color system is a helpful system for patients and families to use to describe wounds to the home health care nurse because colors are easily recognized and understood by most people.

LEARNING TIP
Pressure injuries may be described according to a three-color system:

• *Black* wounds indicate tissue necrosis.
• *Yellow* wounds have slough, which is a layer of dead tissue. It is usually yellow, creamy, or tan in color. It may have exudate and may be infected.
• *Red* wounds are pink or red. These are in the healing stage.

These are guidelines. A full assessment is necessary to determine actual cause of color changes.

Complications

Wound infection is a common complication. New pressure injuries can also appear, and the present injury can progress to a deeper wound. Some wounds take a prolonged time to heal or may never heal.

Diagnostic Tests

All open pressure injuries are considered to be colonized with bacteria. This means that bacteria are present, but the wound is not necessarily infected. In most cases, adequate cleansing and débridement can prevent bacterial colonization from advancing to clinical infection. Culture and sensitivity tests may be done to identify the causative organism in suspected infection sites. (See Chapter 53 for instructions for obtaining a culture.) Results need to be interpreted to distinguish between true wound infection and bacterial colonization. If the wound is healing by secondary intention, it becomes colonized by bacterial flora from the skin and from the environment. If, however, the wound is extensive, bacterial growth may exceed the defenses of the local tissue, and a true wound infection will result.

If the wound does not show signs of healing or if an ischemic wound is suspected, noninvasive (e.g., Doppler studies) or invasive (e.g., arteriogram) arterial blood supply studies are recommended. Biopsies may be performed for large, extensive unhealing wounds to be sure a cancer is not a complicating factor.

Therapeutic Measures

Treatment varies according to the size, depth, and stage of the pressure injury; the special needs of the patient; and health care provider (HCP) preference. All pressure must be removed from the affected area for healing to occur. Cleanliness must be maintained. Basic treatment includes débridement, cleansing, and dressing of the wound to provide a moist and healing environment.

Débridement

Débridement is the removal of dead or nonviable tissue from a wound to help clean the wound and facilitate formation of granulation tissue. It may be done with or without surgery. Nonsurgical débridement includes mechanical, enzymatic, and autolytic methods. Surgical débridement is used only if the patient has sepsis or cellulitis or to remove extensive eschar. **Eschar** is a black or brown hard scab or dry crust, or thick, black, leatherlike tissue that forms from necrotic tissue. It may hide the true depth of the wound and must be removed for the wound to heal.

MECHANICAL DÉBRIDEMENT. Scissors and forceps can be used for mechanical débridement to selectively remove nonviable tissue. Dextranomer beads, another method of mechanical débridement, can be sprinkled over the wound to absorb exudate and all other products of tissue breakdown as well as surface bacteria. Whirlpool baths and wet-to-dry saline gauze dressings may also be used for mechanical débridement. For wet-to-dry dressings, the wet gauze is placed directly on the wound (avoiding surrounding healthy tissue) and allowed to dry completely. The drying process causes the gauze to adhere to the wound; when it is pulled off, tissue is pulled off with it. This results in nonselective débridement because viable tissue may also be removed in this process. These methods are painful, so the patient should be premedicated for pain and assessed often.

ENZYMATIC DÉBRIDEMENT. Enzymatic débridement involves application of a topical enzyme débriding agent. These agents vary as to application methods, so careful reading of instructions is necessary. Most débriding agents are proteolytic enzymes that selectively digest necrotic tissue. Be careful to apply them only to the wound and to avoid contact with healthy tissue.

AUTOLYTIC DÉBRIDEMENT. Autolytic débridement is the use of a synthetic dressing or moisture-retentive dressing over the injury. The eschar then self-digests via the action of the enzymes that are present in the fluid environment of the wound. This method is not used for infected wounds, because the infection would worsen.

SURGICAL DÉBRIDEMENT. Surgical débridement involves the removal of devitalized tissue, slough, or thick, adherent eschar with a scalpel, scissors, or other sharp instrument. *Slough* is loose, yellow to tan stringy necrotic tissue. Slough, like eschar, can be tightly adhered to the wound bed.

Depending on the amount of débridement to be done, surgical débridement may be performed in the operating room, a treatment room, or the patient's room. Following surgical débridement, grafting may be required to close the wound. This becomes necessary if it is a full-thickness injury, if there is loss of joint function, or for cosmetic purposes. For procedures performed without anesthesia, be sure to premedicate the patient for pain. Continually monitor for pain during the procedure, especially if there is a donor site for grafting.

Wound Cleansing

A pressure injury should be thoroughly cleansed using a whirlpool, a handheld showerhead, or an irrigating system with a pressure between 4 and 15 pounds per square inch (psi). A 30-mL syringe with an 18-gauge needle works well for this purpose. Pressure less than 4 psi does not adequately cleanse the wound, and pressure greater than 15 psi may damage tissue. If an irrigating system is used, 250 mL of normal saline solution (or sometimes tap water for home care) should be used to thoroughly cleanse the wound. If the wound is red, gentle irrigation with a needleless 30- to 60-mL syringe should be used to prevent trauma and bleeding. However, if the wound has been diagnosed as being infected, flushing with a 30- to 60-mL syringe and an 18-gauge needle provides the pressure needed to help remove bacteria.

> **LEARNING TIP**
> Dilution is the solution to wound pollution!

Once the wound has been cleansed and débrided, apply a dressing. Wounds heal more rapidly in a moist environment, with minimal bacterial colonization and a healing temperature. This takes 12 hours to occur after the wound is covered with an occlusive dressing. If a dressing is frequently removed, the wound may not reach its healing temperature, and healing may be impaired. When possible, the dressing should be left in place for extended periods. Draining wounds may require frequent dressing changes.

> **LEARNING TIP**
> The epidermis "skates" on moisture, so wounds must be kept moist to heal.

• WORD • BUILDING •
eschar: eschara—scab

Wound Dressings

Dressings vary according to size, location, depth, stage of injury, and preference of the ordering practitioner. Commonly used dressing materials include hydrogel dressings, polyurethane films, hydrocolloid wafers, biological dressings, alginates, and cotton gauze. See Chapter 53 for more information on dressing types. The use of an appropriate dressing promotes an optimum healing environment. Hypoallergenic tape should be used to secure dressings if tape is necessary. Protective paste may be applied to protect unaffected tissue from topical agents. In all cases, pressure should be kept off the wound. No treatment will be effective if pressure continues to damage the tissue.

Negative Pressure Wound Therapy

Negative pressure wound therapy (NPWT) may be effective for healing large open pressure injuries (Fig. 54.1). In NPWT, a wound is packed loosely with a sterile sponge and then covered with an occlusive dressing. A vacuum source is placed in the wound, and gentle negative pressure is applied. The negative pressure allows excess drainage and infectious material to be removed, which reduces pressure on delicate new tissue. With small vessels decompressed, circulation is increased, and healing is accelerated. NPWT also maintains a moist environment for optimal healing. Evidence strongly supports NPWT for nonischemic diabetic foot pressure injuries. It is also effective for other deep wounds (Vig et al., 2011). Risks of NPWT include bleeding in patients at risk, such as those on anticoagulant therapy.

Other Therapies

Much research is ongoing in the field of wound healing. Some success has been shown with the following therapies: biological or biological skin equivalent dressings, collagen application, platelet-rich plasma application, platelet-derived growth factor application, silver-based products, hyperbaric oxygen therapy, and ozone-oxygen treatments.

Nursing Process for the Patient With a Pressure Injury

Data Collection

Collaborate with the registered nurse to evaluate the status of the pressure injury often as well as underlying causes and barriers to healing. Monitor for risk factors for impaired healing, such as prolonged immobility, incontinence, and inadequate nutrition and hydration. Also monitor intact skin to prevent development of new pressure injuries.

Use transparent film or a disposable ruler to measure the diameter of the injury in centimeters. Imagine a clock superimposed over the wound, with 12 o'clock at the head and 6 o'clock at the feet. Measure in centimeters from 12 to 6 o'clock and from 9 to 3 o'clock. Depth can be measured with a cotton-tipped applicator. Also, gently probe a cotton-tipped applicator under the skin edges to detect tunneling and measure lateral tissue destruction.

Several staging systems are available for pressure injuries based on the depth of tissue destroyed. Most staging systems categorize wounds from stage 1 to stage 4. Additional categories may include deep tissue injury and an unstageable

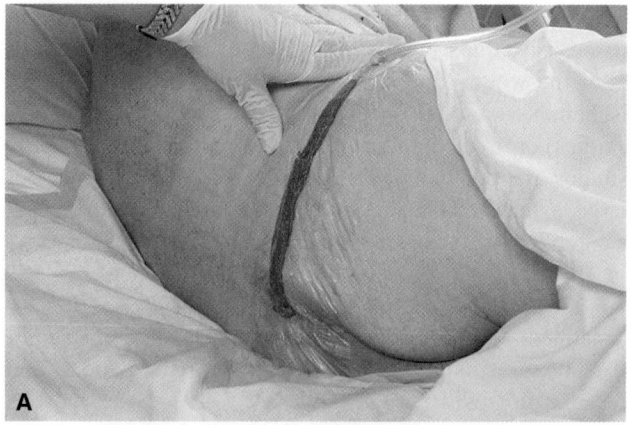

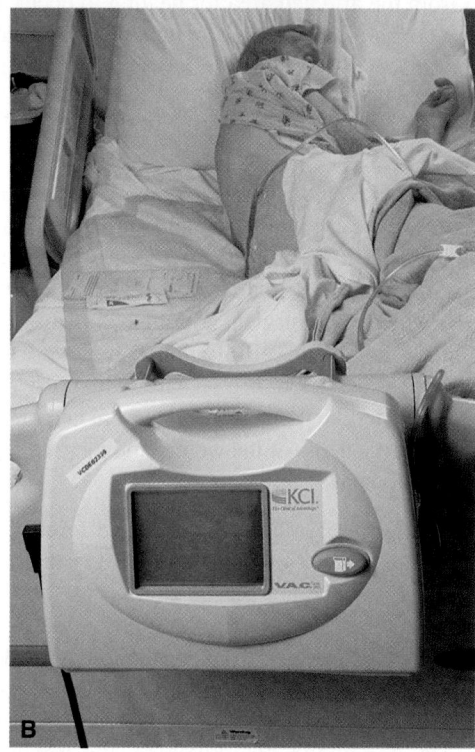

FIGURE 54.1 Negative pressure wound therapy. (A) Occlusive dressing is applied to wound with tubing to vacuum source. (B) Vacuum source exerts gentle negative pressure.

injury (Table 54.2). An unstageable pressure injury typically must be débrided in order to allow healing. One exception to débridement is stable, dry, intact eschar on the heels or ischemic limb (National Pressure Ulcer Advisory Panel, 2016). Eschar serves as the body's natural (biological) cover and should not be removed.

Observe wound exudate. Two common types of wound exudate are serosanguineous and purulent. *Serosanguineous* exudate is fluid consisting of serum and blood. It is blood-tinged, amber-colored fluid. **Purulent** fluid contains pus. It can vary in color and have different odors, depending on which bacteria are present. Creamy yellow pus may indicate

• WORD • BUILDING •

purulent: purulentus—pus

Table 54.2
Pressure Injury Stages

Stage 1: The skin is still intact, but the area is red and does not blanch when pressed. There may also be warmth, hardness, and discoloration of the skin.

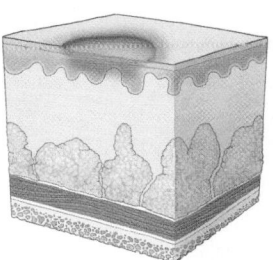
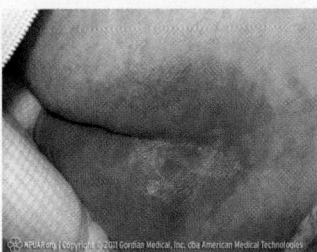

Stage 2: Partial-thickness skin loss with exposed dermis. The wound bed is pink or red and moist; it may appear as an intact or ruptured blister. Skin loss may result from shearing.

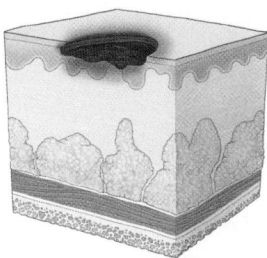
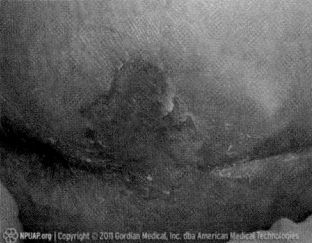

Stage 3: Full-thickness skin loss with visible fat showing. Granulation, slough, and/or eschar may be seen. Undermining and tunneling may occur.

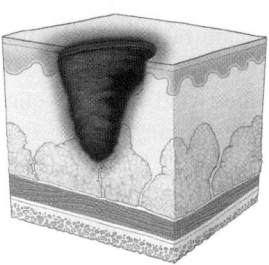
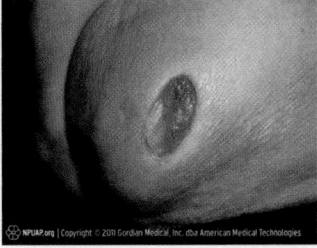

Stage 4: Full-thickness skin loss with exposed muscle, bone, and/or tendons. Slough or eschar may be present.

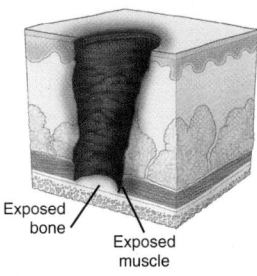

Exposed
bone
Exposed
muscle

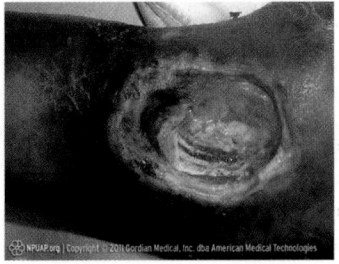

Continued

Table 54.2

Pressure Injury Stages—cont'd

Unstageable: Full-thickness skin and tissue loss is hidden by slough or eschar so that the depth cannot be evaluated. A Stage 3 or Stage 4 pressure injury may be revealed once the wound bed is débrided.

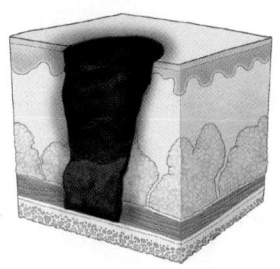
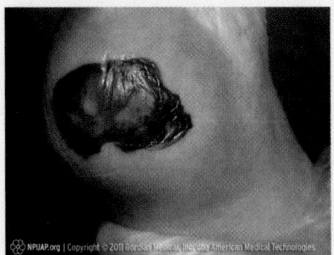

Deep Tissue Injury: Intact or nonintact skin area with persistent, nonblanchable, dark red-maroon-purple discoloration or epidermal separation revealing a dark wound bed or blood-filled blister.

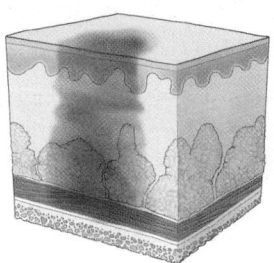
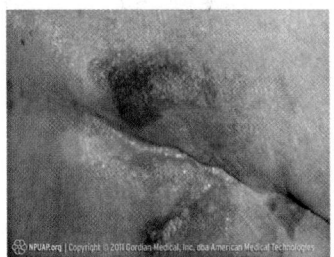

Staphylococcus. Beige pus that has a fishy odor may suggest *Proteus.* Green-blue pus with a fruity odor may indicate *Pseudomonas.* Brown pus with a fecal odor may suggest *Bacteroides.* The wound must be cultured to accurately identify bacteria.

Gently palpate the wound with a gloved hand to determine the texture of granulations. Granulation tissue has a budding appearance from the development of tiny new capillaries. If the granulations are healthy, they have a slightly spongy texture.

Document all findings carefully in the medical record, so all health care team members can monitor progress of healing. Many institutions have specific forms for drawing pictures of the locations and sizes of wounds and for photographs to monitor the healing process. Follow policy at the institution where you work.

Nursing Diagnoses, Planning, Implementation, and Evaluation

See "Nursing Care Plan for the Patient With a Pressure Injury."

Nursing Care Plan for the Patient With a Pressure Injury

Nursing Diagnosis: *Impaired Skin Integrity* related to pressure on skin surface, reduced circulation, or immobility
Expected Outcomes: The patient's skin integrity will be improved as evidenced by a decrease in wound size and depth, and no development of additional pressure injuries.
Evaluation of Outcomes: Is there a decrease in wound size? Are there any new pressure injuries?

Intervention	Rationale	Evaluation
Monitor status of pressure injury according to stage, color, exudate, texture, size, and depth.	*Assessment provides data on which care is based.*	What stage is pressure injury? Is it improving or worsening?
Determine and remove cause of pressure (e.g., immobility, friction, shearing).	*This allows for correction and prevents further trauma.*	What is the cause of the pressure injury? Is cause removed?

Nursing Care Plan for the Patient With a Pressure Injury—cont'd

Intervention	Rationale	Evaluation
Cleanse wound gently with warm water; rinse; pat dry gently with gauze. Do not rub the area.	*Reduces number of bacteria. Drying prevents maceration of skin. Gentle handling prevents further trauma.*	Is wound clean and dry?
Débride or assist with débridement of wound as prescribed.	*Débridement removes drainage and wound debris, and permits granulation of tissue.*	Does wound look clean and free of debris?
Apply topical agents and/or dress wound as prescribed. Make sure dressing stays intact with movement and edges do not roll, causing more pressure.	*Protects underlying wound and helps promote healing.*	Is dressing applied appropriately?
Position patient off the pressure injury.	*Prevents further pressure and trauma on the injured area.*	Is patient positioned off the pressure injury?
If the pressure injury is on the leg, provide for frequent rest periods with leg elevated; if immobile, reposition every 2 hours.	*Prevents further tissue breakdown.*	Is leg elevated? Is patient repositioned every 2 hours?

Nursing Diagnosis: *Risk for Infection* related to open wound
Expected Outcomes: The patient will not experience wound infection or systemic sepsis as evidenced by clean wound bed and by temperature and white blood cell count within normal limits.
Evaluation of Outcomes: Is the patient free from signs and symptoms of local and systemic infection?

Intervention	Rationale	Evaluation
Examine wound at every dressing change. Check for areas of tenderness, swelling, redness, heat, and drainage. Report changes.	*Allows for early recognition of infection and response to treatment.*	Are signs of infection present? Are they reported promptly?
Monitor temperature at least every 12 hours.	*Elevated body temperature is one sign of infection.*	Is patient afebrile?
Provide meticulous wound care (see *Impaired Skin Integrity*).	*Helps decrease the level of contamination and prevent infection.*	Is wound showing signs of healing without purulent drainage?
Use thorough hand hygiene technique. Use sterile technique for dressing changes.	*Prevents cross-contamination.*	Does nurse take proper precautions?

Nursing Diagnosis: *Acute Pain* related to injury and treatments as evidenced by pain rating on 0-to-10 scale
Expected Outcomes: The patient will be as comfortable and as pain free as possible as evidenced by statement of decreased pain and ability to sleep at night.
Evaluation of Outcomes: Does the patient express comfort? Does the patient express a decrease in pain? Is the patient able to sleep?

Intervention	Rationale	Evaluation
Assess level of pain using a pain scale and by observing facial expressions and positioning of body.	*Monitors level of pain and response to therapy.*	At what level is pain? Is it better or worse with treatment?

(nursing care plan continues on page 1170)

Nursing Care Plan for the Patient With a Pressure Injury—cont'd

Intervention	Rationale	Evaluation
Offer analgesics as prescribed. Request order for topical analgesics as needed with dressing changes and cleaning of the wound.	*Analgesics help relieve pain.*	Are analgesics effective?
Decrease anxiety with relaxation techniques (e.g., distraction, music).	*Relaxation can lessen pain intensity.*	Is patient less anxious? Does patient verbalize less pain?
Maintain a comfortable environment (e.g., provide for privacy, position in good alignment and comfortably, maintain a comfortable room temperature).	*Relaxes patient and lessens intensity of discomfort.*	Does patient express an increase in comfort?

NURSING CARE TIP

Many institutions now have nurses who have been specially trained in wound care. Consult one of these nurses for expert wound assessment and treatment recommendations.

CRITICAL THINKING

Mr. Russ is an 84-year-old man who was admitted from home to the medical-surgical unit after a fall that fractured his femur. He has a history of type 2 diabetes. He had an open reduction and internal fixation of his femur and is now in a brace. He is 6 feet tall and weighs 160 pounds. His appetite is poor; his wife states he has lost 15 lb in the past 3 months. He is occasionally incontinent of urine.

1. How can you be vigilant in identifying risks and preventing skin breakdown in Mr. Russ?
2. What other members of the health care team might you collaborate with when planning care for Mr. Russ?

Suggested answers are at the end of the chapter.

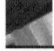 INFLAMMATORY SKIN DISORDERS

Dermatitis
Pathophysiology and Etiology
Dermatitis is inflammation of the skin. It is characterized by itching, redness, and skin lesions, with varying borders and distribution patterns. There are three common types of dermatitis: contact dermatitis, atopic dermatitis, and seborrheic dermatitis. Contact dermatitis is caused by exposure to an allergen or irritant such as soap, perfume, or poison ivy. Atopic dermatitis tends to be hereditary and is associated with allergies, asthma, and hay fever. Seborrheic dermatitis

occurs most often on the scalp, usually in individuals with oily skin. All types tend to be chronic and respond well to treatment but are prone to recur. Table 54.3 lists common types of dermatitis.

Prevention
The patient should prevent irritation to the skin by avoiding irritants, allergens, and excessive heat and dryness and by controlling perspiration. Baths should be short, in tepid water. Deodorant soaps should be avoided; mild superfatted soaps are recommended instead. Dry skin can be lubricated with creams, oils, or ointments as appropriate. Itching and scratching should be prevented as much as possible.

Signs and Symptoms
Itching and rashes or lesions are the main clinical manifestations of dermatitis. The lesions vary depending on the type and location of dermatitis. Rashes and lesions may present as dry and flaky scales, yellow crusts, redness, fissures, macules, papules, and vesicles. (These are described in Chapter 53.) Scratching can make any of these lesions worse.

NURSING CARE TIP

Itching and scratching can occur during sleep, causing the rash to worsen. Have the patient wear cotton gloves at night to prevent scratching.

Complications
The lesion or rash worsens with continued irritation, exposure to offending agents, or scratching. Infections of the skin are common and may be due to the many open areas and

• WORD • BUILDING •
dermatitis: derma—skin + itis—inflammation

Table 54.3
Common Types of Dermatitis

Type	Description
Contact	Acute or chronic condition; caused by contact with irritant or allergen
Irritant contact	Caused by direct contact with an irritating substance, such as soap, detergent, strong medication, astringent, cosmetic, or industrial chemical
Allergic contact	From contact with an allergen, such as perfume, tanning lotion, medication, hair dye, poison ivy, poison oak; contact results in cell-mediated immune response
Atopic	Chronic inherited condition; may be associated with respiratory allergies or asthma; can vary between bright red maculas, papules, oozing, and **lichenified** or hyperpigmented areas
Seborrheic	Chronic, inflammatory disease usually accompanied by scaling, itching, and inflammation; **seborrhea** is excessive production of sebaceous secretions; found in areas with abundant sebaceous glands (e.g., scalp, face, axilla, groin) and where there are folds of skin; can appear as dry, moist, or greasy scales, yellow or pink-yellow crusts, redness, and dry flakiness; can be associated with emotional stress; genetic predisposition may exist

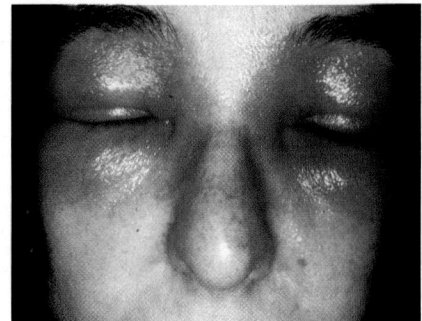

Contact dermatitis caused by nail polish.

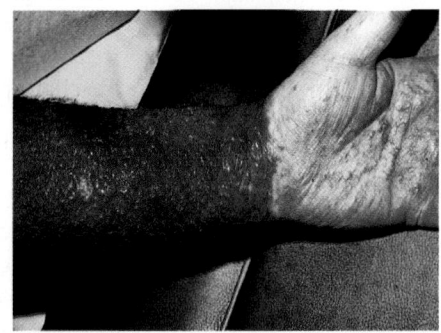

Contact dermatitis caused by topical anesthetic

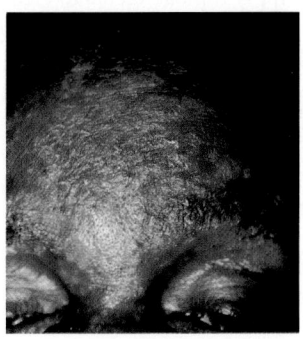

Seborrheic dermatitis.

breaks in the skin. They may also occur due to the patient's reluctance to properly wash the affected area because of pain from the lesions. Some infections can become systemic.

Diagnostic Tests
Diagnosis is usually based on history, symptoms, and clinical findings. If infection is suspected, cultures of the lesions may be ordered to identify the infecting agent.

Therapeutic Measures
Treatment varies according to symptoms. Basic treatment objectives are to control itching, alleviate discomfort and pain, decrease inflammation, control or prevent crust formation and oozing, prevent infection, prevent further damage to the skin, and heal the lesions as much as possible.

Itching, or **pruritus,** and discomfort can be somewhat relieved by antihistamines, analgesics, and antipruritic medications as ordered. Colloidal oatmeal preparations added to baths may also help.

Steroids such as hydrocortisone or methylprednisolone may be used to suppress inflammation. They can be administered as topical, intralesional, or systemic agents. The specific type used depends on the type of lesion, the body area involved, and the extent of the lesion. Topical administration is preferred if possible because systemic steroids can cause serious side effects, including adrenal suppression.

Tub baths and wet dressings help control oozing and prevent further crust formation; they also serve to loosen exudates, scales, and other wound debris, providing a clean area for topical application of medication. Protect the skin by lightly patting dry, avoiding friction, and avoiding hot water. Advise the patient to use a sunscreen agent when outdoors.

Nursing Process for the Patient With Dermatitis
DATA COLLECTION. Use the *WHAT'S UP?* format to assess the rash, as described in Chapter 53. Also refer to Chapter 53, Table 53.1, for specific questions to ask. Observe the rash or

• WORD • BUILDING •
lichenified: leichen—scaly growth + facere—to make
seborrhea: sebum—tallow + rhoia—flow
pruritus: prur—itch + itis—condition

lesions for character, distribution, description, tenderness, signs of scratching, and other associated problems.

NURSING DIAGNOSES, PLANNING, AND IMPLEMENTATION.

Impaired Skin Integrity related to rash, lesions, and scratching

EXPECTED OUTCOME: The patient's skin integrity will improve as evidenced by reduction in lesions and absence of signs or symptoms of infection.

• Monitor skin condition regularly *to determine whether treatment is working.*
• Cleanse the area as ordered by the HCP, taking care not to irritate the skin further, *to keep area clean and prevent infection.*
• Provide cool moist compresses, dressings, or tepid tub baths *to help relieve inflammation and itching, débride lesions, and soften crusts and scales.*
• Pat the skin dry rather than rubbing *to prevent further trauma.*
• Apply topical agents to clean skin as ordered *to help suppress inflammation and itching.*
• Provide skin care at bedtime *to help promote comfortable sleep.* Many antihistamines also have a sedative effect.
• Encourage patient to eat a high-protein diet *to promote healing and replace lost protein.* If lesions are generalized, protein can be lost through oozing of serum. Confirm appropriateness of high-protein diet with HCP.
• Encourage use of gloves or mitts, especially at night, *to help prevent scratching.*
• Advise the patient to keep fingernails short *to prevent scratching.*
• Teach the patient that application of slight pressure with a clean cloth *may help relieve itching.*
• Teach relaxation exercises *to help the patient cope with distressing symptoms.*

Disturbed Body Image related to visible rash or lesions

EXPECTED OUTCOME: The patient will have improved body image as evidenced by a statement of acceptance of the condition and ability to socialize with others.

• Allow patients to verbalize concerns if they wish to do so. Talking about concerns may help the patient to begin *to work through feelings about body image* but should not be forced.
• Refer to a support group, if available, *to receive support from others in similar circumstances.*
• Display an accepting attitude while caring for skin lesions. *The patient will be quick to pick up your reaction to the lesions, especially if it is negative.*
• Encourage the patient to participate in skin care *to allow more control over the situation.*
• Encourage the patient to wear long sleeves or other appropriate covering if the patient desires *to make the lesions less noticeable.*

Deficient Knowledge related to disease and treatment

EXPECTED OUTCOME: The patient will verbalize understanding of the condition and demonstrate ability to perform self-care measures.

• Determine the patient's baseline knowledge of condition and treatment. *Teaching should build on baseline understanding.*
• Instruct the patient in application of topical agents and dressings. *Overuse of medications can further traumatize skin; be sure to follow package or prescription directions.*
• Instruct the patient in how to recognize changes, improvement, or flare-ups of the disorder and what symptoms to report to the HCP. *Because most skin conditions are cared for at home, it is important for the patient to have the skills needed to monitor the condition and carry out treatment appropriately.*
• Advise the patient to avoid overexposure to sun and to use sunscreen agents when outdoors *to prevent skin damage.*
• Encourage use of a humidifier in the home *to help maintain hydration of skin and control itching during dry weather, especially in winter.*
• Teach the patient measures to prevent future flare-ups if possible. *Flare-ups may be avoided if the patient understands what triggers them.*

NURSING CARE TIP

Teach patients that, when applying topical medications, more is not better!

EVALUATION. If medical and nursing care have been effective, the lesions will be controlled or in remission, the patient will state that itching and other discomforts are controlled, the patient will be able to socialize without undue difficulty, and the patient will be able to describe and demonstrate self-care measures.

Psoriasis
Pathophysiology and Etiology

Psoriasis is a chronic inflammatory skin disorder in which the epidermal cells proliferate abnormally fast. Usually, epidermal cells take about 27 days to shed. With psoriasis, the cells shed every 4 to 5 days. The abnormal keratin forms loosely adherent scales with dermal inflammation.

The exact cause is not known; however, it is autoimmune in nature, with T cells attacking healthy skin cells, causing an increase in skin cell, T-cell, and white cell production. Often there is a family history of psoriasis. The average age at onset is 27 years, although it can begin at any age. The condition can be severe if the onset is in childhood.

• WORD • BUILDING •
psoriasis: psor—itch + iasis—inflammation

Psoriasis is characterized by exacerbations and remissions. Many factors influence the suppression and outbreak of lesions, which varies from individual to individual. Sun and humidity may suppress lesions. Aggravating factors include streptococcal pharyngitis, emotional upset, stress, hormonal changes, cold weather, skin trauma, smoking, alcohol, and certain drugs (e.g., antimalarial agents, lithium, beta blockers).

Prevention

Because the exact etiology is not known, measures to prevent exacerbation of symptoms are specific to the patient's circumstances. General preventive measures include avoiding upper respiratory infections, especially streptococcal infections; coping with emotional stress; avoiding skin trauma, including sunburns; and avoiding medications that can precipitate a flare-up.

Signs and Symptoms

Signs and symptoms vary according to the patient and the particular type of psoriasis. Lesions are red papules that join to form plaques with distinct borders (Fig. 54.2). Silvery scales develop on untreated lesions. Areas most often affected are the elbows and knees, scalp, umbilicus, and genitals. Other signs and symptoms include nail involvement, involvement in the gluteal fold (called intergluteal pinking), itching, and dry or brittle hair.

Complications

Because of the nature of the disease with its lesions and itching, secondary infections can occur. Psoriatic arthritis can develop after the psoriasis has developed, with nail changes and

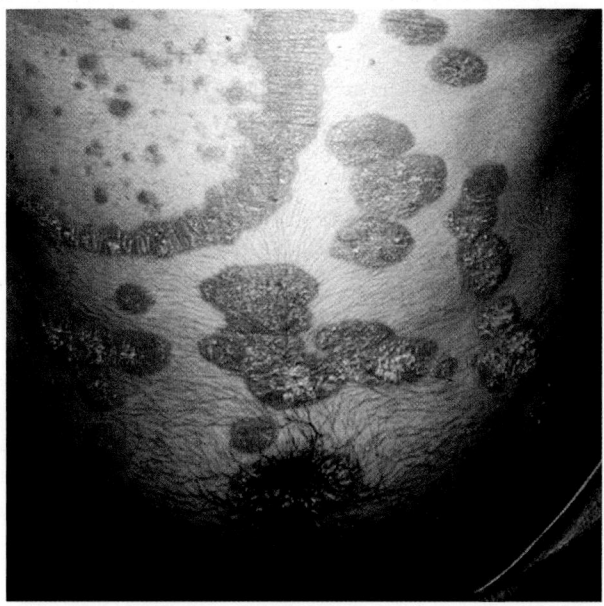

FIGURE 54.2 Psoriasis. Note bright red scaly plaque with silvery scales.

destructive arthritis of large joints, the spine, and interphalangeal joints. If the psoriasis becomes severe and widespread, fever, chills, increased cardiac output, and benign lymphadenopathy can result.

Diagnostic Tests

Testing depends on the severity of the psoriasis. Usually, diagnosis is based on physical assessment alone. Skin biopsy or other diagnostic tests may be performed to rule out concurrent disease or secondary infection.

Therapeutic Measures

Treatment varies according to the type and extent of the disease as well as patient preference. Psoriasis is a chronic disease with remissions and exacerbations. Basic treatment objectives are to decrease the rapid epidermal proliferation, inflammation, and itching and scaling. The patient may be instructed to bathe daily in a tub, using a soft brush to help remove scales.

A variety of topical and systemic agents are used to treat psoriasis. Topical corticosteroids may be used for their anti-inflammatory effect. Occlusive dressings are commonly used to enhance penetration of medications (see Chapter 53). Salicylic acid can help loosen or remove scales. Synthetic vitamin D cream slows the proliferation of skin cells. Fish oil supplements may reduce inflammation in some patients.

Tar preparations may be prescribed along with corticosteroids. The tar acts as an antimitotic, slowing the epidermal cell division. Occlusive dressings are not used with tars. Anthralin is a substance extracted from coal tar that suppresses mitotic activity. Anthralin may be mixed with salicylic acid in a stiff paste. The patient must be closely observed because anthralin is a strong irritant and can cause chemical burns. It is usually applied for no longer than 2 hours. Both coal tar and anthralin are commonly used in combination with ultraviolet (UV) light. They are usually administered in inpatient settings or specialized outpatient clinics.

Topical preparations for the scalp are used in shampoo form. Teach the patient to read package instructions; these preparations generally need to be left in the hair for a period of time to work.

UV light may be designated as UVB (shorter wavelength) or UVA (longer wavelength). UVA is from an artificial source, such as special mercury vapor lamps. The amount of exposure depends on the patient's condition, pigmentation, and susceptibility to burning. The patient must wear eye guards during treatments. Oral psoralen tablets (a photosensitizing agent) followed by exposure to UVA is called PUVA therapy. PUVA therapy temporarily inhibits DNA synthesis, which is antimitotic. Because psoralen is a photosensitizing agent, the patient must wear dark glasses not only during the treatment period but also for the entire day after a treatment. The long-term safety of PUVA therapy is still unknown. Possible side effects include increased skin carcinomas, premature skin aging, and actinic keratosis (premalignant lesions of the skin). The patient should be observed closely for redness, tenderness, edema, and eye changes. Initial and follow-up eye examinations, skin biopsies, urinalysis, and blood tests may be ordered.

Retinoids are oral agents such as acitretin (Soriatane) that promote skin cell differentiation and inhibit malignancies from forming in the skin. They may be used in combination with UV therapy.

Antimetabolites, usually used for cancer chemotherapy, are reserved for the most severe cases. Methotrexate is the most common agent given. Because of its hepatotoxicity, it is contraindicated in patients with liver disease, alcoholism, renal disease, and bone marrow suppression. Other systemic agents, such as cyclosporine and etanercept (Enbrel), work by altering the immune system.

Nursing Care

Nursing care for the patient with psoriasis is the same as nursing care for the patient with dermatitis. Teach the patient how to use prescribed medications and how to identify and avoid triggers. Explain that drinking alcohol can interfere with some treatments. In addition, consult with the HCP about recommending small amounts of sunlight to help improve skin lesions.

CRITICAL THINKING

Mrs. Long arrives at the health care clinic stating that the shampoo prescribed for her scalp psoriasis is not working. She says that she washes her hair thoroughly with the medicated shampoo and then rinses completely. She wants to know why her scalp shows no signs of improvement.

1. What additional information should you collect?
2. What can you teach her?

Suggested answers are at the end of the chapter.

INFECTIOUS SKIN DISORDERS

A variety of infections can affect the skin. The most common disorders are discussed in this section. Table 54.4 provides a summary of additional skin infections.

Herpes Simplex
Pathophysiology and Etiology

Herpes simplex virus (HSV) infection is a common viral infection that tends to recur repeatedly. There are two types of herpes simplex: that caused by type 1 virus (HSV-1), which

Table 54.4
Infectious Skin Disorders

Type	*Description*	*Complications*	*Treatment/Nursing Care*
Impetigo Contagiosa Impetigo on the face 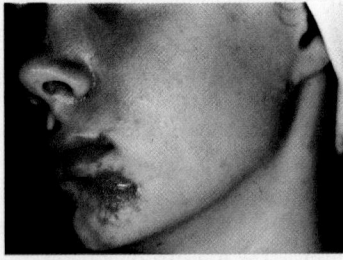 Impetigo contagiosa.	Common contagious, infectious, inflammatory skin disorder usually caused by *Streptococcus* or *Staphylococcus aureus;* sources of infection include swimming pools, pets, dirty fingernails, beauty and barber shops, and contaminated clothing, towels, and sheets; may occur secondary to scrapes, cuts, insect bites, burns, dermatitis, poison ivy. Rash appears as oozing, thin-roofed vesicle that rapidly grows and develops a honey-colored crust; crusts are easily removed, and new crusts appear; lesions heal in 1 to 2 weeks if allowed to dry. Rash is contagious until all lesions are healed.	Glomerulonephritis may occur up to 6–7 weeks after infection. Lesions may spread. Lesions may persist if not permitted to dry. Secondary **pyoderma,** or acute inflammatory purulent dermatitis, can occur if lesions are unresponsive to treatment.	Administer systemic antibiotics as prescribed. Apply topical antibiotics after crust removal. Wash gently with a mild soap or soak with warm, moist compresses to aid in removal of crusts and debris, and to provide a clean bed for topical therapy. Keep fingernails short and clean, and use gloves or hand mitts as necessary to prevent scratching. Teach proper disposal or washing of any material that comes in contact with lesions.

Table 54.4

Infectious Skin Disorders—cont'd

Type	Description	Complications	Treatment/Nursing Care
Furuncles and Carbuncles 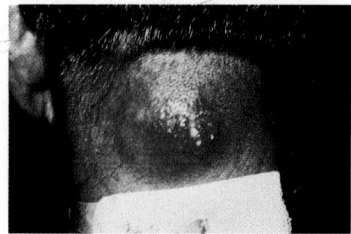 Furuncles and carbuncles.	Furuncle: small, tender boil that occurs deep in one or more hair follicles and spreads to surrounding dermis; usually caused by *Staphylococcus;* usually on body areas prone to excessive perspiration, friction, and irritation (e.g., buttocks, axillae); can recur; eventually comes to a soft yellow, black, or white head with localized pain and surrounding cellulitis; lymphadenopathy may be present. Carbuncle: an abscess of skin and subcutaneous tissue; deeper than a furuncle; usually caused by *Staphylococcus;* usually appears where skin is thick, fibrous, and inelastic (e.g., back of neck, upper back, and buttocks); associated symptoms may include fever, pain, leukocytosis, and prostration.	Furuncles may progress to more severe carbuncles. Carbuncles may progress to infection of bloodstream. Further spread of infection can occur to self and others.	Administer antibiotics as ordered. Prevent trauma; avoid squeezing or irritation. Cleanse surrounding skin with antibacterial soap, followed by application of antibacterial ointment. Surgical incision and drainage may be performed. Cover draining lesions with dressings. Follow standard precautions to prevent cross-contamination. Cover mattress and pillows with plastic and wipe daily with a disinfectant. Wash all linens, towels, and clothing after each use. Properly discard razor blades after each use.

occurs above the waist and causes a fever blister or cold sore (Fig. 54.3), and that caused by type 2 virus (HSV-2), which occurs below the waist and causes genital herpes. See Chapter 44 for information on genital herpes.

The primary infection occurs through direct contact, respiratory droplet, or fluid exposure from another infected person. Following the initial infection, the virus lies dormant in nerve ganglia near the spinal column, where the immune system cannot destroy it. The patient is asymptomatic at this time.

Recurrence of symptomatic infection can happen spontaneously or may be triggered by stressors such as fever, sunburn, illness, menses, fatigue, or injury. The secondary lesion may appear isolated or as groups of small vesicles or pustules on an erythematous base. Crusts eventually form, and the lesions heal in about 1 week. The lesions are contagious for 2 to 4 days before dry crusts form.

Prevention

Avoidance of contact with a known infected lesion during the blistering phase can prevent the primary lesions. Patients should also be taught to avoid sharing contaminated items such as toothbrushes, lipsticks, and drinking glasses. This disease can recur spontaneously. Avoidance of stressors may delay a

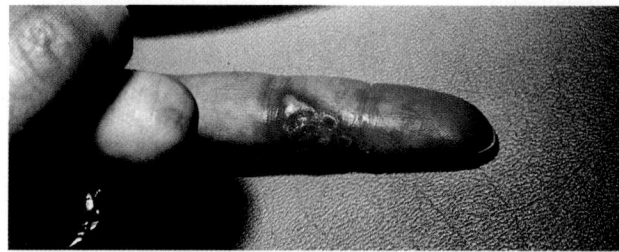

FIGURE 54.3 Herpes simplex.

recurrence. The use of sunscreens, especially on the lips, may be helpful.

Signs and Symptoms

Some patients have a prodromal phase of burning or tingling at the site for a few hours before eruption. The area becomes erythematous and swollen. Vesicles and pustules erupt in 1 to 2 days. There may also be redness with no blistering. Lesions can burn, itch, and be painful. The attacks vary in frequency but diminish with age. The patient is contagious with each outbreak until scabs are formed.

Complications

If HSV is present in the vagina at childbirth, the newborn may be infected (meningoencephalitis or a panvisceral infection may occur). If the person touches the affected area and then rubs the eyes, the eyes can become severely infected. Secondary bacterial infection of lesions can occur. Rarely, herpes encephalitis can occur. This is deadly if not treated promptly.

Diagnostic Tests

Cultures of the lesions provide a definitive diagnosis. Most lesions are diagnosed on the basis of history, signs, and symptoms.

Therapeutic Measures

There is no complete cure for HSV. Recurrences will happen. Topical acyclovir (Zovirax) ointment is the drug of choice for primary lesions, to suppress the multiplication of vesicles. Docosanol (Abreva) is an over-the-counter topical antiviral agent that may be effective. Oral antivirals (acyclovir, famciclovir, or valacyclovir) may be recommended for severe or frequent attacks (i.e., six or more attacks per year) or for patients who are immunosuppressed. Various lotions, creams, and ointments may be prescribed to accelerate drying and healing of lesions (e.g., camphor, phenol, alcohol). Antibiotics may be indicated for secondary infections.

Herpes Zoster (Shingles)
Pathophysiology and Etiology

Herpes zoster, or shingles, is an acute inflammatory and infectious disorder that produces a painful vesicular eruption of bright red edematous plaques along the distribution of nerves from one or more posterior ganglia. This eruption follows the course of the cutaneous sensory nerve and is almost always unilateral (one sided) (Fig. 54.4).

Herpes zoster is caused by the varicella zoster virus, the same virus that causes chickenpox. After a case of chickenpox, the virus remains dormant in nerve tissue near the brain and spinal cord. Herpes zoster is a reactivation of this latent varicella virus. The incubation period of herpes zoster is 7 to 21 days. Vesicles appear in 3 to 4 days. Eruption usually occurs posteriorly and progresses anteriorly and peripherally along the dermatome. The total duration of the outbreak can vary from 10 days to 5 weeks.

This disease occurs most commonly in older adults or in those who have a diminished resistance, such as the patient

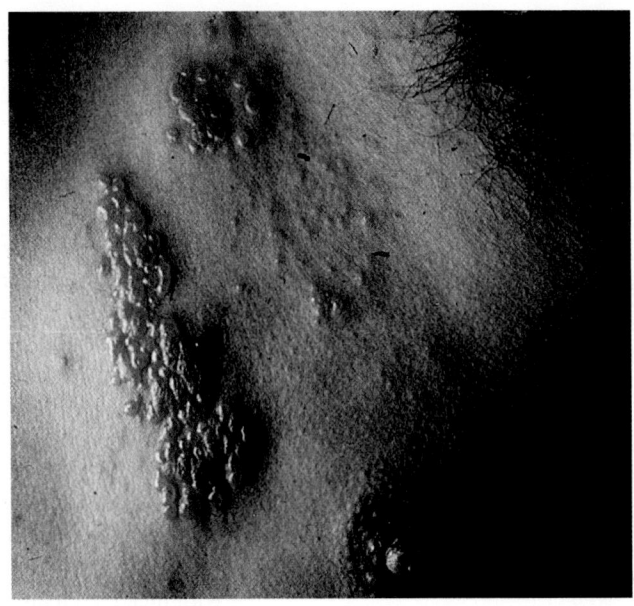

FIGURE 54.4 Herpes zoster (shingles).

with AIDS, the patient on immunosuppressant agents, or the patient with a malignancy or injury to the spine or a cranial nerve.

Prevention

Avoidance of persons with herpes zoster during the contagious phase (a few days before eruption until vesicles dry or scab) is the best prevention. Varicella vaccine (Varivax) in children and adults who have not had chickenpox can reduce the risk of becoming infected with varicella. Another vaccine, Zostavax, is recommended for all patients over age 60 who have had chickenpox. It reduces the risk of shingles outbreak and reduces the severity if it does occur.

Signs and Symptoms

In addition to the vesicles and plaques, there may be irritation, itching, fever, malaise, and, depending on the location of lesions, visceral involvement. Lesions may be very painful; the incidence of pain increases with age.

Complications

Postherpetic neuralgia, persistent dermatomal pain, and hyperesthesia are common in older adults and can last for weeks to months after the lesions have healed. The incidence and severity of these complications increase with age.

Ophthalmic herpes zoster affects the fifth cranial nerve and can be a serious complication. Consultation with an ophthalmologist is essential because this complication can affect eyesight. Other complications can occur with facial and acoustic nerve involvement, including hearing loss, tinnitus, facial paralysis, and vertigo. Full-thickness skin necrosis and scarring can occur if lesions do not heal properly; systemic infection can occur from scratching, causing the virus to enter the bloodstream.

Diagnostic Tests

Diagnosis is usually confirmed by history and physical examination of the patient and associated signs and symptoms. Cultures may be ordered if secondary bacterial infections are suspected.

Therapeutic Measures

Treatment is aimed at controlling the outbreak, reducing pain and discomfort, and preventing complications. Mild cases may heal without medication. Antiviral agents such as acyclovir are used for more severe cases. They are most effective if started within 72 hours of the onset of the rash. Analgesics may be prescribed for pain and discomfort. Anticonvulsants (e.g., gabapentin [Neurontin]) or antidepressants (e.g., amitriptyline [Elavil]) may also be effective for neuropathic pain.

Use of corticosteroids is controversial, but they may help reduce discomfort and improve quality of life when used with antiviral agents. Topical steroids should not be applied if a secondary infection is present because they suppress the immune system. Antihistamines can be administered to control itching. Antibiotics are prescribed for secondary bacterial infections.

In addition to medications, cool compresses or baths may help with pain and itching. Topical agents containing calamine or lidocaine may also be helpful.

Fungal Infections

Pathophysiology and Etiology

Dermatomycosis, or a fungal infection of the skin, occurs when there is an impairment of the skin integrity in a warm, moist environment. This infection occurs through direct contact with infected humans, animals, or objects. *Tinea* is the term used to describe fungal skin infections; the name used after tinea indicates the body area affected. For example, tinea capitis is a fungal infection of the scalp, and tinea pedis is the term used for athlete's foot. The term *candidiasis* is used when *Candida* is the infecting organism. Common fungal infections and treatments are described in Table 54.5.

Table 54.5
Fungal Infections

Type	Description	Treatment/Nursing Care
Tinea Pedis (Athlete's Foot)	Common fungal infection, most frequently seen in those with warm, diaphoretic feet; occlusive shoes; or friction/trauma to the feet. Four types: interdigital (between the toes), chronic hyperkeratotic (chronic plantar erythema and scaling), inflammatory/vesicular (vesicles on plantar surface), and ulcerative (vesicular lesions and ulcers between toes and on plantar surface).	Administer topical antifungal agents as ordered; may be oral in more severe or unresponsive cases. Apply topical agents in a thin layer; treat for time specified, even after apparent clearing. Wet dressings or vinegar soaks may be ordered to dry blisters. Teach patient prevention measures: keep feet dry; dry carefully between toes; apply foot powder and wear cotton socks to absorb perspiration; if weather permits, use perforated shoes or sandals; avoid plastic or rubber-soled shoes; wear water shoes in public showers and near swimming pools.
Tinea Capitis (Ringworm of Scalp) 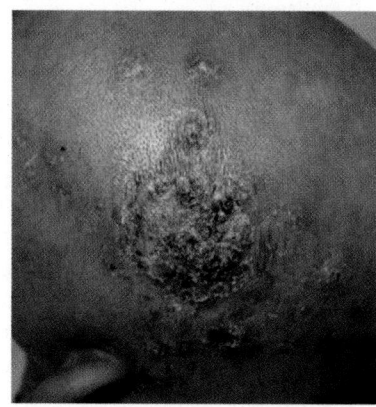 Tinea capitis (ringworm of scalp).	Contagious fungal infection of the scalp; commonly causes hair loss in children. Appears as scattered round, red, scaly patches; small papules or pustules may be evident at edges of patches; hair is brittle at site, breaks off, and temporary areas of baldness result; mild itching, tenderness, and pain may be present. Kerion is a severe inflammation of the scalp with resulting alopecia that sometimes occurs with tinea capitis.	Administer systemic antifungals as prescribed; relapse rate is high with topical agents. Oral corticosteroids are indicated for kerion inflammation to help prevent alopecia. Instruct family on contagious aspect of disease; assess other family members and pets for organism. Teach prevention measures: never share combs, brushes, pillowcases, or headgear.

Continued

Table 54.5

Fungal Infections—cont'd

Type	Description	Treatment/Nursing Care
Tinea Corporis (Tinea Circinata, Ringworm of Body)	Fungal infection of the body that appears as an erythematous macule; progresses to rings of vesicles or scale with a clear center that appears alone or in clusters; usually occurs on exposed areas of body; can be moderately to intensely itchy.	Administer topical or systemic antifungal agents as prescribed. Infected pet is common source of infection. Teach patient prevention measures: avoid heat, moisture, and friction; keep skin areas, especially folds, dry; use clean towel and washcloth daily; wear cotton clothing, especially on hot, humid days.
Tinea Cruris (Ringworm of Groin, Jock Itch) 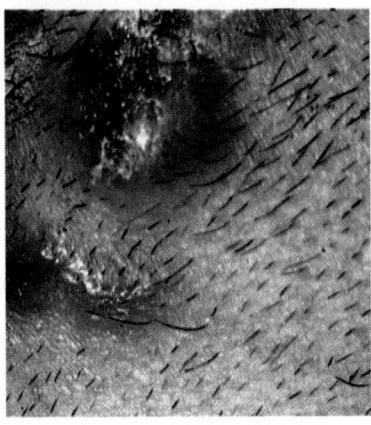 Tinea cruris (ringworm of groin, jock itch).	Infection of groin, inner thighs, and buttocks area; may occur with tinea pedis; often in obese people who are participate in athletics. Lesion first appears as a small red scaly patch and then progresses to a sharply demarcated plaque with elevated scaly or vesicular borders; itching can range from minimal to severe.	Topical antifungals are prescribed; apply in a thin layer to rash and a few centimeters beyond border. Unresponsive cases may require oral antifungal agent. Teach patient prevention measures: bathe daily and change to clean underwear. Avoid tight clothing. Do not share personal items. Treat tinea pedis to prevent spread.
Tinea Unguium (Ringworm of Nails, Onychomycosis) 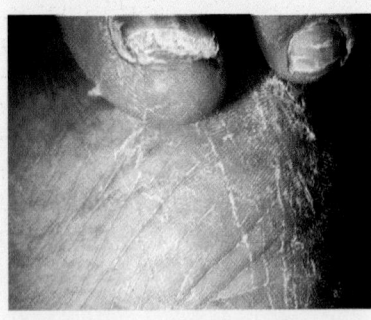 Tinea unguium (ringworm of nails, onychomycosis).	Chronic fungal infection of nails, usually the toenails; a lifelong disease. There is yellow thickening of nail plate; it is friable and lusterless. Eventually crumbly debris accumulates under free edge of the nail and causes nail plate to become separated; over time, the nail may become thickened, painful, and destroyed.	Systemic antifungals are rarely given for toenail involvement but may be prescribed for fingernail involvement. Topical antifungals are usually ineffective because they do not penetrate nails. Nail may have to be surgically removed (nail avulsion). Keep nails neatly trimmed and buffed flat; gently scrape out any nail debris.

• **WORD** • **BUILDING** •

onychomycosis: onycho—fingernail or toenail + myco—
fungus + osis—condition

Table 54.5
Fungal Infections—cont'd

Type	Description	Treatment/Nursing Care
Candidiasis/Thrush 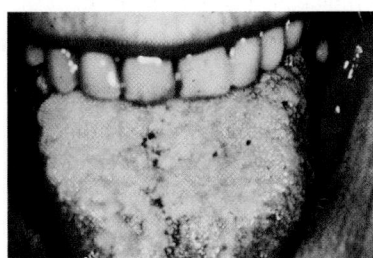 Candidiasis/thrush.	Oral candidiasis is called thrush. Infection of skin or mucous membranes with *Candida*. Grows in warm moist areas such as under breasts, in groin, vagina, or oral mucous membranes. Appears as white patches in mouth, white vaginal discharge, or red irritated areas in skinfolds. May occur as a result of antibiotic therapy because normal flora that usually keep *Candida* in check are destroyed, or with corticosteroid therapy.	Administer oral or topical antifungal agents as ordered. Examples include nystatin "swish and swallow" or lozenges for oral thrush, nystatin powder or ointment for skin infection, or vaginal suppositories or creams. Teach patient to keep skin clean and dry, especially in skinfold areas. Treatment is important to prevent systemic infection.

Cellulitis
Pathophysiology and Etiology
Cellulitis is inflammation of the skin and subcutaneous tissue resulting from infection, usually with *Staphylococcus* or *Streptococcus* bacteria. Methicillin-resistant *Staphylococcus aureus* (MRSA) is a common cause and is resistant to many antibiotics. Cellulitis can occur as a result of skin trauma or as a secondary bacterial infection of an open wound, such as a pressure injury. It also may be unrelated to skin trauma. It most often occurs in the extremities, especially the lower legs.

Prevention
Good hygiene and prevention of cross-contamination are important. If an open wound is present, preventing infection and promoting healing are critical.

Signs and Symptoms
The initial sign of cellulitis is a localized area of inflammation that may become more generalized if not treated promptly. Common clinical manifestations include warmth, redness, localized edema, pain, tenderness, fever, and lymphadenopathy. The infection can worsen rapidly and become systemic if not treated effectively.

Diagnostic Tests
Culture and sensitivity testing of any pustules or drainage is necessary to identify the infecting organism. Blood cultures may also be indicated to rule out bacteremia.

Therapeutic Measures
Topical and systemic antibiotics are prescribed according to culture and sensitivity test results. Débridement of nonviable tissue is necessary if an open wound is present. Systemic antibiotics are indicated if fever and lymphadenopathy are present.

Elevation of the extremity can reduce pain and swelling. Monitor vital signs and report hypotension and tachycardia, because such changes can indicate systemic infection. Measure the extremity daily and document to monitor progress. Outlining the affected area with a marker can also help monitor progress but may be difficult if the borders are not clear.

Acne Vulgaris
Pathophysiology, Etiology, and Signs and Symptoms
Acne vulgaris is a common skin disorder of the sebaceous glands and their hair follicles that usually occurs on the face, chest, upper back, and shoulders. The most common cause is hormonal changes during puberty. The initial lesions are called comedones (singular: **comedo**). Closed comedones, or whiteheads, are small white papules with tiny follicular openings. These may eventually become open comedones, or blackheads. The color is not caused by dirt but by lipids and melanin pigment. Scarring occurs as a result of significant skin inflammation; picking can worsen inflammation and lead to further scarring. The resulting inflammation can lead to papules, pustules, nodules (Fig. 54.5), cysts, or abscesses.

Therapeutic Measures
Medical treatment helps control current lesions and helps prevent new lesions. Effective topical agents include benzoyl peroxide, an antibacterial agent that may help prevent pore plugging; antibiotics (e.g., erythromycin, tetracycline) to kill

• **WORD • BUILDING** •
cellulitis: cellu—cell + itis—inflammation

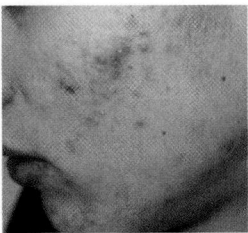

FIGURE 54.5 Acne vulgaris.

bacteria in follicles; and vitamin A acid (Retin-A, tretinoin) to loosen pore plugs and prevent occurrence of new comedones. Topical agents may be used alone or in combination. It may take 3 to 6 weeks before improvement is seen.

Systemic antibiotics (long-term and low dose) and isotretinoin (Accutane) are usually reserved for severe cases of acne. The patient must be closely monitored for side effects. Estrogen therapy (oral contraceptives) may also be prescribed for young women; however, the risks often outweigh the benefits. Women should be aware that some antibiotics reduce the effectiveness of oral contraceptives.

Nursing Process for the Patient With a Skin Infection
Data Collection
Subjective data collection regarding a skin infection can begin with the *WHAT'S UP?* acronym:

- **W**here is the skin infection located?
- **H**ow does it feel? Does it itch, burn, or hurt?
- What **A**ggravates or **A**lleviates the symptoms?
- **T**iming: How long has it been present?
- How **S**evere is it?
- **U**seful other data: Is there swelling, drainage, or fever?
- **P**atient's **P**erception: What does the patient think caused the infection?

Collection of objective data includes observing the affected area and describing the infection in terms of type and configuration of lesions, color, size, and presence of drainage. Also observe for swelling, and check for elevated temperature. If the patient has cellulitis of an extremity, measure and document the circumference of the extremity daily and as needed.

Determine the patient's understanding of the cause of the infection and of infection control measures.

Nursing Diagnoses, Planning, and Implementation

Risk for Infection (spread to surrounding or other areas)

EXPECTED OUTCOME: The infected area will not spread to other areas on the patient or to other individuals.

- Monitor and document size and location of infected area daily and as needed *to identify improvement or new spread of infection.*

- Monitor temperature every 8 hours and prn. *An increasing temperature can indicate worsening or systemic infection.*
- Monitor for signs and symptoms of systemic spread of infection, such as hypotension, tachycardia, and increasing temperature. Systemic infection must be reported and treated promptly *to prevent complications, including sepsis.*
- Use standard precautions, including careful hand hygiene, when providing patient care *to prevent transmission to yourself or to others.*
- Implement appropriate isolation precautions for the patient with a contagious infection. Contact precautions are usually sufficient, although airborne precautions may be necessary if immunocompromised individuals are present. *Isolation reduces spread of infection.*
- Instruct the patient on wound care, appropriate hand hygiene, and disposal of soiled dressings. The patient must follow precautions *to protect self and others.*
- Instruct the patient on use of prescribed anti-infective agents, including the importance of taking it exactly as directed *to prevent development of a resistant infection.*
- For the patient with acne, advise keeping hands away from the face and avoiding touching or squeezing pimples. Keep hair clean and off the face. These measures help *to prevent spread, secondary infection, and scarring.*

Acute Pain related to inflammation as evidenced by patient rating on appropriate pain scale

EXPECTED OUTCOME: The patient will state that pain is controlled at an acceptable level.

- Monitor pain (if present) using a pain scale. *Pain assessment provides a basis for nursing intervention.*
- Administer analgesics as ordered, especially before dressing changes or treatments. *Analgesics relieve pain and help prevent pain during dressing changes.*
- For the patient with shingles, apply cool, moist compresses to painful or itching lesions *to help cleanse and dry lesions and reduce itching.*
- For the patient with shingles, apply firm dressings such as wraps, stockings, or a snug T-shirt *to reduce pain from post-herpetic neuralgia.*
- For the patient with cellulitis, elevate affected extremity as ordered *to reduce swelling and increase comfort.*

Evaluation
If interventions have been effective, the skin lesions will improve and will not spread to new areas or to others. The patient will state that pain is manageable.

PARASITIC SKIN DISORDERS

Pediculosis
Pathophysiology and Etiology
Pediculosis is an infestation by lice. There are three basic types: pediculosis capitis (head lice), pediculosis corporis

(body lice), and pediculosis pubis (pubic, or crab, lice). Generally, the lice bite the skin and feed on human blood, leaving their eggs and excrement, which can cause intense itching. The lice are oval and are approximately 2 mm in length.

In pediculosis capitis, the female louse lays eggs (nits) close to the scalp, where the nits become firmly attached to hair shafts. The most common areas of infestation are the back of the scalp and behind the ears. The nits are about 1 to 5 mm in length and appear silvery white and glistening. Transmission is by direct contact or contact with infested objects, such as combs, brushes, wigs, hats, and bedding. It is most common in children and in people with long hair.

Pediculosis corporis is caused by body lice that lay eggs in the seams of clothing and then pierce the skin. Areas of the skin usually involved are the neck, trunk, and thighs.

Pediculosis pubis is caused by pubic, or crab, lice. It is generally localized in the genital region, but it can also be seen on hairs of the chest, axillae, and beard and on eyelashes. The lice are about 2 mm in length and have a crablike appearance. It is chiefly transmitted through sexual contact or, to a lesser degree, by infested bed linens.

Prevention

Prevention involves avoidance of contact with an infected person or object. Brushes, combs, hats, and other personal items should not be shared. Good personal hygiene and routine clothes washing are other preventive measures; however, even someone with meticulous hygiene can develop an infestation if there is contact with the organism.

Signs and Symptoms

Pediculosis capitis can result in no itching or intense itching and scratching, especially at the back of the head. Nits may be noticeably attached to hair. A papular rash may be seen.

Pediculosis corporis may appear as tiny hemorrhagic points. Excoriations may be noted on the back, shoulders, abdomen, and extremities. It may also cause intense itching.

Pediculosis pubis results in mild to severe itching, especially at night. Black or reddish brown dots (lice excreta) may be noted at the base of hairs or in underclothing. Gray-blue macules may also be noted on the trunk, thighs, and axillae; this is the result of the insects' saliva mixing with bilirubin.

Complications

Secondary bacterial infections can occur with pediculosis capitis, resulting in impetigo, furuncles, pustules, crusts, and matted hair. Complications of pediculosis corporis include secondary infection and hyperpigmentation. Most important, body lice may be vectors for rickettsial or other systemic disease. Complications with pediculosis pubis include dermatitis and the coexistence of other sexually transmitted infections.

Diagnostic Tests

Diagnosis is made through history and physical examination. The patient may also be tested for other sexually transmitted infections if pediculosis pubis is present.

Therapeutic Measures

Medical treatment is aimed at killing the parasites and mechanically removing nits. Over-the-counter pediculicides containing pyrethrins or permethrin are the most commonly recommended compounds. These agents should kill the lice and nits, although some lice develop pesticide resistance, making mechanical removal necessary. Permethrin (Nix) remains active for about a week, killing the adult lice immediately and the nits when they hatch days later. Pyrethrins (RID, A-200 Pyrinate) must be reapplied in 1 week to kill newly hatched lice. Prescription treatments include benzyl alcohol lotion (Ulesfia), ivermectin lotion (Sklice), malathion lotion (Ovide), and spinosad (Natroba).

If initial treatment is not effective, lindane may be prescribed. Lindane is a controversial, highly toxic topical medication that is only used as a second-line agent.

Complications are treated, as appropriate, with antipruritics, topical corticosteroids, and systemic antibiotics. Physostigmine ophthalmic ointment is applied to affected eyebrows and eyelashes. Other medications should not be applied to eyebrows or eyelashes.

Patient Education

Reassure the patient and family that head lice can happen to anyone and that it is not a sign of uncleanliness. Lice infestations are treated on an outpatient basis, so patient education is important. Package instructions should be followed for correct usage of all medications.

Instruct the patient to bathe with soap and water and to disinfect combs and brushes in hot, medicated soapy water. A fine-toothed comb dipped in vinegar can be used to remove nits from hairy areas. Nits can be removed from eyebrows and eyelashes with a cotton-tipped applicator after treatment. Clothing, linens, and towels should be laundered in hot water and detergent; unwashable clothing should be dry cleaned or sealed in a plastic bag for 10 days. Treatment should be started immediately to prevent rapid spread. Family members and close contacts (sexual contacts with pediculosis pubis) should be examined for infestation and should put on clean clothing.

Shampoos and lotions kill nits, but they do not remove them. To loosen nits from the scalp, the hair may be soaked in a solution of equal parts vinegar and water and a shower cap worn for 15 minutes. Then comb the hair with a fine-toothed comb and thoroughly rinse or shampoo to mechanically remove the nits. Infested children should avoid direct contract with other children. Children may not need to be removed from class because, by the time of diagnosis, the infestation has already been present for a month or more (Simmons, 2015).

> **NURSING CARE TIP**
>
> It is not possible to dry clean or wash all items infected with lice, such as mattresses and upholstered furniture. Teach patients to thoroughly vacuum upholstered furniture. The lice die in 3 to 4 days without human contact.

Scabies
Pathophysiology and Etiology
Scabies is a contagious skin disease caused by the mite *Sarcoptes scabiei*. It results from intimate or prolonged skin contact or prolonged contact with infected clothing, bedding, or animals (e.g., dogs, cats, other small animals). The parasite burrows into the superficial layer of the skin (Fig. 54.6). These burrows appear as short, wavy, brownish black lines. The patient is asymptomatic while the organism multiplies, but it is most contagious at this time. Symptoms do not occur until almost 4 weeks after the time of contact.

Prevention
All persons (and animals) in intimate contact with an infected patient should be treated at the same time to eliminate the mites. The mites survive less than 24 hours without human contact. Therefore, bed linens, clothes, and towels should be washed in hot water and dried at high heat, but furnishings need not be cleaned. Clean clothing and linens should be applied.

Signs and Symptoms
The major complaints are itching and rash. Itching can be intense, especially at night. Itching begins about 1 month after infestation and may persist for days to weeks after treatment. The rash appears as small, scattered erythematous papules, concentrated in finger webs, axillae, wrist folds, umbilicus, groin, and genitals. Crusts and scales may be present. Male patients may have excoriated papules on the penis and groin area.

Complications
Hypersensitivity reactions to the mite can result in crusted lesions, vesicles, pustules, excoriations, and bacterial superinfections.

Diagnostic Tests
Diagnosis is confirmed by a superficial shaving of a lesion and microscopic evaluation for adult mites, eggs, or feces.

Therapeutic Measures
Topical scabicides (e.g., permethrin [Elimite], crotamiton [Crotan]) are used for chemical disinfection. Package instructions should be followed for each medication. Antipruritics may be prescribed for itching.

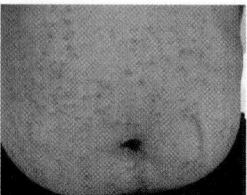

FIGURE 54.6 Scabies.

Patient Education
A warm soapy bath or shower removes scales and skin debris. Advise the patient to apply the topical medication as ordered, follow medication directions, treat family members and close contacts simultaneously to eliminate mites, wear clean clothing, and use clean linens. Remind the patient that itching may continue for up to 2 weeks after treatment until the allergic reaction subsides. (Dead mites remain in the epidermis until exfoliated.)

> **NURSING CARE TIP**
> Animals infested with scabies should be treated by a veterinarian so that they won't infect humans.

◢ SKIN LESIONS

Skin lesions can be either benign (noncancerous) or malignant. Benign lesions are described in Table 54.6. Malignant lesions are discussed next. Also see "Cultural Considerations."

> ### Cultural Considerations
> • Darker-skinned people have a tendency toward an overgrowth of connective tissue components concerned with the protection against infection and repair after injury. Keloid formation is one example of this tendency toward overgrowth of connective tissue. Lymphoma and systemic lupus erythematosus may also occur due to this overgrowth of connective tissue.
> • Some African American men have facial hair that curls back on itself and penetrates the skin, which can result in pustules and small keloids. Many use depilatories or electric razors to prevent nicking the skin, which can also cause keloids.
> • Darker-skinned people have an increased incidence of birthmarks and Mongolian spots compared with lighter-skinned people. Mongolian spots disappear over time. The nurse must be cautious not to mistake these spots for bruising, which can indicate injury or abuse.
> • For people with light skin, such as those of German, Polish, and Irish descent, prolonged exposure to the sun may increase the incidence of skin cancer. Teach patients to protect themselves from sun exposure to reduce their risk of skin cancer. Nevi (freckles and skin discolorations) occur more often in lighter-skinned individuals. They are most common in European Americans, followed by Asians and darker-skinned African Americans.

Malignant Skin Lesions
Pathophysiology and Etiology
The most common type of cancer in the United States is skin cancer, which includes basal cell carcinoma, squamous cell carcinoma, and malignant melanoma. Most cases of skin

Table 54.6

Benign Skin Lesions

Type	Description	Treatment
Cyst 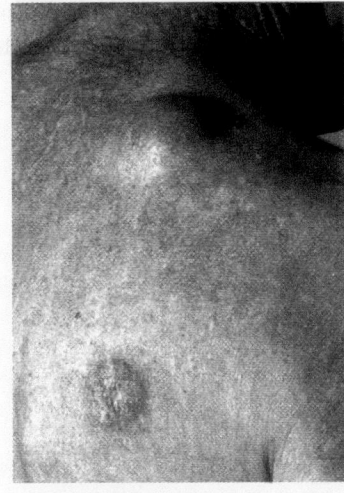 Epidermoid cyst.	A saclike growth with a defined wall that may contain liquid, semifluid, or solid material. An epidermoid cyst is the most common type of cyst. It results from proliferation of epidermal cells in the dermis. Rarely, it is associated with carcinoma development.	Not all cysts need to be treated. Treatments include intralesional steroid therapy and antibiotics, if indicated. If excision is done, the entire cyst wall is removed to prevent recurrence.
Seborrheic Keratosis 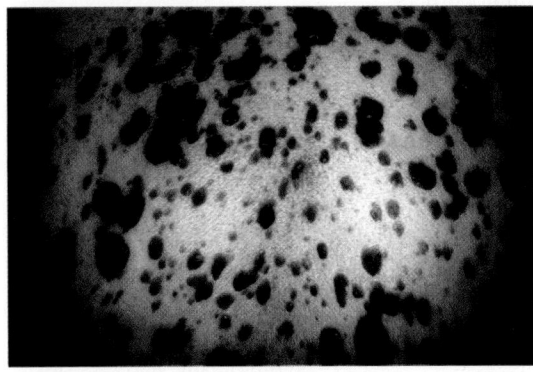 Seborrheic keratosis.	A benign skin lesion with pigmented light tan to dark brown patches. The plaques or papules have a "stuck-on" appearance caused by the proliferation of epidermal cells and keratin piled on the skin surface. Cause is unknown, but it tends to occur in middle-aged to older patients, most commonly on the trunk, scalp, face, and extremities.	Treatment is cosmetic only, or if lesion becomes irritated from friction. Topical agents may be used to reduce lesion size or height. Liquid nitrogen cryotherapy or light curettage may be performed if necessary for removal.
Keloid 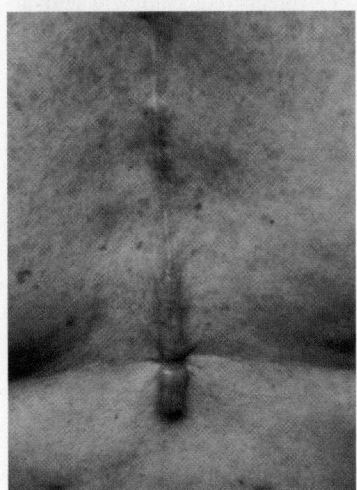 Keloid.	A benign growth of fibrous tissue (scar formation) at the site of trauma or surgical incision; occurs in various sizes. Growth of tissue is out of proportion to what is needed for normal healing. The lesion extends beyond the original injury and occurs mainly in middle-aged and older adult patients and darker-skinned patients.	Treatment varies and is not always successful; a larger scar may ensue. Some treatment options include compression therapy, corticosteroid injections into lesions, excision, and laser therapy.

Continued

Table 54.6
Benign Skin Lesions—cont'd

Type	*Description*	*Treatment*
Pigmented Nevus (mole) 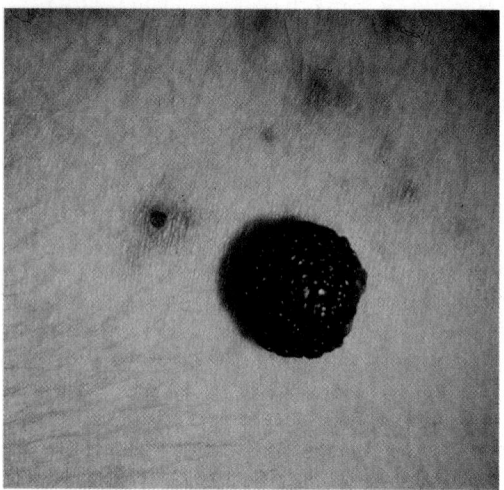 Dermal mole.	A benign, flesh-colored to dark brown macule or papule located randomly over the entire skin surface of the body. Can be inherited or acquired and occurs mostly in light-skinned patients. Usually begin to appear between 1 and 4 years of age, increasing in number into adulthood. Some contain a few hairs. There are many variations. Rate of transformation to a malignant melanoma is higher in congenital moles and larger lesions. Clinical signs of melanoma include change in color or size; inflammation of surrounding skin; irregular or spreading borders; variegated colors, especially a bluish pigmentation; bleeding; and oozing, crusting, and itching. Usually nevi larger than 1 cm should be carefully examined.	Treatment is indicated for risk of melanoma, unsightly nevi (cosmetic), repeated irritation (rubbing from belt, bra), trauma, large moles, and patient report of a change in the mole. Surgical removal can include excision (preferred) or surgical shave. All excised moles should be sent for histological examination.
Wart 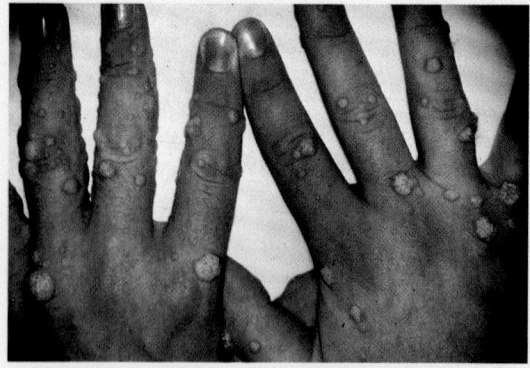 Warts.	Small, common, benign growth of the skin resulting from the hypertrophy of the papillae and epidermis; caused by a virus. Common warts, often seen on hands and fingers, appear as raised, flesh-colored papules that have a rough surface. May crack, fissure, bleed, and be painful to lateral pinching and direct, firm pressure. Plantar warts occur on the sole of the foot. They may appear granular, pitted, or protuberant, with a callous of surrounding normal skin. Incubation period can be several weeks to months. Virus is spread by direct contact.	Patient should be cautioned not to spread lesions by picking or biting them. Treatment is indicated for symptomatic warts and for cosmetic purposes. General treatments include keratolytic agents (e.g., salicylic acid plasters) to soften and reduce keratin; cryotherapy (liquid nitrogen); and light electrodesiccation and curettage (requires local anesthesia).

Table 54.6
Benign Skin Lesions—cont'd

Type	Description	Treatment
Hemangioma (Angioma)	Benign vascular tumor of dilated blood vessels that can have varied clinical manifestations Nevus flammeus involves mature capillaries on the face and neck. It is a congenital neoplasm that appears as a pink-red to bluish purple macular patch. Port-wine stains or port-wine angiomas appear as violet-red macular patches, usually singular lesions, growing proportionately as the child grows. These lesions can persist indefinitely. Cherry hemangiomas are commonly seen in older adults. They appear as small round papules that can vary in color from red to purple.	Nevus flammeus is usually treated for cosmetic reasons. Port-wine stains, if large enough, may be treated surgically or with pulse-dye laser therapy. Cosmetics to camouflage the affected area are also available. Treatment for cherry hemangiomas is usually not prescribed, except for cosmetic purposes.

cancer are preventable. The major cause of skin malignancies is overexposure to ultraviolet rays, most commonly sunlight. Other risk factors include being fair skinned and blue eyed, having multiple moles, family history, history of x-ray therapy, exposure to certain chemical agents (e.g., arsenic, coal tar), burn scars, and immunosuppressive therapy.

Basal cell carcinoma arises from the basal cell layer of the epidermis. It is the most common type of skin cancer. This tumor is mainly seen on sun-exposed areas of the body. The lesion appears as a small pearly or translucent papule with a rolled and waxy edge, depressed center, telangiectasia (lesion formed by dilation of vessels), crusting, and ulceration (Fig. 54.7). Metastasis is rare, although it may be locally invasive.

Squamous cell carcinoma arises from the epidermis. It can occur on sun-exposed areas of the skin and mucous membranes. It is mainly seen on the lower lip, neck, tongue, head, and dorsal surfaces of the hands. The lesion appears as a single, crusted, scaled, eroded papule, nodule, or plaque (Fig. 54.8). A neglected lesion appears more rough, scaly, and darker colored. The lesion is fragile and prone to oozing and bleeding. Untreated squamous cell carcinoma can metastasize to distant areas of the body.

Malignant melanoma, as the name implies, is a malignant growth of pigment cells (melanocytes; Fig. 54.9). It is highly metastatic, with a higher mortality rate than basal or squamous cell carcinomas. It can occur anywhere on the body;

about half arise from preexisting nevi or moles. There are three general types: lentigo maligna, superficial spreading, and nodular.

Lentigo maligna melanoma appears as a slow-growing dark macule on exposed skin surfaces (especially the face) of older adults (Fig. 54.10). The lesion has irregular borders and brown, tan, and black coloring. Prognosis is good if treated early.

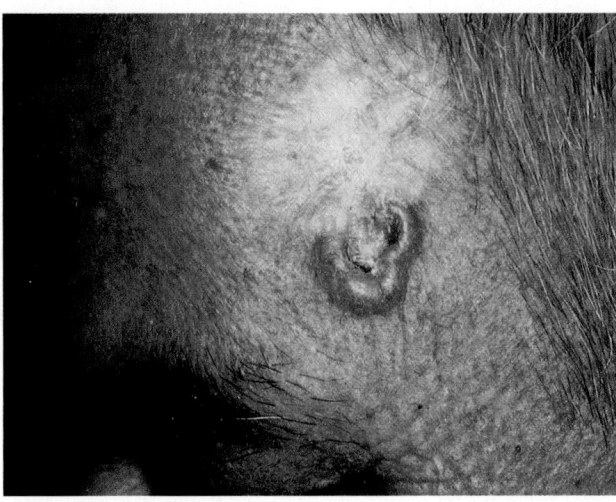

FIGURE 54.7 Basal cell carcinoma.

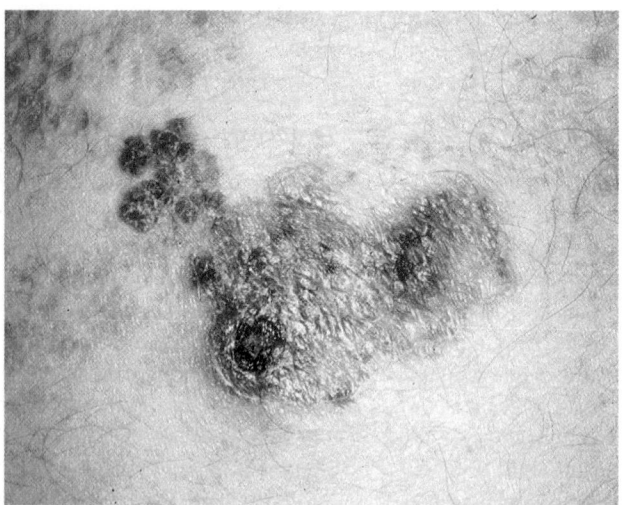

FIGURE 54.8 Squamous cell carcinoma. Surface is fragile and bleeds easily.

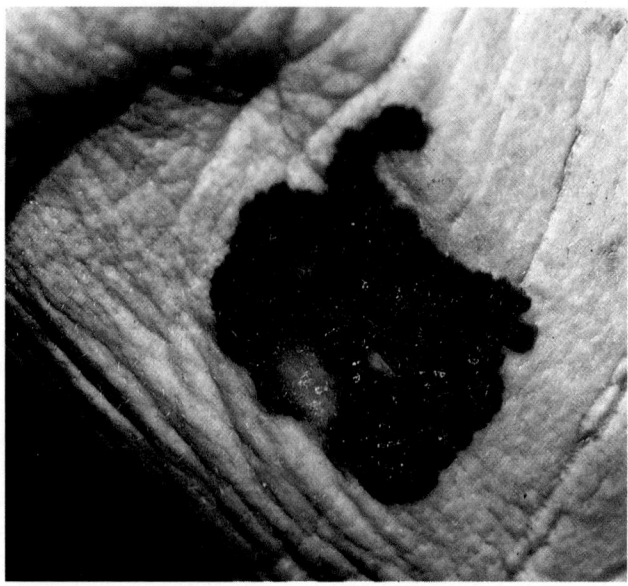

FIGURE 54.10 Lentigo maligna.

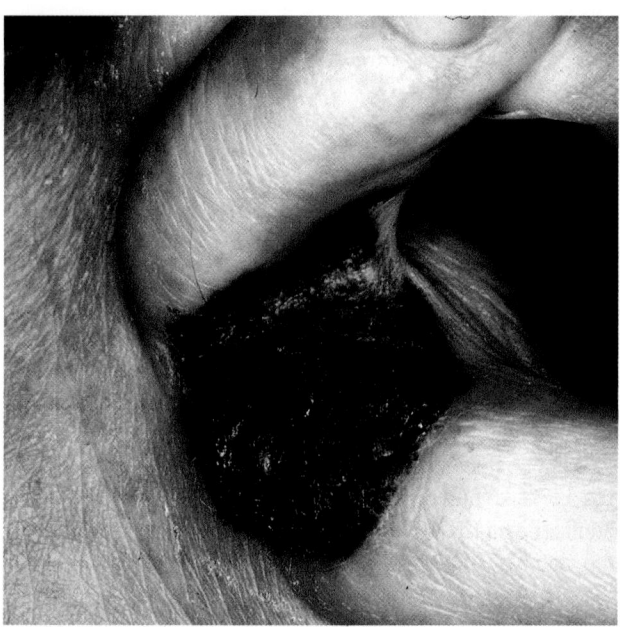

FIGURE 54.9 Malignant melanoma.

NURSING CARE TIP

To help patients find melanomas as early as possible, encourage them to examine their skin regularly and report any lesions that fit this profile:

- Asymmetrical shape
- Irregular or poorly defined border
- Variable color
- Diameter larger than that of a pencil eraser
- Changing appearance

Prevention

Risk of most types of skin cancer can be reduced by limiting or avoiding direct exposure to UV rays (e.g., sun, tanning booths). If exposure to the sun is necessary, exposure should be avoided during the time of its highest intensity (between 1000 and 1600). The patient should use a protective sunscreen with sun protection factor (SPF) of 15 or more, and wear sun-protective clothing such as hats and long sleeves. The patient should seek medical advice if there is a change in color, size, shape, sensation, or character of a lesion or mole.

Diagnostic Tests

A definitive diagnosis is made by biopsy. Other tests may be performed based on the results of the pathological examination.

Therapeutic Measures

Medical treatment depends on the type, thickness, and location of the lesion; the stage of the disease; and the age and general health of the patient. Generally, lesions are surgically excised with a 1- to 2-cm margin to make sure no cancer cells remain. Lymph nodes may also be removed. Mohs surgery is a technique in which the surgeon removes layers

Superficial spreading melanoma is the most common melanoma. It can occur anywhere on the body and is usually seen in middle-aged persons. The lesion appears as a slightly elevated plaque with an irregular border. Coloring varies in combinations of black, brown, and pink. The fragile surface may bleed or ooze. Eventually the plaque develops into a nodule. The cure rate is excellent when it is in the plaque phase; prognosis is poor in the nodular phase.

Nodular melanoma occurs suddenly as a spherical papule or nodule on the skin or in a mole. Coloration is blue-black, blue-gray, or reddish blue color that may have a rim of inflammation. The lesion is fragile and bleeds easily. Metastasis occurs rapidly. This type of melanoma has the least favorable prognosis. Early diagnosis and treatment are important.

of cancerous skin, which is then examined; additional layers are removed until no cancerous cells remain.

Grafting may be necessary for closure or repair. Chemotherapy may be used if metastasis is present. Radiation therapy may be used as adjunct treatment or may be recommended for patients with a deeply invasive tumor or those who are poor surgical risks. Other therapies include cryosurgery or curettage and electrodesiccation.

Nursing Care

Perform a complete skin examination. Palpate lesions to determine texture, size, and firmness. Document size, location, color, surface characteristics, pain, discomfort, itching, and bleeding. Note when the patient first discovered the lesion.

Nursing care of the patient with cancer is covered in Chapter 11. Specific nursing care related to cryosurgery includes preparing the patient for the procedure. Explain that minor discomfort can be expected. Expect swelling, local tenderness, and hemorrhagic blister formation 1 to 2 days after the procedure. After the procedure, the area is cleansed as ordered and prescribed ointments are applied.

Specific nursing care for curettage and electrodesiccation includes preparing the patient for the procedure. After local anesthesia, a dermal curette is used to scrape away the lesion, followed by electrodesiccation of the remaining wound; the wound heals by secondary intention, usually with minimal scarring. After the procedure, the wound is cleansed and dressed as prescribed.

 DERMATOLOGICAL SURGERY

Plastic or reconstructive surgery is performed to correct defects, scars, and malformations and to restore function or prevent further loss of function. This type of surgery is usually an elective procedure; it may be prescribed by the HCP, or it may be the wish of the patient hoping to improve body image. Common types of plastic surgical procedures are listed in Table 54.7. Care of the surgical patient is covered in Chapter 12.

Table 54.7
Common Plastic Surgical Procedures

Operation	Description	Purpose	Possible Complications	Postoperative Nursing Care Considerations
Rhinoplasty (Nose)	Removal of excessive nasal cartilage, tissue, or bone; reshaping of nose	Correct congenital or acquired septal defects; improve cosmetic shape of nose	Hemorrhage, hematoma; temporary ecchymosis and edema; infection, septal perforation	Monitor dressing and packing for bright-red bleeding; monitor vital signs and level of consciousness; maintain semi-Fowler position to minimize edema.
Blepharoplasty (Eyelid)	Incisions on upper and lower lids with excision of fat and skin and primary closure	Removal of bags under eyes and wrinkles and bulges	Corneal injury; hematoma; ectropion; rarely visual loss and wound infection	Administer antibiotic ointment as ordered; maintain eye dressings; maintain semi-Fowler position to minimize edema.
Rhytidoplasty (Facelift)	Incision anterior to ear with removal of excessive skin and tissue; the subcutaneous tissue and fascia are folded and stretched	Removal of excessive wrinkling or sagging skin	Hemorrhage; hematoma; ecchymosis, and edema (temporary); wound infection, facial nerve damage	Surgical improvement lasts from 5 to 10 years; apply antibiotic ointment to suture line; maintain semi-Fowler position to minimize edema.
Otoplasty (Ear)	Incision of ear for correction of defect	Correct congenital defects; correct deformities; improve cosmetic shape of ear	Hemorrhage; hematoma; edema; wound infection	Maintain ear dressing for about 1 week; protect ear at times of sleep for about 3 weeks.

Home Health Hints

- Measure wounds weekly with a disposable centimeter measuring guide.
- Sanitary pads make great cushions for bony prominences. You can also place them in a cotton sock for better molding.
- SurgiNet, or a similar stretchy cover, can be used to cover dressings for patients with tape sensitivities or fragile skin. They are also good for additional support to prevent a dressing from falling off.
- Ask the health care provider for an order for a surgical stockinette for patients with edema who cannot tolerate or apply compression stockings but need some gentle compression to promote wound healing.
- A special pressure-reducing mattress and hospital bed may be necessary for patients with pressure injuries.

- Teach patients dietary measures to promote healing, including adequate protein intake.
- Teach patients to prevent pressure injuries by keeping skin well lubricated with unscented lotions, changing position frequently, and changing briefs when damp. Teach patients in wheelchairs to use their armrests to shift their weight every 15 minutes.
- Teach patients with dressings to keep them clean and dry. Unless the patient or caregiver has been instructed on how to perform the dressing change and has performed a return demonstration, inform him or her to contact the home health care agency if the dressing falls off.
- Teach patients to wear a cast shoe over a dressing on the foot. This will help protect the dressing and provide additional support for the patient while ambulating.

SUGGESTED ANSWERS TO CRITICAL THINKING

Mr. Russ

1. You can do the following:
   - Perform a Braden Scale assessment. A specialty pressure-relieving bed may be appropriate for Mr. Russ.
   - Change Mr. Russ's position at least every 2 hours if not more frequently. Keep his heels off of the bed at all times by propping them on pillows.
   - Request a dietary consult because the body cannot meet the increased healing demands if there is an albumin deficiency. Mr. Russ may need increased protein (contraindicated in kidney failure). He may also need fats, carbohydrates, vitamins, and minerals for wound healing. A dietitian can help determine the amounts of calories and types of foods for the best prevention and/or healing.
   - If Mr. Russ is able to sit up in a chair, provide a chair cushion to prevent skin breakdown and have him shift his weight every 15 minutes.

- Mr. Russ is wearing a brace, so examine the underlying tissue for pressure areas. Braces and splints must be padded to avoid skin breakdown.
- Involve the health care provider, dietitian, wound nurse, registered nurse, physical therapist, and nursing assistant. The nursing assistant is one of the most important members of this team because he or she is often responsible for bathing and turning patients. Ask to be called to examine Mr. Russ's skin during bathing, and teach the assistant warning signs to report.

Mrs. Long

1. Ask how long she is leaving the shampoo in her hair. For medicated scalp shampoos to work properly, they must remain on the scalp for several minutes.
2. Teach Mrs. Long to read the package instructions carefully for each product because they vary from product to product.

Review Questions

1. The nurse notes scratch marks on a patient with psoriasis. What interventions can the nurse teach the patient that will decrease itching and protect the skin? **Select all that apply.**
   1. Apply pressure to the itchy area with a clean cloth.
   2. Encourage use of gloves at night.
   3. Bathe daily in a hot soapy bath.
   4. Consider taking an antihistamine at bedtime.
   5. Use a room humidifier.

2. What information is most important for the nurse to teach patients about avoiding malignant skin lesions?
   1. Shower or bathe daily.
   2. Avoid contact with allergens and irritants.
   3. Avoid overexposure to ultraviolet rays.
   4. Avoid others with malignant lesions.

3. The nurse notes a pressure injury on a newly admitted patient's ischial tuberosity, with a thick, tough black center. Which intervention is most appropriate first?
   1. Coat the wound with antibiotic ointment.
   2. Snip away the black tissue with sterile scissors.
   3. Flush the wound with sterile saline.
   4. Talk to the health care provider about débridement.

4. A patient develops pressure injuries on the sacrum and buttocks despite being turned and repositioned regularly. Which factors may have contributed to the patient's skin breakdown? **Select all that apply.**
   1. The patient is 20 pounds overweight.
   2. The patient commonly slides down in the chair.
   3. Staff use a lift sheet to move the patient in bed.
   4. The patient sits in a chair most of the day.
   5. The patient is often diaphoretic.
   6. The patient is incontinent of urine and stool.

5. Which instruction should the nurse provide to the patient being treated for scabies?
   1. "Dry clean all linens, towels, and clothes."
   2. "Wash linens, towels, and clothes."
   3. "Discard infested mattresses."
   4. "Remove infested pets from the home."

6. A patient diagnosed with impetigo contagiosa wants to know when the disease will no longer be contagious. Which response by the nurse is correct?
   1. "One week after treatment is started."
   2. "After the spread of lesions has stopped."
   3. "After all the lesions crust over."
   4. "When all lesions are healed."

Answer rationales available in your online resources.

ANSWERS 1. 1, 2, 4, 5; 2. 3; 3. 4; 4. 2, 4, 5, 6; 5. 2; 6. 4

Key Points

Find the chapter key points in your online resources available through Davis Edge.

Additional Resources

Study Guide

CHAPTER 55

Nursing Care of Patients With Burns

Rita Bolek Trofino

KEY TERMS

autograft (AW-toh-graft)
epithelialization (ep-ih-THEE-lee-al-eye-ZAY-shun)
escharotomy (es-kar-AHT-oh-mee)
hemochromogen (HEEM-oh-KROH-moh-jen)

CHAPTER CONCEPT

Tissue Integrity

LEARNING OUTCOMES

1. Explain the pathophysiology of burns.
2. Describe current therapeutic measures used for burns.
3. List data to collect when caring for patients with burns.
4. Plan nursing care for patients with burns.
5. Explain how you will know whether your nursing interventions have been effective.

Many people are hospitalized each year for burns. Burns affect not only the skin but also every major body system. Smoke inhalation and wound infections complicate care of the patient who has been burned.

 ## PATHOPHYSIOLOGY AND SIGNS AND SYMPTOMS

Burns are wounds caused by an energy transfer from a heat source to the body, heating the tissue enough to cause damage. Locally, the heat denatures cellular protein and interrupts the blood supply. The three zones of tissue damage that occur with burns are described in Figure 55.1.

The amount of skin damage is related to: (1) the temperature of the burning agent, (2) the burning agent itself, (3) the duration of exposure, (4) the conductivity of tissue, and (5) the thickness of the involved dermal structures. Alterations in normal skin function resulting from a major burn injury include loss of protective functions, impaired ability to regulate temperature, increased risk of infection, changes in sensory function, loss of fluids, impaired skin regeneration, and impaired secretory and excretory functions.

Systemic Responses

Alterations in the functional capacity of the skin in response to a burn affect virtually all major body systems.

Fluid Balance

Following a major burn, damaged cells release inflammatory mediators. The resulting inflammation causes increased capillary permeability, which in turn leads to the leakage of plasma and proteins into the tissue. This results in blisters and edema with a loss of intravascular volume. Water loss by evaporation through the burned tissue can be 4 to 15 times the normal amount. Increased metabolism leads to further water loss through the respiratory system.

Cardiac Function

A burn is followed by an initial decrease in cardiac output. This is further compromised by the loss of circulating plasma volume. Severe hematologic changes resulting from tissue damage and vascular changes occur in patients with major burns. Plasma moves into the interstitial space because of increased capillary permeability. In the first 48 hours after a burn, fluid shifts lead to hypovolemia and, if untreated, hypovolemic shock. Loss of intravascular fluid causes a relative increase in hematocrit, and red blood cells are destroyed. The intense heat decreases platelet function and half-life. Leukocyte and platelet aggregation may progress to thrombosis.

Metabolic Changes

Metabolic demands are very high in patients with burns. A high metabolic rate proportional to the severity of the burn

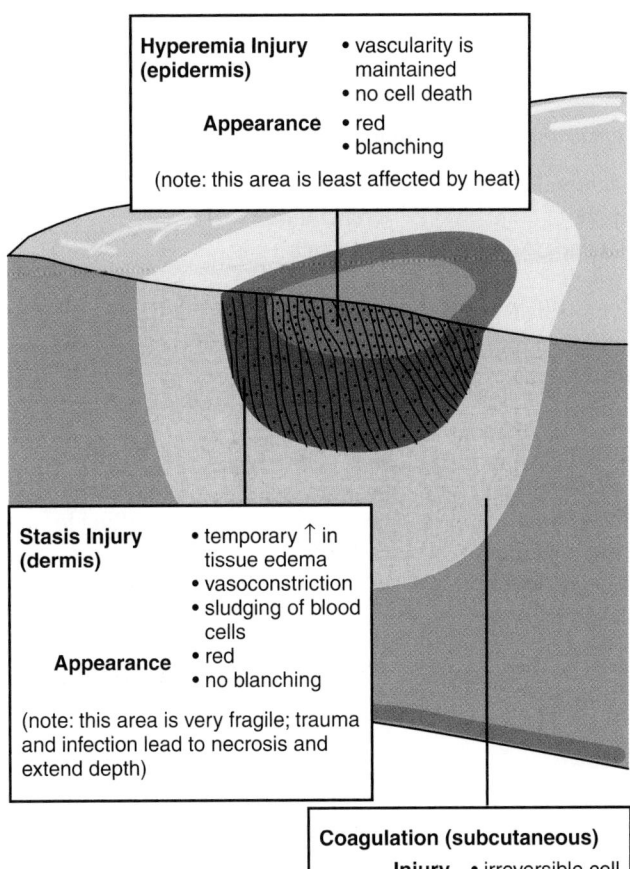

Hyperemia Injury (epidermis)
- vascularity is maintained
- no cell death

Appearance
- red
- blanching

(note: this area is least affected by heat)

Stasis Injury (dermis)
- temporary ↑ in tissue edema
- vasoconstriction
- sludging of blood cells

Appearance
- red
- no blanching

(note: this area is very fragile; trauma and infection lead to necrosis and extend depth)

Coagulation (subcutaneous)

Injury
- irreversible cell death

Appearance
- white or gray
- no blanching

FIGURE 55.1 Three zones of tissue damage.

is usually maintained until wound closure. This hypermetabolism is further compromised by associated injuries, surgical interventions, and the stress response. Severe catabolism also begins early. It is associated with a negative nitrogen balance, weight loss, and decreased wound healing. Elevated catecholamine (epinephrine, norepinephrine) levels are triggered by the stress response. This, along with elevated glucagon levels, can stimulate hyperglycemia.

Gastrointestinal Problems

Some gastrointestinal (GI) problems that can develop with a major burn include gastric dilation, peptic ulcers, and paralytic ileus. Most of these problems occur in response to fluid shifting, dehydration, opioid analgesics, immobility, depressed gastric motility, and the stress response.

Renal Function

Acute renal insufficiency can occur as a result of hypovolemia and decreased cardiac output. Fluid loss and inadequate fluid replacement can lead to decreased renal blood flow and glomerular filtration rate. Extensive burns can cause destruction of muscle, creating myoglobin casts that can block renal tubules and lead to renal failure.

Pulmonary Effects

Pulmonary effects are mostly related to smoke inhalation. However, hyperventilation may occur with any moderate to major burn injury, usually proportional to the severity of the burn. Oxygen consumption increases because of the hypermetabolic state, fear, anxiety, and pain.

> ### BE SAFE!
> ***BE VIGILANT!*** It is not uncommon to administer massive volumes of intravenous fluids to severely burned patients. The patient must be closely monitored with hemodynamic monitoring to avoid fluid overload.

Immune Function

With the skin destroyed, the body loses its first line of defense against infection. Major burns also depress immunoglobulin (Ig)A, IgG, and IgM.

> ### BE SAFE!
> ***BE VIGILANT!*** You must be vigilant in monitoring for infection, as infection is a real and life-threatening risk to severely burned patients.

Evaluation of Burn Injuries

The severity of a burn injury is determined by the depth of tissue destruction (Table 55.1 and Fig. 55.2), percentage of body surface area injured, cause of the burn, age of the patient, related injuries, medical history (e.g., heart disease, diabetes), and location of the burn wound.

The size of a burn wound is estimated based on parts of the body affected. A quick and common method is the Rule of Nines. This method divides the body into segments whose areas are either 9% or multiples of 9% of the total body surface, with the perineum being counted as 1% (Fig. 55.3). This formula is easy, but it is not as accurate when assessing children. A more accurate method uses a table with a relative anatomical scale or diagram that estimates total burned area by ages and by smaller anatomical areas of the body.

> ### NURSING CARE TIP
> For a quick estimation of percentage of burn injury on an adult patient, the palm of your hand is about 1%.

CRITICAL THINKING

Mr. Weinberg is admitted to the hospital with superficial and deep partial-thickness burns. His wife asks how long it will take for the burns to heal. What should you tell her?

Suggested answers are at the end of the chapter.

Table 55.1

Classification of Burn Depth

Classification	Formerly	Areas Involved	Appearance	Sensitivity	Healing Time
Partial thickness (superficial)	First to second degree	Epidermis Papillae of dermis	Bright red to pink Blanches to touch Serum-filled blisters Glistening, moist	Sensitive to air, temperature, and touch	7–10 days
Partial thickness (deep)	Second degree	Epidermis, half to seven-eighths of dermis	Blisters may be present Pink to light red to white Soft and pliable Blanching present	Pressure may be painful because of exposed nerve endings	14–21 days; may need grafting to decrease scarring
Full thickness	Third to fourth degree	Epidermis Dermis Tissue Muscle Bone	Snowy white, gray, or brown Texture is firm and leathery Inelastic	No pain because nerve endings are destroyed, unless surrounded by areas of partial-thickness burns	Grafting necessary to complete healing

Source: Trofino, R. B. (1996). Nursing management of the patient with burns. In S. Ruppert, J. Kernick, & J. Dolan (Eds.), *Dolan's critical care nursing* (p. 943). Philadelphia, PA: F.A. Davis.

 ## ETIOLOGY

Burn injuries have many causes. The most common causes include flames, contact burns, scalding, and chemical, electrical, and radiation burns. Table 55.2 summarizes common causes; see also "Gerontological Issues."

Gerontological Issues

Burn Injury and the Older Adult. Older adults face the greatest threat of dying in a fire as a result of several factors. Older adults have thinner skin. In addition, many suffer from comorbidities, such as diabetes and hypertension, that can increase recovery time and lead to a longer hospital stay.

Prevention measures for older adults should consider vision and hearing impairments as well as limited mobility. Individuals must be able to evacuate in case of a fire and seek help if a burn injury occurs. Nurses should target prevention measures toward the most common activities that can lead to fire or burn injury: smoking and cooking.

BE SAFE!

BE VIGILANT! Most burns are preventable. Prevention should focus on all areas, including electrical safety, fire safety, cooking safety, and scald prevention, especially in the very young and in older adults.

BE SAFE!

BE VIGILANT! Teach patients to keep the temperature of their hot water heater at 120°F or just below the medium setting—a safe bathing temperature—and to check water temperature before entering a bath or shower.

 ## COMPLICATIONS

A major complication with a flame burn in an enclosed space is inhalation injury. An inhalation injury is a major cause of morbidity and mortality associated with burn injuries. Treatment of an inhalation injury takes precedence

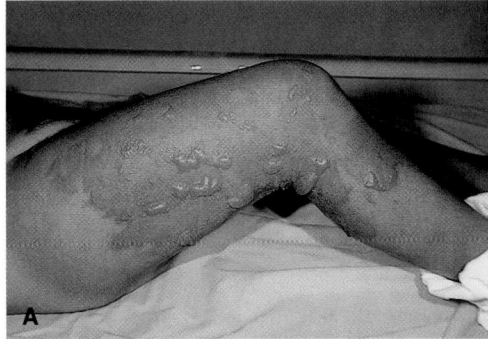

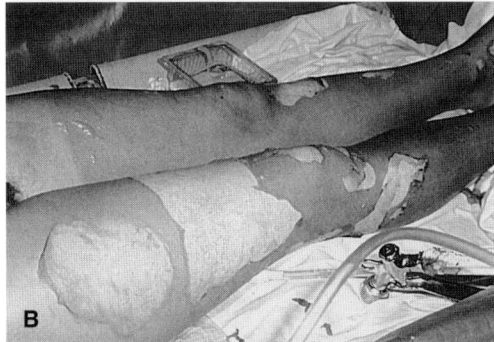

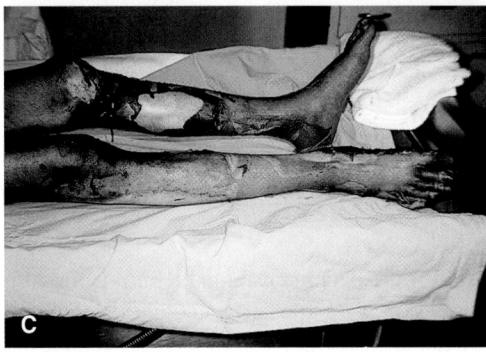

FIGURE 55.2 (A and B) Partial-thickness burns. (C) Full-thickness burn.

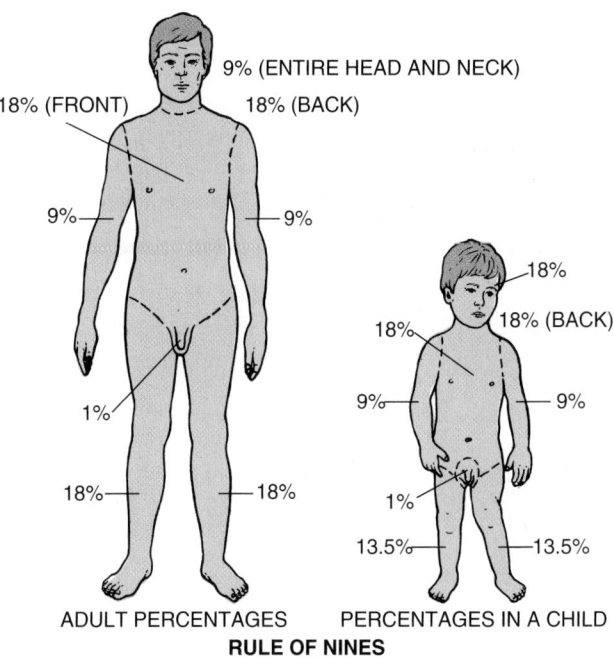

FIGURE 55.3 Estimation of extent of burn injury.

CRITICAL THINKING

Mrs. Rivera is admitted to the emergency department after sustaining injuries from a house fire. Both arms and hands are burned, she has a right leg fracture and a possible neck fracture, her lips are swollen, her face is sooty, and she is spitting up grayish-blackish sputum.

1. What is your priority concern with all of these injuries?
2. An intravenous line with normal saline is ordered at 1 L over 6 hours. How many milliliters per hour should be set on the controller?
3. Approximately what percent of her body is burned?
4. What members of the health care team will collaborate on Mrs. Rivera's care?

Suggested answers are at the end of the chapter.

over other injuries. (Remember your ABCs? Airway always comes first.) Infection is another common complication with a major burn. The incidence of infection increases with the size of the burn wound because the skin is the first line of defense against microorganisms.

Neurovascular compromise can also occur with a major burn. Eschar formation creates pressure and contributes to decreasing blood flow to areas distal to the burned area. Other systemic complications were reviewed in the "Systemic Responses" section earlier in this chapter.

DIAGNOSTIC TESTS

Burns are diagnosed by physical assessment. Various diagnostic tests are performed for systemic reactions, infection, and other complications. Common laboratory tests include complete blood count (CBC) and differential, blood urea nitrogen (BUN), serum glucose and electrolytes, serum protein and albumin levels, urinalysis, urine cultures, and clotting studies. If an inhalation injury is suspected, arterial blood gases, bronchoscopy, and carboxyhemoglobin levels are tested. X-rays, electrocardiogram, and wound cultures are completed if indicated.

THERAPEUTIC MEASURES

Therapeutic interventions vary according to the severity of the burn and the stage the patient is in. Treatment is managed across three overlapping stages (Table 55.3).

Emergent Stage
At the time of injury, the burning process must be stopped. Clothes are removed. The wound is cooled with tepid water.

Table 55.2

Common Causes of Burns

Flame	House fire is a common cause.
	Usually associated with an inhalation injury.
	Flash injury occurs from a sudden ignition or explosion.
Contact	Hot tar, hot metals, or hot grease produce a full-thickness injury on contact.
Scald	A burn from hot liquid.
	More common in children younger than age 5 and adults older than age 65.
	With an immersion scald, there are usually no splash marks; usually involves lower regions of body.
Chemical	Usually occurs in an industrial setting.
	Extent and depth of injury are directly proportional to concentration and quantity of agent, duration of contact, and chemical activity and penetrability of agent.
Electrical	One of the most serious types of burn injury; can be full thickness with possible loss of limbs; can cause internal injuries.
	Entry wound is usually ischemic, charred, and depressed.
	Exit wound may have an explosive appearance.
	Extent of injury depends on voltage, resistance of body, type of current, amperage, pathway of current, and duration of contact.
	Bones offer greatest resistance to the current, resulting in great damage.
	Tissue fluid, blood, and nerves offer least resistance; therefore, the current travels this path.
Radiation	Can occur in an industrial setting, as a result of treatment of disease, or from ultraviolet light (sun or tanning salons).
	Severity depends on type of radiation, duration of exposure, depth of penetration, distance from source, and absorbed dose.

Table 55.3

Stages of Burn Care

Stage	*Duration*
I: Emergent	From onset of injury to completion of fluid resuscitation
II: Acute	From start of diuresis to near completion of wound closure
III: Rehabilitation	From wound closure to return of optimal level of physical and psychosocial function

Source: Trofino, R. B. (1996). Nursing management of the patient with burns. In S. Ruppert, J. Kernick, & J. Dolan (Eds.), *Dolan's critical care nursing* (p. 948). Philadelphia, PA: F.A. Davis.

The patient is covered with clean sheets to decrease shivering and contamination. The burn wound itself is a lower priority than the ABCs (airway, breathing, circulation) of trauma resuscitation. Emergency rescuers at the scene will stabilize the victim by establishing an airway, ensuring oxygenation, inserting an intravenous (IV) line, and stabilizing fractures, hemorrhage, and spinal and other injuries. Inhalation injury is suspected if the patient sustained a burn from a fire in an enclosed space or was exposed to smoldering materials, if the face and neck are burned, if there are vocal changes, or if the patient is coughing up carbon particles. IV fluids are given to prevent and treat hypovolemic shock. The patient is treated for pain with IV opioid analgesics.

An accurate history of the injury is obtained to determine severity, potential complications, and any associated trauma. The patient's medical history is also obtained. Admission to the facility and burn care treatment are explained to the patient and family.

NURSING CARE TIP

If the patient is unable to communicate effectively, interview all involved witnesses to determine the cause of the injury as well as past and current medical history and medications the patient is taking. Getting a full description of the cause of the injury may lead to the detection of other injuries that may not be readily visible.

Acute Stage

If the patient is in a facility with a special burn unit, multidisciplinary care from a burn team is provided during the acute stage. Management goals include wound closure with no infection, minimum scarring, maximum function, maintenance of comfort as much as possible, adequate nutritional support, and maintenance of fluid, electrolyte, and acid–base balance. The patient continues to be medicated for pain as needed, especially before painful treatments. Patient-controlled analgesia (PCA) is very effective. Nutritional support may be maintained via nasogastric enteral feeding ("Nutrition Notes").

Nutrition Notes

Burns. The goals of nutritional support in burned patients are to (1) meet metabolic needs, (2) promote wound healing, (3) promote resistance to infection, and (4) reduce protein loss.

Early (within 4 to 6 hours of injury) use of nasogastric enteral feeding has been shown to reduce the incidence of mortality and infectious morbidity. Indirect calorimetry (IC) should be utilized to determine caloric needs, and needs should be reevaluated more than once per week. If IC is unavailable, caloric needs should be calculated at 25 to 30 kilocalories/kilogram per day. Protein needs are 1.5 to 2 grams/kilogram of body weight per day. A standardized polymeric formula should be utilized for enteral feeding. A combination of antioxidant vitamins (vitamins E and C) and trace minerals (selenium, zinc, and copper) improve patient outcomes and are recommended for burn patients.

When oral intake is possible, supplemental enteral feeding should be used if intake is inadequate. Because of infection risks, parenteral nutrition is reserved for those in whom enteral feeding is not feasible or at least 60% of calorie and protein needs are not met enterally.

Reference
Taylor, B. E., McClave, S. A., Martindale, R. G., Warren, M. M., Johnson, D. R., Braunschweig, C., … Compher, C. (2016). Guidelines for the provision and assessment of nutrition support therapy in the adult critically ill patient: Society of Critical Care Medicine (SCCM) and American Society for Parenteral and Enteral Nutrition (ASPEN). *Journal of Parenteral and Enteral Nutrition, 40*(2), 390–438.

The wound is cleansed and débrided daily to promote healing, prevent infection, and provide a clean bed for grafting. Wound cleansing is achieved by showering (using a shower trolley or shower chair) and bedside care.

Débridement, or the removal of nonviable tissue (eschar), can be done mechanically, surgically, with chemicals, or using a combination of these methods. Mechanical débridement can involve the use of scissors and forceps to manually excise loose, nonviable tissue or the use of wet-to-moist or wet-to-dry fine-mesh gauze dressings (see Chapter 54). Chemical débridement involves the use of a proteolytic enzymatic agent that digests necrotic tissue. Surgical débridement is the excision of full-thickness and deep

partial-thickness burns. This method is followed by application of a skin graft.

If the patient has a circumferential burn (one that surrounds an extremity or area), an increase in tissue pressure secondary to tissue edema occurs. The burn then acts like a tourniquet, impeding arterial and venous flow and impairing distal pulses. Common sites for these burns are the extremities, trunk, and chest. If this occurs on the chest and trunk, respiratory insufficiency can occur as a result of restricted chest expansion. An **escharotomy** may be immediately needed to relieve pressure. An escharotomy is a linear excision through the eschar to the superficial fat that allows for expansion of the skin and return of blood flow or chest expansion (Fig. 55.4).

NURSING CARE TIP
Remember to provide adequate padding of the bed before an escharotomy because this procedure can be accompanied by copious amounts of drainage. Provide for appropriate disposal of the drainage. For an extremity escharotomy, monitor the patient for return of distal pulses.

After the area is cleaned, the burn dressing and topical treatment are prescribed. The type of dressing and topical agent are chosen depending on the area involved, the extent and depth of injury, and health care provider (HCP) preference. Several common topical agents are listed in Table 55.4.

Dressings may be open, closed, biological, synthetic, or a combination. The open method is the use of a topical agent without any dressing. The closed method involves the use of an occlusive dressing over the wound. General principles for dressings include the following:

1. Limit the bulk of the dressing to facilitate range of motion.
2. Never wrap skin-to-skin surfaces (e.g., wrap fingers or toes separately; place a donut gauze dressing around the ear).
3. Base dressings on the size of wounds, absorption, protection, and type of débridement.
4. Wrap extremities from distal to proximal to promote venous return.
5. Do not wrap dressings too tightly. Check peripheral pulses often.
6. Elevate affected extremities.

The term *biological dressing* refers to a dressing that uses tissue from living or deceased humans (cadaver skin) or deceased animals (e.g., pigskin). It also refers to cellular dressings that may use animal tissue, human tissue, or synthetics. Biological dressings help with wound healing and stimulate

• WORD • BUILDING •
escharotomy: eschara—scab + otomy—incision

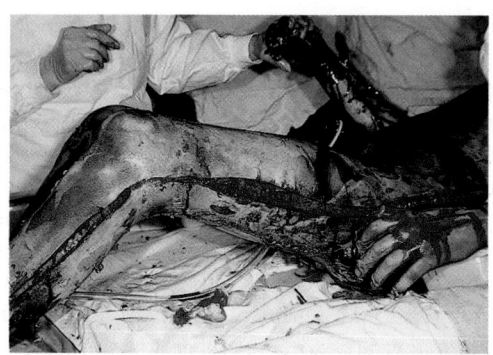

FIGURE 55.4 Escharotomy.

Table 55.4

Common Topical Broad-Spectrum Antibiotic Agents

Examples	Nursing Implications
silver sulfadiazine 1% cream (Silvadene)	Intermediate penetration of eschar. Butter on in thick layer. Cover with light dressings once or twice a day.
mafenide acetate (Sulfamylon)	Premedicate for pain. Butter on. Open exposure method. Apply three to four times daily. Keeps eschar soft for easier débridement.
silver nitrate solution 0.5%	Poor penetration of eschar. Ineffective on established wound infections. Apply with wet dressings, and change twice daily. Soak every 2 hours.
bacitracin (Baciguent)	Poor penetration of eschar. Butter on. Reapply every 4 to 6 hours.
gentamicin (Garamycin)	Painful on application. Apply gently three to four times daily.
mupirocin (Bactroban)	May cause burning, itching, and pain on application. Apply three times daily.
neomycin/ bacitracin/ polymyxin (Neosporin)	Apply one to three times daily.

epithelialization. These dressings may be used as donor site dressings, to manage a partial-thickness burn, or to cover a clean, excised wound before autografting. Some cellular wound dressings have varied layers that form a matrix onto which the patient's own cells migrate over a few weeks to form a new dermis. A very thin layer of the person's own skin is then grafted onto this new dermis.

Synthetic dressings are used in the management of partial-thickness burns and donor sites. Synthetic dressings are more readily available, less costly, and easier to store than biological dressings. They are made from a variety of materials and come in many sizes and shapes. Most of these dressings contain no antimicrobial agents.

Biological and synthetic dressings are used as temporary wound coverings over clean partial- and full-thickness injuries. They act as skin substitutes to help maintain the wound surface until healing occurs, a donor site becomes available, or the wound is ready for autografting.

Skin Grafts

AUTOGRAFT. An **autograft** is a skin graft from the patient's unburned skin that is placed on the clean, excised burn. The two common types of autografts are the split-thickness skin graft (STSG), which includes the epidermis and part of the dermis, and the full-thickness skin graft (FTSG), which includes the epidermis and entire dermal layer.

SPLIT THICKNESS SKIN GRAFT. An STSG (0.006 to 0.016 inch or 0.15 to 0.41 mm) may be applied as a sheet graft or a meshed graft. A sheet graft is used for cosmetic effect, such as for a face, neck, upper chest, breast, or hand burn. It is placed on the area as a full sheet. A meshed graft is passed through a "mesher" that produces tiny splits in the skin, similar to a fishnet, with openings in the shape of diamonds (Fig. 55.5). This permits the skin to expand one and a half to nine times its original size. The meshing allows for coverage of a large burn area with a small piece of skin by stretching it and securing it with sutures or staples. A mesh graft is especially useful when a patient's burns are extensive, resulting in few available donor sites. Graft "take," or vascularization, is complete in about 3 to 5 days.

FULL THICKNESS SKIN GRAFT. An FTSG (0.035 to 0.040 inch or 0.9 to 1.02 mm) can be a sheet graft or pedicle flap. These grafts are used over areas of muscle mass, soft tissue loss, hands, feet, and eyelids. They are not used for extensive wounds because the donor sites usually require an STSG for closure or closure from the wound edges. A pedicle graft or flap is a skin flap and subcutaneous tissue that is still attached at one corner by a "pedicle" to a blood supply (artery and vein); it is then attached to an adjacent area in need of

• WORD • BUILDING •

epithelialization: epi—over + thele—nipple + ization—condition
autograft: auto—self + graft—tissue transplant

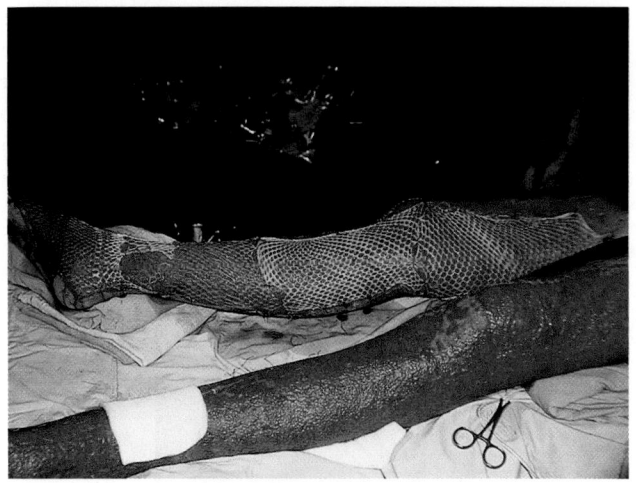

FIGURE 55.5 Meshed graft.

trauma and infection. Use of semiocclusive, transparent dressings (e.g., OpSite, Biobrane, Tegaderm) allows for a moist healing environment and is associated with reduced risk of infection. The donor site is very painful. Appropriate pain medications are provided, along with nonpharmacologic measures (e.g., back rubs or distraction).

With any type of graft, the patient must keep the graft site immobilized until the graft takes, to prevent movement or slippage of the grafted skin. Dressings may be bulky to assist in immobilization. These dressings must not be disturbed. The involved area requires frequent circulatory checks, including assessment of color, warmth, sensation, pulses, and capillary refill. Any involved extremities must be elevated to maintain circulation. A graft has been successful if there is good adherence of the graft to the wound with no evidence of necrosis or infection.

Rehabilitation Stage

The therapy started during the acute phase continues in the rehabilitation phase. There is wound closure, and the goal is to return the patient to an optimum level of physical and psychosocial function. This may take months to years to accomplish, depending on the extent of the injury. Reconstructive surgeries may be ongoing for many years.

Two things to keep in mind when caring for the patient with a major burn are: (1) the most comfortable position (flexion) is the position of contracture, and (2) the burn wound will shorten until it meets an opposing force. Have you ever seen a contracture? They are uncomfortable and debilitating. To avoid contractures (Fig. 55.6), a specific exercise program is begun 24 to 48 hours after injury, along with the use of splinting devices to maintain proper positioning

grafting. Once the distal part of the graft takes, it remains in place and the flap is divided, with the remainder returning to the original site. Pedicle flaps are not as popular as free skin flaps because they require more than one surgery, and it takes longer for the graft site and donor site to heal. Table 55.5 provides a comparison of split-thickness and full-thickness skin grafts.

Donor sites are considered partial-thickness wounds. They usually heal in 10 to 14 days, but this depends on the thickness and method of grafting and the general health of the patient. Treatment for the donor site varies with the individual patient, the area of the body, and HCP preference. Considerations for care include promoting comfort and preventing

Table 55.5
Comparison of Split-Thickness and Full-Thickness Skin Grafts

	Split-Thickness Skin Graft	*Full-Thickness Skin Graft*
Layers	Epidermis Partial layer of dermis	Epidermis Entire dermal layer
Advantages	Donor site may be reused. Healing of donor site is more rapid; results in a good "take."	Allows more elasticity over joints. Can reconstruct cosmetic defects. Soft, pliable. Gives full appearance. Provides good color match. Less hyperpigmentation. May allow hair growth.
Disadvantages	Prone to chronic breakdown. Likely to hypertrophy. More likely to contract.	Donor site takes longer to heal. Requires split-thickness skin graft to heal or closure from wound edges.

Source: Konop, D. (1991). General local treatment. In R. B. Trofino (Ed.), *Nursing care of the burn-injured patient* (p. 61). Philadelphia, PA: F.A. Davis.

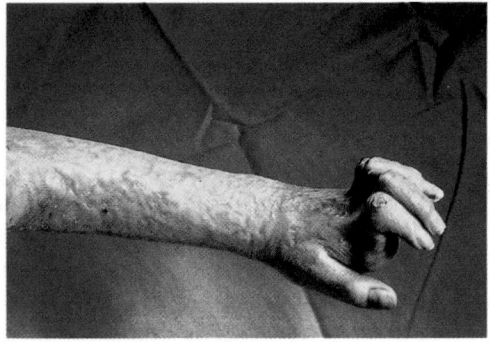

FIGURE 55.6 Burn deformity: contracture.

and stretching. Hypertrophic scarring, or a proliferation of scar tissue, can be minimized or prevented through the use of a pressure garment (Fig. 55.7).

As the burn heals, itching may occur and be intense at times. It is important to control itching, because scratching can impair healing and increase risk of infection ("Evidence-Based Practice").

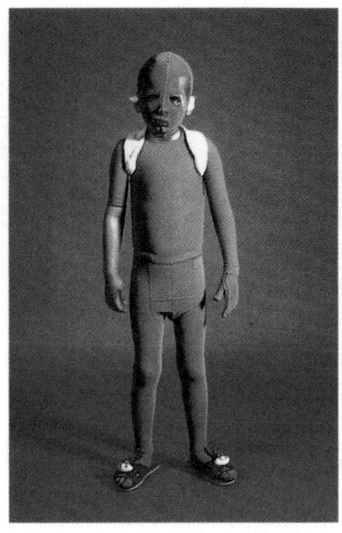

FIGURE 55.7 Full-body pressure garment.

Evidence-Based Practice

Clinical Question
What interventions are helpful for treating itching in a healing burn?

Evidence
Itching (pruritis) can interfere with activities of daily living. Treatment of itching can include pharmacological and nonpharmacological approaches. Some treatments shown to be helpful include cimetidine (an oral antihistamine) and colloidal oatmeal baths. Nonpharmacological techniques include massage in combination with hydrating lotions, application of cold (cool) cloths, and transcutaneous electrical nerve stimulation (TENS) (International Society for Burn Injury, 2016).

Implications for Nursing Practice
Postburn itching affects about 87% of patients. Assessment of postburn itching should be a part of routine care. Pruritus can increase pain and cause insomnia. Assess for the intensity and impact of itching on a 0-to-10 scale and advocate for appropriate orders.

Reference
International Society for Burn Injury. (2016). ISBI practice guidelines for burn care. *Burns, 42*(5), 953–1021.

Psychosocial Effects of Burn Injury
A burn affects the patient's psychosocial status in many ways. The magnitude of these effects is related to the age of the patient, location of the burn (e.g., face, hands) and changes in body image, recovery from injury, cause of the injury (especially if related to negligence or a deliberate act), and ability to continue at the preburn level of normal daily activities. The

patient may experience a disruption of role function and general health and coping ability. Treatment involves the patient and family members. Referrals to support groups, counselors, and psychiatrists are important during this stage.

CRITICAL THINKING

Mrs. Potter is recovering from partial-thickness burns and skin grafts. She mentions that she and her family will be going on a much-needed vacation to the shore. What concerns do you have?
   Suggested answers are at end of the chapter.

NURSING CARE TIP
Use caution with heating pads, water temperature, and electrical equipment when working with your patients. Burns are considered serious reportable events because they can be prevented, and thus hospitals will not be paid by Medicare for treating burns acquired during hospitalization.

NURSING PROCESS FOR A PATIENT WITH A BURN INJURY

Data Collection
A major burn is painful and frightening for the patient as well as for the family. Obtain information from the patient, family, and rescuers. If the injury occurred in an enclosed space with flames or smoldering materials, suspect an inhalation injury. If an electrical injury has occurred, ask about voltage, duration of contact, host susceptibility (wet or dry skin), entry and exit sites, and associated falls. With chemical burns, determine the type of agent and duration of exposure.

General information to collect for all burns (in addition to normally collected data, such as medical history, allergies, and current medications) includes extent, depth, type, and location of the burn; burn agent; duration of contact with the burning agent; severity and location of pain; and associated injuries. Determine the immediate first aid treatment provided at the scene. Obtain psychosocial information, including other people injured, additional losses (e.g., home, pets), whether the patient was at fault, and how this injury affects the patient's role function.

Nursing Diagnoses, Planning, Implementation, and Evaluation

See "Nursing Care Plan for the Patient With a Major Burn Injury" and Table 55.6. Priority nursing diagnoses are presented here. Additional diagnoses such as *Body Image Disturbance* become important during the rehabilitation stage. For more information on burns, go to the American Burn Association web site at www.ameriburn.org.

Nursing Care Plan for the Patient With a Major Burn Injury

Nursing Diagnosis: *Impaired Gas Exchange* related to upper airway edema, carbon monoxide (CO) poisoning, and edema of alveolar capillary membranes, as evidenced by abnormal arterial blood gases (ABGs) and elevated CO level
Expected Outcomes: The patient's gas exchange will be improved as evidenced by patent airway, CO level less than 10%, clear lung sounds, partial pressure of oxygen (Pao_2) 80 to 100 mm Hg, partial pressure of carbon dioxide ($Paco_2$) 35 to 45 mm Hg, oxygen saturation (Spo_2) 95%, responsiveness, and awareness.
Evaluation of Outcomes: Are oxygenation levels improved? Do the lungs sound clear on auscultation? Is the patient aware of his or her surroundings? Are signs of respiratory distress absent (e.g., retractions, nasal flaring, use of accessory muscles)?

Intervention	Rationale	Evaluation
Assess respiratory status; auscultate breath sounds every 15 minutes or as needed. Note any adventitious breath sounds. Observe for chest excursion. Monitor ability to cough.	*Assessment detects changes in pulmonary function for planning care.*	What is patient's respiratory status? Are any adventitious lung sounds noted?
Monitor ABGs and Spo_2 and CO levels.	*Assesses level of oxygenation and helps guide oxygen therapy.*	Is oxygenation adequate?
Monitor for nasal flaring, retractions, wheezing, and stridor.	*Stridor may signal upper airway involvement. Nasal flaring, retractions, and wheezing may indicate lower airway involvement.*	Does patient exhibit signs of upper or lower airway involvement?
Administer humidified 100% oxygen via tight-fitting facemask as ordered.	*Provides oxygen for adequate gas exchange.*	Is oxygen administered appropriately? Are ABGs improving?
Elevate head of bed (if no cervical spine injuries or no history of multiple trauma).	*Decreases swelling of face and neck. Increases ability to expand lungs.*	Is head of bed elevated? Is there any change in facial or neck swelling?
Provide appropriate pulmonary care: turn, cough, deep breathe every 2 to 4 hours.	*Mobilizes secretions and promotes lung expansion.*	Is patient receiving vigorous pulmonary care? Is it affecting outcomes?
Provide incentive spirometer every 2 to 4 hours.	*Promotes lung expansion to prevent atelectasis and mobilize secretions.*	Is patient able to take deep breaths? Are lungs clear?
Suction frequently as needed.	*Keeps airways free of secretions.*	Is suctioning effective? Are lungs clear?
Obtain sputum cultures as ordered. Note amount, color, and consistency of pulmonary secretions.	*Carbonaceous sputum indicates smoke inhalation injury. Infection changes color, amount, and consistency of sputum. Culture and sensitivity (C&S) assists in selection of appropriate antibiotic.*	Is patient coughing up any sputum? Has character of sputum been reported and documented?

(nursing care plan continues on page 1200)

Nursing Care Plan for the Patient With a Major Burn Injury—cont'd

Intervention	Rationale	Evaluation
Administer bronchodilators and antibiotics as prescribed.	*Bronchodilators decrease bronchospasms and edema. Antibiotics fight infection.*	Are medications effective?

Nursing Diagnosis: *Impaired Skin Integrity* related to thermal injury as evidenced by presence of burn lesions
Expected Outcomes: The patient's skin integrity will be improved as evidenced by the stopping of burning process and healing of burned areas with no infection present.
Evaluation of Outcomes: Did burning process stop? Is burned area healed and free from infection?

Intervention	Rationale	Evaluation
Obtain history of burning agent.	*Provides information related to depth, duration of contact, and resistance of tissues. If fire scenario, consider possible inhalation injury.*	What caused this thermal injury? How long was patient in contact with agent?
Assess burning process. If heat is felt on wound, cool with tepid tap water or sterile water, while keeping patient from chilling.	*Depth of injury increases with length of exposure to burning agent.*	Is heat felt over wounds? Has burn process been effectively stopped?
Remove clothing and jewelry.	*These items can retain heat and thermal agent, therefore increasing depth of injury. Jewelry can be constrictive when edema develops.*	Are clothing and jewelry removed and constriction avoided?
Do not apply ice.	*Ice causes vasoconstriction, further increasing skin damage. Ice also causes a decrease in core body temperature, which may promote shock.*	Is burning stopped without the use of ice?
Cover patient with clean sheet or blanket.	*Prevents excessive heat loss. Decreases pain from air exposure. Protects patient from environmental contamination.*	Is patient covered and protected?
For all chemical burns, initiate immediate copious tepid water lavage for 20 minutes along with simultaneous removal of contaminated clothing. Do not neutralize chemical because this takes too much time, and resulting reaction may generate heat and cause further skin injury.	*Dilution and removal of chemical agent halts burning process. Lavage dissipates heat.*	Has lavage been initiated?
Brush off dry chemicals before lavage.	*To prevent further burn damage due to reaction of dry chemical with water.*	Are dry chemicals removed?
Use heavy rubber gloves or thick gauze for removal of clothing.	*Protects health care workers from injury.*	Do health care workers remain safe?
Cleanse wound at bedside or via showering.	*Promotes healing and helps decrease infection.*	Is burn wound clean and free of wound debris?

Nursing Care Plan for the Patient With a Major Burn Injury—cont'd

Intervention	Rationale	Evaluation
Assist registered nurse (RN) or health care provider (HCP) to assess the burn area for extent (percentage) and depth (partial thickness, full thickness) of injury.	*Provides basis for triage of care. Important for calculating resuscitation fluid therapy.*	What is the estimation of percentage of burn injury? What is depth of injury?
Assist RN or HCP with débriding wound via surgical, chemical, or mechanical means. Apply topical agent as prescribed.	*Promotes healing and healthy granulation bed. Most agents prevent infection and promote healing.*	Is eschar present? Is wound free of wound debris? Is agent applied as directed?
Apply dressing as prescribed.	*Dressing types vary and are influenced by area, extent, and depth of injury as well as by topical agent used. Dressing protects burn area and promotes healing.*	Is dressing applied appropriately?
Do not wrap skin surface to skin surface (e.g., wrap fingers and toes separately; donut bandage around ears).	*Wrapping separately prevents webbing and contractures.*	Are skin surfaces separated? Are webbing and contractures avoided?
Limit bulk of dressings.	*Mobility is enhanced with less bulky dressing.*	Is patient's mobility maximized?
Wrap extremities from distal to proximal.	*Circulation is increased when extremities are wrapped distal to proximal.*	Is wrapping done correctly? Is edema of distal extremity avoided?

Nursing Diagnosis: *Deficient Fluid Volume* related to evaporative losses from wound, capillary leak, and decreased fluid intake as evidenced by urine output less than 30-50 mL per hour, hypotension, tachycardia, and weight loss
Expected Outcomes: The (adult) patient will maintain adequate circulating volume as evidenced by urine output of 30-50 mL/hr, blood pressure within normal limits, heart rate between 60 and 100 beats per minute, and stabilized body weight.
Evaluation of Outcomes: Is urine output maintained at least at 30-50 mL/hr? Are blood pressure and heart rate within normal limits? Is the patient's weight stable?

Intervention	Rationale	Evaluation
Obtain admission weight, and monitor weight daily.	*Helps measure fluid loss or gain.*	Is patient's weight documented? Is it stable?
Record intake and output (I&O) hourly.	*Serves as guide for fluid loss and replacement.*	Is urine output adequate?
Examine for signs and symptoms of hypovolemia (e.g., hypotension, tachycardia, tachypnea, extreme thirst, restlessness, disorientation).	*Fluid volume loss is multifocal (e.g., through increased capillary permeability, insensible loss).*	Does patient exhibit any signs or symptoms of hypovolemia?
Monitor electrolytes and complete blood count (CBC), and report abnormal results to HCP.	*Serves as guide for electrolyte replacement and blood product replacement.*	What are patient's lab values? Are abnormal results reported?
Administer or monitor intravenous (IV) fluids as ordered via large-bore IV catheter.	*Fluid replacement begins immediately to prevent hypovolemia. Large vessels are needed for rapid delivery of fluids.*	Is patient's fluid replacement adequate? Is catheter patent?

(nursing care plan continues on page 1202)

Nursing Care Plan for the Patient With a Major Burn Injury—cont'd

Intervention	Rationale	Evaluation
Insert indwelling urinary catheter.	*Accurate urine output measurement is essential for fluid replacement calculation.*	Is catheter patent and output recorded?
Monitor urine for amount, specific gravity, and **hemochromogen.**	*Specific gravity helps predict volume replacement. Hemochromogen can cause renal tubular damage.*	What are patient's urine values?
Administer osmotic diuretics as ordered; monitor response to therapy.	*Decreased urine output can be caused by decreased renal flow (due to myoglobin in urine).*	What is urine output? Has it changed due to therapy?
Assess gastrointestinal function for absence of bowel sounds. Maintain nasogastric tube as ordered.	*Splanchnic constriction due to hypovolemia can cause a paralytic ileus.*	Are patient's bowel sounds within normal limits? Is nasogastric tube patent?

Nursing Diagnosis: *Acute Pain* related to burns or graft donor sites as evidenced by patient's rating on appropriate pain scale, restlessness, and sleeplessness
Expected Outcomes: The patient will experience pain control as evidenced by pain rating acceptable to patient and nonverbal cues, such as less restlessness and ability to rest or sleep.
Evaluation of Outcomes: Does the patient verbalize pain control? How many hours of rest/sleep does the patient get in 24 hours? Does the patient state she or he feels rested?

Intervention	Rationale	Evaluation
Assess pain using *WHAT'S UP?* mnemonic. Rate pain on appropriate pain scale.	*Provides baseline to monitor response to therapy.*	Is patient's individual response to pain documented?
Observe for varied responses to acute pain: increase in blood pressure, pulse, and respirations; increased restlessness and irritability; increased muscle tension; facial grimaces; guarding.	*Responses to pain are variable. These parameters change in response to pain.*	What are patient's responses to pain? Do responses change with treatment?
Acknowledge presence of pain. Explain causes of pain.	*Encourages trust and understanding.*	Is patient more trusting of the nurse and the treatments?
Administer opioids as ordered. Use patient-controlled analgesia (PCA) as appropriate.	*Opioids are needed for severe burn pain. PCA allows patient more control.*	Is patient being medicated for pain appropriately?
Offer diversional activities (e.g., music, TV, books, games, relaxation techniques).	*Helps patient focus on something other than pain.*	Does patient use diversional activities? Do they help?
Position patient for comfort in good body alignment.	*Increases comfort.*	Is patient positioned as comfortably as possible?
Elevate burned extremities.	*Elevation decreases edema and pain.*	Are extremities elevated? Is pain reduced?

• WORD • BUILDING •
hemochromogen: hemo—blood + chromo—color + gen—producing

Nursing Care Plan for the Patient With a Major Burn Injury—cont'd

Intervention	Rationale	Evaluation
Maintain comfortable environment (e.g., bed cradle, comfortable environmental temperature of 86–91.4°F (30–33°C), quiet environment).	*Pressure from bed linens may cause discomfort; with loss of integument, body cannot self-regulate temperature.*	Does patient verbalize comfort of environment?

Nursing Diagnosis: *Impaired Physical Mobility* related to burn healing, pain, and contractures
Expected Outcomes: The patient will maintain adequate physical mobility as evidenced by ability to ambulate, move in bed, and tolerate activity.
Evaluation of Outcomes: Is the patient able to sit? Is the patient able to get out of bed? Is the patient able to walk with or without assistance?

Intervention	Rationale	Evaluation
Encourage ambulation as able.	*Helps prevent atelectasis and pneumonia.*	Is patient optimally mobilized?
Perform active and passive range of motion exercises on affected areas.	*Prevents contractures and hypertrophic scarring.*	Do affected areas remain mobile?
Provide support above and below affected joints. Apply splints and functional devices as ordered.	*Maintains functional position of extremities.*	Are immobilized joints in a functional position?
For lower extremity burns, apply bandages and elastic bandages before patient is in upright position.	*Promotes venous return and minimizes edema formation.*	Does patient tolerate being upright? Is edema minimized?

Nursing Diagnosis: *Ineffective Peripheral Tissue Perfusion* related to circumferential burns, blood loss, and decreased cardiac output as evidenced by weak pulses, cool extremities, limited movement, and sensation
Expected Outcomes: The patient will maintain adequate tissue perfusion as evidenced by presence of peripheral pulses, minimal edema, intact sensation and motion, and warm extremities.
Evaluation of Outcomes: Are peripheral pulses present? Are extremities warm, with adequate sensation, movement, and circulation? Is edema decreased?

Intervention	Rationale	Evaluation
Assess pulses on burned extremities every 15 minutes until stable, then every hour.	*If pulses diminish, an escharotomy may be indicated.*	Are pulses present and documented?
Use Doppler as needed to detect weak pulses. Assess capillary refill, sensation, color, swelling, and movement.	*Assesses peripheral perfusion.*	Is the extremity warm, with adequate color, sensation, movement, and capillary refill?
Monitor for numbness, tingling, and increased pain in burned extremity.	*Can be indicative of increased pressure from edema.*	Does patient report numbness, tingling, or pain?
Measure circumference of burned extremities.	*Monitors edema formation.*	Is there evidence of edema? Is it getting better or worse?
Report changes in assessment promptly.	*Emergency intervention may be indicated.*	Does patient require an emergency intervention?
Elevate burned extremity above level of the heart.	*Enhances venous return and decreases edema formation.*	Are all burned extremities elevated above heart level? Is edema decreasing?

(nursing care plan continues on page 1204)

Nursing Care Plan for the Patient With a Major Burn Injury—cont'd

Intervention	Rationale	Evaluation
Apply burn dressing loosely.	*Prevents constriction and allows for expansion as edema forms.*	Is dressing limiting circulation?
Assist with muscle compartment pressure measurement.	*Helps determine need for escharotomy (if pressure exceeds 25 mm Hg).*	What is patient's pressure?
Assist with escharotomy as needed.	*If indicated, removal of eschar allows for edema expansion and permits peripheral perfusion.*	Does patient require an escharotomy? Is edema relieved?

Nursing Diagnosis: *Risk for Infection*
Expected Outcome: The patient will not develop a wound infection or sepsis.
Evaluation of Outcome: Is there healthy granulation tissue on unhealed areas with no evidence of infection? Are donor sites free of infection? Have skin grafts taken? Is there absence of clinical manifestation of infection (e.g., temperature 98.6°F [37°C], normal white blood cell [WBC] count)?

Intervention	Rationale	Evaluation
Use sterile technique with wound care.	*The unhealed burn wound is an excellent culture medium for bacterial growth.*	Is sterile technique used for all wound care?
Maintain protective isolation with careful hand hygiene.	*Prevents spread of bacteria from patient to patient or nurse to patient.*	Do all persons in contact with patient maintain proper precautions?
Administer immunosupportive medications as prescribed (tetanus and gamma globulin).	*Immunoglobulins are depressed at time of severe burn injury.*	Have medications been administered if indicated?
Perform wound care as prescribed, which may include the following: inspect and débride wounds daily; culture wound three times a week or at sign of infection; shave hair at least 1 inch around burn areas if necessary (excluding eyebrows); inspect invasive line sites for inflammation (especially if line is through a burn area).	*Provides quick identification of bacterial wound invasion and decreases incidence of infection. Presence of hair increases medium for bacterial growth.*	What does wound look like? Is it débrided? What are culture results? Does hair present a risk for infection?
Continually assess for and report signs and symptoms of sepsis (e.g., temperature elevation, change in sensorium, changes in vital signs and bowel sounds, decreased output, positive blood and wound cultures).	*The burn patient is at risk for sepsis until wound is healed.*	Does patient exhibit any signs or symptoms of sepsis?
Administer systemic antibiotics and topical agents as prescribed.	*Antibiotics prevent or treat infection.*	Does patient require systemic antibiotics? Are topical agents applied appropriately? Is wound healing?

Table 55.6
Burn Summary

Signs and Symptoms	Pain Superficial partial-thickness burn: pink to red skin, blisters Deep partial-thickness burn: pink to light red or white skin, blisters, blanching Full-thickness burn: white, gray, or brown color; firm and leathery
Diagnostic Tests	Wound cultures Complete blood count (CBC), blood urea nitrogen (BUN), glucose, electrolytes, urine studies
Therapeutic Measures	Intravenous fluid replacement Antibiotic/antimicrobial agents Analgesics
Complications	Shock Wound infection
Priority Nursing Diagnoses	*Impaired Gas Exchange* *Impaired Skin Integrity* *Deficient Fluid Volume* *Acute Pain* related to burns or graft donor sites *Impaired Physical Mobility* *Ineffective Peripheral Tissue Perfusion* *Risk for Infection*

SUGGESTED ANSWERS TO CRITICAL THINKING

Mr. Weinberg
Superficial partial-thickness burns usually heal in 7 to 10 days. Deep partial-thickness burns may take up to 3 weeks. All of this depends on the location of the injury, the health of the patient, and if he remains infection free.

Mrs. Rivera
1. Mrs. Rivera has an inhalation injury. This takes precedence over the burn and other injuries.
2.

$$\frac{1\,L}{6\,hr} \cdot \frac{1{,}000\,mL}{1\,L} = 167\,mL/hr$$

3. Approximately 18%.

4. Burn care requires a true interdisciplinary approach. She has a major burn, so the burn nurse will collaborate with a burn physician, plastic surgeon, pulmonary physician, orthopedic surgeon, physician assistant or nurse practitioner, physical therapist, occupational therapist, and dietitian.

Mrs. Potter
The burned and graft areas will be sensitive to sunlight for up to 1 year. These areas should be covered, and she needs to use sunscreen anytime she is out in the sun. Her health care provider should offer guidance as to whether any exposure is safe and, if so, what type of sunscreen agent is recommended. In addition, if any areas are not completely healed, she will be at risk for infection.

Review Questions

1. A patient is brought to the emergency department after a house fire. The patient has extensive trunk and lower extremity burns and is diagnosed with a deep partial-thickness burn. What assessment findings does the nurse expect?
   1. Snowy white, painless lesions
   2. Blistered, pinkish-white, painful lesions
   3. Blackened, painful lesions
   4. Bright-red, moist lesions

2. Which of the following actions is appropriate initial treatment of a chemical burn?
   1. Lavage with water.
   2. Neutralize the chemical.
   3. Apply the prescribed topical agent.
   4. Wrap the patient in sterile sheets.

3. A patient is admitted to the emergency department with flame burns to the entire chest, abdomen, back, and upper extremities. Using the Rule of Nines, what approximate percentage of burns should the nurse document?
   1. 36%
   2. 45%
   3. 54%
   4. 64%

4. Which nursing interventions are appropriate for a patient with a circumferential burn to an extremity? **Select all that apply.**
   1. Apply compression bandages starting at the distal end of the extremity.
   2. Administer analgesics if numbness or tingling occur.
   3. Check neurovascular status hourly.
   4. Assist with escharotomy if indicated.
   5. Elevate the extremity.

5. How will the nurse know if interventions for impaired gas exchange related to smoke inhalation have been effective?
   1. Partial pressure of carbon dioxide ($Paco_2$) is greater than 45 mm Hg.
   2. Oxygen saturation (Spo_2) is less than 90%.
   3. pH is 7.34.
   4. Partial pressure of oxygen (Pao_2) is 88 mm Hg.

Answer rationales available in your online resources.

ANSWERS 1. 2; 2. 1; 3. 4; 4. 3, 4, 5; 5. 4

Key Points

Find the chapter key points in your online resources available through Davis Edge.

Additional Resources

DAVIS
edge.

◀ Use the scratch off code on the inside front cover of your book to access online quizzes that will help you to improve your scores on course exams and prepare for the NCLEX-PN®.

Study Guide

CHAPTER 56

Mental Health Function, Assessment, and Therapeutic Measures

Marina Martinez-Kratz

KEY TERMS

adaptation (a-dap-TAY-shun)
affect (AF-ekt)
anxiety (ang-ZY-uh-tee)
cognitive (KOG-nih-tiv)
coping (KOH-ping)
electroconvulsive therapy (ee-LEK-troh kun-VUL-siv THER-uh-pee)
imagery (IM-ij-ree)
insight (IN-site)
mental health (MEN-tuhl HELTH)
mental illness (MEN-tuhl ILL-ness)
milieu (meel-YOO)
psychoanalysis (SY-koh-uh-NAL-ih-sis)
psychopharmacology (SY-koh-FAR-mah-KAWL-luh-jee)
psychotherapy (SY-koh-THER-uh-pee)
stress (STRESS)
stressor (STRESS-ur)

LEARNING OUTCOMES

1. Define mental health and mental illness.
2. Describe the components of a mental health status assessment.
3. Describe the *Diagnostic and Statistical Manual of Mental Disorders* (5th ed.; *DSM-5*) as a tool to diagnose mental illness.
4. Identify common ego defense mechanisms.
5. Describe characteristics of a therapeutic milieu.
6. Explain how psychoanalysis, behavior management, cognitive behavioral therapy, counseling, group therapy, electroconvulsive therapy, and relaxation therapy are carried out.
7. Describe the role of the licensed practical nurse/licensed vocational nurse (LPN/LVN) in mental health nursing.

CHAPTER CONCEPTS

Cognition
Communication
Mood
Neurologic Regulation
Stress

REVIEW OF NEUROLOGIC ANATOMY AND PHYSIOLOGY

When studying mental illnesses, it is important to review and understand the anatomy and physiology of the brain and central nervous system (CNS). The brain is involved in many functions, including thinking, decision making, speaking, emotion, memory, motor and sensory activity, and the basic functions of temperature regulation and breathing. Refer to Chapter 47 to review the nerves, structure of neurons, synapses, neurotransmitters, and the autonomic nervous system as well as the structure and function of the brain. Table 56.1 presents the hypothesized roles of CNS neurotransmitters in mental illness.

MENTAL HEALTH AND MENTAL ILLNESS

Opinions within the mental health community differ as to what mental health and mental illness are. **Mental health** has been defined in many ways. These definitions include the ability to do the following:

• Be flexible.
• Take responsibility for own actions.
• Form close relationships.
• Make appropriate judgments.
• Solve problems.
• Cope with daily **stress.**
• Have a positive sense of self.

Table 56.1

Neurotransmitters in the Central Nervous System

Location/Function	Possible Implications for Mental Health
Cholinergics	
Acetylcholine	
Autonomic nervous system (ANS): sympathetic and parasympathetic presynaptic nerve terminals, parasympathetic postsynaptic nerve terminals Central nervous system (CNS): cerebral cortex, hippocampus, limbic structures, basal ganglia *Functions:* sleep, arousal, pain perception, movement, memory	*Decreased levels:* Alzheimer disease, Huntington disease, Parkinson disease *Increased levels:* depression
Monoamines	
Norepinephrine	
ANS: sympathetic postsynaptic nerve terminals CNS: thalamus, hypothalamus, limbic system, hippocampus, cerebellum, cerebral cortex *Functions:* mood, cognition, perception, locomotion, cardiovascular functioning, sleep and arousal	*Decreased levels:* depression *Increased levels:* mania, anxiety states, schizophrenia
Dopamine	
Frontal cortex, limbic system, basal ganglia, thalamus, posterior pituitary, spinal cord *Functions:* movement and coordination, emotions, voluntary judgment, release of prolactin	*Decreased levels:* Parkinson disease, depression *Increased levels:* mania, schizophrenia
Serotonin	
Hypothalamus, thalamus, limbic system, cerebral cortex, cerebellum, spinal cord *Functions:* sleep and arousal, libido, appetite, mood, aggression, pain perception, coordination, judgment	*Decreased levels:* depression *Increased levels:* anxiety states
Histamine	
Hypothalamus	*Decreased levels:* depression
Amino Acids	
Gamma-Aminobutyric Acid (GABA)	
Hypothalamus, hippocampus, cortex, cerebellum, basal ganglia, spinal cord, retina *Functions:* slowdown of body activity	*Decreased levels:* Huntington disease, anxiety disorders, schizophrenia, various forms of epilepsy
Glycine	
Spinal cord, brainstem *Functions:* recurrent inhibition of motor neurons	*Toxic levels:* "glycine encephalopathy"; decreased levels are correlated with spastic motor movement
Glutamate and Aspartate	
Pyramidal cells of the cortex, cerebellum, and primary sensory afferent systems; hippocampus, thalamus, hypothalamus, spinal cord *Functions:* relay of sensory information and in the regulation of various motor and spinal reflexes	*Increased levels:* Huntington disease, temporal lobe epilepsy, spinal cerebellar degeneration

Table 56.1

Neurotransmitters in the Central Nervous System—cont'd

Location/Function	*Possible Implications for Mental Health*
Neuropeptides	
Endorphins and Enkephalins Hypothalamus, thalamus, limbic structures, midbrain, brainstem; enkephalins are also found in the gastrointestinal tract *Functions:* modulation of pain and reduced peristalsis (enkephalins)	Modulation of dopamine activity by opioid peptides may indicate some link to the symptoms of schizophrenia
Substance P Hypothalamus, limbic structures, midbrain, brainstem, thalamus, basal ganglia, spinal cord; also found in gastrointestinal tract and salivary glands *Function:* regulation of pain	*Decreased levels:* Huntington disease and Alzheimer disease *Increased levels:* depression
Somatostatin Cerebral cortex, hippocampus, thalamus, basal ganglia, brain stem, spinal cord *Function:* inhibits release of norepinephrine; stimulates release of serotonin, dopamine, acetylcholine	*Decreased levels:* Alzheimer disease *Increased levels:* Huntington disease

Source: Townsend, M. C., & Morgan, K. I. (2017). *Essentials of psychiatric mental health nursing: Concepts of care in evidence-based practice* (7th ed.). Philadelphia, PA: F.A. Davis.

Mental illness can be defined as experiencing the following:

- Impaired ability to think
- Impaired ability to feel
- Impaired ability to make sound judgments
- Impaired ability to adapt
- Difficulty in **coping** or inability to cope with reality
- Difficulty in forming or inability to form strong personal relationships

It is important to remember that mental health and mental illness exist on a continuum. It is natural for emotions to ebb and flow from day to day in response to the degree of stress experienced. People who remain mentally healthy can cope with and keep their stress in perspective. Others are not able to do so and over time may develop physical or emotional illnesses because of present and past life stresses.

Etiologies

The line between mental illness and other brain or neurologic disorders is being erased as we learn more about how the brain functions. As scientists study the brains of people who have mental illnesses, they are concluding that mental illness is caused by a variety of biological, genetic, and environmental factors. Changes in the brain's structure, chemistry, and function are associated with expressions of mental illness.

However, it is important to note that, while mental illnesses can be categorized as brain diseases, not all brain diseases are mental illnesses.

Explanations of mental illness in this unit include concepts from the psychological and the psychobiological (or biological) theories. When pertinent, other theories (e.g., behavioral, environmental) are also presented. Most mental illnesses have no identifiable cause. Some etiological theories have stronger positive correlations to illnesses than others. When appropriate, this unit gives the most current or most widely accepted view of an etiology.

Social and Cultural Environments

Many behavioral health professionals believe that social and cultural environments have a great influence on the way people develop and process life experiences. It is part of the nurse's role to take time to learn about traits that are common among cultures and traits that differ. It is essential to understand that each person is a unique individual; but it is also important to understand broad customs and beliefs to avoid unrealistic expectations of patients.

Spirituality and Religion

Spirituality and religion are extremely important to some patients and unimportant to others. A person's success in recuperating from physical or emotional illness may be deeply tied to spiritual beliefs. It is necessary to be comfortable talking to the patient about spiritual needs while being careful not to impose personal values on the patient. If you are not comfortable in these situations, you should offer to call the spiritual or religious leader of the patient's choice.

For more information about mental health and illness, visit the web sites of the National Institute of Mental Health at www.nimh.nih.gov, the American Psychological Association at www.apa.org, the American Psychiatric Nurses Association at www.apna.org, and the International Society of Psychiatric-Mental Health Nurses at www.ispn-psych.org.

NURSING ASSESSMENT OF MENTAL HEALTH

During the assessment phase of the nursing process, a mental status examination is performed. This is a series of questions, activities, and observations that evaluate the following eight areas:

- Appearance and behavior
- Level of awareness and reality orientation
- Thinking/content of thought
- Memory
- Speech and ability to communicate
- Mood and **affect**
- Judgment
- Perception

Many tools of varying names, lengths, and formats are used to evaluate mental capabilities. Table 56.2 is a sample mental status examination.

After data have been collected, the licensed practical nurse/licensed vocational nurse (LPN/LVN) collaborates with the registered nurse (RN) to develop nursing diagnoses (Box 56.1).

DIAGNOSTIC TESTS

Physicians use diagnostic criteria to diagnose mental illness. It is important to rule out physical illness as a cause of symptoms. A health care provider (HCP) may choose to refer a patient to a psychiatrist or other mental health professional for further testing and diagnosis.

The diagnostic tool that is used most widely by psychiatrists and other mental health professionals is the *Diagnostic and Statistical Manual of Mental Disorders,* fifth edition, or *DSM-5* (American Psychiatric Association, 2013). *DSM-5* groups illnesses into categories of clinical disorders. This is a complex diagnostic tool. Although as an LPN/LVN, you will not be responsible for completing the assessment or making a diagnosis, you can contribute valuable information to the diagnostic process.

There are also batteries of psychological tests that can be administered and interpreted by psychiatrists, psychologists, social workers, or advanced practice nurses. Age, hand tremors, vision, language barriers, educational background, and the interpretation of the HCP are some factors that can influence the results of these tests.

Some disorders can mimic mental health disorders, so the following diagnostic tests may be performed to either confirm or rule out a diagnosis of a mental illness:

- Laboratory tests can rule out problems such as electrolyte imbalances, hypothyroidism, infections, dehydration, drug toxicity, or pregnancy.
- Computed tomography (CT) scans or magnetic resonance imaging (MRI) can rule out tumors, lesions, or other physical problems.
- Positron emission tomography (PET) scans can identify how brain areas are functioning by showing chemical activity or metabolism.

COPING AND EGO DEFENSE MECHANISMS

"Oh, just learn to cope with it." "Get a grip." "Don't make a mountain out of a molehill." These are pieces of advice that people may have heard or given at some point. But what do they mean? What is coping? Coping is the way one adapts psychologically, physically, and behaviorally to a **stressor.** People have different ways of coping with their stressors. Culture, religion, individual belief systems, experience, and personal choice influence a person's responses to stress. It is not the value of a behavior that we assess as nurses; it is the desired outcome that is important. What is an effective coping skill? Is it healthy? Does it work? How do we as nurses observe and measure it?

Effective Coping Skills

Effective coping skills offer healthy choices for dealing with stressors. Individuals might use humor, prayer, exercise, or problem-solving, for example. Effective coping skills are also conscious mechanisms. Hospitalization is stressful for patients and families. Many things are unknown and unfamiliar. The patient may not understand the illness or the implications of the treatment plan. It is common for patients to use coping mechanisms during hospitalization. The process of effective coping is sometimes called **adaptation.** Allowing the patient to practice new coping techniques will give him or her confidence. This will decrease the stress that can accompany change.

Often, mild **anxiety** can be positive. A little anxiety can make people more alert and ready to respond. The *fight-or-flight mechanism* can help one adapt to (or escape from) a dangerous situation. However, too much anxiety can cloud the consciousness and interfere with the ability to make appropriate choices or recall new adaptive tools that

Table 56.2

Sample Mental Status Examination

Type of Examination	Normal Parameters	Alterations From Normal
Appearance and Behavior		
Observations about dress, hygiene, posture, and appearance and about the patient's actions and reactions to health care personnel.	Clean, combed hair. Clothing intact and appropriate to weather or situation. Teeth/dentures in good repair. Posture erect. Cooperates with health care personnel.	Displays either unusual apathy or concern about appearance. Displays uncooperative, hostile, or suspicious behaviors toward health care personnel.
Subjective and objective assessment of patient's degree of alertness (wakefulness) and degree of patient's knowledge of self.	Awareness is measured on a continuum that ranges from unconscious to manic. "Normal alertness" is the desired behavior. Facilities may provide a standard format for this assessment, but observations can be documented as well if the patient is not able to stay awake for even short intervals or if the patient is overly active and has difficulty staying in one place. Orientation is assessed by asking the patient questions relating to person, place, and time, such as, "Who is this sitting next to you?" or "Where are you right now?" or "What year is it?"	Outcome is not considered within accepted normal limits if the patient is difficult to arouse and keep awake or if the patient has difficulty feeling calm. Abnormal results of orientation are the patient's inability to correctly answer orientation questions or inability to answer commonly known questions, such as "Who is the president?"
Thinking/Content of Thought		
Subjective assessment of what the patient is thinking and the process the patient uses in his or her thinking.	Formal testing may be done by a psychologist or psychiatrist to determine the patient's general thought content and pattern. Nurses may contribute to the assessment of thought by documenting statements the patient makes regarding daily care and routines.	Abnormal behaviors include flight of ideas, loose associations, phobias, delusions, and obsessions.
Memory		
Subjective assessment of the mind's ability to recall recent and remote (long-term) information.	*Recent memory:* recall of events that are immediately past or within 2 weeks before the assessment, such as a recent news event. One measurement technique is to ask the patient what they had for breakfast that day or what they did yesterday afternoon *Remote memory:* recall of events of the past beyond 2 weeks before assessment. Patients may be asked where they were born, where they went to grade school, etc.	Inability to accurately perform recent or remote (long-term) recall exercises within parameters. May indicate symptom of delirium or dementia.

Continued

Table 56.2

Sample Mental Status Examination—cont'd

Type of Examination	Normal Parameters	Alterations From Normal
Speech and Ability to Communicate		
Objective and subjective assessment of how the patient uses verbal and nonverbal communication. Stuttering, repetition of words, and words that the patient makes up (neologisms) are also assessed.	Patient can coherently produce words appropriate to age, education, and life experience. Rate of speech reflects other psychomotor activity (e.g., faster if the patient is agitated). Volume is not too soft or too loud. Speech is fluid and appropriate.	Limited speech production. Rate of speech is inconsistent with other psychomotor activity. Volume is not appropriate to situation (speaks louder or softer than appropriate). Presence of stuttering, word repetition, or neologisms may indicate physical or psychological illness.
Mood and Affect		
Objective and subjective assessment of the patient's stated feelings and emotions. Affect measures the outward expression of those feelings.	Mood is the stated emotional condition of the patient and should reflect situations as they occur. Facial expression and body language (affect) should match (be congruent with) the stated mood. Affect should change to fluctuate with the changes in mood.	Mood and affect do not match (e.g., facial expression does not appear sad while the patient is expressing sad feelings).
Judgment		
Subjective assessment of a patient's ability to make appropriate decisions about his or her situation or to understand concepts.	When given a proverb or situation to solve, such as "You can't teach an old dog new tricks," the patient should be able to give some sort of acceptable interpretation, such as, "Old habits are hard to break" or "It is hard to learn something new."	Patient cannot interpret the sayings or complete problem-solving questions appropriately. The patient might answer very literally, "Dogs can't learn anything when they get old."
Perception		
Assessment of the way a person experiences reality. Observation of the patient's statements about his or her environment and the behaviors expressed in association with those statements. Assessment of the patient's insight into his or her condition.	All five senses are monitored for the patient's perception of reality. Perceptions of environment are accurate. Insight into condition is appropriate.	Hallucinations (false sensory perceptions) may occur with schizophrenia. Illusions are misperceptions of reality. The patient is unable to state understanding of the origin of the illness; associated behaviors are inappropriate. Many people with schizophrenia or mania have poor insight because of impairment of prefrontal cortex functioning during psychosis.

Box 56.1

Nursing Diagnoses Commonly Used to Address Mental Health Problems

Anxiety (mild to panic)
Body Image, Disturbed
Chronic Sorrow
Community Health, Deficient
Compromised Human Dignity, Risk for
Coping, Compromised Family
Coping, Defensive
Coping, Disabled Family
Coping, Ineffective
Decision-Making, Readiness for Enhanced
Decisional Conflict
Denial, Ineffective
Family Processes, Dysfunctional
Fear
Grieving
Grieving, Risk for Complicated
Health Behavior, Risk-Prone
Hope, Readiness for Enhanced
Impaired Resilience
Impaired Resilience, Risk for
Impulse Control, Ineffective
Injury, Risk for
Mood Regulation, Impaired
Moral Distress
Personal Identity, Disturbed
Post-trauma Syndrome, Risk for
Power, Readiness for Enhanced
Powerlessness
Powerlessness, Risk for
Rape-Trauma Syndrome
Relationship, Risk for Ineffective
Religiosity, Impaired
Religiosity, Readiness for Enhanced
Religiosity, Risk for Impaired
Relocation Stress Syndrome, Risk for
Resilience, Readiness for Enhanced
Role Performance, Ineffective
Self-Care Deficit (Bathing, Dressing, Feeding, or Toileting)
Self-Esteem, Chronic Low
Self-Esteem, Risk for Low (Chronic or Situational)
Self-Mutilation
Sexual Dysfunction
Sleep Pattern, Disturbed
Social Interaction, Impaired
Social Isolation
Spiritual Well-Being, Readiness for Enhanced
Stress Overload
Suicide, Risk for
Violence, Risk for (Self-Directed or Other-Directed)

have been learned. Helpful roles you can perform include actively listening to the patient's thoughts and feelings about the stressor, assisting with identifying precipitating factors and patterns to stress, encouraging the patient to problem-solve, and helping develop alternative solutions to a problem.

CRITICAL THINKING

Mr. Joseph is noted wailing loudly and continuously after the death of his wife. It is disturbing the other patients on the hospital wing. One of the nurses comments, "He is a real nut case. Get him out of here." What is an appropriate response to this nurse? To the husband? How would you document his behavior?

Suggested answers are at the end of the chapter.

Ineffective Coping Skills

Sometimes coping behaviors are ineffective. When conscious techniques are not successful, people may unconsciously fall into habits that give the illusion of coping. These habits are called *ego defense mechanisms*. Ego defense mechanisms act as mental pressure valves. Their purpose is to reduce or eliminate anxiety. They give the impression that they are helping alleviate the stress level. Sometimes ego defense mechanisms can be helpful. When they are overused or are the only means used to deal with anxiety, however, they can become ineffective and unhealthy. People are not born with these coping behaviors; they are learned as responses to stress. Often they develop by age 10. They may appear to be conscious, but they are, for the most part, unconscious mechanisms. Some commonly used ego defense mechanisms are listed in Table 56.3.

CRITICAL THINKING

Mrs. Beison, a 44-year-old mother of three teenagers, is diagnosed with breast cancer. She is refusing treatment because she does not believe she has cancer. She says if anything is wrong, her vitamins will take care of it. What ego defense mechanism is Mrs. Beison using? Is it effective or ineffective? Why? How can you help? Are there other health care providers who could provide assistance?

Suggested answers are at the end of the chapter.

 THERAPEUTIC MEASURES

People who experience alterations in their mental health have special treatment needs. When emotional health is threatened, many other daily activities can be altered as well. **Cognitive** ability (the ability to think rationally and to process thoughts) can be impaired. Emotional responses can be decreased or even absent in some conditions. This can be extremely frightening and can lead to a worsening of the mental disorder

Table 56.3

Ego Defense Mechanisms

Mechanism	Description	Examples
Denial	Usually the first defense learned and used. Unconscious refusal to see reality; not conscious lying.	The alcoholic states, "I can quit any time I want to."
Repression (stuffing)	An unconscious "burying" or "forgetting" mechanism. Excludes or withholds from consciousness events or situations that are unbearable.	A step deeper than "denial." A patient may "forget" about an appointment he or she does not want to keep.
Rationalization	Using a logical-sounding excuse to cover up true thoughts and feelings. The most frequently used defense mechanism.	"I made a medication error because the doctor's orders were confusing." "I failed the test because the teacher wasn't clear about what would be on it."
Compensation	Making up for something perceived as an inadequacy by developing some other desirable trait.	The small boy who wants to be a basketball center instead becomes an honor roll student. The physically unattractive person who wants to model instead becomes a famous designer.
Reaction formation (overcompensation)	Similar to compensation, except the person usually develops the exact opposite trait.	The small boy who wants to be a basketball center becomes a political voice to decrease the emphasis on sports in the elementary grades. The physically unattractive person who wants to be a model speaks out for eliminating beauty pageants.
Regression	Emotionally returning to an earlier time in life when the patient experienced far less stress. Commonly seen in patients while hospitalized.	Children who are toilet trained begin to wet the bed after the birth of a younger sibling. Adults who have a "temper tantrum."
Projection	Ascribing one's own unacceptable qualities or feelings to someone else. May lead to scapegoating.	A patient might state: "My sister is so jealous of me," when actually the patient is jealous of her sister. An anxious patient may say to the nurse, "Why do I make you so nervous?"
Displacement (transference)	"Kick-the-dog syndrome," or transferring anger and hostility to another person or object that is perceived to be less powerful than oneself.	Parent loses job without notice and then goes home and verbally abuses spouse, who unjustly punishes child, who slaps the dog.
Restitution (undoing)	Make amends for a behavior one thinks is unacceptable. Makes an attempt at reducing guilt.	A person gives a treat to a child who is being punished for a wrongdoing. The person who sees someone lose a wallet with a large amount of cash does not return the wallet but puts extra in the collection plate at the next church service.
Conversion reaction	Anxiety is channeled into physical symptoms. Often, the symptoms disappear soon after the threat is over.	Nausea develops the night before a major exam, causing the person to miss the exam. Nausea may disappear soon after the scheduled test is finished.
Avoidance	Unconsciously staying away from events or situations that might cause feelings of aggression or anxiety.	"I can't go to the class reunion tonight. I'm just so tired, I have to sleep."

or even the development of another disorder. This section provides an overview of selected therapies to help patients deal with alterations in mental health.

Therapeutic Communication

Many people take communication for granted. In the mental health setting, communication is a tool used to relate therapeutically with patients. It is important to be intentional about the messages we communicate to patients. Therapeutic communication is accomplished through the deliberate use of verbal and nonverbal techniques. Other areas to consider when communicating are the patient's personal values, attitudes, beliefs, culture, religion, social status, gender, and age or developmental level.

Verbal therapeutic communication techniques can help facilitate an interpersonal interaction. For instance, if you ask a patient to explain something to you in more detail, you are using the verbal therapeutic communication technique of *exploring*. Verbal communication is also influenced by the tone, pitch, speed, and volume of speech. Some commonly used therapeutic communication techniques are listed in Table 56.4.

Table 56.4
Verbal Therapeutic Communication Techniques

Technique	Description	Examples
Encouraging descriptions of perceptions	Asking the patient what he or she is seeing or hearing	"Tell me what the voices are saying to you."
Encouraging comparison	Asking the patient to compare similarities or differences	"How is this medication working for you compared to the last time you used it?"
Exploring	Looking deeper into a subject, idea, or experience	"Tell me more about the last time you were depressed."
Focusing	Concentrating on a single idea or event	"Tell me more about how your divorce made you feel."
Formulating a plan of action	Assisting the patient to come up with a plan to cope with stress	"When this happens in the future, how could you handle it more constructively?"
Giving broad openings	Allowing the patient to steer the interaction	"What would you like to work on today?"
Giving recognition	Acknowledging or showing awareness	"I see you went to your therapy group today."
Making observations	Verbalizing what is observed	"I noticed you seemed upset after your visit."
Offering self	Extending one's presence	"I am available to talk whenever you would like."
Offering general leads	Giving the patient encouragement to continue	"I see …" "Go on …"
Placing event in time or sequence	Clarification of events in time	"Was this before or after your first hospitalization?"
Presenting reality	Defining reality in simple terms	"The voices may seem real to you, but they are a symptom of your illness."
Restating	Repeating the main idea of what the patient has verbalized	"It sounds as if you are feeling frustrated."
Reflecting	Statements, questions, or feelings are stated back to the patient	"What do you think you should do?"
Seeking clarification	Searching for understanding of what was said	"Tell me if this is what you meant when you said …"
Verbalizing the implied	Putting into words what the patient has implied or said indirectly	"You must be feeling very sad right now."

Components of *nonverbal communication* include physical appearance, dress, body movement and posture, touch, facial expression, and eye contact. It is believed that most communication takes place nonverbally, so it is possible that while you are saying one thing to a patient, your body language could be saying something else. Silence is also useful as it gives both the nurse and the patient a chance to collect their thoughts and organize what they are going to say.

There are also barriers to effective communication, commonly called *communication blocks.* A nurse who tells a patient, "Don't worry, everything will be all right" has just given the patient false reassurance. This communicates to the patient that his or her concerns are not being taken seriously. Some common communication blocks are listed in Table 56.5.

Milieu

One area over which you can have some control is the therapeutic environment. In the mental health setting, this therapeutic environment is called the **milieu** or therapeutic milieu. It is believed that environment influences behavior. Milieu therapy is the systematic management of the social environment as a treatment modality.

A therapeutic milieu is an environment that provides containment, support, structure, involvement, and validation during the patient's stay. The goals of milieu therapy are resocialization, ego development, and prevention of regression. Resocialization occurs when patients help govern the running of the mental health unit and attend regular meetings to set rules and assign tasks. Ego development is fostered with structured activities that are provided to assist the patient to learn coping and social skills. Regression is discouraged when patients help with washing dishes or other small jobs that foster independence. Common milieu interventions include role modeling, positive reinforcement, a schedule of events, consistent expectations and rules for behavior, and unit meetings. Milieu therapy is difficult in this era of managed care because of shorter hospital stays.

Psychopharmacology

Psychopharmacology is the use of medications to treat psychological disorders. Since the introduction of the phenothiazine class of drugs in the 1950s, the number of medications available for treating mental health disorders has increased greatly, with newer medications having fewer side effects. The reason for using medications is twofold: First, the medications manage the symptoms, helping the patient feel more comfortable emotionally. Second, the patient is generally more receptive and able to focus on other types of therapy if medications are effective. More information on psychoactive drugs is provided in Chapter 57.

Psychotherapy

Psychotherapy is the term used to describe the form of treatment chosen by the psychologist, psychiatrist, social worker, or advanced practice mental health nurse. The goals of psychotherapy include the following:

- Reduce the patient's emotional discomfort.
- Increase the level of the patient's social functioning.

- Increase the ability of the patient to behave or perform in a manner appropriate to the situation.

Several specific types of therapy that are typically used are described next.

Psychodynamic Therapy

Psychodynamic therapy is based on **psychoanalysis.** It consists of clarifying the meaning of events, feelings, and behavior, thereby gaining **insight** into them. Psychoanalysis was developed from Sigmund Freud's psychoanalytic theory. Freud believed that anxiety was the primary motivation for behavior and that all behavior had meaning. The role of the patient is to provide the therapist with clues to the unconscious source of problems and to try to develop insights into behavior. The role of the therapist is to uncover these unconscious experiences and interpret their meanings to the patient. Some believe that psychodynamic therapy will lose popularity as we gain a better understanding of the role of the brain, neurotransmitters, and genetics in mental health.

Behavior Management

Behavior management (also called behavior modification) is a treatment method that stems from the studies of behavioral theorists, such as B. F. Skinner and Ivan Pavlov. It is a common treatment modality used in long-term care facilities, with children and adolescents, and with individuals who have a low level of cognitive functioning.

According to behavior management theory, all behavior is learned; therefore, it can be unlearned. The belief is that behavior can be shaped by either positive or negative reinforcement. *Positive reinforcement* is the act of rewarding the patient with something pleasant when the desired behavior has been performed. For instance, if a patient has a habit of using foul language to obtain what he or she needs, the desired behavior change might be to go to a staff member and ask appropriately for what he or she needs. If this patient loves to be outside but is not allowed out except at supervised times, then a suitable positive reinforcement might be to allow 15 more minutes outdoors when the desired behavior is exhibited.

Negative reinforcement is the act of responding to the undesired behavior by taking away a privilege or adding a responsibility. Negative reinforcement can be misinterpreted as punishment. Parents who "ground" their children for unacceptable behavior are using negative reinforcement; requiring the child to perform extra household tasks for a stated period is reinforcing the fact that the behavior has consequences. The child may not repeat the undesired behavior after negative reinforcement has been used.

· WORD · BUILDING ·

psychopharmacology: psycho—soul or mind + pharmaco—drug or medicine + ology—study of

psychotherapy: psycho—soul or mind + therapy—treatment

psychoanalysis: psycho—soul or mind + analysis—dissolving

Table 56.5
Communication Blocks

Mechanism	Description	Examples to Avoid
Agreeing/disagreeing	Implies that the patient's ideas or feelings are somehow right or wrong	"That is right on target. I agree 100%."
Asking "why" questions	Implies that the patient knows the reason for his or her behavior and feelings	"Why were you feeling so angry?"
Changing the subject	Takes control of the conversation away from the patient	Patient: "I am feeling so hopeless." Nurse: "Did you go to group therapy today?"
Giving advice	Implies that the nurse knows what is best	"I think you should ..."
Giving approval or disapproval	Passes judgment on the patient's ideas or opinions	"That sounds like a bad idea."
Giving false reassurance	Devalues the patient's feelings	"Everything will be all right."
Self-focusing behavior	Focuses on nurse's own feelings at the expense of the patient's	"That happened to me once. Let me tell you about it."
Double-bind messages	When the nonverbal message doesn't match the verbal message	"I'm listening," as the nurse fidgets in her chair, doesn't make eye contact, and then coughs.

It is necessary to avoid violating the Patient's Bill of Rights when performing behavior management with patients. A signed consent from the patient is advised when using this form of therapy. The patient must understand the consequences of the behavior to be changed and the purpose for the type of consequence that is chosen. If the person is not capable of understanding the situation or is not able to remember the consequences, behavior management may not be the best form of treatment.

Cognitive Behavioral Therapy

Jean Piaget and Aaron T. Beck are cognitive theorists who have greatly contributed to modern cognitive behavioral therapy. Cognitive behavioral therapists believe that people experience mental illness due to cognitive distortions about their situations. Cognitive behavioral therapy stresses ways of rethinking situations. The therapist confronts the patient with certain distortions of thinking and then helps the patient to work out ways of thinking about them differently. This type of treatment is used frequently for affective or mood disorders.

Feeling sad about an unpleasant experience (such as the death of a loved one) is acceptable and normal. However, long-term depression about the death is an extreme emotion and, therefore, considered to be unhealthy. In this situation, the patient might be helped to see the death as a sad loss. Behavioral techniques are also often used with phobias or panic disorders, in which fear may interfere with reasoning.

Cognitive behavioral therapy is gaining in popularity because it is usually significantly shorter term than other types of therapy and, therefore, less costly to the patient. Patients are given "homework" that is specific to their needs; they practice their assignments between sessions. Cognitive behavioral therapy in combination with medications can provide effective treatment for depression.

Counseling

Counseling is the provision of help or guidance by a health care professional. The profession of counseling is licensed and regulated differently by state and sometimes also by municipality. Nurses prepared at an LPN/LVN level or at an RN level, in some areas and with special advanced education, can practice some forms of counseling.

You may be asked or expected to accompany patients to counseling sessions or even to facilitate a group discussion. Remember that these are confidential sessions, even if they are group-oriented. Patients are there to work; others are there by invitation for special reasons.

Group Therapy

Therapy groups are formed for many reasons; they can be ongoing or short-term depending on the needs of the patients or the type of disorder. Group therapy is a cost-effective means of providing treatment. For example, Alcoholics Anonymous (AA) and similar 12-step, self-help groups are well-established, ongoing groups formed around treatment of a specific problem. Family counseling sessions may occur with individual therapists with a specialty in the problem area for that family. Marriage counseling may be done in a group with other couples. Often, peer counselors are used.

Therapists and counselors are tools, or facilitators, in the therapeutic process. Patients must take the suggestions given by the therapist, try them, and see what works for them. You can help by reinforcing the work patients do to learn to stay mentally healthy and develop more effective life skills.

Electroconvulsive Therapy

Electroconvulsive therapy (ECT) is a form of treatment that is used for severely depressed patients who have not responded to psychotropic medications. ECT passes an electric current through the brain to produce a tonic-clonic (grand mal) seizure. Most mental health professionals believe ECT stimulates an increase in circulating levels of the neurotransmitters serotonin, norepinephrine, and dopamine in the brain. Essentially, ECT affects neurotransmitter activity much like antidepressant medications. ECT may be frightening to patients; it is important for the nurse to provide education and information to the patient and family. Many changes have been made in this form of therapy since the 1940s, and ECT is currently a safe and effective treatment for resistant depression.

Procedure

ECT often takes place in the recovery room of an operating suite, where there is ready access to emergency equipment. Informed consent must be obtained by the HCP. About 30 minutes before the procedure, the patient is given a medication to dry secretions and counteract stimulation of the vagus nerve, which can cause bradycardia and syncope. Patients are given a short-acting anesthetic before the treatment and a smooth muscle relaxant to minimize injury. Before giving the muscle relaxant, a blood pressure cuff is placed on one of the patient's lower limbs and inflated. This is to ensure that the seizure activity can be visually monitored in this limb. Blood pressure and pulse are carefully monitored before and after the treatment. The patient is oxygenated with pure oxygen during and after the seizure until spontaneous respirations return. During treatment, an electrical stimulus is delivered to the brain via unilateral or bilateral electrodes. The amount of electrical energy used is individualized to the patient. The seizure must last at least 30 seconds to be effective. The seizure activity is monitored with an electroencephalogram (EEG) and in the cuffed limb.

Side Effects

Side effects of ECT can be unpleasant but are usually temporary. The patient may feel confused and forgetful immediately after the treatment. This can be from both the ECT and the medication that was used before the treatment. If the seizure was severe, the patient may have some muscle soreness.

ECT is not used indiscriminately. It is used when other therapies have not been helpful and is usually reserved for treatment-resistant depression ("Patient Perspective").

Patient Perspective

Ethel. My mom is 83 years old and has had a total of 35 electroconvulsive therapy (ECT) treatments for severe depression in her lifetime. If you met her, you'd never know; you'd find her delightful. She's a sweet, little, plump German lady with a big heart. I am a nurse, and, when I tell fellow nurses about my mom, they often ask me why I didn't get her on antidepressants. I want to scream, "How dumb do you think I am?!" Of course Mom is on antidepressants. But at intervals they don't work, and she sinks into severe depression. My choice then is to help her have ECT or let her stay depressed and miserable and put her in a nursing home. And she would soon die because, when she is depressed, she refuses to move, doesn't sleep, and is horribly miserable.

The first time my mom was scheduled for ECT, one of the nurses in our local community hospital told her to refuse it, that no one should have to go through that. It was a cruel thing to do. My mom doesn't do well in counseling; she doesn't believe in it. In her mind, you don't talk about your "dirty linen." My mom was in an abusive relationship with my father for 47 years, and she hid all the problems away and doesn't talk about them to this day. I'm so grateful to have my mom doing okay and grateful that ECT treatments exist. With ECT, my mother is doing well and enjoying life. Without treatment, she would be gone. Please understand that there are times when ECT treatments are the best thing for severely depressed people, when other treatments have been ineffective.

Nursing Care

The patient should receive nothing by mouth (NPO) for at least 4 hours before a treatment. Remind the patient to empty his or her bladder and to remove dentures, contact lenses, hair pins, and other items on the body. Following ECT, carefully monitor vital signs and document the patient's subjective and objective responses to the treatment. Stay with the patient until he or she is oriented and able to care for him or herself. Withhold oral medications and food until the gag reflex returns. Ensure that the patient is kept safe after ECT therapy.

Relaxation Therapy

A variety of relaxation techniques can be taught to help patients manage their responses to stress. Relaxation exercises such as deep, rhythmic breathing can increase oxygenation and provide distraction from stressors. Breathing exercises may be coupled with progressive muscle relaxation exercises. For this technique, patients are taught to start at the head and neck and systematically tense and then relax muscle groups as they progress toward the lower extremities. Soft music may enhance the patient's ability to fully relax.

Guided **imagery** is the use of the imagination to promote relaxation. For this technique, the patient is assisted to imagine a pleasurable experience from his or her past, such as lying on a beach or soaking in a warm bath. Use of all senses is encouraged: for a beach image, the patient might see a beach, feel the warm sun, smell salt air, and hear waves crashing against the shore. The patient might also be taught to visualize being successful in a problem situation.

Relaxation techniques may be used individually, but they are often used in combination with each other or with other therapies for maximum effect. See Chapter 5 for more information on relaxation and imagery.

Home Health Hints

- Observe for indications that the patient is at risk of falls, especially if the patient is experiencing orthostatic hypotension from medications.
- Reconcile medications at each visit, checking for missed doses, compliance, and new or discontinued medications.
- Ask depressed patients about suicide ideations at every visit. Report to registered nurse or health care provider if needed.
- Maintain a calm demeanor if the patient is agitated, and always have a clear path to an exit in the event the agitation escalates.

SUGGESTED ANSWERS TO CRITICAL THINKING

Mr. Joseph

Different people cope in different ways. This may be a healthy way to cope in this grieving husband's culture. Gently guide him to a room where he can express his emotions without disturbing others. Ask if he would like you to contact someone to come help support him. Document objectively: "Patient's husband weeping loudly; guided to consultation room for privacy." As a licensed practical nurse/licensed vocational nurse, your best course of action may be to report the registered nurse's comment objectively to your supervisor.

Mrs. Beison

Mrs. Beison is overusing the ego defense mechanism denial to cope with her cancer diagnosis. Although at times denial can be an effective coping mechanism, if Mrs. Beison continues to deny her disease and refuse treatment, her life will be in danger. You can help Mrs. Beison verbalize her fears about cancer and cancer treatment, and provide accurate information to help her make wise choices. If needed, a psychiatric evaluation can be requested. If she is found to be mentally competent, then her wishes must be respected.

Review Questions

1. Which patient behavior requires additional mental health assessment?
   1. Patient is always happy and smiling.
   2. Patient can verbalize emotions.
   3. Patient can cope with bad news.
   4. Patient maintains some close, personal relationships.

2. Which data are important to collect during a mental health assessment? **Select all that apply.**
   1. Orientation to reality
   2. Mobility
   3. Ability to communicate clearly
   4. Heart sounds
   5. Memory
   6. Appearance

3. A patient being evaluated for depression asks why blood must be drawn. Which response by the nurse is best?
   1. "Your physical illnesses must be under control before your depression can be treated effectively."
   2. "The provider needs to rule out physical causes for your symptoms."
   3. "Many mental health disorders can be identified with blood tests."
   4. "If your lab work is out of balance, then correcting the imbalance will reverse your depression."

4. The nurse recognizes that the patient who always seems to be making excuses is displaying which ego defense mechanism?
  1. Denial
  2. Fantasy
  3. Rationalization
  4. Transference

5. Which of the following milieus would be most therapeutic for a patient experiencing severe anxiety?
  1. An environment that provides for all the patient's physical and emotional needs
  2. An environment that is locked and supervised at all times
  3. An environment that is structured to reduce stress and encourage coping behaviors
  4. An environment that eliminates all anxiety-producing stimuli

6. Which explanation of psychopharmacology by the nurse is best for the patient starting on medication for a mental health disorder?
  1. "Medication can potentially cure a mental illness."
  2. "Medication will help you control your behavior."
  3. "Medication is used to block emotional responses in your brain."
  4. "Medication can reduce your symptoms so you can focus on other therapies."

7. Which statement by the patient with a substance abuse disorder indicates that interventions have been effective?
  1. "I know I have a problem, and I have a lot of work to do to get better."
  2. "If I don't think about my problem, eventually it will fade from my memory."
  3. "I no longer have a substance abuse problem. My treatment has been effective."
  4. "Now that I know that my family is the cause of my problem, I can move on."

8. A patient shares some very traumatic life experiences. What is the best response by the nurse?
  1. Assure the patient that staff will not allow such experiences to happen again.
  2. Ask probing questions about the patient's emotional responses to the experiences.
  3. Encourage the patient to forget the experiences and move on with life.
  4. Listen attentively to the patient and show empathy.

Answer rationales available in your online resources.

ANSWERS 1. 1; 2. 1; 3. 5; 4. 2; 5. 3; 6. 4; 7. 1; 8. 4

Key Points

Find the chapter key points in your online resources available through Davis Edge.

Additional Resources

DAVIS edge.   Use the scratch off code on the inside front cover of your book to access online quizzes that will help you to improve your scores on course exams and prepare for the NCLEX-PN®.

    Study Guide

CHAPTER 57

Nursing Care of Patients With Mental Health Disorders

Marina Martinez-Kratz

KEY TERMS

abuse (uh-BYOOS)
addiction (ah-DIK-shun)
alogia (ah-LOH-jee-uh)
anhedonia (AN-heh-DOH-nee-uh)
anorexia nervosa (AN-uh-REK-see-ah nur-VOH-sah)
avolition (A-voh-LISH-un)
bipolar (bye-POH-lur)
bulimia nervosa (buh-LEE-mee-ah ner-VOH-sah)
codependence (KOH-dee-PEN-dense)
compulsion (kum-PUHL-shun)
delirium tremens (dee-LEER-ee-um TREE-menz)
delusions (dee-LOO-zhuns)
dependence (dee-PEN-dense)
displacement (dis-PLACE-ment)
dysfunctional (dis-FUNK-shun-uhl)
eustress (YOO-stress)
hallucinations (hah-LOO-sih-NAY-shuns)
illusions (ih-LOO-zhuns)
mania (MAY-nee-ah)
obsession (ob-SESH-un)
phobia (FOH-bee-ah)
tolerance (TALL-er-ense)
withdrawal (with-DRAW-ul)

CHAPTER CONCEPTS

Addiction and Behaviors
Family Dynamics
Mood
Neurologic Regulation
Self
Stress
Trauma

LEARNING OUTCOMES

1. Identify etiological theories for common mental health disorders.
2. Describe signs and symptoms of common mental health disorders.
3. Describe therapeutic management for each of the disorders.
4. Identify actions, side effects, and nursing considerations for selected classifications of psychoactive medications.
5. Plan nursing interventions for patients with mental health disorders.
6. Discuss the role of the licensed practical nurse/licensed vocational nurse in the care of patients with mental health disorders.

As we saw in the last chapter, people with mental health problems may experience impaired ability to think, feel, make sound judgments, adapt to changes, cope with stressors, and form strong relationships with others. This chapter covers some of the more common mental health disorders you will see in medical, surgical, and long-term care settings. Patients with mental health disorders may need modified care planning to help them manage both mental and physiological illnesses.

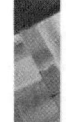

ANXIETY DISORDERS, OBSESSIVE-COMPULSIVE AND RELATED DISORDERS, AND TRAUMA- AND STRESSOR-RELATED DISORDERS

Anxiety Disorders

Do you ever feel stressed? How does it make you feel? Is it possible to live a completely stress-free existence? Stress is everywhere in our society. Stress produces anxiety. Most often, stress is associated with negative situations. However, the good things that happen to us, such as a marriage or a job promotion, also produce stress. The stress from positive experiences is called **eustress.** Eustress can produce just as much anxiety as negative stressors. A *stressor* is

• WORD • BUILDING •
eustress: eu—normal or good + stress

any person or situation that produces an anxiety response. Stress and stressors are different for each person; therefore, it is important to ask patients what their personal stress producers are.

Anxiety is the uncomfortable feeling of dread that occurs in response to extreme or prolonged periods of stress. It is commonly ranked as mild, moderate, severe, or panic. It is believed that mild anxiety is a normal part of being human and is necessary to change and develop new ways of coping with stress.

Anxiety may also be influenced by one's culture. It may be acceptable for people in certain cultures to acknowledge and discuss stress, while those in other cultures may believe that discussing personal problems is inappropriate. Cultural behavior can be a challenge for the nurse when attempting to collect assessment data.

Anxiety is usually referred to as either *free-floating anxiety* or *signal anxiety*. Free-floating anxiety is described as a general feeling of impending doom. The person cannot pinpoint the cause but might say something like, "I just know something bad is going to happen if I go on vacation." Signal anxiety, on the other hand, is an uncomfortable response to a known stressor ("Finals are only a week away, and I've got that nausea again"). Both types of anxiety are involved in the various anxiety disorders.

Etiological Theories

Psychoanalytical theorists believe that anxiety is a conflict between the *id* (the "all for me" part of the personality) and the *superego* (the conscience), which is repressed in early development but emerges again in adulthood.

Biological theorists view anxiety differently. One biological theory points to the sympathoadrenal (fight-or-flight) responses to stress to explain signs and symptoms of anxiety. This theory notes that blood vessels constrict because epinephrine and norepinephrine have been released, causing blood pressure to rise. Another biological theory implicates a lack of the neurotransmitter gamma-aminobutyric acid (GABA) in the etiology of anxiety. GABA is an inhibitory neurotransmitter that prevents postsynaptic excitation.

If the body adapts to the stress, hormone levels adjust and body functions return to a homeostatic state. If the body does not adapt to the stress, the immune system is challenged and risk for physical illness increases.

You may observe psychological responses to physical illness. It is important to recognize the relationship between physical and emotional responses to stress. Some examples of medical conditions that occur because of the body's response to stress are shown in Table 57.1.

Diagnosis

Because there are so many symptoms associated with anxiety disorders, it is important for patients to have a complete physical examination before an anxiety disorder is diagnosed. Some medical disorders, such as hyperthyroidism, can mimic anxiety; hypothyroidism can mimic depression.

Types of Anxiety

SPECIFIC PHOBIA. Specific **phobias** are the most common of the anxiety disorders. There are more than 700 documented phobias. Specific phobias are defined as irrational fears of distinct objects or situations, such as snakes, bridges, or flying. The person is very aware of the fear, and even the fact that it is irrational, but is unable to gain control over the stressor. Therefore, the fear continues.

The psychoanalytic view implies that it really is not the object that is the source of the fear but rather that the fear is a result of a defense mechanism called **displacement.** For example, the person with a phobia of snakes may have seen a frightening movie in which someone died from a snakebite. The stated object of the phobia would be interpreted as a symbol for the underlying cause of the fear, such as fear of dying.

SOCIAL ANXIETY DISORDER (SOCIAL PHOBIA). Social anxiety disorder is a social phobia characterized by a persistent fear of behaving or performing in a way that will be humiliating or embarrassing to the individual. Examples include public speaking, eating in front of others, or using public restrooms. The fear or anxiety is out of proportion to the situation.

PANIC DISORDER. Panic is a state of extreme fear that cannot be controlled; it may be referred to as a panic attack. Panic episodes are recurrent and occur unpredictably. Patients may present themselves at the emergency room because they believe they are having a heart attack or other significant physical illness. Patients must exhibit several episodes within a specified time frame to be given the diagnosis of panic disorder. Some of the symptoms associated with panic disorder include the following:

- Fear (usually of dying, losing control of self, or "going crazy")
- Feelings of impending doom
- Dissociation (feeling that it is happening to someone else or not happening at all)
- Nausea
- Diaphoresis
- Chest pain
- Palpitations
- Shaking

GENERALIZED ANXIETY DISORDER. In generalized anxiety disorder (GAD), the anxiety itself (also referred to as excessive worry or severe stress) is the expressed symptom. Patients with GAD worry about everything. Symptoms that may be present in GAD include the following:

- Restlessness or feeling "on edge"
- Shaking
- Palpitations
- Dry mouth
- Nausea and/or vomiting
- Being easily frightened
- Hot flashes
- Chills

Table 57.1

Responses to Stress

Stress-Related Medical Condition	Pathophysiology	Outcome of Stress on the Body
Lowered immunity	Interferes with effectiveness of antibodies. Possibly related to interactions among the hypothalamus, pituitary gland, adrenal glands, and immune system.	Increased susceptibility to colds and other viruses and illnesses
Burnout	Stress- or work-related emotional exhaustion and depression.	Emotional detachment
Migraine, cluster, and tension headaches	Tightening of skeletal muscles. Dilating of cranial arteries.	Nausea, vomiting, tight feeling in or around head and shoulders, tinnitus, inability to tolerate light, weakness of a limb
Hypertension	Role of stress not positively known. Thought to contribute to hypertension by negatively interacting with kidneys, autonomic nervous system, and endocrine system.	Resistance to blood flow through the cardiovascular system, causing pressure on the arteries Can lead to stroke, heart attack, and kidney failure
Coronary artery disease	Not fully understood. Stress may be associated with behavioral factors such as overeating, physical inactivity, and obesity.	Hypertension, hypercholesterolemia, atherosclerosis, diabetes
Cancer	Stress lowers the immune response.	Lowered immunity may allow for overcolonization of opportunistic cancer cells.
Asthma	Autonomic (parasympathetic) nervous system stimulates mucus, increases blood flow, and constricts airways. May be associated with other stress-related conditions such as allergy and viral infection.	Wheezing, coughing, dyspnea, apprehension May lead to respiratory infections, respiratory failure, or pneumothorax

- Muscle aches
- Hypervigilance (excessive attention to stimuli)
- Polyuria
- Difficulty swallowing

Nursing care of patients with anxiety is discussed after "Trauma- and Stressor-Related Disorders."

Obsessive-Compulsive and Related Disorders

The *Diagnostic and Statistical Manual of Mental Disorders, Fifth Edition*, or *DSM-5* (American Psychiatric Association, 2013), groups obsessive-compulsive and related disorders together in a distinct category separate from the anxiety disorders. Disorders grouped in this new category have common features such as an obsessive preoccupation and repetitive behaviors. Disorders include obsessive-compulsive disorder, body dysmorphic disorder, and trichotillomania (hair-pulling

disorder) as well as two new disorders: hoarding disorder and excoriation (skin-picking) disorder.

Obsessive-Compulsive Disorder

Obsessive-compulsive disorder (OCD) occurs in 2% to 5% of the population. It is the fourth most common psychiatric diagnosis. It consists of two parts: the **obsession** (repetitive thought, urge, or images) and the **compulsion** (an excessive or unrealistic repetitive act that the individual feels driven to perform in response to the obsession). An example of OCD is the need to check that the doors are locked numerous times before one is able to sleep or leave the house. This need may prevent the person from sleeping or leaving the house at all. Some individuals wash their hands compulsively to the point of having raw and bleeding hands. Behaviors become ritualistic. The person with OCD is unable to stop the thought or the action. Performing the action (such as checking the locks or hand washing) is the mechanism that reduces the anxiety. Although as the nurse you should not interfere with these repetitive acts, OCD patients can be helped by therapeutic interventions such as cognitive behavioral therapy or medications such as fluoxetine (Prozac). Nursing care of patients with OCD is discussed after "Trauma- and Stressor-Related Disorders."

Trauma- and Stressor-Related Disorders

The *DSM-5* created a category to group trauma- and stressor-related disorders. Patients diagnosed with these disorders have been exposed to a traumatic or stressful event, such as war or natural disasters, and experience specific symptoms. The disorders included in this new category are posttraumatic stress disorder, reactive attachment disorder, disinhibited social engagement disorder, acute stress disorder, and adjustment disorders.

Posttraumatic Stress Disorder

Posttraumatic stress disorder (PTSD) develops in response to some unexpected emotional or physical trauma when there was the *real threat of death or harm* and the patient was helpless to do anything about it. People who have fought in wars, been raped, or survived violent storms or acts (such as terrorist acts) are examples of those who are susceptible to suffering from PTSD.

An associated condition is *survivor guilt.* This is the feeling of guilt expressed by those who have survived a tragedy. A survivor of an airline crash may say, "Why me? Why did I make it? I should have died too!" This is especially true if a loved one died in the tragedy.

Symptoms may appear immediately or may not appear until years later. A key symptom of PTSD is *flashbacks* in which the person may relive the traumatic event as if it were happening at that moment. Sounds and smells associated with the trauma may trigger the flashback.

Signs and symptoms of PTSD include the following:

- Flashbacks or dissociative reactions
- Recurrent intrusive memories of the traumatic event
- Recurrent intrusive dreams/nightmares related to the traumatic event
- Intense psychological distress at exposure to internal or external cues that resemble an aspect of the traumatic event
- Marked physical reaction to internal or external cues that resemble an aspect of the traumatic event
- Persistent avoidance of stimuli associated with the traumatic events
- Social withdrawal
- Feelings of low self-esteem
- Changes in relationships with significant others
- Difficulty forming new relationships
- Hypervigilance
- Irritability and outbursts of anger seemingly for no obvious reason
- Depression
- Chemical dependency

Therapeutic Measures for Patients With Anxiety, Obsessive-Compulsive, or Trauma-Related Disorders

Treatment for these disorders is individualized. Treatment may include one or more of the following: medications (psychopharmacology), individual psychotherapy, group therapy, systematic desensitization, hypnosis, imagery, relaxation exercises, and biofeedback.

Psychopharmacology may involve benzodiazepines, an antianxiety classification of medications. Alprazolam (Xanax) or lorazepam (Ativan) are commonly used and are effective in most cases. Benzodiazepines are used for short-term treatment because of the strong potential for chemical dependency. Individuals who need long-term therapy for anxiety or who have chemical dependency tendencies may be treated with buspirone (BuSpar), the selective serotonin reuptake inhibitors (SSRIs) paroxetine (Paxil) or sertraline (Zoloft), the antihistamine hydroxyzine hydrochloride (Atarax) or hydroxyzine pamoate (Vistaril), or the antihypertensive agent clonidine (Catapres). Table 57.2 provides a review of medications.

In *systematic desensitization,* the patient is exposed gradually (rating the fear on a scale from 1 to 10) to the object that causes the anxiety. *Hypnosis* places the patient in a subconscious state and then helps the patient recall events that may be producing anxiety so they can be dealt with. Additional therapies are discussed in Chapter 56.

Nursing Process for the Patient With an Anxiety, Obsessive-Compulsive, or Trauma-Related Disorder

DATA COLLECTION. Observe the patient's anxiety level and level of functioning. Ask about triggers of anxiety and coping mechanisms that have been successful or unsuccessful in the past. Stay alert for physical symptoms, such as changes in vital signs, diaphoresis, or tremor. Assess for the presence of suicidal thoughts, and observe for suicidal behavior. It is important to identify anxiety and intervene at lower levels, before escalation to severe or panic anxiety levels (Table 57.3).

NURSING DIAGNOSES, PLANNING, AND IMPLEMENTATION.

Anxiety related to response to stressors

EXPECTED OUTCOME: The patient will verbalize that anxiety is controlled. The patient will identify triggers and patterns for anxiety and demonstrate techniques to control anxiety. Physical signs of anxiety, such as tremors or changes in vital signs, will be absent.

- Assist the patient to identify triggers of and patterns to anxiety. *Recognition of patterns can help guide care and allow the patient to initiate measures to stop anxiety from progressing.*
- Maintain a calm milieu and manner. *A chaotic environment can increase the patient's anxiety. Anxiety is contagious and may be transmitted from staff to patient.*

Table 57.2
Medications Used for Alterations in Mental Health

Medication Class/Action

Typical Antipsychotics

Block mainly D$_2$ dopamine receptors (used less often because of serious extrapyramidal side effects).

Examples	Nursing Implications
chlorpromazine (Thorazine)	For short-term use because of side effects. Monitor for extrapyramidal side effects.
haloperidol (Haldol)	Have patient rise slowly to counter orthostatic hypotension.
fluphenazine (Prolixin)	Offer ice chips, gum, or hard candy for dry mouth.
trifluoperazine (Stelazine)	Monitor urinary and bowel elimination.
	Do not use/take with alcohol or other central nervous system (CNS) depressants.
	Teach:
	Use sunscreen when outside.

Atypical Antipsychotics

Block multiple dopamine and serotonin receptors.

Examples	Nursing Implications
asenapine (Saphris)	Monitor complete blood count for clozapine.
clozapine (Clozaril)	Monitor for weight gain.
lurasidone (Latuda)	Monitor glucose level for onset of type 2 diabetes.
risperidone (Risperdal)	Use gloves when administering risperidone.
olanzapine (Zyprexa)	*Teach:*
quetiapine (Seroquel)	Take lurasidone with food.
ziprasidone (Geodon)	Sublingual forms can dissolve in hands; make sure hands are dry, and take imme-
aripiprazole (Abilify)	diately. Do not eat or drink for 10 minutes.
paliperidone (Invega)	

Antidepressants

Selective Serotonin Reuptake Inhibitor (SSRIs)
Block the reuptake of serotonin at the presynaptic receptor.

Examples	Nursing Implications
fluoxetine (Prozac)	Allow time for side effects to subside.
sertraline (Zoloft)	Do not administer after 1500 to keep excitation from affecting sleep.
paroxetine (Paxil)	*Teach:*
escitalopram (Lexapro)	Take 6–8 weeks for therapeutic effects to occur.
citalopram (Celexa)	Do not stop drug abruptly.
fluvoxamine (Luvox)	Do not take with other serotonin-type medications including St. John's wort
trazodone (Desyrel)	and S-adenosyl-L-methionine (SAMe).

Tricyclic Antidepressants
Partially block the reuptake of serotonin and norepinephrine at the presynaptic receptor; used infrequently because of side effects.

Examples	Nursing Implications
amitriptyline (Elavil)	Decreases effects of antihypertensives.
nortriptyline (Pamelor)	Lowers seizure threshold.
imipramine (Tofranil)	Will affect oral contraceptives.
	Teach:
	Takes 6–8 weeks for therapeutic effects to occur.
	Do not stop drug abruptly.
	Overdose can cause fatal arrhythmias.

Continued

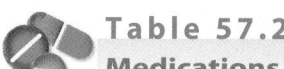

Table 57.2
Medications Used for Alterations in Mental Health—cont'd

Medication Class/Action

Selective Serotonin Norepinephrine Reuptake Inhibitors (SNRIs)
Block the reuptake of serotonin and norepinephrine.

Examples	Nursing Implications
venlafaxine (Effexor, Effexor XR)	Monitor blood pressure for systolic hypertension.
duloxetine (Cymbalta)	*Teach:*
desvenlafaxine (Pristiq)	Do not take with other serotonin-type medications, including St. John's wort and SAMe.
	Do not stop drug abruptly.

Tetracyclic Antidepressants
Block multiple serotonin and histamine receptors; adreno receptor antagonist.

Examples	Nursing Implications
mirtazapine (Remeron)	Administer at bedtime to counteract sedating effects.
maprotiline (Ludiomil)	*Teach:*
	Do not take with alcohol or other CNS depressants.

Norepinephrine-Dopamine Reuptake Inhibitor (NDRI)
Inhibits reuptake of norepinephrine and dopamine.

Examples	Nursing Implications
bupropion (Wellbutrin, Zyban)	May be prescribed for smoking cessation.

Antianxiety Agents

Benzodiazepines
Potentiate effects of gamma-aminobutyric acid (GABA), which causes a calming effect.

Examples	Nursing Implications
alprazolam (Xanax)	For short-term use only; can be addictive.
diazepam (Valium)	Use cautiously in older adults.
lorazepam (Ativan)	Do not use in pregnant patients.
clonazepam (Klonopin)	*Teach:*
	Do not operate heavy machinery.
	Do not stop drug abruptly.

BuSpar
Action is unknown.

Examples	Nursing Implications
buspirone (BuSpar)	Non–habit-forming with little sedating effect.
	Teach:
	Take 3–6 weeks for drug to work.

Anticonvulsant Mood Stabilizers

Antikindling effect; affect GABA receptors.

Examples	Nursing Implications
carbamazepine (Tegretol)	Loading dose may be ordered for acute mania.
lamotrigine (Lamictal)	Monitor for bleeding.
valproic acid (Depakote)	Use cautiously in older adults and in patients with liver or renal disease.
	Do not use in pregnant or breastfeeding patients.
	Teach:
	Use sunscreen.
	Report any signs of rash immediately.

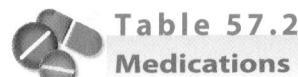

Table 57.2
Medications Used for Alterations in Mental Health—cont'd

Medication Class/Action

Antimanic Agent	

Lithium
Decreases postsynaptic receptor sensitivity.

Examples	**Nursing Implications**
lithium carbonate (Eskalith)	Narrow therapeutic range increases risk of toxicity.
	Monitor blood levels.
	Do not use in cardiac or renal disease.
	Do not use with diuretics.
	Do not use in pregnant patients.
	Check interactions with other medications.

Antiparkinsonian Agents	

Restore the natural balance of acetylcholine and dopamine in the CNS to manage extrapyramidal side effects.

Examples	**Nursing Implications**
benztropine (Cogentin)	Caution in patients with hypersensitivity, glaucoma, or history of urine retention.
trihexyphenidyl (Artane)	
diphenhydramine (Benadryl)	

Table 57.3
Anxiety Summary

Signs and Symptoms	*Phobia:* irrational fear of object or situation
	Panic disorder: extreme fear, feelings of impending doom, palpitations
	Generalized anxiety disorder: worry, restlessness, palpitations
Diagnosis	History of symptoms; physical causes for symptoms must be ruled out first
Therapeutic Measures	Antianxiety medication
	Selective serotonin reuptake inhibitors
	Systematic desensitization
	Psychotherapy
	Relaxation exercises
Primary Nursing Diagnosis	*Anxiety*

• Maintain open communication. Encourage the patient to verbalize thoughts and feelings. Observe nonverbal communication. *Honesty in dealing with patients helps them learn to trust others and enhances their self-esteem.*

• Encourage the patient to use positive self-talk, such as, "I can do this. Anxiety can't kill me." *This helps the patient replace negative anxious thoughts with positive statements to reduce anxiety.*

• Report and document any changes in behavior, such as positive or negative alterations in the way a patient responds to the nursing staff, the treatment plan, or other people and situations. *Any change can be significant to the patient's care.*

• Encourage activities but avoid placing the patient in a competitive situation. *Activities that are enjoyable and nonstressful provide diversion and give staff members an opportunity to provide positive feedback about the progress the patient is making. Competitive situations can produce anxiety.*

• Encourage problem-solving and assist to develop alternative solutions. Help the patient to identify what has worked in the past. *This can help the patient focus on strategies that were effective in the past and eliminate those that are not effective.*

• Stay with a patient during acute severe or panic levels of anxiety. *Feelings of being abandoned can increase* anxiety. *The nurse's presence provides a feeling of safety for the patient.*

• Implement suicide precautions if indicated. *The patient may need to be protected from self-harm until treatment is effective.*

• Assess your own level of anxiety. *An anxious nurse may make the patient more anxious.*

EVALUATION. The patient will be able to implement strategies to control anxiety, recognize triggers of anxiety, and state he or she feels less anxious. Physical signs, such as tremors or changes in vital signs, will be improved.

CRITICAL THINKING

Tommy has come to the clinic with numerous cracks on his hands. They are bleeding and very sore. Tommy tells you that he has to wash his hands all the time. His mother says he washes for 2 to 3 hours at a time, and he will not stop when she tells him to. The doctor has diagnosed Tommy with obsessive-compulsive disorder and has explained the illness to Tommy and his mother. When the doctor leaves the room, Tommy's mother begins to cry. "What did he just say? What am I supposed to do? What did I do wrong that Tommy got this illness?"

How can you respond therapeutically? What team member would you use as a resource?

Suggested answers are at the end of the chapter.

◼ MOOD DISORDERS

Mood disorders (also called affective disorders) are disorders in which the major symptom is extreme changes or instability in mood (emotions) and affect (the outward expression of the mood). Moods involving both highs and lows are bipolar disorders; low moods without any highs are described as depressive disorders. Mood disorders are diagnosed when symptoms begin to interfere with normal day-to-day functioning. People of all age groups and all ethnic and socioeconomic groups can develop mood disorders. Healthy People 2020 (Office of Disease Prevention and Health Promotion, 2017) has objectives to reduce major depressive episodes in both adolescents and adults and to reduce the rate of suicides and suicide attempts.

> **BE SAFE!**
> ***BE VIGILANT!*** Find out which individuals served are most likely to try to commit suicide. (The Joint Commission's 2018 National Patient Safety Goals © The Joint Commission, 2018. Reprinted with permission.)

Etiological Theories

Psychoanalytic theory explains that people who have suffered loss in their lives are at risk for developing depression. Depression is also associated with unresolved anger and has been described as "anger turned inward." In other words,

people who cannot or do not deal appropriately with situations that anger them may repress the anger (turn it inside) and become depressed.

Cognitive theorists believe that the way people perceive events and situations may lead to depression. Instead of thinking about failing an examination as being unfortunate and disappointing, some people with tendencies toward depression may exaggerate the emotion and turn the situation into something much deeper, such as thoughts of "I'm stupid" or "I'll never get anywhere."

Biological theories offer genetic links and neurotransmitter dysfunctions as two etiologies. Serotonin, norepinephrine, and dopamine have an effect on mood. If these neurotransmitters are elevated, mood is elevated; if they are low, mood is low. Some biological theorists also believe that there is a connection between these neurotransmitters and female hormones.

Differential Diagnosis

Symptoms of depression may occur in conjunction with other disorders, such as schizophrenia or drug side effects or overuse. Heart failure, nutritional deficiencies, drug toxicity, thyroid disease, fluid and electrolyte imbalances, infections, and diabetes can be associated with depression.

Types of Mood Disorders

Major (Unipolar) Depression

Major depression is an episodic condition. Its symptoms interfere with the person's usual social or occupational functioning. Depressed people may be described as viewing the world through "gray-tinted glasses." The *DSM-5* specifies that symptoms of major depression include either depressed mood or **anhedonia** (the loss of pleasure in things that are usually pleasurable) along with at least five of the following symptoms:

• Significant weight loss or gain—more than 5% in a month
• Increase or decrease in appetite
• Sleep pattern disturbances—insomnia or hypersomnia
• Increased fatigue or loss of energy
• Increased agitation or psychomotor retardation
• Decreased ability to think, remember, or concentrate
• Feelings of guilt or hopelessness
• Indecisiveness
• Suicidal ideation

Bipolar Disorder

About 2 million people in the United States have **bipolar** disorder. Formerly called *manic depressive illness,* bipolar disorder is a mood disorder in which patients experience the mood states of **mania** (extreme elation or agitation) and extreme depression. Bipolar disorder is more severe than major depression. Affected people stay depressed longer, relapse more often, display more depressive symptoms, have more delusions and hallucinations, commit suicide more often, require more hospitalizations, and overall experience more disability.

• WORD • BUILDING •
anhedonia: an—not + hedonia—pleasure

Affected people can cycle slowly (over weeks, months, or even years), or they can be "rapid cyclers" who can change moods several times in an hour. Research indicates that individuals with bipolar disorder do not experience periods of normal mood alternating with periods of abnormal mood as previously believed. Instead, bipolar illness is characterized by frequent mood lability, with both manic and depressive symptoms, that are sometimes milder and sometimes more severe (Beddes, 2013).

Common signs of major depression were covered in the preceding section. Common signs of mania include the following:

- Excessive high (euphoric) moods lasting at least 1 week
- Increased energy, activity, and restlessness
- Decreased need for sleep
- Grandiosity (unrealistic belief in one's abilities or powers)
- Extreme irritability and distractibility
- Uncharacteristically poor judgment
- Pressured and rapid speech
- Flight of ideas or subjective experience that one's thoughts are racing
- Increase in goal-directed behavior
- Excessive involvement in pleasurable activities that have a high potential for unpleasant consequences, such as sex, substance abuse, or shopping sprees
- Obnoxious, provocative, or intrusive behavior

Therapeutic Measures for Patients With Mood Disorders

About 80% of people with major depression respond to treatment. Bipolar disorder is more difficult to treat. Some common medical treatments for *all* mood disorders include the following:

- Antidepressant medications
- Mood stabilizers
- Psychotherapy
- Electroconvulsive therapy (ECT)

Lithium was once the drug of choice for treating bipolar disorder. It is an antimanic medication with a very narrow therapeutic range, which means that toxic drug levels can easily develop. Blood must be drawn regularly to assess that serum lithium levels are in the therapeutic range.

Mood stabilizers, such as the anticonvulsants valproic acid (Depakote) and lamotrigine (Lamictal), are now more commonly used than lithium to treat bipolar disorder. Atypical antipsychotics are also commonly used with a mood stabilizer when the patient is in an acute manic state. Antidepressant agents, if used, should be monitored carefully because they can trigger a manic episode. See Table 57.2 for a summary of medications. Also see "Nutrition Notes."

Psychotherapy for the patient and family may be helpful for any type of mood disorder. It can help the patient understand the illness and learn problem-solving and other new adaptive coping behaviors. For young children, play therapy is the most common and effective form of therapy. ECT is an option for individuals with rapid-cycling bipolar disorder or major depression that is not responsive to conventional treatment.

Nutrition Notes

Food-Drug Interactions in Patients Taking Lithium. Lithium carbonate (Eskalith), used to treat bipolar disorder, is absorbed, distributed, and excreted alongside sodium. Fluctuations in sodium and caffeine intake may affect lithium metabolism and should remain consistent while a patient is being treated with lithium:

- Decreased sodium and caffeine or caffeine intake with decreased fluid intake may lead to retention of lithium and overmedication.
- Increased sodium or caffeine intake from food or medications and increased fluid intake may hasten excretion of lithium, resulting in worsening signs and symptoms of mania.

Reference

National Institutes of Health Clinical Center Drug-Nutrient Interaction Task Force. (2011). Important drug and food information: Lithium. Retrieved from www.cc.nih.gov/ccc/patient_education/drug_nutrient/lithium1.pdf

BE SAFE!

BE VIGILANT! When collecting data from your patient, be sure to ask about herbal supplements and over-the-counter (OTC) medications the patient may use in addition to prescription medications. Many people take St. John's wort, an OTC herbal supplement, for depression. Although it may be effective for some people with mild depression, it can interact with many prescribed medications that influence serotonin levels. If combined with prescription serotonin-type antidepressants, it can cause serotonin syndrome, an excess of serotonin resulting in agitation, confusion, diarrhea, muscle spasms, and even death (Bartlett, 2017).

CRITICAL THINKING

Mr. Zenz is the director of nursing at a long-term care facility. His usual behavior is rather sullen, and he comes across as quiet or sad to various members of the staff. His management style at the facility is to let people do their jobs; he rarely interferes, unless staff let him know of a problem. Recently, however, staff members have noticed a change in Mr. Zenz. He spends more time interacting with staff and residents. He moves quickly, speaks loudly, and has set unrealistic goals for the staff. He frequently says he has called the owner of the facility to tell him of his new ideas. He says he has not slept in several days, and he feels terrific. He has changed his wardrobe and has begun pointing out specific performance issues to staff. He jokes with staff. Staff members are made aware that he has bipolar disorder and has quit taking his medications.

His wife has asked for the staff's help. Remember: He is your boss.

How do you respond to Mrs. Zenz? How do you approach Mr. Zenz?

Suggested answers are at the end of the chapter.

Nursing Process for the Patient With a Mood Disorder

See "Nursing Care Plan for the Patient With Depression." Also see Table 57.4.

Nursing Care Plan for the Patient With Depression

Nursing Diagnosis: *Ineffective Coping*
Expected Outcomes: The patient will cope effectively as evidenced by verbalizing the ability to cope and asking for help when needed and by demonstrating new effective coping strategies.
Evaluation of Outcomes: Does the patient exhibit increased ability to problem-solve and cope with stressors?

Intervention	Rationale	Evaluation
Use therapeutic communication techniques to allow patient to verbalize feelings.	*Verbalization of feelings in a supportive environment can assist patient to work through issues.*	Does patient verbalize feelings to nursing staff?
Assist patient to describe stressors and identify his or her existing coping skills and knowledge.	*Providing validation of actual stress and available coping resources and strategies aids in positive adaptation to stress.*	Is patient able to identify stressors? Does patient have some effective coping skills on which to draw?
Help patient set realistic goals.	*Achievement of small steps toward a goal can help the patient feel empowered.*	Does patient set realistic goals?
Encourage patient to make choices and participate in care.	*Active involvement in care increases the possibility of positive adjustment.*	Is patient actively involved in care?

Nursing Diagnosis: *Powerlessness*
Expected Outcomes: The patient will have reduced feelings of powerlessness as evidenced by verbal expression of having control over life, situation, or care and by participation in care or decision making when opportunities are provided.
Evaluation of Outcomes: Does the patient identify feelings of powerlessness? Does the patient identify factors that are controllable and actively participate in care?

Intervention	Rationale	Evaluation
Assess for factors contributing to powerlessness.	*Correct identification of actual or perceived problems is essential to providing appropriate support.*	Is patient able to identify factors contributing to powerlessness?
Help patient to identify factors that are or are not under his or her control.	*Identifying factors within patient's control encourages patient to take some control over the situation.*	Is patient able to identify what is controllable and what is not controllable in his or her life?
Allow ventilation of powerless feelings.	*Sharing feelings in groups can lead to the realization that similar feelings are experienced by others and reduce feelings of powerlessness.*	Is patient sharing feelings with nursing staff and in therapeutic groups?
Encourage patient to actively participate in care with goal-directed activities.	*Goal-directed behavior increases self-efficacy and empowerment.*	Does patient set realistic goals daily and achieve them daily?

Nursing Care Plan for the Patient With Depression—cont'd

Nursing Diagnosis: *Risk for Suicide*
Expected Outcome: The patient will not harm himself or herself.
Evaluation of Outcome: Did the patient remain free from self-harm during hospitalization? Does the patient have ongoing support following discharge?

Intervention	Rationale	Evaluation
Ask patient directly about suicidal ideations each shift.	*Ongoing assessment of suicidal risk is essential to patient safety.*	Is patient verbalizing warning signs of suicide?
Create a safe environment for patient.	*Patient safety is a nursing priority.*	Are means of harming self kept from patient?
Initiate suicide precautions according to agency protocol.	*Patient must be protected until risk is reduced.*	Is increased surveillance of patient implemented and communicated to all staff?
Encourage patient to seek out nursing staff when experiencing suicidal thoughts.	*Active listening and therapeutic communication by staff provide patient with empathy and alternatives to acting on suicidal thoughts.*	Does patient seek out nursing staff when experiencing suicidal thoughts?

 SCHIZOPHRENIA

Schizophrenia is becoming more widely viewed as a group of illnesses rather than a single condition. The term *schizophrenia* (which means "split mind") was first used by a Swiss psychiatrist, Eugene Bleuler (1911). Schizophrenia is a serious disorder of thought and association. It is characterized by inability to distinguish between what is real and what is

Table 57.4
Depression Summary

Signs and Symptoms	*Unipolar (major):* depressed mood, weight changes, anhedonia, sleep disturbance, social withdrawal *Bipolar:* signs and symptoms of depression cycling with euphoria, delusions, hallucinations
Diagnosis	History; physiological causes must be ruled out
Therapeutic Measures	Antidepressant medication, mood stabilizers (anticonvulsants), psychotherapy, electroconvulsive therapy
Primary Nursing Diagnoses	*Ineffective Coping* *Powerlessness* *Risk for Suicide*

Evidence-Based Practice

Clinical Question
How do young people living with mental illness view their lives and manage their health?

Evidence
A systematic review of qualitative literature included 54 research papers and 304 study findings. They were combined into nine categories and four synthesis statements (Woodgate et al., 2017). Young people living with mental illness expressed the need for a different way of being, felt challenged to get through difficult times, and yearned for acceptance. There are numerous barriers for accessing help.

Implications for Nursing Practice
Young people living with mental illness need continuous support and plans of care with multiple coping strategies, using a collaborative interdisciplinary approach. Decreasing barriers to accessing help as well as offering a therapeutic approach when interacting with this population is important.

Reference
Woodgate, R. L., Sigurdson, C., Demczuk, L., Tennent, P., Wallis, B., & Werner, P. (2017). The meanings young people assign to living with mental illness and their experiences managing their health and lives: A systematic review of qualitative evidence. *JBI Database of Systematic Reviews and Implementation Reports, 15*(2), 276–401. doi:10.11124/JBISRIR-2016003283

not as well as by hallucinations, delusions, and limited socialization. People who have schizophrenia may not be able to differentiate between what is "theirs" and what is "everybody else's" in relation to social functioning. Poor self-esteem may be present. It is difficult for them to focus on one topic for any length of time. Schizophrenia is not the same as dissociative identity disorder (once called multiple personality disorder). Schizophrenia often begins during adolescence or young adulthood. It develops over time, and symptoms may go unnoticed for a time before diagnosis. There are four phases of schizophrenia:

1. *Schizoid personality.* Those in this phase are perceived as being indifferent, cold, and aloof. They are often described as loners and don't seem to enjoy close relationships with others. In adolescence, these behaviors may be dismissed as normal for age. Not all individuals with schizoid personality go on to develop schizophrenia.
2. *Prodromal phase.* Affected people continue to be socially withdrawn and begin to show behavior that is peculiar or eccentric. Role functioning is impaired, personal hygiene is neglected, and disturbances are evident in communication, ideation, and perception.
3. *Schizophrenia.* This is the third and active phase of the disorder. Psychotic symptoms are prominent and include delusions, hallucinations, and impairment in work, social relations, and self-care.
4. *Residual phase.* Symptoms are like the prodromal phase, with flat affect and impairment in role functioning.

Positive and Negative Symptoms

Positive symptoms of schizophrenia can be thought of as those symptoms that reflect an "excess" or distortion of normal functioning. Patients are usually hospitalized for exacerbation of positive symptoms, which include hallucinations, delusions, disorganized thinking, and disorganized behavior. **Delusions** are fixed, false beliefs that cannot be changed by logic or factual proof. Patients may exhibit delusions of grandeur, persecution, or guilt. **Hallucinations** are false sensory perceptions. They can affect any of the five senses; auditory and visual delusions are most common. For example, a person might see a person no one else sees or hear voices that no one else hears. In contrast, **illusions** are mistaken perceptions of reality. For example, a person may see a glowing sunset and think the horizon is on fire. Both typical and atypical antipsychotic medications work well to manage the positive symptoms of schizophrenia.

Negative symptoms of schizophrenia can be thought of as a loss of normal functioning. Negative symptoms include affective blunting or flattening, **alogia, avolition,** apathy, anhedonia, and social isolation. It is thought that these are the most debilitating symptoms of schizophrenia because they keep the individual from living a normal life. These symptoms respond to atypical antipsychotic medications but not the typical antipsychotic agents.

Pathophysiology and Etiology

The causes of schizophrenia are widely believed to be a combination of neurobiological and environmental factors. Psychological factors as the cause of schizophrenia are no longer considered valid because most researchers and clinicians consider schizophrenia to be a brain disease.

The role of genetics in schizophrenia (neurobiological or nature theory) has been examined in twin studies, family studies, and adoption studies for more than 75 years. Studies of identical twins show that if one twin has schizophrenia, the other has about a 50% chance of developing it. In fraternal twins, the percentage drops to about 10%. It is believed that the more genes twins or family members have in common, the greater the probability of the second twin developing schizophrenia. Additional support for the role of genetics is demonstrated by adoption studies. Research indicates that children born to mothers with schizophrenia are more likely to develop the disorder even when raised in adoptive families.

Other studies have examined brain structure and the relationship between neurotransmitters and schizophrenia. Patients with a diagnosis of schizophrenia typically have elevated dopamine levels or a brain that overreacts to the amount of dopamine present. Glutamate is an excitatory neurotransmitter that also appears to be related to schizophrenia. The glutamate theory proposes that there is an excess of glutamate of the brain (Howes, McCutcheon, & Stone, 2015). The brains of patients with a diagnosis of schizophrenia show a significant loss of gray matter, enlarged ventricles, and diminished prefrontal cortex functioning. Today, schizophrenia is primarily thought of as a series of brain disorders characterized by brain abnormalities and neurotransmitter dysfunction.

Environmental factors that increase risk of schizophrenia include such things as central nervous system damage during childbirth, some infections, and substance abuse.

Symptoms

Patients with paranoid symptoms tend to exhibit unusual suspicions and fears. The person may also be hostile and aggressive or have delusions of persecution or grandeur. Those with persecutory delusions may state that they feel tormented or followed by people. Patients often integrate people around them into their delusions. They may feel that nursing staff, relatives, or announcers on the radio or television are trying to harm them. In delusions of grandeur, patients might state that they are God or the president of the United States.

Hallucinations often accompany delusions and can affect any of the five senses. The most common hallucinations are auditory, followed by visual. Patients diagnosed with schizophrenia talk about hearing voices. These voices are frightening

---

• WORD • BUILDING •

alogia: a—not + logia—(able to) speak

avolition: a—not + volition—energy or initiative to do something

and derogatory to the patient and are responsible for many of the actions performed by people with paranoid schizophrenia. Patients experience increased fear, anxiety, and suicidal ideation as a result of the voices. You may see or hear patients arguing with what at first appears to be themselves. Actually, the patient is arguing with the voices. Describing the voices is difficult, but imagine that you are in a room with six televisions on different stations at the same time. This example comes close to what some patients have described.

Therapeutic Measures

Medications, social skills training, and individual and family psychotherapy are indicated for patients with schizophrenia. Among the classifications of medications that may be prescribed are the typical and atypical antipsychotics, which block dopamine action in the brain. There are different dopamine tracts in the brain. Typical antipsychotics have a greater effect on the D_2 dopamine receptors of the motor function tract, resulting in extrapyramidal side effects such as parkinsonism (see Table 57.2). Anticholinergic medications such as benztropine (Cogentin) or trihexyphenidyl (Artane) are used to combat the extrapyramidal side effects of the typical antipsychotic by helping return balance among dopamine, acetylcholine, and other neurotransmitters. Newer, atypical antipsychotic medications such as lurasidone (Latuda) and risperidone (Risperdal) have fewer extrapyramidal side effects but have other side effects. Atypical antipsychotics are effective in treating both the positive and negative symptoms of schizophrenia.

Psychotherapy can include individual, group, and family therapy (Table 57.5). ECT is used in some severe cases; it is not usually used until other methods of therapy have been exhausted. Referral of the patient and family to organizations such as the National Alliance on Mental Illness (www.nami.org) provides helpful education and support. Table 57.6 provides suggestions for responding to patients experiencing hallucinations.

Nursing Process for the Patient With Schizophrenia

DATA COLLECTION. Observe the patient with schizophrenia for positive and negative symptoms, including hallucinations, delusions, and illusions. Observe interactions with others. Monitor the patient for response to medications, including side effects. Determine the person's ability to function and manage activities of daily living (ADLs).

NURSING DIAGNOSES, PLANNING, AND IMPLEMENTATION.

Social Isolation related to inability to trust and delusional thinking

EXPECTED OUTCOME: The patient will willingly attend milieu activities and initiate interactions with staff and peers.

• Establish a therapeutic rapport with the patient. *This will help the patient learn to interact with others.*

Table 57.5
Schizophrenia Summary

Signs and Symptoms	Disorganized speech and behavior Ineffective thinking and decision making Trouble functioning at school and work; self-care deficits *Positive symptoms:* hallucinations, delusions *Negative symptoms:* apathy, flat affect, anhedonia
Diagnosis	History Psychiatric evaluation *DSM-5* criteria
Therapeutic Measures	Antipsychotic medications Anticholinergic agents to control side effects Psychotherapy Family education Social skills training and therapy
Primary Nursing Diagnoses	*Social Isolation* *Impaired Verbal Communication*

• Convey acceptance and unconditional positive regard for the patient. *An accepting attitude may facilitate trust and increase feelings of self-worth.*
• Assure the patient of his or her safety. *An isolative patient may be fearful of the other patients or staff members.*
• Offer to accompany patient to milieu activities. *An isolative patient may be more likely to be present in the milieu if accompanied by a supportive individual.*
• Acknowledge the patient's efforts to interact and attend activities. *Positive reinforcement may encourage the patient's attempts at interaction.*

EVALUATION. If interventions have been effective, the patient will participate in therapy and interact with other staff and patients.

CRITICAL THINKING

Anne is a young woman receiving chemotherapy on your oncology unit. While preparing to invite her to a movie in the day room, you observe her standing in the corner of her room, trembling. You ask her what's wrong, and she responds that she's talking to the woman in the wall. Your first instinct is to giggle, but you ask her, "What woman?" She tells you that you wouldn't understand and says, "You helped put her there, and you told me that it is my job to be sure she can't get out." You report this to the charge nurse, who calls the physician. Tests are run, and it is determined that Anne is not experiencing side effects from the chemotherapy. Further workup delivers the diagnosis of schizophrenia for Anne.

1. What therapeutic responses are appropriate for this situation? How will you get Anne to the movie or to participate in other care activities?
2. What special needs might Anne now experience relating to her chemotherapy, if any?
3. What actions can team members take to promote trust with Anne?

Suggested answers are at the end of the chapter.

 PERSONALITY DISORDERS

How many times have you heard, "She has such a good personality"? What is it that determines an individual's personality? Personality is composed of enduring patterns or traits that determine how an individual perceives, relates to, and thinks about the environment and self. An individual's personality develops as the person adjusts to physical, emotional, social, and spiritual environments. Personality traits or patterns are reflected in how individuals cope with feelings and impulses, see themselves and others, respond to their surroundings, and find meaning in relationships.

Etiology

The causes of personality disorders are unknown. Genetic and family environmental factors as well as neurobiological and other social factors are thought to play a role.

Diagnosis

Personality disorders are diagnosed when the personality patterns or traits are inflexible, enduring, pervasive, and maladaptive and cause significant functional impairment or subjective distress. In the United States, 9.1% of the population has been diagnosed with a personality disorder (National Institute of Mental Health, 2017).

Personality disorders are characterized by the following:

• *Behavioral manifestations:* Dysfunctional patterns of day-to-day behavior and impulse control
• *Affective manifestations:* Inappropriate range, intensity, mood lability, and emotional response
• *Cognitive manifestations:* Inaccurate interpretation of self, others, and events
• *Sociocultural manifestations:* Ineffective interpersonal functioning

Patients with personality disorders exhibit common problem behaviors that create difficulty in daily living. *Manipulation* is a control behavior that uses and exploits others for personal gain. *Narcissism* is self-centered behavior in which the individual feels entitled to special favors or feels justified in not obeying authority and rules. *Impulsive behavior* creates difficulties for those patients who act without considering the consequences of their own behavior.

The *DSM-5* lists 10 personality disorders that are organized into three diagnostic clusters: Cluster A: Odd and Eccentric, Cluster B: Dramatic and Erratic, and Cluster C: Anxious and Fearful. This text covers two of the more common personality disorders in Cluster B: borderline personality disorder and antisocial personality disorder.

Table 57.6

Suggested Interventions for Patients With Schizophrenia Who Are Hallucinating

Suggested Action	Rationale
"Mr. R., I don't see any snakes. It is time for lunch. I will walk to the dining room with you."	Lets the patient know you heard him, but brings him immediately into the reality of time of day and need to go to the dining room.
"I see a crack in the wall, Mr. R. It is harmless; you are safe. Susan is here to take you down to occupational therapy now."	This is in response to a probable illusion. It lets the patient know that you see something. It validates his fear, but it tells him what you see and then moves him into the here and now.
"I know that your thoughts seem very real to you, Ms. C., but they do not seem logical to me. I would like for you to come to your room and get dressed now, please."	Again, you are validating the patient's concern without exploring and focusing on the delusion.
"Ms. C., it appears to me that you are listening to someone. Are you hearing voices other than mine?"	This is a method of validating your impression of what you see. This is as far as you will go into exploring what she may be hearing.
"Thank you, Ms. C. I want to help you focus away from the other voices. I am real; they are not. Please come with me to the reading room."	Responds to her in the present and reinforces her response to you. Attempts to redirect her thinking.

Borderline Personality Disorder

Individuals with borderline personality disorder (BPD) display a pattern of instability of interpersonal relationships, self-image, and affect. There is marked impulsivity. The personality pattern is present by early adulthood and occurs across a variety of situations. Other symptoms may include intense fear of abandonment, anger and irritability, chronic feelings of emptiness, and transient paranoia or dissociative symptoms. Patients with BPD often engage in idealization and devaluation of others, alternating between high positive regard and great disappointment. This is a defense mechanism referred to as *splitting*. Self-mutilation and recurrent suicidal behavior, gestures, and threats are common.

Antisocial Personality Disorder

Antisocial personality disorder (ASPD) is characterized by a pervasive pattern of disregard for and violation of the rights of others. This begins in childhood or early adolescence and continues into adulthood. Individuals with ASPD have a lack of empathy and/or remorse for their actions. There is a failure to conform to social norms, which often leads to a history of legal problems or criminal behavior. Behavior can be impulsive and aggressive, with a reckless disregard for the safety of self or others. Deceitfulness and consistent irresponsibility are common.

Therapeutic Measures
Psychotherapy

Psychotherapy is the primary way to treat personality disorders. Using the insight and knowledge gained in psychotherapy, patients can learn healthy ways to manage their illness. Types of psychotherapy used to treat personality disorders include cognitive behavioral therapy and psychoeducation. *Cognitive behavioral therapy* helps patients identify unhealthy, negative beliefs and behaviors and replace them with healthy, positive ones. *Dialectical behavior therapy* is a type of cognitive behavioral therapy that teaches behavioral skills to help patients tolerate stress, regulate their emotions, and improve their relationships with others. *Psychodynamic psychotherapy* focuses on increasing the patient's awareness of unconscious thoughts and behaviors, developing new insights and motivations, and resolving conflicts. Psychoeducation teaches the patient and family members about their illness, including treatments, coping strategies, and problem-solving skills.

There are no medications specifically approved to treat personality disorders. However, several types of psychiatric medications may help with various common symptoms. Antidepressant medications are used to treat depressed mood, anger, impulsivity, irritability, or hopelessness. Mood-stabilizing medications are used to help even out mood swings or reduce irritability, impulsivity, and aggression. Antianxiety medications can address anxiety, agitation, or insomnia. Antipsychotic medications can help with paranoia, aggression, anger, and impulsiveness.

Nursing Process for the Patient With a Personality Disorder

DATA COLLECTION. A priority nursing action is assessment of suicidal or homicidal ideation. Mood and affect should also be assessed as depressed, angry, or labile. Mood can indicate a higher risk for self-injury. Assess for paranoia, manipulative behaviors, and impulsiveness as well as history of violence. It will also be necessary to obtain a medical history, psychiatric history, developmental history, and information about sociocultural background.

NURSING DIAGNOSIS, PLANNING, AND IMPLEMENTATION.

Risk for Other-Directed Violence related to impulsivity, impaired judgment, and disregard for the rights of others

EXPECTED OUTCOME: The patient will not harm self or others. The patient will discuss feelings with staff instead of acting on them. The patient will verbalize adaptive coping strategies for use when hostile or suicidal feelings occur.

- Monitor the patient's behavior frequently. *Close monitoring is required so that intervention can occur if required to ensure safety.*
- Remove all dangerous objects from the patient's environment (e.g., sharp items, belts, ties, straps, breakable items, smoking materials). *Safety is a nursing priority.*
- Redirect violent behavior by means of physical outlets for the patient's anxiety (e.g., exercise machines, walking). *Physical activity can be an effective way of relieving tension and stress.*
- Maintain a calm attitude toward the patient. *Anxiety is contagious and can be transmitted from staff members to patient.*
- Encourage appropriate verbal expression of emotions. *Verbalization of feelings in a nonthreatening environment may assist the patient to develop insight into the situation.*

EVALUATION. The patient will be able to discuss anger with staff, engage in physical activity to cope with tension, and act responsive to calm interaction. The patient and others are safe from harm, and environmental safety has been maintained.

AUTISM SPECTRUM DISORDERS

Autism spectrum disorders (ASDs) are lifelong neurodevelopmental disabilities that are typically recognized during the second year of life. ASD prevalence is believed to occur in about 1% of the population in the United States. ASDs are diagnosed four times more in males than in females.

Etiology

ASDs are characterized by abnormal brain development and function. Although the specific causes are unknown, an ASD is likely to have multiple etiologies, including genetic factors. A range of studies has found that, in 10% to 37% of cases, there may be an associated medical condition such as maternal rubella or Angelman syndrome. Current research is also showing that the frontal lobe and amygdala appear to have abnormal growth patterns in patients with ASDs. One study showed that the amygdala, which controls emotions, undergoes disproportionate enlargement by 37 months of age in ASDs (Nordahl et al., 2012). Hereditary estimates range from 37% to higher than 90% based on twin studies. Environmental risk factors include advanced parental age, low birth weight, and fetal exposure to valproate, an anticonvulsant medication.

Signs and Symptoms

An ASD is characterized by (1) deficits in social communication and social interaction and (2) restricted and repetitive behaviors (RRBs), interests, and activities.

Patients with ASDs tend to have communication deficits, such as responding inappropriately in conversations, misreading nonverbal cues, or having difficulty building friendships appropriate to their age. Patients with ASDs may desire friendship and interaction with others, but their inability to understand the emotions, motivations, and perspectives makes relationships difficult. In addition, patients with ASDs may be overly dependent on routines, highly sensitive to changes in their environment, or intensely focused on inappropriate items.

Therapeutic Measures

Early intervention services can greatly improve a child's development and can help children from birth to 3 years learn important skills. Such services include therapy to help the child talk, walk, and interact with others.

The various treatments are targeted toward addressing deficits in communication, social interaction, and behaviors. Applied behavior analysis (ABA) has become widely accepted among health care professionals and is used in many schools and treatment clinics. ABA encourages positive behaviors and discourages negative behaviors to improve a variety of skills.

Occupational therapy teaches skills that help the patient with ADLs such as dressing, eating, bathing, and relating to people. Sensory integration therapy helps the patient cope with sensory information, including sights, sounds, and smells. Sensory integration therapy may help a patient who cannot tolerate certain sounds or physical touch. Speech therapy helps to improve the patient's communication skills either verbally or by using sign language, gestures, or picture boards. The Picture Exchange Communication System uses picture symbols to teach communication skills.

Medications do not provide a cure for ASDs and do not address the key symptoms. Some medications can help people with ASDs function better by managing high energy levels, inability to focus, depression, or seizures. The U.S. Food and Drug Administration has approved the use of the antipsychotic medications risperidone (Risperdal) and aripiprazole (Abilify) to treat patients with ASDs who exhibit behavioral problems such as tantrums, aggression, or self-injurious behaviors. Referral of the patient and family to organizations such as Autism Speaks (www.autismspeaks.org/family-services/resource-guide) can provide helpful education and support.

Nursing Process for the Patient With an Autism Spectrum Disorder

DATA COLLECTION. Assess the patient for developmental spurts or lags or loss of previously acquired skills. Observe the caregiver–patient relationship for bonding, anxiety, tension, and difficult fit. Discuss the patient's social, communication, and behavioral strengths and limitations with the caregiver. Assess the patient for communication style and verbal and nonverbal skills. Assess for risk of injury to self and others, and be alert for the potential for abuse.

NURSING DIAGNOSIS, PLANNING, AND IMPLEMENTATION.

Impaired Social Interaction related to neurological alterations

EXPECTED OUTCOME: The patient will interact appropriately and develop a trusting relationship with at least one staff member. The patient will function appropriately in the inpatient milieu.

- Assign consistent staff to the patient. *This is essential to the development of trust.*
- Provide positive reinforcement for the patient's voluntary interactions with others. *Positive reinforcement enhances self-esteem and encourages repetition of desirable behaviors.*
- Provide direct feedback about the patient's interactions with others in a nonjudgmental manner. *Direct feedback from a trusted individual may help to alter behaviors in a positive manner.*
- Help the patient learn how to respond more appropriately in interactions with others. Practice new skills through role-play. *Practicing skills in role-play facilitates use in real situations.*
- Give positive feedback when eye contact is used. *Positive reinforcement enhances self-esteem and encourages repetition of desirable behaviors.*

EVALUATION. The patient will be able to establish trust with at least one staff member, engage in voluntary interaction with others, be responsive to feedback regarding interactions, be responsive to role-plays, and make eye contact.

 EATING DISORDERS

Anorexia Nervosa

Anorexia nervosa is an eating disorder recognized by the American Psychiatric Association. This disease most commonly occurs in females between ages 12 and 30. Males account for less than 10% of those with anorexia nervosa. Depression and anxiety often are also present. Anorexia nervosa is thought to be multifactorial in origin. Patients may have a phobia about weight gain, be afraid of a loss of control, and be mistrusting.

Signs and Symptoms

The *DSM-5* criteria for anorexia nervosa include restriction of energy intake, an intense fear of gaining weight, and a disturbance in the way one's body weight or shape is experienced. The *DSM-5* further specifies whether the disorder is a restricting type (dieting, fasting) or binge-eating/purging type (self-induced vomiting; misuse of laxatives, diuretics, or enemas). The severity of the disorder is determined by current body mass index. As the disease progresses, additional symptoms appear, including electrolyte imbalance, cardiac arrhythmias, constipation, dry skin, lanugo (downy hair covering body), bradycardia, hypothermia, hypotension, muscle wasting, and facial puffiness. Often, patients with anorexia nervosa deny the existence of any problem. They may develop bizarre food rituals and sometimes weigh themselves several times a day.

Complications

Chronic poor nutrition takes its toll on the body. Complications from starvation occur as the body tries to conserve energy. Pulse and blood pressure fall. Heart and kidney failure are a risk. Osteoporosis and muscle loss occur. Vitamin and electrolyte imbalances result. Diabetes may develop.

Therapeutic Measures

Treating this disorder is complex and requires a multidisciplinary approach. Patients often do not see the need for medical intervention. They do not usually seek help on their own and are often resistant to treatment. When treatment is sought, often through a concerned person's urgings, a medical and psychological workup is necessary. Nutritional status is also evaluated to determine the urgency of intervention. Establishing a trusting relationship, which can be difficult, is a key element in initiating treatment. Early treatment results in a better prognosis.

The first priority is restoration of nutritional health. Up to 18% of anorexia nervosa patients eventually die because of starvation and complications. Hospitalization and re-feeding are indicated for those who are underweight with severe weight loss, life-threatening electrolyte imbalances, and arrhythmias or other symptoms. Nutrition is supplied by intravenous infusions containing electrolytes. Oral food supplements may also be given. Restoring normal weight is a long, slow process. Gains may be small, with setbacks along the way. Praise and rewards for small achievements in weight gains (not food intake) are positive reinforcements that aid recovery. Programs that treat eating disorders are often set up on a reward system, with privileges being increased as progress occurs.

The patient's distorted self-image and need for control are underlying causes of the disorder that must be addressed in conjunction with the nutritional aspect. Psychotherapy and behavior modification that include participation of the patient's family members are used in treatment of anorexia nervosa. Restoration of control and development of a healthy self-image are the main focuses of therapy. Educating the patient on normal body weight, symptoms of the illness, effects of the illness on the body, and methods to feel more control can be helpful. Individual or group therapy is often used. The Maudsley approach is an evidence-based treatment for adolescents with anorexia nervosa (Treasure et al., 2015). During treatment, a support system is vital to success. Visit www.nationaleatingdisorders.org for resources for patients and families.

Bulimia Nervosa

Bulimia nervosa criteria is identified by the *DSM-5* as recurrent episodes of binge eating and recurrent inappropriate compensatory behaviors (purges) to avoid weight gain. Behaviors can include self-induced vomiting, misuse of laxatives or diuretics, fasting, or excessive exercise. The binging and purging both occur at least once a week for 3 months or more and do not occur exclusively during episodes of anorexia nervosa. The individual's self-evaluation is unduly influenced by body shape and weight. Severity is specified by the number of purges per week. Individuals with bulimia nervosa are often within a normal weight range.

Signs and Symptoms

Patients with bulimia nervosa exhibit many of the same signs and symptoms as patients with anorexia nervosa, with a few exceptions. Bulimic patients often have enamel erosion of the front teeth and staining caused by the acid content of the emesis. They also spend a great deal of time locked in the bathroom vomiting, especially after meals. Their knuckles may be calloused or have small cuts from the self-induced vomiting. They may have a chipmunk appearance from enlarged parotid glands secondary to the self-induced vomiting. Electrolyte imbalances occur from dehydration. The loss of potassium and sodium may result in arrhythmias, heart failure, and death. As the electrolyte imbalance worsens, metabolic alkalosis develops because of the loss of gastric acid in the stomach contents. Signs of metabolic alkalosis include hypokalemia and hypocalcemia. Laxative use results in irregular bowel movements.

Therapeutic Measures

Treatment for bulimia nervosa is essentially the same as for the patient with anorexia nervosa.

Nursing Process for the Patient With an Eating Disorder

Caring for patients with eating disorders is challenging. Gaining the patient's genuine cooperation by using therapeutic communication and setting realistic, mutual goals are important for establishing trust and preventing relapse. To work with patients with an eating disorder, a therapeutic relationship must be developed to facilitate effective interactions. Empathy, acceptance of the patient, trust, warmth, and unconditional positive regard are important.

Data Collection

Data are collected related to inadequate nutrition. Note changes in weight (15% or more below expected weight), poor skin turgor, poor muscle tone, lanugo, amenorrhea, electrolyte imbalances, swollen parotid glands, and hypothermia. Data collection findings may also include a normal weight, enamel erosion of front teeth, and metabolic alkalosis for the patient with bulimia. Note abnormal diagnostic studies such as anemia, electrolyte imbalances, altered endocrine studies, and electrocardiogram changes.

Nursing Diagnoses, Planning, and Implementation

Imbalanced Nutrition: Less Than Body Requirements related to inadequate food intake and/or inappropriate compensatory behaviors

EXPECTED OUTCOME: The patient will establish a dietary pattern and gain weight toward desired individual weight range.

- Monitor the patient's weight *to determine baseline* and monitor the patient's progress *toward goal.*
- Monitor vital signs and laboratory studies *to detect changes in cardiac function related to electrolyte imbalances.*
- Promote a consistent approach *to enhance acceptance by the patient and to build trust.*
- Promote a pleasant eating environment and record intake *to enhance patient intake.*
- Provide six small meals and snacks *to prevent gastric dilation.*

Disturbed Body Image related to psychosocial or cognitive/perceptual changes

EXPECTED OUTCOME: The patient will verbalize satisfaction with body appearance.

- Assess and document the patient's verbal and nonverbal responses to own body *to provide baseline understanding of the patient's perceptions of body image.*
- Listen to the patient and acknowledge reality of concerns regarding treatment and progress *to establish therapeutic relationship.*
- Monitor frequency of negative statements about self *to determine whether interventions are helping the patient.*
- Assist with referrals to social services or counseling *to help the patient overcome psychosocial issues.*
- Provide care in a nonjudgmental manner *to maintain the patient's dignity.*
- Use positive praise when the patient verbalizes positive comments about own body. *Praise reinforces the behavior and increases likelihood of repeating the desired behavior.*
- Encourage the patient to verbalize consequences of an eating disorder that have influenced self-concept *to help the patient realize the negative impact of the eating disorder.*

Evaluation

The patient's goals are met if the patient gains weight toward expected weight goal and if the patient verbalizes satisfaction with body appearance and increases the number of positive statements about own appearance.

SUBSTANCE USE DISORDERS

Substance (alcohol and drug) use disorders are serious conditions. People start using alcohol and drugs for many reasons, but often it is to feel accepted by a peer group or to feel comfortable and reduce anxiety in a social situation. People mistake the temporary high as a stimulant. In reality, alcohol is a depressant. Any chemical can be potentially dangerous.

It is important to understand the following terms and their definitions:

- **Addiction:** repeated compulsive use of a substance that continues despite negative consequences (physical, social, legal).
- **Tolerance:** a condition in which increased amounts of a substance are needed over time to achieve the same effect as that previously obtained with smaller doses.
- Physical **withdrawal** syndrome: a physiological response to the abrupt stopping or reduction of a substance used (usually) for a long time. Withdrawal symptoms are specific to the substance used.

Substance use disorders are conditions in which the patient does the following:

- Takes more of the substance or takes it over a longer period of time than intended (**abuse**)
- Has a persistent desire to or unsuccessful efforts to cut down or control use
- Experiences strong craving for the substance
- Is unable to fulfill major role obligations at home, work, or school
- Needs more of the substance and at more frequent intervals to achieve the same "high," or desired effect of the substance (tolerance)
- Spends significant time obtaining the substance
- Gives up important social or professional functions to use the substance
- Has tried at least once to quit but still obsesses about the substance
- Experiences difficulty with job, family, or social activities because of use or withdrawal symptoms
- Uses the substance regardless of the problems it causes
- Experiences the substance-specific withdrawal syndrome
- Uses the substance to avoid withdrawal symptoms

Nurses need to be informed about substance use disorders for several reasons. First, many patients on medical-surgical units have substance use-related disorders. This affects their healing and the effect of their medications. Second, as part of the human experience, your chance of being in a close personal relationship with a person who has a substance use disorder is great. Third, and perhaps most important, you are part of a profession whose members are statistically high users and abusers of drugs and alcohol (see "Ethical Considerations" on Davis Edge). According to the National Council of State Boards of Nursing (2011), between 6% and 15% of nurses in the United States are impaired.

Substance use disorders are not a one-person illness; they affect personal and professional relationships with people who are associated with the user. The term **dysfunctional** is often used to refer to the relationships in a family or work environment with a substance abuser. Dishonesty and inability to discuss the situation are strong components of the disease. Many times, people who live or work in the dysfunctional group begin to cover up for the substance user's behaviors and lack of responsibility. Family members or friends may take sides, begin to be dishonest with each other, and erode the bond within that group. Eventually this leads to a condition called **codependence,** which can be as serious as the substance use. Codependent members of a group begin to lose their own sense of identity and purpose and exist solely for the abuser. Their actions take away the opportunity for the user to take responsibility for his or her own actions. This is called *enabling.*

Denial is a common ego defense mechanism used by people who are substance abusers. The person who is dependent on a substance often uses statements such as, "I can quit anytime I want to" or "I just need a little bump to loosen me up."

Sometimes patients who are actively using drugs or alcohol when admitted to an inpatient setting or who are cut off from substances abruptly experience physiological withdrawal. Withdrawal from alcohol specifically can progress to a condition called **delirium tremens** (DTs). DTs develop when alcohol intake is significantly reduced and the neurotransmitters previously suppressed by alcohol are no longer suppressed. They rebound, resulting in a phenomenon known as brain hyperexcitability. Hyperexcitability can cause visual hallucinations, tremors, and possibly tonic-clonic seizures. Elevated blood pressure and pulse and cardiac arrhythmias also may occur. Symptoms of withdrawal begin within 4 to 12 hours after the patient has stopped drinking and will peak in 24 to 48 hours. Hospitalization is needed to maintain the patient's safety.

Types of Substance Use Disorders
Alcohol Use Disorders
Alcohol use disorders are present in all walks of life, at all economic levels, and in both genders. Sometimes a fine line exists between a person who is a social drinker and a person who has an **abuse** condition. One factor used to make that differentiation is the degree of need or compulsion to drink. There is a high incidence of alcohol use and abuse among older adults, teenagers, and even younger children. Alcoholism either directly or indirectly decreases a person's life expectancy by an average of 10 to 12 years.

Patients with alcohol use disorders may experience:

• Binges usually lasting 2 days or more
• Blackouts (unable to recall what happened during a period of drinking)

• Vomiting and dehydration
• Disorientation
• Increased vulnerability to infections, accidents, and other injuries.

Other Substance Use Disorders
Many substances other than alcohol can be addictive. Caffeine and nicotine are two that are readily available. Coffee, tea, soda, and cigarettes are everywhere in our society and are very addicting. Many experts believe that the single most difficult addiction to overcome is to nicotine.

Illegal substances such as marijuana (in some states), heroin, cocaine, crack, phencyclidine (more commonly known as PCP), and prescription medications for pain and mental health treatment are also potentially addictive. The United States is in the midst of an opioid epidemic that is shifting from prescription medications to heroin (Maxwell, 2015). Deaths from heroin and prescription opioid overdoses are occurring in record numbers. Methamphetamine (meth) abuse is a major problem affecting families and society. Inhalants such as lighter fluid, paint, paint thinners, and gasoline also can be used to get high; in the United States, these substances are mainly used by teenagers. The term for their use is *huffing.* These are highly neurotoxic substances, potentially lethal, and usually available in the house or garage.

The signs and symptoms of drug abuse and dependence can be similar to those of alcohol abuse. Additional signs of drug abuse include the following:

• Red, watery eyes
• Runny nose
• Hostile behavior
• Paranoia
• Needle tracks on arms or legs

Etiological Theories
Why do some people develop substance use disorders and others do not? Is it the substance, or is it the person? Some theorists believe in the existence of an addictive personality, which may begin to explain addictions to food, sex, and gambling as well as alcohol, drugs, and other dependencies.

Psychoanalytical theorists believe that people who develop substance use disorders are people who failed to successfully pass through the "oral" stage of development.

Biological theories include numerous studies that imply some sort of genetic metabolic disorder. Many of these studies were done on twins born to an alcoholic parent or parents and who were separated from the parents at or shortly after birth. The number of twins who were born of alcoholic parents but raised by nonalcoholic adoptive or foster parents and yet developed alcohol use disorder was consistently elevated.

Cognitive behavioral theorists suggest the way in which a person perceives being high may influence the act of becoming

• WORD • BUILDING •
dysfunctional: dys—bad or difficult + functional—performance

high. It can be an innocent beginning: obtaining relief from valid prescription medications can, according to cognitive theory, leave people perceiving that the drugs offer a miracle cure. It becomes appealing to want that kind of relief again; soon a pattern is formed, and other substances may be added.

Differential Diagnosis

A patient with a substance use disorder may be admitted to the hospital for medical problems associated with the substance use (e.g., dehydration, liver failure) or for unrelated problems (e.g., cancer, diabetes). Nursing assessment, unexplained tolerance to pain medication, or symptoms of withdrawal may lead you or the physician to pursue the possibility of substance dependency. Laboratory tests can rule out physiological problems. Blood levels of alcohol or drugs can also be measured. A patient who is uncommonly anxious for early discharge should also be further assessed.

Therapeutic Measures

Treatment for and recovery from a substance use disorder is a slow process. With few exceptions, a person who has a substance use disorder and who is recovering cannot ever use that substance again or he or she will risk the chance of returning to previous patterns of use. Some treatment options are described next. Several forms of treatment may be used together.

SUPPORT GROUPS. A common and effective treatment for substance use disorder is support groups. For, alcoholism, the most famous is Alcoholics Anonymous (AA), a 12-step program that offers support through others who have stopped drinking. For more information on AA, go to www.aa.org. Another program for women dealing with alcoholism is Women for Sobriety (www.womenforsobriety.org). For those who abuse drugs, Narcotics Anonymous (NA; www.na.org) is a well-known support group.

COGNITIVE BEHAVIORAL THERAPY. Cognitive behavioral therapy is used as an adjunct therapy for control of substance abuse. Cognitive behavioral therapists believe that with homework and practice, a person can learn to think differently about the event that led to the substance abuse. When the person changes the belief system about the activating event, he or she can practice more positive thoughts and behaviors.

THERAPY. Psychotherapy provides one-to-one therapy. Because substance use affects an entire family, family or group therapy is important in reinstating honest communication. A commitment to stop the substance abuse is required. Therapy will only help with some of the issues resulting from substance abuse.

SCREENING, BRIEF INTERVENTION, AND REFERRAL TO TREATMENT. Screening, Brief Intervention, and Referral to Treatment (SBIRT) is an evidence-based practice used to identify, reduce, and prevent health problems related to the use, abuse, and dependence on alcohol and illicit drugs (Aldridge, Linford, & Bray, 2017). SBIRT consists of three parts: screening, brief intervention, and referral to treatment. This approach combines screening with brief behavioral counseling interventions. SBIRT is like other preventative health screening measures in that it provides an effective way to identify patients who are at risk for substance use. However, it also offers an appropriate intervention.

MEDICATIONS. In the United States, to treat alcohol use disorders, aversion and anticraving medications have been approved. If a comorbid anxiety or depressive disorder accompanies the alcohol abuse, other medications may be prescribed. Antidepressant or nonaddictive antianxiety drugs are most often prescribed.

The aversion medication disulfiram (Antabuse) is sometimes prescribed as a deterrent to using alcohol. Disulfiram should never be administered without the patient's full informed consent. If a patient taking disulfiram ingests alcohol, a severe reaction causes chest pain, nausea, vomiting, confusion, and other symptoms. Those taking disulfiram also can be adversely affected if they use products that contain alcohol, such as cologne, mouthwash, aftershave, or cough syrup. The effects of disulfiram last 2 to 3 weeks after the last dose.

The medication acamprosate (Campral) is thought to work by helping to restore GABA-glutamate equilibrium. Acamprosate may help combat cravings and is specifically indicated for maintenance of abstinence from alcohol in patients who have stopped drinking. Naltrexone (ReVia) may reduce the urge or desire to drink. Naltrexone helps patients remain abstinent and can interfere with the tendency to want to drink more if a recovering patient relapses and ingests alcohol.

Use of benzodiazepines such as diazepam (Valium) and lorazepam (Ativan) can help prevent symptoms of DTs during acute withdrawal by neurotransmitter action but are not used long term because of risk for **dependence.**

To treat abuse of opioids, a combination of the drugs buprenorphine and naloxone (Suboxone) provides relief from withdrawal symptoms and opioid cravings. It works by binding with the same receptor sites as opioids. If Suboxone is taken correctly, the individual will experience no drug cravings and no withdrawal symptoms and will feel drug free.

Methadone acts as a sort of "step down" for people addicted to certain opioid drugs. It can be legally prescribed and dispensed. Methadone is also potentially addicting, and its critics believe it is only a substitute for heroin. It is typically given once a day. Psychotherapy is also provided for patients in methadone programs.

HOSPITALIZATION. Therapy may range from inpatient hospitalization to halfway houses to eventual independence, usually with attendance at AA or NA meetings. Hospitalization may be necessary during the acute withdrawal stage. It is common for patients to seek treatment multiple times. This should not be interpreted as a weakness in the patient or the treatment program. It is only a sign that the person is learning more about the disorder and the need to help him or herself. People with all kinds of chronic diseases experience relapse at times.

Nursing Process for the Patient With Substance Use Disorders

Nursing care for people who have drug use disorders is essentially the same as for those who are alcohol use disorders. It is important to remember that nurses and physicians cannot "fix" the patient who uses substances. The desire to not use a substance must come from the person who is using it. Table 57.7 provides a substance use summary.

DATA COLLECTION. For patients suspected of alcohol use disorder, a common screening tool to determine whether a patient has a drinking problem is the CAGE questionnaire (Ewing, 1984):

- Have you ever felt you should *Cut down* on your drinking?
- Have people *Annoyed* you by criticizing your drinking?
- Have you ever felt bad or *Guilty* about your drinking?
- Have you ever had a drink first thing in the morning (as an "*Eye opener*") to steady your nerves or get rid of a hangover?

A "yes" answer to two or more questions suggests a drinking problem. Some organizations also use the CAGE questionnaire to screen for substance abuse, although it has not been validated for use in substance use disorders.

Alcohol also can have many physiological effects. See Chapter 32 for assessment of patients with liver disorders.

NURSING DIAGNOSES, PLANNING, AND IMPLEMENTATION.

Ineffective Coping related to lack of effective coping mechanisms as evidenced by abuse of a substance

EXPECTED OUTCOME: The patient will accept responsibility for her or his behavior, verbalize acceptance of the relationship between substance abuse and personal problems, and identify effects of the substance on the body.

- Help the patient to identify recent behavior while under the influence of the substance. *Patients need to see the relationship between their substance abuse and their personal problems.*
- Expect sobriety. *This establishes sobriety as the norm.*
- Teach about the physical impact of drugs and alcohol on the body. *Many patients lack accurate information about the effects of substance abuse on the body.*
- Be honest, and be aware of your own thoughts and feelings about addictions. *Effective communication is essential for a therapeutic relationship.*
- Provide group support such as a 12-step program. *Peer support is an effective treatment that is often more acceptable to patients than other treatments.*
- Confront the patient immediately if projection, rationalization, or denial behaviors are noted. *Projection, rationalization, and denial are ego defense mechanisms that discourage the patient from accepting responsibility for behavior.*
- Use positive reinforcement. *Positive reinforcement for successes is important when helping a person with an addiction. Every step is a big one in this field; every step taken is a new one.*
- Provide a safe environment. *Patients who are chemically addicted may become suicidal or display other bizarre behavior, especially during withdrawal. A patient under the influence of alcohol or another chemical may have poor impulse control or judgment. Maintaining a safe milieu and calm demeanor will help the patient through this difficult time.*
- Remain alert to the possibility that the patient may be using a substance even in the hospital. Report and document all findings and behaviors that may be potential safety hazards for the patient. *The fact that a patient is hospitalized does not guarantee that he or she has no access to the chemical or way of using it in your presence. Unfortunately, family members or friends sometimes smuggle in drugs or alcohol to patients.*
- Practice "tough love." "Doing for" patients may be tempting, but it is not in the patient's best interest most of the time. *This encourages patients to be responsible for their own healing.*

Table 57.7

Substance Abuse Summary

Signs and Symptoms	Inability to fulfill obligations at work, school, or home Recurrent legal or interpersonal problems Continued use despite social and interpersonal problems Participation in physically hazardous situations while impaired
Diagnosis	History Liver function studies Serum drug or alcohol levels Evaluate for other coexisting disorders (bipolar disorder)
Therapeutic Measures	12-step programs Cognitive behavioral therapy Psychotherapy *For alcohol use:* disulfiram (Antabuse), acamprosate (Campral), naltrexone (ReVia) *For opioid use:* buprenorphine and naloxone (Suboxone), methadone Benzodiazepines for acute withdrawal
Primary Nursing Diagnoses	*Ineffective Coping* *Ineffective Denial*

EVALUATION. Does the patient verbalize acceptance of responsibility for own behavior? Does the patient understand the relationship between personal problems and substance abuse? Does the patient understand the effects of substance abuse on the body?

For additional information, visit the web sites of the National Institute on Alcohol Abuse and Alcoholism (www.niaaa.nih.gov) and the National Institute on Drug Abuse (www.drugabuse.gov).

CRITICAL THINKING

Maria, a 17-year-old student, is behaving oddly. She has always been rather loud and even has been referred to as "obnoxious" by several of her peers. You are the school nurse and have observed her sitting alone, as if waiting for someone, but when you approach her, she barely greets you and then moves away. What are your concerns about Maria? What are some of the possibilities that might be affecting her? How can you approach her more effectively the next time you see her?

Suggested answers are at the end of the chapter.

MENTAL ILLNESS AND THE OLDER ADULT

It is not uncommon for older adults to be admitted to the hospital with a tentative diagnosis of "change in mental status." It is important to distinguish between physical and mental disorders in these circumstances. Some neurocognitive disorders that affect older adults' mental status are as follows:

- *Major neurocognitive disorder* is an impairment of mental functioning that interferes with daily activities and relationships. Causes of major neurocognitive disorder include Alzheimer disease, Lewy body disease, vascular disease, Huntington disease, and HIV, among others.
- *Delirium* is an acute change in mental status needing immediate evaluation and treatment. This is often due to a physiological condition such as an infection. It typically can be reversed if recognized and the underlying cause removed. Read more about dementia and delirium in Chapter 48.
- *Pseudodementia* is a condition in which the patient appears to have a major neurocognitive disorder but is really experiencing depression. Treating the depression can help reverse the mental status changes.
- *Depression* in older adults should not be viewed as a normal part of aging; it should be diagnosed and treated. Older adults may be dealing with physical and mental decline, loss of function, isolation, and loss of a marriage partner and friends Their depression may be expressed through bodily symptoms such as pain. If not evaluated and treated, depression can lead to suicide ("Gerontological Issues"). Be sure to review Chapter 15, "Nursing Care of Older Adult Patients."

Older adults often need assistance to develop or enhance skills required to cope with life events. Self-care and personal independence in care choices can be encouraged.

Gerontological Issues

Suicide and the Older Adult. Older adults are not immune to suicidal thoughts. In North America, white men older than age 75 have an especially high suicide rate. Comments by any older adult referring to hopelessness or desire to die must be explored to assess suicide risk. Comments such as, "I am useless. I can't do anything anymore" should be taken seriously. If an older adult is thought to be depressed, the Geriatric Depression Scale (GDS) can be used to assess further risk (Greenberg, 2012).

To adequately assess suicide potential, ask questions that establish whether the older adult has done the following:

- Thought about ending his or her life
- Attempted to end his or her life in the past
- Developed a plan to end his or her life
- Has started to give away as "gifts" his or her personal prized objects
- Set the plan into action (i.e., bought a gun, has a full bottle of pills in the bedside table)

Any older adult who has a plan to end his or her life and has the ability or resources to do so must be immediately referred for psychological evaluation. Never leave a person with suicidal thoughts alone.

If necessary, crisis intervention for a suicidal older adult should include the following:

- Remove any items that the older adult could use to inflict an injury or end his or her life, such as razors, jewelry with pins or sharp points, and mirrors.
- Make arrangements for direct supervision and observation that are reliable, considering personnel and family resources. Often, hospital admission is the most appropriate intervention for a person at high risk for suicide.
- Help the older adult talk about the crisis or life event that has devastated his or her desire to live. For example, encourage reminiscence about the patient's spouse or allow the person to express the frustration of being unable to physically meet the daily demands of life.
- Develop a "do no harm" or suicide contract with the older adult. Outline a short-term, structured plan to keep the older adult safe. Focus on decreasing social isolation by requiring personal social contacts. These could include staying at a daughter's home for a weekend, going to the senior center for lunch, calling a specific person who is willing and wants to listen to feelings and concerns, exercising, taking a walk outside, or volunteering at a nursing home, hospital, or school.

Reference

Greenberg, S. A. (2012). The Geriatric Depression Scale. *Try This: Best Practices in Nursing Care to Older Adults, 4,* 1–2. Retrieved from https://consultgeri.org/try-this/general-assessment/issue-4.pdf

Home Health Hints

- Observe family members for evidence of caregiver role strain.
- Connect patients and families with pharmacies that will deliver medications to the home.
- Set up medications using a system the patient can easily follow.

- Maintain communication with and act as a liaison between the psychiatrist and primary care provider as needed.
- Assist the patient and family to identify community resources such as support groups and respite care.
- Teach patients about their illness and medications and how to manage their symptoms.

SUGGESTED ANSWERS TO CRITICAL THINKING

Tommy

You can reassure Tommy's mother that his obsessive-compulsive disorder is not her fault. Tell her that Tommy can learn to control his illness with medications and therapy. The family must be part of the therapy, for both Tommy's and the family's sake. Positive communication between Tommy and his family is encouraged. Tommy's mother can also be encouraged to attend a support group herself. Suggest to Tommy's mother that she meet with a counselor or behavioral therapist to learn more about the causes and treatment of the disorder.

Mr. Zenz

It is important to be supportive of Mrs. Zenz while maintaining her husband's confidentiality and privacy. Encouraging Mrs. Zenz to talk to Mr. Zenz's health care provider is appropriate. Showing empathy with statements such as, "It must be confusing and difficult to watch your husband change moods so quickly" are good tools to use. It may be a bit more challenging to approach him directly. Ask him if you can speak frankly and share specific observations (e.g., "The residents appear frightened when you approach them quickly and speak loudly"). This may help him to reflect. Chances are, however, that if he is in a manic stage he will not hear your concern. Advise his wife to speak with the next person in the chain of command.

Anne

1. Appropriate communication skills include being positive, reassuring, and not reinforcing the hallucinations. "I don't see or hear a woman, Anne. It is time for the movie. I'd like you to come with me for a while at least" is an example of an appropriate verbal interaction. Reinforcing expectations is also appropriate; you might say, "Anne, part of your care plan includes attending one unit activity each day. This is the last opportunity for you to meet your care plan objective for today."

2. At all times, nurses need to be aware of drug interactions. Anne will most likely be medicated for her schizophrenia, and those medications can interact unfavorably with her chemotherapy. If she is receiving oral medications, it may be necessary to check her mouth to ensure she is swallowing them.

3. Work with team members to provide a therapeutic and low stimulus environment for Anne. Good nursing data collection skills are essential.

Maria

Several things may explain Maria's behavior, including depression, drug use, schizophrenia, or an eating disorder. Next time you see Maria, you might try constructively confronting her behavior by saying something like, "Maria, you used to be much more outgoing. We always were friendly, and now you leave when I'm near. That change in you concerns me. I'm here if you want to talk." Or "Maria, I noticed your behavior is changing. You are loud one moment and very quiet the next. That is unusual for you. What's happening?"

Review Questions

1. Which statement by a depressed patient causes the nurse to contact the registered nurse or health care provider immediately?
   1. "Everyone is out to get me."
   2. "I have tried to kill myself three times."
   3. "I feel so hopeless."
   4. "My friend is bringing me a gun."

2. A patient states, "My doctor says I have obsessive-compulsive disorder. What does that mean?" Which response by the nurse is best?
   1. "It means that you have experienced a major life stress and will need therapy to help you manage the symptoms."
   2. "You can expect to experience periods of high energy and anxiety, alternating with periods of feeling very low."
   3. "You may experience involuntary, intrusive thoughts and feel compelled to respond with seemingly meaningless actions."
   4. "People with obsessive-compulsive disorder are very organized. This is a good disorder to have."

3. A patient is experiencing extrapyramidal side effects while taking antipsychotic medication. Which of the patient's medication orders will help reduce these effects?
   1. benztropine (Cogentin)
   2. chlorpromazine (Thorazine)
   3. haloperidol (Haldol)
   4. lithium carbonate (Eskalith)

4. A patient who is a veteran of the Gulf War hears the hospital fire alarm go off during a drill and cries, "There are people hiding behind the pillars! They have guns! Be careful!" What action should the nurse take first?
   1. Tell the patient that his behavior is inappropriate and that he is frightening the other patients.
   2. Administer an as-needed antipsychotic medication as ordered.
   3. Ask him whether he is afraid of the guns.
   4. Stay with the patient while calmly reorienting him.

5. A patient is being treated on the mental health unit for an anxiety disorder. The patient approaches the nurse and reports feeling dizzy and weak, with a sensation of a racing heart. The nursing care plan includes interventions of imagery exercises and as needed lorazepam (Ativan) for symptoms of anxiety. What should the nurse do first?
   1. Instruct the patient to sit and breathe deeply.
   2. Give the patient the prescribed as needed lorazepam.
   3. Obtain the patient's vital signs.
   4. Instruct the patient in an imagery exercise.

6. A patient reports seeing children playing on the floor in the hallway of the mental health unit. There are no children anywhere on the unit. Which response by the nurse is best?
   1. "The children are fine there. They are just playing."
   2. "I don't see any children, and there haven't been any children on the unit today. Would you like to walk with me?"
   3. "Children are not allowed on this unit. I will ask them to leave."
   4. "You know there are no children here. It must be time for your medication."

7. The nurse is planning care for a patient with an eating disorder. The patient is 40 kg and 68 inches tall. Serum laboratory data is potassium 2.6 mEq/dL, sodium 126 mEq/dL, chloride 95 mEq/dL, and calcium 10.8 mg/dL. Which of these is the priority intervention for this patient?
   1. Weigh the patient daily at the same time.
   2. Maintain an intravenous line of dextrose and electrolytes.
   3. Praise intake of any type of food.
   4. Document intake and output.

Answer rationales available in your online resources.

ANSWERS 1. 4; 2. 3; 3. 1; 4. 4; 5. 3; 6. 2; 7. 2

Key Points

Find the chapter key points in your online resources available through Davis Edge.

Additional Resources

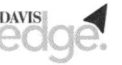 Use the scratch off code on the inside front cover of your book to access online quizzes that will help you to improve your scores on course exams and prepare for the NCLEX-PN®.

 Study Guide

APPENDIX A
Diagnostic Tests

This is intended to be a quick reference only. Please check a diagnostic test reference manual for comprehensive information.

 GENERAL CONSIDERATIONS FOR ALL TESTS:

- Ensure that an informed consent form is signed before any invasive procedure.
- Check orders for need to withhold food or fluids before test.
- Preparation if contrast media will be used to prevent reaction or nephrotoxicity: (1) Check for and report allergies to iodine or contrast media; (2) report low glomerular filtration rate (GFR) or elevated creatinine/blood urea nitrogen (BUN) levels because contrast media is nephrotoxic and excreted by the kidneys; (3) consider patient risk factors for contrast-induced nephropathy (renal disease, diabetes, hypertension, chemotherapy) and discuss with health care provider (HCP) prophylaxis orders such as providing intravenous (IV) hydration or prophylactic pre-medication such as acetylcysteine (Mucomyst); (4) if patient is taking metformin, hold it as ordered before the test (typically 1 or 2 days) and then for 48 hours as ordered after test until renal function is determined to be normal to reduce risk for lactic acidosis if acute renal failure develops due to the contrast media; (5) teach that the patient may experience a feeling of warmth or experience a salty or metallic taste when contrast media is injected; (6) encourage increased fluids after test to promote excretion of contrast media.
- Reinforce patient education for test.

Test or Procedure	Description	Reasons Done	Preprocedure Nursing Considerations	Postprocedure Nursing Considerations
Angiography • abdominal • adrenal • carotid • coronary • pulmonary • renal	Contrast media is injected through a catheter, usually via femoral artery or vein, and then radiographs are taken at intervals to view vasculature.	To view patency and distribution of blood vessels.	See General Considerations for precare for contrast media. Report history of bleeding/clotting disorders. Medications that interfere with clotting are stopped about 1 week before examination. Ensure patent IV is in place.	See General Considerations for postcare for contrast media. Monitor vital signs and circulatory status as ordered. Maintain pressure on insertion site as ordered. Report bleeding or hematoma formation.
Biopsy	Removal of tissue for microscopic examination. May be done with needle, punch, incision, or endoscopically.	To diagnose cancerous or other lesions.	Premedicate for pain relief.	Monitor vital signs and biopsy site as ordered.

Continued

Test or Procedure	Description	Reasons Done	Preprocedure Nursing Considerations	Postprocedure Nursing Considerations
Computed axial tomography (CAT), computed tomography (CT)	Multiple x-ray beams provide three-dimensional cross-section visualization of internal structures. Contrast media may be used.	To visualize abnormal structures or masses.	Assess for claustrophobia (depending on scanner); patient could be in scanner for up to 1 hour. Premedicate anxious or claustrophobic patients as ordered. See General Considerations for precare for contrast media.	See General Considerations for postcare for contrast media.
Electrocardiography (ECG, EKG)	Electrodes provide a graphic display of the electrical current during the cardiac cycle.	To evaluate electrical function of the heart; diagnose arrhythmias.	Explain test to patient.	None specific.
Electroencephalography (EEG)	Electrodes on scalp evaluate electrical activity of the brain.	To evaluate brain activity, lesions, and seizures.	Ensure patient's hair is clean and dry. Check orders for drugs such as sedatives or stimulants that may need to be weaned or withheld before test.	Wash adhesive from hair before it hardens and becomes difficult to remove. Oil or witch hazel may make removal easier. Instruct patient about resuming medications as ordered.
Endoscopy • bronchoscopy • colonoscopy • colposcopy • gastroscopy • sigmoidoscopy	A flexible fiber-optic tube and camera are inserted into a body cavity to observe structures.	To observe for abnormalities, remove polyps, obtain biopsy specimens, suction secretions, coagulate bleeding sites, and more.	Check orders for preparation such as NPO (nothing by mouth), laxatives, and enemas. Premedicate as ordered.	Check for swallow and gag reflexes after upper endoscopy before offering food or fluids.
Lumbar puncture (spinal tap)	A small needle is used to withdraw cerebrospinal fluid for examination. The needle is typically inserted between the L3–4 or L4–5 vertebrae.	To diagnose infection, central nervous system (CNS) disease, or cancers. Sometimes used to inject medication.	Premedicate as ordered. Assist patient to sit leaning forward or lay curled up on side according to HCP preference. Be prepared to assist with procedure.	Label specimens and take to laboratory. Monitor site. Implement activity restrictions if ordered. Encourage fluids.

Test or Procedure	Description	Reasons Done	Preprocedure Nursing Considerations	Postprocedure Nursing Considerations
Magnetic resonance imaging (MRI)	Magnetic field and radiofrequency energy are used to obtain a detailed image of tissues. Contrast media may be used.	To visualize structural abnormalities in organs and tissues.	Because powerful magnets are used, question patient about metallic foreign bodies, implants, pacemakers (some new models are MRI compatible), or tattoos with metal-based inks, which are contraindications for this test. Ask if claustrophobic; patient will be in scanner for up to 1 hour. Consider open MRI availability. Request order for sedative or analgesic to be given 1 hour before test if necessary. Explain that patient must lie still in an enclosed area for prolonged period. Remove all jewelry. Teach patient to expect loud knocking sounds during test (headphones with music can be requested). Teach relaxation and deep-breathing exercises. See General Considerations for precare for contrast media.	See General Considerations for postcare for contrast media.
Myelography	Contrast media is injected into cerebrospinal space following lumbar puncture. Radiographs are then taken to outline the vertebrae.	Identifies spinal column abnormalities.	Same as lumbar puncture.	Maintain bedrest with head elevated less than 30 degrees. Monitor for seizures. See General Considerations for post care for contrast media.

Continued

Test or Procedure	Description	Reasons Done	Preprocedure Nursing Considerations	Postprocedure Nursing Considerations
Nuclear scan • heart • lungs • CNS • thyroid • bone • other	Radioactive substances are administered (orally, inhaled, or IV), and then a special scanner observes where the substance is distributed.	To show both structure and function abnormalities.	Check HCP orders for preparation, which may differ for each scan type. Teach patient that the amount of radioactive material is very small, and no special precautions are needed.	Encourage hydration to promote excretion of radioactive material.
Radiograph (x-ray)	X-ray beams identify internal structures, especially high-density structures such as bone. Contrast media may be used with some tests.	To identify differences in tissue densities. Can help diagnose a variety of structural or other disorders.	Have patient remove jewelry from area to be x-rayed. For bowel prep, laxatives or enemas may be ordered before some gastrointestinal x-rays.	If barium has been used as contrast media to outline the bowel, administer laxative as ordered and increase fluid intake to help evacuate barium before it hardens. See General Considerations for post care for contrast media.
Ultrasonography endoscopic ultrasound • transesophageal echocardiogram • transrectal ultrasound • transvaginal	High-frequency sound waves are passed through soft tissues to outline tissues and masses. Gel is used on skin and transducer to improve conduction of sound waves.	To identify alterations in soft tissues and organs.	Check orders for preparation if ultrasound will be done endoscopically.	None specific.

APPENDIX B
Normal Adult Reference Common Laboratory Values

BLOOD, PLASMA, OR SERUM VALUES

	Reference Range	
Determination	*Conventional*	*SI*
Albumin	3.4–4.8 g/dL	34–48 g/L
Aldolase	Less than 8.1 units/L	12–55 micromol/L
Ammonia	15–60 mcg/dL	41–80 micromol
Amylase	100–300 units/L	
Atrial natriuretic peptide	20–77 pg/mL	20–77 ng/L
B-type natriuretic peptide (BNP)	Less than 100 pg/mL	Less than 100 ng/L
Pro-BNP (N-Terminal)	*Age 0–74:* Less than 125 pg/mL	*Age 0–74:* Less than 125 ng/L
	Age 75 and older: Less than 449 pg/mL	*Age 75 and older:* Less than 449 pg/mL
Bilirubin (total)	Less than 1.2 mg/dL	Less than 21 micromol/L
Calcium, total	8.2–10.2 mg/dL	2.1–2.6 mmol/L
Carbon dioxide, plasma or serum (venous)	23–29 mEq/L	23–29 mmol/L
Chloride	97–107 mEq/L	97–107 mmol/L
Creatine kinase (CK)	*Male:* 50–204 units/L	
	Female: 36–160 units/L	
CK isoenzymes		
CK-BB	Absent	
CK-MB	0%–4%	
CK-MM	96%–100%	
CK-MB by immunoassay	0–5 ng/mL	
Creatinine		
Male	0.6–1.21 mg/dL	54–107 micromol/L
Female	0.5–1.11 mg/dL	45–98 micromol/L
d-Dimer	*Semiquantitative:* No fragments detected.	
	Quantitative: Less than 500 ng/mL fibrinogen equivalent units	
Erythrocyte sedimentation rate (ESR) (Westergren method)		
Male	*Under age 50:* Less than 15 mm/hr	
	Over age 50: Less than 20 mm/hr	
Female	*Under age 50:* Less than 25 mm/hr	
	Over age 50: Less than 30 mm/hr	

Continued

Determination	*Conventional*	*SI*
Glucose, Fasting	Less than 100 mg/dL	Less than 5.6 mmol/L
Iron		
Male	65–175 mcg/dL	11.6–31.3 micromol/L
Female	50–170 mcg/dL	9–30.4 micromol/L
Iron-binding capacity	250–450 mcg/dL	45–81 micromol/L
Lactate dehydrogenase	90–176 units/L	
Lipase	0–60 units/L	
Lipids (desirable)		
Cholesterol	Less than 200 mg/dL	Less than 5.2 mmol/L
Low-density lipoprotein (LDL)	Less than 100 mg/dL	Less than 2.59 mmol/L
High-density lipoprotein (HDL)	Greater than 60 mg/dL	Greater than 1.55 mmol/L
Triglycerides	Less than 150 mg/dL	Less than 1.7 mmol/L
Magnesium	1.6–2.2 mg/dL	0.66–0.91 mmol/L
Myoglobin		
Male	28–72 ng/mL	1.6–4.1 nmol/L
Female	25–58 ng/mL	1.4–3.3 nmol/L
Osmolality	275–295 mOsm/kg	275–295 mmol/kg
Blood Gases, Arterial		
O_2 Saturation	95–100%	
PCo_2	35–45 mm Hg	4.7–6 kPa
Blood Gas Value (pH)	7.35–7.45	7.35–7.45
PO_2	80–100 mm Hg	10.6–12.6 kPa
Phosphatase (prostatic acid)	Less than 2.1 ng/mL	
Phosphatase (alkaline)		
Male	35–142 units/L	
Female	25–125 units/L	
Phosphorus, Blood	2.5–4.5 mg/dL	0.8–1.4 mmol/L
Potassium	3.5–5.3 mEq/L	3.5–5.3 mmol/L
Protein, Total	6–8 g/dL	60–80 g/L
Sodium	135–145 mEq/L	135–145 mmol/L
Transaminase, alanine amino-transferase (ALT)		
Male	19–36 units/L	Same
Female	24–36 units/L	Same
Transaminase, aspartate amino-transferase (AST)		
Male	20–40 units/L	0.34–0.68 microkat/L
Female	15–30 units/L	0.26–0.51 microkat/L
Troponin I	Less than 0.05 ng/mL	Less than 0.05 mcg/L
Troponin T	Less than 0.2 ng/mL	Less than 0.2 mcg/L
Urea Nitrogen, Blood (BUN)	8–21 mg/dL	2.9–7.5 mmol/L

Determination	Conventional	SI
Uric Acid		
Male	4–8 mg/dL	0.24–0.47 mmol/L
Female	2.5–7 mg/dL	0.15–0.41 mmol/L

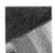

URINALYSIS REFERENCE VALUES

Dipstick pH	4.5–8
Protein	Less than 20 mg/dL
Glucose	Negative
Ketones	Negative
Hemoglobin	Negative
Bilirubin	Negative
Urobilinogen	Up to 1 mg/dL
Nitrite	Negative
Leukocyte esterase	Negative
Microscopic examination	
Red blood cells (RBCs)	Less than 5/hpf
White blood cells (WBCs)	Less than 5/hpf
Renal cells	None seen
Transitional cells	None seen
Squamous cells	Rare; usually no clinical significance
Casts	Rare hyaline; otherwise, none seen
Crystals in acid urine	Uric acid, calcium oxalate, amorphous urates
Crystals in alkaline urine	Triple phosphate, calcium phosphate, ammonium biurate, calcium carbonate, amorphous phosphates
Bacteria, yeast, parasites	None seen

HEMATOLOGIC VALUES

Determination	Conventional	SI
Coagulation screening tests		
Bleeding time (template)	2.5 to 10 minutes	
Prothrombin time (PT)	10 to 13 seconds	
International normalized ratio (INR)	0.9 to 1.1 for patients not receiving anticoagulation therapy	
	2 to 3 for patients receiving treatment for venous thrombosis, pulmonary embolism, or valvular heart disease	
	2.5 to 3.5 for patients with mechanical heart valves and/or treatment for recurrent systemic embolism	

Continued

Determination	*Conventional*	*SI*
Partial Thromboplastin Time, activated (aPTT)	25–35 seconds	
Complete blood count (CBC)		
Hematocrit		
Male	42–52	0.42–0.52
Female	36–48	0.36–0.48
Hemoglobin		
Male	14–17.3 g/dL	140–173 mmol/L
Female	11.7–15.5 g/dL	117–155 mmol/L
Platelet count	$140–400 \times 10^3$/microL	$140–400 \times 10^9$/L
Red Blood Cell (Erythrocyte) Count		
Male	4.21–5.81 million cells/microL	4.21–5.81 trillion cells/L
Female	3.61-5.11 million cells/microL	3.61-5.11 trillion cells/L

Red Blood Cell (RBC) Indices

	Mean Corpuscular Volume (fl)	Mean Corpuscular Hemoglobin (pg/cell)	Mean Corpuscular Hemoglobin Concentration (g/dL)	RBC Distribution Width Index
Male	77–97	26–34	32–36	11.6–14.8
Female	78–98	26–34	32–36	11.6–14.8

Platelet count	$140–400 \times 10^3$/microL	$140–400 \times 10^9$/L

White Blood Cell (WBC) Count and Differential

Conventional Units WBC × 10^3/microL	Neutrophils Total (Absolute and %)	Lymphocytes Bands (Absolute and %)	Monocytes Segments (Absolute and %)	Basophils (Absolute and %)	Eosinophils (Absolute and %)
4.5–11.1	2.7–6.5	1.5–3.7	0.2–0.4	0.05–0.5	0–0.1
	40%–75%	12%–44%	4%–9%	0%–5.5%	0%–1%

THERAPEUTIC DRUG LEVELS

	Reference Range	
Determination	*Conventional*	*SI*
Carbamazepine	4–12 mcg/mL	17–51 micromol/L
Digoxin	0.5–2 ng/mL	0.6–2.6 nmol/L
Ethanol	0 mg/dL	0 mmol/L
Lithium	0.6–1.2 mEq/L	0.6–1.2 mmol/L
Phenobarbital	15–40 mcg/mL	65–172 micromol/L
Phenytoin (Dilantin)	10–20 mcg/mL	40–79 micromol/L
Salicylate, anti-inflammatory	15–30 mg/dL	0.7–2.2 mmol/L

MISCELLANEOUS VALUES

Determination	*Conventional*	*SI*
Carcinoembryonic antigen (CEA)		
Smoker	Less than 5 ng/mL	Less than 5 mcg/L
Nonsmoker	Less than 2.5 ng/mL	Less than 2.5 mcg/L
Gastrin	Less than 100 pg/mL	Less than 48.1 pmol/L
Immunological tests		
Alpha-1-antitrypsin (a-1)	126–226 mg/dL	1.26–2.26 g/L
Antinuclear antibodies (ANA)	Negative at a 1:40 and 1:160 dilution of serum	

Reference range values may differ from one institution to another. hpf = high-power field; SI = International System of Units.

Source: Most data from Van Leeuwen, A. M., & Poelhuis-Leth, D. J. (2017). *Davis's comprehensive handbook of laboratory and diagnostic tests with nursing implications* (7th ed.). Philadelphia, PA: F.A. Davis.

Glossary

ablation: Removal of part, pathway, or function by surgery, chemical electrocautery, or radio-frequency.

abrasion: A scraping away of skin or mucous membrane as a result of injury or by mechanical means.

abuse: Misuse; excessive or improper use. May refer to substances or individuals.

accommodation: A reflex action of the eye for focusing.

acidosis: An actual or relative increase in the acidity of blood caused by an accumulation of acid or a loss of base.

acquired immunodeficiency syndrome (AIDS): Suppression or deficiency of the cellular immune response, acquired by exposure to human immunodeficiency virus (HIV).

active immunity: Acquired immunity attributable to the presence of antibodies or of immune lymphoid cells formed in response to antigenic stimulus.

activities of daily living (ADLs): Those activities and behaviors that are performed in the care and maintenance of self (e.g., bathing, dressing, eating).

acupuncture: Technique using needles inserted at specific points to create anesthesia or treat certain conditions.

acute coronary syndromes: Group of conditions, including unstable angina, non-Q-wave myocardial infarction, and ST segment elevation myocardial infarction, caused by a lack of oxygen to the heart muscle.

acute pulmonary hypertension: An excessive buildup of pressure in the pulmonary arteries caused by sudden obstruction of the pulmonary artery.

adaptation: Adjustment to changes in internal or external conditions or circumstances; coping.

addiction: Psychological dependence characterized by drug seeking and craving for an opioid or other substance for effects other than the intended purpose of the substance.

adjunct: An addition to the principal procedure or course of therapy.

adjuvant: Something that assists something else, such as a second form of treatment added to treat a disease.

administrative law: Establishes the licensing authority of the state to create, license, and regulate the practice of nursing.

adnexa: Appendages or accessory organs.

advance medical directive: A set of documents (living will and durable medical power of attorney) that explain a person's end-of-life wishes and direct care when the patient is no longer able to do so.

adventitious: Abnormal or extra; often refers to extra breath sounds, such as wheezes or crackles.

advocate: Someone who makes sure a person's wishes are adhered to; someone who represents the best interests of the patient.

aerobic: Living only in the presence of oxygen.

affect: Emotional tone.

afterload: The forces impeding the blood flow out of the heart (vascular pressure, aortic compliance, blood mass, and viscosity).

agenesis: Failure of an organ or part to develop or grow.

agonist: A type of opioid that binds to opioid receptors in the central nervous system to relieve pain.

akinesia: Absence or loss of the power of voluntary movement.

alkalosis: An actual or relative decrease in the acidity of blood caused by loss of acid or accumulation of base.

allograft: Transplanted organ, tissue, or cells from one individual to another of the same species who is not genetically identical. Donors can be living (related or unrelated) or cadaveric.

allopathic: Method of treating disease with remedies that produce effects different from those caused by the disease.

alopecia: The loss of hair from the body and the scalp.

alternative modality: Refers to a therapy used *instead* of a conventional modality. An example is using acupuncture instead of analgesics for pain.

amenorrhea: The absence or suppression of menstruation. Amenorrhea is normal before puberty, after menopause, and during pregnancy and lactation.

amputation: The removal of a limb or other appendage or outgrowth of the body.

anaerobic: Able to live without oxygen.

analgesic: A drug that relieves pain.

anaphylactic shock: Systemic reaction that produces life-threatening changes in the circulation and bronchioles.

anaphylaxis: A sudden severe allergic reaction to an allergen.

anastomosed: To surgically connect two parts.

anemia: A condition in which there is reduced delivery of oxygen to the tissues as a result of reduced numbers of red cells or hemoglobin.

anergic: Related to the diminished ability of the immune system to react to an antigen.

anesthesia: Lack of feeling or sensation; artificially induced loss of ability to feel pain.

anesthesiologist: A physician who specializes in anesthesiology.

aneurysm: A sac formed by the localized dilation of the wall of an artery, a vein, or the heart.

angina pectoris: Severe pain and pressure in the chest caused by insufficient supply of blood and oxygenation to the heart.

angioedema: A localized edematous reaction of the deep dermis or subcutaneous or submucosal tissues appearing as giant wheals.

anion: Electrolyte that carries a negative electrical charge.

anisocoria: Inequality in size of the pupils of the eyes.

ankylosing spondylitis: Inflammatory disease of the spine causing stiffness and pain.

annuloplasty: Repair of a cardiac valve.

anorexia: Absence or loss of appetite for food. Seen in depression, with illness, and as a side effect of some medications.

anorexia nervosa: Refusal to maintain body weight over a minimal normal weight for age and height.

antagonist: Medication used to counteract the effects of an opioid (e.g., naloxone).

anteflexion: The abnormal bending forward of part of an organ.

anteversion: A tipping forward of an organ as a whole, without bending.

anthrax: A disease caused by the spore-forming bacterium *Bacillus anthracis* that has three clinical forms in humans: inhalational, cutaneous, and gastrointestinal. It can be used as a biological weapon.

antibodies: Immunoglobulin molecules having a specific amino acid sequence that gives each antibody the ability to adhere to and interact only with the antigen that induced the synthesis.

anticholinesterase: A substance that breaks down acetylcholinesterase.

antidiuretic: Lessening urine excretion.

antigens: Protein markers on the surface of cells that identify the type of cell.

antitussive: An agent that prevents or relieves cough.

anuria: Complete suppression of urine formation by the kidney.

anxiety: The uncomfortable feeling of apprehension or dread that occurs in response to a known or unknown threat.

aphasia: Defect or loss of the power of expression by speech, writing, or signs, or of comprehension of spoken or written language, caused by disease or injury of the brain centers, such as stroke syndrome.

aphthous stomatitis: Small, white, painful ulcers (also known as canker sores) that appear on the inner cheeks, lips, gums, tongue, palate, and pharynx. They tend to recur.

apnea: Temporary absence of breathing.

appendicitis: Inflammation of the vermiform appendix.

arcus senilis: A benign white or gray opaque ring in the corneal margin of the eye.

arrhythmia: Irregular rhythm, especially heartbeat.

arteriosclerosis: Term applied to a number of pathological conditions in which there is gradual thickening, hardening, and loss of elasticity of the walls of the arteries.

arthritis: Inflammation of a joint.

arthrocentesis: Puncture of a joint space with a needle to remove fluid accumulated in the joint.

arthrogram: X-ray examination, with air or a contrast medium injected, of a synovial joint, often the knee and shoulder.

arthroplasty: Repair of a joint. Also called joint replacement.

arthroscopy: Examination of the interior of a joint with an arthroscope.

articular: Pertaining to a joint.

artificial feeding: Feeding via a tube into the stomach or intestine when a person is unable to take oral nutrition.

artificial hydration: Administration of water via intravenous (IV) or gastric tube when a person is unable to take oral fluids.

ascites: Abnormal accumulation of fluid in the peritoneal cavity.

asepsis: A condition free from germs, infection, and any form of life.

aseptic: Free of pathogenic organisms; asepsis.

asphyxia: A condition in which there is a deficiency of oxygen in the blood and an increase in carbon dioxide in the blood and tissues.

aspiration: Accidental drawing in of foreign substances into the trachea and lungs during inspiration.

assessment: An appraisal or evaluation of a patient's condition.

asterixis: Hand-flapping tremor and involuntary movements of tongue and feet; may be present in hepatic encephalopathy.

astigmatism: An error of refraction in which a ray of light is not sharply focused on the retina but is spread over a more or less diffuse area.

ataxia: Failure of muscular coordination; irregularity of muscular action.

atelectasis: Collapsed or airless condition of the lung or portion of lung, caused by obstruction or hypoventilation.

atheroma: Fatty deterioration or thickening of the walls of the larger arteries occurring in atherosclerosis.

atherosclerosis: A form of arteriosclerosis characterized by accumulation of plaque, blood, and blood products lining the wall of the artery, causing partial or complete blockage of an artery.

atrial depolarization: Electrical activation of the atria.

atrial systole: The contraction of the atria.

atrioventricular (AV) node: Located in lower right atrium; receives an impulse from the sinoatrial (SA) node and relays it to the ventricles.

atrophy: Without nourishment; wasting.

atypical: Deviating from normal.

augmentation: The act or process of increasing in size, quantity, degree, or severity.

auscultation: Process of listening for sounds within the body, usually sounds of thoracic or abdominal viscera, to detect an abnormality.

autograft: A graft of tissue from one part of an individual's body to another part of the same individual's body.

autoimmune: A condition in which the body does not recognize itself and the immune system attacks normal cells.

Ayurvedic: An ancient Hindu system of medicine that improves health by harmonizing mind and body.

azotemia: An increase in nitrogenous bodies in the blood, especially urea, as measured by the serum blood urea nitrogen (BUN) level.

bacteria: One-celled organisms that can reproduce but need a host for food and supportive environment. Bacteria can be harmless, normal flora, or disease-producing pathogens.

balanitis: Inflammation of the skin covering the glans penis.

bariatric: Branch of medicine that deals with the prevention, control, and treatment of obesity.

basal cell secretion test: Part of a gastric analysis; measures the amount of gastric acid produced in 1 hour.

behavior management: Treatment method that uses positive and negative reinforcement to alter behavior.

belief: Something accepted as true. Does not have to be proven.

beneficence: To provide good care; to do good for patients. One of the oldest requirements for health care providers.

benign: Not progressive; for example, a tumor that is not cancerous.

beta-hemolytic streptococci: Gram-positive bacteria that, when grown on blood-agar plates, completely hemolyze the blood and produce a clear zone around the bacteria colony. Group A beta-hemolytic streptococci cause disease in humans.

bigeminy: Occurring every second beat, as in bigeminal premature ventricular contractions.

bimanual: With both hands.

biofeedback: A form of therapy that uses provision of visual or auditory evidence to a person of the status of an autonomic body function such as heart rate, blood pressure, or respiratory rate.

bioprosthesis: Prosthesis consisting of an animal part or containing animal tissue (e.g., porcine heart valve).

biopsy: A sample of tissue removed for examination.

bioterrorism: Biological agent use or threat of use with a pathological organism for terrorist purposes.

bipolar: Having two poles or pertaining to both poles. Bipolar disorder is characterized by episodes of manic and depressive behavior.

blanch: To lose color.

blebs: Irregularly shaped elevations of the skin, such as a blister. May also occur in lung tissue.

blepharitis: Inflammation of the glands and lash follicles along the margin of the eyelids.

blindness: Lack or loss of ability to see.

bolus: A dose of intravenous (IV) medication injected all at once.

bone: The hard, rigid form of connective tissue constituting most of the skeleton of vertebrates, composed chiefly of calcium salts.

botulism: A paralytic illness caused by a potent neurotoxin produced by *Clostridium botulinum,* an anaerobic, spore-forming bacterium. It can be used as a biological weapon.

bradycardia: A slow heartbeat characterized by a pulse rate below 60 beats per minute.

bradykinesia: Abnormal slowness of movement; sluggishness.

breakthrough pain: Pain that occurs while medicated with long-acting analgesics.

bronchiectasis: Chronic dilation of a bronchus or bronchi, usually associated with secondary infection and excessive sputum production.

bronchitis: Inflammation of the mucous membrane of the bronchial airways; may be viral or bacterial.

bronchodilator: A drug that expands the bronchial tubes by relaxing bronchial smooth muscle.

bronchospasm: Spasm of the bronchial smooth muscle resulting in narrowing of the airways; associated with asthma and bronchitis.

bruit: A humming heard when auscultating a blood vessel that is caused by turbulent blood flow through the vessel.

bulimia nervosa: Recurrent episodes of binge eating and self-induced vomiting.

bulla: Large blisters or skin lesions filled with fluid. May also occur in lung tissue.

bundle of His: A bundle of fibers of the impulse-conducting system of the heart. Originates in the atrioventricular (AV) node.

bursae: A small fluid-filled sac or saclike cavity situated in tissues such as joints where friction would otherwise occur.

calculi: An abnormal concentration, usually composed of mineral salts, occurring within the body, chiefly in the hollow organs or their passages. Also called stones, as in kidney stones and gallstones.

cancer: A general name for more than 100 diseases in which abnormal cells grow out of control; a malignant tumor.

cannula: A flexible tube that can be inserted into the body and guided by a stiff, pointed rod. For example, an intravenous (IV) cannula is guided by a metal needle.

capillary permeability: The ability of substances to diffuse through capillary walls into tissue spaces.

capillary refill: The amount of time required for color to return to the nailbed after having been compressed, normally 3 seconds or less. Indicator of peripheral circulation.

caput medusae: Dilated veins around the umbilicus, associated with cirrhosis of the liver.

carbuncle: A necrotizing infection of skin and subcutaneous tissue composed of a cluster of boils.

carcinoembryonic antigens (CEA): A class of antigens normally present in fetal cells; CEA level is elevated in many cancers and is measured to guide cancer treatment.

carcinogen: Specific agent known to promote the cancer process.

cardiac output: A measure of the pumping ability of the heart; amount of blood pumped by the heart per minute.

cardiac tamponade: The life-threatening compression of the heart by the fluid accumulating in the pericardial sac surrounding the heart.

cardiogenic shock: Occurs when the heart muscle is unhealthy and contractility is impaired.

cardiomegaly: Enlargement of the heart.

cardiomyopathy: A group of diseases that affect the myocardium's (heart muscle's) structure or function.

cardioplegia: Arrest of myocardial contraction, as by use of chemical compounds or cold temperatures in cardiac surgery.

cardioversion: An elective procedure in which a synchronized shock is delivered to attempt to restore the heart to a normal sinus rhythm.

cartilage: Flexible connective tissue in joints between bones that cushions the joint and reduces friction.

cataract: Opacity of the lens of the eye.

cation: Electrolyte that carries a positive electrical charge.

ceiling effect: The dose of medication at which the maximum therapeutic effect is achieved. Increasing the dose beyond the therapeutic dose will not result in increased relief and may result in undesirable side effects.

cell-mediated immunity: Production of lymphocytes by thymus in response to antigen exposure.

cellulitis: Inflammation of cellular or connective tissue.

cerebrovascular: Pertaining to the blood vessels of the cerebrum or brain.

cervicitis: Inflammation of the cervix.

chalazion: A small eyelid mass resulting from chronic inflammation of a meibomian gland.

chancre: A hard, syphilitic primary ulcer, the first sign of syphilis, appearing approximately 2 to 3 weeks after infection.

chemotherapy: The treatment of disease with medication; often refers to cancer therapy.

chiropractic: Treatment modality that uses manual adjustment of the vertebral column and extremities to remove interference with nerve function.

cholecystitis: Inflammation of the gallbladder.

choledocholithiasis: Gallstones in the common bile duct.

choledochoscopy: An endoscopic test of the gallbladder and common bile duct.

cholelithiasis: Gallstones in the gallbladder.

chorea: A nervous system condition marked by involuntary muscular twitching of the limbs or facial muscles.

chronic illness: An illness that is long lasting or recurring and usually interferes with a person's ability to perform activities of daily living. Medical care and hospitalization are often required on an ongoing basis.

circumcise: Surgical removal of the foreskin covering the head of the penis.

cirrhosis: Chronic disease of the liver, associated with fat infiltration and development of fibrotic tissue.

civil law: Provides the rules by which individuals seek to protect their personal and property rights.

claudication: Severe pain in the calf muscle from inadequate blood supply.

clubbing: A condition in which the ends of the fingers and toes appear bulbous and shiny, most often the result of lung disease.

cochlear implant: A device consisting of a microphone, signal processor, external transmitter, and implanted receiver to aid hearing.

codependence: A situation in which the significant others in a family group begin to lose their own sense of identity and purpose and exist solely for the abuser.

cognitive: The ability to think rationally and to process thoughts.

colectomy: Excision of the colon or a portion of it.

colic: Spasm of a hollow organ or duct, causing pain.

colitis: Inflammation of the colon.

collateral circulation: Small branches off of larger blood vessels that will increase in size and capacity next to a main blood vessel that is obstructed.

colonization: The presence of pathogenic microbes in the body, without development of a symptomatic infection.

colonoscopy: Examination of the upper portion of the rectum with a colonoscope.

colostomy: An artificial opening (stoma) created in the large intestine and brought to the surface of the abdomen for evacuating the bowels.

colporrhaphy: Surgical repair of the vagina.

colposcopy: Examination of the vulva, vagina, and cervix by means of a magnifying lens and a bright light.

comedone: Skin lesion that occurs in acne vulgaris (closed form: whitehead; open form: blackhead).

commissurotomy: Surgical incision of any commissure, as in cardiac valves to increase the size of the orifice.

complementary modality: Refers to a therapy used *in addition* to a conventional modality. For example, a nurse might suggest guided imagery or relaxation techniques for pain control in addition to prescribed drug therapy.

compliance: The ability to alter size or shape in response to an outside force; the ability of the lungs to distend.

compulsion: A recurrent, unwanted, and distressing urge to perform an act.

conductive hearing loss: Impaired transmission of sound waves through the external ear canal to the bones of the middle ear.

condylomata acuminata: Warts in the genital region caused by the human papillomavirus (HPV); a contagious sexually transmitted infection.

condylomatous: Pertaining to a condyloma.

confidentiality: Maintaining privacy of patient information. The patient and his or her care can be discussed only in the professional setting.

congestive heart failure: Results from inability of heart to pump sufficient amounts of blood because of impaired pumping function and sodium and water retention. Congestion refers to the buildup of fluid that ranges from mild to life threatening (pulmonary edema). With left-sided heart failure, the fluid buildup occurs in the lungs, and, if severe, immediate treatment is required or death can occur. With right-sided heart failure, the fluid buildup is seen systemically (lower legs/feet, sacral area in bedridden persons, jugular veins, liver, spleen).

conization: The removal of a cone of tissue, as in partial excision of the cervix uteri.

conjunctivitis: Inflammation of the conjunctiva of the eye.

consensual response: Reaction of both pupils when one eye is exposed to greater intensity of light than the other.

constipation: A condition of sluggish or difficult bowel action/evacuation.

contraceptive: Any process, device, or method that prevents conception.

contractures: Abnormal accumulations of fibrosis connective tissue in skin, muscle, or joint capsule that prevent normal mobility at that site.

contralateral: Originating in or affecting the opposite side of the body.

conversion disorder: An illness that emerges from overuse of the conversion reaction defense mechanism, in which there is impaired physical functioning that appears to be neurologic, but no organic disease can be identified.

coping: The process of contending with the stresses of daily life in an effort to overcome or work through them.

cor pulmonale: Hypertrophy or failure of the right ventricle from disorders of the chest wall, lungs, and pulmonary vessels, as with increased pulmonary pressure caused by chronic obstructive pulmonary disease (COPD).

coronary artery disease: Narrowing of the coronary arteries sufficient to prevent adequate blood supply to the myocardium.

craniectomy: Excision of a segment of the skull.

cranioplasty: Any plastic repair operation on the skull.

craniotomy: Any incision through the cranium.

crepitation: A crackling sound such as that heard in the chest with pneumonia or other lung diseases or with grating of the ends of a fractured bone.

crepitus: *See* crepitation.

criminal law: Regulates behaviors for citizens within a country.

critical thinking: Use of knowledge and skills to make the best decisions possible in patient care situations.

cryotherapy: The therapeutic use of cold.

cryptorchidism: A birth condition in which one or both of the testicles has or have not descended into the scrotum.

culdocentesis: The procedure for obtaining material from the posterior vaginal cul-de-sac by aspiration or surgical incision through the vaginal wall, performed for therapeutic or diagnostic reasons.

culdoscopy: Direct visual examination of the female viscera through an endoscope introduced into the pelvic cavity through the posterior vaginal fornix.

culdotomy: Incision or needle puncture of the cul-de-sac of Douglas through the vagina.

cultural awareness: Being aware of history and ancestry and having an appreciation of and attention to the crafts, arts, music, foods, and clothing of various cultures.

cultural competence: Having an awareness of one's own culture and not letting it have an undue influence over another person's culture. Having the knowledge and skills about a culture that are required to provide care.

cultural diversity: Representing two or more cultures; the differences among cultures. For example, the United States includes people from many countries.

cultural sensitivity: Being aware of and sensitive to cultural differences. Avoiding behavior or language that may be offensive to another person's cultural beliefs.

culture: The socially transmitted behavior patterns, beliefs, values, customs, arts, and all other characteristics of people that guide their worldview.

curet: A loop, ring, or spoon-shaped instrument, attached to a handle and having sharp or blunt edges; used to scrape tissue from a surface.

customs: The usual ways of acting in a given circumstance or something that an individual or group does out of habit. For example, many people in the United States eat turkey on Thanksgiving.

cyanosis: Slightly bluish, grayish, or dark purple discoloration of the skin caused by the presence of abnormal amounts of reduced hemoglobin in the blood.

cystic: Pertaining to cysts or the urinary bladder.

cystitis: Inflammation of the urinary bladder.

cystocele: A bladder hernia that protrudes into the vagina.

cystoscopy: A diagnostic procedure using an instrument (cystoscope) via the urethra to view the bladder.

cytomegalovirus: Species-specific herpesvirus; usually harmless to those with functional immune systems. May cause fatal pneumonia in those who are immunocompromised. Affects retina and may cause blindness in those with acquired immunodeficiency syndrome (AIDS).

cytotoxic: Destructive to cells.

data: A group of facts or statistics.

data, objective: *See* objective data.

data, subjective: *See* subjective data.

débridement: The removal of foreign material and contaminated and devitalized tissues from or adjacent to a traumatic or infected area until surrounding healthy tissue is exposed.

decerebrate: Abnormal extension posture indicating brainstem damage.

decorticate: Abnormal flexion posture indicating cerebral damage.

defibrillation: Use of an electrical device that applies countershock to the heart through electrodes placed on the chest wall to stop fibrillation of the heart.

degeneration: Deterioration.

dehiscence: A splitting open (i.e., rupture) of an incision.

dehydration: A condition resulting from excessive loss of body fluid that occurs when fluid output exceeds intake.

delirium: Acute, reversible state of disorientation and confusion with difficulty focusing attention, inability to sleep, and hyperactivity due to an underlying cause. A fairly common acute condition in older hospitalized adults.

delirium tremens: An acute alcohol withdrawal syndrome marked by acute, transient disturbance of consciousness.

delusions: False beliefs that are firmly maintained despite incontrovertible proof to the contrary.

dementia: A broad term that refers to cognitive deficit, including memory impairment.

demyelination: Loss of myelin from neurons.

deontology: The study of moral obligations and commitments, including medical ethics.

dependence: A state of reliance on something. Psychological craving for a drug that may or may not be accompanied by a physiological need.

depression: A mental disorder marked by altered mood with loss of interest.

dermatitis: Inflammation of the skin.

dermatomycosis: A fungal infection of the skin.

dermoid: Resembling the skin.

developmental stage: An age-defined period with specific psychological tasks that need to be accomplished to maintain ego as proposed by Erik Erikson, a psychoanalyst.

diabetes mellitus: A chronic disease characterized by impaired production or use of insulin and high blood glucose levels.

diaphysis: Long bone shaft.

diarrhea: Passage of fluid or unformed stools.

diastolic blood pressure: The amount of pressure exerted on the wall of the arteries when the ventricles are at rest. The bottom number in a blood pressure reading.

diffusion: The tendency of molecules of a substance (gaseous, liquid, or solid) to move from a region of high concentration to one of lower concentration.

dilation and curettage: A surgical procedure that expands the cervical canal of the uterus (dilation) so that the surface lining of the uterine wall can be scraped (curettage).

diplopia: Double vision.

displacement: Transference of emotion from the original idea with which it was associated to a different idea, allowing the patient to avoid acknowledging the original source.

disseminated intravascular coagulation: A pathological form of coagulation that is diffuse (widespread) rather than localized, as would be the case in normal coagulation. Clotting factors are consumed to such an extent that generalized bleeding may occur.

distributive shock: Excessive dilation of the venules and arterioles, leading to decreased distribution of blood, resulting in shock.

diverticulitis: Inflammation of a diverticulum (a sac or pouch in the walls of a canal or organ, usually the colon), especially inflammation involving diverticula of the colon.

diverticulosis: The presence of diverticula in the absence of inflammation.

do not resuscitate (DNR): An order not to do cardiopulmonary resuscitation (CPR) at the end of life.

dormant: Condition of greatly reduced metabolic activity permitting long-term survival and possible reactivation of bacterial endospores, protozoan cysts, larval stages of worm parasites, and viruses.

Dressler syndrome: Postmyocardial infarction syndrome; pericarditis. Also called Dressler's syndrome.

durable power of attorney: Person legally designated to speak for a patient when the patient is no longer able to speak for himself or herself.

dysrhythmia: Another name for arrhythmia.

dysarthria: Imperfect articulation of speech caused by disturbances of muscular control resulting from central or peripheral nervous system damage.

dysfunctional: Family or work environment that does not function effectively, sometimes because of other problems of members.

dysmenorrhea: Pain in association with menstruation.

dyspareunia: Occurrence of pain in the labia, vagina, or pelvis during or after sexual intercourse.

dysphagia: Inability to swallow or difficulty swallowing.

dysplasia: Abnormal development of tissue.

dyspnea: Subjective sense of labored breathing that occurs because of insufficient oxygenation.

dysreflexia: State in which an individual with a spinal cord injury at or above T6

experiences an uninhibited sympathetic response to a noxious stimulus.

dysuria: Difficult or painful urination.

ecchymoses: A bruise of varying size, the color of which may be blue-black, changing to greenish yellow or yellow with time.

ectasia: Replacement of normal tissue with fibrous tissue.

ectopic: Out of normal position. For example, ectopic hormones are secreted from sites other than the gland where they would normally be found.

edema: Collection of excess fluid in body tissues.

ejaculation: The release of semen from the male urethra.

electrocardiogram (ECG): A recording of the electrical activity of the heart.

electrocautery: Cauterization using platinum wires heated to red or white heat by an electric current, either direct or alternating.

electrocoagulated: Coagulation of tissue by means of a high-frequency electric current.

electroconvulsive therapy (ECT): A type of somatic therapy in which an electric current is used to produce convulsions to treat such conditions as depression.

electroencephalogram: A record produced by electroencephalography; tracing of the electrical impulses of the brain.

electrolytes: Substances that when dissolved in water can conduct electricity.

electroretinography: Measurement of the electrical response of the retina to light stimulation.

elopement: Leaving a facility unsupervised when unable to protect oneself.

emboli: Solid, liquid, or gaseous masses of undissolved matter traveling with the fluid current in a blood or lymphatic vessel.

embolism: Foreign substance or blood clot that travels through the circulatory system until it obstructs a vessel.

emphysema: Distention of interstitial tissue by gas or air; chronic pulmonary disease marked by terminal bronchiole and alveolar destruction and air trapping.

empyema: Pus in a body cavity, especially the pleural space.

encephalitis: Inflammation of the brain.

encephalopathy: Dysfunction of the brain.

endarterectomy: Excision of thickened atheromatous areas of the innermost coat of an artery.

endogenous: Produced or originating from within a cell or organism.

endometritis: Inflammation of the endometrium of the uterus.

endorphins: Naturally occurring opioids in the body, many times more potent than analgesic medications.

endoscope: A device consisting of a tube and optical system for observing the inside of a hollow organ or cavity. Can be flexible or rigid.

endothelium: A single layer of squamous epithelium cells that line the blood vessels, heart, and lymphatic vessels; it is very smooth to prevent abnormal clotting.

enkephalins: One type of endorphin.

enteral nutrition: Feeding using the gastrointestinal tract, including an oral diet or a tube feeding.

enteritis: Inflammation of the intestines, particularly of the mucosa and submucosa of the small intestine.

enucleation: Removal of an organ or other mass intact from its supporting tissues, as of the eyeball from the orbit.

epidemiological: The study of the distribution and determinants of health-related states and events in populations and the application of this study to the control of health problems.

epididymitis: Inflammation or infection of the epididymis.

epidural: Situated on or outside the dura mater.

epinephrine: A hormone secreted by the adrenal medulla in response to stimulation of the sympathetic nervous system.

epiphyses: Ends of long bone.

epispadias: A congenital male defect in which the opening of the urethra is on the dorsum of the penis, instead of the tip.

epistaxis: Nosebleed.

epithelialization: The growth of skin over a wound.

equianalgesic: Drugs having equal pain-killing effect. The same degree of pain relief may require different doses when different medications are given or medications are given by different routes.

erectile dysfunction: Inability to have an erection sufficient for sexual intercourse.

erection: Enlargement and hardening of the penis caused by engorgement of blood.

erythema: Diffuse redness over the skin.

eschar: Hard scab or dry crust that results from necrotic tissue.

escharotomy: Removal of a slough or scab formed on the skin and underlying tissue of severely burned skin.

esophagogastroduodenoscopy: An endoscopic procedure that allows the physician to view the esophagus, stomach, and duodenum.

esophagoscopy: Examination of the esophagus using an endoscope.

esotropia: Strabismus in which there is deviation of the visual axis of one eye toward that of the other eye, resulting in diplopia. Also called cross-eyed.

essential hypertension: Chronic elevation of blood pressure resulting from an unknown cause.

ethical: Describes behavior guided by a system of moral principles or standards.

ethics: Branch of philosophy that answers questions about morality such as good and bad or right and wrong.

ethnic: Pertaining to a religious, racial, national, or cultural group. For example, individuals may identify with the Jewish, Catholic, or Islamic religions.

ethnocentrism: The tendency to think that one's own ways of thinking, believing, and acting are the only right ways. People who are different are seen as strange or bizarre. An example is one who believes that his or her religious beliefs are the only right beliefs and other religions are wrong.

eustress: Stress from positive experiences.

euthyroid: Normal thyroid function.

evaluation: The judgment of something.

evisceration: Extrusion of viscera outside the body, especially through a surgical excision.

exacerbation: Aggravation of symptoms.

exophthalmos: Abnormal protrusion of the eyeball.

exotropia: Abnormal turning outward of one or both eyes; divergent strabismus.

expectorant: Agent that promotes removal of pulmonary secretions.

expectorate: The act or process of coughing up materials from the air passageways leading to the lungs.

external otitis: Inflammation of the external ear.

extracardiac: Outside the heart.

extracellular: Outside the cell.

extracorporeal shock-wave lithotripsy (ESWL): Noninvasive treatment using shock waves to break up gallstones or kidney stones.

extravasation: The escape of fluids into surrounding tissue.

extrinsic factors: External variables.

exudate: Accumulated fluid in a cavity; oozing of pus or serum; often the result of inflammation.

fasciculation: Twitching.

fasciotomy: Incision of fascia.

fetor hepaticus: Foul breath associated with liver disease.

fibrocystic: Consisting of fibrocysts, which are fibrous tumors that have undergone cystic degeneration or accumulated fluid.

fidelity: Obligation to be faithful to commitments made to self and others.

filtration: The process of removing particles from a solution by allowing the liquid portion to pass through a membrane or other partial barrier.

fissure: A narrow slit or cleft, especially one of the deeper or more constant furrows separating the gyri of the brain.

fistula: Any abnormal, tubelike passage within body tissue, usually between two internal organs, or leading from an internal organ to the body surface.

flaccid: Weak, lax, soft muscles.

flail chest: Condition of the chest wall caused by two or more fractures on each affected rib resulting in a segment of rib that is not attached on either end; the flail portion moves paradoxically in with inspiration and out with expiration.

fluoroscope: A device consisting of a fluorescent screen suitably mounted, either separately or in conjunction with an x-ray tube, by means of which the shadows of objects interposed between the tube and the screen are made visible.

fluoroscopy: The use of a fluoroscope for medical diagnosis or for testing various materials by roentgen rays.

full-thickness burn: Burn in which all of the epithelializing elements and those lining the sweat glands, hair follicles, and sebaceous glands are destroyed.

fungi: A general term for a group of eukaryotic organisms (e.g., mushrooms, yeasts, molds).

furuncle: An acute circumscribed inflammation of the subcutaneous layers of the skin or of a gland or hair follicle.

gastrectomy: Any surgery that involves partial or total removal of the stomach.

gastric acid stimulation test: A test that measures the amount of gastric acid for 1 hour after subcutaneous injection of a drug that stimulates gastric acid secretion.

gastric analysis: A test performed to measure secretions of hydrochloric acid and pepsin in the stomach.

gastric lavage: Washing out of the stomach; used to empty the stomach when the contents are irritating.

gastritis: Acute—The inflammation of the stomach mucosa; also known as heartburn or indigestion. Chronic—Gastritis that is recurrent; classified as type A (asymptomatic) or type B (symptomatic).

gastroduodenostomy: Excision of the pylorus of the stomach with anastomosis of the upper portion of the stomach to the duodenum.

gastroepiploic: Pertaining to the stomach and greater omentum.

gastrojejunostomy: Subtotal excision of the stomach with closure of the proximal end of the duodenum and side-to-side anastomosis of the jejunum to the remaining portion of the stomach.

gastroparesis: Paralysis of the stomach, resulting in poor emptying.

gastroplasty: Plastic surgery of the stomach. Used to decrease the size of the stomach to treat morbid obesity.

gastroscopy: Examination of the stomach and abdominal cavity by use of a gastroscope.

gastrostomy: Surgical creation of a gastric fistula through the abdominal wall.

gavage: Feeding with a stomach tube or with a tube passed through the nares, pharynx, and esophagus into the stomach. The food is in liquid or semiliquid form at room temperature.

glaucoma: A group of eye diseases characterized by increased intraocular pressure.

glomerulonephritis: A form of nephritis in which the lesions involve primarily the glomeruli.

glossitis: An inflammation of the tongue.

glycosuria: Abnormal amount of glucose in the urine, often associated with diabetes mellitus.

goitrogens: Foods or medications that cause a goiter.

gout: A common group of arthritic disorders marked by deposition of monosodium urate crystals in joints and other tissues.

gravida: Number of times a woman has been pregnant.

gummas: A soft granulomatous tumor of the tissues characteristic of the tertiary stage of syphilis.

gynecomastia: Excessive breast tissue on a male.

hallucinations: False perceptions having no relation to reality and not accounted for by any exterior stimuli.

hand hygiene: Cleansing of the hands with hand washing as defined by the Centers for Disease Control and Prevention or an alcohol-based hand sanitizer solution.

health: A condition in which all functions of the body and mind are normally active.

health literacy: Degree to which a person has the capacity to obtain, process, and understand basic health information and services to make the best-informed health decisions.

hearing aid: An instrument to amplify sounds for those with hearing loss.

heatstroke: An acute and dangerous reaction to heat exposure, characterized by high body temperature, usually higher than 105°F (40.5°C).

Helicobacter pylori: Bacterium that causes some peptic ulcers.

hemarthrosis: Bleeding into a joint.

hematochezia: Blood in the feces.

hematoma: A localized collection of extravasated blood, usually clotted, in an organ, space, or tissue.

hematuria: Blood in the urine.

hemiparesis: Weakness affecting one side of the body.

hemipelvectomy: The surgical removal of half of the pelvis and the leg.

hemiplegia: Paralysis of only one side of the body.

hemodialysis: A method for replacing the function of the kidneys by circulating blood through tubes made of semipermeable membranes.

hemolysis: The destruction of the membrane of red blood cells with the liberation of hemoglobin, which diffuses into the surrounding fluid.

hemophilia: A hereditary blood disease marked by greatly prolonged coagulation time, with consequent failure of the blood to clot and abnormal bleeding.

hemoptysis: Coughing up of blood from the respiratory tract.

hemorrhoids: A mass of dilated, tortuous veins in the anorectum involving the venous plexuses of that area.

hemothorax: Blood in the pleural space; may be associated with trauma, tuberculosis, or pneumonia.

hepatitis: Inflammation of the liver, most often viral.

hepatomegaly: Enlargement of the liver.

hepatorenal syndrome: A deadly kidney failure that sometimes accompanies liver disease.

hepatosplenomegaly: Enlargement of the liver and spleen.

hernia: The protrusion or projection of an organ or a part of an organ through the wall of the cavity that normally contains it.

herpetic: Pertaining to herpes.

heterograft: Graft from one species to another species (animal to man). Another name for xenograft.

hiatal hernia: A condition in which part of the stomach protrudes through and above the diaphragm.

high-density lipoprotein (HDL): Plasma lipids bound to albumin consisting of lipoproteins. It has been found that those with high levels of HDL have less chance of having coronary artery disease.

histamine: A substance produced in the body that increases gastric secretion, increases capillary permeability, and contracts the bronchial smooth muscle. Plays a role in allergic reaction.

holistic: The view that people and other organisms function as complete units that cannot be reduced to the sum of their parts. In health care, holistic care encompasses the person's body, mind, and spirit along with the environment and society in which the person lives.

homeopathy: System of medicine based on the theory that "like cures like" and uses tiny doses of a substance that create the symptoms of disease.

homeostasis: Maintaining a constant balance, especially whenever a change occurs.

homograft: Graft from a donor of the same species as the recipient.

hopelessness: Subjective state in which a person sees limited or unavailable alternatives; lacking energy.

hordeolum: Sty.

hospice: A service provided to patients and their families in the last 6 months of life to manage pain and provide emotional support.

host: The organism from which a parasite obtains its nourishment.

human immunodeficiency virus (HIV): A retrovirus that causes acquired immunodeficiency syndrome (AIDS).

human trafficking: The act of recruiting, harboring, transporting, providing, or obtaining a person for labor or as a sex worker though the use of force, fraud, or coercion.

humoral: Pertaining to body fluids or substances contained in them.

hydrocele: A collection of fluid in the scrotal sack.

hydrocephalus: A condition caused by enlargement of the cranium caused by abnormal accumulation of cerebrospinal fluid within the cerebral ventricular system.

hydronephrosis: Abnormal dilation of kidneys caused by obstruction of urine flow.

hydrostatic: Pertaining to the pressure of liquids in equilibrium and to the pressure exerted by liquids.

hyperalgesia: Increased sensitivity to pain.

hypercalcemia: An excessive amount of calcium in the blood.

hyperglycemia: Excess glucose in the blood.

hyperkalemia: An excessive amount of potassium in the blood.

hyperlipidemia: Excessive quantity of fat in the blood.

hypermagnesemia: Excess magnesium in the blood.

hypernatremia: Excess sodium in the blood.

hyperopia: Farsightedness.

hyperplasia: Excessive increase in the number of normal cells.

hypertension: Abnormally elevated blood pressure.

hypertensive emergency: Systolic blood pressure above 180 mm Hg and diastolic blood pressure above 120 mm Hg.

hypertensive urgency: Occurs when blood pressure is as elevated as in a hypertensive emergency but without progression of target-organ dysfunction.

hypertonic: Exerts greater osmotic pressure than blood.

hypertrophy: An increase in the size of an organ or structure, or of the body, owing to growth rather than tumor formation.

hyperuricemia: An excess of uric acid or urates in the blood.

hyperventilation: Increased ventilation that results in a lowered carbon dioxide (CO_2) level (hypocapnia).

hypervolemia: An abnormal increase in the volume of circulating blood.

hypocalcemia: Reduced amount of calcium in the blood.

hypoglycemia: Below-normal amount of glucose in the blood.

hypokalemia: Reduced amount of potassium in the blood.

hypomagnesemia: Reduced amount of magnesium in the blood.

hyponatremia: Reduced amount of sodium in the blood.

hypoperfusion: Low blood flow that occurs when the circulatory system cannot deliver adequate oxygenated blood to the organs and tissues, as in shock.

hypophysectomy: Surgical removal of the pituitary gland.

hypoplasia: Underdevelopment of a tissue organ or body.

hypospadias: A congenital male defect in which the opening of the urethra is on the underside of the penis, instead of the tip.

hypotension: Abnormally low blood pressure below 90 mm Hg systolic.

hypothermia: Body temperature below 95°F (35°C).

hypotonic: Pertaining to defective muscular tone or tension; having a lower concentration of solute than intracellular or extracellular fluid.

hypotropia: Downward deviation of the eye away from the visual axis.

hypovolemia: The most common form of dehydration resulting from the loss of fluid from the body; results in decreased blood volume.

hypovolemic: Low volume of blood in the circulatory system.

hypovolemic shock: Shock that occurs when blood or plasma is lost in such quantities that the remaining blood cannot fill the circulatory system despite constriction of the blood vessels.

hypoxemia: Deficient oxygenation of the blood.

hypoxia: Diminished availability of oxygen to the body tissues.

hysterectomy: Surgical removal of the uterus through the abdominal wall or vagina.

hysterosalpingogram: Radiograph of the uterus and fallopian tubes.

hysteroscopy: Endoscopic direct visual examination of the canal of the uterine cervix and the cavity of the uterus.

hysterotomy: Incision of the uterus.

icterus: Yellowing of the skin and the sclera of the eye.

idiopathic thrombocytopenic purpura: The total number of circulating platelets is greatly diminished, even though platelet production in the bone marrow is normal, resulting in slowed blood clotting.

ileostomy: An artificial opening (stoma) created in the small intestine (ileum) and brought to the surface of the abdomen for the purpose of evacuating feces.

illness: The state of being sick.

illusions: Mistaken perceptions of reality.

imagery: The use of the imagination to promote relaxation.

immunocompromised: Having an immune system that is not capable of reacting to a pathogen or tissue damage.

impaction: An immovable accumulation of feces in the bowels.

imperforate: Without an opening.

in situ: Localized, not invading surrounding tissue.

in vitro fertilization: Fertilization in a test tube.

incontinence: *See* urinary incontinence.

induction: The process or act of causing to occur, as in anesthesia induction.

induration: Area of hardened tissue.

infective endocarditis: Inflammation of the heart lining caused by microorganisms.

infiltration: The accumulation of an external substance (such as intravenous [IV] fluids) within tissues.

informatics: The study of information.

inspection: Use of observation skills to systematically gather data that can be seen.

insufficiency: The condition of being inadequate for a given purpose, such as heart valves that do not close properly.

insufflation: Used to inflate the abdomen during laparoscopic or endoscopic procedures to enhance visualization of structures.

intermittent claudication: A symptom associated with arterial occlusive disease. It refers to pain in the calf of a lower extremity, usually brought on by activity or exercise, and ceases with rest.

international normalized ratio: The World Health Organization's standard for reporting the prothrombin time assay test when the thromboplastin reagent developed by the first International Reference Preparation is used. The reagent was developed to prevent variability in prothrombin time testing results and provide uniformity in monitoring therapeutic levels for coagulation during oral anticoagulation therapy.

interstitial: Fluid between tissues.

intervention: One or more actions taken in order to modify an effect.

intracellular: Fluids located within the blood cell.

intracranial: Within the cranium or skull.

intraoperative: Occurring during a surgical procedure.

intravascular: Fluids located within the blood vessels.

intravenous: Within or into a vein.

intrinsic factors: Internal variables.

intussusception: The slipping of one part of an intestine into another adjacent to it.

ipsilateral: On the same side; affecting the same side of the body.

ischemia: Condition of inadequate blood supply.

isoelectric line: The period when the electrical tracing is at zero and is neither positive nor negative.

isolated systolic hypertension: The systolic pressure is 160 mm Hg or more, but the diastolic pressure is lower than 95 mm Hg.

isotonic: A fluid that has the same osmolarity as the blood.

jaundice: Yellowing of the skin and the sclera of the eye.

joint: An articulation. The point of juncture between two bones.

Kaposi sarcoma: A vascular malignancy that is often first apparent in the skin or mucous membranes but may involve the viscera. Also called Kaposi's sarcoma.

ketoacidosis: A condition in which fat breakdown produces ketones, which cause an acidic state in the body; may be associated with weight loss or diabetes mellitus.

Kussmaul respirations: Term describing deep respirations of an individual with ketoacidosis. Also called Kussmaul's respirations.

laceration: A wound or irregular tear of the flesh.

lactic acid: By-product of anaerobic metabolism.

laminectomy: The excision of a vertebral posterior arch, usually to remove a lesion or herniated disk.

laparoscopy: Exploration of the abdomen with an endoscope.

laparotomy: The surgical opening of the abdomen; an abdominal operation.

laryngeal edema: Sudden swelling of the larynx occurring with severe allergic reactions.

laryngectomy: Surgical removal of the larynx.

laryngitis: Inflammation of the larynx.

laser ablation: Therapeutic destruction of a growth or part of a growth by laser treatment.

lavage: Washing out of a cavity.

law: The further formalization of moral considerations.

leadership: The process of socially influencing others to obtain their assistance and support to accomplish a common task.

leiomyoma: A myoma consisting principally of smooth muscle tissue.

leukemia: A malignancy of the blood-forming cells in the bone marrow.

leukocytosis: An increase in the number of leukocytes in the blood, generally caused by the presence of infection and usually transient.

leukopenia: Abnormal decrease of white blood cells, usually below 5,000/mm³.

liability: The level of responsibility that society places on individuals for their actions.

libido: Sexual drive, conscious or unconscious.

lichenified: Thickened or hardened from continued irritation.

ligament: Fibrous connective tissue that connect bone to bone.

limitation of liability: Steps that health care professionals can take to limit their liability.

living will: A document instructing health care workers about a patient's preferences when he or she is no longer able to communicate. Implementation of living wills varies by state.

lobectomy: Surgical removal of a lobe of any organ or gland.

low-density lipoprotein (LDL): A lipoprotein that transports cholesterol and triglycerides from the liver to peripheral tissues. LDL allows fats and cholesterol to move within the water-based solution of the blood. Increased LDL cholesterol is associated with cardiovascular disease, so it is often referred to as "bad cholesterol."

lower gastrointestinal (GI) series: The use of barium sulfate as an enema to facilitate x-ray and fluoroscopic examination of the colon.

lymphadenopathy: Any disorder of the lymph nodes.

lymphangitis: Inflammation of lymphatic channels or vessels.

lymphedema: An abnormal accumulation of tissue fluid (potential lymph) in the interstitial space.

lymphocytes: Cells present in the blood and lymphatic tissue that provide the main means of immunity for the body; white blood cells.

lymphoma: A usually malignant lymphoid neoplasm.

macrodrop: A large drop (typically 15–20 drops per mL). In intravenous (IV) therapy, may refer to an administration device used to deliver large drops of IV solution.

macular degeneration: Age-related breakdown of the macular area of the retina of the eye.

maleficence: Committing harm or evil.

malignant: Growing, resisting treatment; used to describe a tumor of cancerous cells.

malingerer: Someone who pretends to be in pain.

malpractice: A breach of duty arising out of the relationship that exists between the patient and the health care worker.

mammography: Use of radiography of the breast to diagnose breast cancer.

mammoplasty: Plastic surgery of the breast.

mania: Mental disorder characterized by excessive excitement.

marsupialization: Process of raising the borders of an evacuated tumor sac to the edges of the abdominal wound and stitching them there to form a pouch.

mastalgia: Pain in the breast.

mastectomy: Excision of the breast.

mastitis: Inflammation of the breast.

mastopexy: Correction of a pendulous breast by surgical fixation and plastic surgery.

mediastinum: A septum or cavity between two principal portions of an organ.

megacolon: Extremely dilated colon.

melena: Black, tarry feces caused by action of intestinal secretions on free blood.

menarche: The initial menstrual period, normally occurring between the ninth and 17th year.

Ménière disease: A recurrent and usually progressive group of symptoms including progressive deafness, ringing in the ears, dizziness, and a sensation of fullness or pressure in the ears. Also called Ménière's disease.

meningitis: Inflammation of the membranes of the spinal cord and brain.

menopause: The period that marks the permanent cessation of menstrual activity, usually occurring between the ages of 35 and 58.

mental health: State of being adjusted to life; able to be flexible, successful, maintain close relationships, solve problems, make appropriate judgments, and cope with daily stresses.

mental illness: Any illness that affects the mind or behavior.

metastasis: Movement of bacteria or body cells (especially cancer cells) from one part of the body to another.

microbiota: Microorganisms inhabiting a bodily organ or part such as the gut or skin.

microdrop: A small drop (60 drops per mL). In intravenous (IV) therapy, may refer to an administration device used to deliver small drops of IV solution.

milieu: Environment.

miotic: An agent that causes the pupil to contract.

moral distress: Distress experienced when the right thing to do cannot be carried out because of institutional constraints.

morbidity: State of being diseased.

mortality: Condition of being mortal; number of deaths in a population.

mucolytic: Agent that liquefies sputum.

mucopurulent cervicitis: Inflammation of the cervix producing mucus and purulent discharge.

mucositis: Inflammation of a mucous membrane.

multifocal: Many foci (areas) or sites.

murmur: An abnormal sound heard on auscultation of the heart and adjacent large blood vessels.

muscle: A bundle of long slender cells or fibers that have the power to contract and hence to produce movement.

myalgia: Muscle pain or tenderness.

myectomy: Surgical removal of a hypertrophied muscle.

myelogram: The film produced by radiography of the spinal cord after injection of a contrast medium into the subarachnoid space.

myocardial infarction: Death of cells of an area of the myocardium (heart muscle) as a result of oxygen deprivation, which in turn is caused by obstruction of the blood supply. Commonly referred to as a heart attack.

myocarditis: The inflammatory process that causes nodules to form in the myocardial tissue; the nodules become scar tissue over time. Inflammation of the heart muscle.

myocardium: Heart muscle.

myomectomy: Removal of a portion of muscle or muscular tissue.

myopia: The error of refraction in which rays of light entering the eye parallel to the optic axis are brought to a focus in front of the retina; nearsightedness.

myringoplasty: Surgical reconstruction of the tympanic membrane.

myringotomy: Incision of the tympanic membrane, usually performed to relieve pressure and allow for drainage of either serous or purulent fluid in the middle ear behind the tympanic membrane.

myxedema: Condition resulting from hypofunction of the thyroid gland.

nasoseptoplasty: Surgical correction of the nasal septum.

naturopathy: System of medicine that uses natural therapies such as nutrition, herbs, hydrotherapy, counseling, physical medicine, and homeopathy to treat disease, promote healing, and prevent illness.

negligence: An unintentional tort.

neoplasm: New abnormal tissue growth, as in a tumor.

nephrectomy: Surgical removal of a kidney.

nephrogenic: Caused by the kidneys.

nephrolithotomy: Incision of a kidney for removal of kidney stones.

nephropathy: Any disease of the kidney.

nephrosclerosis: Hardening of the kidney associated with hypertension and disease of the renal arterioles.

nephrostomy: Creation of a permanent opening into the renal pelvis.

nephrotoxin: A toxin having a specific destructive effect on kidney tissue.

neuralgia: Nerve pain.

neurogenic: Originating in the nervous system.

neuropathic: Resulting from peripheral nerve injury.

neuropathy: A general term denoting functional disturbances and pathological changes in the peripheral nervous system.

neutrophils: Granular leukocytes (white blood cells) having a nucleus with three to five lobes connected by threads of chromatin and cytoplasm containing very fine granules.

nociception: Refers to the body's normal reaction to noxious stimuli, such as tissue damage, with the release of pain-producing substances.

nociceptive: Pain sensitive.

nocturia: Excessive urination at night.

nodal or junctional rhythm: A cardiac rhythm with its origin at the atrioventricular (AV) node.

nonmaleficence: The requirement that health care providers do no harm to their patients, either intentionally or unintentionally.

norepinephrine: A hormone produced by the adrenal medulla, similar in chemical and pharmacological properties to epinephrine, but chiefly a vasoconstrictor with little effect on cardiac output.

normoglycemia: Normal blood glucose.

nosocomial infection: Infection acquired in a health care agency.

nuchal rigidity: Rigidity of the nape, or back, of the neck.

numeracy: Ability to understand and use numbers in everyday life.

nursing diagnosis: A standardized label placed on a patient's problem to make it understandable to all nurses.

nursing process: An orderly, logical approach to administering nursing care so that the patient's needs for such care are met comprehensively and effectively.

nystagmus: Involuntary, cyclical, rapid movement of the eyes in response to vertical, horizontal, or rotary movement.

obesity: Abnormal amount of fat on the body ranging from 20% to 30% above average weight for age, sex, and height.

objective data: Factual data obtained through physical examination and diagnostic tests; objective data are observable or knowable through the five senses.

obsession: Repetitive thought, urge, or emotion.

obstipation: Intractable constipation.

obstructive shock: Shock caused by indirect pump failure.

occult blood: Blood not seen by the naked eye.

oliguria: Diminished urination.

oncology: The study of cancer and cancer treatment.

oncovirus: Viruses linked to cancer in humans.

onychomycosis: Disease of the nails caused by fungus.

oophorectomy: Surgical removal of the ovaries. the fallopian tubes

ophthalmia neonatorum: Conjunctivitis in the newborn resulting from exposure to infectious or chemical agents.

ophthalmologist: A physician who specializes in the treatment of disorders of the eye.

ophthalmoscope: An instrument used for examining the interior of the eye, especially the retina.

opioid: A narcotic drug with morphine-like effects. True opioids are derived from opium.

optician: One who specializes in filling prescriptions for corrective lenses for eyeglasses and contact lenses.

optimum level of functioning: Highest level of patient activity considering the patient's condition.

optometrist: A doctor of optometry who diagnoses and treats conditions and diseases of the eye per state laws.

orchiectomy: Removal of one or both testicles; a treatment for prostate cancer.

orchitis: Inflammation of a testis.

orgasm: Pleasurable physical release sensation related to physical, sexual, and psychological stimulation.

orientation: The ability to comprehend and to adjust oneself in an environment with regard to time, location, and identity of persons.

orthopnea: Labored breathing that occurs when lying flat; relieved when sitting up; associated with left ventricular heart failure.

osmolality: Osmotic concentration; ionic concentration of the dissolved substances per unit of solvent.

osmolarity: Concentration of the substances in body fluids.

osmosis: The passage of solvent through a semipermeable membrane that separates solutions of different concentrations.

osteoblast: Produce bone matrix during growth and replace matrix during normal remodeling or in repair of fractures.

osteoclast: Resorb bone matrix when more calcium is needed in the blood or during repair.

osteomyelitis: Inflammation of bone, especially the marrow, caused by a pathogenic organism.

osteopathic: Related to the system of medicine emphasizing the interrelationship of the body's nerves, muscles, bones, and organs; involves treating the whole person, and stresses the importance of diet, exercise, and fitness, with a focus on prevention.

osteoporosis: A condition in which there is a reduction in the mass of bone per unit volume.

osteosarcoma: A malignant sarcoma of a bone.

otalgia: Pain in the ear.

otorrhea: Inflammation of the ear with purulent discharge.

otosclerosis: A condition characterized by chronic, progressive deafness, especially for low tones.

ototoxic: Having a detrimental effect on the eighth cranial nerve or the organs of hearing.

pain: An unpleasant sensory and emotional experience associated with actual or potential tissue damage, or described in terms of such damage. Pain is whatever the patient says it is whenever the patient says it occurs.

palliation: The relief of symptoms without the intent to cure disease.

palpation: Use of the fingers or hands to feel something.

pancreatectomy: Removal of all or part of the pancreas.

pancreatitis: Inflammation of the pancreas.

pancytopenia: Abnormal depression of all of the cellular elements of the blood.

panhysterectomy: Excision of the entire uterus, including the cervix uteri.

panmyelosis: Increased level of all bone marrow components, red blood cells, white blood cells, and platelets.

para: Number of deliveries a woman has had from pregnancies after 20 weeks' gestation.

paradoxical respiration: Chest movement on respiration that is opposite to that expected.

paranoia: Behavior that is marked by delusions of persecution or delusional jealousy.

paraparesis: Partial paralysis of the lower extremities.

paraphimosis: Uncircumcised foreskin that has swollen and stuck behind the head of the penis.

paraplegia: Paralysis of the lower body, including both legs, resulting from a spinal cord lesion.

parenteral: A medication delivery route that is "beside" rather than in the intestine, such as intramuscular, intravenous (IV), or subcutaneous.

parenteral nutrition: Nutrition by intravenous (IV) route, either centrally or peripherally.

paresis: Weakness; incomplete paralysis.

paresthesia: A heightened sensation, such as burning, prickling, or tingling.

paroxysmal nocturnal dyspnea: Sudden attacks of shortness of breath that usually occur during sleep. Person wakes gasping for breath and sits up to relieve symptoms; associated with left ventricular heart failure.

partial-thickness burn: Burn in which the epithelializing elements remain intact.

passive immunity: Reinforcement of the immune system with immune serum for such conditions as tetanus, diphtheria, and venomous snake bite.

paternalism: A unilateral and sometimes unreasonable decision by health care providers that implies they know what is best, regardless of the patient's wishes.

pathogen: A microorganism or substance capable of producing a disease.

pathological fracture: Fracture resulting from weakening of the bone structure by pathological processes such as neoplasia or osteomalacia.

patient-controlled analgesia (PCA): An apparatus that delivers an intravenous (IV) analgesic to relieve pain, which is controlled by the patient.

pedicle: The stem that attaches a new growth.

pediculosis: Infestation with lice.

pemphigus: Acute or chronic serious skin disease characterized by the appearance of bullae (blisters) of various sizes on normal skin and mucous membranes.

penumbra: An area of brain tissue surrounding damage from a stroke that may be revived if the brain is reperfused quickly.

peptic ulcer disease: A condition in which the lining of the esophagus, stomach, or duodenum is eroded.

perception: A unique impression of events by an individual. These impressions are strongly influenced by personality, cultural orientation, attitudes, and life experiences.

percussion: A tapping technique used by physicians and advanced practice nurses to determine the consistency of underlying tissues.

percutaneous: Through the skin; may refer to an injection, a medication application, or a biopsy.

perfusion: Supplying an organ or tissue with blood.

pericardial effusion: A buildup of fluid in the pericardial space.

pericardial friction rub: Friction sound heard over the fourth left intercostal space near the sternum; a classic sign of pericarditis.

pericardial tamponade: Compression of the heart by an abnormal filling of the pericardial sac with blood.

pericardiectomy: Excision of part or all of the pericardium.

pericardiocentesis: Surgical perforation of the pericardium.

pericardiotomy: Incision of the pericardium.

pericarditis: Inflammation of the pericardium (two thin layers of a saclike membrane surrounding the heart).

perimenopausal: The phase before the onset of menopause, during which the cycle of a woman with regular menses changes, perhaps abruptly, to a pattern of irregular cycles and increased periods of amenorrhea.

perinatal: Concerning the period beginning after the 28th week of pregnancy and ending 28 days after birth.

perioperative: Occurring in the period immediately before, during, and after surgery.

periosteum: Connective tissue covering all outer bone surfaces except at joints that protects, is involved in bone growth and repair, and participates in the blood supply of bone.

peripheral arterial disease: Disease of the peripheral arteries that interferes with adequate flow of blood.

peripheral vascular resistance: Opposition to blood flow through the vessels.

peristalsis: Progressive, wavelike movement that occurs involuntarily in hollow tubes of the body such as the alimentary (digestive) canal; causes contents of tube to be moved onward.

peristomal: Area around a stoma.

peritoneal dialysis: The employment of the peritoneum surrounding the abdominal cavity as a dialyzing membrane for the purpose of removing waste products or toxins accumulated as a result of renal failure.

peritonitis: Inflammation of the peritoneum.

personal protective equipment: Items worn to protect oneself and one's patients from direct transmission of organisms (including gloves, surgical masks, goggles, gowns, and shoe booties) based on the task to be performed and the type of isolation precautions in use.

petechiae: Small, purplish, hemorrhagic spots on the skin that appear in certain illnesses and bleeding disorders.

phagocytosis: Ingestion and digestion of bacteria and particles by phagocytes, cells that have the ability to ingest and destroy particulate substances such as bacteria, protozoa, and cell debris.

pharyngitis: Inflammation of the mucous membranes and lymph tissues of the pharynx, usually caused by infection.

pheochromocytoma: Rare tumor of the adrenal system that secretes catecholamines.

phimosis: Uncircumcised foreskin that cannot be moved down from the head of the penis.

phlebitis: Inflammation of a vein; may be due to irritating intravenous fluids or thrombosis.

phlebotomy: Entry into a vein for the removal or withdrawal of blood.

phobia: A persistent, irrational, intense fear of a specific object, activity, or situation.

photophobia: Abnormal visual intolerance to light.

physical dependence: A pharmacological phenomenon characterized by signs and symptoms of withdrawal when medication is withdrawn.

phytoestrogens: Naturally occurring plant sterols that have an estrogen-like effect.

pinocytosis: Reabsorption of small proteins from renal filtrate by attachment to the membranes of the tubule cells and then engulfment and digestion.

plague: A severe febrile illness caused by the gram-negative coccobacillus *Yersinia pestis* that is usually transmitted by the bite of an infectious flea. It can also be used as a biological weapon in which primary pneumonic plague would likely occur.

plaque: A deposit of fatty material on the lining of an artery.

plasmapheresis: Removal of blood to separate cells from plasma.

pleurodesis: Creation of adhesions between the parietal and visceral pleura to treat recurrent pneumothorax.

pneumocystis pneumonia (PCP): An acute pneumonia caused by the fungus *Pneumocystis jiroveci.*

pneumonectomy: Surgical removal of all or part of a lung.

pneumothorax: Air in the pleural space.

poikilothermy: The absence of sufficient arterial blood flow, causing the extremity to become the temperature of the environment.

point of maximum impulse (PMI): The area of the chest where the greatest force can be felt with the palm of the hand when the heart contracts or beats. Usually at the fourth to fifth intercostal space in the midclavicular line.

polycythemia: Excessive red cells in the blood.

polydipsia: Excessive thirst.

polyneuropathy: A disease involving multiple nerves.

polyphagia: Excessive eating.

polyuria: Excessive urination.

portal hypertension: Persistent blood pressure elevation in the portal circulation of the abdomen.

postcoital: After sexual intercourse.

postictal: Occurring after a sudden attack, such as an epileptic seizure.

postmortem care: Care after death.

postoperative: Following a surgical operation.

postprandial: After a meal.

powerlessness: Perceived lack of control over a situation.

preload: End-diastolic stretch of cardiac muscle fibers; equals end-diastolic volume.

preoperative: Preceding an operation.

preprandial: Before a meal.

presbycusis: Progressive, bilaterally symmetrical perceptive hearing loss occurring with age; usually occurs after age 50 and is caused by structural changes in the organs of hearing.

presbyopia: Diminution of accommodation of the lens of the eye occurring normally with aging, and usually resulting in hyperopia, or farsightedness.

pressure injury: An open sore or lesion of the skin that develops because of prolonged pressure against an area.

priapism: Erection that lasts too long.

primary hypertension: Abnormally elevated blood pressure of unknown cause. Also called essential hypertension.

probiotics: Supplements of live bacteria or yeast that assist the body's naturally occurring gut microbiota. Often recommended after antibiotic therapy to reestablish the normal microbiota.

proctitis: Inflammation of the rectum and anus.

proctosigmoidoscopy: Visual examination of the rectum and sigmoid colon by use of a sigmoidoscope.

prodrome: A symptom indicating the onset of a disease.

prostaglandins: Chemical neurotransmitters usually associated with pain at the site of an injury, periphery.

prostatectomy: Removal of the prostate gland.

prostatitis: Inflammation or infection of the prostate gland.

protozoa: Single-celled parasitic organisms that can move and live mainly in the soil.

pruritus: Severe itching.

pseudoaddiction: Syndrome in which behaviors similar to addiction appear as a result of inadequate pain control and patients fear not receiving adequate pain medications and pain relief.

psoriasis: Chronic inflammatory skin disorder in which epidermal cells proliferate abnormally fast.

psychoanalysis: Form of therapy based on the theories of Sigmund Freud, regarding the dynamics of the unconscious.

psychogenic: Of mental origin.

psychological dependence: Obsession of obtaining drugs for use other than medicinal; addiction.

psychopharmacology: The study of the action of drugs on psychological functions and mental states.

psychosomatic: Having bodily symptoms of psychological, emotional, or mental origin; illness traceable to an emotional cause.

psychotherapy: A method of treating disease (especially mental illness) by mental rather than pharmacological means.

ptosis: Drooping of eyelid.

puerperal: Concerning the puerperium, or period of 42 days after childbirth.

pulmonary edema: Acute heart failure in which there is severe fluid congestion in the alveoli of the lungs; life threatening.

pulse deficit: A condition in which the number of pulse beats counted at the radial artery is less than those counted in the same period of time at the apical heart rate.

purpura: Hemorrhage into the skin, mucous membranes, internal organs, and other tissues.

purulent: Fluid that contains pus.

pyelogram: A diagnostic procedure involving x-ray of the kidneys; may be done after injection of a dye into the bloodstream or directly into the kidneys.

pyelonephritis: Inflammation of the kidney and renal pelvis.

pyoderma: Any acute, inflammatory, purulent bacterial dermatitis.

QSEN project: Quality and Safety Education for Nurses project; focuses on nursing education that promotes the continual improvement of quality and safety in patient care.

quadrigeminy: PVC occurs every fourth beat (three normal beats and then a PVC).

quadriparesis: Weakness involving all four limbs caused by spinal cord injury.

quadriplegia: Paralysis of all four limbs caused by spinal cord injury.

radiation therapy: Cancer treatment with ionizing radiation.

range of motion (ROM): The range of movement of a body joint.

Raynaud disease: A primary or idiopathic vasospastic disorder characterized by bilateral and symmetrical pallor and cyanosis of the fingers. Also called Raynaud's disease.

reality orientation: A process to orient a person to facts such as names, dates, and time, through the use of verbal and nonverbal repeating messages.

rectocele: Protrusion or herniation of the posterior vaginal wall with the anterior wall of the rectum through the vagina.

red blood cells: Erythrocytes; circulating blood cells that contain hemoglobin and carry oxygen to tissues.

regurgitation: A backward flowing, as in the backflow of blood through a defective heart valve.

reminiscence therapy: Use of life reflection with a therapist to resolve conflicts or bring closure to life events.

remyelination: Replacement of myelin or neurons.

replantation: The replacement of an organ or other structure, such as a digit, limb, or tooth, to the site from which it was previously lost or removed.

reservoir: A person, animal, arthropod, plant, soil, or substance in which an infectious agent normally lives and multiplies, on which it depends for survival.

resorption: To absorb again, as in removal of bone tissue by absorption.

respiratory excursion: Downward movement of the diaphragm with inspiration.

respite care: Short-term, intermittent care for the chronically ill; provides rest for the family members or caregivers from the stress of sustained caregiving.

respondeat superior: An institution that employs a worker may be liable for the acts or omissions of its employees.

retinopathy: Disease of the retina of the eye.

retroflexion: A bending or flexing backward.

retrograde: Moving backward; degenerating from a better to a worse state.

retrograde cholangiopancreatography: An endoscopic procedure that permits the physician to visualize the liver, gallbladder, and pancreas using an endoscope, dye, and x-ray examinations.

retroversion: A turning, or a state of being turned back; the tipping of an entire organ.

rhabdomyolysis: Rapid skeletal muscle tissue breakdown that releases damaged cell contents, such as myoglobin, into the bloodstream, which are harmful to the kidneys and can lead to kidney damage.

rheumatic carditis: Serious complication of rheumatic fever in which all layers of the heart become inflamed.

rheumatic fever: A hypersensitivity reaction to antigens of group A beta-hemolytic streptococci.

rhinitis: Inflammation of the nasal mucosa, usually associated with congestion, itching, sneezing, and nasal discharge.

rhinoplasty: Plastic surgery of the nose.

rickettsia: A genus of bacteria of the tribe rickettsiae that multiply only in host cells.

Rinne test: A test of hearing made with tuning forks.

Romberg test: A test to determine if a person has the ability to maintain body balance when the eyes are shut and the feet are close together. Also called Romberg's test.

Roux-en-Y: Gastric bypass surgery. A small stomach pouch the size of a thumb is created with staples, then a Y-shaped section of the small intestine is attached to the pouch to allow food to bypass the lower stomach and duodenum.

rule of nines: A formula for estimating percentage of body surface area, particularly helpful in judging the percentage of skin that has been burned.

sacral radiculopathy: Pathology of sacral nerve roots.

salpingectomy: Surgical removal of the fallopian tubes.

salpingitis: Inflammation of a fallopian tube.

salpingoscopy: Endoscopic visualization of the fallopian tubes.

scleroderma: A chronic manifestation of progressive systemic sclerosis in which the skin is taut, firm, and edematous, limiting movement.

sclerosis: A hardening or induration of an organ or tissue, especially from excessive growth of fibrous tissue.

seborrhea: Disease of the sebaceous glands marked by increase in the amount and often alteration of the quality of sebaceous secretions.

secondary hypertension: High blood pressure that is a symptom of a specific cause, such as a kidney abnormality.

semipermeable: Partly permeable; said of a membrane that will allow fluids but not the dissolved substance to pass through it.

sensorineural: Hearing loss caused by impairment of a sensory nerve.

sensory deprivation: No or minimal stimulation of the senses that creates the potential for maladaptive coping.

sensory overload: Excessive stimulation of the senses that creates the potential for maladaptive coping.

sepsis: Systematic infection caused by microorganisms in the bloodstream.

serologic: Study of substances present in blood serum.

sanguineous: Bloody.

serosanguineous: Fluid consisting of serum and blood.

serous: Watery fluid resembling serum.

serotonin: A chemical neurotransmitter important in sleep/wake cycles. Reduced serotonin levels are associated with depression.

shock: A clinical syndrome in which the peripheral blood flow is inadequate to return sufficient blood to the heart for normal function, particularly transport of oxygen to all organs and tissues.

sinoatrial (SA) node: Node at the junction of the superior vena cava and right atrium, regarded as the starting point of the heartbeat.

sinusitis: Inflammation of the sinuses; may be due to viral or bacterial infection, or to allergies.

Snellen chart: A chart imprinted with lines of black letters graduating in size from smallest on the bottom to largest on top; used for testing visual acuity.

somatoform: Denoting psychogenic symptoms resembling those of physical disease; psychosomatic.

spider angioma: Thin reddish-purple vein lines close to the skin surface.

spirituality: Sense of connectedness with all of life and the universe.

splenectomy: Excision of the spleen.

splenomegaly: Enlargement of the spleen.

standard precautions: Guidelines recommended by the Centers for Disease Control and Prevention to reduce the risk of the spread of infection.

stapedectomy: Excision of the stapes to improve hearing, especially in cases of otosclerosis.

Staphylococcus: A genus of gram-positive bacteria; they are constantly present on the skin and in the upper respiratory tract and are the most common cause of localized suppurating infections.

status asthmaticus: Prolonged period of unrelieved asthma symptoms.

steatorrhea: Fat in the stools; may be associated with pancreatic disease.

stenosis: The constriction or narrowing of a passage or orifice, such as a cardiac valve.

stent: Any mold or device used to hold tissue in place or to provide a support, graft, or anastomosis while healing is taking place.

stereotype: An opinion or belief about an individual or group that may not be true.

sternotomy: The operation of cutting through the sternum.

stoma: A mouth, small opening, or pore.

stomatitis: Inflammation of the mouth.

stress: The physical (gravity, mechanical, pathogenic, injury) and psychological (fear, anxiety, crisis, joy) forces that are experienced by individuals.

stressor: Any person or situation that produces an anxiety response.

striae: A line or band of elevated or depressed tissue; may differ in color or texture from surrounding tissue.

subarachnoid: Below or under the arachnoid membrane and the pia mater of the covering of the brain and spinal cord.

subdural: Beneath the dura mater.

subjective data: Information that is provided verbally by the patient.

suffering: A state of severe distress associated with events that threaten the intactness of the person. Emotional pain associated with real or potential tissue damage.

summons: A notice of suit.

suprapubic: Bone of the groin (or region) located above the pubic arch.

surgeon: A medical practitioner who specializes in surgery.

synarthrosis: Immovably fixed joint between bones connected by fibrous tissue (sutures of the skull).

synovitis: Inflammation of the synovial membrane that may be the result of an aseptic wound, a subcutaneous injury, irritation, or exposure to cold and dampness.

systolic blood pressure: Maximal pressure exerted on the arteries during contraction of the left ventricle of the heart. The top number of a blood pressure reading.

tachycardia: An abnormal rapidity of heart action, usually defined as a heart rate greater than 100 beats per minute in adults.

tachydysrhythmia: An abnormal heart rhythm with rate greater than 100 beats per minute in an adult.

tachypnea: Abnormally rapid respiratory rate.

tamponade: Compression of a part.

telenursing: Delivering nursing care from a distance with the use of telecommunications.

tendon: Fibrous connective tissue which connects muscle to bone.

tension pneumothorax: Abnormal accumulation of air with buildup of pressure in the pleural space.

teratoma: A congenital tumor containing one or more of the three primary embryonic germ layers.

terminal illness: An illness that will probably cause death in 6 months or less.

tetanus: A highly fatal disease caused by the bacillus *Clostridium tetani* and characterized by muscle spasm and convulsions.

tetany: Muscle spasms, numbness, and tingling caused by changes in pH and low serum calcium.

therapeutic privilege: Limitation for veracity used by health care providers when telling patients the truth would cause them greater harm.

thoracentesis: Insertion of a large-bore needle into the pleural space to remove fluid.

thoracotomy: Surgical incision into the chest wall.

thrill: Palpation of a vibration on the surface of the skin. Can be caused by turbulent blood flow through a blood vessel (as with a fistula or graft) or cardiac abnormalities.

thrombi: Blood clots.

thrombocytopenia: Abnormal decrease in the number of blood platelets.

thrombolytic: Agent that dissolves or splits up a thrombus, an aggregation of blood factors.

thrombophlebitis: The formation of a clot and inflammation within a vein.

thrombosis: Formation, development, or presence of a thrombus, an aggregation of blood factors.

tidaling: Rise and fall; may refer to water in water-seal chamber of a chest drainage system.

titration: Adjustment of medication up or down to meet patient needs.

tolerance: The response of the body to medication that requires increased medication administration to achieve the same effect. Often refers to opioids.

torts: Lawsuits involving civil wrongs.

toxemia: Spread of the poisonous products of bacteria throughout the body.

tracheostomy: A surgical opening in the neck into the trachea to provide an airway when the trachea is obstructed.

tracheotomy: An opening in the neck into the trachea.

traditions: Practices and customs handed down through the generations, often by word of mouth.

transcellular: Across cell membranes.

transdermal: Entering through the dermis, or skin, as in administration of a drug applied to the skin in ointment or patch form.

transillumination: The passage of strong light through a body structure to permit inspection of an observer on the opposite side.

transjugular intrahepatic portosystemic shunt (TIPS): Shunt that sidetracks venous blood around the liver to the vena cava for treatment of ascites.

transmyocardial: Across all layers of the heart.

trauma: Physical injury caused by an external force.

trauma-informed care: Special care based on knowing trauma survivors' (such as those of abuse, Holocaust survivors, veterans, or victims of large-scale disasters) personal experiences to avoid triggers that could cause re-traumatization.

Trendelenburg position: A position in which the patient's head is low and the body and legs are on an elevated and inclined plane. Also called Trendelenburg's position.

triage: The assignment of degrees of urgency to wounds or illnesses to decide the order of treatment of patients or casualties.

trichinosis: A disease caused by the roundworm *Trichinella spiralis,* which is spread by eating raw or undercooked meat from pigs or wild animals that contains *Trichinella* larvae.

trigeminy: Occurring every third beat, as in trigeminal premature ventricular contractions.

tropia: A manifest deviation of an eye from the normal position when both eyes are open and uncovered.

tumor: An abnormal growth of cells or tissues; tumors may be benign or malignant.

turbid: Cloudy.

turgor: The resistance of the skin to being grasped between the fingers. Dehydration causes poor skin turgor.

unifocal: Coming or originating from one site or focus.

upper gastrointestinal (GI) series: X-ray and fluoroscopic examinations of the stomach and duodenum after the ingestion of a contrast medium.

uremia: An excess in the blood of urea, creatinine, and other nitrogenous end products of protein and amino acid metabolism.

urethritis: Inflammation of the urethra.

urethroplasty: Plastic repair of the urethra.

urinary incontinence: Inability to control urine excretion creating accidental urinary leakage.

urodynamic: The study of the holding or storage of urine in the bladder, the facility with which it empties, and the rate of movement of urine out of the bladder during urination.

urosepsis: Sepsis resulting from urinary tract infection.

urticaria: Hives signifying an allergic reaction.

utilitarian: Consequences or outcomes of a dilemma are the most important element.

vaginitis: Inflammation of the vagina.

vaginosis: Inflammation of the vagina caused by *Gardnerella vaginalis.*

values: Ideals or concepts that give meaning to an individual's life.

valvotomy: Cutting through a valve.

valvuloplasty: Plastic or restorative surgery on a valve, especially a cardiac valve.

varices: Dilated veins.

varicocele: Varicose veins of the scrotum; can lead to infertility.

varicose veins: Swollen, distended, and knotted veins, usually in the subcutaneous tissue of the leg.

vasculitis: Inflammation of a vessel.

vasectomy: Surgically cutting and sealing the vas deferens to prevent sperm from getting outside the body. Used as a birth control method for men.

vector: Living organism that transmits disease.

venous stasis ulcers: Poorly healing ulcers that result from inadequate venous drainage.

ventricular diastole: The period of relaxation of the two ventricles.

ventricular escape rhythm: The naturally occurring rhythm of the ventricles when the rest of the cardiac conduction system fails.

ventricular repolarization: Reestablishment of the polarized state of the muscle after contraction.

ventricular systole: The contraction of the two ventricles.

ventricular tachycardia: A series of at least three beats arising from a ventricular focus at a rate greater than 100 beats per minute.

veracity: Truthfulness.

verrucous: Wartlike, with raised portions.

vertebrae: Any of the 33 bony segments of the spinal column: 7 cervical, 12 thoracic, 5 lumbar, 5 sacral, and 4 coccygeal vertebrae.

vesicant: Agent that causes blistering of tissue.

vesicular: Pertaining to vesicles or small blisters.

virulence: The power of an organism to cause disease.

virus: The smallest organism identified by use of electron microscopy; intracellular parasites that may cause disease.

viscosity: Thickness, as of the blood.

vulvovaginitis: Inflammation of the vulva and vaginitis.

volvulus: A twisting of the bowel on itself, causing obstruction.

Weber test: A test for unilateral deafness.

white blood cells: Leukocytes; the body's primary defense against infection.

withdrawal: Symptoms caused by cessation of administration of a drug, especially a narcotic or alcohol, to which the individual has become either physiologically or psychologically addicted.

worldview: The way individuals look on the world to form values and beliefs about life and the world around them.

xenograft: Graft from one species to another species (animal to man).

xerostomia: Dry mouth caused by reduction in secretions.

Photo & Illustration Credits

Chapter 2
Fig 2.1: From Ackley, B. J., Ladwig, G. B., Swan, B. A., & Tucker, S. J. (2008). *Evidence-based nursing care guidelines: Medical-surgical interventions.* Philadelphia: Elsevier, with permission.
Fig 2.2: Courtesy of Sage Products, Cary, Illinois.

Chapter 4
Fig 4.1: Adapted from United States Census Bureau. (2017). QuickFacts: Population estimates, July 1, 2017: People: Race and Hispanic origin. Retrieved from www.census.gov/quickfacts/fact/table/US/PST045217

Chapter 7
Fig 7.2: Courtesy of Deb Richardson & Associates.
Figs 7.4B, 7.4C: Modified from Phillips, L. D., & Gorski, L. A. (2014). *Manual of IV therapeutics: Evidence-based practice for infusion therapy* (6th ed.). Philadelphia: F.A. Davis.

Chapter 8
Fig 8.1: Adapted from Wilkinson J. M., & Treas, L. S. (2016). *Fundamentals of nursing: Theory, concepts & applications.* (3rd ed., Vol. 1). Philadelphia: FA Davis.

Chapter 10
Fig 10.3: From the International Association for the Study of Pain, with permission.
Fig 10.4: From Warden, V., Hurley, A. C., & Volicer, L. (2003). Development and psychometric evaluation of the Pain Assessment in Advanced Dementia (PAINAD) Scale. *Journal of the American Medical Directors Association, 4*(1), 9–15. Developed and tested by clinicians and researchers at the New England Geriatric Research Education and Clinical Center, a Department of Veterans Affairs center of excellence with divisions at EN Rogers Memorial Veterans Hospital, Bedford, MA, and VA Boston Health System. www.amda.com
Fig 10.5: From the Purdue Frederick Company, Norwalk, CT.

Chapter 11
Figs 11.1, 11.2, 11.3: Modified from Thompson, G. C. (2015). *Understanding anatomy and physiology* (2nd ed.). Philadelphia: F.A. Davis.
Figs 11.5, 11.6, 11.7, 11.9, 11.12: Photo courtesy of Dinesh Patel, MD, Medical Oncology, Internal Medicine, Zanesville, OH.
Fig 11.8: Data from the American Cancer Society. (2017). *Cancer facts and figures 2017.* Atlanta: Author. Accessed from www.cancer.org/content/dam/cancer-org/research/cancer-facts-and-statistics/annual-cancer-facts-and-figures/2017/cancer-facts-and-figures-2017.pdf
Fig 11.10: Photo courtesy of National Cancer Institute (NCI).

Chapter 12
Fig 12.1: Courtesy of © 2017 Intuitive Surgical, Inc., Sunnyvale, CA.

Chapter 13
Fig 13.5: From the Centers for Disease Control and Prevention, Public Health Image Library, #1809.
Fig 13.6: From the Centers for Disease Control and Prevention, Public Health Image Library, #1934.

Chapter 14
Fig 14.2: Modified from Miller, J. (2000). *Coping with chronic illness: Overcoming powerlessness* (3rd ed.). Philadelphia: F.A. Davis.

Chapter 15
Fig 15.3: Courtesy of Sammons Preston, Inc., Bolingbrook, IL.

Chapter 17
Fig 17.1: From Emanuel, L. L., von Gunten, C. F., & Ferris, F. D. (Eds.). (1999). *The Education for Physicians on End-of-Life Care [EPEC] curriculum.* Chicago: The EPEC Project. Copyright Robert Wood Johnson Foundation.

Chapter 18
Figs 18.2, 18.5: Adapted from Scanlon, V., & Sanders, T. (2019). *Essentials of anatomy and physiology* (8th ed.). Philadelphia: F.A. Davis.
Figs 18.3, 18.4: From Thompson, G. S. (2015). *Understanding anatomy and physiology* (2nd ed.). Philadelphia: F.A. Davis.

Chapter 19
Fig 19.3: From Scanlon, V., & Sanders, T. (2019). *Essentials of anatomy and physiology* (8th ed.). Philadelphia: F. A. Davis.
Fig 19.6: From Goldsmith, L. A., Tharp, M., & Lazarus, G. (Eds.). (1997). *Adult and pediatric dermatology.* Philadelphia: F.A. Davis.

Chapter 20
Fig 20.1: Modified from United States Department of Health and Human Services. (2017). The HIV life cycle. Retrieved from https://aidsinfo.nih.gov/understanding-hiv-aids/fact-sheets/19/73/the-hiv-life-cycle/#

Chapter 21
Figs 21.1, 21.2, 21.5: From Scanlon, V., & Sanders, T. (2019). *Essentials of anatomy and physiology* (8th ed.). Philadelphia: F.A. Davis.
Figs 21.3, 21.4: From Thompson, G. S. (2015). *Understanding anatomy and physiology* (2nd ed.). Philadelphia: F.A. Davis.
Fig 21.11: From McKinnis, L. N. (2014). *Fundamentals of musculoskeletal imaging* (4th ed.). Philadelphia: F.A. Davis.
UNFig 21.1: From Thompson, J. (2018). *Essential health assessment.* Philadelphia: F.A. Davis.

Chapter 23
Figs 23.5, 23.6: From Goldsmith, L. (1997). *Adult and pediatric dermatology.* Philadelphia: F.A. Davis.

Chapter 25
Fig 25.1: From Scanlon, V. C., & Sanders, T. (2019). *Essentials of anatomy and physiology* (8th ed.). Philadelphia: F.A. Davis.
Figs 25.10, 25.11, 25.12, 25.13, 25.15, 25.16, 25.17, 25.18: Modified from Jones, S. A. (2008). *ECG success: Exercises in ECG interpretation.* Philadelphia: F.A. Davis.

Chapter 27
Figs 27.1, 27.2, 27.3, 27.4, 27.5: From Thompson, G. S. (2015). *Understanding anatomy and physiology* (2nd ed.). Philadelphia: F.A. Davis.

Chapter 28

Fig 28.1: From Harmening, D. M. (2009). *Clinical hematology and fundamentals of hemostasis* (5th ed.). Philadelphia: F.A. Davis.

Fig 28.2: From Goldsmith, L. A., Lazarus, G. S., & Tharp, M. D. (1997). *Adult and pediatric dermatology*. Philadelphia: F.A. Davis.

Fig 28.4: Courtesy of Sandoz Pharmaceutical Corp., East Hanover, NJ.

Fig 28.6: From Huether, S. E., & McCance, K. L. (1996). *Understanding pathophysiology*. St. Louis, MO: Mosby, p. 548, with permission.

Figs 28.7ABC: From del Regato, J. A., Spjut, H. J., & Cox, J. D. (1985). *Cancer: Diagnosis, treatment, and prognosis* (6th ed.). St. Louis, MO: Mosby, with permission.

Chapter 29

Figs 29.1, 29.2, 29.3, 29.4, 29.5, 29.6: From Thompson, G. S. (2015). *Understanding anatomy and physiology* (2nd ed.). Philadelphia: F.A. Davis.

Fig 29.21, 29.28: Modified from Barnes, T. A. (1991). *Respiratory care principles*. Philadelphia: F.A. Davis.

Fig 29.23: Courtesy of Axcan Scandipharm, Birmingham, AL.

Fig 29.24: Courtesy of Deknatel Snowden Pencer, Inc., Tucker, GA.

Fig 29.27: Courtesy of Passy-Muir, Inc., Irvine, CA.

Chapter 30

Fig 30.1: Courtesy of ArthroCare, Inc., Austin, TX.

Figs 30.2AB: Courtesy of Philips Respironics, Murrysville, PA.

Fig 30.4A: Courtesy of UltraVoice Ltd., Newtown Square, PA.

Fig 30.4B: Courtesy of InHealth Technologies, Carpinteria, CA.

Chapter 31

Fig 31.5: From Hoffman, J., & Sullivan, N. (2017). *Medical-surgical nursing: Making connections to practice*. Philadelphia: F.A. Davis.

Fig 31.6: From U.S. Department of Health & Human Services, *Get on a Path to a Healthier You (Quitting)*. Retrieved from https://betobaccofree.hhs.gov/gallery/quit.html

Fig 31.13: From the National Cancer Institute, June 1998.

Chapter 32

Figs 32.1, 32.2, 32.3: From Thompson, G. S. (2015). *Understanding anatomy and physiology* (2nd ed.). Philadelphia: F.A. Davis.

Figs 32.6AB: Courtesy Dr. Russell Tobe.

Fig 32.8: Modified from Watson, J., & Jaffe, S. (1995). *Nurse's manual of laboratory and diagnostic tests* (2nd ed.). Philadelphia: F.A. Davis.

Chapter 34

Figs 34.9, 34.10: Reproduced with permission of Hollister Inc., Libertyville, IL.

Fig 34.11: Courtesy ConvaTec, a Bristol-Myers Squibb Company, Princeton, NJ, with permission.

Chapter 35

Fig 35.1: From the Centers for Disease Control and Prevention/Dr. Thomas F. Sellers; Emory University, 1963.

Chapter 36

Figs 36.1, 36.2, 36.3: From Thompson, G. S. (2015). *Understanding anatomy and physiology*. Philadelphia: F.A. Davis.

Chapter 38

Figs 38.1, 38.2, 38.3, 38.4, 38.5, 38.6AB, 38.7, 38.8, 38.9: From Thompson, G. S. (2015). *Understanding anatomy and physiology* (2nd ed.). Philadelphia: F.A. Davis.

Chapter 39

Fig 39.1: From Tamparo, C. D. (2000). *Diseases of the human body* (3rd ed.). Philadelphia: F.A. Davis.

Fig 39.2AB: From Chanson, P., & Salenave, S. (2008). Acromegaly. *Orphanet Journal of Rare Disease, 3*(17). Published online 2008 June 25, PMCID. © 2008 Chanson and Salenave, licensee BioMed Central Ltd.

Fig 39.4: From Tamparo, C. D. (2005). *Diseases of the human body* (4th ed.). Philadelphia: F.A. Davis.

Fig 39.5: Courtesy of the CDC Public Health Image Library (PHIL), #15470.

Chapter 40

Fig 40.1: Adapted from Thompson, G. S. (2015). *Understanding anatomy and physiology* (2nd ed.). Philadelphia: F.A. Davis.

Fig 40.5: From Hoffman, J., & Sullivan, N. (2016). *Medical-surgical nursing*. Philadelphia: F.A. Davis.

Fig 40.6: Courtesy of Roche Diabetes Care, Inc.

Fig 40.8: From Goldsmith, L. A., Lazarus, G. S., & Tharp, M. D. (1997). *Adult and pediatric dermatology*. Philadelphia: F.A. Davis.

Chapter 41

Figs 41.1, 41.2, 41.3, 41.4, 41.5, 41.6: Adapted from Thompson, G. S. (2015). *Understanding anatomy and physiology* (2nd ed.). Philadelphia: F.A. Davis.

Figs 41.8, 41.10: From Dillon, P. M. (2007) *Nursing health assessment: A critical thinking, case studies approach* (2nd ed.). Philadelphia: F.A. Davis.

Fig 41.9: From National Cancer Institute, created by Rhoda Baer (Photographer).

Figs 41.11, 41.12: Modified from Cavanaugh, B. M. (2003). *Nurse's manual of laboratory and diagnostic tests* (4th ed.). Philadelphia: F.A. Davis.

Chapter 42

Figs 42.1, 42.2, 42.3: Modified from Love, S. M. (2000). *Dr. Susan Love's breast book* (3rd ed.). Cambridge, MA: Perseus Publishing, with permission.

Chapter 44

Figs 44.1, 44.2: From Reeves, J. R. T., & Maibach, H. (1991). *Clinical dermatology illustrated: A regional approach*. Philadelphia: F.A. Davis.

Fig 44.3: From Lemone, P., & Burke, K. M. (1996). *Medical-surgical nursing: Critical thinking in client care*. Menlo Park, CA: Addison-Wesley, with permission.

Chapter 45

Figs 45.1, 45.2, 45.3, 45.4, 45.5: From Thompson, G. S. (2015). *Understanding anatomy and physiology* (2nd ed.). Philadelphia: F.A. Davis.

Figs 45.7, 45.8: From McKinnis, L. N. (2014). *Fundamentals of musculoskeletal imaging* (4th ed.). Philadelphia: F.A. Davis.

Chapter 46

Figs 46.4, 46.6, 46.12: From McKinnis, L. N. (2014). *Fundamentals of musculoskeletal imaging* (4th ed.). Philadelphia: F.A. Davis.

Fig 46.8: From Goldsmith, L. A., Lazarus, G. S., & Tharp, M. D. (1997). *Adult and pediatric dermatology*. Philadelphia: F.A. Davis.

Fig 46.14: From Hoffman, J., & Sullivan, N. (2017). *Medical-surgical nursing: Making connections to practice*. Philadelphia: F.A. Davis.

Chapter 47

Figs 47.1, 47.2, 47.3, 47.4, 47.5, 47.6, 47.7, 47.8, 47.9: From Thompson, G. S. (2015). *Understanding anatomy and physiology* (2nd ed.). Philadelphia: F.A. Davis.

Fig 47.12: From Wijdicks, E. F. M., Bamlet, W. R., Marmatton, B. V., Manno, E. M., & McClelland, R. L. (2005). Validation of a new coma scale: The FOUR Score. *Annals of Neurology, 58*, 585–593. doi:10.1002/ana.20611. Figure 1 and Table 1. Used with permission. © Mayo, 2005.

Fig 47.14: Adapted from Thompson, J. (2018). *Essential health assessment.* Philadelphia: F.A. Davis.

Chapter 48

Fig 48.11: Modified from Scanlon, V. C., & Sanders, T. (2019). *Student workbook of essentials of anatomy and physiology* (8th ed.). Philadelphia: F.A. Davis.

Fig 48.15: From Spillane, J. D. (1968). *An atlas of clinical neurology.* New York: Oxford University Press, p. 219, with permission.

Chapter 49

Fig 49.2: From the National Stroke Association, © 2015. Reprinted by permission of National Stroke Association. Please visit www.stroke.org for stroke education resources.

Fig 49.4: Modified from National Institutes of Health, National Institute of Neurological Disorders and Stroke. Stroke Scale. http://www.ninds.nih.gov/doctors/NIH_Stroke_Scale.pdf

Chapter 50

Figs 50.1, 50.2: Modified from Scanlon, V. C., & Sanders, T. (2019). *Workbook for essentials of anatomy and physiology* (8th ed.). Philadelphia: F.A. Davis.

Chapter 51

Figs 51.1, 51.2, 51.3, 51.4, 51.5, 51.6, 51.7, 51.11, 51.12, 51.13: From Thompson, G. S. (2015). *Understanding anatomy and physiology* (2nd ed.). Philadelphia: F.A. Davis.

Chapter 53

Figs 53.1, 53.2, 53.3: From Thompson, G. S. (2015). *Understanding anatomy and physiology* (2nd ed.). Philadelphia: F.A. Davis.

Chapter 54

Figs 54.2, 54.3, 54.4, 54.7, 54.8, 54.9, 54.10; UNFig 54.21: From Goldsmith, L. A., Lazarus, G. S., & Tharp, M. D. (1997). *Adult and pediatric dermatology.* Philadelphia: F.A. Davis.

Figs 54.5, 54.6; UNFig 54.18: From Barankin, B., & Frieman, A. (2006). *Derm notes: Clinical dermatology pocket guide.* Philadelphia: F.A. Davis.

UNFigs 54.1, 54.3, 54.5, 54.7, 54.9, 54.11: From Hoffman, J. J., & Sullivan, N. J. (2017). *Medical-surgical nursing.* Philadelphia: F. A. Davis.

UNFigs, 54.2, 54.4, 54.6, 54.8, 54.10, 54.12: National Pressure Ulcer Advisory Panel Copyright. Reprinted with permission of the copyright holder, Gordian Medical, Inc. dba American Medical Technologies.

UNFig 54.24: From Venes, D. (Ed.). (2017). *Taber's cyclopedic medical dictionary* (23rd ed.) Philadelphia: F.A. Davis.

Chapter 55

Fig 55.1: Modified from Ruppert, S. D., Kernick, J. G., & Dolan, J. T. (1996). *Dolan's critical care nursing.* Philadelphia: F.A. Davis, p. 942.

Figs 55.2, 55.4, 55.5, 55.6, 55.7: From Trofino, R. B. (1991). *Nursing care of the burn-injured patient.* Philadelphia: F.A. Davis, plates 1–3, 16, 17, 36, 19, with permission.

Fig 55.3: From Venes, D. (Ed.). (2009). *Taber's cyclopedic medical dictionary* (21st ed.) Philadelphia: F.A. Davis.

Index

Note: Page numbers followed by f refer to figures; page numbers followed by t refer to tables; page numbers followed by b refer to boxes; **medication entries are in boldfaced type.**

Medical Abbreviations

Although it is still important to know medical abbreviations, many can increase risk of errors. Check www.jointcommision.org for a list of abbreviations to avoid.

ABG	arterial blood gas	g, gm	gram
ac	before a meal	GERD	gastroesophageal reflux disease
AD	advance directive		
ad lib	freely; as desired	GI	gastrointestinal
ALT	alanine aminotransferase	gr	grain
AM	morning	gt	drop
A-P	anterior-posterior	gtt	drops
AST	aspartate aminotransferase	GYN	gynecology
		h, hr	hour
AV	atrioventricular	Hgb	hemoglobin
bid	twice a day	hor som, hs	bedtime
BM	bowel movement	IM	intramuscular
BP	blood pressure	in.	inch
BUN	blood urea nitrogen	IUD	intrauterine device
C	Celsius/centigrade	IV	intravenous
c̄	with	IVP	intravenous pyelogram
cap	a capsule	J	joule
CBC	complete blood count	kg	kilogram
cc	cubic centimeter	KUB	kidney, ureter, and bladder
cm	centimeter	L	liter
CNS	central nervous system	lb	pound
CSF	cerebrospinal fluid	lmp	last menstrual period
CV	cardiovascular	mEq	milliequivalent
D & C	dilation and curettage	mg	milligram
dc	discontinue	mL	milliliter
dL	deciliter	mm	millimeter
DNR	do not resuscitate	MRI	magnetic resonance imaging
DOA	dead on arrival		
dr	dram	MS	mitral stenosis; multiple sclerosis
Dx	diagnosis		
ECF	extracellular fluid	μ	"micro" symbol*
ECG	electrocardiogram	microEq	microequivalent
ECT	electroconvulsive therapy	microg	microgram
ED	emergency department	npo	nothing by mouth
EEG	electroencephalogram	NSAID	nonsteroidal anti-inflammatory drug
EKG	electrocardiogram		
EMG	electromyogram	NSR	normal sinus rhythm
EMS	emergency medical service	OB	obstetrics
		O.C.	oral contraceptive
ENT	ear, nose, and throat	O.D.	right eye
EOM	extraocular muscles	O.S.	left eye
ER	emergency room	O.U.	both eyes
ESR	erythrocyte sedimentation rate	oz	ounce
		p̄	after
F	Fahrenheit	pc	after meals

PCo₂	carbon dioxide pressure		
PERRLA	pupils equal, regular, react to light and accommodation		
pH	hydrogen ion concentration		
PM	afternoon/evening		
PMI	point of maximal impulse		
post	posterior		
pr	through the rectum		
prn	as needed		
qhr	every hour		
q2hr	every 2 hours		
q3hr	every 3 hours		
qid	four times a day		
qs	as much as is needed		
RBC	red blood cell; red blood count		
s̄	without		
SA	sinoatrial		
SC, sc	subcutaneous(ly)		
SOB	shortness of breath		
s.o.s.	if necessary		
sq	subcutaneous(ly)		
STAT	immediately		
STI	sexually transmitted infection		
T	temperature		
tab	medicated tablet		
temp	temperature		
tid	three times a day		
top	topically		
URI	upper respiratory infection		
USP	United States Pharmacopeia		
UTI	urinary tract infection		
WBC	white blood cell; white blood count		
WF/BF	white female/black female		
WM/BM	white male/black male		
wt.	weight		

*The United States–based Institute for Safe Medication Practices (ISMP) and the U.S. Food and Drug Administration (FDA) recommend that the symbol μg should not be used when communicating medical information due to the risk that the prefix μ (micro-) might be misread as the prefix m (milli-), resulting in a thousandfold overdose. The non-SI symbol mcg is recommended instead.

Adapted from Venes, D. (2017), *Taber's cyclopedic medical dictionary* (23rd ed.). Philadelphia, PA: F.A. Davis.

Prefixes, Suffixes, and Combining Forms

a-, an-. Without; away from; not

ab-, abs-. From; away from; absent

abdomin-, abdomino-. Abdomen

-ad. Toward; in the direction of

aden-, adeno-. Gland

adip-, adipo-. Fat

-aemia. Blood

aer-, aero-. Air

-algesia, -algia. Suffering; pain

andro-. Man; male; masculine

angi-, angio-. Blood or lymph vessels

aniso-. Unequal; asymmetrical; dissimilar

ankyl-, ankylo-. Crooked; bent; fusion or growing together of parts

ant-, anti-. Against

ante-. Before

antero-. Anterior; front; before

arteri-, arterio-. Artery

arthr-, arthro-. Joint

-ase. Enzyme

-asis, esis, -iasis, -isis, -sis. Condition; pathological state

aut-, auto-. Self

axo-. Axis; axon

bacteri-, bacterio-. Bacteria; bacterium

bi-, bis-. Two; double; twice

bili-. Bile

bio-. Life

blast-, -blast. Germ; bud; embryonic state of development

blephar-, blepharo-. Eyelid

brady-. Slow

bronch-, bronchi-, broncho-. Airway

cardi-, cardio-. Heart

cat-, cata-, cath-, kat-, kata-. Down; downward; destructive; against; according to

cent-. Hundred

cephal-, cephalo-. Head

cervic-, cervice-. Head; the neck of an organ

chrom-, chromo-. Color

-cide. Causing death

contra-. Against; opposite

crani-, cranio-. Skull; cranium

cry-, cryo-. Cold

cyan-, cyano-. Blue

cyst-, cysto-, -cyst. Cyst; urinary bladder

cyt-, cyto-, -cyte. Cell

derm-, derma-, dermato-, dermo-. Skin

di-. Double; twice; two; apart from

dors-, dorsi-, dorso-. Back

-dynia. Pain

dys-. Difficult; bad; painful

ec-, ecto-. Out; on the outside

-ectomy. Excision

ef-, es-, ex-, exo-. Out

electr-, electro-. Electricity

-emesis. Vomiting

-emia. Blood

en-. In; into

end-, endo-. Within

ent-, ento-. Within; inside

enter-, entero-. Intestine

ep-, epi-. Upon; over; at; in addition to; after

erythr-, erythro-. Red

eury-. Broad

ex-. Out; away from; completely

exo-. Out; outside of; without

extra-. Outside of; in addition; beyond

-facient. Causing; making happen

-ferous. Producing

ferri-, ferro-. Iron

fluo-. Flow

fore-. Before; in front of

-form. Form

-fuge. To expel; to drive away; fleeing

gaster-, gastero-, gastr-, gastro-. Stomach

gen-. Producing; forming

-gen, -gene, -genesis, -genetic, -genic. Producing; forming

glosso-. Tongue

gluc-, gluco-, glyc-, glyco-. Sugar; glycerol or similar substance

gyn-, gyne-, gyneco-, gyno-. Woman; female

hem-, hema-, hemato-, hemo-. Blood

hemi-. Half

hepat-, hepato-. Liver

heter-, hetero-. Other; different

histo-. Tissue

homo-. Same; likeness

hydra-, hydro, hydr-. Water

hyp-, hyph-, hypo-. Less than; below; under

hyper-. Above; excessive; beyond

hyster-, hystero-. Uterus

-ia. Condition, esp. an abnormal state

-iasis. SEE -asis

-iatric. Medicine; medical profession; physicians

in-. In; inside; within; intensive action; negative

infra-. Below; under; beneath; inferior to; after

inter-. Between; in the midst

intra-, intro-. Within; in; into

ipsi-. Same

irid-, irido-. Iris

-ism. Condition; theory

iso-. Equal

-itis. Inflammation of

kera-, kerato-. Horny substance; cornea

kolp-, kolpo, colp-, colpo-. Vagina

kypho-. Humped

leuk-, leuko-. White; colorless; rel. to a leukocyte

lip-, lipo-. Fat

-lite, -lith, lith-, litho-. Stone; calculus

-logia, -logy. Science of; study of

lumbo-. Loins

-lysis. 1. Setting free; disintegration; 2. In medicine, reduction of; relief from

macr-, macro-. Large; long

mal-. Ill; bad; poor

med-, medi-, medio-. Middle

mega-, megal-, megalo-. Large; of great size

-megalia, -megaly. Enlargement of a body part

melan-, melano-. Black

mening-, meningo-. Meninges

-meter. Measure

metr-, metra-, metro-. Uterus

micr-, micro-. Small

mon-, mono-. Single; one

muc-, muci-, muco-, myxa-, myxo-. Mucus

multi-. Many; much

musculo-, my-, myo-. Muscle

my-, myo-. SEE *musculo-*

myel-, myelo-. Spinal cord; bone marrow

naso-. Nose

necr-, necro-. Death; necrosis

neo-. New; recent

nephr-, nephra-, nephro-. Kidney

neur-, neuri-, neuro-. Nerve; nervous system

non-. No

normo-. Normal; usual

oculo-. Eye

-ode, -oid. Form; shape; resemblance

-odynia, odyno-. Pain

olig-, oligo-. Few; small

-ology. Science of; study of

-oma. Tumor

onco-. Tumor; swelling; mass

oo-, ovi-, ovo-. Egg; ovum

oophor-, oophoro-, oophoron-. Ovary

ophthalm-, ophthalmo-. Eye

-opia. Vision

optico-, opto-. Eye; vision

orchi-, orchid-, orchido-. Testicle

orth-, ortho-. Straight; correct; normal; in proper order

os-. Mouth; bone

-osis. Condition; status, process; abnormal increase

oste-, osteo-. Bone

ostomosis, -ostomy, -stomosis, -stomy. A created mouth or outlet

ot-, oto-. Ear

-otomy. Cutting

-ous. 1. Possessing; full of; 2. Pertaining to

pan-. All; entire

para-, -para. 1. Prefix: near; alongside of; departure from normal; 2. Suffix: Bearing offspring

path-, patho-, -path, -pathic, -pathy. Disease; suffering

ped-, pedi-, pedo-. Foot

-penia. Decrease from normal; deficiency

peri-. Around; about

perineo-. Perineum

phaco-. Lens of the eye

phag-, phago-. Eating; ingestion; devouring

-phil, -philia, -philic. Love for; tendency toward; craving for